SECTION 6
Advanced Administrative Skills

S0-AFT-637

UNIT THREE
CLINICAL PRINCIPLES: PATIENT CARE: LABORATORY TECHNIQUES: ADVANCED SKILLS

SECTION 7
Fundamental Principles of Patient Care

SECTION 8
The Protocols of Patient Care

SECTION 9
Understanding and Performing Diagnostic Orders and Tests

SECTION 10
Advanced Clinical Care Techniques

The Medical Assistant

ADMINISTRATIVE AND CLINICAL

MARY E. KINN, CPS, CMA-A

Assistant Professor, Health Technologies, Retired
Long Beach City College
Long Beach, California

Member of California Certifying Board for Medical Assistants

Past President, American Association of Medical Assistants

Former Chairman, American Association of Medical Assistants Certifying Board

MARYANN WOODS, PHD, RN, CMA

Professor, Health Sciences and the Arts Division, and
Director of the Medical Assistant–Clinician Program,
Fresno City College, Fresno, California

Member of California Association for Medical
Assistant Instructors

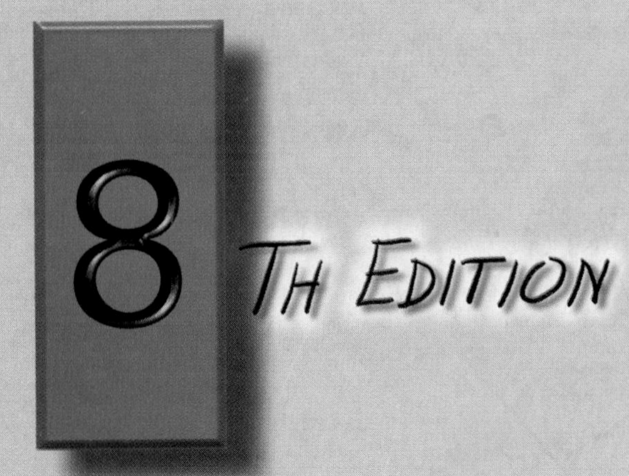

W.B. SAUNDERS COMPANY
A Division of Harcourt Brace & Company
Philadelphia London Toronto Montreal Sydney Tokyo

W.B. SAUNDERS COMPANY
A Division of Harcourt Brace & Company

The Curtis Center
Independence Square West
Philadelphia, Pennsylvania 19106

Library of Congress Cataloging-in-Publication Data

Kinn, Mary E.
The medical assistant: administrative and clinical/Mary E. Kinn, MaryAnn Woods.—8th ed.

p. cm.

Includes bibliographical references and index.

ISBN 0-7216-7299-X

1. Medical assistants. I. Woods, MaryAnn. II. Title.
[DNLM: 1. Medical Secretaries. 2. Allied Health Personnel.
W 80K55m 1999]

R728.8.K493 1999 610.69′53—dc21

DNLM/DLC 98-36106

THE MEDICAL ASSISTANT: Administrative and Clinical ISBN 0-7216-7299-X

Copyright © 1999, 1993, 1988, 1981, 1974, 1967, 1960, 1956 by W.B. Saunders Company.
Copyright renewed 1988 by Genevieve Hanacock.

All rights reserved. No part of this publication may be reproduced or transmitted in any form or by any means, electronic or mechanical, including photocopy, recording, or any information storage and retrieval system, without permission in writing from the publisher.

Printed in the United States of America.

Last digit is the print number: 9 8 7 6 5 4 3 2 1

Contributors and Reviewers

Contributors

MYRA M. DeWULF, MT (ASCP), MHA
Blood Banking Department
St. Agnes Hospital
Fresno, California
College Instructor and Organizational Lecturer on Process of Aging
Assisting with the Older Patient

LANCE GRANUM, LVN, CHHA
Trauma Room
Emergency Department
University Medical Center
Fresno, California
Assisting in Urology and Male Reproduction

SUE A. HUNT, MA, RN, CMA
Coordinator
Medical Assisting Program
Middlesex Community College
Lowell, Massachusetts
Health Insurance and Managed Care; Coding and Claims Processing

MARY JANE McCLAIN, RN, BSN, AORN
Inservice Educational Director and Surgical Nurse
Fresno Surgical Center
Instructor in the Surgical Technician Program
Training Institute
Fresno City College
Fresno, California
Preparing for Surgery; Surgical Methods; Assisting with Surgical Procedures

MARY AGNES TAYLOR, RN
Instructor
Advanced Medical/Surgical Nursing
Fresno City College
Fresno, California
Applying the Principles of Pharmacology; Administering Medications

Editorial Review Board

JUDITH BELL, BA, RT, CMA-C
Director, Allied Health
Midstate College
Peoria, Illinois

REV. DR. GENEVA BEURCH
West Virginia Northern Community College
Benwood, West Virginia

KATHERINE BLANKENSHIP
San Antonio College
San Antonio, Texas

TRISH BOUDRIA, CMA-RMA
Department of Medical Assisting
Ultrasound Diagnostic School
Irving, Texas

BONNY MARIE BUTCHY, BA, MLT (ASCP), CMA (AAMA)
California Vocational Credentialed Teacher
Eden Area ROP
Hayward, California

PAMELA J. CARLTON
Director, Medical Assistant Program
Assistant Professor of Biology and Certified Paramedic
The College of Staten Island
Staten Island, New York

DEBBIE CUNNINGHAM
Medix School
Baltimore, Maryland

BARBARA M. DAHL, CMA
Whatcom Community College
Bellingham, Washington

VERA DAVIS, RN, CMA
Harper College
Palatine, Illinois

BONNIE DEISTER, MS, MA, BSN, RN, CMA-C
Broome Community College
Binghamton, New York

BARBARA F. ENSLEY, MS, RN, CMA-C
Haywood Community College
Clyde, North Carolina

LINDA FARRELL
Tidewater Tech–Virginia Beach
Virginia Beach, Virginia

MARGARET SCHELL FRAZIER, RN, CMA, BS
Program Chair, Medical Assisting Program
Ivy Tech State College, Northeast
Fort Wayne, Indiana

THERESA GAVAZZI, MS, BS, CMA
Delaware Technical and Community College
Dover, Delaware

MICHELLE GREEN, MPS, RRA, CMA
Alfred State College
Alfred, New York

DEBORAH HECHT
Akron Medical and Dental Institution
Cuyahoga Falls, Ohio

MARSHA HEMBY, BA, RN, CMA
Medical Assisting Department Chair
Pitt Community College
Greenville, North Carolina

JEANNE HOWARD, CMA, AAS
Department of Medical Assisting Technology
El Paso Community College
El Paso, Texas

SUE A. HUNT, MA, RN, CMA
Middlesex Community College
Lowell, Massachusetts

KAREN A. KITTLE, CMA, AAS
Department of Medical Assisting
Oakland Community College
Waterford, Michigan

CAROL LIGON, BS, RT (ARRT) (R), CMA
Ivy Tech State College
Evansville, Indiana

ANNE L. LILLY, RN, MVED
Curriculum Consultant, Allied Health, Adult Education
Professor, Retired
Santa Rosa Junior College
Santa Rosa, California

PATTY J. LYNCH, MED
Bellingham, Washington

DEBORAH MONTONE, BS, RN, RMA
Dean of Academics
HoHoKus School of Medical Science
Ramsey, New Jersey

JANET R. SESSER, RMA (AMT), CMA, BS, Educational Administration
High Tech Institute, Inc.
Phoenix, Arizona

DIANE J. TRAMA, MT(ASCP)
Allied Medical and Technical Careers
Scranton, Pennsylvania

LORI WRIGHT, CMA, RMA, ART
Ultrasound Diagnostic School
Pittsburgh, Pennsylvania

CAROL ZEGLIN
Mt. Pleasant, Pennsylvania

Preface

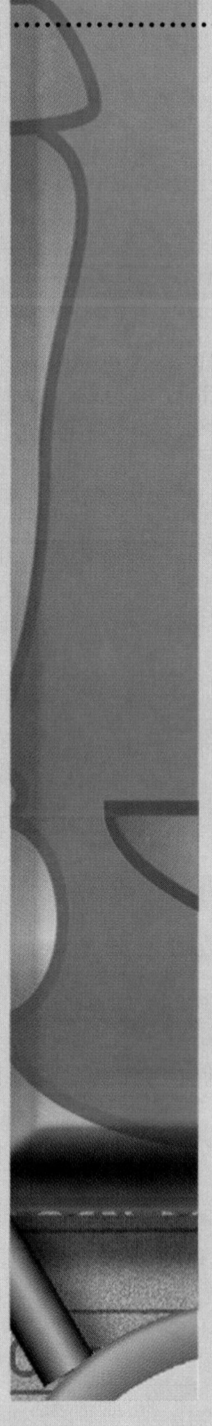

The delivery of health care has been revolutionized since the previous edition of *The Medical Assistant: Administrative and Clinical,* and this eighth edition recognizes these changes. The newly developed AAMA Entry-Level Medical Assisting Curriculum with its content and competency guidelines, has been incorporated in each chapter as the authors strive to maintain the student-friendly level of presentation that has been the hallmark of this text since its inception in 1956.

As with all previous editions, this book remains designed for use in community colleges, vocational/technical schools, medical offices or clinic inservices, cross-training programs, and independent study programs. Key AAMA Curriculum content and competency guidelines are listed on each section introductory page and are covered in the appropriate chapters. Additionally, the text has been reorganized into a more logical presentation to be easier to use and better help students prepare for certification examination.

UNIT I (Chapters 1 to 7) guides the student through the basics, beginning with professionalism, education, and the history from which modern medicine has evolved. The cornerstones of medical ethics from historical codes to the AMA Principles of Medical Ethics are presented in some detail. The legal responsibilities as well as the limitations of practicing medical assistants are addressed in each chapter. This unit concludes with a discussion of the importance of personal communications in every encounter.

UNIT II (Chapters 8 to 24) addresses in detail the procedural steps in performing the administrative functions in a medical facility, from the role of receptionist to the responsibilities of office management. Special attention is directed to the evolution of managed care and the changes that are taking place in the administrative aspects of medical assisting.

UNIT III, Clinical Medical Assisting (Chapters 25 to 52), begins with the philosophy that health assessment forms the foundation of all clinical care. Whether the person whose health status is being assessed is young or old, well or ill, the medical assistant is an asset to the ongoing process of whole-person physical, psychosocial, and functional evaluation. Each chapter embraces a dual focus, based on the art of medical assisting and the science of caring. Each chapter uses one body system as its theme, emphasizing the anatomy and physiology of the system, possible diseases and disorders to be aware of, and the skills needed to assist in the examination and treatment of that particular system. This style has been used to provide well-organized information that may be easily read and assimilated, empowering readers as educated assistants in decision making and developing skills of analysis and critical thinking. Practicing medical assistants will find this systems approach helpful as a review of the protocols and skills needed in each specialty. Medical assistant students will welcome the clear presentation as they learn the basic skills of assisting the physician in general and specialty practices.

Many pedagogical features are included to enhance the learning process. Outstanding photographs and drawings highlight administrative skills, including scheduling, financial managing, and organizing of the office, and clinical assisting, which includes techniques and procedures, anatomy and physiology, and normal and abnormal findings. Each chapter opens with an outline of the chapter, introducing the material to be learned; a vocabulary with definitions, introducing the terminology used in the chapter; and learning objectives, targeting the main areas in each chapter to master. Key terms are in boldface type the first time they are used in the chapter text. Memory jogger questions are inserted throughout each chapter to help the student focus on the primary issues emphasized within each topic section. Legal and ethical issues are discussed at the end of each chapter relevant to the medical assistant's responsibilities in this highly sensitive area of medical practice. Throughout the text, many examples of essential information are highlighted and summarized in boxed format to emphasize the varying qualities, responsibilities, and skills required to become a successful Medical Assistant. Boxed examples illustrate ways of approaching different situations that arise daily and should stimulate the student to think of other solutions. These examples also act as a handy guide to use when encountering similar problems in real life. Appendices contain materials to broaden the student's understanding of clinical language. The Glossary at the end of the book defines all key terms used in the text and serves as a comprehensive resource for study and review. An index facilitates access to material.

As we enter the new millennium, the entire health care system is facing multiple changes in techniques, patient involvement, and the health care delivery system. The eighth edition of *The Medical Assistant: Administrative and Clinical* forms the foundation to meet these challenges. From cover to cover our focus has been on the advances in the technology of equipment and educational methodology as well as an emphasis on new medical achievements and procedures.

Finally, this eighth edition is accompanied by a complete supplemental package that has been developed with the major text to achieve two primary goals:

1. To assist students in mastering essential skills and information needed to secure a career as a medical assistant
2. To assist instructors in planning and implementing their programs for the most efficient use of time and available resources

The authors and editors sincerely hope that students are stimulated and motivated to learn and educators to teach because of access to a complete and innovative educational package.

MARY E. KINN, CPS, CMA-A
MARYANN WOODS, PHD, RN, CMA

Acknowledgments

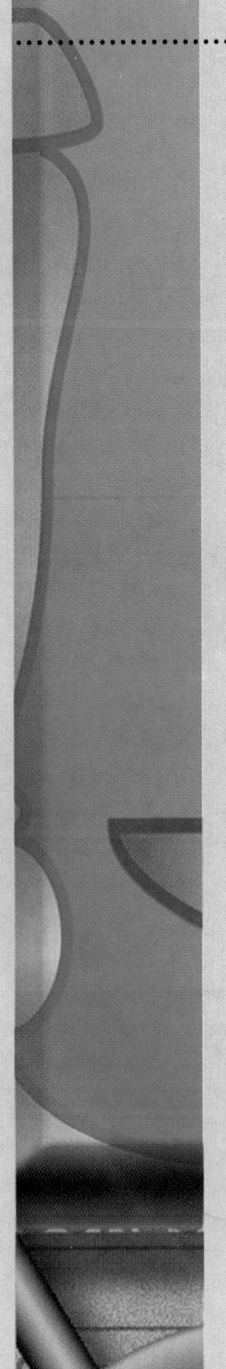

Over the span of more than 30 years that I have been involved with this text, hundreds of individuals have contributed ideas, knowledge, encouragement, praise, and—best of all—their hands in friendship. I acknowledge and express thanks to all of you.

Specifically I am deeply grateful to my editors:

Margaret Biblis and Shirley Kuhn for their innovative suggestions during the planning stage of this edition
Helaine Barron for her creative editing, patience, and devotion to the project
Adrianne Williams for her foresight, marketing talents, and personal touches.

I give special thanks to the Center for Women's Medicine in San Diego for the privilege of photographing in their beautiful facility, and especially to Arlene Saunders, Clinic Manager, for her cheerful cooperation.

I am grateful to:

Sue Hunt for rescuing the insurance and coding chapters
Bibbero Systems in Petaluma, California, and Colwell Systems, Inc., in Champaign, Illinois, for their continued support in providing sample forms for illustrating various administrative procedures

For the privilege of membership, for the sharing of their friendship and accumulated knowledge, and for fostering the challenge of excellence, I acknowledge the officers and members of the American Medical Writers Association (AMWA), the American Association of Medical Assistants (AAMA), the California Medical Assistants Association (CMAA), and the California Association of Medical Assistant Instructors.

MARY E. KINN, CPS, CMA-A

This textbook is the product of many dedicated, knowledgeable, and hardworking individuals. First, I want to thank all of the contributors who worked so diligently to add their technical expertise to make this book an outstanding production. Their talents radiate from cover to cover.

Thanks are also due to the editorial and production staffs at the W.B. Saunders Company, who kept the project on track. One individual that I would like to single out for her tremendous assistance is Helaine Barron, our development editor. This person is the unsung hero of this project. She took pages of typed manuscript and turned them into a work of art. Likewise, I want to thank all of the reviewers who thoughtfully read and commented on the manuscript. Their attention to detail and suggestions strengthened each chapter.

Special appreciation goes to the photographers David Graham and Lionel Bernal. They were there to help whenever I called, and their artistry captured concepts that I marvel at. Of course, special thanks also go to the medical assistants who gave their Saturdays to "picture taking" and to my precious grandchildren who, as the patients, allowed themselves to be probed and positioned hundreds of times to achieve the best lighting. In addition, many of the pictures had to be taken during actual events. I want to express special thanks to the Adult Day Health Care at Saint Agnes and Somerford Place for the pictures of our eldercare and to Dr. Sam Borno, who allowed us to photograph an actual treadmill testing in his cardiology office.

Last, but certainly very important, my husband and family gave me comfort and support when I was having difficulties and shared in the enthusiasm and thrill of accomplishment. I love you all.

MARYANN WOODS, PHD, RN, CMA

The authors wish to acknowledge the helpful and talented production team at the W.B. Saunders Company: Ellen Zanolle, designer, for the interior and cover designs; Sharon Iwanczuk, illustrator, for the creation of the collages and the interior art; Jeanne Carper, for copy editing; and Frank Polizzano, for overseeing the production process.

The Publisher wishes to acknowledge the permission of the AAMA to use the interim language of the AAMA medical assisting curriculum. The language used for the curriculum content and competencies topics is adapted from the *AAMA Role Delineation Study: Occupational Analysis of the Medical Assisting Profession,* published by the American Association of Medical Assistants (AAMA), Chicago, IL. The AAMA does not endorse the language nor is the language the official, or taken from the official, AAMA medical assisting curriculum document.

Contents

UNIT ONE

PROFESSIONALISM: LEGAL CONCEPTS: COMMUNICATION SKILLS

SECTION 1

The Medical Assisting Profession

SECTION 2
Understanding the Protocols of Medical Practice

SECTION 3
Communicating with Patients and Colleagues

UNIT TWO
ADMINISTRATIVE PROCEDURES: PRACTICE FINANCE: ADVANCED ADMINISTRATION SKILLS

SECTION 4
Written Communications and Record Keeping

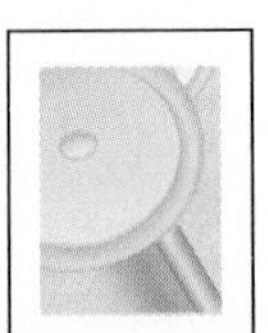

UNIT THREE
CLINICAL PRINCIPLES: PATIENT CARE: LABORATORY TECHNIQUES: ADVANCED SKILLS

SECTION 7
Fundamental Principles of Patient Care

SECTION 8
The Protocols of Patient Care

NOTICE

Medical assisting is an ever-changing field. Standard safety precautions must be followed, but as new research and clinical experience broaden our knowledge, changes in treatment and drug therapy become necessary or appropriate. Readers are advised to check the product information currently provided by the manufacturer of each drug to be administered to verify the recommended dose, the method and duration of administration, and the contraindications. It is the responsibility of the treating physician, relying on experience and knowledge of the patient, to determine dosages and the best treatment for the patient. Neither the publisher nor the editor assumes any responsibility for any injury and/or damage to persons or property.

THE PUBLISHER

List of Procedures

TO THE STUDENT

Learning and mastering all the information in a textbook can seem like a daunting task. This is why the authors and editors have built in many helpful features throughout each chapter of the new The Medical Assistant: Administrative and Clinical, eighth edition. *These features, when used in conjunction with the* Student Mastery Manual *and* Virtual Medical Office CD-ROM, *are designed to enhance the lessons and assignments of your instructor to ensure a successful learning experience. Take a moment now to review these features, and keep them in mind as you move through the textbook and through your medical assisting curriculum.*

1 Section Openers

Each section opener identifies all the current content and competencies from the Medical Assisting Entry-Level Curriculum that can be found in that section of the book. These are listed by chapter below the section title.

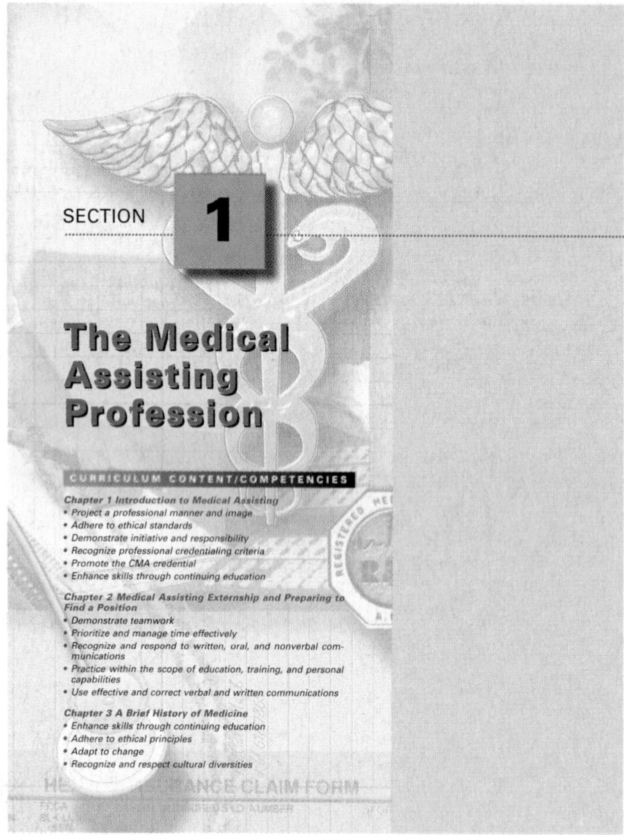

SECTION 1

The Medical Assisting Profession

CURRICULUM CONTENT/COMPETENCIES

Chapter 1 Introduction to Medical Assisting
- *Project a professional manner and image*
- *Adhere to ethical standards*
- *Demonstrate initiative and responsibility*
- *Recognize professional credentialing criteria*
- *Promote the CMA credential*
- *Enhance skills through continuing education*

Chapter 2 Medical Assisting Externship and Preparing to Find a Position
- *Demonstrate teamwork*
- *Prioritize and manage time effectively*
- *Recognize and respond to written, oral, and nonverbal communications*
- *Practice within the scope of education, training, and personal capabilities*
- *Use effective and correct verbal and written communications*

Chapter 3 A Brief History of Medicine
- *Enhance skills through continuing education*
- *Adhere to ethical principles*
- *Adapt to change*
- *Recognize and respect cultural diversities*

2 Chapter Openers

A detailed *Chapter Outline* introduces you to the material as a whole, allowing you to see at a glance how the subject material is organized. It will also help you focus on one topic at a time by showing you the relationship and placement of topics.

Learning Objectives list all the theoretical (cognitive) and procedural (performance) objectives you will be expected to meet on completion of the chapter.

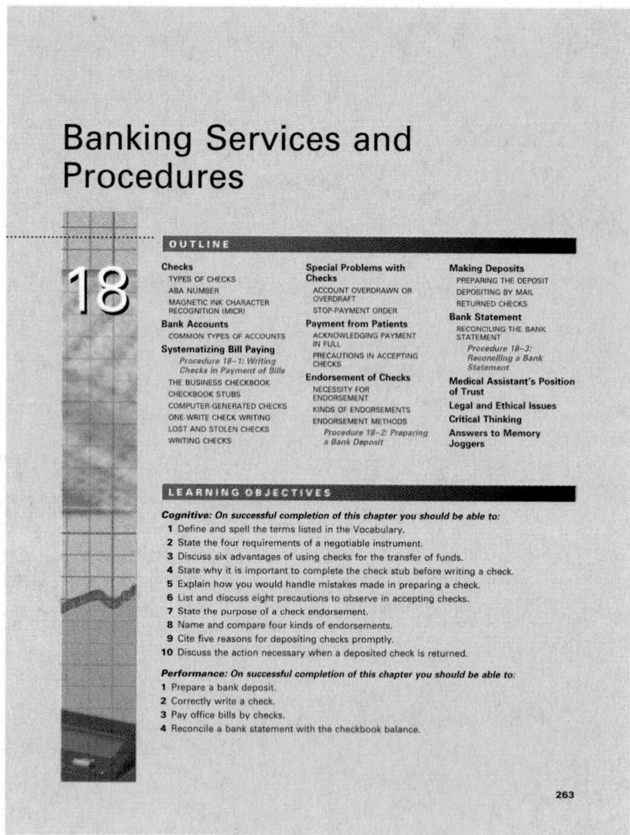

Banking Services and Procedures

18

OUTLINE

Checks
TYPES OF CHECKS
ABA NUMBER
MAGNETIC INK CHARACTER RECOGNITION (MICR)
Bank Accounts
COMMON TYPES OF ACCOUNTS
Systematizing Bill Paying
Procedure 18–1: Writing Checks in Payment of Bills
THE BUSINESS CHECKBOOK
CHECKBOOK STUBS
COMPUTER-GENERATED CHECKS
ONE-WRITE CHECK WRITING
LOST AND STOLEN CHECKS
WRITING CHECKS

Special Problems with Checks
ACCOUNT OVERDRAWN OR OVERDRAFT
STOP-PAYMENT ORDER
Payment from Patients
ACKNOWLEDGING PAYMENT IN FULL
PRECAUTIONS IN ACCEPTING CHECKS
Endorsement of Checks
NECESSITY FOR ENDORSEMENT
KINDS OF ENDORSEMENTS
ENDORSEMENT METHODS
Procedure 18–2: Preparing a Bank Deposit

Making Deposits
PREPARING THE DEPOSIT
DEPOSITING BY MAIL
RETURNED CHECKS
Bank Statement
RECONCILING THE BANK STATEMENT
Procedure 18–3: Reconciling a Bank Statement
Medical Assistant's Position of Trust
Legal and Ethical Issues
Critical Thinking
Answers to Memory Joggers

LEARNING OBJECTIVES

Cognitive: On successful completion of this chapter you should be able to:
1 Define and spell the terms listed in the Vocabulary.
2 State the four requirements of a negotiable instrument.
3 Discuss six advantages of using checks for the transfer of funds.
4 State why it is important to complete the check stub before writing a check.
5 Explain how you would handle mistakes made in preparing a check.
6 List and discuss eight precautions to observe in accepting checks.
7 State the purpose of a check endorsement.
8 Name and compare four kinds of endorsements.
9 Cite five reasons for depositing checks promptly.
10 Discuss the action necessary when a deposited check is returned.

Performance: On successful completion of this chapter you should be able to:
1 Prepare a bank deposit.
2 Correctly write a check.
3 Pay office bills by checks.
4 Reconcile a bank statement with the checkbook balance.

263

Vocabulary Lists define all pertinent medical terminology you will be expected to master throughout the chapter, in one easy-to-find location.

3 Special Focus

Sidebars contain information that focuses on professional topics that transcend chapters and reflect material that will be important to you as a student entering the real world of medical assisting. *Personal Qualities* highlight skills that are particularly essential to communicating and interacting effectively with people in general and patients and co-workers specifically. *Skills and Responsibilities* highlight important elements of your job that will be vital to your success and growth within the medical profession. *Patient Education* discussions offer tips and strategies for effectively implementing this important aspect of your job.

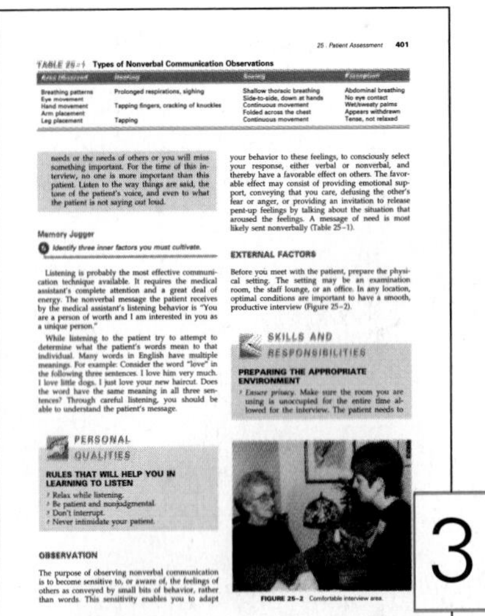

Legal and Ethical Issues (located at the end of each chapter) focus on areas of your job responsibility of which you will need to become keenly aware in order to protect yourself, your patients, and the practice for which you work.

Full Color Artwork

4

All photos and illustrations have been replaced for this new edition. Over 950 pieces of full color artwork throughout the text will help you clearly envision important concepts and skills.

Safety Alerts

These serve as a ready reminder of the many times when—and how—safety must be observed in order to protect you and others in the medical office.

Memory Jogger/How Did I Do?

Questions appear at intervals throughout the body of the text and are intended to intermittently check your understanding of the content. Answers to the questions are provided at the end of each chapter.

Examples

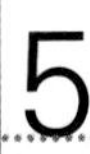

The highlighted examples bring the real world into your learning experience by discussing how the material you are mastering is directly and practically applied to the workplace.

Critical Thinking

Retaining content is not enough to completely master the material successfully. The scenarios presented in these boxes at the end of each chapter reinforce the content while also applying it to the real world through problem-solving and decision-making exercises of situations you could easily encounter on the job.

References

Located at the end of some chapters, references and resources provide you with a listing of other sources of information to help you further your understanding of chapter content.

Procedural Icons

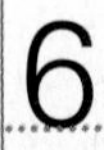

These pictures serve as a reminder of those important safety precautions that are required before performing the procedure.

Student Mastery Manual

7

This supplement to the eighth edition of *The Medical Assistant: Administrative and Clinical* tests your knowledge of chapter content, mastery of chapter skills, and ability to apply what you've learned in that chapter to a clinical situation.

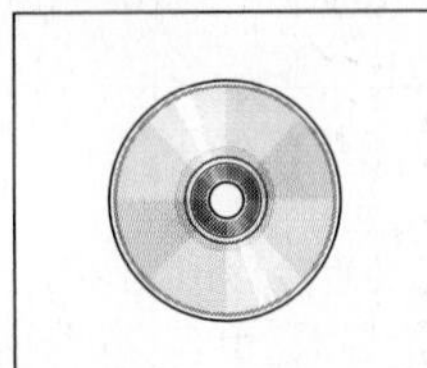

The Virtual Medical Office CD-ROM

This innovative product, bound free in the back of the textbook, lets you "put it all together" in a reality-based environment that makes learning challenging and fun.

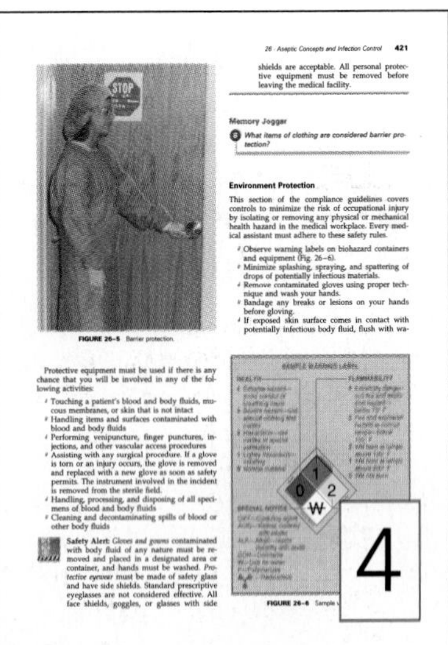

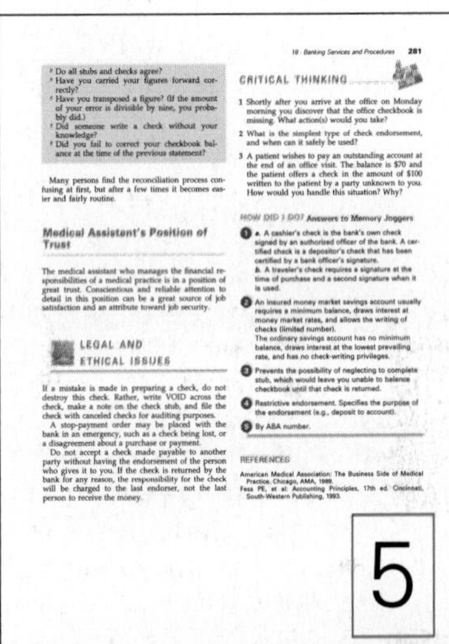

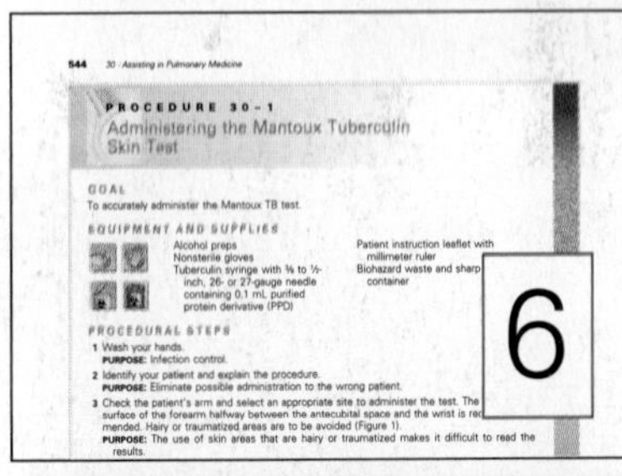

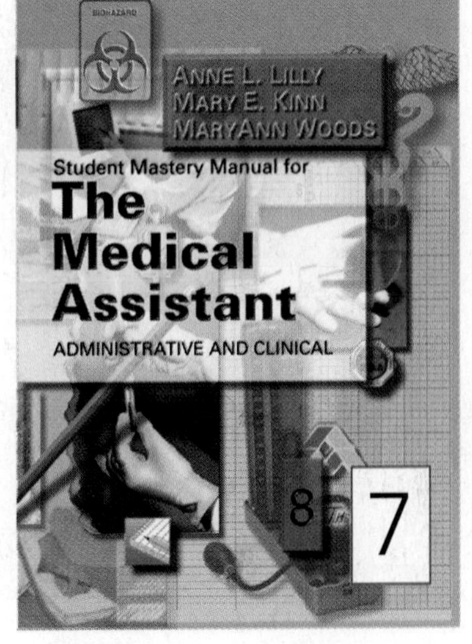

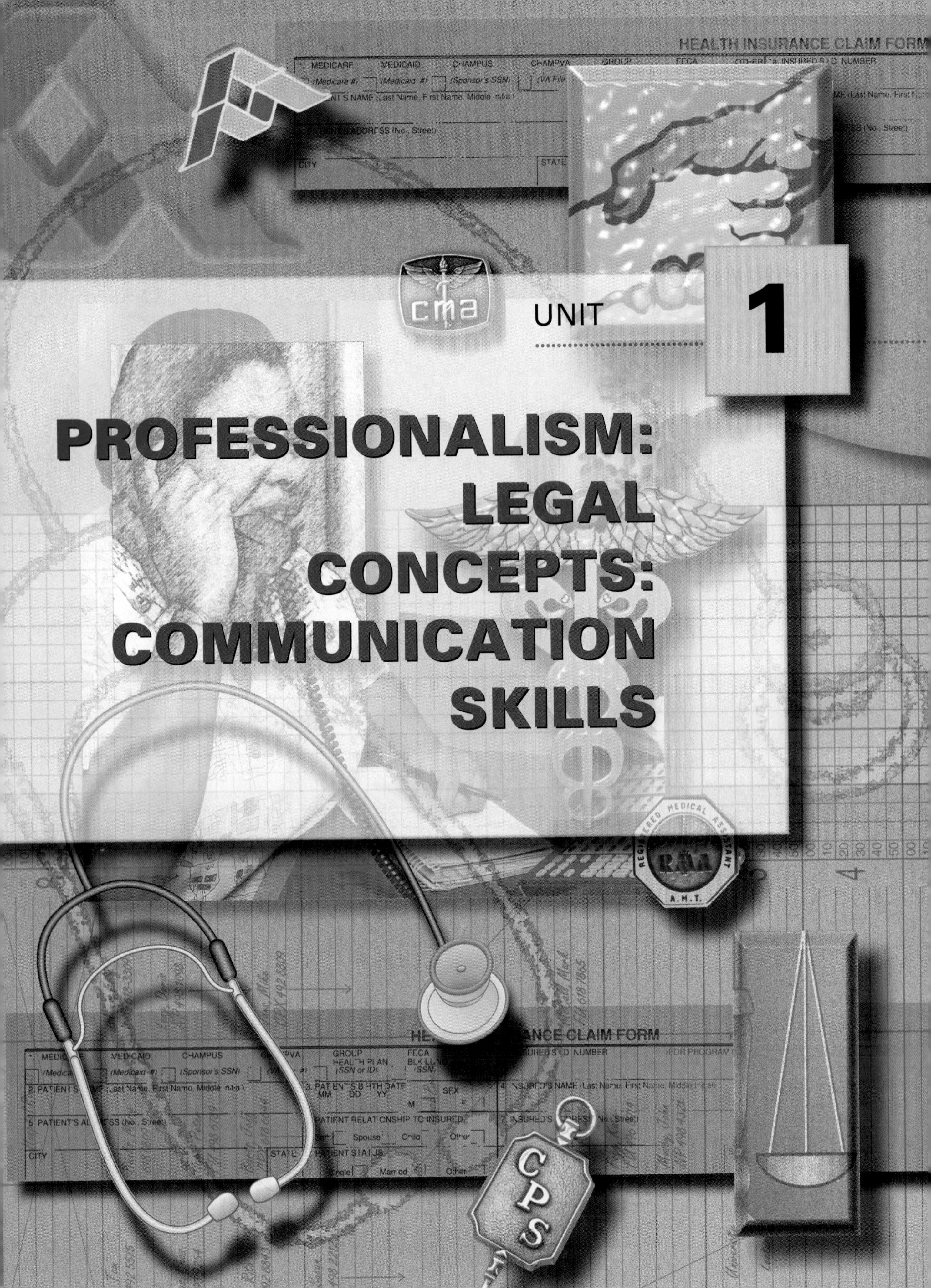
UNIT 1
PROFESSIONALISM: LEGAL CONCEPTS: COMMUNICATION SKILLS

SECTION 1

The Medical Assisting Profession

CURRICULUM CONTENT/COMPETENCIES

Chapter 1 Introduction to Medical Assisting

- Project a professional manner and image
- Adhere to ethical standards
- Demonstrate initiative and responsibility
- Recognize professional credentialing criteria
- Promote the CMA credential
- Enhance skills through continuing education

Chapter 2 Medical Assisting Externship and Preparing to Find a Position

- Demonstrate teamwork
- Prioritize and manage time effectively
- Recognize and respond to written, oral, and nonverbal communications
- Practice within the scope of education, training, and personal capabilities
- Use effective and correct verbal and written communications

Chapter 3 A Brief History of Medicine

- Enhance skills through continuing education
- Adhere to ethical principles
- Adapt to change
- Recognize and respect cultural diversities

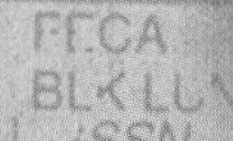

Introduction to Medical Assisting

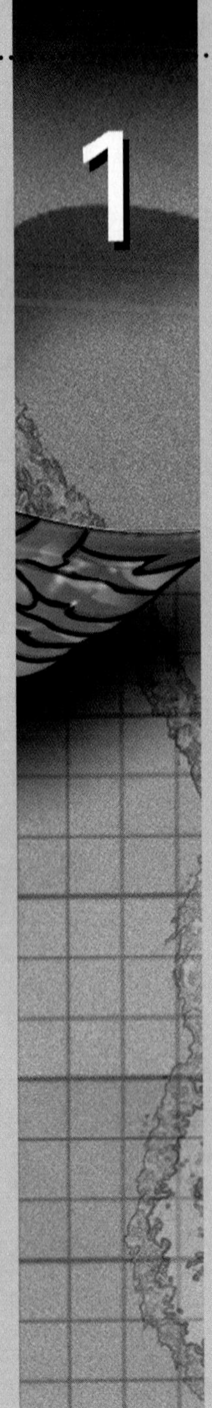

OUTLINE

LEARNING OBJECTIVES

Cognitive: On successful completion of this chapter you should be able to:

1 Identify 10 career opportunities that are available to the trained medical assistant.

2 Identify at least five general knowledge areas in which the medical assistant should be proficient.

3 Differentiate between administrative and clinical responsibilities of a medical assistant.

4 List five personality traits that are beneficial to the successful medical assistant.

5 Briefly describe the training programs that are available for medical assistants.

6 Name four professional organizations that provide educational opportunities and certification examinations.

VOCABULARY

administrative Having to do with management duties; in medical assisting, refers to all "front office" activities

clinical Pertaining to actual observation and treatment of patients

discretion Quality of being discreet, tactful, or prudent

ethnic Pertaining to large groups of people classed according to cultural origin or background

externship The practice of receiving employment experience in qualified health care facilities under the cooperative supervision of the medical staff and the program instructor as part of the educational curriculum

freestanding emergency center An emergency facility not associated with a hospital

group practice The provision of services by a group of at least three practitioners

health maintenance organization (HMO) An organization that provides comprehensive health care to an enrolled group for a fixed periodic payment

mandatory In the nature of a mandate or command; obligatory

paradox A statement that seems to be contradictory and yet is perhaps true

regional Pertaining to a region or territory; local

rural Pertaining to the country, as distinguished from a city or town

solo private practice One physician practicing alone

urban Characteristic of or pertaining to a city or town

A career as a medical assistant is challenging and offers variety, job satisfaction, opportunity for service, commensurate financial reward, and possibility for advancement. It is open to both men and women. Entering the field of medical assisting is a significant decision. Medical assisting is a career requiring dedication, integrity, and a commitment to continuing education.

Past, Present, and Future

The first medical assistant was probably a neighbor of a physician who was asked to help when an extra pair of hands was needed. As the practice of medicine became more complicated, some physicians hired registered nurses to help in their office practices. Gradually, record keeping, data reporting, and an increasing number of business details began to be burdensome, and physicians realized a need for an assistant with business training. Community and junior colleges began offering training programs that focused on both administrative and clinical skills in the late 1940s.

Medical assistant organizations on county and state levels began developing around 1950. A national organization for medical assistants was formed in 1957, and, a few years later, national certification for medical assistants became possible. In recent years, legislation regarding the scope of practice of medical assistants has been enacted in some states.

Career Advantages

A trained medical assistant is equipped with a flexible, adaptable career. The skills acquired by the medical assistant can be carried throughout life, and employment is readily available anywhere in the world that medicine is practiced. Although medical assisting holds many opportunities for both men and women, it is one career that usually does not have a mandatory retirement age. Medical assisting attracts the nontraditional student who may be older than the average postsecondary student by a decade or more. Many medical assistants pursue their careers far beyond the usual retirement age because physicians realize the value of experienced, mature employees.

CAREER OPPORTUNITIES

The practice of medicine has changed dramatically in the past two decades. Increasing costs have created a trend away from hospital-based treatment and toward the delivery of care in physicians' offices and in outpatient centers. Although doctors have employed assistants in their practices for many years, computerization and technologic advances have created more opportunities for qualified medical assistants and increased their responsibilities. The result is an increase in the need for professional training. More clearly defined educational needs of medical assistants have resulted in improvement in both quality and accessibility of training courses. Medical assisting is recognized as an important allied health care profession. Employment opportunities in allied health for the medical assistant are abundant and extremely varied. More medical assistants are employed by practicing physicians than any other type of allied health care personnel.

Memory Jogger

1 *Why is it increasingly important for medical assistants to receive formal training before employment?*

A medical assistant's work can be **administrative** or **clinical.** Training for medical assisting has become a paradox. Leaders in the profession as well as employers are emphasizing the need for multiskilled medical assistants. At the same time, job descriptions are becoming more specialized. Employment can be as a receptionist in a hospital or physician's office, transcriptionist, insurance specialist, financial secretary, billing and collection specialist, clinical assistant involved in patient care, or emergency technician, to name just a few. The medical assistant may choose to work for a physician in **solo private practice,** for a medical partnership or **group practice,** for a **health maintenance organization (HMO),** for a hospital, or for a **freestanding emergency center.** The physician(s) may be engaged in general practice or a specialty such as surgery, internal medicine, dermatology, obstetrics, pediatrics, or psychiatry. The choices are almost limitless.

ADDITIONAL OPPORTUNITIES

Career opportunities abound in public health facilities, hospitals, laboratories, medical schools, research centers, voluntary health agencies, and medical firms of all kinds. Opportunities for work are also available with such federal agencies as the Department of Veterans Affairs, the United States Public Health Service, and Armed Forces clinics or hospitals.

This text is designed primarily for the student who is in training for employment in a private health care facility. It is also valuable as a reference after employment and as a review resource for the medical assistant in preparing for certification.

Earnings

What kind of earnings can the medical assistant expect? As in any other career field, there are **regional** differences, particularly between earnings in **rural** and in **urban** areas. Overall, the medical assistant can generally expect a satisfactory return on the investment in training, experience, and skill. Most physicians realize that a good medical assistant is worth a good salary. Many have learned through bitter experience that "bargain help" is often the most expensive.

The job turnover among medical assistants is surprisingly low. This fact may show that medical assistants derive a high degree of satisfaction from their work. Many instances have been reported of medical assistants who were hired when a physician started practice and remained until the physician's retirement.

Knowledge and Skills

Ideally, the medical assistant should have both administrative and clinical skills, although he or she may have a personal preference for one or the other. The physician's staff must be able to handle all responsibilities of the office except those requiring the services of a physician or other licensed personnel. Where there are several assistants, each should be able and willing to substitute in an emergency for any of the others. Teamwork is a very important part of any occupation. Few physicians in private practice attempt to serve their patients without at least one assistant. The great majority have at least two assistants, and many have five or more.

Certain knowledge and skills are expected of a trained medical assistant. The skills listed here are not intended to be all inclusive but suggest what may be expected on entry to employment as a medical assistant.

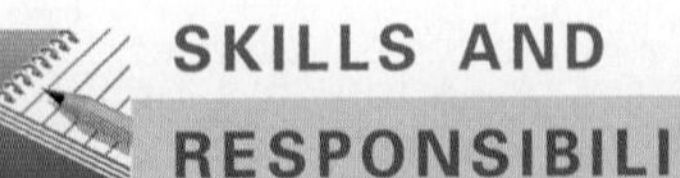

SKILLS AND RESPONSIBILITIES

GENERAL SKILLS

- Medical terminology usage and spelling
- Basics of medical law and ethics
- Human relations and personal communications
- Computer literacy
- Documentation of health information
- Cardiopulmonary resuscitation
- Emergency first aid
- Legible handwriting

ADMINISTRATIVE SKILLS

- Telephone skills and scheduling
- Proficiency in typing and keyboarding
- Communication, written and spoken
- Electronic dictation and word processing
- Health information management
- Patient and insurance billing

CLINICAL SKILLS

- Application of aseptic technique and infection control
- Testing for vital signs
- Interviewing and recording of patient history
- Patient instruction
- Specimen collection and handling
- Performance of selected tests

Memory Jogger

Why is it important for a medical assistant to have both administrative and clinical skills?

Personal Attributes

The professional services of a medical assistant are extremely personal. Therefore, the manner in which these services are performed can affect the health and welfare of a patient in either a positive or negative way.

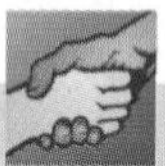

PERSONAL QUALITIES

HOW DO YOU INTERACT WITH PATIENTS?

- Do you have a friendly and pleasant attitude?
- Are you able to maintain confidentiality?
- Are you courteous?
- Are you considerate, respectful, and kind?
- Can you control your temper?
- Can you view a situation through the eyes of others?

You may be called on to assume charge of the office when the doctor is out. The doctor must depend on the medical assistant's good judgment when he or she is left alone.

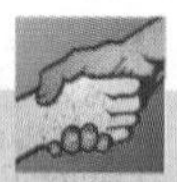

PERSONAL QUALITIES

CAN YOU TAKE CHARGE?

- Are you attentive to details?
- Are you accurate?
- Are you dependable?
- Can you remain calm and accept responsibility during an emergency?

Discretion and concern for the patient are very important. Patients might choose another physician because of the seeming lack of concern by a medical assistant. The patient who feels comfortable with the medical assistant will probably feel comfortable with the doctor.

Memory Jogger

Name at least 10 desirable personal attributes that would enhance the medical assistant's success.

Training

CLASSROOM EDUCATION

Medical assistants who were self-trained and already employed in the field were among the first to recognize the need for formally trained personnel in medical offices. Through chapters of the American Association of Medical Assistants (AAMA) and aided by local medical societies, established medical assistants have strongly influenced the rapidly accelerating development, refinement, and accessibility of such training. Formal training is essential for today's medical assistant.

Many community colleges and private vocational schools offer courses in medical assisting. After satisfactory completion of a program, the student receives a certificate, diploma, or, from some community colleges, an associate degree. Courses in a community college take 10 months to 2 years to complete. Students are usually admitted only once or twice per year. Private schools more frequently have open enrollment, and some programs are completed in 7 months. Currently, the trend is toward offering training in modules, thereby including the individual who may have limited time or who needs the opportunity for upgrading skills and specialty courses (Fig. 1–1).

ON-THE-JOB TRAINING

Effective training also includes an **externship** of at least several weeks to provide practical experience in physicians' offices, accredited hospitals, or other health care facilities. The success of a physician's practice is highly dependent on teamwork of the staff members. Furthermore, the physician, probably more than any other employer, expects employees to carry out their duties independently, with little or no direct supervision.

As a new employee, you should

- Be told exactly what your duties are
- Read your job description as it appears in an

TYPICAL CURRICULUM FOR MEDICAL ASSISTANT PROGRAM

anatomy and physiology
medical terminology
medical law and ethics
human relations
oral and written communications
computer skills, electronic transcription
financial record keeping
insurance coding and billing
health information management
clinical procedures, such as preparation, assisting, and follow-up of patients for medical examinations
first aid
principles of CPR
pharmaceutical principles and medication administration
specimen collection and processing
basic office diagnostic procedures

FIGURE 1–1 Typical curriculum for medical assistant program.

office procedure manual and then discuss it with the physician or your supervisor
- Ask for direction if it is not offered
- Show that you are responsible and dependable

The new employee brings many intangibles to the job that are not found in the job description. Courtesy toward others and a capacity for teamwork, a positive attitude, enthusiasm, initiative, and dedication are important personal attributes. After becoming comfortably acquainted with what is expected of your position, you will probably want to learn what other employees are doing so that you can offer them assistance when needed. In this way, you become a full member of the health care team.

CONTINUING EDUCATION

Education does not end with the completion of formal training. The amount of medical knowledge gained since the beginning of medical history is said to double every 5 years. The practicing medical assistant must keep current with the rapid changes within the profession. Most physicians appreciate the medical assistant who asks questions about unfamiliar conditions or procedures.

Much can be learned by reading or at least briefly reviewing the medical literature that arrives in the daily mail or the articles that appear in newspapers, news magazines, and specialized newsletters. The medical assistant who wishes to advance becomes an active member of a professional organization, has an inquisitive mind, and attends available professional seminars and workshops.

Memory Jogger

4 *Explain the statement "Education does not end with the completion of formal training."*

Responsibilities

The responsibilities of the medical assistant vary from one facility to another, because the position must be geared to the type of practice and the working habits of the individual physician. In the office with only one employee, the medical assistant's time is divided between administrative and clinical duties. In the multiple-employee office, positions generally are more specialized, but each employee has to have the ability to "pitch in" and help in any position.

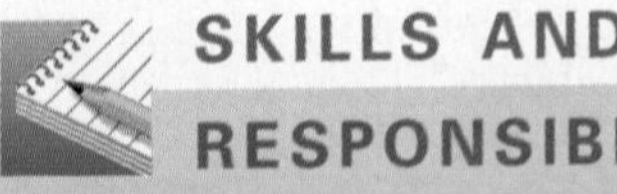

SKILLS AND RESPONSIBILITIES

ADMINISTRATIVE RESPONSIBILITIES

The administrative (sometimes called *front office*) responsibilities of a medical assistant are similar to those of any administrative assistant to a top executive, but they have specific medical aspects.

- Answering telephones
- Scheduling appointments
- Interviewing and instructing new patients
- Explaining fees
- Opening and sorting mail
- Answering routine correspondence
- Transcribing electronic dictation
- Pulling patient charts for scheduled appointments
- Filing reports and correspondence
- Arranging for patient admission to a hospital and instructing the patient regarding admission
- Planning financial arrangements with patients
- Coding and transmitting insurance claims
- Maintaining financial records and files

- Preparing and mailing statements
- Collecting delinquent accounts
- Preparing checks for employer's signature
- Reconciling bank statements
- Maintaining files of paid and unpaid invoices
- Preparing and maintaining employees' payroll records (or supplying payroll information to an outside accountant)
- Supervising personnel
- Helping in the preparation of manuscripts or speeches
- Clipping articles from professional journals
- Assisting with the maintenance of the physician's professional library

CLINICAL RESPONSIBILITIES

The duties of a clinical assistant are also varied.

- Helping the patient prepare for examinations and other procedures
- Recording the medical history
- Assisting in the examination when requested to do so
- Cleaning and sterilizing instruments and equipment
- Instructing patients regarding preparation for radiologic and laboratory examinations
- Keeping supply cabinets well stocked
- Conforming with Occupational Safety and Health Administration (OSHA) requirements
- Supplying patient education
- Performing a variety of laboratory tests such as urinalysis and blood studies
- Performing electrocardiography and, depending on state regulations, assisting in radiography
- Taking of vital signs
- Preparing treatment or surgical trays

Professional Commitment

APPEARANCE

A well-groomed assistant in professional attire has a good psychologic effect on patients. The essentials of a professional appearance are good health, good grooming, and appropriate dress.

Good health requires getting adequate sleep, eating balanced meals, and exercising enough to keep fit. Medical assistants can set a good example by following a sensible and healthful lifestyle that includes regular checkups of their own physical condition. A radiantly healthy office staff promotes the best possible public relations image for the physician.

Good grooming is little more than attention to the details of personal appearance. Personal cleanliness, which includes taking a daily bath or shower, using a deodorant, and practicing good oral hygiene, is vital. Use of perfume or aftershave should be avoided; patients and co-workers may be allergic to some scents. The female medical assistant's makeup should be carefully selected and applied. Heavy or exaggerated makeup is out of place in the professional office. Subtle eye makeup and clear or natural shades of nail polish may enhance the assistant's appearance. Both male and female medical assistants should be sure that their hair is clean, neatly styled, and off the collar.

The medical assistant usually wears a uniform or laboratory coat, which not only presents a professional appearance but also identifies the assistant as a member of the health care team. Synthetic fabrics and fashionable styling make it possible for the medical assistant's uniform to be both practical and attractive.

Women may choose to wear pantsuits, which are available in white or a variety of colors; a two-piece dress uniform in white or a color; or an attractively styled traditional white uniform. Men usually wear white slacks with a white or light-colored shirt, jacket, or pullover top. A laboratory coat may be worn over casual street clothes by men or women if this is within the facility's dress code. Today's easy-care fabrics make it unthinkable to wear a uniform more than one day without laundering. Even accidental spills and spots that occur during the working day can usually be rinsed out immediately. Uniforms that are worn where people are ill should be considered contaminated.

The shoes the assistant wears should be appropriate for a uniform and be spotless and comfortable. White shoes must be kept white by daily cleaning. Remember that if a laced shoe is worn, the laces also need cleaning.

In some facilities, the physician prefers that the staff not wear uniforms. Some psychiatrists and some pediatricians, for example, believe that the clinical appearance of a uniform may affect patients adversely. Nevertheless, the medical assistant who does not wear a uniform should follow the dictates of good taste and propriety in choosing a professional wardrobe. The garments worn while on duty must be comfortable, allow easy movement, and still look fresh at the end of a busy day.

Whatever uniform style the assistant chooses, it should be personally becoming and worn over appropriate undergarments. The lines, colors, and ornamentation of undergarments should not be seen through the uniform; therefore, it is best to wear a neutral color without ornamentation. When wearing a uniform, jewelry should be limited to an engagement ring, wedding band, and professional pin (Fig. 1–2). A name badge worn on the right shoulder will help patients to identify each staff person by name.

Follow these guidelines in maintaining a professional appearance.

1. Appear ready to work, in a fresh, clean, and pressed professional uniform.
2. When wearing white, be careful that undergarments do not show through uniform.
3. Clean and polish your shoes daily.
4. Wear your name badge on the right side of your uniform where it can be easily read, and wear your professional pin on the left collar or pocket.
5. Use an unscented deodorant daily and pay particular attention to **oral hygiene**.
6. Style your hair so that it is up and off your collar.
7. Trim your nails and polish them as appropriate.
8. Keep jewelry to a minimum.
9. Be aware of personal habits that may be unacceptable or unprofessional, e.g., smoking and gum chewing.

Female Assistants

1. Wear full-length, neutral shade, run-free hosiery.
2. Apply makeup conservatively and use no cologne or perfume.

Male Assistants

1. Wear socks that are compatible with your shoes and uniform.
2. The face should be clean-shaven, or if you have a mustache or beard, it should be clean and neatly trimmed.

FIGURE 1–2 Guidelines for maintaining a professional appearance.

ATTITUDE

Getting along with people is essential to success in the medical field. The person who can preserve his or her own positive self-image and the individual self-images of others has achieved the first step in human relations. Patients appreciate a reception that is polite and cordial. Establish rapport with the patient on the first encounter. In some areas a wide assortment of geographic and cultural customs exists throughout the population. The person suffering from an illness is often highly sensitive to any violation of ethnic customs, so violations should be avoided whenever possible.

TEAM DYNAMICS

The new employee must be exceptionally considerate of those who are experienced on the job. A natural tendency exists for the trainee just completing formal medical assisting training to want to share this new knowledge with others. This is not always what the established employee wants to hear. The new assistant should emphasize willingness to follow instructions and show appreciation for what others are doing until a firm relationship is in place. Team dynamics include working together, offering to do a colleague's work when he or she cannot be in the office, and being willing to help others when your work is caught up.

INITIATIVE AND RESPONSIBILITY

Responsibility is shown by arriving on time and being available for the full time agreed on. You should know what is expected in the regular course of employment and, if time permits, volunteer to help others who may have an overload if it is within your scope of education. Show a willingness to learn additional skills and show initiative by finding things to do when the office is less busy. Responsibility also includes calling your superior any time you will be unavoidably late or absent or alerting a co-worker when you will be absent from your work station.

Memory Jogger

5 *Can you recall an ethnic custom that would affect your contact with a patient?*

JOIN YOUR PROFESSIONAL ORGANIZATION

You may have become a student member of the local medical assistants association and advanced to an active member after your employment. Membership in your professional association shows a dedication to your career and establishes your identity as a medical assistant. Attending chapter meetings provides a source of continuing education. Participating in organization activities and being involved in the planning and action within the chapter develops your "people skills" and teaches leadership. Each individual can influence the future of the profession.

Being a medical assistant is more than just a job. It is a way of life.

Professional Organizations

BENEFITS OF MEMBERSHIP IN A PROFESSIONAL ORGANIZATION

By joining a professional organization and participating in the activities it affords, a medical assistant can grow personally and professionally and keep abreast of current trends. Most organizations give continuing education events resulting in continuing education units (CEUs) being recorded and reported that can be applied to a recertification program. Participation in a recognized professional organization shows that the employee is serious about his or her career and an asset to the employer. Dedicated medical assistants will attest to its rewards.

American Association of Medical Assistants

The AAMA was formally organized in 1956 as a federation of several state associations that had been functioning independently. In 1997, the AAMA had affiliated societies in more than 40 states, with national headquarters in Chicago, Illinois. It has been a continuing force behind establishing a national certifying program for medical assistants, the accrediting of medical assisting training programs in community colleges and private schools, and setting minimum standards for the entry-level medical assistant.

AAMA members have the opportunity to attend local, state, regional, and national meetings, where they can participate in workshops, learn of educational advances in their field, hear prominent speakers, and establish a networking system with other medical assistants.

The AAMA publishes a bimonthly journal, the *PMA (Professional Medical Assistant),* which includes articles with tests that may be submitted for CEUs. Members may wear the AAMA insignia (Fig. 1–3). Since 1963, the AAMA has administered a certifying examination, with successful completion leading to a certificate and recognition as a certified medical assistant (CMA). Examinations are given in January and June of each year at designated centers throughout the United States. Certification is available to students or graduates of programs accredited by the Commission on Accreditation of Allied Health Education Programs (CAAHEP). Recertification is required every 5 years and can be accomplished through CEUs or reexamination. A certified medical assistant is permitted to wear the CMA pin (Fig. 1–4).

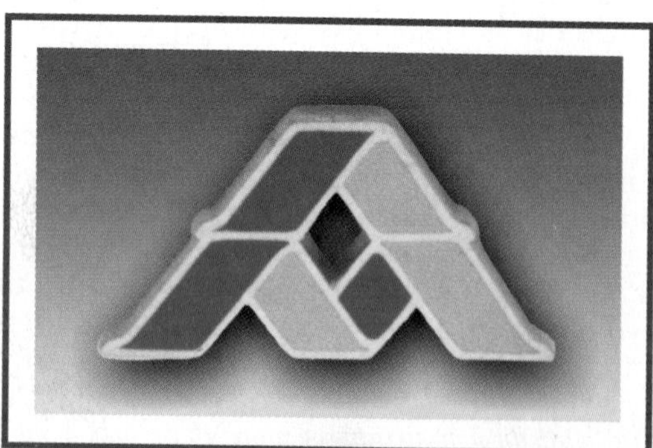

FIGURE 1–3 Insignia of the American Association of Medical Assistants. (Courtesy of the American Association of Medical Assistants, Chicago, IL.)

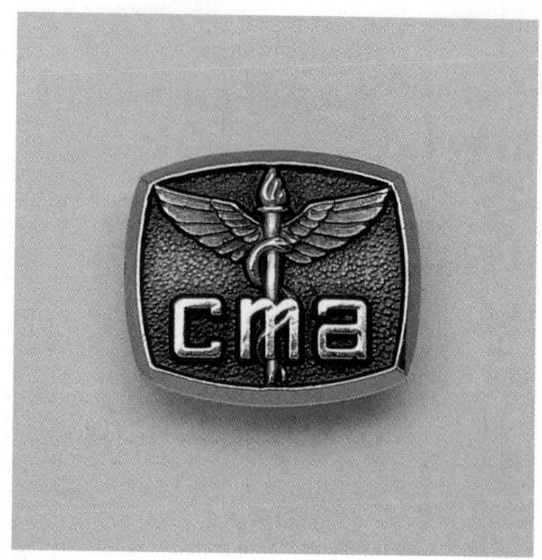

FIGURE 1–4 Pin worn by the certified medical assistant. (Courtesy of the American Association of Medical Assistants, Chicago, IL.)

REGISTERED MEDICAL ASSISTANTS OF THE AMERICAN MEDICAL TECHNOLOGISTS In the early 1970s, the American Medical Technologists (AMT), a national certifying body for laboratory personnel since 1939, began offering an examination for medical assistants. The solid success of this project brought about the formulation of the registered medical assistant (RMA) program within AMT in 1976. Since that time, the RMAs have earned great respect in their own right. They have played an active role in public relations and professional recognition, protective legislation, improvements in training programs, and the provision of continuing education materials and opportunities.

The RMA certification examination is given in June and November of each year throughout the United States and as needed at schools accredited by the Accrediting Bureau of Health Education Schools (ABHES). Applicants must be graduates of a medical assisting course accredited by ABHES, a regional accrediting commission, or other acceptable agency or must meet certain experience requirements. All RMA members of the AMT Registry are certified medical assistants by examination and are entitled to wear the RMA insignia (Fig. 1–5). RMA headquarters is located in Park Ridge, Illinois.

Independent unaffiliated medical assistant organizations in some states offer professional participation at the local and state level as well as continuing education opportunities.

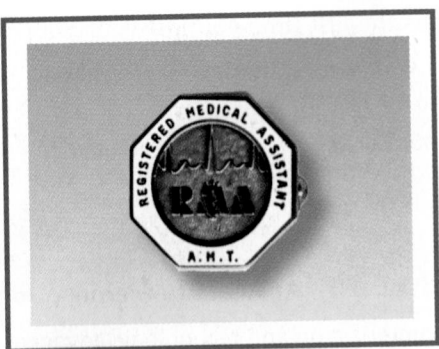

FIGURE 1–5 Pin worn by the registered medical assistant. (Courtesy of the RMA/American Medical Technologists, Park Ridge, IL.)

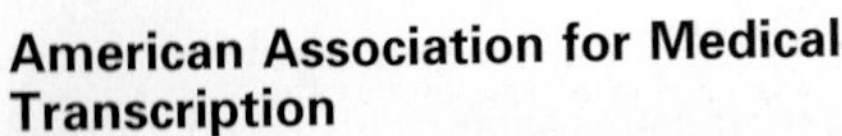

American Association for Medical Transcription

Many medical offices employ medical language specialists as medical transcriptionists; such professionals will find membership in the American Association of Medical Transcription (AAMT) valuable. The association was incorporated in 1978 with headquarters in Modesto, California. Voluntary certification by successful completion of an examination has been offered since 1981 and may be maintained through continuing education (Fig. 1–6). The AAMT publishes a professional journal six times per year. It offers outstanding education materials and holds an annual national convention.

Professional Secretaries International, the Association for Office Professionals

The administrative medical assistant may profit from membership in Professional Secretaries International (PSI), which was founded in 1942 as The National Secretaries Association (International) and is headquartered in Kansas City, Missouri. Through its Institute for Certifying Secretaries, PSI sponsors the Certified Professional Secretary (CPS) Examination, which covers Finance and Business Law (accounting, economics, business law); Office Systems and Administration (office technology, office administration, business communications); and Management (behavioral science in business, human resources management, organizations and management). The rating of CPS is obtained by meeting educational and work experience requirements and by passing the three-part examination (Fig. 1–7). The organization publishes *The Secretary* magazine nine times per year, sponsors Collegiate Secretaries International and the Future Secretaries Association in colleges and high schools, respectively, and holds an annual CPS seminar each June and an international convention each July.

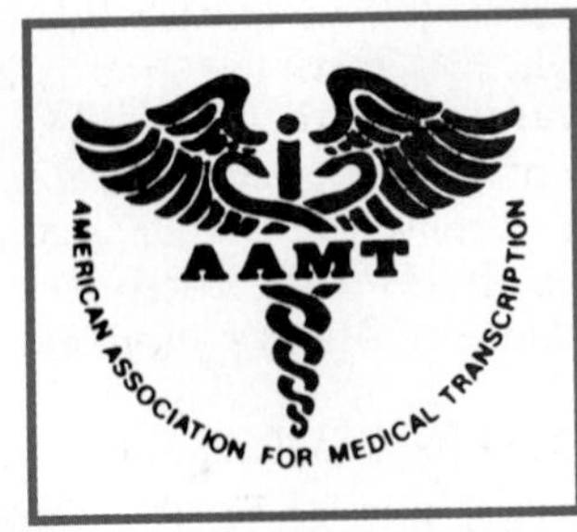

FIGURE 1–6 Insignia of American Association for Medical Transcription. (Courtesy of American Association for Medical Transcription, Modesto, CA.)

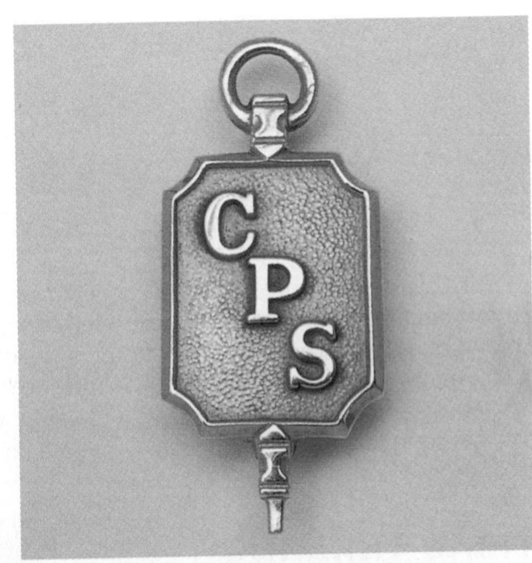

FIGURE 1–7 Pin worn by the certified professional secretary. (Courtesy of Professional Secretaries International.)

Overview

This introductory chapter has presented the advantages of becoming a trained medical assistant and some of the many career opportunities available. Emphasis was placed on the necessary skills that must be developed and the general knowledge that must be acquired to function successfully in the medical arena. However, skills and knowledge alone do not bring success to the aspiring medical assistant. Therefore, personality traits and professional appearance have also been emphasized in this introductory chapter. The importance of getting the right start when entering new employment and the necessity for continuing education was discussed. Reviewing the development of the rapidly changing career of medical assisting highlights the importance of each individual in upholding the established professional standards.

Although this introduction to the profession precedes the presentation of performance skills, it is recommended that the student review it immediately before interviewing for a position in this fascinating field of health care.

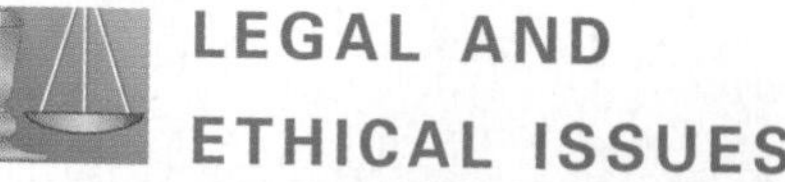

LEGAL AND ETHICAL ISSUES

As a medical assistant you will be exposed to a vast amount of personal and intimate knowledge of the patients who entrust their care to your physicians. Such information must be held in confidence and never discussed or relayed to others, including your professional associates.

CRITICAL THINKING

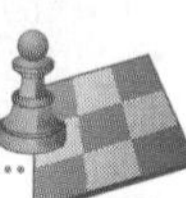

Medical assisting is a serious and rewarding career for both women and men. Persons involved in health care are highly respected in the community and provide an essential service. The expected qualifications are demanding but attainable. The woman or man who accepts this career must be willing to accept the responsibilities inherent in its standards.

1 Do you have a preference for either administrative or clinical duties? If you do, do you know why?

2 When is the last time you lost your temper?

3 Have you ever divulged information someone asked you not to tell?

4 Do you know any medical assistants who have attained certification status? How did they feel about it?

HOW DID I DO? Answers to Memory Joggers

1. Computerization and technologic advances in the practice of medicine require more training, and physicians expect this when hiring.
2. The physician's staff must be able to handle all responsibilities of the office except those requiring the services of licensed personnel.
3. Individual responses.
4. The practicing medical assistant must keep current with changes within the profession to function effectively.
5. *Example:* The Hmong people from Laos believe the head is sacred because that is where the soul resides. A Hmong child would be very distressed if you patted him or her on the head even in an affectionate way.

Medical Assisting Externship and Preparing to Find a Position

2

OUTLINE

LEARNING OBJECTIVES

Cognitive: On successful completion of this chapter you should be able to:

1 Define and spell the terms listed in the vocabulary.
2 Explain the essentials of an externship.
3 Briefly explain four responsibilities of the student during externship.
4 Describe the responsibilities of an externship office or agency.
5 Explain how a student will benefit from externship experience.
6 List the three steps in applying for a position.
7 Identify the five essential parts of a personal inventory.
8 List seven basic items that should be included in every resumé.
9 Specify five items that must *not* be inserted in a resumé.
10 Cite five sources of leads for employment as a medical assistant.
11 List three avenues of evaluation that an interviewer may use in selecting an employee.

Performance: On successful completion of this chapter you should be able to perform the following activities:

1 Prepare a personal inventory.
2 Prepare two examples of a resumé.
3 Demonstrate a telephone request for an interview.
4 Write a letter in response to a newspaper help-wanted ad.
5 Compose a follow-up letter of thanks after an interview for a position.

VOCABULARY

avocational Pertaining to a subordinate occupation or a hobby

chronologic In the order of time

externship The practice of receiving employment experience in qualified health care facilities under the cooperative supervision of the medical staff and the program instructor as part of the educational curriculum

extracurricular Relating to those activities that form part of the life of students but are not part of the courses of study

format Shape, size, and general makeup of a publication, such as a resumé

objective Something toward which effort is directed; an aim or end of action

personal inventory A complete summary of pertinent information about oneself

re-entry student One who has been away from formal education or employment for several years and who is now preparing to re-enter the workplace

resumé A *selective* summary of one's education and employment record tailored to the position being sought

seminar A group of students meeting regularly and informally with a professor to discuss ideas and problems

Externship

As you progress in your training, you will be giving thought to just how and where you will fit into the health care world, and you will undoubtedly have acquired certain preferences.

One aid in defining and focusing your interests is experiencing an **externship** program that provides practical experience in a variety of qualified physicians' offices, accredited hospitals, or other health care facilities. Externship experience is included by most schools and colleges that have a complete curriculum for medical assisting. In those programs accredited by the Council on Accreditation of Allied Health Education Programs (CAAHEP) in collaboration with the American Medical Association and the American Association of Medical Assistants, an externship is mandatory. A minimum of 160 hours is recommended.

WHAT IS AN EXTERNSHIP?

The externship phase of your training may also be known as *work experience* or *on-the-job* training and is done without pay. The externship is planned and supervised by the instructor in collaboration with local employers. The medical offices and health care facilities serve as an extension of the college when physicians and administrators accept students for the externship. You may be expected to carry malpractice insurance during the externship. You will probably be required to undergo a physical examination, chest x-ray, appropriate serologic tests, and hepatitis vaccine.

During the very important weeks of your externship, you will have an opportunity to apply your administrative and clinical skills under the supervision of a practicing medical assistant. You will be expected to responsibly carry through with the assigned tasks. Your supervisor and the physician(s) at the externship site will be evaluating your personal qualities as well as the skills you have learned in the classroom.

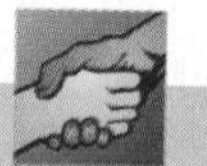

PERSONAL QUALITIES

- Grooming
- Poise
- Integrity
- Punctuality
- Relations with co-workers and patients
- Reaction to criticism and direction
- Respect for ethical standards
- Consideration for others

The on-site supervisor and physician assume responsibility for continual evaluation of your performance, as directed by your instructor, and this evaluation becomes a part of your student record.

DURATION AND TIME OF EXTERNSHIP

The duration of the externship and the time at which it is introduced into the program will vary, depending on the school or college. Some schools have the student spend 1 or 2 days in a health care

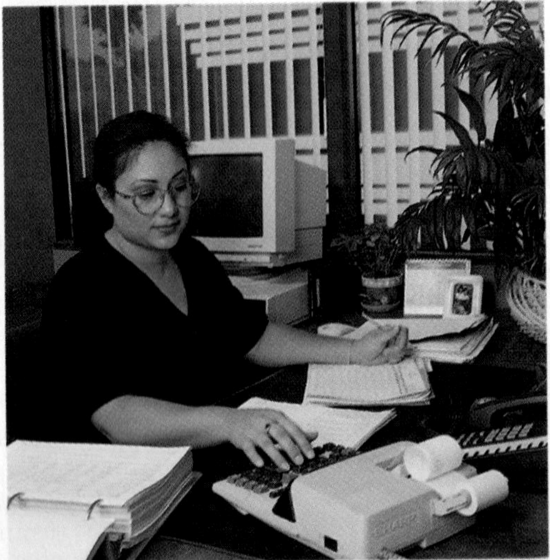

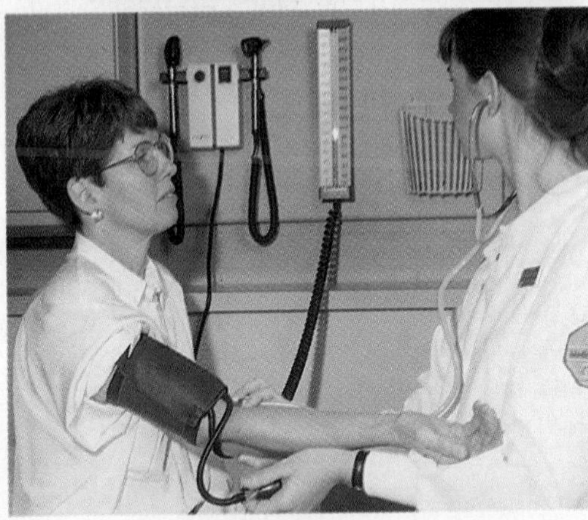

FIGURE 2–1 Medical assisting externship includes both administrative and clinical duties. (Bottom photo from Chester GA: Modern Medical Assisting. Philadelphia, WB Saunders, 1998, p 445.)

facility early in the training to provide a frame of reference for later instruction. Others combine work experience with classroom instruction throughout the training period. The majority of schools prefer a concentrated period of externship near the conclusion of the classroom instruction (Fig. 2–1).

STUDENT RESPONSIBILITIES

During the externship, both your appearance and actions must be according to accepted professional standards. You will report to work at a specified time on specified days, just as if you were a regular employee, but you will not be paid by the training facility. You may spend all your externship in one facility, but it is usually preferable to rotate among several types of practice for a well-rounded experience. Do not be surprised if you are expected to apply and be interviewed for the position just as you will later on when you are seeking employment. This is valuable experience and should be welcomed.

You, as a student, should recognize that a health care agency that cooperates with your education is accepting a great responsibility. You will require continual supervision, and your questions must be answered. You must be aware of ethical and legal concerns and of the potential for a claim of medical malpractice. One large concern is that of patient privacy. You must reveal no information concerning a patient or the practice to persons outside the facility. Some agencies may ask you to sign an oath of privacy while in that facility.

EXTERNSHIP SITES

The school or college will designate a specific individual to be your externship coordinator, who will carefully choose and screen suitable training facilities. The supervising staff at the health care facility must agree to complete an evaluation of your performance while providing ample opportunity for you to practice your skills. Quite often, the coordinator will seek out offices where former graduates of the program are employed. This ensures greater understanding and cooperation as well as the assurance that work habits and procedures meet the standards promoted in the classroom. In rare instances, a student may feel that the training facility is taking advantage of a situation and simply using the student to perform menial tasks. If you do have such an experience, it should be reported to your instructor.

The value of the externship is enhanced when the training program includes a weekly **seminar** at which all the students serving externship and their instructor may share experiences, problems, and solutions. All three parties to the agreement—the school, the externship agency or facility, and the trainee—benefit from the experience.

BENEFITS FROM AN EXTERNSHIP

- The school has a line of communication to the community and is better able to assess the needs and expectations of the public for which it is training prospective employees.
- The externship agency benefits from the new ideas and methods that the trainee may introduce. If the facility is looking for additional help, this is an ideal way to evaluate the performance of a trainee without involvement in the hiring process.
- The trainee benefits most of all by exposure to practical experience in a variety of settings. This experience in the real world removes a great deal of the anxiety that might otherwise be present in a first employment situation.

If the student performs well during the externship, he or she may be offered a permanent job with the facility, but it should not be assumed that this will happen. The externship facility may also be used as a reference when seeking a permanent position. When you are confident that you have performed well and have a comfortable relationship with the supervisory staff in the training facility, you may ask for a reference to be used later on when interviewing for employment.

Memory Jogger

Explain the similarities and the differences between externship and regular employment.

Finding the Right Position

After you have completed your classroom training and externship, the next step will be to find the right position. Your aptitudes and skills must be matched with the requirements of a physician or facility in need of an employee. Whether you are seeking your first position or are returning to the field after an absence of several years, or even if you are an experienced medical assistant preparing to change employers, the steps in applying for a position are essentially the same:

- Preparing for the interview
- Locating prospective employers
- Interviewing

Looking for work is a job in itself. Approach it as a job, establish a schedule, and stick to it.

PREPARING FOR THE INTERVIEW

Preliminary Steps

Before seeking an interview, you should give yourself a "preinterview" self-test:

- What type of work do I really want?
- Where can I function best?
- Do I prefer clinical or administrative functions?
- What are my best skills?
- Do I prefer to work in a small practice or in a large medical group?
- Would I enjoy the variety of a general practice or the concentration of a specialty?
- How important to me are salary, hours, and location?

In your externship experience, you may have formed some rather definite preferences, or you may feel absolutely certain of some things that would cause you to be dissatisfied. Include these judgments in your search.

Personal Inventory

It sometimes happens that your first position is so ideally suitable that you will accept and stay in it for the remainder of your working years. More than likely, however, you will have to make several changes of employment during your lifetime.

A **personal inventory,** to which you will add as you gain additional experience, will prove invaluable to you later as well as now. The personal inventory is for your own information and reference—rather like keeping a journal. It will be a ready source of information in preparing and updating your resumé. The personal inventory is *complete* information about your working life; a resumé is *selected* information tailored to the position you are seeking. Five steps are involved: (1) biographical data, (2) employment history, (3) educational data, (4) extracurricular interests, and (5) activities and personal goals.

Step 1. Start with a page for biographical data: your name, birth date, Social Security number, address, and telephone number.

BIOGRAPHICAL DATA

Name ____________ Birth Date ____________

Address ______________________________

Tel. No. ____________ Soc. Sec. No. ____________

Step 2. Prepare a separate page for your employment history. This is especially important for the **re-entry student.** Not all students enter vocational training directly from high school or early in their employment careers. Many have spent intervening years as full-time homemakers or in other employment. The experience gained during these years should be included in your personal inventory. It could be important in future situations. If you have never been employed but have done volunteer work requiring personal responsibility, list that here. The employment history should include dates of employment, name of employer, type of business, your position title, and major duties. Because this will be a continuing record that you will add to as you gain experience, it is prepared in **chronologic** order, starting with the first major job you held. However, when you use this information in a resumé it will be listed in reverse chronologic order, beginning with the latest position.

EMPLOYMENT HISTORY

June 19xx June 19xx
Month Year to Month Year

Employer XXXXXXXXXXX

Type of Business Women's clothing

Position Held Part-time sales clerk

Major Duties: Assisting customers in their selections, registering sales, closing out register at end of day.
Satisfactions: Enjoyed personal contacts
Learned to accept responsibility
Dissatisfactions: Not related to my goals

Step 3. Next, record your educational data, beginning with high school. List the dates, the institution attended, and the year of graduation, plus the diploma or degree earned. Make note of the areas of study you enjoyed most and list special competencies, awards, or honors. As time goes by, it may be difficult to recall these details, and you never know what will be important to an employer in the future. Remember, you are starting a permanent record for your own information and as a handy reference tool when needed. As with the employment history, the educational data are listed here in chronologic order but will appear in reverse chronologic order in a resumé, starting with the highest degree or certificate.

EDUCATIONAL DATA

Dates	Institution Attended	Year Graduated/ Degree
19xx–19xx	Valley High School Ola Vista	19xx Diploma
19xx–19xx	Ola Vista Community College	19xx Associate in Science, Medical Assisting

Special Competencies:
Typing Certificate (70 wpm)
Limited X-ray permit, 19xx
CPR Certificate, 19xx, renewed annually
Fluency in Spanish
Awards:
Dean's list, all four semesters in college

Step 4. You may wish to include a page for your extracurricular interests and activities. List organization memberships and activities and any positions of leadership you held. Your volunteer activities and any significant hobbies might be included here if they are not in your employment record. Mention significant skills obtained while performing these activities. Many of these skills are important assets to a medical facility.

EXTRACURRICULAR INTERESTS AND ACTIVITIES

Organization Memberships	Year	Personal Participation
Associated Women Students	19xx	Secretary 19xx–19xx
American Association of Medical Assistants	19xx	Student Member
	19xx	Page, 19xx convention
Girl Scouts of the U.S.A.	19xx	Brownie group leader, 19xx

Hobbies
Oil painting, backpacking

Step 5. Have a page for your personal goals. What are your *immediate* goals? your *long-term* goals? What concessions are you willing to make in order to reach your goals (e.g., working nonconventional hours)?

PERSONAL GOALS

Date	Immediate Goals	Long-Term Goals
19xx	Medical assistant position preferably in pediatric practice	Bachelor of Science degree in Business Administration
		Administrative position in large group practice or HMO

Resumé

The final and most important step in preparing for an interview is producing a **resumé** that will arouse the interest of a prospective employer.

THERESA O'SULLIVAN

233 Wentworth Street, San Diego, CA 92100 **Telephone (619) 222-3333**

EDUCATION	**Associate in Science**, Ola Vista Community College June 19xx (Dean's List, four semesters) **Diploma**, Valley High School, June 19xx
CERTIFICATES	**CPR** certificate (renewed annually since 19xx) **Certificate in Medical Assisting**, Ola Vista Community College
SPECIAL COMPETENCIES	Speak Spanish fluently Hold Limited X-ray Permit
EMPLOYMENT	**Part-Time Medical Assistant**, June 19xx to June 19xx Duties included: preparing patients for examination in general practice office; taking height, weight, and vital signs; answering the telephone and reception; and appointment scheduling. **Part-Time Sales**, Baxter Department Store, June 19xx to June 19xx Duties included: assisting customers in making their selections; registering sales; and closing out register at end of day.
AVOCATIONAL INTERESTS	**Student Member**, American Association of Medical Assistants **Secretary**, Associated Women Students OVCC
REFERENCES	Furnished upon request.

FIGURE 2–2 Sample chronologic resumé.

If you do not feel confident in doing this yourself, get help. If you are a student in a 2-year college, there is probably a career center on campus where you can ask for assistance. There are also many guidebooks in public libraries and in bookstores where you can find ideas (see the references at the end of this chapter). Computer software that provides guidelines, formatting, and suggestions for preparing the resumé is plentiful and easily located.

The purpose of the resumé is to get an interview, not to get a job. This should be kept in mind as you decide what to include. Using your personal inventory, you can select the information that applies to the position you have in mind. The **format** should be attractive, and the information typed on one sheet of paper with absolutely no errors or misspelled words (Figs. 2–2 and 2–3). Tinted paper will make the resumé more distinctive, but bright

THERESA O'SULLIVAN

233 Wentworth Street, San Diego, CA 92100 **Telephone (619) 222-3333**

STATEMENT OF EMPLOYMENT ASSETS
FOR A CAREER IN MEDICAL ASSISTING

GENERAL	Take pride in appearance Display professionalism Recognize and respond to verbal and nonverbal communication Apply legal and ethical concepts Work as a team member Speak Spanish fluently
ADMINISTRATIVE	Appointment scheduling, filing, pegboard and electronic billing systems, account collections, insurance billing, coding, record keeping, bank deposits and statement reconciliation, patient histories, medical terminology, machine transcription, word processing
CLINICAL	Understanding of anatomy and physiology, symptoms and diseases, collecting and handling specimens, procedures for assisting with physical examination, emergency first aid and CPR, injections, sterile techniques, ECG, inventory and supplies
REFERENCES	Furnished upon request.

FIGURE 2–3 Sample skills resumé.

colors or "arty" headings should be avoided. The resumé gives you an opportunity to display the qualifications that enhance your appeal to prospective employers. Anything that cannot help you or anything that would detract from your image should be omitted. Once you are in the interview, you can clarify any item not entirely explained on the resumé.

Memory Jogger

 *Why is it better to have a prepared resumé rather than just a discussion of your qualifications during an interview?*

Writing the Resumé

There is no standard format for a resumé, but it should be typewritten on $8\frac{1}{2} \times 11$ good-quality paper. It should be concise and honest and have a professional look. Appearance and accuracy cannot be overemphasized. An employer may interview several acceptable candidates and will be looking for a reason to exclude one or more. Don't allow a "typo" to deny your possible acceptance.

HEADING At the top of the paper should be the necessary personal information: name, address, and telephone number. This is displayed prominently so that it stands apart and can be easily identified (it may be centered).

OBJECTIVE The current trend is to omit reference to an **objective,** particularly if your qualifications are vocationally specific. If you do include an objective, such words as *challenge* or *opportunity* should be avoided because this focuses on what the applicant wants instead of showing understanding of what the employer wants and needs.

EDUCATION AND EXPERIENCE If you are a recent graduate with little or no experience, your education should be listed first and then your employment, if any. College graduates need not include high school information. If you have a good history of recent employment, this is the first item, followed by education. In both cases, you should start with your most recent position and list the rest in *reverse* chronologic order. This is opposite to the order suggested for the personal inventory.

PROFESSIONAL LICENSES Any professional licenses or certificates are included along with memberships in professional organizations.

EXTRACURRICULAR ACTIVITIES Any **extracurricular** or **avocational** interests that would be applicable to the position sought are listed.

REFERENCES You should state on your resumé that references will be furnished on request. (Do not list names and addresses of references on the resumé.) Be prepared to furnish the names of at least three references at the time of your interview. These should have been typewritten on a separate page in the same style as your resumé. The permission of the persons you are listing should be obtained before you provide their names.

ITEMS TO EXCLUDE Do not include

- Your photograph
- Names of spouse and/or children
- Reasons for terminating previous position, if any
- Past salaries or present salary requirements
- Names and addresses of references

Memory Jogger

 *List seven items to be included in your resumé and five items to exclude.*

LOCATING PROSPECTIVE EMPLOYERS If you are a student in an accredited school, your instructor or the school may be able to give you names of prospective employers. Other good sources for leads are the local medical society, other medical assistants, the local chapter of a professional medical assistants association, branches of the United States Employment Service, and state-operated employment offices.

You may also wish to check the classified advertisements in your local newspaper or place your name with an employment agency. Private employment agencies generally charge a fee equivalent to 2 to 4 weeks' salary to successful applicants. This fee is sometimes paid by the employer after a probationary period.

If you are responding to an advertisement that lists a telephone number, telephoning to request an interview is preferable to writing a letter, but an unsolicited telephone call may be disruptive and destroy the opportunity for an interview. If no telephone number is included in the advertisement, there will be an address listed (usually a box number) to which you may direct a letter requesting an interview. A cover letter responding to an advertisement should include

- A reference to the advertisement, including name of newspaper, date of publication, and position title. The employer may be running more than one recruitment ad.
- An enthusiastic expression of interest in the position.
- A comparison of your own qualifications with those of the position to be filled.
- Information about where you can be contacted.
- A request for a response or interview.
- Thanks for considering your request.

PROCEDURE 2–1

Preparing a Resumé

GOAL

To prepare a resumé of education and experience that will be informative to a prospective employer and create interest in arranging an interview for employment.

EQUIPMENT AND SUPPLIES

Summary of personal data
Quality stationery
Typewriter or computer

PROCEDURAL STEPS

1 Assemble all personal data necessary for resumé.

2 Arrange in reverse chronologic order.
PURPOSE: To enable you to proceed in orderly fashion in preparing the resumé and to check accuracy of dates.

3 Typewrite heading that includes your name, address, and telephone number.
PURPOSE: For easy identification by reader.

4 List highest education degree or diploma, including name of institution and year. Include high school if you are not a college graduate.
PURPOSE: Training may be important to your employability.

5 List all work experience in reverse chronologic order.
PURPOSE: To demonstrate transferable experiences toward future employment.

6 Include any professional licenses, certificates, and memberships in professional organizations.
PURPOSE: Indicates employability and personal interest in profession.

7 List any extracurricular or avocational interests applicable to the position sought.

8 State that references will be furnished on request.
PURPOSE: Prospective employers may wish to verify your experience and character. *Note:* Obtain permission before listing anyone as a reference.

9 Review resumé for accuracy, completeness, and attractive format.

10 If mailing, place in No. 10 envelope on which you have typed the address and your return address. Include a cover letter.

UNSOLICITED INTERVIEW REQUEST You may decide to canvass a number of medical facilities to determine whether there are openings for a medical assistant. A letter such as the one shown in Figure 2–4 can be written and your resumé enclosed. Then you should follow up with a telephone call in about 1 week.

INTERVIEWING

Application Form

Completing an application for employment is not standard procedure in small medical practices, but you should be prepared for complying if requested (see Management Responsibilities). Larger health agencies such as hospitals and health maintenance organizations will definitely ask you to fill out their application form.

You should have readily available your Social Security number, driver's license, and telephone numbers where you can be reached. Your resumé should have the information you will need regarding education and employment. You need to be prepared to furnish telephone numbers for previous employers, if any, and have available the names, addresses, and telephone numbers of three references who have given you their permission to list them.

The appearance and completeness of your filled-in application will be considered in your overall evaluation. By law, employers cannot require you to answer questions regarding your place of birth, ethnic origin or religious preference, or your age, marital status, or number of children. If these questions are on the application, you may choose to leave them blank, but all allowable questions should be an-

PROCEDURE 2-2
Answering a Help-Wanted Advertisement

GOAL

To write a letter in response to a newspaper advertisement that will relay your qualifications and generate interest in arranging an interview.

EQUIPMENT AND SUPPLIES

Recent newspaper with classified employment ads
Stationery
Typewriter or computer
Pen

PROCEDURAL STEPS

1 Review letter writing information in Chapter 11, Correspondence and Mail Processing.

2 Draft a letter to include
- Name of newspaper, date of publication, and title of position for which you are applying.
PURPOSE: Employer may be running more than one advertisement.
- Information about where you can be contacted.
PURPOSE: To enable interested employer to reach you.

3 Express enthusiastic interest in the position offered, and state your qualifications.

4 Request a response to your letter by telephone or mail.
PURPOSE: So that an interview can be arranged if position is still open and employer is interested in your qualifications.

5 End the letter with an expression of thanks for considering your request.
PURPOSE: To demonstrate your knowledge of courtesy.

6 Review the letter for content and accuracy.
PURPOSE: To make certain that you have included all essential information and that the letter is free of errors.

swered honestly and completely. Print your answers or write as plainly as possible. *Hint:* Have your own favorite pen with you.

Day of the Interview

Your appearance is extremely important. Clothing should be conservative, neat, and well pressed. Women should wear a dress or suit with a skirt. Slacks or pantsuits and open sandals are considered inappropriate for a job interview. Men should wear a suit and tie and appropriate dress shoes.

Hair should be well groomed and worn in a professional-looking style. Jewelry should be kept to a minimum and heavy scents of perfume or antiperspirants avoided. Women should be careful and conservative in applying makeup and should carry a modest purse that is not bulging with unnecessary items.

You should take a critical look at yourself in the mirror before leaving home and again just before entering the prospective employer's office (see Interviewing Tips).

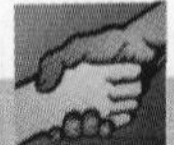

PERSONAL QUALITIES

INTERVIEWING TIPS

- *Be prompt.* Arrive promptly for the interview. Under no circumstances should you be even so much as 1 minute late and then have to make a weak excuse.
- *Be prepared.* Bring two copies of your resumé, one to give to the interviewer and one to refer to in case you get nervous.
- *Be self-sufficient.* Go alone. You may want moral support, but you will be more relaxed if there is no one waiting for you.
- *Be poised.* Enter the office confidently and without appearing rushed.
- *Be polite.* Introduce yourself to the receptionist, and then express appreciation when you are asked to be seated.
- *Be patient.* If you must wait, try to relax, but avoid slouching in your chair.
- *Be considerate and composed.* Do not smoke or chew gum.

Theresa O'Sullivan
233 Wentworth Street, San Diego, CA 92100
Telephone (619) 222-3333

June 15, 19xx

Arthur M. Blackburn, MD
2200 Broadway
Any Town, US 98765

Dear Doctor Blackburn:

In a few weeks, I will complete my formal training in medical assisting with an Associate in Science degree from Ola Vista Community College.

The medical assisting program at Ola Vista includes theory and practical application in both administrative and clinical skills. My six-week supervised externship gave me additional practical experience in two specialty practices.

While studying at Ola Vista, I also worked part-time for a physician in family practice, while maintaining a 3.5 grade point average. My experience as Dr. Madden's employee is outlined on the enclosed resumé. I have enjoyed my work in Dr. Madden's office and am now seeking full-time employment.

If you will require a replacement or addition to your staff in the near future, may I be considered as an applicant? I will follow up with a telephone call within a week.

Sincerely yours,

Theresa O'Sullivan

Enc. Resumé

FIGURE 2–4 Sample cover letter.

When you prepared your resumé, you listed your job skills, your education, or both. The interviewer already knows how well you ought to be able to do the job. However, you will be judged in at least two other areas of evaluation:

- *What kind of co-worker you will be.* Working in a health care facility requires team effort, and your ability to work in cooperation and coordination with others bears heavily on how well you will do your job, apart from the excellence of your job skills.
- *What kind of employee you will be.* Dependability, trustworthiness, dedication, loyalty, and other personal characteristics are always important to an employer.

During the Interview

When you are ushered into the interviewer's room, wait to be seated until you are invited to do so. Let the interviewer lead the conversation. Be prepared to answer such questions as "Tell me about yourself," and "Why do you want to work here?" One reason for an opening such as this is to provide a little time to relax and get acquainted. You might start out by reviewing your professional background and training and then progress to personal interests, hobbies, and so forth (Fig. 2–5).

The interviewer will be observing your body language, your manners, poise, speech, alertness, and ability to give direct answers. A relaxed, friendly

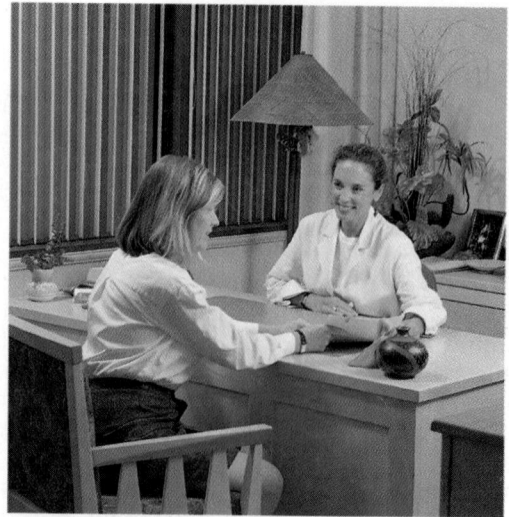

FIGURE 2–5 Student being interviewed for a job.

manner with good eye contact is important—look directly at the person to whom you are speaking. Your sense of humor may be tested as well, and questions may be directed to you that will test your common sense and frankness. You can promote yourself honestly and graciously by showing that you enjoy others, that you are willing to work and accept responsibility, and that you have an open mind about the position and are willing to learn.

Legislation affecting employment practices has influenced hiring practices nationwide. (See discussion of Americans with Disabilities Act of 1990 in Chapter 6.) Employers are restricted in the information that can be required on an application or asked in an interview. Although you may not be *required* to answer questions, such as your age, birthplace, and marital status, a prospective employer might appreciate your mentioning any such pertinent information in conversation. Remember that your objective is to obtain a position.

At the end of the interview, if the interviewer has not mentioned hours and salary, you may properly inquire about these subjects at this time. If you are not really interested in the position, do not bother to ask; but if the position sounds satisfactory and is one that you would like to accept, you may then ask if the interviewer wishes to discuss the salary. This should be enough of a lead, because it was probably an oversight on the interviewer's part. If the interviewer seems reluctant to discuss it, however, do not press the issue, because this may be an indication that your qualifications do not fit the position and there is no reason to pursue the interview further.

If you have been given a tour of the office, you may make some pleasant observations and comments but do not be falsely overenthusiastic. When you are introduced to the staff, be gracious and friendly. Try to remember their names so that you can thank them later. Show enthusiasm, but do not overdo it because it may appear to others that you are putting on an act.

Closing the Interview

The interviewer will usually take the initiative in closing the interview, perhaps by sliding back the chair and asking whether you have further questions. Do not show disappointment if the position is not offered to you at the time of the interview. There may be other applicants to see, or the interviewer may wish to check your references before making a commitment. Express your thanks for the interview as you leave, and remember, too, to thank the receptionist and say a friendly good-bye.

Follow-Up Activities

A brief, well-worded letter of thanks sent to the interviewer immediately after the interview could be crucial in deciding whether you will be hired. This is one of the most essential steps in the entire job-seeking process, and the one most overlooked by job-seekers. Simply write a brief note expressing appreciation for the interview and interest in the position (Fig. 2–6).

After a few days, you may call the office and ask if the position has been filled and tell them you are interested because you enjoyed your interview and the office staff. If the position is still open, ask

Theresa O'Sullivan
233 Wentworth Street, San Diego, CA 92100
Telephone (619) 222-3333

June 16, 19xx

Arthur M. Blackburn, MD
2200 Broadway
Any Town, US 98765

Dear Doctor Blackburn:

Thank you for taking the time to talk with me today about the medical assistant position in your office and for considering my qualifications for filling that position.

I would be pleased to accept your offer if you should decide that I meet your requirements.

Sincerely yours,

Theresa O'Sullivan

FIGURE 2–6 Sample of thank-you letter after interview.

whether you may inquire again in a few days. Be brief and thank the person with whom you are speaking.

If you are not hired, ask yourself some pertinent questions:

- Did I look my best?
- Did I show enthusiasm for the job?
- Did I listen carefully during the interview?
- Did I say or do something I should not have said or done?

Even if you are not hired, you should never feel that an interview is a waste of time. You learn from each experience, and with experience you are better able to promote your qualifications in future interviews.

If you are hired, ask the interviewer if you may borrow the office policy and procedure manual to review before you report to work. If this is allowed, jot down items that you find important to remember in your own notebook or questions that you need to ask when reporting to work.

On your first day of work, arrive promptly and eager for your new experience. And remember to bring your notebook!

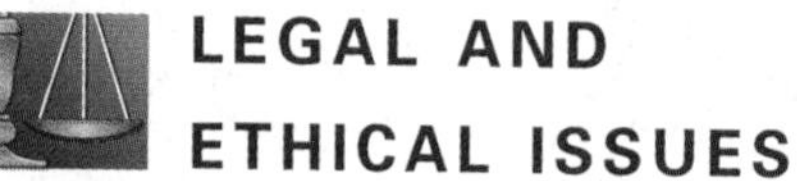

LEGAL AND ETHICAL ISSUES

Expect to observe all the office protocols of regular attendance, being on time and in appropriate attire. Do not expect or ask for payment for your services as an extern.

During your externship practice you are bound by the same regulations as the regular staff. Be punctual in your attendance. Restrict your performance to those areas in which you have been trained. If the state in which you live has a scope of practice for medical assistants, know the boundaries within which you can perform and do not exceed them. You may be expected to carry malpractice insurance. Some schools provide a blanket policy for their students.

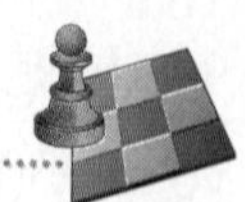

CRITICAL THINKING

Observe your surroundings and make a mental note of situations or practices that could be improved. Offer suggestions only when asked.

HOW DID I DO? Answers to Memory Joggers

1. *Similarities:*
   Appearance and actions meet professional standards.
   Regular hours are observed.
   Differences:
   Short term, may be part-time.
   All activities will be supervised and evaluated.
   No payment.
   May report to several different agencies.
2. The purpose of the resumé is to provide preliminary information that will assist in arranging an interview. The resumé allows the interviewer to determine whether the applicant meets basic requirements.
3. *Include* name, address, telephone number, education, experience, licenses and certificates, and extracurricular activities.
   Exclude photo, names of spouse and/or children, reasons for terminating previous position, past salaries or present salary requirements, and names and addresses of references.

REFERENCE

Bolles RN: What Color Is Your Parachute? Berkeley, CA, Ten Speed Press, revised annually. *Resumé Expert* software.

A Brief History of Medicine

3

OUTLINE

Medical Language and Mythology
Medicine in Ancient Times
Early Development of Medical Education
Early Pioneers
Scientific Advances (18th and 19th Centuries)
Nineteenth Century Women in Medicine
Twentieth Century Medicine
National Institutes of Health
Centers for Disease Control and Prevention
Overview
Legal and Ethical Issues
Critical Thinking
Answers to Memory Joggers

LEARNING OBJECTIVES

Cognitive: On successful completion of this chapter you should be able to:

1. Define and spell the terms listed in the Vocabulary.
2. Identify the two ancient mythologies that contributed a major portion of our medical terminology.
3. Distinguish between and describe the two medical symbols in general use today.
4. Name the oath that has been administered to new physicians for more than 2000 years.
5. Name the medical school that was the most famous in the world at the end of the 19th century.
6. Name a 20th century educator who played a major role in the development of medical education in the United States.
7. Identify the important discovery made by William Harvey that was only substantiated 200 years later.
8. Name the 18th century English surgeon who was declared the Founder of Scientific Surgery.
9. Name the Hungarian physician who earned the title Savior of Mothers.
10. List the names of five 19th century women who contributed significantly to medical history.
11. Name the surgeon who performed the first human heart transplant.
12. Name two agencies of the U.S. Department of Health and Human Services that play an important role in the advancement of health in the United States and the world.

VOCABULARY

anesthetic Agent that causes loss of sensation with or without loss of consciousness

anthrax An acute infectious disease caused by a bacillus. Humans contract the disease from animal hair, hides, or waste matter.

aphonia Loss of the ability to speak

aphrodisiacs Drugs that cause sexual arousal

attenuated Made thin or weaker

auscultation The act of listening for sounds within the body, normally with a stethoscope

bacteria Single-celled microscopic organisms

catheterization The act of passing a tube through the body for removing fluids or injecting them into body cavities

cervical vertebrae The upper seven bones of the spinal column; the skeleton of the neck

chemotherapy The treatment of disease using chemical agents

cholera An acute, infectious, bacillus-caused disease involving the entire small bowel; *chicken cholera*—cholera that affects chickens

contamination The act of soiling, staining, or polluting; especially the introduction of infectious materials or germs that produce disease

cyanosis A bluish discoloration of the skin

dissection The process of cutting apart or separating tissues for anatomic study

embryology The science or study of the development of living organisms during the embryonic stage

fallopian tubes The tubes that carry the ovum from the ovary to the uterus; the oviducts

hemiplegia Paralysis of one side of the body

histologist One who specializes in the study of the minute structure, composition, and function of the tissues

immunology A science that deals with the phenomena and causes of immunity and immune responses

innovation Act of introducing something new or novel

invulnerable Incapable of being injured or harmed

isolation The act of placing alone apart from others

ligation Something that binds

microorganisms Organisms of microscopic or ultramicroscopic size

millennia Thousands of years (*mille* = thousand)

mons veneris The rounded, elevated area overlying the symphysis pubis that is covered with hair after puberty

mysticism The experience of seeming to have direct communication with God or ultimate reality

mythology A branch of knowledge that deals with the interpretation of myths

neophyte A new convert or novice

oviducts The pair of tubes in the female that carry the egg from the ovary to the uterus; fallopian tubes

pandemic Affecting the majority of the people in a country or a number of countries

pathologic Altered or caused by disease

percussion The act of striking a part of the body with short, sharp blows as an aid in diagnosing the condition of the underlying parts by the sound obtained

perfusion The passing of a fluid through spaces

periphery The external surface or boundary of a body

phagocytosis The engulfing of microorganisms, other cells, and foreign particles by phagocytes

placenta The vascular structure that develops within the uterus during pregnancy and through which a fetus receives nourishment

protozoa Primitive animal organisms, each of which consists of a single cell

puerperal fever The fever that accompanies an infection of the birth canal following delivery of a child; childbed fever

purulent Consisting of or containing pus

pustule A raised pus-filled area or sac

putrefaction Decomposition of animal matter that results in a foul smell

rabies An acute infectious disease of the nervous system caused by a virus, usually communicated to humans through animal bite

rete mucosum The innermost layer of the epidermis (*rete* = network of nerves or vessels)

spermatozoa Mature male germ cells

statutory body A part of the legislative branch of a government

stethoscope An instrument for listening to sounds within the body

swine erysipelas A contagious disease affecting young swine in Europe

syphilitic chancre The primary sore of syphilis

vagina The canal in the female that extends from the vulva to the cervix

virulent Exceedingly pathogenic, noxious, or deadly

vivisection Operation or cutting on a living animal for research purposes

Learning the history of the development of modern medicine is not necessary to perform your duties as a medical assistant, just as a study of the genealogy of your family is not necessary for you to live a full life. However, both of these pursuits add interest and a uniqueness to the quality of life.

Modern medicine reflects its history in the names given to anatomic and physiologic phenomena, medications, diseases, instruments, and specialties. Even the latest medical discoveries often have names drawn from the ancients. When we live in the world of medicine and speak its language we are constantly touched by this fascinating past. The rich cultural heritage of medicine is interesting to study and provides a perspective and understanding of its impact on the present. It is also a history of hardships and disappointment that were pushed aside by determined men and women who wanted to pursue their dreams and goals. Learning about these pioneers (Table 3–1) is inspiring as we realize that we, too, can be a part of the heritage of caring and discovery that continues to improve health care throughout the world.

Medical Language and Mythology

Borrowing so liberally from ancient **mythology,** and so actively using the classical language that most civilizations abandoned centuries ago, may seem strange. Yet today's medicine uses words whose origins stem from the romance and fantasy of this long "dead" world. Anatomy, especially, seems to reach back to the dawn of history. Many early anatomic terms have reached modern times almost unchanged, although some terms are false when translated literally (because the ancients did not correctly understand body functions). *Example:* "artery," which comes from the Greek word *arteria,* literally "a windpipe"—the Greeks believed that the artery carried air, not blood.

Greek and Roman mythology have contributed a major portion of our medical terminology, but we have also borrowed liberally from Arabic, Anglo-Saxon, and German sources, with a heavy dash of the Bible added. A few of the many examples of medical terms derived from the classical past are presented.

ATLAS, the anatomic name for the first **cervical vertebrae** upon which the head rests, is aptly named for the famous Greek titan, who, according to mythology, was condemned by Zeus to bear the heavens on his shoulders. The tendon of ACHILLES (ah-kil'ēz) reminds us of the story of the youth whose mother held him by the heel and dipped him into the river Styx to make him **invulnerable.** This tendon was not immersed. Later, a mortal wound was inflicted in Achilles' heel. A common expression used today to show a point of weakness is "your Achilles heel." APHRODITE (af'ro-dī-te), the Greek goddess of love and beauty, gave her name to the sex-arousing drugs known as **aphrodisiacs.** The equivalent Roman goddess of love, VENUS (vē'nus), has distinctions paid to her not so much as the goddess of love but of lust. A portion of the female anatomy, the **mons veneris,** was dedicated to her memory. Venereal diseases are also named after Venus.

AESCULAPIUS (es"-ku-la'pe-us), the son of Apollo, was revered as the god of medicine. The early Greeks worshiped the healing powers of Aesculapius and built temples in his honor, where patients were treated by trained priests. His daughters were HYGEIA (hi-jé-ah), goddess of health, and PANACEA (pan"ah-se"-ah), goddess of all healing and restorer of health. Our modern word "hygiene," the science of health maintenance, has its origin in Hygeia, and the modern meaning of "panacea" is "a remedy for all ills or difficulties." The staff of Aesculapius, which is a staff encircled by one serpent, is used to signify the art of healing and has been adopted by the American Medical Association as the symbol of medicine. The mythological staff belonging to Apollo, the caduceus, which is a staff encir-

TABLE 3–1 Milestones in the History of Medicine

Dates	Person	Achievement
1205 BC	Moses (First "Public Health Officer")	Incorporated rules of health into the Hebrew religion
460–377 BC	Hippocrates (Father of Medicine)	Gave scientific basis to medicine Hippocratic Oath
131–201 AD	Galen (Father of Experimental Physiology)	First to describe cranial nerves and sympathetic system
1514–1564	Andreas Vesalius (Belgian anatomist; Father of Modern Anatomy)	Corrected some of Galen's errors Published *De Corporis Humani Fabrica* describing structure of human body
1578–1657	William Harvey	Described pumping action of heart and circulation of the blood
1628–1694	Marcello Malpighi (First histologist)	Pioneered microscopic anatomy Identified the taste buds; described minute structures of brain and optic nerve
1632–1723	Anton van Leeuwenhoek	Discovered lens magnification First to observe bacteria and protozoa through a lens Made first accurate description of red blood cells
1722–1809	Leopold Auenbrugger	Developed the use of percussion in diagnosis
1728–1793	John Hunter (Founder of Scientific Surgery)	Introduced artificial feeding by insertion of flexible tube into stomach Made classic description of syphilitic chancre (hunterian chancre)
1745–1813	Benjamin Rush	Published first American treatise on psychiatry in 1812
1749–1823	Edward Jenner	Discovered smallpox vaccine
1781–1826	René Laënnec	Invented the stethoscope
1818–1865	Ignaz Philipp Semmelweis (Savior of Mothers)	Developed theory of childbed (puerperal) fever
1820–1910	Florence Nightingale (Lady with the Lamp)	Founder of nursing
1821–1912	Clara Barton	Founder of American Red Cross
1821–1910	Elizabeth Blackwell	First woman in United States to receive Doctor of Medicine degree from a medical school
1822–1895	Louis Pasteur (Father of Bacteriology)	Developed germ theory of disease and destruction of microorganisms through use of heat
1827–1912	Joseph Lister	Applied Pasteur's theories and developed sterile techniques in surgery
1843–1910	Robert Koch	Bacteriologist who developed culture-plate method for isolation of bacteria Set down Koch's postulates
1845–1922	Wilhelm Konrad Roentgen	Discovered x-ray in 1895
1854–1915	Paul Ehrlich	Began the use of injecting chemicals into the body to destroy a specific organism Developed drug used to fight syphilis
1867–1940	Lillian Wald	New York City nurse who operated a visiting nurse service and helped establish the world's first public school nursing system

cled by two serpents, is the medical insignia of the United States Army Medical Corps and is often misused as a symbol of the medical profession (Fig. 3–1).

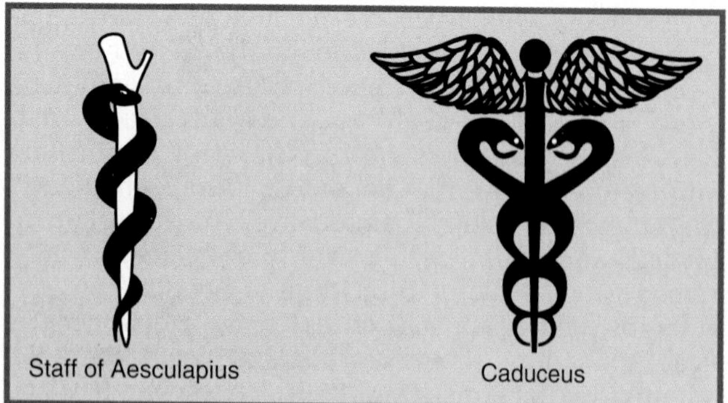

FIGURE 3–1 Symbols of medicine.

Memory Jogger

 *How does the caduceus differ from the staff of Aesculapius?*

Medicine in Ancient Times

Although religion and myth were the basis of care for the sick for **millennia,** there is evidence of drugs, surgery, and other treatments based on theories about the body from as early as 5000 to 2000 BC. In the well-developed societies of the Egyptians, Babylonians, and Assyrians, certain men acted as physicians and used their scant knowledge to try to treat illness and injury.

MOSES incorporated rules of health into the Hebrew religion around 1205 BC. He was thus the first

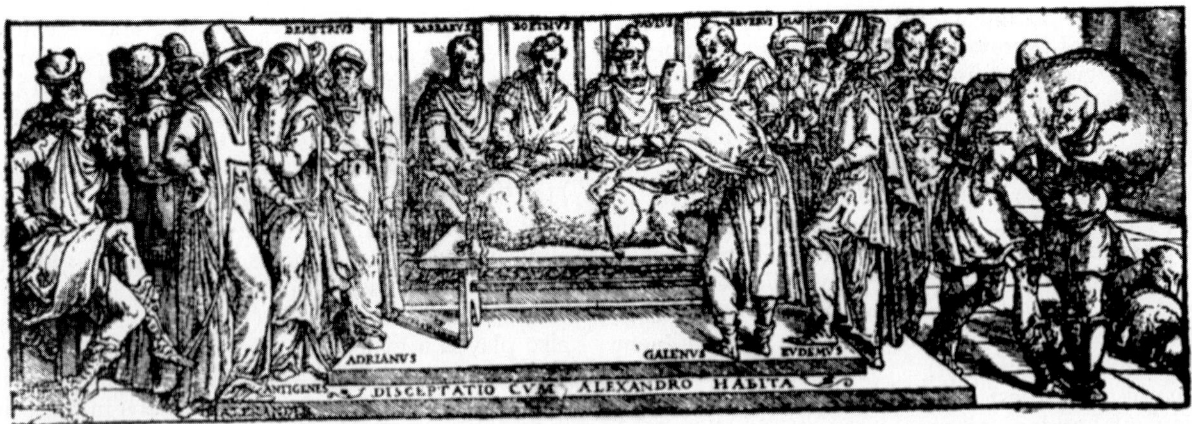

FIGURE 3–2 Demonstration of Galen performing surgery on a live pig. (Courtesy of the National Library of Medicine.)

advocate of preventive medicine and could even be called the first public health officer. Moses knew that some animal diseases might be passed on to humans and that **contamination** might linger on unclean dishes. Consequently, it became a religious law that no one was permitted to eat animals that were not freshly slaughtered or to eat or drink from dirty dishes, lest they become defiled and lose their souls.

HIPPOCRATES (hip-pok'rah-tēz) (460–377 BC) is the most famous of the ancient Greek physicians and is known as the Father of Medicine. He did much to separate medicine from **mysticism** and gave it a scientific basis. He is best remembered for the Hippocratic Oath (see Chapter 5) exacted from his pupils. This oath has been administered to physicians for more than 2000 years. Hippocrates' astute clinical descriptions of diseases and his voluminous writings on epidemics, fevers, epilepsy, fractures, and instruments were studied for centuries. He believed that the body tends to heal itself and that it is the physician's responsibility to help nature. In Hippocrates' time, very little was known about anatomy, physiology, and pathology, and no knowledge of chemistry existed. In spite of these handicaps, many of his classifications of diseases and his descriptions of symptoms are being used today.

Memory Jogger

2 *Why was Moses called the "first public health officer"?*

Many Greek physicians practiced, studied, and taught in Rome in the time after Hippocrates. One was GALEN (131–201 AD), who came to Rome in 162 AD and became known as the Prince of Physicians (Fig. 3–2). Galen is said to have written 500 treatises on medicine. He wrote an excellent summary of anatomy as it was known at that time. Nevertheless, his work was faulty and inaccurate, because it was based largely on the **dissection** of apes and swine. He is considered the Father of Experimental Physiology and the first experimental neurologist. He was the first to describe the cranial nerve and the sympathetic nervous system, and he made the first experimental sections of the spinal cord, producing **hemiplegia.** Galen also produced **aphonia** by cutting the recurrent laryngeal nerve, and he gave the first valid explanation of the mechanism of respiration.

The profound influence of the writings of Hippocrates and Galen on the course of medicine gives praise to these great thinkers, but their unquestioned authority actually had a negative effect on the progress of science throughout the Dark Ages. Their theories and descriptions were held to as law, so **innovation** was rarely attempted. Experimenters were scoffed at by their contemporaries. Later, the Christian religion taught people to care for the sick and encouraged the establishment of institutions where the sick could find help. This provided an opportunity for physicians to observe, analyze, and discuss the progress of a variety of patients. The establishment of universities led more to a study of theories of disease rather than to observation of the sick. It was not until the 16th century that Andreas Vesalius began to correct some of Galen's errors.

Early Development of Medical Education

In early times medical knowledge developed slowly, often in **isolation,** and distribution of knowledge was poor. Before the invention of the printing press there was very little exchange of scientific knowledge and ideas, and scientists were not well informed about the works of others.

In the middle of the 15th century, Johann Gutenberg's invention of movable type and adaptation of a certain kind of press for printing marked a turning point in history. Gutenberg's invention resulted in a faster way to produce multiple identical copies of any single text. Printing rapidly replaced the laborious method of scribes, who had to copy manuscripts by hand. The greater availability of books increased the number of literate people throughout Europe. In turn, ever greater refinements in the printing press were developed to meet the growing demand for books.

Another development important to science occurred in the 17th century with the establishment in Europe of academies or societies consisting of small groups of men who met to discuss subjects of mutual interest. The academies provided freedom of expression that, with the stimulus of exchanging ideas, contributed significantly to the development of scientific thought.

One of the earliest of the academies was the Royal Society of London, an organization formed in 1662 by the incorporation of several smaller groups under one royal charter. A significant aspect of these societies was their publications, such as the Royal Society of London's *Philosophical Transactions.*

The development of communications was improving. Society was becoming more complex and the need for regulation becoming greater. The passage of the Medical Act of 1858 in Great Britain was considered one of the most important events in British medicine. It established a **statutory body,** the General Medical Council, which controlled admission to the medical register and had great power over medical education and examinations.

In the United States, medical education was greatly influenced by the example set in 1893 by the Johns Hopkins University Medical School in Baltimore. It admitted only college graduates with a year's training in the natural sciences. Its clinical work was superior because the school was supplemented by the Johns Hopkins Hospital, which had been created expressly for teaching and research by members of the medical family. The first four professors at Johns Hopkins were SIR WILLIAM OSLER, professor of medicine; WILLIAM H. WELCH, chief of pathology; HOWARD A. KELLEY, chief of gynecology and obstetrics; and WILLIAM D. HALSTED, chief of surgery. Together, these four men transformed the organization and curriculum of clinical teaching and made Johns Hopkins the most famous medical school in the world.

ABRAHAM FLEXNER (1866–1959), an educator, also played a major role in the development of medical education in the United States. After publishing an appraisal of educational institutions in the United States in 1908, Flexner received a Carnegie Foundation commission to study the quality of medical colleges in the United States and Canada. The Flexner report, published in 1910, rated 155 schools according to the quality of instruction and facilities available to the students. The publication of this report resulted in the closure of many low-ranking schools and the upgrading of many others.

Memory Jogger

Why did the Johns Hopkins Medical School become the most famous in the world?

Early Pioneers

ANDREAS VESALIUS (an'drē-as ve-sa'le-us) (1514–1564), a Belgian anatomist, is known as the

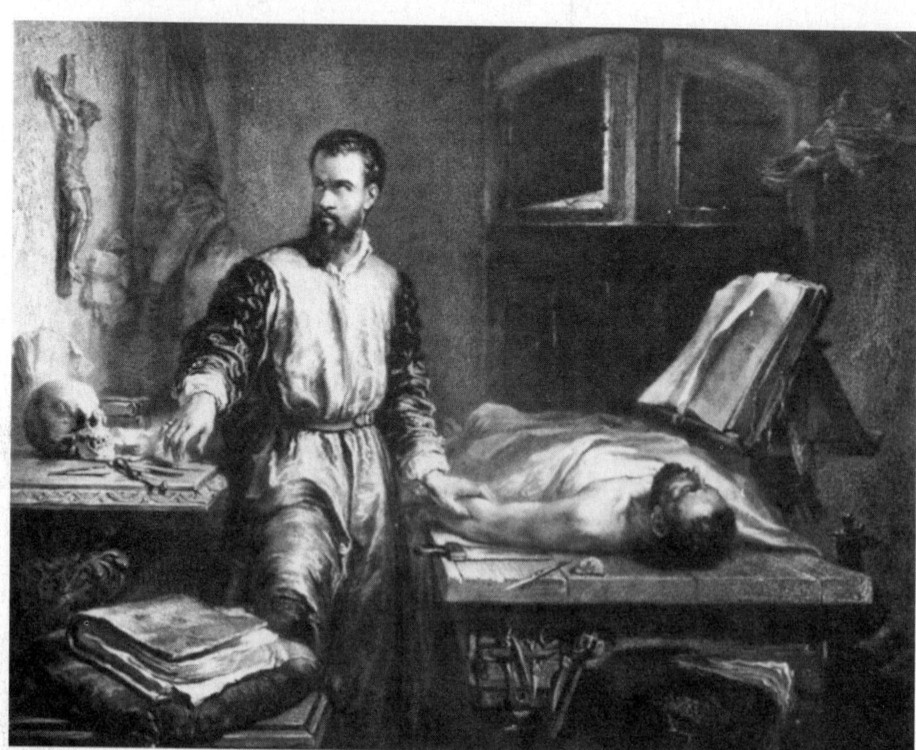

FIGURE 3–3 Andreas Vesalius. (Courtesy of the National Library of Medicine.)

Father of Modern Anatomy (Fig. 3–3). At the age of 29, he published his great *De Corporis Humani Fabrica,* in which he described the structure of the human body. This work marked a turning point by breaking with the past and throwing overboard the Galen tradition. Vesalius introduced many new anatomic terms, but because of his radical approach he was subjected to some persecution from his colleagues, his teachers, and his pupils. Despite his great contributions to the science of anatomy, his name is not used to identify any important anatomic structures.

GABRIELE FALLOPIUS (gā′brē-el fal-ōp′-e-us) (1523–1562), a student of Vesalius, was also an accurate and detailed dissector who described and named many parts of the anatomy. He gave his own name to the **oviducts,** known as the **fallopian tubes.** He also named the **vagina** and the **placenta.**

In 1628, WILLIAM HARVEY (1578–1657) made his pronouncement that the heart acts as a muscular force-pump in propelling the blood along and that the blood's motion is continual and continuous in a cycle or circle (Fig. 3–4). Harvey based his conclusion on his experimental **vivisection, ligation,** and **perfusion** as well as brilliant reasoning. The work of this English physician was not fully recognized until 1827, when the full importance of his work was substantiated. Harvey's writings were recognized in Germany before the English permitted their publication at home. Modern England now considers Harvey to be its medical Shakespeare.

Great advances in medicine were somewhat stilled for a century or so, but the unseen world of **microorganisms** was opened as ANTON VAN LEEUWENHOEK (ăn′tōn van lu′-en-hōk) (1632–1723), a Dutch linen draper and haberdasher by trade, pursued his hobby of grinding lenses. He ground over 400 lenses during his lifetime, most of which were very small—some no larger than a pinhead—and usually mounted between two thin brass plates that were riveted together. In grinding lenses Leeuwenhoek discovered how to use a simple biconvex lens to magnify the minute world of organisms and structures that had never been seen before.

Leeuwenhoek was the first man ever to observe **bacteria** and **protozoa** through a lens. His accurate interpretations of what he saw led to the sciences of bacteriology and protozoology. He described for the first time the **spermatozoa** from insects, dogs, and men. He studied the structure of the optic lens, striations in muscles, and the mouthparts of insects. Leeuwenhoek extended Marcello Malpighi's demonstration in 1661 of the blood capillaries by giving (in 1684) the first accurate description of red blood cells. From 1673 until 1723, he communicated by means of informal letters most of his discoveries to the Royal Society of England, to which he was elected as a fellow in 1680. Leeuwenhoek's advances have been further developed, and, with modern refinements, magnification now allows visualization of the smallest organisms with chemical structures.

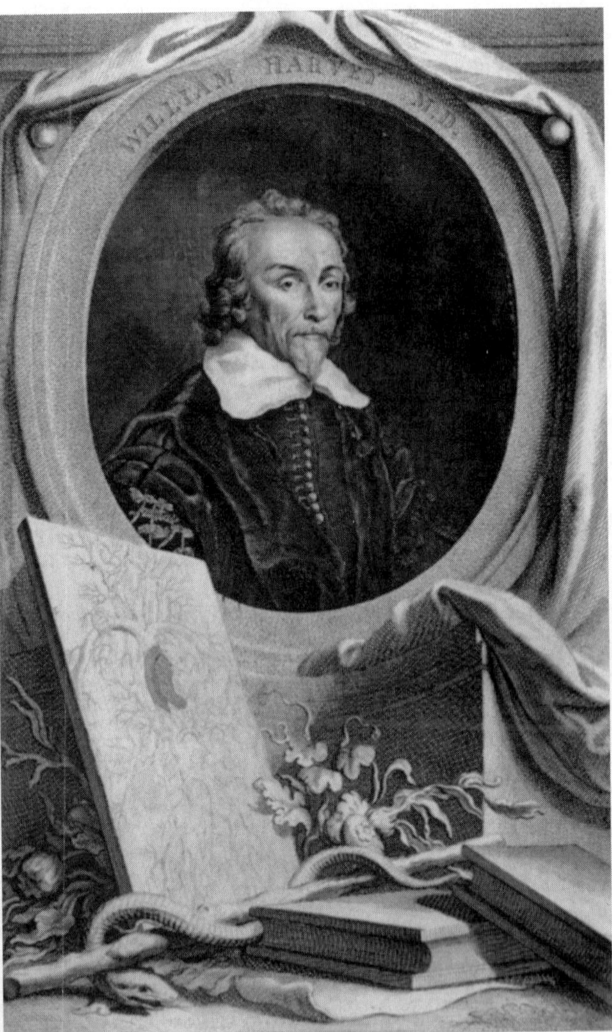

FIGURE 3–4 William Harvey. (Courtesy of the National Library of Medicine.)

Memory Joggers

 How were the lenses produced by Leeuwenhoek used in the advancement of medicine?

MARCELLO MALPIGHI (mar-chel′-o mahl-pe′-ge) (1628–1694), the greatest of the microscopists, was born near Bologna, Italy; entered the University of Bologna in 1646; and, in 1653, was granted doctorates in both medicine and philosophy. Malpighi pioneered the use of the microscope in the study of plants and animals, after which microscopic anatomy became a prerequisite for advances in physiology, **embryology,** and practical medicine. He may be regarded as the first **histologist.** In 1661, he identified and described the pulmonary and capillary network connecting the small arteries with small veins, one of the most important discoveries in the history of science. When Malpighi found that the blood passed through the capillaries, it meant that Harvey was right—that blood was not transformed into flesh in the **periphery,** as the ancients had thought.

Malpighi continued to pursue his studies with the microscope while teaching and practicing medicine. He identified the taste buds and described the minute structure of the brain and the optic nerve. He was the first to see the red blood cells and to attribute the color of blood to them. He discovered the **rete mucosum** or malpighian layer of the skin. His work on the structure of the liver, spleen, and kidney is recalled today when we speak of the malpighian bodies of the kidney and spleen, Malpighi's pyramids (pyramides renales), and Malpighi's vesicles (alveoli pulmonis).

Scientific Advances (18th and 19th Centuries)

JOHN HUNTER (1728–1793), the famous English surgeon and anatomist, was born a few years after Leeuwenhoek's death (Fig. 3–5). Hunter has been given the title Founder of Scientific Surgery because his surgical procedures were soundly based on **pathologic** evidence. He was the first to classify teeth in a scientific manner. In 1778, he introduced artificial feeding by means of a flexible tube passed into the stomach. His description of the **syphilitic chancre** is classic, and the lesion is sometimes called the hunterian chancre.

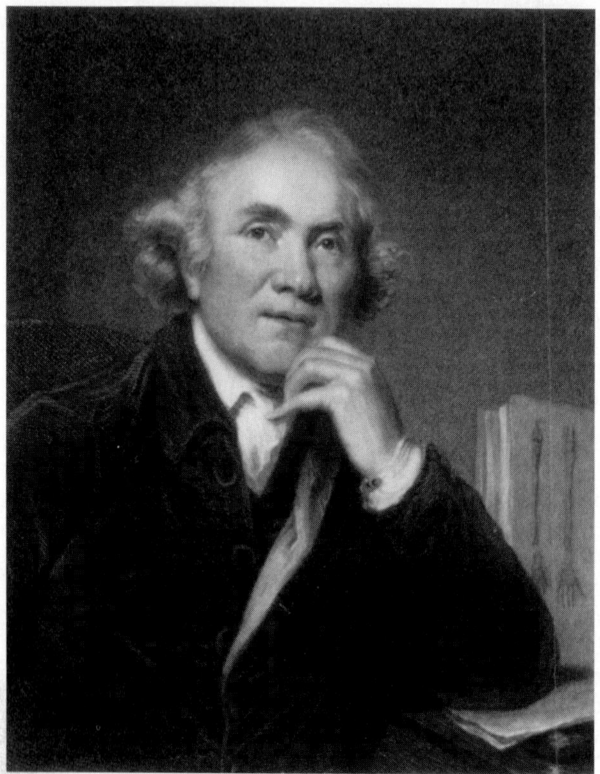

FIGURE 3–5 John Hunter. (Courtesy of the National Library of Medicine.)

In an unsuccessful attempt to differentiate gonorrhea from syphilis, Hunter inoculated himself with what he thought was gonorrhea, but instead he acquired syphilis. Hunter's results increased the confusion, because he concluded that gonorrhea was a symptom of syphilis. This confusion continued until the beginning of the 20th century.

Hunter's great collection of anatomic and animal specimens formed the basis for the museum of the Royal College of Surgeons. He was also a member of the Royal Society of Medicine and the Royal Academy of Surgery in Paris.

Memory Jogger

5 *Why was Hunter given the title "Founder of Scientific Surgery"?*

Hunter wrote many papers on anatomy and physiology; he was a brilliant lecturer and teacher. Among his many students was one who would become famous and well loved—Edward Jenner.

EDWARD JENNER (1749–1823) was a country physician in Dorsetshire, England (Fig. 3–6). He is listed among the immortals of preventive medicine for his discovery of the smallpox vaccine. The story goes that one day, while Jenner was serving as an apprentice in the office of Daniel Ludlow, a dairy maid was being given treatment. Smallpox was mentioned, and she said, "I cannot take that disease, for I have had cowpox." Smallpox at that time was a deadly **pandemic.** Jenner observed that farmers and dairy maids who once had cowpox never contracted smallpox. Later, as a practicing physician, Jenner continued investigating the relationship between cowpox and smallpox, to the extent that other medical society members became bored by him and threatened to expel him from their ranks.

On May 14, 1796, Dr. Jenner took some **purulent** matter from a **pustule** on the hand of Sarah Nelmes, a dairy maid, and inserted it through two small superficial incisions into the arm of James Phipps, a healthy 8-year-old boy. This was the first vaccination. Later, on July 1, a **virulent** dose of smallpox matter was given to young Phipps in the same arm. It had no effect: Phipps had been vaccinated and was safe from the dreaded disease. Edward Jenner's method of vaccination spread throughout the world. The results of his methods and experiments were published in 1798. He called this method of protection "vaccination" because the Latin word *vacca* means "cow." Cowpox was called vaccinia. Pasteur applied the term "vaccine" to suspensions of dead bacteria or **attenuated** bacteria. This term has come to be used in reference to other immunizing antigens not derived from cows. Today smallpox is extinct throughout the world due to a planned program of world vaccination.

Victor Robinson, in *Pathfinders in Medicine,* said of Dr. Jenner, "He died where an intellectual man

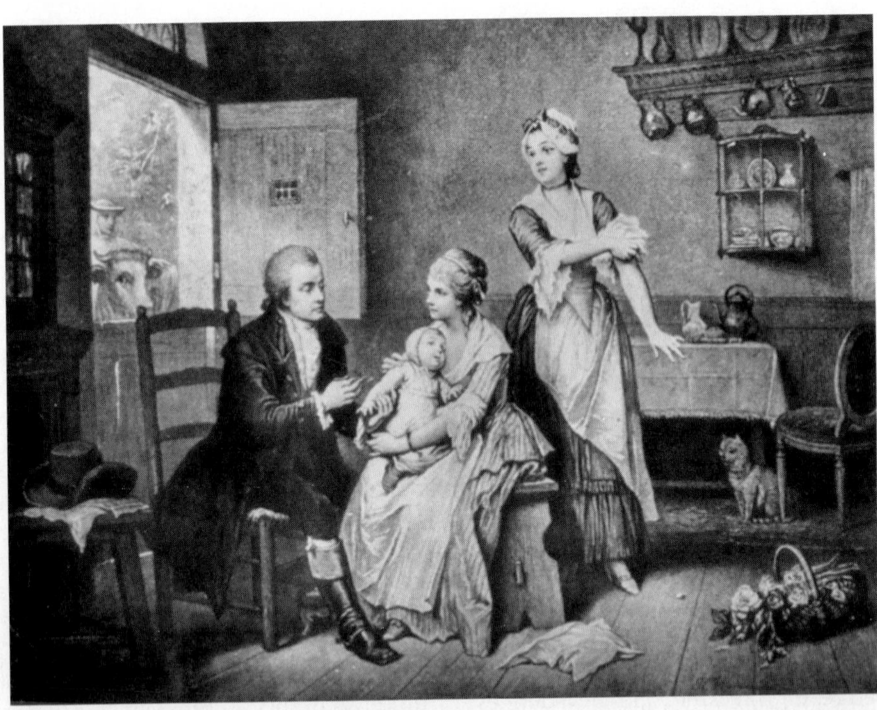

FIGURE 3–6 Edward Jenner vaccinating an infant. (Courtesy of the National Library of Medicine.)

should die (in his library)." The village that gave him birth received his illustrious ashes. When his worn-out body was laid to rest, it would not be surprising if some humble woman, whose child he had saved from smallpox, imagined that Edward Jenner had gone to heaven—to vaccinate the angels.

Memory Jogger

 *What is the origin of the word* vaccination?

Percussion and **auscultation** have been the very basics of physical examination for many years. But no physician had a real understanding of what went on inside the body until anatomists had paved the way for an Austrian physician, LEOPOLD AUENBRUGGER (le'-a-pōld Ow-en-broog'-er) (1722–1809), who developed the use of percussion in diagnosis, and a French physician, RENÉ LAËNNEC (re-na' La'-en-nek) (1781–1826), who developed the **stethoscope.** Auenbrugger became physician-in-chief to the Hospital of the Holy Trinity at Vienna in 1751, and it was there that he tested his discovery, which afterward made him famous but which was generally ignored and scorned by his contemporaries. Laënnec invented the stethoscope in 1819, but at first it was only a cylinder of paper in his hands. His book concerning the stethoscope was readily accepted and translated into many languages. It is said to be the most important treatise in diseases of the thoracic organs ever written.

The first American treatise on psychiatry, *Medical Inquiries and Observations upon the Diseases of the Mind,* published in 1812, was written by BENJAMIN RUSH (1745–1813), a member of the Continental Congress in 1776 and a signer of the Declaration of Independence.

In the early 1800s, there were several men who are remembered for their fight against **puerperal fever** and for their concern for women's health. Puerperal fever, an infectious disease of childbirth, is also known as puerperal sepsis or childbed fever. This term is from *puerpera,* denoting a woman in childbed, from the Latin *puer,* a child, and *pario,* to bring forth. The word "puerperium" now designates the period from delivery to the time the uterus returns to normal size (about 42 days).

The best known of these men is the Hungarian physician IGNAZ PHILIPP SEMMELWEIS (ig'näts fil'-ip sem'-el-vīs) (1818–1865).* History has called him the Savior of Mothers. His fight against puerperal fever is a sad story of hardships, and resistance, especially from his instructor in Vienna, Professor Klein. Semmelweis noted the terrible results of puerperal fever in lying-in hospitals and observed that it occurred with special frequency in cases delivered by medical students who came directly from the autopsy or dissecting room. Semmelweis directed that in his wards the students were to wash and disinfect their hands with a solution of chloride of lime after leaving the dissection room and before going to the wards to examine a woman and deliver her child. This brought about a marked reduction of cases of childbed fever on his ward, but violent opposition was given by the hospital's medical men, and especially by Dr. Klein. As his theories were proven correct, Semmelweis began to feel the horror

*For a riveting novel about Semmelweis's life and career, read *"Not as a Stranger"* by Morton Thompson.

of the deaths that had been caused in the past by doctors themselves.

At the age of 47 years, Semmelweis died, ironically from the very infection he had fought, which was brought on by a cut in his finger while he was doing an autopsy. A monument to Semmelweis in Budapest is given great care, and it has been said that if people had been as tender to the man as they are to his statue, his career would have been happier.

Surely Semmelweis's death was a matter of tragic timing, for his grave had hardly been closed when the causes of this deadly disease were beginning to be understood as a result of the works of two great men, Louis Pasteur and Joseph Lister.

LOUIS PASTEUR (loo'is pas-ter') (1822–1895), a Frenchman, did brilliant work as a chemist, but his studies in bacteriology made him one of the most famous men in medical history and earned him the title of Father of Bacteriology (Fig. 3–7). He has also sometimes been honored with the name Father of Preventive Medicine. His skills and studies reached far beyond the outermost boundaries of the knowledge of the time. He pursued everything with the fire of genius.

Pasteur's adventures included studying the difficulties in the fermentation of wine. He saved the most important industry of France at that time from disaster by a process now called pasteurization, immortalizing his name. By this process of supplying enough heat to destroy microorganisms, wine was prevented from turning into vinegar. This made great improvements in spirit and malt liquors.

The French people called on Pasteur again to help the ailing silkworm industry. The silkworm epidemic in the south of France had reached such proportions that whole plantations were ruined. Pasteur devoted 5 years to the conquest of the two diseases that infected the silkworm. His work was interrupted only when he was stricken with hemiplegia. But after a long, difficult recovery when his mind was always fully active, he continued his work with a stiff hand and a limping foot.

With the conviction that the infinitely small world of bacteria held the key to the secrets of contagious diseases, Pasteur again left chemistry, this time to become a medical man. Many renowned scientists denied the germ theory of disease and devoted themselves to degrading Pasteur. In the midst of all this controversy he became involved in the prevention of **anthrax,** which threatened the health of the cattle and sheep of France as well as of the world. Pasteur's name was also honored for work on many other diseases, such as **rabies,** chicken cholera, and **swine erysipelas.** Pasteur died in 1895, with his family at his bedside. His last words were said to be, "There is still a great deal to do."

Memory Jogger

Which of Pasteur's major accomplishments reflects his name?

JOSEPH LISTER (1827–1912) was to revolutionize surgery through the application of Pasteur's discoveries. He saw the similarity between the infections that were taking place in postsurgical wounds and the processes of **putrefaction,** which Pasteur had proved were caused by microorganisms. Before this time, surgeons accepted infection in surgical wounds as inevitable. Lister reasoned that microorganisms must be the *cause* of infection and must, therefore, be kept out of wounds. Lister's own colleagues were

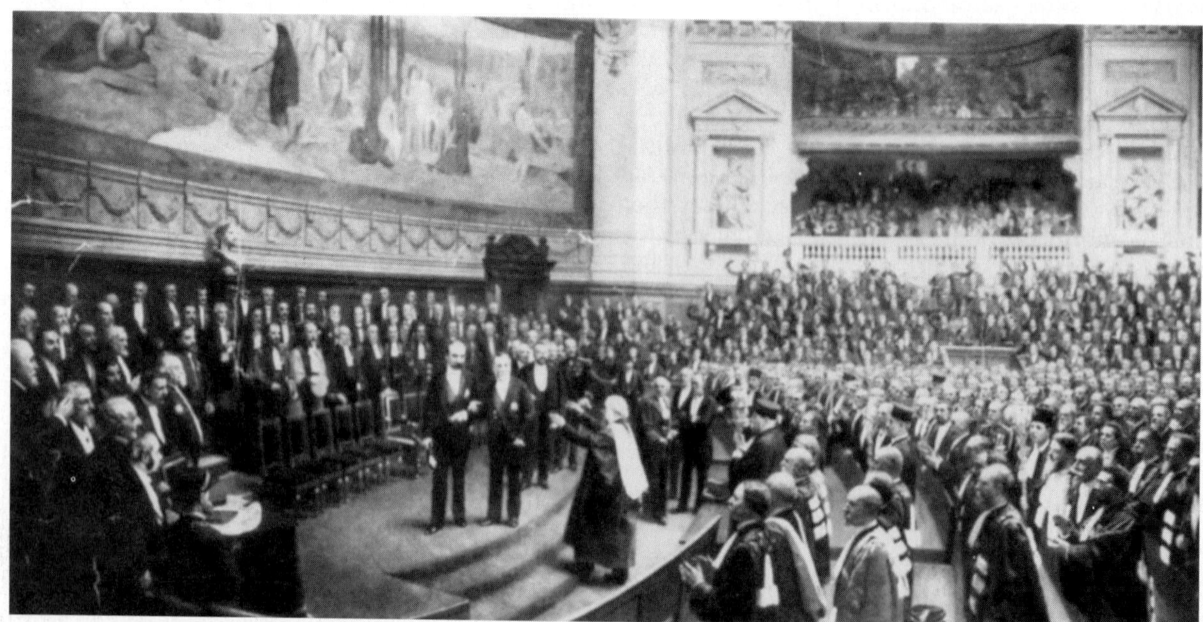

FIGURE 3–7 Louis Pasteur being honored at the Sorbonne. (Courtesy of the National Library of Medicine.)

quite indifferent to his theories, because they felt infections were God given and natural. Lister had once seen pain quelled by the administration of an anesthetic, and pain had been thought to be God given and inevitable also. He developed antiseptic methods by using carbolic acid for sterilization. By spraying the room with a fine mist of the acid, by soaking the instruments and ligatures, and by washing his hands in carbolic solutions, Lister proved his theory. He is honored with the title of Father of Sterile Surgery.

Pasteur and Joseph Lister met at the Sorbonne after years of great mutual admiration. The meeting was filled with emotion, and Robinson, in *Pathfinders in Medicine,* has said that a new star should have appeared in the heavens to commemorate the event. Only a small percentage of the human race entertains any adequate realization of how much we really owe to the combined labors of Louis Pasteur and Joseph Lister.

Memory Jogger

8 *What modern product reflects the name of Joseph Lister?*

ROBERT KOCH (Kok) (1843–1910) is a familiar name to all bacteriologists, because the first law learned as a **neophyte** in this microscopic world is Koch's postulates, which state rules that must be followed before an organism can be accepted as the causative agent in a given disease.

Koch was a German physician who truly earned great honors in bacteriology and public health. He gave the bacteriology laboratory many of its tools, such as the culture-plate method for isolation of bacteria. He discovered the cause of **cholera** and demonstrated its transmission by food and water. This discovery completely transformed health departments and proved the importance of bacteriology. It also established a place of great respect for Koch in the scientific world. A great disappointment in Koch's career was his failure to find a cure for tuberculosis. In this attempt, however, he isolated tuberculin, the substance produced by tubercle bacteria. Its use as a diagnostic aid proved to be of immense value to medicine.

Koch's work took him throughout the world. He traveled to America, Africa, Bombay, Italy, and anywhere nations sought his help in ridding themselves of feared diseases. He was investigating anthrax at the same time as Pasteur, but the ill-concealed animosity between the two men prevented any cooperative effort. In 1885, the University of Berlin created the Chair of Hygiene and Bacteriology in honor of Robert Koch. He became the Nobel Laureate in 1905.

Memory Jogger

9 *Define Koch's Postulates.*

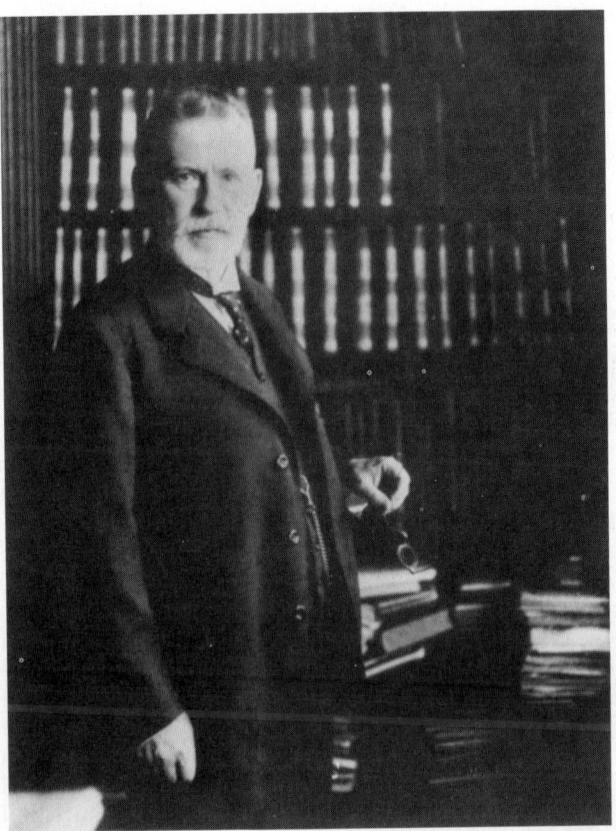

FIGURE 3–8 Paul Ehrlich. (Courtesy of the National Library of Medicine.)

While Robert Koch's brilliant career was nearing an end because of advanced age and illnesses, the work of PAUL EHRLICH (Ār'lik) (1854–1915) was reaching its zenith (Fig. 3–8). Ehrlich had been greatly honored when Koch had invited him to work in his laboratory. Koch had known Ehrlich well, since he had been a distinguished student of his and had already made a place for himself in scientific circles.

Ehrlich was a German physician, and one of the pioneers in the fields of bacteriology, **immunology,** and especially **chemotherapy,** a fairly new science. He was only 28 years old when he wrote his first paper on typhoid, but his greatest gift to humanity was to be called his *magic bullet,* or 606, which was designed to fight the terrible disease, syphilis. Only 3 years before, Bordet and Wasserman had identified the organism and devised a test that would smoke it out of hiding. With the offending germ identified, Ehrlich set out to find a chemical that would destroy the organism but not harm the germ's host, the human body. The search was long and tedious, and history tells us it was the 606th drug that Ehrlich tried that finally did the healing. He called the drug *salvarsan* because he believed it offered humankind salvation from this disease. This also was the beginning of the practice of injecting chemicals into the body to destroy a specific organism. Later, in 1912, Ehrlich discovered a less toxic drug, called neosalvarsan, to replace the original

606. The new drug bore the number 914. In 1908, Ehrlich shared the Nobel Prize with ELI METCHNIKOFF, who is remembered for his theory of **phagocytosis** and immunology.

EMIL ADOLPH VON BEHRING (ba'ring) (1854–1917), a German bacteriologist and Nobel laureate, was born in Prussia (now Poland) and educated at the University of Berlin. In 1890, while working in the laboratory of German bacteriologist Robert Koch in Berlin, Behring and a Japanese bacteriologist Kitasato Shibasaburo discovered that injecting the blood serum of an animal that has tetanus into another animal produces an immunity against the disease in the second animal. On Behring's suggestion, and working with Paul Ehrlich, this principle was applied the following year to fight diphtheria in children, with highly successful results. Behring was awarded the first Nobel Prize in physiology or medicine in 1901.

CRAWFORD WILLIAMSON LONG (1815–1878) was the first to employ ether as an **anesthetic** agent. Early in 1842, after lectures on chemistry, a group of students would have a social gathering and inhale ether as a form of amusement. At one of these so-called "ether frolics," Dr. Long observed that people under the influence of ether did not seem to feel pain. After considerable thought, Dr. Long decided to use ether for a surgical operation. In March of 1842, he removed a tumor from the neck of James M. Venable after placing him under the influence of ether. Long did not report this operation or his discovery until 1848.

DR. HORACE WELLS, a dentist, reported discovering the use of nitrous oxide as an anesthetic in 1844. Another dentist, DR. WILLIAM T. G. MORTON, reported using ether in 1846 when he extracted a tooth from a patient, and also at Massachusetts General Hospital for a surgical procedure.

Surgery owes much to WILHELM KONRAD ROENTGEN (rent'gen) (1845–1922), a professor of physics at the University of Würzburg, Germany, who discovered the x-ray in 1895 while experimenting with electrical currents passed through sealed glass tubes (cathode-ray tubes). Roentgen was awarded the Nobel Prize in Physics in 1901. Although he called his ray the x-ray, science has honored him by calling it the roentgen ray.

Anyone who has had a radiograph or has received radium therapy should know the long struggle of MARIE and PIERRE CURIE leading to the discovery of radium in 1898.

Nineteenth Century Women in Medicine

Much attention is given to honoring great men in medical history, but women have also played important roles, which during those times was not an easy thing to do. Two famous women, in particular, are Florence Nightingale (1820–1910) and Clara Barton (1821–1912). You may notice that their careers overlap almost to the year.

FLORENCE NIGHTINGALE has been honored and known far and wide as "The Lady with the Lamp" and is immortalized as the founder of nursing (Fig. 3–9). She was of noble birth, and somewhat late in life she sought nurse's training in both England and Europe. By the time of the Crimean War in 1854, she already had a reputation for her work in hospital organization. She was invited by the Secretary of War to visit the Crimea to correct the terrible conditions that existed in caring for the wounded. She created the Women's Nursing Service at Scutari and Balaklava. The doctors at Scutari re-

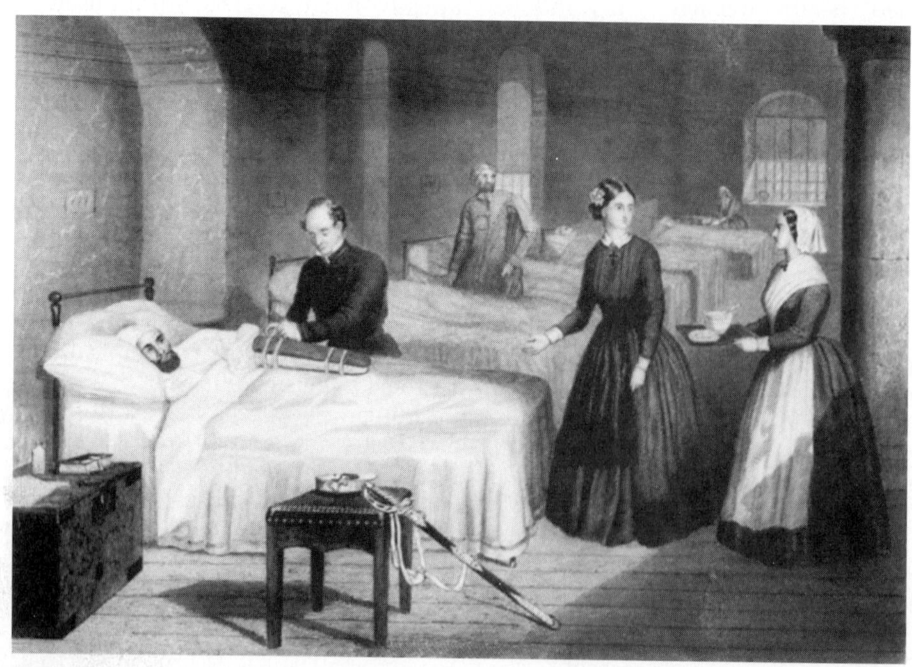

FIGURE 3–9 Florence Nightingale in the hospital at Scutari. (Courtesy of the National Library of Medicine.)

garded Florence Nightingale as a troublesome female intruder and treated her and her nurses quite shabbily. Only a crisis that brought thousands of wounded and sick soldiers to army hospitals persuaded the doctors to accept help from her and her nurses.

Miss Nightingale ruled her nurses with an iron hand. Aside from the practical work she did, it was she who insisted the nursing profession get public recognition and that nursing require special training and experience. From donated funds she organized a school of nursing that bears her name. The modern concept of nursing is based largely on the foundations laid by Florence Nightingale.

CLARA BARTON (Fig. 3–10) is the American counterpart to Florence Nightingale. Miss Barton was a nurse and philanthropist whose work during the American Civil War led her to recognize that very poor records, if any at all, were kept in Washington to aid in the search for missing men wounded or killed in combat. This led to the formation of the Bureau of Records. Clara Barton's fame spread as a result of her organization and recruitment of supplies for the wounded. In 1870, she observed the work of the Red Cross in the Franco-Prussian War; and in 1881, she organized a Red Cross Committee in Washington, forming the American Red Cross, of which she served as the first president from 1881 to 1904.

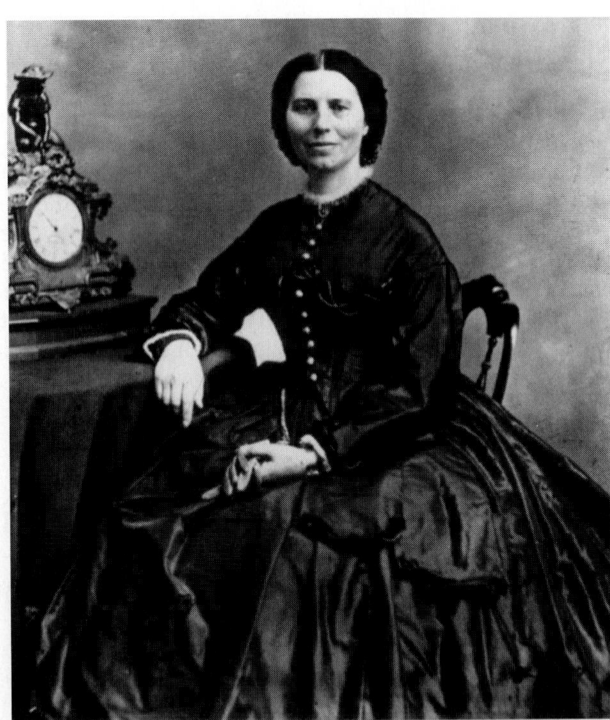

FIGURE 3–10 Clara Barton. (Courtesy of the National Library of Medicine.)

ELIZABETH BLACKWELL (1821–1910) was the first woman in the United States to receive the Doctor of Medicine degree from a medical school. Blackwell's family immigrated to New York from England in 1832. Young Elizabeth began her medical education by reading medical books and later on had private instruction. Medical schools in New York and Pennsylvania refused her applications for formal study, but, finally, in 1847, she was accepted at the Geneva (New York) Medical College. Ten years later, when Blackwell was practicing medicine in New York City, she established the New York Infirmary for Indigent Women and Children (now New York Infirmary), the first hospital staffed entirely by women. In 1869, Dr. Blackwell returned to her native England and became professor of gynecology (1875–1907) at the London School of Medicine for Women, of which she was a founder.

LILLIAN WALD (1867–1940), a social worker and nurse, made a great contribution to medical care when she founded the internationally known Henry Street Settlement at 265 Henry Street, New York City. Wald operated a visiting nurse service from this establishment. When one of her nurses was assigned to the city's public schools in 1902, the New York City Municipal Board of Health established the world's first public school nursing system.

MARGARET SANGER (1883–1966) was born in Corning, New York, on September 14, 1883, and trained as a nurse at the White Plains (New York) Hospital. Women all over the world can give thanks to Margaret Sanger, who became the American leader of the birth control movement. While working among the poor in New York City, she became aware of the need for information concerning contraception. She abandoned nursing to devote herself to the promotion of that objective. In 1873, federal legislation, known as the Comstock Law, had made it a crime to import or distribute any device, medicine, or information designed to prevent conception or induce abortion, or to mention in print the names of sexually transmitted diseases. Nurses and physicians were legally barred from providing this information to their patients. In 1914, Sanger was indicted for circulating through the mails a magazine called *The Woman Rebel,* in which she attacked the legislative restrictions of the Comstock Law. The case was dismissed 2 years later. In this same year she established the first American birth control clinic in Brooklyn, New York, for which she was charged and convicted and spent time in the county penitentiary. Sanger continued in her work, and when the Planned Parenthood Federation of America, Inc. was formed in 1941, she was named honorary chairperson.

Memory Jogger

a. Who founded the American Red Cross?
b. What 19th century woman was called "the Lady with the Lamp"?
c. Who was the inspiration for founding the first public school nursing system?
d. Why should women all over the world give thanks to Margaret Sanger?

Twentieth Century Medicine

Coca-Cola was first used toward the end of the 19th century as a therapeutic agent and general tonic, containing cocaine. It also contained an extract of the kola nut, which is high in caffeine. When the Pure Food and Drug Law was passed in 1906 the makers of Coca-Cola were using decocainized coca leaves, but the caffeine remained.

WALTER REED, a United States Army pathologist and bacteriologist, in 1900, proved that yellow fever is transmitted by the bite of a mosquito. In 1901, action by U.S. military engineers in Cuba freed Havana from the disease by eliminating the mosquitoes.

Diabetics should be grateful to SIR FREDERICK GRANT BANTING, a Canadian physician, and CHARLES HERBERT BEST, a Canadian physiologist, both Nobel laureates, who isolated insulin for the treatment of diabetics in 1922.

In 1928, SIR ALEXANDER FLEMING (1881–1955), a British bacteriologist, discovered penicillin. This discovery came about accidentally while Fleming was researching influenza and working with staphylococcal bacteria. On investigation, he found a substance in the mold that prevented growth of bacteria even when the substance was diluted 800 times. He called it penicillin. His discovery remained a laboratory curiosity until World War II. In 1945, the Nobel Prize for Physiology and Medicine was awarded to Alexander Fleming, Howard Florey, and Ernst Chain for the "discovery of penicillin and its curative effect in various infectious diseases."

Children born with **cyanosis** due to a malformed heart (tetralogy of Fallot) owe thanks to HELEN B. TAUSSIG (tau'sig), of Baltimore, Maryland, who, together with ALFRED BLALOCK developed the lifesaving operation for so-called "blue babies." Although the Blalock-Taussig procedure, first performed in 1944 at Johns Hopkins University Hospital, may seem simple today, in 1944 it was revolutionary and led to a major change of direction in the treatment of heart disease.

During the 1950s the vaccines developed by JONAS EDWARD SALK and ALBERT SABIN almost eradicated poliomyelitis, once the killer or crippler of thousands in the United States. Dr. Salk's work in the 1940s on an anti-influenza vaccine led him and his colleagues to develop an inactivated vaccine against polio in 1952. Following wide-scale testing in 1954, the vaccine was distributed nationally and greatly reduced the disease. In the mid 1950s, Albert Sabin, an American virologist, developed an oral, live vaccine, which with Salk's discovery brought polio under control.

WEERNER FORSSMANN (fors'man) (1904–1979), a Berlin surgeon, originated a cardiologic technique, called **catheterization,** that is used in the diagnosis and treatment of heart disease, for which he was awarded a Nobel Prize in physiology or medicine. He first demonstrated the technique by experimenting on himself by making an incision in a vein in his right arm and maneuvering a catheter up the vessel and into the right auricle of his heart while observing via a mirror the fluoroscoped image of the instrument as it traveled through his body.

CHRISTIAAN N. BARNARD (1922–), a South African surgeon, performed the first human heart transplant operation on December 3, 1967, when he transferred the heart of a 25-year-old woman into the body of a 55-year-old man. This patient died 18 days later. The second patient, who received a transplant on January 2, 1968, lived for 563 days after the operation. Since then bypass surgery has made thousands of hearts more functional and organ transplants are becoming almost commonplace.

In 1972, British engineers invented the computed tomography (CT) scanner; in 1978, the first test tube baby was born (in England); in 1982, the U.S. Food and Drug Administration approved the first drug developed with recombinant-DNA technology (a form of human insulin); in 1995, a Duke University surgeon successfully transplanted a heart from a genetically altered pig into a baboon; and in 1997, a sheep was cloned in Great Britain. What will follow?

National Institutes of Health

The National Institutes of Health (NIH) observed its centennial anniversary in the year 1987. It began as a one-room laboratory in the marine hospital on New York's Staten Island in 1887. Tuberculosis was the number-one cause of death at that time. There were few drugs that could alleviate or cure disease. There were no vaccines except for smallpox. There were no antibiotics. Doctors could diagnose some conditions but fell short on treatment. And there was not even aspirin. Morphine was injected for severe pain. In 1891, the laboratory moved from Staten Island to Washington, DC. In 1902 the Marine Hospital Service became the Public Health Service and in 1930 became the National Institutes of Health, an agency of the U.S. Department of Health and Human Services. As a part of the Public Health Service, it seeks to improve the health of the American people, supports and conducts biomedical research into the causes and prevention of diseases, and uses a modern communications system to furnish biomedical information to the health care professions.

The Institutes moved from Washington, DC, to Bethesda, Maryland, in 1938, where it occupied 3 buildings. It remains in Bethesda today but occupies more than 60 buildings covering 30 acres. It consists of 13 research institutes, four divisions, and the National Library of Medicine. Thousands of research projects are under way in NIH laboratories and clinics at any given time.

Centers for Disease Control and Prevention

The CDC is an agency of the United States Public Health Service, headquartered in Atlanta, Georgia. It was established in 1946 as the Communicable Disease Center, and became the Centers for Disease Control in 1970; "and Prevention" was added in 1992, but Congress requested that "CDC" remain the agency's initials. The agency conducts research into the origin and occurrence of diseases and develops methods for their control and prevention. Additionally, it develops immunization services, provides public health information, and aids in the training of health workers. The CDC also conducts international programs. In recent years the agency has been deeply involved in the battle against human immunodeficiency virus infection and acquired immunodeficiency syndrome (AIDS) through arranging educational programs to help prevent future outbreaks. The agency has developed guidelines that emphasize that *standard blood and body-fluid precautions* be consistently used for all patients in all situations where the risk of contamination by body fluids exists. The precautions are enforced by the Occupational Safety and Health Administration (OSHA).

Memory Jogger

11 *What is the basic purpose of the CDC?*

Overview

The nature of this text does not permit the exploration of every one of the medical miracles of the past century. It is tremendously exciting simply to be open to such advancements and to be aware of their potential. The supportive role of medical assisting is very important in maintaining the quality of medical service and in making today a strong foundation for the progress of tomorrow. If you have been enlightened by this brief history of medicine, further attention to medical discoveries as they occur will add an extra dimension to your study of medical assisting. Perhaps you will contribute some miracles of your own.

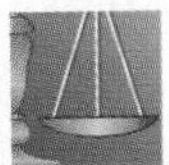

LEGAL AND ETHICAL ISSUES

As you advance in this exciting profession of health care, you will do well to review the efforts (sometimes lives) expended by those who pushed on to achieve today's level of care and to respect the standards achieved. Think positive, and expect a miracle.

CRITICAL THINKING

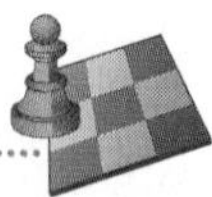

The historical legacy that is taken for granted by most people in our society represents enormous sacrifices by the discoverers of new principles and treatments in past centuries. The last half of the 20th century has completely changed the possibilities of diagnosis and treatment.

Let us be respectful of the efforts of our forefathers and be grateful for the added quality of life available at the beginning of the 21st century.

HOW DID I DO? Answers to Memory Joggers

1 The caduceus has two serpents; the staff of Aesculapius has only one.

2 Moses was called the "first public health officer" because he was an advocate of preventive medicine.

3 The university (a) acquired prior training in the natural sciences, and (b) had the advantages of Johns Hopkins Hospital close by as a training site.

4 The lenses ground by Leeuwenhoek magnified the minute world of organisms and led to the sciences of bacteriology and protozoology.

5 Hunter was given the title "Founder of Scientific Surgery" because his procedures were based on pathologic evidence.

6 The origin of the word *vaccination* is *vacca,* meaning "cow."

7 The process *pasteurization.*

8 Listerine.

9 Koch's postulates are laboratory rules that must be followed before an organism can be accepted as the causative agent in a given disease.

10 a. Clara Barton
b. Florence Nightingale
c. Lillian Wald
d. Sanger fought for the advancement of planned parenthood.

11 Research into the origin and occurrence of diseases and developing methods for their control and prevention.

REFERENCES

Bullock A, Woodings R (eds): Twentieth Century Culture, New York, Harper & Row, 1983.

Garrison FH: History of Medicine, 4th ed. Philadelphia, WB Saunders, 1929.

Magner LN: A History of Medicine. New York, Marcel Dekker, 1992.

Robinson V: Pathfinders in Medicine. New York, Medical Life Press, 1979.

SECTION 2

Understanding the Protocols of Medical Practice

CURRICULUM CONTENT/COMPETENCIES

Chapter 4 Medical Practice Systems

- Work as a team member
- Locate community resources and disseminate information

Chapter 5 Medical Ethics

- Practice within the scope of education, training, and personal capabilities
- Use appropriate guidelines when releasing information
- Maintain awareness of federal and state health care legislation and regulations
- Explain office policies and procedures

Chapter 6 Medicine and the Law

- Follow federal, state, and local legal guidelines
- Maintain and dispose of regulated substances in compliance with government guidelines
- Prepare and maintain medical records
- Document accurately
- Comply with established risk management and safety procedures

Medical Practice Systems

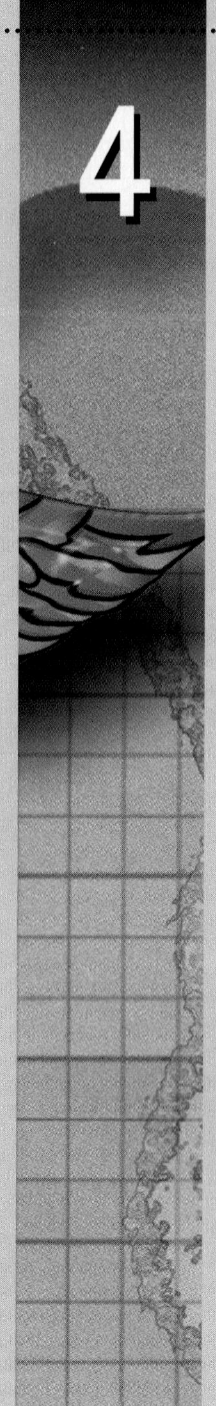

OUTLINE

LEARNING OBJECTIVES

Cognitive: On successful completion of this chapter you should be able to:

1 Define and spell the terms listed in the Vocabulary.

2 Name the system of medical care delivery that has brought about a significant change in medical practice in the past decade.

3 State the principal difference between the training of the MD and the DO.

4 List the three medical practice business structures discussed in the chapter.

5 Name and compare the two principal methods of paying for medical care.

6 Identify 10 or more allied health occupations that might be represented in a medical practice.

VOCABULARY

accelerating Causing to act or move faster
maladies Diseases or disorders of the body
manipulative Treating or operating with the hands in a skillful manner
overutilization Excessive use
puerperium The period between childbirth and the return of the uterus to its normal size
rehabilitation Restoration of normal form and function after injury or illness
substantiated Having been established as true by proof of competent evidence; verified

The Business Structure of Medical Practices

Three general types of business structure exist in medical practice: sole proprietorship, partnership, and corporation. Sole proprietorship, or solo practice, consisting of one physician only, dominated medical practice until the last quarter of the 20th century. Solo practice is steadily declining.

SOLE PROPRIETORSHIP

A sole proprietor is an individual who holds exclusive right and title to all aspects of the medical practice. The sole proprietor may employ other physicians to participate in the practice. The employed physician is entitled to employee fringe benefits, but the owner is not so entitled. Additionally, the owner would be potentially liable for all of the acts of his professional employees. Earlier physicians enjoyed the flexibility and independence of practicing alone. Disadvantages are that the physician is totally responsible 24 hours a day, and the potential earnings are limited. In an unincorporated solo practice, the practice dies with the owner.

Memory Jogger

 *Why do you think sole proprietorship is declining?*

Associate Practice

Often two or more physicians agree to share office space and employees but conduct their practice as sole proprietors. They have an agreement among themselves as to the manner in which the practice is to operate.

PARTNERSHIP

When two or more physicians elect to associate in the practice of medicine, they may draw up a partnership agreement, which should show all the rights, obligations, and responsibilities of each partner. The partners have more potential for profit than they would have if practicing as individuals. Each has more freedom by having another physician available in emergencies. One major disadvantage of partnership is the liability of each for the acts and conduct of other partners unless otherwise specified in the partnership agreement. In a partnership practice the death or retirement of a partner requires a new agreement.

PROFESSIONAL CORPORATION

A *corporation* may be defined as an artificial entity having a legal and business status that is independent of its shareholders or employees. Corporations are regulated by statutes of the state in which the incorporation takes place.

The physician shareholders are employees of the corporation. Even one physician in solo practice can incorporate. All employees of the corporation receive income and tax advantages. An attractive fringe benefit package is usually offered to the employees and may include pension and profit-sharing plans, medical expense reimbursement, life insurance, disability income insurance, and employee death benefit. Fringe benefits to the corporate employee are separate from salary; that is, they are tax deductible to the corporation and not taxable to the employee.

Professional employees of a corporation are liable only for their own acts. Another advantage of the corporate entity is the continuous life of the corporation. The corporation is an entity unto itself and does not end with a change in shareholders.

Group Practice

The governing bodies of the American Medical Association (AMA), the American Group Practice Association, and the Medical Group Management Association have formally adopted the following definition of medical group practice:

> *Medical Group Practice is the provision of health care services by a group of at least three licensed physician-practitioners, engaged full-time in a*

formally organized and legally recognized entity; sharing the group's income and expenses in a systematic manner; and sharing facilities, equipment, common records, and personnel, involved in both patient care and business management.

A small or medium-sized group may be a single-specialty group with all the physicians engaged in the same specialty. Family practice and anesthesia services are two common examples. A large group would more likely be a multispecialty practice. Group practice usually takes the legal form of a partnership or a corporation.

Memory Jogger

 *What are the three general business practice structures in medicine and how do they differ?*

Delivery of Medical Care

By the mid-20th century, medical practice was experiencing many changes. Rapid developments in medical science encouraged more specialization. The **accelerating** cost of maintaining an office was becoming prohibitive for a solo practitioner, especially the new graduate. Medical insurance for the patient became the rule rather than the exception. More government programs, with their accompanying regulations, were developing, and the management of a medical practice required more and better-trained personnel. These developments brought many changes in the delivery of medical care and the payment for those services.

FEE-FOR-SERVICE

Before July 1, 1966, when Medicare under Social Security for the patient older than age 65 years went into effect, payment for medical care was accomplished on a fee-for-service arrangement. The physician established the fee for his or her services. Fees for surgery or an extensive series of visits were usually discussed and agreed on by the patient before service. The patient was billed direct and was responsible for payment, irrespective of any reimbursement from insurance. Traditional fee-for-service plans now serve less than a fourth of insured workers in the United States.

MANAGED CARE

Managed care is difficult to define because it is still evolving. By general definition, the intent of managed care is a streamlining of the system of delivering medical care so that patients receive appropriate care in an appropriate setting at the least possible cost. In 1993, about half the Americans insured through employers were in managed care. That figure jumped to 73% by 1995 and is still rising. In 1997, there were 158 million members enrolled in managed care health plans.

Health Maintenance Organization (HMO)

An HMO is an organization that provides for comprehensive health care to an enrolled group for a fixed periodic payment. In the early 1970s, the federal government, which bears a great percentage of the costs of medical care, took action to contain the potential abuses of overtreatment and **overutilization** of health care services. The enactment of Public Law 93-222, the HMO Assistance Act, in December 1973, created Title XIII of the Public Health Service Act. Title XIII is intended to encourage and promote the growth of HMOs resulting in cost containment. HMOs function in a variety of ways within a federally regulated environment. The methods of delivering care vary, but the basic characteristics are similar.

As the name implies, the HMO concept emphasizes the maintenance of health and preventive medicine. Insured members of HMOs, because their contracts provide for comprehensive care, are more inclined to visit their physicians before major and more costly problems arise. An employer who provides health care benefits to employees may be required to offer federally qualified HMOs as an option. Managed care is discussed in more detail in a later chapter.

PREVENTIVE CARE AND PUBLIC HEALTH

The practice of medicine does not always involve patient care. General preventive medicine involves the relation of environment to health with special concern for the health requirements of population groups. The community is the public health physician's patient. Public health is a special field of preventive care embodying the use of medical and administrative methods to prevent disease and improve general health through community efforts in areas such as sanitation and education. The United States Public Health Service and the World Health Organization (WHO) are both concerned with preventive medicine. All branches of medicine are committed to preventive medicine.

SPECIALTY PRACTICE

Many physicians have a special interest in a specific branch of medical practice and eventually direct their efforts to becoming expert in their chosen field. Physicians who decide to limit their practice to a specialized field will spend an additional 3 to 6 years in a residency program after completion of internship and will probably seek certification by one of the specialty boards.

Memory Jogger

 *Give a general definition of managed care.*

American Board of Medical Specialties

Twenty-four specialty boards exist under the umbrella of the American Board of Medical Specialties. These specialty boards help improve the quality of medical education by elevating the standards of graduate medical education and approving facilities for specialty training. The primary function of each approved specialty board is to evaluate the qualifications of candidates in its field who apply voluntarily for examination and to certify as diplomates those who are qualified. Qualifications vary with the various boards.

In accomplishing the described function, specialty boards determine whether candidates have received adequate preparation according to established educational standards; they provide comprehensive examinations to such candidates; and they issue certificates to those physicians who have satisfied the requirements. Those physicians who are board certified are known as diplomates of a specific specialty board (e.g., Fredrick B. Mears, MD, Diplomate of the American Board of Surgery).

A listing of the 24 specialty boards is shown here. The American Board of Medical Specialties is at One American Plaza, Suite 805, Evanston, IL 60201. It regularly publishes a directory listing all physicians certified as diplomates by the specialty boards, including biographical sketches detailing their educational qualifications. Many physicians consult the directory in making referrals.

APPROVED SPECIALTY BOARDS OF THE UNITED STATES

American Board of Allergy and Immunology
American Board of Anesthesiology
American Board of Colon and Rectal Surgery
American Board of Dermatology
American Board of Emergency Medicine
American Board of Family Practice
American Board of Internal Medicine
American Board of Medical Genetics
American Board of Neurological Surgery
American Board of Nuclear Medicine
American Board of Obstetrics and Gynecology
American Board of Ophthalmology
American Board of Orthopaedic Surgery
American Board of Otolaryngology
American Board of Pathology
American Board of Pediatrics
American Board of Physical Medicine and Rehabilitation
American Board of Plastic Surgery
American Board of Preventive Medicine
American Board of Psychiatry and Neurology
American Board of Radiology
American Board of Surgery
American Board of Thoracic Surgery
American Board of Urology

American College of Surgeons

The American College of Surgeons, located at 55 East Erie Street, Chicago, IL 60611 may also confer a degree on an applicant from a surgical specialty. The applicant is required to have completed a course of postgraduate training equivalent to "board requirements" and to have submitted 50 detailed, **substantiated** case reports of varied surgical procedures in which the applicant has been the chief surgeon during the past 3 years of practice before application. Successful applicants are identified as a Fellow of the American College of Surgeons (FACS).

American College of Physicians

The American College of Physicians issues a similar fellowship degree (FACP) to applicants who have completed approved postgraduate training and have exhibited special interest and competence in one nonsurgical specialty.

Osteopathic Medicine

Osteopathic medicine is a complete school of medical practice that began in the United States in the 19th century. Its founder was Andrew Taylor Still, an American Civil War army physician. Dr. Still established the first College of Osteopathic Medicine in 1892 at Kirksville, Missouri.

The Doctor of Osteopathy (DO) differs from the Doctor of Medicine (MD) in placing more emphasis on the relationship between the musculoskeletal structure and organ function. The use of **manipulative** therapy in diagnosis and treatment is an integral part of osteopathy. The DO is a graduate of a college of osteopathy and is a fully trained physician, qualified to be licensed as a physician and to practice all branches of medicine and surgery.

Colleges of osteopathy are accredited by the Bureau of Professional Education of the American Osteopathic Association (AOA), which is recognized by the U.S. Department of Education and the Council on Postsecondary Accreditation. Four academic years of study are required, which include the basic sciences of anatomy, physiology, biochemistry, pathology, microbiology, and pharmacology and a wide range of clinical subjects. Integrated throughout the curriculum is special instruction in osteopathic principles dealing with the interrelationship of all body systems in health and disease. After graduation, DOs participate in a 12-month rotating internship. Those who wish to become specialists serve an additional 2 to 6 years of residency or fellowship training.

Osteopathic physicians are licensed to practice medicine in all states of the United States. Requirements for licensure for both DOs and MDs are very similar, and after licensure both provide the same range of professional services. More than half of active DOs provide primary health care; the remainder are specialists practicing in such fields as internal medicine, surgery, psychiatry, and obstetrics. DOs are more prevalent in towns and cities having fewer than 50,000 inhabitants.

Memory Jogger

How does the education of a DO differ from that of an MD?

Specialties of Medicine

AEROSPACE MEDICINE Aerospace medicine is the specialty concerned with the physiologic, pathologic, and psychologic problems encountered by humans in space. This field is mostly confined to the space agencies of the federal government.

ALLERGY AND IMMUNOLOGY An allergy is an abnormal reaction to substances that are harmless to most people. Substances that frequently bother the allergic person include pollens from grass, weeds, and trees; molds; house and other dusts; dog and cat danders; certain foods and medications; and the stings of insects.

There are many kinds of medicines and treatments that can help relieve the allergic symptoms, but it is essential first to identify the cause. The allergist is specially trained to diagnose and treat allergy problems with a high degree of accuracy and success.

The American Board of Allergy and Immunology is a conjoint board of the American Board of Internal Medicine and the American Board of Pediatrics. To become an allergist, the pediatrician or internist must take several years of additional specialty training and pass another certifying examination.

ANESTHESIOLOGY An anesthesiologist is a physician who administers local and general anesthesia, usually to prepare and maintain a patient for surgery and in some cases for relief of pain. An anesthesiologist monitors the surgical patient through the surgical process until stable consciousness returns postoperatively.

DERMATOLOGY Dermatologists are medical doctors who have extensive specialized training in the medical and surgical treatment of disorders of the skin, hair, and nails.

Because of specific training, the dermatologist is able to determine the best treatment approach to skin disorders. This approach may involve the use of medicines, both internal and external, or it may involve skin surgery. In addition to common dermatologic procedures such as removal of moles, warts, cysts, benign tumors, and skin cancers, many dermatologists are also trained in certain surgical and cosmetic procedures. These include skin grafts and flaps, hair transplants, dermabrasion, and collagen implants.

EMERGENCY MEDICINE The emergency medicine specialist is a physician who specializes in the immediate recognition and treatment of acute illnesses and injuries. These specialists may also be involved in the administration, teaching, and research of systems designed to help patients seeking emergency care. Qualifications for this specialty include a formal emergency medicine residency training or experience and continuing medical education.

Traditionally, specialists in emergency medicine provide 24-hour coverage of emergency departments in acute care hospitals, making emergency care available at all times. These specialists also provide the authority and license under which paramedic prehospital care is provided.

FAMILY PRACTICE Family or general practice encompasses the care of all members of the family regardless of age or sex and covers a vast range of medical problems. This allows for continuity of care for the individual and integration of care for the family as a whole.

INTERNAL MEDICINE Internal medicine is the specialty concerned with the complete nonsurgical care of the adult. Internists are experts in the medical diagnosis and treatment of adult disorders as well as in the areas of health maintenance and wellness. General internists are responsible for a broad range of adult medical problems. Internal medicine comprises multiple subspecialties including allergy, cardiology, endocrinology, gastroenterology, gerontology, hematology, infectious disease, nephrology, oncology, pulmonary diseases, and rheumatology.

MEDICAL GENETICS The specialty of medical genetics is concerned with the study of heredity and its effects on individuals in health and disease.

NEUROLOGY Neurology is concerned with the nonsurgical management of neurologic disease. Generally, the neurologist manages infectious, metabolic, degenerative, and systemic involvement of the nervous system.

NUCLEAR MEDICINE Nuclear medicine is a specialty field in which radioactive substances are used for the diagnosis and treatment of disease.

OBSTETRICS AND GYNECOLOGY Obstetrics is the specialty involved in the care and management of women during pregnancy, labor, delivery, and the **puerperium.** Gynecology is the specialty devoted to the medical and surgical treatment of diseases of women, especially diseases affecting the reproductive organs and functions.

OPHTHALMOLOGY Ophthalmology involves the diagnosis and treatment of eye and vision disorders, utilizing surgery and other corrective techniques. The testing of visual acuity is a basic procedure. The ophthalmologist treats glaucoma, strabismus, astigmatism, and cataracts and is skilled in surgical procedures and laser techniques.

OTOLARYNGOLOGY Otolaryngology is professionally known as Otolaryngology/Head and Neck Surgery, whereas the community may think of the specialty as ENT. Otolaryngology is broadly based, encompassing medical and surgical treatment of ear, nose, and throat disorders, allergy therapy, facial cosmetic and reconstructive surgery, and tumor problems in the head and neck. Otolaryngology is advancing in the fields of microsurgery and laser surgery.

PATHOLOGY Pathology is the science that deals with the causes, mechanisms of development, and effects of disease. The pathologist seeks to detect the actual nature of disease—not just the physical symptoms or how it feels to the patient but what the disease is from a biologic standpoint, that is, what visible or measurable changes it produces in the cells, fluids, and life processes of the entire body.

The practice of pathology is divided into two major areas, Anatomic Pathology and Clinical Pathology, and these areas are further subdivided into many subspecialties. The function of the anatomic pathologist is to render a diagnosis based on examination of a tissue specimen and to learn as precisely as possible the extent of the disease. The clinical pathologist is in charge of the medical laboratory, in which a variety of diagnostic studies are done. Forensic pathology is a subspecialty dealing with various aspects of medicine and the law.

PEDIATRICS Caring for the health of children from birth to adolescence is the unique purpose of pediatrics. The pediatrician continually strives to prevent and treat all aspects of childhood diseases. The extent of the pediatrician's interest and responsibilities spans such areas as infectious diseases, newborn care, hospital care of children, environmental hazards, school health problems, nutrition, accident prevention, children with disabilities, drugs, allergy, cardiology, and pediatric pharmacology. The pediatric specialist can handle the problems of acutely ill children and provide guidance to parents regarding the development and preventive care of children who are well. The neonatologist treats the diseases and abnormalities of the newborn.

PHYSICAL MEDICINE AND REHABILITATION The specialty of Physical Medicine and Rehabilitation is concerned with the diagnosis and treatment of disorders and disabilities of the neuromuscular system. A physician in this specialty is called a *physiatrist.* The physiatrist uses the physical elements such as heat, cold, water, electricity, and exercise to help restore physical function and independence.

PREVENTIVE MEDICINE Preventive Medicine is concerned with preventing the occurrence of both mental and physical illness and disability. Analysis of present health services and planning for future medical needs are part of Preventive Medicine, as are Occupational Medicine and Public Health.

HOLISTIC HEALTH AND HOLISTIC MEDICINE Holistic health requires total cooperation of the patient. It is a philosophy of life that encompasses lifestyle, attitudes, and everyday events, all of which affect the physical response of the body—for good or for ill. Holistic medicine is not a specific method of treatment but includes all safe methods, as appropriate for the situation. The dominant factor is the acceptance, by the patient, of personal responsibility to cooperate with the chosen practitioner in achieving a reasonable state of well-being.

PSYCHIATRY A psychiatrist is a physician whose specialty is the diagnosis and treatment of persons with mental, emotional, or behavioral disorders. The psychiatrist is qualified to conduct psychotherapy and to prescribe medications when necessary. This allows the psychiatrist comprehensively to treat complex interactions of biologic, psychologic, and social factors that affect patients.

RADIOLOGY Radiology is a specialty in which x-rays (roentgen rays) are used for diagnosis and treatment of disease. A diagnostic radiologist specializes in using x-rays, ultrasound, nuclear medicine, computed tomography (CT), and magnetic resonance imaging (MRI) for detection of abnormalities throughout the body. Therapeutic radiology involves the use of ionizing radiation in the treatment of cancer and other tumors.

SURGERY Surgery is the correction of deformities, defects, diseases, or injured parts of the body by means of operative treatment. By making an incision into body tissue or by passing instruments through the skin, the diseased or injured tissues or organs can be corrected, modified, removed, or replaced. The various specializations contained within the broad field of surgery are listed below.

GENERAL SURGERY General Surgery may include all aspects of surgery other than those included under special groups. Many general surgeons restrict their practice to surgery of abdominal conditions, traumatic situations, or tumor conditions. However, there is no restriction on the general surgeon's scope of activities, and many general surgeons take on additional fields as their training, interest, and capabilities dictate.

COLON AND RECTAL SURGERY Colon and Rectal Surgery is a surgical subspecialty that concentrates on surgical treatment of the lower intestinal tract, which includes the colon and rectum.

NEUROSURGERY A neurosurgeon specializes in the diagnosis and surgical treatment of the nervous system (the brain, spinal cord, and nerves) and the surrounding bony structures.

ORAL SURGERY Oral Surgery is a branch of dentistry dealing with the extraction of teeth and the treatment of fractures of the jaws and adjacent facial bones. The oral surgeon may also do other surgical procedures on the jaws, oral tissues, and adjacent tissues to treat or correct abnormal conditions.

ORTHOPEDIC SURGERY The orthopedic surgeon treats not only **maladies** of the musculoskeletal system but also congenital and acquired deformities, including spinal curvatures and arthritis. Orthopedic techniques are also used to treat sports injuries, including arthroscopic techniques, to maximize **rehabilitation.** Although orthopedics is a branch of surgery, many conditions are treated without surgery, including most fractures and muscle and tendon infirmities.

PLASTIC SURGERY Plastic Surgery includes the operative repair of defects by graft, tissue transfer, or cosmetic alteration of tissue. A plastic surgeon specializes in burns, congenital defects, hand and extremity reconstruction, the treatment of skin wounds and lesions, the performance of aesthetic surgery of the face, and body contouring.

THORACIC (CARDIOVASCULAR) SURGERY This surgical subspecialty is concerned with the operative treatment of the chest and chest wall, lungs, and respiratory passages. Specialists in this field are involved with heart surgery, including both valvular and coronary heart surgery.

UROLOGY Urology is a medical specialty concerned with the treatment of diseases and disorders of the urinary tract of men, women, and children and of the male genitalia.

Related Health Care Specialists

CHIROPRACTOR (DC) The practice of chiropractic is based on the premise that disease is caused by abnormal functioning of the nervous system. The chiropractor attempts to restore normal function by manipulation, especially of the spinal column. The practitioner earns the degree of Doctor of Chiropractic and is licensed by the state.

OPTOMETRIST (OD) The optometrist is trained and licensed to examine the eyes to test visual acuity and to treat defects of vision by prescribing and adapting correctional lenses and other optical aids. He or she may also plan programs of exercise for the patient's eyes. An optician fills optical prescriptions for both ordinary eyeglasses and contact lenses.

PODIATRIST (DP) Podiatrists are educated in caring for the feet, including the anatomy, pathology, medical, and surgical treatment. They earn the degree of Doctor of Podiatry and are licensed practitioners.

Support Personnel

In the complex delivery of 20th century medical care, the physician is the maestro, but for every practicing physician there are many behind-the-scenes support persons. As the delivery of medical

TABLE 4–1 Allied Health Professions for Which the AMA Has Collaborated in Establishing Accreditation of Educational Programs

Credential	Profession
AA	Anesthesiologist's Assistant
AT	Athletic Trainer
CVT	Cardiovascular Technologist
CLS	Clinical Laboratory Scientist
CLT	Clinical Laboratory Technician
CT	Cytotechnologist
DMS	Diagnostic Medical Sonographer
EEG-T	Electroneurodiagnostic Technologist
EMT-P	Emergency Medical Technician–Paramedic
RRA	Health Information Administrator
ART	Health Information Technician
HT	Histologic Technician/Technologist
CMA	Medical Assistant
MI	Medical Illustrator
NMT	Nuclear Medicine Technologist
OMT	Ophthalmic Medical Technician/Technologist
OP	Orthotist/Prosthetist
OT	Occupational Therapist
OTA	Occupational Therapy Assistant
PERF	Perfusionist
PA	Physician's Assistant/Surgeon's Assistant
RAD	Radiographer
RADT	Radiation Therapist
RRT	Respiratory Therapist
CRTT	Respiratory Therapy Technician
SBB	Specialist in Blood Bank Technology
ST	Surgical Technologist

TABLE 4–2 Health Care Occupations Accredited by the Commission on Accreditation of Allied Health Education Programs (CAAHEP)

Occupation	Credential	Brief Job Description
Anesthesiologist Assistant	AA	Functions under the direction of a licensed and qualified anesthesiologist. Assists in developing and implementing the anesthesia care plan.
Athletic Trainer	AT	Functions under supervision of attending and/or consulting physician. Provides a variety of services, including injury prevention, recognition, immediate care, treatment, and rehabilitation after physical trauma.
Cardiovascular Technologist	CVT	Performs diagnostic examinations at the request or direction of a physician in one or more of three areas: (1) invasive cardiology, (2) noninvasive cardiology, and (3) noninvasive peripheral vascular study.
Cytotechnologist	CT	Works with pathologist. Prepares cellular samples for study under the microscope and assists in the diagnosis of disease by examining the samples.
Diagnostic Medical Sonographer	DMS	Provides patient services using medical ultrasound under the supervision of a physician. Assists in gathering sonographic data necessary to diagnose a variety of conditions and diseases.
Electrodiagnostic Technologist	EEG-T	Works in collaboration with the electroencephalographer. Possesses the knowledge, attributes, and skills to obtain interpretable recordings of patients' nervous system function.
Emergency Medical Technician–Paramedic	EMT-P	Works under the direction of a physician—often through radio communication—and is able to recognize, assess, and manage medical emergencies of acutely ill or injured patients in prehospital care settings.
Health Information Administrator	RRA	Manages health information systems consistent with the medical, administrative, ethical, and legal requirements of the health care delivery system. Works with medical and hospital administrative staff involving medical records.
Health Information Technician	ART	Maintains components of health information systems in all types of facilities including hospitals and ambulatory health care centers. Processes, maintains, compiles, and reports patient data.
Medical Assistant	CMA	Multiskilled practitioner who works primarily in ambulatory settings such as physicians' offices and clinics, performing both administrative and clinical procedures.
Medical Illustrator	MI	Working with many different media, medical illustrators create visual material designed to facilitate the recording and dissemination of medical, biological, and related knowledge.
Ophthalmic Medical Technician/ Technologist	OMT	Renders supportive services to the ophthalmologist. Administers diagnostic tests, takes ocular measurements, tests ocular functions, and performs other tasks assigned by the ophthalmologist.
Orthotist/Prosthetist	OP	Both the orthotist and the prosthetist work directly with the physician in the rehabilitation of the physically challenged. The orthotist designs and fits orthoses to provide care to patients who have disabling conditions of the limbs and spine. The prosthetist designs and fits devices for patients who have partial or total absence of limb.
Perfusionist	PERF	A perfusionist operates extracorporeal circulation equipment during any medical situation in which it is necessary to support or temporarily replace the patient's circulatory or respiratory function (e.g., cardiopulmonary bypass).
Physician Assistant	PA	The physician assistant is academically and clinically prepared to practice medicine with the supervision of a licensed doctor of medicine or osteopathy. The functions of the physician assistant include performing diagnostic, therapeutic, preventive, and health maintenance services.
Respiratory Therapist	RRT	The respiratory therapist working under the supervision of a physician evaluates all data to determine the appropriateness of the prescribed respiratory care and participates in the development of the respiratory care plan.
Respiratory Therapy Technician	CRTT	The respiratory therapy technician works under the supervision of the respiratory therapist and a physician in administering general respiratory care.
Specialist in Blood Bank Technology	SBB	Specialists in blood bank technology perform both routine and specialized tests in blood bank immunohematology in technical areas of the modern blood bank and perform transfusion services.
Surgical Technologist	ST/CST	Works in the surgical suite with surgeons, anesthesiologists, registered nurses, and other surgical personnel.

From Allied Health and Rehabilitation Professions Education Directory, 24th ed. American Medical Association, Chicago, IL, 1996–1997.

TABLE 4–3 Health Care Occupations Accredited by Agencies Other Than CAAHEP Under the AMA Umbrella

Occupational Therapist
Occupational Therapy Assistant
Dietetic Technician
Dietitian/Nutritionist
Dental Assistant
Dental Hygienist
Dental Laboratory Technician
Audiologist
Speech-Language Pathologist
Radiation Therapist
Radiographer
Nuclear Medicine Technologist
Clinical Laboratory Technician/Medical Laboratory Technician—Associate Degree
Clinical Laboratory Technician/Medical Laboratory Technician—Certificate
Clinical Laboratory Scientist/Medical Technologist
Histologic Technician/Technologist
Pathologists' Assistant

From Allied Health and Rehabilitation Professions Education Directory, 24th ed., American Medical Association, Chicago, IL, 1996–1997.

care has become more fragmented, the close relationship that formerly existed between family physician and patient has diminished, and the specialist often enters the picture as a complete stranger. The medical assistant is the professional who can bridge this gap. Familiarity with the training and scope of practice of other allied health occupations can help the medical assistant in this role.

For more than 50 years, the AMA has been involved in the setting of standards and the accreditation of allied health education programs. In 1935, the training of the occupational therapist was the first in allied health education to be accredited by the AMA. By 1997, the AMA Council on Medical Education was accrediting the training of nearly 30 health care professions (Table 4–1). The medical assisting program was accredited in 1969. Table 4–2 defines various members of the health care team and their functions. Table 4–3 lists health care occupations accredited by agencies other than the Commission on Accreditation of Allied Health Education Programs.

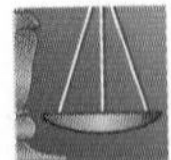

LEGAL AND ETHICAL ISSUES

During the era when sole proprietorship dominated medical care, practices were smaller and patients enjoyed an intimate climate of health care. Managed care has "depersonalized" the patient's care. The medical assistant has the unique opportunity to ensure that the patient feels comfortable and appropriately cared for.

CRITICAL THINKING

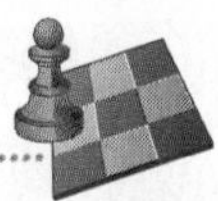

1 Briefly explain the two principal methods of paying for medical care and how it is changing.

HOW DID I DO? Answers to Memory Joggers

1. Sole proprietorship is declining because of the changes in the economic structure of medical practice.
2. *Sole proprietorship:* one individual holds exclusive ownership.
   Partnership: two or more owners, with a legal agreement outlining their rights and responsibilities.
   Corporation: the corporation is the legal owner, regulated by the state. The physician is an employee of the corporation.
3. A system by which patients receive appropriate care in an appropriate setting at the least possible cost.
4. A DO places more emphasis on the relationship between the musculoskeletal structure and organ function.

Medical Ethics

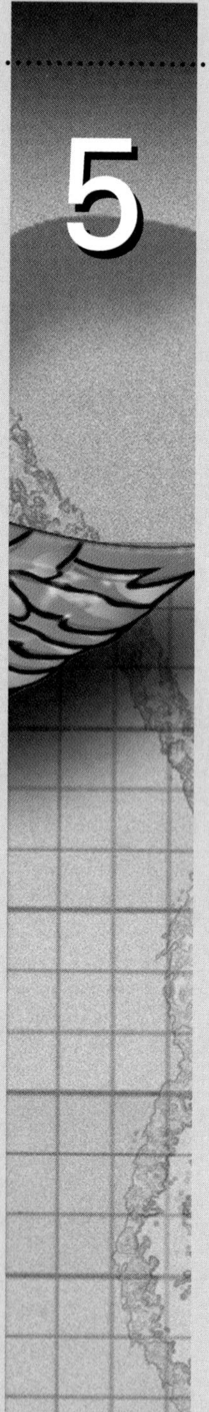

OUTLINE

LEARNING OBJECTIVES

Cognitive: On successful completion of this chapter you should be able to:

1. Define and spell the terms listed in the Vocabulary.
2. Differentiate between the terms *ethics* and *etiquette*.
3. Identify the earliest written code of ethical conduct for medical practice.
4. Name the ancient Greek oath that remains an inspiration to physicians today.
5. Identify a code that was an example for the AMA Principles of Medical Ethics.
6. State a significant reason for the 1980 revision of the AMA Principles.
7. State the maximum penalty that a medical society can impose on a member for unethical conduct.
8. Discuss what and to whom information about a patient may be released.
9. Discuss the application of ethics in dealing with fees and charges.
10. Discuss the medical assistant's ethical obligations and restrictions.

VOCABULARY

abetting Encouraging or supporting

access Freedom to obtain or make use of

allocation Apportioned for a specific purpose or person

artificial insemination The introduction of semen into the vagina or cervix by artificial means

censure The act of blaming or condemning sternly

compulsory Obligatory; enforced

contingent Dependent on or conditioned by something else

culminate To reach a high or decisive point

deceptive Misleading; having the power to deceive

ethics A set of moral principles or values

expulsion Act of expelling or forcing out

fee splitting Sharing a fee with another physician, laboratory, or drug company not based on services performed

genetic Pertaining to the branch of biology dealing with heredity and variation among related organisms

ghost surgery A situation in which a patient has consented to have surgery done by one surgeon but, without the patient's knowledge or consent, the surgery is actually performed by another surgeon

preamble An introductory portion; a preface

precepts Practical rules guiding behavior or technique

public domain The realm embracing property rights that belong to the community at large and that are subject to appropriation by anyone

resident A graduate and licensed physician receiving training in a specialty in a hospital

suspension The act of interrupting or discontinuing temporarily, but with an expectation or purpose of resumption

Ethics concerns the thoughts, judgments, and actions on issues that have the greater implications of moral right and wrong. A morally right attitude is usually understood to be directed toward an ideal form of human character or action, which should **culminate** in the highest good for humanity. From the desire to achieve this good comes the sense of moral duty and a system of interpersonal moral obligations.

Medical ethics should not be confused with medical etiquette. *Etiquette* deals with courtesy, customs, and manners; *ethics* concerns itself with the underlying philosophies in the ideal relationships of humans. These relationships are often formally set forth in social contracts and codes.

Historical Codes

Ethics—judgments of right and wrong—have always been a concern of humans. It is not surprising that for centuries the medical profession has set for itself a rigid standard of ethical conduct toward patients and colleagues. The earliest written code of ethical conduct for medical practice was conceived around 2250 BC by the Babylonians and was called the Code of Hammurabi. It went into much detail regarding the conduct expected of a physician, even prescribing the fees that could be charged. Probably because of its length and detail, it did not survive the ages. See Evolution of Modern Code of Ethics.

About 400 BC, Hippocrates, the Greek physician known as the Father of Medicine, developed a brief statement of principles that has come down through history and remains an inspiration to the physician of today. The Oath of Hippocrates has been administered to medical graduates in many European universities for centuries (Fig. 5–1).

The most significant contribution to ethical history subsequent to Hippocrates was made by Thomas Percival, a physician, philosopher, and writer from Manchester, England. In 1803, he published his Code of Medical Ethics. Percival's personality, his interest in sociologic matters, and his close association with the Manchester Infirmary led to the preparation of a "scheme of professional conduct relative to hospitals and other charities," from which he drafted the code that bears his name.

In 1846, as the American Medical Association (AMA) was being organized in New York City, medical education and medical ethics were being

THE OATH OF HIPPOCRATES

I swear by Apollo, the physician, and Aesculapius, and Health, and Allheal, and all the gods and goddesses, that, according to my ability and judgment, I will keep this oath and stipulation, to reckon him who taught me this art equally dear to me as my parents, to share my substance with him and relieve his necessities if required; to regard his offspring as on the same footing with my own brothers, and to teach them this art if they should wish to learn it, without fee or stipulation, and that by precept, lecture, and every other mode of instruction, I will impart a knowledge of the art to my own sons and to those of my teachers, and to disciples bound by a stipulation and oath, according to the law of medicine, but to none other.

I will follow that method of treatment which, according to my ability and judgment, I consider for the benefit of my patients, and abstain from whatever is deleterious and mischievous. I will give no deadly medicine to anyone if asked, nor suggest any such counsel; furthermore, I will not give to a woman an instrument to produce abortion.

With purity and holiness, I will pass my life and practice my art. I will not cut a person who is suffering with a stone, but will leave this to be done by practitioners of this work. Into whatever houses I enter I will go into them for the benefit of the sick and will abstain from every voluntary act of mischief and corruption; and further from the seduction of females or males, bond or free.

Whatever, in connection with my professional practice, or not in connection with it, I may see or hear in the lives of men which ought not to be spoken abroad, I will not divulge, as reckoning that all such should be kept secret.

While I continue to keep this oath unviolated, may it be granted to me to enjoy life and the practice of the art, respected by all men at all times, but should I trespass and violate this oath, may the reverse be my lot.

FIGURE 5–1 The Oath of Hippocrates.

considered from a national point of view. At the first AMA annual meeting in Philadelphia in 1847, a Code of Ethics was formulated and adopted. It specifically acknowledged Percival's Code as its basic example and became a part of the fundamental standards of the AMA and of its component parts.

Memory Jogger

 *How does ethics differ from etiquette?*

EVOLUTION OF MODERN CODE OF MEDICAL ETHICS

2250 BC	Code of Hammurabi
400 BC	Oath of Hippocrates
1803	Percival's Code of Medical Ethics
1847	First AMA Principles of Medical Ethics
1980	AMA Principles of Medical Ethics (latest revision)

AMA Code of Ethics

The AMA's Code of Ethics has four components:

- Principles of Medical Ethics
- Fundamental Elements of the Patient–Physician Relationship
- Current Opinions with Annotations
- Reports of the Council on Ethical and Judicial Affairs

The publication *Code of Medical Ethics, Current Opinions with Annotations,* contains the first three components, with discussion of more than 135 ethical issues encountered in medicine. A separate publication, the *Reports of the Council on Ethical and Judicial Affairs,* discusses the rationale of the Council's opinions.

Principles of Medical Ethics

The AMA Principles of Medical Ethics has been revised on several occasions to keep it consistent with the times, but there has never been change in the moral intent or overall idealism. Major revisions were made in 1903, 1912, and 1947. In 1957, the AMA Principles of Medical Ethics was condensed to a **preamble** and 10 sections, a major change in format from the 1847 code. The 1980 revision of the code, which contains a preamble and seven sections, was done to clarify and update the language, to eliminate reference to gender, and to seek a proper and reasonable balance between professional standards and contemporary legal standards in our changing society (Fig. 5–2).

AMA Council on Ethical and Judicial Affairs

The Council on Ethical and Judicial Affairs of the AMA consists of nine active members of the AMA, including one resident physician member and one medical student member, and is charged with interpreting the Principles as adopted by the House of Delegates of the AMA. Although the code and the interpretations are directed specifically toward physicians, the medical assistant, as a member of the medical team, must be familiar with these principles and cooperate with the physician in practicing within their concepts.

Current Opinions with Annotations

The opinions of the Council elaborate and expand the **precepts** in the Principles of Medical Ethics. These opinions are continually updated to encompass developing situations, and they reflect the changing challenges and responsibilities of medicine.

Current Opinions with Annotations, 1996–1997, is presented in nine parts; selected portions are briefly summarized in the following pages. For a more detailed coverage, a copy of the publication may be ordered from the American Medical Association, 515 North State Street, Chicago, IL 60610.

INTRODUCTION

As stated in the Preamble, the AMA Principles are not laws but standards. Laws vary from state to state and from community to community. Ethical standards are universal and are never less than the standards required by law; frequently they are greater. Violation of the ethical standards of an association or society may result in **censure, expulsion,** or **suspension** of membership.

If a physician violates ethical standards involving a breach of moral duty or principle, the maximum penalty that the medical society can impose is expulsion. If there is alleged criminal conduct relating to the practice of medicine, the medical society is obligated to report it to the appropriate governmental body or state board. Violation of a law followed by conviction may result in punishment by fine, imprisonment, or revocation of license.

OPINIONS ON SOCIAL POLICY ISSUES

Abortion

The physician is not prohibited by ethical considerations from performing a lawful abortion in accordance with good medical practice and under circumstances that do not violate the law.

Abuse

Discovery that a patient is abusing a child, spouse, or parent creates a difficult situation for the physician. The patient may be the object of abuse but deny its existence in fear of further attacks. The law requires that such abuse be reported. If the physician does not report such suspected or discovered abuse, as required by the law, an added ethical violation is created that may result in continued abuse to the victim. The medical assistant is frequently the

AMA PRINCIPLES OF MEDICAL ETHICS

PREAMBLE

The medical profession has long subscribed to a body of ethical statements developed primarily for the benefit of the patient. As a member of this profession, a physician must recognize responsibility not only to patients, but also to society, to other health professionals, and to self. The following Principles adopted by the American Medical Association are not laws, but standards of conduct which define the essentials of honorable behavior for the physician.

I. A physician shall be dedicated to providing competent medical service with compassion and respect for human dignity.

II. A physician shall deal honestly with patients and colleagues, and strive to expose those physicians deficient in character or competence, or who engage in fraud or deception.

III. A physician shall respect the law and also recognize a responsibility to seek changes in those requirements which are contrary to the best interests of the patient.

IV. A physician shall respect the rights of patients, of colleagues, and of other health professionals, and shall safeguard patient confidences within the constraints of the law.

V. A physician shall continue to study, apply and advance scientific knowledge, make relevant information available to patients, colleagues and the public, obtain consultation, and use the talents of other health professionals when indicated.

VI. A physician shall, in the provision of appropriate patient care except in emergencies, be free to choose whom to serve, with whom to associate, and the environment in which to provide medical services.

VII. A physician shall recognize a responsibility to participate in activities contributing to an improved community.

FIGURE 5–2 AMA Principles of Medical Ethics. (From Code of Medical Ethics. Current Opinions with Annotations of the Council on Ethical and Judicial Affairs of the American Medical Association. Copyright 1997, American Medical Association.)

first to notice symptoms of abuse and should report this to the physician or act as required by law.

Memory Jogger

Why should the medical assistant report any symptoms of patient abuse to the physician?

Allocation of Health Resources

Society must sometimes decide who will receive care, when serving all who need it is not possible. In organ transplantation, for example, several need the transplant and only one donor is available. Who shall be the recipient? Kidney dialysis is another situation in which the demand is greater than the supply. This creates a conflict for the physician, who has the duty to do all that can be done to benefit the patient. The attending physician must remain a patient advocate and therefore should not make **allocation** decisions. Procedures for such allocations are determined in an objective manner by the institutions involved.

Artificial Insemination

Informed consent for **artificial insemination** should include disclosure of risks, benefits, likely success rate of the method proposed, and potential alternative methods.

If the donor is married to the recipient, the resultant child will have all the rights of a child naturally conceived. Artificial insemination by an anonymous donor requires the informed consent of the recipient and consent of the husband if he is to become the legal father of the resultant child. Anonymous donors do not have the rights or responsibilities of parenthood.

If the donor and recipient are not married, the recipient would be considered the sole parent, unless both parties agree to recognize a paternity right.

Clinical Investigation

Without clinical investigation, no new drugs or procedures would be developed. However, all such investigation must follow a competently designed systematic program with due concern for the welfare, safety, and comfort of patients. The physician–patient relationship does exist in clinical investigation; and when treatment of the patient is involved, voluntary written consent must be obtained from the patient or the patient's legally authorized representative. Additional restrictions apply when the subject is a minor or a mentally incompetent adult. When participating in the clinical investigation of new drugs and procedures, physicians should show the same concern for the welfare and safety of the person involved as they would have if the person were a private patient.

Cost

Concern for the quality of patient care should be the physician's first consideration. However, the physician should be conscious of costs and not provide or prescribe unnecessary services.

Provision of Adequate Health Care

Access to an adequate level of health care for all members of our society is now a moral expectation. The following ethical principles should be considered in determining whether particular procedures or treatments should be included in an adequate level of health care:

- Degree of benefit
- Likelihood of benefit
- Duration of benefit
- Cost
- Number of people who will benefit

Genetic Counseling

Genetic counseling and organ transplantation may require personal and ethical decisions concerning the quality of the life that is to be saved.

Organ Donation

The physician should encourage the donation of organs when it is appropriate. However, it is considered unethical to participate in proceedings in which the donor receives payment, except reimbursement of expenses directly incurred in the removal of the donated organ.

The rights of both the donor and the recipient must be equally protected. In a case involving the transplantation of a vital, single organ, the death of the donor must be determined by a physician other than the recipient's physician.

Quality of Life

Physicians must sometimes participate or advise on decisions affecting the fate of a person whose future is dim, such as a deformed newborn or a person of advanced age with many physical problems. The first thought may be the burden to be borne by the family or by society in caring for this person. Ethically, the physician's primary consideration must be what is best for the patient.

Withholding or Withdrawing Life-Prolonging Medical Treatment

A physician is committed to *saving life* and *relieving suffering*. Sometimes these two goals are incompatible, and a choice between them must be made. If possible, the patient may decide. Often, the patient makes his or her wishes known to a responsible relative or other representative in the event that he or she becomes incapacitated. Patients who live in a state that has living will statutes may have some choice if a living will has been established. The living will is a document that states the wishes of that person in case of terminal illness. Usually, it is done to prohibit heroic measures being taken in a situation in which the patient would be unable or incompetent to make a decision. Without preplanning, the physician must act in the best interest of the patient. If it has been determined beyond a doubt that the patient is permanently unconscious, cutting off life-prolonging treatment is ethical.

Euthanasia

Euthanasia is the administration of a lethal agent by another person to a patient for the purpose of relieving the patient's intolerable and incurable suffering. Euthanasia is fundamentally incompatible with the physician's role as healer.

Memory Jogger

What is the physician's primary consideration in deciding the fate of a deformed newborn?

Interprofessional Relations

The interprofessional relations of the physician are mostly governed by ethics; however, some legal restrictions do exist. State laws may prohibit a physician from aiding and **abetting** an unlicensed person in the practice of medicine. Such laws also forbid aiding and abetting a person with a limited license in providing services beyond the scope of that license.

If a nurse or medical assistant recognizes or suspects an error in a physician's orders, it is his or her obligation to report this to the physician. Questioning a possible error is necessary even if it means risking the displeasure of the physician. It may possibly save a life or save the physician from a lawsuit if there is an error. For example, the person initiating a drug administration order should always check the dosage in the *Physician's Desk Reference (PDR)*.

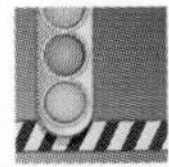

Safety Alert: If the dosage is suspected of being wrong, it should always be questioned.

Physicians often refer a patient to another physician for diagnosis or treatment when it is beneficial to the patient. The physician should make these referrals only when confident that the patient will receive competent treatment.

Lacking legal restrictions, a physician in private practice is free to choose whom to serve. Although private practitioners may refuse certain patients, patients who have already been accepted in the practice cannot be neglected.

The sports physician must keep in mind that the professional responsibility at a sporting event is to protect the health and safety of the participants, with personal judgments being governed only by medical considerations.

Hospital Relations

Most practicing physicians have staff privileges at one or more hospitals. It is considered unethical for a physician to charge a separate fee for the routine, nonmedical services performed in admitting a patient to a hospital. The physician may ethically bill a patient for services rendered the patient by a **resident** under the physician's personal observation, direction, and supervision, if the physician assumes responsibility for the services. The granting of hospital privileges should be based on the training, competence, and experience of the applicant—never on the condition of **compulsory** assessments for any purpose, such as a fee of $1000 for staff membership. Self-imposed assessments by vote of the medical staff are acceptable.

Confidentiality, Advertising, and Communications Media Relations

MINORS

When minors request confidential services, physicians should encourage them to involve their parents. If the minor does not wish to involve the parents, and the law does not require otherwise, physicians should permit a competent minor to consent to medical care and should not notify parents without the patient's consent.

For minors who are mature enough to be unaccompanied by their parents for their examination, confidentiality should be maintained, and information relayed to the parents only with consent of the patient.

ADVERTISING

The only restrictions on advertising by physicians are those that specifically protect the public from

deceptive practices. Standards regarding advertising and publicity have been liberalized over the years, but any advertisement or publicity must be true and not misleading. Testimonials of patients, for instance, should not be used in advertising, because they are difficult to verify or measure by objective standards. The physician can safely include information on educational background, fees, available credit, and any other nondeceptive information, but statements regarding the quality of medical services are highly subjective and difficult to verify.

Health maintenance organizations routinely seek members through advertising. Physicians who practice in such prepaid plans must abide by the same principles of ethics as do other physicians. Any deceptive advertising—for example, any that would be misleading to patients or prospective subscribers—is unethical.

COMMUNICATIONS WITH MEDIA

Although information regarding some patients, such as celebrities and politicians, may be considered news, the physician may not discuss a patient's condition with the press without authorization from the patient or the patient's lawful representative. The physician may release only authorized information or that which is public knowledge. Certain kinds of news are a part of the public record. News in this category is known as news in the **public domain** and includes births, deaths, accidents, and police cases.

Memory Jogger

 What about sharing information about a celebrity with just a few close friends?

The medical assistant must be aware that only the physician is authorized to release information, and under no circumstances should the medical assistant violate the confidential nature of the physician–patient relationship.

An item of specific interest to the medical assistant is *what information may be revealed* by the physician's office to the representatives of insurance companies. The history, diagnosis, prognosis, and other information acquired during the physician–patient relationship may be disclosed to an insurance company representative only if the patient or the patient's lawful representative has consented to the disclosure by signing a release form. It is unethical even to certify that the individual was under the physician's care without the patient's permission. The same restriction applies to discussions with the patient's lawyer. However, a physician may testify in court or before a workers' compensation board in any personal injury or related case.

COMPUTERS

The expanding uses of computer technology permit the accumulation and storage of an unlimited amount of medical information. With the use of computers in the physician's office and the employment of computer service organizations, confidentiality becomes more difficult.

> *All individuals and organizations with some form of access to the computerized databases, and the level of access permitted, should be specifically identified in advance. Full disclosure of this information to the patient is necessary in obtaining informed consent to treatment. Patient data should be assigned a security level appropriate for the data's degree of sensitivity, which should be used to control who has access to the information.*

Detailed guidelines have been developed by the AMA and are included in the *Current Opinions with Annotations.* These guidelines should be followed by physicians and any employed computer service organizations in maintaining the confidentiality of information in medical records when that information is stored in computerized databases.

Fees and Charges

Charging or collecting an illegal or excessive fee is unethical. Illegal charges may occur through ignorance of the law when billing for treatment of Medicaid or Medicare patients. A medical assistant has the responsibility to keep informed on current regulations and to see that they are conscientiously followed.

FEE SPLITTING AND CONTINGENT FEES

If a physician accepts payment from another physician solely for the referral of a patient, both are guilty of an unethical practice called **fee splitting.** Fee splitting, whether with another physician, a clinic or laboratory, or a drug company, is unethical.

Lawyers often accept cases on a contingency basis, that is, the fee is **contingent** on a successful outcome. A physician's fee is always based on the value of the service provided to the patient. Charging a fee based on the successful outcome of the medical care would be considered unethical.

INSURANCE FORMS

An attending physician should expect to complete one simplified insurance claim form for the patient without charge. Multiple or complex forms for the same patient may warrant a charge if this is in conformity with local custom.

INTEREST AND FINANCE CHARGES

Requesting that payment be made at the time of treatment is entirely appropriate, particularly if the patient has a history of making late payments. If the patient is notified in advance, adding interest or other reasonable charges to delinquent accounts is also proper. Advance notice can be accomplished by posting this information in the reception office or by notations on the billing statements. A more effective approach is the use of a Patient Information Folder that includes billing information; such a folder is provided for every new patient on the initial visit. Federal laws and regulations applicable to the imposition of interest charges are addressed in Chapter 16, Professional Fees and Credit Arrangements. Accounting and collection policies should be regularly reviewed with the physician to ensure that no patient's account is sent to collection without the physician's knowledge.

WAIVER OF INSURANCE COPAYMENTS

Physicians frequently write off or waive copayments to facilitate patient access to medical care. If access to care is directly threatened because the patient cannot make the copayment, the physician may forgive the copayment. Routine or consistent forgiveness or waiver of copayments may constitute fraud under state and federal laws. The forgiveness or waiver of copayments may violate the policies of some insurers, both public and private. Physicians should ensure that their policies on copayments are consistent with applicable law and with the requirements of their agreements with insurers.

PROFESSIONAL COURTESY

Professional courtesy (the provision of medical care to physician colleagues or their families free of charge or at a reduced fee) is a long-standing tradition. It is not an ethical requirement, and this decision is made on an individual basis.

Physician's Records

OWNERSHIP AND ACCESS

Notes made by the physician while treating a patient are made for the physician's own use and are considered the physician's personal property. On request of the patient, the physician should provide a summary of the record to the patient, to another physician, or to a person designated by the patient. Original records should not be released except on the physician's retirement or sale of the medical practice.

In some states, a patient is authorized by law to have **access** to his or her medical records. Health care professionals should familiarize themselves with the laws in their own states. Of primary concern regarding all records is the authorization of the patient before releasing any information, unless the release is required by law. A reasonable charge may be made for the cost of duplicating records.

RECORDS OF PHYSICIANS ON LEAVING A GROUP, RETIREMENT, OR DEATH

A patient may, for a variety of reasons, need access to his or her health records after a physician leaves a group, retires, or dies. The records may be necessary for employment, insurance, litigation, or other reasons.

The patients of a physician who leaves a group practice should be notified that the physician is leaving the group. They should also be notified of the physician's new address and offered the opportunity to have their medical records forwarded to the departing physician at his or her new address.

When a physician retires or dies, patients should be notified and encouraged to find another physician. They should be informed that, on their authorization, their records will be forwarded to the new physician. Records that are not forwarded to another physician should be retained by a custodian of the records in compliance with any legal requirements.

Practice Matters

APPOINTMENT CHARGES

May a physician charge for a missed appointment or one that was not canceled within a stated time? Yes, but only if the patient has been fully advised in advance that such charge will be made. Discretion should be used, however, in applying such charges.

CONSULTATION

Physicians should obtain consultation whenever they believe that it would be medically indicated in the care of the patient or when requested by the patient. When a patient is referred to a consultant, the referring physician should provide a history of the case to the consultant. The consultant should communicate the results of the consultant's examination to the referring physician.

DRUGS AND DEVICES: PRESCRIBING

A physician should not be influenced in the prescribing of drugs, devices, or appliances by a direct or indirect financial interest in the supplier. A physician may own or operate a pharmacy but generally may not refer his or her patients to the pharmacy. Patients should enjoy the same freedom of choice in deciding who will fill a prescription as they have in choosing a physician. A prescription is an essential part of a patient's record, and the patient is entitled to a copy.

HEALTH FACILITY OWNERSHIP BY A PHYSICIAN

A physician may ethically own or have a financial interest in a for-profit hospital or other health care facility such as a freestanding clinic. However, before admitting or referring a patient to that facility, the physician has an ethical obligation to reveal such ownership to the patient. In general, physicians should not refer patients to a health facility that is outside their office practice and at which they do not directly provide care or services.

GHOST SURGERY

The substitution of another surgeon without the patient's consent is called **ghost surgery.** The patient has a right to choose his or her own physician or surgeon. To make a substitution without consulting the patient is deceitful and unethical.

Professional Rights and Responsibilities

DISCIPLINE AND MEDICINE

A physician should expose incompetent, corrupt, dishonest, or unethical conduct on the part of members of the profession, without fear of loss of favor.

A physician may be subject to civil or criminal liability for violation of governmental laws. Expulsion from membership is the maximum penalty that may be imposed by a medical society for violation of ethical standards.

FREE CHOICE

The concept of free choice ensures the right of every individual generally to choose or change at will his or her physician. Likewise, a physician in private practice may decline to accept that individual as a patient.

PATENTS

A physician may ethically patent a surgical or diagnostic instrument that he or she has discovered or developed, based on the doctrine that one is entitled to protect one's discovery. The patenting of medical procedures could pose substantial risk to the practice of medicine by limiting the availability of new procedures. It is unethical for a physician to patent medical procedures.

PHYSICIAN–PATIENT RELATIONSHIP

The physician–patient relationship is a form of contract. Both parties are free to enter into or decline the relationship. For example, a physician may decline to accept a patient whose medical condition is not within the physician's line of practice. However, physicians who offer their services to the public may not decline to accept patients because of race, color, religion, national origin, or any other discriminatory basis. The physician–patient relationship does not exist until the physician undertakes care of the patient (Fig. 5–3).

PHYSICIANS AND INFECTIOUS DISEASE

A physician who knows that he or she has an infectious disease, which if contracted by a patient would pose a significant risk to the patient, should not engage in any activity that creates an identified risk of transmission of that disease to the patient.

SUBSTANCE ABUSE

It is unethical for a physician to practice medicine while under the influence of a controlled substance, alcohol, or other chemical agents that would impair the ability to practice medicine.

Ethics for the Medical Assistant

The Code of Ethics of the American Association of Medical Assistants (AAMA) is an honorable standard for all medical assistants to observe. The Code is patterned after the AMA Principles and is adapted to the professional medical assistant who accepts this discipline as a responsibility of trust (Fig. 5–4).

FUNDAMENTAL ELEMENTS OF THE PATIENT-PHYSICIAN RELATIONSHIP

From ancient times, physicians have recognized that the health and well-being of patients depends upon a collaborative effort between physician and patient. Patients share with physicians the responsibility for their own health care. The patient-physician relationship is of greatest benefit to patients when they bring medical problems to the attention of their physicians in a timely fashion, provide information about their medical condition to the best of their ability, and work with their physicians in a mutually respectful alliance. Physicians can best contribute to this alliance by serving as their patients' advocates and by fostering these rights:

1. The patient has the right to receive information from physicians and to discuss the benefits, risks and costs of appropriate treatment alternatives. Patients should receive guidance from their physicians as to the optimal course of action. Patients are also entitled to obtain copies or summaries of their medical records, to have their questions answered, to be advised of potential conflicts of interest that their physicians might have, and to receive independent professional opinions.
2. The patient has the right to make decisions regarding the health care that is recommended by his or her physician. Accordingly, patients may accept or refuse any recommended medical treatment.
3. The patient has the right to courtesy, respect, dignity, responsiveness, and timely attention to his or her needs.
4. The patient has the right to confidentiality. The physician should not reveal confidential communications or information without the consent of the patient, unless provided for by law or by the need to protect the welfare of the individual or the public interest.
5. The patient has the right to continuity of health care. The physician has an obligation to cooperate in the coordination of medically indicated care with other health care providers treating the patient. The physician may not discontinue treatment of a patient as long as further treatment is medically indicated, without giving the patient reasonable assistance and sufficient opportunity to make alternative arrangements for care.
6. The patient has a basic right to have available adequate health care. Physicians, along with the rest of society, should continue to work toward this goal. Fulfillment of this right is dependent on society providing resources so that no patient is deprived of necessary care because of an inability to pay for the care. Physicians should continue their traditional assumption of a part of the responsibility for the medical care of those who cannot afford essential health care. Physicians should advocate for patients in dealing with third parties when appropriate.

FIGURE 5–3 Fundamental Elements of the Patient–Physician Relationship. (From Report of the Council on Ethical and Judicial Affairs of the American Medical Association. Updated June 1994.)

AAMA CODE OF ETHICS

The Code of Ethics of AAMA shall set forth principles of ethical and moral conduct as they relate to the medical profession and the particular practice of medical assisting.

Members of AAMA dedicated to the conscientious pursuit of their profession, and thus desiring to merit the high regard of the entire medical profession and the respect of the general public which they serve, do pledge themselves to strive always to:

A. render service with full respect for the dignity of humanity;
B. respect confidential information obtained through employment unless legally authorized or required by responsible performance of duty to divulge such information;
C. uphold the honor and high principles of the profession and accept its disciplines;
D. seek to continually improve the knowledge and skills of medical assistants for the benefit of patients and professional colleagues;
E. participate in additional service activities aimed toward improving the health and well-being of the community.

AAMA CREED

I believe in the principles and purposes of the profession of medical assisting.
I endeavor to be more effective.
I aspire to render greater service.
I protect the confidence entrusted to me.
I am dedicated to the care and well-being of all people.
I am loyal to my employer.
I am true to the ethics of my profession.
I am strengthened by compassion, courage and faith.

FIGURE 5–4 AAMA Code of Ethics and AAMA Creed. (Courtesy of the American Association of Medical Assistants.)

A PATIENT'S BILL OF RIGHTS

This policy document presents the official position of the American Hospital Association as approved by the Board of Trustees and House of Delegates

The American Hospital Association presents a Patient's Bill of Rights with the expectation that observance of these rights will contribute to more effective patient care and greater satisfaction for the patient, his physician, and the hospital organization. Further, the Association presents these rights in the expectation that they will be supported by the hospital on behalf of its patients, as an integral part of the healing process. It is recognized that a personal relationship between the physician and the patient is essential for the provision of proper medical care. The traditional physician-patient relationship takes on a new dimension when care is rendered within an organizational structure. Legal precedent has established that the institution itself also has a responsibility to the patient. It is in recognition of these factors that these rights are affirmed.

1. The patient has the right to considerate and respectful care.
2. The patient has the right to obtain from his physician complete current information concerning his diagnosis, treatment, and prognosis in terms the patient can be reasonably expected to understand. When it is not medically advisable to give such information to the patient, the information should be made available to an appropriate person in his behalf. He has the right to know, by name, the physician responsible for coordinating his care.
3. The patient has the right to receive from his physician information necessary to give informed consent prior to the start of any procedure and/or treatment. Except in emergencies, such information for informed consent should include but not necessarily be limited to the specific procedure and/or treatment, the medically significant risks involved, and the probable duration of incapacitation. Where medically significant alternatives for care or treatment exist, or when the patient requests information concerning medical alternatives, the patient has the right to such information. The patient also has the right to know the name of the person responsible for the procedures and/or treatment.
4. The patient has the right to refuse treatment to the extent permitted by law and to be informed of the medical consequences of his action.
5. The patient has the right to every consideration of his privacy concerning his own medical care program. Case discussion, consultation, examination, and treatment are confidential and should be conducted discreetly. Those not directly involved in his care must have the permission of the patient to be present.
6. The patient has the right to expect that all communications and records pertaining to his care should be treated as confidential.
7. The patient has the right to expect that within its capacity a hospital must make reasonable response to the request of a patient for services. The hospital must provide evaluation, service, and/or referral as indicated by the urgency of the case. When medically permissible, a patient may be transferred to another facility only after he has received complete information and explanation concerning the needs for and alternatives to such a transfer. The institution to which the patient is to be transferred must first have accepted the patient for transfer.
8. The patient has the right to obtain information as to any relationship of his hospital to other health care and educational institutions insofar as his care is concerned. The patient has the right to obtain information as to the existence of any professional relationships among individuals, by name, who are treating him.
9. The patient has the right to be advised if the hospital proposes to engage in or perform human experimentation affecting his care or treatment. The patient has the right to refuse to participate in such research projects.
10. The patient has the right to expect reasonable continuity of care. He has the right to know in advance what appointment times and physicians are available and where. The patient has the right to expect that the hospital will provide a mechanism whereby he is informed by his physician or a delegate of the physician of the patient's continuing health care requirements following discharge.
11. The patient has the right to examine and receive an explanation of his bill regardless of source of payment.
12. The patient has the right to know what hospital rules and regulations apply to his conduct as a patient.

No catalog of rights can guarantee for the patient the kind of treatment he has a right to expect. A hospital has many functions to perform, including the prevention and treatment of disease, the education of both health professionals and patients, and the conduct of clinical research. All these activities must be conducted with an overriding concern for the patient, and, above all, the recognition of his dignity as a human being. Success in achieving this recognition assures success in the defense of the rights of the patient.

FIGURE 5–5 A Patient's Bill of Rights. (Courtesy of the American Hospital Association.)

Patient's Bill of Rights

The Patient's Bill of Rights developed and approved by the American Hospital Association in 1973 should also be the credo of the practicing medical assistant (Fig. 5–5).

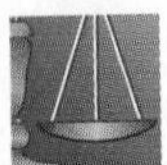

LEGAL AND ETHICAL ISSUES

The prime objective of the medical profession is to render service to humanity, and this must be the medical assistant's first concern as well. The importance of respecting the confidentiality of information learned from or about patients in the course of employment cannot be overemphasized. It is unethical to reveal patient confidences to *anyone*—this includes family, spouse, best friends, and other medical assistants. Do not even mention the names of patients outside the place of employment, because sometimes the doctor's specialty reveals the patient's reason for consultation.

Never discuss one patient's case with another patient; if curious patients ask questions about another, simply change the subject. A patient who asks questions of a medical nature about his or her own case should be referred to the physician for information. The medical assistant must avoid giving advice of a personal nature to any patient, because patients tend to identify remarks from any of the personnel as reflecting the advice of the physician. By remaining silent in these situations, the physician, the medical assistant, and the patient are protected. Confidential papers, case histories, and even the appointment book should be kept out of sight of curious eyes to protect the patient as well as the physician and office staff.

The medical assistant has an obligation to keep abreast of current developments that affect the practice of medicine and care of the patients. Membership in a professional organization provides access to continuing education for maintaining knowledge and skills pertaining to the performance of medical assisting.

In rare instances, a medical assistant is faced with a situation in which the physician-employer's conduct appears to violate established ethical standards. Before making any judgments, the medical assistant must be absolutely sure of all the information and circumstances. If there are, in fact, occurrences of unethical conduct, the medical assistant must then make some decisions.

Is it wise to remain under these circumstances?
Would it be better to seek other employment?
Will a decision to remain adversely affect future opportunities for employment with another physician?

These decisions are difficult to make, especially if the relationship and employment conditions have been satisfactory and congenial. A medical assistant is not legally obliged to report questionable actions of the physician or to attempt to alter the circumstances. However, an ethical medical assistant will not wish to participate in the continuance of known substandard or unlawful practices that may be harmful to patients. The medical assistant is bound to ethical practices as are all health care providers.

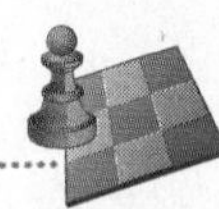

CRITICAL THINKING

1 Give an example showing the difference between ethics and etiquette.

2 What symptoms of patient abuse would a medical assistant be likely to observe?

3 Have you read any articles in the news about "assisted suicide" or other ethical issues?

4 While assisting a patient in interpreting a prescription written by the physician you notice that the instructions specify taking the medication three times a day. Usually the drug is taken only once a day. How would you handle this?

5 A mother accompanies her teenage daughter to the doctor's office but remains in the reception area. While the patient is with the physician the mother engages you, the medical assistant, in discussion of the patient. How would you respond?

HOW DID I DO? Answers to Memory Joggers

1 Ethics concerns the issues of moral right or wrong. Etiquette deals with courtesy, customs, and manners.

2 The law requires that abuse noted must be reported.

3 The physician's primary consideration is what is best for the patient.

4 Only authorized information may be released. It is best to not even mention the case outside the office.

REFERENCE

American Medical Association: Code of Medical Ethics, Current Opinions with Annotations. Chicago, AMA, 1997.

Medicine and the Law

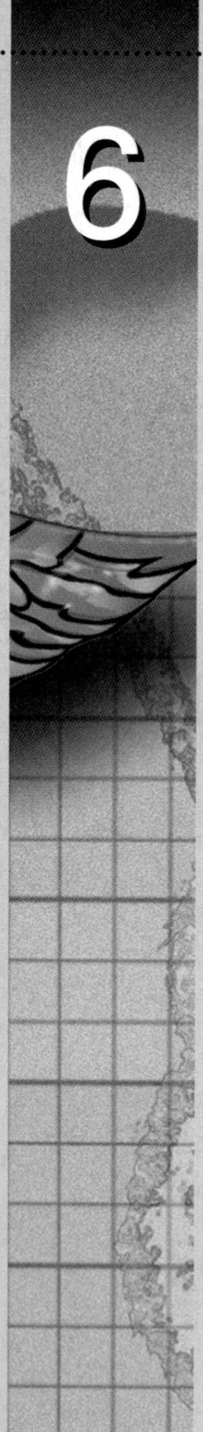

OUTLINE

LEARNING OBJECTIVES

Cognitive: On successful completion of this chapter you should be able to:

1. Define and spell the terms listed in the Vocabulary.
2. State the purpose of medical practice acts and how they are established.
3. List the three methods by which licensure may be granted.
4. List the general categories of cause for revocation or suspension of a license.
5. Explain the difference between *criminal* and *civil* law.
6. Define a contract and explain its importance in a health care facility.
7. Outline the correct way for a physician to terminate the physician–patient relationship.
8. State the four "Ds of Negligence" as published by the American Medical Association.
9. Briefly describe the *arbitration* procedure, and identify three advantages.
10. List the six components of *informed consent.*
11. Explain the purpose of Good Samaritan Acts.
12. State two restrictions imposed on physicians by the Anatomical Gift Act.
13. Explain the medical assistant's role in claims prevention.

14 State the meaning of *administrative law.*
15 Discuss the importance of compliance with OSHA regulations.
16 Explain the essential difference between a living will and a durable power of attorney.

VOCABULARY

administering Instilling a drug into the body of a patient

administrative law Regulations set forth by government agencies

allegation A statement of what a party to a legal action will undertake to prove

arbitration The hearing and determination of a cause in controversy by a person or persons either chosen by the parties involved or appointed under statutory authority

arbitrator A neutral person chosen to settle differences between two parties in a controversy

assault An intentional, unlawful *attempt* of bodily injury to another by force

battery A willful and unlawful use of force or violence upon the person of another

biennially Occurring every 2 years

communicable Capable of being transmitted from one person to another

compensatory damages General or special damages without specific monetary value

concurrently Occurring at the same time

contagious Transmitted readily from one person to another by direct or indirect contact

contract law Enforceable promises

deposition Oral testimony taken from a party or witness to the litigation and is not limited to parties named in the lawsuit.

dispensing Giving drugs, in some type of bottle, box, or other container, to the patient. (Under the Controlled Substances Act of 1970, the definition of "dispense" includes the administering of controlled substances.)

emancipated minor A person under legal age who is self-supporting and living apart from parents or a guardian

endorsement To express approval publicly and definitely

exemplary Serving as a warning

expert witness Professional who belongs to a certifying or qualifying organization and who is called to testify in court

felony A crime of a graver nature than one designated as a misdemeanor; generally, an offense punishable by imprisonment in a penitentiary

infectious Capable of causing infection

informed consent A consent in which there is understanding of what treatment is to be undertaken and of the risks involved, why it should be done, and alternative methods of treatment available (including no treatment) and their attendant risks

infraction Breaking the law; a minor offense of the rules

liability Subject to some adverse action

litigation Contest in a court of justice for the purpose of enforcing a right

living will A document in which an individual expresses wishes regarding medical treatment at or near the end of life

malfeasance The doing of an act that is wholly wrongful and unlawful

malpractice Professional misconduct, improper discharge of professional duties, or failure to meet the standard of care by a professional that results in harm to another

misdemeanor A crime less serious than a felony

misfeasance The improper performance of a lawful act

nominal Existing in name only

nonfeasance The failure to do something that should have been done

perjured testimony Telling what is false when sworn to tell the truth

prescribing Issuing a prescription for the patient; directing, designating, or ordering use of a remedy

prudent Marked by wisdom or circumspection

punitive Inflicting punishment

quackery The pretension of curing disease
reciprocity A mutual exchange of privileges
respondeat superior Let the master answer
revoked Annulled by recalling or taking back
subpoena A writ commanding a person to appear in court
suspended Debarred temporarily from a privilege
tort law Governs acts that bring harm to a person or damage to property, caused negligently or intentionally
treason A crime against the United States
trespass To exceed the bounds of what is lawful, right, or just

A graduate of a medical school must be licensed before beginning the practice of medicine. Licensure is regulated by state statutes by their medical practice acts. It is important for the medical assistant to understand licensing and other laws and regulations that are intended to protect patients, physicians, medical assistants, and other health care workers.

Licensure and Registration

MEDICAL PRACTICE ACTS

Medical practice acts existed as early as colonial days. However, these acts were later repealed, and in the mid-19th century practically none of the states had laws governing the practice of medicine. As one might expect, a rapid decline in professional standards followed. The general welfare of the people was endangered by medical quackery and inadequate care; by the beginning of the 20th century, medical practice acts were established by statute and were again in effect in every state. Their purpose is to

- Define what is included in the practice of medicine within that state
- Govern the methods and requirements of licensure
- Establish the grounds for suspension or revocation of license

LICENSURE

A doctor of medicine (MD) degree or a doctor of osteopathy (DO) degree is conferred on graduation from medical school. The license to practice medicine is granted by a state board, frequently known as the Board of Medical Examiners or Board of Registration. Licensure may be accomplished by any of the following procedures:

- Examination
- Reciprocity
- Endorsement

EXAMINATION Every state requires medical doctors to pass a written examination. The Federation of State Medical Boards and the National Board of Medical Examiners agreed in 1990 to establish a single licensing examination—the Federation Licensing Examination (FLEX)—for graduates of accredited medical schools.

RECIPROCITY Some states grant the license to practice medicine by **reciprocity;** that is, they automatically recognize that the requirements of the state in which the license was granted meet the standards required by the second state.

ENDORSEMENT Most graduates of medical schools in the United States have been licensed by **endorsement** of the National Board certificate. Licensure by endorsement is granted on a case-by-case basis. Those graduates who have not been licensed by endorsement are required to pass a state board examination.

In all states, graduates of foreign medical schools who are seeking licensure by endorsement must meet the same requirements as graduates of medical schools in the United States, in addition to various other qualifying factors.

EXEMPTIONS Some graduates may not wish to engage in the practice of medicine. Their interests may lie in research or administration, or even in the practice of law with a special interest in medical liability. In such instances licensure is not required. Licensed physicians in the Armed Forces, Public Health Service, or Veterans Administration facilities need not be licensed in the state where they are employed.

Memory Jogger

 *What are the three ways by which a physician might seek licensure?*

REGISTRATION AND RE-REGISTRATION

After a license is granted, periodic re-registration is necessary annually or **biennially.** A physician can be **concurrently** registered in more than one state.

The issuing body notifies the physician when reregistration is due.

The medical assistant can aid the physician by being aware of when the registration fees are due, thus preventing a possible lapsing of the registration. Many states require proof of continuing education besides payment of a registration fee.

Continuing education units (CEUs) are granted to physicians for attending approved seminars, lectures, scientific meetings, and formal courses in accredited colleges and universities. A total of 50 hours a year is the average requirement for license renewal. The medical assistant may be expected to help the physician arrange for completing the required units for license renewal.

REVOCATION OR SUSPENSION

Under certain conditions, the license to practice medicine may be **revoked** or **suspended.** Grounds for revocation or suspension of the license to practice medicine generally fall within one of three categories:

1. Conviction of a crime. This may include felonies such as murder, rape, larceny, and narcotic violations.
2. Unprofessional conduct. Failure to uphold the ethical standards of the medical profession is indicated, for example, by betrayal of patient confidence, giving or receiving rebates, and excessive use of narcotics or alcohol.
3. Personal or professional incapacity. This is difficult to label or prove. For example, advanced age or an injury may reduce the apparent capacity of some physicians. Certain illnesses can affect the memory or judgment necessary to practice medicine.

Categories of Legal Environment

When the physician enters the practice of medicine certain medicolegal principles must be considered in the daily operation of the health care facility. Law is the system by which society gives order to our lives. For our purposes, the law may be divided into two general categories: criminal law and civil law.

CRIMINAL LAW

Criminal law governs violations of the law that are punishable as offenses against the state or government. Such offenses involve the welfare and safety of the public as a whole rather than of one individual. Criminal offenses are classified as

- **Treason**—A crime against the United States
- **Felony**—A major crime, such as robbery, arson, issuing bad checks, forgery, and using the mail to defraud. Conviction may result in imprisonment for 1 year or more.
- **Misdemeanor**—A lesser offense that might result in imprisonment for 6 months to 1 year. An example of a misdemeanor is possession of a hypodermic syringe or needle by an unauthorized person.
- **Infraction**—A minor offense, such as traffic or drug violations, that usually result in a fine only.

CIVIL LAW

This chapter is mainly concerned with civil law affecting the practice of medicine, which is explained in the following pages. Civil law is concerned with the relations of individuals with other individuals, with corporations or other organizations, or with government agencies. Classifications of civil law that might affect the practice of medicine are

- **Contract law,** which governs enforceable promises.
- **Tort law,** which governs acts, intentional or unintentional, that bring harm to a person or damage to property
- **Administrative law,** which involves regulations set forth by government agencies, for example, the Internal Revenue Service

Contract Law

The law of contracts touches our lives in many ways practically every day, but usually we do not give it much thought. The patient–physician relationship is governed by the law of contracts, and the medical assistant must be aware of what constitutes a contract.

A *contract* is an agreement creating an obligation. An *express contract* is a verbalized agreement between two or more parties, containing explicit terms of the agreement, either orally or in writing. An *implied contract* is a conclusion drawn from actions of the two parties, for example, when a patient seeks care by a physician and the physician undertakes care of the patient. To be valid or enforceable, a contract must have the following four basic elements:

1. Manifestation of assent (an offer and an acceptance). The parties to the contract must understand and agree on the intent of the contract. The party making the offer is known as the *offeror,* and the party to whom the offer is made is the *offeree.*
2. Legal subject matter. An obligation that requires an illegal action is not an enforceable contract.
3. Legal capacity to contract. Both parties to the

contract must be adults of sound mind. The emancipated minor may contract for medical care.
4. Consideration. There must be an exchange of something of value.

If any of these four elements is missing, there is no contract.

The physician–patient relationship is generally held by the courts to be a contractual relationship that is the result of three steps:

1. The physician invites an offer by establishing availability.
2. The patient makes an offer by arriving for treatment (offeror).
3. The physician accepts the offer by undertaking treatment of the patient (offeree).

Before accepting the offer, the physician is under no obligation, and no contract exists. However, once the physician has accepted the patient an implied contract does exist that the physician (1) will treat the patient, using reasonable care, and (2) possesses the degree of knowledge, skill, and judgment that might be expected of another physician in the same locality and under similar circumstances. It is extremely important that no express promise of a cure be made, for this then becomes a part of the contract.

The patient's part of the agreement includes the liability for payment for services and a willingness to follow the advice of the physician. Most physician–patient relationships are implied contracts. After the physician–patient relationship has been established, the physician is obligated to attend the patient as long as attention is required, unless a special arrangement is made. The physician–patient relationship may be terminated by the physician or the patient.

Memory Jogger

What are the four basic elements of a binding contract?

Termination by Physician

Before withdrawing from the relationship, the physician may wish to take into consideration the condition of the patient, the size of the community, and the availability of other physicians. When a physician does terminate the relationship, the patient must be given notice of the physician's intention to withdraw so that the patient may secure another physician.

The physician may write a letter of withdrawal from the case to the patient, similar to the one shown in Figure 6–1. The letter should state that

- Professional care is being discontinued
- The physician will turn over the patient's records to another physician
- The patient should seek the attention of another physician as soon as possible

The letter should be delivered by certified mail with a return receipt requested and a copy of the letter placed in the patient's medical record. When the return receipt is received, it should be attached to the copy of the letter and retained permanently.

To protect the physician against a lawsuit for abandonment, the details of the circumstances under which the physician is withdrawing from the case are included in the patient's medical record.

Termination by Patient

In the event that the patient terminates the relationship, the termination of the contract and the circum-

.... Date

Dear (Patient):

I find it necessary to inform you that I am withdrawing from providing you with medical care for the reason that ____________________

____

As your condition requires medical attention, I suggest that you promptly place yourself under the care of another physician. If you do not know of other physicians, you may wish to contact the county medical society for a referral.

If you so desire, I shall be available to attend you for a reasonable time after you have received this letter, but in no event for more than 15 days.

When you have selected a new physician, I would be pleased to make available to him or her a copy of your medical chart or a summary of your treatment.

Very truly yours,

FIGURE 6–1 Letter of withdrawal from a case.

Date

Dear (Patient):

This will confirm our telephone conversation of today in which you discharged me from attending you as your physician in your present illness.

In my opinion, your condition requires continued medical treatment by a physician. If you have not already done so, I suggest that you employ another physician without delay.

At your request, I would be pleased to make available to him or her a summary of the diagnosis and the treatment you have received from me.

Very truly yours,

FIGURE 6–2 Physician confirmation of patient discharge.

stances surrounding it should be carefully documented in the physician's records. This may be accomplished by the physician's confirming the discharge by a certified mail letter similar to the one shown in Figure 6–2.

Statute of Frauds

In 1677, a statute was adopted in England aimed at reducing the evil of **perjured testimony,** by providing that certain contracts could not be enforced if they depended on the testimony of witnesses alone and were not evidenced in writing. The provisions of this English statute have been closely followed by statutes adopted in all the states of this country. Under the Statute of Frauds, some contracts, to be enforceable, must be in writing.

The promise to pay the debts of another is an example of this provision. If a third party who is not otherwise legally responsible for the person's debts agrees to pay a patient's medical bills, the agreement cannot be enforced unless it is in writing.

Another example is a contract that cannot be completed within a year. If the physician entered into an agreement to perform a series of treatments for a given sum, and this series covered a time span of more than 1 year, it would have to be in writing to be enforceable.

Tort Law

Medical professional liability is governed by the law of torts. The term *medical professional liability* encompasses all possible civil liability that can be incurred during the delivery of medical care. Medical professional liability is more easily prevented than defended.

All medical professional liability claims fall into one of three classifications:

- **Malfeasance**—the performance of an act that is wholly wrongful and unlawful
- **Misfeasance**—the improper performance of a lawful act
- **Nonfeasance**—the failure to perform an act that should have been done

Any and all of these situations are considered *professional negligence.*

Negligence Defined

When applied to the medical profession, negligence is called **malpractice.** *Negligence* is generally defined as the doing of some act that a reasonable and **prudent** physician or other health care provider would not do or the failure to do some act that such a person should or would do. The standard of prudent conduct is not defined by law but is left to the determination of a judge or jury.

A physician who performs an operation carelessly or contrary to accepted standards, or performs an unnecessary operation, or fails to render care that should have been given may be found guilty of negligence or malpractice.

A medical assistant whose responsibilities are clearly set forth in a policy and procedure manual may be found guilty of negligence through failure to carry out these responsibilities or to exercise reasonable and ordinary care in so doing. The medical assistant must also avoid rendering any care to a patient that might be construed as the practice of medicine, for example, giving an injection of penicillin without detaining the patient for several minutes in case of an allergic reaction.

Memory Jogger

3 *List the three classifications of professional liability.*

The Four Ds of Negligence

In a report by the Committee on Medicolegal Problems of the American Medical Association (AMA), it was stated that:

To obtain a judgment against a physician for negligence, the patient must present evidence of what has been referred to as the "four Ds." He must show: (1) that the physician owed a duty *to the patient, (2) that the physician was* derelict *and breached that duty by failing to act as the ordinary, competent physician in the same community would have acted under the same or similar circumstances, (3) that such failure or breach was the* direct cause *of the patient's injuries, and (4) that* damages *to the patient resulted therefrom.*

DUTY Duty exists when the physician–patient relationship has been established; that is, the patient has sought the assistance of the physician and the physician has knowingly undertaken to provide the needed medical service.

DERELICT (NEGLECTFUL OF OBLIGATION) Proof of dereliction, or proof of negligence of an obligation, must be shown in obtaining a judgment for malpractice.

DIRECT CAUSE There must be proof that the injury or death was directly caused by the physician's actions or failure to act and that it would not otherwise have occurred.

DAMAGES There are three kinds of damages recognized by the law:

- **Nominal** (existing in name only) damages are a token compensation for the invasion of a legal right in which no actual injury was suffered.
- **Punitive** (inflicting punishment) or **exemplary** (serving as a warning) damages require **allegations** and proof of willful misconduct and are unusual in lawsuits against physicians.
- **Compensatory** or actual **damages** are most frequently involved in professional liability cases and may be general or special. Compensatory or actual damages for injuries or losses that are the natural and necessary consequences of the physician's negligent act or omission are referred to as *general damages.* General damages include compensation for pain and suffering, for loss of a bodily member or faculty, for disfigurement, or for other similar direct losses or injuries. The fact of the losses must be proved—the monetary value need not be proved.

Memory Jogger

4 *What are the 4 Ds of negligence?*

Special damages are those injuries or losses that are not a necessary consequence of the physician's negligent act or omission. These may include the costs of medical and hospital care, loss of earnings, cost of travel, and so forth. Both the fact of these injuries or losses and the monetary value must be proved. Some states limit the award amounts of nominal and punitive damages.

The Committee on Professional Liability of the California Medical Association in 1971 called these same four elements the "ABCDs" of negligence in medical practice.

ABCDs OF NEGLIGENCE IN MEDICAL PRACTICE

Acceptance of a person as a patient
Breach of the physician's duty of skill or care
Causal connection between the breach by the physician and the damage to the patient
Damage of a foreseeable nature—such as injury, pain, or loss of earnings—that could reasonably have been foreseen to result

Standard of Care

If a physician were to be held legally responsible for every unsuccessful result occurring in the treatment of a patient, no person would undertake the responsibility of practicing medicine. The courts hold that a physician must

- Use reasonable care, attention, and diligence in the performance of professional services
- Follow his or her best judgment in treating patients
- Possess and exercise the best skill and care that are commonly possessed and exercised by other reputable physicians in the same type practice in the same or a similar locality

Physicians who represent themselves as specialists must meet the standards of practice of their specialty. Whether or not they have met these requirements in treating a particular patient is generally a matter for the court to decide on the basis of testimony provided by an **expert witness.** Expert witnesses are members of the profession involved—in this case, medicine. To be considered an expert witness, the person must belong to a certifying or qualifying organization against which the qualities of the defendant may be compared. *Negligence is not presumed; it must be proved.*

Physicians are not required to possess extraordinary learning and skill, but they must keep abreast of medical developments and techniques, and they cannot experiment. They are also bound to advise their patients if they discover that the condition to be treated is one beyond their knowledge or technical skill.

Importance of the Physician–Patient Relationship

When injury results to a patient as a result of a physician's negligence, the patient can legally initiate a malpractice suit to recover financial damages. However, experience has shown that the incidence of malpractice claims is directly related to the personal relationship existing between the physician and the patient. Deterioration of the physician–patient relationship is a frequently demonstrated reason for a patient's initiating a malpractice suit, even though there was no real injury to the patient.

Medical Assistant's Role in the Physician–Patient Relationship

The medical assistant acts as the physician's agent and has an important role in forming and maintaining a favorable physician–patient relationship. For example, a patient who is kept waiting for an inexcusably long time without explanation or reassurance has developed some feeling of hostility before ever seeing the physician. A few words from the medical assistant at the appropriate time may forestall hostility and promote understanding.

When reassuring an apprehensive patient, the medical assistant must be very careful in the choice of words. Rather than saying, "I'm sure you will soon be entirely well," a friendly smile will comfort the patient but be noncommittal. Any time a medical assistant has reason to believe that a patient is dissatisfied, it is the medical assistant's duty to pass along such information to the physician.

Administrative Law

Administrative law involves the rights and powers of government agencies. The Workers' Compensation Insurance laws and the Family and Medical Leave Act are examples related to employees.

Workers' Compensation

Workers' compensation insurance is mandated by federal and state law. It becomes effective when a worker is injured on the job or suffers an incapacity as a result of the employment. The purpose of the insurance is to provide medical care and compensation during the period of disablement and to provide rehabilitation if necessary.

Family and Medical Leave Act, 1993

The Family and Medical Leave Act requires employers covered by the act to provide 12 weeks per year of unpaid, job-protected leave to eligible employees for some family and medical reasons. Employees must have worked for the employer at least 1 year and for 1250 hours during the previous 12 months. The reasons for the leave and conditions of employment are clearly outlined in the law. The United States Department of Labor is authorized to settle any violation.

There are many other mandated regulations, for example, the Internal Revenue Service, Social Security Act of 1935, and state medical practice acts. Other more recent federal regulations are discussed more fully later in this chapter.

When the Physician Is Sued

Malpractice suits are far from rare, and every physician faces the probability of being sued at least once during his or her career. When a suit is filed, the medical assistant may become involved in scheduling depositions or court appearances and in preparing materials for court.

INTERROGATORY

Before the trial, the physician may be requested to complete an *interrogatory*, which is a list of general questions from another party to the lawsuit. Answers to the interrogatory must be provided within a specified time and must be answered under oath. Interrogatories are limited to parties named in the lawsuit.

DEPOSITION

There may be a request for a **deposition.** A deposition is oral testimony taken from a party or witness to the litigation and is not limited to parties named in the lawsuit. A witness who is not a party to the lawsuit will be summoned by **subpoena** for the deposition. The deposition is usually taken in an attorney's office in the presence of a court reporter and must be taken under oath to tell the truth, just as in a court of law. The person giving the deposition is called the *deponent*. The transcribed deposition is sent to the deponent for review, and the deponent is at liberty to make any necessary changes or corrections. Only deponents who are not parties to the suit are compensated for their time.

SUBPOENA

A subpoena is a document issued by the court requiring the person to whom it is directed to be in court at a given time and place to testify as a witness in a lawsuit.

SUBPOENA DUCES TECUM

A subpoena duces tecum is an order to provide records or documents of some sort and is usually addressed to the custodian of the records. This may be the medical assistant. The custodian of the records may expect to be compensated for the time spent in compiling the records and for photocopying charges. The fee must be demanded at the time the

Physician's Copy

PATIENT-PHYSICIAN ARBITRATION AGREEMENT

1. It is understood that any dispute as to medical malpractice, that is as to whether any medical services rendered under this contract were unnecessary or unauthorized or were improperly, negligently or incompetently rendered, will be determined by submission to arbitration as provided by California Law and not by a lawsuit or resort to court process except as California Law provides for judicial review of arbitration proceedings. Both parties to this contract, by entering into it, are giving up their constitutional right to have any such dispute decided in a court of law before a jury, and instead are accepting the use of arbitration.

2. I have read and understood Article 1 above and I voluntarily agree, for myself and all persons identified in Article 3 below, to submit to arbitration any and all claims involving persons bound by this Agreement whether those claims are brought in tort, contract or otherwise. This includes, but is not limited to, suits for personal injury, actions to collect debts, or any other kind of civil action.

3. I understand and agree that this Arbitration Agreement binds me and anyone else who may have a right to assert a claim on my behalf. I further understand and agree that if I sign this Agreement on behalf of some other person for whom I have responsibility (including my spouse or children, living or yet unborn) then, in addition to myself, such person(s) will also be bound, along with anyone else who may have a right to assert a claim on their behalf. I also understand and agree that this Agreement relates to claims against the physician and any consenting substitute physician, as well as his/her partnership, professional corporation, employees, partners, heirs, assigns or personal representatives. I also hereby consent to the intervention or joinder in the arbitration proceeding of all parties relevant to a full and complete settlement of any dispute arbitrated under this Agreement, as set forth in the Medical Arbitration Rules and/or CHA-CMA Rules for the Arbitration of Hospital and Medical Fee Disputes.

4. I agree to accept medical services from the undersigned physician and to pay therefor. I UNDERSTAND THAT I DO **NOT** HAVE TO SIGN THIS AGREEMENT TO RECEIVE THE PHYSICIAN'S SERVICES, AND THAT IF I DO SIGN THE AGREEMENT AND CHANGE MY MIND WITHIN 30 DAYS OF TODAY, THEN I MAY REVOKE THIS AGREEMENT BY GIVING WRITTEN NOTICE TO THE UNDERSIGNED PHYSICIAN WITHIN THAT TIME STATING THAT I WANT TO WITHDRAW FROM THIS ARBITRATION AGREEMENT. I further understand that after those 30 days, this Agreement may be changed or revoked only by a written revocation signed by both parties.

5. On behalf of myself and all others bound by this Agreement as set forth in Article 3, agreement is hereby given to be bound by the Medical Arbitration Rules of the California Hospital Association and California Medical Association and the CHA-CMA Rules for the Arbitration of Hospital and Medical Fee Disputes, as they may be amended from time to time, which are hereby incorporated into this Agreement.

6. I have read and understood the attached explanation of the Patient-Physician Arbitration Agreement and I have read and understood this Agreement, including the Rules. I understand and agree that this writing makes up the entire arbitration agreement between me and/or the person(s) on whose behalf I am signing and the undersigned physician and/or consenting substitute physicians.

NOTICE: BY SIGNING THIS CONTRACT YOU ARE AGREEING TO HAVE ANY ISSUE OF MEDICAL MALPRACTICE DECIDED BY NEUTRAL ARBITRATION AND YOU ARE GIVING UP YOUR RIGHT TO A JURY OR COURT TRIAL. SEE ARTICLE 1 OF THIS CONTRACT.

Dated: ______________________, 19 __ ______________________
(Patient)

Physician's Agreement to Arbitrate

In consideration of the foregoing execution of this Patient-Physician Arbitration Agreement, I likewise agree to be bound by the terms set forth in this Agreement and in the Rules specified in Article 5 above.

Dated: ______________________, 19 __ ______________________
(Physician)

______________________ ______________________
(Name of partnership or professional corporation) (Title—e.g., Partner, President, etc.)

© California Medical Association, 1977, 1981

FIGURE 6–3 Arbitration agreement between patient and physician. (Copyright, California Medical Association. Reprinted by permission of the Western Journal of Medicine.)

subpoena is served, or it is considered to be waived. The medical assistant never copies or releases records without physician approval. Often private services bring the subpoena duces tecum and make an appointment to copy the records.

Some states have laws that permit patients to obtain a copy of their records on request, although a photocopying charge may be made. It is never wise to release the original records.

Memory Jogger

How does a subpoena *differ from a* subpoena duces tecum?

Arbitration

Arbitration is the settlement of a dispute by a third party or parties who have been selected because of their familiarity with the practices involved. It is common in modern business life. **Arbitration** is established by statute and is available to the medical profession in many states. It affords an alternative method of resolving legal disputes between doctor and patient. Many physicians and lawyers see it as one way to help solve the malpractice crisis. Instead of taking the disagreement through the long and expensive process of court litigation, which may take as long as 7 or 8 years, the patient and the physician (or hospital) agree in advance to submit the dispute informally to a neutral person or persons. After an informal hearing, a binding decision is rendered by the arbitrator(s) based on very specific rules of arbitration, as to any award. Arbitration applies essentially the same rights and the same measure of damages as a court. Arbitration is fair, less expensive, faster, and more confidential than court litigation.

DEVELOPING AN ARBITRATION AGREEMENT

An arbitration agreement is a contract and is subject to the judgment of the courts only as to the fairness of the agreement. The agreement is precisely worded by an attorney and should not be paraphrased when explaining it to a patient (Fig. 6–3). Signing the agreement is a voluntary act on the part of the patient, who has a period of grace in which to revoke the agreement if he or she later decides against it.

SELECTING AN ARBITRATOR

Both the patient and the physician have the opportunity to agree on who will arbitrate the case, so that it does not favor one side over the other. By prior agreement, the **arbitrator(s)** may be appointed by or from the American Arbitration Association, which is a neutral, private, nonprofit association dedicated solely to the advancement of out-of-court remedies. Its panels of arbitrators are made up of persons from business, the professions, and public interest groups.

THE MEDICAL ASSISTANT'S ROLE IN ARBITRATION

If an arbitration statute exists in your state, you should get details of the procedure from your state or local medical society. If a physician elects to implement the procedure, every member of the physician's staff should know the details of the agreement, how to sign up patients, and how to answer the patient's questions. The fairness with which the physician's personnel present the program to the patient and the willingness with which the personnel answer the patient's questions largely determine whether the court will uphold the arbitration agreement. Furthermore, when the physician's personnel "speak for the physician," any representations made by the personnel could be held against the physician.

Securing a Patient's Informed Consent or Informed Refusal

A physician must have consent to treat a patient even though this consent is usually implied by virtue of the patient's having come to that physician for treatment. This implied consent is sufficient for common or simple procedures that are generally understood to involve little risk. A blood screen, chest radiograph, and electrocardiogram are examples. When more complex procedures are anticipated, the physician must obtain the patient's **informed consent** for each procedure. A physician who fails to secure some formal expression of consent could be charged with **trespass** or with **assault** and **battery.**

A number of states have passed specific laws that require the written informed consent of a patient before a test for the acquired immunodeficiency virus (AIDS) antibody may be performed by a health care facility, physician, or other health care provider.

Even in cases in which the treatment was not negligent, the physician can be sued for failing to obtain an informed consent. Under such circumstances, the physician must be prepared to prove in court that a full explanation was given to the patient before obtaining the patient's consent. Informed consent implies an understanding of

- What is to be done
- Why it should be done
- The risks involved

- Expected benefits of recommended treatment
- Alternative treatments, including the failure to treat
- Attendant risks of alternative treatment

The informed consent is not satisfied merely by having the patient sign the form. A discussion must occur during which the physician provides the patient or the patient's legal representative with enough information to decide whether to undergo the proposed therapy. After such a discussion, the patient either consents or refuses to consent to the proposed therapy and may be required to sign a consent form. If the patient signs with an "X," the medical assistant should write beside the "X" the words "patient's mark" and have a family member witness the signature. In any event, the discussion should be fully documented in the patient's medical record. If a form is used, a copy of the signed form should also be included in the patient's record. Treatment may not exceed the scope of the consent.

Forms on which a patient can grant written consent for operations or other procedures are kept in most physicians' offices. Many procedures are performed in the medical office that may require a consent form.

Who May or May Not Give Consent

MENTALLY COMPETENT ADULTS

If a mentally competent adult expressly indicates assent to a particular form of treatment, then consent has been obtained. If the act consented to is unlawful—for instance, an abortion in states where abortion is prohibited—the consent is invalid. The consent is also invalid if it is given by a person unauthorized to do so or if it is obtained by misrepresentation or fraud.

IN EMERGENCIES

In an emergency, one may render aid or care to prevent loss of life or serious illness or injury. However, implied consent in this circumstance lasts only as long as the emergency, and formal consent must be obtained for follow-up procedures done after the emergency has passed.

Good Samaritan Acts

The purpose of a Good Samaritan Act is to provide immunity from liability to volunteers at the scene of an accident for any civil damages as a result of rendering emergency care. Physicians are sometimes reluctant to fulfill an ethical obligation to render aid in an emergency to someone who is not their patient for fear they may later be charged with negligence or abandonment by a total stranger. In 1959, California passed the first *Good Samaritan Act,* and today all 50 states have Good Samaritan statutes. Although there are minor variations in the state statutes, their purpose is to provide immunity from liability to volunteers at the scene of an accident for any civil damages as a result of rendering emergency care to accident victims, provided that such care is given in good faith and with due care under the circumstances. There is no creation of a contract in giving emergency care (Fig. 6–4).

INCOMPETENT ADULTS

Adults who have been found by a court to be insane or incompetent usually cannot consent to medical treatment. Consent must be obtained from the guardian.

MINORS

Generally, when the patient is a minor, consent for surgery or treatment must be obtained from a parent or guardian except in an emergency requiring immediate treatment. If the parents are legally separated or divorced, consent should be obtained from the parent who has legal custody. There are exceptions to necessary consent.

Consent for treatment is not required when

- Consent may be assumed, such as in a life-threatening emergency
- A certain treatment is required by law, such as vaccination or x-ray for school entry or safety
- A court order has been issued, as in a situation in which parents withhold consent for a necessary treatment because of religious reasons

Treatment of sexually transmitted disease, drug abuse, alcohol dependency, or pregnancy usually does not require parental consent.

Emancipated Minors

Emancipation is defined by statute and varies from state to state. An emancipated minor is a person younger than the age of majority (usually 18 or 21 years) who meets one or more of the following conditions:

- Is married
- Is in the armed forces
- Is living separate and apart from parents or a legal guardian
- Is self-supporting

Some statutes include a minimum age for emancipation.

Unless a statute declares otherwise, a minor who has the right to consent to treatment is entitled to

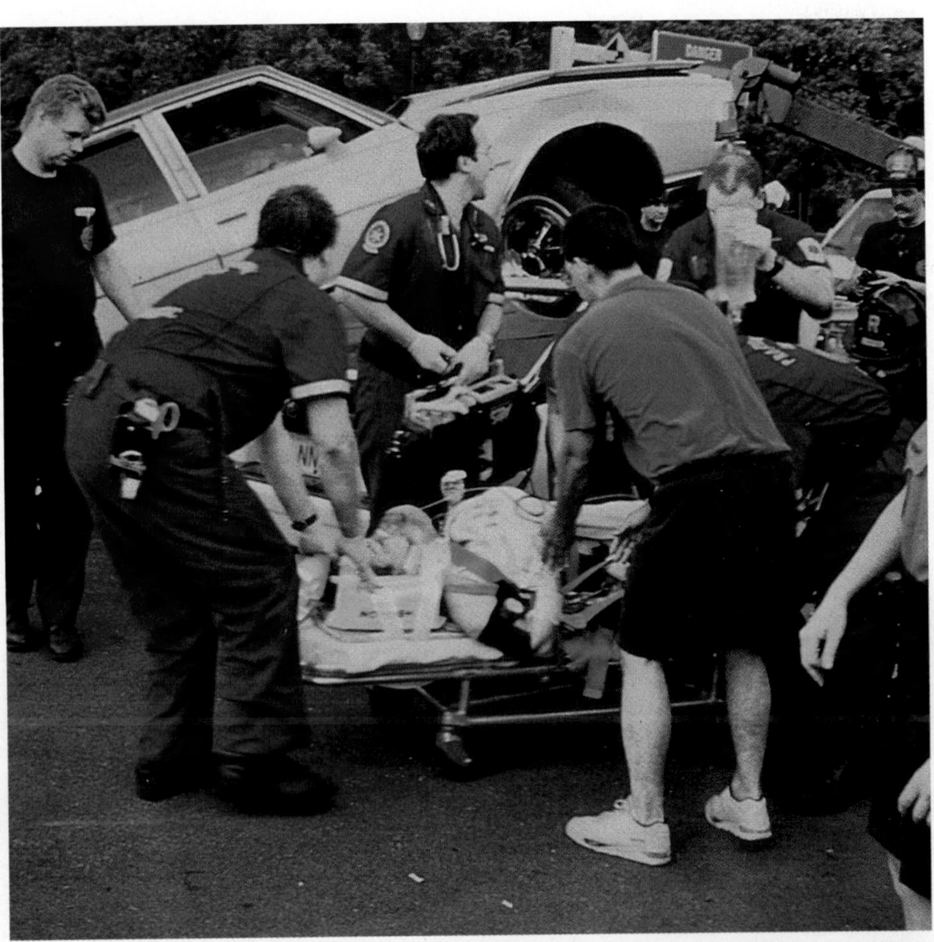

FIGURE 6–4 The Good Samaritan Act protects medical professionals from liability for any civil damages as a result of rendering emergency care. (From Henry M, Stapleton ER: EMT Prehospital Care, 2nd ed. Philadelphia, WB Saunders, 1997.)

the protection of his or her confidences, even from parents.

Memory Jogger

 *What is the purpose of the Good Samaritan Act?*

Federal Regulations

The following is a brief overview of laws and regulations affecting the medical office environment. A fuller discussion will be found in the clinical coverage in Unit 3.

OCCUPATIONAL SAFETY AND HEALTH ACT (OSHA)

The Occupational Safety and Health Act was established by the federal government in 1970 to set standards and protocols for occupational health and safety. OSHA is a part of the Department of Labor. The involvement of OSHA with medical practices accelerated during the 1980s, partly because of the risk of exposure to the hepatitis B virus and later because of the spread of AIDS. As a result of the increasing danger of exposure to the AIDS virus, bloodborne pathogen regulations were introduced in 1991.

OSHA regulations are critically important to all health care facilities. Medical office managers must know the regulations and follow them explicitly. The regulations include

- A hazard communications plan
- An exposure plan
- A medical waste management plan
- Housekeeping facilities
- Personal protective measures
- General safety precautions
- Fire safety plan
- Staff development/in-service training program

Training sessions must be provided to every employee who is at risk of exposure to blood or other infectious materials. The training session must be provided during working hours and before a new employee begins the job.

The health care facility is subject to an OSHA compliance inspection at any time during regular office hours.

CLINICAL LABORATORY IMPROVEMENT AMENDMENTS OF 1988 (CLIA '88)

The Clinical Laboratory Improvement Act was first enacted in 1967, then amended in 1988. Its purpose was to establish performance requirements for all laboratories within the United States and its territories. In-office laboratories are subject to both state and federal regulations. Inspections of the laboratories are conducted by regional surveyors from the Health Care Financing Administration (HCFA) and state agency representatives. Physicians' office laboratories are included under these regulations.

AMERICANS WITH DISABILITIES ACT OF 1990 (ADA)

Employers with 15 or more employees are subject to ADA regulations. The ADA prohibits covered employers from discriminating against a person with a mental or physical disability in any aspect of employment merely because the person has such a disability. This affects the employment process, hiring, job training, promotion or advancement, compensation, termination, and any other aspect of the employment relationship.

The ADA protects all *qualified* individuals with a disability from employment discrimination. A qualified individual is a person (1) who satisfies the prerequisites for the position, such as educational background, employment experience, skills, or licenses and (2) who, *with or without reasonable accommodation*, can perform the essential functions of the job. An example of reasonable accommodation is *making all facilities readily accessible to, and usable by, individuals with disabilities.* The act also includes a *public access* requirement for service establishments, for example, a health care provider, that would focus on making the place physically accessible from public sidewalks, public transportation, or parking areas. Examples of structural and nonstructural alterations might be adding grab bars, lowering telephones, creating a ramp, adding raised letters or braille markings to elevator control buttons, and widening doors.

PATIENT SELF-DETERMINATION ACT, 1991

This law requires that medical care facilities such as hospitals, nursing homes, personal care facilities, hospices, home health care agencies, and health maintenance organizations ask patients whether they have prepared an advance directive for guidance in the event they are terminally ill or in a vegetative state. The directive may be a living will or a durable power of attorney for health care.

The term **living will** generally refers to any document in which an individual expresses his or her wishes regarding medical treatment at or near the end of life. A durable power of attorney for health care (DPAHC) must meet certain statutory requirements. A valid DPAHC document must specifically authorize the agent to make health care decisions for the patient.

Each state has its specific regulations on what is acceptable and the wording that must be used. Some states do not accept the living will. The health care facility performs a service for its patients by having copies of acceptable forms available for patients and being willing and informed enough to explain them.

Controlled Substances Act of 1970

On May 1, 1971, the Controlled Substances Act of 1970 became effective, replacing the former Narcotic Acts and the Drug Abuse Control Amendments. In October 1973, the regulatory agency became known as the Drug Enforcement Administration (DEA) within the U.S. Department of Justice.

REGISTRATION

Before **administering, prescribing,** or **dispensing** any of the scheduled drugs, a physician is required to register with the Registration Branch, Drug Enforcement Administration, PO Box 28083, Central Station, Washington, DC 20038-8033, or with the nearest regional office. The registration is renewable every 3 years. The medical assistant should take note of the renewal date and make certain that the renewal is filed. If a physician administers or dispenses any of the drugs listed in the five schedules at more than one office, he or she must register each office. Regulations regarding the writing, telephoning, and refilling of prescriptions vary according to which schedule is involved.

SCHEDULES

Under the Controlled Substances Act, drugs are categorized into Schedules I, II, III, IV, and V. Drugs in schedule I have the highest potential for abuse and addiction, and those in Schedule V have the least potential.

Schedule I substances are those that have no accepted medical use in the United States and have a high potential for abuse. Examples include heroin and LSD. Only the physician who is involved in conducting research with such drugs is concerned with Schedule I substances.

Schedule II substances have a high abuse potential with severe psychic or physical dependence liability. They include certain narcotic, stimulant, and depressant drugs. Examples are opium, morphine, and codeine. Controlled substances in Schedule II can be obtained only with a Federal Triplicate Order form obtained from the DEA. A special inventory must be maintained on controlled substances and retained for 2 years. Some states require the inventory to be kept 3 years. When a controlled substance is removed from the inventory it must be recorded. The record must show the date, the name of the drug, the dosage, and the names of the patient, the physician, and the employee involved.

Schedule III substances have an abuse potential that is lesser than that of the first two schedules. They include compounds that contain limited quantities of certain narcotic drugs combined with nonnarcotic substances. Paregoric, Empirin Compound with Codeine, and Tylenol with Codeine are examples.

Schedule IV substances have still less potential for abuse. Phenobarbital, diazepam (Valium), and propoxyphene (Darvon) are examples.

Schedule V substances have less abuse potential than those in Schedule IV but still warrant control. They include preparations that contain moderate quantities of certain narcotics such as may be found in cough medicines and antidiarrheal products.

WRITTEN PRESCRIPTIONS

Schedule III, IV, and V substances do not require triplicate forms but are subject to the following prescription requirements.

PRESCRIPTION REQUIREMENTS FOR SCHEDULE III, IV, AND V SUBSTANCES

- The prescription must be signed and dated by the prescriber.
- It must contain the name and address of the person for whom the controlled substance is prescribed, the name and quantity of the substance, and the directions for its proper use.
- For all controlled substances classified in Schedules III and IV, the signature, date, and information described above must be written in ink or indelible pencil in the handwriting of the prescriber.
- These substances may not be refilled in an amount exceeding a 120-day supply unless the prescription is renewed by the prescriber.
- The prescription must contain the name, address, telephone number, category of professional license, and DEA registration number of the prescriber.

Schedule V prescriptions must be signed and dated by the prescriber and must also include the name of the patient, name and quantity of the controlled substance prescribed, and the directions for use.

Memory Jogger

 *Which schedule of controlled substances has the highest potential for abuse?*

ORAL PRESCRIPTIONS

The physician may dispense any Schedule III, IV, or V controlled substance by an oral prescription, but the prescription must be put in writing by the pharmacist who fills it. With permission from the physician, any employee may orally transmit a prescription for controlled substances *only* in Schedules III, IV, or V, again with the prescription being put in writing by the dispensing pharmacist. An employee cannot, under any circumstances, orally transmit a prescription for a controlled substance classified in Schedule II.

NONNARCOTIC DRUGS

A physician who regularly engages in dispensing any of the nonnarcotic drugs listed in the schedules as a regular part of the professional practice and who charges for the drugs either separately or together with other professional services must keep records of all such drugs received and dispensed. The records must be kept for a period of 2 years and are subject to inspection by the DEA. If the physician only occasionally dispenses a nonnarcotic controlled drug to a patient (such as a physician's sample), he or she is not required to maintain a record of such dispensing.

SECURITY

Stored controlled substances must be kept in a locked cabinet or safe. Any loss of controlled drugs by theft must be reported to the regional office of the DEA at the time the theft is discovered. If a physician discovers that his or her DEA number is being used in the unauthorized prescribing of controlled substances, he or she should report the incident to the DEA, the state regulatory agency, and to the local police authorities.

DISCONTINUANCE OF PRACTICE

A physician who discontinues medical practice must return his or her registration certificate and any unused order forms to the nearest office of the DEA. The regional DEA office will advise on the disposition of any controlled drugs still on hand.

Uniform Anatomical Gift Act

The Uniform Anatomical Gift Act was approved by the National Conference of Commissioners on Uniform State Laws in 1968. Although many states had passed laws before this time that permitted living persons to make a gift of their body or portions of it after death, the laws were so different from state to state that arrangements for a donation in one state might not be recognized in another. All states have adopted the Uniform Anatomical Gift Act or similar legislation.

Essentially, the model law for donation states that

- Any person of sound mind and 18 years of age or older may give all or any part of his or her body after death for research, transplantation, or placement in a tissue bank.
- A donor's valid statement of gift is paramount to the rights of others except when a state autopsy law may prevail.
- If a donor has not acted during his or her lifetime, his or her survivors, in a specified order of priority, may do so.
- Physicians who accept organs or tissues, relying in good faith on the documents, are protected from lawsuits. The physician attending at the time of death, if acquainted with the donor's wishes, may dispose of the body under the Uniform Anatomical Gift Act.
- The time of death must be determined by a physician who is not involved in the transplantation, and the attending physician cannot be a member of the transplant team.
- The donor may revoke the gift, or the gift may be rejected.

The most important clause permits the donation to be made by a will (without waiting for probate) or by other written or witnessed documents, such as a card designed to be carried on the person (Fig. 6–5). The Uniform Donor Card is considered a legal document in all 50 states.

The provisions of the Uniform Anatomical Gift Act are so designed that the offer is exercised only after death. Therefore, the donors should reveal their intentions to as many of their relatives and friends as possible and to their physician. Because the human body or its parts are not commodities in commerce, no money can be exchanged in making an anatomic donation.

Legal Disclosures

The physician is charged with safeguarding patient confidences within the constraints of the law, but according to state laws, which vary somewhat throughout the nation, certain disclosures must be made. Frequently it is the medical assistant who has the responsibility of reporting these events.

UNIFORM DONOR CARD

OF____________________

Print or type name of donor

In the hope that I may help others, I hereby make this anatomical gift, if medically acceptable, to take effect upon my death. The words and marks below indicate my desires.

I give: (a)____ any needed organs or parts

(b)____ only the following organs or parts

____

Specify the organ(s) or part(s)

for the purposes of transplantation, therapy, medical research or education;

(c)____ my body for anatomical study if needed.

Limitations or special wishes, if any:____________________

Signed by the donor and the following two witnesses in the presence of each other:

Signature of Donor — Date of Birth of Donor

Date Signed — City and State

Witness — Witness

This is a legal document under the Uniform Anatomical Gift Act or similar laws.

FIGURE 6–5 Uniform Donor Card.

Births and deaths must be reported. Births out of wedlock must be reported on special forms in some states; some states require detailed information about stillbirths.

Physicians are required to report cases that may have been a result of violence, such as gunshot wounds, knife injuries, or poisonings. They must also report deaths from accidental or unexplained causes.

In some states, occupational diseases must be reported within specific time lines.

Sexually transmitted diseases are reportable in every state. All fifty states require that confirmed cases of AIDS be reported to state public health officials. In at least 13 states, a seropositive test result is also a reportable condition. Individuals are reported either by name or by patient identifiers.

Child abuse is a leading cause of death among children younger than 5 years of age, and health care professionals are required by law to report any suspected cases of child abuse. This should be done as soon as evidence is discovered. Suspected elder abuse often creates a dilemma for the physician and other health care personnel. The older adult may deny the abuse in fear of further mistreatment if it is made known. The law requires that suspected cases of physical abuse to children, the elderly, or any others at risk be reported to the authorities.

The physician must report any cases of **contagious, infectious,** or **communicable diseases.** Local health departments publish lists of diseases that are reportable as well as the method of reporting. Often, the report may be made by telephone. When reporting by mail, the appropriate forms, which are supplied by the health department, must be used. In many areas, the county health department issues regular bulletins that are sent to all physicians in the county. Check with the local authorities for specific procedures in your area.

Memory Jogger

8 *How many required legal disclosures of patient information can you list?*

Legal Responsibilities of the Medical Assistant

Generally, the law holds that every person is liable for the consequences of his or her own negligence when another person is injured as a result. In some situations, this liability also extends to the employer. Physicians may be held responsible for the mistakes of those who work in the health care facility, and sometimes they must pay damages for the negligent acts of their employees.

Physicians are legally responsible for the acts of their employees when the employees are acting within the scope of their duties or employment. Physicians are also responsible for the acts of assistants who are not their own employees if they commit acts of negligence in the presence of the physician while under the physician's immediate supervision. For example, a medical assistant who is a clinic employee makes an error in a procedure while acting under a physician's direction. The court may determine that the medical assistant came so completely under the direction and supervision of the physician that the physician is liable for the medical assistant's negligence. This is known as the doctrine of **respondeat superior** (let the master answer). On the other hand, if a registered nurse is employed by the patient, the physician is not usually held liable for negligent acts of the registered nurse. When physicians practice as partners, they are liable not only for their own acts and those of their partner but also for the negligent acts of any agent or employee of the partnership. The medical assistant, while acting within the scope of the employment contract, is considered an agent of the employer.

A physician who properly writes a prescription is not liable for a pharmacist's negligence in compounding it but may be liable in cases in which there is misunderstanding as to the ingredients when the prescription is ordered over the telephone.

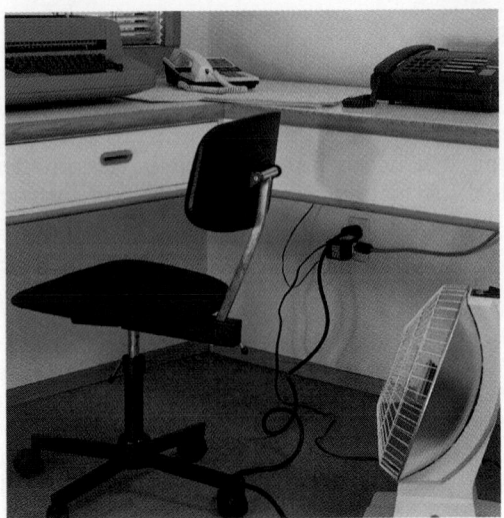

FIGURE 6–6 Example of potential hazard from exposed electrical cord.

NEED FOR EXTREME CARE

Medical assistants who are guilty of negligence are liable for their own actions, but the injured party generally sues the physician because there is a better chance of collecting damages. However, even an assistant who has no money can still be liable for any negligent action. This fact illustrates the continuing importance of exercising extreme care in performing all duties in the professional office.

While working under pressure, there is always the danger of interchanging blood, serum, or medications or of mixing names or improperly preparing labels. Medication and treatment solutions should be labeled clearly and their expiration dates checked. Never proceed with administration of a medication or treatment without checking all details at least three times. It is an accepted rule that the medication label should be read three times: (1) when you remove the container from its storage place; (2) when you are preparing the medication; and (3) when you return the medication to the storage place before patient administration.

RECHECKING EQUIPMENT

One person in the facility should be designated to make periodic safety checks of reception room and treatment room furniture and of the condition of instruments and supplies. Every person on the staff should be alert for potential hazards, such as slipping rugs, exposed telephone and light cords, highly waxed floors, and protruding objects, because patients who are harmed as a result of these conditions can sue for damages (Fig. 6–6).

ILLEGAL PRACTICE OF MEDICINE

A physician studies many years to learn the profession before becoming licensed by the state to practice medicine. The medical assistant is not licensed to practice medicine and must never prescribe or attempt to diagnose a patient's ailment. This is the *illegal practice of medicine.* For this reason, it is not good policy for the medical assistant to discuss patients' complaints with them because patients tend to identify the medical assistant's remarks as being the opinion of the physician.

ASSISTING AT PATIENT EXAMINATIONS

Except in an actual emergency, the male physician should not examine a female patient unless a third person is present. Allegations of sexual misconduct are made against physicians of all specialties. The charge of undue familiarity against a physician is very damaging. For this reason, the assistant generally stands by during examinations.

EMERGENCY AID

The question sometimes arises of whether a medical assistant should give emergency care to a patient brought into the office during the physician's absence. In a medical emergency, the medical assistant, like any other layperson, may do whatever is reasonably necessary, provided the action taken is within that person's skill and competence. The physician should instruct the medical assistant regarding what course of action to take in such instances. The medical assistant must immediately get in touch with a physician to care for the patient once any emergency measures have been performed.

The Medical Assistant's Role in Claims Prevention

The majority of patients never entertain the thought of taking legal action against their physicians, and the medical assistant should not develop an attitude of skepticism. However, the medical assistant can play a role in preventing legal claims.

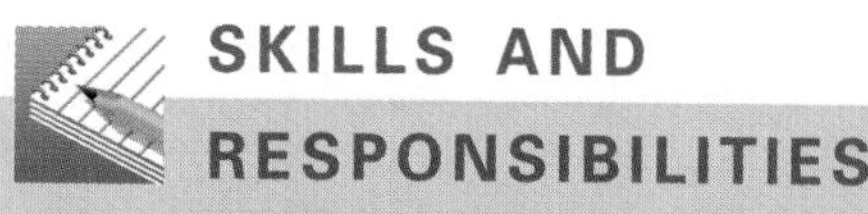

SKILLS AND RESPONSIBILITIES

PREVENTION OF LEGAL CLAIMS AGAINST THE PRACTICE

Give scrupulous attention to the needs of each patient.
Avoid leaving patients alone (especially children and elderly patients).
Avoid destructive and unethical criticism of the work of other physicians.
Do not give out information either orally or in writing without the patient's consent.
Verify the identity of anyone requesting information.
Use discretion in telephone and office conversations.
Be aware of your tone of voice and attitude during spoken communications.
Communicate office policies and procedures to patients in advance of treatment whenever possible.
Keep records that clearly show what was done and when it was done.
Record all patient interactions on the patient's chart.
Make no promises as to outcome of treatment.
Record canceled appointments.
Record the facts if a patient discontinues treatment or fails to follow instructions.
Avoid making any statement that might be construed as an admission of fault.
Check the office equipment regularly to see that it is operating properly and safely.
Make periodic safety inspections of furniture.
Keep toxic substances out of reach of patients and clearly labeled.
Keep drug samples and prescription pads out of sight.
Never diagnose, prescribe, or offer a prognosis.
Perform only those tasks that are within your scope of knowledge and training.
Keep abreast of new procedures and technical advances in health care.
Correctly follow all federal and state recordkeeping and reporting requirements.

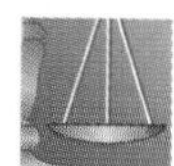

LEGAL AND ETHICAL ISSUES

Both the physician and the medical assistant must be thorough when giving instructions to patients. Written instructions should be provided whenever possible. A patient might forget oral instructions, resulting in drug-related injuries stemming from poor understanding of the proper use of the medications, their limitations, and their contraindications.

An efficiently operated medical practice will have a policy and procedure manual describing the office policies and including a designated procedure section for each personnel position in the practice. A medical assistant who fails to carry out the written instructions or who failed to exercise reasonable and ordinary care in doing so may be found guilty of negligence. The medical assistant who renders any care to a patient that might be deemed the practice of medicine is also subject to malpractice liability.

A physician must have consent to treat a patient. When complex procedures are planned, a discussion must occur between the patient and the physician whereby the physician provides enough information for the patient to decide whether or not to go ahead with the proposed therapy. Discussion between the patient and the medical assistant is not sufficient to satisfy this requirement.

Regulations of the Drug Enforcement Administration require a federal triplicate order and prohibit the oral transmittal of prescriptions for Schedule II substances, which have a high abuse potential.

If you will be at risk of exposure to blood or other infectious materials, make certain that you go through a training session in OSHA regulations before you begin the job.

A "medical assistant" is an unlicensed health professional who performs noninvasive routine technical support services under the supervision of a licensed physician and surgeon or a licensed podiatrist in a medical office or clinic setting.

"Technical supportive services" means simple routine medical tasks and procedures which may be performed by a medical assistant with limited training who functions under the supervision of a physician or podiatrist. For example, a medical assistant may administer certain medications; perform electrocardiograms or electroencephalograms; apply and remove bandages and dressings; apply orthopedic appliances; select crutches; perform automated visual field testing; remove sutures, and so forth.

CRITICAL THINKING

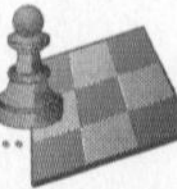

1 For what reasons might a medical assistant be accused of negligence?

2 What is the meaning of *prudent* conduct? How is it determined?

3 Why would the attending physician of a deceased patient whose organs are being donated be prohibited from being a member of the transplantation team?

4 Who is responsible for a mistake made by a medical assistant during the course of his or her employment? Give examples.

5 Why is it dangerous for a medical assistant to discuss a patient's complaint with the patient?

HOW DID I DO? Answers to Memory Joggers

1 A physician may be licensed by
a. Examination
b. Endorsement
c. Reciprocity

2 The basic elements of a binding contract are
a. Offer and acceptance
b. Legal subject matter
c. Legal capacity to contract
d. Consideration

3 The three classifications of professional liability are
a. Malfeasance
b. Misfeasance
c. Nonfeasance

4 The four Ds of negligence are
a. Duty
b. Derelict
c. Direct cause
d. Damages

5 A *subpoena* requires a person to appear in court. *Subpoena duces tecum* is an order to provide records or documents.

6 The Good Samaritan Acts are designed to provide immunity from liability to volunteers at the scene of an accident for any civil damages as a result of rendering emergency care.

7 Schedule I drugs have the highest potential for abuse.

8 State laws vary, but many are common to all states (e.g., births, deaths, out of wedlock births, injuries resulting from violence, gunshot, knifings, poisonings, venereal diseases).

REFERENCES

Andress A: Saunders Manual of Medical Office Management. Philadelphia, WB Saunders, 1996.

Flight MR: Law, Liability, and Ethics. Albany, NY, Delmar Publishers, 1988.

SECTION 3

Communicating with Patients and Colleagues

CURRICULUM CONTENT/COMPETENCIES

Chapter 7 Interpersonal Skills and Human Relations
- *Treat all patients with compassion and empathy*
- *Recognize and respect cultural diversities*
- *Recognize and respond to verbal and nonverbal messages*
- *Serve as liaison*

Chapter 8 Patient Reception
- *Adapt communications to individual's ability to understand*
- *Promote the practice through positive public relations*
- *Instruct patients according to their needs*

Chapter 9 Telephone Techniques
- *Use professional telephone techniques*
- *Project a professional manner and image*
- *Use medical terminology appropriately*
- *Receive, organize, prioritize, and transmit information*

Chapter 10 Appointment Scheduling and Time Management
- *Schedule, coordinate, and monitor appointments*
- *Schedule inpatient/outpatient admissions and procedures*
- *Use professional telephone techniques*
- *Prioritize and perform multiple tasks*
- *Explain office policies and procedures*

Interpersonal Skills and Human Relations

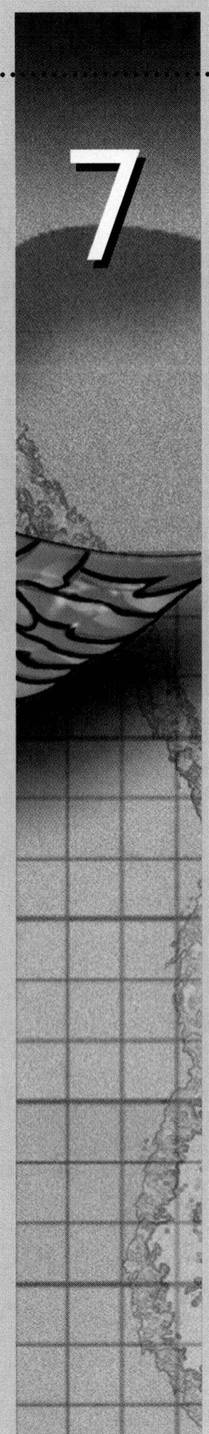

OUTLINE

LEARNING OBJECTIVES

Cognitive: On successful completion of this chapter you should be able to:

1. Define and spell the terms listed in the Vocabulary.
2. State the factors that most influence the formation of a first impression.
3. List three distinct steps in communicating with the patient.
4. Name the three components of listening.
5. List four possible barriers to communication.
6. Briefly describe the paths of communication.
7. List seven rules of good team cooperation.
8. List and briefly describe the three styles of management.
9. Explain the meaning of being a patient advocate.

VOCABULARY

advocate A person who leads the cause of another
authority The quality of being in command
autocratic Ruling with unlimited authority
barrier A factor that restricts free movement
body language Gestures and mannerisms that influence communication
categorically Applied to a limited classification
caustic remark Biting comment
congruency The quality of agreeing
conversely Something reversed in order
democratic Relating to social equality
discernible To see or understand a difference between two or more things
discrimination Different treatment on a basis other than individual merit
empathy Intellectual and emotional awareness of another person's thoughts, feelings, and behavior
feedback Letting people know how you feel about them at a given moment
gesture The use of motions as a means of expression
harmony Having an atmosphere of cordiality
impartiality The quality of treating or affecting all equally
laissez-faire Management style of "hands off" when dealing with employees
listening An active process of receiving information and examining one's reaction to the messages received
litigious Tending to engage in lawsuits
nonconsensual Not having received consent
observation An inference from what has been seen or heard
physical impairment A lessening of physical capabilities
pitch Highness or lowness of sound
response Something constituting a reply or reaction
self-concept A mental picture of one's self
steepling Upward position of hands together with fingertips touching

The interpersonal skills of the medical assistant set the tone of the human relations in the medical establishment. Greeting the patient pleasantly starts the process. Every ensuing encounter of the patient with a staff member adds to that first impression. If these encounters are consistently pleasant and positive, the patient will tell the world how wonderful the doctor is. The medical assistant is the key person in helping the physician make the patient feel comfortable and important.

First Impressions

Physical appearance is the first attribute to be noticed and is probably the most influential factor in forming that first impression. The successful medical assistant presents the best appearance that he or she can. A clean appropriate uniform, good grooming and personal hygiene, and a warm greeting, all combined with a healthful energetic attitude, set the stage for a positive patient experience.

Communicating with the Patient

To be an effective communicator you must understand the underlying cause-and-effect process. Several steps are involved.

OBSERVATION

Notice how the patient approaches the first station, which is probably a "sign-in" window or reception desk. Look the patient in the eye when you extend your greeting. Does the patient seem apprehensive, seriously ill, or carefree?

LISTENING

True listening includes hearing, understanding, and responding. The main reason for the patient's appointment has probably been noted on the daily schedule. Acknowledge to the patient that you are aware of his or her needs, while at the same time preserving the patient's privacy. Speak quietly. Give the patient an opportunity to ask questions or convey any problems. If there are questions to be answered, make sure that the patient understands.

> PATIENT: Will you be billing my insurance?
> MEDICAL ASSISTANT: We will be glad to do that, but first you must sign this form.
> PATIENT: Why do I need to sign a form?
> MEDICAL ASSISTANT: This is called a consent form. By signing here you give us permission to release confidential information to your insurance company.

A good listener helps the speaker to clarify or modify his or her ideas in the course of expressing them, by responding with meaningful questions and comments, eye contact, and appropriate smiles.

RESPONSE

Responding is both verbal and nonverbal. There needs to be an exchange of information. Is the patient responding in the way you expected? Does he or she seem hesitant? Try to find a way to ensure there is no lack of understanding.

Every patient should be treated with **empathy** and **impartiality.** This does not mean that every patient is treated exactly the same.

Memory Jogger

 *As an appointed patient approaches the reception desk, what observations should the medical assistant make?*

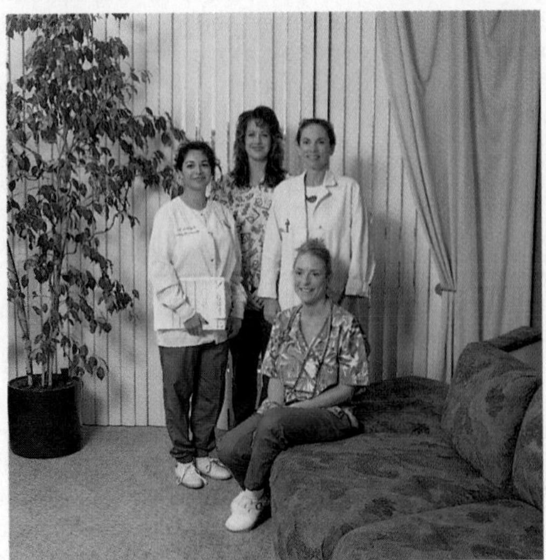

FIGURE 7–1 Colleagues who represent an ethnic mix.

Barriers to Communication

PHYSICAL IMPAIRMENT

Does the patient have a vision problem? This need is usually readily discernible. Try to use more descriptive language in your communication with this patient.

The person with diminished hearing may be very sensitive and in denial of this condition. Be certain that you have his or her attention and that you are face to face with the person while speaking. The hearing impaired are often very dependent on lip reading for comprehension.

Being elderly is not an impairment. Many of your older patients will be physically able and mentally alert and will not expect special treatment.

LANGUAGE

With non–English-speaking patients you may need to use **gestures** and body language to convey your message. In such cases you must be extra alert to the possibility of misunderstanding. Confirm that the message you are sending is the message that the listener is receiving. A response with **feedback** is necessary.

BIAS

Personal and social bias brings about discrimination. **Discrimination** is a word that is used to **categorically** describe unfair treatment of a person because of race, gender, religious affiliation, or handicap. Discrimination is unethical, morally and socially wrong, and in many situations illegal. It prevents us from effectively communicating.

Another type of discrimination is often referred to as *subtle discrimination.* It is not obvious and seldom expressed openly. Subtle discrimination is based on a person's appearance, values, or lifestyle or on some other personal factor. Examples include discrimination against obesity, divorce, homosexuality, welfare recipients, and victims of sexually transmitted diseases. Sometimes we may not even be aware that our words or actions reflect subtle discrimination against another.

Recognize your personal prejudices in order to change them. Medical personnel are exposed to a great variety of persons who need care. You cannot allow prejudice to affect the care of any individual (Fig. 7–1).

Memory Jogger

 *Describe what is meant by "subtle discrimination."*

Communication Paths

In the medical arena, much of the communication is accomplished through talking. We also communicate through writing, by gesturing, by facial expression, and much more. *Verbal communication* in its strictest sense means "relating to or consisting of words." In this chapter we will use verbal communication in the context of talking (Table 7–1).

TABLE 7–1 Therapeutic Communication Techniques

Technique	Therapeutic Value
Acknowledgment	Emphasizes the importance of the patient in the communication process
Establishing guidelines	Helps patients to know what is expected of them
Focusing	Directs the conversation toward important topics
Listening	Communicates your interest in the patient
Open-ended comments	Helps patients to decide what is relevant and encourages them to continue discussion
Reducing distance	Communicates your involvement to the patient
Reflecting	Shows the patient the importance of his or her ideas and feelings
Restating	Lets the patient know how you interpreted the message that he or she communicated
Seeking clarification	Demonstrates your desire to understand what the patient is communicating
Silence	Communicates your acceptance of the patient

VERBAL COMMUNICATION

Verbal communication depends on words and sounds. The messages are conveyed by the use of language, which may be written or spoken. While you may function comfortably in your familiar surroundings, try to put yourself in the place of the new patient who is entering unknown territory. As the "resident" medical assistant you are in familiar surroundings and already have some information about the new patient but he or she knows nothing of you or the other staff members. The very best first step in breaking that barrier is to have all staff members wear name badges, with letters large enough to be read at a distance of three feet. Include the staff position if there are several divisions of responsibility (e.g., medical assistant, nurse, laboratory assistant). When the patient approaches, even though you are wearing a name badge, stand and introduce yourself in the way you wish to be addressed. If your badge reads DOROTHY OWEN and you like to be on a first name basis, say, "Good morning, Mr.—, my name is Dorothy," while you smile with both your mouth and your eyes. This small effort will put the patient at ease in your environment.

The **pitch** of the voice is a part of verbal communication. The voice lifts at the end of a question. It drops at the end of a statement. Usually, when a speaker intends to continue a statement, the voice will hold the same pitch, the head will remain straight, the eyes and hands will be unchanged. This is not an appropriate time to interrupt. If the message is interrupted before its time, it may never be completed. The tone of voice and choice of words also affect the message.

Medical assistants must become aware of how they express themselves and how they affect the feelings of others. There is no place for sarcasm or a **caustic remark** in the medical facility. For example, "I hope you can manage to be on time for your next appointment," "I don't understand why you are late," or "Late people lose their appointment times."

NONVERBAL COMMUNICATION

Nonverbal communications are messages conveyed without the use of words. They are transmitted by body language, which is partly instinctive, partly taught, and partly imitative. Nonverbal communication, or **body language,** as it is sometimes called, involves grooming, dress, eye contact, facial expression, hand gestures, space, tone of voice, posture, the way we walk, ethnic customs, and much more. We are usually unaware of our own nonverbal signals and recognize only a small number of the signals sent by others. Our ability to help others increases greatly as we increase our own skills in interpreting nonverbal communication.

Appearance is a part of nonverbal communication. This emphasizes the message presented in an earlier paragraph that your appearance is influential. The successful person expresses self esteem, confidence, and ability to perform the job by appropriate clothing, stance, vocabulary, facial expression, and a caring attitude.

If you have ever had the experience of speaking to a person who does not make eye contact, you will realize the importance of greeting the patient with your eyes as well as your voice or body language. Facial expressions usually convey our true feelings and are not masked by the words we use.

Our need for personal space is demonstrated by how patients in the reception area will choose a seat. You will seldom see a person sit in an adjoining seating space with a stranger, if there is an option. Although the need for space varies with the individual culture, some might even remain standing to satisfy the need for personal space. Imagine how those patients feel when you touch them, especially when the patient does not know your name.

GENERALLY ACCEPTED PERSONAL AND SOCIAL SPACE DISTANCES

Intimate: physical contact
Personal: 1.5 to 4 feet
Social: 4 to 12 feet
Public: 12 to 25 feet

Posture can signal depression, excitement, anger, or even an appeal for help. When the physician sits at the front of the chair and leans forward, he or she is giving the message of caring.

Positioning is also important. Sitting behind a desk gives the message of **authority.** Standing or sitting across a room may convey a negative message of denying involvement.

The interchange of warmth by touching can have a dynamic effect on people. Until recent years, touching was acceptable in a medical setting. In the **litigious** atmosphere of the modern world, any nonconsensual touching may be deemed battery, and it is best avoided or used with discretion.

Congruency

Nonverbal and spoken language are dependent on each other. They must be in harmony to convey a definite message. If they are not harmonious, the nonverbal is usually dominant and expresses the true message.

Some believe that crossed arms mean "I will not let you in" and that **steepling** of the fingers means a feeling of superiority. Sometimes these gestures are true and sometimes they are not. They are only true in the context of the entire behavior pattern of the person (Table 7–2).

WRITTEN COMMUNICATIONS

The medical assistant may be asked to give instructions to a patient regarding medication, exercise, diet, and many other topics. This is best done through written instructions that are read and orally explained to the recipient. Use common uncomplicated language that is not likely to be misinterpreted or confusing. Make certain that the instructions are correctly understood before the patient leaves the premises (Fig. 7–2).

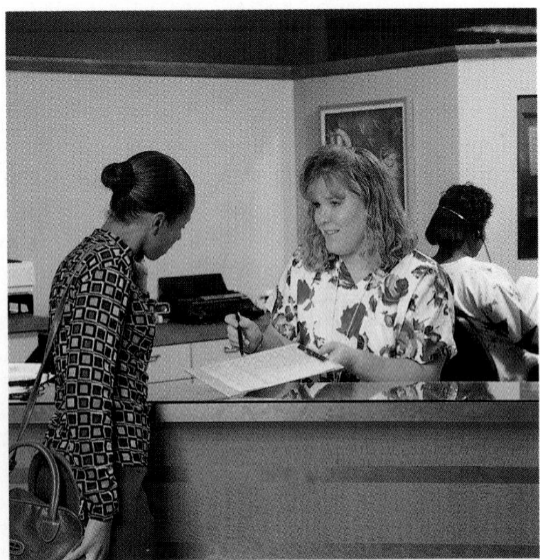

FIGURE 7–2 Medical assistant explaining instructions to a patient.

MEDICAL ASSISTANT: (handing prescription to patient) Dr. . . . wants you to take this medication for 2 weeks.

PATIENT: When do I take it?

MEDICAL ASSISTANT: Under the directions, you see "1 tab h.s." This means that you will take one tablet at bedtime.

PATIENT: Do I take it every night?

MEDICAL ASSISTANT: Yes, the prescription is for 14 tablets. You will take one each night until they are all gone.

CULTURAL DIFFERENCES

Body language is not universal in the messages conveyed. Cultural differences are responsible for many misunderstandings unless we make an attempt to understand them. As a medical assistant you need to be aware of the nonverbal messages being sent by

TABLE 7–2 Nonverbal Communication

Message	Low-Level Behavior	High-Level Behavior
Empathy	Frown resulting from lack of understanding	Positive head nods; facial expressions that reflect the content of the conversation
Respect	Mumbling; patronizing tone of voice	Devoting one's full attention
Warmth	Apathy; fidgeting; signs indicating a desire to leave	Smiling; physical contact
Genuineness	Avoidance of eye contact	Congruence between verbal and nonverbal behavior
Self-disclosure	Bragging gestures; pointing to oneself	Gestures that minimize references to oneself
Confrontation	Pointing a finger or shaking one's fist; speaking in a loud tone of voice	Speaking in a natural tone of voice

the persons with whom you interact, as well as of the messages you are returning. In our society a simple up-and-down nod of the head means yes and a side-to-side shake means no, but in Bulgaria and among the Eskimos these signals have the opposite meaning. See Examples of Various Cultural Traditions for other traditions that illustrate the importance of being sensitive to and aware of beliefs of the many cultures that will be represented in your patient population.

EXAMPLES OF VARIOUS CULTURAL TRADITIONS

- A husband speaks for his wife. The wife does not speak to the physician.
- The palm of the hand, facing down, is used to beckon someone. The hand motion signaling one to come or follow, performed with the back of the hand toward the patient, is used only when calling an animal. An open hand is used to point, rather than one finger.
- A female's clothing is not removed without the presence of another female family member.
- Emotional crying and sobbing denote femininity.
- Going to the doctor is a sign of weakness.
- The female medical assistant never touches the male patient.
- Acquaintances are not permitted to stand within 3 feet of the patient; only immediate family members are permitted to stand within this space.
- The Chinese do not like to be touched by people they do not know.
- The Laotian's "yes" response may not mean "yes," because it is considered rude to say "no" to others or to cause conflict.
- A native of Cambodia, as well as a Laotian, will not look into the eyes of the person being addressed because long eye contact means disrespect and is impolite.
- Cambodians do not like to have their blood drawn because they believe it will weaken them.
- Afghans and Mexicans have a concept of time that is less precise than in the United States.
- Vietnamese consider the head to be a sacred part of the body and are offended by being touched on the head or shoulders. Only the elderly may touch the head of a child without giving offense.

If you work in a practice that predominantly serves a distinct ethnic group, discuss possible cultural differences with the physician and with influential people within the cultural group. Learning to understand cultural differences helps you to gain the confidence and respect of patients.

Memory Jogger

Can you list additional signs of nonverbal communication not discussed previously?

Communicating with Staff Members

SETTING THE TONE

Patients are usually quite sensitive to the degree of **harmony** that exists in the medical facility, and it is important to their well-being that they be treated in a harmonious atmosphere. The tone of the medical establishment is determined by the interpersonal skills demonstrated by the employees toward one another. When personality problems exist among staff members, these problems should be openly discussed so that they can be resolved. Care must be taken to avoid constantly criticizing others and participating in office gossip. Liking a person is not a requirement for acceptance of that person as a working colleague. Try addressing yourself to the situation rather than to the person's character or personality.

A successful medical assistant must have the knowledge to understand what he or she is expected to do and the skills to perform the assigned tasks. This is essential in today's busy and multiskilled offices. With this assumption, the success of the medical assistant is almost always dependent on how he or she responds to patients, staff, and the physicians.

SELF-CONCEPT

Your self-concept is composed of all the attitudes you have about yourself. Understanding yourself and feeling good about yourself are important. Confidence and self-esteem can affect your success, and feeling down on yourself can lead to failure. When you expect to fail, it is almost inevitable that you will. However, when you believe in yourself and expect to succeed, the likelihood of your success is greatly improved.

Many of the perceptions you have about yourself are based on the feedback you have received from others. Keep in mind that you, too, affect others in the way they perceive themselves. This is especially true when people are involved in a team effort, as you will be in the medical facility. In other words, the self-concept has a circular effect.

COOPERATION

Cooperation is the ability to work with others effectively. It requires your extending yourself to be helpful to others. You learn cooperation not by thinking of your immediate comfort but rather of the ultimate success of your medical facility and of your patients. Cooperation is actually an expression of self-interest and unselfishness. It demands that you adjust your own immediate pleasure to benefit the interests of others.

As a medical assistant, you will be expected to cooperate often and in many ways. You will need to keep your work place and belongings neat and orderly, assume additional duties and responsibilities without complaint, work overtime when there is a need, and *offer your services even when you are not obligated to do so.* Share ideas and listen when others are trying to help you. Work harmoniously with others to advance the interests of the medical facility.

Teamwork is based on the ability of one worker to depend on another. Every person on the team is important and must complete his or her share of the workload if the team is to succeed.

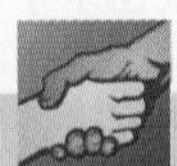

PERSONAL QUALITIES

BEING A TEAM MEMBER

- Act with initiative about getting the job done; don't wait to be told what to do.
- Avoid being rigid about procedures; be flexible and receptive to doing things the way another person might want them done.
- Try never to take advantage of co-workers.
- Think before you speak.
- Never let your emotions take control over you.
- Don't make hasty judgments about others.
- Share the sense of accomplishment from a job well done.
- Don't expect others to do things "your way."

Little phrases such as *please, thank you, good morning,* and *good night* are very powerful in the work environment. Comments of politeness let others know that you care about them and appreciate them. A simple "good morning" may minimize the impact of an unpleasant event that occurred the previous workday and contribute to a cooperative working atmosphere.

Not everyone catches on to new ideas and routines at the same rate. It is important that you remain calm when helping a co-worker perform a new routine. Be patient when you are asked questions. A negative attitude can quickly lead to conflict and a breakdown of communication. Remember that someone took the time to teach you, so when the time comes for you to be the teacher, you should do the very best job you can.

When you have a difficult situation, or do not know how to solve a problem, invite your co-workers to assist in the solution. Be prepared to share the successful resolution when it occurs. A word of caution—ask for advice only when you are willing to consider hearing something with which you may disagree. If all you are seeking is confirmation of what you already have decided, you are not being fair to ask for advice. When you do receive help, be certain to say *thank you* and be sincere when saying it.

FEEDBACK

Feedback is letting people know how you feel about them at a given moment. When a co-worker does something you like, tell him or her. It will make both of you feel good. **Conversely,** sometimes you will need to give negative feedback. A co-worker does something that is not acceptable. Instead of harboring ill feelings, be open and honest about it. Your comments should refer to the situation—not to the co-worker's character.

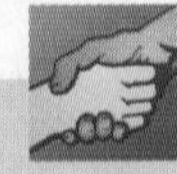

PERSONAL QUALITIES

RULES IN CONVEYING NEGATIVE FEEDBACK

- Give it as soon as possible after the event at a mutually agreeable time.
- Keep it friendly and nonthreatening.
- Give it in the appropriate place, in private.
- Deal only with facts, and how the behavior affects you.
- Avoid appearing judgmental.

If you are the recipient of negative feedback, learn to accept it in the same manner as you would any constructive information. The goal for every staff member is to deliver the best possible health care.

Relating to Management Style

A medical facility with three or more employees usually has a supervisor who manages the staff under the direction of the physician(s). In a few instances this may be an informal arrangement, but inevitably someone must be in charge. The supervisor may be one of the medical assistants. In any event, a supervisor has personality traits, strengths and weaknesses, good days and bad days, hopes and fears, just as you do. Learn to respect the manager's style and respond to him or her as another human being.

The three basic styles of management are **autocratic, democratic,** and **laissez-faire.** An awareness of these different management styles will aid your relationship. Remember that you cannot change the supervisor's style of management. After you discover which style of management inspires your best efforts, you should direct any future search for employment toward a facility that has the management style you prefer.

AUTOCRATIC

This supervisor is a strong leader who dictates procedure, policy, and assignments, including directions for when and how things should be done. The autocrat does not delegate easily and seldom welcomes initiative or creativity in the staff. If your supervisor fits into this category, be sure to follow directions and strictly adhere to the rules.

DEMOCRATIC

In contrast to the autocrat, the democratic supervisor encourages participation in the management process and exercises only a moderate degree of control over the employees' performance. This supervisor will be quick to explain policies and procedures when needed. Staff members will be encouraged to make suggestions and participate as a member of the management team. A democratic environment will allow you to "stretch your wings."

LAISSEZ-FAIRE

The highly confident medical assistant will blossom under this supervisor, who provides only general guidance and allows staff members to work independently. Initiative and creativity are encouraged. Employees are free to complete their tasks relying on their own training and past experience. The "down side" is that it requires more self-discipline from the employee. People may not work together because there is little direction. If you are not a self-starter you may not succeed in this environment.

Memory Jogger

 *Name the three basic styles of management.*

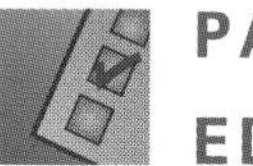

PATIENT EDUCATION

The medical assistant has the opportunity to provide an educational service to every patient who enters the medical facility. If patients feel uneasy about asking the physician questions, let them know that you are available to transmit their questions to the physician. You might suggest that they prepare a list of their questions before their appointments and that they give this list to the physician when they come to the office.

When patients experience anxiety about why a procedure is necessary or how it will be accomplished, the medical assistant can often explain. He or she can help by alerting the physician to the patient's concerns or by encouraging the patient to speak to the physician directly. By acting as the patient's **advocate,** the medical assistant helps to establish a positive rapport between the patient and the physician.

Patients have many questions about medical care facilities and providers of medical services such as laboratories, therapeutic facilities, and hospitals. Medical information and new treatment methods are favorite topics for coverage by the news media. Patients often ask questions about medical news that they have heard.

The entire staff should work as a team to create an atmosphere of patient confidence and trust. Offer information regarding appointment schedules, billing, insurance services, telephone hours, office hours, and emergency coverage. Information about fees for services, office policy, and Medicare should be readily available to patients.

The medical assistant is the front door to the practice. In this role, expect to have contact with outside physicians, staff members, salespersons, supply company representatives, and service representatives. Courtesy, patience, and effective communication skills help to promote a positive public image of the facility.

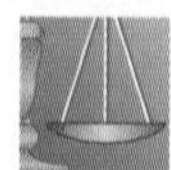

LEGAL AND ETHICAL ISSUES

The physical appearance of the medical assistant has a profound effect on the patient's appraisal of medical care received.

When personality problems exist among staff members, an attempt should be made to resolve them. Address yourself to the existing situation—not to the person's character or personality.

Study the cultural differences of ethnic groups served by your facility for a better understanding of their behavior.

CRITICAL THINKING

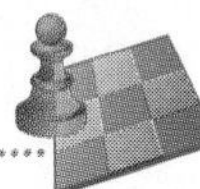

1 Patients often will express their fear of a situation by exhibiting anger. A patient is early for his appointment but is becoming abusive and making unreasonable demands. In your position as medical assistant, how will you react to this patient?

2 The patient often loses the sense of privacy while in a health care facility. As a medical assistant, what can you do to diminish this loss to the patient?

3 List some possible reasons that a patient might feel apprehensive about visiting the physician.

4 Have you ever been a victim of discrimination? Have you felt discrimination toward another person? Describe your feelings.

5 Which of the three described management styles would you find most comfortable as a working environment? Why?

HOW DID I DO? Answers to Memory Joggers

1 Is the patient relaxed? Apprehensive? Obviously ill? Assertive? Defensive? Add your own suggestions.

2 Subtle discrimination is based on the observer's personal experience and expectations.

3 Some additional signs of nonverbal language: playing with a finger ring, moving restlessly, tapping of the foot, a wink of the eye, crossing the legs, turning the head, pulling one's hair.

4 Autocratic, democratic, laissez-faire.

REFERENCES

Dresser N: Multicultural Manners. New York, John Wiley & Sons, 1996.

Fast J: Body Language. New York, Pocket Books, 1970.

Peterson A, Allen R: Human Relations for the Medical Office. Chicago, AAMA, 1978.

Patient Reception

8

OUTLINE

LEARNING OBJECTIVES

Cognitive: On successful completion of this chapter you should be able to:

1 Define and spell the words listed in the Vocabulary.
2 List six considerations in keeping a reception room comfortable for patients.
3 State two reasons for checking supplies at the beginning of each day.
4 Identify and discuss the importance of the three components of greeting an arriving patient.
5 Instruct a new patient about providing personal data for the records and completing a registration form.
6 List three actions a medical assistant might take to reduce stress caused by a delayed schedule.
7 Discuss ways a medical assistant might help a physically impaired, uncomfortable, or ill patient.
8 Suggest a way to successfully handle an angry patient.

Performance: On successful completion of this chapter you should be able to perform the following activities:

1 Follow correct procedure for reviewing patient charts for the day's appointments.
2 Supervise completion of a new patient's registration form.

VOCABULARY

augment To make greater or more effective
flagged Using something to signal or attract attention
harmonious All parts are agreeably related or in accord
intercom (intercommunication system) A direct telephone line from one station to another
pediatrician A physician who specializes in the care of children
perception A mental image
phonetic Alteration of ordinary spelling that better represents the sounding of a word
responsible person One who is responsible for payment, usually the patient if an adult
sequentially Following one another in an orderly plan

A first impression is lasting. Nowhere is this more important than in the health care facility, where the environment must appear orderly and faultlessly clean. The facility may be a physician's office, a hospital, a health maintenance organization, an insurance company, or one of the many other health care sources. No matter what facility is involved, the appearance of the reception room and the front desk, and a cordial greeting by the receptionist, influence a patient's **perception** of the entire facility and the care that he or she will receive.

The Reception Room

The *reception room* is just that—a place to *receive* patients. The area should be planned for the patients' comfort, made as attractive and cheerful as possible, and kept clean and uncluttered (Fig. 8–1). Often the medical assistant has the opportunity to assist in decorating or re-decorating this very important room.

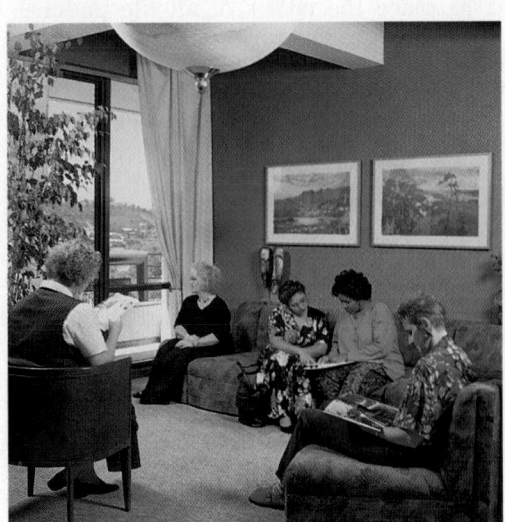

FIGURE 8–1 A comfortable, tasteful reception room.

Fresh **harmonious** colors and cleanliness are the basis of an attractive room. Add comfortable furniture that is adequate to accommodate the peak load of patients seen each day and arrange it in conversational groups. Individual chairs are best. People sometimes prefer to stand rather than sit next to a stranger on a sofa. Provide good lighting, ventilation, and a regulated temperature for additional comfort, and you have the essentials of an attractive reception room that tells the patient you care. A place to hang coats, rainwear, and umbrellas helps reduce reception room clutter. Professional designers can be consulted regarding reception room improvements when there is a problem area. See Features of Reception Area.

FEATURES OF RECEPTION AREA

- Cleanliness
- Restful colors
- Adequate seating
- Lighting to read by
- Good ventilation
- Regulated temperature

Most physicians' offices are well supplied with recent magazines in washable plastic covers. Patients seem to enjoy looking at pictures rather than something that requires concentrated reading. Pictorial travel books and magazines with short items of popular interest are favorites. The reception room, incidentally, is *not the place* for the physician's professional journals.

A writing desk and writing paper in the reception area for the convenience of patients are a nice touch, as is restful music via a concealed speaker. Even such additions as a television, available coffee or a cool drink, a lighted aquarium, or an educational display of some sort will enhance the attractiveness and individuality of the reception area of the professional practice. See Added Attractions for Reception Area.

For the **pediatrician,** a children's corner, equipped with small-scale furniture and some playthings, works well. Youngsters who might otherwise get into mischief are kept pleasantly occupied. Toys should be easily cleanable; plastic washable items are especially good. Take extra care to ensure that no toy has sharp corners that could injure a child, and that it has no small parts that could be swallowed. Also, in selecting toys, make certain that they will not stimulate the child toward noisy activity. And no rubber balls, for obvious reasons!

Take an objective look around the reception room periodically. Could it use a little brightening or freshening up? Try to look at it as if you were seeing it for the first time. The receptionist is at least partly responsible for the appearance of the area by making certain that the room remains neat and orderly throughout the day. Check the temperature and lighting for comfort. Scanning the room at intervals during the day and 1 to 2 minutes devoted to putting the room in order aid in keeping it at its best.

If the medical assistant's desk is in the reception area or in open view of the patients, it should be free of clutter. In particular, patients' charts and financial records should not be in sight. Personal articles, coffee cups, and so forth should not be on the receptionist's desk. Computer monitors should not be in view of patients, to protect the confidentiality of records (Fig. 8–2).

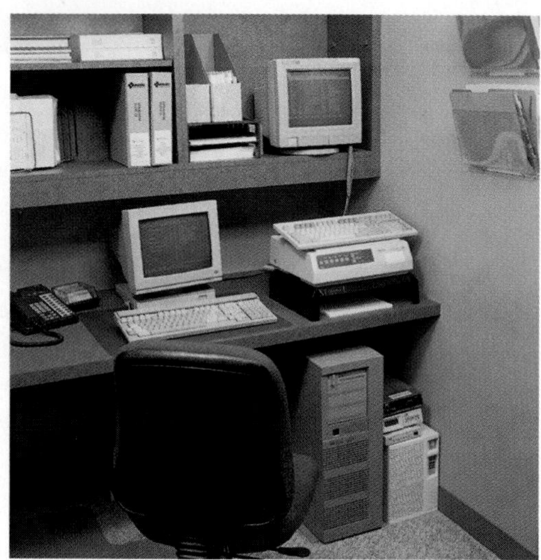

FIGURE 8–2 A neat, well-organized reception desk.

ADDED ATTRACTIONS FOR RECEPTION AREA

Plants, fresh or artificial; if artificial arrangements are used, make sure they are dusted and cleaned
Pictures
Travel posters
Bulletin board displays
Recent general interest magazines
Pictorial travel books
Coffee, or cool drink
Aquarium (built-in for safety)
Safe toys for children's corner

Preparing for Patient Arrival

Advance preparation helps to make the day go smoothly and contributes toward a more relaxed atmosphere for all concerned.

KNOW WHO THE PATIENTS ARE

Patients like to be acknowledged when they arrive. All staff members should review the day's schedule in the morning to be prepared to greet patients by name, and to know whether the patient is *new* or *established.* Patients should not be expected to provide details of the reason for their visit in a public area. Remember to ask *about the patient* before you ask about insurance.

REVIEW THE PATIENTS' CHARTS

Pull the charts for the day, checking the patient's name on your day list for accuracy (see Procedure 8–1). Occasionally, more than one patient may have the same or a similar name. Review each chart to verify that any recently received information, such as laboratory reports and radiograph readings, has been correctly entered and that each chart is current. Arrange the charts **sequentially** in the order the patients are scheduled to be seen. You may be expected to place the charts of all the patients to be seen that day on the physician's desk. It is more likely that the physician will prefer to receive a patient's chart just before seeing him or her.

REPLENISH SUPPLIES

Supplies at the reception desk need to be replenished regularly. Stationery, appointment cards, charge slips, sharpened pencils, and any items likely to be needed during the day should be on hand when the day begins. Discovering depleted supplies during a busy day can seriously interrupt the flow of patient care. One person can be in charge of checking the inventory of supplies on a regular basis and of ordering as necessary (see Inventory Control in Chapter 23).

In a multiple-employee practice, a clinical assistant usually has the responsibility of checking clinical supplies. However, in a small practice there may be

PROCEDURE 8–1

Preparing Charts for Scheduled Patients

GOAL

To prepare patient charts for daily appointment schedule and have them ready for the physician before patients' arrival.

EQUIPMENT AND SUPPLIES

Appointment schedule for current date
Patient files
Clerical supplies (e.g., pen, tape, stapler)

PROCEDURAL STEPS

1 Review the appointment schedule.

2 Identify full name of each scheduled patient.

3 Pull patients' charts from files, checking each patient's name on your list as each chart is pulled.
PURPOSE: To determine that the correct charts have been pulled and that none have been omitted.

4 Review each chart.
PURPOSE: To reaffirm that:
- All information has been correctly entered.
- Any previously ordered tests have been performed.
- The results have been entered on the chart.

5 Annotate the appointment list with any special concerns.
PURPOSE: To alert the physician regarding matters that should be checked or discussed with the patient.

6 Arrange all charts sequentially according to each patient's appointment.

7 Place the charts in the appropriate examination room or other specified location.

only one assistant in charge. Before patients start arriving, *everything should be ready for the day* so that the physician and medical assistant can give undivided attention to the patients' needs.

Check all rooms to make certain that

- Everything is clean
- Cabinets are well stocked
- Drugs have been counted with narcotics checked off and locked if appropriate

Memory Jogger

1 *Why is it important to* preview *the day's schedule of patients to be seen that day?*

Greeting the Patient

Every patient has the right to expect courteous treatment in the physician's office. No matter what the patient's economic or social status may be, each individual who enters the reception room should receive a cordial, friendly greeting. Using the personal touch in receiving patients is important.

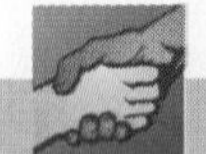

PERSONAL QUALITIES

GREETING THE PATIENT

Cultivate the habit of greeting each patient immediately in a friendly, self-assured manner. Establish eye contact, smile, and introduce yourself to the *new patient*, giving your name and job title: "Good morning, I'm Elizabeth Parr, Dr. Wade's medical assistant."

Greet the *established patient* by name. Learn how to pronounce each patient's name correctly, because incorrect pronunciations may offend and irritate some people. If the name is unusual, write the **phonetic** spelling on the record for reference.

Try to remember the patients' names and something personal about each one. Jot down key words on the patient's chart that will provide reminders for future conversations. Most patients appreciate the interest of the physician and the staff in their families, hobbies, and work.

The reception desk is usually placed for a clear view of all visitors who come into the office. If there is only one medical assistant, it is sometimes impossible for each new caller to be welcomed personally. In this situation, some announcement system must be worked out. The patient who enters an empty reception room does not know whether to sit down, knock on the glass partition, or try to announce his or her presence in some way. A bell at the desk or window that the patient can ring is one solution.

Sometimes a register is placed in the reception room with a sign above it reading:

PLEASE SIGN THE REGISTER WHEN YOU ARRIVE. THE DOCTOR WILL SEE YOU SHORTLY.

This is a makeshift arrangement and *should be avoided* because patient confidentiality is violated when others can read the register. It is preferable to hand the register to the patient if this system must be used.

PROCEDURE 8-2
Registering a New Patient

GOAL

To complete registration form for a new patient with information for credit and insurance claims, and to inform and orient patient to facility.

EQUIPMENT AND SUPPLIES

Registration form
Clerical supplies (pen, clipboard)
Private conference area

PROCEDURAL STEPS

1 Determine whether the patient is new.
2 Obtain and record the necessary information:
   - Full name, birth date, name of spouse (if married)
   - Home address, telephone number (include ZIP and area codes)
   - Occupation, name of employer, business address, telephone number
   - Social Security number and driver's license number, if any
   - Name of referring physician, if any
   - Name and address of person responsible for payment
   - Method of payment
   - Health insurance information (photocopy both sides of insurance ID card)
   - Name of primary carrier
   - Type of coverage
   - Group policy number
   - Subscriber number
   - Assignment of benefits, if required

   PURPOSE: This information is necessary for credit and insurance claims
3 Review the entire form and confirm patient eligibility for insurance coverage
   PURPOSE: To verify that information is complete and legible
4 Determine that required referrals have been received if applicable.
   PURPOSE: Insurance coverage may not be valid without referral.
5 Explain medical and financial procedures to patient.
   PURPOSE: Patient develops comfort level and knows what to expect
6 Collect copays or balance payment charges.
   PURPOSE: Keeps accounts current and prevents the necessity of mailing statements

Today's Date ______________________

PATIENT INFORMATION SHEET

Patient's Name ______________________ First Middle Last Date of Birth ___/___/___ Mo Day Year

Responsible Person's Name ______________________ First Middle Last ________ Relationship

Address ______________________ Number Street City State Zip ___/______ Area Phone

Employer ______________________ Department or Occupation ______________________

Address ______________________ Number Street City State Zip ___/______ Area Phone

Social Security Number ______________________ Driver's License Number ______________________

Spouse of Resp. Person ______________________ First Middle Last ___/______ Area Phone

Employer ______________________ Department or Occupation ______________________

Address ______________________ Number Street City State Zip ___/______ Area Phone

Social Security Number ______________________ Driver's License Number ______________________

Nearest relative (not living with you) ______________________ ________ Relationship

Address ______________________ Number Street City State Zip ___/______ Area Phone

Patient referred to this office by ______________________

AUTHORIZATION TO PAY BENEFITS TO PHYSICIAN: I hereby authorize payment of any insurance benefits covering these medical charges directly to the physician/surgeon.
Signature of the Insured ______________________ Date ________

AUTHORIZATION TO RELEASE INFORMATION: I hereby authorize the physician/surgeon to release any medical information to my insurance company.
Responsible person's signature ______________________ Date ________

STATEMENT OF FINANCIAL RESPONSIBILITY: I, ______________________, do hereby agree to pay all medical charges incurred by the above listed patient. I further understand that these charges are my responsibility regardless of insurance coverage.
Responsible person's signature ______________________.

FIGURE 8–3 Patient information sheet and credit application. (Courtesy of Credit Service Systems, Anaheim, CA.)

Introductory Procedures

REGISTRATION

Certain introductory procedures are required on a patient's first visit to the facility (see Procedure 8–2). Most physicians use a Patient Information Form of some kind to gather subjective information about the patient (Fig. 8–3). The medical assistant may complete the form while interviewing the new patient or have the patient complete the form on arrival for the first appointment. The form may be attached to a clipboard and handed to the patient with instructions to complete all parts of the form, with assurance that the assistant is ready and willing to answer any questions.

The patient's name and date of birth should appear prominently at the top of the form, followed by the name of the **responsible person** and pertinent facts in logical order. See Information Contained in a Patient Information Form.

INFORMATION CONTAINED IN A PATIENT INFORMATION FORM

- Patient's name and date of birth
- Responsible person's name
  Relationship to patient
  Address and telephone number
  Name, address, and telephone number of employer
  Occupation
  Social Security number
  Driver's license number
- Name of responsible person's spouse
  Related information, same as for responsible person (in some community property states, both spouses are equally responsible)
- Nearest relative not living with patient, and his or her relationship
- Source of referral, if any

When the completed form is returned to the medical assistant, it must be checked carefully to verify that all the necessary information has been included.

Memory Jogger

It is not uncommon to find a patient registration form at the reception desk for patients to sign in. Why is this practice discouraged?

OBTAINING PATIENT HISTORY

The personal and medical history, and the patient's family history, may be obtained by asking the patient to complete a questionnaire; the physician can augment this information during the patient interview. The *experienced medical assistant* may be expected to conduct the interview for the patient's personal and medical history, family history, and chief complaint. This is a very specialized procedure, and the interviewer must be specifically trained for the individual practice.

Consideration for Patients' Time

Once the preliminaries have been completed, the patient will expect to see the physician or practitioner at the appointed time. The medical assistant should get the patient in for treatment or consultation as near the appointment time as possible or explain any potential delay to the patient. All patients want to be kept informed about how long to expect to wait. Almost all patients will respond positively when the physician or the assistant comes to the reception area to apologize for any delay. *Consideration for the patient's time* is the keyword.

Most experts will agree that in a solo or small practice, there should seldom be more than three to five patients in the reception room. "Too long a wait in the doctor's office" is one of the most frequently heard criticisms of the medical profession. The patient who complains about medical fees or the care received may actually be complaining about the long wait or discourteous service. Most patients are fearful and tense, but the medical assistant can often put them in a better frame of mind with just a friendly smile and a show of concern.

A crowded reception room is not always an indication of a physician's popularity. It may simply mean that the physician or the assistant is inefficient in scheduling patients. Business people, for example, who are in the habit of making the most of their time, are particularly displeased at what may appear to them to be inefficient scheduling of appointments. Any delay of longer than 15 minutes should be explained to the person waiting. Some personal attention, such as offering a drink of water, a cup of coffee, or a new magazine, may help to calm a patient who appears irritated with the delay.

Patients with Special Needs

Some patients will be physically challenged, some will be very ill, and some will be severely uncomfortable. There may be language or cultural barriers.

Observe the patient's appearance and behavior. Is the patient pale or drawn looking? Do the eyes or voice reflect pain or discomfort? Find out how the patient is feeling before you suggest that he or she be seated to wait for the physician. The patient may need to lie down in a cool room or perhaps should be seen as an emergency.

The patient who is in a wheelchair or using a walker or crutches may need personal attention. Some patients may need help in disrobing even when a disability is not obvious. Ask if you can be of assistance. The medical assistant must use good judgment in helping disabled patients, perhaps even bypassing some of the usual routines.

Escorting and Instructing the Patient

Sometimes we become so accustomed to our own surroundings that we forget that the stranger may be confused or disoriented by all the hallways, doors, and rooms. Uncertainty creates anxiety. Do take the time to personally escort the patient to the appropriate examination or treatment room. This is usually the responsibility of the clinical medical assistant. If a urine specimen is to be obtained, direct the patient to the rest room.

If the patient is to disrobe, explain what garments, if any, can be left on, whether shoes are to be removed, that he or she must remove jewelry if an x-ray film is to be taken, and so forth. If a gown is to be worn, specify whether the opening should be in front or back, and tell the patients where they can hang their clothes if this is not obvious. All instructions must be clear. *Do not assume* that patients will know what you want if you have not told them.

Be equally clear when the examination has been completed: "You can get dressed now and return to the consultation room," or "After you are dressed, please stop by the desk to make your next appointment," or "Have you any questions?"

The medical assistant can help keep the schedule operating smoothly by immediately tidying each examination room and moving the next patient in so that the physician need have no idle moments waiting for a patient to be prepared. Try not to place a patient in an examination room just to clear out the reception area. It is especially inconsiderate to keep the patient waiting after being gowned, draped, and positioned on the examining table. A magazine rack on the wall of the treatment room is a welcome addition in some practices.

Handling Complaints

Even under the best of conditions, there will at times be complaints from patients. Remember that the practice of medicine is a personal service for individual personalities, and the medical assistant must cultivate the skill of listening (see Chapter 7). Each patient is a very important person, and any complaint should be taken seriously. Try to resolve the matter if it is within your realm of responsibility. Otherwise, assure the patient of your concern and explain that you will try to find a solution. Then be sure to carry through.

Problem Situations

THE TALKER

There can be certain problem patients in any professional office. The *talker,* for example, takes up far more of the physician's time than is justified. An alert medical assistant can usually spot this tendency during the initial interview. The patient's history can be **flagged** with a symbol to alert the physician. A prearranged agreement to contact the physician on the **intercom** at the end of the allotted time, with the message that the next patient is waiting, gives the physician an opportunity to conclude the interview. Once you have learned which patients take extra time, you can book them for the end of the day or simply allow more time for them.

CHILDREN

Children sometimes present special management problems. It is often advisable to escort the younger patients into the treatment room *without the parent.* This, of course, should be at the discretion of the physician.

While this practice of separating children from their parents to treat their needs is not always feasible, it sometimes can be applied with great success. In some offices, a token of the physician's friendship, such as a trinket or toy, is given to the child at the completion of the visit.

THE ANGRY PATIENT

Every medical assistant at some time will be confronted by an angry patient. The anger may simply be a reflection of the patient's pain or fear of what the physician may discover on the examination. If possible, invite the patient into another room out of the reception area. Usually it is best to let the patient talk out his or her anger. A calm attitude on the part of the medical assistant, with a few remarks interjected in a low voice, will often pacify the patient. Under no circumstances should the assistant return the anger or become argumentative.

PATIENT'S RELATIVES

A patient will sometimes be accompanied by a relative or well-meaning friend who may become restless while waiting for the patient and attempt to discuss the patient's illness. The medical assistant should sidestep any discussion of a patient's medical care, except by direction of the physician. Also avoid a too casual attitude, such as "I'm sure there's nothing to worry about." A show of moderate concern and offering reassurance that "the patient is in good hands" usually takes care of the situation.

Friendly Farewell

As soon as the visit with the physician has been completed the medical assistant should be ready to take charge by assisting the patient in dressing, if necessary, and by making sure that any questions that the patient may have are answered. In a small practice, this may be the responsibility of the administrative medical assistant.

If the patient has *nontechnical* questions that the assistant can capably and ethically answer, the assistant should answer them clearly and note this on the patient's chart. Some questions can be answered only by the physician; in such cases the assistant can offer to get answers for the patient.

The assistant can help convey the impression of *caring* by terminating the patient's visit cordially. If the patient is returning for another visit, the assistant can say something like "We'll see you next week." If it is the patient's last visit, a pleasant "I certainly hope you'll be feeling fine from now on" is appropriate. The assistant may wish to tell a patient on his (or her) last visit that he has been a fine patient and that it has been a pleasure to serve him. Whatever words of good-bye are chosen, all patients should leave the facility with the feeling that they have received top-quality care and were treated with friendliness and courtesy.

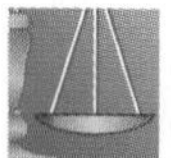

LEGAL AND ETHICAL ISSUES

Use the personal touch in receiving patients.

Try to remember the patients' names and something personal about each one.

Greet the established patient by name.

The registration form may be considered an application for credit and is subject to the regulations of the Equal Credit Opportunity Act of 1975. If you ask for the marital status, avoid using the terms *divorced* or *widowed*.

When a patient complains, listen carefully and resolve the problem or assure the patient that you will try to find a solution.

If someone other than the patient asks for information regarding that patient, refrain from discussion except by direction of the physician.

CRITICAL THINKING

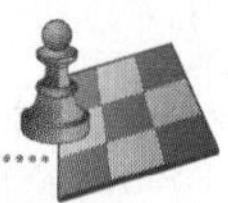

1 Role-play with another student in the various patient situations (talker, children, angry patient, relatives) described in this chapter.

2 Calm an angry patient who is complaining about a long wait. The physician has been delayed by an emergency at the hospital.

3 Recall your latest visit to a medical facility and consider how the reception area could have been more attractive or more comfortable.

4 Based on your own experience or other information, describe what you believe to be a good system of handling patient arrival.

HOW DID I DO? Answers to Memory Joggers

1 Patients like to be acknowledged on arrival. You need to be able to identify *new patients* who will usually require more time and attention.

2 A sign-in sheet at the reception desk violates patient confidentiality.

Telephone Techniques

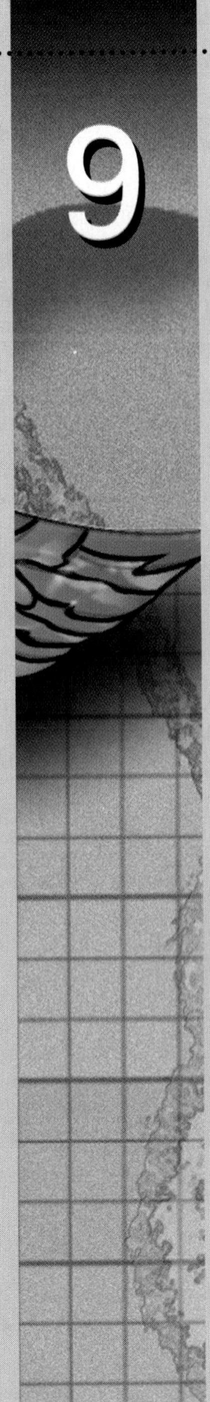

OUTLINE

LEARNING OBJECTIVES

Cognitive: On successful completion of this chapter, you should be able to:

1 Define and spell the terms in the Vocabulary.
2 Discuss the importance of telephone communications.
3 List ways by which the medical assistant can develop a pleasing telephone personality.
4 Cite seven items to be included in taking a complete telephone message.
5 Identify 10 kinds of telephone calls that the medical assistant should be able to handle successfully.
6 Identify six kinds of telephone calls that will need to be referred to the physician for response.
7 Explain what is involved in monitoring telephone calls.
8 Explain what is meant by *preplanning a call.*
9 Explain the ways in which an operator-answered telephone answering service can benefit a medical practice.

Performance: On successful completion of this chapter, you should be able to:

1 Demonstrate the appropriate method of placing and receiving telephone calls.
2 Using a multiple-line telephone, demonstrate the correct handling of two incoming calls, one of which must be transferred to another person.
3 Correctly record a telephone message from a laboratory facility reporting test results on a patient.
4 Respond to a call from a pharmacist regarding a request for a prescription refill, demonstrating appropriate precautions and completing necessary information.
5 Using a list of local social service agencies, respond to telephone calls for emergency treatment (at a poison or burn center) and for nonemergency services (at a facility for crippled children or a cancer-screening center).

VOCABULARY

appease To make peaceful or quiet
clarity The quality or state of being clear
confidential Containing information that requires authorization for disclosure
copay A flat fee payable by the insured in most health maintenance organization plans
diction Choice of words to express ideas, especially with regard to correctness, clearness, or effectiveness
enunciation The act of pronouncing words distinctly
flourishing Achieving success
inflection Change in pitch or loudness of the voice
monitor To listen to a matter transmitted by telephone as a third party
noncommittal Not revealing any specific attitude or opinion
overaccentuate Greatly emphasize
pitch The vibratory frequency of a tone or sound
practitioner One who practices a profession
pronunciation The act or manner of pronouncing words
salutation Expression of greeting (e.g., *good morning*)
screen The act of determining to whom a telephone call is to be directed
tedious Tiresome because of length or dullness
transmitter The part of telephone into which one speaks

General Guidelines

The telephone is the lifeline of a medical practice as well as a powerful public relations instrument. Ninety percent of the patients who are seen in a medical facility make their initial appointments by telephone. When used appropriately, the telephone can help build a beginning medical practice; if used inappropriately, it can do much to destroy even a **flourishing** practice. A physician's office without one or more telephones is impossible to imagine, and the medical assistant who regards the telephone as a nuisance has no place in a medical practice.

The majority of telephone contacts are incoming calls from

- Established patients calling for appointments or to seek advice
- Individuals reporting emergencies
- Other physicians who are making referrals
- Laboratories reporting vital information regarding a patient
- New patients making a first contact

Although great emphasis is placed on rules for speaking, the importance of active listening is often overlooked. The same attention should be given a telephone conversation that would be given a face-to-face conversation. Concentration is not always easy; it must be practiced. Effective active listening is vital to the medical assistant.

YOUR TELEPHONE PERSONALITY

When you receive a telephone call from a stranger, you probably try to visualize that person's appearance. You also form some opinion of his or her personality (e.g., he or she is a mature adult, is somewhat worried, thinks quickly, is well educated). The caller responds to your voice in the same way. To the caller, your voice is your entire personality. The caller cannot see you, your smile, or your facial expression. The caller's total impression of you and of the facility is formed from hearing your voice. What image do you create with your telephone personality?

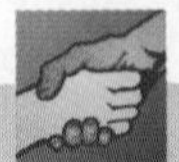

PERSONAL QUALITIES

IS THIS YOUR TELEPHONE PERSONALITY?

- Your voice is warm and friendly.
- Your tone is confident.
- Your conversation is courteous and tactful.
- Your words are well chosen.

Every caller should be made to feel that you have time to attend to his or her wishes. A small mirror, placed near the telephone, will remind you to smile. Smiling helps to relax your facial muscles and improves your tone of voice. If you are rushed when you pick up the telephone, wait a few seconds until you are able to answer graciously without seeming breathless or impatient.

CONFIDENTIALITY

Keep in mind that all communications in a health care facility are **confidential.** This means that if others are within hearing range of your voice, you are to use discretion when mentioning the name of the caller. You must also be careful about being overheard when you repeat any symptoms or other information you are receiving by telephone.

EXAMPLES OF SENSITIVE PHONE CALLS

A woman calls about being struck by her husband, resulting in injuries that need to be treated.

An established patient believes he may have been exposed to the human immunodeficiency virus.

HOLDING THE TELEPHONE HANDSET CORRECTLY

You may have developed some very casual personal habits when using the telephone that will need correction in the professional office. How do you hold the telephone handset? Is it placed so that your voice is relayed distinctly and accurately?

Practice holding the handset around the middle, with the mouthpiece about 1 inch from your lips and directly in front of your teeth. Never hold it under your chin. You can check the proper distance by taking your first two fingers and passing them

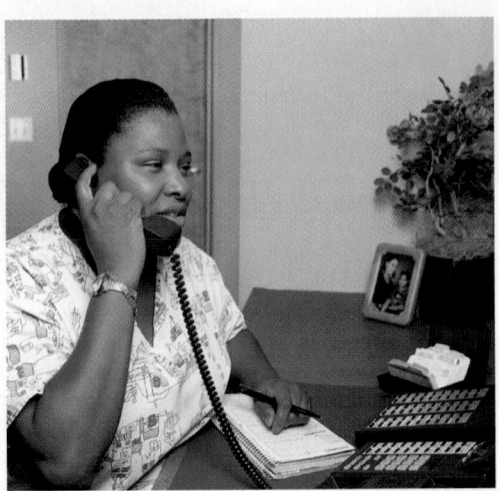

FIGURE 9–1 Correct way to hold telephone.

through sideways in the space between your lips and the mouthpiece. If your fingers just squeeze through, your lips are the correct distance from the telephone and your voice will go over the line as close to its natural tone as possible (Fig. 9–1).

Speak directly into the telephone immediately after removing it from its cradle. If you turn to face a window or another part of the room, make sure the telephone transmitter moves, too; otherwise, your voice will be lost.

DEVELOPING A PLEASING TELEPHONE VOICE

What are the qualities of a good telephone voice? How do you cultivate good voice quality? Some general tips are presented.

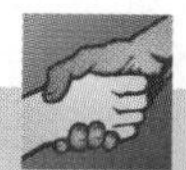

PERSONAL QUALITIES

TIPS ON DEVELOPING A PLEASING TELEPHONE VOICE

- Stay alert. Be alert and interested in the person who is calling. Let the caller know that he or she has your full attention
- Be pleasant. Build a pleasant, friendly image for you and your office. Be the voice with a smile.
- Talk naturally and be yourself. Use your own words and expressions. Avoid repetition of mechanical words or phrases (e.g. "you know," "uh huh," "like"). Avoid the use of professional jargon, such as referring to *otalgia* when the patient is reporting an *earache.*
- Speak distinctly. Clear, distinct pronunciation and enunciation are vital. Move the lips, tongue, and jaw freely. Talk directly into the transmitter. Never answer the telephone when you are *eating, drinking,* or *chewing gum.*
- Be expressive. A well-modulated voice carries best. Use a normal tone of voice, neither too loud nor too soft. Talk at a moderate rate, neither too quickly nor too slowly. Vary your tone. It will bring out the meaning of sentences and add color and vitality to what you say.

HOW IS YOUR DICTION?

Everyone should have the experience of hearing his or her own voice; it reveals immediately the importance of careful **diction.** Try putting your voice on tape and listening to a playback. Each word and each sound must be given individual attention to achieve **clarity.** Slurring your words or dropping your voice too much at the end of a sentence can place a strain on your listener.

TABLE 9–1 Key Words to Verify Letters

A as in Adams	J as in John	S as in Samuel
B as in Boston	K as in Katie	T as in Thomas
C as in Charles	L as in Lewis	U as in Utah
D as in David	M as in Mary	V as in Victor
E as in Edward	N as in Nellie	W as in William
F as in Frank	O as in Oliver	X as in x-ray
G as in George	P as in Peter	Y as in Young
H as in Henry	Q as in Queen	Z as in Zebra
I as in Ida	R as in Robert	

Memory Jogger

1 *There will be days when you are not feeling your best. What one exercise can you use to relax facial muscles and improve the tone of your voice?*

Do not **overaccentuate;** it causes you to sound artificial. Use a friendly natural style. Few words need to be spelled over the telephone if a person speaks slowly and clearly. Table 9–1 lists key words commonly used when it is necessary to verify letters in spelling over the telephone.

Try to avoid the habit of dropping "ers," "uhs," and long pauses into your conversation. Also, remember that it is seldom necessary to raise the **pitch** of your voice to be heard. If you have trouble being understood on the telephone you probably are

- Speaking too fast
- Enunciating poorly
- Failing to speak into the transmitter

Incoming Telephone Calls

You will be receiving many calls during the course of a single day. Each one deserves your most competent attention. See Procedure 9–1, Answering the Telephone, and also Professional Office Telephone Communication for a summary of how to communicate effectively on the telephone. Carefully review Pitfalls to Avoid to help you side-step problems with telephone communications.

PERSONAL CALLS

Because the telephone is so vital to the medical practice, personal calls should not be allowed to keep a line busy. Physicians usually are understanding about occasional urgent calls from the medical assistant's family, but casual calls should be discouraged.

PROCEDURE 9-1

Answering the Telephone

GOAL

To answer the telephone in a physician's office in a professional manner, respond to a request for action, and accurately record a message.

EQUIPMENT AND SUPPLIES

Telephone
Message pad
Pen or pencil
Appointment book
Script for conversation

PROCEDURAL STEPS

1 Answer the telephone on the first ring, speaking directly into the transmitter, with the mouthpiece positioned 1 inch from the mouth.
PURPOSE: Answering promptly conveys interest in the caller. Proper positioning of the handset carries the voice best.

2 Speak distinctly with a pleasant tone and expression, at a moderate rate, and with sufficient volume for the calling party to understand every word.

3 Identify the office and yourself.
PURPOSE: The caller will know that the correct number has been reached and the identity of the staff member.

4 Verify the identity of the caller.
PURPOSE: To confirm the origin of the call.

5 Provide the caller with the requested information or service, if possible.
PURPOSE: The medical assistant can handle many calls and conserve the time and energy of the physician or other staff members.

6 Take a message for further action, if required.
PURPOSE: Not all calls can be responded to immediately.

7 Terminate the call in a pleasant manner and replace the receiver gently.
PURPOSE: To promote good public relations.

A medical assistant who is active in a professional organization sometimes finds it necessary to take calls from colleagues or others involved in the profession. Although these communications are not considered entirely personal, they, too, should be kept to a minimum. The physician's telephone lines should be clear to receive all professional calls.

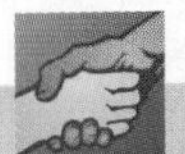

PERSONAL QUALITIES

PROFESSIONAL OFFICE TELEPHONE COMMUNICATION

- Answer promptly.
- Visualize the person to whom you are speaking.
- Hold the instrument correctly.
- Develop a pleasing telephone voice.
- Identify your office and yourself.
- Identify the caller.
- Offer assistance.
- Screen incoming calls.
- Minimize waiting time.
- Identify the caller when transferring a call.
- When answering a second call, identify the caller, then return to the first call.
- End each call pleasantly and graciously.

PITFALLS TO AVOID

- **Having too few telephone lines.** On request, the telephone company will do a traffic survey to determine how many busy signals are occurring and advise you as to whether you need additional lines. If collections and insurance processing require extensive use of the telephone, a special line just for this purpose may be advisable.

- **Having too few assistants to handle the existing lines.** One assistant can handle two incoming lines, but three lines are probably too many for one person. Another assistant should be assigned to pick up the phone after a specified number of rings.
- **Wasting time looking up frequently called numbers.** Keep these in a personal directory where they can be quickly and easily located or use speed dialing.
- **Incoming or outgoing personal calls by employees, except in emergencies.** Most physicians have an unlisted private line to take care of their own personal and priority calls.
- **Using the telephone to give travel directions to new patients** (except for short notice appointments). This information should be included in a patient information sheet or folder sent to every new patient.
- **Taking extensive patient histories by telephone.** This can be done more efficiently at the time of the patient visit.
- **Diagnosing or giving medical advice without authorization from the physician.**
- **Releasing patient information without authorization.**

ANSWERING PROMPTLY

Whenever possible, answer the telephone on the first ring, and always by the third ring. If your facility has several incoming lines or more than one telephone, it will sometimes be necessary for you to interrupt a conversation to answer another call. It is courteous to

- Excuse yourself by saying, "Pardon me just a moment; the other line is ringing."
- Answer the second call, determine who is calling, and, if it is not an emergency, ask that person to hold while you complete the first call. Do not make the mistake of continuing with this call while the first caller waits.
- Return to your first call as soon as possible, and apologize briefly for the interruption.

Think of what you would do if there were a face-to-face conversation. You would not allow a second person to just interrupt a conversation and then ignore the *one you* were speaking with first.

If the second call is an emergency, you can still take a moment to return to the first line and alert the caller that you will have to keep him or her waiting or call back.

Never answer a call by saying, "Hold the line, please," without first finding out who is calling. It could be an emergency, and it is extremely discourteous. It takes only a moment to be courteous, and this courtesy could save a life.

Memory Jogger

Recall at least 7 of the 12 rules for Professional Office Telephone Communication.

PERSONALIZING THE CALL

Try to use the caller's name three times during the conversation. Use other courtesy expressions, such as *thank you, please,* and *you're welcome,* as often as possible.

IDENTIFYING THE FACILITY AND YOURSELF

Your response to an incoming call should be to *first identify the facility* and then *yourself.* Numerous telephone greetings can be used. You will probably wish to discuss which are best with the physician or office manager. Your response might be something like this:

"This is Dr. Black's office—Miss Anderson."

Answering a professional office telephone merely by repeating the telephone number or saying "Hello" is unsatisfactory. The caller will invariably ask:

"Is this Dr. Black's office?"

Rarely can a person immediately recall the number that he or she has just dialed. Time is wasted, the caller is psychologically rebuffed, and you have lost another opportunity to create a favorable impression of your facility.

The use of a **salutation** in telephone identification is optional. Sometimes the addition of "Good morning" or "Good afternoon" to the identification is awkward. A rising **inflection** or a questioning tone in your voice indicates interest and a willingness to assist and eliminates the need for an additional greeting.

When you have decided on the greeting to be used, practice it until you can say it easily and smoothly without having to think about what you are saying.

IDENTIFYING THE CALLER

If the caller does not identify himself or herself, you should ask to whom you are speaking. Repeat the caller's name by using it in the conversation as soon as possible; if patients are within the range of your voice, remember that the caller's privacy should be respected.

OFFERING ASSISTANCE

You can offer assistance both by the *tone of your voice* and by the *words you use.*

"May I help you?" or "How may I help you?" will open the conversation and assure the caller that you are both willing and capable of being of service.

SCREENING INCOMING CALLS

Most physicians expect the medical assistant to **screen** all telephone calls. Good judgment in deciding whether to put a call through to the physician comes with experience.

Do put through calls from other physicians at once. If your physician is busy and cannot possibly come to the telephone, explain this briefly and politely and then say that you will ask the physician to return the call as soon as possible.

Many callers will ask, "Is the doctor in?" Avoid answering this question with a simple "Yes" or "No" or by responding with the question, "Who is calling, please?" *If the physician is not in,* say so *before* asking the identity of the caller. Otherwise, you may create the impression that the physician is just not willing to talk with this person.

If the *physician is away* from the office, the rule of offering assistance still holds. You can say

> "No, I am sorry, Dr. Black is not in. May I take a message?" *or*

> "No, I am sorry, but Dr. Black will be at the hospital most of the morning. May I ask her to return your call after 1 o'clock?"

If the *physician is in* and is available for telephone calls, a typical response would be

> "Yes, Dr. Black is in; may I say who is calling, please?"

When physicians prefer to keep telephone calls to a minimum, you might say

> "Yes, Dr. Black is here, but I am not sure whether she is free to come to the phone. May I say who is calling, please?"

By responding in this way, the physician is not committed to taking the call.

During the time that a physician is examining a patient, he or she will not wish to be interrupted with a routine call. In such cases, you might say

> "Yes, Dr. Black is in but is with a patient right now. May I help you?" *or*

> "Yes, Dr. Black is in but is with a patient right now. Is there anything you would like me to ask her?"

Try to guard against being overprotective. A patient should be able to talk with the physician when necessary; but unless it is an emergency, the patient is probably willing to do so at the convenience of the physician. Don't let it be said of your physician, "He's a good doctor, but you can never talk to him." The medical assistant who answers the telephone acts as a screen, not a roadblock.

Find out exactly how calls are to be handled when the physician is out of the office and under what circumstances you can interrupt when the physician is on the premises. Be firm in your commitment to those preferences and cultivate a reputation for being helpful and reliable. You will save the physician many interruptions if patients develop confidence in your ability to help them and have faith in your promise to take their messages and deliver them properly.

MINIMIZING WAITING TIME

When a call cannot be put through immediately, ask

> "Will you wait, or shall I call you back when Dr. Black is free?"

If the caller elects to wait, remember that waiting with a silent telephone can be **irritating** and **tedious.** The waiting time, no matter how brief, always seems long. *Let no more than 1 minute pass* without breaking in with some reassuring comment, for instance

> "I'm sorry, Dr. Black is still busy."

If the wait is longer than expected, the caller may wish to reconsider and call back at another time or have the call returned, but he or she needs to communicate this to you. By going back on the line at frequent intervals, you give the caller an opportunity to express such concerns. In fact, you may ask the caller if he or she wishes to continue waiting. Say something like the following:

> "I'm sorry to keep you waiting so long, Mr. Hughes. Would you prefer to have me return your call when Dr. Black is free?"

Try to give the caller some estimate of when he or she may expect the return call. In any event, irritation can be lessened by your consideration in saying

> "Thank you for waiting, Mr. Hughes."

When it is necessary that you leave the telephone to obtain information, ask the caller

> "Will you please wait while I get the information?"

Wait for a reply. If it will take longer than a few seconds to get the information, give some estimate of the time required and offer to call back. When you return to the telephone, thank the caller for waiting. Requests that might require pulling the patient's chart from the files may best be handled with a call back to the patient.

Memory Jogger

What is the maximum time a caller should wait on a telephone line without being able to communicate?

TRANSFERRING A CALL

Always identify the person who is calling when you transfer a call to the physician or another person in the facility. Any person who refuses to give a name should not be put through unless you have been instructed to do so.

When the caller is a patient, the physician will probably need the patient's chart at hand during the conversation. If there is no concern about others hearing your conversation, you can announce the caller's name on the intercom and tell the physician that you will bring the chart. If there are others within hearing range, you might simply take the chart to the physician and say

> "Dr. Black, this party is waiting on the telephone to speak with you."

In this way, the patient's right to privacy is protected.

ENDING A CALL

When a caller's requests have been satisfied, do not encourage needless chatting or permit the call to monopolize your time unnecessarily. The telephone lines should be cleared for other calls.

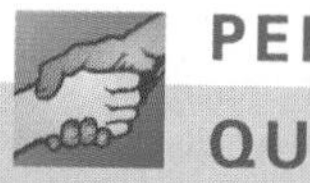

PERSONAL QUALITIES

HOW TO END A CALL

- End the call pleasantly.
- Allow the person who placed the call to hang up first.
- Thank the person for calling.
- Close the conversation with some form of good-bye; do not just abruptly hang up.
- Replace the telephone on its cradle as gently as if you were closing a door.

Taking a Telephone Message

BE PREPARED

Always have a pen or pencil in your hand and a message pad nearby when you answer the telephone. You may be answering several calls before you have an opportunity to relay a message or carry out a promise of action. The *written message* is vital.

What kind of message pad will you use? An ordinary spiral-bound stenographer's notebook is inexpensive, sturdy, and well proportioned; lies flat on a desk; and can be filed for future reference if desired. Never use small scraps of paper for messages. They are too easily lost.

Date the bottom of the first blank page in your notebook at the beginning of each day. You will then have a permanent record that can be referred to later if the need arises. If you will draw a half-inch column down one side of each page, you can use this area to check off each message as it is delivered or taken care of. This creates a good reminder system.

MINIMUM INFORMATION REQUIRED FROM EACH CALL

- Name of the person to whom the call is directed
- Name of the person calling
- Caller's daytime telephone number
- Reason for the call
- Action to be taken
- Date and time of the call
- Your initials

TRANSMITTING AND RECORDING THE MESSAGE

Messages that are to be transmitted to another person may be rewritten on individual message slips and delivered or posted on a message board later. Message pads that provide for a carbon copy of each page are good insurance that no message will be forgotten. The nature of the message will determine whether you must report it immediately. Figure 9–2 illustrates a model message log that can be adapted to the practice by inserting the patient symptoms and requests you hear most often. The person who completes the call must sign and date it. If the call is from a patient and relates in any way to the medical history, or if any instructions were given or queries answered, this information should be placed in the patient's chart. Message forms that have a self-adhesive backing and can be placed permanently in the patient's case history (Fig. 9–3) are readily available.

TAKING ACTION

The message procedure is not complete until the necessary action has been taken. Notations on the memo pad should be carried over to the following day if they have not been attended to. Just place an

TELEPHONE MESSAGE LOG

Date: ____________ Time: ____________ Taken by: ____________

Caller: ____________ Patient: ____________ Age: ____________
Phone # Day: ____________ Evening: ____________
Address: ____________

Complaint: ____________ How long: ____________
Pain: ____________ Location: ____________
Any treatment: ____________
Temperature: ____________

___ Cough
___ Sore throat
___ Vomiting
___ Diarrhea
___ Bleeding

___ Return call

___ Lab results
___ Rx refill
___ Appointment
___ Insurance
___ Billing

___ Will call back

Message: ____________

Action taken: ____________ Date: ____________ Signature: ____________

FIGURE 9–2 Telephone message log.

"X" in front of the item and move it onto the next page. Sometimes a notation will be carried over for several days until action can be completed. Do not trust to memory messages unattended to from previous days; always carry them forward in writing.

Make brief notations of patients' reactions while you are talking to them on the telephone. The physician does not require a character study, but it is helpful to know when a patient appears fearful, apprehensive, or nervous. If a patient shows such symptoms, it may be wise to transfer the call to the physician.

When your employer is talking to another physician about a referral, you may sometimes be requested to take down a brief outline of the patient's case history by listening on the extension telephone. This information can be typewritten and incorporated with the patient's chart and handed to the physician before the patient is seen.

Memory Jogger

4 *List the seven bits of information that are basic in recording a telephone memorandum.*

Incoming Calls the Medical Assistant Can Handle

One reason for having a medical assistant answer the incoming calls is to spare the physician unnecessary interruptions during visits with patients. Additionally, many calls relate to the administrative aspects of the office and can actually be better handled by the medical assistant. The policy regarding how calls are to be handled should be clearly set forth in the office procedure manual. Figure 9–4 shows how the instruction page might be arranged in the manual. Listed below are some kinds of calls that can be handled by the medical assistant in most offices.

NEW PATIENT AND RETURN APPOINTMENTS

Procedures for handling appointments for new patients and scheduling return appointments are discussed in the previous chapter.

INQUIRIES ABOUT BILLS

A patient may request to speak with the physician about a recent bill. Ask the caller to hold for a moment while you pull the ledger. If you find nothing irregular on the ledger, you can return to the telephone and say

> "I have your account in front of me now. Perhaps I can answer your question."

Most likely, the caller will have some simple inquiry, such as

> "Is that my total bill?"
>
> "Has my insurance paid anything?"
>
> "May I wait until next month to make a payment?"

Not all patients realize that the medical assistant

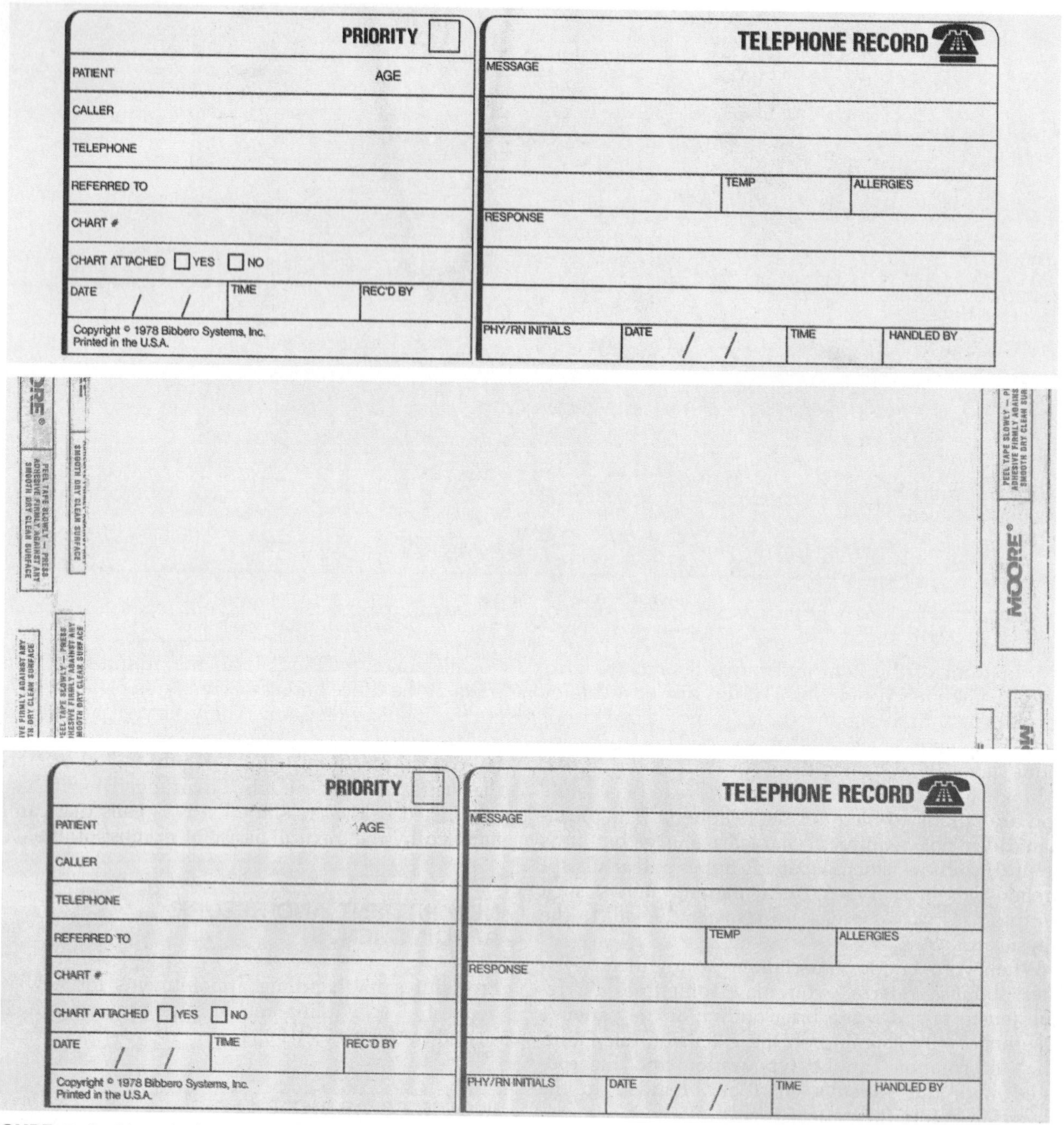

PRIORITY

PATIENT AGE

CALLER

TELEPHONE

REFERRED TO

CHART #

CHART ATTACHED ☐ YES ☐ NO

DATE / / | TIME | REC'D BY

Copyright © 1978 Bibbero Systems, Inc.
Printed in the U.S.A.

TELEPHONE RECORD

MESSAGE

TEMP | ALLERGIES

RESPONSE

PHY/RN INITIALS | DATE / / | TIME | HANDLED BY

PEEL TAPE SLOWLY — PRESS ADHESIVE FIRMLY AGAINST ANY SMOOTH DRY CLEAN SURFACE

MOORE®

PRIORITY

PATIENT AGE

CALLER

TELEPHONE

REFERRED TO

CHART #

CHART ATTACHED ☐ YES ☐ NO

DATE / / | TIME | REC'D BY

Copyright © 1978 Bibbero Systems, Inc.
Printed in the U.S.A.

TELEPHONE RECORD

MESSAGE

TEMP | ALLERGIES

RESPONSE

PHY/RN INITIALS | DATE / / | TIME | HANDLED BY

FIGURE 9–3 Message form with self-adhesive backing. (Courtesy of Bibbero Systems, Inc., Petaluma, California, (800) 242-2376, Fax (800) 242-9330.)

STANDARD PROCEDURE FOR TELEPHONE CALLS IN THE OFFICE OF

______________________________:

CALLS THE ASSISTANT CAN HANDLE:

Appointments for New Patients

Office Administration Problems

CALLS TO BE PUT THROUGH IMMEDIATELY:

Calls from Other Physicians

Emergency Calls

CALLS TO BE REFERRED TO PHYSICIAN:

Unsatisfactory Progress Reports

Third Party Requests for Information

FIGURE 9–4 Page from procedure manual showing standard procedure for incoming telephone calls.

usually makes such decisions and is the best person with whom to discuss these matters.

INQUIRIES ABOUT FEES

In some offices, the medical assistant is instructed *not to quote fees.* For example, a caller may inquire

> "How much does Dr. Arnold charge for an examination?"

He or she may not be pleased to hear

> "That's impossible to say—it depends on how extensive an examination is required."

The following response is equally noncommittal but far more satisfying to the caller.

> "Mr. Barker, the fee usually varies with the nature of the problem. An uncomplicated physical examination without any laboratory tests or x-rays might run as low as $ ______. On the other hand, the fee could be considerably higher if special tests are required."

If fees are regularly discussed on the telephone, write a suggested script in the policy manual. Do not be evasive. Have a schedule of fees available.

REQUESTS FOR INSURANCE ASSISTANCE

Not too many years ago, many patients completed and mailed their own insurance claims. In today's environment of managed care, copay, Medicaid, and Medicare, insurance claims will more than likely be completed and filed by the health care facility. Still, patients may call to inquire about their coverage or ask whether there has been any response to the filing of the claims. The medical assistant or a member of the staff whose sole responsibility is filing of insurance claims will have the knowledge to answer these inquiries.

RADIOLOGY AND LABORATORY REPORTS

Laboratory and radiologic findings may be telephoned to the physician's office on the day the procedures are performed when they are urgent. The medical assistant can take these reports and relay them to the physician. More often the report is faxed to the physician if it is a stat report. Original reports will be delivered by mail for the permanent record. Some facilities are equipped to receive laboratory results directly from the laboratory via computer and electronic media.

SATISFACTORY PROGRESS REPORTS FROM PATIENTS

Physicians sometimes ask a patient "Phone and let me know how you are feeling in a few days." The medical assistant can take such calls and relay the information to the physician if the report is satisfactory. Assure the patient that you will inform the physician about the call by saying, for example,

> "I will relay this information as soon as Dr. Wright is available."

ROUTINE REPORTS FROM HOSPITALS AND OTHER SOURCES

There may be routine calls from a hospital and other sources reporting a patient's progress. If it is only a reporting procedure, take the message carefully, make sure that the physician sees it, and then place the message in the patient's medical record.

OFFICE ADMINISTRATION MATTERS

Not all calls concern patients. There may be calls from the accountant or auditor or calls regarding banking procedures, office supplies, or office maintenance, most of which the medical assistant can handle or refer to the appropriate person. For some of these calls, the medical assistant may need to gather additional information and return the call.

REQUESTS FOR REFERRALS

Physicians who are liked and respected by their patients frequently will be called for referrals to other specialists. If the physician has furnished the medical assistant with a list of practitioners for this purpose, these inquiries can usually be handled without consulting the physician. However, the physician should always be informed of such requests.

PRESCRIPTION REFILLS

If the physician has placed a note on the patient's chart indicating that a prescription may be filled a certain number of times, the medical assistant can give an okay to the pharmacist after determining the number of times it has already been filled. This information should appear on the patient's chart, but it is always best to double check. If there is any question, tell the pharmacist that you will have to check with the physician and call back.

Memory Jogger

 *Name 10 categories of calls that a medical assistant should be able to handle without assistance.*

Incoming Calls That Require Transfer to the Physician or Call Back

PATIENTS WHO WILL NOT REVEAL SYMPTOMS

Occasionally, patients will call and wish to talk with the physician about symptoms that they are reluctant to discuss with a medical assistant. Do not make the mistake of pressing for details. Even though you may not be embarrassed, patients have the right to privacy. Put these calls through or offer to have the physician call back.

UNSATISFACTORY PROGRESS REPORTS

If a patient under treatment reports that he or she "still is not feeling well" or that the "prescription the doctor gave me makes me feel sick," do not try to practice medicine by telling the patient that this is to be expected. Even though you think the physician will say the same thing, the patient should hear it directly from the physician for reassurance.

REQUESTS FOR TEST RESULTS

When the physician orders special tests for the patient, the patient may be told to call the office in a couple of days for the results. Never assume that the patient will call for results. It is ultimately the responsibility of the physician to notify the patient of test results. Be certain that the physician has seen the results and has given you permission to tell the patient before giving out any information. Particularly if the result is unfavorable, the physician should be the one to inform the patient and give further instructions. This call must be handled tactfully; otherwise, the patient may get the feeling that you are concealing information.

Patients do not always understand that the medical assistant does not have the privilege of giving out information without the permission of the physician. You might answer an inquiry in this manner:

"Dr. Wright has not seen the report yet; will you please call back after 2 o'clock? I will try to have the information for you then."

Alternatively, you might offer to call the patient as soon as you have the necessary information. Never call the patient with laboratory results unless specifically directed to do so.

THIRD-PARTY REQUESTS FOR INFORMATION

If there is no legal requirement for disclosure of information, you must have the written permission of the patient before giving information to third-party callers. This includes insurance companies, attorneys, relatives, neighbors, employers, or any other third party.

COMPLAINTS ABOUT CARE OR FEES

You may be able to offer a satisfactory explanation to a patient who complains about the care he or she received or the fee charged. If a patient seems angry, you may say that it will take a few moments to pull the chart and offer to call back. This reassures the patient that someone is willing to talk about the problem and also gives the patient a chance to cool off. However, if you are unable to appease the patient easily, the physician would probably prefer to talk directly to the patient.

UNIDENTIFIED CALLERS

Although it will rarely happen, you will sometimes encounter individuals who refuse to give you their name or business but are insistent on speaking with the physician. Such callers frequently are salespersons who are fully aware that if their identity is revealed they will never get the opportunity to speak to the physician. Your own course in such instances is to say firmly,

"Dr. Jones is very busy with a patient and has asked me to take all messages. If you will not give me a message, I suggest you write a letter to Dr. Jones and mark it *personal.*"

CALLS FROM FAMILY AND FRIENDS

Personal calls to the physician from family members or friends are handled in accordance with instructions from the physician. If the physician does not wish to take the calls, the medical assistant must deal with it. You can say,

"Dr. Wilson is with a patient now and cannot be disturbed. We are booked rather heavily this afternoon, and you may have more time to talk with Dr. Wilson if you call at home this evening."

Occasional Situations

ANGRY CALLERS

No matter how efficient you are on the telephone or how well liked your employer may be, sooner or later you will have an angry caller on the line. There may be a legitimate reason for the anger, or it may have resulted from a misunderstanding. It is a real challenge to handle such calls. First, take the required action—even if it is to say that you will take the matter up with your employer as soon as possible and call back later. If answers are not readily available, a friendly assurance that you will find the answer and call back will usually calm the angry feelings.

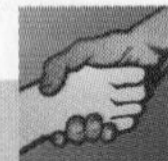

PERSONAL QUALITIES

HOW TO RESPOND TO AN ANGRY CALLER

- Avoid getting angry yourself.
- Try to find out what the real problem is.
- Provide the answers, if possible.
- Actively listen while you let the caller talk.
- Express interest and understanding.
- Do not pass the buck.
- Take careful notes.
- Maintain your own poise.

MONITORING CALLS

Occasionally you may be asked to **monitor** a telephone call. You will be expected to listen from an extension phone and take notes on the conversation. It is possible to record both sides of a telephone call by placing a tape recorder close to the telephone receiver. However, you should be aware that this is illegal unless the other person is told that the conversation is being recorded.

REQUESTS FOR HOUSE CALLS

Scheduling house calls is discussed in Chapter 10. In responding to a telephone request for a home visit, be sure to inquire as to the nature of the illness. Certain conditions are impossible to treat at home, and time will be saved if the patient is sent directly to the hospital where the doctor can meet him or

EMERGENCY CALL PROCEDURES					
When the physician is not in the office, follow these emergency procedures:					
				Have Patient	
Patient Complaint	Refer to Physician Below	Call RN	Call Paramedics	Go to Hospital	Come to Office
Severe bleeding Head injury Severe chest pain Broken bone Severe laceration Unconscious High fever Difficulty in breathing					

FIGURE 9–5 Form for instructions on emergency call procedures (when physician is not in office).

ASSISTANT'S GUIDE FOR HANDLING ROUTINE TELEPHONE CALLS	Refer immediately to physician	Physician will call back	Refer to clinical personnel: RN, CMA, PA	Other
New patient—ill and wants to talk to physician				
Established patient—wants to talk to physician				
Patient—request for lab results				
Family requesting patient information				
Patient or pharmacy—regarding Rx refill				
Another physician—wants to talk to physician				
Hospital—regarding a patient				
Insurance carrier or attorney requesting patient information				
Business calls for physician (attorney, accountant, broker)				
Professional society calls for physician				
Personal calls for physician (family, friends)				

FIGURE 9–6 The new assistant needs a guide for handling even routine calls.

her. Alternatively, you might urge the patient to come to the office. You can point out that the health care facility is better equipped to give the best medical care and that office visits are more economical.

Consult the physician, if possible, before scheduling a house call. In most cases, you can explain to the patient that you will check with the physician and call back immediately. If making the house call is not possible, you should attempt to find other assistance for the patient. It is easier for one of the office staff to call another physician than it is for the distraught patient to do so. One of the most common complaints of patients about the medical profession is that patients are unable to get help in an emergency. In communities that have paramedic teams, this is not such a problem.

RESPONDING TO EMERGENCY CALLS

The handling of telephone calls involving possible emergency situations is briefly discussed in Chapter 10. According to the American Medical Association's *The Business Side of Medical Practice:*

> *Many emergency calls are judgment calls on the part of the person answering in the medical practice. Good judgment only comes from proper training by the physician in what constitutes a real emergency in your type of practice and how such calls should be handled. If you are not immediately available, what should your staff do?*

The person answering the telephone should first determine, "Is it urgent?" If the physician is in, the call should probably be transferred immediately. Some plan for the action to be taken when the physician is not present should be agreed on (Fig. 9–5). The physician and medical assistant may also jointly develop typical questions to ask the caller to determine the validity and disposition of an emergency.

EXAMPLES OF QUESTIONS TO ASK TO DETERMINE AN EMERGENCY CALL

- At what telephone number can you be reached?
- What are the chief symptoms?
- When did they start?
- Has this happened before?
- Are you alone?
- Do you have transportation?

TRIAGE GUIDELINES

In the facility with multiple employees, the physician may designate one individual as the triage nurse or assistant. Within the environment of managed care, the physician would be wise to have a written telephone protocol for handling urgent situations and emergencies. The protocol should state that the employees are bound by the written guidelines and that any giving of advice by unauthorized personnel may be grounds for dismissal.

A special sheet of instructions listing specific medical emergencies such as chest pain, heavy bleeding, fainting, seizure, and poisoning should be posted by each telephone. Include the phone number for the nearest poison control center, hospital, and ambulance. Such calls would be routed to a physician immediately. Additional instructions should include what action to take if no physician is available, for example, sending the patient to an emergency department or calling an ambulance or 911.

Routine but Troublesome Calls

Many of the so-called routine calls coming into the physician's office will be difficult for a new medical assistant to handle (Fig. 9–6). Although no stock answer can be phrased for these calls, a gracious and prompt reply paves the way for a quicker handling of a call, because it lets the caller know that you are capable, pleasant, and willing to offer assistance.

Following are a few typical calls that any medical assistant might receive:

APPOINTMENT CHANGES

THE CALL: "I have an appointment with the doctor this morning and I cannot keep it. May I come in this afternoon?"

THE ANSWER: Even though this type of call throws the appointment book into confusion, showing irritation with the patient will not help the situation. Make a sincere effort to help the caller make a new appointment.

STATEMENTS

THE CALL: "I received my statement this morning, and I don't understand why it is so high."

THE ANSWER: If billing matters are handled by another employee, tell the patient that you will transfer his or her call to the billing office. If you are responsible for billing, politely *ask the patient to hold the line* while you pull the patient ledger. When you return to the line, *thank the patient* for waiting and *explain the charges* carefully. If there is an error, apologize and say a corrected statement will be sent out at once. *Thank the patient for calling.* If patients are properly advised about charges at the time that services are rendered, the number of these calls will be considerably reduced.

PRESCRIPTION REFILL

THE CALL: "The last time I had an office visit, the doctor gave me a prescription for some sleeping tablets. Please call the druggist and okay a refill."

THE ANSWER: Ask the patient for the *prescription number and date,* the *name* and *telephone number of the pharmacy,* and the *patient's phone number.* Explain that you will give the message to the physician as soon as possible. Pull the patient's chart and have it ready with the message when the physician is available. If the physician okays the refill, you may be asked to phone the pharmacy and the patient with the information.

PHYSICIAN "SHOPPING"

THE CALL: "Does the doctor treat stomach trouble?"

THE ANSWER: The answer depends on the physician's field of practice. Many people do not understand the various medical specialties, and this call may come from a person referred to the physician by a friend who did not explain that your physician is an orthopedist. In situations in which your physician would be unable to handle the case, you may have to refer the patient to another physician. Give the patient the *names of at least three physicians,* when possible; these should be only names that your employer has had you place on the referral list. Do not presume to make a diagnosis when a patient calls in with bizarre complaints; transfer the call to the physician or take the caller's name and number and have the physician return the call later.

UNAUTHORIZED INQUIRY

THE CALL: "My next-door neighbor is a patient of the doctor's, and I am quite concerned about her. Could you tell me what is wrong with her?"

THE ANSWER: Confidentiality is a legal and ethical issue here. It is not the role of the medical assistant to give out any information about a patient's condition, except information that the physician has specifically okayed for release. The caller in this case may be merely curious or may actually be a kindly neighbor who wishes to help a friend. Your possible response might be

"I'm unable to answer your question because information about a patient cannot be released without that person's authorization. I will relay your message of concern to the doctor if you wish."

Telephone Answering Services

Because a physician's telephone is an all-important tool of the practice, it must be constantly *covered;* that is, there must be someone to answer it at all times—day and night, weekends and holidays. This presents no problem during weekdays, but nights and weekends require special attention. Most physicians subscribe to telephone answering services that provide round-the-clock coverage. Alternatively, the physician may use an automatic answering device.

OPERATOR-ANSWERED SERVICES

There are two types of operator-answered services.

Type 1

Doctor-subscribers leave messages with, or obtain patients' messages from, a service whose number appears in the local telephone directory in this way,

After ____ PM, call ____ (number) *or*
If no answer, call ________ (number).

Such listings are placed immediately below the physician's own telephone number in the directory. This form of service is somewhat inconvenient for the patient but is far better than no coverage at all.

Type 2

The answering service has a direct connection with the office telephone. When the telephone rings in the physician's office or at home, it also signals on the switchboard of the answering service. As long as the telephone is ringing, it will continue to signal at the answering service. If no one answers within a certain agreed-on number of rings, the answering service operator takes the call. This method provides continuous live telephone coverage.

Even during the day, such an answering service can function effectively. There may be times when you are assisting the physician and it is impossible for you or anyone else to answer the telephone. Not answering the telephone is extremely poor policy, but if you have an agreement with the answering service (sometimes referred to as "the exchange"), its operators will accept calls for you in such situations. With this direct-wire answering method, the operator answers the telephone in your employer's name, as you would in the office, explaining "This is Dr. Wilson's exchange. May I take a message?"

The answering service will greatly appreciate your cooperation if you call them every day before leaving the office and tell them where the physician will be during the evening or give them other special messages. Then, in the morning when you return to the office, call the exchange and ask for any messages they may have taken. Usually there will be messages from patients who called after office hours but whose calls were not urgent enough to merit an emergency call to the doctor. An exchange can act as a buffer for the physician and help eliminate too frequent, unnecessary calls during the late evening or night hours.

Here is how the system works: During the hours that the office is closed, the exchange will answer the telephone, take a message, and relay it to the physician. If it is urgent, the physician will then return the call to the patient; if not, the exchange will call the patient and explain that the physician will call the first thing in the morning. Emergency calls, of course, are immediately put through by the exchange to the doctor.

Occasionally, it is a good idea to check up on your answering service by placing a few random calls at various hours. It may be that now and then the service does not answer the calls or the response may not meet your standards. The service may be enhanced by inviting the manager of the answering service in to see the office or by the medical assistant going to the exchange facility to meet with the manager and staff. This personal contact frequently improves the rapport and quality of service you may expect.

ELECTRONIC ANSWERING DEVICES

Some physicians use an answering device after office hours. Callers who dial the office number hear a recorded message either telling them how to reach the physician (or a colleague who may be covering the practice) or inviting the caller to leave a message. The caller's message is recorded for later checking by the physician or a staff member.

Most electronic answering devices are equipped with remote control to allow the subscriber to operate them from any Touch-Tone telephone. By using a personal code number, it is possible to

- Retrieve messages, including the times at which they were recorded
- Reset the tape for future messages
- Change the outgoing message when necessary

VOICE MAIL

Voice mail is a computer system that operates much like the answering devices that we have incorporated into our home telephone systems. In large facilities it is an integral part of the private system. For individuals or small groups voice mail is available by subscribing to a service. By dialing a personal code, the subscriber can record, send, or receive messages.

AUTOMATIC ROUTING

The call is answered by an automated operator that presents a list of options, such as *If you are calling about your account, push 1; to make an appointment, push 2;* and so forth. The impersonal nature of automation does not lend itself well to answering the telephone in a private physician's office, but the medical assistant will encounter it frequently when placing outgoing calls.

Placing Outgoing Calls

PREPLANNING THE CALL

Before placing a call, make certain you have the correct telephone number and the information you will need during the call at your fingertips.

If you are reporting a patient's history, have the complete record before you, including all the latest laboratory and radiology reports.

If you are placing a call to order supplies, have the catalog in front of you, along with any previous order sheets or invoices. Also have a list of the items desired, the specifications for the items, and any questions you may have regarding them.

Apply this rule to every call you make. You will save a great deal of time and prevent errors.

PLACING THE CALL

Lift the receiver, listen for the dial tone, and then start dialing your number. It sometimes happens that just as you pick up the telephone to place a call, an incoming call has reached your line but you lifted the receiver before the telephone had time to ring. If you start dialing without listening for the dial tone, you will not only fail to reach your number, you will have offended the ear of the party trying to reach you.

CALLING ETIQUETTE

When placing a call, at your employer's request, to a patient or any other person, your physician should be ready to speak as soon as the call goes through. Physicians, because of their busy schedules, sometimes are negligent in this respect. The telephone company's courtesy rule is that the person placing the call should be on the line and ready to speak when the called party answers.

If you are calling a patient to change an appointment, be ready to offer a new appointment time. Also, give the patient a logical reason for the inconvenience of having to change the original appointment. This change may cause considerable disruption of plans, and the patient is fully entitled to an explanation.

Remember that if your telephone is within hearing range of office patients, you should be careful when mentioning names or diagnoses.

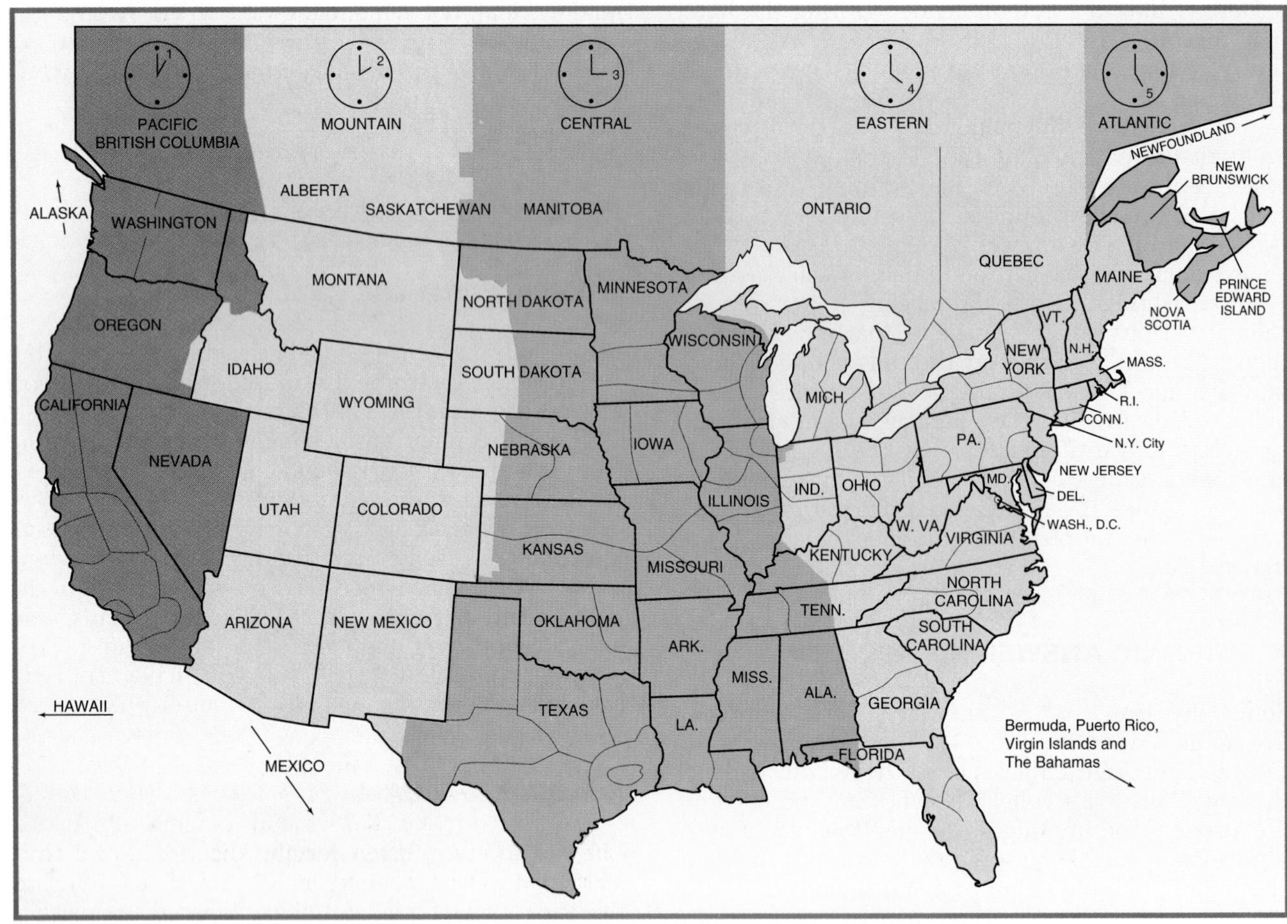

FIGURE 9–7 Time zones across the United States.

LONG DISTANCE SERVICE

Long distance calls are simple to place, inexpensive, and efficient. When information is needed in a hurry, it is much more expedient to telephone rather than wait for an exchange of letters.

Before placing a long distance call, have the correct number ready. This number often may be obtained from a letterhead or from other records. If you do not have the number, you may obtain directory assistance by dialing the area code of the party you are calling, followed by 555-1212. In some areas you must dial 1 before the area code. Directory assistance is now an automated service and you will be asked for the name of the city and the person you are calling.

TIME ZONES

The continental United States is divided into four standard time zones: Pacific, Mountain, Central, and Eastern (Fig. 9–7). When it is noon Pacific time, it is 3 PM Eastern time. If you are calling from San Francisco to New York, you will probably plan to make the call no later than 2 PM when calling a business or professional office. When it is 2 PM on the West Coast it is 5 PM on the East Coast.

DIALING DIRECT

By dialing your own long distance calls, you will pay the lowest rate and pay for only the minutes you talk (minimum, 1 minute). Use direct dialing when you are willing to talk with anyone who answers the phone and you want the call charged to the number from which you are calling.

OPERATOR-ASSISTED CALLS

Operator-assisted calls include calls such as

- Person-to-person
- Bill to a third party
- Collect calls
- Requests for time and charges
- Certain calls placed from hotels

There is a 1-minute initial period charge through most servers. The rates are equal to the direct-dial rates plus a service charge.

INTERNATIONAL SERVICE

International Direct Distance Dialing (IDDD) is available in many areas. International dialing codes are the same for all companies offering IDDD. Depending on your long distance company, additional numbers or codes may preface the international access, country, and city codes. IDDD is still not available in all areas. If it is available, you may place international station-to-station calls by dialing in sequence

1. International Code 011
2. Country Code
3. City Code
4. Local telephone number
5. # button if your telephone is Touch-Tone

If you were to place a call to London you would dial:

International Access Code		Country Code		City Code
011	+	44	+	1

plus the local telephone number and # if Touch-Tone dialing

After dialing any international code, allow at least 45 seconds for the ringing to start.

WRONG NUMBERS

One slip in direct distance dialing can give you Los Angeles or New York instead of Dallas. If you reach a wrong number when dialing long distance, be sure to obtain the name of the city and state you have reached. By reporting this information promptly to the operator in your own city, you will not be charged for the call. If you are cut off before terminating your call, this, too, should be reported to the operator, who will either reconnect your call or make an adjustment of the charge.

CONFERENCE CALLS

Conference telephone service is of great value to the medical profession in notifying and explaining to a family how a patient is progressing. It has exceptional value in family conferences, at which a quick decision by the entire family regarding a patient's condition is required.

This service can connect from 3 to 14 points for a two-way conference in which each person can hear or talk to all others participating. Conference calls may be local or long distance. Charges are added for the number of places connected, mileage, and the length of the conversation.

To place a call, dial the operator and say you wish to make a conference call. Give the operator the names and telephone numbers of the people you want to connect. If prior arrangements are made with all parties, there is a better chance of reaching everyone at a given time.

Telephone Equipment and Services

NUMBER AND PLACEMENT OF TELEPHONES

Familiarity with a multiple-line telephone is a must for the medical assistant. Few health care facilities can get along with just one telephone line. Two incoming lines along with a private outgoing line with a separate number for the physician's exclusive use is the minimum recommended.

One medical assistant can handle no more than two incoming lines, so the addition of more lines may also involve additional staffing. If there is a staff member assigned solely to dealing with insurance and billing, a separate line and listing in the telephone directory for this service may considerably lessen the load on the main incoming lines.

Telephones should be placed where they are accessible but private. Rather than placing telephones in the examining rooms, many practices have a wall telephone placed near a stand-up desk top outside the examining room. Some facilities place a telephone in the reception room for the convenience of patients and to prevent their asking to use the facility's phones.

Recent trends suggest a separate telephone line with a limited calling area for the convenience of patients who need to call out. This telephone should not be in the reception room but in an area available to patients on request. It should be placed low enough for use by patients in wheelchairs. Wherever possible, telephones should be placed on the wall to conserve desk space.

EQUIPMENT SELECTION

Selection of telephone equipment and services offers many options. The *six-button key set* with several incoming lines, an intercom line, and a hold button has been the standard business phone for decades. It is still being used in many offices. Lights within the buttons flash slowly for incoming calls and blink rapidly to remind of calls being held; a steady light indicates that the line is in use.

A popular modern system is the two-line speaker phone that has distinctive ringing and flashing indicators that let you know which line is receiving a call. It also has other features, including:

- Last number redial
- Volume control on the receiver, ringer, and speaker

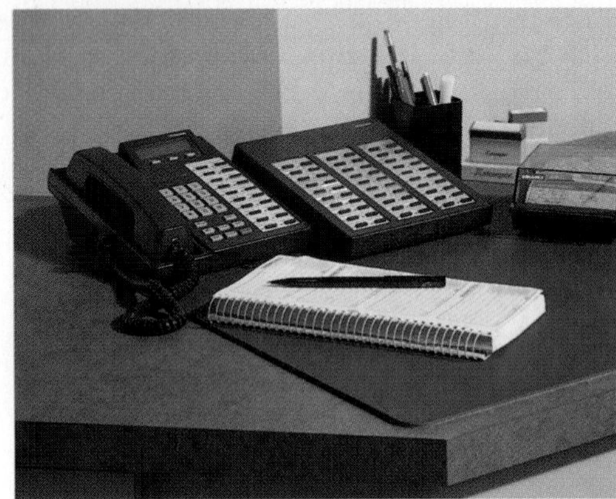

FIGURE 9–8 Multi-line telephone.

- Memory for frequently dialed numbers
- Intercom paging

Another available feature, *ring back on HOLD,* allows the caller who dials a busy number to place it on hold. When the called line is free, the connection is completed and the caller is reminded.

Larger facilities tend to select small switchboard-type equipment. One system can start with as few as 2 lines and 6 extensions and expand to a maximum of 8 outside lines and 24 extensions (Fig. 9–8).

HEADSETS

A popular headset is a very lightweight plastic earphone and microphone combination that allows the wearer to move about the room and to have the hands free. One brand name is StarSet. Originally designed for the astronauts, it weighs less than 1 ounce and is worn behind the ear or clipped to the wearer's glasses. The headset can be equipped with a cord up to 10 feet long for easy mobility. It also has an optional quick-disconnect feature that allows the user to separate the headset even during a call without breaking the connection.

FACSIMILE (FAX) MACHINES

A FAX machine can be a great time and labor saver in conveying patient information from physician to physician or from physician to hospital. It allows its user to send and receive copies of printed documents over telephone lines to other facilities that have FAX machines. Most offices find this machine indispensable. Unless precautions are taken to ensure security of information arriving by FAX, there is some danger of loss of confidentiality. When sending sensitive material it is wise to telephone ahead to alert the receiver that this information will be arriving so that the appropriate person will be on hand to receive it (Fig. 9–9).

CELLULAR PHONES AND PAGERS

Many physicians have a mobile phone installed in their automobiles for communication with their office or the hospital while they are traveling by car. Most carry a personal pager that can be activated by the medical assistant or the answering service by calling a special number.

Using the Telephone Directory

The primary purpose of the telephone directory, of course, is to provide lists of those who have telephones, their telephone numbers, and, in most cases, their addresses. Additionally, the directory is an aid in checking the spelling of names and in locating certain types of businesses (through the yellow pages). Some directories are color coded (e.g., residences are on white pages, business numbers on pink pages, business by categories and advertisements on yellow pages). Directories are usually organized into three sections:

- Introductory pages
- Alphabetical pages (white pages)
- Yellow pages

The introductory pages are sometimes entirely overlooked by the subscribers. This section precedes the white alphabetic pages and provides basic information concerning the telephone services in the area, including

- Emergency services (fire, police, ambulance, and highway patrol)
- Service calls
- Dialing instructions for local and out-of-town calls
- Area codes for some cities

The introductory pages may also include

- A survival guide
- Community service numbers
- Prefix locations

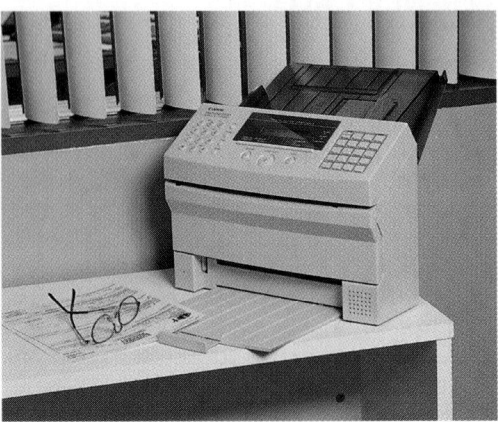

FIGURE 9–9 Facsimile machine.

- Rates
- Long distance calling information
- International calling information
- Time zones
- Government listings

Some directories include ZIP code maps for the local area. Take a few moments to familiarize yourself with your local directory; then use it frequently for getting information fast.

The white pages are an alphabetical listing of telephone subscribers with their telephone numbers and, in most cases, their addresses.

The yellow pages directory, sometimes published separately, contains listings for businesses arranged by the product or services they sell. Physicians are listed alphabetically, usually under the heading *Physicians and Surgeons,* and have the option of another listing by type of practice.

In some metropolitan areas, a street address telephone directory is published that is arranged by street address, followed by the name and telephone number of the person or business at that address.

Organizing a Personal Telephone Directory

Organize your telephone numbers in an indexed 3 × 5-inch desktop file or a rotary file. Emergency numbers might be typed on a colored card or flagged with a color tab. Your personal directory of telephone numbers should include all the numbers that you frequently call.

FREQUENTLY CALLED NUMBERS

- Specialists to whom your employer refers patients
- Professional facilities, such as hospitals, the Poison Control Center, pharmacies, ambulance companies, and laboratories
- Special duty nurses, along with their specialties and other pertinent information
- Administrative contacts, such as stationers, equipment dealers and repair services, laundry and maintenance services, and surgical supply houses
- Personal numbers, such as the physician's family, special friends, insurance agent, stockbroker, accountant, and lawyer

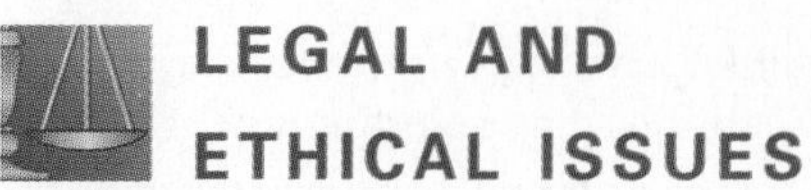

LEGAL AND ETHICAL ISSUES

Use discretion when mentioning the name of a caller. All communications in a health care facility are confidential. Discourage personal phone calls. Encourage friends and family to call you at home. When answering an incoming call, identify the facility and then yourself. Transfer calls from other physicians at once if possible. If you are requested to furnish names of other specialists, refer these requests to the physician unless you have been given a list of preferred practitioners from which to choose. When a patient calls for results of a test, the physician should be the one to inform the patient unless you have been given permission to do so. Never give unfavorable results to a patient over the telephone.

CRITICAL THINKING

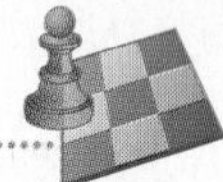

1 Develop a dialogue for responding to a telephone call from a patient who is complaining about a fee.

2 Use a situation to illustrate the meaning of triage.

HOW DID I DO? Answers to Memory Joggers

1. Smile
2. Seven of these 12 rules:
   Answer promptly.
   Visualize the persons to whom you are speaking.
   Hold the instrument correctly.
   Develop a pleasing telephone voice.
   Identify your office and yourself.
   Identify the caller.
   Offer assistance.
   Screen incoming calls.
   Minimize waiting time.
   Identify the caller when transferring a call.
   When answering a second call, identify the caller, then return to the first call.
   End each call pleasantly and graciously.
3. One minute
4. Name of person to whom call is directed
   Name of the person calling
   Caller's daytime telephone number
   Reason for the call
   Action to be taken
   Date and time of the call
   Your initials
5. New patient and return appointments
   Inquiries about bills
   Inquiries about fees
   Requests for insurance assistance
   Radiology and laboratory reports
   Satisfactory progress reports from patients
   Routine reports from hospitals and other sources
   Office administration matters
   Requests for referrals
   Prescription refills

Appointment Scheduling and Time Management

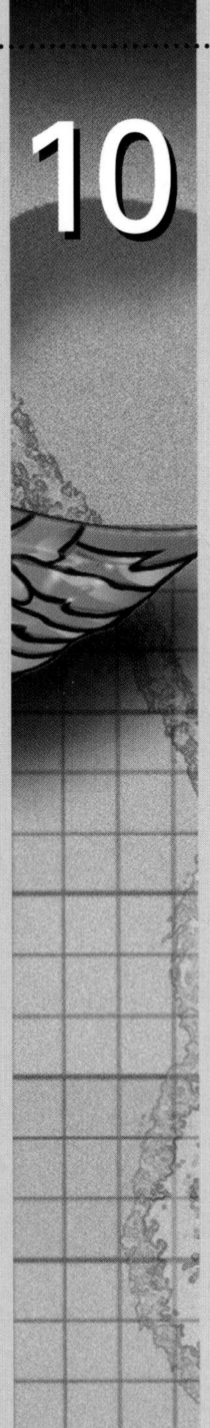

OUTLINE

LEARNING OBJECTIVES

Cognitive: On successful completion of this chapter, you should be able to:

1. Define and spell the terms listed in the Vocabulary.
2. Describe four important features of an appointment book.
3. List and explain the three basic guidelines to follow in scheduling appointments.
4. Identify and discuss the advantages of wave scheduling.
5. Cite three common situations that would require adjusting the appointment schedule.
6. Describe how you would determine whether a request for an appointment is an emergency.
7. State the reason for recording a failed appointment in the patient's chart.

8 Discuss the handling of cancellations and delays brought about by office situations.
9 List the seven points of information that will be necessary in scheduling surgery with a hospital.
10 State four items of information that must be available before arranging an outside laboratory appointment for a patient.

Performance: On successful completion of this chapter, you should be able to:

1 Select an appropriate appointment book to suit a given type of practice.
2 Demonstrate the advance preparation that must be done before using a new appointment book.
3 Schedule patients according to the urgency of their complaints and the anticipated treatment time.
4 Rearrange the schedule in the event that the physician's arrival is delayed.
5 Explain the physician's unavailability to patients in the reception room.
6 Arrange a referral appointment for a patient.
7 Schedule a patient for a diagnostic test as indicated by the physician.
8 Schedule a surgery with the hospital, notifying all the persons and departments concerned.
9 Instruct a patient regarding preadmission requirements, hospital stay, and insurance information needed.
10 Arrange for a patient's admission to a hospital as ordered by the physician.

VOCABULARY

disruption A breaking down or upset

expediency A situation requiring haste or caution

integral Essential; being an indispensable part of a whole

interaction A two-way communication

intermittent Coming and going at intervals, not continuous

matrix Something in which something else originates, develops, takes shape, or is contained; a base upon which to build

no-show A person who fails to keep an appointment without giving advance notice of that failure

proficiency Competency as a result of training and practice

socioeconomic Relating to a combination of social and economic factors

stat report An immediate report (from the Latin *statim,* meaning "at once"

tickler (file) A chronologic file used as a reminder that something must be taken care of on a certain date

triage Responding to requests for immediate care and treatment after evaluating the urgency of the need and prioritizing the treatment

The most valuable asset within a medical practice is the physician's time. It follows that the person who schedules this time must understand the practice, be familiar with the working habits of the physicians, and have clear guidelines for time management within the practice.

Management of Office Hours

Appointment scheduling is the process that determines which patients will be seen by the physician, dates and times of the appointments, and how much time will be allotted to each patient based on his or her complaint and the practitioner's availability. Time management involves the realization that there will always be unforeseen interruptions and delays. Most providers of medical care find that efficient scheduling of appointments is one of the most important factors in the success of the practice. There are many approaches to scheduling and each facility must find what suits it best.

OPEN OFFICE HOURS

Few health care facilities in metropolitan areas have open office hours with no *scheduled* appointments, but this system is still found in some rural areas, where the way of life is governed not so much by the clock as by the sun and the seasons. With *open office hours*, the facility is open at given hours of the day or evening, and the patients are "scheduled" by the physician or the medical assistant by saying something such as, "Come back in a couple of weeks." At a convenient time, the patients come in, knowing in advance that they will be seen in their order of arrival. Physicians who use this method say that it eliminates the annoyance of broken appointments and of the office "running late." The open office hours method has been referred to as *tidal wave scheduling*. There can be many disadvantages to open office hours:

- The office may already be crowded when the physician arrives, resulting in extremely long waits for some patients.
- There is danger of rushing some patients through without giving them full attention.
- Few, or possibly no, patients will arrive before noon, and both the physician and the staff will need to stay late to accommodate everyone.
- Without planning, the facilities as well as the staff can be overburdened.

Other types of practices that have open hours are emergency centers, many of which are open on a 24-hour basis. Although they are frequently referred to as "emergicenters," they may in reality deal with many general practice types of care.

SCHEDULED APPOINTMENTS

Studies have shown that practitioners are able to see more patients with less pressure when their appointments are scheduled. If appointments are made by telephone, that first telephone interaction creates the patient's impression of the practice (Fig. 10–1). Unfortunately, the skill required for the scheduling of appointments is often not fully appreciated by the practitioner or practice manager, resulting in this responsibility being delegated to perhaps the least qualified medical assistant. But while the skill and attitude of the assistant who manages the appointment schedule is very important, the ultimate success of the system lies in the cooperation of the practitioner(s).

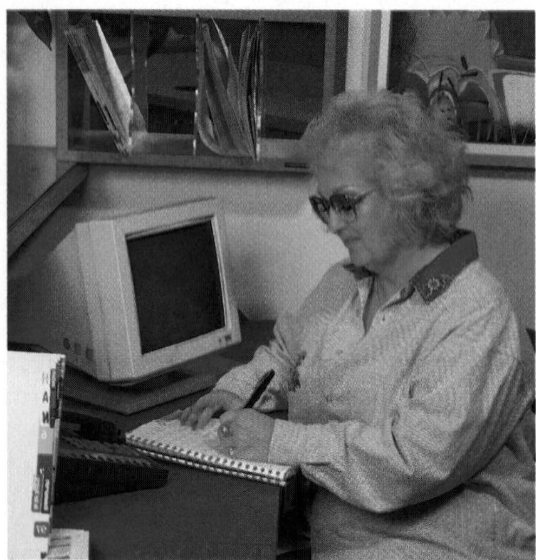

FIGURE 10–1 Receptionist with appointment book.

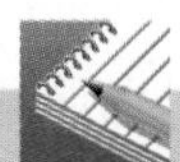

SKILLS AND RESPONSIBILITIES

GUIDELINES FOR EFFICIENT SCHEDULING

Understand the nature of the practice.

Consider the personality and habits of the medical staff.

Be aware of the time needed for each patient.

The key to planning appointments efficiently is planning realistically.

Scheduling with this in mind (1) pleases the patients, (2) results in economic gain, and (3) ensures a more regular schedule for the staff and the physicians.

FLEXIBLE OFFICE HOURS

Most scheduling practices are carryovers from the days when expectant mothers or families with young children relied on one wage earner—the father. Today, families commonly have two working parents. As a result, many health care providers, especially family practice, pediatricians, obstetricians, gynecologists, and ophthalmologists, are turning to *extended-day* and *flexible office hours*. Staff hours are affected by these changes.

EXAMPLE OF A FACILITY'S SCHEDULE	
Monday	7 AM–3 PM
Tuesday	8 AM–5 PM
Wednesday	8 AM–5 PM
Thursday	NOON–8 PM
Friday	8 AM–5 PM

Evening and weekend hours are frequently scheduled, as well. With a schedule such as this, a variety of options are made available to patients.

Memory Jogger

Why is efficient scheduling of patient appointments so important? What one factor most influences the success of the scheduling?

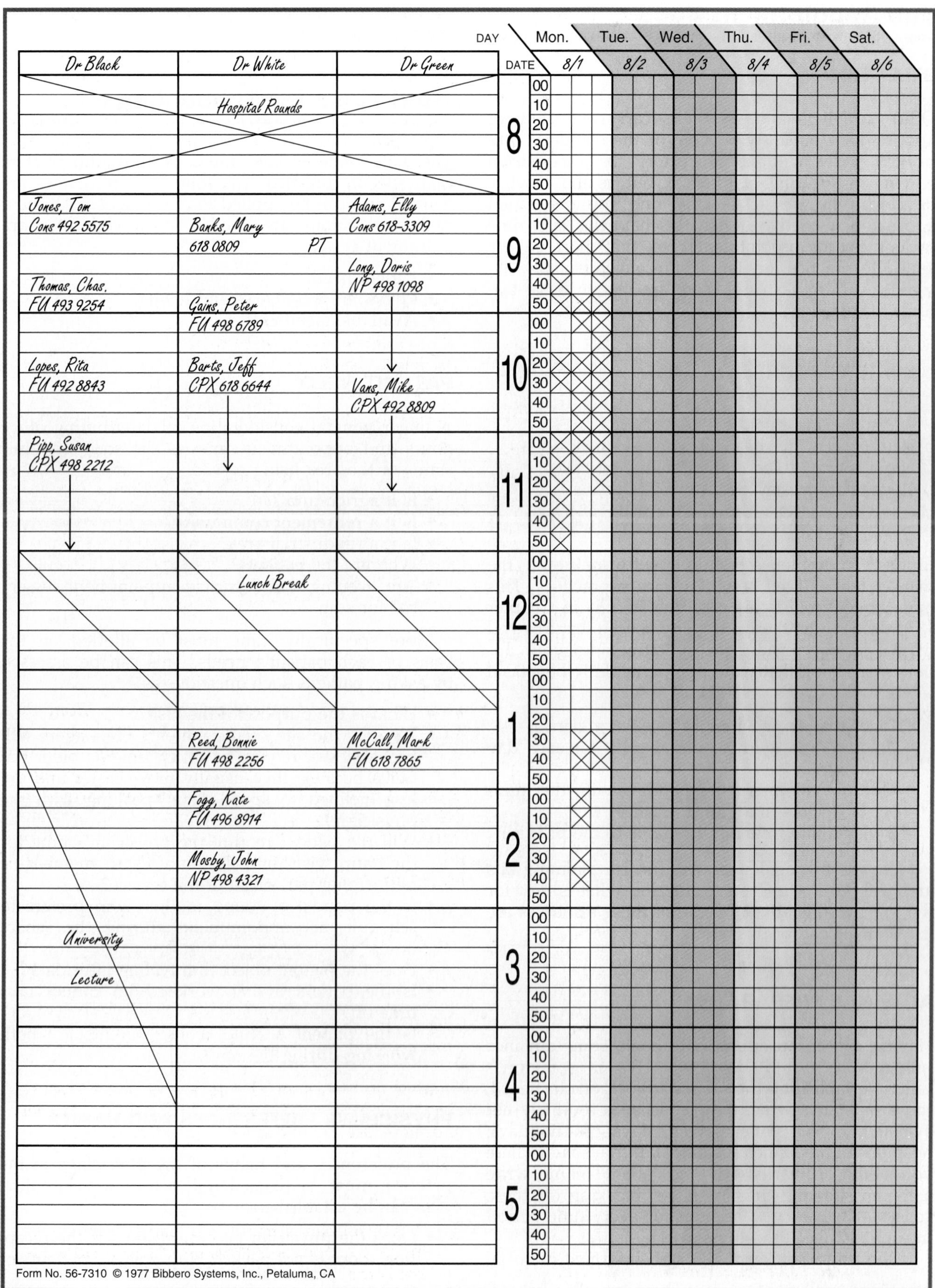

DAY	Mon.	Tue.	Wed.	Thu.	Fri.	Sat.
DATE	8/1	8/2	8/3	8/4	8/5	8/6

Time	Dr Black	Dr White	Dr Green
8 00–50		Hospital Rounds	
9 00	Jones, Tom		Adams, Elly
9 10	Cons 492 5575	Banks, Mary	Cons 618-3309
9 20		618 0809 PT	
9 30			Long, Doris
9 40	Thomas, Chas.		NP 498 1098
9 50	FU 493 9254	Gains, Peter	
10 00		FU 498 6789	
10 20	Lopes, Rita	Barts, Jeff	
10 30	FU 492 8843	CPX 618 6644	Vans, Mike
10 40			CPX 492 8809
11 00	Pipp, Susan		
11 10	CPX 498 2212		
12 10		Lunch Break	
1 30		Reed, Bonnie	McCall, Mark
1 40		FU 498 2256	FU 618 7865
2 00		Fogg, Kate	
2 10		FU 496 8914	
2 30		Mosby, John	
2 40		NP 498 4321	
3 10	University		
3 30	Lecture		

Form No. 56-7310 © 1977 Bibbero Systems, Inc., Petaluma, CA

FIGURE 10–2 Sample appointment book. (Courtesy of Bibbero Systems, Inc., Petaluma, California, (800) 242-2376, Fax (800) 242-9330.)

The Appointment Book

SELECTION

Office suppliers and stationers carry a variety of appointment book styles. One of the standard preprinted styles will be satisfactory for a physician who is just starting a practice, but as the practice develops, the physician may find the preprinted books too restrictive. When this happens, it is time to look for an appointment book that more closely suits the practice, or, failing this, to personally design one. In either case, there are certain basic features to consider.

BASIC FEATURES OF AN APPOINTMENT BOOK

Size conforms to the desk space available
Large enough to accommodate the practice
Opens flat for easy writing and reference
Allows space for writing when, who, and why

Efficient computer scheduling software is on the market that is well suited to larger practices. This management tool is discussed more fully in Chapter 13. Additionally, there are many special features you may want to consider incorporating into your appointment book that would be particularly beneficial to your employer's practice.

- Pages that show an entire week at a glance
- Color coding, with a special color for each day of the week
- Multiple columns corresponding with the number of doctors in a group practice
- Division into time units suitable to the practice

Many professional stationers furnish planning kits and will work with you to develop what is best for the practice (Fig. 10–2). Some of these resources are listed at the end of this book.

ADVANCE PREPARATION

Having chosen an appropriate book, some advance preparation should be done. This is sometimes called "establishing the matrix." Block off, in pencil, those time slots when the physician is routinely not available to see patients (e.g., days off, holidays, hospital rounds, lunch meetings). In the space where you would ordinarily write the patient's name, write a memo showing the reason for blocking off these spaces. Always try to account for every time period in each day (see Procedure 10–1).

If the physician keeps the staff informed of social or family engagements, also make a note of these on the appointment book as a reminder.

Guidelines for Scheduling

The scheduling system must be individualized to each specific practice. The following guidelines are general and can be applied to any practice. All these recommendations are similar for a computer appointment system.

- Patient need
- Physician preferences and habits
- Available facilities

PATIENT NEED

A major general consideration in determining office hours and appointment times is the socioeconomic status of the area being served.

- Is it agricultural?
- Is it a retirement community?
- Is it an industrial area?
- Who are the patients?
- Are evening and Saturday appointments essential for some?

More specifically, time must be allotted on the basis of each patient's needs. This can be assessed by asking patients such questions as

- What is the purpose of the visit?
- What is the age of the patient? (Teenagers will probably not require as much time as older patients because they usually move faster and are less inclined to spend time speaking with the physician.)
- Will the patient require the physician's time for the entire visit, or will another staff member be performing part or all of the service?
- Is the patient a young mother who prefers to schedule her appointments during the school hours?
- Does the patient object to traveling after dark?
- Is the patient a day worker who cannot take time off?
- Is the patient a child whose parents are both working during the day?

PHYSICIAN'S PREFERENCES AND HABITS

The preferences and habits of the physicians in the practice must be considered before a scheduling plan can be established.

- Does the physician become restless if the reception room is not packed with waiting patients or

PROCEDURE 10 – 1

Preparing and Maintaining the Appointment Book

GOAL

To establish the matrix of the appointment page, arrange appointments for 1 day, and enter information according to office policy

EQUIPMENT AND SUPPLIES

Page from appointment book
Office policy for office hours, and doctor' availability
Clerical supplies
Calendar
Description of patients to be scheduled

PROCEDURAL STEPS

1 Determine the hours that the physician will not be available.
PURPOSE: To block out those hours on the appointment page.

2 Establish the matrix of the appointment page for the day.
PURPOSE: To leave available only those time slots that can be used for patient appointments.

3 Identify each patient's complaint.
PURPOSE: This information is necessary in allotting time and space for the appointment.

4 Consult guidelines to determine the length of time necessary for each patient.

5 Allot appointment time according to the complaint and facilities available.

6 Enter information in the appointment book.
NOTE: A telephone number must follow the patient's name. If the patient is new, add the letters N.P. (new patient) after his or her name.

7 Allow buffer time in the morning and afternoon.
PURPOSE: To allow the physician and staff a short rest period and catch-up time.

does the physician worry if even one patient is kept waiting?

- Is the physician methodical and careful about being in the facility when patient appointments are scheduled to begin, or is the physician habitually late?
- Does the physician move easily from one patient to the next, or does the physician require a "break time" between patients?
- Would the physician rather see fewer patients and spend more time with each one?

All of these preferences and habits become an **integral** part of the scheduling process.

Keep in mind that the physician cannot spend every moment of the day with patients. There are telephone calls to make and receive, reports to examine and dictate, meetings to attend, mail to answer, and many other business items that require the physician's attention. The experienced staff can handle many, but not all, of these tasks.

AVAILABLE FACILITIES

There is no point in getting a patient into the office at a time when no facilities are available for the services needed. For example, suppose that in a two-physician office there is only one room that can be used for minor surgery. You would not schedule two patients requiring minor surgery for the same time block even though both doctors could be available. If there is only one electrocardiograph, you would not book two electrocardiograms at the same time. As you gain proficiency in scheduling, you should be able to pair patients' needs with the available facilities.

Memory Jogger

What are the three basic guidelines that determine the system of scheduling? Why are they important?

APPOINTMENT TIME ANALYSIS				
NAME	ARRIVED	BEGIN TREATMENT	END TREATMENT	SERVICE CODE

SUMMARY		
SERVICE	AVERAGE WAITING TIME	AVERAGE TREATMENT TIME

FIGURE 10–3 Form for determining appointment pattern.

Planning a Time Pattern

The physician is the person who should decide how much time each type of visit usually requires, and an estimated time schedule should be posted at the appointment desk. The physician who has been in practice for years knows how much time he or she needs for the various kinds of office visits: complete physical, presurgery workup, well-child visit, eye examination, and so forth. However, because a physician's timing does change through the years owing to experience or changes in the practice, an annual review of the scheduling pattern should be made to accommodate these changes as well as changes in the patient profile.

It may be that a time pattern has never been determined. The medical assistant can do the preliminary work on this through an informal practice analysis, noting the arrival time, treatment or conference time, departure time, and service performed (Fig. 10–3). After a few weeks, a definite time pattern should be distinguishable for each type of service. When possible, smooth out the schedule by having some long and some short appointments and go over the schedule with the physician at the beginning of each day.

BUFFER TIME

Every medical practice should have at least one, or preferably two, appointment slots open each day. These slots are usually referred to as *buffer time.* Family practitioners may leave as much as 25% of their time open for emergencies and walk-in patients. Many find that reserving one time slot at the end of the morning and one at the end of the afternoon works well and causes the least **disruption** of a schedule.

Time studies have shown that in the average medical practice, Mondays and Fridays are the most hectic days of the week. Patients may have waited the whole weekend to call for an appointment and expect to be seen immediately on Monday. Similarly, toward the end of the week, small problems that could magnify if left unattended over the weekend may prompt anxious emergencies on Friday. Consequently, incorporating more buffer time on these 2 days can be worthwhile.

Time Management

WAVE SCHEDULING

Many scheduling systems lack flexibility. *Wave scheduling* is an attempt to include short-term flexibility within each hour by allowing for such variables as

- Late arrival of one patient
- A patient who needs more time or less time than expected
- Failed appointments
- Unscheduled interruptions

When all patients are assigned the same length of time, for instance, 20 minutes each, the schedule might look like this:

EXAMPLE OF WAVE SCHEDULING APPOINTMENTS EVERY 20 MINUTES

10:00 Barker, Alicia
10:20 Davies, Colleen
10:40 Farber, Edna
11:00 Havens, Gertrude
11:20 Jackson, Irene
11:40 Lambert, Katherine

Barker, the first patient is late, arriving at 10:15. The physician has already lost 15 minutes. The patient needs 25 minutes instead of the allotted 20 minutes.

Davies, the second patient, also arrived at 10:15, five minutes early for her appointment, but is kept waiting until 10:40, the time that Farber, the third patient, was to have been seen.

Farber is on time but will also be kept waiting. Fortunately, Davies actually needs only 10 minutes, so Farber can be seen at 10:50, but if she requires the allotted 20 minutes, Havens, the fourth patient, will also have to wait, and so on throughout the day.

Wave scheduling assumes that the actual time needed will average out. If the average time is 20 minutes per patient, three patients will be scheduled for each hour and will be seen in order of arrival. Thus, one person's late arrival will not disrupt the entire schedule. The appointment schedule would then look like this:

EXAMPLE OF WAVE SCHEDULING AVERAGING OUT

10:00 Barker, Alicia
Davies, Colleen
Farber, Edna
11:00 Havens, Gertrude
Jackson, Irene
Lambert, Katherine

Given the circumstances illustrated above, Davies would have arrived first (5 minutes early), Farber would be next (on time), and Barker would be third (15 minutes late). All could have been seen within the hour, with no delay affecting the patients scheduled for the next hour.

MODIFIED WAVE SCHEDULING

There are several ways of modifying the wave schedule. One method is to have two patients scheduled to come in at 10:00 and the third at 10:30, with this hourly cycle repeated throughout the day. Another application is to have patients scheduled to arrive at given intervals during the first half of the hour, and none scheduled to arrive during the second half of the hour.

DOUBLE BOOKING

Booking two patients to come in at the same time, both of whom are to be seen by the physician, is poor practice. Of course, if each is expected to take only 5 minutes or so, there is no harm in telling both to come at 2:00 and in reserving a 15-minute period for the two. This is one application of wave scheduling. However, if each patient requires 15 minutes, two will require 30 minutes; this should be reflected in the scheduling. It is not considered double booking if a patient comes to the office to receive a treatment or injection from a member of the staff other than the physician.

GROUPING PROCEDURES

Another method of time management that appeals to some practitioners is the grouping or *categorization* of procedures

EXAMPLES OF GROUPING CATEGORIES

An internist might reserve all morning appointments for complete physical examinations.

A surgeon whose practice depends on referrals might reserve 1 day of each week or specific hours of each day for referrals.

A pediatrician might have well-baby hours.

By experimenting with different groupings, the plan that works best for the practice will eventually become evident. In applying a grouping system of appointments, the medical assistant may find it helpful to lightly color-code those sections of the appointment book being reserved for special procedures.

ADVANCE BOOKING

When booking appointments weeks or months ahead, make it a policy to leave some open time during each day's schedule. Then, if a patient calls with a special problem that is not an immediate emergency, you will be able to book the patient for at least a brief visit. A busy physician will always be able to fill these open slots, and the patients will appreciate being able to book an appointment within a reasonable time when the circumstances warrant it. Some authorities recommend that appointments not be scheduled more than 3 months in advance.

If possible, set aside time in the morning and afternoon for a *breather,* or work break. Even 15 minutes will give the physician an opportunity to return calls from patients, verify prescription calls, or answer questions you may have that were not an emergency.

Details of Arranging Appointments

ARRANGEMENTS BY TELEPHONE

It is as important for the medical assistant to express pleasantness and a desire to be helpful when using the telephone as it is when meeting patients face to face. This is especially essential in the arranging of appointments. It is often the manner in which the booking is made rather than the convenience of the appointment time that makes a lasting impression.

Be especially considerate if you must refuse an appointment for the time requested. Explain why and offer a substitute time and date. It should also be determined whether the patient has been in before and whether any necessary insurance information has been obtained. Comply with the patient's desires as much as possible and do not show annoyance if a patient is not understanding of the problems involved in scheduling appointments. Most people do appreciate the need for a well-managed office and are willing to cooperate.

End the conversation pleasantly with something like this:

> "Thank you for calling, Mrs. Albright. Dr. Wright will see you next Wednesday, August 28, at 2:30. Goodbye."

This little courtesy adds to the patient's feeling of esteem and additionally reinforces the time of the appointment. While you are saying this, you should be rechecking your appointment page to be certain that you have written it in the right time slot on the right day.

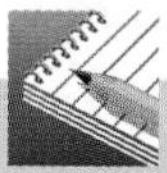

SKILLS AND RESPONSIBILITIES

PROFESSIONAL APPROACH TO TELEPHONE APPOINTMENTS

- Write legibly when making entries in the appointment book.
- Check off the patients' names as they arrive.
- Note any appointment failure or cancellations in ink on the appointment schedule.
- Always *immediately* write the patient's name in full, last name first, together with the reason for the appointment. *Do not trust the information to memory.*
- Reserve sufficient time for the appointment.
- Form the habit of entering the patient's daytime telephone number after every entry in the appointment book. It may become necessary to cancel or rearrange that day's schedule in a hurry, and many precious minutes can be saved if you have the telephone number handy.

APPOINTMENTS FOR NEW PATIENTS

Arranging the first appointment for a new patient requires time and attention to detail (see Procedure 10–2). At this first encounter you are, in a sense, extending a welcome to the practice. The patient will form a first impression of the office, of you, and of the physician from that first telephone contact. Tact and courtesy are extremely important.

ESSENTIAL QUESTIONS TO ASK WHEN SCHEDULING A NEW PATIENT

- Patient's full name (verify the spelling)
- Date of birth
- Complete address
- Daytime telephone number
- Pager number, if appropriate
- Source of referral, if any
- General type of examination required
- Insurance coverage, especially in a managed care practice

During this conversation request preliminary information to assist you in deciding how much time to allot on the appointment schedule. The physician may also expect you to give general instructions to patients seeking care for specific complaints; for example, to request the patient to bring in a urine specimen or to make certain that laboratory work is done before the appointment.

After you have recorded the necessary data, you may ask the patient, "Do you prefer morning or afternoon?" and then offer the first available date. Make certain that the patient knows where the office is located and, if necessary, how to get there. If there are special parking conveniences, tell the patient. Before concluding the conversation, repeat the appointment date and time agreed on and thank the person for calling.

If the appointment is several days away, mail to the patient a patient information brochure (see Chapter 24), a registration form, and a "welcome" letter. The brochure should provide advance information to the patient about the nature of the practice, introduce the medical staff, and explain appointment policies and financial arrangements.

If another physician has referred the patient, the medical assistant may need to call the referring physician's office and obtain additional information before the patient's appointment. This information should be printed out and given to the attending physician in advance of the patient's arrival.

In some offices, the medical assistant calls all patients the day before their appointment as a reminder. This takes time but can be done during slow periods, and many patients appreciate this service.

PROCEDURE 10–2
Scheduling a New Patient

GOAL
To schedule a new patient for a first office visit.

EQUIPMENT AND SUPPLIES
Appointment book
Scheduling guidelines
Appointment card
Telephone

PROCEDURAL STEPS
1 Obtain the patient's full name, birth date, address, and telephone number.
NOTE: Verify the spelling of the name.

2 Determine whether the patient was referred by another physician.
PURPOSE: You may need to request additional information from the referring physician, and your physician will want to send a consultation report.

3 Determine the patient's chief complaint and when the first symptoms occurred.
PURPOSE: To assist in determining the length of time needed for the appointment and the degree of urgency.

4 Search the appointment book for the first suitable appointment time and an alternate time.

5 Offer the patient a choice of these dates and times.
PURPOSE: Patients are better satisfied if they are given a choice.

6 Enter the mutually agreeable time in the appointment book followed by the patient's telephone number.
NOTE: Indicate that the patient is new by adding the letters "N.P."

7 If new patients are expected to pay at the time of visit, explain this financial arrangement when the appointment is made.
PURPOSE: The patient will be aware of the payment policy and can come prepared to pay at the time of the visit.

8 Offer travel directions for reaching the office as well as parking instructions.
PURPOSE: To relieve any anxiety about being able to find the medical facility.

9 Repeat the day, date, and time of the appointment before saying good-bye to the patient.
PURPOSE: To verify the patient understands the date and time of the appointment.

SCHEDULING RETURN APPOINTMENTS

In Person

Many return appointments are arranged while a patient is in the office. The physician will probably ask the patient to stop at the desk and make another appointment before leaving. While you reach for your pencil and the appointment book, look at the patient and say something such as

> "We have Tuesday and Thursday morning or evening available. Do you have a preference?"

If the patient asks for a time that is not available, this places the medical assistant in a negative position by having to refuse a request.

Enter the patient's name and telephone number in the slot agreed on and give the patient a completed appointment card that you have verified with the book entry, along with your best smile. Give the patient any necessary instructions at this time.

By Telephone

Usually it is necessary only to determine when the patient is expected to return and then to find a suitable time on the schedule. It is not necessary to give extensive explanations about the location of the office and parking facilities. However, if there has been a lengthy interval since the patient's last visit, the medical assistant should recheck certain information and enter any changes on the patient's chart.

Don't Forget... Your Appointment

Name: __________

Date: __________

Time: __________

MARYLAND FAMILY CARE
0890 CLARENDON AVENUE
RAYBURN, TEXAS 32150
(123) 987-6543

Please give us 24 hours notice in case of cancellation. Thank you.

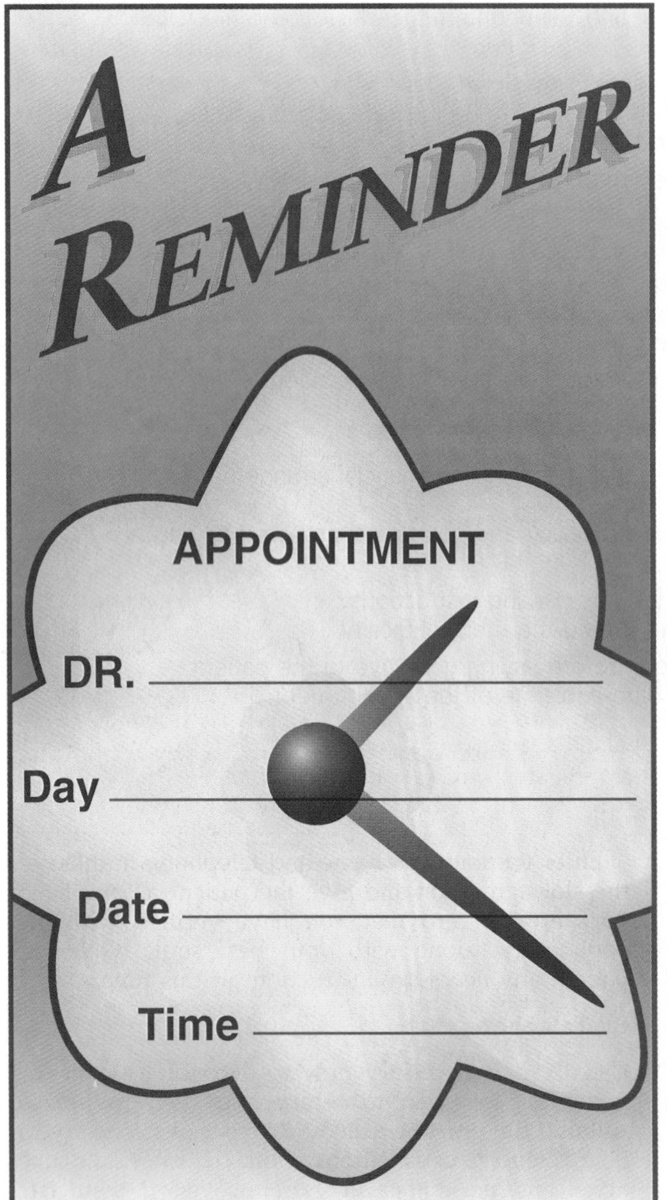

M __________

HAS AN APPOINTMENT ON

DATE __________ AT __________ A.M. P.M.

EDWARD W. WATLOW, M.D.

241 RAINSET BLVD.
Urban, Texas 77700

TELEPHONE:
(555) 999-8888

24 HOURS NOTICE IS APPRECIATED IF YOU ARE UNABLE TO KEEP YOUR APPOINTMENT.

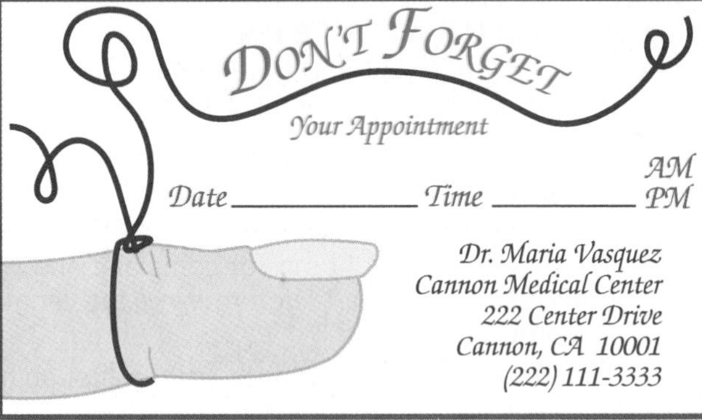

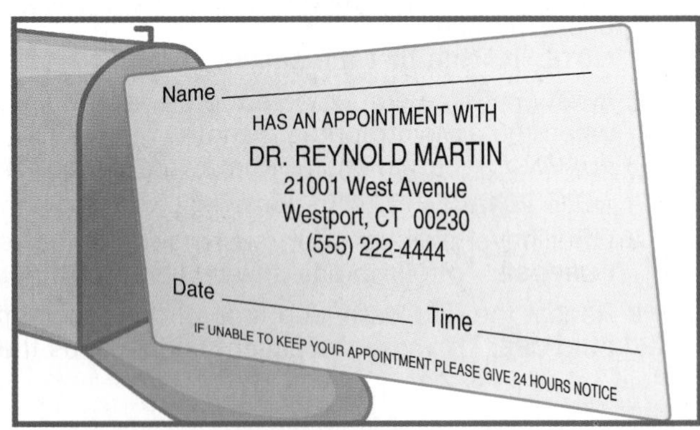

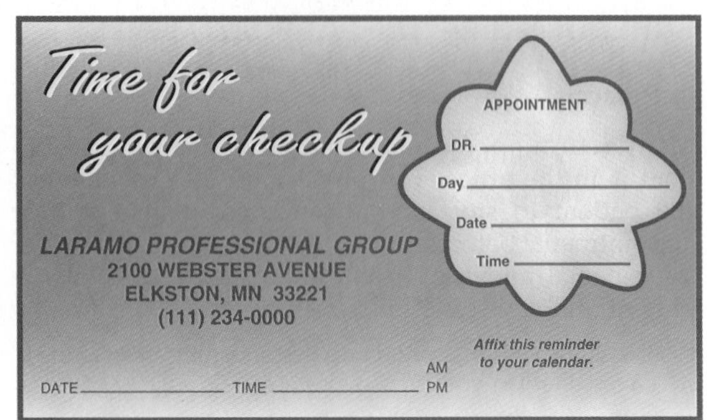

FIGURE 10–4 Examples of appointment cards.

ESSENTIAL QUESTIONS TO ASK A PATIENT BETWEEN LENGTHY INTERVALS

- Patient's current address
- Daytime telephone number
- Current insurance coverage
- Employment information
- Nature of the current complaint

Memory Jogger

What are the seven items of information that you must obtain from each new patient?

Appointment Cards and Reminders

APPOINTMENT CARDS

Most health care facilities use cards to remind patients of scheduled appointments, as well as to eliminate misunderstandings about dates and times (Fig. 10–4).

Make a habit of reaching for an appointment card while writing an entry in the appointment book. After you have written the date and time on the appointment card, double-check with the book to see that the entries agree. Patients who have made appointments in advance may be sent a reminder card or notified by telephone near the time of the appointment.

REMINDERS

A patient who is due for an appointment but has not yet arranged a date and time may be sent a *recall reminder.* A simple way of handling this is to have a supply of postal cards on hand; while the patients are still in the office, have them write their name and address on a card. Then place the card in a file box under the date it is to be mailed.

Special Circumstances

LATE PATIENTS

Probably every medical practice has a few patients who are habitually late for appointments. This seems to be a problem for which no cure has been found; consequently, you must find a way of booking such patients as the last appointments of the day. Then, if closing time arrives before the patient does, you need feel no obligation to wait. Some medical assistants simply tell the patient to come in 30 minutes earlier than the time they actually write in the book. The point to remember is that you must learn to work around this patient, with the realization that in all likelihood he or she is not going to change.

RESCHEDULING A CANCELED APPOINTMENT

Sometimes changes must be made in the appointment schedule. For example, the patient who has a 3 PM appointment next Monday calls and asks to have this postponed to 1 week later. You find an opening at 3 PM on the following Monday and write in the patient's name, but in your haste you fail to cross out the first appointment. Someone else looking at the appointment book (or possibly even yourself a couple of days later) will either expect the patient on both days or be unable to determine which day is correct. Avoid this embarrassing situation by making it a habit to cross out the first appointment before writing in the new one.

You may have a patient who requires a series of appointments, for example, at weekly intervals. Try to set up the appointments on the same day of each week at the same time of day, if possible. This considerably reduces the risk of a forgotten appointment. A calendar that shows the dates several months in advance at a glance is useful to have on or near the appointment desk.

EMERGENCY CALLS

Calls for appointments may be categorized as *emergencies, urgent,* or *routine.* **Triage** in responding to requests for immediate care and treatment puts the responsibility of evaluating the urgency of the need and prioritizing the treatment on the medical assistant who answers the telephone. Triage is an extremely important function that requires experience and tact.

Emergencies may include emotional crises as well as the more obvious physical problems, and patients having emergencies generally should be seen the same day. The calling patient may have an emotionally charged issue such as "I just found a lump in my breast" or "I can't urinate or get an erection." The urgency of the call can be initially determined by having available a list of questions previously prepared with the help of the physician and posted near the telephone for easy reference. The physician should define what is to be considered *urgent* as well as the time frame for scheduling urgent appointments (probably within 1 to 4 days). Try to have a list of questions to ask the caller appropriate to the situation.

RESPONDING TO AN EMERGENCY CALL

1 Is there bleeding?
2 From where is the blood coming?
3 What is the patient's temperature?
4 Are there chills?
5 Is there nausea or vomiting?
6 If there is pain, is it steady or intermittent?
7 Is the pain severe? sharp? dull?
8 How long have the symptoms been present?

In many cases the caller will consider the situation more urgent than his or her responses to the medical questions would indicate. Skillful handling of these situations requires considerable tact by the medical assistant. Maintaining a caring and reassuring response will frequently alleviate the fear being evidenced by the caller.

ACUTELY ILL PATIENTS

Patients cannot always give advance notice of when they will need medical care. There is sometimes a very fine line between an emergency patient and the acutely ill patient, but the latter should be seen as soon as possible. At the very least, let the physician decide whether the patient should be seen immediately or whether an appointment should be made for another day.

For example, a patient may report having had flu symptoms for several days and now has an elevated temperature. The physician will probably want more information before deciding whether the patient should be seen immediately or whether some other course of action is appropriate. The 15- to 20-minute breather time you saved in the middle of the morning and the afternoon may rescue your schedule. Patients with symptoms of contagion should be placed so as to discourage patient cross-contamination.

PHYSICIAN REFERRALS

If another physician telephones and requests that a patient be seen by your physician today, this is another exception you will have to make. Most physicians recognize the importance of keeping a schedule and will not be inconsiderate in this respect.

Memory Jogger

 *How can the medical assistant determine the urgency of a call when the physician is not present?*

Failed Appointments

REASONS FOR FAILED APPOINTMENTS

Why do patients fail to keep appointments? Some are simply forgetful. If you detect this tendency in a patient, form the habit of telephoning a reminder the day before the appointment or send a postcard timed to arrive 1 or 2 days in advance of the appointment.

If your office consistently runs behind schedule, with patients being kept waiting for more than 20 to 30 minutes, the patient whose own time is well planned may simply elect not to run the risk of losing so much valuable time. Perhaps you gave a patient an appointment at a time that really was not agreeable to him.

A patient who has been pressed for payment may stay away because of being unable to pay on that day.

It is extremely important that you determine the reason for failed appointments and do what you can to remedy the situations. Telephone the patient to be sure there was no misunderstanding. If the patient's health is such that medical treatment must continue, write a letter explaining this to the patient. Send the letter by certified mail with return receipt requested and keep this letter in the chart for legal protection.

NO-SHOW POLICY

Some patients may not realize the importance of keeping their appointments. A busy practice must have a very specific policy on appointment no-shows and enforce it effectively. A suggested **no-show** policy may be as follows: The first time a patient fails to show, note the fact on the medical record or ledger card. The second time this happens, you'll have a warning, and if the patient is more than a half-hour late, call his or her home. The third time a patient fails to show without good reason, consider dropping the patient by using the customary methods that avoid legal problems.

CHARGING FOR FAILED APPOINTMENTS

Legally, a patient may be charged for failing to keep an uncanceled appointment if the patient was informed in advance about this policy and if it can be shown that this time was not used for another patient. However, few physicians attempt to collect for such occasions. The risk of poor public relations is too great; it generally results in a lost patient. Some other way must be found to handle failed appointments if they become a problem.

RECORDING THE FAILED APPOINTMENT

Whenever a patient fails to keep an appointment, a notation should be made in the patient's chart as well as in the appointment book. If the patient is seriously ill, the physician should also be told about the failure. This may be a legal consideration at some later date. In some cases, it may be necessary for the physician or the medical assistant to call and remind the patient that an unkept appointment may have serious effects on the patient's health.

Handling Cancellations and Delays

WHEN THE PATIENT CANCELS

Inevitably some cancellations will occur. If you keep a list of patients with advance appointments who would like to come in sooner, get busy on the telephone and try to get one of them in to fill the available opening. By placing a colored dot alongside their names in the appointment book where the first appointment was made, you can readily identify which patients to call to fill the vacancy.

WHEN THE PHYSICIAN IS DELAYED

There will be days when the physician(s) is delayed in reaching the office. If you have advance notice of the delay, you can start calling those patients with early appointments and suggest that they come later. If some patients have already arrived before you learn of the delay, you will have to explain that an emergency has detained the physician.

Show concern for the patient, but avoid being overly apologetic, which might imply some degree of guilt. Most patients realize that a physician has certain priorities. The patient who is in the office may be *inconvenienced,* but it is not a *life-or-death* matter. If this kind of situation occurs frequently, however, you may have to devise a different scheduling system.

WHEN THE PHYSICIAN IS CALLED OUT ON EMERGENCIES

Physicians are conscious of their responsibilities for responding to medical emergencies, and most patients will be sympathetic to such occurrences if the medical assistant takes the time to explain what has happened. You may say something like,

> "Dr. Wright has been called away to answer an emergency. She asked me to tell you she is very sorry to keep you waiting. There will be at least a 1-hour delay."

Ask the patient,

> "Do you wish to wait? If it is inconvenient, I'll be glad to give you the first available appointment on another day. Or perhaps you'd like to have some coffee or do some shopping and return in an hour."

As quickly as possible, call the patients who are scheduled for a later hour. In many offices, especially those of obstetricians, surgeons, and general practitioners, it sometimes is necessary to cancel a whole day's appointments. For this reason, it is particularly important that you have the daytime telephone number of each patient available so that you can cancel the appointment and make a new one without delay. If it is at all possible, cancel appointments *before* the patient arrives in the office to find that the doctor is not available.

WHEN THE PHYSICIAN IS ILL OR IS CALLED OUT OF TOWN

Physicians get ill, too, and the patients who are scheduled to be seen during the course of the physician's expected recovery period must be informed of this. They need not be told the nature of the illness. When the physician is called out of town for personal or professional reasons, the appointments will have to be canceled or rescheduled. It is customary to give the patient the name of another physician, or possibly a choice of several, who will be providing care during such absences. For security reasons, it is best to merely state that the doctor is unavailable. Stating over the telephone that the physician is out of town could lead to attempted burglary or other unauthorized intrusion of the premises.

Patients Without Appointments

What will you do with *walk-in* patients, that is, those who arrive without a scheduled appointment? There must be a policy agreed on by the physician and then carried out by the medical assistant.

The patient who requires immediate attention will most likely be accommodated into the schedule somehow. If the patient does not need immediate care, a brief visit with the physician and a scheduled appointment at a later time may be the answer. You may simply have to turn down the request. Follow the established office policy.

The medical assistant should always make it clear, even when accommodating patients without appointments, that the office runs on an appointment basis. You might say, for example:

> "Dr. Wright will be able to see you today, but we would appreciate it very much if you would make an appointment for your next visit."

Or,

> "Dr. Wright can see you now and I am sorry you had to wait so long. Perhaps it would be possible for you to make an appointment the next time."

Try to convey the message that appointments save not only the physician's time but also the patient's time. Emphasize that the physician is able to give the patient full attention and more time if an advance appointment is made.

Preplanning for the Next Day

Before leaving at the end of the day, look over the appointments scheduled for the next day. Review the charts for scheduled patients. If laboratory tests or other procedures were scheduled on the patient's last visit, determine that the reports are available in the chart. If the patient is scheduled for specific procedures on this visit, make certain that everything that will be needed for the procedure is on hand and available. Preplanning can save many precious moments at the time of the patient visit.

Scheduling Outside Appointments

There are other appointments that the medical assistant will make and that will appear on the appointment book, such as *scheduled surgery* at a hospital, *consultations* at a hospital or at another physician's office, and *house calls* at extended-care facilities or in the home. The physician must have time to get from one place to another, so allowance must be made for traveling time when arranging these appointments.

SURGERIES

You may be responsible for scheduling surgeries. In scheduling with most hospitals, you should call the secretary in surgery first when your physician plans an operation. Give the surgical secretary the necessary information. Explain any special requests the physician may have, such as the amount of blood to have available. Be certain that you have all this information at hand before placing the call.

ESSENTIAL INFORMATION TO GIVE FOR SCHEDULING SURGERY

- Preferred date and time
- Type of surgery to be scheduled
- Approximate time required

After the date and hour have been established, give

- Patient's full name
- Sex
- Age
- Telephone number

Some hospitals request that the patient complete a preadmittance form so that all records can be processed before the patient is admitted. In such cases it may be the medical assistant's responsibility to see that this is done. These are general guidelines only, because procedures will vary in different areas and different hospitals.

HOUSE CALLS

If the physician regularly makes *house calls* or sees patients in *convalescent homes,* you will probably set aside a special block of time for this on your appointment schedule. In arranging such appointments, be sure to get all the pertinent details.

ESSENTIAL INFORMATION TO GIVE PHYSICIAN

- Name and address of patient
- Telephone number
- Best route to reach the home
- Nearest cross street
- Name of person making the request

Again, traveling time must be allowed for. Many physicians never make house calls, believing that the patient can best be examined and treated in the medical facility or in a hospital.

OUTSIDE APPOINTMENTS FOR PATIENTS

The medical assistant is often requested to arrange laboratory or x-ray appointments for patients (see Procedure 10–3). Before calling you need to know certain facts.

ESSENTIAL INFORMATION IN ARRANGING LABORATORY APPOINTMENTS

- Exact procedure required
- Whether **expediency** is a factor
- Whether the insurance plan requires notification and determination of medical necessity

PROCEDURE 10-3

Scheduling Outpatient Diagnostic Tests

GOAL

To schedule a patient for outpatient diagnostic test ordered by physician within the time frame needed by physician, confirm with the patient, and issue all required instructions.

EQUIPMENT AND SUPPLIES

Diagnostic test order from physician
Name, address, and telephone number of diagnostic facility
Patient chart
Test preparation instructions
Telephone

PROCEDURAL STEPS

1 Obtain an oral or written order from the physician for the exact procedure to be performed and the time frame for results.
PURPOSE: The urgency of the test results affects the time and date of the appointment needed.

2 Determine the patient's availability.
PURPOSE: To be certain that the patient will be able to comply with the arrangements for the test.

3 Telephone diagnostic facility:
- Order the specific test needed.
- Establish the date and time.
- Give the name, age, address, and telephone number of the patient.
- Determine any special instructions for the patient.
- Notify the facility of any urgency for test results.

4 Notify the patient of arrangements, including:
- Name, address, and telephone number of the diagnostic facility
- Date and time to report for the test
- Instructions concerning preparation for the test (e.g., eating restrictions, fluids, medications, enemas)
- Ask the patient to repeat the instructions.

PURPOSE: To be certain that the patient understands the preparation necessary and the importance of keeping the appointment. If time permits, issue written instructions to the patient.

5 Note arrangements on the patient's chart.
PURPOSE: To ensure follow-up on diagnosis and/or treatment.

6 Place reminder on a tickler or desk calendar.
PURPOSE: To check whether the appointment was kept and report was received from the testing facility.

- Which laboratory or facility must be used to qualify for insurance payment
- Whether a **stat report** is necessary
- Patient's availability

With this information before you, you can set up the appointment with confidence. When you inform the patient of the time and place for the appointment, you can also relay any special instructions that may be necessary. Then note these arrangements on the patient's chart and place a follow up reminder on your **tickler** or desk calendar.

Other Callers

There will be a wide range of other unscheduled callers with whom the physician will need to meet.

PHYSICIANS

Another physician dropping in to your facility should be ushered in to see the physician as soon as possible regardless of the appointment schedule. If your physician is seeing a patient, explain the situation and, if possible, take the visiting physician into a private room to wait. Then notify your employer as soon as possible. Visits from other physicians are usually brief and do not appreciably affect your schedule.

PHARMACEUTICAL REPRESENTATIVES

Also known as *detail persons* or *reps,* representatives from pharmaceutical houses are frequent visitors to physicians' offices and are generally welcomed when the schedule permits. They are well trained and bring valuable information on new drugs to the physician. The medical assistant is often expected to screen such visitors and turn away those whose products would not be used in that practice. If you do not know the representative or the pharmaceutical company, ask for a business card, then check with the physician, who will decide whether or not to see the caller.

Specialists usually limit their conferences with pharmaceutical representatives to their line of practice. The medical assistant, together with the physician, can prepare a list of those representatives with whom the physician is willing to spend time, and then let the list be the determining factor in future conferences.

The medical assistant can say whether the physician will be available that day and give an estimate of the waiting time or suggest a later time at which to return. The caller can then make a decision regarding whether to wait or return later. The pharmaceutical representative is usually quite understanding and cooperative and is willing to wait patiently a long while for just a brief visit with the physician. The medical assistant should in turn treat the representative with courtesy, showing as much cooperation as possible.

In some cases, the representative will just leave literature or materials for the physician with the medical assistant. The detail person who is not on the calling list for a particular physician will also appreciate the saving in time by knowing this in advance. Most representatives say they would rather be told outright if the physician does not wish to see them than to be given some evasive reply.

SALESPERSONS

Salespersons from medical, surgical, and office supply houses call regularly at physicians' offices. Sometimes they will want to see the physician, but the office manager or the medical assistant who is in charge of ordering supplies usually is able to handle these calls.

Unsolicited salespersons can sometimes present a problem in the professional office. If the physician does not wish to see such callers, the medical assistant must firmly but tactfully send them away. You can suggest that they leave their literature and cards for the physician to study and say that the physician will contact them if further information is desired. Persistent callers who ignore a polite "No" can be discouraged by the suggestion that perhaps they would like to schedule an appointment, at the physician's customary fee.

MISCELLANEOUS CALLERS

From time to time, other callers appear in the medical office. Some are civic leaders seeking the physician's aid in community projects. Others may be church leaders, insurance representatives, solicitors for fund drives, and so forth. A general policy regarding seeing such callers should be established so that each incident does not require a separate discussion and decision.

Civic leaders should be treated with courtesy and consideration when they telephone or come into the office. Most physicians feel a responsibility to take an active part in community affairs, but no one can participate in all activities. The responsibility for accepting or refusing such community appointments is sometimes delegated to the office manager or medical assistant. In this event, one should use discretion and exercise great tact and courtesy. Turning away community leaders with a blunt refusal does not create good medical public relations.

When it is necessary to refuse requests for community projects, the medical assistant can explain that the physician is already participating in such community projects as, for example, the Boy Scouts, Girl Scouts, Kiwanis, and the Health Council (naming specific activities or organizations) and cannot accept additional responsibilities at this time. The practice of tact, courtesy, and consideration applies to *every caller* in the health care facility.

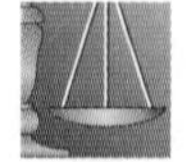

LEGAL AND ETHICAL ISSUES

When scheduling appointments be especially considerate of complying with the patient's wishes when possible. Explain any refusal and offer a substitute time and date.

If a patient fails to appear for a scheduled appointment, note this in the patient's chart and in the appointment book. Always determine the reason for failed appointments and attempt to remedy anything that can be changed.

CRITICAL THINKING

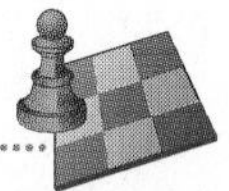

1 List the three premises that determine an efficient scheduling system.

2 When entering an appointment in the daily schedule, what two items will you include in addition to the patient's name?

3 Recall some of the reasons that patients fail to keep appointments and describe how you would handle each situation.

4 Discuss the meaning and reason for buffer time?

HOW DID I DO? Answers to Memory Joggers

1 Efficient scheduling is important because the most valuable asset within the medical practice is the physician's time. Its success ultimately depends on the cooperation of the physician.

2 The nature of the practice, the personality and habits of the medical staff, and time needed by each patient. Be able to discuss the reasons for their importance.

3 Patient's full name, date of birth, complete address, daytime telephone number, source of referral, if any, general type of examination required, and insurance coverage.

4 Refer to a list of questions approved by the physician and the action to follow based on the answers.

REFERENCES

American Medical Association: Managing the Medical Practice. Chicago, AMA, 1996.

Conomikes Associates: Medical Office Management Institute, 1996.

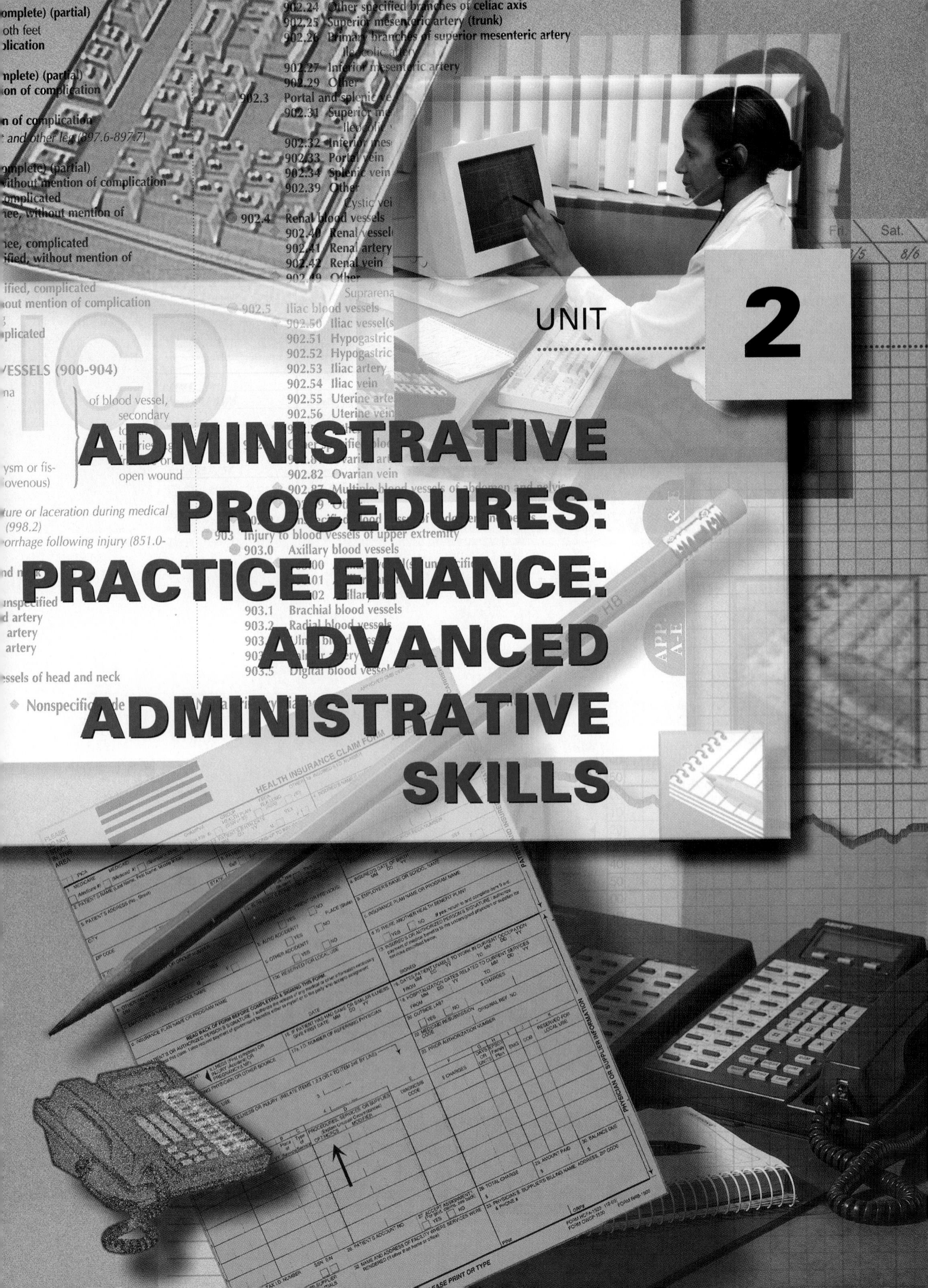

UNIT 2

ADMINISTRATIVE PROCEDURES: PRACTICE FINANCE: ADVANCED ADMINISTRATIVE SKILLS

SECTION 4

Written Communications and Record Keeping

CURRICULUM CONTENT/COMPETENCIES

Chapter 11 Correspondence and Mail Processing

- *Perform basic clerical functions*
- *Recognize and respond to verbal and nonverbal communications*
- *Receive, organize, prioritize, and transmit information*
- *Promote the practice through positive public relations*

Chapter 12 Dictation and Transcription

- *Perform medical transcription*
- *Manage time effectively*
- *Use medical terminology appropriately*
- *Prepare and maintain medical records*

Chapter 13 The Computer in Medical Practice

- *Apply computer techniques to support office operations*
- *Obtain reimbursement through accurate claims submission*
- *Practice within the scope of education, training, and personal capabilities*
- *Evaluate and recommend equipment and supplies*

Chapter 14 Filing Methods and Record Keeping

- *Receive, organize, and prioritize information*
- *Document accurately*
- *Perform basic clerical functions*

Chapter 15 Health Information Management

- *Prepare and maintain health information records*
- *Document accurately*
- *Maintain confidentiality*
- *Perform basic clerical functions*
- *Use appropriate guidelines when releasing information*

Correspondence and Mail Processing

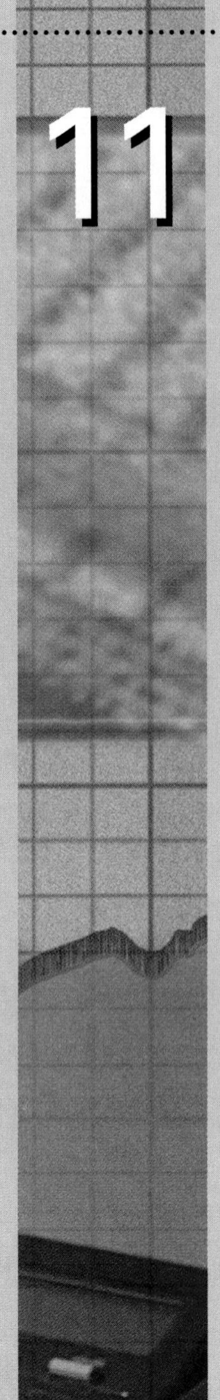

OUTLINE

LEARNING OBJECTIVES

Cognitive: On successful completion of this chapter, you should be able to:

1. Define and spell terms listed in the Vocabulary.
2. Discuss the responsibility of the medical assistant with respect to office equipment.
3. Select stationery suitable for producing professional correspondence.
4. List the three basic sizes of letterhead stationery.
5. Name three types of essential references for the medical assistant's library.
6. Explain the five steps in getting ready to answer a letter.
7. Discuss the process of developing and the value of a correspondence portfolio.
8. Name four letter styles and discuss their differences.
9. List the four standard parts of a business letter.
10. Explain how using ZIP codes can save money for the mailer.

Performance: On successful completion of this chapter, you should be able to:

1 Open, sort, and annotate incoming mail.
2 Prepare a response to an inquiry letter.
3 Compose original letters.
4 Correctly address envelopes for optical scanning.
5 Fold outgoing mail for insertion into three styles of envelopes.

VOCABULARY

academic degree A title conferred by a college, university, or professional school on completion of a program of study

annotating To furnish with notes, which are usually critical or explanatory

categorically Placed in a specific division of a system of classification

clarity The state of being clear or lucid

concise Expressing much in brief form

continuation pages The second and following pages of a letter

intrinsic Inward; indwelling

portfolio A set of documents either bound in book form or loose in a folder

Correspondence and mail processing can consume a large part of the administrative medical assistant's day. Many physicians, when queried about the skills they most desire in an administrative assistant, have said, "Send me someone who can write a good letter." Or they may say, "My spelling is atrocious; I need help!" When a physician delegates to the medical assistant the responsibility of composing letters or reports that have the potential to reflect positively or negatively on the practice, he or she is expressing confidence in the assistant.

Public Relations Value

Written communications offer the perfect opportunity for making a good impression on others, but they don't just happen. They require thought, preparation, skill, and a positive attitude. Written communications take many forms in the medical office. The medical assistant may be required to be skilled in creating various forms of communication.

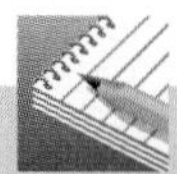

SKILLS AND RESPONSIBILITIES

WRITTEN COMMUNICATION SKILLS

- Transcribe from machine or shorthand dictation
- Type consultation and surgical reports
- Compose original letters
- Reply to inquiries
- Respond to requests for information
- Write collection letters
- Order supplies
- Write instructions for patients
- Process a variety of other communications

The form and process of letter writing are discussed in this chapter. Transcription will be covered in Chapter 12.

Written communications should be *courteous* to the reader, *correct* in content, and **concise** without being curt. Communication is an art as well as a skill: The ability to communicate effectively is extremely important to the administrative medical assistant who wants to succeed and advance in his or her career.

Equipment and Supplies

To create a good impression with your letters, you must use good equipment and quality supplies.

EQUIPMENT

Whatever kind of equipment is available for your use, it is your responsibility to know how to use it to the best advantage and keep it in good working condition. If the equipment manual is available, study it and keep it handy for reference when problems occur. Know how to maintain your equipment so that your best efforts always result in a quality appearance.

COMPUTER OR WORD PROCESSOR If you are unfamiliar with the specific model supplied, study the manual so that you know how to format documents, make corrections, and print the necessary copies.

TYPEWRITER Most typewriters use correctable film ribbon that passes through the spool only one time. However, if your typewriter uses a cotton or silk ribbon that becomes lighter with use, be sure to change the ribbon before the resulting type impression becomes too light. Typewriters that use a cotton ribbon also need frequent cleaning of the typewriter keys.

COPIER If you are composing with a typewriter, you are probably using a copier for making any necessary copies of the original. Here, too, maintain the copier so that copies are crisp and clear.

STATIONERY

QUALITY The quality of paper unquestionably affects the reader's total impression of the communication. Your stationer or printing company is qualified to advise on the selection of paper, which can range from all-sulfite (a wood pulp) to all-cotton fiber (sometimes called *rag*). Letterhead paper is usually on bond with a 25% or higher cotton fiber content.

The weight of paper is described by a *substance number*. This number is based on the weight of a ream consisting of 500 sheets of 17 × 22-inch paper. The larger the substance number, the heavier the paper. If the ream weighs 24 pounds, the paper is referred to as Sub 24 or 24-pound weight. Letterhead stationery and matching envelopes are usually 16-, 20-, or 24-pound weight.

SIZES Letterhead paper is available in three basic sizes:

- Standard — 8½ × 11 inches
- Monarch or executive — 7¼ × 10½ inches
- Baronial — 5½ × 8½ inches

Standard letterhead is used for general business and professional correspondence. *Monarch* is often used by professional persons for informal business and social correspondence. *Baronial*, which is a half-sheet of Standard, is used for very short letters or memoranda. Each size letterhead should have its matching envelope.

CONTINUATION PAGES The second and continuing pages of a letter or report are placed on plain bond that matches the letterhead in weight and fiber content.

Bond paper has a *felt* side and a *wire* side. Printing and typing are done on the felt side. Pick up a sheet of letterhead and hold it to the light; you will see a design or letters that can be read from the printed side. This design is called a *watermark* and is an indication of quality. The side from which you can read the watermark is the felt side of the paper and is the side on which typing should be done. Always have the watermark read across the page in the same direction as the typing.

Memory Jogger

 *You may see the notation Sub 24 on a package of paper. What does this tell you?*

Your Personal Tools

Competent handling of written communications requires a basic knowledge of composition (i.e., sentence structure, spelling, and punctuation; see Chapter 12). You will also need a personal reference library that includes an up-to-date standard dictionary, a medical dictionary, and a secretary's manual. Some suggestions are included in the reference list at the end of this chapter.

If you have difficulty with spelling (many people do), you may wish to keep a small looseleaf indexed notebook or card index of words that are troublesome. Whenever it is necessary to look up a word in the dictionary for spelling, record it in the notebook or card index for quick reference.

Your physician or a medical assistant who is familiar with the practice might compile a basic list of frequently used medical terms and abbreviations as a reference for the trainee.

Table 11–1 lists 150 frequently misspelled or misused English words. Table 11–2 lists 100 frequently misspelled medical terms. Your list may be entirely different, depending on your capabilities and the branch of medicine in which you are involved.

Memory Jogger

 *One of the most frequently misspelled medical words describes the study of the eye. Can you spell this word?*

Composing Tips

WRITING SKILLS

If your only experience in letter writing has been social correspondence, you will have a new set of rules to learn. Social letters tend to be long and chatty, "I" oriented, and do not necessarily follow any organized plan. Most business letters should be less than one page in length, "you" oriented, and carefully organized. This takes practice and preparation.

TABLE 11–1 150 Frequently Misspelled or Misused English Words

absence	corroborate	inimitable	persistent	ridiculous
accede	definitely	inoculate	personal	sacrilegious
accessible	description	insistent	personnel	seize
accommodate	desirable	irrelevant	possession	separate
achieve	despair	irresistible	precede	siege
affect	development	irritable	precedent	similar
agglutinate	dilemma	judgment	predictable	sizable
all right	disappear	labeled	predominant	stationary
altogether	disappoint	led	predominate	stationery
analyses (pl.)	disastrous	leisure	prerogative	subpoena
analysis (s.)	discreet	license	prevalent	succeed
analyze	discrete	liquefy	principal	suddenness
anoint	discriminate	maintenance	principle	superintendent
argument	dissatisfaction	maneuver	privilege	supersede
assistant	dissipate	miscellaneous	procedure	surprise
auxiliary	drunkenness	mischievous	proceed	tariff
balloon	ecstasy	misspell	professor	technique
believe	effect	necessary	pronunciation	thorough
benefited	eligible	newsstand	psychiatry	tranquility
brochure	embarrass	noticeable	psychology	transferred
bulletin	exceed	occasion	pursue	truly
category	exhilaration	occurrence	questionnaire	tyrannize
changeable	existence	oscillate	rearrange	unnecessary
clientele	February	paid	recede	until
committee	forty	pamphlet	receive	vacillate
comparative	grammar	panicky	recommend	vacuum
concede	grievous	parallel	referring	vicious
conscientious	height	paralyze	repetition	warrant
conscious	incidentally	pastime	rheumatism	Wednesday
coolly	indispensable	perseverance	rhythmical	weird

TABLE 11–2 Frequently Misspelled Medical Words

abscess	defibrillator	intussusception	parietal	pruritus
additive	desiccate	ischemia	paroxysmal	psoriasis
aerosol	ecchymosis	ischium	pemphigus	pyrexia
agglutination	effusion	larynx	percussion	respiratory
albumin	epididymis	leukemia	perforation	rheumatic
anastomosis	epistaxis	malaise	pericardium	roentgenology
aneurysm	eustachian	malleus	perineum	sagittal
anteflexion	fissure	melena	peristalsis	sciatic
arrhythmia	flexure	mellitus	peritoneum	scirrhous
bilirubin	glaucoma	menstruation	petit mal	serous
bronchial	gonorrhea	metastasis	pharynx	sessile
cachexia	graafian	neurilemma	pituitary	sphincter
calcaneus	hemorrhage	neuron	plantar	sphygmomanometer
capillary	hemorrhoids	occlusion	pleura	squamous
cervical	homeostasis	optic chiasm	pleurisy	staphylococcus
chromosome	humerus	oscilloscope	pneumonia	suppuration
cirrhosis	idiosyncracy	osseous	polyp	trochanter
clavicle	ileum	palliative	prophylaxis	venous
curettage	ilium	parasite	prostate	wheal
cyanosis	infarction	parenteral	prosthesis	xiphoid

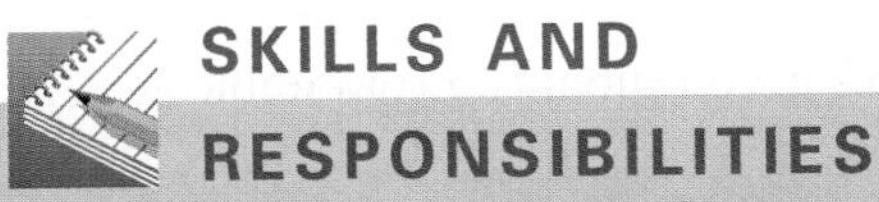

SKILLS AND RESPONSIBILITIES

PLANNING BEFORE ANSWERING A LETTER

1 Carefully read the letter you are to answer.
2 Make note of, or underline, any questions asked or materials requested.
3 Decide on the answers to the questions and verify your information. This is called **annotating.**
4 Draft a reply, using the tools you are most comfortable with (e.g., the computer, typewriter, longhand, or shorthand).
5 Rewrite for **clarity.**

Keep most of your sentences short. Put only one idea in each sentence. Eliminate superfluous words. Be careful about using medical terms in correspondence with patients; use only language that the reader will easily understand.

Every person who writes letters develops his or her own personal style. Most physicians conform to a highly professional and formal style in their dictation.

The medical assistant who is given the responsibility of composing correspondence for the medical office should strive for the same degree of formality used by the physician. It would be inappropriate for the assistant to write in a breezy, informal style when acting as the representative of an employer who is more formal in his or her approach.

The principal point to remember is that every letter produced in your office should project the image of the physician regardless of who composes or signs the letter.

Memoranda are usually intended for interoffice correspondence. Larger facilities often have printed forms that merely require filling in the date, the receiver and sender, and the topic. You can easily prepare a memo in an accepted form. If you are using a computer or word processor, you will probably find a preformatted memorandum already prepared for you. When starting with only plain paper, set the side margins for 1-inch. Begin typing the memo heading 2 inches from the top of the page (line 13). Set up the heading with the words: TO, FROM, DATE, and SUBJECT. Setting a tab stop 10 spaces in from the left margin will enable you to tab to each entry, clearing the headings.

You may start the body of your memorandum at the left margin or set your margin 10 spaces in so that your text starts directly beneath the typed headings. No salutation is necessary in a memorandum. The purpose is to expedite the communication of a message in a manner that provides a record without becoming cumbersome (Fig. 11–1).

INTEROFFICE MEMORANDUM

TO All Staff

FROM Office Manager

DATE December 1

SUBJECT Holiday Schedule

Our entire facility will be closed on December 24, December 25, December 31, and January 1. The office will be on reduced staff during the days of December 26, 27, 28, 29, and 30. Assignments will be based on seniority of staff members. Please submit your preferences as soon as possible.

A

MEMO TO: George Walker

FROM: Stanley Barr

DATE: February 8, 1999

SUBJECT: Office rental

We are experiencing unexpectedly rapid growth in our business office and will soon need additional space for our increased number of employees. Do you have a larger facility available in this building? If so, I would like to hear from you regarding the location, square footage, and anticipated rental costs.

B

FIGURE 11–1 *A* and *B*, examples of memoranda.

DEVELOPING A PORTFOLIO

Letter composition can be sped up by developing a **portfolio** of sample letters to suit the various situations that frequently arise. As the physician approves your letters you can add them to your portfolio. Suppose, for instance, you need to write to a patient to change an appointment. Compose the very best letter you can—one that is clear, concise, and courteous—and make an extra copy to place in your portfolio of letters. Alternatively, if you are using a computer, store the letter on a disk. Do this each time you write a new kind of letter. Soon you will be able to select a letter from your portfolio and change it slightly to suit the current situation. You will have your letters written in no time!

Watch for sample letters that appear from time to time in the physician's business journals and clip them for your portfolio. Scan the textbooks and office manuals on the market or in your public library for additional help.

OTHER WRITTEN FORMS OF COMMUNICATION

Written communications include more than letters and memoranda. For example, consider telephone messages that you record. Are you sure that they are clearly stated and convey to the reader what you intend? You may need to mail a prescription to a patient, with instructions from the physician. Make sure that the patient will be able to read and understand what you intend to communicate.

Memory Jogger

Describe the difference between a formal letter and a memorandum.

Letter Styles

A business letter is usually arranged in one of three styles: *block, modified block (standard),* or *modified block indented.* A fourth style, called *simplified,* is occasionally used. The block and modified block (standard) styles are most commonly used in the physician's office.

BLOCK LETTER STYLE All lines start flush with the left margin. This style is considered the most efficient but is less attractive on the page (Fig. 11–2).

MODIFIED-BLOCK LETTER STYLE (STANDARD) The date line, the complimentary closing, and the typewritten signature all begin at the center. All other lines begin at the left margin (Fig. 11–3).

MODIFIED-BLOCK WITH INDENTED PARAGRAPHS This style is identical to the block style except that the first line of each paragraph is indented five spaces (Fig. 11–4).

Elizabeth Blackwell, M.D.
223 Orange Avenue, N.W.
Cottonwood, UT 84121

January 26, 19—

Mr. Richard Fluege
3678 North Willow Avenue
Palm Beach, FL 33480

Dear Mr. Fluege:

Please send me full particulars on the professional suites you expect to offer for sale or rent in the Medical Arts Professional Annex.

In about six months, I will be ready to open my practice, and I am interested in locating in Florida. My preference is a street-level suite of approximately 2,000 square feet.

After I have had an opportunity to study the information you send me, I will write or telephone you if I have further questions.

Very truly yours,

Elizabeth Blackwell, M.D.

EB:mek

FIGURE 11–2 Block letter style.

MEDICAL ARTS PROFESSIONAL ANNEX
3678 North Willow Avenue
Palm Beach FL 33480

January 29, 19—

Elizabeth Blackwell, M.D.
223 Orange Avenue, N.W.
Cottonwood, UT 84121

Dear Doctor Blackwell:

We have two remaining street-level suites available for occupancy about July 1. These are marked on pages 3 and 4 of the enclosed descriptive brochure. If one of these suites appeals to you, we will be pleased to customize it for your practice.

Please feel free to call me collect at the number on the brochure for further discussion of your needs.

Sincerely yours,

Richard Fluege
Business Manager

RF:ab
Enclosure

FIGURE 11–3 Modified block letter style (standard).

WILLIAM OSLER, M.D.
1000 South West Street
Park Ridge, NJ 07656

January 26, 19—

Robert Koch, M.D.
398 Main Street
Park Ridge, NJ 07656

Dear Doctor Koch:

Mrs. Elaine Norris

Thank you for referring your patient, Mrs. Elaine Norris, for consultation and care. She was examined in my office today.

FINDINGS: The patient complained of pain in the left lower quadrant and some abdominal tenderness. She had a temperature of 100.2 degrees.

RECOMMENDATIONS: The patient was placed on a soft, low-residue, bland diet, antibiotics, and bed rest for a few days. Upper and lower gastrointestinal x-rays will be performed next week.

TENTATIVE DIAGNOSIS: Diverticulitis of large bowel.

Mrs. Norris has been asked to return here for reevaluation in about ten days.

Sincerely yours,

William Osler, M.D.

WO:gm

FIGURE 11–4 Modified block letter style with indented paragraphs.

ROBERT KOCH, M.D.
398 Main Street
Park Ridge, NJ 07656

January 30, 19—

William Osler, M.D.
1000 South West Street
Park Ridge, NJ 07656

ANNABELLE ANDERSON

You will be pleased to know, Bill, that Mrs. Anderson is progressing nicely. Her wound is healing. Her temperature has returned to normal, and she is beginning to resume her usual activities.

Mrs. Anderson has an appointment to return here for one more visit next week. At that time, I will ask her to return to you for any further care.

ROBERT KOCH, M.D.

RK:hb

FIGURE 11–5 Simplified letter style.

SIMPLIFIED LETTER STYLE All lines begin flush with the left margin. The salutation is replaced with an all-capital subject line on the third line below the inside address. The body of the letter begins on the third line below the subject line. The complimentary closing is omitted. An all-capital typewritten signature is entered on the fifth line below the body of the letter (Fig. 11–5).

Punctuation

Traditionally, the punctuation pattern is selected on the basis of letter style. Normal punctuation is always used *within the body* of a business letter. The other parts use either *standard* or *open* punctuation.

STANDARD (MIXED) PUNCTUATION A colon is placed after the salutation, and a comma is placed after the complimentary closing. This is the punctuation pattern most commonly used. It is appropriate with the block or modified-block letter styles.

OPEN PUNCTUATION No punctuation is used at the end of any line outside the body of the letter unless that line ends with an abbreviation. This pattern is always used with the simplified letter style.

Spacing and Margins

Generally, a letter centered on a page is the most attractive. Accomplishing this requires experience, but a few guidelines with which to start are helpful.

SPACING Business letters are almost always single spaced. If a letter consists of only a few lines, you can double-space both the inside address and the message. In this case, you should indent the first line of each paragraph five spaces.

TOP MARGIN The first typed entry (the date) is usually placed on the third line below the letterhead or on line 13 (two inches) if there is no letterhead. Continuation pages begin 1 inch from the top (line 7).

SIDE MARGIN On standard letterhead, the 6½-inch line is common and leaves 1-inch margins on each side. The appearance of a very short letter is improved by increasing the width of all margins.

BOTTOM MARGIN A 1-inch bottom margin is the minimum. This can be increased if the letter is to be carried over to a second page. *Note:* Never use a second page to type only the complimentary closing and signature. Carry over a minimum of two lines of the body of the letter.

Memory Jogger

Why is it important to carry over a minimum of two lines from the body of the letter?

Parts of Letters

The structure of a letter and its placement on a page have been fairly well standardized into four main parts:

Heading
Opening
Body
Closing

HEADING

The heading includes the *letterhead* and the *date line.*

The printed letterhead is usually centered at the top of the page and includes the name of the physician or group and the address. It may include the telephone number and the medical specialty (or specialties). In a group or corporate practice, the names of the physicians may also be listed. Occasionally, the heading also includes the name of an office manager.

The date line consists of the name of the month written in full, followed by the day and year. The date should not be abbreviated, nor should ordinal numbers (i.e., 1st, 2nd, and 3rd) be used after the name of the month.

OPENING

The opening consists of the *inside address,* the *salutation,* and the *attention line,* if there is one.

The inside address has two or more lines, starts flush with the left margin, and contains at least the name of the individual or firm to whom the letter is addressed and the mailing address. When the letter is addressed to an individual, the name is preceded by a courtesy title, such as Dr., Mr., Mrs., Miss, or Ms. When addressing a letter to a physician, omit the courtesy title and type the physician's name followed by his or her **academic degree.** (Herbert H. Long, MD). Do not use both a courtesy title and a degree that mean the same thing (e.g., Dr. Herbert H. Long, MD).

The salutation is the letter writer's introductory greeting to the person being addressed. It is typed flush with the left margin on the second line below the last line of the address and is followed by a colon unless open punctuation is used. The words in the salutation vary depending on the degree of formality of the letter.

The attention line, if used, is placed on the second line below the inside address. If you know the name of the person for whom the letter is intended, use that person's name in the inside address and address him or her personally. If the letter is being addressed to a company or organization and directed to a division or department within the company, place the division or department name on the attention line.

BODY

The body of a letter includes the *subject line,* if one is used, and the *message.*

Frequently in medical office correspondence, the subject of a letter is a patient. The patient's name is used as the *subject line.* Because the subject line is considered to be a part of the body of the letter, it is placed on the second line below the salutation. It may start flush with the left margin or at the point of indentation of indented paragraphs, or it may be centered. The word *subject,* followed by a colon, may be used or omitted entirely.

Begin typing the *message* on the second line below the subject line, or on the second line below the salutation if there is no subject line. The first line of each paragraph may be indented five spaces or may start flush with the left margin, depending on the chosen letter style.

CLOSING

The closing includes the *complimentary closing,* the *typewritten signature,* the *reference initials,* and any *special notations.*

The complimentary closing is the writer's way of saying good-bye. It is placed on the second line below the last line of the body of the letter and is followed by a comma unless open punctuation is used. Only the first word is capitalized. The words used are determined by the degree of formality in the salutation. For example, if the salutation is "Dear Herb:" the closing might be "Cordially" or "Sincerely yours" with consistent punctuation. If the letter is addressed to a business, the complimentary closing most used is "Very truly yours."

A typewritten signature is a courtesy to the reader, especially if the name does not appear on the printed letterhead or when the personal signature is difficult or impossible to decipher. Place the typewritten signature on the fourth line directly below the complimentary closing.

Reference initials that identify the typist are placed flush with the left margin on the second line below the typewritten signature. If the writer's name is included on the signature line, the writer's initials need not be included in the reference block unless desired. The writer's initials, if used, should precede the typist's initials and be separated by a colon or diagonal: mek or GB:mek or GB/mek

Special notations are sometimes needed to indicate that enclosures are included with the letter or that copies of the letter are being distributed to others. If the letter indicates an enclosure, type the word *Enclosure* or *Enc.* on the first line below the reference initials. If there is more than one enclosure, specify the number (e.g., Enclosures 3). If copies are to be sent to others, type this notation in the same manner as the enclosure notation or following it if both notations are needed. The copy notation is usually written as cc: or c: or copy to: followed by the name or names of those to whom a copy will be sent. If the person to whom the letter is addressed is not to know that copies are being distributed to others, use the notation bcc: for *blind carbon copy,* on all copies *except* the original. Place this notation either in the upper left of the letter at the margin or below the last notation at the lower left margin.

POSTSCRIPTS

Although a postscript may sometimes be used to express an afterthought, it is more often used to *place emphasis* on an idea or statement.

Begin the postscript on the second line below the last special notation. Follow the style of the letter, indenting the first line if paragraphs were indented in the body of the letter or starting at the margin if indentation was not used in the letter.

Memory Jogger

List the parts of a letter and describe what is included in each part.

Continuation Pages

If the letter requires one or more **continuation pages,** the heading of the second and subsequent pages must contain three items of information: (1) the name of the addressee, (2) the page number, and (3) the date.

The heading should begin on the 7th line (1 inch) from the top of the page. Continuation of the body of the letter begins on the 10th line or the 3rd line below the heading. There are three accepted forms for the continuation page heading.

Elizabeth Blackwell, M.D.   -2-   July 4, 2000

William Osler, M.D.
Page 2
July 4, 2000

William S. Halsted, M.D.
Page 2
July 4, 2000
Subject: Susan Barstow

Signing the Letter

Some physicians prefer to compose and sign all letters that leave their offices. The majority are more than pleased to delegate to a competent assistant the responsibility of composing and signing letters of a business nature.

Although not all authorities agree on the form to be followed, most recommend that a woman's typewritten signature include a courtesy title (Miss, Mrs., or Ms.) and that the title not be enclosed in parentheses. It is not necessary to include the courtesy title in the handwritten signature.

How will you know which letters to sign? In general, the physician signs all of the following:

- Letters that deal with medical advice to patients
- Letters to officers or committees of the medical society
- Referral and consultation reports to colleagues
- Medical reports to insurance companies
- Personal letters

The medical assistant usually composes and signs letters dealing with the following matters:

- Routine matters such as arranging or rescheduling appointments
- Ordering office supplies
- Notifying patients of surgery or hospital arrangements
- Collecting for delinquent accounts
- Letters of solicitation

The steps in composing business correspondence and an example using composing and writing instructions are given in Procedures 11–1 and 11–2.

PROCEDURE 11–1
Composing Business Correspondence

GOAL

To compose and type a letter ordering medical and office supplies using tabular placement of items and following the guidelines of a commonly used business letter style.

EQUIPMENT AND SUPPLIES

Typewriter or computer
Draft paper
Letterhead paper
Pen or pencil
"Want" list of supplies needed
Medical and office supply catalog
Correction tape (optional)

PROCEDURAL STEPS

1 Locate items from "want" list in catalog.

2 Note the catalog number of each item; the unit price, size, and color; and any special information requirements.
EXPLANATION: Compare this information with the "want" list to confirm the correctness of the order.

3 Prepare a draft of the letter by hand or machine, tabulating the items ordered.
PURPOSE: To provide practice in composing a letter and the use of tabulation. (With sufficient experience, preparation of a draft can be eliminated.)

4 Edit the draft carefully for correct information, grammar, spelling, and punctuation.

5 Set line and margins for attractive placement of the letter.

6 Prepare final letter from the corrected draft.

7 Type your signature and identification initials.
EXPLANATION: The medical assistant signs letters ordering supplies.

8 Proofread the letter for composition errors and accuracy of the order before removing it from typewriter or sending to print.

9 Sign letter in preparation for mailing.

PROCEDURE 11-2
Composing and Writing Instructions

GOAL

To inform new patient of most desirable automobile route to physician's office, including any known landmarks, and description of parking facilities at destination.

EQUIPMENT AND SUPPLIES

Local map
Name and address of patient
Typewriter or word processor
Draft paper
Pen or pencil
Bond paper
Envelope
Dictionary
Correction tape (optional)

PROCEDURAL STEPS

1 Locate the physician's office on the map.

2 Locate the patient's address on the map.
PURPOSE: To determine the most desirable route between these two points.

3 On draft paper, using a pencil or typewriter, compose directions, using street names and including any prominent intersections, right or left turns, landmarks just preceding the destination, and means of identifying the destination.
PURPOSE: To create a mental picture of a route and directions that can easily be followed.

4 Read your copy for clarity and recheck with the map for accuracy.
PURPOSE: Note the spelling of street names and check for the accuracy of direction turns.

5 Describe parking facilities and their utilization.
EXPLANATION: Include information about meters, validation, time limit, and so forth.

6 Describe route to physician's office entrance from the parking facility.
PURPOSE: To provide peace of mind to patients who feel apprehensive about traveling to an unfamiliar location.

7 Check the complete draft for clarity and detail.
PURPOSE: It is very important that directions be accurate, clear, and complete.

8 Prepare directions in narrative form on bond paper.

9 Proofread and make any necessary corrections.

10 Prepare an envelope using the format for optical scanning.

Preparing the Outgoing Mail

ADDRESSING THE ENVELOPE

Mailing Address

The U.S. Postal Service attempts to have all mail (in No. 10 and No. 6¾ envelopes) read, coded, sorted, and canceled automatically at regional sorting stations where mail can be processed at a rate of 30,000 letters per hour. The success of automatic sorting depends on the cooperation of mailers in preparing envelopes in a format that can be read by automatic equipment. Key points are as follows:

- Use dark type on a light background; black on white is best.
- Do not use script or italic type; these cannot be read by an electronic scanner.
- Type all addresses in block format and in the area on the envelope that the scanner is programmed to read.
- Capitalize everything in the address.
- Eliminate all punctuation in the address.
- Use the standard two-letter state code instead of the spelled out name of the state (Table 11–3).
- The last line of the address must contain the city, state code, and ZIP code, and it must not exceed 27 characters in length.

TABLE 11–3 Two-Letter Abbreviations to Be Used with Zip Codes

United States and Territories			
Alabama	AL	Montana	MT
Alaska	AK	Nebraska	NE
Arizona	AZ	Nevada	NV
Arkansas	AR	New Hampshire	NH
California	CA	New Jersey	NJ
Canal Zone	CZ	New Mexico	NM
Colorado	CO	New York	NY
Connecticut	CT	North Carolina	NC
Delaware	DE	North Dakota	ND
District of Columbia	DC	Ohio	OH
Florida	FL	Oklahoma	OK
Georgia	GA	Oregon	OR
Guam	GU	Pennsylvania	PA
Hawaii	HI	Puerto Rico	PR
Idaho	ID	Rhode Island	RI
Illinois	IL	South Carolina	SC
Indiana	IN	South Dakota	SD
Iowa	IA	Tennessee	TN
Kansas	KS	Texas	TX
Kentucky	KY	Utah	UT
Louisiana	LA	Vermont	VT
Maine	ME	Virgin Islands	VI
Maryland	MD	Virginia	VA
Massachusetts	MA	Washington	WA
Michigan	MI	West Virginia	WV
Minnesota	MN	Wisconsin	WI
Mississippi	MS	Wyoming	WY
Missouri	MO		
Canadian Provinces and Territories			
Alberta	AB	Nova Scotia	NS
British Columbia	BC	Ontario	ON
Manitoba	MB	Prince Edward Island	PE
New Brunswick	NB	Quebec	PQ
Newfoundland	NF	Saskatchewan	SK
Northwest Territories	NT	Yukon Territory	YT

The characters should be distributed so that they will not exceed the following limits:

Allowance for city name	13
Space between city name and state code	1
Allowance for state code	2
Space between state code and ZIP code	1
Space for basic ZIP code	5
Space for hyphen and four additional characters	5
	27

If a city name contains more than 13 characters, you must use the approved code for that city as shown in the Abbreviations Section of the National Zip Code Directory.

The Postal Service provides three special sets of abbreviations: (1) state names; (2) long names of cities, towns, and places; and (3) names of streets and roads and general terms, such as University or Institute. You can obtain this information from the Postal Service or purchase a program for the computer. By using these abbreviations, it is possible to limit the last line of any domestic address to 27 strokes. The next-to-last line in the address block should contain a street address or post office box number.

MEDICAL ASSOCIATES INCORPORATED
4444 AVENIDA WILSHIRE
SAN CLEMENTE CA 92672-1500

HENRY B TURNER MD
PO BOX 845
JACKSONVILLE FL 32232-9950

The address block should start no higher than 2¾ inches from the bottom. Leave a bottom margin of at least ⅝ inch and left and right margins of at least 1 inch. Nothing should be written or printed below the address block or to the right of it.

The regulations for addressing envelopes were developed mainly for volume mailers with computerized mailing lists. Some exceptions are acceptable to the Postal Service and its scanning equipment. For example, the traditional style of typing an address in lower case with initial capital letters is readable by the optical scanners. Also, if you cannot fit the ZIP code on the line with the city and state, you can place it on the line immediately below.

Memory Jogger

What information should appear on the next-to-last line of an address block on the envelope?

Return Address

Always place a complete return address on your envelope. The US Postal Service will not deliver mail without postage; and if you should forget to stamp the envelope or if the stamp should fall off and there is no return address, it will go to the dead letter office. There the postal employees will open the mail in an attempt to identify the sender.

If they find an address for the sender, they will return the mail in an official envelope with a notice of postage due. If they do not find an address for the sender, the mail is destroyed and you may never know what happened to it. At best, it causes a great delay.

Notations

Any notations on the envelope directed toward the addressee, such as *Personal* or *Confidential*, should be typed and underlined on line 9 or on the third line below the return address, whichever is lower. Align it with the return address on the left edge of the envelope.

Any notations directed toward the postal service, such as SPECIAL DELIVERY or CERTIFIED MAIL,

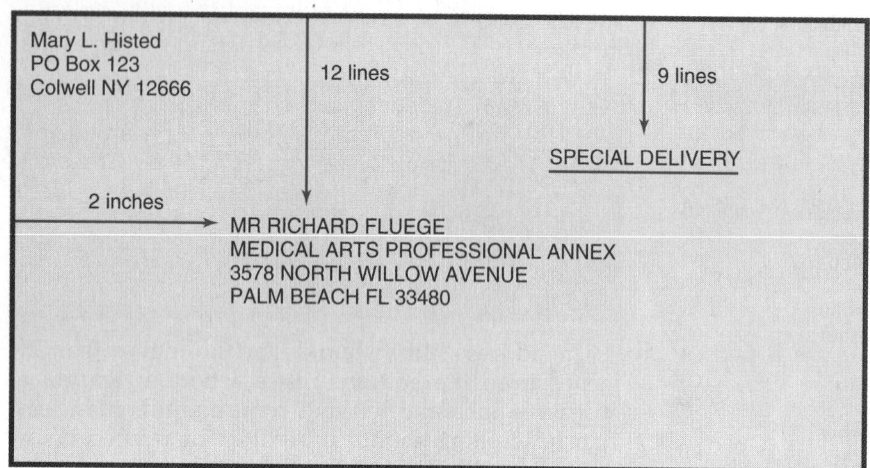

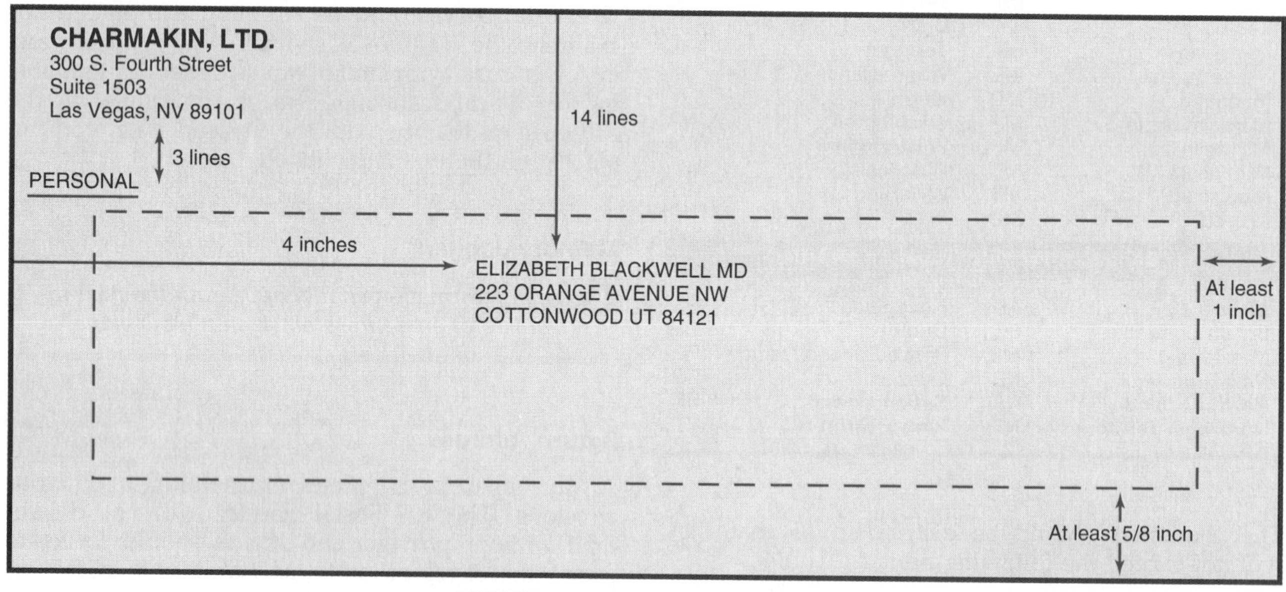

FIGURE 11–6 Addressing envelopes.

should be typed in all capital letters on the upper right side of the envelope immediately below the stamp area. If an address contains an attention line, it should be typed above the organization line, or on the line immediately above the street address or post office box number (Fig. 11–6).

Folding and Inserting Letters

Standard ways of folding and inserting letters are used so that the letter fits properly into the envelope and so that it an be easily removed without damage (Fig. 11–7).

NO. 10 ENVELOPE For a standard-size letter, bring the bottom third of the letter up and make a crease. Fold the top of the letter down to within about ⅜ inch of the creased edge and make a second crease. The second crease goes into the envelope first.

NO. 6¾ ENVELOPE For a standard-size letter, bring the bottom edge up to within about ⅜ inch of the top edge and make a crease. Then, folding from the right edge, make a fold a little less than one third of the width of the sheet and crease it. Folding from the left edge, bring the edge to within about ⅜ inch of the previous crease. Insert the left creased edge into the envelope first.

WINDOW ENVELOPE To fold a letter for insertion into a window envelope, bring the bottom third of the letter up and make a crease, then fold the top of the letter back to the crease you made before. (The inside address should now be facing you.) This method is often followed for mailing statements.

Sealing and Stamping Hints

Here's a suggestion for speeding up the sealing of a number of envelopes; at statement time, for example, many envelopes go into the mail at one time:

- Fan out unsealed envelopes, address side down, in groups of 6 to 10.
- Draw a damp sponge over the flaps and, starting with the lower piece, turn down the flaps and seal each one.

Do not use too much moisture because this may cause the glue to spread and several envelopes to stick together. A similar process simplifies stamping several letters at one time if you are not using a postage meter. If possible, purchase your stamps by the roll.

- Tear off about 10 stamps from the roll.
- Fanfold the stamps on the perforations so that they separate easily.
- Fan the envelopes address side up.
- Wet a strip of stamps with the sponge and, starting at one end of the fanned envelopes, attach the stamp at the end of the strip, tear it off, and proceed to the next envelope.

Automated sealer/stampers are also available.

Cost-Saving Mailing Procedures

USING ZIP CODES

The ZIP code is a very important part of an address, just as the area code is a very important part of a

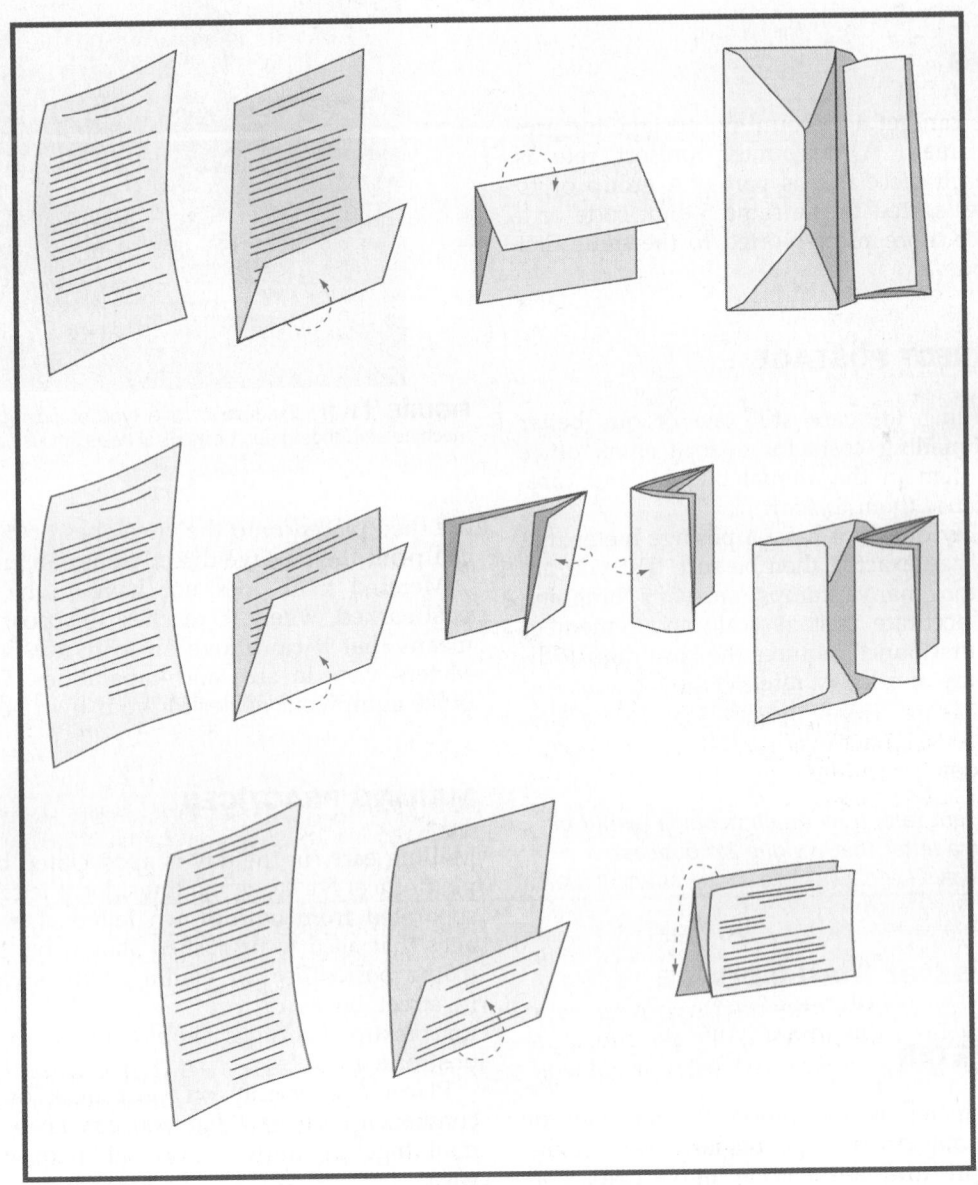

FIGURE 11–7 Correct methods of folding letters.

telephone number. ZIP codes start with the number 0 on the East Coast and gradually increase to number 9 on the West Coast and Hawaii.

The 5-digit ZIP code was introduced in 1961. The first three digits identify a major city or distribution point, and all five digits identify an individual post office, zone of a city, or other delivery unit. Later on the Postal Service added the 9-digit ZIP code, consisting of the original five digits followed by a hyphen and four additional digits that further identify the addressee's street location. The ZIP code is electronically transformed into a bar code. Your office computer may have this capability. The Postal Code claims that the ZIP-plus-4, when used with the automated letter-sorting machinery, can eliminate 20 mail handling steps and result in considerable savings. This saving is passed on to large mailers on mailings of 250 or more pieces of mail that have typewritten addresses in machine-readable format along with the 9-digit ZIP code.

PRESORTING

Large mailers can get a discount on postage for presorting their mail. A discounted presort rate is charged on each piece that is part of a group of 10 or more pieces sorted to the same 5-digit code or a group of 50 or more pieces sorted to the same first 3-digit ZIP code.

USING CORRECT POSTAGE

Although mailing fees are still one of our better bargains, the mailing costs for even a small office are a sizable item in the annual budget, and carelessness can cause them to soar.

If your facility does not have a postage meter that dispenses postage exactly, then be sure that you are not putting too many stamps on your outgoing mail. Use an accurate postage scale and remember that only the first ounce requires the base rate; additional ounces are at a lower rate.

Memory Jogger

At the current rate, how much postage would be needed on a letter that weighs 2¼ ounces?

Getting Faster Mail Service

POSTAGE METER

The postage meter is the most efficient way of stamping the mail in a large business office (Fig. 11–8). It can print postage onto adhesive strips that are then placed onto the envelopes or packages, or it can print the postage directly onto an envelope.

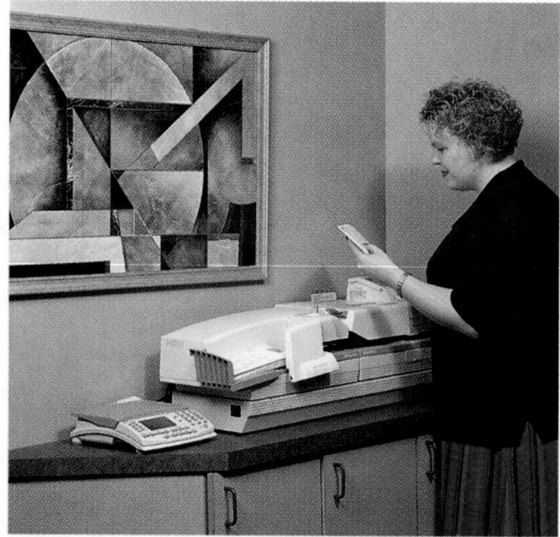

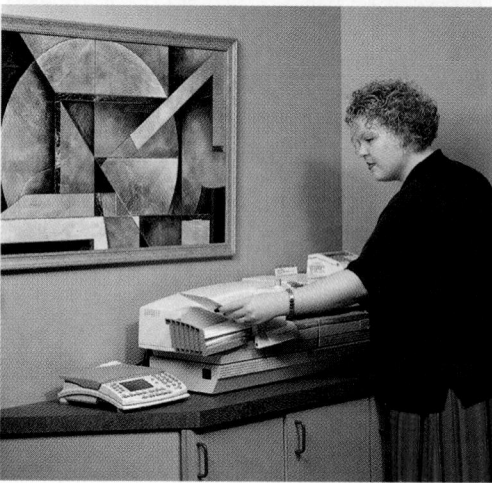

FIGURE 11–8 Example of one type of postage meter-mailing machine and photograph of medical assistant using the machine.

Metered mail does not have to be canceled or postmarked when it reaches the post office. This means that it can move on to its destination faster. Meters vary in size and capabilities. Consult your office equipment dealer for your own needs.

MAILING PRACTICES

Mailing early in the day is appreciated by your local post office. For large mailings, local letters should be separated from out-of-town letters. Letters or packages that need to be rushed should be taken directly to the post office for mailing. Others can be placed in street boxes or your own building's mail chute for pickup. Packages should always be taken to a post office.

Place a letter tray on your desk or some other convenient place so that you can keep all outgoing mail together until you are able to send it on its way.

Classifications of Mail

Mail is classified according to *type*, *weight*, and *destination*. The ounce and pound are the units of measurement.

EXPRESS MAIL NEXT-DAY SERVICE

Express Mail is available 7 days per week, 365 days per year for mailable items weighing up to 70 pounds and measuring 108 inches in combined length and girth. Service features include

- Noon delivery between major business markets
- Merchandise and document reconstruction insurance
- Express mail shipping containers
- Shipment receipt
- Optional return receipt service
- Optional COD service
- Waiver of signature option
- Collection boxes
- Optional pickup service

FIRST CLASS MAIL

This includes sealed or unsealed handwritten or typed material, such as letters, postal cards, postcards, and business reply mail. Postage for letters weighing 11 ounces or less is based on weight, in 1-ounce increments.

Envelopes larger than the standard No. 10 business envelope should have the green diamond border to expedite First Class delivery.

PRIORITY MAIL

First class mail weighing over 11 ounces is classified as priority mail, and the postage is calculated on the basis of weight and destination, with the maximum weight being 70 pounds. Flat-rate envelopes (9½ × 12¼) that can be packed with mailable materials and mailed at a 2-pound postage rate regardless of weight are available from the post office. The amount of postage is predetermined, and the filled envelope can be mailed without having to be weighed.

SECOND CLASS MAIL

Regular and preferred second class rates are available only to newspapers and periodicals that have been authorized to receive Second Class mail privileges. Copies mailed by the public are charged at the applicable express mail, priority mail, or single piece first, third, or fourth class rate.

THIRD CLASS MAIL

Third Class includes such items as catalogs, circulars, books, photographs, and other printed matter. Pieces should be sealed or secured so that they can be handled by machine but must be clearly marked with the words "Third Class."

FOURTH CLASS MAIL

Fourth Class consists of merchandise, books and printed matter that are not included in first or second class and that weigh 16 ounces or more but do not exceed 70 pounds. There are size limitations on fourth class mail; check with your post office regarding regulations on very large parcels. Rates are determined on the basis of *weight* and *destination*. Such mail may be sealed or unsealed.

Domestic Mail

MINIMUM SIZE STANDARDS

All mail must be at least 0.007-inch thick. Mail that is ¼ inch or less in thickness must be rectangular and at least 3½ inches in height and 5 inches long.

NONSTANDARD MAIL

It is important to use a standard size envelope. For each piece of nonstandard mail, the Postal Service assesses a surcharge in addition to the applicable postage and fees. Envelope sizes were standardized when the Postal Service began sorting mail by machine. The following material is considered nonstandard mail: first class mail (except presort first class and carrier route first class) weighing 1 ounce or less and all single-piece rate third class mail weighing 1 ounce or less if

1. Any of these dimensions are exceeded:

   Length—11½ inches
   Height—6½ inches
   Thickness—¼ inch

2. The length divided by the height is not between 1.3 and 2.5.

SPECIAL SERVICES

INSURANCE Insurance for coverage against loss or damage is available in amounts up to $600 for priority mail, first class, or parcel post.

REGISTRY Mail of all classes, particularly that of unusually high value, can be additionally protected by registering it. Evidence of its delivery may be requested by the sender. Registering a piece of mail also helps to trace delivery, if necessary.

When sending a registered letter, it is necessary to go to the post office and fill in the required forms. All articles to be registered must be thoroughly sealed with U.S. Postal Service tape (do not use cellophane tape) and have postage paid at first class rates.

On receipt of the item, the recipient is required to sign a form that acknowledges delivery. A registered letter may be released to the person to whom it is addressed or to his or her agent. For an additional fee, a personal receipt may be requested. This ensures that the letter will be released only to the individual to whom it is addressed. Such pieces bear the label *To Addressee Only.*

Registered mail is accounted for by number from the time of mailing until delivery and is transported separately from other mail under a special lock. In case of loss or damage, the customer may be reimbursed up to $25,000, provided that the value of the registered article has been declared at the time of mailing and that the appropriate fee has been paid.

POSTAL MONEY ORDERS Postal money orders are a convenient way of mailing money, especially for the individual who does not have a personal checking account. They may be purchased in amounts as high as $700. If a sum greater than $700 is needed, additional money orders must be purchased in amounts of $700 or less.

SPECIAL DELIVERY Mail of any class that has been marked SPECIAL DELIVERY is charged at the Special Delivery rate. Such pieces may be regular First or Second Class mail, registered, insured, or COD (Collect on Delivery) pieces. The Special Delivery designation generally does not speed up the normal travel time between two cities but does ensure immediate delivery of the item when it arrives at the designated post office.

Special delivery stamps may be purchased at the post office. Alternatively, the equivalent value in regular stamps may be affixed to the envelope, which should always be clearly marked Special Delivery. Use Special Delivery when you need delivery of an item the same day as it is received at the addressee's post office (including weekend delivery that is not available with regular mail). A fee based on the weight of the item is required in addition to the required postage. *Do not* use Special Delivery for mail addressed to a post office box or military installation.

SPECIAL HANDLING Third and Fourth Class mail sent by Special Handling receives the fastest service and ground transportation practicable—about the same as that for First Class mail. The Special Handling fee is in addition to required postage and is determined according to weight. This fee does not include insurance or Special Delivery at the destination, but Special Delivery, if desired, is available at an added cost. If a parcel is sent by Priority Mail, Special Handling is of no additional advantage because it is already traveling at the greatest possible speed.

CERTIFIED MAIL Any piece of mail without **intrinsic value** and on which postage is paid at the First Class rate will be accepted as Certified Mail. Such items as contracts, deeds, mortgages, bank books, checks, passports, insurance policies, money orders, and birth certificates that are not themselves valuable but that would be difficult to duplicate if lost should be certified. Certified Mail is also often used as an aid in collections.

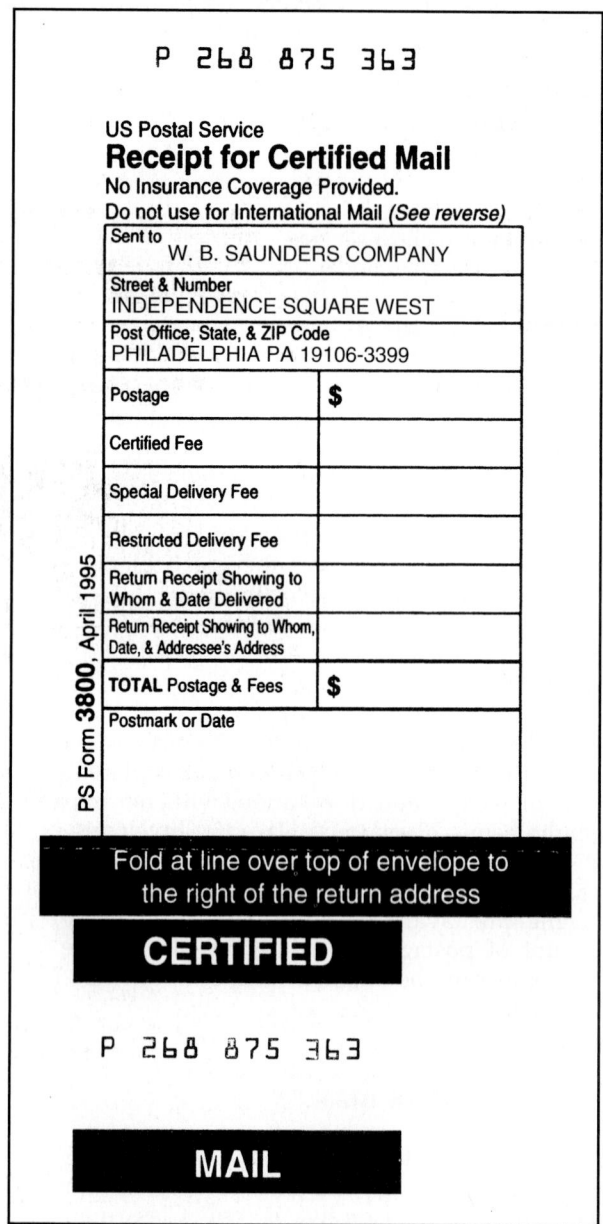
P 268 875 363

US Postal Service
Receipt for Certified Mail
No Insurance Coverage Provided.
Do not use for International Mail *(See reverse)*

Sent to W. B. SAUNDERS COMPANY	
Street & Number INDEPENDENCE SQUARE WEST	
Post Office, State, & ZIP Code PHILADELPHIA PA 19106-3399	
Postage	$
Certified Fee	
Special Delivery Fee	
Restricted Delivery Fee	
Return Receipt Showing to Whom & Date Delivered	
Return Receipt Showing to Whom, Date, & Addressee's Address	
TOTAL Postage & Fees	$
Postmark or Date	

PS Form **3800**, April 1995

Fold at line over top of envelope to the right of the return address

CERTIFIED

P 268 875 363

MAIL

FIGURE 11–9 Example of receipt for certified mail. Attach at top of envelope to the right of return address.

Regular postage in addition to a Certified Mail fee must be affixed. For an additional fee, a receipt verifying delivery can be requested. Certified Mail can be sent Special Delivery if the prescribed Special Delivery fees are paid. A record of delivery of Certified Mail is kept for 2 years at the post office of delivery; however, no record is kept at the post office of origin. Furthermore, this type of mail does not provide insurance coverage.

The medical assistant should keep a supply of Certified Mail forms and return receipts on hand (Figs. 11–9 and 11–10). These may be obtained at any post office. Full instructions are included on the forms. Fees and postage may be paid using ordinary postage stamps, meter stamps, or permit imprint. Certified Mail can be mailed at any post office, station, or branch or can be deposited in mail drops or in street letter boxes if specific instructions are followed.

CERTIFICATE OF MAILING If a sender needs proof of mailing but is not especially concerned with proof of receipt of an item, the most economic method is to obtain a Certificate of Mailing. Obtain this form at your post office and fill in the required information. Attach a stamp for the current fee and hand the form to the postal clerk along with the piece of mail. The clerk will postmark the receipt, initial it, and hand it back as acknowledgment of having received the piece of mail at the post office. This is sometimes used when mailing tax reports or other items that must be postmarked by a certain date.

Memory Jogger

Explain the basic differences between Certified Mail and Certificate of Mailing.

International Mail

Letters to distant points of the globe are in almost all cases sent by air and can be expected to reach their destination within a very few days. The rates for international mail are based on increments of one-half ounce. A table of rates can be obtained from your post office. If you wish to supply a foreign correspondent with reply postage, international reply coupons may be purchased at the post office and sent to other countries.

Private Delivery Services

Not all mail is delivered by the U.S. Postal Service. Many private services pick up and deliver mail overnight. Among these are Federal Express, United Parcel Service, Emery, and DHL. These services are highly advertised and competitive. All large cities and many smaller communities have centralized points where packages can be dropped off for the service of the sender's choice. Pickup service is also available in many communities.

Handling Special Situations

FORWARDING MAIL

First Class mail only may be forwarded from one address to another without payment of additional postage. Simply cross out the printed address and write in the address to which it should be delivered.

OBTAINING CHANGE OF ADDRESS

If the mailer wants to know an addressee's new address, this service can be obtained from the post office by placing the words *Address Correction Requested* beneath the return address on the envelope. This can be handwritten, stamped, typewritten, or printed. The post office charges a postage-due fee for this service. For First Class mail, the post office will forward the piece of mail and return a card to the sender showing the forwarding address of the addressee. The card will have a postage due stamp on it for the amount of the required fee.

RECALLING MAIL

If you have dropped a letter in the mailbox and want it back, do not ask the mail collector to give it to you; he or she is not permitted to do this. However, mail can be recalled by making written application at the post office, together with an envelope addressed identically to the one being recalled. If your letter has already left the local post office, the postmaster, at the sender's expense, can notify the postmaster at the destination post office to return the letter.

RETURNED MAIL

If a letter is returned to the sender after an attempt has been made to deliver it, it cannot be remailed without new postage. It is best simply to prepare a new envelope with the correct address, affix the proper postage, and remail.

TRACING LOST MAIL

Receipts issued by the post office, whether for money orders, registered mail, certified mail, or in-

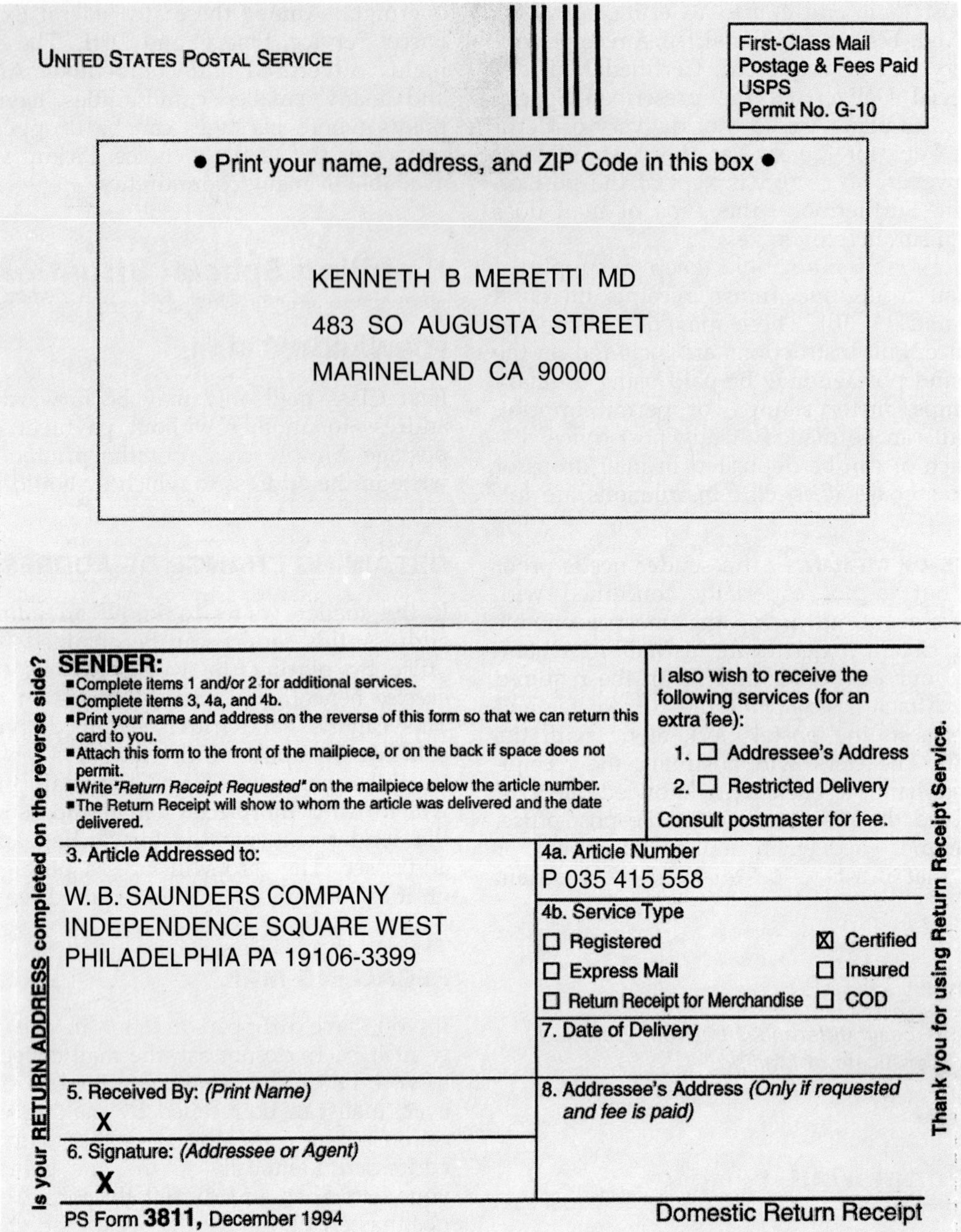

UNITED STATES POSTAL SERVICE

First-Class Mail
Postage & Fees Paid
USPS
Permit No. G-10

• Print your name, address, and ZIP Code in this box •

KENNETH B MERETTI MD
483 SO AUGUSTA STREET
MARINELAND CA 90000

Is your RETURN ADDRESS completed on the reverse side?

SENDER:
- Complete items 1 and/or 2 for additional services.
- Complete items 3, 4a, and 4b.
- Print your name and address on the reverse of this form so that we can return this card to you.
- Attach this form to the front of the mailpiece, or on the back if space does not permit.
- Write *"Return Receipt Requested"* on the mailpiece below the article number.
- The Return Receipt will show to whom the article was delivered and the date delivered.

I also wish to receive the following services (for an extra fee):
1. ☐ Addressee's Address
2. ☐ Restricted Delivery

Consult postmaster for fee.

3. Article Addressed to:
W. B. SAUNDERS COMPANY
INDEPENDENCE SQUARE WEST
PHILADELPHIA PA 19106-3399

4a. Article Number
P 035 415 558

4b. Service Type
☐ Registered ☒ Certified
☐ Express Mail ☐ Insured
☐ Return Receipt for Merchandise ☐ COD

7. Date of Delivery

5. Received By: *(Print Name)*
X

6. Signature: *(Addressee or Agent)*
X

8. Addressee's Address *(Only if requested and fee is paid)*

PS Form **3811,** December 1994 — **Domestic Return Receipt**

Thank you for using Return Receipt Service.

FIGURE 11–10 Examples of receipts for delivery of certified, registered, or insured mail. Attach to front of article if space permits. Otherwise, attach to back of article and endorse front of article with "return receipt requested" adjacent to the number.

sured mail, should be retained until receipt of the item has been acknowledged. If, after an adequate time elapses, no acknowledgment of receipt for such mailing arrives, notify the post office to trace the letter or package. Regular First Class mail is not easily traced, but the post office will make every attempt to find it for you. In tracing a lost letter or package, the post office requires that a special form be filled out; data from any original receipt should be written along with any other identifying information on this form.

Incoming Mail

Each day, a great variety of mail comes into the professional office and must be processed. There may be

- General correspondence
- Payments for services
- Bills for office purchases
- Insurance claim forms to be completed
- Laboratory reports

V-693 686 598

Receipt for Insured Mail
(Domestic or International)

UNITED STATES POSTAL SERVICE™

If Your Article is Lost or Damaged, See Instructions on the Reverse.
SAVE THIS RECEIPT UNTIL ARTICLE IS ACCOUNTED FOR

Sent To		
Street & No.		
PO, State, & ZIP Code		
Postage	Airmail ☐	$
Insurance Coverage		Fee
Special Handling		
Domestic Only	Special Delivery	
	Restricted Delivery	
Return Receipt (Except Canada)		
☐ Fragile ☐ Liquid	☐ Perishable	Total $
Postmark		Postmaster (by)

PS Form 3813-P, September 1991

U S Insured Mail

V-693 686 598

NOTE: You must present the article, container, and packaging when filing a claim for damage.

Registered No.

Date Stamp

To Be Completed By Post Office

Reg. Fee $	Special Delivery $
Handling Charge $	Return Receipt $
Postage $	Restricted Delivery $
Received by	

To Be Completed By Customer (Please Print)
All Entries Must Be in Ballpoint or Typed

Customer Must Declare Full Value $

☐ With Postal Insurance
☐ Without Postal Insurance

Domestic Insurance Is Limited To $25,000; International Indemnity Is Limited *(See Reverse)*

FROM

TO

PS Form **3806,** February 1995 **Receipt for Registered Mail** *(Customer Copy)* *(See Information on Reverse)*

FIGURE 11–10 *Continued*

- Hospital reports
- Medical society mailings
- Professional journals
- Promotional literature and samples from pharmaceutical houses
- Advertisements

In large clinics and medical centers, the mail is opened by specially designated persons in a central department to speed up this daily task. But in the average professional office, a medical assistant opens the mail using the ordinary letter-opener method.

MAIL PROCESSING

Before opening any mail, the medical assistant should have an agreement with the physician as to what procedure to follow regarding incoming mail—in other words, what letters should be opened and what pieces, if any, the physician prefers to open personally. For example, the physician may prefer to open any communications from an attorney or accountant, even when they are not marked *Personal.* If there is any doubt in regard to opening an envelope, the best rule to follow is, "Don't." Treat your physician's mail with the same consideration that you expect others to exercise toward your own. Even a simple procedure such as opening the daily mail can be done with more efficiency if a good system is followed. Have a clear working space on your desk or countertop, and proceed as follows:

Assemble the equipment and supplies you will need:

1. Letter opener
2. Paper clips
3. Stapler
4. Transparent tape
5. Date stamp

Sort the mail according to importance and urgency:

1. Physician's personal mail
2. Ordinary First Class mail
3. Checks from patients
4. Periodicals and newspapers
5. All other pieces, including drug samples

Open the mail neatly and in an organized manner:

1. Stack the envelopes so that they are all facing in the same direction.
2. Pick up the top one and tap the envelope so that when you open it you will not cut the contents.
3. Open all envelopes along the top edge for easiest removal of contents.
4. Remove the contents of each envelope and hold the envelope to the light to see that nothing remains inside.
5. Make a note of the postmark when this is important.
6. Discard the envelope after you have checked to see that there is a return address on the message contained inside. Some offices make it a policy to attach the envelope to each piece of correspondence until it has received attention.
7. Date stamp the letter and attach any enclosures.
8. If there is an enclosure notation at the bottom of the letter, check to be certain that the enclosure was included. Should it be missing, indicate this on the notation by writing the word *no* and circling it. This may be as far as your employer will want you to proceed with handling the correspondence.

ANNOTATING

If you have to **annotate** the mail, you can perform an additional service by reading each letter through, underlining the significant words and phrases, and noting in the margin any action required. If it is a letter that needs no reply, you can code it for filing at this time. A nonprint pencil that does not photocopy may be used for the annotating, if desired.

When mail refers to previous correspondence, obtain this from the file and attach it. Or if the patient's chart is needed in replying to an inquiry, pull the chart and place it with the letter.

A specific place should be agreed on for placing the opened and annotated mail. This will probably be some area on the physician's desk. When you have completed the sorting, opening, and annotating of the mail, place those items that the physician will wish to see in the established place, with the most important mail on top.

Personal mail, of course, is to remain unopened. Should you in error open a piece of personal mail addressed to your employer, fold and replace it inside the envelope, and write across the outside *Opened in Error,* followed by your initials. Use the same procedure with a piece of mail addressed to another office that may have been opened in error. In such cases, reseal the envelope with transparent tape and hand it to your carrier.

RESPONDING TO THE MAIL

In some offices, the physician and the medical assistant go over the mail together. As you gain confidence, you will find that you can draft a reply to some inquiries. Most physicians are very pleased to delegate this responsibility, especially on matters that do not relate to patient care.

Letters of referral from other physicians should be carefully noted so that an answer may be sent after the patient has been seen and the physician can give a report. If considerable time may pass before such information can be sent, it is a courteous gesture to write a thank-you note to the referring physician advising that a detailed letter will follow. Some physicians send printed cards expressing thanks for referrals; others prefer to write thank-you letters to professional colleagues.

Mail the Assistant Can Handle

CASH RECEIPTS

There will be some mail that the medical assistant can handle alone, for instance, payments from patients and insurance forms to be completed. All cash and checks should be separated and recorded immediately in the day's receipts.

INSURANCE FORMS

Insurance forms for completion should be put in a predetermined place for handling at the appropriate time. If there is an insurance clerk or other individual who processes the claims, they should be passed along to that person immediately.

DRUG SAMPLES

Sample drugs and related literature may arrive in the mail. Determine from the physician what types of literature and samples should be saved. Most physicians keep pertinent new samples in their desks, along with the accompanying literature for immediate reference. Other drug samples are **categorically** stored. Drugs should never be tossed into the trash.

Vacation Mail

When the physician is away from the office, it is generally the responsibility of a medical assistant to handle all mail. In this event, all pieces should be examined carefully. The medical assistant can then make a decision in regard to handling each piece on the basis of the following questions:

- Is this important enough that I should phone or FAX the physician?
- Shall I forward this for immediate attention?
- Shall I answer this myself or send a brief note to the correspondent, explaining that there will be a slight delay because the physician is out of the office?
- Can this wait for attention until the physician returns without appearing negligent?

If you are unable to contact the physician or to forward important mail, always answer the sender immediately, explaining the delay and requesting cooperation. Most offices have a copy machine as part of the office equipment. Instead of forwarding an original piece of mail and risking possible loss, make a copy for forwarding. Then, if the physician wishes you to answer the letter, notations can be made on the copy and returned to you without defacing the original letter.

When your employer is traveling from place to place, the envelope on each communication should be numbered consecutively. Doing this enables the physician to easily determine whether any mail has been lost or delayed. By keeping your own record of each piece of mail sent out, with its corresponding number, anything that might be lost can be identified and remailed if necessary.

Correspondence not requiring immediate action that the medical assistant is unable to answer until the physician returns should be placed in a special folder marked *Requires Attention* and placed on top of other accumulated mail. Mail that the medical assistant can compose but that requires the physician's approval before mailing, should be put into another special folder marked *For Approval*. When the physician returns, these letters can be rapidly checked and signed.

Any letters marked *Personal* that you hesitate to open and are unable to forward may be acknowledged to the return address on the envelope. The brief acknowledgment should state that the physician is out of town for a certain length of time and will attend to the letter immediately on returning. Your acknowledgment should also offer your help in any way possible in the meantime.

Discard any mail that you would ordinarily not bring to the physician's attention. Some promotional literature falls into this category. (Make certain that mailings from professional organizations, whether they are First, Second, Third, or Fourth Class, are saved.)

There may be rare periods when the entire facility is closed. In such cases, the local post office should be notified to forward all First Class mail to an address supplied by the physician, if possible. Your postal carrier cannot accept an oral request to leave the mail with another person or at another address. A formal request must be made. If forwarding is out of the question, place a request with the post office to hold the mail until a specified date when someone will again be on duty. Never leave mail unattended to gather outside a mailbox or clutter up a doorway in a hall. Even mail slots may become filled or magazines may become stuck in them, causing important mail to pile up outside the slot. Far too much money and mail of a confidential nature is sent to physicians' offices to take chances on mail theft or destruction.

Systematizing your routine for processing all incoming and outgoing mail can put you in control of the paper blizzard!

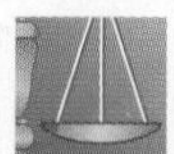

LEGAL AND ETHICAL ISSUES

Every letter sent out from your facility should project a professional image.

The U.S. Postal Service requires that all volume mailers follow a special format in addressing envelopes so that they can be read, coded, sorted, and canceled automatically. Private mailers are requested to follow the same format.

The Postal Service will not deliver mail without postage attached. If there is no return address the mail goes to the dead letter office, where postal employees will open the mail in an attempt to identify the sender.

CRITICAL THINKING

1 What could be a negative effect of poorly written communications?

2 Visit a store that sells office stationery and observe the quality of the various offerings.

3 Examine a few of the promotional letters that arrive in your mail. Think about what is pleasing or not pleasing about their look and content.

4 Can you suggest the reason that volume mailers

would need special regulations for addressing envelopes?

HOW DID I DO? Answers to Memory Joggers

1. Sub 24 is an abbreviation for substance number or weight of a ream of 17 × 22-inch paper. Heavier weight paper has a higher substance number.
2. Ophthalmology
3. Memorandum is less formal. No salutation or complimentary closing is used.
4. The pages could become separated and difficult to identify.
5. *Heading*—letterhead and date line
   Opening—inside address, salutation, and attention line, if used.
   Body—subject line and message
   Closing—complimentary closing, typed signature, reference initials, special notations.
6. Either the street address or the post office box number.
7. At this writing the postage would be 32¢ + 23¢ + 23¢, a total of 78¢. Rates are periodically changed.
8. The post office keeps a record of delivery of Certified Mail, and the sender may request a receipt verifying delivery. A Certificate of Mailing provides only proof of mailing.

REFERENCES

Sabin W: The Gregg Reference Manual, 7th ed. New York, Glencoe/McGraw-Hill, 1994.

Schwager E: Medical English Usage and Abusage. Phoenix, AZ, The Oryx Press, 1991.

Taber's Cyclopedic Medical Dictionary, 18th ed. Philadelphia, FA Davis, 1997.

The Postal Manual. Washington, DC, US Government Printing Office.

Dictation and Transcription

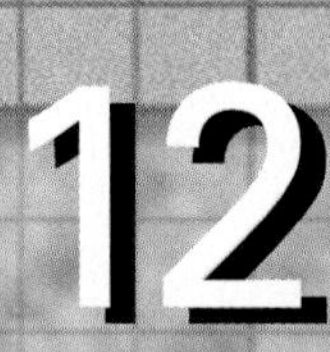

OUTLINE

LEARNING OBJECTIVES

Cognitive: On successful completion of this chapter, you should be able to:

1. Define and spell the terms listed in the Vocabulary.
2. List six basic educational requirements for the medical transcriptionist.
3. Name two primary requisites for the independently practicing transcriptionist.
4. List the three steps of activity in the machine transcription process.
5. List five functional features of a typical transcribing unit.
6. State the principal differences between a *dedicated word processor* and a *computer.*
7. Name three kinds of frequently dictated reports in the average physician's office.

Performance: On successful completion of this chapter, and given the necessary equipment, you should be able to:

1. Estimate the length of a finished document before transcribing it.
2. Make any necessary corrections in keyboarding before removing the document from the machine.
3. Correctly utilize basic rules of capitalization.
4. Follow the rules for word division.
5. Determine when to use figures for numbers.
6. Correctly format medical reports.
7. Proofread and edit a transcribed document.

VOCABULARY

alignment The state of being in the correct relative position

cassette A magnetic tape wound on two reels and encased in a plastic or metal container; *microcassette* A very small cassette tape that may be used in a hand-held dictating unit

consultation report A report of the findings of the consulting physician to be sent to the referring physician

CPT manual *Current Procedural Terminology* manual

daisy wheel A printing element made of plastic or metal used on some typewriters and impact printers that derives its name from its shape, which is like that of a daisy

dictation The process of recording the spoken word onto a storage medium from which a printed copy will be produced

editing The process of examining text to determine accuracy and clarity

flagging A way of bringing attention to a blank space for possible correction in a transcribed page (also called tagging, carding, or marking)

fonts Sets of printing type that are of one size and style

HCPCS Acronym for HCFA's Common Procedure Coding System, used in determining Medicare fees

ICD manual International Classification of Diseases manual

indicator strip A charted strip that is inserted into the dictation unit and on which the dictator marks the beginning and end point of each document and any corrections to be made

keyboarding The process of entering characters into the memory of a word processor

progress notes Records of patient visits, telephone calls, progress, and treatment that are inserted into the patient's chart

proofreading Checking a document for spelling, sentence structure, punctuation, capitalization, style, and format

subscripts Symbols or numbers written immediately below another character

superscripts Symbols or numbers written immediately above another character

transcription Listening to recorded dictation and translating it into written form

A medical transcriptionist is a highly skilled professional whose educational background is similar in some respects to that of the administrative medical assistant. The medical transcriptionist must demonstrate many skills and qualities.

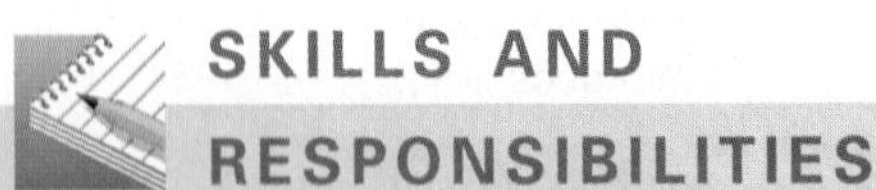

SKILLS AND RESPONSIBILITIES

ESSENTIAL SKILLS OF THE MEDICAL TRANSCRIPTIONIST

- Above-average typing and word processing skills
- Understanding of human anatomy and physiology and of the pathologic conditions that affect the human body
- Knowledge of medical terminology used in medical records, medical and surgical procedures, and laboratory tests
- Superior command of grammar, sentence structure and style, and spelling
- **Editing** and **proofreading** skills
- Ability to use a medical dictionary and other standard reference materials

Administrative medical assistants may find that transcribing **dictation** is one of their job requirements. Transcribing can be performed from handwritten notes, such as those in shorthand, or from machine dictation. In the health care facility the medical transcriptionist is a part of the team. Smooth operation of the facility may depend on the timely and accurate performance of assigned responsibilities, such as record documentation and the preparation of special reports.

Many professional medical transcriptionists practice independently and may affiliate with the American Association for Medical Transcription and become certified (see Chapter 3). The independent transcriptionist will find that *accuracy* and *speed* are primary requisites. Income depends on the transcriptionist's productivity, which may be measured by the number of pages, characters, or lines typed. The person who intends to do transcribing exclusively would do well to take a special course in transcription techniques.

Machine Transcription

Three stages of activity are involved in the process of dictation and transcription:

- Dictating into a dictation unit
- Listening to what has been dictated
- **Keyboarding** the dictated text to a printed document using correct format and required punctuation

Memory Jogger

It is understood that accuracy is essential in preparing medical reports. Why is speed also important to the independent transcriptionist?

DICTATION UNIT

The dictation unit is used by the physician to record material to be typed. Dictation units vary in design and capabilities. The desktop dictation unit is common in an office setting. This may be a combination unit used for both dictation and transcription. Alternatively, a machine used only for dictation may remain at the physician's desk; a separate **transcription** unit, including headphones and a foot pedal, remains at the transcriptionist's station. A lightweight portable hand-held dictation unit may be used for times when the physician (dictator) wishes to dictate while traveling or attending meetings away from the office. Physicians in a larger setting may install transcribing equipment that they can access by telephone wherever they may be. Many hospitals have this arrangement. All produce a recording that the transcriptionist listens to while keyboarding the text.

TRANSCRIBER UNIT

The unit operated by the transcriptionist may use magnetic tape, a **cassette,** or a disk. A desk-top unit using mini-, micro-, or standard cassettes is typical in the physician's office (Fig. 12–1).

There are many types and manufacturers of transcribing equipment, but most units contain certain standard features. Before using any equipment, the medical assistant should study the manufacturer's instruction manual. Most transcription units have a minimum of the following features:

- Stop and start control, with back-up and fast-forward ability
- Speed control
- Volume control
- Tone control
- Indicator for locating special instructions and determining the document length

STOP AND START CONTROL A foot pedal allows the transcriptionist to start, stop, back up, or fast forward the unit. He or she may wish to stop the unit while catching up with the typing, back up to replay a portion that was not understood, pause to insert additional matter from another source, or stop to check spelling. Most have an optional adjustment so that a slight rewind of the tape occurs when the machine is stopped and restarted. This prevents the loss of any dictated material in the process.

SPEED CONTROL The speed control feature can be used to slow down the recording of a fast dictator or speed up that of a slow dictator to match the speed of the transcriptionist.

VOLUME CONTROL The volume control in the headset can be adjusted to suit each unit of transcription. The headset also serves as a sound barrier by shutting out extraneous office sounds and preserving the confidentiality of the dictation.

TONE CONTROL The tone control feature allows the transcriptionist to increase or decrease the bass or treble to the pitch most understandable and pleasing to the ear.

INDICATOR STRIP For many years, dictating and transcribing machines have had **indicator strips** that could be inserted into the machine to allow the dictator to mark the point at which each item begins and ends and where corrections, if any, are needed. These strips are then attached to the transcribing machine to aid the typist. All too often the dictator refuses or neglects to use these indicators. When this happens, the transcriptionist should courteously remind the dictator of the importance of using this device.

Instead of an indicator strip, the machine may have a display window or cue-tone indexing capability that provides this same information. All of these features assist the transcriptionist in planning his or her transcribing duties.

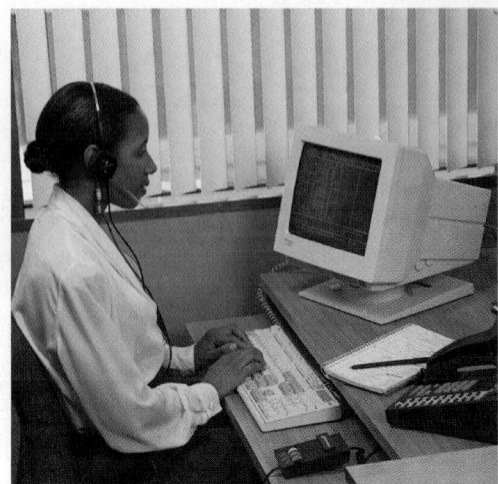

FIGURE 12–1 Transcriptionist.

The beginning transcriptionist tends to listen to a few words, stop the machine, type those words, and then restart the transcriber unit. Through practice, the transcriptionist learns to coordinate keyboarding activity with listening skills and listen ahead, thereby retaining in memory more and more of the dictated material so that it becomes unnecessary to stop and start the machine for this purpose.

Memory Jogger

 *What feature of a transcribing unit prevents the loss of dictated material when the machine is stopped and restarted?*

KEYBOARDING UNIT

The most important piece of equipment for the transcriptionist is the typewriter or computer on which the printed text will be produced. Many improvements have occurred within the past few years.

The manual typewriter is now virtually a museum piece. The electric typewriter appears to be on its way out as well, having been replaced by the electronic typewriter. The machines of choice in the modern office are the electronic typewriter, with or without memory; the dedicated word processor (display text editor); and the desk-top computer with word processing software.

ELECTRONIC TYPEWRITER

The electronic typewriter improves on the features of the electric typewriter by having the ability to automatically perform many tasks that save time and produce a more pleasing result. It is sometimes referred to as the *intelligent typewriter.* Instead of noisy keys, it has a single element, which is most likely a **daisy wheel.** With a daisy wheel, the typist may choose from among many kinds of type styles and sizes by simply removing one wheel and substituting the one of choice. Automatic features, such as number **alignment,** automatic centering, underlining, indenting, caps lock, and carrier return, are accomplished with the stroke of a key. Most have the capability of storing a limited amount of text and may have a display screen and spell-check capability (see Procedure 12–1).

PROCEDURE 12–1

Transcribing a Machine-Dictated Letter Using a Typewriter

GOAL

To transcribe a machine-dictated letter into a mailable document without error or detectable corrections, using a typewriter.

EQUIPMENT AND SUPPLIES

Transcribing machine	Letterhead Paper
Typewriter	Correcting Supplies
Draft paper	Reference Manual

PROCEDURAL STEPS

1. Assemble supplies
2. Turn on the transcription equipment
3. Set *line* for double spacing
   PURPOSE: To allow room for making changes or corrections
4. Type a draft of the letter
5. Edit the draft for spelling, insertions, and sentence structure
6. Note any necessary corrections
7. Set *line* and *margins* for attractive placement of the letter
8. Retype the draft on letterhead paper
9. Proofread the letter for content and errors before removing it from the typewriter

PROCEDURE 12-2
Transcribing a Machine-Dictated Letter Using a Computer or Word Processor

GOAL

To transcribe a machine-dictated letter into a mailable document without error or detectable corrections, using a computer or word processor.

EQUIPMENT AND SUPPLIES

Transcribing machine
Word processor or computer with appropriate software
Stationery
Reference Manual

PROCEDURAL STEPS

1 Assemble supplies
2 Set up the format for selected letter style
3 Keyboard the text while listening to the dictated letter
4 Edit the letter on the monitor
PURPOSE: The letter should be in mailable form before printing
5 Execute a spell check
6 Direct the letter to the printer

DEDICATED WORD PROCESSOR

The term *word processing* was coined by IBM in the 1960s to describe its innovative Magnetic Tape Selectric Typewriter (MT/ST). The MT/ST was costly and met with some resistance because it required special training. Word processors today are much simpler. The word processor is a computer that is especially designed to perform one function only—word processing. It is more expensive than the electronic typewriter, but in situations that require a great amount of word processing it is a good investment.

COMPUTER

A desk-top computer with word processing software is a third type of keyboarding equipment (Fig. 12–2). The principal difference between it and the dedicated word processor is that other tasks can be performed on the computer.

The person who uses a word processor or computer can throw away the eraser and correcting fluid because the entire text can be edited on the monitor, any necessary corrections or changes made, and a perfect copy obtained before any printing is done (see Procedure 12–2). Revisions can be made easily without retyping a whole document. Blocks of text can be moved from one section of the document to another with just a few keystrokes. Even whole sections of text can be inserted into a document easily and quickly. Paragraphs or statements that are used frequently in letters or reports can be saved as *macros* and with a stroke or two on the keyboard can be retrieved and inserted in the appropriate place without retyping.

Most word processing programs can instruct the printer to print in boldface or in alternate type **fonts.** Some can create **subscripts** and **superscripts.**

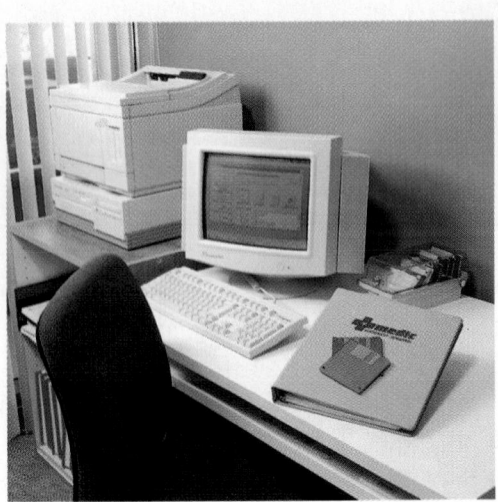

FIGURE 12–2 Desk-top computer.

HISTORY AND PHYSICAL EXAMINATION

CHIEF COMPLAINT: Severe pain, left hip area, duration for the past couple of years.

PRESENT ILLNESS: The patient in 1950 was involved in a severe auto accident, at which time he sustained injury to his back and leg as well as to his right shoulder and left hip. He subsequently had back surgery performed as well as a fusion, which was performed at St. Francis Hospital in Yourtown. The patient, however, has had continue sciatica and has been seen by Dr. Thomas Brown. Appropriate studies have been done. It was felt that there is nothing from the neurosurgical standpoint which could be of benefit to his left leg sciatic-type pain.

In June 1990, the patient underwent insertion of a total right shoulder because of severe progressive degenerative osteoarthritis of the right shoulder. He has done quite well with that, has improved his range of motion, and has minimal to no pain. The patient, however, has had progressive pain about his left hip that has not responded to anti-inflammatory medications. X-rays reveal a progressive degenerative osteoarthritis with cystic formation.

FORMER SURGERIES:
1. Removal of right kidney in 8/85.
2. Former back surgeries in the 1940s.
3. Right total shoulder in 7/90.

SERIOUS ILLNESSES: None.

MEDICATIONS: Occasional Darvocet for pain.

HABITS: Patient does not smoke.

REVIEW OF SYSTEMS:
HEENT: Patient denies any recent URIs or chronic sore throat.
CV: Patient denies history of chest pain or heart disease.
GI: Patient denies nausea, vomiting, diarrhea.
GU: Patient denies dysuria or frequency.
MS: See Present Illness.
HEM: Patient denies any bleeding tendencies.

VITAL SIGNS: Blood pressure 132/72.

GENERAL APPEARANCE: Patient appears to be in good health for his stated age.

HEENT: PERRL. Funduscopic examination within normal limits. Ears are clear, mouth negative.

NECK: Supple, Thyroid is not enlarged.

LYMPHADENOPATHY: None.

HEART: Regular rate, no murmurs. Patient has good bilateral carotid pulsations.

PHYSICAL EXAMINATION:
ADBOMEN: Soft, no abnormal masses.

GENITALIA: Normal male.

RECTAL: Prostate is somewhat firm; however, there are no changes from 1992 exam.

EXTREMITIES: Patient has 0 internal rotation of the left hip. He has abduction approximately 10 degrees, flexion marked pain about 70 degrees. Patient has a very mild left hip flexion contracture.

IMPRESSION:
1. Severe degenerative osteoarthritis, left hip.
2. Postoperative right total shoulder replacement.
3. Residual sciatica, left leg.

____
xxxx, M.D.

FIGURE 12–3 History and physical examination report.

A *spell-check* feature can proofread a lengthy document in minutes with complete accuracy. One disadvantage of the spell checker is that it can determine only whether a word is spelled correctly. If an incorrect word that is correctly spelled is typed, the checker will not pick it up (e.g., the use of *ilium* instead of *ileum*). With the text stored in memory or on a diskette, additional editing can be done and a corrected copy printed out almost effortlessly at any future time.

Preparation of Reports

The scope of a transcriptionist's duties is determined by each specific employer. In most instances, the preparation of medical reports is a large part of the professional assignment. The reports most frequently dictated in the physician's office are

- History and Physical
- Progress Notes
- Consultation Reports
- Correspondence

TURN-AROUND TIME

Specific time limits may be established for the completion of a variety of reports, with a designation of STAT (abbreviation for the Latin *statim,* meaning *immediate*), CURRENT, or OLD.

EXAMPLES OF HOW TO USE TIME LIMITS

STAT: Radiology, Pathology, and Laboratory Reports, which should be reported in 12 hours or less
CURRENT: History and Physical, Consultation, and Operation Reports due within 24 hours
OLD: Discharge Summaries and Emergency Department notes due within 72 hours

Memory Jogger

What reports are most frequently dictated in a physician's office?

HISTORY AND PHYSICAL

The History and Physical (H & P) may be dictated as the basis for the new patient's chart. When a patient is to be admitted to a hospital for treatment or observation, the physician will dictate an H & P before admitting the patient, and this becomes a part of the patient's hospital chart. No universal standard form exists for the H & P, but Figure 12–3 is a typical example.

Many sections of this report have a standard response that occurs over and over, depending on the patient's complaint and condition. These responses can be stored in memory as macros and used as needed with one or two strokes of the keyboard.

PROGRESS NOTES

The physician who sees many patients during a day does not have the time to handwrite **progress notes** on the medical chart after each patient visit. The physician will either dictate notes in the presence of the patient or immediately after the visit. The transcriptionist will then prepare these notes as an addition to the chart (Fig. 12–4).

By using continuous pages of pressure-sensitive paper, a great deal of time and motion can be saved. The paper is inserted only once and is later separated for the appropriate charts. Some papers have interval perforations that expedite the separation of entries. When typing these progress notes, space is left at the end for the physician's signature. The notes should never be entered into the chart without the physician's approval and signature.

PROGRESS NOTES

1. Brought back to ofc. regarding wart, left dorsal hand, of about 6 mo duration.
   EXAM: 5-mm diameter raised, round, sharply marginated, gray-pink, finely papillomatous and keratotic lesion, left dorsal hand.
   IMP: Verruca vulgaris.
   DISP: 1) Discussed treatment by electrosurgery vs. cryotherapy with father, including scarring with electrosurgery.
   2) Lesion removed by D & C under local anesth with Xyl. + Epi.
   3) Monsels, DSD, H_2O_2 t.i.d.
   4) See prn
2. Has been treating superficial multicentric BCCA, distal left mandible, with Efudex 5% cream b.i.d. for 3 wks. See inflammation with central erosion and peripheral crusting in involved area. Response appears appropriate.
   DISP: 1) Cont Efudex 5% cream b.i.d.
   2) See in 3 wks.
3. Pt. points out very small, quiescent-appearing actinic keratosis—inferior right lateral arm x 1 and proximal left extensor forearm x 1. Discussed nature of lesions with pt. L N2 about 10 sec. each. Re/ck prn persistence.
4. Pt. inquires about lesion, medial right leg. Possibly present since birth. No change in size or color over time. No tmt to date.
   EXAM: Inferior right medial leg: 17 x 15-mm diameter round, sharply marginated, macular, uniformly medium-brown lesions; a few terminal hairs penetrate surface of lesion.
   IMP: Benign pigmented macule.
   DISP: 1) Discussed benign appearance of lesion with pt.
   2) No tmt at this time.
   3) Re/ck prn change.

FIGURE 12–4 Progress reports.

CONSULTATION REPORTS

Physicians who act as consultants are expected to prepare a detailed report of their findings and recommendations and send it to the referring physician. The **consultation report** is dictated by the consulting physician to be transcribed within the office or by an independent transcriptionist if outside services are used. The report may have the same general form as the H & P or may be in correspondence form as the one in Figure 12–5.

OPERATION REPORT

The operation report is dictated by the surgeon immediately after surgery. The heading will show the patient's name, date, hospital code number and room number, plus names of the surgeon, any assistants, and the anesthetist. The report includes a preoperative diagnosis, postoperative diagnosis (these may be identical), the name of the procedure done, and a detailed narrative of the procedure accomplished. The surgeon must sign the report before it

December 2, 200x

Thomas Brown, M.D.
234 Maine Avenue
Yourtown, USA

Dear Doctor Brown:

Re: Rebecca Bloom

Rebecca Bloom is a 79-year-old, right-handed lady with known asthma who was seen in neurological consultation for progressive weakness in her legs.

She has had a prior neurological consultation, which suggested motor neuron disease. A muscle biopsy was consistent with neurogenic atrophy, and an EMG revealed positive sharp waves and fibrillation potentials in the quadriceps bilaterally and, to a lesser degree, in the distal groups of both legs below the knees. EMG of the upper extremities was normal.

Chemistry studies were unremarkable.

She denies any exposure to heavy metals or other neurotoxins. She has noted weakness in her legs for the past two years, initially above the knees, left greater than right. The problem has been slowly progressive, but she does not experience any weakness below the knees. She feels that her arms are strong, and she has experienced no difficulty with speech, swallowing, or eye movements. She has lost approximately 20 pounds in the last two years, which she attributes to nausea and poor dentures. She denies any significant muscle wasting or muscle twitching in the thigh muscles. She notes that her feet feel "abnormal," but she does not describe true numbness or tingling. Bowel/bladder function is intact. She has had a vertebral compression fracture due to osteoporosis because of her chronic prednisone therapy for asthma.

Her past medical history is significant for right hip surgery; ectopic pregnancy; status post bladder repair; history of asthma-COPD; status post muscle biopsy; history of mild enlargement of her heart with a valvular dysfunction.

Her medications include prednisone, 7.5 mg q.d. for several years; Brethine; TheoDur, 150 mg p.o. bid; Lanoxin, 0.125 mg p.o. every day; supplemental folic acid; daily Coumadin therapy; Premarin; vitamin D, 50,000 units two times per week; as well as an Alupent Inhalor and Intal; Dyazide, 1 p.o. qd.

Allergies: None known.

The patient denies tobacco or ethanol use. In the past six months, she has required the use of a cane to ambulate.

On physical exam, she is a well-developed, well-nourished female in no acute distress. She is oriented x three with an intact mental status exam. Speech is normal. Blood pressure is 120/80. Neck is supple. Carotids are 2+ bilaterally without bruits over the carotids or the supraclavicular region. Spine is nontender to percussion, HEENT: Normocephalic; atraumatic. Chest is clear to auscultation. Heart has a regular rate and rhythm; S1 and S2 without murmur. Cranial nerves: Olfactory sense is intact. Right disc is sharp with an intraocular lens present; left disc is nonvisible secondary to the presence of a cataract. The right pupil is greater than the left pupil by 0.5 mm; both are round and reactive to light. Visual fields are full. Extraocular movements are intact without nystagmus. Corneal reflexes are intact bilaterally, and there is normal facial symmetry and expression. Hearing is intact bilaterally, and the uvula is midline and upgoing. Sternocleidomastoid function is symmetric, and the tongue is midline.

Motor exam displays strength to be intact in the upper extremities bilaterally. The lower extremities display 3 4/5 strength in the iliopsoas and quadriceps bilaterally. There is trace weakness in the adductors and abductors, as well as hip extensors bilaterally. There is trace weakness of the hamstrings. There is no notable atrophy or fasciculation. The patient is unable to squat and has difficulty arising from a chair. Strength in the musculature distal to the knees is intact. There are no notable fasciculations. Thigh diameter is 33 mm on the right and 34 mm on the left, and the calves are both 30 mm in diameter. Sensory exam displays diminished vibratory and pinprick response in the feet, with position and soft touch intact. Finger-to-nose and heel-to-shin are intact. Fine motor movements and rapid alternating hand movements are normal. Deep tendon reflexes for the bicep, tricep, brachioradialis are 1-2+ bilaterally, with absent knee and ankle jerks; and the toes are downgoing. Gait and tandem are fair. Straight leg raise testing is unremarkable, as is bilateral hip rotation. Pedal pulses are 2+; the feet are cool in temperature, slightly erythematous, and swollen, with evidence of venous stasis.

FIGURE 12–5 Consultation report.

Thomas Brown, M.D. -2- December 2, 200x

Data Base: Nerve conduction studies of the lower extremities suggested a peripheral polyneuropathy, and an EMG of the upper extremities was normal. EMG of the left lower extremity revealed denervation to a greater extent in the left quadriceps and, to a minimal extent, in the left gastrocnemius. Some polyphasic small amplitude motor unit potentials were noted in the quadriceps that can be seen in myopathies.

Impression: Rebecca Bloom has evidence of proximal muscle weakness in her lower extremities with associated sensory deficits, including diminished vibratory and pinprick response in her feet and has been on chronic steroid therapy for her asthma-COPD. Her clinical picture, correlating with the electrical studies, suggests a peripheral polyneuropathy and possibly a proximal myopathy from chronic steroid use, rather than a motor neuron disorder, considering the lack of development of symptoms in the bulbar musculature or the upper extremities and the slow rate of progression.

Chemistry studies were unremarkable other than an elevated calcium of 11.3, and this will be further evaluated with the appropriate ionized calcium and PTH level.

I have recommended that we observe her over a period of time to document any evolution of her illness. I have referred her to physical therapy and pointed out that any reduction in her steroid use would be of value.

Further recommendations include a pelvic examination in view of the proximal muscle weakness in the lower extremities.

Her prior records will be reviewed, and the appropriate chemistry studies will be ordered.

Thank you for referring this pleasant lady for neurological evaluation.

Very truly yours,

Oliver South, M.D.

FIGURE 12–5 *Continued*

REGIONAL MEDICAL CENTER
YOURTOWN, USA

REPORT OF OPERATION

DATE: 12/05/99

PREOPERATIVE DIAGNOSIS: MASS, LEFT CALF

POSTOPERATIVE DIAGNOSIS: SAME, PROBABLY DEGENERATIVE MUSCLE DISEASE, LEFT CALF

PROCEDURE: OPEN BIOPSY LEFT CALF MUSCLE

SURGEON: XXXX, M.D.
ASST. SURGEON: XXXX, M.D.
ANESTHESIA: XXXX, M.D. General endotracheal anesthesia

FINDINGS: Under general anesthetic, the patient's left lower extremity was prepped and draped in the usual manner. The left leg was isolated in a sterile field, a well-padded thigh tourniquet was inflated to 300 mm of mercury after elevating and exsanguinating the leg with an Esmarch bandage. Linear incision was made over the posterior medial aspect of the calf, and dissection was carried out through the skin and subcutaneous tissue and superficial fascia. The gastrocnemius muscle was opened posteromedially. It was obvious that the muscle appeared to be rather firm and woody in consistency with infiltrating lighter tissue consistent with fatty tissue throughout the muscle fibers. The muscle fibers also appeared to be essentially relatively avascular and did not contract with direct stimulation. Samples of tissue were sent for frozen section, which indicated both degenerative and reparative process within the muscle without evidence of any tumor infiltration or evidence of infection. The specimens were sent for permanent section. At this point, the wound was thoroughly irrigated with normal saline solution containing bacitracin and neomycin. Previously, the wound was cultured, aerobic and anaerobically. The tourniquet was deflated at 10 minutes of tourniquet time. The wound was closed in layers with 0 and 2-0 Dexon followed by closure of the skin with subcuticular 4-0 Dexon followed by Steri-Strips and dry sterile compression dressings. The patient tolerated the procedure well; she was awakened from the anesthetic and went to the recovery room in good condition. EBL less than 20 mL.

______________________ M.D.

NAME: XXXX
HOSPITAL NO. XXXX
ROOM NO. OP
ATTENDING: XXXX, M.D.

mek

FIGURE 12–6 Operation report.

is placed in the permanent record. It is important that this report be completed and filed currently, because there may be other physicians attending the patient who were not present during the surgery (Fig. 12–6).

PATHOLOGY REPORT

When tissue or fluid is removed by the surgeon it is examined by the pathologist, who reports on the findings. If a malignancy is suspected, the completion of the surgery may be delayed pending the pathologist's findings. The pathology report will include the usual heading, followed by a notation of the tissue submitted, with a gross description (meaning as seen by the naked eye), the microscopic description, and the pathologic diagnosis. The pathologist usually dictates the report simultaneously with the examination. As you will note in Figure 12–7, the narrative is dictated in the present tense. The report is signed by the pathologist and becomes a permanent part of the patient's record.

REGIONAL MEDICAL CENTER

PATHOLOGY REPORT

Name: ____________ **Pathology No.** ____________
Hospital No.: ________ **Sex:** ________ **Age:** ________ **Room No.:** ________ **Date Received:** ____________
Physicians: ____________
Preoperative Diagnosis: Mass of left calf
Postoperative Diagnosis: Pending
Procedure: Open biopsy, left calf muscle
Specimens: (1) Left calf mass-f/s
(2) Left calf mass-f/s
(3) Left calf mass

GROSS:

1. The specimen consists of 3 irregularly shaped fragments of dark maroon-brown muscle tissue measuring in aggregate 1.5 x 1 x 0.3 cm. No discrete lesions are identified. A minimal amount of adipose tissue is present in the largest fragment. The entire specimen is submitted for frozen section diagnosis.

FROZEN SECTION DIAGNOSIS: Benign muscle tissue showing degenerative and regenerative changes.

After frozen section, the tissue submitted is resubmitted and labeled F/S.

2. The specimen consists of 2 fragments of maroon-brown muscle tissue measuring in aggregate 1 x 0.7 x 3 cm. One of the fragments is submitted for frozen section diagnosis.

FROZEN SECTION DIAGNOSIS: Benign muscle tissue showing degenerative and regenerative changes.

After frozen section, the tissue submitted is resubmitted and labeled F/S.

3. Received is a wedge of grossly recognizable muscle tissue, brown-tan, and measuring 2.1 x 1.2 x 0.8 cm in size. On sectioning, this is moderately firm and focally only slightly discolored. All processed.

MICROSCOPIC:

Sections from all three parts show skeletal muscle. There is variable fiber morphology ranging from severely atrophic to markedly hypertrophic. There are abnormal numbers of central nucleoli, and some muscle fibers are vacuolated. In the interstitium there is fatty infiltration but no significant inflammatory infiltrate. No vasculitis is noted.

DIAGNOSIS:

NONSPECIFIC DEGENERATIVE AND HYPERTROPHIC CHANGES CONSISTENT WITH SEQUELA OR PREVIOUS TRAUMATIC INJURY, LEFT LEG MUSCLE BIOPSY.

NOTE: The morphology is somewhat similar to a muscular dystrophy, but the clinical presentation is incompatible. Denervation myopathy could account for some of the features seen. An inflammatory myopathy such as polymyositis is excluded based on the hypertrophic fibers present.

____
Pathologist

mek

FIGURE 12–7 Pathology report.

RADIOLOGY MEDICAL GROUP, INC.

Name: ______________ Age: ______ X-ray No. ______________
Doctor: ______________ Date ______________

DOUBLE-CONTRAST ARTHROGRAM OF THE RIGHT KNEE:

Double-contrast arthrography of the right knee was performed under local anesthesia following intra-articular injection of Conray contrast medium and air.

Multiple views of the medial meniscus in various degrees of internal and external rotation demonstrate a faintly outlined vertically directed linear tear involving primarily the posterior horn and mid segment of the medial meniscus.

The lateral meniscus is intact with no evidence of tear or disruption. Overhead views show normal smooth synovial lining and articular surfaces. No popliteal cyst is demonstrated.

OPINION:

Faintly outlined vertically directed linear tear involving primarily the posterior horn and mid segment of the medial meniscus.

Normal lateral meniscus.

____
Radiologist

mek

FIGURE 12–8 Radiology report.

RADIOLOGY REPORT

A radiology report contains the usual heading, including the date, name, and age of the patient, and the name of the referring physician. It will describe the radiographic findings and the resulting impression by the radiologist who signs the report (Fig. 12–8).

DISCHARGE SUMMARY

The final progress report for a hospital patient is the discharge summary, which will include the admission date and the date of discharge; admitting diagnosis and principal or discharge diagnosis; history of present illness; hospital course; and disposition and condition at time of discharge. The summary is dictated and signed by the attending physician (Fig. 12–9).

OTHER APPLICATIONS

The office that regularly sends out identical letters, such as recall notices or collection letters, will find word processing very helpful. Form letters can be stored in memory and personalized as needed.

A physician who does academic writing will want a program that can create footnotes, bibliographies, indexes, and so forth.

Transcribing: The Process

In most cases, the transcriptionist aims for finished copy and takes certain preliminary steps toward reaching this goal.

HOW TO PLAN FOR FINISHED COPY

1 Estimate the length of the finished document by first checking the indicator slip or electronic cuing. This makes it possible to decide what margins and spacing to use to produce the desired end product.
2 Look for any special instructions or corrections from the dictator.
3 Try to listen ahead so as to sense the meaning of a sentence and determine the punctuation necessary (some dictators include the punctuation marks).
4 When keyboarding directly on paper, as with a typewriter, it is important to type correctly the first time, whereas with a computer or word processor it is possible to go back and change punctuation, paragraphing, and so forth.
5 Before removing a page from the typewriter or before printing out the document, check the document for any errors.

Hospital No.: ______
Patient Name: ______
Physician: ______
Date of Discharge: ______

YOURTOWN
HOSPITAL

DISCHARGE SUMMARY

DATE OF ADMISSION: 12/15/200X

DATE OF DISCHARGE: 12/19/200X

ADMITTING DIAGNOSIS: 1. TEAR OF THE RIGHT ROTATOR CUFF

PRINCIPAL DIAGNOSIS:
1. TEAR OF THE RIGHT ROTATOR CUFF
2. HYPERTENSION
3. ALLERGIC REACTION

OPERATION:

BRIEF HISTORY: Patient came in for an elective surgery on the right rotator cuff. He had injured his shoulder while playing football; and because of continuing pain, an ultrasound vasogram was performed, which revealed a tear of the right rotator cuff.

HOSPITAL COURSE: Approximately 24 hours following surgery, the patient was provided with patient-controlled anesthesia with intravenous morphine and also received 1 g Ancef every eight hours. Patient developed rather severe itching and subsequent facial flush and mild rash. Both medications were discontinued. It is unknown which medication was the cause of his apparent allergic reaction.

Patient also had a very mild hypertension upon admission. During his admission, at times, blood pressure was as high as 190/116, and he ran a rather consistently elevated blood pressure for systolic and diastolic. Dr. Tom Brown was called for consultation because of both the allergic reaction and the hypertension, and initial studies were started concerning the hypertension. Patient was placed on Benadryl and responded rather appropriately to this treatment as far as allergic reaction was concerned.

DISPOSITION: Patient was discharged home in a sling and strap. He is to remain in this until I see him in approximately two weeks. He will also be followed up with Dr. Tom Brown concerning his hypertension in approximately two weeks, when all studies have been completed.

______
Signature

mek

FIGURE 12–9 Discharge summary.

ABBREVIATIONS

If transcribing for a hospital, use only abbreviations approved by the hospital for which the reports are intended. The Joint Commission on Accreditation of Healthcare Organizations requires that any abbreviations or symbols used in its medical records be from a list approved by that specific hospital. Progress notes done in the physician's office are less formal, and the physician's personally approved abbreviations are used to conserve space. There are entire books published on abbreviations, and most terminology books contain a list of frequently used abbreviations (see References at the end of this chapter).

CAPITALIZATION

Capitalize the first word of

- Every sentence
- An expression used as a sentence
- Each item in a list or outline
- The salutation and complimentary closing of a letter
- A drug brand name, such as Bufferin. The first letter of a generic name, such as aspirin, is not capitalized.
- The official name of a specific person, place, or thing, for example:

  Andrew Jackson
  New York City
  World Trade Center

- A common noun when it is part of a proper name:

  Give the paper to Professor Claudia Lane.
  But Give the paper to the professor.
  The parade traveled along Madison Avenue.
  But: The parade traveled along the avenue.

TABLE 12–1 Basic Rules of Forming Plurals

	Singular	Plural
Nouns ending in	a	ae
	is	es
	um	a
	us	i
	ix, ex	ces

TABLE 12–2 Proper Aligning in Number Systems

Arabic	Decimal	Roman
1	1.23	I
5	3.25	II
13	8.05	III

WORD DIVISION

Avoid excessive division of words at the end of a line. Word divisions clutter a page and may even confuse a reader. Basic rules of word division include

- Dividing words only between syllables
- Never dividing a one-syllable word
- Never setting off a one-letter syllable at the end or beginning of a word
- Never dividing abbreviations or contractions
- Never dividing a word unless you can leave a syllable of at least three characters (including the hyphen) on the upper line and carry a syllable of at least three characters (may include a punctuation mark) to the next line

PLURALS

Some basic rules for forming plurals are

- Plurals of nouns are usually formed by adding *s* or *es* to the singular form.
- Plurals of abbreviations are formed by adding *s* (e.g., ECGs and CVAs); some use an apostrophe before the *s*, but this is unnecessary and losing popularity.
- Medical terms: Many medical terms have Latin roots; the plural of a Latin noun is determined by its gender (masculine, feminine, or neuter) (Table 12–1).

APOSTROPHE

The apostrophe is used to

- Form contractions—It's a sunny day (it is a sunny day).
- Form possessives—the patient's chart (*Exception:* The apostrophe is *omitted* in the possessive form of *it*—its color; not it's color)
- Show omissions in dates—the year '99

NUMBERS

Spell out numbers from 1 to 10. Use figures for numbers greater than 10 except at the beginning of a sentence.

- Use only figures (including 1 through 10) in tables and statistical matter and in expressing dates, money, clock time, and percentages.
- Express related numbers the same way.
- Express measurements in figures.
- Always use figures with AM and PM.
- Do not use zeros with on-the-hour time (e.g., 9 AM, *not* 9:00 AM).
- Always write decimals in figures, without commas in the decimal part of the number.
- Write percentages in figures and spell out *percent* (e.g., 10 percent).
- When typing figures in columns, Arabic numbers (e.g., 1, 2, and 3) are aligned on the right, decimal amounts (e.g., 1.23) are aligned on the decimal, and Roman numerals (e.g., I, II, and III) are aligned on the left (Table 12–2).

Proofreading and Editing

As a final step, the finished printed page should be checked twice—once for typing accuracy and once to be sure that the text makes sense. Never present material for signature unless it makes sense to you and is free of errors.

Proofreading is the process by which you determine whether the copy is exactly what was intended by the dictator and that all words are correctly interpreted and accurately spelled. Be especially careful to watch for sound-alike words, such as site/cite, ilium/ileum, right/write, and anti-/ante- (Table 12–3). Proofreading usually includes checking for sentence structure, correct punctuation, capitalization, style, and format (Table 12–4). Watch for repeated words, substitutions that might change the meaning, the transposition of numbers, and inconsistencies of any kind.

Because you do not have another document with which you can compare the current document, it is your responsibility to make any necessary corrections or, if you are unsure, to mark any questionable area for checking by the dictator. A reliable office worker's reference manual can be your guide in these matters. If you plan to specialize in transcription, a proofreading class is essential.

Editing is the process of questioning the transcribed material for accuracy and clarity. Medical reports generally do not require extensive editing, but as you check for typing accuracy, you should

TABLE 12–3 Sound-Alike Words

addiction adduction abduction	diaphysis diastasis diathesis	mastitis mastoiditis
alveolus alveus alvus	epigastric epispastic	menorrhea menorrhagia metrorrhagia
amenorrhea dysmenorrhea	embolus thrombus	mucous mucus
antidiarrheic antidiuretic	endemic epidemic pandemic	nephrosis neurosis
antiseptic aseptic asepsis	facial fascial	palpation palpitation
arteritis arthritis	foci fossae	precardiac pericardium
aural oral	gavage lavage	perineal peroneal
bradycardia tachycardia	hypertension hypotension	perineum peritoneum
callus callous	hypocalcemia hypokalemia	perivascular perivesical
carbuncle caruncle furuncle	ileum ilium	stasis staxis
carpus corpus	infection infestation	sycosis psychosis
chronic chromic	insulin inulin	tenia tinea
contusion concussion convulsion	keratosis ketosis	trachelotomy tracheotomy
corneal cranial	larynx pharynx	ureter urethra
cocci coxa	lymphangitis lymphadenitis	vesical vesicle
cystostomy cystotomy cystoscopy	maco micro	xerosis cirrhosis

also check the clarity of the text. In making corrections, be careful not to change the meaning. Always check with the dictator when making any changes in what was dictated. Questions to the dictator are done by **flagging** the place in question. Leave a blank space sufficient for insertion of correction. Attach a memo on a Post-it or other adhesive backed note. Include the page number, subject's name, the paragraph and line of the word or sentence in question, and your name if there is more than one transcriptionist in the facility.

Memory Jogger

In editing the final copy of a report, certain parts are unclear to the transcriptionist. What action should be taken?

Reference Sources

OFFICE WORKERS' REFERENCE MANUAL

A good reference manual can serve as a ready source of information when you are transcribing. In it, you will find in-depth information on punctuation, capitalization, writing numbers, the use of abbreviations, and plurals and possessives as well as spelling guides. It is also a source of information on typing manuscripts, reports, and bibliographies as well as other information that you may use only occasionally.

ENGLISH LANGUAGE DICTIONARY

Keep a good dictionary near your desk for those times when you are unsure of your spelling or of the meaning of a word (especially one that sounds like another).

MEDICAL DICTIONARY

Not all medical dictionaries have the same arrangement of entries. No matter which one you have available, you will soon become accustomed to finding what you need. In one popular dictionary, terms consisting of two words are primarily defined under the second word—usually the noun. For example, to find *acetic acid*, you would look under the noun *acid* and then for the subheading *acetic;* to find *splenic vein*, you would first find the noun *vein*, and then the subentry *splenic*. *Syndrome* is a main entry; the many names of syndromes are shown as subentries. Other examples are *tests, disease, culture,* and *method*. Just remember that whenever you must find a two-word entry, you will probably find it under the second word.

A specialized dictionary is available for almost every medical specialty. The transcriptionist in a specialty practice will find it worthwhile to invest in a reference for that specialty.

PHYSICIANS' DESK REFERENCE (PDR)

An unknown drug is difficult to spell, and the spelling must be verified by the transcriptionist. A drug

TABLE 12–4 Proofreader's Marks

Proofreader's Mark	Draft Copy	Finished Copy
ss [Single space	ss [Read a good book every day	Read a good book every day
ds [Double space	ds [Where will you go on your vacation?	Where will you go on your vacation?
⌐2 Indent two spaces	His address is ⌐2 450 Newport Avenue	His address is 450 Newport Avenue
⊙ Insert period	Mr⊙Herbert Hoover	Mr. Herbert Hoover
^ Insert comma	Marysville^Indiana	Marysville, Indiana
⊙ Insert colon	Dear Mr. Adams^	Dear Mr. Adams:
;/ Insert semicolon	letter of March 6^ your question	letter of March 6; your question
?/ Insert question mark	Will he come^	Will he come?
∨ Insert apostrophe	the captains ship	the captain's ship
∨∨ Insert quotation marks	his remark, don't be late	his remark, "don't be late"
=/ Insert hyphen	a one^time thing	a one-time thing
# Insert space	townhouse	town house
^ Caret—to mark exact position of error	Insert caret toshow error	Insert caret to show error
Delete	It may ~~not~~ be yours	It may be yours
⌒ Close up	Cl ose	Close
Delete and close up	Meerry Christmas	Merry Christmas
¶ Begin new paragraph	¶ At the time	At the time
no ¶ No paragraph	no ¶ This is correct	This is correct
// Align vertically	Ellen Peters Alice Brown	Ellen Peters Alice Brown
= Align horizontally	Dear Doctor Roberts	Dear Doctor Roberts
⊐ Move right	$10,000	$10,000
⊏ Move left	⊏ Read a book	Read a book
⊓ Move up	Move	Move
⊔ Move down	Move	Move
⊐⊏ Center	⊐ $10,000 ⊏	$10,000
∿ Transpose	resileint	resilient
(sp) Spell out	(3) years ago	three years ago
stet..... Let it stand	They were ~~very~~ sad	They were very sad
lc Lower case	It is a Big house	It is a big house
≡ Upper case	Robert birch	Robert Birch
sc Set in small capitals	Regional	REGIONAL
ital Set in italic	special	*special*
bf Set in bold	federal government	**federal government**
wf Wrong font	investment	investment
∨3 Superscript	reference number 3	reference number^3
^7 Subscript	reference number 7	reference number$_7$
⌒ Ligature Æ	aesop	æsop

may have three types of names: chemical, generic, and trade. The chemical name of a drug represents its exact formula, the generic name is the common name of the chemical or drug, and the trade name is the name by which a manufacturer identifies the drug.

The *PDR* is the reference of choice for checking the names and spelling of drugs. It is published each year; and during the year, supplements are published to keep the reference up-to-date. The PDR contains seven different color-coded indexes:

- Alphabetical by Manufacturer
- Alphabetical by Brand Name
- Product (Drug) Category
- Generic and Chemical Name
- Product Identification
- Product Information
- Diagnostic Information

If the dictation contains an unfamiliar drug name, look in the Alphabetical Index for the correct spelling. If this search is unsuccessful, try the Generic and Chemical Name index. In typing the names of drugs, it is important to know whether it is a brand name or a generic name, because brand names are capitalized whereas generic names are not. In addition to being helpful as a source for the spelling and capitalization of drug names, the *PDR* contains a vast amount of information about drugs and their specific uses.

Names of over-the-counter drugs can be found in the *Physicians' Desk Reference for Nonprescription Drugs*, issued annually by the same publisher.

STANDARD ABBREVIATIONS

Except for the physician's own records, any abbreviations used in transcription should be standard and not subject to interpretation. If in doubt, it is always best to check. In some cases there is a difference in meaning if the letters are capitalized or in lower case. Many good books are available for checking abbreviations and should be consulted when the meaning of an abbreviation is in doubt.

CODING BOOKS

If your transcription involves procedural or diagnostic coding, you should have copies of the most recent editions of *Current Procedural Terminology* (**CPT Manual**), the Health Care Financing Administration's Common Procedure Coding System **(HCPCS)**, and the *International Classification of Diseases* (**ICD Manual**) in your reference library. Internet sites and CD-ROM databases are available for information about medications and medical terms. Medical spellers can be installed to check spelling of medical terms before a document is printed.

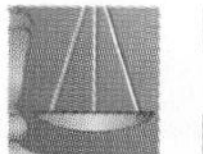

LEGAL AND ETHICAL ISSUES

If you are transcribing for a hospital, remember that the Joint Commission on Accreditation of Healthcare Organizations requires that any abbreviations or symbols used must be from a list approved by that specific hospital.

CRITICAL THINKING

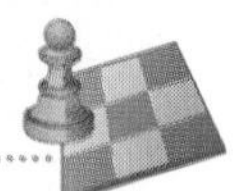

1 Discuss the educational requirements for a medical transcriptionist.

2 Explore some of the published volumes of medical abbreviations and note the similarities/differences of many. How might the use of an incorrect abbreviation affect the patient's care?

3 Discuss the legal aspects of medical reports and the need to be aware of the importance of confidentiality.

4 Can you suggest reasons that a STAT report would be expected for radiology, pathology, and laboratory results?

HOW DID I DO? Answers to Memory Joggers

1 Independent transcriptionists are usually paid on the basis of productivity, and their income depends on the number of pages, characters, or lines typed.

2 A slight rewind of the tape occurs when the machine is stopped and restarted.

3 History and Physical (H & P), Progress Notes, Consultation Reports, Correspondence.

4 Answer depends somewhat on the nature and extent of the lack of clarity. If it is a grammatical error, correct it. If a specific word is in question, consult the dictator before changing it.

REFERENCES

Diehl MO, Fordney MT: Medical Keyboarding, Typing and Transcribing: Techniques and Procedures, 4th ed. Philadelphia, WB Saunders, 1997.

Fordney MT, Diehl MO: Medical Transcription Guide: Do's and Don'ts. Philadelphia, WB Saunders, 1990.

Sabin WA: The Gregg Reference Manual, 7th ed., Lake Forest, IL, Gregg/McGraw-Hill, 1994.

Schwager E: Medical English Usage and Abusage. Phoenix, AZ, The Oryx Press, 1991.

Sloane SB: Medical Abbreviations and Eponyms, 2nd ed. Philadelphia, WB Saunders, 1997.

Strunk W Jr, White EB: The Elements of Style, 3rd ed. New York, Macmillan, 1979.

Tessier C: The AAMT Book of Style for Medical Transcription. Modesto, CA, American Association for Medical Transcription, 1995.

The Computer in Medical Practice

13

OUTLINE

LEARNING OBJECTIVES

Cognitive: On successful completion of this chapter you should be able to:

1. Define and spell the terms listed in the Vocabulary.
2. Distinguish between the three types of computers.
3. List the four general categories of computer hardware devices.
4. Name and state the functions of the most important computer hardware devices.
5. Name the pointing device that controls the cursor.
6. Explain the function of the *Enter* key.
7. Describe the cursor-control keys.
8. Name the output devices.
9. Explain the purpose of diskettes.
10. List 10 administrative tasks in a medical practice that might utilize a computer.

Performance: On successful completion of this chapter, and given the necessary equipment, you should be able to:

1. Start the computer
2. Load a program
3. Format a disk
4. Make a back-up copy of a document
5. Generate a patient record
6. Prepare a billing statement
7. Complete a patient insurance form
8. Personalize a computerized form letter
9. Access, add, correct, and delete information on the computer
10. Shut down the computer

VOCABULARY

applications Software programs designed to perform specific tasks

back-space key Key at upper right of keyboard with left arrow that deletes characters as it is struck

back-up A tape or floppy disk for storage of files to prevent their loss in the event of hard disk failure

CD-ROM Compact disk—read-only memory command; an instruction telling the computer to do something with a program

computer A machine that is designed to accept, store, process, and give out information

CPU Central processing unit; the part of a computer system that processes information

cursor A symbol appearing on the monitor that shows where the next character to be typed will appear

cursor-control keys Keys that have an arrow pointing up, down, left, or right that are used to move a cursor

database A collection of related files that serves as a foundation for retrieving information

demographics Relating to the statistical characteristics of populations, such as births, marriages, mortality, and health

disk A magnetic surface that is capable of storing computer programs that sometimes is flexible (*floppy disks*) and sometimes is hard (*hard disks*)

disk drives Devices that load a program or data stored on a disk into a computer

dot matrix printer An impact printer that forms characters using patterns of dots

electronic mail (E-mail) Communications transmitted via computer using a telephone modem

Enter key Key that performs same function as the Return key on a typewriter

floppy disk (diskette) A thin disk (diskette) of magnetic material capable of storing a large amount of information

format To magnetically create tracks on a disk where information will be stored; to initialize

hard copy The readable paper copy or printout of information

hardware Computer components that perform the four main functions

input Information entered into and used by the computer

letter-quality printer A printer that resembles a typewriter and which may be either mechanical or electronic

main memory Section of the computer where information and instructions are stored

modem Acronym for modulator demodulator; a device that enables data to be transmitted over telephone lines

monitor A device used to display computer-generated information; a video screen; a CRT

mouse Pointing device that controls the cursor

output Information that is processed by the computer and transmitted to a monitor, printer, or other device

printout The output from a printer, also called *hard copy*

provider One who provides medical service (e.g., a physician)

random access memory (RAM) The computer's temporary memory that stores data and programs that are input

read-only memory (ROM) Memory that can be altered only by changing the physical structure of the computer chip and that is used to store information essential to the operation of the computer

scanner An input device that converts printed matter into a computer-readable format

software The programming necessary to direct the hardware of a computer system; computer programs

telecommunication The science and technology of communication by transmission of information from one location to another via telephone, television, or telegraph

word processing System used to process written communications

Little more than 50 years ago, in 1946, the first electronic computer (ENIAC) was completed after 2½ years in the making. It weighed 30 tons, required a space of 15,000 square feet, and cost over 1 million dollars. Since that time, a computer explosion has taken place, brought about at first by the application of the transistor, then integrated circuits, and now silicon chips. A compact personal computer in the home and a desk-top monitor in the office are now commonplace.

For many years, the computer has been used in hospitals and large group practices, but the proliferation of software, the decrease in cost of hardware, and the sharp increase in paperwork that must be done in the medical marketplace have brought computerization into private medical practices. The computer is now standard equipment in all health care facilities. Consequently, it is now essential that any person looking toward a medical assisting career must become computer literate.

The development of computers, their programming, and internal operation is extremely complicated. Entire volumes have been written on the minute technical details of the computer. Fortunately, this technical knowledge is not necessary to use the computer, just as it is not necessary to be a mechanic to drive an automobile or to be an electrician to operate a light switch. But a knowledge of the functions that a computer can perform, how it influences our lives, and how it is used to perform tasks in the workplace has become a necessary part of the general education of all students. This chapter is intended to deal only with the use of the computer by the medical assistant as a tool in a medical facility. We will first examine the equipment, and then discuss its applications.

What Is a Computer?

A **computer** is a machine that is designed to accept, store, process, and give out information (Fig. 13–1). The general categories of microcomputer hardware units serve the following functions:

- Processing
- Input
- Output
- Storage

CENTRAL PROCESSING UNIT

The **CPU** is the most important piece of hardware. Acting as the brain of the computer, it interprets the instructions from a program. Although you cannot see it, within the CPU is the memory consisting of electronic and magnetic cells, each of which contains information.

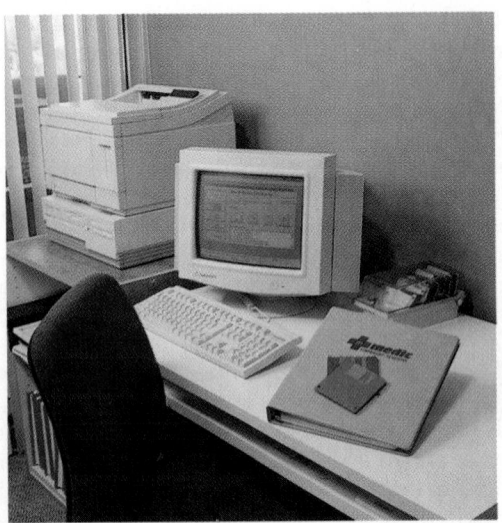

FIGURE 13–1 Microcomputer with software package.

There are two kinds of memory: **read-only memory (ROM)** and **random access memory (RAM).** ROM is internal memory that contains the entire operating system and a computer language. It is also known as the **main memory.** With this permanent memory, much less information has to be transferred from a disk to start the computing process. The ROM cannot be overwritten and is not erased when the power is shut off. RAM can be thought of as the internal scratch pad of the computer. It contains the program instructions and the data that it is currently processing. RAM is normally erased automatically when the power is shut off.

INPUT DEVICES

Information input to the computer is accomplished by means of a keyboard or other input device such as a mouse, scanner, or voice-activated device. The computer keyboard looks very much like an ordinary typewriter keyboard but has a few extra keys, which are called *special function keys.* These special function keys are numbered F1 to F12 and are used to perform specific **word processing** or computer-related operations. Used alone, a function key may create bold print, underline, indent, or call up a HELP screen, as well as other functions. Used in conjunction with the *Ctrl, Alt, or Shift* keys, function keys can produce other desired results, such as activating the printer, inserting the current date into a document, retrieving a file, and moving a designated block of text. A **mouse** is a pointing device with a ball on the bottom that is moved by rolling on a flat table top or mouse pad. Some computers, especially laptops, have a built-in mouse called a trackball that is moved by rotating the ball with the thumb. Others may have a touchpad, which is stroked by the thumb to move the cursor, or a track-point that is manipulated like a joy stick. The mouse controls the **cursor,** which is a flat bar or pointer appearing on the monitor that shows where the next character will appear.

At the right end of the keyboard is a numeric keypad, which has keys that resemble the keypad of a calculator. The numeric keypad is normally not in use during word processing. The *NumLock* key must be pressed to activate this feature.

The *Enter* key performs the same function as the *Return* key on the typewriter but is not used at the end of a line. The computer senses when the next word will not fit on the line and performs a *soft return.* The *Enter* key is used to start a new paragraph or an intentional (or hard) return. The left arrow key at the upper right of the keyboard is the **backspace key** and deletes characters as you move it to the left.

Cursor-control keys have an arrow that points up, down, left, right, and in some cases diagonally.

Memory Jogger

What is ROM, and why is it important?

OUTPUT DEVICES

Monitor

The monitor, which looks very much like a television screen, is a device used to display computer-generated information. Some monitors are black and white only but may be adjusted for screen brightness and contrast. Color monitors allow the operator to choose the background color that is most pleasing to the eye and easiest to read (Fig. 13–2). A blinking marker on the screen, called the cursor, indicates the position where the next information can be added or inserted. By watching the monitor you have instant feedback on your entries.

Printer

Printers are also **output** devices. Documents appearing on the monitor may be directed to a printer to produce what is called a **printout** or **hard copy** (paper). Four types of printers are commonly used with computers:

- Dot matrix
- Letter-quality or print wheel
- Ink jet
- Laser

Many printers print bidirectionally (i.e., they print both from left to right and from right to left). Some are capable of both draft-quality and correspondence-quality printing. Dot matrix and letter-quality printers are impact printers, using an inked ribbon; ink jet and laser printers are nonimpact and use an ink cartridge.

A **dot matrix printer** is the least expensive of the four types of printer. They are used in many classrooms. Dot matrix printers form the letters or shapes that they are directed to print by arranging patterns of dots on the paper. They operate more quickly than do letter-quality machines, but their print lacks the clarity generally desired for a professional look.

A **letter quality printer** may be either mechanical or electronic. The electronic letter-quality printer generally uses a print wheel, or daisy wheel, that is interchangeable for variations in print style or size. Many printers have 10-, 12-, and 15-pitch typing capability as well as proportional spacing capability.

Ink jet printers use an ink cartridge that feeds an array of nearly microscopic tubes, each of which has a heating element that is energized during the printing process. The ink cartridge may be black-and-white or color. Ink jet printers cost less than laser printers, but the ink cartridges they use are fairly expensive and bring up the operating cost.

Laser printers use xerographic technology similar to that in photocopiers, so the laser printer is able to produce an almost limitless variety of type forms

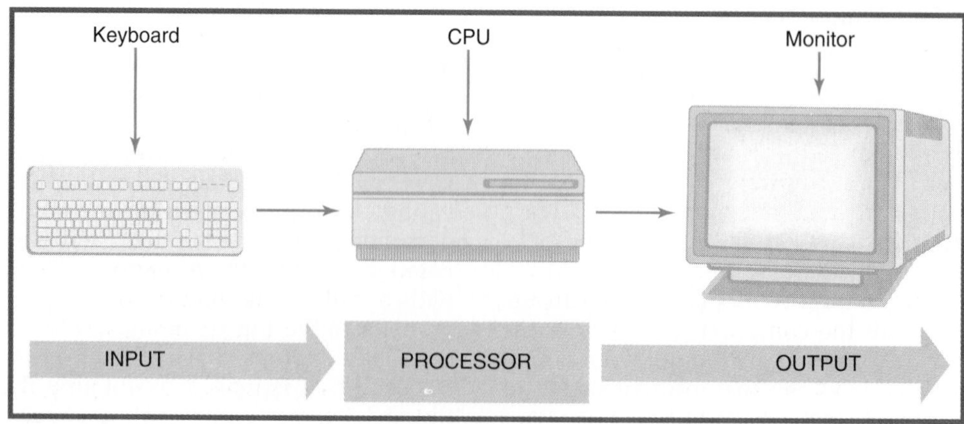

FIGURE 13–2 Input device (keyboard), central processing unit (CPU), and output device (monitor).

and sizes as well as complex graphics. One disadvantage of ink jet and laser printers is that they are incapable of producing multiple copies with carbon sets or multicopy forms, such as many types of insurance forms.

STORAGE

Information may be saved (stored) on a disk for future reference or printing. The amount of information that can be stored depends on the type of **disk** the system uses. Storage is achieved on either a hard disk or **floppy disk (diskette)** or both. The hard disk is inside the computer and you do not see it. The hard disk contains the operating system and the information on all the programs you use. Hard disks store much more information than do diskettes and make possible faster information access. There is a wide variation in the space capacity of hard disks. The disk must be large enough to hold all the programs you use as well as the information that you will store. Diskettes are used principally as an auxiliary storage medium and **back up** for the hard disk. They can also be used for transmitting information between computers. The size of the disk needed depends on the type of drive being used. Older computers used the 5¼-inch floppy, but most computers being sold today accommodate only the 3½-inch floppy. The term *floppy* is misleading, because the disk is quite firm and does not "flop."

A computer may have four or more **disk drives.** There may be two drives for diskettes. Drive A is used for the smaller 3½-inch diskette and drive B for the 5¼-inch diskette. Drive C is the hard disk and Drive D accommodates the CD-ROM. There may also be a ZIP or back-up drive.

Memory Jogger

2 *If your computer is intended principally for insurance billing, what kind of printer would you need? Why?*

Diskette Files

Before information can be stored on a diskette, the diskette must be initialized, or formatted. When correctly instructed your computer will **format** the diskette by creating magnetic tracks (recording bands) on the diskette where information is to be stored. Diskettes that are preformatted are also available at slightly higher cost than nonformatted diskettes. After a diskette has been formatted, the disk operating system (DOS) can both read data from the diskette and write data onto the diskette. When information is stored only on diskettes, it is always wise to make back-up or duplicate diskettes in case the original diskettes are lost or damaged. These back-up diskettes must be kept in a secure location for protection against fire or theft. Floppy diskettes are more easily damaged than are hard disks (a type of floppy disk different in texture, size, and capacity) and must be carefully stored, always in a jacket, and filed for easy reference. For tips on the proper care of diskettes, see the Care of Diskettes chart. A more dependable system for backing up files is by subscribing to an online backup service on the Internet. The service keeps a copy of your files in two separate locations. For privacy protection your files are encrypted before being transmitted, and a password is needed to retrieve them.

CD-ROM

The **CD-ROM** (compact disk–read-only memory) at this writing is becoming standard equipment on all computers and is increasingly popular as a means of providing programs for installation on computers. The CD-ROM requires a separate disk drive and is able to store much more information than an ordinary diskette. In the medical office it might be used to store a medical dictionary or a medical reference library. It is not used for storing information created on your computer.

CARE OF DISKETTES

- Avoid exposing the diskette to extremes of temperature.
- When the diskette is not in use always return it to its storage envelope, where it will not collect dust.
- Avoid placing a diskette on top of the monitor because this could scramble information on the diskette.
- Keep your fingers off the surface of the diskette, especially around the window in the jacket. Body oils can permanently destroy data.
- Hold the diskette with your thumb on the label.
- Write or type on the label before attaching it to the diskette, if possible, or write with a soft felt-tipped pen. Never write with a ballpoint pen or pencil on a label that is on a diskette. Also, do not erase on a diskette label. All of these can cause impressions in the diskette, and the ink can run.
- Do not force a diskette into a disk drive or its storage envelope. If there is resistance, pull it out and try again. Bending or folding a diskette will render it useless.
- Store the diskettes vertically in dust-tight containers.
- Keep smoke, food, and drink away from the area of use.

Hard Disk Management

The hard disk is the filing cabinet of the computer. Thousands of files can be placed on a hard disk and retrieved with a few specific keystrokes. A hard disk system usually comprises two or more rigid metal plates enclosed in a sealed case. It stores data by magnetic encoding similar to that when using a floppy disk or cassette tape. Hard disks provide much greater storage capacity than do floppy diskettes.

For efficiency in retrieving a given piece of information, a directory is established for each main topic; subdirectories can be set up within directories. Computer files are organized in much the same fashion as ordinary files that contain paper records (Fig. 13–3). When a disk becomes overcrowded, more time is required for the system to retrieve a specific file. The hard disk needs to be periodically purged of files that are outdated or no longer useful just as does any other filing system.

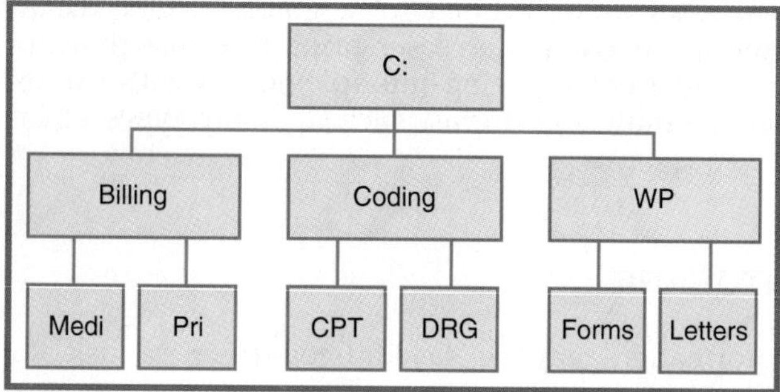

FIGURE 13–3 Organization of files into directories and subdirectories.

Software

Software consists of sets of instruction placed on magnetic disks. Software is necessary for a computer to function. The operating system, which is preinstalled on your computer, is one kind of software. In operating the computer you will be selecting and using **applications.** Application programs are designed to perform specific tasks such as word processing, patient billing, accounting, appointment scheduling, insurance form preparation and processing, payroll, and database management. Many software applications are available for complete medical practice management. Some health care facilities have software designed specifically for their practices, but this is usually unnecessary in today's market.

Getting Started

Even with some basic knowledge of computer components and of what computers can do, if you have not had any hands-on experience with a computer, you may feel some initial fear—fear of the unknown, fear of machines, or fear of being unable to master the computer. You will soon overcome any such fears if you will remember that you really are smarter than the computer. It is only a machine. All it can do is perform the tasks that you tell it to do. It cannot think. It cannot make decisions, and it will wait for your commands. What it can do is

- Relieve you of repetitive clerical tasks
- Reduce errors
- Speed up production
- Recall information on command
- Save time
- Reduce paperwork
- Allow more creative use of your time

As you begin your familiarization with the computer, you may key in some wrong information. As a result, the computer will become confused and will respond with a question mark or a comment such as

FILE NOT FOUND or INVALID DRIVE SPECIFICATION or SYNTAX ERROR

The computer will allow you the opportunity and time to figure out the correct information and input it. Look at the monitor screen. Most of the time it will indicate what to do next. If the answer is not readily available on the monitor, pull down the *Help* menu. Your next resort will be the program instruction manual.

You cannot break the computer simply by hitting the wrong keys. It is unlikely that you will destroy records accidentally; a specific command is necessary. However, if you shut off the computer without saving the information on disk or tape you will lose what you have put in. By using a computer in the classroom, you will gain familiarity with computer operation and confidence that you can master it. Mastery is accomplished only through practice.

The computer that you will encounter on the job is likely to be different from the one on which you will learn in the classroom. The programs and tasks performed may also be different, but you will be given training with that specific system, either by the vendor or by a member of the staff. It is important to keep an open mind while learning to operate any system.

With a knowledge of computer terms, the ability to follow step-by-step instructions, and reasonable expertise with a typewriter keyboard, you should have no problem with learning and using any computer system. In fact, many computer users consider the computer to be their best friend. You probably will, too.

Memory Jogger

Explain the meaning of application program *and give an example.*

Common Computer Applications

PROCESSING INSURANCE CLAIMS

Claims information can be sent from the physician's office directly to the computer of an insurance company using a **modem,** which transmits information over telephone lines. Electronic processing of insurance claims not only saves transit time but also provides immediate information as to whether a given claim will be accepted. Errors in coding or procedure are immediately evident, and such errors result in the rejection of the claim by the insurance company's computer. Corrections can then be made instantly using the computer.

The codes that are most commonly used for claims processing can be stored on the computer disk and retrieved when needed (Fig. 13–4).

Many insurance companies give preferential treatment to providers who file claims electronically (Fig. 13–5; see p. 188). By the year 2000 all providers of care under *Medicare* and *Medicaid* will be required to file their claims electronically.

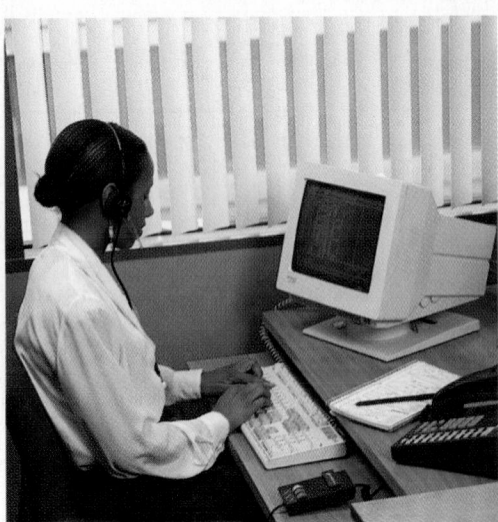

FIGURE 13–4 Computer operator.

In medical offices that do not file insurance claims for patients, a computer can generate a *superbill* for the patient to attach to his or her own insurance form. The superbill gives information about diagnosis and procedures that is needed to file a claim.

PATIENT LEDGER

The **demographics** about a patient (e.g., his or her name, address, telephone, number, and insurance carrier) will appear on the patient's computerized ledger (Fig. 13–6; see p. 189). As services are rendered, all charges and payments are entered into the computer. This results in the availability of a current balance at all times.

BILLING AND COLLECTION

At the appropriate time, the computer can print a patient's billing statement that shows detailed charges, payments, adjustments, and a balance (Fig. 13–7; see pp. 190–191). Additionally, the computer can be programmed to age the accounts according to any criteria selected and to include this information on the billing statement. A series of collection letters can also be developed and personalized for individual patients as they are needed.

BOOKKEEPING ENTRIES

With the appropriate software, the computer can easily handle all bookkeeping processes.

EXAMPLES OF SOFTWARE BOOKKEEPING PROCEDURES

- Recording payables and receivables
- Computing the payroll
- Keeping track of bills to be paid
- Generating checks
- Producing a deposit slip for the bank
- Reconciling bank statements
- Preparing daily, monthly, and annual financial and statistical reports

DATABASE MANAGEMENT

Database software makes it possible to organize a large volume of information that can be used in a number of ways. One of the most practical uses is organization of identifying information on each patient, which would include name, address, date of

APPROVED OMB-0938-0008

PLEASE DO NOT STAPLE IN THIS AREA

CARRIER

PICA

HEALTH INSURANCE CLAIM FORM

PICA

1. MEDICARE X (Medicare #) MEDICAID (Medicaid #) CHAMPUS (Sponsor's SSN) CHAMPVA (VA File #) GROUP HEALTH PLAN (SSN or ID) FECA BLK LUNG (SSN) OTHER (ID)

1a. INSURED'S I.D. NUMBER (FOR PROGRAM IN ITEM 1)

2. PATIENT'S NAME (Last Name, First Name, Middle Initial)

3. PATIENT'S BIRTH DATE MM DD YY 08 27 25 SEX M F X

4. INSURED'S NAME (Last Name, First Name, Middle Initial)

5. PATIENT'S ADDRESS (No., Street)

6. PATIENT RELATIONSHIP TO INSURED Self X Spouse Child Other

7. INSURED'S ADDRESS (No., Street)

CITY STATE CA

8. PATIENT STATUS Single Married X Other

CITY STATE

ZIP CODE 92683 TELEPHONE (Include Area Code) (714)

Employed Full-Time Student Part-Time Student

ZIP CODE TELEPHONE (INCLUDE AREA CODE) ( )

9. OTHER INSURED'S NAME (Last Name, First Name, Middle Initial)

10. IS PATIENT'S CONDITION RELATED TO:

11. INSURED'S POLICY GROUP OR FECA NUMBER NONE

a. OTHER INSURED'S POLICY OR GROUP NUMBER

a. EMPLOYMENT? (CURRENT OR PREVIOUS) YES NO X

a. INSURED'S DATE OF BIRTH MM DD YY 08 27 1925 SEX M F X

b. OTHER INSURED'S DATE OF BIRTH MM DD YY 08 27 1925 SEX M F X

b. AUTO ACCIDENT? YES NO X PLACE (State)

b. EMPLOYER'S NAME OR SCHOOL NAME

c. EMPLOYER'S NAME OR SCHOOL NAME RETIRED

c. OTHER ACCIDENT? YES NO X

c. INSURANCE PLAN NAME OR PROGRAM NAME

d. INSURANCE PLAN NAME OR PROGRAM NAME METLIFE-IL 5090

10d. RESERVED FOR LOCAL USE

d. IS THERE ANOTHER HEALTH BENEFIT PLAN? X YES NO *If yes, return to and complete item 9 a-d.*

READ BACK OF FORM BEFORE COMPLETING & SIGNING THIS FORM.

12. PATIENT'S OR AUTHORIZED PERSON'S SIGNATURE I authorize the release of any medical or other information necessary to process this claim. I also request payment of government benefits either to myself or to the party who accepts assignment below.

SIGNED Signature on File DATE 03/12/98

13. INSURED'S OR AUTHORIZED PERSON'S SIGNATURE I authorize payment of medical benefits to the undersigned physician or supplier for services described below.

SIGNED Signature on File

PATIENT AND INSURED INFORMATION

14. DATE OF CURRENT: MM DD YY ILLNESS (First symptom) OR INJURY (Accident) OR PREGNANCY (LMP)

15. IF PATIENT HAS HAD SAME OR SIMILAR ILLNESS. GIVE FIRST DATE MM DD YY

16. DATES PATIENT UNABLE TO WORK IN CURRENT OCCUPATION FROM MM DD YY TO MM DD YY

17. NAME OF REFERRING PHYSICIAN OR OTHER SOURCE

17a. I.D. NUMBER OF REFERRING PHYSICIAN

18. HOSPITALIZATION DATES RELATED TO CURRENT SERVICES FROM MM DD YY TO MM DD YY

19. RESERVED FOR LOCAL USE

20. OUTSIDE LAB? YES NO X $ CHARGES

21. DIAGNOSIS OR NATURE OF ILLNESS OR INJURY. (RELATE ITEMS 1,2,3 OR 4 TO ITEM 24E BY LINE)

1. 362.51
2. 365.11
3.
4.

22. MEDICAID RESUBMISSION CODE ORIGINAL REF. NO.

23. PRIOR AUTHORIZATION NUMBER

24.	A DATE(S) OF SERVICE From MM DD YY	To MM DD YY	B Place of Service	C Type of Service	D PROCEDURES, SERVICES, OR SUPPLIES (Explain Unusual Circumstances) CPT/HCPCS	MODIFIER	E DIAGNOSIS CODE	F $ CHARGES	G DAYS OR UNITS	H EPSDT Family Plan	I EMG	J COB	K RESERVED FOR LOCAL USE
1	03 12 98	03 12 98	11		92012		1	43.30	1				
2													
3													
4													
5													
6													

PHYSICIAN OR SUPPLIER INFORMATION

25. FEDERAL TAX I.D. NUMBER SSN EIN X

26. PATIENT'S ACCOUNT NO.

27. ACCEPT ASSIGNMENT? (For govt. claims, see back) X YES NO

28. TOTAL CHARGE $ 43.30

29. AMOUNT PAID $ 0.00

30. BALANCE DUE $ 43.30

31. SIGNATURE OF PHYSICIAN OR SUPPLIER INCLUDING DEGREES OR CREDENTIALS (I certify that the statements on the reverse apply to this bill and are made a part thereof.)

SIGNED DATE 03/12/98

32. NAME AND ADDRESS OF FACILITY WHERE SERVICES WERE RENDERED (If other than home or office)

33. PHYSICIAN'S, SUPPLIER'S BILLING NAME, ADDRESS, ZIP CODE & PHONE #

SANTA ANA, CA 92704

PIN# GRP#

(APPROVED BY AMA COUNCIL ON MEDICAL SERVICE 8/88) *PLEASE PRINT OR TYPE* FORM HCFA-1500 (12-90) FORM OWCP-1500 FORM RRB-1500

WHCFA-1500-2-90

FIGURE 13–5 Computer-generated insurance claims form.

```
                                SMITH, JANE A                               PAGE   1
                               PATIENT LEDGER
                                  03/12/99

CHART           DATE  PROV LOC   BILLING        DIAGNOSIS  PROCEDURE          AMOUNT
----------- ------ ---- ----  ------------ ------------ ----------- -------------
973944-00                                          0
               (INSURANCE ID:                 INSURANCE PHONE: (714)261-6700)
               11/11/97 02    11    11564       365.04     92004              105.00
               11/11/97 02    11    11564       365.04     PCP                -10.00
               02/19/98 02          11564                  IP                 -22.00
               02/19/98 02          11564                  WO                 -73.00
               (INSURANCE 1 BILLED 11/20/97)
               01/20/98 02    11    11983       365.04     92083              120.00
               01/20/98 02          11983                  PCP                -10.00
               (INSURANCE 1 BILLED 01/29/98)
                                                                       -------------
                                                PATIENT DEBITS....            225.00
                                                PATIENT CREDITS...           -115.00
                                                                       -------------
                                                BALANCE...........            110.00
                                                                       =============
SMITH, JANE A                                   PROVIDER DEBITS...            225.00
                                                PROVIDER CREDITS..           -115.00
                                                                       -------------
                                                PROVIDER BALANCE..            110.00
                                                                       -------------
                                                REPORT DEBITS.....            225.00
                                                REPORT CREDITS....           -115.00
                                                                       -------------
                                                REPORT BALANCE....            110.00
                                                                       =============
```

FIGURE 13–6 Computerized patient ledger.

birth, Social Security number, daytime telephone number, insurance information, and place of employment. The amount and character of information that can be stored on a computer **database** about patients, procedures, diagnoses, and other topics is limitless. After the data are recorded onto the disk, the information can be sorted into any chosen order and retrieved as desired (Fig. 13–8; see p. 192).

HEALTH INFORMATION RECORDS

Computer systems can store clinical information about patients using much less space and with greater security than can papers in a patient chart. Anyone who has worked in a medical office understands the problems that a lost or misfiled patient chart can cause. The chart stored on the computer can be set up in such fashion that a printout of only the most important information can be reviewed by the physician at the time of the patient's visit; as a result, he or she does not have to thumb through an ever-growing stack of papers. Reports from outside sources can be added to the computer record using a scanner. Access to records can be limited with passwords.

APPOINTMENT SCHEDULING

The computer has replaced the appointment book in many medical practices. Software for appointment scheduling ranges from relatively simple programs that merely display available and scheduled times to sophisticated systems into which the operator may enter information such as the length and type of appointment required and day and time preferences of the patient; the computer then selects the best appointment time based on inputted information.

The computer can also be used to keep track of future appointments. For example, when a patient calls and inquires about an appointment, the system can search by his or her name to find the time and date. The computer can provide printouts of the daily schedule that include the patients' names and telephone numbers and the reason for their visiting. Multiple copies of these schedules can be made according to the needs of the practice.

A big advantage of computer scheduling is that more than one person can access the system at one time, and the information is available to all operators. The medical assistant can generate a hard copy of the next day's appointments before leaving for the day. In some facilities, employees still maintain

```
                                                              PAGE   1

                                                   Tax ID
                                                   95-2585978




                                       June 10 , 1999

    To:


                                              Patient   :
    Diagnosis:                                Acct #    :
    1 4659   UPPER RESPIRATORY INFECTI        SS#       :
    2 4959   ALLERGIC ALVEOLITIS & PNE        D.O.B.    :
    3 7856   LYMPHADENOPATHY                  Phone     :
                                              Employer  :
                                              Claim No.:
                                              Group     :


 #     Date   Dr Pl Svc       Description  Bil  Charge   Credit    Bal    Prev
-------------------------------------------------------------------------------
 1.  052999             777   COURTESY ADJU B             -30.50   0.00   30.50
 2.  052999             742   DEBIT ADJUSTM B              97.50  30.50  -67.00
 3.  043099  INSURANCE BILLED        B/C PRUDE 0401-0430(  30.50)
 4.  043099  INSURANCE BILLED        RISK MANA 0401-0430(  30.50)
 5.  040699   9  1 8706000  NOSE\THROAT C *    30.50             -67.00  -97.50
 6.  093098             751   COURTESY DISC B             -97.50 -97.50    0.00
                                            2/11-2/14/98
 7.  053098             751   COURTESY DISC B            -235.75   0.00  253.75
                                                  4/23/98
 8.  043098  INSURANCE BILLED        B/C PRUDEN 0401-0430   253.75
 9.  043098  INSURANCE BILLED        RISK MANAG 0401-0430   253.75
10.  042398   9  1 9902301  LABORATORY DR *     5.75             253.75  248.00
11.  042398   9  1 8444300  TSH           *    35.00             248.00  213.00
12.  042398   9  1 8425100  T4R           *    21.00             213.00  192.00
13.  042398   9  1 8425000  T3 RESIN      *    21.00             192.00  171.00
14.  042398   9  1 8429500  SODIUM        *     9.25             171.00  161.75
15.  042398   9  1 8413200  POTASSIUM     *     9.25             161.75  152.50
16.  042398   9  1 8371800  HDL CHOLESTER *    27.50             152.50  125.00
17.  042398   9  1 8011200  CHEM PANEL 12 *    42.50             125.00   82.50
18.  042398   9  1 8272800  FERRITIN,EIA  *    47.00              82.50   35.50
19.  042398   9  1 8565100  WESTERGREN SE *    13.50              35.50   22.00
20.  042398   9  1 8502400  CBC           *    22.00              22.00    0.00
21.  041998             751   COURTESY DISC B             -41.00   0.00   41.00
                                            BAL APPLD TO DED
22.  022898  INSURANCE BILLED        B/C PRUDEN 0201-0228    97.50
23.  022898  INSURANCE BILLED        RISK MANAG 0201-0228    97.50
24.  022198             751   COURTESY DISC B             -56.50  41.00   97.50
                                            D.O.S.    11/12/97
25.  021498   4  1 9006000  OFFICE VISIT- *    48.75              97.50   48.75
26.  021198   4  1 9006000  OFFICE VISIT- *    48.75              48.75    0.00
27.  013198             751   COURTESY DISC B             -56.50   0.00   56.50
                                            TO DEDUCTIBLE
```

FIGURE 13–7 Patient's billing statement.

```
                                                                    PAGE   2
28.  112397  INSURANCE BILLED       AETNA LIFE 1001-1123  56.50
29.  111297  10  1 8720503  10% KOH PREP  *    10.50           56.50   46.00
30.  111297   6  1 9006000  OFFICE VISIT- *    46.00           46.00    0.00
31.  053197          751    COURTESY DISC B                     0.00  220.25
32.  022897  INSURANCE BILLED      AETNA LIFE 0201-0228  178.00
33.  020297   6  1 9902200  ALLIED CLINIC *     8.00          220.25  212.25
                                               \FERRITIN
34.  020297   6  1 8444300  TSH           *    33.00          212.25  179.25
35.  020297   6  1 8425100  T4R           *    19.75          179.25  159.50
36.  020297   6  1 8425000  T3 RESIN      *    19.75          159.50  139.75
37.  020297   6  1 8371800  HDL CHOLESTER *    26.00          139.75  113.75
38.  020297   6  1 8011200  CHEM PANEL 12 *    38.00          113.75   75.75
39.  020297   6  1 8565100  WESTERGREN SE *    12.75           75.75   63.00
40.  020297   6  1 8502400  CBC           *    20.75           63.00   42.25
41.  093096  INSURANCE BILLED      AETNA LIFE 0901-0930   42.25
42.  091996   3  1 8565100  WESTERGREN SE *    12.00           42.25   30.25
43.  091996   3  1 8503100  Not in ISAM   *    19.50           30.25   10.75
44.  091996   3  1 9902201  ALLIED SPECIM *    10.75           10.75    0.00
                                               /FER,IBC,SE IRON
45.  010096   3  1 9999900  BALANCE FORWA B     0.00            0.00    0.00
                                               COMPRESSED TO BALF

                 Current     30-day     60-day     90-day     120 + Balance
Bal Fwd Age:        0.00       0.00       0.00       0.00       0.00    0.00

Treatment Rendered by:

Referring Physician    : NO REFERRAL

Please Make Check Payable to:
```

FIGURE 13–7 *Continued*

an appointment book as a back-up to computer scheduling.

WORD PROCESSING

Word processing software is available for all desktop computers. The latest software is very sophisticated with the capability to create footnotes, bibliographies, indexes, graphics, and much more. Formatting processes are quick and easy, and error detection is continuous. A word processing applications program is used in transcription and preparing written communications such as correspondence and reports, as well as many other tasks.

Styles and formatting of all kinds can be established and stored in the application program for use as needed. Formatting includes setting margins, determining line spacing, justification, setting tabs, pagination, page breaks, and so forth. If the document is to be saved, you must first assign a file name and complete the "save" process before exiting the item or turning off the computer.

NETWORKING

With the exception of the very small facility, the computer system will be set up to communicate with other systems or individuals via networks and telecommunication systems. The network will link one or more computers in the same facility or farther away, such as with a hospital or the home of one or more physicians, via modem and special software.

Clinical Research

Patient information stored in a database can be used by the physician to develop research reports from this source. For example, if a study were being done on the results of a specific treatment, the physician could gather the needed information from the database.

```
DATE : 00/00/00 TIME : 08:37 AM                                          PAGE    1

LIST OF PATIENTS

                              R E G I S T R A T I O N
06/10/92
 1.CHART #:                                        10.RESP PARTY:
 2.NAME    :                                       11.ADDRESS    :
 3.ACCT # :                                        12.CITY/STATE:
 4.DR/PL #: 03/01                                  13.ZIP        :
 5.SEX    : F                                      14.RELATION   :
 6.MARITAL: M                                      15.PHONE RES  :
 7.BIRTH  :   7/22/57                              16.PHONE BUS  :
 8.REF DOC:     1  NO REFERRAL                     17.EMPLOYER   :
 9.ACC DAY:     /  / 0                             18.SSN        :
- - - - - - - - - - - - - - - - - - - I N S U R A N C E - - - - - - - - - - - - - - -
 20.CODE    : 851                                  26.CODE       : 856  B/C PRUDENT BUYER
 21.PRIMARY: RISK MANAGEMENT RESO                  27.SECONDARY :
 22.ID #    : 429-27-7469                          28.ID #       :
 23.GROUP  : 664-626                               29.GROUP      : 336631/101/3
 24.ASSN:1              25.STAT: 0                 30.ASSN:0          31.STAT: 0
- - - - - - - - - - - - - - - - - - - - - - - - - - - - - - - - - - - - - - - - - - -
 32.NOTE 1: PARENTS      524-8240 34.RECALL DATE:08/18/88 36.RECALL TYPE:  0
 33.NOTE 2: SISTER      -524-6995 35.RECALL DONE:08/30/88 37.PAN:NEW INS 1/91
- - - - - - - - - - - - - - - - - - - - - - - - - - - - - - - - - - - - - - - - - - -
 38.ICD #1:4659    39.DESC:UPPER RESPIRATORY INFECTI    44.ADMITTED    :00/00/00
 40.ICD #2:4959    41.DESC:ALLERGIC ALVEOLITIS & PNE    45.DISCHARGED :00/00/00
 42.ICD #3:7856    43.DESC:LYMPHADENOPATHY              46.LAWYER      :    0


SECPAG - Extra Patient Information

 1. Pat Address :                             10. Family Planning    :
 2.     Address :                             11. Other Accident     :
 3.     City St :                             12. Patient Employed   : Y
 4.         Zip :                             13. Patient P/T Std.   :
 5. O.I. Emp/Sch:                             14. Patient F/T Std.   :
 6. Time of Inj.:                             15. Insured's Sex      : F
 7. Active/Ret. :                             16. Other Ins. Sex     : M
 8. Date to Clinic     :                      17. Insured's D.O.B.   : 07/22/57
 9. Discharge Date     :                      18. Other Ins. D.O.B.  : 10/21/45

19. Refered Out :                             25. Auto Accident    :
20.     Contact :                             26. Work Related     :
21.     Address :                             27. Return Mod Work:
22.     City St :                             28. Return Reg Work:
23.         Zip :                             29. Claim #          :
24.       Phone :                             30. Examiner         :

31. Extra Info 1:

             Change what # ( 0 for none ) :
```

FIGURE 13–8 Patient registration information stored in a database.

Electronic Mail (E-Mail)

Telecommunication (or **electronic mail**) software allows one computer to communicate with another computer via telephone lines through the use of a modem. Letters and reports travel along telephone lines to your computer, which can provide a printout in a manner not unlike that previously discussed concerning the electronic transmission of insurance claims.

Electronic Signature

Physicians are sometimes negligent about signing clinical reports generated in the hospital as well as those reports originating in the private office. Recently introduced on the market is the electronic signature option. Electronic signature programs are offered both as stand-alone products and as part of a computerized medical record system. After the dictated report is transcribed, the physician by using a password and personal identification number (PIN) can log on to the patient record system by computer. The physician accesses and reviews a report, makes any necessary changes or additions, then "signs" the report by clicking on an icon. Once the record has been signed it cannot be altered; only addenda are allowed.

Ergonomic Work Areas

The increase in utilization of computers in the workplace has emphasized the need to choose and arrange furniture and equipment that employees use to maintain comfort and safety. Repetitive strain injury (RSI) accounts for a majority of job-related injuries. RSI includes a number of conditions that are caused by repeatedly straining certain nerves, muscles, or tendons. Carpal tunnel syndrome is one example of RSI.

To avoid such injuries it is very important that posture chairs support the lumbar section of the back with correct angle of the knee and the feet resting on the floor. Many designs for keyboards are available and every effort should be made to choose a keyboard height that allows a right angle at the elbow with the wrist being held in a neutral position. Extensive studies have been done to ensure the comfort and safety of employees. Prevention of RSI is possible; a cure is sometimes not possible.

Eyestrain is another danger arising from continuous use of a computer. The monitor should be just below eye level and at an arm's length away. At least once each hour take a break from looking at the monitor to rest your eyes.

Security Guidelines for Computerized Data

As we learned in an earlier chapter, the patient is entitled to utmost confidentiality with respect to his or her medical records and the release of any information of a personal nature. Computer technology allows the accumulation and storage of a vast amount of data that may be accessible to a variety of individuals, making it imperative that guidelines be set up for the protection of that data. Security guidelines have been established by the Council on Ethical and Judicial Affairs of the American Medical Association and are included in the 1996–1997 edition of the *AMA Code of Ethics* (see Chapter 5).

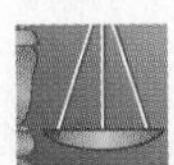

LEGAL AND ETHICAL ISSUES

The patient is entitled to complete confidentiality of his or her records. Follow the security guidelines that have been established by the Council on Ethical and Judicial Affairs of the American Medical Association.

CRITICAL THINKING

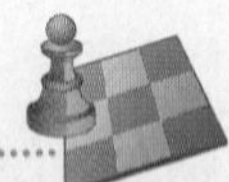

1 Why are security guidelines so important for computerized data?

2 Is security more important for medical records than it is for other kinds of data?

HOW DID I DO? Answers to Memory Joggers

1. ROM (read-only memory) is the internal memory of the computer that contains the entire operating system and computer language. It remains stored in the computer when the power is off and is present to start the computer process when the power is turned on.
2. Dot matrix and letter-quality printers are impact printers and can generate multiple form copies.
3. Application program is software designed to perform specific tasks (e.g., Word Perfect, a word processing program).

REFERENCES

American Medical Association: Code of Medical Ethics, 1996–1997 edition. Chicago, AMA 1996.

Gylys BA: Computer Applications for the Medical Office. Philadelphia, FA Davis, 1997.

Filing Methods and Record Keeping

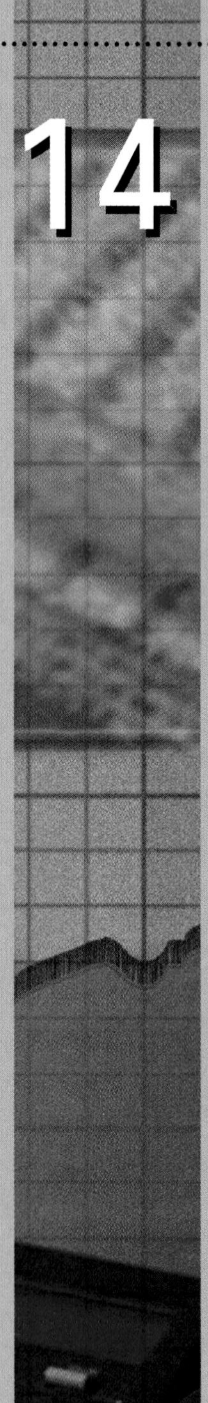

OUTLINE

LEARNING OBJECTIVES

Cognitive: On successful completion of this chapter, you should be able to:

1 Define and spell the terms listed in the Vocabulary.
2 List and discuss the basic equipment and supplies in a filing system.
3 Describe the seven sequential steps in filing a document.
4 List and discuss application of the four basic filing systems.
5 Explain how color coding of files can be advantageous in a health care facility.

Performance: On successful completion of this chapter, you should be able to:

1 Type a list of names in indexing order and arrange them alphabetically for filing.
2 Arrange a group of patient numbers in filing sequence for a terminal digit filing system.
3 Using the color key in this chapter, state the tab color to be used for a given list of names.

VOCABULARY

alphabetic filing Any system that arranges names or topics according to the sequence of letters in the alphabet

alphanumeric Systems made up of combinations of letters and numbers

caption A heading, title, or subtitle under which records are filed

direct filing system A filing system in which materials can be located without consulting an intermediary source of reference

indirect filing system A filing system in which an intermediary source of reference, such as a card file, must be consulted to locate specific files

numeric filing The filing of records, correspondence, or cards by number

OUTfolder A folder used to provide space for the temporary filing of materials

OUTguide A heavy guide that is used to replace a folder that has been temporarily moved from the filing space

shelf filing A system that uses open shelves (rather than cabinets) for storing records

subject filing Arranging records alphabetically by names of topics or things rather than by names of individuals

tab The projection on a file folder or guide on which the caption is written

tickler file A chronologic file used as a reminder that something must be taken care of on a certain date

transfer Removing inactive records from the active file

unit Each part of a name that is used in indexing

A filing system is only as good as the ease of retrieval of everything in the files. A modern filing system should have three key components: (1) a symbol on the outside of the jacket or folder indicating the active or inactive status of the record, (2) safeguards to prevent misfiling, and (3) a filing technique that allows quick, accurate retrieval and refiling. Files may be kept as hard copy (on paper) or on the computer disk. Most medical facilities use a combination, with the patients' notes as hard copy.

Filing Equipment

The vertical four-drawer steel filing cabinet, used with manila folders with the patient's name on the tab, was the traditional system of choice for years. The most popular system today is color coding on open shelves. There are also rotary, lateral, compactable, and automated files. Some records are kept in card or tray files. Regardless of the type or style of equipment, the best quality is always an economy.

Some of the considerations in selecting filing equipment are

- Office space availability
- Structural considerations
- Cost of space and equipment
- Size, type, and volume of records
- Confidentiality requirements
- Retrieval speed
- Fire protection

DRAWER FILES

Drawer files should be full suspension; they should roll easily, close securely, and be equipped with a locking device. The best cabinets have a center trough at the bottom of each drawer with a rod for holding divider guides. Floor space of twice the depth of the drawer must be allowed so that the drawer can be pulled out to its full extent. A drawback of the vertical four-drawer files is that only one person can use a file cabinet at any given time. Filing is also slower because the drawer must be opened and closed each time a file is pulled or filed. Drawer files are relatively easy to move, but for safety reasons they should be bolted to the wall or to each other.

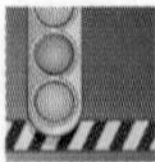

Safety Alert: File drawers are heavy and can tip over, causing serious damage or injury unless reasonable care is observed. Open only one file drawer at a time and close it when the filing has been completed. A drawer left even slightly open can cause injury to a passerby.

SHELF FILES

Shelf files should have doors to protect the contents. A popular type of shelf file has doors that slide back

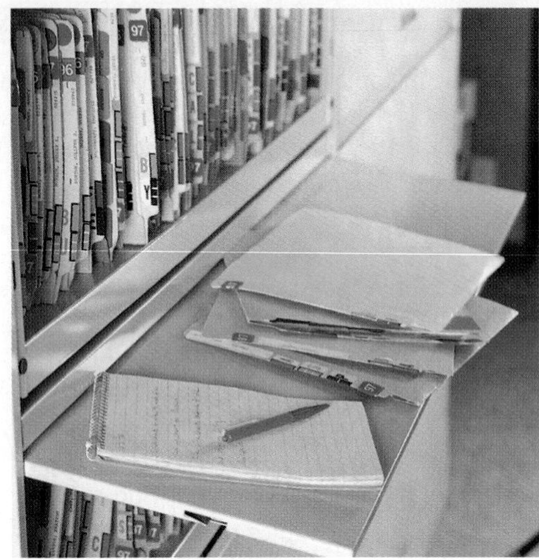

FIGURE 14–1 Open shelf filing using shelf door as work space.

into the cabinet; the door from a lower shelf may be pulled out and used for work space (Fig. 14–1). About 50% more material per square foot of floor space may be filed in shelf files as compared with the four-drawer file. Open shelf units hold files sideways and can go higher on the wall because there is no drawer to pull out. File retrieval is faster because several individuals can work simultaneously.

Open shelf units without doors are the most economical but offer little protection or confidentiality to the records. They are susceptible to water and fire damage. Shelf files are available in many attractive colors and can add a decorative note to the business office.

Special storage or shelf space should be provided for x-ray films if many films are stored.

ROTARY CIRCULAR FILES

Rotary circular files can hold a large volume of records. They save space and clerical motion. The files revolve easily; some come with push-button controls. Several persons can work at one rotary file and use records at the same time. One disadvantage is that they afford less privacy and protection than files that can be closed and locked.

LATERAL FILES

Lateral files are good for personal files and are especially attractive for the physician's private office. They use more wall space than the vertical file but do not extend out into the room so far. The folders are filed sideways in the lateral file, left to right, instead of front to back as in a vertical file. Some have a pull-out drawer, as the vertical file does; others have doors that slide into the cabinet, exposing the filing space.

COMPACTABLE FILES

The office with little space and a great volume of records might use compactable files, which are a variation of open shelf files. The files are mounted on tracks in the floor, and the units slide along the tracks so that access is gained to the needed records. They may be either automated or manual. One drawback is that not all records are available at the same time.

AUTOMATED FILES

Automated files are very expensive initially and require more maintenance than do the other types of filing equipment. They will probably be found only in very large installations such as clinics or hospitals. These files bring the record to the operator instead of the operator going to the record. When the operator presses a button indicating the appropriate shelf, the shelf automatically moves into position in front of the operator for record retrieval. The automated or power file is fast and can store large amounts of records in a small amount of space. Only one person can use the unit at one time.

CARD FILES

Almost every office has some occasion to use a card file. This may be for patient ledgers, a patient index, library index, index of surgical tray setups, telephone numbers, or numerous other records. A good-quality steel box or tray is a sound investment.

SPECIAL ITEMS

Metal framework is available that can convert a regular drawer file into suspension-folder equipment. The assistant with a great deal of filing may wish to purchase a portable filing shelf that fits on the side of an opened drawer and can be moved from place to place as needed. Another special filing item is a sorting file, which can be a great time saver. A portable file cart for the temporary filing of unbilled insurance claims may be quite useful. It may also be used for the preliminary sorting of charts to be refiled. This is sometimes called a suspense file.

Memory Jogger

 *Discuss the various styles of file storage, noting their advantages and disadvantages.*

Supplies

DIVIDER GUIDES

Each file drawer or shelf should be equipped with plenty of dividers or guides. Some authorities recommend one guide for approximately each inch and a half of material, or every 8 to 10 folders. Guides should be of good-quality pressboard. Economy guides will soon become bent and frayed and have to be replaced. Divider guides have a protruding tab, which may be either an integral part of the card or may be made of metal or plastic. The guides reduce the area of search and serve as supports for the folders. They are available in single, third, or fifth cut (one, three, or five different positions). The guide may have a projection at the bottom edge with a ring or hole through which a rod may go. This type of guide card is used in drawers that have a trough for the projection and a rod to hold the guides in place.

OUTGUIDES

An **OUTguide** is a heavy guide that is used to replace a folder that has been temporarily removed. It should be of a distinctive color for quick detection. This makes refiling simpler and alerts the file clerk that a file is missing. Several colors may be used, each color designating the temporary location of the file. The OUTguide may have lines for recording information, or it may have a plastic pocket for inserting an information card (Fig. 14–2).

CHART COVERS OR FOLDERS

Most records to be filed are placed in covers or tabbed folders. The most commonly used is a general-purpose third-cut manila folder that may be expanded to ¾ inch. These are available with a double-thickness reinforced tab that will greatly lengthen the life of the folder. Folders kept in drawers have tabs at the top; those kept on shelves have tabs at the side. There are many variations of folder styles obtainable for special purposes:

- A classification folder separates the papers in one file into six categories yet keeps them all together.
- An **OUTfolder** is used like the OUTguide and provides space for temporary filing of materials.
- The vertical pocket, which is heavier weight than the general purpose folder, has a front that folds down for easy access to contents and is available with up to 3½ inch expansion. These are used for bulky histories or correspondence.
- Hanging or suspension folders are made of heavy stock and hang on metal rods from side to side of a drawer. They can be used only with files equipped with suspension equipment.
- Binder folders have fasteners with which to bind papers within the folder. These offer some security for the papers but are time consuming in filing the materials.

The number of papers that will fit in one folder depends on the thickness of the papers. Near the bottom edge of most folders are one or more score marks, which should be used as the contents of the folders expand. If folders are refolded at these score marks, the danger of their bending and sliding under other folders is reduced, and a neater file results. Papers should never protrude from the folder edges, and they should always be inserted with their tops to the left. When papers start to ride up in any folder, the folder is overloaded.

Memory Jogger

Describe an OUTguide and its uses.

LABELS

The label is a necessary filing and finding device. Use labels to identify each shelf, drawer, divider guide, and folder.

A label on the drawer or shelf identifies the nature of its contents. It should also indicate the range (alphabetic, numeric, or chronologic) of the material filed in that space.

EXAMPLES OF TYPES OF LABELS

PATIENT HISTORIES (ACTIVE)
A–F

OR

GENERAL CORRESPONDENCE
1997–1998

The label on the divider guide identifies the range of folder headings following that divider guide up to the next divider, for example, Ba–Bo.

The label on the folder identifies the content of that folder only. This may be the name of the patient, subject matter of correspondence, a business topic, or anything at all that needs to be filed. You will need to label a folder when a new patient is seen or existing folders are full or when you need to **transfer** materials within the filing system.

Paper labels may be purchased in rolls of gummed tape or have adhesive backs that are peeled from a protective sheet. They are available in

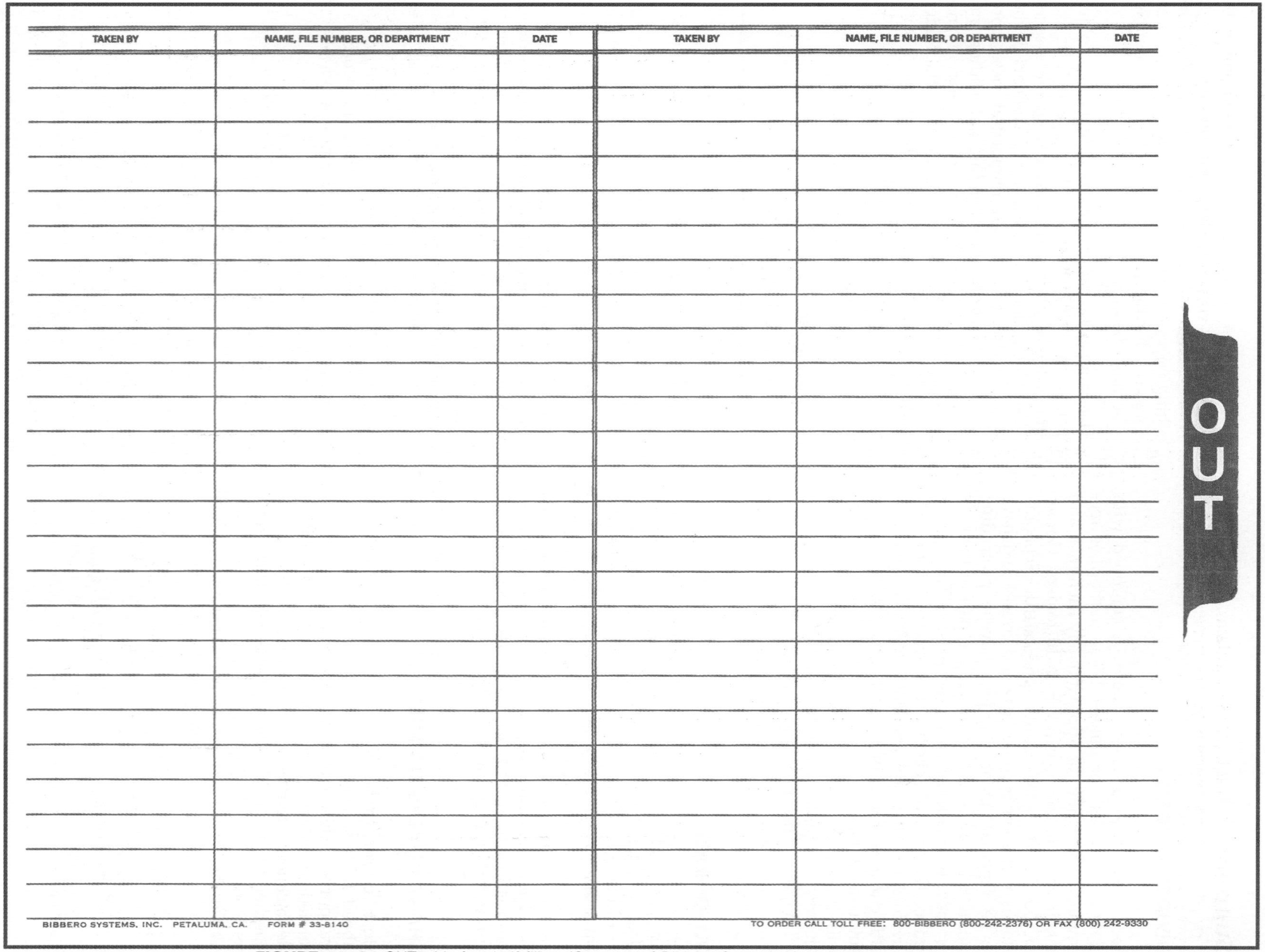

OUT

TAKEN BY	NAME, FILE NUMBER, OR DEPARTMENT	DATE	TAKEN BY	NAME, FILE NUMBER, OR DEPARTMENT	DATE

BIBBERO SYSTEMS, INC. PETALUMA, CA. FORM # 33-8140

TO ORDER CALL TOLL FREE: 800-BIBBERO (800-242-2376) OR FAX (800) 242-9330

FIGURE 14–2 OUTguide for shelf filing. (Courtesy of Bibbero Systems, Inc., Petaluma, CA.)

TABLE 14–1 Application of Indexing Rules

Indexing Rule	Name	Unit 1	Unit 2	Unit 3
1	Robert F. Grinch	Grinch	Robert	F.
	R. Frank Grumman	Grumman	R.	Frank
2	J. Orville Smith	Smith	J.	Orville
	Jason O. Smith	Smith	Jason	O.
3	M. L. Saint-Vickery	Saint-Vickery	M.	L.
	Marie-Louise Taylor	Taylor	Marielouise	
4	Charles S. Anderson	Anderson	Charles	S.
	Anderson's Surgical Supply	Andersons	Surgical	Supply
5	Ah Hop Akee	Akee	Ah	Hop
6	Alice Delaney	Delaney	Alice	
	Chester K. DeLong	Delong	Chester	K.
7	Michael St. John	Stjohn	Michael	
8	Helen M. Maag	Maag	Helen	M.
	Frederick Mabry	Mabry	Frederick	
	James E. MacDonald	Macdonald	James	E.
9	Mrs. John L. Doe (Mary Jones)	Doe	Mary	Jones (Mrs John L.)
10	Prof. John J. Breck	Breck	John	J. (Prof.)
	Madame Sylvia	Madame	Sylvia	
	Sister Mary Catherine	Sister	Mary	Catherine
	Theodore Wilson, M.D.	Wilson	Theodore (M.D.)	
11	Lawrence W. Sloan, Jr.	Sloan	Lawrence	W. (Jr.)
	Lawrence W. Sloan, Sr.	Sloan	Lawrence	W. (Sr.)
12	The Moore Clinic	Moore	Clinic (The)	

almost any size, shape, or color to meet the individual needs of any facility. Visit your stationer and study the catalogs to find the best product for you.

A narrow label applied to the front of the folder tab is the easiest to use and is satisfactory for folders kept in a drawer file. Labels for shelf filing should be identifiable from both front and back. Always type the label before separating it from the roll or protective sheet. Type the **caption** on the label in indexing order (see Indexing Rules and Table 14–1).

Filing Procedures

Filing of all materials involves five basic steps: conditioning, releasing, indexing and coding, sorting, and storing and filing.

CONDITIONING

Conditioning of papers involves (1) removing all pins, brads, and paper clips, (2) stapling related papers together, (3) attaching clippings or items smaller than page size to a regular sheet of paper with rubber cement or tape, and (4) mending damaged records.

RELEASING

The term *releasing* simply means that some mark is placed on the paper indicating that it is now ready for filing. This will usually be either the medical assistant's initials or a FILE stamp placed in the upper left corner.

INDEXING AND CODING

Indexing means deciding where to file the letter or paper, and coding means placing some indication of this decision on the paper. This may be done by underlining the name or subject, if it appears on the paper, or writing in some conspicuous place the indexing subject or name. If there is more than one logical place to file the paper, the original is coded for the main location and a cross-reference sheet prepared, indicating this location and coded for the second location. Every paper placed in a patient's chart should have the date and name of the patient on it, usually in the upper right corner.

SORTING

Sorting is arranging the papers in filing sequence. Sort papers before going to the file cabinet or shelf. Do any necessary stapling of papers at your desk or filing table. Invest in a desktop sorter with a series of dividers between which papers are placed in filing sequence. One general-purpose sorter has six means of classification: alphabetic sections, numbers 1 to 31, days of the week, months of the year, numbers in groups of five, and space on the tabs for special captions to be taped when desired. In the preliminary sorting you place the papers in the appropriate division in the sorter. Then it is comparatively simple to arrange these groups into the proper sequence for filing.

PROCEDURE 14-1

Initiating a Medical File for a New Patient

GOAL

To initiate a medical file for a new patient that will contain all the personal data necessary for a complete record and any other information required by the agency.

EQUIPMENT AND SUPPLIES

Computer or Typewriter
Clerical supplies (pen, clipboard)
Information on agency's filing system
Registration form
File folder
Label for folder
ID card if using numeric system
Cross-reference card
Financial card
Routing slip
Private conference area

PROCEDURAL STEPS

1 Determine that the patient is new to the office.

2 Obtain and record the required personal data.
PURPOSE: Complete information is necessary for credit and insurance claim processing.

3 Type the information onto the patient history form.

4 Review the entire form.
PURPOSE: To confirm that the information is complete and correct.

5 Select a label and folder for the record.
EXPLANATION: If color coding is used, a decision must be made regarding the appropriate color for the patient name.

6 Type the caption on the label and apply to the folder.
EXPLANATION: Use patient's name for alphabetic filing or appropriate number for numeric filing.

7 For numeric filing system, prepare a cross-reference card and a patient ID.
PURPOSE: Numeric filing is an indirect system and requires a cross-reference to a patient's name for locating a chart. The patient will use the number of the ID card when arranging appointments or making inquiries.

8 Prepare the financial card, or place the patient's name in the computerized ledger.

9 Place the patient's history form and all other forms required by the agency into the prepared folder.

10 Clip a routing slip on the outside of the patient's folder.

STORING AND FILING

In storing or filing papers in the folder, items should be placed face up, top edge to the left, with the most recent date to the front of the folder. Lift the folder 1 or 2 inches out of the drawer before inserting new material, so that the sheets can drop down completely into the folder.

If you are refiling completed folders, arrange them in indexing order before going to the file cabinets. Procedure 14-1 provides the steps for initiating a new patient file.

Memory Jogger

List and describe the five steps in filing.

Locating Misplaced Files

Unless files are promptly replaced after use, they may become lost. Papers may be misfiled, requiring a thorough search to find them. After you have made a methodical and complete search through the proper folder, there are several places you may look for a misplaced paper: (1) in the folder in front of and behind the correct folder; (2) between the folders; (3) on the bottom of the file under all the folders; (4) in a folder of a patient with a similar name; or (5) in the sorter.

Indexing Rules

Indexing rules are fairly well standardized, based on current business practices. The Association of Records Managers and Administrators takes an active part in updating the rules. Some establishments adopt variations of these basic rules to accommodate their needs. In any case the practices need to be consistent within the system.

1. Last names of persons are considered first in filing; given name (first name), second; and middle name or initial, third. Compare the names beginning with the first letter of the name. When you find a letter that is different in the two names, that letter determines the order of filing. Example:

   ab*e*
   ab*i*
   ab*x*
   acl
   ac*m*
   ada
   ad*e*
   ad*i*

2. *Initials* precede a *name* beginning with the same letter. This illustrates the librarian's rule, "Nothing comes before something." Example:

   Smith, J.
   Smith, Jason

3. *Hyphenated personal names.* The hyphenated elements of a name, whether first name, middle name, or surname, are considered to be one **unit.** Example:

   Carlotta Freeman-Duque is filed as
   Freemanduque, Carlotta
   Cindy-Jean Green is filed as
   Green, Cindyjean

4. The apostrophe is disregarded in filing. Example:

   Andersons' Surgical Supply
   Andersons Surgical Supply

5. When you are indexing a foreign name and *cannot* distinguish the first and last name, you should index each part of the name in the order in which it is written:

   Cau Liu
   Talluri Devi

   If you *can* make the distinction, you should use the last name as the first indexing unit:

   Liu, Jason

6. Names with prefixes are filed in the usual alphabetic order with the prefix being considered as part of the name. Example:

   DeLong is filed as Delong
   LaFrance is filed as Lafrance
   von Schmidt is filed as Vonschmidt

7. Abbreviated parts of a name are indexed as written if that is the form generally used by that person. Example:

   Ste. Marie is filed as Stemarie
   St. John is filed as Stjohn
   Wm. is filed as Wm
   Edw. is filed as Edw
   Jas. is filed as Jas

8. Mac and Mc are filed in their regular place in the alphabet:

   Maag
   Mabry
   *Mac*Donald
   Machado
   *Mac*Hale
   Maville
   *Mc*Aulay
   *Mc*Williams
   Meacham

   If your files contain a great many names beginning with Mac or Mc, you may, for convenience, wish to file them as a separate letter of the alphabet.

9. The name of a married woman is indexed by her legal name (her husband's surname, her given name, and her middle name or maiden surname). Example:

   Doe, Mary Jones (Mrs. John L.)
   not Doe, Mrs. John L. (unless first name is unknown)

10. Titles, when followed by a complete name, may be used as the *last* filing unit if needed to distinguish from another identical name. Example:

Dr. James D. Conley	Conley James D Dr.
Mr. James D. Conley	Conley James D Mr.

Titles without complete names are considered the *first* indexing unit:

Madame Sylvia
Sister Theresa

11. Terms of seniority, or professional or academic degree, are used only to distinguish from an identical name. Example:

Theodore Wilson, Sr.
Theodore Wilson, Jr.
Theodore Wilson, MD
Theodore Wilson, PhD

would be filed in the following order

Theodore Wilson, Jr.
Theodore Wilson, MD
Theodore Wilson, PhD
Theodore Wilson, Sr.

12. Articles such as *The* or *A* are disregarded in indexing:

Moore Clinic (The)

Filing Methods

The three basic methods of filing used in health care facilities are

- Alphabetic by name
- Numeric
- Subject

Patient charts are filed either alphabetically by name or by one of several numeric methods. Subject filing is used for business records, correspondence, and topical materials.

ALPHABETIC FILING

Alphabetic filing by name is the oldest, simplest, and most commonly used system. It is the system of choice for filing patient records in the majority of physicians' offices. If you can find a word in the dictionary or a name in the telephone directory, you already know some of the rules.

The alphabetic system of filing is traditional and simple to set up, requiring only a file cabinet or shelf, folders, and some divider guides. It is a **direct filing system** in that you need only know the name in order to find the desired file.

Alphabetic filing does have some drawbacks:

- You must know the correct spelling of the name
- As the number of files increases, more space is needed for each section of the alphabet. This results in periodic shifting of folders from drawer to drawer or shelf to shelf to allow for expansion.
- As the files expand, more time is required for filing or retrieving each folder because of the greater number of folders involved in the search. The time can be greatly reduced by color coding, which is discussed in detail later in this chapter. Procedure 14–2 explains how to add material to existing patient files.

NUMERIC FILING

Some form of **numeric filing** combined with color and **shelf filing** is used by practically every large clinic or hospital. Management consultants differ in their recommendations; some recommend numeric filing only if there are more than 5,000 charts, more than 10,000 charts, or in some cases more than 15,000 charts. Others recommend nothing but numeric filing. Numeric filing is an **indirect filing system,** requiring the use of an alphabetic cross-reference in order to find a given file. Some people object to this added step and overlook the advantages, which are that it

- Allows unlimited expansion without periodic shifting of folders, and shelves are usually filled evenly
- Provides additional confidentiality to the chart
- Saves time in retrieving and refiling records quickly. One knows immediately that the number 978 falls between 977 and 979. By contrast, an alphabetic system, even with color coding, requires a longer search for the exact spot.

There are several types of numeric filing systems. In the *straight* or *consecutive* numeric system, patients are given consecutive numbers as they visit the practice. This is the simplest of the numeric systems and works well for files of up to 10,000 records. It is time consuming, and there is a greater chance for error when filing documents with five or more digits. Filing activity is greatest at the end of the numeric series (Table 14–2).

In the *terminal digit* system, patients are also assigned consecutive numbers, but the digits in the number are usually separated into groups of twos or

PROCEDURE 14–2
Adding Supplementary Items to Established Patient File

GOAL

To add supplemental documents and progress notes to patient histories, observing standard steps in filing, while creating an orderly file that will facilitate ready reference to any item of information.

EQUIPMENT AND SUPPLIES

Assorted correspondence, diagnostic reports, and progress notes
Patient files
Computer or typewriter
Mending tape
FILE stamp or pen
Sorter
Stapler

PROCEDURAL STEPS

1 Group all papers according to patients' names.
PURPOSE: Some related papers may require stapling.

2 Remove any pins or paper clips.
PURPOSE: Pins in file folders are hazardous; paper clips are bulky and may become inadvertently attached to other materials.

3 Mend any damaged or torn records.

4 Attach any small items to standard-size paper.
PURPOSE: Small items are easily lost or misplaced in files.

5 Staple any related papers together.

6 Place your initials or FILE stamp in the upper left corner.
PURPOSE: To indicate that the document is released for filing.

7 Code the document by underlining or writing the patient's name in the upper right corner.
PURPOSE: To indicate where the document is to be filed.

8 Continue steps 2 through 7 until all documents have been conditioned, released, indexed, and coded.

9 Place all documents in the sorter in filing sequence.
EXPLANATION: Sorter can be taken to file cabinet or shelf for placing documents in patient folders.

threes and are read in groups from right to left instead of from left to right. The records are filed backward in groups. For example, all files ending in 00 are grouped together first, then those ending in 01, etc. Next the files are grouped by their middle digits so that the 00 22s come before the 01 22s. Finally the files are arranged by their first digits, so that 01 00 22 precedes 02 00 22 (Table 14–3).

Middle digit filing begins with the middle digits, followed by the first digit and finally by the terminal digits.

Some practices use the last four digits of each patient's Social Security number to file patient records. However, there is no legal requirement that every United States resident have a Social Security

TABLE 14–2 Consecutive Sequencing

Morales, Maria	012479
Rees, Charles	012480
Dreis, Patrick	012481

TABLE 14–3 Terminal Digit Sequence

Carter, John	01 99 00
Delgado, Juan	00 73 01
Geiselmann, Troy	05 55 11
Herr, Leonard	01 68 21
Julian, Bruce	01 68 22
Grissom, Randal	88 34 23
Cook, Robert	90 34 23

number, in which cases a "pseudo number" would have to be issued.

Numeric filing requires more training, but once the system is mastered, fewer errors occur than with alphabetic filing.

SUBJECT FILING

Subject filing can be either alphabetic or **alphanumeric** (A 1-3, B 1-1, B1-2, etc.) and is used for general correspondence. The main difficulty with subject filing is indexing, or classifying—deciding where to file a document. Many papers require cross-referencing. All correspondence dealing with a particular subject is filed together. The papers within the folders are filed chronologically, the most recent on top. The subject headings are placed on the tabs of the folders and filed alphabetically.

Memory Jogger

a. Name the three most commonly used systems of filing.
b. Which of the three is the simplest?
c. Which is an indirect system?

Color Coding

When a color coding system is used, both filing and finding are easier, and misfiled folders are kept to a minimum. The use of color visually restricts the area of search for a specific record. A misfiled chart is easily spotted even from a distance of several feet. In color coding, a specific color is selected to identify each letter of the alphabet. The application of the principle may be through using colored folders, adhesive colored identification labels, or various combinations of these (Fig. 14–3; Procedure 14–3). Any selection of colors may be used, and the division of the alphabet is determined by one's own needs. However, studies have shown that there is wide variation in the frequency with which different letters occur. One division that has been used successfully is shown in Table 14–4. Experience has proved that this breakdown results in almost equal representation of the five colors.

TABLE 14–4 Division of Letters in Color Coding

Color of Label	Letters of Alphabet
Red	A B C D
Yellow	E F G H
Green	I J K L M N
Blue	O P Q
Purple	R S T U V W X Y Z

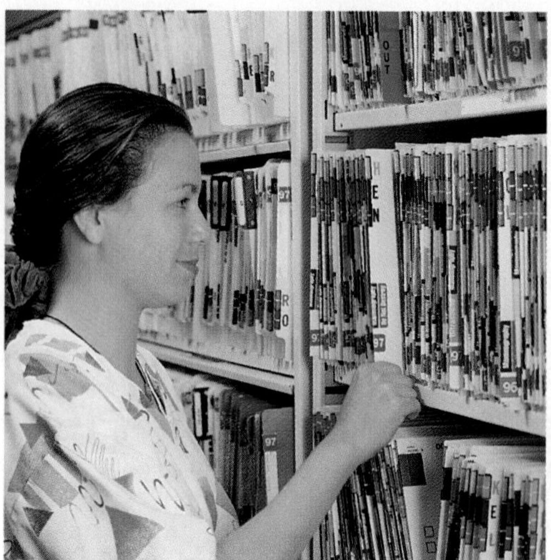

FIGURE 14–3 Application of color coding.

ALPHABETIC COLOR CODING

There are several ways of color coding files. One alphabetic system utilizes five different colored folders, with each color representing a segment of the alphabet. The *second* letter of the patient's last name determines the color, as shown in Table 14–5.

As medicine continues to consolidate into larger facilities, with more patients under one management, the filing of patient charts becomes more complicated and color coding becomes more useful. Sev-

TABLE 14–5 Division of Alphabet in 5-Color System

RED FOLDER (second letters a, b, c, d)	C*a*nfield E*b*erhart A*c*kerman A*d*ams
YELLOW FOLDER (second letters e, f, g, h)	V*e*nable E*f*fron I*g*awa T*h*ill
GREEN FOLDER (second letters i, j, k, l, m, n	H*i*sted B*j*ork A*k* U*l*lman I*m*hoff A*n*derson
BLUE FOLDER (second letters o, p, q)	G*o*rdon E*p*perley A*q*uino
PURPLE FOLDER (second letters r, s, t, u, v, w, x, y, z)	T*r*out O*s*terberg A*t*herton A*u*er U*v*ena O*w*sley O*x*ford N*y*e A*z*zaro

PROCEDURE 14-3

Color Coding Patient Charts

GOAL

To color code patient charts using the agency's established coding system to effectively facilitate filing and finding.

EQUIPMENT AND SUPPLIES

20 patient charts
Information on agency's coding system
20 file folders
Full range of color labels

PROCEDURAL STEPS

1 Assemble patient charts.

2 Arrange charts in indexing order.
PURPOSE: When charts have been color coded, they will be in filing order.

3 Pick up the first chart and note the second letter of the patient's surname.
EXPLANATION: For purpose of this activity, the color coding system in the text will be used.

4 Choose a folder and/or caption label of the appropriate color.

5 Type patient's name on label in indexing order and apply to folder tab.
PURPOSE: To identify sequence of folder in filing system.

6 Repeat steps 4 and 5 until all charts have been coded.

7 Check entire group for any isolated color.
PURPOSE: If the order and color of the folders is correct, all charts of the same color within each letter of the alphabet will be grouped together.

eral color-coding systems use two sets of 13 colors—one set for letters A–M, and a second set of the same colors on a different background for the letters N–Z.

There are many ready-made systems available (e.g., Bibbero, Colwell, Kardex, Remington Rand, Smead, TAB, VisiRecord). Self-adhesive colored letter blocks with either two or three letters in the specific colors are supplied in rolls. The color blocks with the appropriate letter are placed on the index tab of the folder, along with the patient's full name. The letters are in pairs so that they can be seen from either side of the chart. Strong, easily differentiated colors are used, creating a band of color in the files that makes it easy to spot out-of-place folders.

NUMERIC COLOR CODING

Color coding is also used in numeric filing. Numbers 0 through 9 are each assigned a different color. In a terminal digit filing system, the colors for the last two numbers would be affixed to the tab. If the number 1 is red and 5 is yellow, all files with numbers ending in 15 form a red and yellow band. Usually a predetermined section of the number is color coded.

OTHER COLOR CODING APPLICATIONS

There are many other ways to make color work for you. Small pressure-sensitive tabs in a variety of colors may be used to identify certain types of insured patients and other specific information. For example, a red tab over the edge of the folder may identify a patient on Medicaid, a blue tab may identify a CHAMPUS patient; a green tab may identify a Workers' Compensation patient; matching tabs may be attached to the insured's ledger card; research cases may be identified by a special color tab; and brightly colored labels on the outside of a patient chart can indicate certain health conditions, such as drug allergies. In a partnership practice, a different color folder or label may identify each physician's patients. Color can also be used to differentiate dates—one color for each month or year.

Business records may also utilize color coding. Main divider guide headings may be of one color, subheadings in a second color, and subdivisions in a

TABLE 14–6 Color Coding for Business Records

Main Heading:	DISBURSEMENTS	Red label
Subheading:	Equipment	Blue label
Subdivisions:	Typewriter	Yellow label
	Copier	Yellow label
	Calculator	Yellow label

third color (Table 14–6). A fourth color might be used for personal items.

The use of color in filing is limited only by the imagination. One word of caution: Every person in the facility who uses the files must know the key to the coding, and the key should also be written in the facility's procedures manual.

Organization of Files

PATIENT HEALTH INFORMATION

It is very difficult for a physician to study a disorganized history. Some systematic method must be followed in placing items in the patient folder. The content of the patient record has already been discussed. From the filing standpoint, it should be emphasized that when a patient record is not in actual use, there is only one place it should be—in the filing cabinet or shelf. Many precious hours can be lost in searching for misplaced or lost records that were carelessly left unfiled.

The patient's full name, in indexing order, should be typed on a label and attached to the folder tab. A strip of transparent tape can be placed on the label to prevent smudging if this is a problem. The patient's full name should also be typed on each sheet within the folder.

HEALTH-RELATED CORRESPONDENCE

Correspondence pertaining to patients' medical records should be filed with the case history. Other medical correspondence should probably be filed in a subject file.

GENERAL CORRESPONDENCE

The physician's office operates as a business as well as a professional service. There will be correspondence of a general nature pertaining to the operation of the office. In all likelihood, a special drawer or shelf is set aside for the general correspondence. The correspondence is indexed according to subject matter or names of correspondents. The guides in a subject file may appear in one, two, or three positions, depending on the number of headings, subheadings, and subdivisions. Examples are shown in Table 14–6.

PRACTICE MANAGEMENT FILES

The most active financial record is, of course, the patient ledger. In facilities that still use a manual system, this will be a card or vertical tray file, and the accounts will be arranged alphabetically by name. There will be at least two divisions:

- Active accounts
- Paid accounts

MISCELLANEOUS FOLDER

Papers that do not warrant an individual folder are placed in a miscellaneous folder. Within the folder, all papers relating to one subject, or with one correspondent, are kept together in chronologic order, the most recent on top, and then filed alphabetically with other miscellaneous material. Related materials may be stapled together. Never use paper clips for this purpose. When as many as five papers accumulate with one correspondent or subject, a separate folder should be prepared.

EXAMPLES OF SPECIAL CATEGORIES THAT MAY BE SET UP

Government-sponsored insurance
Workers' Compensation
Delinquent accounts
Collection accounts

Other business files include records of income and expense, financial statements, income and payroll tax records, canceled checks, and insurance policies. These papers may be filed chronologically.

TICKLER OR FOLLOW-UP FILE

The most frequently used follow-up method is that of a **tickler file,** so called because it tickles the memory that something needs to be done or followed up on a particular date. The tickler file is always a chronologic arrangement. In its simplest form, it consists of notations on the daily calendar. If information, such as an x-ray report or laboratory report, is expected concerning a patient who has an appointment to come in, the medical assistant might make a note on the calendar or tickler file a day ahead to check on whether the report has arrived.

The tickler file is often a card file with 12 guides for the names of the months and 31 guides printed with numbers 1 through 31 for the days of the month. The guide for the current month, followed by the 31 day guides, is placed at the front of the file. Notations of actions to be taken are placed behind the guides for specific days of the current month. Notations for future months are placed behind the guide for that month. To be effective, the tickler file must be checked the first thing each day.

There are many ways to use the tickler file. It is a useful reminder for recurring events such as payments, meetings, and so forth. On the last day in each month, all the notations from behind the next month's guide are distributed among the daily numbered guides, and the guide for the month just completed is placed at the back of the file.

TRANSITORY OR TEMPORARY FILE

Many papers are kept longer than necessary because no provision is made for segregating those that have a limited usefulness. This situation is avoided by having a *transitory* or *temporary* file. For example, if the medical assistant writes a letter requesting a reprint, the file copy is placed in the transitory folder. When the reprint is received, the file copy is destroyed. The transitory file is used for materials having no permanent value. The paper may be marked with a T and destroyed when the action is completed.

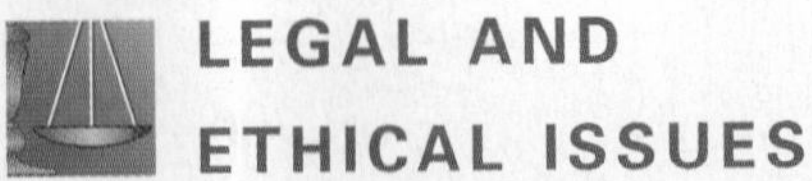

LEGAL AND ETHICAL ISSUES

Shelf units with doors afford the best protection of confidentiality of patient records. Make certain that every paper placed in a patient's chart carries the date and name of the patient.

CRITICAL THINKING

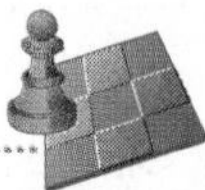

1 Explain why the number of patient records might determine the method of filing.

2 Discuss the difference between a direct filing system and an indirect system. What is the determining factor?

3 Explain how color coding can speed up filing and retrieval.

HOW DID I DO? Answers to Memory Joggers

1. Answers will vary but should include six styles.
2. An OUTguide is used to indicate the place of a file that has been temporarily removed. It also avoids unnecessary search for a missing file.
3. Conditioning, releasing, indexing and coding, sorting, storing, and filing
4. a. alphabetic, numeric, subject
   b. alphabetic
   c. numeric

REFERENCES

Huffman EK: Health Information Management, 10th ed. Berwyn, IL, Physicians' Record Company, 1994.

Sabin WA: The Gregg Reference Manual, 7th ed. New York, Glencoe Division, McGraw-Hill, 1994.

Health Information Management

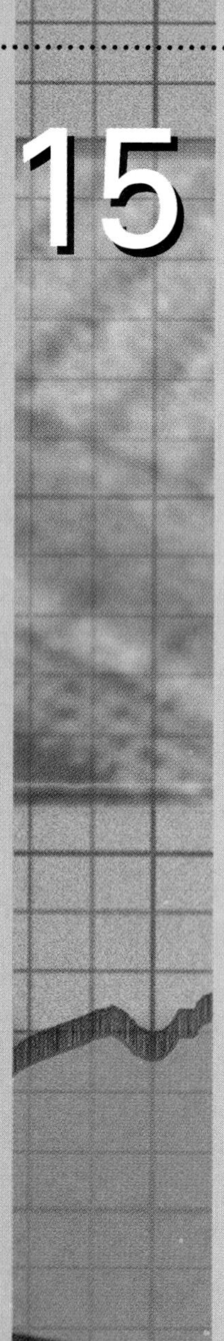

OUTLINE

LEARNING OBJECTIVES

Cognitive: On successful completion of this chapter, you should be able to:

1 Define and spell the terms listed in the Vocabulary.
2 State five important reasons for keeping good medical records.
3 Explain ownership of the record.
4 List three advantages of the POMR.
5 Explain the basic differences between a traditional medical record and a problem-oriented record.
6 Illustrate the meaning of *subjective* and *objective* information in a medical record.
7 List four categories each of *subjective* and *objective* information contained in a complete case history.
8 List 15 items of personal data needed on a patient history.
9 Discuss changing an entry in the medical record and the importance of following correct procedure.
10 List and describe the three classifications of patient files.

Performance: On successful completion of this chapter, you should be able to:

1 Initiate a medical record for a new patient.
2 Add reports and correspondence into the patient's file in the correct manner and sequence.
3 Make a correction in a patient's chart in a manner affording legal protection.

VOCABULARY

augment To make larger or more intense

chronologic order In the order of time

continuity The quality or state of being continuous

correlation To show a mutual relationship

demographic Relating to the statistical characteristics of populations, such as births, marriages, mortality, health, and so forth

litigation Contest in a court of justice for the purpose of enforcing a right

microfilming Photographic records in reduced size on film.

objective information Perceptible to the external senses (e.g., conclusions reached by a physician after listening to body sounds with a stethoscope)

obliteration To remove from existence; destroy

OUTfolder A folder used to provide space for the temporary filing of materials

parlance Manner or mode of speech

pejorative Having negative connotations; a deprecatory word

POMR Problem-oriented medical record

procrastination The intentional putting off of doing something that should be done

retention schedule A listing of dates until which records are to be kept, based on statutes of limitation, tax regulations, and other factors

sequential Succeeding or following in order or as a result

statute of limitations The time limit within which an action may legally be brought upon a contract

subjective information Findings perceptible only by the affected person (the patient) (e.g., pain experienced in a specific area under certain circumstances)

Complete and accurate records are essential to a well-managed medical practice. They provide a continuous story of a patient's progress from the first visit to the last. The treatment and therapy prescribed are noted, along with regular reports on the patient's condition. When a patient is discharged, the degree of improvement is noted in the record. Health information management includes not only the assembling of the medical record for each patient but also having an efficient system for the saving, retrieval, transferring, protection, retention, storage, and destruction of these records.

SKILLS AND RESPONSIBILITIES

OBJECTIVES OF GOOD INFORMATION MANAGEMENT

- Save space
- Reduce the creation of unnecessary records
- Retrieve information fast
- Comply with legal safeguards
- Save time for the physician and the patient

Ownership of the Record

The information in a medical record is private and confidential. The medical record should be kept away from patient care areas. Its contents should not be made public. Authority to release information from the medical record lies solely with the patient unless required by law. The *record* belongs to the physician; the *information* belongs to the patient.

Reasons for Health Information Records

The three traditionally important reasons for careful recording of health information are to

- Provide the best medical care
- Supply statistical information
- Provide legal protection

PROVIDE THE BEST MEDICAL CARE

The physician examines the patient and enters the findings on the patient's medical record. These findings are the clues to diagnosis. The physician may order many types of tests to confirm or **augment** the clinical findings. As the reports of these tests come in, the findings fall into place like the pieces of a jigsaw puzzle. Now, with the confirmation data to support the diagnosis, the physician can prescribe treatment and form an opinion about the patient's chances of recovery, assured that every resource has been used to arrive at a correct judgment.

Keeping good medical records helps a physician provide **continuity** in a patient's care. Earlier illnesses and difficulties that appear on the patient's record may supply the key to current medical problems. For example, information that the patient was treated for rheumatic fever as a child can be extremely important in determining the course of treatment the physician prescribes for that patient when an illness develops a number of years later.

SUPPLY STATISTICAL INFORMATION

Medical records may be used to evaluate the effectiveness of certain kinds of treatment or to determine the incidence of a given disease. **Correlation** of such statistical information may result in a new outlook on some phases of medicine and can lead to revised techniques and treatments. The statistical data from medical records are also valuable in the preparation of scientific papers, books, and lectures.

PROVIDE LEGAL PROTECTION

Sometimes a physician must produce case histories and medical records in court. For example, a patient may wish to substantiate claims made to an insurance company for damages resulting from an accident in which he or she was injured and required medical treatment. The physician's record can be a help or a hindrance, depending on the care with which the record is kept.

In recent years other increasingly important reasons for keeping adequate health information records have affected the practice of medicine: financial reimbursement and participation in managed care.

FINANCIAL REIMBURSEMENT

Those who pay the bills require complete data to evaluate the necessity for care and the level and quality of that care before reimbursing the provider. Services must be carefully documented to justify insurance billing. The motto is "If it is not documented, it was not done (even if it was done)."

PARTICIPATION IN MANAGED CARE

Managed care organizations randomly conduct chart reviews and judge the physician on the quality of his or her documentation. The managed care organization must be able to assure its members that the physician is providing appropriate care.

Memory Joggers

1. Discuss the statement "If it is not documented, it was not done."
2. How would you answer the question "Who owns the medical record?"

Form and Quality of the Record

A record is any form of documented information. It may be kept on paper, film, or magnetic medium, such as computer tapes or disks.

FACTORS IN CREATING A USEFUL RECORD

- Easily retrievable
- Orderly
- Timely
- Legible
- Complete
- Understandable by anyone who needs to use it

Using shortened forms of words in records may be a timesaver, but any such system should be clearly understandable by anyone who needs to consult the chart. If the short forms vary from standard abbreviations (e.g., inf. could mean *infirm, inform,* or *information*), an explanation should be prepared and placed in the front of the files for immediate reference (Table 15–1).

If a record is to be *helpful,* it must be completely accurate. To be *good,* the record must be brief.

Style of the Record

NATURE OF PRACTICE

The style selected by a physician for recording case histories depends partly on the nature of the practice. General practitioners and some specialists keep

TABLE 15-1 Abbreviations Commonly Used in Patient History and Physical Examination

Abbreviation	Meaning
A&W	Alive and well
CC	Chief complaint
CNS	Central nervous system
CR	Cardiorespiratory
CV	Cardiovascular
Dx	Diagnosis
FH	Family history
GI	Gastrointestinal
GU	Genitourinary
GYN	Gynecology
HEENT	Head, ears, eyes, nose, throat
MM	Mucous membrane
PH	Past history
PI	Present illness
prn	As necessary *(pro re nata)*
ROS/SR	Review of systems/Systems review
TPR	Temperature, pulse, respirations
UCHD	Usual childhood diseases
VS	Vital signs
w/d	Well developed
w/n	Well nourished
WNL	Within normal limits

very detailed records. A specialist who sees patients only on a consultant basis, or a specialist who is likely to see a patient only once, such as a radiologist or an anesthesiologist, need not keep complex records.

NATURE OF PATIENT'S COMPLAINT

The nature of the patient's complaint is also a factor in determining how detailed a record should be. If a patient comes into a physician's office to have a foreign body removed from an eye or to have some minor injury such as a cut finger treated, a less detailed past medical history or family history is required. In contrast, the patient who is being treated for cardiac, hypertensive, or diabetic symptoms requires a complete examination and a detailed history.

USE OF SIMPLIFIED FORM

In some health care facilities where detailed histories are less common, a simple patient registration form (Fig. 15-1) can be used to record personal data and a plain sheet of paper used to record the complaint and treatment rendered. The physician who uses a plain sheet of paper for the patient record generally develops an outline that serves as a guide to taking down the information required for a history. The physician then dictates the history, and the medical assistant types it according to an established format and places it in the patient's folder after having it read and initialed by the physician. In every medical facility certain technical terms are used frequently in the physician's reports. The medical assistant who types the reports should become familiar with the correct spelling and meaning of the medical terms. Because of the close similarity in sound and spelling of some medical terms it is also wise to check the definition to verify that the word fits the context in which it is used.

STRUCTURED FORMAT

For the physician who wishes to use a more structured format, there are many different types of forms available from professional suppliers: forms for general practice, obstetrics, surgery, pediatrics, internal medicine, or any other of the established specialties. Some physicians design their own forms to suit their particular practice and have them printed to order.

Suppliers that specialize in medical forms sometimes provide a planning kit for the physician to use. Local printers, too, often can be very helpful with form design. The record may be **sequential,** or it may be separated into problems, as described later in the section on the problem-oriented medical record. Regardless of the form used, the record will contain certain basic information (see Legal Considerations of the Patient Record).

LEGAL CONSIDERATIONS OF THE PATIENT RECORD

For adequate legal protection, the patient record should include the following:

- Patient's name and the date on every page
- Patient's medical history
- Specific quotes of comments made by the patient about symptoms or reasons for consultation
- Physician's response to any such comments
- Results of examinations
- All notations of vital signs, dated and initialed
- Records of treatment, including all possible complications that might arise
- Any failed appointments, dated and initialed by receiver
- Copies of laboratory reports
- Notations of all instructions given

Thank you for selecting our health care team!
To help us meet all your health care needs, please fill out this form completely in ink. If you have any questions or need assistance, please ask us - we will be happy to help.

Welcome

Patient # ______
Soc. Sec. # ______
Date ______

Patient Information (CONFIDENTIAL)

Name ______ Birth date ______ Home phone ______
Address ______ City ______ State ______ Zip ______
Check appropriate box: ☐ Minor ☐ Single ☐ Married ☐ Divorced ☐ Widowed ☐ Separated
If student, name of school/college ______ City ______ State ______ ☐ Full time ☐ Part time
Patient's or parent's employer ______ Work phone ______
Business address ______ City ______ State ______ Zip ______
Spouse or parent's name ______ Employer ______ Work phone ______
Whom may we thank for referring you? ______
Person to contact in case of emergency ______ Phone ______

Responsible Party

Name of person responsible for this account ______ Relationship to patient ______
Address ______ Home phone ______
Driver's license # ______ Birth date ______ Financial institution ______
Employer ______ Work phone ______ SSN# ______
Is this person currently a patient in our office? ☐ Yes ☐ No

Insurance Information

Name of insured ______ Relationship to patient ______
Birth date ______ Social Security # ______ Date employed ______
Name of employer ______ Union or local # ______ Work phone ______
Address of employer ______ City ______ State ______ Zip ______
Insurance company ______ Group # ______ Policy/ID # ______
Ins. co. address ______ City ______ State ______ Zip ______
How much is your deductible? ______ How much have you used? ______ Max. annual benefit ______

DO YOU HAVE ANY ADDITIONAL INSURANCE? ☐ Yes ☐ No IF YES, COMPLETE THE FOLLOWING:

Name of insured ______ Relationship to patient ______
Birth date ______ Social Security # ______ Date employed ______
Name of employer ______ Union or local # ______ Work phone ______
Address of employer ______ City ______ State ______ Zip ______
Insurance company ______ Group # ______ Policy/ID # ______
Ins. co. address ______ City ______ State ______ Zip ______
How much is your deductible? ______ How much have you used? ______ Max. annual benefit ______

I authorize release of any information concerning my (or my child's) health care, advice and treatment provided for the purpose of evaluating and administering claims for insurance benefits. I also hereby authorize payment of insurance benefits otherwise payable to me directly to the doctor.

X ______
Signature of patient or parent if minor ______ Date ______

FIGURE 15–1 Patient registration form.

- Documentation of information disclosed during the informed consent process when applicable
- Any correspondence that relates to the patient's diagnosis or treatment
- Any other data pertinent to the patient's health

When a patient fails to follow instructions or refuses recommended treatment, a letter to this effect should be sent to the patient by certified, return-receipt mail and a copy retained in the patient record. A similar type of letter should be sent if the patient leaves the physician's care or if the physician feels it is necessary to withdraw from the case (Fig. 15–2).

EXAMPLES OF ITEMS TO EXCLUDE FROM THE RECORD

- Reports from consulting physicians *should not* be placed in the record until they have been carefully reviewed to ensure that the overall diagnostic and treatment plan is consistent or that any inconsistencies have been identified and justified. If the report contains confidential data from another source, release of such data without authorization can lead to legal difficulties.
- Transferred records from the patient's previous physicians should never be added to the patient's new record until the physician has reviewed them. The same advice would apply to records received from any outside source (e.g., hospital emergency departments or free-standing urgent-care clinics).
- **Pejorative** or flippant comments should never be entered in the record. For example, after seeing a patient who tended toward hypochondria, a physician might be tempted to enter only one note, such as "new verse, same refrain." This comment would reflect negatively on the physician in court. In some states, patients or their representatives have the legal right to a copy of their medical records.

Date

Dear (Patient):

I find it necessary to inform you that I am withdrawing from providing you medical care for the reason that ____________.

Because your condition requires medical attention, I suggest that you promptly seek the care of another physician. If you do not know of another physician, you may wish to contact the county medical society for a referral.

If you so desire, I shall be available to provide care to you for a reasonable time after you have received this letter, but in no event for more than 15 days.

When you have selected a new physician, I would be pleased to make available to him or her a copy of your medical chart or a summary of your treatment.

Very truly yours,

FIGURE 15–2 Letter of withdrawal from a case.

Organization of the Record

SOURCE-ORIENTED RECORD

The traditional patient record is *source oriented;* that is, observations and data are catalogued according to their source—physician, laboratory, x-ray, nurse, technician—with no recording of a logical relationship between them. Forms and progress notes are filed in reverse **chronologic order** (most recent on top) and filed in separate sections of the record by the type of form or service rendered—all laboratory reports together, all x-ray reports together, and so forth.

PROBLEM-ORIENTED RECORD

The problem-oriented medical record **(POMR)** is a radical departure from the traditional system of keeping patient records. It is sometimes referred to as the Weed system because it was originated by Dr. Lawrence L. Weed, a professor of medicine at the University of Vermont's College of Medicine. The POMR is a record of clinical practice that divides medical action into four bases:

- The *database* includes chief complaint, present illness, and patient profile and also a review of systems, physical examination, and laboratory reports.
- The *problem list* is a numbered and titled list of every problem the patient has that requires management or workup. This may include social and **demographic** troubles as well as strictly medical or surgical ones.
- The *treatment plan* includes management, additional workups needed, and therapy. Each plan is titled and numbered with respect to the problem.
- The *progress notes* include structured notes that are numbered to correspond with each problem number.

One company, which designed the Andrus/Clini-Rec Charting System, has developed a file folder for

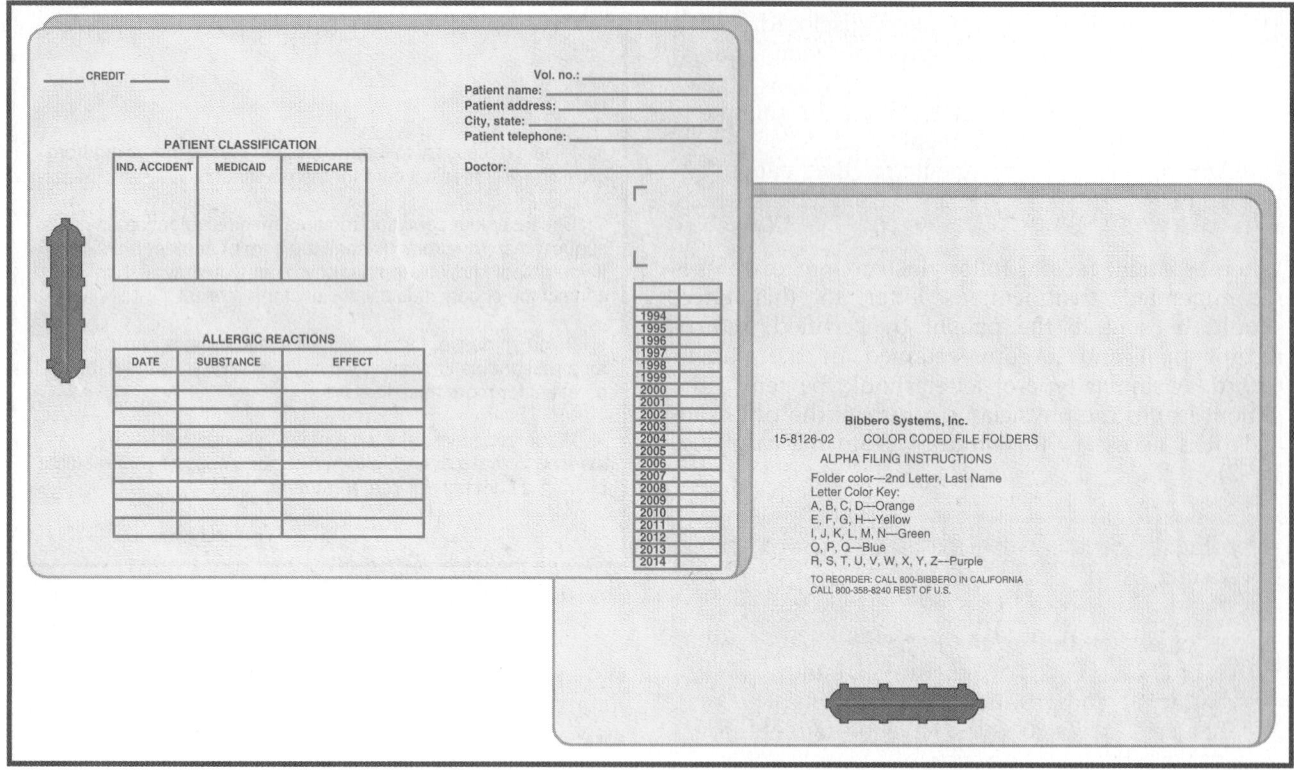

FIGURE 15–3 File folder for organization of patient data. (Courtesy of Bibbero Systems, Inc., Petaluma, CA.)

its recommended organization of patient data. The folder is preprinted on the front for age dating and easy access to basic information. With the calendar years printed on the cover, it is simple to keep track of when the patient was last seen. On the initial visit, the year, say 1998, is checked on the cover. If the patient appears again in 2000, and the year 1999 is not checked, it is immediately evident that more than a year has elapsed since the last visit (Fig. 15–3). The system includes dividers for laboratory reports, consultations, hospital reports, and radiologic and electrocardiograph reports (all scientific information) on the left side and database and progress notes (communication and supervision) on the right side.

The chart is begun by obtaining a patient-completed database system record, which contains family and past medical history together with many carefully selected screening questions (Fig. 15–4). There are also questionnaires designed for screening problems in specialty practices.

The problem list is entered on the divider cover for laboratory reports. Special sections are provided for current major and chronic problems and for inactive major or chronic problems. The divider cover for progress notes is a chart for listing medications and other therapeutic modalities. Progress notes follow the SOAP approach (Fig. 15–5).

SOAP APPROACH

- *S*ubjective impressions
- *O*bjective clinical evidence
- *A*ssessment or diagnosis
- *P*lans for further studies, treatment, or management

The POMR has the advantage of imposing order and organization on the information added to a patient's medical record. The records are more easily reviewed, and the likelihood of overlooking a problem is greatly reduced. The SOAP approach essentially forces a rational approach to patient problems and assists in formulating a logical and orderly plan of patient care.

Popularity of the POMR has continued to grow since its introduction in the 1960s, and it is especially advantageous in clinics, group practices, and hospitals, where more than one person must be able to find essential information in the chart.

Memory Jogger

3 *Explain the SOAP* approach.

PART A – PRESENT HEALTH HISTORY (continued)

IV. GENERAL HEALTH, ATTITUDE AND HABITS (continued)

Have you recently had any changes in your: If yes, please explain:

Marital status? No ___ Yes ___

Job or work? No ___ Yes ___

Residence? No ___ Yes ___

Financial status? No ___ Yes ___

Are you having any legal problems or trouble with the law? No ___ Yes ___

CONFIDENTIAL

PART B – PAST HISTORY

I. FAMILY HEALTH

Please give the following information about your immediate family:

Relationship	Age, If Living	Age At Death	State of Health Or Cause of Death
Father			
Mother			
Brothers and Sisters			
Spouse			
Children			

Have any **blood relatives** had any of the following illnesses? If so, indicate relationship (mother, brother, etc.)

Illness	Family Members
Asthma	
Diabetes	
Cancer	
Blood Disease	
Glaucoma	
Epilepsy	
Rheumatoid Arthritis	
Tuberculosis	
Gout	
High Blood Pressure	
Heart Disease	
Mental Problems	
Suicide	

II. HOSPITALIZATIONS, SURGERIES, ...

Please list all times you have been hospitalize...

Year Operation...

III. ILLNESS AND MEDICAL PROBLE...

Please mark with an (X) any of the following ill...
If you are not certain when an illness started, w...

Illness	(X)
Eye or eye lid infection	
Glaucoma	
Other eye problems	
Ear Trouble	
Deafness or decreased hearing	
Thyroid trouble	
Strep throat	
Bronchitis	
Emphysema	
Pneumonia	
Allergies, asthma or hay fever	
Tuberculosis	
Other lung problems	
High blood pressure	
Heart attack	
High cholesterol	
Arteriosclerosis (Hardening of arteries)	
Heart murmur	
Other heart condition	
Stomach/duodenal ulcer	
Diverticulosis	
Colitis	
Other bowel problem	
Hepatitis	
Liver trouble	
Gallbladder trouble	

Page 2 © 1979, 1983 Bibbero Systems Inter... (REV. 6/92)

PART C – BODY SYSTEMS REVIEW

MEN: Please answer questions 1 through 12, then skip to question 18.
WOMEN: Please start on question 6.

...N ONLY

Have you had or do you have prostate trouble? No ___ Yes ___

Do you have any sexual problems or with impotency? No ___ Yes ___

Have you ever had sores or lesions on your penis? No ___ Yes ___

Have you ever had any discharge from your penis? No ___ Yes ___

Do you ever have pain, lumps or swelling in your testicles? No ___ Yes ___

...k here if you wish to discuss any special problems with the doctor. ☐

Rarely/Never Occasionally Frequently

Is it sometimes hard to start your urine flow?

CONFIDENTIAL

...RN THIS PAGE 19-711-4 5/83 Page 3

Chart No. ___

ANDRUS/CLINI-REC® HEALTH HISTORY QUESTIONNAIRE

Identification Information Today's Date ___

Name ___ Date of Birth ___

Occupation ___ Marital Status ___

PART A – PRESENT HEALTH HISTORY

I. CURRENT MEDICAL PROBLEMS

Please list the medical problems for which you came to see the doctor. About when did they begin?

Problems	Date Began

What concerns you most about these problems?

If you are being treated for any other illnesses or medical problems by another physician, please describe the problems and write the name of the physician or medical facility treating you.

Illness or Medical Problem	Physician or Medical Facility	City

II. MEDICATIONS

Please list all medications you are now taking, including those you buy without a doctor's prescription (such as aspirin, cold tablets or vitamin supplements)

III. ALLERGIES AND SENSITIVITIES

List anything that you are allergic to such as certain foods, medications, dust, chemicals, or soaps, household items, pollens, bee stings, etc., and indicate how each affects you.

Allergic To:	Effect	Allergic To:	Effect

IV. GENERAL HEALTH, ATTITUDE AND HABITS

How is your overall health now?	Health now:	Poor___ Fair___ Good___ Excellent___
How has it been most of your life?	Health has been	Poor___ Fair___ Good___ Excellent___
In the past year:		
Has your appetite changed?	Appetite:	Decreased___ Increased___ Stayed same___
Has your weight changed?	Weight:	Lost___ lbs. Gained___ lbs. No change___
Are you thirsty much of the time?	Thirsty:	No___ Yes___
Has your overall 'pep' changed?	Pep:	Decreased___ Increased___ Stayed same___
Do you usually have trouble sleeping?	Trouble sleeping:	No___ Yes___
How much do you exercise?	Exercise:	Little or none___ Less than I need___ All I need___
Do you smoke?	Smokes:	No___ Yes___ If yes, how many years?___
How many each day?		___Cigarettes ___Cigars ___Pipesfull
Have you ever smoked?	Smoked	No___ Yes___ If yes, how many years?___
How many each day?		___Cigarettes ___Cigars ___Pipesfull
Do you drink alcoholic beverages?	Alcohol:	No___ Yes___ I drink___ Beers___ Glasses of Wine ___ Drinks of hard liquor - per day
Have you ever had a problem with alcohol?	Prior problem:	No___ Yes___
How much coffee or tea do you usually drink?	Coffee/Tea:	___ cups of coffee or tea a day.
Do you regularly wear seatbelts?	Seatbelts:	No___ Yes___

DO YOU:	Rarely/Never	Occasionally	Frequently	DO YOU:	Rarely/Never	Occasionally	Frequently
Feel nervous?				Ever feel like committing suicide?			
Feel depressed?				Feel bored with your life?			
Find it hard to make decisions?				Use marijuana?			
Lose your temper?				Use "hard drugs"?			
Worry a lot?				Do you want to talk to the doctor about a personal matter? No___ Yes___			
Tire easily?							
Have trouble relaxing?							
Have any sexual problems?							

CONFIDENTIAL

Created and Developed by "Medical Economics" Professional Systems
Copyright © 1979, 1983 Bibbero Systems International, Inc. STOCK NO. 19-711-4 5/83 Page 1

FIGURE 15–4 Database self-administered general health history questionnaire. (Courtesy of Bibbero Systems, Inc., Petaluma, CA.)

OUTLINE FORMAT PROGRESS NOTES

Patient Name *Fletcher, LeRoy*

Prob. No. or Letter	DATE	S Subjective	O Objective	A Assess	P Plans	Page 1
2	01/26/00	*Patient complains of two days of severe high epigastric pain and burning, radiating through to the back. Pain accentuated after eating.*				
			On examination there is extreme guarding and tenderness, high epigastric region. No rebound. Bowel sounds normal. BP 110/70			
				R/O gastric ulcer, pylorospasm.		
					To have upper gastrointestinal series. Start on Cimetidine, 300 mg. q.i.d. Eliminate coffee, alcohol, and aspirin. Return in two days.	

Start each Progress Note (Subjective, Objective, Assessment and Plans) at the appropriate shaded column to create an outline form. Write through the intervening columns to the right margin of the page.

ANDRUS/CLINI-REC® PRIMARY CARE CHARTING SYSTEM FORM NO. 26-7115, ©1976 BIBBERO SYSTEMS, INC., PETALUMA, CA.

FIGURE 15–5 SOAP progress note form. (Courtesy of Bibbero Systems, Inc., Petaluma, California (800) 242-2376, Fax (800) 242-9330.)

Contents of the Complete Case History

The medical case history is the most important record in a physician's practice. For completeness, each patient's record should contain **subjective information** provided by the patient and **objective information** provided by the physician. If all entries are completed, the case history will stand the test of time. No branch of medicine is exempt from the necessity of keeping records. Records aid the physician in the practice of medicine, as well as provide legal protection.

SUBJECTIVE INFORMATION

Routine Personal Data

The patient's case history begins with routine personal data, which the patient usually supplies on the first visit. The basic facts needed are

- Patient's full name, spelled correctly
- Names of parents if patient is a child
- Patient's sex
- Date of birth
- Marital status
- Name of spouse, if married
- Number of children, if any
- Home address and telephone number
- Occupation
- Name of employer
- Business address and telephone number
- Employment information for spouse
- Health care insurance information
- Source of referral
- Social Security number

Personal and Medical History

This portion of the medical record, which is often obtained by having the patient complete a questionnaire, provides information about any past illnesses or surgical operations that the patient may have had and includes data about injuries or physical defects, whether congenital or acquired. It also includes information about the patient's daily health habits.

Patient's Family History

The family history comprises the physical condition of the various members of the patient's family, any past illnesses or diseases that individual members may have suffered, and a record of the causes of death. This information is important, because a hereditary pattern may be present in the case of certain diseases.

Patient's Chief Complaint

This is a concise account of the patient's symptoms, explained in the patient's own words. It should include

- Nature and duration of pain, if any
- Time when the patient first noticed symptoms
- Patient's opinion as to the possible causes for the difficulties
- Remedies that the patient may have applied before seeing the physician
- Other medical treatment received for the same condition in the past

OBJECTIVE INFORMATION

Objective findings, sometimes referred to as signs, become evident from the physician's examination of the patient.

Physical Examination and Findings and Laboratory and Radiology Reports

This section of the case history varies greatly with the specialty of the physician and the complaint of the patient. After the physician has examined the patient, the physical findings are recorded on the history. Results of other tests or requests for these tests are then recorded or, if they appear on separate sheets, attached to the history.

Diagnosis

The physician, on the basis of all evidence provided in the patient's past history, the physician's examination, and any supplementary tests, places the diagnosis of the patient's condition on the medical record. If there is some doubt, it may be termed *provisional diagnosis.*

Treatment Prescribed and Progress Notes

The physician's suggested treatment is listed after the diagnosis. Generally, instructions to the patient to return for follow-up treatment in a specific period of time are noted here as well.

On each subsequent visit, the date must be entered on the chart and information about the patient's condition and the results of treatment added to the history, on the basis of the physician's observations. Notations of all medications prescribed or instructions given, as well as the patient's own progress report, should be placed in the record. Any home visits are noted. If the patient is hospitalized, the name of the hospital, the reason for the admission, and the dates of admission and discharge are recorded. Much of this information may be obtained from the hospital discharge summary.

Condition at Time of Termination of Treatment

When the treatment is terminated, the physician will record that information, for example, *August 18, 1999. Wound completely healed. Patient discharged.*

Memory Joggers

 *Explain the difference between* subjective *and* objective *information.*

Obtaining the History

The medical assistant usually secures the routine personal data. The personal and medical history and the patient's family history may be secured by asking the patient to complete a questionnaire, with the physician **augmenting** the information provided during the patient interview.

BY THE MEDICAL ASSISTANT

When the medical assistant is responsible for recording the patient's history, care must be exercised to ensure that the patient's answers are not heard by others in the reception room. If privacy is not possible, it is better to give the patient a form to fill out and then transfer this information to permanent records later. When privacy is available, the medical assistant may ask the patient questions and at the same time type the answers directly on the record. This method offers an opportunity to become better acquainted with the patient while completing the necessary records. In facilities where lengthy questionnaires are to be completed by the new patient, the questionnaire is mailed to the patient with a request that it be completed and returned to the physician before the appointment. If the record is to be computerized, requesting the information ahead of time gives the office staff the opportunity to transfer information to the computer before the new patient's visit.

BY THE PHYSICIAN

The patient's chief complaint may have been indicated to the medical assistant, but the physician will question the patient in more detail. Many practitioners write their own entries on the chart in longhand. Some may keyboard the findings direct into the computer. Others may dictate the material, either directly to the medical assistant or by using a recording device. If the material is dictated and typed, the physician should check each entry and then initial the entry to verify accuracy. Although the physician may find this a "bother," it should be encouraged. For a chart to be admissible as evidence in court, the person dictating or writing the entries must be able to attest that they were true and correct at the time they were written. The best indication of that is the physician's signature or initials on the typed entry.

Making Additions

As long as the patient is under the physician's care, the medical history is building. Each laboratory report, radiology report, and progress note is added to the record with the latest information always on top. Although each item is important, the most recent is usually of greatest significance to the patient's care. Again, the physician should read and initial each of these reports before it is placed in the record.

LABORATORY REPORTS

Different colors of paper are often used for reporting different procedures. For example, urinalysis report forms may be yellow, blood count forms pink, and so forth. When laboratory slips are smaller than the history form, they should be placed on a standard 8½ × 11-inch sheet of colored paper. Type the patient's name in the upper right corner, and then, with transparent tape, fasten the first report even with the bottom of the page. The second laboratory report will be taped or glued in place on top of and about ½ inch above the first slip, allowing the date to show on the first report. By this method, called shingling, the latest report always appears on top. When checking previous reports, it is necessary only to run your finger down the slips until you find the desired date; then flip up the slips above. Laboratory report carrier forms with adhesive strips may be purchased (Fig. 15–6).

RADIOLOGY REPORTS

Radiology reports are usually typed on standard letter-size stationery. They are placed in the patient's history folder, with the most recent report on top. All radiology reports may be stapled together or kept behind a special divider in the chart.

PROGRESS NOTES

Reports on the patient's progress are continually being added to the case history. Each visit of the patient should be entered on the chart, with the date preceding any notations about the visit. The medical

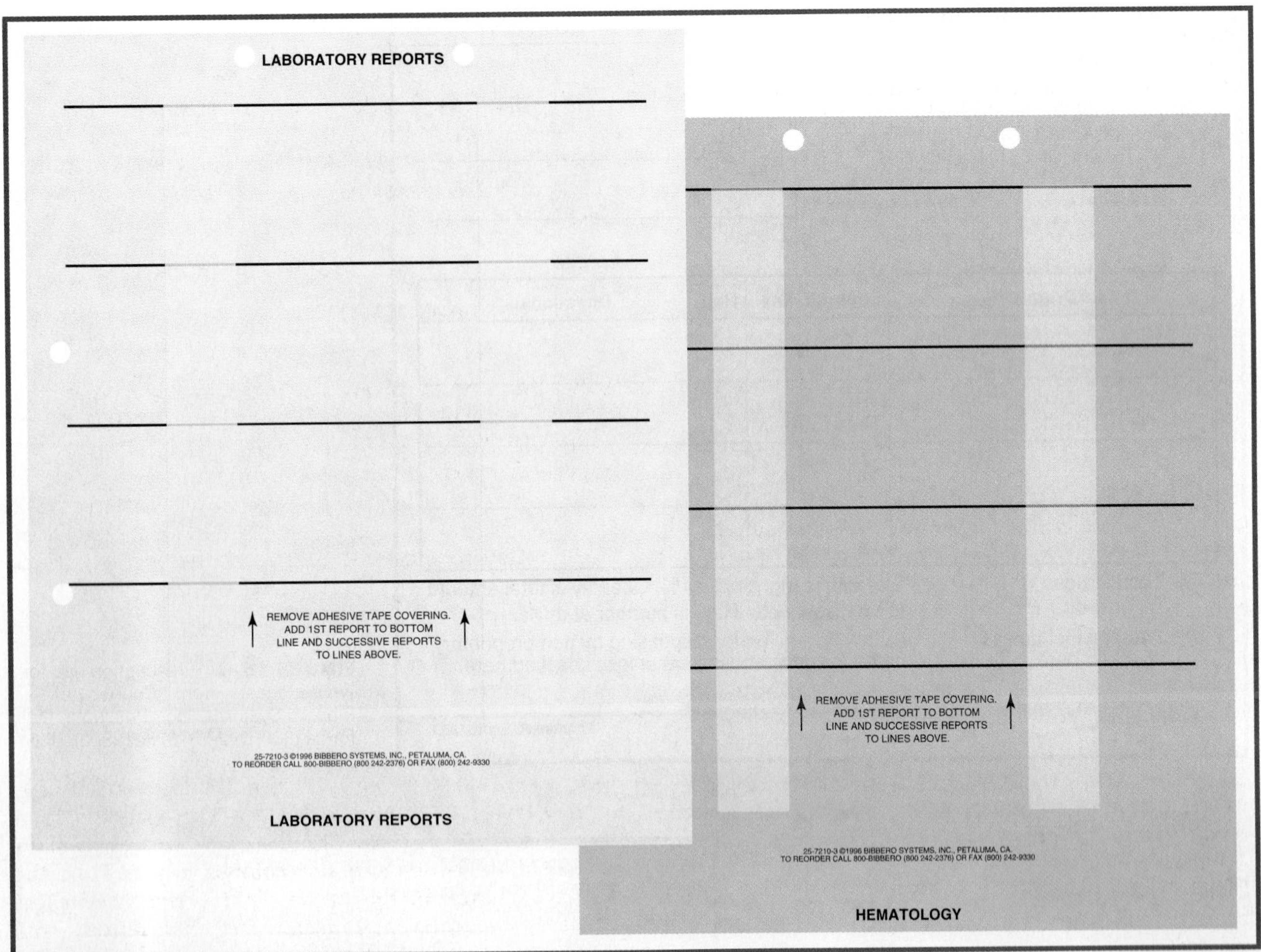
LABORATORY REPORTS
REMOVE ADHESIVE TAPE COVERING. ADD 1ST REPORT TO BOTTOM LINE AND SUCCESSIVE REPORTS TO LINES ABOVE.
25-7210-3 ©1996 BIBBERO SYSTEMS, INC., PETALUMA, CA.
TO REORDER CALL 800-BIBBERO (800 242-2376) OR FAX (800) 242-9330
LABORATORY REPORTS
REMOVE ADHESIVE TAPE COVERING. ADD 1ST REPORT TO BOTTOM LINE AND SUCCESSIVE REPORTS TO LINES ABOVE.
25-7210-3 ©1996 BIBBERO SYSTEMS, INC., PETALUMA, CA.
TO REORDER CALL 800-BIBBERO (800 242-2376) OR FAX (800) 242-9330
HEMATOLOGY

FIGURE 15–6 Quick-stick color-coded lab carriers. (Courtesy of Bibbero Systems, Inc., Petaluma, California (800) 242-2376, Fax (800) 242-9330.)

assistant can type or stamp the date on the chart when readying the charts for the patient's visits. Every instruction, prescription, or telephone call for advice should be entered with the correct date. If several persons are handling and making entries on a patient's record, it is advisable to initial each entry. This aids in tracing entries about which there may be some question.

Making Corrections

Sometimes it is necessary to make corrections on medical records. Erasing and **obliteration** must be avoided. To correct a handwritten entry, follow these three steps:

1. Draw a line through the error
2. Insert the correction above or immediately after the error.
3. In the margin, write correction or *Corr.*, your initials, and the date.

Errors made while typing are corrected in the usual way. However, an error discovered in a typed entry at a later date is corrected in the same manner as described for a handwritten entry.

Keeping Records Current

One of the greatest dangers to good record keeping is **procrastination.** The record must be methodically kept current. It is the medical assistant's responsibility to see that this is done.

The case histories and reports may accumulate on the physician's or the medical assistant's desk during the day. After the last patient has gone, check each history to make certain that all necessary information has been recorded and that each entry is sufficiently clear for future understanding. Give the physician all extra reports, such as laboratory and radiology reports, to read and initial so that they may be filed in the patient's case history folder.

While the physician is reviewing these reports,

THOMAS A. SCOTT
General Practice
135 SO. ELM STREET
DALLAS, TEXAS 75019
TELEPHONE: (214) 340-9999

TX. LIC. #6099914 DEA #AK08888888

Name
Address
City
Date

Rx Drug	Strength	Qty.	Rep.	Directions

☐ Total Drugs

☐ Please label unless checked here

Strength is Mg. Units or %; Quantity is total amount to be dispensed. Rep. is number of refills.
Authority is given for dispensing by non proprietary name (generic equivalent) unless checked here. ☐

FORM #25-8298

Thomas A. Scott, M.D.

FIGURE 15–7 Prescription pad for write-it-once system. (Courtesy of Bibbero Systems, Inc., Petaluma, California (800) 242-2376, Fax (800) 242-9330.)

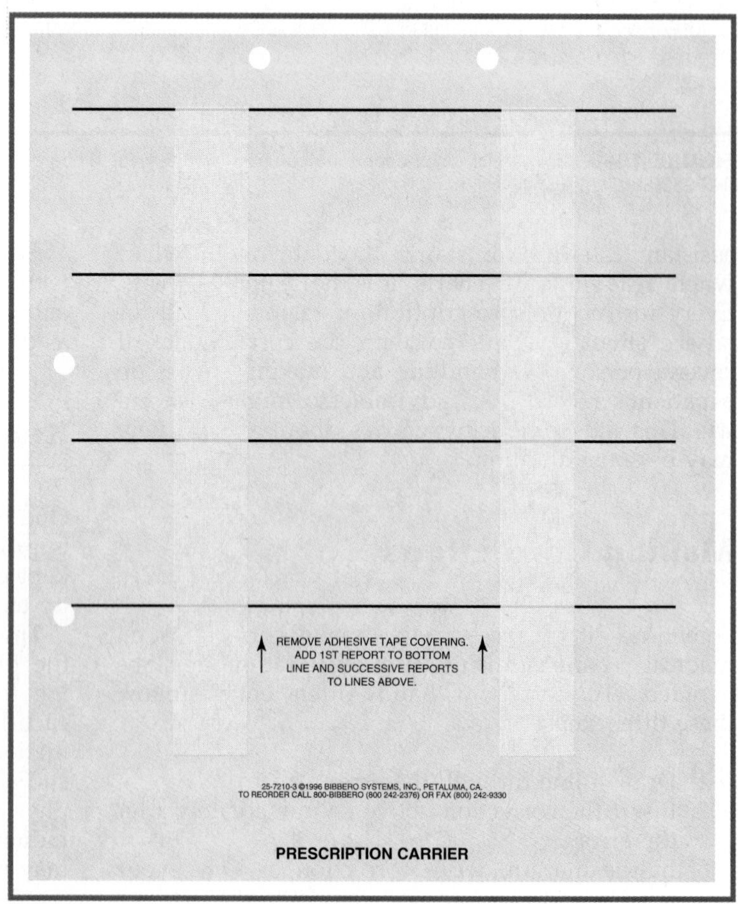
REMOVE ADHESIVE TAPE COVERING.
ADD 1ST REPORT TO BOTTOM
LINE AND SUCCESSIVE REPORTS
TO LINES ABOVE.
25-7210-3 ©1996 BIBBERO SYSTEMS, INC., PETALUMA, CA.
TO REORDER CALL 800-BIBBERO (800 242-2376) OR FAX (800) 242-9330
PRESCRIPTION CARRIER

FIGURE 15–8 Quick-stick prescription carrier. (Courtesy of Bibbero Systems, Inc., Petaluma, California (800) 242-2376, Fax (800) 242-9330.)

you can pull the histories of any patients seen outside the office that day, as well as those of patients who have been given special instructions by telephone or for whom prescriptions were ordered. These entries are made in the same manner as for an office visit, but the type of call is explained in parentheses after the date.

EXAMPLE OF A HOME VISIT ENTRY

May 23, 1998 (Res.). Routine PX. Temp 98.6. Chest clear.
Cont. Rx. May now eat semi-bland diet.

EXAMPLE OF A TELEPHONE CALL TO PHYSICIAN

June 26, 1998 (Tel.). To change Rx (Vit. B Comp) to one b.i.d.
Force fluids. Feeling much better.

EXAMPLE OF CHARTING TESTS ORDERED FOR PATIENT

April 10, 1999. Consultation. Bil. mammograms scheduled at SJH on April 17. Scheduled with Dr. Abbot for office consultation on April 26.

EXAMPLE OF CHARTING PRESCRIPTIONS

April 25, 1999. Refill Tylenol c Cod. #25

A prescription pad, printed on no-smear, spot carbon paper, is available for a timesaving, write-it-once system. By placing the prescription blank over the patient's record, the prescription is automatically copied on the record as it is written (Fig. 15–7). Prescription carriers with adhesive strips are also available for the physician who uses duplicate prescription blanks (Fig. 15–8).

The patient record should not leave the office. A physician's pocket call record, as shown in Figure 15–9, can be used for outside calls, and the information can be transferred to the chart in the office.

Notations should be made of any unkept appointments or of refusals to cooperate with instructions as they occur.

After all records have been reviewed, they should be placed in a file tray and locked away for the night, if there is insufficient time to file them the same day. Do not leave histories out in view at night, especially if the facility has a night cleaning service.

On arrival the next morning, the medical assistant can index the histories for filing. Attach extra reports and information sheets (do not simply drop them into the folders). When this has been done, the records are ready for filing.

The physician may prefer to dictate progress notes rather than write them in longhand. At appropriate times during the day, everything is dictated: patient histories, physical examination findings, medications prescribed, follow-up findings, summaries of telephone conversations. At the end of the day the recorded information is given to the medical assistant for transcribing onto the records.

A great deal of time may be saved in transcribing these notes by using a continuous roll or pages of

PHYSICIANS POCKET CALL RECORD DATE________

NAME	ADDRESS OR REMARKS	SYMBOL	MONEY RECEIVED	HOME CHARGES	HOSPITAL CHARGES
	Post these TOTALS to office book daily. ☛				

FIGURE 15–9 Physician's pocket call record.

self-adhesive strips (Fig. 15–10). When the transcription has been completed, the physician may wish to check the notes, underline important points, and initial each entry before returning the notes to the medical assistant for insertion into the charts to verify that they are correct in the event of audit or **litigation.** The use of self-adhesive strips saves removing the sheet from a chart that may be bound with metal fasteners, inserting the sheet into the typewriter, and putting the sheet back into the

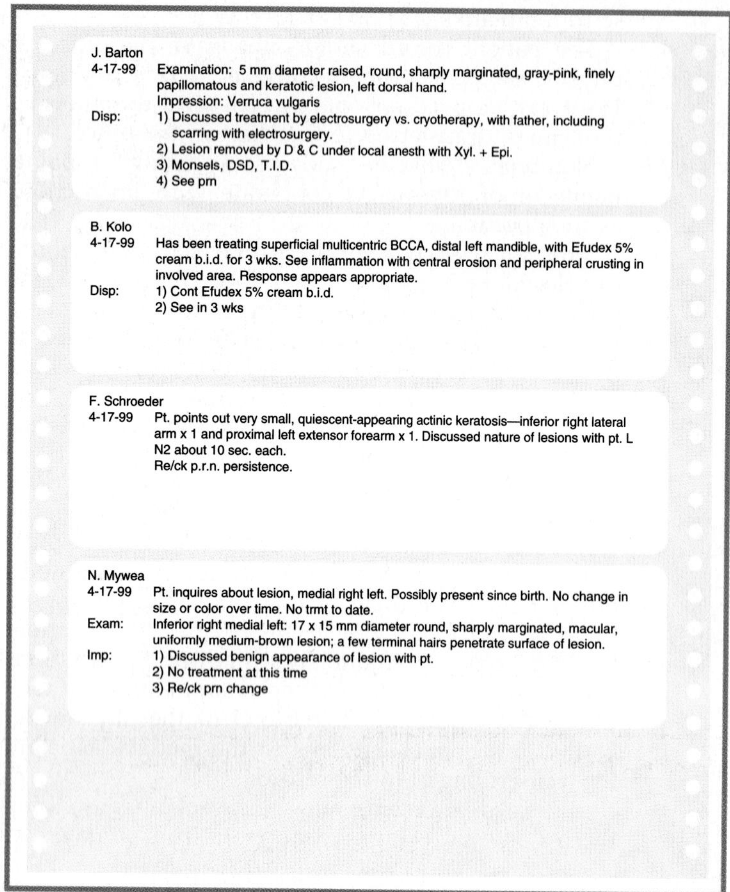

J. Barton
4-17-99 Examination: 5 mm diameter raised, round, sharply marginated, gray-pink, finely papillomatous and keratotic lesion, left dorsal hand.
Impression: Verruca vulgaris
Disp: 1) Discussed treatment by electrosurgery vs. cryotherapy, with father, including scarring with electrosurgery.
2) Lesion removed by D & C under local anesth with Xyl. + Epi.
3) Monsels, DSD, T.I.D.
4) See prn

B. Kolo
4-17-99 Has been treating superficial multicentric BCCA, distal left mandible, with Efudex 5% cream b.i.d. for 3 wks. See inflammation with central erosion and peripheral crusting in involved area. Response appears appropriate.
Disp: 1) Cont Efudex 5% cream b.i.d.
2) See in 3 wks

F. Schroeder
4-17-99 Pt. points out very small, quiescent-appearing actinic keratosis—inferior right lateral arm x 1 and proximal left extensor forearm x 1. Discussed nature of lesions with pt. L N2 about 10 sec. each.
Re/ck p.r.n. persistence.

N. Mywea
4-17-99 Pt. inquires about lesion, medial right left. Possibly present since birth. No change in size or color over time. No trmt to date.
Exam: Inferior right medial left: 17 x 15 mm diameter round, sharply marginated, macular, uniformly medium-brown lesion; a few terminal hairs penetrate surface of lesion.
Imp: 1) Discussed benign appearance of lesion with pt.
2) No treatment at this time
3) Re/ck prn change

A

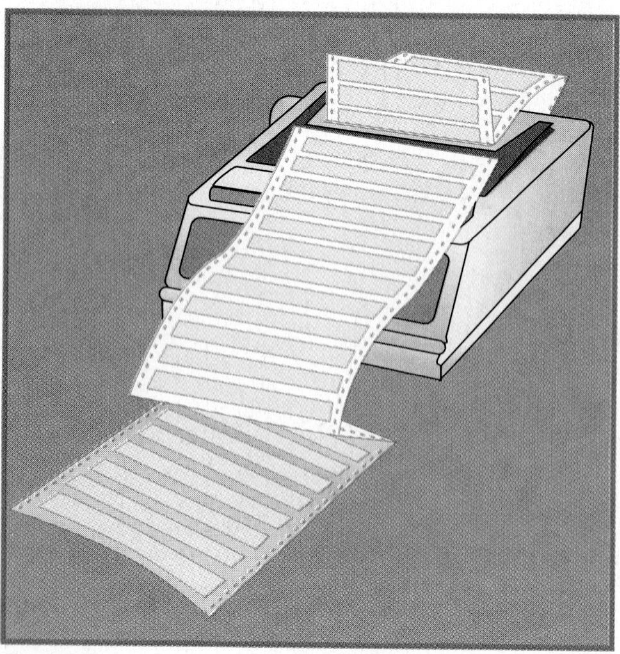

B

FIGURE 15–10 *A* and *B*, Self-adhesive strip and continuous roll used to transcribe notes.

folder. It also simplifies the physician's part in checking and initialing the notes, because only the transcribed material is handled, not the bulky charts.

Memory Jogger

Why is it important for the physician to sign or initial typewritten progress notes?

Regular Transfer of Files

In most medical offices, records are filed according to three classifications:

- *Active files* are those of patients currently receiving treatment.
- *Inactive files* generally are those of patients whom the doctor has not seen for 6 months or longer. When such individuals return for care, their folders are replaced in the active file.
- *Closed files* are records of patients who have died, moved away, or otherwise terminated their relationship with the physician.

Some system must be established for regular transfer of files from active to inactive status or possibly destruction. The yearly expansion of charts and the file space available can influence the transfer period. Charts for patients who are currently hospitalized may be kept in a special section for quick reference, then placed in the regular active file when the patient is discharged from the hospital. In a surgical practice, there frequently is a specific date on which the patient is discharged from the physician's care and the notation made on the chart "Return prn" (for the Latin *pro re nata:* as the occasion arises). This record may safely be placed in the inactive file. In a general practice office, the outside of the folder may be stamped with the date of the visit each time the patient is seen. It will then be a simple matter to determine when the chart should be transferred to the inactive status. In the **parlance** of filing, this is called the *perpetual transfer method.*

Retention and Destruction

Physicians have an obligation to retain patient records that may reasonably be of value to a patient, according to the AMA Council on Ethical and Judicial Affairs. There is no standard rule to follow in establishing a records **retention schedule**.

- Medical considerations are the primary basis for deciding how long to retain medical records. For example, operative notes and chemotherapy records should always be part of the patient's chart.
- If a particular record no longer needs to be kept for medical reasons, the physician should check state law to see if there is a requirement that records be kept for a minimum length of time (most states do not have such a provision). The time is measured from the last professional contact with the patient.
- In all cases, medical records should be kept for at least as long as the length of time of the **statute of limitations** for medical malpractice claims, which may be 3 or more years, depending on the state law. In the case of a minor, the statute of limitations may not apply until the patient reaches the age of majority.
- The records of any patient covered by Medicare or Medicaid must be kept at least 5 years.
- Before discarding old records, patients should be given an opportunity to claim the records or have them sent to another physician, if it is feasible to give the patient that opportunity.
- To preserve confidentiality when discarding old records, the documents should be destroyed.

Protection of Records

Releasing original case histories to anyone outside the health care facility should be avoided if possible. Instead, prepare a summary or photocopy the materials needed for reference and retain the original in the physician's office. With the facsimile machine becoming standard equipment in business facilities, as well as in many of our homes, the transfer of information is simplified and the records remain in safekeeping. Often only certain aspects of the record are requested by colleagues or others, and these can easily be supplied by faxing the required pages, observing precautions for confidentiality.

Occasions may arise when records are temporarily out of the office. Some physicians release case histories to their colleagues, or an original record may be subpoenaed by the court. In such instances, a colored **OUTfolder** should be inserted in the file in place of the regular folder and a notation made of the name, date, and to whom the record was released. Interim papers may be placed in the OUTfolder until the original is returned.

Long-Term Storage

Large health care facilities may find it advisable to microfilm records for storage. Another option is the transfer of paper records by laser beam onto optical disks. **Microfilming** and optical disk technology are both very expensive and probably are not practical for any but the very large group practice or health maintenance organization.

Facilities that have computerized the patient records will be able to keep those records indefinitely on disk. Scanners can convert a paper record into an image on the computer screen resulting in an electronic medical record. The bulky paper files can then be put in storage or eliminated. There is no longer a need to fill hundreds of square feet of storage space or search through stack upon stack of storage file boxes for an inactive or closed file.

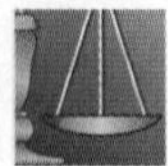

LEGAL AND ETHICAL ISSUES

Authority to release information from the medical record lies solely with the patient unless required by law.

Ownership of the record is often a subject of controversy. The record belongs to the physician; the information belongs to the patient.

When the physician withdraws from the care of a patient, or if the patient leaves the physician's care, a letter acknowledging this situation should be sent by the physician to the patient by certified, return-receipt mail.

When a medical chart is used as evidence in a court case, the person dictating or writing the entries must be able to attest to their authenticity.

The person making corrections to a medical record always must follow the steps as outlined in this chapter.

The records of any patient covered by Medicare or Medicaid must be kept at least 5 years. All records should be kept until the statute of limitations for medical malpractice claims has expired.

CRITICAL THINKING

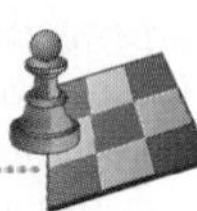

1 Interview a fellow student and create a patient history using 15 items of personal data.

2 Using the Discharge Summary in Chapter 12, demonstrate the correct method of making an alteration in the record.

HOW DID I DO? Answers to Memory Joggers

1 Example: In performing a physical examination, the physician may actually examine every body system but may record information about only those systems that are abnormal. This record would not stand up in court.

2 The answer should explain the ownership of both the physician and the patient.

3 *S*ubjective impressions
*O*bjective clinical evidence
*A*ssessment or diagnosis
*P*lans for further studies, treatment, or management.

4 Subjective information is supplied by the patient and includes personal data, past medical history, family medical history, and the patient's current complaint (symptoms). Objective information is what the physician notes on examination of the patient (signs).

5 It is important for the physician to initial typewritten notes to verify that they are correct, in the event of audit or litigation.

REFERENCES

American Medical Association: Current Opinions with Annotations of the Council on Ethical and Judicial Affairs, 1996–97 edition. Chicago, AMA, 1997.

Huffman EK: Health Information Management, 10th ed. Berwyn, IL, Physician Record Company, 1994 (revised by American Health Information Management Association).

Notes

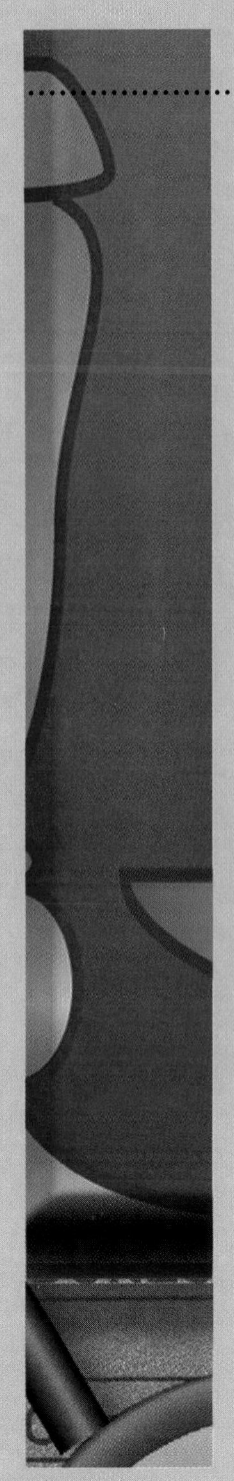

SECTION 5

Financial Management

CURRICULUM CONTENT/COMPETENCIES

Chapter 16 Professional Fees and Credit Arrangements

- *Understand and apply third-party guidelines*
- *Understand and adhere to managed care policies and procedures*
- *Explain office policies and procedures*
- *Follow employer's established policies dealing with the health care contract*

Chapter 17 Managing Practice Finances

- *Apply bookkeeping principles*
- *Manage accounts receivable*
- *Manage accounts payable*

Chapter 18 Banking Services and Procedures

- *Document and maintain accounting and banking records*
- *Maintain confidentiality*
- *Manage accounts payable*
- *Comply with established risk management and safety procedures*

Chapter 19 Billing and Collecting Procedures

- *Obtain reimbursement through accurate claims submissions*
- *Monitor third-party reimbursement*
- *Understand and adhere to managed care policies and procedures*
- *Manage accounts receivable*

Chapter 20 Health Insurance and Managed Care

- *Understand and adhere to managed care policies and procedures*
- *Understand and apply third-party guidelines*
- *Obtain reimbursement through accurate claims submission*

Chapter 21 Coding and Claims Processing

- *Perform procedural and diagnostic coding*
- *Document accurately*
- *Obtain reimbursement through accurate claims submission*
- *Apply computer techniques to support office operations*

Professional Fees and Credit Arrangements

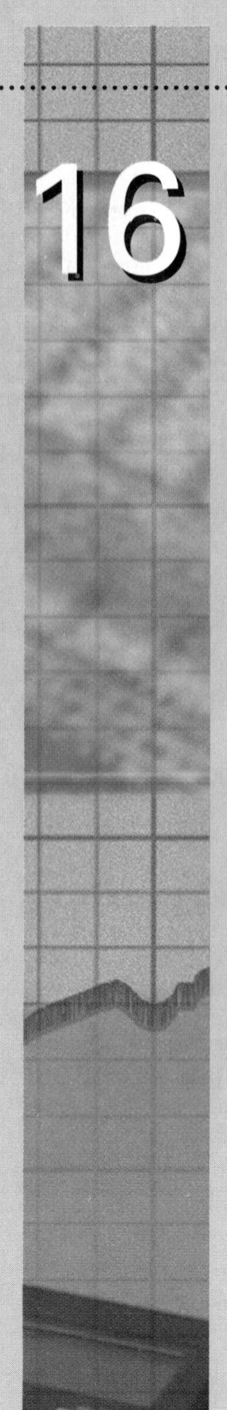

OUTLINE

LEARNING OBJECTIVES

Cognitive: On successful completion of this chapter you should be able to:

1. Define and spell the terms listed in the Vocabulary.
2. Discuss how fees are determined.
3. List three values that are considered in determining professional fees.
4. Give an example of usual and customary fee.
5. Explain how a physician's fee profile is determined.
6. List three reasons for giving patients an estimate slip.
7. Discuss the concept of professional courtesy.
8. List four kinds of charges that should be avoided.
9. List the items to be included on a credit form.
10. Explain what is meant by third-party liability.
11. Identify the three items of information that can be released in response to a request for credit information.
12. State three items that should be *excluded* in replying to a request for credit information.
13. Discuss the Truth in Lending Regulation.
14. Discuss how confidentiality relates to credit.

Performance: On successful completion of this chapter you should be able to:

1. Make financial arrangements with a patient requesting credit.
2. Prepare a Truth in Lending form.
3. Respond to patient's request for explanation of the physician's fee.

VOCABULARY

assignment of benefits Statement authorizing the insurance company to pay benefits directly to physician

capitation System of payment in which providers are paid a fixed per capita fee for each enrolled patient, not dependent on the services rendered

fee profile Compilation of a physician's fees over a given period of time

fee schedule Compilation of preestablished fee allowances for given services or procedures.

fiscal agent An organization under contract to the government as well as some private plans to act as financial representative in handling insurance claims from providers of health care; also referred to as fiscal intermediary

medically indigent Able to take care of ordinary living expenses but cannot afford medical care

professional courtesy Reduction or absence of fee to professional associates

third-party payer Someone other than the patient, spouse, or parent who is responsible for paying all or part of the patient's medical costs

usual, customary, and reasonable A formula for determining medical insurance benefits payable

The practice of medicine is a business as well as a profession, and the details of conducting the business aspects are often the responsibility of the medical assistant. While service to the patient is the primary concern of the medical profession, a physician must charge and collect a fee for such services to continue providing medical care. The physician is one of many contributors in determining the amount of the fees. The medical assistant usually has the responsibility of informing the patient on financial matters, collecting the payment, and, in some cases, making arrangements for deferred payment.

How Fees Are Determined

Setting fees is no simple matter. The physician has three commodities to sell—time, judgment, and services. Yet the value of these commodities is never exactly the same to any two individuals. Medical care has little value except to the patient, and the value to the patient may not be consistent with the ability to pay. In every case, the physician must place an estimate on the value of the services. Such an arrangement is known as fee for service. This value may then be modified by other considerations.

THE EFFECTS OF MANAGED CARE

An important consideration in today's atmosphere of managed care is the preponderance of patients who are enrolled in health maintenance organization (HMO)-type insurance contracts. Under managed care the physician agrees to accept predetermined fees for specific procedures and services instead of the fee-for-service arrangement described in the preceding paragraph. The patient may be subject to a copay that is determined by the insurance contract and is collected at the time of service. When payment is made on a **capitation** basis the records of all patients in each plan are kept together and billed collectively.

- In 1993 only about half the Americans insured through employers were in managed care.
- In 1995 three of four insured U.S. workers had health coverage through managed care.
- In 1997 fewer than one fourth of U.S. workers had fee-for-service plans.

PREVAILING RATE IN THE COMMUNITY

One of the bases for determining charges on the fee-for-service basis is the economic level of the community. Different communities reflect different living scales, and this situation is reflected in medical fees as well. Consequently, the prevailing rate in the community—the average composite fee—must be taken into consideration by each individual physician. Strangely enough, fees that are too low drive patients away just as quickly as do fees that are too high because the average person tends to judge worth of a product on its cost—low cost translates as low value.

USUAL, CUSTOMARY, AND REASONABLE FEE

Most insurance plans base their payments on what has become known as a usual and customary fee for a given procedure. Some include the word "reasonable," that is, **usual, customary, and reasonable:**

- **usual**—The physician's usual fee for a given service is the fee that that an individual physician most frequently charges for the service.
- **customary**—The customary fee is a range of the usual fees charged for the same service by physicians with similar training and experience practicing in the same geographic and socioeconomic area. There is now a growing tendency for fees to be determined by national trends rather than by local custom.
- **reasonable**—The term *reasonable* usually applies to a service or procedure that is exceptionally difficult or complicated, requiring extraordinary time or effort on the part of the physician.

It should be noted that under Medicare Part B, *customary and prevailing* corresponds to *usual and customary* as defined here.

To illustrate, let us suppose that Dr. Wallace usually charges private patients $100 for a first office visit. The usual fees charged for a first visit by other physicians in the same community with similar training and experience range from $75 to $125. Dr. Wallace's fee of $100 is within the customary range and would therefore be paid by an insurance plan that pays on a usual and customary basis. If, on the other hand, the range of usual fees in the community is from $60 to $85, the insurance plan would allow only the maximum within the range, or $85, to Dr. Wallace.

FEE SETTING BY THIRD-PARTY PAYERS

The physician does not act alone in determining fees. A **third-party payer** may provide the physician with a predetermined **fee schedule** that it will approve for payment. Some require preapproval of the fee before service is rendered. A third-party payer may require precertification before it will pay for a specific service. Government programs such as Medicare and Medicaid (see Chapter 20) have strict guidelines regarding reimbursement for fees and the raising of fees.

PHYSICIAN'S FEE PROFILE

The **fiscal agent,** or **fiscal intermediary,** for government-sponsored insurance programs as well as some private plans keeps a continuous record of the usual charges submitted for specific services by each individual physician. By compiling and averaging these fees over a given period, usually a year, the physician's **fee profile** is established. This fee profile is then used in determining the amount of third-party liability for services under the program. One of the objections voiced by physicians is the lag between the time of a private fee increase and the time it is reflected in payments by an insurance carrier. It may be as long as 2 to 3 years.

INSURANCE ALLOWANCE

In some individual cases, the physician may not wish to charge the patient in addition to what will be allowed by the patient's insurance. This is often a professional courtesy for other health care professionals. The full fee should be quoted to the patient and charged to the account, with the understanding that after the insurance allowance has been received, the balance may be discounted. If a smaller fee is quoted and charged, several problems may arise:

- The lower fee will alter the physician's fee profile.
- If it should become necessary to bring suit for payment of the fee, only the reduced fee can be recovered.
- If the insurance allowance is paid on the basis of a certain percentage of the physician's fee and a lower fee is charged, the insurance allowance will be correspondingly lower. Also, if the physician does this with many patients, the insurance company may take the position that the reduced fee is the physician's usual fee and base its payments accordingly. It may even be considered fraudulent in some instances.

Explaining Costs to Patient

It is natural for the patient, particularly one new to the practice, to wonder, "How much is this going to cost?" However, some patients may be reluctant to voice this concern.

RESPONSIBILITY TO DISCUSS FEES

It is the responsibility of the physician or the medical assistant to raise the discussion of fees if the patient does not do so (see Procedure 16–1). Be prepared to discuss fees with any patient who is interested, but do not assume that you must do so with everyone. You might open the discussion of fees with something like this: "Mr. Willardson, do you have any questions about the costs of your operation? If you do, I'll be glad to review them." On the other hand, in this preliminary discussion of fees, the physician must not sidestep the issue by saying, "Don't worry about the bill, let's just get you well first." Avoid attempting to calm a worried patient about to undergo surgery by saying, "There's

PROCEDURE 16-1
Explaining Professional Fees

GOAL

To explain the physician's fees so that the patient understands his or her obligations and rights for privacy.

EQUIPMENT AND SUPPLIES

Patient's statement
Copy of physician's fee schedule
Quiet private area where the patient feels free to ask questions

PROCEDURAL STEPS

1 Determine that the patient has the correct bill.
PURPOSE: To make certain that the bill belongs to this patient and that the insurance numbers, the address, and the telephone number are correct.

2 Examine the bill for possible errors.
PURPOSE: To demonstrate that the patient's concerns are important and that you are willing to make any necessary adjustments.

3 Refer to the fee schedule for the services rendered.
PURPOSE: To explain how physicians determine their fees. If an error has occurred, correct it immediately with a sincere apology.

4 Explain itemized billing:
- Date of each service
- Type of service rendered
- Fee

PURPOSE: To make certain that the patient realizes the number and extent of services rendered.

5 Display professional attitude toward the patient.
PURPOSE: To reassure the patient that you have a thorough understanding of the fee schedule and show willingness to answer questions politely and completely.

6 Determine whether the patient has specific concerns that may hinder payment.
PURPOSE: To provide an opportunity for making special arrangements if needed.

7 Make appropriate arrangements for a discussion between the physician and patient if further explanation is necessary for resolution of the problem.

really nothing to it." The patient may later complain loudly about the bill because he or she misunderstood the complexity of the service.

Even in those cases in which the physician quotes a fee, the medical assistant often has the responsibility of explaining the physician's fees to the patient. The medical assistant must know how fees are determined and why charges vary, as well as have a thorough knowledge of the physician's practice and policies to handle perplexing situations involving fees.

As the medical assistant's understanding of the practice increases, he or she can build respect for the physician's services by educating patients that money spent for medical care is an excellent investment in the future. It is a rare patient who understands the intricate procedures involved in diagnosis and treatment.

ADVANCE DISCUSSION OF FEES

Advance fee discussions help the patient to plan ahead for medical expenditures. Most patients want to pay their financial obligations but rightly insist on an accurate estimate of those obligations before they contract for purchase of goods or services. When a physician frankly discusses fees in advance with patients, even to the point of describing how a fee is established, misconceptions and complaints about overcharging and fee discrepancies are usually eliminated.

Memory Jogger

List and explain six factors that may affect the determination of the fee for a given service.

EXPLAINING ADDITIONAL COSTS

Explanations of medical costs should extend beyond the physician's own charges. For example, if a patient is to undergo surgery, the physician should also explain the costs of the operation, the anesthesiologist's and radiologist's charges, the laboratory fees, and the approximate hospital bill. The importance of calling in another physician for consultation should be explained to patients when consultation becomes necessary. It should be made clear, in advance, that there will be a separate bill submitted by the consulting physician. Patients do not always understand that the consultation is for the benefit of the patient, not the physician.

ESTIMATE SLIPS

Some physicians give patients an estimate of medical expenses before hospitalization (Fig. 16–1). A few medical societies cooperatively develop such estimate sheets with local hospitals. Individual physicians occasionally work up their own estimate forms when a patient is embarking on long-term treatment. The physician should, however, emphasize that it is an estimate only and that the actual cost may vary somewhat.

Estimate slips should be prepared in duplicate so that the patient may have a copy and the original is retained in the patient's file. Duplicate estimate slips may help to

- Avoid your forgetting that a fee was quoted
- Eliminate the possibility of later misquoting the fee
- Simplify collection by preventing misunderstanding and confusion over charges

Adjusting or Canceling Fees

CARE FOR THOSE WHO CANNOT PAY

The medical profession has traditionally accepted the responsibility of providing medical care for individuals unable to pay for these services. In spite of the increased scope of government-sponsored care for the **medically indigent,** physicians still donate thousands of dollars' worth of such medical services each year.

In many instances, medical care of the indigent is available through social service agencies. The medical assistant should learn about any local organizations and agencies that can aid the patient in obtaining the necessary assistance. The physician can provide only medical services. Other agencies must provide hospitalization, for example, or arrange for

SURGICAL COST ESTIMATE

Name of Patient: ______________________ Date: ______________
Procedure: ____

Your surgery has been scheduled at ______________ Hospital on ______________.
You should report to the Admitting Office between the hours of ______ (AM) (PM) and ______ (AM) (PM).

Although medical and hospital expenses are seldom welcome, knowing in advance what expenses to expect and how to plan for them can lessen the burden. This estimate is prepared to assist you in budgeting your surgical costs.

PROFESSIONAL FEES

When you have major surgery, the surgical team includes the operating surgeon, the assistant surgeon, and the anesthetist. Each has an important part in your care, and each will render a separate statement for services. While each doctor will independently set his/her own fee, it is usually possible to estimate in advance an approximate range of fees. Assuming an uncomplicated course for your surgery, the charges are estimated as follows:

Operating Surgeon $ ________ to $ ________
Assistant Surgeon ________ to ________
Anesthetist ________ to ________

The assistant surgeon and the anesthetist usually base their fees on the operating time; consequently, if a surgical procedure turns out to be more complicated than was expected, their fees may be correspondingly increased.

The estimated duration of your hospital stay is ______ days at $ ______ per day for a (semi-private) (private) room. During your hospital stay there will be charges for laboratory tests, medications as required, and other services. It is impossible to estimate in advance what these charges will be; they will be itemized on your hospital bill. If you have health insurance, please take the appropriate forms and I.D. information with you on the day of your admittance.

PLEASE KEEP IN MIND THIS IS ONLY AN ESTIMATE

FIGURE 16–1 Form for surgical cost estimate.

paying the costs of special therapy, rehabilitation, or medications. Unfortunately, there is still another segment of the population that consists of uninsured employees who are not eligible for public assistance, are not covered under a group policy, and cannot afford the high premiums for private medical insurance. Special attention must be given to helping these persons arrange to pay their medical bills.

If a physician accepts a case for which a fee will not be paid, complete records must still be kept on the patient. The only deviation in procedure is that the financial record indicates no charge (n/c) in the debit column.

FEES IN HARDSHIP CASES

Sometimes a physician is faced with the problem of deciding whether to reduce or cancel a fee in a hardship case. Before adjusting or canceling a fee, the physician or the medical assistant should engage in a frank discussion of the patient's financial situation. Find out whether the patient is entitled to an insurance settlement of some kind. Circumstances may qualify the patient for local or state public assistance. If so, the assistant may direct the patient to the appropriate agency.

If the circumstances of hardship are known before the services are rendered, thorough discussion of what the fee will be and how it will be paid should take place at that time. In most cases, it is far better to adjust a fee before rather than after treatment. The physician may suggest that a medically indigent patient seek care at a county hospital with public assistance. A physician should be free to choose his or her form of charity and not feel obligated to substantially reduce or cancel a fee when the circumstances are known in advance.

After the physician and patient have agreed on a fee, special circumstances may arise that create a hardship. If the physician then agrees to reduce the fee, the patient should be told that the reduction will be effective only after the adjusted amount is paid in full. For instance, if a fee of $500 is reduced to $350, the full amount of the $500 charge should appear on the ledger and when $350 has been received the remainder can be written off as an adjustment.

PITFALLS OF FEE ADJUSTMENTS

Great care should be taken in reducing the fee for care of a patient who dies. The physician's sympathy is with the family in such instances, but the physician's generosity in reducing a fee could be misinterpreted and result in a suit for malpractice.

If the physician agrees to settle for a reduced fee in a situation in which the patient is disputing the fee, care should be taken to make certain the negotiations are *without prejudice.* By taking this precaution, the physician protects the right to collect the original sum should the patient refuse to pay the lowered fee. The offer of a discount, therefore, should be made in writing, with the insertion of the words "without prejudice" and a definite time limit for making payment stated. Prepare two copies of the agreement and have the signatures witnessed. Keep the original for the physician and give a copy to the patient.

A fee should never be reduced on the basis of a poor result or as a means of obtaining payment to avoid the use of a collection agency. A reduction for these reasons degrades the physician and the practice of medicine.

PROFESSIONAL COURTESY

Traditionally, physicians do not charge professional colleagues or their immediate dependents for medical care. Although the concept of **professional courtesy** is often attributed to Hippocrates, the foundations of professional courtesy today are derived from Thomas Percival's Code of 1803.

In some cases, the giving of professional courtesy represents the loss of a large amount of potential income. If there is a substantial outlay in the cost of materials, the professional colleague will probably wish to reimburse the physician for the materials used. Most physicians today subscribe to a health insurance plan. If the care they receive is covered by insurance, it is entirely ethical for the attending physician to accept the insurance benefits in payment for services.

If the services are frequent enough to involve a significant portion of the physician's professional time, or extend over a long period of time, the physician may wish to charge on an adjusted basis.

When professional courtesy has been offered and the recipient still insists on paying, the physician need not hesitate on ethical grounds to accept a fee for service.

Professional courtesy is often extended beyond fellow physicians and their dependents. Most physicians treat their own medical assistants without charge and grant discounts to nurses and medical assistants not in their direct employ. Professional courtesy is sometimes extended to others in the health care field, for instance pharmacists and dentists. There is a growing sentiment that professional courtesy has outlived its usefulness and should be abandoned.

Charges to Avoid

TELEPHONE CALLS

It is generally considered inadvisable to charge for telephone calls. Some physicians, especially pediatricians, find they must give considerable advice over the telephone. However, many of these calls are fairly routine to the office—although not to the worried mother or patient—and an able medical assistant can be trained to answer many of the questions or a special time can be set aside for telephone calls.

LATE PAYMENTS

Levying late charges on fees for professional services not paid within a prescribed time is usually not in the best interest of the public or the profession. However, the physician who has experienced problems with delinquent accounts may properly choose to request that payment be made at the time of treatment or add interest or other reasonable charges to delinquent accounts. The physician must comply with state and federal regulations applicable to the imposition of such charges (see Truth in Lending Act).

MISSED APPOINTMENTS

Most physicians believe that charging for a missed appointment or for one not canceled 24 hours in advance, although not unethical if the patient is fully advised, is nevertheless not in the best interest of their patients or their practices.

FIRST INSURANCE FORM

If the patient has multiple insurance forms to be completed, the physician is justified in making a charge but should be willing to complete the first standard form without charge. Exceptions are Medicare and Medicaid, which prohibit charging for completing forms.

Credit Arrangements

EXTENDING CREDIT

Whenever a service is rendered before payment is received, an extension of credit has been made. If payment is collected on completion of the service, no problem exists. But if payment is deferred, credit arrangements are best made during the patient's initial visit (see Procedure 16–2). Successful collection of an account may depend on the skill and tact with which the medical assistant conducts the first interview.

Under the Federal Equal Credit Opportunity Act of 1975, once you agree to extend credit to one patient, you must offer the same arrangement to any other patient who requests it. You can refuse to do so only on the basis of ability or inability to pay. One way to avoid involvement with the credit laws is to accept bank credit cards. The Equal Credit Opportunity Act bars discrimination in all areas of credit, with the purpose of ensuring that credit is made available fairly and impartially, and specifies prohibited bases under the law. The law prohibits discrimination against any applicant for credit because (1) of race, color, religion, national origin, sex, marital status, or age; (2) the applicant receives income from any public assistance program, and (3) he or she has exercised rights under consumer credit laws.

Many medical assistants inform a patient who is telephoning for a first appointment that new patients are expected to pay cash for their first visit, at which time credit arrangements can be established if further care is needed. For example:

> Mr. Barrington, your appointment is scheduled for 9:30 AM, Tuesday, September 25, with Dr. Newhouse. The usual charge for a first office visit is about XX dollars, and we ask that payment for a first visit be made at the time of service. If you wish to establish credit arrangements in case further care is needed, please plan to be here 15 minutes early so that the necessary papers can be completed.

This approach informs the patient in advance that he or she will be expected to complete a credit application.

Information from the Patient

Maintaining records is essential to the follow-up of collections. It is extremely important that the medical assistant get adequate information about the patient's ability to pay—on the first visit, if possible. It is neither unprofessional nor time consuming to get full credit information from patients. The public is conditioned to supplying such information and respects a business-like approach if it is done tactfully and without apology. Although a patient needing medical care is rarely turned away because of a credit risk, the information provided on the initial visit may alert the medical assistant to be cautious about allowing an account to fall in arrears.

The medical assistant should check the completed form carefully, to make certain that nothing was overlooked. The new patient will view these questions as reasonable, but the established patient may resent such an inquiry. Consequently, it is important that the form be completed on the first visit.

Although the registration form the patient completes in the physician's office is usually not as detailed as an application for credit in, for example, a department store, it must establish an information base, should future collection steps become necessary.

Many printed forms are available, but some physicians design their own to include specific information desired in their practices. Whatever form is used, it should include certain basic information and

PROCEDURE 16-2
Making Credit Arrangements with a Patient

GOAL
To assist the patient in paying for services by making mutually beneficial credit arrangements according to established office policy.

EQUIPMENT AND SUPPLIES
Patient's ledger
Calendar
Truth in Lending form
Assignment of Benefits form
Patient's insurance form
Typewriter
Private area for interview

PROCEDURAL STEPS
1 Answer thoroughly and kindly all questions about credit.
2 Inform the patient of office policy regarding credit:
- Payment at the time of first visit
- Payment by bank card
- Credit application

PURPOSE: To ensure complete understanding of mutual responsibilities.

3 Have the patient complete the credit application.
PURPOSE: To comply with office practices on the extension of credit.

4 Check the completed credit application.
PURPOSE: To confirm that all necessary information is included.

5 Discuss with the patient the possible arrangements and ask the patient to decide which of those arrangements is most suitable.
PURPOSE: Better compliance can be expected when the patient makes the choice.

6 Prepare the Truth in Lending form and have the patient sign it if the agreement requires more than four installments.
PURPOSE: To comply with Regulation Z.

7 Have the patient execute an assignment of insurance benefits.
PURPOSE: To comply with credit policy.

8 Make a copy of the patient's insurance ID and have the patient sign a consent for release of the information to insurance company.
PURPOSE: Consent for the release of information is necessary on most insurance forms before a claim can be processed

9 Keep credit information confidential.

not ask for information that is disallowed under the 1977 Federal Equal Credit Opportunity Act (ECOA). For instance, under the ECOA "marital status" can be requested only as *married, unmarried,* or *separated.* Terms such as *divorced, single,* or *widow/er* are illegal. *Age* is also forbidden, but *date of birth* is acceptable.

INFORMATION FROM PATIENT

Patient's full name. The patient's first, middle, and last names, correctly spelled, should be at the top of the form.

Patient's birth date. With this information, the patient's age can be calculated at any time.

Telephone number

Social Security number

Responsible person's full name. Relationship to the patient, his or her address, telephone number, Social Security number, and driver's license number should be included.

Responsible person's employer. Name, address, and telephone number of the employer and the responsible person's occupation or department

Insurance information
Spouse of responsible person. Same information as for responsible person. (Community property laws in some states make each and both responsible.)
Nearest relative. Name, relationship to patient, address, and telephone number
Referral. Name of physician or other person who referred the patient (see Fig. 8–3)

An individualized form can ask for further specific information appropriate for a particular practice. When a patient applies for credit you may *not* ask for the patient's race, color, religion, or national origin. It is also illegal to gather information on the patient's birth control practices or plans to have children. Those questions may be asked when it is part of a medical history but not when it is related to granting credit.

Third-Party Liability

If financial responsibility is attributed to an individual other than the patient, spouse, or parent, be sure to obtain full name, address, employment data, and other credit information about that person. Also, contact the named individual for verification of the obligation. If a third-party payer's agreement to pay is contingent on the patient's failure to pay, such an agreement must be in writing to be enforceable and must be made before treatment. Any agreement made after completion of treatment could be considered as a moral obligation only. The guarantee of a person to pay the account of another may be very simple. It may be typewritten or handwritten, stating:

I, the undersigned, do promise to pay for the medical services rendered by Theodore Wilson, MD, to my nephew, Robert L. Smith.
Date:
Signed: ______________________________

or

I, the undersigned, promise to pay the medical bill of Robert L. Smith, if his mother, Mrs. Lydia Smith, does not pay by the 15th of July, 19xx.
Date:
Signed: ______________________________

Accounts for services rendered to a spouse or child should always carry full data about the party responsible, which in most cases is the other spouse or the parent. Generally, a responsible spouse or parent pays the account without any follow-up collection procedures. In the case of a minor, it is generally held that the parent accompanying the child to the medical facility is responsible for paying. Any agreement between divorced or separated parents is solely between them and does not affect the obligation to the physician.

If you foresee legal difficulties in collecting an account in which divorce, legal guardianship, or the involvement of an emancipated minor complicates the matter, it is best to contact the physician's attorney for advice. The laws governing such matters vary according to each state. One regulation is that you must always have the signature of the third party responsible for the debt if he or she is not otherwise obligated by law. An oral agreement in this case is not binding.

Memory Jogger

What is the purpose of the Equal Credit Opportunity Act of 1977? What are its restrictions?

Health Insurance Information

The initial interview is the best time to get full information on the patient's insurance coverage. The patient registration form usually provides a place for the name of the insurance company. Ask to see the patient's identification card and make a photocopy for your records. The card usually shows the name of the subscriber and the group and member number and often includes a service code indicating the patient's coverage. Also obtain information on any supplementary coverage—for instance, a plan in which the spouse is the subscriber and the patient is covered as a dependent. There may also be major medical or supplementary benefits to the patient's policy. Verify this information on each visit.

Assignment of Benefits

Many physicians ask the patient to execute an **assignment of benefits** at this time. The assignment, authorizing the insurance company to pay benefits directly to the physician, may be stamped on the insurance form or may be subsequently attached to a completed insurance form.

Consent for Release of Information

Use a standard claim form or the form the patient has brought to the office. Have the patient sign the consent for release of the information that is on the claim form. In this way, the insurance billing can be processed without delay as services are performed. Some states require a special form for release of information separate and apart from the insurance claim form itself. The medical assistant should check local regulations.

INSTALLMENT BUYING OF MEDICAL SERVICES

Because installment buying is so much a part of our economic system today, the physician's office must be prepared to help patients budget for their medical care. Patients expect to use their credit resources and appreciate business-like assistance in establishing a payment plan. The medical profession has too long suffered a poor collection record because of its fear of appearing too commercial. The physician should be ready to arrange credit when medical bills will be high or when a patient for some reason is unable to pay at the time of service. In general, fees for routine office calls and small medical bills should be kept on a pay-as-you-go basis.

Credit Cards

The acceptance of credit cards, sometimes called bank cards, has become commonplace in medical practice. Patients appreciate the convenience, and paying by credit card may help to improve collections. The signed credit card voucher is deposited to the physician's bank account. The card company deducts a percentage (from 1% to 5% depending on volume) for the collection service. The patient may pay the full amount when billed by the card company or may pay a portion and be charged interest on the balance.

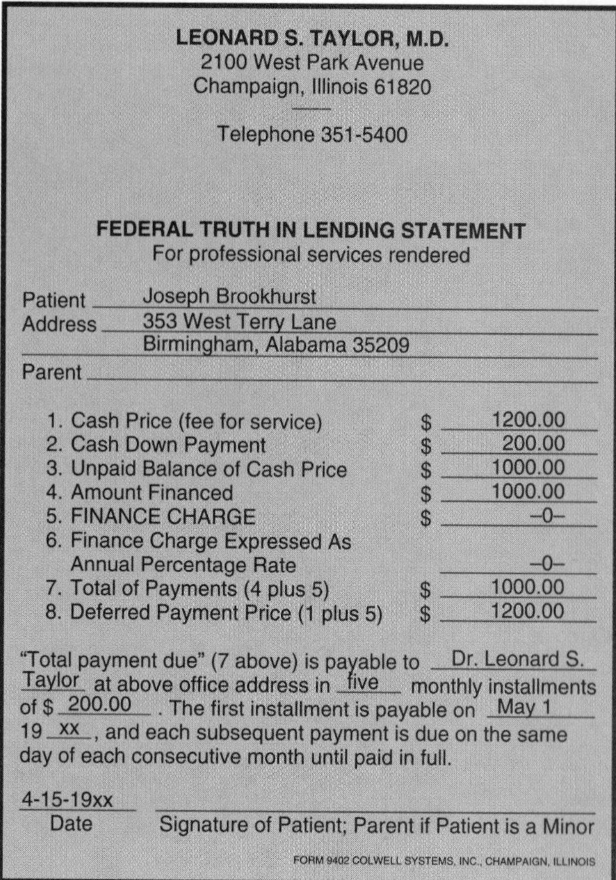
LEONARD S. TAYLOR, M.D.
2100 West Park Avenue
Champaign, Illinois 61820

Telephone 351-5400

FEDERAL TRUTH IN LENDING STATEMENT
For professional services rendered

Patient Joseph Brookhurst
Address 353 West Terry Lane
Birmingham, Alabama 35209
Parent

1. Cash Price (fee for service)	$	1200.00
2. Cash Down Payment	$	200.00
3. Unpaid Balance of Cash Price	$	1000.00
4. Amount Financed	$	1000.00
5. FINANCE CHARGE	$	-0-
6. Finance Charge Expressed As Annual Percentage Rate		-0-
7. Total of Payments (4 plus 5)	$	1000.00
8. Deferred Payment Price (1 plus 5)	$	1200.00

"Total payment due" (7 above) is payable to Dr. Leonard S. Taylor at above office address in five monthly installments of $ 200.00 . The first installment is payable on May 1 19 xx , and each subsequent payment is due on the same day of each consecutive month until paid in full.

4-15-19xx
Date

Signature of Patient; Parent if Patient is a Minor

FORM 9402 COLWELL SYSTEMS, INC., CHAMPAIGN, ILLINOIS

FIGURE 16–2 Disclosure statement. (Courtesy of Colwell Systems, Inc., Champaign, IL.)

Special Budget Plans

If a patient appears concerned about the ability to meet his financial obligations, the physician or the medical assistant can suggest in a tactful way:

> Mr. Elwood, if you think you will have difficulty paying for your treatments at one time, we can work out some special arrangement.

This allows the patient to ask what sort of plan you have in mind, and the discussion progresses very easily into various payment plans. Generally, it is better to let the patient decide what arrangements are best rather than to suggest a plan. However, if the patient has no suggestion, the medical assistant can say:

> Mr. Elwood, would you be able to pay $50 each month until the account is paid in full?
>
> or
>
> Usually an account of this size can be settled in 3 to 4 months. Would you be able to pay $100 now, then $50 a month until the account is paid in full?

When the amount of each installment has been agreed on, it is then wise to establish definite dates on which the payments will be expected. Strive for an arrangement that will result in the balance being paid within a reasonable time, generally within 6 months.

Truth in Lending Act

Regulation Z of the Truth in Lending Act, which is enforced by the Federal Trade Commission, requires that when there is a bilateral agreement between physician and patient to accept payment in more than four installments, the physician is required to provide disclosure of information regarding finance charges. Even if there are no finance charges involved, the form must be completed stating this fact. A copy of the form is retained by the physician, and the original is given to the patient. Specific wording is required in the disclosure. The form in Figure 16–2 meets the requirements. Have the patient sign the agreement in your presence, because you must have proof of signing. The disclosure statement must be kept on file for 2 years. Although the disclosure statement is designed as protection for the debtor, it can be a good collection tool for the creditor.

It is recognized that physicians generally permit their patients to pay in installments, and as long as there is no specific agreement on the part of the physician for payment to be made in more than four installments, and no finance charge is made, the account is not subject to the regulation. If the patient chooses to pay in installments instead of the full amount, this is considered a unilateral action. The physician, in accepting such payments, probably would not be subject to the provisions of the regulation. The physician's office, however, must be certain to bill for the full balance each time. If the statement is for only a partial payment, it then becomes a bilateral agreement and as such is subject to Regulation Z.

Helping patients budget their medical expenses is a rather new aspect of the business side of medical practice. However, it is a real service to patients and demonstrates that the physician and the office staff are sincerely anxious to help patients pay their own way. It may also prevent many collection problems.

Memory Jogger

What is the purpose of Regulation Z of the Truth in Lending Act and when is it applied?

CONFIDENTIALITY

Obtaining Credit Information

Credit information is confidential. It should be guarded as carefully as a confidential medical history and should be disclosed to no one. When you ask for credit information from patients in the office, do so in a private area where others cannot overhear the conversation. A desk or table away from the reception area where a patient can sit in total privacy and complete a credit application is a great asset. Credit information is personal—it should be kept that way.

Credit Bureaus

Some physicians join a credit bureau, particularly in large cities where it is more difficult to gauge informally the patients' ability to pay. Credit bureaus gather credit information from many sources, pool it, and make it available to dues-paying bureau members. If you receive a request for credit information about one of your patients, it is permissible to furnish it because the debtor, by giving the physician's name as a reference, has given implied consent; otherwise, the credit bureau would not have contacted you. According to the Fair Credit Practices Act Amendments of 1975, you can reply by giving ledger information only, including

- When the account was opened
- How much the patient now owes
- The highest amount of the account at any time

You should avoid any reference to

- Character
- Paying habits
- Credit rating

Medical-Dental-Hospital Bureaus

The Medical-Dental-Hospital Bureaus of America (MDHBA), with headquarters in Chicago, is a national organization of agencies serving physicians, dentists, and hospitals. It seeks to maintain the highest standards among its members and is committed to following the collection methods most acceptable to physicians. Members who use their collection services have access to credit information on accounts assigned by other clients. Member bureaus of the MDHBA frequently assist the medical assistant by sponsoring collection seminars as well as by providing speakers for medical assistant society meetings.

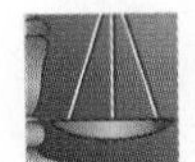

LEGAL AND ETHICAL ISSUES

Government plans such as Medicare and Medicaid have strict guidelines regarding setting fees and reimbursement.

If a physician allows or suggests to a patient that the insurance payment will be considered payment in full, discounting the deductible, the physician may be judged guilty of fraud.

The tradition of not charging professional colleagues (professional courtesy) is diminishing because most physicians today carry health insurance, and it is entirely ethical for the attending physician to accept the insurance in payment of services.

The Federal Equal Credit Opportunity Act of 1977 bars discrimination in all areas of credit. If the physician agrees to extend credit to one patient, then the same arrangement must be offered to any other patient who requests it.

If both the physician and the patient agree that payment for services may be made in more than four installments, the physician must complete a Federal Truth in Lending Statement and have it signed by the patient.

CRITICAL THINKING

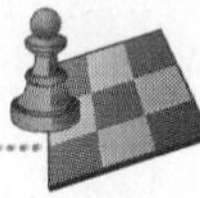

1 Explain the meaning of "bilateral agreement."

2 When does the matter of third-party liability become an issue?

3 How would the medical assistant know when it is ethical to release credit information about a patient? What information can be released?

HOW DID I DO? Answers to Memory Joggers

a. Managed care participation
b. Prevailing rate in the community

c. Usual, customary, and reasonable fee
d. Third-party fee schedule
e. Physician's fee profile
f. Insurance allowance

2 The purpose of the Equal Credit Opportunity Act is to bar discrimination in all areas of credit, ensuring that credit is available fairly and impartially. It prohibits discrimination because of race, color, religion, national origin, sex, marital status, or age or because applicant receives public assistance or has exercised rights under consumer credit laws.

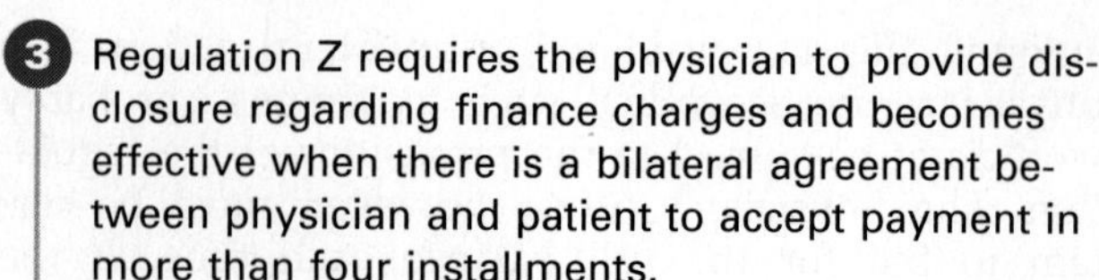
3 Regulation Z requires the physician to provide disclosure regarding finance charges and becomes effective when there is a bilateral agreement between physician and patient to accept payment in more than four installments.

REFERENCES

Federal Reserve Board: Equal Credit Opportunity Act, October 28, 1977.
Truth in Lending Act, 1968.

Managing Practice Finances

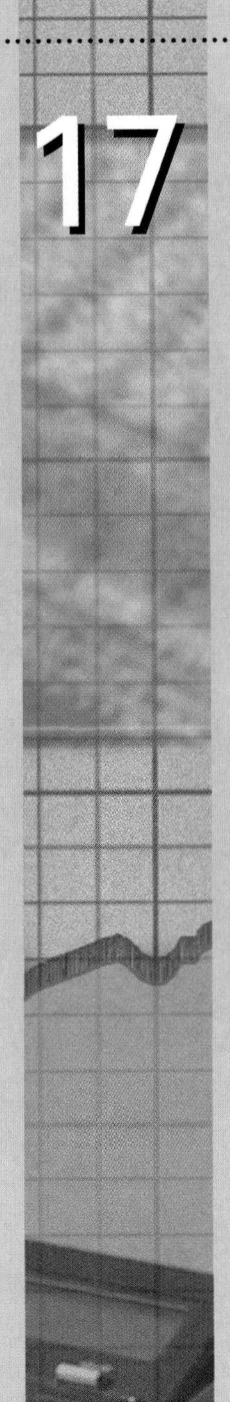

OUTLINE

LEARNING OBJECTIVES

Cognitive: On successful completion of this chapter you should be able to:

1. Define and spell the terms listed in the Vocabulary.
2. Name the two bases of accounting and explain their differences.
3. State the four kinds of information that the financial records of any business should show at all times.
4. Differentiate between a debit balance and a credit balance.
5. Describe and demonstrate the entry for a credit balance.
6. List six kinds of bookkeeping records.
7. Compare the three most common systems used in the professional office.
8. State the basic accounting equation.
9. Discuss the importance of a trial balance.
10. Describe how to maintain a petty cash fund.
11. List and state the purpose of the five common periodic accounting reports.

Performance: On successful completion of this chapter you should be able to:

1 Prepare a ledger account for a new patient.
2 Prepare a patient charge slip.
3 Journalize service charges and payments using a single-entry system.
4 Post the entries from the daily journal to patient ledger cards.
5 Prepare a daily proof of posting.
6 Prepare a daily proof of cash control.
7 Prepare a monthly trial balance.
8 Establish and maintain a petty cash fund.
9 Post service charges and payments using a pegboard.

VOCABULARY

account A single financial record.

account balance The debit or credit balance remaining in the account

accounting equation Assets = Liabilities + Proprietorship (Capital)

accounts payable Debts incurred and not yet paid

accounts receivable Amounts owed to the physician

accounts receivable control A summary of unpaid accounts

accounts receivable ledger The combined record of all patient accounts

accounts receivable trial balance A method of determining that the journal and the ledger are in balance

accrual basis of accounting Income is recorded when earned, and expenses are recorded when incurred

adjustment column An account column, sometimes included to the left of the balance column, that is used for entering discounts

balance The difference between the debit and credit totals

balance column The account column on the far right that is used for recording the difference between the debit and credit columns

balance sheet A financial statement for a specific date that shows the total assets, liabilities, and capital of the business

bookkeeping The recording part of the accounting process

cash basis of accounting Income is recorded when received, and expenses are recorded when paid

cash flow statement A financial summary for a specific period that shows the beginning balance on hand, the receipts and disbursements during the period, and the balance on hand at the end of the period

cash payment journal A record of all cash paid out

credit The record of a payment received

credit balance The amount of advance payment or overpayment on an account (amount of receipts exceeding amount chargeed)

credit column The account column to the right of the debit column that is used for entering funds received

daily journal The book in which all transactions are first recorded; the book of original entry, or general journal

debit The record of a charge or debt incurred

debit column The account column on the left that is used for entering charges

disbursements Money paid out

disbursements journal A summary of amounts paid out

discounts Subtractions from the patient's balance

general journal The book of original entry in bookkeeping

in balance Total ending balances of patient ledgers equal total of accounts receivable control

invoice A paper describing a purchase and the amount due
packing slip An itemized list of objects in a package
payables Amounts owed to others
petty cash fund A fund maintained to pay small unpredictable cash expenditures
posting The act of transferring information from one record to another
receipts Money received
receivables Amounts owing from others
statement A request for payment
statement of income and expense A summary of all income and expenses for a given period
superbill A combination charge slip, statement, and insurance reporting form
transaction The occurrence of a financial event or condition that must be recorded
trial balance A method of checking the accuracy of accounts

A physician's business records are the key to good management practice. The medical assistant who can keep accurate financial records and who will conduct the nonclinical side of the practice in a business-like fashion is genuinely needed and appreciated.

Financial records that are complete, correct, and current are essential for

- Prompt billing and collection procedures
- Professional financial planning
- Accurate reporting of income to federal and state agencies

What Is Accounting?

Accounting is a system of recording, classifying, and summarizing financial transactions.

Bookkeeping is mainly the recording part of the accounting process. The bookkeeping must be done daily and is the responsibility of the administrative medical assistant in a small practice. In a larger practice, the office manager or financial manager assumes this responsibility.

ACCOUNT BASES

There are two general bases for accounting: the cash basis and the accrual basis (Table 17–1). Most physicians use the **cash basis of accounting.** Expressed simply, this means that (1) charges for services are entered as income when payment is received and (2) expenses are recorded when they are paid. Merchants, on the other hand, generally use an **accrual basis of accounting.** Income is considered earned when services have been performed or goods have been sold, even though payment may not have been received. Expenses are recognized and recorded when incurred, even though they have not been paid.

TABLE 17–1 Accounting Bases

	Cash Basis	Accrual Basis
Income is recorded	When received	When service is performed or goods are sold
Expense is recorded	When paid	When incurred (even if not paid)

FINANCIAL SUMMARIES

The financial records of any business should at all times show

- How much was earned in a given period
- How much was collected
- How much is owed
- The distribution of expenses incurred

From the daily entries, the accountant can prepare monthly and annual summaries that provide a basis for comparing any given period with another similar period.

Periodic analyses of the financial records can result in improved business practices, better management of time, curtailment or elimination of unprofitable services, and better budgeting of expenses. With the appropriate software these analyses can be accomplished using the computer.

Bookkeeping

A willingness to pay attention to detail, good organizational skills, and the ability to concentrate and maintain consistency in working patterns and procedures are all necessary qualifications for the person who has the responsibility of keeping financial records.

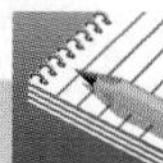

SKILLS AND RESPONSIBILITIES

BOOKKEEPING PROCEDURES

- Use good penmanship.
- Use the same pen style and ink consistently.
- Keep columns of figures straight.
- Write well-formed figures (a careless 9 may look like a 7; an open 0 may resemble a 6).
- Carry decimal points correctly.
- Do not erase, write over, or blot out figures. If an error is made, a straight line should be drawn through the incorrect figure and the correct figure written above it.

Bookkeeping procedures are not difficult or complicated, but they do require concentration to avoid errors. There is no such thing as *almost* correct financial records. The books either balance, or they do not balance. The bookkeeping is either right or wrong. This is not the place to be creative or take shortcuts.

The medical assistant should set aside a certain time each day for bookkeeping tasks, if possible. Do not attempt to work on financial records when you are busy attending patients or when there are other distractions.

CARDINAL RULES OF BOOKKEEPING

- Enter all charges and receipts immediately in the daily record or journal.
- Write a receipt in duplicate for any currency received. Writing receipts for checks is optional, but a consistent pattern should be followed.
- Post all charges and receipts to the patient ledger daily.
- Endorse checks for deposit as soon as received.
- Deposit all receipts in the bank.
- Verify that the total of the deposit plus the amount on hand equals the total to be accounted for in the daily journal.
- Use a petty cash fund to pay for small unpredictable expenses. Pay all other expenses by check (a cancelled check is the best proof of payment).
- Pay all bills before their due dates, after checking them for accuracy. Place date of payment and number of check on paid bills.

Memory Jogger

1 *What four items of information must be available from the financial records of a business at all times?*

Terminology of Accounts

To understand and perform bookkeeping procedures, it is first necessary to learn some of the terminology of accounts.

A business **transaction** is the occurrence of an event or of a condition that must be recorded.

EXAMPLES OF BUSINESS TRANSACTIONS

- A service is performed for which a charge is made.
- A debtor makes a payment on account.
- A piece of equipment is purchased.
- The monthly rent is paid.

Each example is a transaction that must be recorded within the accounting system. You will very likely encounter various other business transactions as you become more familiar with the individual needs of your employer's practice.

The **daily journal** is called the book of original entry because this is where all transactions are first recorded (Fig. 17–1).

A patient's financial record is called an **account**. All of the patients' accounts together constitute the **accounts receivable ledger.**

Account cards vary in design, but all will have at least three columns for entering figures. In the manual system these are

- **Debit** (abbreviation: Dr) **column** on the left is used for entering charges and is sometimes called the charge column
- **Credit** (abbreviation: Cr) **column** to the right, sometimes headed Paid, is used for entering payments received
- **Balance column** on the far right is used for recording the difference between the debit and credit columns

An **adjustment column** is available in some systems and is used for entering professional discounts, write-offs, disallowances by insurance companies, and any other adjustments (Fig 17–2).

In a computer system, when you call up a patient by name or ID you will get the patient's balance. This is the individual patient's ledger.

Posting means the transfer of information from one record to another. Transactions are posted from the journal to the ledger (this is accomplished in one writing on the pegboard system).

The **account balance** is normally a debit balance (charges exceed payments). A **debit** balance is entered by simply writing the correct figure in the balance column.

A **credit balance** exists when payments exceed charges; for example, when a patient pays in advance. This is common in obstetric practices. To

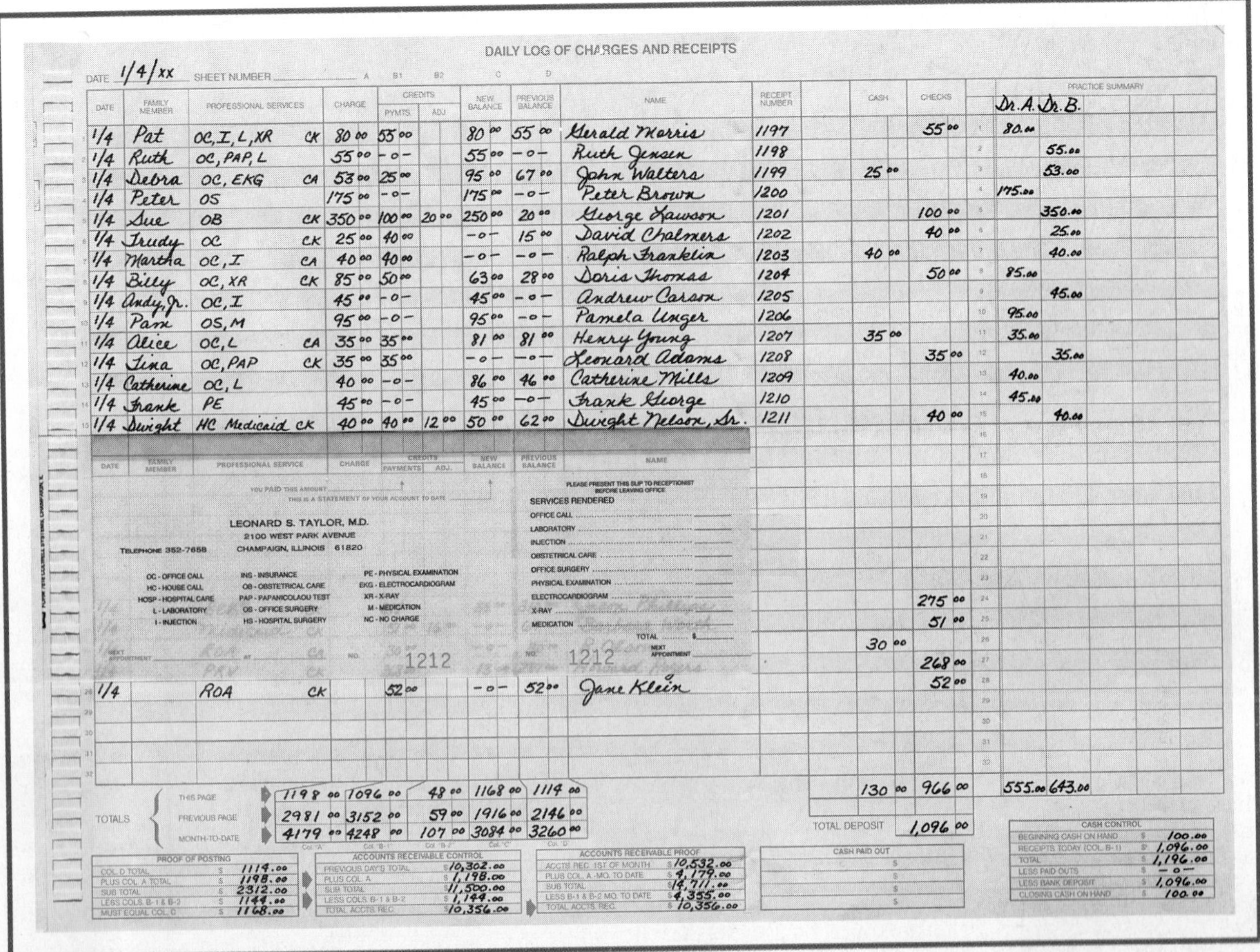

DAILY LOG OF CHARGES AND RECEIPTS

DATE 1/4/xx SHEET NUMBER

	DATE	FAMILY MEMBER	PROFESSIONAL SERVICES		CHARGE	CREDITS PYMTS.	CREDITS ADJ.	NEW BALANCE	PREVIOUS BALANCE	NAME	RECEIPT NUMBER	CASH	CHECKS		PRACTICE SUMMARY Dr. A.	Dr. B.
1	1/4	Pat	OC, I, L, XR	CK	80.00	55.00		80.00	55.00	Gerald Morris	1197		55.00	1	80.00	
2	1/4	Ruth	OC, PAP, L		55.00	-0-		55.00	-0-	Ruth Jensen	1198			2		55.00
3	1/4	Debra	OC, EKG	CA	53.00	25.00		95.00	67.00	John Walters	1199	25.00		3		53.00
4	1/4	Peter	OS		175.00	-0-		175.00	-0-	Peter Brown	1200			4	175.00	
5	1/4	Sue	OB	CK	350.00	100.00	20.00	250.00	20.00	George Lawson	1201		100.00	5		350.00
6	1/4	Trudy	OC	CK	25.00	40.00		-0-	15.00	David Chalmers	1202		40.00	6		25.00
7	1/4	Martha	OC, I	CA	40.00	40.00		-0-	-0-	Ralph Franklin	1203	40.00		7		40.00
8	1/4	Billy	OC, XR	CK	85.00	50.00		63.00	28.00	Doris Thomas	1204		50.00	8	85.00	
9	1/4	Andy, Jr.	OC, I		45.00	-0-		45.00	-0-	Andrew Carson	1205			9		45.00
10	1/4	Pam	OS, M		95.00	-0-		95.00	-0-	Pamela Unger	1206			10	95.00	
11	1/4	Alice	OC, L	CA	35.00	35.00		81.00	81.00	Henry Young	1207	35.00		11	35.00	
12	1/4	Tina	OC, PAP	CK	35.00	35.00		-0-	-0-	Leonard Adams	1208		35.00	12		35.00
13	1/4	Catherine	OC, L		40.00	-0-		86.00	46.00	Catherine Mills	1209			13	40.00	
14	1/4	Frank	PE		45.00	-0-		45.00	-0-	Frank George	1210			14	45.00	
15	1/4	Dwight	HC Medicaid	CK	40.00	40.00	12.00	50.00	62.00	Dwight Nelson, Sr.	1211		40.00	15		40.00
24													275.00	24		
25													51.00	25		
26												30.00		26		
27													268.00	27		
28	1/4		ROA	CK		52.00		-0-	52.00	Jane Klein			52.00	28		

DATE | FAMILY MEMBER | PROFESSIONAL SERVICE | CHARGE | CREDITS PAYMENTS ADJ. | NEW BALANCE | PREVIOUS BALANCE | NAME

YOU PAID THIS AMOUNT — THIS IS A STATEMENT OF YOUR ACCOUNT TO DATE

LEONARD S. TAYLOR, M.D.
2100 WEST PARK AVENUE
CHAMPAIGN, ILLINOIS 61820
TELEPHONE 352-7658

OC - OFFICE CALL · INS - INSURANCE · PE - PHYSICAL EXAMINATION
HC - HOUSE CALL · OB - OBSTETRICAL CARE · EKG - ELECTROCARDIOGRAM
HOSP - HOSPITAL CARE · PAP - PAPANICOLAOU TEST · XR - X-RAY
L - LABORATORY · OS - OFFICE SURGERY · M - MEDICATION
I - INJECTION · HS - HOSPITAL SURGERY · NC - NO CHARGE

NEXT APPOINTMENT ______ AT ______ NO. 1212

PLEASE PRESENT THIS SLIP TO RECEPTIONIST BEFORE LEAVING OFFICE
SERVICES RENDERED: OFFICE CALL · LABORATORY · INJECTION · OBSTETRICAL CARE · OFFICE SURGERY · PHYSICAL EXAMINATION · ELECTROCARDIOGRAM · X-RAY · MEDICATION · TOTAL $ · NEXT APPOINTMENT · NO. 1212

TOTALS	Col. "A"	Col. "B-1"	Col. "B-2"	Col. "C"	Col. "D"
THIS PAGE	1198.00	1096.00	48.00	1168.00	1114.00
PREVIOUS PAGE	2981.00	3152.00	59.00	1916.00	2146.00
MONTH-TO-DATE	4179.00	4248.00	107.00	3084.00	3260.00

Cash 130.00 · Checks 966.00 · Practice summary 555.00, 643.00

TOTAL DEPOSIT 1,096.00

PROOF OF POSTING	
COL. D TOTAL	$ 1114.00
PLUS COL. A TOTAL	$ 1198.00
SUB TOTAL	$ 2312.00
LESS COLS. B-1 & B-2	$ 1144.00
MUST EQUAL COL. C	$ 1168.00

ACCOUNTS RECEIVABLE CONTROL	
PREVIOUS DAY'S TOTAL	$ 10,302.00
PLUS COL. A	$ 1,198.00
SUB TOTAL	$ 11,500.00
LESS COLS. B-1 & B-2	$ 1,144.00
TOTAL ACCTS. REC.	$ 10,356.00

ACCOUNTS RECEIVABLE PROOF	
ACCTS. REC. 1ST OF MONTH	$ 10,532.00
PLUS COL. A - MO. TO DATE	$ 4,179.00
SUB TOTAL	$ 14,711.00
LESS B-1 & B-2 MO. TO DATE	$ 4,355.00
TOTAL ACCTS. REC.	$ 10,356.00

CASH PAID OUT	
	$
	$
	$
	$

CASH CONTROL	
BEGINNING CASH ON HAND	$ 100.00
RECEIPTS TODAY (COL. B-1)	$ 1,096.00
TOTAL	$ 1,196.00
LESS PAID OUTS	$ -0-
LESS BANK DEPOSIT	$ 1,096.00
CLOSING CASH ON HAND	$ 100.00

FIGURE 17–1 Sample day sheet for pegboard bookkeeping system, with deposit list of checks and optional business analysis summaries. (Courtesy of Colwell Systems, Inc., Champaign, IL.)

show a credit balance, record the figures in one of the following two ways:

- Write the credit balance on the card in regular ink and enclose the figure in parentheses or circle it.
- Write the credit balance in red ink (this cannot be done on the pegboard system).

Discounts are also credit entries and are entered in the adjustment column, or, if there is no adjustment column, the discount is entered in the debit column in red ink or enclosed in parentheses. By making the entry this way, it is recognized as a subtraction from the charges. When totaling columns, any figure in red or in parentheses is always *subtracted.*

Receipts are cash and checks taken in payment for professional services. **Receivables** are charges for which payment has not been received—amounts that are owing. **Disbursements** are cash amounts paid out. **Payables** are amounts owed to others but not yet paid.

Kinds of Financial Records

DAILY JOURNAL

The daily journal day sheet is the chronologic record of the practice—the financial diary. All information regarding services rendered, charges, and receipts is first recorded in the general journal. It is important that every transaction be recorded.

In addition to professional services rendered in and out of the office, there may be income from other sources, such as rentals, royalties, interest, and so forth. Usually a special place is provided in the journal for such income. Any income that is not practice related should be recorded separately from patient receipts.

LEDGER

The accounts receivable ledger comprises all the individual patients' financial accounts on which there is a balance.

BILLING NAME	NAMES OF OTHER FAMILY MEMBERS
PATIENT'S NAME	
RES. PHONE / BUS. PHONE	
OCCUPATION	RELATIVE OR FRIEND
EMPLOYED BY	REFERRED BY
INS. INFORMATION	SOC. SEC. NUMBER
FORM NO. MDP. 8550	1976 BIBBERO SYSTEMS, INC. SAN FRANCISCO

GEORGE D. GREEN, M.D.
JOHN F. WHITE, M.D.
Family Practice
100 MAIN STREET, SUITE 14
ANYTOWN, CALIFORNIA 90000
TELEPHONE: (999) 399-6000

STATEMENT TO:

JANE L JONES
1211 EAST FIRST AVENUE
ANYWHERE US 10000

TEAR OFF AND RETURN UPPER PORTION WITH PAYMENT

19XX DATE	PROFESSIONAL SERVICE	FEE	PAYMENT	ADJUST-MENT	NEW BALANCE
03/04	99202	125 00			125 00
04/20	99213	50 00	175 00		–0–
04-21	4/20 VISIT, NO CHARGE			50 00	(50 00)
	DEBIT COLUMN →				
	CREDIT COLUMN →				
	ADJUSTMENT COLUMN →				
	BALANCE COLUMN SHOWING CREDIT BALANCE →				

PROFESSIONAL SERVICE CODES:
1. OFFICE VISIT
2. HOME VISIT
3. HOSPITAL VISIT
4. EMERGENCY ROOM
5. CONSULTATION
6. IMMUNIZATION
7. INJECTION
8. DRUGS/SUPPLIES/MATERIALS
9. COLLECTION OF LAB. SPEC.
10. SPECIAL REPORTS
11. OTHER SERVICES
12. SPEC. DIAGNOSTIC SERVICES
13. SPEC. THERAPEUTIC SERV.
14. EXTENDED CARE FACILITY
15. CUSTODIAL CARE
16. OBSTETRICAL CARE
17. SURGICAL
18. CASTS
19. LABORATORY
20. X-RAY
21. ALLERGY TEST.
22. NO CHARGE
23. ADJUSTMENTS OR CORRECTIONS
24. TOTAL CARE

GEORGE D. GREEN, M.D.
CAL. LIC. # 6-2856

JOHN F. WHITE, M.D.
CAL. LIC. # G-5281

FIGURE 17–2 Account card/statement showing debit, credit, adjustment, and credit balance. (Courtesy of Bibbero Systems, Inc., Petaluma, California (800) 242-2376, Fax (800) 242-9330.)

Manual Posting

All charges and payments for professional services are posted to the ledger daily. The ledger then becomes a reliable source of information for answering all inquiries from patients about their accounts.

A separate account card or page is prepared for each patient (or each family) at the time of the first visit or service (Fig. 17–3). The heading of the account should include all information pertinent to collecting the account:

- Name and address of person responsible for payment
- Insurance identification

STATEMENT

LEONARD S. TAYLOR, M.D.
2100 WEST PARK AVENUE
CHAMPAIGN, ILLINOIS 61820

TELEPHONE 351-5400

DATE	FAMILY MEMBER	PROFESSIONAL SERVICE	CHARGE	CREDITS		BALANCE
				PAYMENTS	ADJ.	
		BALANCE FORWARD				
5/13/00		Office consult	60–	60–		0
		99203				

Form 1625 PAY LAST AMOUNT IN THIS COLUMN

OC - OFFICE CALL
HC - HOUSE CALL
HOSP - HOSPITAL CARE
L - LABORATORY
I - INJECTION
INS - INSURANCE
OB - OBSTETRICAL CARE
PAP - PAPANICOLAOU TEST
OS - OFFICE SURGERY
HS - HOSPITAL SURGERY
PE - PHYSICAL EXAMINATION
EKG - ELECTROCARDIOGRAM
XR - X-RAY
M - MEDICATION
NC - NO CHARGE

FIGURE 17–3 Sample of an account card for a patient. (Courtesy of Caldwell Systems, Inc., Champaign, IL.)

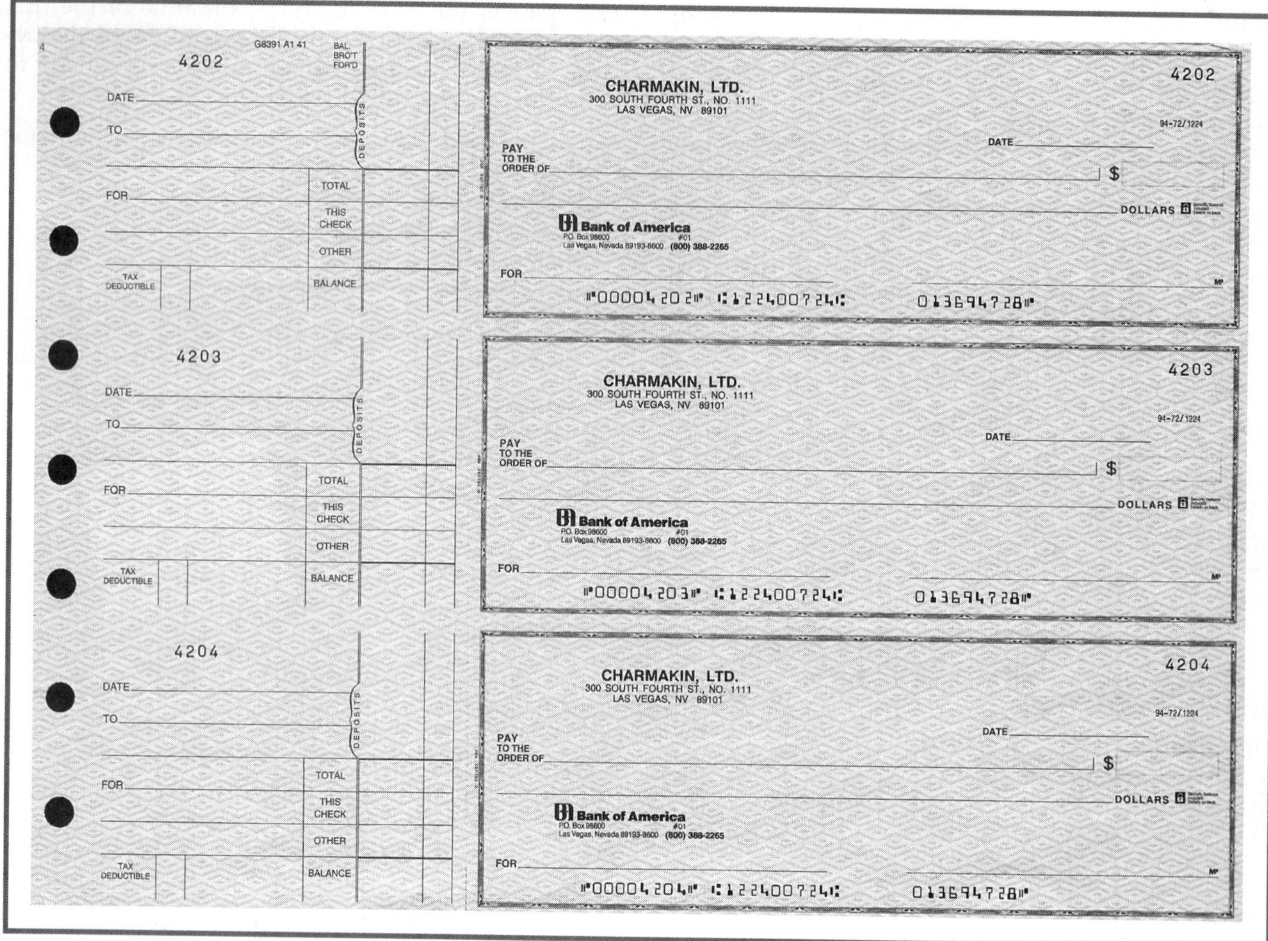
G8391 A1 41

4202

BAL BRO'T FOR'D

DATE

TO

DEPOSITS

FOR

TOTAL

THIS CHECK

OTHER

TAX DEDUCTIBLE

BALANCE

CHARMAKIN, LTD.
300 SOUTH FOURTH ST., NO. 1111
LAS VEGAS, NV 89101

4202

94-72/1224

DATE

PAY TO THE ORDER OF $

DOLLARS

Bank of America
P.O. Box 98600 #01
Las Vegas, Nevada 89193-8600 (800) 388-2265

FOR

MP

00004202 122400724 013694728

4203

DATE

TO

DEPOSITS

FOR

TOTAL

THIS CHECK

OTHER

TAX DEDUCTIBLE

BALANCE

CHARMAKIN, LTD.
300 SOUTH FOURTH ST., NO. 1111
LAS VEGAS, NV 89101

4203

94-72/1224

DATE

PAY TO THE ORDER OF $

DOLLARS

Bank of America
P.O. Box 98600 #01
Las Vegas, Nevada 89193-8600 (800) 388-2265

FOR

MP

00004203 122400724 013694728

4204

DATE

TO

DEPOSITS

FOR

TOTAL

THIS CHECK

OTHER

TAX DEDUCTIBLE

BALANCE

CHARMAKIN, LTD.
300 SOUTH FOURTH ST., NO. 1111
LAS VEGAS, NV 89101

4204

94-72/1224

DATE

PAY TO THE ORDER OF $

DOLLARS

Bank of America
P.O. Box 98600 #01
Las Vegas, Nevada 89193-8600 (800) 388-2265

FOR

MP

00004204 122400724 013694728

FIGURE 17–4 Page from a commercial checkbook with end stubs.

- Social Security number
- Home and business telephone numbers
- Name of employer
- Any special instructions for billing

Billing statements to the patient and the patient's insurance carrier are prepared from the ledger.

Computer Posting

The patient's name, date, diagnosis, and procedures are posted when the patient leaves the office. The database will retrieve the correct charges and post the charges on the computerized patient record and the accounts receivable ledger.

CHECKBOOK

All receipts are deposited in the checking account, and a record of the deposit is entered in the journal and on the check stub. A copy of each deposit slip should be kept with the financial records. All bills are paid by check, and a record of the payment is entered on the check stub and in the disbursements section of the general journal (Fig. 17–4).

DISBURSEMENTS JOURNAL

Manual Posting

In simplified accounting systems, the **disbursements journal** usually consists of a section at the bottom of each day sheet and a check register page at the end of each month, plus monthly and annual summaries. It must show

- Every amount paid out
- Date and check number
- Purpose of payment

Disbursements that are not practice related should be recorded separately.

Computer Posting

Use cash or check payments screen. Enter payment information and the computer can print the check, *or* enter information after the check has been manually prepared.

PETTY CASH RECORD

A **petty cash fund** and voucher system should be established to take care of minor unpredictable expenditures such as postage due, parking fees, small contributions, emergency supplies, and miscellaneous small items. In the average facility, $25 to $50 is sufficient for the petty cash fund. If a larger sum is available, there is a tendency to pay too many bills out of petty cash instead of writing a check.

When the check for this fund is exchanged at the bank for small bills and coins, the money is placed in a cashbox or drawer that can be locked or kept in the safe at night. One person only should be in charge of the petty cash fund. This person must be able to account for the full amount of the fund at any time.

PAYROLL RECORD

The payroll record is an auxiliary disbursement record. A separate page or card for each employee, as well as a summary record, should be kept. This procedure is discussed in more detail in Chapter 24 as a management responsibility.

Memory Jogger

Briefly explain the difference between a debit *balance and a* credit *balance.*

Comparison of Common Bookkeeping Systems

Success in bookkeeping requires a thorough understanding of the system and what it is expected to accomplish. There are many variations in bookkeeping systems, from simple to complex, no one of which can meet the needs of every physician. The basic principles are the same for all; only the system of recording varies.

The three most common systems found in the professional office are

- Single-entry
- Double-entry
- Pegboard or write-it-once

An overview of the three systems is presented here (Table 17–2), followed later in the chapter by more detailed instruction for the pegboard system, which is currently the most widely used manual system in medical practices.

TABLE 17–2 Accounting Systems

	Advantages	Disadvantages
Single-entry	Inexpensive Requires little training Simple to use	Provides only simple summaries Errors difficult to locate No built-in controls
Double-entry	Provides comprehensive financial picture Built-in accuracy controls	Requires special training, more time, and greater skill
Pegboard	Generates all records with one writing Daily control on accounts receivable Daily record of bank deposits and cash on hand	Cost of supplies greater than single-entry system Some training required (usually included in medical assistant programs)

SINGLE-ENTRY SYSTEM

Single-entry bookkeeping is inexpensive, is simple to use, and requires very little training. It is the oldest and simplest of bookkeeping systems and includes at least three basic records:

- A **general journal,** which may also be called a daily log, daybook, daysheet, daily journal, or charge journal
- A **cash payment journal,** which in its simplest form is a checkbook
- An accounts receivable ledger, which is a record of the amounts owed by all the patients. The accounts receivable ledger may be a bound book, a loose-leaf binder, a card file, or loose pages in a ledger tray.
- There may also be auxiliary records for petty cash and payroll records.

The records of charges and receipts are usually entered into a bound journal with a page for each day of the year, monthly summary pages, and an annual summary. Daily pages have columns for entering each transaction that show the patient's name, the service performed and the charge, any payments received, and the totals for charges and receipts. The daily totals are entered on the monthly summary, and the monthly totals are carried forward to the annual summary (Figure 17–5).

The same bound book may also have space for recording cash payments, or the checkbook may be the only cash payment journal. Monthly and annual summaries would be done from the checkbook.

The accounts receivable ledger usually consists of an account card for each patient on which are entered the charges and payments from the general

MONTHLY SUMMARY OF PAYMENTS AND FEES

NOTES	YR / Day	BEGINNING VISIT SLIP NUMBER	NUMBER OF PATIENT'S VISITS	FEES COL. A TODAY	PAYMENTS COL. B TODAY	PAYMENTS COL. B MONTH TO DATE	ADJUSTMENTS COL. C TODAY	NET PROFESSIONAL FEES COLUMN A MINUS C TODAY	NET PROFESSIONAL FEES COLUMN A MINUS C MONTH TO DATE	DISTRIBUTION OF NET PROFESSIONAL FEES COL. F TODAY	COL. G TODAY	COL. H TODAY	COL. I TODAY	COL. J TODAY	COL. K TODAY	COL. L TODAY	COL. M TODAY	COL. N TODAY
	1																	
	2																	
	3																	
	4																	
	5																	
	6																	
	7																	
	8																	
	9																	
	10																	
	11																	
	12																	
	13																	
	14																	
	15																	
	16																	
	17																	
	18																	
	19																	
	20																	
	21																	
	22																	
	23																	
	24																	
	25																	
	26																	
	27																	
	28																	
	29																	
	30																	
	31																	
	TOTALS This Month																	
	TOTALS Previous Year-To-Date																	
	TOTALS Year-To-Date																	

#42-9012 © BIBBERO SYSTEMS, INC. SAN FRANCISCO

FIGURE 17–5 Page from a daily log used in single-entry bookkeeping. (Courtesy of Bibbero Systems, Inc., Petaluma, California (800) 242-2376, Fax (800) 242-9330.)

journal. The patients' statements are prepared from these cards (Fig. 17–6).

In a single-entry system, each entry is made separately.

The single-entry system was at one time widely used in health care facilities but has been mostly replaced in favor of more complete accounting systems.

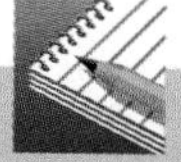

SKILLS AND RESPONSIBILITIES

RECORDING AN ENTRY

1 Record the entry on the daily journal or log.
2 Write a patient receipt if payment was made.
3 Post the transaction to the ledger.
4 Generate a monthly statement from the ledger.

Although the single-entry system may satisfy the requirements for reporting to government agencies, it does have some drawbacks:

- Errors are not easily detected.
- There are no built-in controls.
- Periodic analyses are inadequate for financial planning.

DOUBLE-ENTRY SYSTEM

Double-entry bookkeeping is also inexpensive but requires a trained and experienced bookkeeper or the regular services of an accountant. The transactions may be recorded manually or by computer. In addition to the basic journals used in a single-entry system, there may be numerous subsidiary journals. The system is based on the **accounting equation:**

Assets = Liabilities + Proprietorship (Capital)

Every transaction requires an entry on each side of the accounting equation, and the two sides must always be in balance. For this reason the system is called *double-entry*. It is the most complete of the three systems. An understanding of the basics of double-entry bookkeeping will help to clarify the principles of all systems.

BILLING NAME

NAMES OF OTHER FAMILY MEMBERS

PATIENT'S NAME

RES. PHONE

BUS. PHONE

OCCUPATION

RELATIVE OR FRIEND

EMPLOYED BY

REFERRED BY

INS. INFORMATION

SOC. SEC. NUMBER

THE BIBBERO SYSTEM FORM NO. MDP. 8510

©1965 BIBBERO SYSTEMS, INC. - SAN FRANCISCO

GEORGE D. GREEN, M.D.
JOHN F. WHITE, M.D.
Family Practice
100 MAIN STREET, SUITE 14
ANYTOWN, CALIFORNIA 90000
TELEPHONE: (999) 399-6000

STATEMENT TO:

TEAR OFF AND RETURN UPPER PORTION WITH PAYMENT

DATE	PAYMENTS			PROFESSIONAL SERVICE	FEE	LAST AMOUNT IN THIS COLUMN IS BALANCE DUE
	BANK NUMBER	BY CHECK OR P.M.O.	BY COIN OR CURRENCY			

PROFESSIONAL SERVICE CODES:
1. OFFICE VISIT
2. HOME VISIT
3. HOSPITAL VISIT
4. EMERGENCY ROOM
5. CONSULTATION
6. IMMUNIZATION
7. INJECTION
8. DRUGS/SUPPLIES/MATERIALS
9. COLLECTION OF LAB. SPEC.
10. SPECIAL REPORTS
11. OTHER SERVICES
12. SPEC. DIAGNOSTIC SERVICES
13. SPEC. THERAPEUTIC SERV.
14. EXTENDED CARE FACILITY
15. CUSTODIAL CARE
16. OBSTETRICAL CARE
17. SURGICAL
18. CASTS
19. LABORATORY
20. X-RAY
21. ALLERGY TEST.
22. NO CHARGE
23. ADJUSTMENTS OR CORRECTIONS
24. TOTAL CARE

GEORGE D. GREEN, M.D.
CAL. LIC. # 6-2856

JOHN F. WHITE, M.D.
CAL. LIC. # G-5281

FIGURE 17–6 Combination account card/statement from accounts receivable ledger. (Courtesy of Bibbero Systems, Inc., Petaluma, California (800) 242-2376, Fax (800) 242-9330.)

Assets are the properties owned by a business, such as bank accounts, accounts receivable, buildings, equipment, and furniture. The rights to these assets are called *equities*. The equity of the owner is called *capital, proprietorship,* or *owner's equity*. The equities of the creditors (those to whom money is owed) are called *liabilities*. The owner's equity (capital) is what remains of the value of the assets after the creditor's equities (liabilities) have been subtracted.

For example, if the physician purchased equipment for \$1000, paid \$250 down, and gave a promissory note for \$750, the accounting equation would be:

Assets	\$1000 =	Liabilities	\$ 750
		+	
		Capital	250
	\$1000		\$1000

The total value of the asset is \$1000. The owner's equity is \$250, and the creditor's equity is \$750. The accounting terms *capital, proprietorship, owner's equity,* and *net worth* are used interchangeably.

Few medical assistants are trained in accounting. If a double-entry system is used, it is usually set up by a practice management consultant or the accountant who does most of the actual bookwork and reports. The medical assistant in this instance generally maintains only the daily journal, from which the accountant takes the figures once a month.

The double-entry system provides a more comprehensive picture of the practice and its effect on the physician's net worth. Errors show up readily, and there are many built-in accuracy controls; but because of the time and skill required, it is not frequently used in the small practice.

PEGBOARD OR WRITE-IT-ONCE SYSTEM

The initial cost of materials for the pegboard system is slightly more than that for a single- or double-entry system but is still moderate. The system is simple to operate, and training is included in most medical assisting programs.

The system gets its name from the lightweight aluminum or masonite board with a row of pegs along the side or top that hold the forms in place. The accounting forms are perforated for alignment on the pegs. All of the forms used in any system must be compatible so that they may be aligned perfectly on the board.

The pegboard system generates all the necessary financial records for each transaction with one writing:

- Charge slip and receipt
- Ledger card
- Journal entry

It may also include a statement and bank deposit slip.

The system provides current accounts receivable totals and a daily record of bank deposits and cash on hand, in addition to the record of income and expenses. The need for separate posting to patient accounts is eliminated, and the chance for error is decreased.

Memory Jogger

Compare the advantages and disadvantages of the three bookkeeping systems. Why would pegboard be the most popular of the three?

Using the Pegboard System

The pegboard system provides positive control over cash, collections, and receivables and ensures that every cent is accounted for and properly entered (see Procedure 17–1). It provides a record of every patient, every charge, and every payment, plus a daily recap of earnings—a running record of receivables and an audited summary of cash. The system requires a minimum of time. One writing allows one to

- Enter a transaction on the daysheet.
- Give the patient a receipt for payment.
- Bring the patient's account up to date.
- Provide a current statement of account for the patient.
- Give the patient a notation of the next appointment.

All of these features communicate the money message to patients effectively and courteously and generate good financial records.

MATERIALS REQUIRED

The pegboard may be of inexpensive masonite construction with pegs down the left side, or it may be a more sophisticated aluminum sliding board that allows flexible positioning of materials. The basic forms are

- Day sheet
- Patient ledger
- Patient charge slip/receipt or superbill

All of the forms must be compatible and are available from medical office supply companies. They are customized to the practice, incorporating the usual services and procedure codes of the practice.

PREPARING THE BOARD

At the beginning of each day, place a new daysheet on the accounting board. Some systems have a sheet of clean carbon attached to the daysheet; others use

Ruling and column headings to match your current system.
Please enclose sample of daysheet for an exact match.

LEONARD S. TAYLOR, M.D.
Internal Medicine
2100 WEST PARK AVENUE
CHAMPAIGN, IL 61820
Telephone: (217) 352-5400
Fax: (217) 351-5413

Tax I.D. # 123456
S.S. No. 000-00-0000
UPIN #E00000

IL LIC. #00-00000
MC #TA 000000
BCBS 123-45678-00

OFFICE VISIT - NEW PATIENT	**CPT-4**	**GENERAL SERVICES (Cont.)**	**CPT-4**
Focused	☐ 99201	Sigmoidoscopy, Flexible Fiberoptic	☐ 45330
Expanded	☐ 99202	Cardiovascular Stress Test	☐ 93015
Detailed	☐ 99203	Spirometry	☐ 94010
Comprehensive	☐ 99204	Spirometry with BD	☐ 94060
Complex	☐ 99205	ECG, with Interpre. and Report	☐ 93000
OFFICE VISIT - ESTABLISHED PATIENT		Handing and / or	☐ 99000
Minimal	☐ 99211	Conveyance Specimen	
Focused	☐ 99212	Tuberculosis, Intradermal	☐ 86580
Expanded	☐ 99213	**LABORATORY**	
Detailed	☐ 99214	Routine Venipuncture	☐ 36415*
Comprehensive	☐ 99215	Florescent Antibody, Screen	☐ 86255
Comprehensive Service	☐ 90080	Hemogram (CBC) Manual Differential	☐ 85022
CONSULTATIONS - INITIAL		General Health Screen Panel	☐ 80050
Limited	☐ 90600	Digoxin, RIA	☐ 82643
Intermediate	☐ 90610	Glucose, Blood	☐ 82948
IMMUNIZATION INJECTIONS		Blood; Occult, Feces, Screening	☐ 82270
Diphtheria and Tetanus Toxoids	☐ 90718	Hematocrit	☐ 85014
Influenza Virus Vaccine	☐ 90724	Heterophile Antibodies(Monotype)	☐ 86300
Pneumococcal Vaccine. Polyvalent	☐ 90732	Platelet Count	☐ 85580
Therapeutic Injection	☐ 90782	Potassium: Blood	☐ 84132
Specify Material: ______________		Prothrombin Time	☐ 85610
Therapeutic IV	☐ 90784	Quinidine, Blood	☐ 84230
Specify Material: ______________		Syphilis Test, Qualitative	☐ 86592
Inj., B - 12	☐ J3420	Culture or Direct Bacterial	☐ 87072
Inj. Ampicillin, 500 mg	☐ J0290	Commercial Kit	
GENERAL SERVICES		Urinalysis, by Reagent Strips	☐ 81002
Allergen Immunotherapy,	☐ 95115	______________	☐ ____
Single Injection	☐	______________	☐ ____
Removal Impacted Cerumen	☐ 69210	______________	☐ ____

PATIENT NAME ______________________________

DIAGNOSTIC CODES: ICD-9-CM

☐ 789.0	Abdominal Pain	☐ 401.0	Hypertension, Malignant
☐ 795.0	Abnormal Pap Smear	☐ 402.90	Hypertension, W / O CHF
☐ 706.1	Acne Vulgaris	☐ 244.9	Hypothyroidism, Primary
☐ 477.0	Allergic Rhinitis,	☐ 380.4	Impacted Cerumen
☐ 285.9	Anemia, NOS	☐ 487.1	Influenza
☐ 281.0	Anemia, Pernicious	☐ 564.1	Irritable Bowel Syndrome
☐ 411.1	Angina, Unstable	☐ 464.0	Laryngitis, Acute
☐ 427.9	Arrhythmia, NOS	☐ 454.9	Leg Varicose Veins
☐ 440.9	Arteriosclerosis	☐ 424.0	Mitral Valve Prolapse
☐ 714.0	Arthritis, Rheumatoid	☐ 412	Myocardial Infarction, Old
☐ 414.0	ASHD	☐ 715.90	Osteoarthritis, Unspec. Site
☐ 493.90	Asthma, Bronchial W/O Status. Ast.	☐ 620.2	Ovarian Cyst
☐ 493.91	Asthma, Bronchial W/Status Ast.	☐ 614.9	Pelvic Inflammatory Disease
☐ 466.1	Bronchiolitis, Acute	☐ 685.1	Pilonidal Cyst
☐ 466.0	Bronchitis, Acute	☐ 462	Pharyngitis, Acute
☐ 727.3	Bursitis	☐ 486	Pneumonitis
☐ 786.50	Chest Pain	☐ 627.1	Postmenopausal Bleeding
☐ 574.20	Cholelithiasis	☐ 625.4	Premenstrual Tension
☐ 372.30	Conjunctivitis, Unspecified	☐ 782.1	Rash
☐ 564.0	Constipation	☐ 569.3	Rectal Bleeding
☐ 496	COPD	☐ 398.90	Rheumatic Heart Disease, NOS
☐ 692.9	Dermatitis, Allergic	☐ 461.9	Sinusitis, Acute, NOS
☐ 250.01	Diabetes Mellitus, ID	☐ 782.1	Skin Eruption, Rash
☐ 250.00	Diabetes Mellitus, NID	☐ 845.00	Sprain, Ankle
☐ 558.9	Diarrhea	☐ 848.9	Sprain, Muscle, Unspec. Site
☐ 562.11	Diverticulitis	☐ 785.6	Swollen Glands
☐ 562.10	Diverticulosis	☐ 246.9	Thyroid Disease, Unspecified
☐ 782.3	Edema	☐ 463	Tonsillitis, Acute
☐ 492.8	Emphysema	☐ 474.0	Tonsillitis, Chronic
☐ V18.0	Family History Of Diabetes	☐ 465.9	Upper Respir. Infection, Acute
☐ 780.6	Fever of Undetermined Origin	☐ 599.0	Urinary Tract Infection
☐ 578.9	G. I. Bleeding, Unspecified	☐ V03.9	Vaccination / Bacterial Dis.
☐ 727.41	Ganglion Of Joint	☐ V06.8	Vaccination / Combination
☐ 535.0	Gastritis, Acute	☐ V04.8	Vaccination, Influenza
☐ V72.3	Gynecological Exam	☐ 616.10	Vaginitis, Vulvitis, NOS
☐ 748.0	Headache	☐ 780.4	Vertigo
☐ 785.2	Heart Murmur, Innocent	☐ 787.0	Vomiting, Nausea
☐ 550.90	Hernia, Inguinal, NOS	☐ ____	______________
☐ 054.9	Herpes Simplex	☐ ____	______________
☐ 053.9	Herpes Zoster	☐ ____	______________
☐ 708.9	Hives / Urticaria	☐ ____	______________
☐ 401.1	Hypertension, Benign		

DATE OF SERVICE	CPT CODE	DIAGNOSIS CODE(S)	CHARGE

Place of Service:	TOTAL CHARGE	$
( ) Office	AMOUNT PAID	$
( ) Emergency Room		
( ) In-Patient Hospital	PREVIOUS BALANCE	$
( ) Out-Patient Hospital		
( ) Nursing Home	BALANCE DUE	$

____
Doctor's Signature

FORM 7201 COLWELL SYSTEMS, CHAMPAIGN, IL

065987

FIGURE 17–7 Example of a superbill. (CPT only © American Medical Association. All Rights Reserved.)

special carbon with holes for the pegs; some use NCR (no carbon required) paper. The carbon goes on top of the daysheet. Over the carbon, place the charge slip/receipt or **superbill** (Fig. 17–7). The receipt has a carbonized writing line that should align with the first open writing line on the daysheet. If the slips are shingled, lay the entire bank of receipts over the pegs, with the top one aligned as mentioned. The remainder will be automatically in place. Receipts should be used in numerical order.

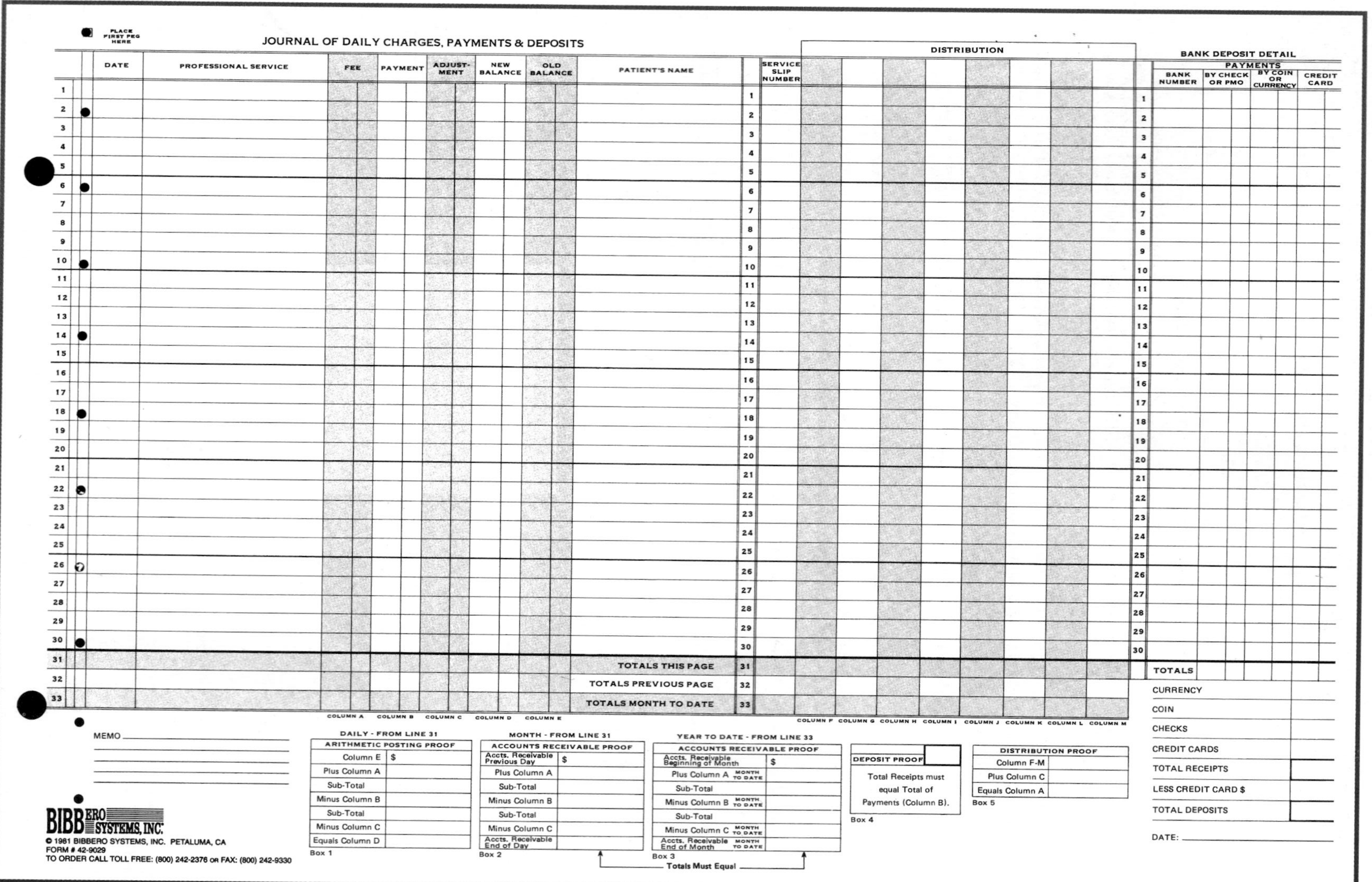

PLACE FIRST PEG HERE

JOURNAL OF DAILY CHARGES, PAYMENTS & DEPOSITS

	DATE	PROFESSIONAL SERVICE	FEE	PAYMENT	ADJUST-MENT	NEW BALANCE	OLD BALANCE	PATIENT'S NAME	SERVICE SLIP NUMBER	DISTRIBUTION	BANK DEPOSIT DETAIL: BANK NUMBER	PAYMENTS: BY CHECK OR PMO	PAYMENTS: BY COIN OR CURRENCY	CREDIT CARD
1														
2														
3														
4														
5														
6														
7														
8														
9														
10														
11														
12														
13														
14														
15														
16														
17														
18														
19														
20														
21														
22														
23														
24														
25														
26														
27														
28														
29														
30														
31								TOTALS THIS PAGE	31		TOTALS			
32								TOTALS PREVIOUS PAGE	32					
33								TOTALS MONTH TO DATE	33					
			COLUMN A	COLUMN B	COLUMN C	COLUMN D	COLUMN E			COLUMN F, COLUMN G, COLUMN H, COLUMN I, COLUMN J, COLUMN K, COLUMN L, COLUMN M				

CURRENCY

COIN

CHECKS

CREDIT CARDS

TOTAL RECEIPTS

LESS CREDIT CARD $

TOTAL DEPOSITS

DATE: ______

MEMO ______

DAILY - FROM LINE 31

ARITHMETIC POSTING PROOF	
Column E	$
Plus Column A	
Sub-Total	
Minus Column B	
Sub-Total	
Minus Column C	
Equals Column D	

Box 1

MONTH - FROM LINE 31

ACCOUNTS RECEIVABLE PROOF	
Accts. Receivable Previous Day	$
Plus Column A	
Sub-Total	
Minus Column B	
Sub-Total	
Minus Column C	
Accts. Receivable End of Day	

Box 2

YEAR TO DATE - FROM LINE 33

ACCOUNTS RECEIVABLE PROOF	
Accts. Receivable Beginning of Month	$
Plus Column A MONTH TO DATE	
Sub-Total	
Minus Column B MONTH TO DATE	
Sub-Total	
Minus Column C MONTH TO DATE	
Accts. Receivable End of Month MONTH TO DATE	

Box 3

Totals Must Equal

DEPOSIT PROOF

Total Receipts must equal Total of Payments (Column B).

Box 4

DISTRIBUTION PROOF	
Column F-M	
Plus Column C	
Equals Column A	

Box 5

BIBBERO SYSTEMS, INC.

© 1981 BIBBERO SYSTEMS, INC. PETALUMA, CA
FORM # 42-9029
TO ORDER CALL TOLL FREE: (800) 242-2376 OR FAX: (800) 242-9330

FIGURE 17–8 Sample daily log of charges and receipts. (Courtesy of Bibbero Systems, Inc., Petaluma, California (800) 242-2376, Fax (800) 242-9330.)

PULLING THE LEDGER CARDS

If a great many patients are to be seen in one day, pulling the ledger cards for all the scheduled patients at the beginning of the day will save time. Keep the cards in the order in which the patients are scheduled to be seen.

ENTERING AND POSTING TRANSACTIONS

As each patient arrives, insert the patient's ledger card under the first receipt, aligning the first available writing line of the card with the carbonized strip on the receipt. Enter the receipt number and date, the account balance in the space labeled previous balance, and the patient's name. The information recorded on the receipt is automatically posted to the ledger and the daysheet (Fig. 17–8).

The charge slip is then detached and clipped to the patient chart to be routed to the physician, who now has an opportunity to see how much the patient owes and can discuss the account in privacy, if desired.

After the service has been performed, the physician enters the service on the charge slip and asks the patient or the nurse to return it to the medical assistant. The assistant then has an opportunity to ask the patient whether this is to be a charge or cash transaction before completing the posting.

Again, insert the ledger card under the proper receipt, checking the number that was previously entered to make sure you have the correct card. Record the service by procedure code, post the charge from the fee schedule, enter any payment made, and write in the current balance. If there is no balance, place a zero or straight line in the balance column. If another appointment is required, enter the date and time at the bottom of the receipt.

The transaction has now been posted to the journal and the ledger, and, if payment was made by the patient, a receipt has been generated. The service receipt is given to the patient; no other receipt is necessary. The ledger card is ready for refiling.

File the charge slips in numerical order for your internal audit. At the end of the month, the total of the charge slips should equal the total of the charges recorded on the daysheets for the month.

RECORDING OTHER PAYMENTS AND CHARGES

Payments will be received in the mail and may be brought in by patients some time after a service was performed. These payments are entered on the daysheet and the ledger card in the same manner as previously explained. Payments by mail do not require a receipt.

The physician may have daily charges for visits to patients in a hospital or convalescent facility. Enter these charges on the daysheet and ledger card only. Surgery fees are usually recorded as one entry that includes the surgery and aftercare.

END-OF-DAY SUMMARIZING

At the end of the day, all columns must be totaled and proved. Although all bookkeeping is done in ink, it is a good idea to write the totals in pencil until they have been proved. If an error is discovered, you must correct the entry in which it occurred. Do not attempt to erase or write over the incorrect entry. Simply draw a line through it and make a new entry on the first open writing line. Remember that you must reinsert the ledger card for these corrections. Also, if the entry included a receipt for the patient, you must make a new receipt and notify the patient of the correction.

The pegboard system provides several ways for proving the arithmetic on the day sheet. Two examples are shown.

EXAMPLE OF POSTING PROOF FOR DAY

Old Balance		$____
Plus total charges		____
	Subtotal	$____
Less payments received		____
	Subtotal	$____
Less adjustments		$____
New Balance		*$____

*This figure is carried forward to next page for "old balance."

EXAMPLE OF CASH CONTROL PROOF

Cash on hand at beginning of day		$____
Cash received		____
	Subtotal	$____
Less cash paid out		____
Less bank deposit		____
Cash on hand at end of day		*$____

*This figure is carried forward to next page for "cash on hand at beginning of day."

Special Bookkeeping Entries

The following special entries are necessary occasionally and may be used with pegboard or any other accounting system.

ADJUSTMENTS

At times, it is necessary to enter a credit adjustment. These could be for (1) professional discounts, (2) insurance disallowances, or (3) writeoffs. If the system has an adjustment column, enter them there. Otherwise, because the adjustment is actually a subtraction from the charge, enter it in the charge column with the figure enclosed in parentheses or circled and an explanation of the entry in the description column. When the column of figures is totaled, the circled figure is *subtracted* rather than added. The learner has a tendency to ignore the circled figures. This is incorrect—they must be subtracted.

CREDIT BALANCES

A credit balance occurs when

- A patient has paid in advance
- There has been an overpayment

For example, an overpayment occurs if the patient made a partial payment and later the insurance allowance was more than the remaining **balance.** The difference between the total amount of money received and the amount owed must be entered in the balance column and enclosed within parentheses or circled. This indicates a credit balance.

The credit balance is money owed to the patient. If the patient has paid in advance or wishes to leave the overpayment in the account in anticipation of future charges, care must be taken in figuring the balance on future transactions. Whereas normally a charge increases the balance, it will decrease a credit balance.

REFUNDS

If a patient wishes to have an overpayment refunded, write a check for the amount due and enter the transaction on the daysheet as shown.

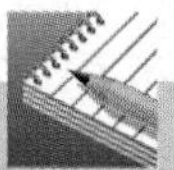

SKILLS AND RESPONSIBILITIES

HOW TO GENERATE A REFUND

1 Place the ledger card on the daysheet.
2 Enter an explanation in the description column.
3 Show the existing credit balance within parentheses or circled.
4 Write the amount of the refund in the payment column within parentheses or circled to show that it is a subtraction.
5 Show a zero balance.

NONSUFFICIENT FUNDS (NSF) CHECKS

Sometimes a patient sends in a check without having sufficient funds to cover it; this check is later deposited to the physician's account. The bank will return the check to you marked NSF. You must now perform two accounting functions as shown.

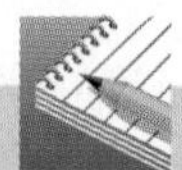

SKILLS AND RESPONSIBILITIES

HOW TO RECORD NSF CHECKS

1 Deduct the amount from your checking account balance.
2 Add the amount back into the patient's account balance by
   - Entering the amount in the paid column in parentheses
   - Increasing the balance by the same amount
3 Write a brief explanation of the transaction in the description column (Fig. 17–9).

ONE-ENTRY CASH TRANSACTIONS

For the transient patient who has no ledger card and pays at the time of service, use a receipt as previously described. Enter the amount of the fee in the charge column and in the paid column and a zero balance. This records the transaction on the journal page and provides a receipt for the patient. There is no need for a ledger card.

COLLECTION AGENCY PAYMENTS

When a collection agency recovers an account for the physician, the agency deducts a commission, usually 40% to 50% of the amount recovered. For example, if the patient had a balance of $100 and pays it in full, the agency will send the physician $50. The patient now has a zero balance and the physician has only $50. This transaction is recorded on the ledger card and the daysheet in the following manner:

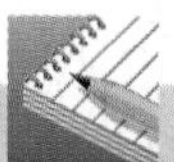

SKILLS AND RESPONSIBILITIES

RECORDING A COLLECTION AGENCY PAYMENT

1 $100 appears in the balance column.
2 Enter $50 in the cash received or paid column.

NAME
BROWN, JOHN S.S.# 000 00 0000
ADDRESS
429 WEST MARKET STREET, LONG DESERT, NV 80056
TELEPHONE 702-345-6789 INSURANCE METROPOLITAN REF. BY BAFFLE

DATE	FAMILY MEMBER	PROFESSIONAL SERVICE	CHARGE	CREDITS PAYMENT	CREDITS ADJ.	BALANCE
2000		BALANCE FORWARD				
10-20	self	99245	200 00	50 –		150 00
11-15		99213	100 00			250 00
11-20		Personal check		100 00		150 00
11-28		Check retd NSF		(100)		250 00

Form 5128 Colwell Systems, Champaign, IL

FIGURE 17–9 Entry for returned NSF (nonsufficient funds) checks.

3 Enter $50 in the adjustment column.
4 Enter zero in the new balance column.
5 If there is no adjustment column, the $50 commission is entered in the charge column in parentheses ($50), so that the total charge is reduced by this amount and the transaction is reflected correctly in the accounts receivable control.

Accounts Receivable Control—Pegboard System

The **accounts receivable control** is a daily summary of what remains unpaid on the accounts.

This is an integral part of the pegboard and double-entry systems but is a separate operation in single-entry accounting. A simple form such as the one

ACCOUNTS RECEIVABLE CONTROL

Month of December, 19___

Accounts receivable at end of last day of preceding month: $37,506

Day	Value of Services Rendered	Received from Patients	Adjustments	+	−	Accounts Receivable Balance
1	785	1098			313	37,193
2	210	630			420	36,773
3	950	510	33	407		37,180
4						

FIGURE 17–10 Accounts receivable control for a single-entry bookkeeping system.

PROCEDURE 17-1

Posting Service Charges and Payments Using Pegboard

GOAL

To post one day's charges and payments and complete the daily bookkeeping cycle using a pegboard.

EQUIPMENT AND SUPPLIES

Pegboard
Calculator
Pen
Daysheet
Carbon
Receipts
Ledger cards
Balances from previous day

PROCEDURAL STEPS

1 Prepare the board:
- Place a new daysheet on the board.
- Cover daysheet with carbon.
- Place bank of receipts over the pegs aligning the top receipt with the first open writing line on the daysheet.

2 Carry forward balances from the previous day.
PURPOSE: To keep all totals current.

3 Pull ledger cards for patients to be seen today.

4 Insert the ledger card under the first receipt, aligning the first available writing line of the card with the carbonized strip on the receipt.
PURPOSE: To ensure that one writing will correctly post the entry to receipt, ledger, and daysheet.

5 Enter the patient's name, the date, receipt number, and any existing balance from the ledger card.

6 Detach the charge slip from the receipt and clip it to the patient's chart.
PURPOSE: The physician will indicate the service performed on the charge slip and return it to you.

7 Accept the returned charge slip at the end of the visit.

8 Enter the appropriate fee from the fee schedule.

9 Locate the receipt on the board with a number matching the charge slip.
PURPOSE: To make certain it is the correct receipt.

10 Reinsert the patient's ledger card under the receipt.

11 Write the service code number and fee on the receipt.

12 Accept the patient's payment and record the amount of payment and new balance.
PURPOSE: Brings patient's account up to date and provides current statement for patient.

13 Give the completed receipt to the patient.

14 Follow your agency's procedure for refiling the ledger card.

15 Repeat steps 4 to 14 for each service for the day.

16 Total all columns of the daysheet at the end of the day.
PURPOSE: To determine total amount of charges, receipts, and resulting balances for the day.

17 Write preliminary totals in pencil.
PURPOSE: To facilitate any necessary changes.

18 Complete proof of totals and enter totals in ink.

19 Enter figures for accounts receivable control.
PURPOSE: To complete daily accounting cycle.

illustrated in Figure 17–10 is useful. Using a separate page or card for each month, proceed as listed below:

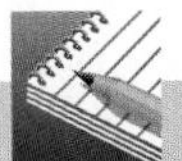

SKILLS AND RESPONSIBILITIES

PERFORMING AN ACCOUNTS RECEIVABLE CONTROL

1 Total the unpaid balances from the entire ledger on the last day of the preceding month and enter this figure at the top of the card or page.
2 Total the charges and receipts at the end of each day and enter these figures in columns 1 and 2.
3 Determine the **accounts receivable** figure as follows:
   - If charges for the day are greater than the receipts, there is an increase in the accounts receivable. Enter this figure in column 4 and add it to the balance in column 6.
   - If receipts for the day are greater than the charges, there is a decrease in the accounts receivable. Enter this figure in column 5 and subtract it from the balance in column 6.

Note that the accounts receivable figure changes at the end of any day on which there is financial activity. The balance consists of the accounts receivable figure from the previous day, plus the charges for the day, minus the day's receipts and adjustments.

The total of the entire file of ledger card balances at the end of any given day should equal the accounts receivable balance shown for that day on the control form.

EXAMPLE OF ACCOUNTS RECEIVABLE CONTROL

Total outstanding A/R balance (from previous day)		$_____
Plus today's charges		_____
	Subtotal	$_____
Less today's payments		_____
	Subtotal	$_____
Less today's adjustments		_____
Balance outstanding		*$_____

*This figure is carried forward to next page for "total outstanding A/R balance."

Trial Balance of Accounts Receivable

A trial balance should be done once per month *after* all posting has been completed and *before* preparing the monthly statements.

The purpose of a trial balance is to disclose any discrepancies between the journal and the ledger. It does not prove the accuracy of the accounts.

For example, if a charge or payment were posted to the wrong account, or if the wrong amount were entered in the journal and then posted to the ledger, the totals would still "balance," but the accounts would not be accurate.

To begin, pull all the account cards that have a balance, enter each balance on the adding machine, and total the figures. This should equal the accounts receivable balance figure on your control.

If you have not kept a daily control, you must total all of the charges, all of the payments, and all of the adjustments for the month, and then do the computation illustrated below.

The end-of-month accounts receivable figure must agree with the figure arrived at by adding all the account card balances. The accounts are then said to be **in balance.** If the two totals do not agree, you must locate the error.

EXAMPLE OF BALANCING END-OF-MONTH ACCOUNTS RECEIVABLE

Accounts receivable at first of month		$_____
Plus total charges for month		_____
	Subtotal	$_____
Less total payments for month		_____
	Subtotal	$_____
Less total adjustments for month		_____
Accounts receivable at end of month		$_____

LOCATING AND PREVENTING ERRORS

After you have checked your tape and verified that you have not made an error in calculation, the first step in locating an error in your trial balance is to find the difference between the two totals. Then search the daily journal pages and the account cards for an entry of the identical amount. Check each one you find, to verify that it was posted correctly. Of course, there may be more than one error that adds up to this amount.

If there is only one error, and the amount of the error is divisible by 9, you may have transposed a figure. For example, if the difference is $81 (a number divisible by 9), you may find that you wrote $209 instead of $290. If the amount of the error is divisible by 2, you may have posted to the wrong column, reversing a debit and a credit.

A common error is made by entering the wrong amount in the previous balance column or in figuring the new balance. This kind of error will show up on the pegboard daily proof but could easily go undetected in the single-entry system.

Another common error is made by carrying forward a wrong total from one day to the next (e.g., carrying forward the beginning accounts receivable total rather than the ending accounts receivable total).

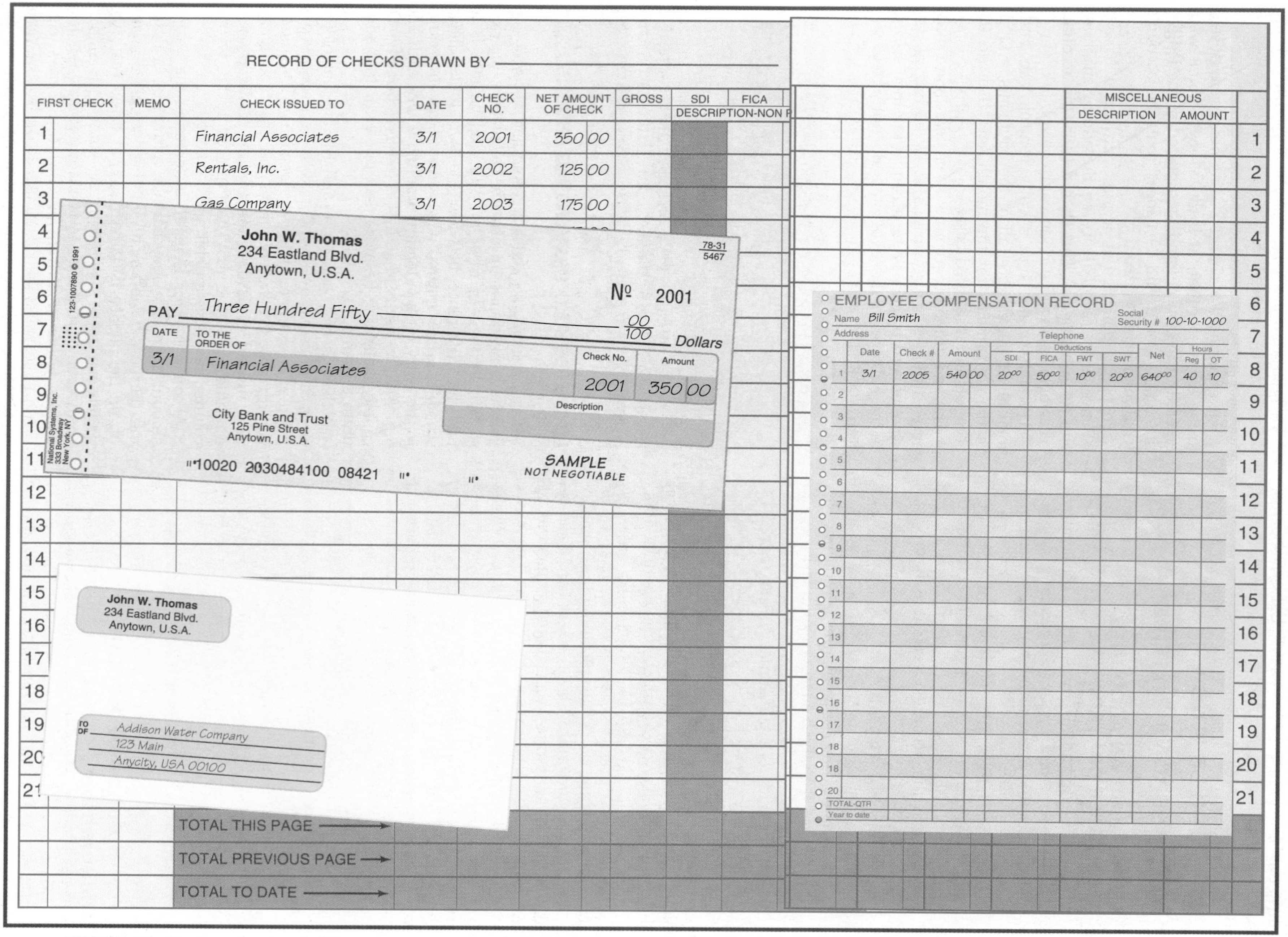

RECORD OF CHECKS DRAWN BY ____________

FIRST CHECK	MEMO	CHECK ISSUED TO	DATE	CHECK NO.	NET AMOUNT OF CHECK	GROSS	SDI	FICA
1		Financial Associates	3/1	2001	350 00			
2		Rentals, Inc.	3/1	2002	125 00			
3		Gas Company	3/1	2003	175 00			
TOTAL THIS PAGE →								
TOTAL PREVIOUS PAGE →								
TOTAL TO DATE →								

MISCELLANEOUS: DESCRIPTION | AMOUNT

John W. Thomas
234 Eastland Blvd.
Anytown, U.S.A.

78-31 / 5467

№ 2001

PAY Three Hundred Fifty 00/100 Dollars

DATE	TO THE ORDER OF	Check No.	Amount
3/1	Financial Associates	2001	350 00

Description

City Bank and Trust
125 Pine Street
Anytown, U.S.A.

⑈10020 2030484100 08421 ⑈

SAMPLE
NOT NEGOTIABLE

National Systems, Inc. 333 Broadway New York, NY
123-1007890 © 1991

John W. Thomas
234 Eastland Blvd.
Anytown, U.S.A.

TO OF Addison Water Company
123 Main
Anycity, USA 00100

EMPLOYEE COMPENSATION RECORD

Name Bill Smith — Social Security # 100-10-1000

Address — Telephone

	Date	Check #	Amount	SDI	FICA	FWT	SWT	Net	Reg	OT
1	3/1	2005	540 00	20 00	50 00	10 00	20 00	640 00	40	10
TOTAL-QTR										
Year to date										

FIGURE 17–11 Payroll and cash disbursement journal showing payroll check that has been prepared for an employee and a window envelope for mailing a check.

There is always a chance of sliding a number, that is, writing the first digit in the wrong column, such as writing 400 for 40 or 60 instead of 600.

Many bookkeepers avoid errors in the cents column by using a line (—) instead of writing two zeros when only even dollars are involved. For example, instead of writing $12.00, the bookkeeper will write $12.—. This eliminates the possibility of misreading zeros as other numbers. It also speeds the adding process when columns must be totaled.

If you are unable to locate any numerical error, there is the possibility that an account card was lost or overlooked or was transferred as paid in full.

Memory Jogger

 *What is the purpose of preparing a trial balance, and what does it reveal? Does it prove the accuracy of the accounts?*

Accounts Payable Procedures

INVOICES AND STATEMENTS

When time purchases are made, that is, the item is not paid for at the time of purchase, the vendor usually includes a **packing slip** with delivery of the merchandise. A packing slip describes the items enclosed. The vendor may also enclose an **invoice.** An invoice describes the items and shows the amount due. Always check to verify that the items listed on the packing slip and invoice are included in the delivery.

Invoices should be placed in a special folder until paid. You may be making more than one purchase from the same vendor during the month. Some vendors request that payment be made from the invoice; others expect to send a **statement** later. A statement is a request for payment.

PAYING FOR PURCHASES

At the time of payment, compare the statement with the invoice(s) to verify accuracy, fasten the statement and invoices together, write the date and check number on the statement, and place it in the paid file.

RECORDING DISBURSEMENTS

Both the pegboard and the single-entry bookkeeping systems provide pages for recording disbursements. This is sometimes called a *check register* (Fig. 17–11). On these pages, disbursements are distributed to specific expense accounts such as

- Auto expense
- Dues and meetings
- Equipment
- Insurance
- Medical supplies
- Office expenses
- Printing, postage, and stationery
- Rent and maintenance
- Salaries
- Taxes and licenses
- Travel and entertainment
- Utilities
- Miscellaneous
- Personal withdrawals

Each check should be entered on the disbursement page, showing the date, to whom the check was written, the number and amount of the check, and the payment allocated to one or more of the expense accounts. It is important to separate personal expenditures from business expenses. Business expenses are tax deductible and are considered in determining net income from the practice, but personal expenditures are not.

RECORDING PERSONAL EXPENDITURES

Some system must be established for transferring funds from the practice account to the physician's personal account. If the practice is incorporated, the physician is paid a salary. In the unincorporated practice, the transfer is usually accomplished through what is known in accounting terms as a *drawing account.*

The physician establishes a personal checking account and perhaps one or more savings accounts. Each month, or at any specified time, the medical assistant writes a check payable to the physician, which is then endorsed and deposited to the physician's personal account. In the disbursements journal, the amount of the check is posted in a special column headed *Personal* or *Drawing.*

Although personal expenses are not deductible in determining net income from the practice, some qualify as personal deductions in computing personal income tax, so a careful accounting should be kept. Deductible expenses would include property taxes, interest paid out, contributions, and so forth.

ACCOUNTING FOR PETTY CASH

The petty cash fund is a revolving fund. It does not change in amount except to increase or decrease the established fund. To establish the petty cash fund, a check is written payable to Cash or Petty Cash and entered in the disbursements journal under Miscellaneous (see Procedure 17–2). This is the *only* time the petty cash check is charged to Miscellaneous.

No.	Date	Description	Amount	Office Exp.	Automobile	Misc.	Balance
	04-01	Fund established					50.00
1	04-02	Postage due	.55	.55			49.45
2	04-08	Parking fee	6.00		6.00		43.45
3	04-10	Delivery charge	2.32			2.32	41.13
4	04-25	Stationery supplies	3.38	3.38			37.75
		TOTAL	12.25	3.93	6.00	2.32	
	05-01	Balance 37.75					
	Ch #	374 12.25					50.00

FIGURE 17–12 Petty cash record.

Each time the fund is replenished, the amount of the check is spread among the various accounts for which the money was used. This is determined from a record of expenditures such as that shown in Figure 17–12. The headings of the columns should correspond to headings in the disbursements journal to which they will be posted.

A pad of petty cash vouchers is kept in or near the cash box. For every disbursement from the fund, the petty cashier should either have a receipt or prepare a voucher similar to the one in Figure 17–13. The total of the petty cash vouchers and receipts plus the amount of cash in the box must always equal the original amount of the fund.

Receipt and voucher total	$12.25
Cash on hand	37.75
Amount of fund	$50.00

Figure 17–12 shows that $50 was received into the fund on April 1. This is entered in the Description column and in the Balance column. On April 2 postage due was paid out, a voucher prepared, the number of the voucher and the amount of 55 cents entered, and a new balance brought down. On April 8, the physician paid a parking fee. The amount of $6 was entered in the record, $6 taken from petty cash to reimburse the physician, and the new balance of $43.45 brought down.

Amount $ 20.00 No. 17

RECEIVED OF PETTY CASH

For Nurses' Benefit, Mercy Hospital

Charge to Miscellaneous

Approved by Received by

FIGURE 17–13 Petty cash voucher.

At the end of the month, or sooner if the fund is depleted, a check is written to Cash for replenishing the fund, but instead of being charged to Miscellaneous as previously, the amount of the check is divided among the various accounts affected. Our record shows that at the end of April, we have $37.75 remaining in the fund and need $12.25 to bring it back to $50.

When the check is written for $12.25, it is accounted for in the monthly distribution of expenditures by posting $3.93 as office expense, $6 as car expense, and $2.32 as a miscellaneous expense. In this way, the expenditures from petty cash are charged to the specific accounts affected.

The accounted-for vouchers are clipped together and placed with paid invoices, the check for $12.25 is cashed, and the money is placed in the petty cash fund. The amount of the check is entered as being received into the fund, and the new balance of $50 is brought down.

Avoid the habit of borrowing from the petty cash fund. This admonition applies to the physician as well as to the medical assistant. If the physician requests cash from the fund, request a personal check or an office check in exchange for cash from the fund.

It is also poor policy to use the petty cash fund for making change. In facilities where patients frequently pay with currency, a separate change fund should be kept.

Periodic Summaries

Financial summaries are compiled on monthly and annual bases. They may be prepared either by the medical assistant or by the accountant (or by computer). Common summary reports include

- Statement of Income and Expense
- Cash Flow Statement
- Trial Balance

PROCEDURE 17–2
Accounting for Petty Cash

GOAL

To establish a petty cash fund, maintain an accurate record of expenditures for 1 month, and replenish the fund as necessary.

EQUIPMENT AND SUPPLIES

Form for petty cash fund
Pad of vouchers
Disbursements journal
Two checks
List of petty cash expenditures

PROCEDURAL STEPS

1 Determine the amount needed in the petty cash fund.

2 Write a check in the determined amount.
PURPOSE: To establish a fund.

3 Record the beginning balance in the petty cash record.

4 Post the amount to miscellaneous on the disbursement record.
PURPOSE: To account for original amount of fund.

5 Prepare a petty cash voucher for each amount withdrawn from the fund.
PURPOSE: Voucher will be used for internal audit.

6 Record each voucher in the petty cash record and enter the new balance.
PURPOSE: To record current balance and determine the need for replenishing the fund.

7 Write a check to replenish the fund as necessary.
NOTE: The total of the vouchers plus the fund balance must equal the beginning amount.

8 Total the expense columns and post to the appropriate accounts in the disbursement record.
PURPOSE: To record expenditures in the correct expense category.

9 Record the amount added to the fund.

10 Record the new balance in the petty cash fund.

- Accounts Receivable Trial Balance and Aging Analysis
- Balance Sheet

The **statement of income and expense** is also known as the profit and loss statement and covers a specific period. It lists all the income received and all expenses paid during the period. The total income is called *gross income* or *earnings*. The income after deduction of all expenses is the *net income*.

A **cash flow statement** starts with the amount of cash on hand at the beginning of the month (or for any specified period). It then lists the cash income and the cash disbursements made throughout the period and concludes with a statement of the amount of cash remaining on hand at the end of the period.

A **trial balance** is necessary to determine that the books are in balance. All of the columns on the disbursements journal must be totaled at the end of the month. The combined totals of all the expense columns must be equal to the total of the checks written. If the figures do not balance, it is necessary to recheck every entry until an error is found.

The **accounts receivable trial balance** is done before sending out the monthly statements. First, record the total of the accounts receivable ledger at the end of the previous month; then add the charges for the current month and subtract the adjustments and the payments received. The remainder should equal the total of the accounts receivable ledger at the end of the current month.

The **balance sheet,** also known as a statement of financial condition, shows the financial picture of the practice on a specific date. Often, it is done only on an annual basis. The balance sheet is set up using the accounting equation: *Assets = Liabilities + Proprietorship.* The title of the statement had its origin in the equality of the elements—the balance between the sum of the assets and the sum of the liabilities and capital.

At the end of the accounting year, it is very simple to combine the monthly reports to compile the annual summaries. The annual summaries simplify the reporting of income for tax returns.

Bookkeeping with the Aid of the Computer

The office with an in-house computer and the appropriate software can accomplish all the described accounting operations and more in a fraction of the time required to do them manually. The role of the computer in the medical practice was discussed in Chapter 13. The office without a computer can still reap some of the benefits by using an outside computer service.

A computer service can relieve the office staff of the repetitive clerical procedures necessary in the recording of charges and in the preparation and mailing of statements and insurance forms. It can produce weekly and monthly financial reports that would be too time-consuming and perhaps beyond the capabilities of the staff to do manually.

Memory Jogger

5 *Name the five periodic financial summaries.*

Payroll Records

The office accounting system must include records of payroll, federal and state tax deductions, Social Security tax information, and quarterly and annual reports. These topics are discussed in Chapter 24, Management Responsibilities.

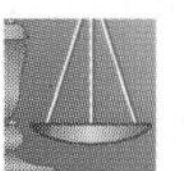

LEGAL AND ETHICAL ISSUES

The keeping of the financial records is a position of great trust and responsibility. The records must be accurate and completed on a daily basis. Daily journal pages should be kept indefinitely in support of tax returns.

CRITICAL THINKING

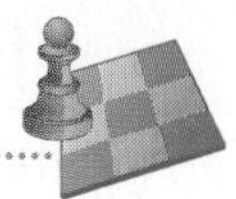

1 Discuss the statement "There is no such thing as almost correct financial records."

2 In what bookkeeping record is all financial information first recorded?

3 What symbol or mark is used to indicate that a figure must be subtracted rather than added?

4 What are the three most common bookkeeping systems used in a professional office?

HOW DID I DO? Answers to Memory Joggers

1
a. How much was earned in a given period
b. How much was collected
c. How much is owed
d. The distribution of expenses incurred

2 A debit balance represents money due to the provider.
A credit balance represents an advance or overpayment.

3 Answers will vary.

4 The purpose of preparing a trial balance is to determine that the journal and ledger are in balance. The trial balance will reveal any discrepancies.

5
a. Statement of income and expense.
b. Cash flow statement
c. Trial balance
d. Accounts receivable trial balance
e. Balance sheet

REFERENCES

Colwell Systems: One-Write Pegboard Bookkeeping System. Champaign, IL, Colwell Systems, 1997.

Fess PE, et al: Accounting Principles, 17th ed. Cincinnati, South-Western Publishing Company, 1989.

Banking Services and Procedures

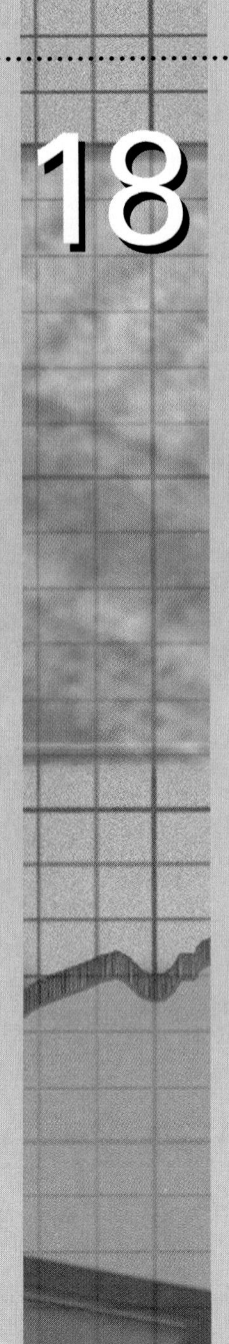

OUTLINE

LEARNING OBJECTIVES

Cognitive: On successful completion of this chapter you should be able to:

1. Define and spell the terms listed in the Vocabulary.
2. State the four requirements of a negotiable instrument.
3. Discuss six advantages of using checks for the transfer of funds.
4. State why it is important to complete the check stub before writing a check.
5. Explain how you would handle mistakes made in preparing a check.
6. List and discuss eight precautions to observe in accepting checks.
7. State the purpose of a check endorsement.
8. Name and compare four kinds of endorsements.
9. Cite five reasons for depositing checks promptly.
10. Discuss the action necessary when a deposited check is returned.

Performance: On successful completion of this chapter you should be able to:

1. Prepare a bank deposit.
2. Correctly write a check.
3. Pay office bills by checks.
4. Reconcile a bank statement with the checkbook balance.

VOCABULARY

disbursements Funds paid out.

endorser Person who signs his or her name on the back of a check for the purpose of transferring title to another person.

maker (of a check) Any individual, corporation, or legal party who signs a check or any type of negotiable instrument.

negotiable Legally transferable to another party.

payee Person named on a draft or check as the recipient of the amount shown.

payer Person who writes a check in favor of the payee.

power of attorney A legal statement in which a person authorizes another person to act as his or her attorney or agent. The authority may be limited to the handling of certain procedures. The person authorized to act as the agent is known as an *attorney in fact.*

reconciliation (of bank statement) The process of proving that the bank statement and the checkbook balance are in agreement.

teller A bank employee who is assigned the duty of waiting on the bank's customers.

third-party check A check written to the order of the person offering payment and unknown to the payee, who is a third party in the process.

Financial transactions in the professional office nearly always involve banking services and the use of checks. Therefore, the medical assistant must understand the responsibilities involved in accepting payments, in endorsing and depositing checks, in writing checks, and in regularly reconciling bank statements.

Checks

A check is a draft or an order on a bank for the payment of a certain sum of money to a certain person therein named, or to the bearer, and is payable on demand. It is considered to be a negotiable instrument. A **negotiable** instrument must

- Be written and signed by **a maker**
- Contain a promise or order to pay a sum of money
- Be payable on demand or at a fixed future date
- Be payable to order or bearer

ADVANTAGES OF USING CHECKS

Using checks for the transfer of funds has many advantages:

- Checks are both safe and convenient, particularly for making payments by mail.
- Expenditures are quickly calculated.
- Specific payments can be easily located from the check record.
- A stop-payment order can protect the payer from loss due to stolen, lost, or incorrectly drawn checks.
- Checks provide a permanent reliable record of disbursements for tax purposes.
- The deposit record provides a summary of receipts.
- Checking accounts protect the money while on deposit.

TYPES OF CHECKS

You are probably already familiar with the standard personal check, but there are many additional types of checks in use in business transactions. You should be familiar with the following:

BANK DRAFT A check is drawn by a bank against funds deposited to its account in another bank.

CASHIER'S CHECK A bank's own check is drawn on itself and signed by the bank cashier or other authorized official. It is also known as an officer's or treasurer's check. A cashier's check is obtained by paying the bank cashier the amount of the check, in cash or by personal check. Some banks charge a fee for this service. Cashier's checks are often issued to accommodate the savings account customer who does not maintain a checking account.

CERTIFIED CHECK This is the depositor's own check, on the face of which the bank has placed the word *certified* or accepted with the date and a bank official's signature. Because the bank deducts the amount of the check from the depositor's account at the time it certifies the check, the bank can guarantee that the amount is available. A certified check, like a cashier's check, can be used when an ordinary personal check might not be acceptable. If not used,

CARB-OUT

Seattle Optical Company
222 Elm
Seattle, WA 90202

_______19___ 093 78-31/5467

Pay to the Order of ______________________ $ [ ]

______________________ **Dollars**

United Trust Company
P.O. Box 327
Anytown, U.S.A.

Sample-VOID

Memo ________

⑆123400051⑆0851⑆038 2948 39⑈

DETACH AND RETAIN THIS STATEMENT

Seattle Optical Company Seattle, WA 90202 — THE ATTACHED CHECK IS IN PAYMENT OF ITEMS DESCRIBED BELOW. IF NOT CORRECT PLEASE NOTIFY US PROMPTLY. NO RECEIPT DESIRED

DATE	INVOICE NO.	AMOUNT	DISC.	NET	DATE	INVOICE NO.	AMOUNT	DISC.	NET

FIGURE 18–1 Page from bank order book showing sample voucher check.

a certified check should be redeposited promptly, so that the funds previously set aside are credited back to the depositor's account.

LIMITED CHECK A check may be limited as to the amount written on it and as to the time during which it may be presented for payment. The limited check is often used for payroll or insurance checks.

MONEY ORDER Domestic money orders are sold by banks, some stores, and the United States Postal Service. The maximum face value varies according to the source. International money orders may be purchased for limited amounts, indicated in U.S. dollars, for use in sending money abroad.

TRAVELER'S CHECK Traveler's checks are designed for persons traveling where personal checks may not be accepted or for use in situations in which it is inadvisable to carry large amounts of cash. Traveler's checks are usually printed in denominations of $10, $20, $50, and $100, and sometimes $500 and $1000. They require two signatures of the purchaser, one at the time of purchase and the other at the time of use. They are available at banks and some travel agencies.

VOUCHER CHECK A voucher check is one with a detachable voucher form. The voucher portion is used to itemize or specify the purpose for which the check is drawn. It is used for the convenience of the **payer** and shows discounts and various other itemizations. This portion of the check is removed before presenting the check for payment and provides a record for the **payee** (Fig. 18–1).

Memory Jogger

a. Explain the difference between a cashier's check and a certified check.
b. What kind of check needs to be signed twice by the payer?

ABA NUMBER

The ABA number is part of a coding system originated by the American Bankers Association. It appears in the upper right area of a printed check. The number is used as a simple way to identify the area where the bank upon which the check is written is located and the particular bank within the area. The code number is expressed as a fraction, for example, $\frac{90\text{-}1822}{1222}$ (Fig. 18–2). In the top part of the fraction, before the hyphen, the numbers 1 to 49 designate cities in which Federal Reserve banks are located or other key cities; the numbers from 50 to 99 refer to states or territories. The part of the number following the hyphen is a number issued to each bank for

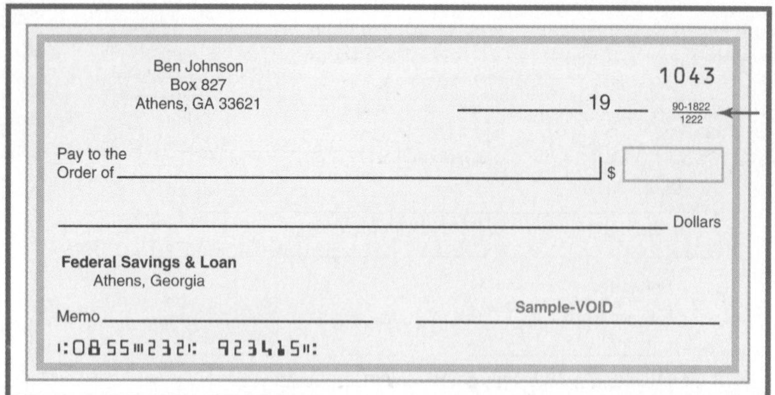

FIGURE 18–2 Sample check. Arrow indicates American Bankers Association number.

its own identification purposes. The ABA number is used in preparing deposit slips, to identify each check. The bottom part of the fraction includes the number of the Federal Reserve district in which the bank is located and other identifying information.

MAGNETIC INK CHARACTER RECOGNITION (MICR)

Characters and numbers printed in magnetic ink are found at the bottom of checks. They represent a common machine language, readable by machines as well as by humans. When a check is deposited, the amount of the check can also be printed in magnetic ink below the signature. MICR identification facilitates processing through a high-speed machine that reads the characters, sorts the checks, and does the bookkeeping.

Bank Accounts

COMMON TYPES OF ACCOUNTS

Checking Accounts

By placing an amount of money on deposit in a bank, a depositor can set up a checking account. Simply stated, a checking account is a bank account against which checks can be written. Many variations in checking accounts have been developed over the years. Instead of a straight non–interest-bearing account, one might have an insured money market checking account, which bears interest at the daily money market rate if a certain minimum balance is retained.

A physician often requires three different checking accounts:

1. An account for personal and family expenses
2. A separate checking account for office expenses
3. A high-yield interest-bearing account for funds reserved for paying insurance premiums, property taxes, and other seasonal expenses

Savings Accounts

Money that is not needed for current expenses can be deposited in a savings account (Fig. 18–3). In most cases, savings accounts earn interest on the amounts deposited; that is, the bank pays the depositor a certain percentage monthly or quarterly for the use of the money in the savings account. The ordinary savings account draws interest at the lowest prevailing rate and has no minimum balance requirement and no check-writing privileges.

Money Market Savings Account

An insured money market savings account requires a minimum balance, frequently $2500, draws interest at money market rates, and allows the writing of a specified number of checks (frequently three) per month. There may be a minimum amount for each transaction. Such checks are usually written for transfer of funds to a checking account.

Memory Jogger

How does an insured money market savings account differ from an ordinary savings account?

Systematizing Bill Paying

A systematic plan should be established for the writing of checks and the paying of bills. Check writing usually is done on a specific day or days of each month. An exception sometimes arises when it is possible to realize a good discount if payment of a bill is made within a specified time, for instance,

Statement of Account 14700 CT

014143759	R		1	12/20/99
Account Number	Type	Items	Page No.	Statement Date

001

Current Balance	Previous Statement Date	Previous Balance
2896.34	11/21/99	2886.59

ANSWERS TO YOUR BANKING QUESTIONS 24 HOURS A DAY,
7 DAYS A WEEK. CALL ANSWERLINE TODAY

**** SUPER INSURED MONEY MARKET ACCOUNT ****

YOUR OPENING BALANCE OF: 2,886.59

NO DEPOSITS LISTED TOTALING: .00

- - - - - - - - - - OTHER CREDITS - - - - - - - - - -

12-20 SUPER INSURED MONEY MKT. INT. PAID 9.75

1 CREDITS LISTED TOTALING: 9.75

NO CHECKS LISTED TOTALING: .00

NO DEBITS LISTED TOTALING: .00

EQUALS YOUR ENDING BALANCE OF: 2,896.34

DAILY ACCOUNT BALANCES

DATE	BALANCE	DATE	BALANCE	DATE	BALANCE
12-20	2896.34				

- - - - - - - - - - SUPER INSURED MONEY MARKET STATEMENT - - - - - - - - - -

DATE	COLLECTED BALANCE	INTEREST RATES	DATE	COLLECTED BALANCE	INTEREST RATES
11-22	2,886.59	04.40	11-25	2,886.59	04.40
11-26	2,886.59	04.40	11-27	2,886.59	04.40
12-02	2,886.59	04.40	12-03	2,886.59	04.40
12-04	2,886.59	04.15	12-05	2,886.59	04.15
12-06	2,886.59	04.15	12-09	2,886.59	04.15
12-10	2,886.59	04.15	12-11	2,886.59	04.15
12-12	2,886.59	04.15	12-13	2,886.59	04.15
12-16	2,886.59	04.15	12-17	2,886.59	04.15
12-18	2,886.59	04.15	12-19	2,886.59	04.15
12-20	2,886.59	04.15			04.15

FIGURE 18–3 Example of a money market account statement. This type of check-writing has limited privileges.

PROCEDURE 18–1

Writing Checks in Payment of Bills

GOAL

To correctly write checks for payment of bills

EQUIPMENT AND SUPPLIES

Checkbook
Bills to be paid

PROCEDURAL STEPS

1 Locate the first bill to be paid. Before writing the check, fill out the stub or the place designated for recording expenditures. Include the date, name of payee, amount of check, the new balance to be carried forward, and usually the purpose of the check.
PURPOSE: To prevent the possibility of delivering or mailing a check without entering the information in the checkbook.

2 Complete both the check and the stub with pen or typewriter.
PURPOSE: To avoid danger of alteration for any reason.

3 Date the check the day it is written (do not postdate).

4 Write the name of the payee after the printed words, "Pay to the Order of ______" with the necessary information following. Do not use abbreviations unless so instructed.

5 Leave no space before the name, and follow it with three dashes if there is space remaining.

6 Omit personal titles from the names of payees.

7 If a payee is receiving a check as an officer of an organization, the name of the office should follow the name. Example: "John F. Jones, Treasurer."

8 Start writing at the extreme left of each space. Leave no blank spaces. Keep the cents notation close to the dollars figure to prevent alteration.

9 Verify that the amount of the check is recorded correctly on the stub, in the box for the dollar ($) amount, and on the line where the amount is written in words.

10 If a check is written for an amount less than one dollar, the figures by the $ sign may be circled or enclosed in parentheses ($0.65) to emphasize the amount.

10 days. Such discounts are usually indicated at the bottom of invoices or billing statements.

When a check is written in payment of a statement or invoice, it is good practice to write on the invoice the number of the check and the date it was paid. Then if any question arises about whether or when the bill was paid, you can readily locate the check stub. The handling and writing of checks must be done with extreme care (see Procedure 18–1).

THE BUSINESS CHECKBOOK

The checkbook most generally used in the professional office has three checks per page with a perforated stub at the left end of the check (Fig. 18–4). The checks may be in a bound soft cover or punched for a ring binder. The check and matching stubs are numbered in sequence and preprinted with the depositor's name and account number and any additional optional information such as address and telephone number. From 100 to 300 checks are usually ordered at one time, and the cost is charged against the account. Numbered deposit slips are also supplied to the depositor.

CHECKBOOK STUBS

The check stub (the part that remains in the book after the check has been written and removed) is the depositor's own record of the checks written, date, amount, payee, and purpose. It is important that the stub be completed before the check is written (Fig. 18–5). This prevents the possibility of writing a

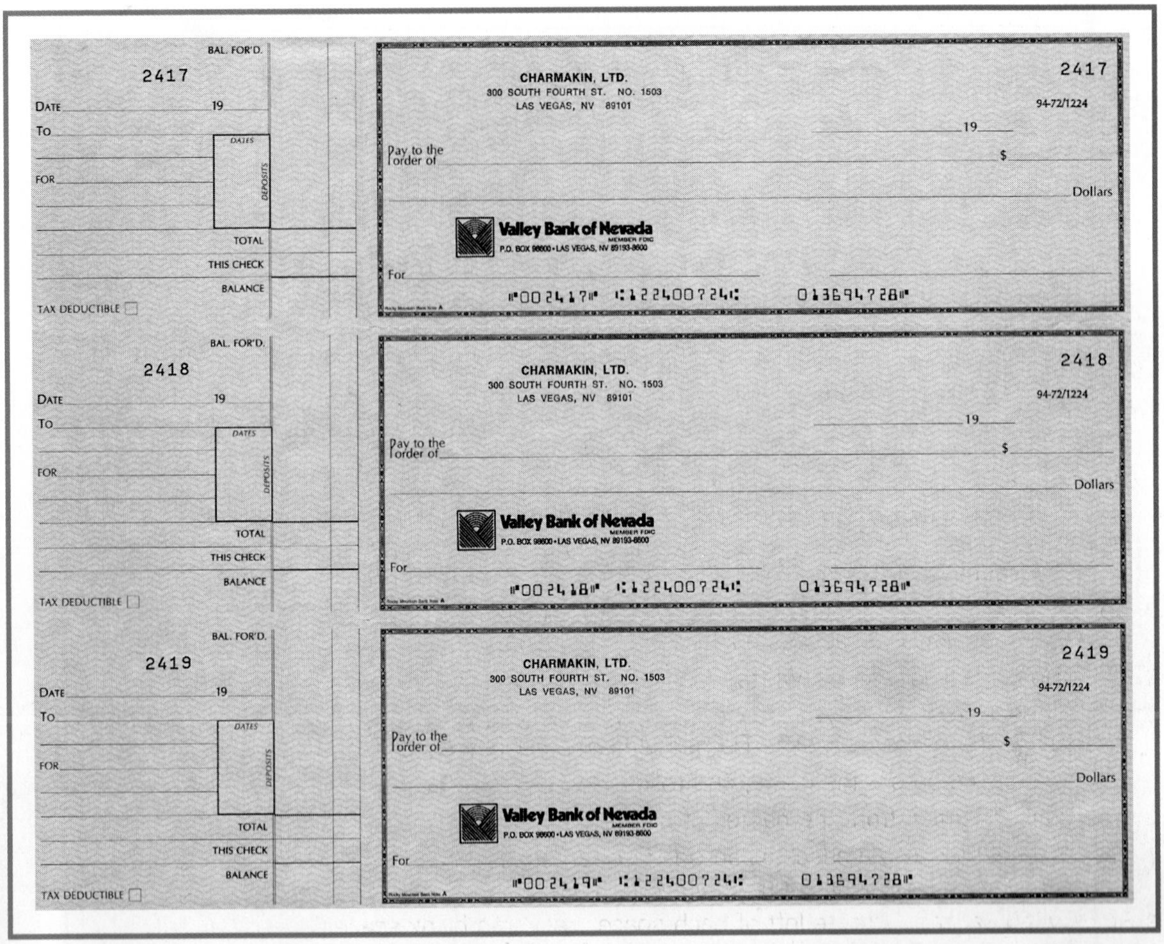

BAL. FOR'D.
2417
DATE ______ 19 ___
TO ______
FOR ______
DATES | DEPOSITS
TOTAL
THIS CHECK
BALANCE
TAX DEDUCTIBLE ☐

CHARMAKIN, LTD.
300 SOUTH FOURTH ST. NO. 1503
LAS VEGAS, NV 89101

2417
94-72/1224
______ 19 ___
Pay to the order of ______ $ ______
______ Dollars
Valley Bank of Nevada
MEMBER FDIC
P.O. BOX 98600 • LAS VEGAS, NV 89193-8600
For ______
002417 122400724 013694728

BAL. FOR'D.
2418
DATE ______ 19 ___
TO ______
FOR ______
DATES | DEPOSITS
TOTAL
THIS CHECK
BALANCE
TAX DEDUCTIBLE ☐

CHARMAKIN, LTD.
300 SOUTH FOURTH ST. NO. 1503
LAS VEGAS, NV 89101

2418
94-72/1224
______ 19 ___
Pay to the order of ______ $ ______
______ Dollars
Valley Bank of Nevada
MEMBER FDIC
P.O. BOX 98600 • LAS VEGAS, NV 89193-8600
For ______
002418 122400724 013694728

BAL. FOR'D.
2419
DATE ______ 19 ___
TO ______
FOR ______
DATES | DEPOSITS
TOTAL
THIS CHECK
BALANCE
TAX DEDUCTIBLE ☐

CHARMAKIN, LTD.
300 SOUTH FOURTH ST. NO. 1503
LAS VEGAS, NV 89101

2419
94-72/1224
______ 19 ___
Pay to the order of ______ $ ______
______ Dollars
Valley Bank of Nevada
MEMBER FDIC
P.O. BOX 98600 • LAS VEGAS, NV 89193-8600
For ______
002419 122400724 013694728

FIGURE 18–4 Example of business check with stub. (Courtesy of Valley Bank of Nevada, Las Vegas, NV.)

check and neglecting to complete the stub. If the stub is not completed and the check is sent out, you will have no record of the payee and the amount taken from the account until the canceled check is returned at a later date. Consequently, you will be unable to balance the account or determine the amount on hand until those canceled checks are returned by the bank. It is possible to get this information from the bank after the check has been cashed. There may be a charge for this service.

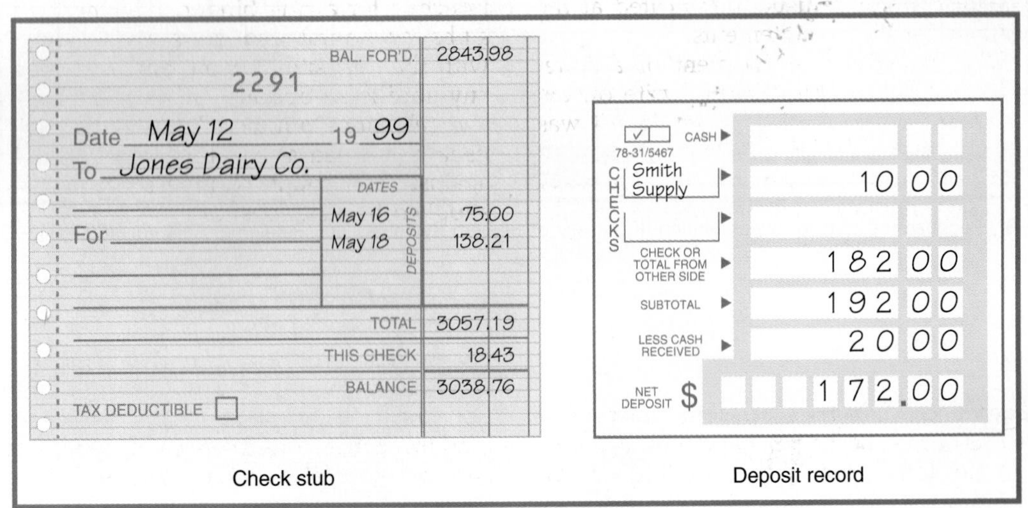

BAL. FOR'D. 2843.98
2291
Date May 12 19 99
To Jones Dairy Co.
For ______
DATES | DEPOSITS
May 16 | 75.00
May 18 | 138.21
TOTAL 3057.19
THIS CHECK 18.43
BALANCE 3038.76
TAX DEDUCTIBLE ☐

Check stub

☑ CASH ▶
78-31/5467
CHECKS
Smith Supply ▶ 10 00
▶
CHECK OR TOTAL FROM OTHER SIDE ▶ 182 00
SUBTOTAL ▶ 192 00
LESS CASH RECEIVED ▶ 20 00
NET DEPOSIT $ 172.00

Deposit record

FIGURE 18–5 Methods of filling out check stubs.

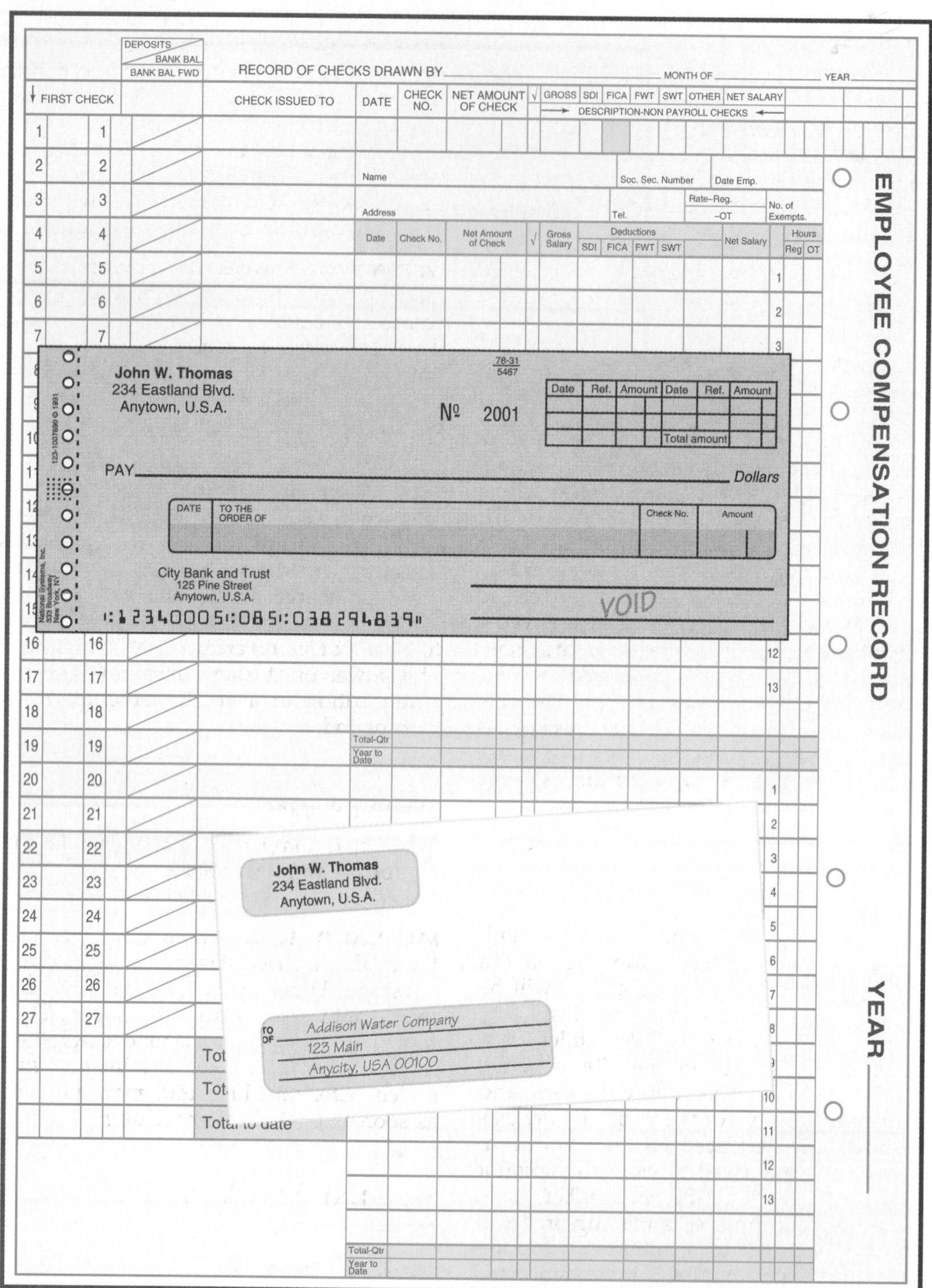

FIGURE 18–6 Pegboard system for check writing. (Courtesy of Bibbero Systems, Inc., Petaluma, California (800) 242-2376, Fax (800) 242-9330.)

COMPUTER-GENERATED CHECKS

Instead of ordering checks to be printed by the bank, personalized checks can be ordered from printing houses to fit your computer financial program (e.g., *Quicken*). Checks can be prepared on the computer in much the same manner as using a typewriter. The checks may have one or more copies that serve as the record of checks written.

ONE-WRITE CHECK WRITING

A one-write system of writing checks can save time and minimize errors in medical office **disbursements.** The office with a pegboard bookkeeping system (see Chapter 17) may wish to include one-write check writing. By using a combination check-writing system, such as the one illustrated in Figure 18–6, one check and one record of checks drawn handle both bill paying and payroll check writing.

When the check is written, a permanent record is created through the carbonized line of the check onto the record of checks drawn and the employee's payroll record, including a record of all deductions. Space is provided for the payee's address so that the check can be mailed in a window envelope. This not only saves time but also ensures that the check goes to the right address. Suppliers of basic pegboard systems can also provide a check-writing system such as the one described.

LOST AND STOLEN CHECKS

If any of the checks are lost, report this to the bank promptly. The bank will place a warning on the account, and signatures on incoming checks will be carefully inspected to detect possible forgeries.

If you suspect that checks have been stolen, first make a report to the police in the city or town where the theft took place. Then notify the bank and relate the time, date, and place the police report was made. A warning will be placed on the account. In some cases, you may be asked to close the account and open a new one under a different number.

As long as the loss of the checks missing or stolen has been reported to the proper authorities, the depositor usually will not be held responsible for losses due to forgery. The bank or merchant who accepts the forged checks will be charged for the loss. For this reason, anyone accepting a check from a person who is not known personally must be very careful about establishing the person's identity.

WRITING CHECKS

HANDLING CORRECTIONS AND MISTAKES Do not cross out, erase, or change any part of a check. Checks are printed on sensitized paper so that erasures are easily noticeable, and the bank has the right to refuse to pay on any check that has been altered. Figures 18–7 and 18–8 show examples of correct and incorrect check writing.

If a mistake is made, write the word **VOID** on the stub and the check, but do not throw out or destroy the check. It should be filed with the canceled checks so that it is available for auditing purposes.

WRITING CASH CHECKS A cash check is a check made payable to cash or bearer. Such checks are completely negotiable. Because these checks are easily cashed without positive identification, it is poor policy to write cash checks unless they are to be cashed at the time they are written. Banks may require that the person receiving the cash endorse the check.

SIGNING CHECKS After all checks have been written, place them, along with the invoices or other verifying information, on the physician's desk for signature. In some practices, the medical assistant who has charge of the financial matters is also allowed to sign the checks. This is accomplished by filing a **power of attorney** at the depositor's bank. The power of attorney may limit the check-signing authorization to a certain amount or to a limited time period.

Memory Jogger

Why is it important to complete the check stub before writing a check?

MAILING CHECKS When checks are sent through the mail, the check should not be visible through the envelope. Either place the check within a letter or fold it into a plain sheet of paper. Checks may be folded at the right end to conceal the amount of money written. Make certain the envelopes are sealed before mailing, and mail all checks yourself as soon as possible after writing.

Special Problems with Checks

Special problems may arise when a check is written on nonexistent funds or when a payer wishes, for a legitimate reason, to prevent the payee from cashing a check.

ACCOUNT OVERDRAWN OR OVERDRAFT

When a depositor draws a check for more than the amount on deposit in the account, the account becomes overdrawn. In most states, it is illegal to issue

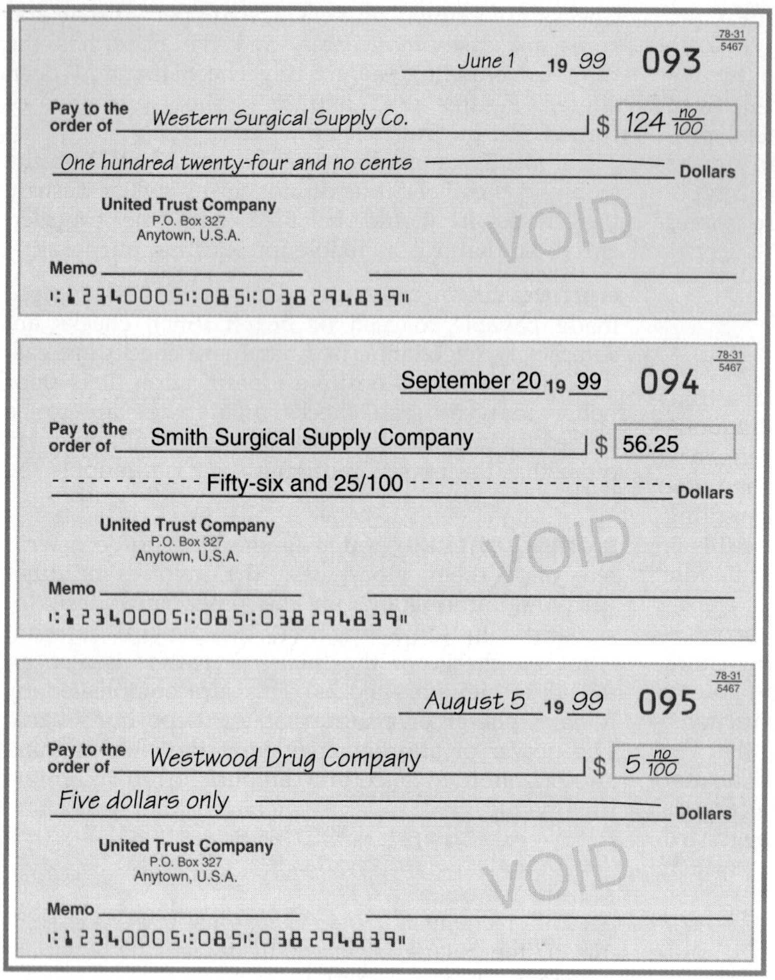

78-31/5467
June 1 19 99 093
Pay to the order of Western Surgical Supply Co. $ 124 no/100
One hundred twenty-four and no cents Dollars
United Trust Company
P.O. Box 327
Anytown, U.S.A.
VOID
Memo
⑆1234000 5⑆085⑆038 294839⑈

78-31/5467
September 20 19 99 094
Pay to the order of Smith Surgical Supply Company $ 56.25
------------ Fifty-six and 25/100 -------------------- Dollars
United Trust Company
P.O. Box 327
Anytown, U.S.A.
VOID
Memo
⑆1234000 5⑆085⑆038 294839⑈

78-31/5467
August 5 19 99 095
Pay to the order of Westwood Drug Company $ 5 no/100
Five dollars only Dollars
United Trust Company
P.O. Box 327
Anytown, U.S.A.
VOID
Memo
⑆1234000 5⑆085⑆038 294839⑈

FIGURE 18–7 Correct methods of writing checks.

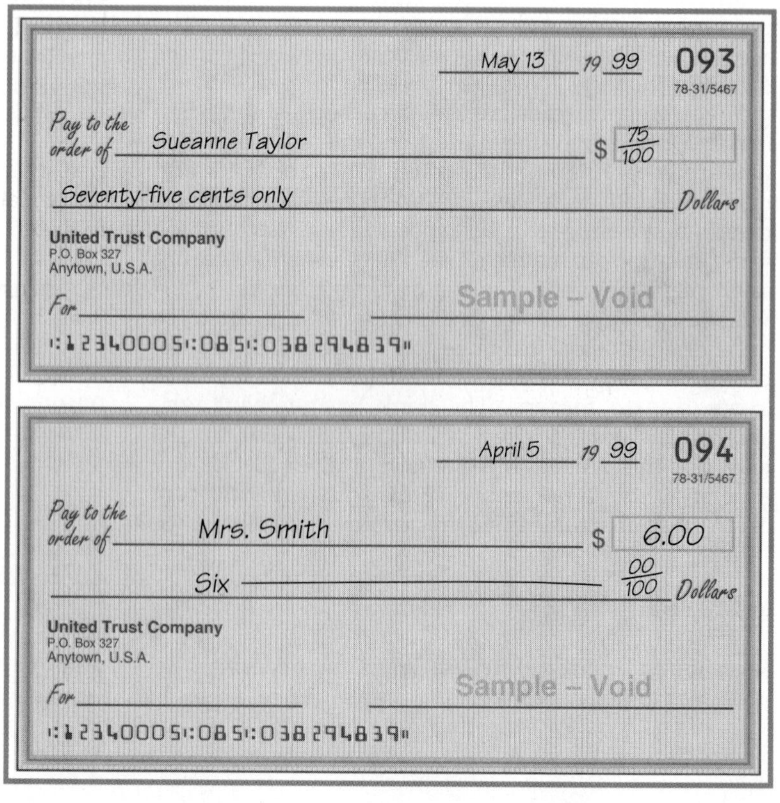

May 13 19 99 093
78-31/5467
Pay to the order of Sueanne Taylor $ 75/100
Seventy-five cents only Dollars
United Trust Company
P.O. Box 327
Anytown, U.S.A.
For
Sample – Void
⑆1234000 5⑆085⑆038 294839⑈

April 5 19 99 094
78-31/5467
Pay to the order of Mrs. Smith $ 6.00
Six 00/100 Dollars
United Trust Company
P.O. Box 327
Anytown, U.S.A.
For
Sample – Void
⑆1234000 5⑆085⑆038 294839⑈

FIGURE 18–8 *Top,* Correct method of writing a check. *Bottom,* Incorrect method of writing a check, with incomplete name and space for altering (e.g., 6.00 could be made into 26.00 or more and 00 could be made into 88).

a check for more than the amount on deposit in the bank. Should this happen through error or oversight, the bank may refuse to honor the check and will return it to the bank that presented it for payment. Such a check is said to "bounce."

If the check is written by an established depositor, the bank may honor the check and notify the depositor that the account is overdrawn. If the bank thus pays or covers the check, it issues an overdraft on the depositor's account.

STOP-PAYMENT ORDER

A depositor or maker of a check who wishes to rescind or stop payment of that check has the right to request the bank to stop payment on it. Stop-payment orders should be used only in emergencies. Reasons for stop-payment requests are

- Loss of a check
- Disagreement about a purchase
- Disagreement about a payment

Payment from Patients

ACKNOWLEDGING PAYMENT IN FULL

If payment in full is to be recognized in regard to a given check, the statement "Payment in Full to Date" must appear *on the back of the check,* above the endorsement, not on the face of the check. Canceled checks are a receipt for the maker of the check, not for the payee.

PRECAUTIONS IN ACCEPTING CHECKS

The medical assistant is frequently presented with checks in payment for the physician's services. In most cases, these are personal checks. See Guidelines for Accepting Checks

GUIDELINES FOR ACCEPTING CHECKS

- Scan the check carefully for the correct date, amount, and signature.
- Do not accept a check with corrections on it.
- If you do not know the person presenting a personal check, ask for identification and compare signatures.
- Accept an out-of-town check, government check, or payroll check only if you are well acquainted with the person presenting it and it does not exceed the amount of the payment.
- Acceptance of a **third-party check** is generally unwise. A third-party check is one made out to your patient by a party unknown to you. A check from the patient's health insurance carrier is an exception.
- When accepting a postal money order for payment, make certain it has only one endorsement. Postal money orders with more than two endorsements will not be honored.
- Do not accept a check marked "Payment in Full" unless it does pay the account in full up to and including the date on which it is received. If a check so marked is less than the amount due, you will be unable to collect the balance on the account once you have accepted and deposited such a check. It is illegal for you to scratch out the words "Payment in Full."
- Accepting checks written for more than the amount due and returning cash for the difference between the amount of the check and the amount owed is poor policy. If the check is not honored by the bank, your office will suffer the loss not only of the amount of the check but also of the amount returned in cash.

Endorsement of Checks

An endorsement is a signature plus any other writing on the back of a check by which the **endorser** transfers all rights in the check to another party. Endorsements are made in ink, with either pen or rubber stamp, on the back of the check across the left (or perforated) end.

NECESSITY FOR ENDORSEMENT

The Uniform Negotiable Instrument Act, applicable in all states, explains the need of an endorsement as follows:

> *An instrument is negotiated when it is transferred from one person to another in such a manner as to pass title to another party. If payable to bearer, it is negotiated by delivery. If payable to order, it is negotiated by the endorsement of the holder completed by delivery.*

The name of the last endorser of the check shows who last received the money. If a check is cashed for someone who did not endorse it and is returned for some reason, the bank will charge the check to the last endorser, not to the last person receiving the money. For this reason, it is not wise to cash a check made payable to another party without having the endorsement of the person who delivered the check to you for cashing.

KINDS OF ENDORSEMENTS

There are four principal kinds of endorsements. Blank and restrictive endorsements are the ones most commonly used.

BLANK ENDORSEMENT The payee signs only his or her name. This makes the check payable to the bearer. It is the simplest and most common type of endorsement on personal checks but should be used only when the check is to be cashed or deposited immediately.

RESTRICTIVE ENDORSEMENT This specifies the purpose of the endorsement. You use a restrictive endorsement in preparing checks for deposit to the physician's checking account. An example is shown in Figure 18–9.

Pay to the Order of
Midwest National Bank
Main Branch
For Deposit Only
CARLOS MACAULEY
301-012697

FIGURE 18–9 Example of restrictive endorsement.

SPECIAL ENDORSEMENT This endorsement includes words specifying the person to whom the endorser makes the check payable. For instance, a check naming Helen Barker as payee may be endorsed to the physician by writing on the back of the check

Pay to the order of
Theodore F. Wilson, M.D.
Helen Barker

The check is still negotiable but requires Dr. Wilson's signature or endorsement.

QUALIFIED ENDORSEMENT The effect of the endorsement is qualified by disclaiming or destroying any future liability of the endorser. Usually the words "without recourse" are written above by an attorney who accepts a check on behalf of a client but who has no personal claim in the transaction.

ENDORSEMENT METHODS

The medical assistant may use a blank endorsement when cashing a check to replenish the petty cash fund. This endorsement should be made only at the time of exchanging the check for cash.

As checks from patients and other sources arrive, they should be recorded on the ledger and immediately stamped with the restrictive endorsement *For Deposit Only*. This is a safeguard against lost or stolen checks.

Any endorsement should agree exactly with the name on the face of the check. If the name of the payee is misspelled, it is usually necessary for the payee to endorse the check the way the name is spelled on the face, followed by the correctly spelled signature. The Uniform Commercial Code, Section 3-203, states

> *Where an instrument is made payable to a person under a misspelled name or one other than his own, he may endorse in that name or his own or both; but signature in both names may be required by a person paying or giving value for the instrument.*

Most banks accept routine stamp endorsement that is restricted to deposit only, if the customer is well known and maintains an established account. Some insurance checks or drafts require a personal signature endorsement; a stamped endorsement is not acceptable. This will be stated on the back of the check. In such cases, ask the payee to endorse the check, then stamp immediately below the signature the restrictive endorsement *For Deposit Only*.

Memory Jogger

Name and describe the endorsement that is usually used in preparing checks for deposits to the physician's checking account.

Making Deposits

Financial duties of the medical assistant include depositing checks and reconciling the bank statements with the checkbook. Checks should be deposited promptly because

- There is the possibility of a stop-payment order.
- The check may be lost, misplaced, or stolen.
- Delay may cause the check to be returned because of insufficient funds.
- The check may have a restricted time for cashing.
- It is a courtesy to the payer.

PREPARING THE DEPOSIT

Deposit slips are itemized memoranda of cash or other funds that a depositor presents to the bank with the money to be credited to the account. All deposits must be accompanied by a deposit slip. A carbon or photocopy of the deposit slip should be kept on file. (See Procedure 18–2.)

There are several types of deposit slips, sometimes

PROCEDURE 18-2

Preparing a Bank Deposit

GOAL

To prepare a bank deposit for the day's receipts and complete appropriate office records related to the deposit.

EQUIPMENT AND SUPPLIES

Currency
Six checks for deposit
Deposit slip
Endorsement stamp (optional)
Typewriter
Envelope

PROCEDURAL STEPS

1 Organize currency.
PURPOSE: To arrange currency in the best order for speedy and accurate presentation to the teller.

2 Total the currency and record the amount on the deposit slip.

3 Place restrictive endorsements on the checks, using an endorsement stamp or the typewriter.
PURPOSE: To transfer the title and protect checks from loss or theft.

4 List each check separately on the deposit slip by ABA number and its amount.

5 Total the amount of currency and checks and enter on the deposit slip.

6 Enter the amount of the deposit in the checkbook.
PURPOSE: To record the current balance in the account.

7 Prepare a copy of the deposit slip for the office record, including the names of the payers.
PURPOSE: For verification of checks deposited, if necessary.

8 Place the currency, checks, and deposit slip in an envelope for transporting to the bank.

called *deposit tickets*. The commercial slip is used for the office checking account. The deposit slips are printed with the number of the account in magnetic ink characters to correspond with the checks. Preprinted deposit slips are ordered along with the checks.

Some write-it-once accounting systems include a deposit slip that the bank will accept as the itemization if it is attached to the customer's numbered deposit slip. The deposit slip should be prepared before you go to the bank, with the money organized and ready to present to the bank **teller.**

Payment on patient accounts is generally made by check, but some payments are made in currency (paper money). Each type of funds is recorded separately on the deposit slip. The currency is usually listed first. Organize the currency so that all of the bills are facing in the same direction—that is, the black side up with the portrait right-side-up. Place the largest bills on top.

Checks are recorded individually by the ABA number. If the checks are arranged alphabetically by the names of the patient accounts, with these names included on your office copy of the deposit slip, you will have a ready reference of checks deposited should a question arise regarding a patient's payment. Follow the procedure listed below for preparing a deposit slip (Fig. 18-10):

1. List all checks on the back of the deposit slip.
2. Transfer the total to the front of the slip.
3. Enter the amount of the total deposit on the deposit slip stub.

Money orders, either postal, express, or others, are identified by PO Money Order or Express MO. Remember that money orders cannot have more than two endorsements.

The deposit slip should be carefully totaled and the total entered in the checkbook. Any torn bills should be mended with transparent tape. Clip the currency together, and clip the checks in a separate packet. Then place the entire amount in a heavy envelope for taking to the bank. Deposit the currency and checks daily if possible.

Memory Jogger

How are checks identified when they are listed on a deposit slip?

FOR DEPOSIT TO THE ACCOUNT OF

Central Electronics, Inc.
111 Central Ave.
Anytown, USA 29042

CASH	CURRENCY	330	00
	COIN	-0-	
LIST CHECKS SINGLY			
TOTAL FROM OTHER SIDE		905	00
TOTAL		1235	00
LESS CASH RECEIVED			
NET DEPOSIT		1235	00

78-31
5467

DATE November 10 19 99

Deposits may not be available for immediate withdrawal

SIGN HERE FOR LESS CASH IN TELLER'S PRESENCE

USE OTHER SIDE FOR ADDITIONAL LISTING

Be sure each item is properly endorsed

City Savings & Loan
PO Box 11100
Anytown, USA 29042

⑆1234000 5⑆085⑆038 294839⑈

PLEASE LIST EACH CHECK SEPARATELY BY BANK NUMBER

CHECKS	DOLLARS	CENTS
1 Blue Shield	535	00
2 Medicare	320	00
3 Thompson, R.J.	15	00
4 Swann, E.B.	20	00
5 Whitt, L.W.	15	00
6		
7		
8		
9		
10		
11		
12		
13		
14		
15		
16		
Please forward total to reverse side		

CASH COUNT—FOR OFFICE USE ONLY

X 100	
X 50	
X 20	
X 10	
X 5	
X 2	
X 1	
TOTAL	$ 905 00

FIGURE 18–10 Front and back of deposit slip.

DEPOSITING BY MAIL

Depositing by mail saves time and is easily accomplished if the deposit consists of checks only. Banks usually supply their customers with special mailing deposit slips and envelopes on request (Fig. 18–11). Some mailing deposit slips have an attached portion that the bank will stamp and return to the customer as a receipt. Others may provide the customer with a receipt card that is sent along with the deposit each time for the bank's notation. The mailer shown in Figure 18–11 has a peel-off receipt for the depositor's records. Mailed deposits are prepared in the same manner as are regular deposits, but certain precautions should be observed.

DEPOSIT BY MAIL PRECAUTIONS

1 Do not send cash or currency by mail. If this is absolutely necessary, then send it by registered mail.
2 Use only a restrictive endorsement; use a deposit stamp or write the notation "For Deposit Only to the account of ______."
3 If you have not obtained mailing deposit slips or your bank does not provide them, make duplicate slips and mail them with your deposit. Ask the bank to stamp one copy and return it to you as a receipt.

RETURNED CHECKS

Occasionally, the bank may return a deposited check because of some irregularity such as a missing signature or missing endorsement. More often, it is because the payer has insufficient funds on deposit to cover the check.

If the check is stamped "NSF," indicating nonsufficient funds, do not delay in contacting the person who gave you the check. If you are unable to contact the maker of a bad check, waste no time in tracking down all leads, such as referrals, numbers you obtained from credit cards, driver's license, and so forth. There are several places to which bad checks may be reported. Credit associations are often a great help when such problems arise. Turn the account over to a qualified collection agency if you do not succeed in collecting on the account yourself within a short time.

If a check is returned to your office marked "No Account," and it is a check that you had deposited promptly, you have obviously been swindled. This check should be given to the police, the local Better Business Bureau, or your collection agency.

Bank Statement

A statement is periodically sent by the bank to the customer; it shows the status of the customer's account on a given date. This statement indicates the

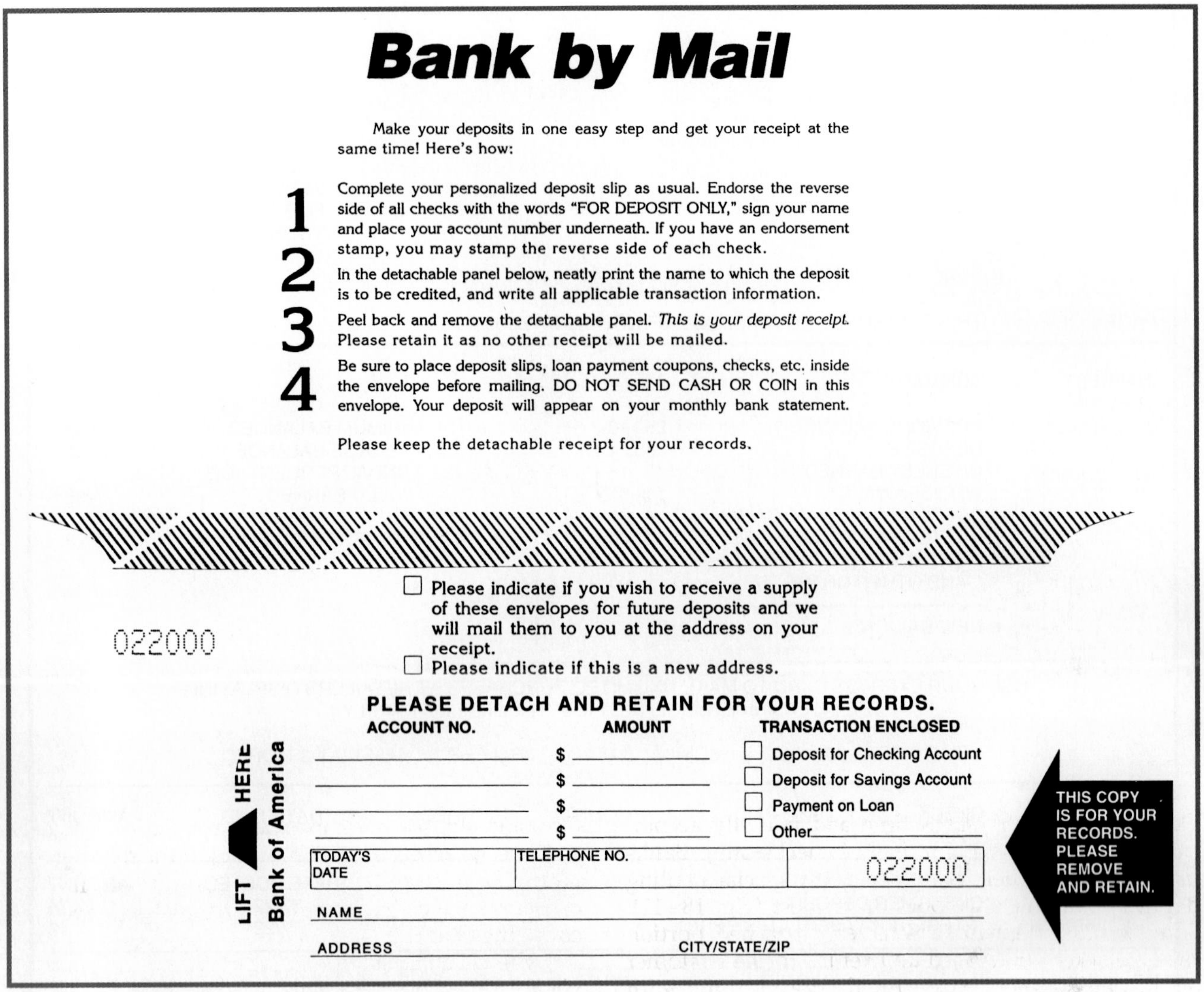

Bank by Mail

Make your deposits in one easy step and get your receipt at the same time! Here's how:

1 Complete your personalized deposit slip as usual. Endorse the reverse side of all checks with the words "FOR DEPOSIT ONLY," sign your name and place your account number underneath. If you have an endorsement stamp, you may stamp the reverse side of each check.

2 In the detachable panel below, neatly print the name to which the deposit is to be credited, and write all applicable transaction information.

3 Peel back and remove the detachable panel. *This is your deposit receipt.* Please retain it as no other receipt will be mailed.

4 Be sure to place deposit slips, loan payment coupons, checks, etc. inside the envelope before mailing. DO NOT SEND CASH OR COIN in this envelope. Your deposit will appear on your monthly bank statement.

Please keep the detachable receipt for your records.

022000

☐ Please indicate if you wish to receive a supply of these envelopes for future deposits and we will mail them to you at the address on your receipt.
☐ Please indicate if this is a new address.

PLEASE DETACH AND RETAIN FOR YOUR RECORDS.

LIFT HERE
Bank of America

ACCOUNT NO.	AMOUNT	TRANSACTION ENCLOSED
	$	☐ Deposit for Checking Account
	$	☐ Deposit for Savings Account
	$	☐ Payment on Loan
	$	☐ Other

TODAY'S DATE	TELEPHONE NO.	022000

NAME

ADDRESS CITY/STATE/ZIP

THIS COPY IS FOR YOUR RECORDS. PLEASE REMOVE AND RETAIN.

FIGURE 18–11 Example of bank-by-mail deposit envelope. (Courtesy of Valley Bank of Nevada, Las Vegas, NV.)

- Beginning balance
- Deposits received
- Checks paid
- Bank charges
- Ending balance

The bank statement (Fig. 18–12) is usually accompanied by the customer's canceled checks. Many banks are now microfilming canceled checks and storing the information in the bank's computer. The customer is asked for permission to use this procedure and has the privilege of requesting a copy of any check when needed. Bank statements are prepared at regular intervals, usually once per month.

RECONCILING THE BANK STATEMENT

The bank statement balance and the customer's checkbook balance will usually be different, except in a relatively inactive account. The two balances must be reconciled. The **reconciliation** discloses any errors that may exist in the checkbook or, on rare occasions, in the bank statement (Fig. 18–13).

The bank statement may include an entry for service charges that must be deducted from the checkbook balance. In all types of accounts, the bank may charge a fee for services. Usually in the case of an individual account, it is a flat fee; in a business account, the fee is based on services rendered. If the average or minimum balance is maintained at an established level, the bank may forego a service charge.

Most banks ask to be notified within 10 days of any error found in the statement. The bank statement should be reconciled as soon as it is received. You will usually find a form to follow in carrying out this procedure on the back of the bank statement.

0821-402054

#821

N
2

CALL (888) 555-2932
24 HOURS/DAY, 7 DAYS/WEEK
FOR ASSISTANCE WITH
YOUR ACCOUNT.

PAGE 1 OF 2 THIS STATEMENT COVERS: 6/22/99 THROUGH 7/22/99

INTEREST CHECKING
0821-402054

SUMMARY

PREVIOUS BALANCE	252.10
DEPOSITS	68.74+
INTEREST EARNED	.18+
WITHDRAWALS	109.55−
CUSTOMER SERVICE CALLS	.00−
INTERLINK/PURCHASE FEE	.00−
MONTHLY CHECKING FEE AND OTHER CHARGES	.00−
▶ **NEW BALANCE**	**211.47**

MINIMUM BALANCE	142.55
AVERAGE BALANCE	220.00
ANNUAL PERCENTAGE YIELD EARNED	.96%
INTEREST EARNED 1994	2.23

USE YOUR EXPRESS CARD TO MAKE UNLIMITED PURCHASES AT RETAILERS DISPLAYING THE INTERLINK SYMBOL. (A $1 MONTHLY FEE MAY APPLY.)

TRY IT TODAY AT ARCO . . . MOBIL . . . LUCKY . . . RALPHS . . . SAFEWAY & MORE!

CHECKS AND WITHDRAWALS

CHECK	DATE PAID	AMOUNT	CHECK	DATE PAID	AMOUNT
202	7/05	15.05	203	7/15	94.50

DEPOSITS

	DATE POSTED	AMOUNT
CUSTOMER DEPOSIT	7/22	68.74
INTEREST PAYMENT THIS PERIOD	7/22	.18

BALANCE INFORMATION

DATE	BALANCE	DATE	BALANCE	DATE	BALANCE
6/22	252.10	7/05	237.05	7/15	142.55
				7/22	211.47

24 HOUR CUSTOMER SERVICE

EACH ACCOUNT COMES WITH 3 COMPLIMENTARY CALLS PER STATEMENT PERIOD.

CALLS TO 24 HOUR CUSTOMER SERVICE THIS STATEMENT PERIOD: 0

INTEREST INFORMATION

FROM	THROUGH	INTEREST RATE	ANNUAL PERCENTAGE YIELD (APY)
6/22	7/22	1.00%	1.01%

INTEREST RATE/APY AS OF 7/22/94 IF YOUR BALANCE IS

$ 0 - 4,999	1.00%	1.01%
$ 5,000 - 9,999	1.00%	1.01%
$ 10,000 AND OVER.	1.00%	1.01%

CALL 1-800-555-2932 IN CALIFORNIA ANYTIME FOR CURRENT RATES.

MEMBER FDIC

STATEMENT

FIGURE 18–12 Example of regular checking account statement.

THIS WORKSHEET IS PROVIDED TO HELP YOU BALANCE YOUR ACCOUNT

1. Go through your register and mark each check, withdrawal, Express ATM transaction, payment, deposit or other credit listed on this statement. Be sure that your register shows any interest paid into your account, and any service charges, automatic payments, or Express Transfers withdrawn from your account during this statement period.

2. Using the chart below, list any outstanding checks, Express ATM withdrawals, payments or any other withdrawals (including any from previous months) that are listed in your register but are not shown on this statement.

3. Balance your account by filling in the spaces below.

ITEMS OUTSTANDING		
NUMBER	AMOUNT	
TOTAL	$	

ENTER

The NEW BALANCE shown on this statement ____________________ $______

ADD

Any deposits listed in your register or transfers into your account which are not shown on this statement.
$______
$______
$______
+$______

TOTAL ________ +$______

CALCULATE THE SUBTOTAL __________ $______

SUBTRACT

The total outstanding checks and withdrawals from the chart at left __________ −$______

CALCULATE THE ENDING BALANCE

This amount should be the same as the current balance shown in your check register ________________ $______

IF YOU SUSPECT ERRORS OR HAVE QUESTIONS ABOUT ELECTRONIC TRANSFERS

If you believe there is an error on your statement or Express ATM receipt, or if you need more information about a transaction listed on this statement or an Express ATM receipt, please contact us immediately. We are available 24 hours a day, seven days a week to assist you. Please call the telephone number printed on the front of this statement. Or, you may write to us at United Trust Company, P.O. Box 327, Anytown, USA.

1) Tell us your name and account number or Express card number.

2) As clearly as you can, describe the error or the transfer you are unsure about, and explain why you believe there is an error or why you need more information.

3) Tell us the dollar amount of the suspected error.

You must report the suspected error to us no later than 60 days after we sent you the first statement on which the problem appeared. We will investigate your question and will correct any error promptly. If our investigation takes longer than 10 business days (or 20 days in the case of electronic purchases), we will temporarily credit your account for the amount you believe is in error, so that you may have use of the money until the investigation is completed.

FIGURE 18–13 Reverse side of bank statement to be used for reconciling checking account.

PROCEDURE 18–3
Reconciling a Bank Statement

GOAL
To reconcile a bank statement with the checking account

EQUIPMENT AND SUPPLIES
Ending balance of previous statement
Current bank statement
Canceled checks for current month
Checkbook stubs
Calculator
Pen

PROCEDURAL STEPS
1 Compare the opening balance of the new statement with the closing balance of the previous statement.
PURPOSE: To determine that the balances are in agreement.

2 Compare the canceled checks with the items on the statement.
PURPOSE: To verify that they are your checks and that they are listed in the right amount.

3 Arrange the canceled checks in numerical order and compare with the checkbook stubs.

4 Place a checkmark (√) on each stub for which a canceled check has been returned.
PURPOSE: To locate any outstanding checks.

5 List and total the outstanding checks.

6 Verify that all previous outstanding checks have cleared.

7 Subtract the total of the outstanding checks from the bank statement balance.
NOTE: Do not include any certified checks as outstanding because their amount has already been deducted from the account.

8 Add to the total in Step 7 any deposits made but not included in the bank statement.
PURPOSE: To correct the credits in the bank statement balance.

9 Total any bank charges that appear on the bank statement and subtract them from the checkbook balance. Such charges may include service charges, automatic withdrawals or payments, and NSF checks.
PURPOSE: To correct the checkbook balance.

10 If the checkbook balance and the statement balance do not agree, match the bank statement entries with the checkbook entries.

The reconciliation procedure may be put in a formula, as shown below:

BANK STATEMENT RECONCILIATION FORMULA

Bank statement balance	$_____	
Less outstanding checks	$_____	
Plus deposits not shown	$_____	
Corrected Bank Statement Balance		$_____
Checkbook balance	$_____	
Less any bank charges	$_____	
Corrected Checkbook Balance		$_____

If the two *corrected balances* agree, you may stop there. If they do not agree, *subtract* the lesser figure from the greater figure; the difference will usually give you a clue to locating the error. (See Procedure 18–3.)

QUESTIONS TO ASK IN SEARCHING FOR A POSSIBLE ERROR

- Is your arithmetic correct?
- Did you forget to include one of the outstanding checks?
- Did you fail to record a deposit or did you record it twice?

- Do all stubs and checks agree?
- Have you carried your figures forward correctly?
- Have you transposed a figure? (If the amount of your error is divisible by nine, you probably did.)
- Did someone write a check without your knowledge?
- Did you fail to correct your checkbook balance at the time of the previous statement?

Many persons find the reconciliation process confusing at first, but after a few times it becomes easier and fairly routine.

Medical Assistant's Position of Trust

The medical assistant who manages the financial responsibilities of a medical practice is in a position of great trust. Conscientious and reliable attention to detail in this position can be a great source of job satisfaction and an attribute toward job security.

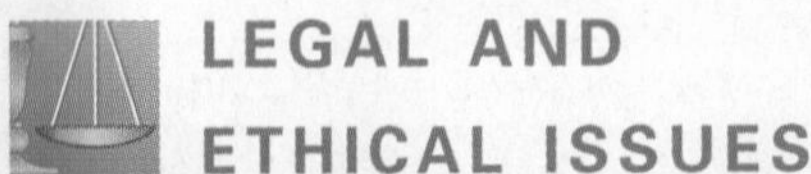

LEGAL AND ETHICAL ISSUES

If a mistake is made in preparing a check, do not destroy this check. Rather, write VOID across the check, make a note on the check stub, and file the check with canceled checks for auditing purposes.

A stop-payment order may be placed with the bank in an emergency, such as a check being lost, or a disagreement about a purchase or payment.

Do not accept a check made payable to another party without having the endorsement of the person who gives it to you. If the check is returned by the bank for any reason, the responsibility for the check will be charged to the last endorser, not the last person to receive the money.

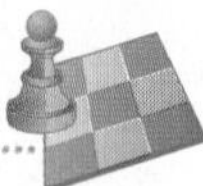

CRITICAL THINKING

1 Shortly after you arrive at the office on Monday morning you discover that the office checkbook is missing. What action(s) would you take?

2 What is the simplest type of check endorsement, and when can it safely be used?

3 A patient wishes to pay an outstanding account at the end of an office visit. The balance is $70 and the patient offers a check in the amount of $100 written to the patient by a party unknown to you. How would you handle this situation? Why?

HOW DID I DO? Answers to Memory Joggers

1 *a.* A cashier's check is the bank's own check signed by an authorized officer of the bank. A certified check is a depositor's check that has been certified by a bank officer's signature.
b. A traveler's check requires a signature at the time of purchase and a second signature when it is used.

2 An insured money market savings account usually requires a minimum balance, draws interest at money market rates, and allows the writing of checks (limited number).
The ordinary savings account has no minimum balance, draws interest at the lowest prevailing rate, and has no check-writing privileges.

3 Prevents the possibility of neglecting to complete stub, which would leave you unable to balance checkbook until that check is returned.

4 Restrictive endorsement. Specifies the purpose of the endorsement (e.g., deposit to account).

5 By ABA number.

REFERENCES

American Medical Association: The Business Side of Medical Practice. Chicago, AMA, 1989.

Fess PE, et al: Accounting Principles, 17th ed. Cincinnati, South-Western Publishing, 1993.

Billing and Collection Procedures

19

OUTLINE

LEARNING OBJECTIVES

Cognitive: On successful completion of this chapter you should be able to:

1. Define and spell the terms listed in the Vocabulary.
2. Name the three ways by which payment for medical services is accomplished.
3. List nine items that should be addressed in developing a credit policy.
4. State three reasons for itemizing billing statements.
5. Describe cycle billing and its advantages.
6. Discuss the significance of determining the collection ratio and the accounts receivable ratio.
7. List the three most common reasons for patients' failure to pay accounts.
8. Discuss the do's and don'ts of telephone collection procedures.
9. Name five sources of information in tracing skips.
10. State the procedure to follow on receiving notice of a debtor's bankruptcy.
11. List three advantages of using small claims courts for collecting delinquent accounts.
12. Discuss five appropriate follow-up actions after assigning accounts to a collection agency.

Performance: On successful completion of this chapter you should be able to:

1. Prepare patients' monthly statements.
2. Calculate a collection ratio and an accounts receivable ratio.
3. Prepare an age analysis of accounts receivable.
4. Initiate proceedings to collect delinquent accounts.
5. Demonstrate telephone collection techniques.

VOCABULARY

accounts receivable ratio A formula for measuring how fast outstanding accounts are being paid

age analysis A procedure for classifying accounts receivable by age from the first date of billing

collection ratio A formula for measuring the effectiveness of the billing system

invasion of privacy Unauthorized disclosure of a person's private affairs

statute of limitations The time limit within which an action may legally be brought upon a contract

subsidize To aid or promote something (such as a private enterprise) with public money

superbill A combination charge slip, statement, and insurance reporting form

In Chapter 16 we discussed how fees are determined, the importance of advance discussion of fees, the adjusting or canceling of fees in hardship cases, and the legal aspects of credit arrangements. We also addressed the importance of getting adequate information on the first visit when it appears that an extension of credit will be necessary. Attention to these details helps immeasurably in the collection efforts that follow.

The collection of fees and account management of the medical practice is often entrusted to the medical assistant.

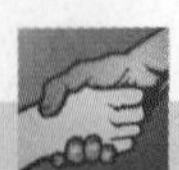

PERSONAL QUALITIES

HOW THE MEDICAL ASSISTANT CAN BE AN EFFECTIVE ACCOUNT MANAGER

- Believe that the physician and the facility have a right to charge for the services provided.
- Do not be embarrassed to ask for payment for the value of the service.
- Possess tact and good judgment.
- Give individual attention and personal consideration to each situation.
- Be courteous and show a sincere desire to help the patient who has financial problems.
- Try to find out the patient's reason for nonpayment when this occurs.

The payment for medical services is accomplished in four ways: (1) payment at time of services, (2) billing when extension of credit is necessary, (3) insurance or other third party, and (4) using outside collection assistance.

Payment at Time of Service

A large percentage of patients will have some type of health insurance for at least major items. Every practice in which there are patient visits should encourage time-of-service collection. It is especially important to collect copayments and payment for office visits not covered by insurance. If patients get into the habit of paying their current charges before they leave the office, there are no further billing and bookkeeping expenses. If patients are informed when making an appointment that payment is expected at the time of service, they are not surprised when you say at the end if the visit,

> Your charge for today is $xx. Will that be cash or check?

Many patients are hesitant to ask about charges and are unsure whether to offer to pay or to wait until asked. You will make it easier for the patients by offering to accept their payments, because most people are prepared to pay small bills on a cash basis. Even if a patient requests to be billed, you can say,

> The normal procedure is to pay at the time of service, but we can make an exception this time.

A patient who may have forgotten his or her checkbook should be given a self-addressed envelope with the charge slip and asked to send the payment in the next mail.

Memory Jogger

What are the benefits of time-of-service collections?

Billing After Extension of Credit

In some types of practice, particularly those involving large fees for surgery or long-term care, it becomes necessary to extend credit and establish a regular system of billing. This requires informing the patient of (1) what the charges will be, (2) what professional services these charges cover, and (3) the credit policy of the office.

CREDIT POLICY

Many practices do not have a true credit policy; thus, each account continues to be evaluated individually. It is almost impossible to judge accounts objectively and equitably under such circumstances.

The physician and the staff should think through their situation, decide what they expect of patients with respect to payments, and how they will inform the patient. Although there will always be exceptions to any rule, there must *be* a rule, which should be in writing and conveyed to the patient at the outset of the relationship.

Some medical practices prepare an information booklet that includes the payment policy. New patients are given a copy of the booklet. Any patient who needs special consideration can be counseled by the medical assistant. (See Issues to be Addressed in Credit Policy.) The medical assistant who has the guidance and support of an established credit policy can perform with confidence when handling patient accounts.

ISSUES TO BE ADDRESSED IN CREDIT POLICY

1 When payment is due from patients
2 When the practice requires payment at time of service
3 When or if assignment of insurance benefits is accepted
4 Whether insurance forms will be completed by the office staff
5 Billing procedures
6 Collection protocol
7 How long an account will be carried without payment
8 Telephone collection protocol
9 Sending accounts to a collection agency

INDEPENDENT BILLING SERVICE

Many health care facilities find it advantageous to refer their billing and collections to an independent billing service. The information related to services and fees is sent to the billing service on a daily or weekly basis. The servicing agent then handles all billing and collections, as well as any telephone inquiries. This system frees the regular office staff for more patient-oriented duties. An added advantage is that any dispute that may arise is handled by a person who is not connected with the patient care on a personal basis.

Memory Jogger

How does having a credit policy benefit the collection of fees?

Internal Billing by the Account Manager

This chapter is directed to billing fee-for-service patients in a private practice. Insurance and managed care billing are addressed in following chapters.

METHODS AND APPEARANCE OF BILLING

In a practice with only a moderate number of accounts, the medical assistant handles the preparation and mailing of statements. This may be accomplished by a (1) computer-generated statement, (2) superbill, (3) typewritten statement, or (4) photocopied statement.

The appearance of the statement carries a visual impact just as a letter does, so the statement heads should be carefully chosen and the typing clean and accurate. Statement heads are usually imprinted with the same information as the physician's letterhead. They should be of good quality and large enough to allow itemization of charges. Envelopes should be imprinted with "Address Correction Requested" under the return address, to maintain up-to-date mailing lists. A self-addressed return envelope included with the statement encourages prompt payment. This is mainly for the convenience of patients who do not always have stationery available for sending a return payment or who are less likely to return a payment immediately if they must address an envelope.

Computer-Generated Statement

Patient accounts are generated and stored in the computer, and a statement can be produced whenever needed. The statement can show the service rendered on each date, the charge for each service, the date on which a claim was submitted to the insurance company, the date of payment, and the balance due from the patient. The computer may also be programmed to print messages on the statement, such as "Balance now 30 days past due," or a selection of other messages.

Superbill

The **superbill** is a combination charge slip, statement, and insurance reporting form. There are variations in style, but they are usually personalized for the practice. Figure 19–1 is an example of a form used in the practice of an endocrinologist. It has space for all the elements required in submitting medical insurance claims:

- Name and address of patient
- Name of insurance carrier
- Insurance identification number
- Brief description of each service by code number

LIC. # 181181
S.S. # 052-56-3472
UPIN # F29065

MARGARET J. NACHTIGALL, M.D.
Reproductive Endocrinology
251 EAST 33RD STREET
NEW YORK, N.Y. 10016

TELEPHONE: (212) 683-0519
FAX: (212) 779-8432

PATIENT INFORMATION

PATIENT'S LAST NAME	FIRST	INITIAL	BIRTHDATE / /	SEX ☑ FEMALE	TODAY'S DATE / /
ADDRESS	CITY	STATE ZIP	RELATION TO SUBSCRIBER	REFERRING PHYSICIAN	
SUBSCRIBER OR POLICYHOLDER			INSURANCE CARRIER		
ADDRESS	CITY	STATE ZIP	INS. ID	COVERAGE CODE	GROUP
OTHER HEALTH COVERAGE? ☐ NO ☐ YES IDENTIFY		DISABILITY RELATED TO: ☐ IND. ☐ ACCIDENT ☐ PREGNANCY ☐ OTHER		DATE SYMPTOMS APPEARED, INCEPTION OF PREGNANCY, OR ACCIDENT OCCURRED: / /	

ASSIGNMENT & RELEASE: I hereby assign my insurance benefits to be paid directly to the undersigned physician. I am financially responsible for non-covered services. I also authorize the physician to release any information required to process this claim.
SIGNED: (Patient, or Parent, if Minor) DATE: / /

✔	DESCRIPTION	CODE	FEE	✔	DESCRIPTION	CODE	FEE	✔	DESCRIPTION	CODE	FEE
	OFFICE VISIT				**OFFICE PROCEDURES**				**LABORATORY - IN OFFICE**		
	New Patient				Sperm Wash	58323			Pregnancy Test	85160	
	Consultation	99204			Cauterization of Cervix	57510			Urinalysis	81002	
	Comprehensive	99205			Cervical Biopsy	57500			Stool Occult Blood	82270	
	OFFICE VISIT				Endocervical Curettage	57505			Lyme Titer	86317	
	Established Patient				Endometrial Biopsy	58100			Estradiol	82670	
	Limited	99211			Office Endometrial Curettage	58102			Chemistry	80019	
	Intermediate	99212			Post Coital Test	89300			CBC, pit., Diff.	85024	
	Extended	99213			Artificial Insemination	58310			T3 Uptake	84479	
	Comprehensive	99214			Pelvic Sonogram	76856			T4	84435	
	Comprehensive	99215			Vulvar Biopsy	56600			TSH	84443	
	SURGERY				Bilateral Mammogram	76091			ESR	85650	
	D & C	58120			Unilateral Mammogram	76090			Pregnancy Test	84702	
	Pregnancy Termination	59840			Breast Ultrasound	76645			FSH	83000	
	Laparoscopy	56305			Abdominal Ultrasound	76700			Prolactin	84146	
	Hysteroscopy	56351			Polypectomy	57500					
	Laporotomy	49000									
	Myomectomy	58140									
	Hysterectomy	58150									

DIAGNOSIS: **ICD-9**

- ☐ Abortion, Incomplete 634.71
- ☐ Abortion, Spontaneous 634.90
- ☐ Alopecia 704.09
- ☐ Amenorrhea 626.0
- ☐ Anemia 285.9
- ☐ Anovulation 628.0
- ☐ Atrophic Vaginitis 627.3
- ☐ Breast Cyst 610.1
- ☐ Breast Mass 611.72
- ☐ Breast Pain 611.71
- ☐ Cervical Polyp 622.7
- ☐ Cervicitis 616.0
- ☐ Condyloma 091.3
- ☐ Cyclic Adrenal Hyperplasia .255.2
- ☐ Cystocele 618.0
- ☐ Cystitis 595.9
- ☐ Diabetes Mellitus 250.0
- ☐ Dysmenorrhea 625.3
- ☐ Dyspareunia 625.0
- ☐ Dysuria 788.1
- ☐ Ectopic Pregnancy 633.9
- ☐ Edema 782.3
- ☐ Endometrial Hyperplasia ..621.3
- ☐ Endometriosis 617.0
- ☐ Fatigue 780.7
- ☐ Fibrocystic Breast Disease .610.1
- ☐ Galactorrhea 676.6
- ☐ Headache 784.0
- ☐ Hemorrhoids 455.6
- ☐ Herpes 054.1
- ☐ Hypercholesterolemia 272.0
- ☐ Hyperprolactinemia 253.1
- ☐ Hypertension 401.9
- ☐ Hyperthyroidism 242.9
- ☐ Hypothyroidism 244.9
- ☐ Infertility 628.9
- ☐ Luteal Phase Insufficiency .628.8
- ☐ Menometrorrhagia 626.2
- ☐ Menopausal Syndrome 627.2
- ☐ Menorrhagia 626.2
- ☐ Monilial Vaginitis 112.1
- ☐ Obesity 278.0
- ☐ Osteoarthritis 715.9
- ☐ Osteopenia 733.9
- ☐ Osteoporosis 733.0
- ☐ Ovarian Cyst 620.2
- ☐ Ovarian Insufficiency 256.3
- ☐ Pelvic Pain 625.9
- ☐ Polycystic Ovary Syndrome 256.4
- ☐ Postmenopausal Bleeding .627.1
- ☐ Pregnancy V22.2
- ☐ Pregnancy Termination ...V72.4
- ☐ Premature Ovarian Failure .256.3
- ☐ Premenopausal Menorrhagia .627.0
- ☐ Prolactinoma 253
- ☐ Prolapsed Uterus 618.1
- ☐ Rectocele 569.1
- ☐ Thyroiditis 245.2
- ☐ Trichomonas 131.0
- ☐ Urinary Tract Infection 599.0
- ☐ Uterine Fibroids 218.9
- ☐ Vasomotor Instability 780.2
- ☐ Vaginitis 616.1
- ☐ Vulvitis 616.1

DIAGNOSIS: (IF NOT CHECKED ABOVE)	ADDITIONAL INFORMATION:	DOCTOR'S SIGNATURE

SERVICES PERFORMED AT: ☐ OFFICE ☐ University Hospital 560 First Avenue N.Y., N.Y. 10016 ☐ Day Surgery / University Hosp. 530 First Avenue N.Y., N.Y. 10016

REFERRING PHYSICIAN:

ACCEPT ASSIGNMENT? ☐ YES ☐ NO

TOTAL TODAY'S FEE	
PREVIOUS BALANCE	
AMT. REC'D. TODAY	
NEW BALANCE	

INSTRUCTIONS TO PATIENT FOR FILING INSURANCE CLAIMS:

1. COMPLETE UPPER PORTION OF THIS FORM; SIGN AND DATE.
2. MAIL THIS FORM DIRECTLY TO YOUR INSURANCE COMPANY. YOU MAY ATTACH YOUR OWN INSURANCE COMPANY'S FORM IF YOU WISH, ALTHOUGH IT IS NOT NECESSARY.

PLEASE REMEMBER THAT PAYMENT IS YOUR OBLIGATION, REGARDLESS OF INSURANCE OR OTHER THIRD PARTY INVOLVEMENT.

INSUR-A-BILL ® BIBBERO SYSTEMS, INC. • PETALUMA, CA • © 5/95 (SB M-N) (REV. 9/96)

FIGURE 19–1 Superbill. (Courtesy of Bibbero Systems, Inc., Petaluma, California (800) 242-2376, Fax (800) 242-9330.)

- Fee for each service
- Place and date of service
- Diagnosis
- Physician's name and address
- Physician's signature

The superbill can be used as a charge slip for office treatments if the physician checks the services performed at the completion of the visit and asks the patient to hand it to the medical assistant when leaving. Either the physician or the medical assistant may write in the amount of the fee. If a payment is made, it can be so indicated. Instructions to the patient for filing insurance claims are on the bottom left. The physician's office keeps one copy, the patient is given the original, and one copy is for filing with the insurance company.

Statements must be correct and must include the

BILLING NAME	NAMES OF OTHER FAMILY MEMBERS
PATIENT'S NAME	
RES. PHONE / BUS. PHONE	
OCCUPATION	RELATIVE OR FRIEND
EMPLOYED BY	REFERRED BY
INS. INFORMATION	SOC. SEC. NUMBER
FORM NO. MDP. 8550	1976 BIBBERO SYSTEMS, INC. SAN FRANCISCO

GEORGE D. GREEN, M.D.
JOHN F. WHITE, M.D.
Family Practice
100 MAIN STREET, SUITE 14
ANYTOWN, CALIFORNIA 90000
TELEPHONE: (999) 399-6000

STATEMENT TO:

TEAR OFF AND RETURN UPPER PORTION WITH PAYMENT

DATE	PROFESSIONAL SERVICE	FEE	PAYMENT	ADJUST-MENT	NEW BALANCE
9-10-94	99213	30 –			30 –
10-8	99215	110 –			140 –
	88151	22 –			162 –
11-15	Insurance		129 60		32 40

PROFESSIONAL SERVICE CODES:
1. OFFICE VISIT
2. HOME VISIT
3. HOSPITAL VISIT
4. EMERGENCY ROOM
5. CONSULTATION
6. IMMUNIZATION
7. INJECTION
8. DRUGS/SUPPLIES/MATERIALS
9. COLLECTION OF LAB. SPEC.
10. SPECIAL REPORTS
11. OTHER SERVICES
12. SPEC. DIAGNOSTIC SERVICES
13. SPEC. THERAPEUTIC SERV.
14. EXTENDED CARE FACILITY
15. CUSTODIAL CARE
16. OBSTETRICAL CARE
17. SURGICAL
18. CASTS
19. LABORATORY
20. X-RAY
21. ALLERGY TEST.
22. NO CHARGE
23. ADJUSTMENTS OR CORRECTIONS
24. TOTAL CARE

GEORGE D. GREEN, M.D.
CAL. LIC. # 6-2856

JOHN F. WHITE, M.D.
CAL. LIC. # G-5281

FIGURE 19–2 Itemized statement. (Courtesy of Bibbero Systems, Inc., Petaluma, California (800) 242-2376, Fax (800) 242-9330.)

patient's name and address as well as the balance owed. If statements are photocopied or microfilmed, special care must be taken that the ledger card is correct because it will be duplicated in the billing process.

Typewritten Statements

The use of continuous form billing statements is a timesaver. The statements are printed in a roll with perforated edges for separation. The roll is fed into the typewriter for the first statement and remains until the last statement is typed, eliminating the time and energy necessary for inserting and removing each statement form from the typewriter.

Another timesaver is the multiple-copy statement. The Colwell Company calls its version "E-Z Statements." The E-Z Statement features three monthly statements plus one patient's ledger card in each set, all in NCR (no carbon required) paper. Services and payments are posted during the month, and at billing time the top sheet is removed, folded, and mailed in a window envelope. If more than three mailings are required, a new set must be headed and the balance forwarded.

Photocopied Statements

Coordinated ledger cards and copy paper are used in preparing photocopied statements. A perfect statement is ready for mailing in minimum time. Extra care must be used in posting the ledgers. A black pen should be used in making entries on the ledger card, because other ink colors do not reproduce well. Writing must be clear and legible. There should be no personal notes made on the ledger cards unless it is something you wish conveyed to the patient. (It is possible to buy pencils with nonreproducible lead if you believe this is necessary for making collection entries.) Usually a window envelope is used for mailing, which means that the name and address on the ledger must be neat, correct, and in the right position for the envelope window.

PROCEDURE FOR INTERNAL BILLING

Itemizing the First Statement

If the medical fee has been explained in advance, as discussed in Chapter 16, the monthly statement is merely a confirmation of what is owed, and there should be no misunderstanding. However, it is good business practice—and a courtesy to the patient—to itemize the charges. This is essential if the statement is to be used for billing the patient's insurance. Patients are entitled to an understanding of the physician's statement for medical services (Fig. 19–2).

Itemizing statements is not difficult. The simplest method is merely to allow space on the original statement, below the "For Professional Services" line, on which to list the separate charges for office, house, or hospital calls or for treatments or tests performed in the medical facility.

Many physicians have devised their own itemized charge slips; these are given to the patient when payment is made at the time of service or later mailed in a combination statement-reply envelope. Use of such charge slips simplifies the itemization procedure, because filling out the slips is usually just a matter of checking the procedures listed. An itemized charge slip is shown in Figure 19–3. Although the itemization of bills may seem an unnecessary waste of time, if you do itemize you will spend less time in explaining services provided, clearing up misunderstandings with patients, and following up on delinquent accounts.

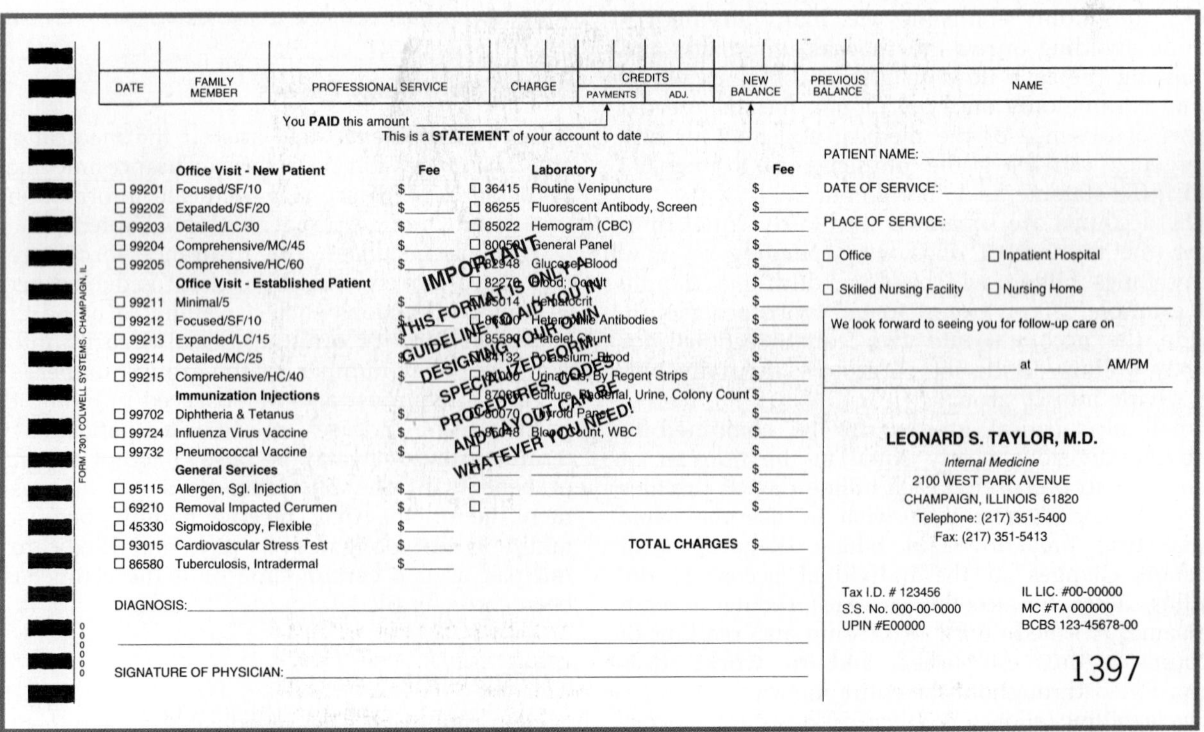

DATE	FAMILY MEMBER	PROFESSIONAL SERVICE	CHARGE	CREDITS		NEW BALANCE	PREVIOUS BALANCE	NAME
				PAYMENTS	ADJ.			

You **PAID** this amount ______

This is a **STATEMENT** of your account to date ______

	Office Visit - New Patient	Fee		Laboratory	Fee
☐ 99201	Focused/SF/10	$____	☐ 36415	Routine Venipuncture	$____
☐ 99202	Expanded/SF/20	$____	☐ 86255	Fluorescent Antibody, Screen	$____
☐ 99203	Detailed/LC/30	$____	☐ 85022	Hemogram (CBC)	$____
☐ 99204	Comprehensive/MC/45	$____	☐ 80050	General Panel	$____
☐ 99205	Comprehensive/HC/60	$____	☐ 82948	Glucose, Blood	$____
	Office Visit - Established Patient		☐ 82270	Blood; Occult	$____
☐ 99211	Minimal/5	$____	☐ 85014	Hematocrit	$____
☐ 99212	Focused/SF/10	$____	☐ [illegible]	Heterophile Antibodies	$____
☐ 99213	Expanded/LC/15	$____	☐ 85590	Platelet Count	$____
☐ 99214	Detailed/MC/25	$____	☐ 84132	Potassium; Blood	$____
☐ 99215	Comprehensive/HC/40	$____	☐ [illegible]	Urinalysis, By Regent Strips	$____
	Immunization Injections		☐ [illegible]	Culture, Bacterial, Urine, Colony Count	$____
☐ 99702	Diphtheria & Tetanus	$____	☐ 80070	Thyroid Panel	$____
☐ 99724	Influenza Virus Vaccine	$____	☐ 85048	Blood Count, WBC	$____
☐ 99732	Pneumococcal Vaccine	$____	☐ ____	____	$____
	General Services		☐ ____	____	$____
☐ 95115	Allergen, Sgl. Injection	$____	☐ ____	____	$____
☐ 69210	Removal Impacted Cerumen	$____	☐ ____	____	$____
☐ 45330	Sigmoidoscopy, Flexible	$____			
☐ 93015	Cardiovascular Stress Test	$____		**TOTAL CHARGES**	$____
☐ 86580	Tuberculosis, Intradermal	$____			

IMPORTANT
THIS FORMAT IS ONLY A GUIDELINE TO AID YOU IN DESIGNING YOUR OWN SPECIALIZED FORM. CODES, PROCEDURES, AND LAYOUT CAN BE WHATEVER YOU NEED!

DIAGNOSIS: ______

SIGNATURE OF PHYSICIAN: ______

FORM 7301 COLWELL SYSTEMS, CHAMPAIGN, IL

PATIENT NAME: ______

DATE OF SERVICE: ______

PLACE OF SERVICE:

☐ Office ☐ Inpatient Hospital

☐ Skilled Nursing Facility ☐ Nursing Home

We look forward to seeing you for follow-up care on ______ at ______ AM/PM

LEONARD S. TAYLOR, M.D.
Internal Medicine
2100 WEST PARK AVENUE
CHAMPAIGN, ILLINOIS 61820
Telephone: (217) 351-5400
Fax: (217) 351-5413

Tax I.D. # 123456
S.S. No. 000-00-0000
UPIN #E00000

IL LIC. #00-00000
MC #TA 000000
BCBS 123-45678-00

1397

FIGURE 19–3 Charge slip. (Courtesy of Colwell Systems, Champaign, IL.)

Time and Frequency of Billing

A regular system of mailing statements should be put into operation. Most people expect to receive statements from their creditors, and they plan their budgets around first-of-the-month bills received. Punctuality in billing encourages prompt payment.

Statements should be sent at least once each month. Some offices send bills immediately after treatment; others bill all patients on the same day each month. Mailing statements twice a month—for example, half of the accounts on the 10th and the remaining half on the 25th—is also common practice.

According to the Fair Credit Billing Act of October 28, 1975, when a billing date for an account has been established, the date of mailing the statement must not vary more than five days without notification to the patient/debtor. If there is a *balance due* or a *credit balance* of one dollar or more, the account must be billed every 30 days.

ONCE-A-MONTH BILLING If a monthly pattern is followed, bills should leave your office in time to reach the patient no later than the last day of each month and preferably by the 25th of the month. Planning ahead for the preparation of statements can lighten the burden of once-a-month billing. The statement can be prepared at the time of service (or during slack periods), postdated, and mailed at the end of the month.

CYCLE BILLING Many physicians prefer to use the cycle billing system, which calls for the billing of certain portions of the accounts receivable at given times during the month instead of preparing all statements at the end of each month. Cycle billing is used in large businesses such as department stores, banks, and utility companies. Its many advantages include avoiding once-a-month peak workloads and stabilizing the cash flow. In a small office in which billing is done only once per month, the unexpected illness or absence of the medical assistant for any emergency can leave the physician in a financial bind if the statements do not go out.

The accounts are separated into fairly equal divisions, the number of divisions depending on how many times billing will be done during a month. For example, if you expect to bill twice per month, divide the accounts into two equal sections; for weekly billing, divide into 4 groups; for daily billing, divide into 20 groups.

Small alphabetical groups can be combined to keep the divisions nearly equal in the number of statements to prepare on each billing day. If the files are color coded, you may wish to use the same alphabetical breakdown in billing. Regardless of constant changes in the individual accounts, the mailing dates for accounts in each section remain the same. A schedule for processing and mailing of accounts is thus established, and the workload is apportioned throughout the entire month.

Cycle billing allows the medical assistant to continue all routine duties each day, handling the statements on a day-to-day or weekly schedule rather than in one intensive period at the end of the month. This means that whole days need not be sacrificed from other duties to get statements in the mail. By spacing the billing throughout the month, more time and consideration can be given to each statement, the itemization of bills is less burdensome, and the likelihood of error is decreased.

Patients generally accept the cycle billing system quickly, often with enthusiasm. However, if your office decides to change from a once-a-month billing system to a cycle billing system, patients should be notified in advance, and the new plan should be explained to them. To explain the new system to established patients, enclose a notice in each statement for 2 months preceding the transfer, describing the plan and indicating the future dates on which each patient will receive the bill.

Before a physician adopts the cycle billing system, particularly in a small community, several factors should be taken into consideration, such as

- What is the general income level of the community, and how and when does the average patient get paid?
- Do local companies pay employees at various times during the month, or are most paychecks handed out at the beginning of the month?
- Would cycle billing benefit patients as well as the overall operation of the office?

Memory Jogger

 *How does the Fair Credit Billing Act affect the frequency or date of mailing statements?*

Billing Third-Party Payers

Collection problems may arise if the medical assistant fails to get the necessary insurance information, particularly Medicare and Medicaid information (see section on Credit Arrangement in Chapter 16).

In some instances, the insurance forms are not completed correctly, and the claim is denied because of minor infractions such as failing to name the responsible party or omitting Social Security information, the policy number, or the group number.

Time limits must also be observed in billing third-party payers. In cases of Medicare patients with a terminal illness, it may be best to accept assignment of benefits. If the physician does not take assignment he or she may receive nothing because the family is not obligated to pay, and Medicare will not pay after a certain time or if the claim has not been correctly filed.

Billing Minors

Minors cannot be held responsible for payment of a bill unless they are emancipated (see Chapter 6).

PROCEDURE 19-1

Preparing Monthly Billing Statements

GOAL

To process monthly statements and evaluate accounts for collection procedures in accordance with the agency's credit policy.

EQUIPMENT AND SUPPLIES

Typewriter or computer
Patient accounts
Agency's credit policy
Statement forms

PROCEDURAL STEPS

1 Assemble all accounts that have outstanding balances
2 Separate accounts that need special attention in accordance with the agency's credit policy.
EXPLANATION: Routine statements should be prepared first, after which special attention can be given to delinquent accounts.
3 Prepare routine statements, including
- Date the statement is prepared
- Name and address of the person responsible for payment
- Name of the patient if different from the person responsible for payment
- Itemization of dates, services, and charges for the month
- Any unpaid balance carried forward (may or may not be itemized, depending on office policy)

4 Determine the action to be taken on accounts separated in step 2.
5 Make a note of the necessary action on the ledger card (telephone call, collection letter series, small claims court, or assignment to collection agency).
PURPOSE: For guidance in executing an action and for later follow-up when necessary.

Bills for minors must be addressed to a parent or legal guardian. If a bill is addressed to a minor, the parent or parents could take the attitude that they are not responsible because they never received the bill.

If the parents are separated or divorced, the parent who brings the child in for treatment is responsible for payment. Whatever financial agreement exists between the parents is strictly their personal business and should not concern the medical office. The responsible parent should be so informed from the beginning.

If an emancipated minor appears in the office and requests treatment and you can ascertain that the person is not living at home, the minor is responsible for the bill. It may be wise to make a determination either with the business manager or with the physician as to whether your office wishes to treat this emancipated minor. (See Procedure 19–1.)

Memory Jogger

When is a minor responsible for paying the cost of medical care?

Payment Collection

COLLECTION GOALS

Management consultants for the medical profession say that if good financial practices are followed, the accounts receivable on a physician's books should equal no more than 2 to 3 months' gross charges, but if the receivables start falling below the average of 1 month's total charges, perhaps the collection procedures are too stringent. Guidelines can be determined by establishing two ratios. Evaluation of collection is based on the **collection ratio** and the **accounts receivable ratio.**

Collection Ratio

The collection ratio measures the effectiveness of the billing system. A minimum of 6 to 12 months' data should be used in computing the collection ratio. The basic formula for figuring the collection ratio is to divide the total collections by the net charges

If you are unable to pay your account this month, please telephone this office (776-4900) before _______________ and let us know how you plan to take care of it.

Your balance due is $350.

FIGURE 19–4 Suggested note to patient for 60-day billing.

(gross charges minus any discounts) to reach a percentage figure. This calculation is illustrated in the following example:

EXAMPLE OF CALCULATING A COLLECTION RATIO

Gross Charges		$125,000
Less:		
Courtesy discounts	$5,000	
Third-party insurance allowance	6,000	
Other adjustments	1,000	
Total Adjustments		12,000
Net charges (gross charges minus adjustments)		
Total Collections		$113,000
$110,000 ÷ $113,000 = 97% collection ratio		110,000

Accounts Receivable Ratio

The accounts receivable ratio measures how fast outstanding accounts are being paid. The formula for figuring the accounts receivable ratio is to divide the current accounts receivable balance by the average gross monthly charges. A desirable accounts receivable ratio is less than 2 months. It is the medical assistant's responsibility to keep both the accounts receivable and collections within normal limits. The method of calculating the accounts receivable ratio is shown in the following example:

EXAMPLE OF CALCULATING ACCOUNTS RECEIVABLE RATIO

Annual Gross Charges	$125,000
Average Monthly Gross Charges (125,000 ÷ 12 months)	10,417
Current Acc/Rec Balance	16,000
Acc/Rec Ratio: 16,000 ÷ 10,417 = 1.54 months	

IMPORTANCE OF COLLECTING DELINQUENT ACCOUNTS

The reasons for pursuing collections go beyond the obvious one that a physician must be paid for services to pay expenses and continue to treat patients. Failure to collect can result in the loss of a patient. A person who owes money to the physician and is not prodded gently into payment may stay away in embarrassment or may even change physicians.

Noncollection of medical bills may also imply guilt. A patient may infer that the physician thought that the patient received inadequate or improper care, and a malpractice suit may result. It is also not fair to paying patients to make no attempt to collect from nonpaying patients. Abandoning accounts without collection follow-up encourages nonpayers, and, as a result, the paying patients indirectly **subsidize** the cost of medical care for those who can pay but do not.

Why Patients Do Not Pay

Most patients are honest. It is estimated that probably fewer than 4% never intend to pay. There may be a larger percentage who are financially "shipwrecked" and temporarily unable to pay. Also, a certain percentage of patients irresponsibly live beyond their incomes. According to the American Medical Association, the three most common reasons for patients' failure to pay are negligence, inability to pay, and unwillingness to pay.

Figures 19–4 and 19–5 illustrate notes that might be sent to patients to remind them of their financial obligations.

Know When to Say No

There must be some limit put on the time, effort, and expense invested in trying to collect an uncollectible account. Under some circumstances, it may be better simply to write off an unpaid account. An example of a letter that might be used to cancel the obligation and at the same time improve the image of the physician is shown in Figure 19–6.

Every courtesy has been extended to you in arranging for payment of your long overdue account. Our auditor suggests that it no longer be carried on our books.

Unless we hear from you by _______________, the account will be turned over to _______________ for collection.

FIGURE 19–5 Suggested final letter to patient.

PROCEDURE 19-2

Collecting Delinquent Accounts

GOAL

To initiate proceedings to collect delinquent accounts.

EQUIPMENT AND SUPPLIES

Typewriter or computer
Telephone
Delinquent accounts
Stationery
Collection letter series
Agency's credit policy

PROCEDURAL STEPS

1 Assemble the delinquent accounts
2 Separate accounts according to the action required.
PURPOSE: It is more efficient to process as a group all accounts requiring the same activity.
3 Make telephone calls to those so designated.
4 Record responses on the ledger cards.
PURPOSE: For further action as necessary.
5 Review the accounts requiring collection letters.
6 Choose an appropriate letter from the collection series and individualize it for the account in question.
PURPOSE: Form letters may be used as a guide but should be individualized to suit the situation.
7 Prepare the collection letter(s).
8 Make a notation of the action taken on the ledger card.
PURPOSE: To avoid repetition of the same letter if further action is necessary.

Date

Patient Name
Street Address
City, State ZIP Code

Dear Patient:

Your balance of $200 has been on our books for 23 months.

In view of the financial circumstances that make payment for these past services difficult for you, Dr. Johnson has instructed me to consider the debt cancelled. We will no longer bill you for it.

Dr. Johnson wants you to feel free to call on him for any future service you may require.

Sincerely yours,

Office Manager for
E. F. Johnson, M.D.

FIGURE 19-6 Example of a letter that cancels a fee.

ACCOUNTS RECEIVABLE AGE ANALYSIS

Dr.____________________

Address ____________________ Date __________

Patient's name	Total account receivable	Distribution of accounts receivable by age				Remarks
		1-2-3 months	4-5-6 months	7-8-9-10-11-12 months	over 1 year	
A	450.00	100.00	350.00			
B	50.00	50.00				
C	100.00		75.00	25.00		
D	200.00		10.00	150.00	40.00	
E	550.00		550.00			
F	42.50	42.50				
G	65.00	20.00	45.00			
H	325.00	325.00				

FIGURE 19–7 Form for accounts receivable age analysis.

AGING ACCOUNTS RECEIVABLE

Aging is a term used for the procedure of classifying accounts receivable by age from the first date of billing. It should be done on a regular basis. Aging of accounts helps collection follow-up, because it enables the medical assistant to tell at a glance what accounts need attention in addition to a regular statement. Computer billing programs usually include this feature. With sufficient time, an **age analysis** may be accomplished manually (Fig. 19–7).

If the patient is billed on the day of service, the aging begins on that day; if the first billing is 30 days after service, the aging begins at 30 days. Some systems use a breakdown of Current, 30 days, 60 days, 90 days, and 90-plus days.

Looking at Figure 19–7, you see that

- Patient A has a balance of $450. Unless regular payments are being made, this account may be heading toward a collection problem because $350 of the balance is more than 3 months old.
- Patient B presents no problem because the entire balance is current.
- Patient C definitely is a potential problem even though the account is small. The entire balance is more than 3 months old, and one fourth of it is more than 6 months old.
- Patient D's account should never have been allowed to reach this stage of delinquency. If there had been a good collection policy established, it would not have happened.

The age analysis is simply a tool to show at a glance the status of each account. There is no need to do this every month if time is at a premium. If the accounts are aged quarterly you will stay on top of the problem. Usually, a coding system with metal clip-on tabs or adhesive peel-off labels on the ledger cards is used in conjunction with the age-analysis system.

To illustrate, after two statements have been sent, a green tab may be placed on the record, indicating that a courteous reminder was sent with the last statement. The following month the green tab may be replaced with a yellow tab to show that a second payment request was sent in the form of a polite letter or printed request. An orange tab may be substituted the next month, indicating that the patient received a letter requesting prompt attention to the account. Red tabs may be reserved for the accounts of patients who, as a last resort, have been notified of a specific time limit in which payment must be made, after which sterner measures will be taken. If you reach this stage in pursuing a particular account, make certain that you record the date of the time limit on the patient's ledger.

The law requires that once you have made a statement indicating that a specific action will be taken, you must follow through or be liable for the consequences under the law (Fair Debt Collection Practices Act 1977).

If you say, for example, "I am going to turn your account over for collection unless it is paid within 10 days," then you must do so. If you state in a collection letter that you will be taking the debtor to small claims court if the account is not paid by a certain date, then you must do as you say. The intent of the law is to prevent the collector from making idle threats or harassing a debtor. A patient may sue for harassment if such idle threats are made.

Memory Jogger

5 *Briefly describe the process and reason for "account aging."*

COLLECTION TECHNIQUES

Persuasive collection procedures include telephone calls, collection reminders and letters, and personal interviews. (See General Rules to Follow in Telephone Collections.)

GENERAL RULES TO FOLLOW IN TELEPHONE COLLECTIONS

What To Do

1 Call the patient when you can do so in privacy.
2 Call between 8 AM and 9 PM.
3 Determine the identity of the persons with whom you are speaking. If you ask, "Is this Mrs. Noble?" and she answers "Yes" it could be the patient's mother-in-law or daughter-in-law, who is also "Mrs. Noble." Use the person's full name.
4 Be dignified and respectful in your attitude. You can be friendly and formal at the same time.
5 Ask the patient if it is a convenient time to talk with you. Unless you have the attention of the called party, there is little to be gained by continuing. If you are told that you have called at an inopportune time, ask for a specific time when you may call back, or get a promise for the patient to call you at a specified time.
6 After a brief greeting, state the purpose of your call. Make no apology for calling but state your reason in a friendly, business-like way. You expect payment and are interested in helping the patient meet the financial obligation. "This is Alice, Dr. Brown's financial secretary. I'm calling about your account." A well-placed pause at this point in the call sometimes gets an immediate response from the debtor in regard to the nonpayment.
7 Assume a positive attitude. For example, convey the impression that you know the patient intended to pay and it is only a matter of working out some suitable arrangements.
8 Keep the conversation brief and to the point, and avoid threats of any kind.
9 Try to get a definite commitment—payment of a certain amount by a certain date.
10 Follow up on promises. This is best accomplished by a tickler file or a note on your calendar. If the payment does not arrive by the promised date, remind the patient with another call. If you fail to do this, your whole effort has been wasted.

WHAT NOT TO DO

1 Do not call between 9 PM and 8 AM. To do so may be considered harassment.
2 Do not make repeated telephone calls.
3 Do not call the debtor's place of work if you know that the employer prohibits personal calls.
4 If you do place a call to the debtor at work and the person cannot take the call, you can leave a message asking the debtor to "call Mrs. Black at 727-9238" without revealing the nature of the call—that is, do not state that the call is from "Dr. Jones's office" or "Dr. Jones's medical assistant."
5 Do not lose your temper or show hostility. An angry patient is a poor-paying patient. Insulted patients often do not pay at all.

Telephone Collection Calls

A telephone call at the right time, in the right manner, is more effective than a collection letter. The personal contact of a telephone call will bring in more money than if a call is not made. In the absence of time to make calls, the collection letter is the next best avenue. If collections are a serious problem, it may pay to hire an extra person to do the telephoning. Written notification is a must before making a final demand for payment indicating that legal or collection proceedings will be started. There are no hard and fast rules for pursuing collections by telephone. You must handle each case individually on the basis of your own acquaintance or experience with the person involved.

Collection Letters

Some consultants believe that a printed collection letter or reminder enclosed with a statement is more effective than a personal letter. Their attitude is that a patient may be embarrassed by a personal letter and feel that he or she has been singled out for attention. An impersonal printed message will probably encourage the debtor to send a payment. The printed form is a time saver and is recommended if a lack of time is contributing to poor collection follow-up. Standard printed forms are readily available; you can also design your own forms.

Letters that are friendly requests for an explanation of why payment has not been made are still effective in many cases. These letters should indicate that the physician is sincerely interested in the patient and wishes to help straighten out the financial obligations. The patient should be invited to visit the office to explain the reasons for nonpayment so that, if possible, special arrangements can be worked out. To give the patient an opportunity to save face, these letters can suggest that the patient may have overlooked previous statements.

On receipt of such a letter, most patients make some effort to explain their failure to make payment. If a patient really is having financial difficulties, the physician may be able to get public assistance for him or her. Or, if it is a temporary financial embarrassment, the physician and the patient may together be able to work out a satisfactory installment plan for payment.

The medical assistant often is given a free hand in designing collection patterns and composing collection letters. Many medical assistants compose a series of collection letters, using model letters that they have found to be effective. Such a series usually includes at least five letters in varying degrees of forcefulness (Fig. 19–8).

Sometimes even the person with poor paying habits will pay the bill if treated with respect and consideration. See Figure 19–9 for a suggested collection program.

OBSERVE ESTABLISHED COLLECTION POLICY The medical assistant should never go beyond the authority granted by the physician in pursuing collections. If you have questions about special collection problems, always check with the physician before proceeding. This is particularly important with patients whom you do not know personally—for example, patients whom the physician has seen in the hospital or at home and others for whom you have no credit history. It is difficult to say whether pressing collections too hard loses more good will of patients than not pursuing collections diligently enough. The physician and the medical assistant together should agree on general collection policies as outlined earlier in this chapter, and then the policies should be followed. In all cases in which an account is to be assigned to a collection agency, be certain that the physician is aware of it.

WHO SIGNS COLLECTION LETTERS? In most medical offices, the medical assistant signs collection letters with the identification "Assistant to Dr.

1. Your account has always been paid promptly in the past, so this must be an oversight. Please accept this note as a friendly reminder of your account due in the amount of $ ________.

2. Since your care in this office in March, we have had no word from you in regard to how you are feeling or your account due. If it is impossible for you to pay the full amount of $ ________ at this time, please call this office before June 15 so that satisfactory arrangements can be worked out.

3. Medical bills are payable at the time of service unless special credit arrangements are made. Please send your check in full or call this office before June 30.

4. If you have some question about your statement, we will be happy to answer it for you. If not, may we have a payment before the end of this month?

5. Unless some definite arrangement is made to reduce your balance of $ ________, we can no longer carry your account on our books. Delinquent accounts are turned over to our collection agency on the 25th of the month.

6. **When a payment plan has been established, it can be reinforced by recognizing the first remittance with a letter of acknowledgment:**

   Thank you for the recent payment of $ ________ on your account. We are glad to cooperate with you in this arrangement for clearing your account. We will look for your next check at about the same time next month, and your final payment the following month.

7. **When a payment schedule has been arranged by a telephone call, it can be confirmed by letter.**

   As agreed upon in our telephone conversation today, we will expect you to mail a payment of $50 on February 10; $50 on March 10; and the balance on April 10. If some emergency should prevent your making one of these payments on time, please notify us immediately by telephone.

DO'S AND DON'TS

DO:

1. Individualize letters to suit the situation.
2. Design your early letters as mere reminders of debt.
3. Always imply that the patient has good intentions to pay, until lack of response over a period of time proves otherwise.
4. Send letters with a firmer tone only after you have sent one or two friendly reminders.

DON'T

1. Use the same collection letter for a patient with good paying habits as for one who is known to neglect financial obligations.
2. Place an overdue notice of any kind on a postcard or on the outside of an envelope. This is an **invasion of privacy.**

FIGURE 19–8 Suggestions for composing collection letters.

GOAL	TIME	PROCEDURE
Inform patient of expected charges	Prior to or at time of service	Personal contact
Confirmation of charges	At time of service or next billing cycle	Billing statement
Reminder of charges or new balance	30 days after first billing	Billing statement with notation "Second Statement"
Determine whether there is a problem with payment or service	Prior to third billing	Telephone patient to arrange payment commitment
If previous step was unsuccessful or not completed	At 60 days	Third billing with note (see Fig. 19-4)
Ask for definite date and dollar amount of payment	Prior to fourth billing	Telephone patient; must have definite plan
Final notice 15 days before sending to collection	At 90 days	Fourth billing; send final notice (see Fig. 19-5) by certified mail with return receipt requested
	At 105 days	Send to collector

FIGURE 19-9 Suggested collection program.

Brown" or "Financial Secretary" below the typewritten signature. Some physicians may wish to personally sign these communications, but generally the medical assistant who handles the accounts also signs the collection letters.

Personal Interviews

Personal interviews with patients can sometimes be more effective than a whole series of collection letters. By talking to a patient face to face, you can come to an understanding of the problem more quickly and reach an agreement about future payment plans.

Occasionally, a patient may undergo a long course of treatment and yet make no attempt to pay anything on account. Perhaps such a patient is only waiting for the physician or the medical assistant to suggest that a payment be made. When there is advance knowledge that the patient will require extensive treatment, the matter of payment should be discussed early in the course of treatment, the credit policy explained, and some agreement reached as to a payment plan.

Because the fee for medical services is far more intangible than that of any commercial account, collection efforts must not be delayed too long. Any responsible, sincere patient will call or write the physician's office after receiving a second statement and explain the delay in payment or ask for a payment plan.

If it becomes necessary to refer the account to a collector, a good agency should have a 35% to 40% recovery rate with an account that is assigned within 4 or 5 months. This may drop to 25% if the account is held only a few more months. If recovery by the agency is greater than 40%, it may indicate that the collection effort by the medical assistant needs to be intensified.

The value of medical accounts diminishes in direct proportion to the length of time that has elapsed since service was rendered. Do not fight the law of diminishing returns. All collection activity is costly. Know when to stop and call on the services of a professional agency.

Memory Jogger

What are the procedural options for the medical assistant in pursuing collections?

SPECIAL COLLECTION SITUATIONS

Tracing "Skips"

When a statement is returned marked "Moved—no forwarding address," you may consider this account as a "skip." This generally is accepted as an indication that the patient is attempting to avoid liability for debts. Some so-called skips are innocent errors. The person may have been careless in not leaving a forwarding address. Or the mistake may have occurred in the physician's office; the wrong name or address may have been placed on the statement.

However, immediate action should be taken in regard to returned statements. Do not wait until the next billing time to attempt to trace the debtor (see Suggestions for Tracing Skips).

SUGGESTIONS FOR TRACING SKIPS

1 Examine the patient's original office registration card.
2 Call the telephone number listed on the card. Occasionally a patient may move without leaving a forwarding address but will transfer the old telephone number. Or the new telephone number will be given when you call the old number.
3 If you are unable to contact the individual by telephone, make a few discreet calls to the references listed on the registration card to get leads.
4 Check the *City Directory* to secure the names and telephone numbers of neighbors or the landlord, and contact these persons to secure information about the debtor's whereabouts.
5 Do not inform a third party that the person owes you money. Simply state that you are trying to locate or verify the location of the individual.
6 Check the debtor's place of employment for information. If the person is a specialist in his or her field of work, the local union or similar organizations may be contacted. Although they may not give you the person's current address, they will relay the message that you are seeking to contact him or her. Often, people will be stirred into paying a bill if they think that their employer may learn of their payment failure.
7 Do not communicate with a third party more than once. This is specifically forbidden by law (Public Law 95-109, Sec. 804) unless the third party requests the collector to do so.

The tracing of skips is a challenge to any medical assistant. A certified letter can be sent; by paying additional fees, you can request the Postal Service to obtain a receipt including the address where the letter was delivered. The certified letter may be sent in a plain envelope so that the patient will not refuse to accept the letter because of the return address.

If all your attempts fail, turn the account over to your collection agency without delay. Do not keep a skip account too long, because the trail may become so cold as time elapses that even collection experts will be unable to follow it.

Claims Against Estates

A bill owed by a deceased patient may be handled a little differently than regular bills. Courtesy dictates that a bill not be sent during the initial period of bereavement, but do not delay more than 30 days. The person responsible for settling the affairs of the estate will be assembling outstanding accounts and will expect to receive the medical bills along with all others. Address the statement to

Estate of (name of patient)
c/o (spouse or next of kin, if known)
Patient's last known address

Do not address the statement to a relative unless you have a signed agreement that that person will be responsible. If for some reason the statement cannot be addressed as just suggested (e.g., if the patient was in a convalescent home and you do not know the name of a relative), you may seek information from the county seat in the county in which the estate is being settled.

A will is generally filed within 30 days of a death. A request to the Probate Department of the Superior Court, County Recorder's Office, will usually provide you with the name of the executor or administrator. The time limits for filing an estate claim are determined by the state in which the decedent resided.

After the name of the administrator or executor of the estate has been obtained, a duplicate itemized statement of the account should be sent to that person by certified mail, return receipt requested, so that you will know who received it. If no response is received in 10 days, you should contact the executor or the county clerk where the estate is being settled and obtain forms for filing claim against the estate. (Some states do not have special claim forms but will accept simple itemized statements.) This claim against the estate must be made within a certain length of time, varying from 2 to 36 months, depending on the state in which it is filed.

The executor of the estate will either accept or reject the claim and, if it is accepted, will send an acknowledgment of the debt. Payment is often delayed, owing to the legal complications in settling an estate, but if the claim has been accepted, you will receive your money in due time. If the claim is rejected and you have full justification for claiming the bill, you must file claim against the executor within a limited time, according to state laws. The time limit in such cases starts with the date on the letter of rejection that was sent you in response to your original claim.

Because states have different time limits and statutes in regard to such matters, it is advisable for the medical assistant to contact the physician's attorney or the local court for the exact procedure to follow.

Bankruptcy

Bankruptcy laws were passed to secure equal distribution of the assets of an individual among the individual's creditors. Bankruptcy laws are federal and are applicable in all states. When you are notified that a patient has declared bankruptcy, you should no longer send statements or make any attempt to collect on the account from the patient.

Chapter VII bankruptcy is usually a "no asset" situation. Because the physician's fee is an unsecured debt, there is little purpose in pursuing collection.

Chapter XIII is known as "Adjustment of Debts of an Individual with Regular Income," according to the Revised Bankruptcy Act of October 1, 1979. Under Chapter XIII, the patient/debtor pays a fixed amount (agreed on by the court) to the trustee in bankruptcy. This is then passed on to the creditors. During this period, none of the creditors can attach the debtor's wages or otherwise attempt to collect the debt. It is sometimes beneficial to file a claim under Chapter XIII because small payments will be made by the debtor under the supervision of the court over a period of 3 years.

STATUTES OF LIMITATIONS

A **statute of limitations** assigns a certain time after which rights cannot be enforced by action.

Malpractice Statutes

In many states, there are statutes of limitations applicable to malpractice lawsuits, which set a limit to the time during which malpractice actions can be filed. It is usually best to wait until this time has passed before pressing the account of a patient who may feel he or she is entitled to sue the physician. However, this should not be made a blanket policy; each case should be judged on its own merit.

Collection Statutes

Statutes of limitations affecting collections prescribe the time within which a legal collection suit may be rendered against a debtor; the term *outlaw* is sometimes used to refer to debts on which the time limit has passed. This legal time limit varies according to the state in which the debt is incurred. Table 19–1 lists the time limits for collections in the various states. It should be noted that if the debtor moves out of state, either temporarily or permanently, the time spent out of state is not included in the time limit. Only the time during which the debtor resides within the state is included in the statute.

The time limit may vary according to the class of account. Generally, accounts may be placed in one of three classes:

- Open book accounts
- Written contracts
- Single-entry accounts

OPEN BOOK ACCOUNTS Open book accounts are accounts on the books that are open to charges made from time to time. The bill for each illness or treatment is computed separately, and the last date of entry—debit or credit—for that specific illness is the time designated by the statute of limitations for starting that specific debt. It is almost impossible to have a time limit on an account of a patient with a chronic condition, because there is no actual termination of the illness or treatment unless the patient changes physicians or dies. When legal time limits

TABLE 19–1 Statute of Limitations

Location	Open Accounts (Years)	Contracts in Writing (Years)
Alabama	3	6
Alaska	6	6
Arizona	3	6
Arkansas	3	5
California	4	4
Colorado	6	6
Connecticut	6	6
Delaware	3	6
District of Columbia	3	3
Florida	4	5
Georgia	4	6
Hawaii	6	6
Idaho	4	5
Illinois	5	10
Indiana	6	10
Iowa	5	10
Kansas	3	5
Kentucky	5	15
Louisiana	3	10
Maine	6	6
Maryland	3	3
Massachusetts	6	6
Michigan	6	6
Minnesota	6	6
Mississippi	3	6
Missouri	5	10
Montana	5	8
Nebraska	4	5
Nevada	4	6
New Hampshire	6	6
New Jersey	6	6
New Mexico	4	6
New York	6	6
North Carolina	3	3
North Dakota	6	6
Ohio	6	15
Oklahoma	3	5
Oregon	6	6
Pennsylvania	6	6
Rhode Island	6	6
South Carolina	6	6
South Dakota	6	6
Tennessee	6	6
Texas	4	4
Utah	4	6
Vermont	6	6
Virginia	3	5
Washington	3	6
West Virginia	5	10
Wisconsin	6	6
Wyoming	8	10
Puerto Rico	15	—

From Summary of Collection Laws published in the American Collectors Association, Inc., 1986 Membership Roster. (Reprinted with permission of American Collectors Association, Inc., Minneapolis, MN.)

are set, they usually refer to these "open book accounts."

WRITTEN CONTRACTS Written contracts often have the same time limit as open book accounts, but in some states they have a longer time limit. The time limit on written contracts starts from the date due.

SINGLE-ENTRY ACCOUNTS Single-entry accounts are accounts with only one entry or charge. These accounts are usually short-lived and are for small amounts. Some states, such as California, place a shorter statute of limitations span on such accounts.

In many states, even though the legal time limit set by the statutes has passed, the account may be reopened and the date extended if you are able to obtain a written acknowledgment of the debt due. For instance, a letter from the patient stating "Yes, I know I owe you $150, but I do not intend paying Dr. Brown" is an acknowledgment of the debt. If this letter is signed and dated, keep it and contact your collector. On the basis of this letter, the collector can then proceed with collection. Also, a small payment on the account will extend the statute expiration date. Photocopy these small checks for proof of payment, should proof become necessary.

Memory Jogger

 *Define statute of limitations.*

Using Outside Collection Assistance

When you have done everything possible internally to follow up on an outstanding account and have not received payment, the question arises as to what step to take next.

- Should your facility sue for the payment?
- Should the account be sent to a collection agency?
- Should the account be written off as a bad debt?

Before forcing an account, you must first consider the time element: Has the patient been given a fair chance to pay this bill? Have you sent statements regularly and used a systematic method of following the account? Ask yourself if there might be a misunderstanding about the fee charged. Did you fully itemize the first statement? A large unexplained bill may frighten a patient into making no payments at all because the whole balance looks too large.

If you have used correct registration forms to secure advance credit information, you should know the financial abilities of the patient to pay. However, illness may have caused a loss of salary and resulted in temporary inability to pay. Try to thoroughly analyze the situation.

Could the patient have been dissatisfied with the care received? For some unknown reason, a patient may feel that he or she was not treated correctly. Perhaps the patient expected a complete cure too soon. Only an explanation of the condition, prognosis, and care can enlighten such patients, and this is best handled by the physician. If payment of a bill is pressed too hard and the patient is dissatisfied for some reason, a malpractice suit may be filed by the patient to "get even."

COLLECTING THROUGH THE COURT SYSTEM

Making the Decision to Sue

Will a physician lose more good will by suing for a bill than by writing it off as a loss? One management official has related that, strangely enough, when a physician-client sued two patients for large amounts, the patients lost the cases, paid up, and were back in the office for treatment very shortly! However, most physicians believe it is unwise to resort to the court to collect medical bills unless there are extraordinary circumstances.

An account must be considered a 100% loss to the physician before legal proceedings are started. Remember that you should never threaten to instigate legal proceedings unless you are prepared to carry out the threat and have the physician's consent to issue such a warning.

If the physician decides in favor of a lawsuit, investigate thoroughly before taking action. Litigation to collect a bill is generally in order when the

1. Patient can afford to pay without hardship.
2. Physician can produce office records that support the bill.
3. Physician can justify the size of the bill by comparison with fee practices in the community.
4. Patient's general condition after treatment is satisfactory.
5. Persuasive powers of an ethical collection agency have been exhausted, and the agency advises suing.
6. Patient can be given ample warning of the physician's intention to sue.
7. Defendant (whether a patient or a parent or legal guardian) is legally liable for the services rendered to the patient.
8. Defendant is not judgment proof.*
9. Statute of limitations has ruled out any possible malpractice action.
10. Physician is not bubbling over with indignation and is not in a "he-can't-do-this-to-me" frame of mind.

*The Soldiers and Sailors Civil Relief Act (1940) protects the rights of servicemen and women on active duty.

The experienced practitioner establishes these 10 "whens" before plunging into costly litigation.

Small Claims Court

Many medical practices find the small claims court a satisfactory and inexpensive way to collect delinquent accounts. The law places a limit on the amount of debt for which relief may be sought in the small claims court. Because this varies from state to state (from $300 to $5000) and in some instances even within a state, this limit should be checked locally before seeking recovery in this manner.

Parties to small claims actions cannot be represented by an attorney at the trial but may send another person to court in their behalf to produce records supporting the claim. Physicians often send their bookkeeper or medical assistant with records of unpaid accounts to show the judge.

If the court awards a judgment for the amount owed, the plaintiff in small claims court may also recover the costs of the suit. For a very small investment in time and money, the physician who uses this method has

- Saved the time of a regular court action
- Had no attorney's fee to pay
- Not sacrificed the commission charged by a collection agency

After being awarded a judgment, you must still collect the money. The only person in a small claims action who has the right of appeal is the defendant. An appeal by the defendant may have the judgment set aside. The plaintiff cannot file an appeal in a small claims action; the decision of the court is final.

The necessary papers for filing action and full instructions on the course to follow may be obtained from the clerk of the small claims court. The medical assistant who has never appeared in the court would probably be wise to attend once as only a spectator, to preview the procedure and feel more at ease when appearing for the physician.

A collection agency to which an account may have been assigned may not file or handle a small claims action. It must either sue in the regular municipal or justice court or attempt to collect the debt in some other manner.

USING A COLLECTION AGENCY

The medical assistant should try every means possible to collect accounts before they become delinquent. But as soon as the account is determined uncollectible through your office—that is, the patient has failed to respond to your final letter or has failed to fulfill a second promise on payment—send the account to the collector without delay. Skips should be assigned immediately.

Even though collection by an agency will mean sacrificing from 40% to 60% of the amount owed, further delay will only reduce the chances of recovery by the professional collector. If the agency finds that the case deserves special consideration, it will seek the physician's advice before proceeding further.

Selecting a Collection Agency

There are a number of agencies either owned and operated as an integral part of the county medical society or operated separately from the medical society but supervised by the medical profession. These bureaus provide specialized medical collection services.

Another type of collection agency is a division of the local credit association, recognized by the National Retail Credit Association. If the local credit association does not maintain a collection department, it will be able to recommend a reputable one. A nationally recognized credit association has considerable responsibility and a high standard to maintain. These factors serve as monitors to its reliability.

The most common type of collection agency throughout the United States is the privately owned and operated agency. Many of these work with the local professional societies and strive to keep their work on a high ethical standard. Because a few bureaus are unethical and unscrupulous in their tactics, care should be taken to be sure that the one you choose is reliable and ethical. For the sake of comparison, many health care facilities use two or three agencies.

Responsibilities to the Collection Agency

When you select a reputable agency and decide to make use of its services, you must be prepared to provide the agency with all the necessary data to enable it to begin prompt collection procedures on overdue accounts. The agency should receive

- Full name of the debtor
- Name of the spouse
- Last known address
- Full amount of the debt
- Date of the last entry on account (debit or credit)
- Occupation of the debtor
- Business address
- Any other pertinent data

After an account has been released to a collection agency, your office makes no further collection attempts. Once the agency has begun its work, follow these guidelines and procedures:

1. Send no more statements.
2. Mark the patient's ledger or stamp it so that you know it is now in the hands of the collector.
3. Refer the patient to the agency if he or she contacts you in regard to the account.
4. Promptly report any payments made directly to

your office (a percentage of this payment is due the agency).

5. Call the agency if you obtain any information that will be of value in tracing or collecting the account.
6. Do not push the agency with frequent calls. The representatives of the agency will report to you regularly and keep you posted on collection progress.

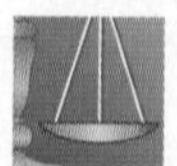

LEGAL AND ETHICAL ISSUES

Regularity in billing accounts is controlled by the Fair Credit Billing Act of October 28, 1975, which states that when a billing date for an account has been established, future mailings must not vary more than 5 days without notification to the debtor (patient). If there is a balance due or a credit balance of one dollar or more, the account must be billed every 30 days .

A bill for a minor must be addressed to a parent or legal guardian unless the minor is emancipated.

A threat to take any action against a debtor that cannot legally be taken or that is not intended to be taken is a violation of the federal Fair Debt Collection Practices Act 1977 Section 807 (5).

A person who has declared bankruptcy is protected from any further attempts to collect a debt, and the physician should discontinue sending bills.

Representation by an attorney is prohibited in actions of the small claims court.

We have checked and verified all statements made in this chapter about collection law and legal procedures. However, laws do change, and it is recommended that you check with your local state regulations and laws to verify points pertinent to your special area. State law takes precedence over federal law if the state law is stronger. For a general textbook of this nature, it is impossible to check each of these state requirements to determine which are stronger and which would prevail over federal Public Law 95–109.

CRITICAL THINKING

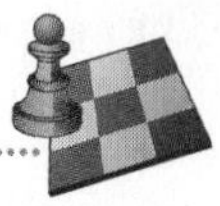

1 Some medical assistants are uncomfortable about asking a patient for payment. Examine your own feelings, leading to ease of making collections. Understand why the physician is justified in the need for payment, and how to explain this to the patient if questioned.

2 Study the age analysis chart in Figure 19–7. Evaluate the accounts of patients E, F, G, H.

HOW DID I DO? Answers to Memory Joggers

1. No further billing and bookkeeping expenses, and no risk of loss.
2. Provides basis for judging accounts objectively and equitably.
3. The Fair Credit Billing Act requires that the date of mailing a statement must not vary more than 5 days without notification to the debtor.
4. When the minor is emancipated.
5. Aging is a procedure of classifying accounts receivable by the length of time they have been owed and the probability of their being collectible.
6. Printed collection letter or reminder, personal letter, personal interview, telephone.
7. A certain time after which rights cannot be enforced by action.

REFERENCES

American Medical Association: The Business Side of Medical Practice, Chicago, AMA, 1989.

Fair Credit Billing Act, October 28, 1975.

Bankruptcy Act (Title II, U.S. Code), October 1, 1979.

Health Insurance and Managed Care

20

Sue Hunt, MA, RN, CMA

OUTLINE

LEARNING OBJECTIVES

Cognitive: On successful completion of this chapter you should be able to:

1. Define the terms listed in the Vocabulary.
2. Cite three advantages of group insurance policies over individual policies.
3. Name seven major types of health insurance benefits.
4. State the meaning of the birthday law.
5. State the basic differences between indemnity and service benefit plans.
6. Describe the major government insurance plans.
7. Discuss the implications of managed care for the medical assistant.
8. Explain the differences between health maintenance organizations (HMOs), independent practice associations (IPAs), and preferred provider organizations (PPOs).
9. Describe the role of the medical assistant in obtaining referrals and authorizations for care.
10. Identify the legal implications of the medical records audit.

VOCABULARY

assignment of insurance benefits Statement authorizing the insurance company to pay benefits directly to the physician

beneficiary Person receiving the benefits of an insurance policy

birthday rule Rule governing the hierarchy of coordination of benefits

capitation Reimbursement to a health care provider as a fixed amount per member in a given time period

claim A demand to the insurer by the insured person for the payment of benefits under a policy

co-insurance Policy provision by which both the insured person and the insurer share in a specified ratio of the expenses resulting from an illness or injury

coordination of benefits The provision in an insurance contract that limits benefits to 100% of the cost

copayment A fixed dollar amount that the insured person must pay each time service is received

deductible A statement in an insurance policy that the insuring company will pay the expenses incurred after the insured person has paid a specified amount

disability The condition resulting from illness or injury that makes an individual unable to be employed

fee schedule A list of services or procedures indemnified by the insurance company and of the specific dollar amounts that will be paid for each service

fringe benefit A benefit granted by an employer that involves a money cost but does not affect the basic wage rates of employees

group policy Policy that covers a group (e.g., all employees of one company) under a master contract

indemnity Benefit paid by an insurer for a loss insured under a policy

individual policy Policy usually held by a person who does not qualify for a group policy

medically indigent Able to take care of ordinary living expenses but unable to afford medical care

member physician A physician who has agreed to accept the contracts of an insurer, usually including accepting the insurance benefits as payment in full

premium The periodic payment required to keep a policy in force

prepaid plan A plan that provides all covered services to a policyholder for payment of a monthly fee

rider Legal document that modifies the protection of a policy

service benefit plan Plan that agrees to pay for certain surgical and medical services and that is not restricted to a fee schedule

subscriber Person named as principal in an insurance contract

utilization review Approval for services by an outside group

Health insurance is an important factor in the practice of medicine. As a medical assistant, you must understand insurance terminology, types of insurance coverage, the importance of obtaining consent for release of information, the effect of **assignment of insurance benefits,** and how to handle a **claim.** You must also be able to communicate with patients about processing their insurance.

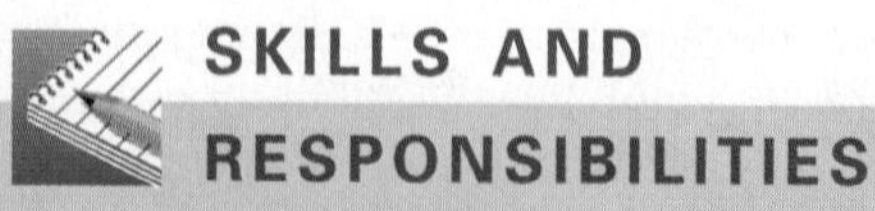

SKILLS AND RESPONSIBILITIES

INSURANCE CLAIM RESPONSIBILITIES

- Obtaining authorizations and referrals
- Preparing insurance claim forms
- Maintaining an insurance claims register
- Tracing unpaid claims
- Evaluating claims rejection
- Reporting procedures to prepaid care plans
- Translating medical terminology into procedural and diagnostic codes

Fifty years ago, health insurance as we know it now was uncommon. Today, most patients who come into a health care facility have some kind of health insurance coverage, either privately or through government-sponsored programs. Although the rapid growth of health insurance coverage is a recent phenomenon brought about by economic necessity, the concept of health insurance is not new.

The first company organized specifically to write

health insurance was founded in 1847. The nation's earliest accident insurance company came into being in 1850 in response to public demand for coverage against frequent rail and steamboat accidents of the mid-19th century. By the turn of the 20th century, 47 American companies were issuing accident insurance.

In its early stages, the emphasis of health insurance was directed toward replacement of income rather than toward hospital or surgical benefits. The early insurance company policy protected the policyholder against loss of earned income due to a limited number of diseases, including typhus, typhoid, scarlet fever, smallpox, diphtheria, diabetes, and a few others. Emphasis on insurance as a means of replacing income lost due to illness continued until 1929, the start of the Great Depression.

At this time, a group of schoolteachers formed an arrangement with Baylor Hospital in Dallas, Texas, to provide themselves with hospital care on a prepayment basis. This was the origin of the Blue Cross service concept for provision of hospital care.

A further major change occurred during World War II when the freezing of industrial wages made the **fringe benefit** a significant element of collective bargaining. Group health insurance became a large part of the fringe benefit package.

Memory Jogger

 *Name seven tasks you may be expected to perform to process insurance.*

The Purpose of Health Insurance

Voluntary health insurance is designed to cover the cost of accidents or illness. In addition, there is an increasing trend for insurance policies to cover services that prevent illness (e.g., immunizations) or lead to early diagnosis (e.g., mammograms). Procedures that are not medically necessary (e.g., cosmetic surgery) or whose effectiveness is not proven (e.g., experimental procedures) are usually not covered.

COST OF COVERAGE

Few insurance policies pay all expenses resulting from accident or illness. The basic cost of health care coverage is a **premium,** monthly or annual, for which the insurer agrees to provide certain benefits. The real cost to the individual at the time of treatment includes

- Deductibles
- Copayment or co-insurance
- Services not covered

The **deductible** is that portion of the bill that a subscriber must pay before insurance coverage is effective. The amount of the deductible is stated in the contract.

A **copayment** is a contribution the subscriber must make to cover some portion of each bill. This could be $2 to $15 for each office visit. **Co-insurance** is a percentage of the total cost. The **subscriber** must also pay for services not covered by the insurance policy, such as eye examinations or dental care.

COORDINATION OF BENEFITS

Coordination of benefits (COB) or provisions to prevent duplicate payments for the same service are included in most group contracts. The purpose of COB provisions is to limit the benefits to 100% of the cost. If a plan does not have COB provisions, it becomes the primary payer and pays benefits first. Laws establishing which payer is primary, including the birthday law, were enacted in January 1987 in many states. In the case of an employed person who is eligible for Medicare benefits, the employer's plan is the primary carrier and Medicare is the supplemental carrier. In many families, both husband and wife are wage earners and, frequently, both are eligible for health insurance benefits through their own employment and that of their spouses.

COB follows the rules of the plan that is the primary payer. If both plans have COB provisions:

- The policyholder's own plan is primary for that individual. An exception occurs if the policyholder is laid off or retired and not a Medicare recipient. In this case, the policyholder's plan pays second.
- The primary coverage for dependents of policyholders is determined by the **birthday rule.** The insurance plan of the policyholder whose birthday comes first in the calendar year (month and day, not year) provides primary coverage for each dependent.
- If neither of the above situations applies, the plan that has been in existence longer is the primary payer.

The primary plan for dependents of legally separated or divorced parents is more complicated.

- The birthday rule is in effect if the parent who has custody of the dependent has not remarried. If the custodial parent has remarried, that parent's plan is primary for that dependent.
- If one parent has been decreed by the court as the responsible party, that parent's policy is primary. This is not always the parent with custody of the child.
- If one of the plans originated in a state that does not have the COB law, the plan that did originate in a state with a COB law will determine the order of benefits.

All of this emphasizes the need to determine whether there is a birthday rule in your state.

Memory Jogger

What are the real costs of coverage to an individual at the time of treatment?

Availability of Health Insurance

Health insurance is available through a **group policy, individual policy,** and subscription to a **prepaid plan.** Many people are covered by government plans.

GROUP POLICIES

Insurance written under a group policy covers a group of people under a master contract, which is generally issued to an employer for the benefit of the employees. The individual employee may be given a certificate of insurance containing information regarding the master policy and indicating that the individual is covered under the policy. Professional associations also frequently offer group insurance as a benefit of membership.

Group coverage usually provides greater benefits at lower premiums, and a physical examination is seldom required for the enrollees. Every person in a group contract has identical coverage.

Memory Jogger

Explain what the birthday rule means.

INDIVIDUAL POLICIES

Individuals who do not qualify for inclusion in a group policy may apply to companies that offer individual policies. The applicant may be required to have a physical examination before acceptance and, if there is an unusual risk, may be denied insurance or may have to accept a **rider** or limitation on the policy. In any event, the individual premium will probably be greater and the benefits less than in a group policy.

GOVERNMENT PLANS

The federal government first became responsible for insuring a large group of people in 1956 with passage of Public Law 569. This law authorized dependents of military personnel to receive treatment by civilian physicians at the expense of the government. We know this today as the Civilian Health and Medical Program of the Uniformed Services (CHAMPUS).

In 1965 the federal government provided for another group, namely, the **medically indigent,** through a program that is still known as Medicaid. Title XIX of Public Law 89–97, under the Social Security Amendments of 1965, provided for agreements with states for assistance from the federal government to provide medical care for people who could not afford it.

Coverage for the patient older than age 65 years, called Medicare, went into effect on July 1, 1966. This plan was established under Social Security. The group of people eligible to receive Medicare was expanded in 1973 to cover disabled persons younger than 65 who had been receiving Social Security benefits, railroad retirement, or civil service retirement. This included disabled workers of any age, disabled widows, disabled dependent widowers and adults disabled before age 18 whose parents are eligible for or are retired on Social Security benefits, children and adults with end-stage renal disease, and kidney donors (including all expenses related to the kidney transplant).

The passage of the Health Maintenance Organization (HMO) Act in 1973 provided for federal aid to health insurance prepayment plans that met certain criteria. This brought about an accelerated growth of HMOs, which are organizations that provide for comprehensive health care to an enrolled group for a fixed periodic payment.

Title VI of the Social Security Amendments Act of 1983 contained the prospective payment system (PPS) for hospitals, which would begin the radical restructuring of the payment system to hospitals for Medicare inpatient services.

The most fundamental change in the determination of physicians' fees under Medicare since its inception was the resource-based relative value scale (RBRVS) reimbursement system put into effect in 1992.

Many large groups of people are covered by governmental insurance plans. The patient who is older than age 65 probably is covered by Part B of Medicare. The medically indigent patient may be eligible for Medicaid with or without Medicare. Dependents of military personnel are covered by CHAMPUS; surviving spouses and dependent children of veterans who died as a result of service-connected disabilities are covered by the Civilian Health and Medical Program of the Veterans Administration (CHAMPVA). Many wage earners are protected against the loss of wages and the cost of medical care resulting from occupational accident or disease through workers' compensation insurance. All of these plans are dealt with in more detail later in this chapter.

Memory Jogger

What does medically indigent mean?

Types of Insurance Benefits

An insurance package is tailored to the needs of each individual or group policy, and the combinations of benefits are limitless. A policy may contain any one or any combination of the following kinds of benefits.

HOSPITALIZATION

Hospital coverage pays the cost of all or part of the insured person's hospital room and board and special hospital services. Hospital insurance policies frequently set a maximum amount payable per day and a maximum number of days of hospital care. Some insurance companies require that the hospital be an accredited or a licensed hospital. Most hospital plans exclude admission for diagnostic studies.

SURGICAL

Surgical coverage pays all or part of the surgeon's fee; some plans also pay for an assistant surgeon. Surgery includes any incision or excision, removal of foreign bodies, aspiration, suturing, and reduction of fractures. The surgery may be accomplished in the hospital, in a doctor's office, or elsewhere. The insurer frequently provides the subscriber with a surgical fee schedule that sets forth the amount the insurer will pay for commonly performed procedures.

BASIC MEDICAL

Medical coverage pays all or part of the physician's fee for nonsurgical services, including hospital, home, and office visits. Usually there is a deductible amount payable by the patient as well as a copayment or co-insurance each time service is received. The insurance plan may include provision for diagnostic laboratory, x-ray, and pathology fees. Some medical plans do not cover routine physical examinations when the patient does not have a specific complaint or illness.

MAJOR MEDICAL

Major medical insurance (formerly called catastrophic coverage) provides protection against especially heavy medical bills resulting from catastrophic or prolonged illnesses. It may be a supplement to basic medical coverage or a comprehensive integrated program providing both basic and major medical protection.

DISABILITY (LOSS OF INCOME) PROTECTION

Weekly or monthly cash benefits are provided to employed policyholders who become unable to work owing to an accident or illness. Many policies do not start payment until after a specified number of days or until a certain number of sick leave days have been used. Payment is made directly to the patient and is intended to replace loss of income resulting from illness. It is not intended for payment of specific medical bills.

Memory Jogger

What does basic medical *mean?*

DENTAL CARE

Dental coverage is included in many fringe benefit packages. Some policies are based on a copayment and incentive program, with the company's copayment increasing each year until 100% coverage is reached.

VISION CARE

Vision care insurance may include reimbursement for all or for a percentage of the cost for refraction, lenses, and frames.

MEDICARE SUPPLEMENT

These are contracts insuring persons 65 years of age or older that supplement the coverage provided by Medicare. Federal regulation now requires these contracts to be uniform in benefits to decrease confusion for the purchaser.

SPECIAL CLASS INSURANCE

Applicants for health insurance who cannot qualify for a standard policy by reason of health may be issued special class insurance with limited coverage.

SPECIAL RISK INSURANCE

This insurance protects a person in the event of a certain type of accident, such as automobile or airplane crashes, or for certain diseases, such as tuberculosis or cancer. There is usually a maximum benefit.

LIABILITY INSURANCE

There are many types of liability insurance, including automobile, business, and homeowners' policies. Liability policies often include benefits for medical expenses payable to individuals who are injured in the insured person's home or car, without regard to the insured person's actual legal liability for the accident.

LIFE INSURANCE

Life insurance policies sometimes provide monthly cash benefits if the policyholder becomes permanently and totally disabled. Sometimes, the proceeds from life insurance are used to meet the expenses of the insured person's last illness.

How Benefits Are Determined

Insurance benefits may be determined and paid in one of several ways:

- By indemnity schedules
- By service benefit plans
- By determination of the usual, customary, and reasonable fee
- By relative value studies

INDEMNITY SCHEDULES

In **indemnity** plans, the insurer agrees to pay the subscriber a set amount of money for a given procedure or service. The insured person is given a schedule of indemnities (**fee schedule**) when the policy is purchased.

Indemnity plans do not agree to pay for the complete services rendered. Often there is a difference in the amount paid by the insurance company and the amount of the physician's fee. For example, the insurer may agree to pay up to $1000 for a specific operation, with no consideration for the time or complications of the surgery. If the physician charges $1200, the difference of $200 is the responsibility of the patient.

This type of plan takes the major expense out of medical bills and helps to keep the premiums down. The amount of the premium often determines the schedule of benefits. Indemnity benefits are usually paid to the person insured unless that person has authorized payment directly to the provider.

SERVICE BENEFIT PLANS

In **service benefit plans,** the insuring company agrees to pay for certain surgical or medical services without additional cost to the person insured. There is no set fee schedule.

In a service benefit plan, surgery with complications would warrant a higher fee than an uncomplicated procedure. Premiums are sometimes higher for this type of coverage, but often payments are larger. Frequently, the payment for benefits is sent directly to the physician and is considered full payment for the services rendered.

USUAL, CUSTOMARY, AND REASONABLE FEE

Some insurance companies agree to pay on the basis of all or a percentage of the physician's usual, customary, and reasonable fee. Charges for a specific service are compared to a database of charges for the same service to other patients by the same physician and to patients by other physicians in the same geographic area. The insurance company determines whether the charge is usual, customary, and reasonable. Any amount over the limit determined by the insurance company will not be paid.

RESOURCE-BASED RELATIVE VALUE SCALE

This is the fee schedule that is the basis for payment to physicians for services provided under Medicare Part B since 1992. This system was implemented to standardize payments with an adjustment for overhead costs in different geographic areas. More specific information regarding RBRVS is provided in Chapter 21.

Memory Jogger

Name four ways benefits are determined.

Kinds of Plans

BLUE CROSS AND BLUE SHIELD

In the early 1930s, hospitals introduced Blue Cross plans to provide coverage for hospital costs. Today, there are local Blue Cross plans operating in all states of the United States, the District of Columbia, Canada, Puerto Rico, and Jamaica.

In 1939, state medical societies in California and Michigan began sponsoring health plans to provide medical and surgical services; these became known as Blue Shield plans. Other states soon followed, and today Blue Shield is the largest medical prepayment system in the country.

Early in its development, Blue Shield was often known as the doctor's plan. A **member physician** agreed to bill Blue Shield for services to subscribers and abide by other prearranged procedures. Under many Blue Shield contracts, physicians accept Blue Shield's payment as payment in full for covered services. Blue Shield and its member physicians agree on methods of reimbursement in advance of the service performed.

In many plans, Blue Shield provides the medical and surgical coverage and Blue Cross provides hospital coverage. However, in some areas, Blue Cross plans write medical and surgical insurance in addition to providing hospital coverage. Conversely, some Blue Shield plans offer hospital insurance as well as medical and surgical coverage.

Blue Cross benefits are normally paid to the provider of service. In some cases, a check issued jointly to the provider and the person insured is sent to the latter, who must then endorse and forward it to the provider. Blue Shield makes direct payment to member physicians. For services of a nonmember physician, the payment is sent to the subscriber.

BC/BS identification cards usually carry the subscriber's name and identification number with a three-character alphabetical prefix. The letters are an important part of the number and must be included on the claim form (Fig. 20–1).

BLUE CARD

The Blue Shield Reciprocity has been replaced by an improved service known as the Blue Card Program. It is designed to serve subscribers while they are traveling or covered by a Blue Plan in another area. The Blue Card may cover Blue Shield only, Blue Cross only, or a combination of the two programs.

FOUNDATIONS FOR MEDICAL CARE

A foundation for medical care is a management system for community health services. It takes the form of an organization created by local physicians through their medical society, and it concerns itself with the quality and cost of medical care. Under the foundation concept, the following procedure occurs:

1. An insurance company sells and negotiates the policy. It collects the premiums, assumes all the risks, and reimburses the foundation for the cost of the claims office.
2. The foundation sets policy standards; receives, processes, reviews, and pays claims to doctors; sets maximum fees based on current fees in the area; elects doctor-members yearly; and continually studies local medical-economic problems.
3. Member doctors agree to accept foundation fees as full payment under foundation-approved policies. The local medical society legally controls the foundation and selects foundation trustees.
4. The patient selects the doctor of his or her own choice; the patient or the patient's union or employer pays the premium directly to the insurance company.

COMMERCIAL INSURERS

Many people are covered by health insurance issued by private (commercial) insurance companies. Physicians and medical societies control neither the premiums paid nor the benefits received from such policies. For traditional types of policies payment is normally made to the subscriber unless the subscriber has authorized that payment be made directly to the physician. For HMOs, payment is made directly to the physician.

GOVERNMENT PLANS

Medicare

There are two distinct parts (A and B) to the Medicare program.

PART A: HOSPITAL INSURANCE Retired people 65 years of age and older and other people who receive monthly Social Security or railroad retirement checks are automatically enrolled for hospital insurance benefits and pay no premiums for this insurance. Part A is financed by special contributions paid by employed individuals as deductions from their salary, with matching contributions from their employers. These sums are collected along with regular Social Security contributions from wages and self-employment income earned during a person's working years. There is a significant deductible that the hospitalized patient must pay toward the hospital expenses.

Medicare health insurance cards identify if a person has Part A alone or has both Part A and Part B insurance. A patient whose Medicare claim number ends in the letter "A" will have the same Social Security number and Medicare number. If the person has different Social Security numbers and Medicare numbers, the Medicare number ends in a "B" or a "D" (Fig. 20–2).

PART B: MEDICAL INSURANCE Those persons who are eligible for Part A are eligible for Part B but must apply for this coverage and pay a monthly premium. Some federal employees and former fed-

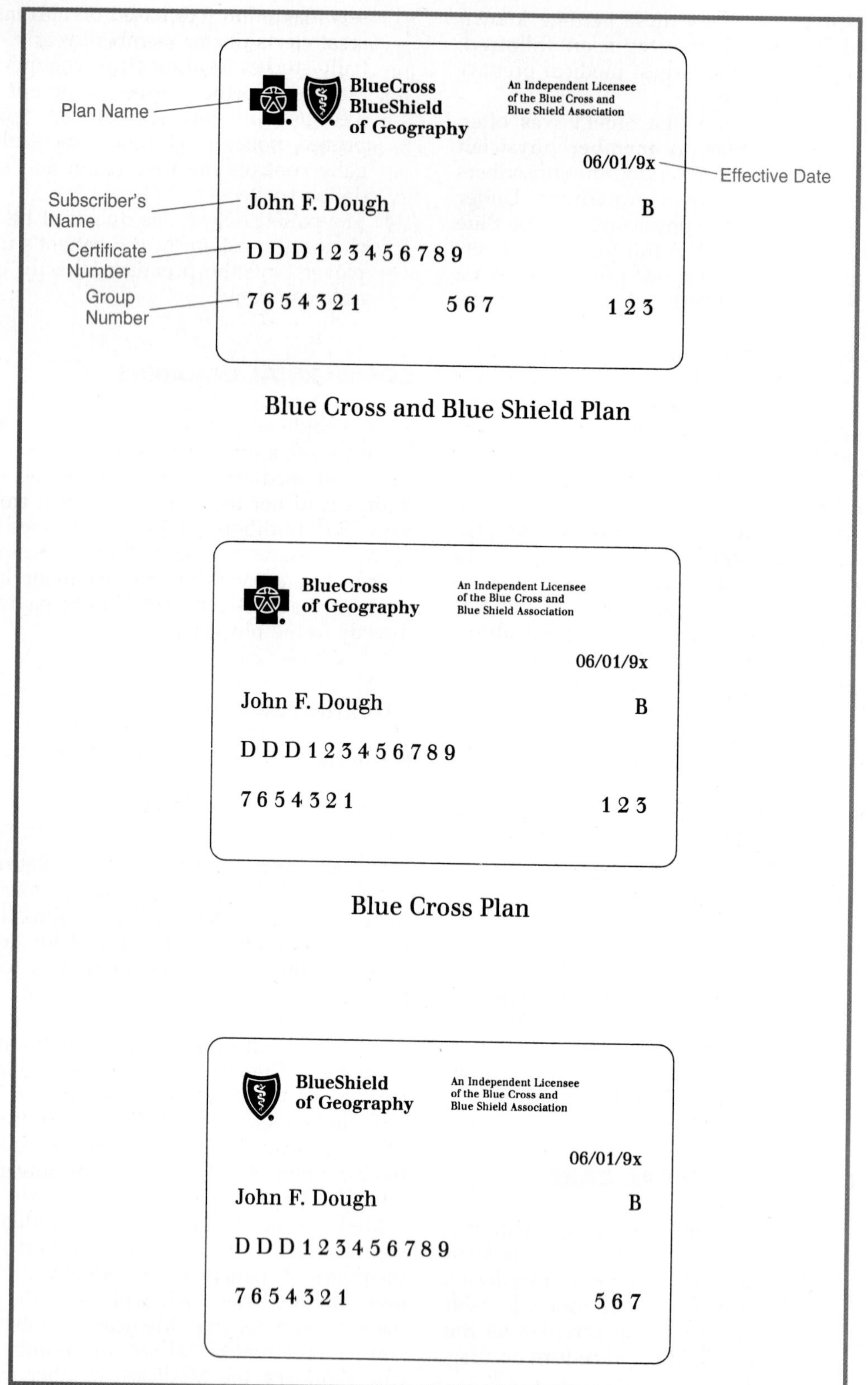

FIGURE 20–1 Typical Blue Cross and Blue Shield identification cards. (Courtesy of Blue Cross/Blue Shield Association, Chicago, Illinois.)

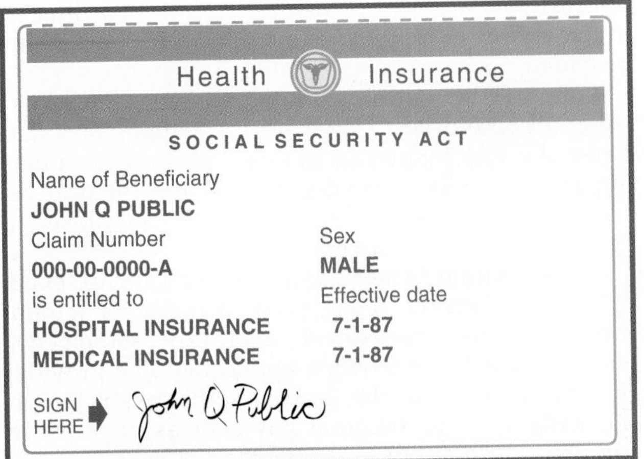

Health Insurance
SOCIAL SECURITY ACT
Name of Beneficiary
JOHN Q PUBLIC
Claim Number
000-00-0000-A
Sex
MALE
is entitled to
Effective date
HOSPITAL INSURANCE 7-1-87
MEDICAL INSURANCE 7-1-87
SIGN HERE
John Q Public

FIGURE 20–2 Medicare identification card.

eral employees who are not eligible for Social Security benefits and Part A may still enroll in Part B. Certain disabled persons younger than age 65 years are also eligible for Medicare.

The patient with Medicare Part B has to meet an annual deductible before benefits become available, after which Medicare pays 80% of the covered benefits. Usually the physician accepts assignment of benefits for Medicare patients and is paid directly. In these cases the physician must accept the payment that Medicare allows and bills the patient for 20% of the charge allowed by Medicare. If the physician does not accept assignment, the patient must pay the entire bill (which cannot be greater than the limit set by Medicare for nonparticipating physicians), and the patient will receive a check from Medicare.

Many Medicare enrollees also carry private supplemental insurance that pays the deductible and the 20% copayment.

Medicaid

Title XIX of Public Law 89–97 under the Social Security Amendments of 1965 provides for agreements with states for assistance from the federal government in providing health care for the medically indigent. All states and the District of Columbia have Medicaid programs, but wide variations may exist among these programs.

The federal government provides basic funding to the state, after which the states individually elect whether to provide funds for extension of benefits. The state determines the type and extent of medical care that will be covered within the minimum requirements established by the federal government. Some local areas and states are developing HMOs that serve only the patients who qualify for Medicaid.

The physician may accept or decline to treat Medicaid patients. The physician who does accept Medicaid patients automatically agrees to accept Medicaid payment as payment in full for covered services. The patient cannot be billed for the difference between the Medicaid fee and the physician's normal fee. The patient can be billed for any services that are not covered by Medicaid. Eligibility for benefits is determined by the respective states.

EXAMPLES OF INDIVIDUALS WHO QUALIFY FOR ELIGIBILITY BENEFITS

- Persons receiving certain types of federal and state aid
- Persons who are medically needy (i.e., they can provide for the expenses of daily living but are unable to afford medical care)
- Recipients of Aid to Families with Dependent Children
- Persons who receive Supplemental Security Income (SSI)
- Qualified Medicare Beneficiaries (QMB) (pays Medicare Part B premiums, deductibles, and co-insurance for qualified low-income elderly)
- Persons in institutions or other long-term care in nursing facilities and intermediate care facilities
- Medicaid purchase of COBRA coverage (low income persons who lose employer health insurance coverage)

A benefits identification card (BIC), which looks like a white credit card, or sticker/label showing proof of eligibility is usually issued to the beneficiary. The BIC is verified by a point of service (POS) device similar to a credit card verification. The medical assistant must verify coverage each time the patient comes into the office before being seen if the state uses a BIC.

Medi/Medi

Some patients who qualify for Medicare are still unable to pay the portion for which they are responsible and may qualify for both Medicare and Medicaid. Medicare is the primary coverage, and any residual is paid by the Medicaid assistance program. Claims submitted for coverage under Medicare and Medicaid are sometimes referred to as crossover claims.

Memory Jogger

What does BIC stand for?

Military Medical Benefits

CHAMPUS In 1956, the passage of Law 569 authorized dependents of military personnel to receive in-hospital treatment by civilian physicians at the expense of the government. This program was first called Medicare but was later changed to CHAMPUS.

On September 30, 1966, the Military Medical Benefits Amendment Act of 1966 became law. This act added outpatient care benefits, including prescription drugs, to the in-hospital benefits previously allowed. Military retirees and their dependents as well as dependents of deceased members became eligible for outpatient benefits in January 1967.

To receive CHAMPUS benefits, eligible persons must be enrolled in the Defense Enrollment Eligibility Reporting System (DEERS), a computerized database that is used for verifying eligibility.

Benefits under CHAMPUS are limited to (1) dependents of active-duty personnel, (2) retirees and their dependents, and (3) dependents of service personnel who have died in active duty.

CHAMPVA In 1973, a program similar to CHAMPUS was established for the spouses and dependent children of veterans suffering total, permanent, service-connected disabilities and for the surviving spouses and dependent children of veterans who have died as a result of service-connected disabilities. This is called the Civilian Health and Medical Program of the Veterans Administration (CHAMPVA).

Eligibility is determined, and identification cards are issued, by the nearest Veterans Affairs medical center. The insured persons then are free to choose their own private physicians. Benefits and cost-sharing features are the same as those for CHAMPUS beneficiaries who are military retirees or their dependents and dependents of deceased members of the military.*

CHAMPUS/TRICARE MANAGED CARE In 1993 the Department of Defense contracted to provide an alternative managed care system for CHAMPUS beneficiaries in the states of California and Hawaii. It has continued to expand to other states and is expected to be available in all 50 states before 2000. Only CHAMPUS-eligible persons have the option of TRICARE Managed Care. It is not available to CHAMPVA or Medicare recipients. CHAMPUS/TRICARE offers three options: TRICARE/PRIME (HMO), TRICARE/EXTRA (PPO), and TRICARE STANDARD, which is the same as standard CHAMPUS.

WORKERS' COMPENSATION

All state legislatures have passed workers' compensation laws to protect wage earners against the loss of wages and the cost of medical care resulting from occupational accident or disease. State laws differ as to the classes of employees included and the benefits provided.

None of the states' workers' compensation laws cover all employees. However, if a patient says that he or she was injured in the workplace or is suffering from a work-associated illness, the medical assistant should check with the patient's employer to verify the insurance coverage.

Compensation benefits include medical care benefits, weekly income replacement benefits for temporary disability, permanent **disability** settlements, and survivor benefits when applicable. The provider of service (e.g., doctor, hospital, therapist) accepts the workers' compensation payment as payment in full and does not bill the patient.

Time limitations are set forth for the prompt reporting of workers' compensation cases. The employee is obligated to promptly notify the employer; the employer, in turn, must notify the insurance company and must refer the employee to a source of medical care. In some states, the employer and the insurance company have the right to select the physician who will treat the patient. In essence, the purpose of workers' compensation laws is to provide prompt medical care to the injured or ill worker so that the person may be restored to health and return to full earning capacity in as short a time as possible.

LIFE INSURANCE

When an individual whom the physician is treating or has treated in the past makes application for life insurance, the insuring company naturally wants to know the current state of the applicant's health and any significant past medical history.

To get an account of the applicant's current state of health, the insurance company authorizes a health care professional (physician or nurse, depending on the state) to perform physical examinations of prospective clients.

The insurance company's agent arranges the applicant's appointment for the physical examination and supplies the necessary forms for completion. After the examination, a report is sent to the insurance company. The company may require that the forms be completed in the examiner's own handwriting. The insurance company pays a stipulated amount on receipt of the report.

For a summary of the applicant's past medical history, the agent asks the applicant to supply the names and addresses of any physicians consulted in the past. The company, in turn, requests reports from these physicians. Your physician may receive a request for such information concerning a current or previous patient. Before completing the form, make certain that the applicant has signed an authorization for release of information to that insurance carrier.

*Further information regarding these military medical benefit programs may be obtained by writing to OCHAMPUS, Aurora, CO 80045-6900.

The request form usually has a voucher check for a minimal fee attached. The physician may accept the proffered fee or, if it is inadequate, may bill the insurance company for balance of fee. If the bill is reasonable, it is paid without question.

DISABILITY INSURANCE

MANDATED Several states require that employees be covered by nonindustrial disability (time loss) insurance. A small percentage (ranging from 0.3% to 1.2%) of the employee's salary may be deducted to cover the cost of this insurance. All regular employees, part or full time, are covered until they retire.

The weekly benefits are based on the employee's salary and calculated using a predetermined formula. There is a waiting period before benefits begin (usually 7 days) and a time limit ranging from 26 to 52 weeks for benefits to continue.

VOLUNTARY In states that do not have mandated disability insurance, employees or groups may seek coverage from a commercial carrier.

Managed Care

What is managed care? *Managed care* is a term used for a variety of prepaid health plans developed to provide health services at low cost. Under managed care, a medical group such as a health maintenance organization (HMO) or an independent practice association (IPA) is contracted to assume some of the responsibilities of the insurance company, that is, claims processing, provider relations, member services, utilization review, and eligibility. The primary care physician (PCP), selected by the patient, manages all patient services.

There has been mass confusion at times of what an HMO is. Some will refer to their insurance company as their HMO, some will refer to their PCP as their HMO, and some will refer to their medical group as their HMO. At first, an HMO and IPA were both simply two entities of medical groups; but with the daily changes of managed care, the entire organization is now considered as an HMO with different functions (Fig. 20–3).

In the traditional type of HMO, the HMO builds a medical group of physicians (PCPs and specialists) who agree to be paid on a per-patient basis instead of a fee-for-service basis. The HMO contracts with employers to provide health service for their employees. The member of an HMO selects a PCP from the medical group. Under an HMO without a foundation, the HMO is responsible for all but limited administrative needs of a PCP, including processing of **capitation** and/or fee-for-service checks.

In an IPA, an organization of physicians (a foundation for medical care) will contract with several employers to provide health services in the same way as an HMO. The IPA contracts with physicians, specialists, hospitals, and laboratories in the community and the member/patient will select a PCP under the IPA. Under an IPA, physicians or group practices will contract to tap into the IPA's health plans (insurance contracts). In return, the IPA will provide member physicians with administrative services either partially or in full. The IPA will receive all capitation monies, keep a contracted percentage for its services, process all the capitation checks, and will forward all the printed checks to the administrator for approval.

EXAMPLE "A"	EXAMPLE "B"
Insurance Company	Insurance Company
	Foundation
Medical Group	Medical Groups
PCP — Specialist	PCP — Specialist
Member/Patient	Member/Patient

FIGURE 20–3 Examples of organizational levels of medical groups. *A*, Without foundation. *B*, With foundation.

INSURANCES ACCEPTED BY PHYSICIAN(S); CREDENTIALED			
NAME	ADDRESS	PR CONTACT NAME AND TELEPHONE #	MS CONTACT NAME AND TELEPHONE #

FIGURE 20–4 Telephone list for provider relations (PR) and member services (MS).

CONTRACTED HOSPITAL(S)				
	NAME	ADDRESS	TELEPHONE	CONTACT
1				
2				
3				
4				

A

CONTRACTED URGENT CARE CENTER(S) - ANCILLARY				
	NAME	ADDRESS	TELEPHONE	CONTACT
1				
2				
3				
4				

B

FIGURE 20–5 *A*, Telephone directory for contracted hospitals. *B*, Telephone directory for contracted urgent care centers.

ANCILLARY PROVIDERS

RADIOLOGY - usually capitated

	NAME	ADDRESS	TELEPHONE	CONTACT
1				
2				
3				

LAB(S) - usually capitated

	NAME	ADDRESS	TELEPHONE	CONTACT
1				
2				
3				

HOME CARE SERVICES - available through medical group

	NAME	ADDRESS	TELEPHONE	CONTACT
1				
2				
3				

FIGURE 20–6 Lists for ancillary providers.

When you work in a physician's office, you will most likely be working with one or more managed care plans. You will need to maintain a list of telephone and fax numbers for the following: provider relations, member services, claims department, utilization review/utilization management, eligibility, and medical director (Figs. 20–4 through 20–6).

HEALTH MAINTENANCE ORGANIZATION

The HMO is what first comes to mind when we speak of prepaid plans. An HMO plan agrees to provide specific services to every enrolled member for a prepaid fee. When a health insurance carrier is involved, it contracts to pay in advance for the full range of health services to which the insured is entitled under the terms of the health insurance contract.

Public Law 93-222, the HMO Assistance Act, was enacted in 1973 to encourage and promote the growth of HMOs as a means of health care cost containment. Many Medicare recipients endorse their benefits over to an HMO for fully prepaid medical care. Employers who provide health care benefits to employees are required to offer federally qualified HMOs as an option.

Several types of HMOs are

- Prepaid group practice model, in which physicians form a group and contract with a health plan. The physicians are not paid by the health plan and, therefore, can concentrate on practicing medicine.
- Staff model, in which a health plan hires physicians directly and pays them a salary.
- Independent practice association, in which the physicians are not employees and are not paid salaries. Instead, they are paid fees for their services out of a fund drawn from the premiums collected by an organization that markets the health plan minus a discount of up to 30% to cover operating deficits. At the end of the year, the physicians share in any surplus or deficit.
- Network HMO, which contracts with two or more group practices to provide health services.

Examples of HMO plans are

Kaiser Permanente

Blue Cross/Blue Shield HMO USA

CHAMPUS/TRICARE Prime, TRICARE/Extra and TRICARE/Standard

Medicare HMO risk plans or HMO cost plans

Medicaid (Medi-Cal in California)

INDEPENDENT PRACTICE ASSOCIATION

An IPA is a closed-panel HMO. Instead of maintaining its own staff and clinic buildings, the IPA contracts with independently practicing physicians who continue to practice in their own offices. The IPA may pay each doctor a set amount per patient in advance (capitation), or the fees charged for services to group members may be billed directly to the IPA rather than to the patient. Fees for services to nonmember patients are handled the same as any other fee for service. The physician may be contracted with several IPAs.

Memory Jogger

8 *Name three HMO plans.*

PREFERRED PROVIDER ORGANIZATION

The PPO preserves the fee-for-service concept that is desirable in the eyes of many physicians. An insurer, representing its clients, contracts with a group of providers (physicians) who agree on a predetermined list of charges for all services, including those for complex and unusual procedures.

The care is not prepaid. Usually, there are deductibles of 20% to 25% of the predetermined charge that the patient pays; the insurer pays the balance. A provider who joins a PPO does not need to alter the manner of providing care and continues to treat and bill the regular patients on a fee-for-service basis. When a patient covered under a PPO plan comes for treatment, the physician treats the patient and bills the PPO.

Working with Managed Care Plans

PRECERTIFICATION OR PREAUTHORIZATION

Most managed care systems require preauthorization for a patient to be referred to a specialist or even for certain laboratory tests or other procedures. It is necessary when a new patient makes an appointment to ask what type of insurance the patient has. If the patient belongs to an HMO you should check that plan contract for precertification or preauthorization requirements. If you are not sure of the requirements, call the plan and keep a record of the requirements on a reference guide that you prepare with the following information:

- Plan name
- Address
- Telephone number(s)
- Name and phone number of contact person
- Copay amount or deductible
- Hospital benefits for inpatient and outpatient surgery
- Second opinion, preauthorization requirements, telephone number, and assistant surgeon with percentage
- Participating hospitals, x-ray providers, laboratories, and physicians

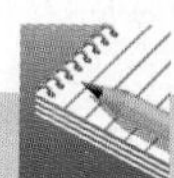

SKILLS AND RESPONSIBILITIES

NEW PATIENT INSURANCE VERIFICATION PROCEDURE

1 When a patient calls for an appointment, identify what type of insurance the patient has or what HMO the patient belongs to.
2 When the patient arrives for the appointment, photocopy both sides of the patient ID card, because amounts to be paid may appear on the back side for hospital, office, or the emergency department.
3 Give the patient a letter to read and sign outlining the plan requirements and possible restrictions or noncovered items.
4 When referrals are required, explain the procedure to the patient so that it is understood that without the referral, it is the patient's responsibility to pay for the physician's services.
5 Collect any copays or deductibles.

PROVIDER RELATIONS

The provider relations department is designed to assist the physician's office with any inquiries he or she may have about capitation, contract, credentialing, physician appeals, formularies, and so forth. Whenever questions arise concerning a member/patient, the physician's office should contact the appropriate department (member services eligibility or the insurance company). *Do not* refer a patient to this department.

MEMBER SERVICES

This department was designed to assist the member/patient with any inquiries and/or concerns that may arise. Some HMOs will have one department that is a combination of provider relations and member services where a physician's office is able to check the status of their claims.

Memory Jogger

List the five steps in new patient procedure under managed care.

CLAIMS DEPARTMENT

Although this department was designed primarily to process all medical claims, the setup will vary from medical group to medical group. *If you provided services that required an authorization, always submit a copy of the authorization.* You need to determine where to forward claims and what kind of documentation is required for each managed care plan with which your office has a contract. Payments for managed care plans may be made either on a capitation basis (that is, a monthly check based on the number of patients in the plan) or based on the services that have been rendered to the patient (that is, a monthly check with an explanation of benefits [EOB] to indicate how much was paid for each service rendered to each patient). The EOB will have all the information from the claim and a code that specifies that the claim was processed and forwarded to the insurance company for processing and payment.

UTILIZATION MANAGEMENT

Review of care by health care professionals who do not provide the care is a necessary component of managed care to control costs. A **utilization review** committee reviews individual cases to make sure that the medical care services are medically necessary and to study how providers use medical care resources. This department reviews all the physician's referrals, emergency department visits, and urgent care. After review, this department will either approve or deny the referral, so it is important to submit exact documentation and precise statements. You will be able to contact this department directly. Never refer a member/patient to this department.

ELIGIBILITY SERVICES

Eligibility services was designed to assist the physician's office in checking eligibility of a patient/member. If the member is not in the database, this department is responsible to contact the insurance company and enter the information into the database.

MEDICAL DIRECTOR

The medical director is a highly qualified physician who works with every department in the medical group, including utilization review management. When certain referrals, questions, and/or concerns arise, the medical director will contact the PCP and will make a final decision based on the information obtained from the PCP.

FORMULARY

A formulary is a list of oral and parenteral medications that are covered by a member's (patient's) health plan. Every physician should have a copy of a formulary (one for every health plan with which he or she is connected). If you do not have one, contact your medical group's provider relations manager.

If a medication is in question, contact the plan's provider relations department and it will either give you an answer or will contact the insurance company.

Referrals and Authorizations

Managed care changes on a day-to-day basis. To compete within this market, some insurance companies have added a benefit that will allow a member/patient to self-refer (an authorization is not required to see a specialist). Many plans for senior citizens now have a self-referral and a copay as well as some other insurance coverage.

The following information will apply if you are working for a primary care physician, internist, family practitioner, general practitioner, pediatrician, and sometimes obstetrician or gynecologist.

Referral is a term used in managed care to refer a patient from the PCP to a specialist (Fig. 20–7). When completing a referral form, it is imperative that all necessary information be included. For example

> Referring physician ⇛ Specialist being referred to ⇛ Diagnosis ⇛ Treatment (medication ⇛ past and present) ⇛ Chart notes (if necessary) ⇛ Minor surgical procedures

If a referral is denied because of insufficient information or no medical necessity, the PCP's office will be notified. Some medical groups will notify both the PCP and the patient. When the PCP's office provides the medical group with the necessary information, the referral will be reviewed again.

A referral can take a few minutes to a few days to be reviewed and approved or denied. There are three types of referrals:

1. *Regular* referral usually takes 3 to 10 working days. This type of referral is used when a patient has not responded to any of a PCP's treat-

LIST OF SPECIALTIES AVAILABLE THROUGH OUR MEDICAL GROUP

		Y	N	
	Acupuncture			Otorhinolaryngology
	Allergy/Immunology			Pathology
	Anesthesiology			Pediatrics
	Cardiovascular Diseases			Pediatric Allergy
	Critical Care Medicine			Pediatric Cardiology
	Dermatology			Pediatric - Dental Trauma
	Dermatopathology			Pediatric Dermatology
	Emergency Medicine			Pediatric Endocrinology
	Endocrinology			Pediatric Gastroenterology
	Family/General Practice			Pediatric Genetics
	Gastroenterology			Pediatric Hematology/Oncology
	Gynecology			Pediatrics, Infectious Disease
	Hematology			Pediatrics, Nephrology
	Hepatology			Pediatric Neurology
	Hyperbaric Medicine			Pediatric Neurosurgery
	Internal Medicine			Pediatric Ophthalmology
	Maternal and Fetal Medicine			Pediatric Orthopedic Surgery
	Neonatal-Perinatal Medicine			Pediatric Otorhinolaryngology
	Nephrology			Pediatric Plastic Surgery
	Neurology			Pediatric Podiatry
	Obstetrics and Gynecology			Pediatric Psychiatry
	Oncology			Pediatric Psychology
	Ophthalmology			Pediatric Pulmonology
	Ophthalmic Plastic Reconstructive and Orbital Surgery			Pediatric Rheumatology
	Orthopedic Surgery			Pediatric Surgery
	Pediatric Urology			Surgery, Colon and Rectal
	Podiatry			Surgery, Head and Neck
	Psychiatry			Surgery, Neurological
	Psychiatry, Child and Adolescent			Surgery, Oncology
	Pulmonary Diseases			Surgery, Maxillofacial
	Radiology, Diagnostic			Surgery, Orthopedic
	Radiology, Oncology			Surgery, Orthopedic/Oncology
	Rheumatology			Surgery, Facial Plastic, and Otorhinolaryngology
	Sleep Disorders			Surgery, General Vascular
	Sports Medicine			Urology
	Surgery, Cardiovascular and Thoracic			
	OTHER			

FIGURE 20–7 Keeping a record of authorized specialty referrals.

ment and/or medication, and the physician believes that the patient needs to see a specialist to continue treatment.
2. An *urgent* referral will usually take 24+ hours. This type of referral is used when an urgent matter occurs and is not life threatening.
3. A *STAT* referral can be approved by telephone immediately after faxing it to the utilization review department. A STAT referral is used in an emergency situation as indicated by the physician, such as a matter of life or death, miscarriage, loss of limb, or other conditions of similar magnitude. Usually the physician will refer the patient by telephone and will fax the information with the referral afterward.

A regular referral is the most common and can be troublesome. Most managed care plans require you to contact the member services department to check the status of a referral. A cardinal rule is to never tell the patient that the referral has been approved unless you have a hard copy of the **authorization.** *Authorization* is a term used by managed care for an approved referral. A referral becomes an authorization after it is reviewed by utilization management/review and/or the medical director and approved.

When a referral is approved the PCP's office will receive by mail or fax a copy of the authorization. Always review the authorization in full. The patient will receive a letter with an authorization number and the approved services. The patient must present the authorization to the specialist's office receptionist on the day the services will be provided. An authorization provides the following information to both the PCP and the specialist:

1. An authorization number, which could be alpha, numeric, or alphanumeric.
2. The date on which it was received by utilization management, the date on which it was approved, and the expiration date.
   a. An authorization is good for 60 days.
   b. If the services are provided after the expiration date, the services will be denied. If this happens, you need to contact utilization management or member services and ask for an extension and answer a few questions. Sometimes you may have to involve the patient and/or specialist's office.
   c. If the authorization expires and services have not been provided, you can request an extension. Utilization management will change the expiration date and will fax a copy to the PCP and specialist or will generate a new authorization with a new number.
3. A diagnosis code.
4. The name, address, and telephone number of the contracted specialist where the services will be provided. Sometimes the PCP will refer the patient to a specialist but will not receive approval for that specialist and must get approval for another. Always be sure that any specialist to whom your physician refers patients is contracted with the same managed care plan as the PCP.
5. The comment(s) section is the most critical area of a referral because this area will designate what services are approved.
   a. The specified number of authorized visits to the specialist.
   b. An authorization may be issued for (1) evaluation only, (2) evaluation and treatment plan, (3) evaluation and biopsy, (4) evaluation and one injection, etc.
   c. Authorization for an evaluation only and/or treatment plan. When this authorization appears, the medical assistant must inform the patient that there will not be any treatment—only an evaluation and/or a treatment plan.

Memory Jogger

Name the three types of referrals.

Guidelines for the Assistant in Specialty Practice

If you work for a specialist you do not have to worry about the referral process—only the authorizations.

SKILLS AND RESPONSIBILITIES

GUIDELINES FOR THE MEDICAL ASSISTANT FOR PROCESSING AUTHORIZATIONS

1 Always review the authorization thoroughly before providing services.
2 Deny services if a patient comes in for an appointment without an authorization. Contact the managed care plan and request a copy of the authorization.
3 If you do provide services to the patient, and then discover that the services were not authorized, you cannot bill the patient for any services provided. You can try to get the service authorized by working with the PCP, the member/patient, and the managed care plan, but most of the time you will eventually have to write off the charges. This will not please your employer.
4 Have the patient sign a form agreeing to pay for any services not covered by insurance.

ALLERGIES: ______

PATIENT NAME: ______
PHONE NO. ______

PRESCRIPTIONS

DATE	MEDICATION	AMOUNT	DOSE	START	STOP	REFILLS	INITIALS

FIGURE 20–8 Form for keeping a record of a patient's prescriptions.

HEALTH INSURANCE AND MANAGED CARE

CHART JACKET (FRONT)

Labeled Properly:

1. Last name, first name, middle initial
2. Account number
3. Stickers
    a. First 2 or 3 initials of last name
    b. Current year
    c. Allergies (in red ink)
    d. Living will
    e. Restrictions

CHART CONTENTS

Left side:

1. Patient information sheet
2. Prescription sheet
3. Assignment of benefits
4. Waivers
5. Treatment authorizations

CHART CONTENTS

Right side:

1. Laboratory reports
2. X-ray reports
3. Diagnostic tests
4. Hospital records
5. Surgery reports
6. Consultations
7. Progress notes (in chronological order). Should be in SOAP format

S **Subjective:** Information obtained from the patient (chief complaint)
O **Objective:** Physician's findings (lab reports x-rays, etc.)
A **Assessment:** Diagnosis
P **Plan:** Treatment

FIGURE 20–9 Chart assembly.

Medical Records Audit

Medical records can be audited at any time by the managed care carrier. The medical record (chart) is a legal document that supports the patient/physician relationship. The managed care carrier has the right to access any chart for audit purposes on demand. Therefore, the medical assistant must be certain that the record is properly assembled and maintained.

Auditors look for the following items:

A. Security of Records
   1. Can records be easily accessed by patients or others?
   2. What procedures are being taken to maintain confidentiality?
   3. Are records kept from harm's way?
   4. Are records in a jacket and the contents secured?
   5. Are active records separate from inactive records?
   6. Can records be easily obtained?

B. Documentation Requirements
   1. Is the chart organized and in chronologic order?
   2. Is the chart complete and does it contain the following information:
      a. Family history
      b. Personal history
      c. Past history
      d. Social history
      e. Menstrual and pregnancy history
   3. Is the patient's name on each page?
   4. Are all entries dated?
   5. Is the chart legible?
   6. Are all entries signed by the person making the entry?
   7. Is there proper documentation of weight, height, blood pressure, vital signs, etc., as mandated by the insurance carrier?
   8. Does the chart reflect the SOAP notes as well as patient education?
   9. Are the sections of the chart separated from one another?
   10. Is there an immunization log?
   11. Is there a chart of current medications?
   12. Are samples given to the patient properly documented?
   13. Are there copies of orders from consulting physicians, for blood work, for x-rays, prescriptions, etc.?
   14. Does the documentation for prescriptions contain the following information (Fig. 20–8):
      a. Name of patient
      b. Date
      c. Drug
      d. Strength of drug
      e. Amount dispensed
      f. Number of refills
      g. Instructions to the patient
      h. Who ordered the prescription
      i. The name of the person calling in the prescription
   15. Are missed appointments documented in the chart?
   16. Are there growth charts for pediatric patients?
   17. Has the physician initialed all reports, tests, procedures, etc., after reviewing them?

See Figure 20–9 for an example of setting up the patient record.

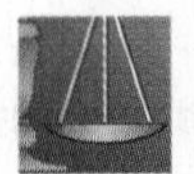

LEGAL AND ETHICAL ISSUES

It is the medical assistant's responsibility to become well acquainted with the various insurance plans utilized by the patients. The medical assistant must be knowledgeable or be able to find the requirements for referral or authorization of patient care. The medical assistant must explain insurance submission policies and patient financial responsibilities before care. Signatures to authorize insurance billing, supplying information to insurance companies, and accepting assignment of benefits (if appropriate) should be obtained from all new patients. Managed care can create a physician/patient barrier that did not exist during the fee-for-service era. An extra effort in human relations on the part of the medical assistant can overcome this barrier and put the patient at ease.

CRITICAL THINKING

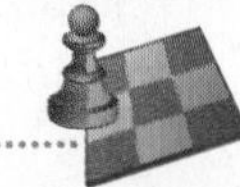

1 A patient enters your office stating she has an HMO of which your physician is not a member. How would you deal with this situation?

HOW DID I DO? Answers to Memory Joggers

1 Seven tasks a medical assistant may have to perform are to
a. Obtain authorizations and referrals
b. Prepare insurance claim forms
c. Maintain an insurance claims register
d. Trace unpaid claims
e. Evaluate claims rejection
f. Report procedures to prepaid care plans
g. Translate medical terminology into procedural and diagnostic codes

2 Deductibles, copayment, and services not covered.

3 The insurance plan of the policyholder whose birthday comes first in the calendar year (month and day, not year) provides primary coverage for each dependent.

4 Medically indigent is someone who is able to take care of ordinary living expenses but is unable to afford medical care.

5 Basic medical means that insurance pays all or part of the physician's fee for nonsurgical services, including hospital, home and office visits, depending on the coverage. It may also include diagnostic laboratory, x-ray, and pathology fees.

6 Benefits are determined by indemnity schedules, by service benefits plans, by determination of the usual, customary and reasonable fee, and by relative value studies.

7 BIC stands for benefits identification card used in California.

8 HMO plans are Kaiser Permanente, Blue Cross/ Blue Shield HMO USA, TRICARE Prime, TRICARE Extra, TRICARE Standard, Medicare HMO risk plans, or HMO cost plans; and Medicaid has various plans.

9 *a.* Verify name of HMO when patient makes appointment.
b. Photocopy ID card.
c. Have patient read and sign a letter outlining plan and or restrictions.
d. Explain the necessity for referral authorization.
e. Collect copay or deductible.

10 *a.* Regular
b. Urgent
c. Stat

REFERENCES

American Medical Association: American Medical News. Chicago, AMA, published weekly.

Fordney M: Insurance Handbook for the Medical Office, 5th ed. Philadelphia, WB Saunders, 1997.

Coding and Claims Processing

21

Sue Hunt, MA, RN, CMA

OUTLINE

LEARNING OBJECTIVES

Cognitive: On successful completion of this chapter you should be able to:

1. Define and spell the terms listed in the Vocabulary.
2. Identify four purposes of numerical diagnostic and procedural coding.
3. Name the principal coding systems that link the medical profession and the insurance system.
4. List 10 reasons for possible rejection of insurance claims.
5. State the maximum billing period for Medicare claims.
6. Explain why a patient's care under workers' compensation should be recorded separately from his or her care as a private patient.
7. List and briefly describe three types of managed care organizations.

Performance: On successful completion of this chapter you should be able to:

1. Identify and complete the appropriate insurance forms for patients covered by
   - a Medicare
   - b CHAMPUS
   - c Workers' compensation
   - d Blue Cross and Blue Shield
2. Calculate the billing for patients whose insurance includes deductibles and copayments or co-insurance.

VOCABULARY

ancillary diagnostic services Services that support patient diagnoses (e.g., laboratory or x-ray)

ancillary therapeutic services Services that support patient treatment (e.g., specialists, surgery)

coding Converting verbal descriptions of diseases, injuries, and procedures into numerical and alphanumerical designations

comorbidities Preexisting conditions that will, because of their presence with a specific principal diagnosis, cause an increase in length of stay by at least 1 day in approximately 75% of the cases

complications Conditions that arise during the hospital stay that prolong the length of stay by at least 1 day in approximately 75% of the cases

crossover claim Claim for benefits under both Medicare and Medicaid

discharge face sheet Summary of the hospital stay prepared at the time of the patient's discharge from the hospital

electronic billing Submission of a claim via computer to computer

established patient A patient who has received care from the physician within the past 3 years or other specified period

etiology Classifying a claim according to the cause of the disorder

fiscal intermediary An organization that handles claims from hospitals, nursing facilities, intermediate and long-term care facilities, and home health care agencies

grouper Computer software program that is used by the fiscal intermediary in all cases to assign discharges to the appropriate DRGs using the following information abstracted from the inpatient bill: patient's age, sex, principal diagnosis, principal procedures performed, and discharge status

International Classification of Diseases, Ninth Revision, Clinical Modification (ICD-9-CM) System for classifying diseases to facilitate collection of uniform and comparable health information

major diagnostic categories (MDCs) Broad clinical categories differentiated from all others based on body system involvement and disease etiology

mandated Required by an authority or law

new patient A patient who has not received any professional services from the physician in the past 3 years or other specified period

nonparticipating provider (non-par) A physician who does not accept assignment under Medicare or the Blue Plans

participating provider (par) A physician who accepts assignment under Medicare or the Blue Plans

peer review organization (PRO) Entity composed of a substantial number of licensed doctors of medicine and osteopathy engaged in the practice of medicine or surgery in the area, or an entity that has available to it the services of a sufficient number of physicians engaged in the practice of medicine or surgery, to assure the adequate peer review of the services provided by the various medical specialties and subspecialties

preauthorization Permission by the insurance carrier obtained before giving certain treatment to a patient

preexisting condition Physical condition of an insured person that existed before the issuance of the insurance policy

principal diagnosis That condition that after study is determined to be chiefly responsible for occasioning the admission of the patient to the hospital

professional standards review organization (PSRO) A group of physicians working with the government to review cases for hospital admission and discharge under government guidelines; sometimes referred to as peer review

Tax Equity and Fiscal Responsibility Act (TEFRA) Signed into federal law in 1982 and contains provisions for major changes in Medicare reimbursement

uniform hospital discharge data set (UHDDS) A minimum data set required to be collected for each Medicare patient on discharge

In recent years the process of submitting insurance claims for payment has become more complicated. After a patient receives service, the office computes charges and adds them to the patient's ledger. If the patient has insurance, a claim is prepared to submit to the insurance company. To facilitate the processing of large numbers of claims insurance companies increasingly require numerical codes for diagnoses and procedures. The insurance company wants to have a means of reviewing quickly that the patient received appropriate services and identifying exactly what services were provided to a given patient. Converting verbal descriptions of diseases, injuries, and procedures into numerical designations is the essence of **coding.**

Numerical diagnostic procedural coding was developed for a number of reasons:

- Tracking disease processes
- Classification of medical procedures
- Medical research
- Evaluation of hospital utilization

This transference of words to numbers also facilitated the use of computers in claims processing. Without the use of computers, it would be impossible to take care of the 60,000 to 65,000 claims processed each day in an average mid-sized claims processing center.

Fee Schedules

RELATIVE VALUE SCALE (RVS)

The RVS was pioneered by the California Medical Association in 1956 to help physicians establish rational, relative fees. Other states soon followed suit. Hundreds of the most commonly performed procedures were compiled, given procedure numbers similar to those in the American Medical Association's *Current Procedural Terminology*, and assigned a unit value. The assigned unit value represented the value of that procedure in relation to other procedures commonly performed. Although no monetary value was placed on the units, many insurance companies used the RVS to determine benefits by applying a conversion factor to assign a monetary value to the unit value. In 1978, the Federal Trade Commission (FTC) interpreted the California RVS as a fee-setting instrument and prohibited its publication and distribution. The FTC was attempting to make medical practice more competitive by ruling against the setting of fees and by encouraging physicians to advertise.

Memory Jogger

 *Name four reasons that coding was developed.*

RESOURCE-BASED RELATIVE VALUE SCALE (RBRVS)

We have now come full circle and are again practicing under relative value scales nationally. The RBRVS is one of the outcomes of the Medicare Physician Payment Reform that was enacted in the Omnibus Budget Reconciliation Act of 1989 (OBRA '89). Since the beginning of Medicare, Part B of the program has paid physicians using a fee-for-service system based on customary, prevailing, and reasonable charges. The RBRVS, effective in 1992, has changed this. The RBRVS consists of three parts:

1. Physician work
2. Charge-based professional liability expenses
3. Charge-based overhead

The physician work component includes the degree of effort invested by the physician in a particular service or procedure and the time it consumed. The professional liability and overhead components are computed by the Health Care Financing Administration (HCFA).

The fee schedule is designed to provide national uniform payments after being adjusted to reflect the differences in practice costs across geographic areas. The fee schedule includes a conversion factor, which is a single national number applied to all services paid under the fee schedule.

Procedural Coding

PHYSICIANS' CURRENT PROCEDURAL TERMINOLOGY (CPT-4)

The *CPT-4 Manual* is a listing of descriptive terms and identifying codes that is used for reporting medical services and procedures performed by physicians. The purpose of the terminology is to provide a uniform language that accurately identifies medical, surgical, and diagnostic services and that can be used as an effective means for reliable, nationwide communication among physicians, patients, and third parties. The *CPT Manual* was developed initially in 1966 by the American Medical Association. There have been several revisions, and it is updated yearly. It is organized into six sections:

1. Evaluation and Management	99201–99499
2. Anesthesiology	00100–01999
3. Surgery	10040–69979
4. Radiology	70010–79999
5. Pathology and Laboratory	80000–89399
6. Medicine	90701–99199

Evaluation and Management has various categories divided into three to five levels based on key components, contributory factors, and the face-to-face time of the services. The three key components the physician uses to select the appropriate level of services are (1) the level of history, (2) the level of examination, and (3) the complexity of medical decision-making. When seeing a **new patient,** all three key components must be met. When seeing an **established patient,** only two of the three components need to be met. Time is considered only if over 50% of the encounter was spent in counseling.

New codes for services and procedures are identified in the *CPT Manual* by the following symbols:

A bullet (●) in front of a code number indicates a new code.

A triangle (▲) in front of a code number indicates that the description for the code has been changed or modified.

A star (★) placed after a code number indicates that a procedure is not subject to the surgical package concept.

The *CPT Manual* is divided into sections, subsections, subheadings, and categories.

Section: Surgery
  Subsection: Respiratory System
    Subheading: Lung
      Category: Excision

An alphabetical index of procedures is located at the back of the *CPT-4 Manual.* At the beginning of each section are guidelines that explain items unique to that section that should be reviewed by the coder. A number of specific code numbers have been designated for reporting unlisted procedures. Use of an unlisted code requires a special report. Two-digit modifiers may be attached to the five-digit code to indicate that the service or procedure has been altered. For example, -50 indicates multiple or bilateral procedures, -52 indicates reduced service, -62 indicates two surgeons, and -80 indicates surgical assistant services.

Books with revised CPT codes are published yearly in the last quarter after Congress has approved the changes and use of new numbers recommended by the American Medical Association.

Memory Jogger

 *Name the six sections of the* CPT-4 Manual.

HCPCS CODING SYSTEM

Medicare carriers have converted to the HCFA's Common Procedure Coding System (HCPCS) (pronounced Hic-Pics). HCPCS, which is based on the current edition of the *CPT,* is a five-digit alphanumerical coding system that can accommodate the addition of modifiers. There are three levels of codes assigned and maintained by Medicare carriers:

- Level I codes include 95% to 98% of all Medicare Part B procedural codes and comprise only CPT codes (excluding those for anesthesiology, which is currently designated by surgery codes).
- Level II codes are assigned by the HCFA and are consistent nationwide. These codes are for physician and nonphysician services not contained in the CPT system; they are alphanumerical, ranging from A0000 to V9999.
- Level III codes are assigned and maintained by each local fiscal intermediary. These codes represent services that are not included in the CPT system and are not common to all carriers. These codes range from W0000 to Z9999.

Diagnostic Coding

INTERNATIONAL CLASSIFICATION OF DISEASES, NINTH REVISION, CLINICAL MODIFICATION (ICD-9-CM)

The ***International Classification of Diseases, Ninth Revision, Clinical Modification (ICD-9-CM)*** is published in three volumes:

Volume 1 (Diseases: Tabular (Numerical) Index)
Volume 2 (Disease: Alphabetical List)
Volume 3 (Tabular List and Alphabetical Index of Procedures)
Volumes 1 and 2 are used in the physician's office to complete insurance claims. Volume 3 is used primarily in hospitals.

The *ICD-9-CM* is used by health care providers in coding and reporting clinical information required for participation in Medicare and Medicaid programs and for statistical tabulation. Each single disease entity has been assigned a three-digit category. A fourth digit is added to provide specificity to the diagnosis regarding **etiology,** site, or manifestations. In certain cases, a fifth digit is required. It is important to use the correct code because the insurance carrier bases its payment for services on their medical justification or necessity. If the claim contains an incomplete or incorrect code, the insurance company may consider the service unnecessary.

The *ICD-9-CM* lists what is wrong with the patient and what initially brought the patient to see the doctor. The list of diagnoses includes

- Diseases
- Conditions
- Accidents
- Injuries
- Poisonings
- All diagnoses

Although diagnostic coding dates back to 17th century England, and the first *International Classifica-*

tion of Diseases (ICD) was published by the World Health Organization (WHO) in 1948, the *ICD-9* took on new significance in 1988 when Congress passed the Medicare Catastrophic Coverage Act. Since 1989, the HCFA has **mandated** the use of *ICD-9-CM* codes on every Medicare Part B claim. New numbers are published yearly.

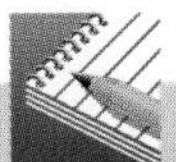

SKILLS AND RESPONSIBILITIES

CODING GUIDELINES

1 Billers must use the appropriate code or codes from 001.0 through V82.9 to identify diagnoses, symptoms, conditions, or other reasons for the encounter/visit.

2 List first the *ICD-9-CM* code for diagnosis, condition, problem, or other reason for encounter/visit shown in the medical record to be chiefly responsible for the services provided. List additional codes that describe any coexisting conditions.

3 Codes must be used at their highest level of specificity, e.g.:

- Assign three-digit codes only if there are no fourth-digit codes within that code category.
- Assign fourth-digit codes only if there is no fifth-digit subclassification for that category.
- Assign the fifth-digit subclassification code for those categories where it exists.

4 Do not code diagnoses documented as Probable, Suspected, Questionable, or Rule Out, as if they are established. Rather, code the condition(s) to the highest degree of certainty for that encounter/visit, such as Symptoms, Signs, Abnormal Test Results, or other reason for the visit (e.g., chest pain, fever).

5 Chronic disease treated on an ongoing basis may be coded and reported as many times as the patient receives treatment and care for the condition(s).

6 For patients receiving **ancillary diagnostic services** only during an encounter/visit, the appropriate V code for the examination is sequenced first and the diagnosis or problem for which the services are being performed is sequenced second.

7 For patients receiving **ancillary therapeutic services** only during an encounter/visit, the appropriate V code for the service is listed first and the diagnosis or problem for which the services are being performed is listed second.

8 For surgery, code the diagnosis for which the surgery was performed. If the postoperative diagnosis is known to be different from the preoperative at the time the claim is filed, select the postoperative diagnosis for coding.

9 Code all documented conditions that coexist at the time of the encounter/visit and that require or affect patient care, treatment, or management. Do not code conditions previously treated and no longer existing.

10 E codes are supplementary and used to describe a variety of external causes of injuries and poisonings.

11 E codes should not be listed as primary diagnoses; they are supplementary. Although not usually required, these codes are sometimes useful to clarify the cause of a disease or injury.

Memory Jogger

3 *Which volume number of the* ICD-9-CM *has the alphabetical listing?*

Guidelines for Claims Processing

GATHERING DATA AND MATERIALS

When the first appointment is made, the medical assistant should ask the patient for all insurance information. The information obtained for the patient record (see Chapter 15) is used for processing the insurance claim. Verify that it is current.

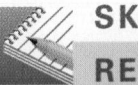

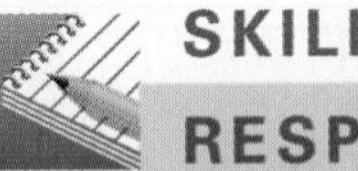

SKILLS AND RESPONSIBILITIES

GUIDELINES FOR THE MEDICAL ASSISTANT FOR CLAIMS PROCESSING

- If the patient has an identification card, it should first be examined to determine that the coverage is current and then photocopied for the office record.
- If more than one insurance policy is involved, obtain the name, address, group, and policy number for each company.
- Obtain the name of the subscriber if it is someone other than the patient.
- Obtain a signed authorization form for releasing information if you are submitting the insurance claim for the patient.

PLEASE DO NOT STAPLE IN THIS AREA

APPROVED OMB-0938-0008

CARRIER

PICA

HEALTH INSURANCE CLAIM FORM

PICA

1. MEDICARE (Medicare #) MEDICAID (Medicaid #) CHAMPUS (Sponsor's SSN) CHAMPVA (VA File #) GROUP HEALTH PLAN (SSN or ID) FECA BLK LUNG (SSN) OTHER (ID)

1a. INSURED'S I.D. NUMBER (FOR PROGRAM IN ITEM 1)

2. PATIENT'S NAME (Last Name, First Name, Middle Initial)

3. PATIENT'S BIRTH DATE MM DD YY SEX M F

4. INSURED'S NAME (Last Name, First Name, Middle Initial)

5. PATIENT'S ADDRESS (No., Street)

6. PATIENT RELATIONSHIP TO INSURED Self Spouse Child Other

7. INSURED'S ADDRESS (No., Street)

CITY STATE

8. PATIENT STATUS Single Married Other

CITY STATE

ZIP CODE TELEPHONE (Include Area Code) ( )

Employed Full-Time Student Part-Time Student

ZIP CODE TELEPHONE (INCLUDE AREA CODE) ( )

9. OTHER INSURED'S NAME (Last Name, First Name, Middle Initial)

10. IS PATIENT'S CONDITION RELATED TO:

11. INSURED'S POLICY GROUP OR FECA NUMBER

a. OTHER INSURED'S POLICY OR GROUP NUMBER

a. EMPLOYMENT? (CURRENT OR PREVIOUS) YES NO

a. INSURED'S DATE OF BIRTH MM DD YY SEX M F

b. OTHER INSURED'S DATE OF BIRTH MM DD YY SEX M F

b. AUTO ACCIDENT? PLACE (State) YES NO

b. EMPLOYER'S NAME OR SCHOOL NAME

c. EMPLOYER'S NAME OR SCHOOL NAME

c. OTHER ACCIDENT? YES NO

c. INSURANCE PLAN NAME OR PROGRAM NAME

d. INSURANCE PLAN NAME OR PROGRAM NAME

10d. RESERVED FOR LOCAL USE

d. IS THERE ANOTHER HEALTH BENEFIT PLAN? YES NO *If yes*, return to and complete item 9 a-d.

READ BACK OF FORM BEFORE COMPLETING & SIGNING THIS FORM.

12. PATIENT'S OR AUTHORIZED PERSON'S SIGNATURE I authorize the release of any medical or other information necessary to process this claim. I also request payment of government benefits either to myself or to the party who accepts assignment below.

SIGNED DATE

13. INSURED'S OR AUTHORIZED PERSON'S SIGNATURE I authorize payment of medical benefits to the undersigned physician or supplier for services described below.

SIGNED

PATIENT AND INSURED INFORMATION

14. DATE OF CURRENT: MM DD YY ILLNESS (First symptom) OR INJURY (Accident) OR PREGNANCY(LMP)

15. IF PATIENT HAS HAD SAME OR SIMILAR ILLNESS. GIVE FIRST DATE MM DD YY

16. DATES PATIENT UNABLE TO WORK IN CURRENT OCCUPATION FROM MM DD YY TO MM DD YY

17. NAME OF REFERRING PHYSICIAN OR OTHER SOURCE

17a. I.D. NUMBER OF REFERRING PHYSICIAN

18. HOSPITALIZATION DATES RELATED TO CURRENT SERVICES FROM MM DD YY TO MM DD YY

19. RESERVED FOR LOCAL USE

20. OUTSIDE LAB? YES NO $ CHARGES

21. DIAGNOSIS OR NATURE OF ILLNESS OR INJURY. (RELATE ITEMS 1,2,3 OR 4 TO ITEM 24E BY LINE)

1. ___ . ___ 3. ___ . ___

2. ___ . ___ 4. ___ . ___

22. MEDICAID RESUBMISSION CODE ORIGINAL REF. NO.

23. PRIOR AUTHORIZATION NUMBER

24. A DATE(S) OF SERVICE From MM DD YY To MM DD YY	B Place of Service	C Type of Service	D PROCEDURES, SERVICES, OR SUPPLIES (Explain Unusual Circumstances) CPT/HCPCS MODIFIER	E DIAGNOSIS CODE	F $ CHARGES	G DAYS OR UNITS	H EPSDT Family Plan	I EMG	J COB	K RESERVED FOR LOCAL USE
1										
2										
3										
4										
5										
6										

25. FEDERAL TAX I.D. NUMBER SSN EIN

26. PATIENT'S ACCOUNT NO.

27. ACCEPT ASSIGNMENT? (For govt. claims, see back) YES NO

28. TOTAL CHARGE $

29. AMOUNT PAID $

30. BALANCE DUE $

31. SIGNATURE OF PHYSICIAN OR SUPPLIER INCLUDING DEGREES OR CREDENTIALS (I certify that the statements on the reverse apply to this bill and are made a part thereof.)

SIGNED DATE

32. NAME AND ADDRESS OF FACILITY WHERE SERVICES WERE RENDERED (If other than home or office)

33. PHYSICIAN'S, SUPPLIER'S BILLING NAME, ADDRESS, ZIP CODE & PHONE #

PIN# GRP#

PHYSICIAN OR SUPPLIER INFORMATION

(APPROVED BY AMA COUNCIL ON MEDICAL SERVICE 8/88)

PLEASE PRINT OR TYPE

FORM HCFA-1500 (12-90) FORM OWCP-1500 FORM RRB-1500

FIGURE 21–1 Health insurance claim form.

CLAIM FORMS

Universal Health Insurance Claim Form

The HCFA designed the basic claim form HCFA-1500 (Fig. 21–1) for the Medicare and Medicaid claims of physicians and other suppliers (see Procedure 21–1). It has also been adopted by the Civilian Health and Medical Program of the Uniformed Services (CHAMPUS) and has received the approval of the American Medical Association Council on Medical Services. Form HCFA-1500 answers the needs of most health care insurers and is referred to as the universal health insurance claim form. One exception is that it is not used to claim reimbursement for ambulance services.

Some commercial insurance companies provide their own forms. When filing a claim with such a company, you can complete the HCFA-1500 form and attach it to the commercial form for submission to the insurance carrier. Because many insurance carriers are using optical character recognition (OCR) scanners to transfer the information on claim forms to their computers' memories, the original form printed in red must be used.

THE SUPERBILL

A private insurance carrier may send its own form to the patient. Rather than completing this form, the office that uses the superbill discussed in Chapter 19 can usually simply attach a copy to the insurance form or give an extra copy of the superbill to the patient if he or she is to submit the claim form. Make certain that the code descriptions on the superbill match those listed in the latest CPT code book.

ASSIGNMENT OF BENEFITS

Some insurance companies honor requests for assignment of benefits to the physician. The medical assistant should request that the patient complete an assignment of benefits form (Fig. 21–2). This is an authorization to the insurance company to make payment directly to the physician. In the case of private insurance it is the patient's responsibility to pay any balance that is not covered by the insurance.

In the case of government-sponsored insurance agreeing to accept assignment of benefits, the physician will accept the fee determination of the plan and the insurance carrier will pay its portion of the fee directly to the physician. The patient can only be billed based on the amount allowed by the insurance plan. See a more complete description below under Medicare billing.

Keeping current with insurance information and changes is no small part of the medical assistant's responsibility. The procedure manual should be updated as changes occur (Fig. 21–3). Government programs are frequently modified, and these changes are reported in bulletins sent to all physicians. *Read these bulletins carefully and save those that contain pertinent information.*

Attend workshops offered to medical assistants and physicians in your area whenever possible and keep the information in a notebook or folder.

TRACKING INSURANCE CLAIMS

Keep a log of insurance claims as they are received and processed (Fig. 21–4). Date-stamp the forms as they are received and enter the information on the log. This log will enable you to determine immediately whether a claim form has been completed and mailed.

- If possible, set aside a definite time for completing insurance claims.
- Have a central location for all insurance forms.
- Have readily available the necessary manuals, code books, and other references needed.
- Create a master list of codes most often used by the practice, including fourth and fifth digits, if appropriate.

ASSIGNMENT OF INSURANCE BENEFITS

I, the undersigned, represent that I have insurance coverage with and do hereby authorize
________________ to pay and assign directly to ________________
(NAME OF COMPANY) (NAME OF DOCTOR)
all surgical and/or medical benefits, if any, otherwise payable to me for services as described on the attached forms hereof, but not to exceed the charges for those services. I understand that I am financially responsible for all charges whether or not paid by said insurance. I hereby authorize said assignee to release all information necessary to secure the payment of said benefits.

Date ________________ Signed ________________

FIGURE 21–2 Assignment of benefits form.

INSURANCE CARRIER Name and Address	Department and Individual to Contact	POLICYHOLDER Individual to Contact	Group or Policy Number	SPECIAL NOTES
BLUE SHIELD PO Box 12345 Anytown, USA	Tom Jones Professional Relations 123-456-7890	Aerospace Industries Joan Crawford 123-888-3030	AI-89037	Tom Jones will speak to groups or give personal assistance in office
		Bell Burgers Nancy Donovan 123-465-2210	BB-3415Z	Scheduled benefits
OCCIDENTAL PO Box 42873 Anytown, USA	Cathy Redding Claims Dept. 213-440-3131	Town School Dist. Mary Embers 312-055-3210	Group No. 4414	Does not pay for assistant surgeon

FIGURE 21–3 Page from procedure manual. Insurance problems can be diminished by knowing whom to contact at the insurance carrier and the policyholder.

- Make it a practice to complete the forms as soon as possible after service is rendered, usually at the end of the day.
- Use the superbill or HCFA-1500 form as often as possible.
- Complete the forms by category (e.g., all Blue Cross, all Medicare).
- Set the tabulator stops on the typewriter or word processor for the form being completed. Make a note of these stops so they can easily be set up when completing the same kind of form again.
- If using a computer billing program to print insurance forms, the computer will store insurance information on outstanding claims that can be printed in batches using the HCFA-1500 forms. Adjust the printer so that the information prints correctly on the form.
- Transmit claims electronically whenever possible.

INSURANCE CLAIM REGISTER

PATIENT	INSURANCE COMPANY	DATE FILED	AMOUNT BILLED	AMOUNT PAID	DIFFERENCE

FIGURE 21–4 Insurance log showing the date each claim was filed, the amount billed, the amount paid, and the difference that must be either discounted or billed to the patient.

RECORDS RELEASE Date ______________

To ____
DOCTOR
____
ADDRESS

I hereby authorize and request you to release

to ____
DOCTOR
____
ADDRESS

the complete medical records in your possession, concerning my illness and/or treatment during

the period from ______________ to ______________

Signed ______________________
(PATIENT OR NEAREST RELATIVE)

______________________ Relationship ______________
WITNESS

FORM 122 - Eastman, Inc.

FIGURE 21–5 Authorization form for release of medical information.

COMPLETING THE HCFA-1500 FORM

1. If you plan to mail the form directly to the insurance company, be sure that the patient has signed the Authorization to Release Information form (Fig. 21–5)
2. Make sure that Medicare patients sign an Extended Signature Authorization form (Fig. 21–6)
3. Typewrite all claim forms and keep a photocopy or computer printout of each.
4. Use accepted diagnostic and procedure codes, and be certain that the procedures are consistent with the diagnoses.
5. List all procedures performed, one procedure per line. Be specific. If a laceration was treated, give the location, length, and depth; the number of sutures required; and the duration of treatment involved. If a sterile surgical tray was used for office surgery, itemize and bill as a separate fee. If a treatment injection was given, state the injected material and the amount given.
6. Attach a copy of the x-ray report, hospital report, and/or consultant's report in complicated cases.
7. State the physician's usual and customary fee on all claim forms, regardless of what payment is expected.

MEDICARE LIFETIME ASSIGNMENT

Name of beneficiary: ______________________

Medicare number: ______________________

I request that payment of authorized Medicare benefits be made to me or on my behalf to (physician/supplier name) for any services furnished me by that provider. I authorize any holder of medical information about me to release to the Health Care Financing Administration and its agents any information needed to determine benefits or the benefits payable for related services.

This authorization is in effect until I choose to revoke it.*

Signed: ______________________ Date: ______________

**If you are a patient in a hospital or skilled nursing facility, this authorization is in effect for the period of your confinement.*

FIGURE 21–6 Patient's extended signature authorization for Medicare claims.

8 Never alter a claim as to services performed, date of service, or fees established.
9 If more than one visit per day was required, state the times of day so that the claims processor will know they were separate procedures and attach a letter of medical necessity on the physician's letterhead.
10 Fill in all blanks. Type DNA (does not apply) or NA (not applicable) or simple dash lines (–) rather than leave an item blank. This is confirmation that the item was not overlooked.

ELECTRONIC CLAIMS SUBMISSION

The medical practice that is computerized probably uses the computer for processing electronic claims (E-claims). This may be handled in several ways (e.g., transmitting data via modem or by recording data on computer disk or tape and sending it to the payer or intermediary).

An obvious advantage of **electronic billing** is the amount of time saved with its use. The system interrupts the transmission of incomplete or incorrect data, giving the biller the opportunity for on-the-spot correction. The sender knows immediately whether the insurance company is accepting the claim. Another advantage of electronic billing is that it speeds up the date of payment, which results in an increase in cash flow to the practice.

Electronic transfer of information is also advantageous to the payer. The HCFA is a strong advocate and has long given preference to the processors of E-claims. By 2000, all providers of Medicare and Medicaid must file their claims electronically.

Not all claims are suitable for electronic submission. For example, those claims that are complicated and require a cover letter or those that require some kind of attachment must be sent on hard copy (paper) by mail or messenger.

CLAIM REJECTION

If a claim form is not sufficiently detailed, complete, and accurate, it may be rejected by the insurance company.

EXAMPLES OF THE REASONS FOR CLAIM REJECTION

- Diagnosis is missing or incomplete
- Diagnosis is not coded accurately
- Diagnosis does not correspond with treatment
- Charges are not itemized
- Patient's group, member, or policy number is missing or incorrect
- Patient's portion of the form is incomplete, or the patient's signature is missing
- Patient's date of birth is missing
- Fee is not listed
- Dates are incorrect or missing
- Physician's signature or address is missing

Memory Jogger

4 *If a diagnosis is missing from an insurance claim, what will be the result?*

Billing Requirements

MEDICARE

Under Medicare, the physician may be a **participating provider** or a **nonparticipating provider** (sometimes referred to as **par** and **non-par providers**). Both are required by law to file the HCFA-1500 insurance claim for all eligible patients. The office may also file for a secondary carrier.

A participating provider accepts assignment on Medicare claims. The allowance payment comes directly to the physician and is accepted as payment in full. The patient is still responsible for paying the deductible and the 20% co-insurance to the physician.

A nonparticipating provider is not required to accept assignment. If such is the case, the patient is responsible for the balance after Medicare makes its payment. The allowable payment to the non-par provider is less than the payment to the par provider.

The non-par provider who plans to perform elective surgery on a Medicare patient that costs $500 or more is subject to Medicare's $500 surgery rule (Fig. 21–7). The provider must prepare a financial statement showing the type of surgery to be performed, the estimated charge, the estimated payment from Medicare, and the patient's probable out-of-pocket expense. This statement must be signed by the patient. Give one photocopy to the patient and file another with the patient's chart.

Claims for Medicare must be filed by December 31 of the year following that in which the services were rendered. For example, care rendered in 1999 must be billed no later than December 31, 2000.

MEDICAID

A physician is free to accept or to refuse to treat a patient under Medicaid. However, if the patient is accepted, requirements for rendering service and billing for services are strict and must be closely followed:

The patient's identification card must be current. Some include labels that must be attached to the

Dear Patient:

I do not plan to accept assignment for your surgery. The law requires that where assignment is not taken and the charge is $500 or more, the following information must be provided prior to your surgery. These estimates assume you have met the annual Part B Medicare deductible.

Type of surgery ______
Estimated charge $ ______
Estimated Medicare payment $ ______
Your estimated payment $ ______
(This includes your Medicare co-insurance)

Physician's Signature ______

I have read and understand the above information.

X ______ (Patient's Signature) ______ (Date)

FIGURE 21–7 Non-par provider's financial statement that is used to comply with Medicare's $500 surgery rule.

billing form. Others have a benefits identification card (BIC) that must be verified before seeing the patient.

Preauthorization may be required for the service, for which a form is completed. For an emergency situation, authorization may be secured by telephone but must be followed up with the appropriate form.

Claims are submitted on the HCFA-1500 form or a similar form required by the individual state for optical scanning. There will be a time limit for billing after the termination of which the claim may be rejected, depending on the state regulations. It is important that the medical assistant check the local regulations and keep current on requirements. Some Medicaid patients have been shifted to HMOs, and their bills should be sent to the HMO not the Medicaid fiscal agent.

Physicians who accept Medicaid are required to accept assignment of benefits and are not allowed to bill the patient beyond what Medicaid allows.

Memory Jogger

 *Describe Medicare's $500 surgery rule.*

MEDI/MEDI

The HCFA-1500 form is used, and the physician must always accept assignment. Failure to indicate acceptance of assignment will result in a Medicare payment going to the patient and in rejection of the claim by Medicaid. A label from the patient's ID card or a photocopy of the current card may be required.

The claim form is first processed through Medicare and is then automatically forwarded to Medicaid. It is not necessary to prepare two claims forms. This is sometimes referred to as a **crossover claim.**

Memory Jogger

 *What does HCPCS stand for?*

BLUE PLANS

When a patient is covered under a Blue Plan, claims should be submitted as soon as possible after the service is provided. Many of the Blue Plans have adopted use of the HCFA-1500 form. Check with the local office or representative in your area.

Like Medicare, the Blue Plans have arrangements with participating and nonparticipating providers. Usually the participating provider is paid directly for covered services and agrees not to bill the patient for any difference between the provider's fee and the allowed fee.

The Blue Plans have provider manuals that describe coverage and coding features of the Plan. These manuals are periodically revised. Contact your local representative if your manual might be outdated.

CIVILIAN HEALTH AND MEDICAL PROGRAM OF THE UNIFORMED SERVICES (CHAMPUS) AND CIVILIAN HEALTH AND MEDICAL PROGRAM OF THE VETERANS ADMINISTRATION (CHAMPVA)

Use form HCFA-1500 for the covered portion of the fee. Like Medicare, if the physician accepts assignment, the patient should be billed for the entire deductible but can only be billed for the co-insurance portion of the charge allowed by CHAMPUS or CHAMPVA. If the physician does not accept assignment, the patient submits claim forms with the physician's itemized statement to the insurance company and is responsible for the total deductible and co-insurance. The claim must be filed no later than December 31 of the year following that in which services were provided.

WORKERS' COMPENSATION

Records for the workers' compensation case (sometimes referred to as an industrial case) should be kept separate from the physician's regular patient histories. If the patient who is seen for an industrial injury has previously been treated as a private patient, a new chart and ledger should be started that will be used only for the treatment rendered under conditions of the workers' compensation law.

The insurance carrier may request and is entitled to receive copies of all records pertaining to the industrial injury but not the records of a private patient. *Information in the records of a private patient is privileged information and may be released only with the patient's consent.* There could be a lawsuit or a hearing before a referee or appeals board for which records are subpoenaed. If separate records are kept, there is no question of privilege involved.

The employer and the physician who sees the injured or ill worker first are required, in most states, to file a report with the insurance carrier within a specified length of time. The medical assistant should make a minimum of five copies of this report. The insurance company usually requires at least two copies. One copy goes to the state regulatory body. The employer may get a copy, and one file copy should remain with the physician's record. This report must be personally signed by the physician and should contain the following information:

- The history of the case as obtained from the patient, with notation of any **preexisting condition** (injuries or diseases)
- The patient's symptoms and physical complaints
- Complete physical findings, including laboratory and x-ray results
- A tentative diagnosis
- An estimate of the type and extent of the disability. In cases in which permanent disability has resulted, there should be a careful survey and the extent of disability should be given.
- Treatment indicated, including type, frequency, and duration. It may be necessary to attach a letter giving more detailed information to assist in making an evaluation of the case.
- If the patient is unable to return to work, the probable date that he or she will be able to return to work

The insurance carrier may supply its own billing forms. Payment is usually made on the basis of a fee schedule. Any charges in excess of the fee schedule must be fully explained and documented. In billing for the service, use the coding system specified in your state. Itemize the statement, including any drugs and dressings used.

In severe or prolonged cases, supplementary reports and billing should be sent to the insurance carrier at least once per month. At the termination of treatment, a final report and bill are sent to the insurance carrier. Do not bill the patient.

PROCEDURE 21-1
Completing Insurance Forms

GOAL

To complete an insurance claim form for services.

EQUIPMENT AND SUPPLIES

Patient chart
HCFA-1500 claim form
Patient ledger
Typewriter or computer

PROCEDURAL STEPS

A Ask for patient's identification card
PURPOSE: To determine whether the patient is insured.

B Photocopy card and place the copy in the patient's file.
PURPOSE: If questions arise, the office has an exact copy of the insurance information.

C Have the patient sign an Extended Signature Authorization form.
PURPOSE: This form grants lifetime authorization for the physician to submit assigned or unassigned claims on the beneficiary's behalf. (It must be canceled on the patient's request.)

D Complete the following entries (blocks 1–33) on the HCFA-1500 form:

Continued

1 Check the appropriate boxes for all types of health insurance coverage applicable to the claim.

1A Enter the insured person's identification number (and all letters) as it appears on the person's insurance card.

2 Enter the patient's full name (last name, then first name and middle initial) exactly as it appears on the insurance card.

3 Enter six-digit birth date and sex.

4 Enter word "SAME" if patient and insured are the same person, or enter the full name of the insured person (last name, then first name and middle initial).

5 Enter the patient's permanent mailing address and telephone number. (Do not use P.O. box for address.)

6 Enter patient's relationship to the policyholder by checking the correct box.

7 Enter the word "SAME" if the patient and insured live at the same address. Otherwise enter the mailing address of the policy holder. If CHAMPUS, put the sponsor's military address.

8 Check the appropriate boxes to identify the patient's marital and employment status.

9 Complete this block only if the patient has other insurance coverage. Otherwise enter NA on the first line of this block. On the first line of the block enter the name of the insured person (last name, then first name and middle initial).
- A Enter the policy or group number including letters.
- B Enter date of birth and sex.
- C Enter employer's name or school name.
- D Enter insurance plan or program name.

10 Check the appropriate boxes (YES or NO).
- A If the patient's condition is related to employment, check YES and submit the claim to workers' compensation.
- B If the patient's condition is related to a vehicular accident, check YES and include the two-letter code for the state where the accident occurred.
- C If the patient's condition is related to an accident other than a vehicular accident, check YES.
- D Generally this box is used exclusively for Medicaid. Enter the patient's Medicaid number preceded by "MCD."

11 This block must be completed for Medicare. If the patient has insurance that is primary to Medicare, complete blocks 11A through 11C. If other insurance is not primary to Medicare, enter "NONE." Indicate "CHAMPUS" in this block if the patient has Medicare. The block should be filled out with the information of the insured person.

12 If the patient has signed an "Authorization for Release of Medical Information," fill in this box with "SIGNATURE ON FILE" or "SOF." If the claim will be filed electronically, it is necessary to have the signature on file. If the claim will be sent through the mail, the patient can sign the form.

13 Reserve for the patient's signature if a Medicare supplement policy is indicated in block 9; or if the patient has signed a separate Medicare or Medigap authorization, enter "SIGNATURE ON FILE." If the claim is to Medicaid, the POE sticker goes here.

14 For Medicare, CHAMPUS, or commercial insurance, enter the date of the patient's current illness; or for pregnancy, enter the date of the last menstrual period.

15 For Medicare, Medicaid, or Blue Cross/Blue Shield, leave blank. For CHAMPUS, workers' compensation, or commercial insurance, fill in if appropriate.

16 For Medicare or commercial insurance, enter the dates the patient cannot work, if employed. This box may also be filled in for workers' compensation.

17 Enter the HCFA-assigned unique provider identification number of the physician. This is written as a 10-digit number: the first seven characters are the provider's number, the next is a check digit, and the last two characters identify the provider's location.

18 Complete this block when the medical service is related to hospitalization (enter admission and discharge dates).

Continued

PROCEDURE 21-1 (CONTINUED)
Completing Insurance Forms

19 Consult the billing manual of the particular insurance to determine what may be needed in this box.

20 Complete when billing for diagnostic tests. Check "NO" if all laboratory tests included on the claim form were completed in the physician's office. Check "YES" if laboratory tests were done outside the office and billed to the physician's office. Fill in the amount of the bill. If "YES" is checked, the charge for each test should be entered in box 24D and the name of the outside laboratory should be entered in block 32.

21 Enter ICD-9-CM diagnosis codes beginning with the primary diagnosis and up to three other diagnoses that justify the procedures entered in block 24. If more than four diagnoses are needed, fill out a second claim form. Do not use decimal points.

22 Complete only for Medicaid.

23 For Medicare, Medicaid and CHAMPUS enter the prior authorization number (PRO), a 10-digit number if required for the procedure.

24 One procedure may be listed per line for blocks 24A through 24K.

- 24A Enter the month, day, and year for each procedure or service. If the from and to dates are the same, enter only the from date. If the same service or procedure with identical charges is provided on consecutive days, both the from and to dates should be entered.
- 24B Enter the code for the place of service.
- 24C Enter CHAMPUS, Medicaid, and workers' compensation service codes.
- 24D Enter procedure codes, either CPT codes or HCPCS codes, depending on the requirements of the insurance. Enter the five-digit code and modifiers if needed, without decimal points.
- 24E Enter the number 1, 2, 3, or 4 that points to the diagnosis code for the procedure in box 21 that justifies the medical necessity for performing the procedure. Do not use the actual codes in this box.
- 24F Enter the fee for each service. Do not enter dollar signs or decimal points.
- 24G Enter the number of days or units being billed.
- 24H This box is used only for Medicaid. EPSDT refers to a Medicaid early, periodic, screening, diagnosis, and treatment. Enter "E" for these services or "F" for family planning.
- 24I Check this box for commercial insurance or Medicaid if care was given in an emergency department.
- 24J For Medicaid, check if coordination of benefits.
- 24K For Medicare, CHAMPUS, and commercial insurance, enter the employer identification number (EIN) or the HCFA-assigned unique provider identification number (UPIN) of the provider when the physician is in a group practice. Enter the first two digits in box 24J and the remaining eight digits in box 24K.

25 Enter the physician's federal tax ID number. This may be the EIN or the Social Security number (SSN).

26 Enter the number assigned to the patient if the practice uses numerical identification numbers or if the claim is filed electronically.

27 For Medicare or CHAMPUS, check "YES" or "NO" to indicate whether the physician accepts assignment of benefits. For Medicaid and Medicare/Medicaid, the physician must check "YES."

28 Enter the total charge for services. This block must be completed.

29 For Medicare, enter the amount paid by the patient with the exception of the 20% co-insurance and deductible. For CHAMPUS, enter the amount paid by the patient or other insurance. For Medicaid, enter payment by insurance other than Medicare.

30 Enter the balance due.

Continued

31 Show the signature of the physician or that of his or her representative. Most insurance companies will accept a stamp if it fits in the box. Type the provider's name underneath (not the practice name.)

32 Enter the name and address of the facility if other than home or office. If you checked "YES" in box 20, you must enter the name and address of the laboratory that performed diagnostic tests billed on this form.

33 Enter the billing name, address and telephone number for the physician. Enter the UPIN number for a physician in solo practice or the group PIN number if the physician practices as part of a group.

Health Care and Cost Containment

HEALTH CARE REFORM

Since World War II, group insurance has been a significant fringe benefit in collective bargaining. In the fee-for-service concept of the 1960s to 1980s, the patient saw the doctor, received care, and then received a bill for the service. Insurance programs were first designed simply to pay those bills. The patient who had insurance paid an annual premium, and in return the insurance company paid at least a portion of the bill. Much of the fee-for-service care has been provided by Medicare, Medicaid, and the Blue Plans, but all of these plans are now utilizing cost-containment alternatives to fee for service.

During the 1990s, a major restructuring of the U.S. health care system was brought about because

- A growing percentage of Americans were not covered by private or government insurance.
- Employers were having to pay escalating health care premiums and did not want to cut wages. They wanted methods to lower the cost of employee health care.
- The government needed to reduce the deficit by keeping down increases in Medicaid and Medicare programs.
- Physicians and hospital costs were soaring out of sight due to inflation, expensive equipment, medications, and so on.
- Patients were reluctant to pay for physical examinations and immunizations, which were not usually covered by traditional insurance policies, and sometimes conditions were not diagnosed as early as desirable.

Over 70% of insurance has become HMO and is no longer fee for service.

MANAGEMENT OF HMO PLANS

If claims are not being paid promptly or correctly, the medical assistant should take steps to resolve the problem.

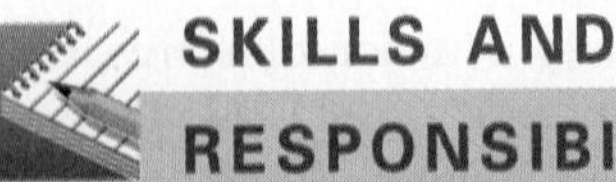

SKILLS AND RESPONSIBILITIES

GUIDE TO RESOLVING UNPAID OR INCORRECTLY PAID CLAIMS

1 Take examples to the next renegotiating session when the physician's contract expires.
2 Send a statement to the director notifying him or her that if the bill is not paid you will contact the employer's benefits manager or patient notifying him or her of the slow payments. Tell that person that the physician may not renew the contract and the director may need to find another physician.
3 Write to the plan representative.

PEER REVIEW ORGANIZATIONS

A **peer review organization (PRO)** is an outgrowth of a 1972 amendment to the Social Security Act that brought about the formation of federal **professional standards review organizations (PSROs),** whose purposes were to monitor the validity of diagnoses and the quality of care and to evaluate the appropriateness of hospital admissions and discharges of patients covered by government-sponsored health insurance. The effectiveness of PSROs was continually debated, and they were gradually phased out.

In 1982 PROs were legislated as part of the **Tax Equity and Fiscal Responsibility Act (TEFRA).** The purpose of a PRO is identical to that of the PSRO. The primary difference is that the PROs are mostly limited to a single group within a state. PRO contracts are awarded by the HCFA to physician-based organizations within each state, and the mechanics of PROs vary slightly from state to state. In an attempt to control costs, an insurance carrier may require prior authorization from the PRO before a patient is hospitalized for elective medical or surgical care. If the patient's condition can be adequately and safely treated on an outpatient basis, payment for hospitalization will not be approved. It is important that the medical assistant be aware of the types of admission cases that require previous authorization and that the authorization be obtained before the admission date.

PROSPECTIVE PAYMENT SYSTEM

In April 1983, the Social Security Amendments Act of 1983 (Public Law 98-21) was signed into law. Title VI of this law contained the prospective payment system (PPS) for hospitals, which would begin the radical restructuring of the payment system to hospitals for Medicare inpatient services.

As identified by HCFA, a major objective of the PPS was to establish the government as a prudent buyer of health care while maintaining beneficiaries' access to quality care. The prudent buyer objective was to be accomplished by paying Medicare providers a predetermined specific rate per discharge for diagnoses rather than on the basis of reasonable costs.

If a hospital does not contract with a PRO, it is not eligible for payment from the Medicare program. The law provides authority to grant waivers from the PPS if a state has an approved hospital reimbursement control system. Additional criteria must be met by a state to receive approval and a waiver from the federal PPS.

Diagnosis-Related Groups (DRGs)

The DRG classification forms the basis for payment under the PPS. It is based on an average cost for the patient's problem, as opposed to the traditional method of payment based on actual costs incurred in the provision of care. Payment to the hospital of a DRG amount generally constitutes payment in full for services rendered to Medicare patients.

The DRG system classifies patients on the basis of diagnosis and was developed by Yale University researchers in the 1970s as a mechanism for utilization review. DRGs are derived from taking all possible diagnoses identified in the ICD-9-CM system, classifying them into 25 **major diagnostic categories** (MDCs) based on organ system, and further breaking them into 495 **distinct groupings,** each of which is said to be medically meaningful. The principal diagnosis is the most critical factor in the assignment of DRGs. All diagnoses must reflect information contained in the patient's medical record.

To assign a case to a DRG, five pieces of information are necessary:

1. Patient's **principal diagnosis** and up to four **complications** or **comorbidities**
2. Treatment procedures performed
3. Patient's age
4. Patient's sex
5. Patient's discharge status

Physician's Responsibility

The major factor determining the assignment of a DRG is the physician's assessment of the principal diagnosis. It is the physician's responsibility to record the principal diagnosis as well as the other determining factors on a **discharge face sheet.** It is extremely important that the principal diagnosis, as stated by the physician, correspond to the various tests, procedures, and notes contained within the complete medical record.

Once the discharge face sheet has been completed by the physician, the chart is forwarded to the hospital's medical records department for review and coding. The codes contained in the *ICD-9-CM* are used for determining the DRG and, therefore, must be entered in the appropriate section of the discharge face sheet.

From the medical records department the information is forwarded to the financial office for completion of the bill to be submitted to the **fiscal intermediary.** The fiscal intermediary, through the use of a **grouper** computer program, determines the appropriate DRG and then calculates the payment to the hospital.

Memory Jogger

7 *What is the major factor in determining the assignment of a DRG?*

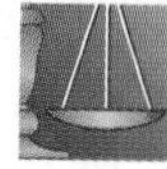

LEGAL AND ETHICAL ISSUES

The practice of medicine and the responsibilities of the medical assistant, are greatly affected by the legislative process. It is extremely important to stay current on the laws that affect medicine, and in particular the coding process.

The person who is responsible for coding procedures must be very careful. It is the physician's responsibility to identify the patient's diagnosis and identify the procedures that have been performed. Often these codes are preprinted on the encounter form or superbill and/or in the computer, but if they are not, the medical assistant must identify the correct code. An incorrect code used for billing a service can be considered a fraud, especially if it is a recurrent offense.

In addition, the medical assistant must be sure to obtain patient signatures permitting insurance billing and to obtain proper authorizations from insurance carriers whenever required.

CRITICAL THINKING

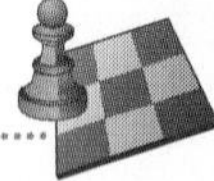

1 Using your *CPT Manual,* code the following: The physician is called to the ICU at the local hospital to see a patient in coronary crisis. The physician spends 1 hour at the patient's bedside stabilizing him.
Code: ______________________

2 An established patient is one who has received professional services from the physician or another physician of the same specialty in the same group within ______________________.

3 Using your *ICD-9-CM Manual,* code the following:
a. Bacterial endocarditis due to AIDS
Code: ______________________
b. Herniated disk, L4S1
Code: ______________________
c. Congestive heart failure with hypertension
Code: ______________________

HOW DID I DO? Answer to Memory Joggers

1 Tracking disease processes, classification of medical procedures, medical research, and evaluation of hospital utilization

2 Evaluation and Management, Anesthesiology, Surgery, Radiology, Pathology and Laboratory, and Medicine

3 Volume 2

4 The claim could be returned or rejected, or the physician could be fined if the claim were for Medicare.

5 If elective surgery is necessary on a Medicare patient, the provider must prepare a financial statement showing the type of surgery to be performed, the estimated charge, the estimated payment from Medicare, and the patient's probable out-of-pocket expenses. This statement must be signed by the patient. Put a copy in the patient's chart and give the patient a copy.

6 Health Care Financing Administration Common Procedure Coding system

7 The principal diagnosis

REFERENCES

American Medical Association: DRGs and the Prospective Payment System: A Guide for Physicians. Chicago, AMA, 1984.

American Medical Association: Physician's Current Procedural Terminology, 4th ed. Chicago, AMA, 1997.

American Medical Association: American Medical News, a weekly newspaper.

Fordney M: Insurance Handbook for the Medical Office, 5th ed. Philadelphia, WB Saunders, 1997.

Gosfield AG: RBRVS Special Report. Salt Lake City, Med-Index Publications, 1991.

HCPCS 1991–1992, 3rd ed. Salt Lake City, Med-Index Publications, 1997.

Reimbursement Strategies. Salt Lake City, Med-Index Publications, 1991.

SECTION 6

Advanced Administrative Skills

CURRICULUM CONTENT/COMPETENCIES

Chapter 22 Editorial Duties and Travel Arrangements

- *Perform basic clerical functions*
- *Schedule, coordinate, and monitor appointments*
- *Develop educational materials*
- *Conduct continuing education activities*

Chapter 23 Facility Environment

- *Maintain supply inventory*
- *Comply with established risk management and safety procedures*
- *Maintain and dispose of regulated substances in compliance with government guidelines*
- *Negotiate leases and prices for equipment and supply contracts*

Chapter 24 Management Responsibilities

- *Orient and train personnel*
- *Interview and recommend job applicants*
- *Supervise personnel*
- *Process payroll*
- *Develop and maintain personnel, policy, and procedure manuals*

Assisting with Library, Research, Travel, and Meetings

22

OUTLINE

LEARNING OBJECTIVES

Cognitive: On successful completion of this chapter you should be able to:

1. Define and spell the terms listed in the Vocabulary.
2. Originate and maintain a card catalog for a personal library.
3. Discuss the nature and importance of an abstract.
4. List the four items to include on a cross-reference card for a general reference file.
5. Name five items of information to include on a diagnostic file card.
6. Name two of the largest medical databases for electronic retrieval of information.
7. List the seven items of information needed for each bibliography reference.
8. Briefly outline the general procedure for preparing a manuscript for publication.
9. List the five items that should be included in the first paragraph of meeting minutes.

Performance: On successful completion of this chapter you should be able to:

1. Prepare cards for an abstract file.
2. Set up a diagnostic file, including subject cards and the necessary subheadings to accommodate the patient charts.
3. Retype a manuscript that has been edited using proofreader's marks.
4. Type a speech in correct format and estimate the time necessary for delivery.
5. Make travel arrangements for a proposed trip.
6. Prepare a typewritten itinerary.
7. Make arrangements for a group meeting.
8. From a rough draft, type the minutes of a meeting in correct form, including the secretary's signature.

VOCABULARY

abstract A written summary of the key points of a book, paper, or case history

agenda A list of the specific items under each division of the order of business that is to be presented at a business meeting

bibliography A list of the works that are referred to in a text or that were consulted by the author in producing a text

colloquialisms Expressions that are acceptable and correct in ordinary conversation or informal speeches but unsuitable for formal speech or writing

draft A preliminary outline or writing that the author expects to amend or revise

footnotes Comments placed at the bottom of a page that would be distracting if placed within the main text

galley proofs Printer's proofs taken from composed type before page composition

legend Heading or title of a figure

manuscript Written or typewritten document, as distinguished from printed copy

monograph Learned treatise on a small area of knowledge; a written account of a single thing or class of things

order of business List of the different divisions of business in the order in which each is to be addressed at a business meeting

periodicals Journals published with a fixed interval (greater than 1 day) between their issues or numbers

reprints Reproductions of printed matter

synopsis Summary of the main points of a longer text

treatise Systematic exposition or argument in writing

The medical profession is unique in that the physician traditionally shares with others, through writing and speaking, the discoveries, information, and observations gained in practice, research, and private study. The medical assistant who becomes proficient in maintaining the physician's personal library and in assisting with the preparation of articles and speeches can be of immeasurable help in these endeavors.

The Physician's Library

The books that a physician acquires while in medical school are the nucleus of a personal library that will grow over the years. New books reflecting the changes in medicine and the physician's special interests are continually added (Fig. 22–1). The physician may accumulate a file of professional journals such as the *Journal of the American Medical Association* (JAMA), the journal of the state medical society, specialty journals, trade journals, and even informative material provided by pharmaceutical companies.

Journals should be bound at regular intervals, generally by volume, to preserve the individual copies. The medical assistant may be responsible for having the journals bound regularly and consistently. Most journals in the medical field publish indexes, annually, semiannually, or quarterly. The index should be bound with the journal pages. In most cities, the binding of **periodicals** can be done locally. The hospital librarian is a good source of information for locating a bookbinder.

ORGANIZING THE LIBRARY

Although the physician's library may not be large, it must be systematically organized so that information is readily accessible.

In setting up or rearranging a small library, books should be classified by subject groupings that reflect

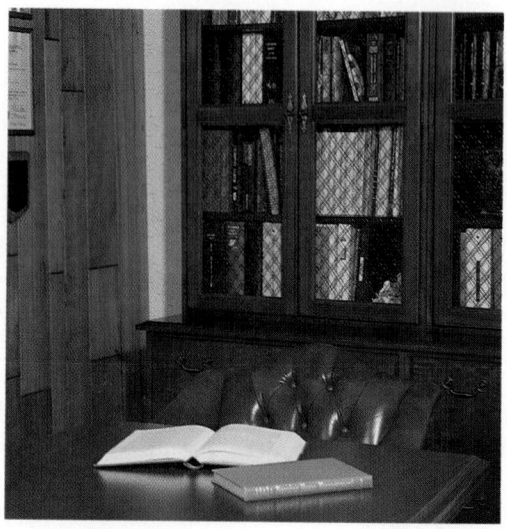

FIGURE 22–1 A physician's library.

medical specialties. Those dealing with related topics should be placed together. Journals and periodicals are usually arranged alphabetically.

CATALOGING OF BOOKS

The books should be indexed, either in a card catalog or in a computer database. A 3 × 5-inch card file is practical for this purpose. Generally, three or more cards should be prepared for each book (Fig. 22–2):

- Title card
- Subject card
- Author card(s)

Here is how to index a book in this manner, using the book you are reading as an example:

1. Prepare a title card with the heading "The Administrative Medical Assistant."
2. Prepare a subject card with the heading "Medical Assisting."
3. Prepare author card with the heading Kinn, Mary E.
4. The cards may then be filed alphabetically or, preferably, in a file divided into sections for title, subject, and author. With such a file and cross-reference system, any book can be located very quickly.

Administrative Medical Assistant, The, 4th Edition

Mary E. Kinn
Philadelphia, W. B. Saunders Company, 1999

Textbook and reference covering all administrative phases of medical assisting in the physician's office

TITLE CARD

Medical Assisting

The Administrative Medical Assistant, 4th Edition,
Philadelphia, W. B. Saunders Company, 1999

Mary E. Kinn

SUBJECT CARD

Kinn, Mary E.

The Administrative Medical Assistant, 4th Edition,
Philadelphia, W. B. Saunders Company, 1999

1. Medical Assisting

AUTHOR CARD

FIGURE 22–2 Title, subject, and author cards for referencing a book in a personal library.

Memory Jogger

What is the purpose of indexing the contents of a personal library?

PERIODICAL FILE

One of the physician's greatest challenges is keeping up with medical literature, particularly the articles that appear regularly in the periodicals. It is unlikely that the physician will want to maintain a complete index of all articles appearing in these periodicals, but most will want to keep track of those articles that are of particular interest. Abstracts are of great value in the continuing task of keeping abreast of scientific developments.

Preparation of an Abstract

An **abstract** is a **synopsis** of a book, paper, or case history. It is brief, indicates the nature of the article, and summarizes the most important points and conclusions. Abstracts prepared by professionals are found in many medical journals as a service to the individual physician.

Many physicians prepare abstracts of the articles that they find of particular value; and in some offices, the medical assistant is trained to do abstracting for the physician. A medical assistant who can prepare a good abstract of an article can save the physician from reading 10 to 20 pages of the original article and can help focus attention on information of particular interest in the article.

Abstracts must clearly indicate the nature of the information contained in the article. Each should note

- Any new procedures
- Results of studies and experiments
- Conclusions noted

The length and character of the article determine the type and length of the abstract. In most scientific articles, the conclusions of the writer are summarized at the end of the piece. This summary is of great help in preparing an abstract.

The abstracts are typed on cards, with the text of the abstract preceded by the following information:

- Title of the article
- Surname and initials of the author
- Name of the publication
- Volume number
- Inclusive page numbers
- Month and year

The cards are then filed. If abstract cards are kept, it is not necessary to clip and file the actual articles separately. The journals in which they appear can be kept in the usual alphabetical order.

Memory Jogger

Name the three classes of information that should be included in an abstract.

OTHER REFERENCE FILES

Physicians frequently need a variety of miscellaneous medical information in addition to book collections and periodicals and their indexes. For this reason, they may develop a separate reference file of valuable information. Often, this consists of pages photocopied from journals or reference books.

The physician and the medical assistant together may set up a subject index for filing the material and a cross-reference card file for easily locating the information. Begin by tabbing file dividers with the main topics and folders with subheadings. When an article or item is photocopied, a card is prepared with the title of the article or chapter, author's name, periodical or book in which it appears, and the date of publication. The copy of the reference material is then filed in the appropriate folder and the card filed by subject for easy reference. As new developments occur, later articles may be filed and the outdated material discarded.

DIAGNOSTIC FILES

Physicians often draw material for their writing and speaking from the case histories of their own patients. For this reason, many physicians like to set up diagnostic files so that they can quickly pull out information on, for example, the incidence of certain side effects among patients treated with a specific medication. The medical assistant must be familiar with medical terminology to maintain this kind of file.

The system used can vary, but subject cards generally have a main heading with the name of the disease or surgical procedure and subheadings for various aspects of the disease or procedure. The patient cards list the patient's name, diagnosis, and type of treatment.

EXAMPLE OF MAIN HEADING WITH SUBHEADINGS

BLOOD DISEASES
Anemia
Granulocytosis
Hemophilia
Leukemia
Polycythemia
Thalassemia
Toxemia

EXAMPLE OF A PATIENT'S CARD FILED UNDER ANEMIA

Anemia
Patient name: Date:
Diagnosis:
Treatment:
Prognosis:
Other pertinent information:

By keeping a file such as this, a physician can readily obtain the charts of all patients with a specified condition from the history files. This is particularly valuable to physicians who do a great deal of teaching, writing, or research. In the physician's office equipped with a computer, it is very easy to keep a detailed diagnostic file using these same principles.

LIBRARY FOR PATIENTS

A small library of educational information for patients may be maintained by the medical assistant. This library generally contains some books written in language that the average patient can understand as well as a number of pamphlets and reprints that the patient can take home. This might include information on such subjects as diabetes, heart disease, skin conditions, the danger signals of cancer, lung disease, first aid, and other subjects of interest to many patients, depending on the type of practice. The specialist may have information dealing specifically with his or her specialty. A library service such as this saves the physician considerable time in repeating simple educational information and is generally welcomed by the patients. Maintaining the library for patients may be a joint effort of physician and staff. Any items added to the library should first be approved by the physician.

Research

The medical assistant who is employed by a physician who teaches, writes, or lectures frequently may be called on to assist with the preparation of papers. The duties might include

- Preparing a list of references for a presentation or a paper for publication
- Doing actual research
- Preparing abstracts

Any medical assistant who is called on to assume such responsibilities must know how to make the best use of the available library and Internet reference facilities.

USING LIBRARY FACILITIES

Almost all physicians, even those practicing in rural areas, have access to medical libraries. The physician who practices in a metropolitan area or near a medical center such as one affiliated with a university is particularly fortunate, because outstanding library facilities are readily at his or her disposal.

All general hospitals maintain medical libraries consisting of a basic collection of carefully selected, authoritative medical textbooks and reference works of the latest edition as well as files of current journals. The Medical Library Association sets standards for member libraries.

A physician usually has access to a county society library or can use the package library services of the state society. In addition, extension library facilities can be used to obtain information from special supplemental collections. The American Medical Association, for example, and some specialty societies, offer periodical lending services and package library services to their members.

The National Library of Medicine has established a system whereby physicians may get materials from a regional medical library program when information is not available locally. In those instances when the regional program cannot satisfy the need, the request is channeled to the National Library of Medicine.

All libraries systematically organize the books, periodicals, and other materials in a fairly uniform manner so that the information can be easily located and is accessible. The medical assistant who finds it necessary to go to a library to do special work should seek out the librarian or an assistant and get an idea of what the library has to offer with respect to materials and their arrangement, privileges, rules, and regulations for use of the library. After a brief discussion, the trained medical librarian usually can suggest shortcuts that are of great help in locating references or doing research.

Memory Jogger

 *List the three research activities that a medical assistant might assume in medical research.*

Card Catalog (Computer)

Any book, monograph, treatise, handbook, dictionary, and encyclopedia contained in a library is indexed by author and subject and sometimes by title in the card catalog. Although we still refer to it as the "card" catalog, in reality, the index is now usually accessed via a computer terminal. This catalog is really an index of the book contents of the library. Cards are arranged alphabetically (with subject, author, and title cards alphabetized in one series) or are alphabetized within separate sections for subject, author, or title.

CLASSIFICATION SYSTEMS There are a number of systems for classifying library books. In library procedure, classification means putting together materials on a given subject with related materials placed nearby. Medical libraries use various classification systems. The two most used systems are the Dewey decimal system and the Library of Congress classification system.

The Dewey decimal system is used not only in medical but also in all types of libraries. This system uses decimal numbers to indicate specific subjects and arranges the book collection in numerical sequence for easy location. For example, "616" indicates "Pathology, Diseases, Treatment."

EXAMPLE OF HOW THE DEWEY DECIMAL SYSTEM WORKS

616.1	Diseases of the cardiovascular system
616.9	Communicable and other diseases
616.96	Parasitic diseases
616.99	Other general diseases
616.992	Neoplasms and neoplastic diseases

The Library of Congress classification system consists of a number of separate, mutually exclusive classifications based on combination of letters of the alphabet and numerals.

EXAMPLE OF LIBRARY OF CONGRESS SYSTEM

QR	Bacteriology
RD	Surgery
RC 321–431	Diseases of the nervous system

HOW THE CARD CATALOG CAN HELP YOU LOCATE BOOKS No matter which system of classification is used, its main purpose is to help those who use the library to locate volumes quickly. The symbol for the particular book, whether it be a numeral, a letter, or a combination of numerals and letters, appears on the entry for the book in the card catalog. This symbol is called a classification mark. It also appears on the spine of the volume.

To locate a volume, check the classification mark on the card catalog entry and, if an open-shelf system is used, find that shelf in the library where corresponding symbols appear. If a closed-shelf system is used in the library, give the number of the book and its title to a librarian who will locate it for you.

Memory Jogger

 *What is the purpose of a card catalog?*

Periodical Indexes

The bulk of current medical literature appears in medical journals, and some reference system for organizing and accessing the thousands of articles is necessary. The majority of journals publish their own indexes, one for each volume, sometimes with an annual index. If you know the name of the journal that published the article you are looking for, this is the fastest way to locate it. Otherwise, composite indexes may be consulted.

CLINICAL MEDICINE The monthly *Index Medicus* and the annual *Cumulated Index Medicus,* published by the National Library of Medicine, include author and subject indexes for over 3000 periodicals. They are international in scope, representing foreign publications and languages as well as publications in English.

The monthly *Abridged Index Medicus* and the annual *Cumulated Abridged Index Medicus* are smaller versions of *Index Medicus* and *Cumulated Index Medicus* and are limited to indexing 100 major periodicals in the medical field. These periodicals are readily available in the majority of medical libraries. The computer equivalent of both the *Index Medicus* and the *Abridged Index Medicus* is MEDLINE.

NURSING AND ALLIED HEALTH The *Cumulative Index to Nursing & Allied Health Literature* is published by Glendale Adventist Medical Center.* This index is very comprehensive and is the only thorough source for coverage of allied health. It is published bimonthly with an annual cumulation. The computer equivalent is Nursing & Allied Health Index on Bibliographic Retrieval System (BRS) and Dialog.

The *International Nursing Index* is published quarterly, with an annual cumulation, by the *American Journal of Nursing.* The computer equivalent is MEDLINE.

*1509 Wilson Terrace, Glendale, CA 91206.

Bibliography Search

Information for a **bibliography** may be obtained either by a manual search through indexes or by a computer search.

For a manual search, you must look under the subject closest to the one on which you need information, then copy down all the information (author, title of journal, and complete bibliographic information, including volume number, pages, and date).

Most of the world's literature is now accessible through various vendors that provide computer access to specialized files. There are thousands of these databases. The major vendors in health care facilities are

- National Library of Medicine
- Dialog Information Services, Inc.
- Bibliographic Retrieval System (BRS)
- Systems Development Corporation (SDC)

The National Library of Medicine is the least expensive of these four vendors.

PREPARING A BIBLIOGRAPHY Utilizing the various reference sources of the medical library, you can make up a bibliography or list of references on a specific topic with comparatively little difficulty. It does take time, and the list of references must be accurate. Many researchers recommend listing each reference separately on a card or in a small looseleaf notebook (Fig. 22–3). This simplifies the actual preparation of the formal bibliography that always accompanies any published medical paper. Note the following information for each reference:

1. Author
2. Subject
3. Title of book or article
4. Publisher or periodical
5. Volume number
6. Date of publication
7. Page numbers

Author ____________ Subject ____________
Title ____________ Available at: ____________
____________ Call no. ____________
Publisher/Journal ____________ Reference: Excellent, good, fair
Copyright date ______ Volume: ______ Pages: ______ Illustrated: ____________
Student's name: ____________

(Summary, including problem, source of data, method, results, quotations, references.)

Summary: ____________

FIGURE 22–3 Card for reporting bibliographic data.

Sometimes card catalogs and other periodical references list brief summaries of the specific reference cited; this information is also helpful in research and should be noted.

Some libraries prepare medical bibliographies free of charge or for a small fee. Some also abstract or review literature, translate articles, and collect case reports. The library of the American College of Surgeons, for example, offers this service at a modest fee to its members. The American Medical Association also offers this service to its members.

ELECTRONIC RETRIEVAL OF INFORMATION

The individual physician or health care facility with a computer, a modem, telecommunications software, and a telephone line may subscribe to one or more information utilities. Some of the medically oriented utilities are

- GTE Medical Information Network (MINET)
- BRS Colleague Medical
- DIALOG

Through GTE access may be made to EMPIRES (Excerpta Medica Physician Information Retrieval and Education Service), the American Medical Association's clinical literature database that contains current and historical citations and abstracts from over 300 key medical journals.

The development of databases and electronic retrieval systems has provided an invaluable service to the medical profession by making possible easy access to references on an unlimited number of medical subjects. It is also possible for subscribers to read the complete text of books, journals, and other publications.

Principal Medical Resources

Two of the largest medical databases are MEDLINE and EMBASE, each of which includes citations and abstracts from thousands of publications.

MEDLINE is one of a family of several databases known as MEDLARS (MEDical Literature Analysis and Retrieval System). It is produced by the National Library of Medicine (NLM), which is part of the National Institutes of Health, a federal agency in Bethesda, Maryland. *Index Medicus* is produced from this computer file.

EMBASE is produced by Excerpta Medica, and the *Excerpta Medica Index* is produced from this database.

Both MEDLINE and EMBASE are bibliographic indexes, not full-text databases. The computer search generates a bibliography of literature. The searcher must then locate a copy of the article. Some files provide abstracts that are available online. Articles not available from a health care library can usually be requested through the library as an interlibrary loan.

AMA/NET The American Medical Association offers an online information service called AMA/Net free to its members. The subscriber to this service has instant access to millions of published documents. MEDLINE and EMPIRES are two of the sources available through this service. AMA/Net also offers continuing medical education programs, several sources of medical news, and an electronic mail system.

AAMA Members of the American Association of Medical Assistants may contact the Association or network with other members nationwide through the Internet at www.aama-ntl.org.

Other Reference Sources

There are a number of other specialized reference volumes that a medical librarian may use to locate literature. The Monthly Catalog of U.S. Government Publications, for example, contains certain medical listings and is sometimes valuable in research work. In securing biographical information about physicians or other professionals, it is often necessary to turn to such books as the *Directory of Medical Specialists, American Men of Science,* the *American Medical Directory,* or *Who's Who Among Physicians and Surgeons.* Encyclopedias such as *Encyclopedia Britannica* and the *Practical Medicine* series also are sometimes helpful in obtaining basic information.

Memory Jogger

5 *Name the two largest medical databases.*

Manuscript Preparation

In most cases, the medical assistant's tasks in connection with the preparation of a lecture or a **manuscript** for publication are mainly the gathering of references and facts; the physician is responsible for the actual writing. However, because some physicians ask their medical assistants to serve in the capacity of editorial assistants and to smooth out and actually edit their copy before submitting it for publication, a basic understanding of the style, format, and characteristics of medical papers is helpful.

SPEECHES

Not all papers are intended for publication. Some are prepared for presentation before medical and scientific meetings. Speeches should be typed and double-spaced; in some offices a jumbo or magna type machine is used so that the speech is easy to read. Special large-type elements, such as the IBM Orator, are available for single-element or daisy wheel typewriters. All computer word processing programs have a vast selection of print type and size.

At the bottom of each page, in the lower right-hand corner, type the first two or three words that appear at the beginning of the next page. The final draft of the paper should be carefully checked for any typographical errors.

The speaker at a large meeting is usually allotted 10 to 20 minutes to present a paper. At county society and small meetings, the speaker may have from 30 minutes to an hour for the presentation. Check in advance to find out exactly how much time will be allowed. The physician or the medical assistant should time the speech. On average, it takes about 2 minutes to read a page of copy on which there are 200 to 250 words. If slides or other exhibits are planned, arrangements for showing this material must be made in advance and the necessary time allowed.

MANUSCRIPT STYLE

Each medical journal has its own style for published papers. The individual hoping to publish in a specific journal should request a copy of the journal's guidelines for manuscripts in advance and then prepare the manuscript accordingly to minimize editorial changes. However, there are certain fairly uniform procedures to be followed in the preparation of a manuscript to be submitted for publication.

A good medical paper must present established new facts, modes, or practices; principles of value; results of suitable original research; or a review of facts on a subject from which the reader can draw a legitimate conclusion. The subject should be limited to a definite area or problem before writing is begun, and the purpose should be determined in advance.

The typical medical article begins with an introductory section outlining the nature of the material or problem to be covered, follows with actual discussion of the subject, and concludes with a summary in which conclusions are usually noted in numerical form. The format for case reports is somewhat similar. Case reports based on clinical information should be written clearly in smooth narrative style and should not read like a collection of telegraphic notes. There should be a clear presentation of the sequence of events. A brief abstract summarizing the article may appear at the beginning or end of any article. This summary should be rigidly condensed and should contain the deductions as well as clearly reflect the author's viewpoint. Only the actual conclusions reached should be numbered.

The writing in a scientific paper should be simple and straightforward. Excess words should be ruthlessly pared from the article. Grammatical construction must facilitate direct, clear expression. The paper should be well organized and proceed smoothly from beginning to end. Slang, **colloquialisms,** personal allusions, and reminiscences should generally be avoided in papers for publication, although they are often acceptable and add a friendly tone to a paper to be delivered in person before a medical meeting.

DRAFTING, REVISING, AND FINAL COPY

A **draft** of a paper may be made before the final copy. Sometimes several drafts are made. Using an electronic word processor or computer can greatly reduce the laborious retyping of manuscripts, but the author may still want a printout of each revision. Sometimes different colors of paper are used to distinguish between each draft. Double- or triple-space drafts to allow plenty of room for the author's revisions.

An important step in the preparation of any manuscript is a careful revision of copy. This is a duty sometimes delegated to the medical assistant or secretary.

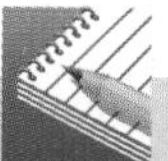

SKILLS AND RESPONSIBILITIES

MAKING REVISIONS TO A SCIENTIFIC PAPER

- Organization—Determine that information moves from topic to topic in an organized, logical sequence.
- Accuracy—Check for accuracy by referring to reference material or querying physician.
- Content—Verify that content is complete by comparing with outline or summary.
- Conciseness—Confirm that explanations are straightforward and free of unnecessary wording.
- Correct sentence construction and grammar—Review for any errors in grammar or awkwardly constructed sentences.
- Clarity and smoothness—Read through for a sense of clarity in the explanation of material and ease in moving from one idea to another.

Check for correct spelling, using the computer spell check, a medical dictionary, and a standard dictionary.

Prepare the final copy using a good-quality $8\frac{1}{2} \times$ 11-inch white paper. Print on one side of the paper only. Double-space the copy, allowing a margin of at least 1 inch at each side and at the bottom. Double-spacing provides space for the editor who receives the manuscript to make corrections or insert instructions for the publisher. Unless otherwise instructed, number each page in the upper right-hand corner.

The original manuscript is submitted to the publisher, and the author should retain one or more copies. If the manuscript is on disk or tape, one printout is sufficient to retain in the file.

FOOTNOTES

When a paper is based on a study of the writing of others, it is necessary to acknowledge the sources used. In medical and scientific papers, **footnotes** usually provide exact references to sources of material. Forms of footnotes differ slightly, depending on the style of the periodical; but, in general, a footnote contains the following information:

- Author's name
- Title of the work cited
- Facts of publication
- Exact page from which the citation was taken

The first time a book or article is mentioned in a footnote, all the information about the publication should appear in the footnote; after that, references to the same source can be shortened to the author's last name and the page number cited. When a periodical is concerned, a later reference need contain only the author's name, the journal name, and the page number.

Detailed information about footnote preparation can be obtained from *The Chicago Manual of Style* or one of several published reference manuals for office workers (Table 22–1).

FINAL BIBLIOGRAPHY

All scientific papers should carry a complete bibliography of source materials. List only those sources that directly pertain to the paper and that were used in its preparation. The form of bibliographies is fairly uniform.

LISTING FOR PERIODICALS

- Author's name and initials
- Title of the article
- Name of the periodical
- Volume number
- Pages cited
- Date of publication

LISTING FOR BOOK REFERENCES

- Author's name and initials
- Title of the book
- Edition (only after the first edition)
- Place of publication
- Name of publisher
- Year of publication

Bibliographies may be arranged alphabetically according to author's name or numerically as the references appear in the text. Whatever form and punctuation are used should be consistent through the entire listing.

TABLE 22–1 Abbreviations Used in Manuscript Preparation

Abbreviation	Meaning
cf.	compare
e.g.	for example
et al.	and other people
ibid.	in the same place
i.e.	that is
loc. cit.	in the place cited
op. cit.	in the work cited
sic	intentionally so written
q.v.	which see

ILLUSTRATIONS

All drawings, photographs, and other illustrative material submitted with a manuscript should be placed on separate sheets and keyed to the manuscript. In other words, illustrations should be numbered and indications should be noted in the manuscript as to where each illustration will be placed. Do not include such materials in the body of the manuscript. The explanation of the drawing or illustration should appear in a caption, or **legend.**

Glossy black and white or color photographs reproduce best. Captions for photographs should be typed on separate sheets or may be attached with rubber cement below the photograph. On the back of the photograph, the author's name and the number of the illustration should be penciled lightly. Do not use paper clips on photographs. Credit lines should be given for copyrighted or commercial photographs or illustrations. If x-ray films are submitted, make sure the prints are shiny; indicate on the back where they may be cropped but leave localizing landmarks.

Charts and line drawings must be carefully prepared to achieve good reproduction. Such drawings preferably should be done with India or black ink on heavy white bond paper. Present-day techniques point to preparation of these items using a computer. Charts should be condensed and simplified as much as possible. Letters and identifying numerals can be placed on the face of the chart with the explanation in the legend below.

Tables should be prepared in a uniform style on separate sheets, using a typewriter or computer. Each table should be numbered consecutively and have a descriptive heading.

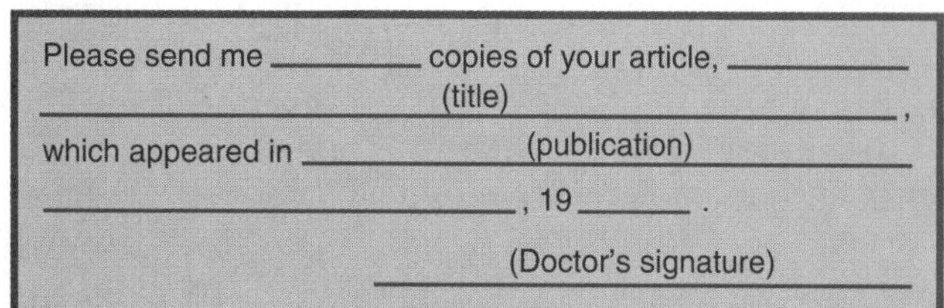
Please send me ________ copies of your article, ________ (title) ________,
which appeared in ________ (publication) ________, 19________.
________ (Doctor's signature)

FIGURE 22–4 Typical card for ordering reprints.

Memory Jogger

List the six items of information that should be included in a bibliographical book reference.

MAILING THE MANUSCRIPT

Generally, manuscripts should not be folded but should be mailed flat in a large envelope. Sometimes a paper of fewer than four pages can be folded twice and mailed in a regular business envelope, or a manuscript of four to eight pages can be folded once and mailed in a 6 × 9-inch envelope. A letter stating that the manuscript is being submitted for publication should be included. Photographs and illustrations should be mailed flat, between sheets of protective cardboard.

GALLEY PROOFS

A paper accepted for publication will be set in type, and proofs of the article will usually be returned by the editor to the author for checking. Because changes in a manuscript once it is set in type are costly, revisions should be limited to correction of errors and minor changes.

If possible, work as a team when checking **galley proofs,** with one person holding the proofs and the other person reading from the original copy. Check for typographic errors, omitted lines and words, and so forth. When correcting proofs, use a different-colored pencil from the one used by the proofreader on the publication. Corrections should be entered in the margins of the proof, next to the line with the error to be corrected. A knowledge of proofreader's marks is helpful (see Chapter 12).

One corrected set of galley proofs should be returned to the editor, and one set of proofs should be retained by the author. If a second set of proofs is sent later, check the first corrected set against the second set to make sure that all corrections have been made.

INDEXING

Often it is necessary to provide an index for a long paper or a book. An author and subject index can be made from page proofs. One system for indexing is to use slips of paper or 3 × 5-inch cards. Each index entry is listed on a separate card or slip; this simplifies alphabetizing under major headings later. The whole index can then be typed from the alphabetized cards. Manuscripts prepared by computer can be indexed quickly and accurately with the necessary software.

REPRINTS

At the time an article is set in type, the author should order all needed **reprints,** because type is often destroyed after the original press run. The medical assistant generally handles the ordering of the reprints, which may be as many as 500 copies or more. The order should be adequate to cover any future needs. Most physicians send copies of their articles to colleagues, to physicians who have evidenced an interest in their work, and to hospitals and teaching institutions with which they have had contact (Fig. 22–4). They probably maintain a card file of names and addresses of those to whom they wish to send reprints.

Addresses in the card file should be checked from time to time in the *American Medical Directory* or by scanning membership and request lists. Some record of reprint mailing should be kept, and acknowledgments should be checked. A person who does not acknowledge two or three reprints should be taken off the mailing list.

An enclosure card, printed in advance, is sent by some authors with a copy of the reprint. Others prefer to enclose a short letter stating that the reprint is a complimentary copy.

Travel and Meeting Arrangements

TRANSPORTATION AND LODGING

The medical assistant may be expected to make transportation and lodging arrangements for the physician for out-of-town meetings (see Procedure 22–1). Although the physician who is located in a

PROCEDURE 22-1
Making Travel Arrangements

GOAL
To make travel arrangements for the physician from his or her city of residence to Toronto, Canada

EQUIPMENT AND SUPPLIES
Travel plan
Telephone
Telephone directory
Typewriter or computer
Typing paper

PROCEDURAL STEPS
1 Verify the details of planned trip:
- Desired date and time of departure
- Desired date and time of return
- Preferred mode of transportation
- Number in party
- Preferred lodging and price range

2 Telephone travel agency to arrange for transportation and lodging reservations.

3 Arrange for traveler's checks if desired.

4 Pick up tickets or arrange for their delivery

5 Check tickets to confirm conformance with the travel plan.
PURPOSE To avoid any error due to misunderstanding and to verify compliance with requests.

6 Check to see that hotel reservations are confirmed.

7 Prepare an itinerary, including all the necessary information:
- Date and time of departure
- Flight numbers or identifying information of other modes of travel.
- Mode of transportation to hotel(s).
- Name, address, and telephone number of hotel(s), with confirmation numbers if available.
- Date and time of return.

8 Place one copy of itinerary in the office file.
PURPOSE It may be necessary to contact the traveler or to forward mail.

9 Give several copies of the itinerary to the traveler.
PURPOSE The traveler may wish to have extra copies for family or friends.

metropolitan area probably uses a travel agent for most travel arrangements, the medical assistant may be responsible for working with the travel agent and preparing the detailed itinerary.

When not working with a travel agent, the medical assistant may be expected to personally make the hotel and transportation arrangements. A person who is sufficiently skilled in computer operations may be able to accomplish both without outside help. One should keep a file of the telephone numbers of airlines and hotels that have been found satisfactory or been recommended. When a reservation has been made, ask for the confirmation number. When traveling by automobile, the literature and maps provided by an auto club can be very useful.

ITINERARY

When all arrangements are final, prepare the itinerary. Keep one copy in the office file. Give the original to the physician plus any copies that may be requested for family members or other individuals. Since it is sometimes necessary to contact the physician while traveling, it is important that the itinerary be carefully prepared, including locations and telephone numbers.

MEETING CALENDAR

A calendar of all meetings that the physician plans to attend should be kept by the medical assistant, with both the physician and the medical assistant retaining a copy. The calendar can be merely a sheet of paper but should include the following information for each event:

- Name of the meeting
- Date
- Place
- Time

Any changes or additions to the calendar should be made on both copies as notices are received. A reminder to the physician a few days in advance of each meeting is usually appreciated.

MEETING RESPONSIBILITIES

A physician often accepts official responsibilities in his or her professional society or on the hospital board. The administrative medical assistant for this physician may be expected to assist in arranging meetings, preparing an agenda, and typing minutes of the meeting dictated by the physician (see Procedure 22–2).

The medical assistant who takes an active part in a professional society for medical assistants will have personal use for these skills as well.

Arranging a Meeting

When arranging a meeting you need to know

- The purpose of the meeting
- The number of persons expected to attend
- Whether a meal is to be included
- The expected duration of the meeting
- The date, time, and place
- The list of persons to be notified

Choosing the Location

Some groups meet regularly and use the same facility each time. In this case, it is necessary merely to confirm the date and time with the facility. If a meal is to be served, the menu, price, and approximate number expected to attend must be determined. If a new location is being used, you need to verify that

- The space is adequate
- Any necessary electronic equipment is available
- Parking facilities are available if needed
- Lighting and ventilation are adequate
- Menus are available if a meal is to be included

Preparing the Notice of Meeting

Meeting notices are usually mailed to all members of the group. For a small committee meeting, the members may be notified by telephone. If there is to be a speaker, the name of the speaker and the topic are included in the meeting notice. The notice must include the date, time, and place of the meeting.

Preparing the Agenda

Organizations whose bylaws specify *Robert's Rules of Order, Newly Revised,* as the parliamentary authority and that have not adopted a special order of business use the following prescribed **order of business:**

1. Reading and approval of the minutes
2. Reports of officers, boards, and standing committees
3. Reports of special (select or ad hoc) committees
4. Special orders
5. Unfinished business and general orders
6. New business

The order of business lists the different divisions of business in the order in which each will be called for at business meetings.

An **agenda** is a list of the specific items under each division of the order of business that the officers or board plan to present at a meeting. The medical assistant who is expected to prepare the agenda should determine what topics are to be discussed, type them in the prescribed order, and duplicate enough copies for the meeting. For a large group, the program is usually printed. For the smaller group, photocopies are satisfactory.

Memory Jogger

How does an agenda differ from an order of business?

Preparing the Minutes

The record of the proceedings of a meeting is called the minutes. The minutes contain mainly a record of what was done at the meeting, not what was said by the members.

The first paragraph of the minutes should contain the following information:

- Kind of meeting (e.g., regular, special)
- Name of the association
- Date, time, and place of the meeting
- The fact that the regular chairman and secretary were present or, in their absence, the names of the persons who substituted for them
- Whether the minutes of the previous meeting were read and approved

The body of the minutes should contain a separate paragraph for each subject matter. It should include all main motions, including (a) the wording in which each motion was adopted or otherwise dis-

PPROCEDURE 22-2
Arranging a Group Meeting

GOAL
To arrange a breakfast meeting for the physician's hospital committee

EQUIPMENT AND SUPPLIES
Directory of committee members
Meeting plan
Telephone
Typewriter or computer
Post cards

PROCEDURAL STEPS
1 Verify the proposed date and time for the meeting.
2 Gather details for meeting arrangements
- Purpose of the meeting
- Expected attendance
- Name of the speaker, if any, and the program topic
- Expected duration of the meeting

3 Arrange for a meeting room based on the requirements
4 Mail notice of the meeting to members and invited guests. Include:
- Date
- Time
- Place
- Name of the speaker and the topic
- Cost, if any
- Registration information

5 Arrange for any necessary equipment (e.g., microphone, projector, and screen).
6 Notify the meeting place of the number of reservations, if required.
7 Arrange for registration check-in.
8 Prepare the agenda.
9 Give the required number of copies of the agenda to physician.

posed of, (b) the disposition of the motion, and (c) the name of the mover. The name of the seconder of a motion should not be entered in the minutes unless ordered by the assembly. The body of the minutes should also include any points of order and appeals, whether they were sustained or lost, and the reasons given by the chair for the ruling. The minutes may include the name and subject of a guest speaker, but no attempt should be made to summarize the speech. The last paragraph should state the hour of adjournment.

The minutes should be signed by the secretary. In some organizations the president also signs the minutes. The practice of including the words "Respectfully submitted" is obsolete and should not be used.

The medical assistant who might be expected to type the minutes of meetings should consult an authoritative book on the subject and prepare a model to follow in typing the minutes of each meeting so that every set of minutes will be in the same style.

Memory Jogger

Under what circumstance is the name of the seconder of a motion included in the minutes?

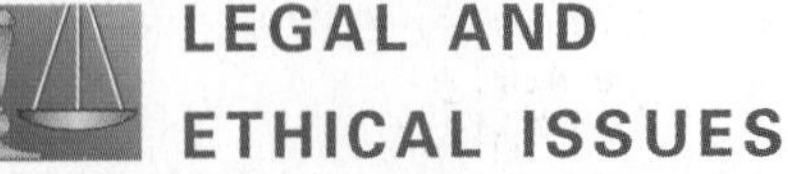

LEGAL AND ETHICAL ISSUES

The medical assistant can provide a significant contribution by helping the physician fulfill his or her obligation to keep current with medical progress. In so doing, the medical assistant is also gaining insight into new developments.

CRITICAL THINKING

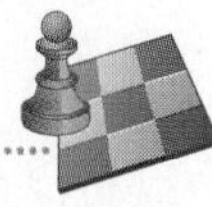

1 Select a short article from a professional journal and prepare an abstract using the suggested form in this chapter.

2 Suggest specific items that might be placed in a library for patients.

3 What items would *not* be displayed?

4 Describe how the typing of a speech that is to be presented at a professional meeting might differ from an ordinary typewritten page.

5 What advance information is needed before arranging a group meeting?

HOW DID I DO? Answers to Memory Joggers

1 The purpose of indexing is to provide ready access to information being sought.

2 *a.* New procedures
b. Results of studies and/or experiments
c. Any conclusions noted

3 *a.* Prepare a list of references
b. Perform actual research
c. Prepare abstracts

4 The purpose of a card catalog is to provide a means of locating information quickly.

5 The two largest medical databases are MEDLINE and EMBASE

6 *a.* Author's name and initials
b. Title of book
c. Edition number (after the first edition)
d. Place of publication
e. Name of publisher
f. Year of publication

7 The agenda is a list of the specific items under each division of the order of business.

8 The name of the seconder of a motion is included in the minutes only when ordered by the assembly.

REFERENCES

Baldwin F, McInerney S: Infomedicine. Boston, Little, Brown & Co., 1996.

Robert's Rules of Order, Newly Revised. Glenview, IL, Scott, Foresman & Co., 1990.

Sabin WA: The Gregg Reference Manual, 7th ed. New York, McGraw-Hill, 1994.

Facility Environment

23

OUTLINE

LEARNING OBJECTIVES

Cognitive: On successful completion of this chapter you should be able to:

1. Define and spell the terms listed in the Vocabulary.
2. List seven items of concern in controlling the general environment of a health care facility.
3. Discuss the utilization of various areas of the facility.
4. Describe how the medical assistant would arrange for and supervise a maintenance service.
5. Explain the inventory process.
6. Explain the importance of the instructions and warranties accompanying new equipment purchases.
7. Cite precautions to be observed in storing poisons, narcotics, acids and caustics, and flammable items.
8. Discuss the procedure for storing supplies and drug samples.
9. List six possible safety hazards in a health care facility.
10. Discuss the importance of and procedures to observe in routine office security.

Performance: On successful completion of this chapter you should be able to:

1. Write instructions for a maintenance service.
2. Set up an equipment inventory.
3. Organize, store, and dispose of drug samples.
4. Establish and maintain a supply inventory and ordering system.

VOCABULARY

capital purchase The purchase of a major item of furniture or equipment

categorically Pertaining to a division in any classification system

caustics Substances that corrode or eat away tissues

expendable Concerning supplies or equipment that is normally used up or consumed in service

inventory A list of articles in stock, with the description and quantity of each

reputable Honorable; having a good reputation

Planning and Organizing Facilities

The same principles of organization and planning that guide the business management of a medical office are essential in the organization and care of the facilities and supplies. A comfortable, attractive, clean environment lifts the spirits of patients and contributes to the efficiency and enthusiasm of the staff.

GENERAL ENVIRONMENT

TEMPERATURE The ideal temperature for a reception room is about 74° F. Working areas can be somewhat cooler. There should be a constant exchange of air by means of open windows or air conditioning. However, you should guard against drafts, because people who are ill are very susceptible to chills.

LIGHTING Working areas need to be well lighted. Fluorescent lights are usually preferable, because their light is uniform and they do not give off heat. Lamps in the reception area can be decorative, but they are useful only if carefully chosen and properly placed. They should be at reading height. If they are too high, they will shine into the eyes of others in the room. Lighting, furnishings, and comfort of the reception room are fully discussed in Chapter 8.

WALLS AND FLOOR COVERINGS Carpeting is usually chosen for floor covering in the reception area and often in the physician's consultation room. Unsecured rugs should never be used in a medical facility. In the clinical areas, a smooth washable floor covering, such as vinyl or tile, is generally more satisfactory. If wax is used on the floor covering, it should be the nonskid variety.

Wallpaper can add a pleasant atmosphere in the reception area. In the administrative and clinical areas, a good quality wall paint in soft colors is attractive, easily cleaned, and long lasting.

TRAFFIC CONTROL The furnishings in the entrance and reception areas should be arranged to allow easy traffic without crowding in any one area. The reception desk must be placed so that anyone coming into the office can easily spot the desk and so that the medical assistant at the desk can view the entire reception area (see Chapter 8). In the inner office, the physician and other members of the staff should be able to pass from one station to another without creating a roadblock.

SOUND CONTROL Walls should be soundproof, if possible, to prevent voices and conversations from being heard from one room to another.

PRIVACY Treatment rooms should be arranged so that the patient is out of view if it should become necessary to open the door to a hallway.

EFFICIENCY The physician and medical assistant must be able to move easily within each room and have access to equipment and supplies as needed.

Memory Jogger

Briefly describe several general features of the medical facility that are essential to a comfortable and efficient working environment.

AREA UTILIZATION AND CARE

The medical facility, whether large or small, is separated by utilization into the following areas:

- Reception
- Administration
- Clinical activities
- Lavatories
- Storage and utility

The overall cleaning and maintenance of these areas is probably being done by an outside service under the direction of the medical assistant or office manager. However, additional individual attention is required by members of the staff. In some instances, particularly in less populated areas, it may be the sole responsibility of the medical assistant.

Good housekeeping begins with having a place

for everything and with keeping everything clean and ready for use. Good housekeeping saves time and energy, conserves property, and eliminates incorrect use of materials. Poor housekeeping holds potential dangers for patients, physicians, and assistants alike.

Reception Area

The importance of a neat, attractive reception room was discussed in Chapter 8. Draperies, carpet, and upholstery should be cleaned at regular intervals in addition to the daily maintenance.

Administration Area

The administration area includes the receptionist desk; the records storage; telephone equipment; business machines such as typewriters, computers, calculators, photocopier, and fax machine; and so forth. This area should be separated from the reception room by a locked door. Records and business papers on the receptionist's desk should be placed in desk trays where they will be safe and out of sight of visitors during the day and in locked files at night. Personal items should be put away in a drawer or locker.

Clinical Area

The clinical area includes the physician's consultation room, which is used for patient interviews and for the physician's private study; patient examination and treatment rooms; and a recovery room where patients may rest after therapy or minor surgery.

CONSULTATION ROOM The physician's consultation room should always be kept neat and clean. Give this room a quick onceover after each patient visit and remove any evidence of the departing patient. Follow the preferences of the physician with respect to straightening the desk or other furnishings.

Memory Jogger

Why is good housekeeping a high-priority item in a health care facility?

EXAMINATION AND TREATMENT ROOMS Examination and treatment rooms are designed for utility; only necessary equipment and supplies should be placed here (Fig. 23–1). Instruments, medications, and other supplies are in cabinets or drawers. Supply cabinets should be checked daily before the first patient arrives (Fig. 23–2). The room must be straightened and all counter tops and the sink wiped clean after each patient. Disposable gowns, towels, and tissues must be discarded, fresh linens provided, and the room left spotless. The temperature in these rooms is crucial to the comfort of the patients, who are often asked to disrobe and put on a gown—and sometimes left waiting.

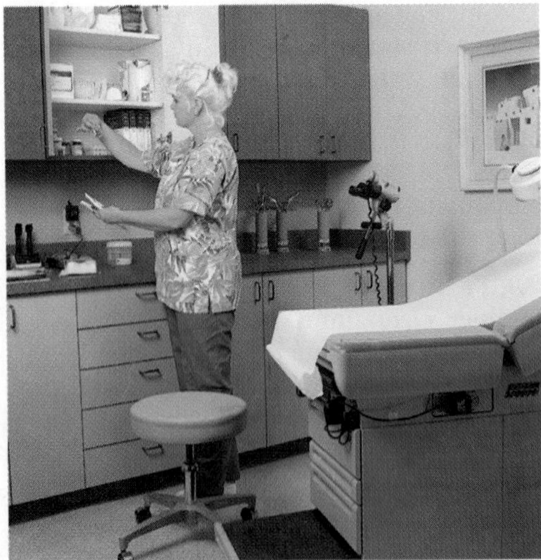

FIGURE 23–1 Patient examination room.

LABORATORY The laboratory may be anything from a small closet to a large room or suite of rooms. It must be kept clean, with everything in its place, for accurate work to be accomplished.

Adequate ventilation in the laboratory is especially important. There are many odors from the laboratory to which the staff becomes accustomed but which may be disagreeable to patients.

Contamination control must be exercised according to the current regulations of the Occupational Safety and Health Administration (OSHA), which are available from the U.S. Department of Labor. The department issues standards that employers and employees must follow, and site visits are made to

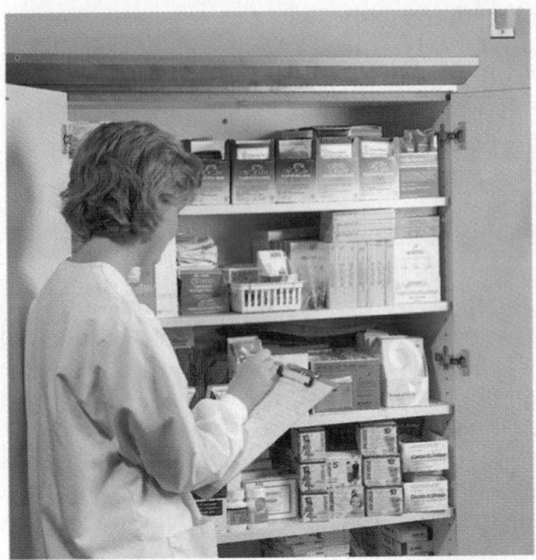

FIGURE 23–2 Example of supply cabinet.

ensure compliance. One of the most important is the exposure control plan. The facility's exposure control plan must be written and available to all employees and should be included in the policy and procedures manual (see Chapter 24). Some states have their own OSHA-approved occupational safety and health regulations, which may be even more stringent than the federal standards.

RECOVERY ROOM The recovery room should be comfortable, clean, and quiet. Facilities should be provided so that patient can relax and keep warm. Interesting reading material will help the time pass more pleasantly. If the patient wishes to sleep, provide a light blanket and see that no one enters the room.

Lavatories

In the small solo practice office, the lavatory may be shared by staff and patients. In this situation, every member of the staff should be instructed to leave the room meticulously clean. Larger medical facilities provide a separate lavatory for patients. This room must be checked by the medical assistant after each use to be certain it is left clean and that all supplies are replenished as needed.

Storage and Utility Rooms

There must be storage space for office and medical supplies, cleaning equipment and supplies, staff lockers or coat hooks, and so forth. The size of these spaces will vary, but whatever area is available must be kept organized and supplies and other items kept in order. Storage and utility rooms are generally kept closed to all except the staff.

Memory Jogger

Name an important part of the OSHA regulations that should be included in the office policy and procedures manual.

Maintenance

RESPONSIBILITIES OF STAFF

One member of the staff, often the administrative medical assistant, is delegated the responsibility of overseeing the maintenance of the premises. The details should be outlined in the office policy and procedures manual (see Chapter 24).

Each staff member will probably wish to tidy and dust his or her own desk or work station, with the administrative medical assistant taking care of the physician's desk.

The clinical medical assistant is usually the one who periodically cleans the interior of cabinets and drawers in the examination and treatment rooms. This should be done only when there is time to complete the job.

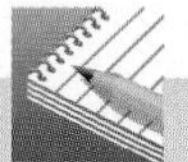

SKILLS AND RESPONSIBILITIES

PROPER METHOD OF CLEANING CABINET AND DRAWER INTERIORS

1 Do one shelf at a time.
2 Start at the top.
3 Remove all items from the shelf and place them on a table in the same order as on the shelf.
4 Wash the shelf with warm water and soap and rinse it well. Dry the shelf.
5 Clean and polish the instruments and check for faults. Examine hinges and blades.
6 Check all labels on containers for clarity. Reglue labels, if necessary. Examine supplies for expiration dates, quantity, and deterioration. Make a list of those items that should be reordered.
7 Replace the supplies in their original places on the shelf.

Clean the tops of cabinets and the undersides of towel and tape dispensers as necessary. These areas are frequently overlooked in the daily cleaning.

Maintenance services do not usually include as part of their service such tasks as cleaning mirrors, replacing light bulbs, cleaning the refrigerator, daily cleaning of sinks, straightening magazines, and watering plants. These and numerous other occasional as well as daily jobs are performed by the office staff.

Memory Jogger

You are assigned to clean the cabinets in an examination room. Where would you start?

INSTRUCTIONS TO MAINTENANCE SERVICE

Every member of the staff must be alert to any problem of cleanliness or safety that might be overlooked by the maintenance service and report the condition to the medical assistant in charge. The staff member who has the responsibility for instructing the maintenance service must be able to plan and be explicit in giving instructions:

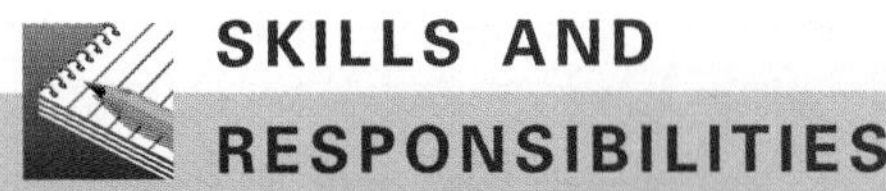

SKILLS AND RESPONSIBILITIES

SYSTEM OF INSTRUCTING MAINTENANCE SERVICES

- Prepare a written list of the service that you expect.
- Go over it with the service people.
- Be specific about any areas that are not to be entered or disturbed.
- Set up a regular schedule.
- Evaluate the service regularly.
- Communicate your pleasure or displeasure promptly to the person in charge of performing the service.

Furniture and Equipment

The physician, individually or as a member of a group practice, has a large investment in the furnishings and equipment necessary to carry on a medical practice. The medical assistant has a responsibility to properly use and care for any piece of equipment to preserve its useful life.

ACQUISITION

When a new piece of equipment is acquired, read the instructions thoroughly and carefully. Do not attempt to assemble or use items before consulting the instructions. Keep the purchase invoice on file. The date of purchase and the cost are required for insurance and for depreciation credit on income tax.

WARRANTY REQUIREMENTS

If there is a warranty card with the item, copy the code number, fill in the blanks, and mail it as instructed.

SERVICE

Keep a service file for equipment that will need regular servicing.

SERVICE FILE CONTENTS

- Warranty dates
- Frequency of service
- When and by whom the unit was last serviced
- Cost of service

File all instructions in a special folder and save them for future reference or for your successors.

INVENTORY

It is good business to **inventory** all equipment and supplies once per year. If you have an office computer, keep the inventory on disk for easy access and updating.

First, list all **capital purchases,** such as furniture, medical and surgical instruments, sterilizers and autoclaves, laboratory equipment, business machines, and any major pieces of artwork or artifacts. These items are permanent and usually expensive. List the date of purchase of each item, along with its original price.

Next, list the smaller, less costly items that are considered **expendable,** such as small instruments, syringes, and thermometers.

Last, estimate the usable supplies and drugs on hand. Keep this inventory to check against the inventory for the coming year. An inventory is valuable in preparing income tax, and especially in case of office burglary or loss from other causes.

Memory Jogger

Why is an annual inventory of equipment and supplies important? What is included?

Supplies

SELECTING SUPPLIES AND SUPPLIERS

Supplies are those items that are expendable and must be ordered fairly frequently.

ADMINISTRATIVE FUNCTION SUPPLIES

- Stationery and filing supplies
- Appointment books and cards
- Accounting supplies
- Small desk items, such as paper clips, staples, typewriter ribbons, pens, and pencils

CLINICAL AREA SUPPLIES

- Examination and treatment items, such as disposable scopes, specula, lubricants, tongue blades, applicators, syringes and needles, dressings, and bandages
- Paper gowns, drapes, towels
- Autoclaving and sterilizing supplies

GENERAL USAGE SUPPLIES

- Soap and towels for lavatories
- Cleaning supplies
- Tissues
- Items for the staff lounge

In general, the person who will use the item is the best person to select what is to be ordered, but it is probably best for only one person to be in charge of ordering all supplies. The purchasing agent in the local hospital is a good source of information on supplies and suppliers.

Because such a variety of supplies is needed, you will probably use more than one supplier. Study the market and find the items that are best suited to the practice with respect to quality and packaging, and order from the suppliers who offer the best service and prices. You should make periodic price checks, but do not sacrifice convenience and service for the sake of saving a few pennies.

RED FLAG RE-ORDER TAG

when this inventory point is reached, its time to reorder

Product Identification

The Colwell Company
Champaign, Illinois

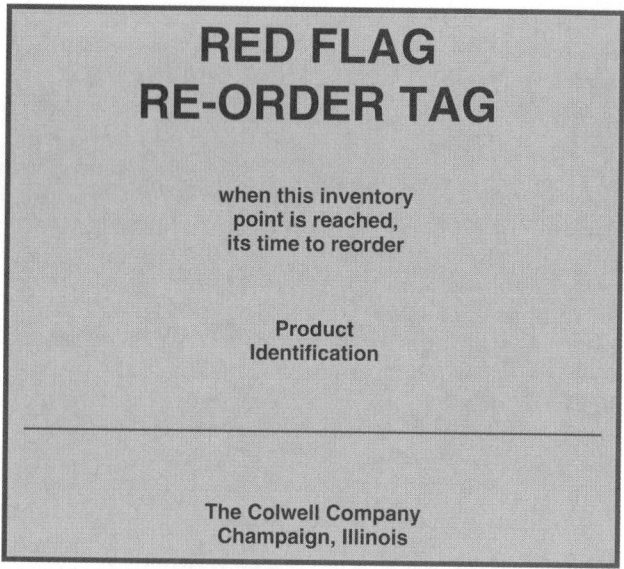

FIGURE 23–4 Reorder flag for low supplies. (Courtesy of Colwell Systems, Champaign, IL.)

ORDERING SUPPLIES

There should be an established method for ordering supplies. Keep a list or running inventory from which you can note diminishing supplies and determine when to reorder (Figs. 23–3 and 23–4; see Procedure 23–1). Representatives of supply houses regularly call at physicians' offices and are often very helpful in suggesting new items and answering questions about what is available to meet your needs. Mail-order houses also send catalogs describing a great variety of equipment and supplies that can be ordered by mail.

ORDER (ITEM NAME) 3-ply Disposable Drape Sheets (white) 7459 **ON ORDER**

ORDER QUANTITY 300 REORDER POINT 100

ORDER	QTY	REC'D	COST	PREPAID	ON ACCT	ORDER	QTY	REC'D	COST	PREPAID	ON ACCT
1/25	300	2/10	64.95	X							

INVENTORY COUNT

	JAN	FEB	MAR	APR	MAY	JUNE	JULY	AUG	SEPT	OCT	NOV	DEC
20 00	200											
20 00												

ORDER SOURCE
The Colwell Company
201 Kenyon Road
Champaign, IL 61820

UNIT PRICE
100 - $23.95
300 - $64.95

FORM 2450 COLWELL CO., CHAMPAIGN, ILLINOIS

FIGURE 23–3 Preprinted form for inventory control. (Courtesy of Colwell Systems, Champaign, IL.)

It is advisable to establish good credit with several reputable supply companies, both local and mail order, to provide a choice of vendors. However, do not shift your purchases from company to company without good reason. The loyal customer usually receives better service and may enjoy special privileges, such as being given the option of trying a piece of equipment before actually agreeing to purchase it.

Attention to detail in ordering will speed delivery and ensure greater accuracy. Use the actual title of the supply being ordered, including any special name, size, color, and so forth. The order should state whether payment is enclosed or whether the purchase is to be charged to the physician's account.

PREVENTION OF WASTE

In some cases, the unit cost of an item may be reduced by purchasing in larger quantities, but this is not always a saving. Make this decision only after considering the following guidelines.

GUIDELINES FOR PURCHASING LARGE QUANTITIES

- Will the supply be used in a reasonable length of time?
- Will it spoil or deteriorate?
- Is there sufficient space for storage?
- Will the practice continue to use the product?

RECEIVING AND STORING

RECEIVING All orders should be placed in the storage area when they arrive and opened only when you have time to check the contents. Compare the items in the package with your original purchase order and the invoice included with the shipment. Check for correct items, sizes, and styles as well as the number or amount received.

If you have any questions regarding the order or if you have a complaint to make, gather the following information before contacting the supplier.

INFORMATION NEEDED TO CORRESPOND WITH A SUPPLIER

- Invoice number
- Date ordered
- Name of person who placed the order

List on paper your questions and the information you desire. If a catalog was used in placing the order, open your copy to the correct page and secure any additional pertinent information. With all this information at hand, you can make a professional inquiry by letter or telephone.

When you are satisfied that the order is correct and complete, make the necessary notations on the inventory and order cards and place the items in their designated storage areas.

Memory Jogger

When a shipment of supplies arrives, what three procedures will you do before placing the items in their designated storage areas?

STORING Follow good housekeeping standards in storing supplies. Place supplies where they are most accessible yet protected from damage and exposure to moisture, heat, light, and air. Most drugs and solutions should be stored in a cool, dark cupboard, because direct light and sunlight cause drug deterioration. If drugs are to be stored for some time, the stoppers should be dipped in paraffin to seal them from the air. Do not fill these bottles to the very top; leave a little room for expansion.

Poisons should be stored in a locked compartment and kept separate from products used routinely. Have a distinct label or cap for poisons. A bright red color for their labels or caps may be useful. Narcotics must be stored in a secure place out of sight. Acids and **caustics** should have special resistant lids; never use metal lids for these substances. Do not store strong acids next to alkalis. Flammable items must be stored away from heat (Fig. 23–5).

PRODUCT	STORAGE	SPECIAL INSTRUCTIONS
Poisons	In locked case	Separate from products used routinely
Narcotics	Secure cabinet	Out of sight
Acids and caustics	Separate from alkalis	Special resistant lid; no metal lids
Inflammables	Away from heat	
Long-term storage solutions	Cool, dark cupboard	1. Dip stoppers in paraffin to air-seal 2. Leave some open space at top for expansion

FIGURE 23–5 Storage of drugs and solutions.

PROCEDURE 23-1

Establishing and Maintaining a Supply Inventory and Ordering System

GOAL

To establish an inventory of all expendable supplies in the physician's office and follow an efficient plan of order control using a card system.

EQUIPMENT AND SUPPLIES

File box
Inventory and order control cards
List of supplies on hand
Metal tabs
Reorder tags
Pen or pencil

PROCEDURAL STEPS

1 Write the name of each item on a separate card.
PURPOSE: To establish a record of all items in inventory.

2 Write the amount of each item on hand in the space provided.
PURPOSE: To establish beginning inventory.

3 Place a reorder tag at the point where the supply should be replenished.
PURPOSE: The tag will serve as an alert that supply is low.

4 Place a metal tab over the *order* section of the card.
PURPOSE: The metal tab will be a reminder to include this item in the next order.

5 When the order has been placed, note the date and quantity ordered and move the tab to the *on order* section of the card.

6 When the order is received, note the date and quantity in the appropriate column, remove the tab, and refile the card.
NOTE: If the order is only partially filled, let the tab remain until the order is complete.

CARING FOR LABELS

If a bottle is to be used for a long time, the label should be indestructible. The original label should be treated for preservation when it is first received. When using the contents of the bottle, pour away from the label side to prevent any dripping on the label. Plastic screw caps protect the lip of the bottle and keep it clean.

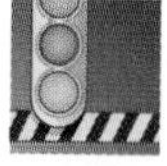

Safety Alert: When a label shows signs of wear or mutilation, or is difficult to read, replace the entire bottle and solution for safety purposes.

DRUG SAMPLES

Samples of drugs and medications that are suitable to the physician's practice should be organized **categorically** in a sample cupboard or drawer.

Place all similar drugs together, preferably in boxes of similar size and shape, with the tops open and plainly labeled on the outside. Clear plastic boxes are excellent for this type of storage. Color-coded labels are an additional help in identification.

Keep all the sedative samples in one box, all stimulant samples in another, and so forth. It is good practice to band together drug samples that have the same code number or expiration date. Rotate the drugs by placing the most recently received items in back of those that were previously on hand. At regular intervals, check all samples for expiration dates, and properly dispose of those that have expired.

Memory Jogger

What action should you take when a drug container label shows signs of wear or mutilation?

The Doctor's Bag

Although the physician who makes house calls has become a rarity, the practice is not entirely extinct and is even making a comeback in some areas. Any

Blood pressure set Stethoscope Thermometers (oral and rectal) Flashlight or penlight Sterile gloves and lubricant Wooden applicators Assorted bandages Adhesive tape (assorted widths) Safety pins Towel Ballpoint pens Prescription pads Sterile hemostatic forceps	Sterile syringes and needles (disposable) Sterile swabs Sterile dressings Tongue depressors Scissors Sterile dressing forceps Aspiration equipment Microscopic slides and fixative Containers for specimens Culture tubes for throat cultures Sterile stuture set Sterile scalpel	Probe Tourniquet Percussion hammer Illuminated diagnostic set (otoscope and ophthalmoscope) Sterile tissue forceps Medications: Epinephrine Digitalis Antibiotics Antihistamines Alcohol and/or skin disinfectant Sterilizing solution Spirits of ammonia

FIGURE 23–6 Basic inventory of items commonly found in a doctor's bag.

medical assistant who is given the responsibility of keeping the doctor's bag ready for use must regard it seriously and give it close and continual attention.

The items that are included in the bag depend on professional requirements, the kinds of emergencies that are responded to, and the personal preferences of the person using it. That person could be the physician, a physician assistant, a nurse practitioner, or an emergency medical technician. A basic inventory of items commonly found in a doctor's bag are listed in Figure 23–6.

As a guide, keep an inventory of the bag's contents posted inside a cupboard above the place where you check and clean the bag. When checking the bag after a patient has been tended to, remove any specimens and see that they are properly labeled with the patient's full name, the date, and the type of test if the specimen is to be sent out for examination.

If any instruments or gloves have been used, remove them and replace with sterile ones. Even if this equipment has not been used, it should be sterilized weekly. Keep the containers of alcohol, germicides, and other substances filled, and check containers often for any leakage. Allow a small space for heat expansion in containers of fluid.

Safety and Security Considerations

DETECTION OF HAZARDS

The physician and every member of the staff should continually monitor possible hazards to themselves and the patients.

The reception room and public areas of the facility are particularly vulnerable. Are the chairs in the reception room safe for children, for an exceptionally heavy patient, or for a physically disadvantaged patient? Are there any exposed telephone or light cords that could cause someone to trip? Are there lamps that could tip?

In the examining rooms, be especially careful to put away any sharp instruments, hazardous liquids, or medications. Any spills on the floor should be wiped immediately to prevent slipping or a fall. Keep prescription pads out of sight.

Are the stairways and entrances to the facility well lighted and safe? Are there any known hazards in the parking area?

DRUG ENFORCEMENT ADMINISTRATION REGULATIONS

A physician who has controlled substances (narcotics) stored on the premises must keep these drugs in a locked cabinet or safe. Any loss of controlled drugs by theft must be reported to the regional office of the Drug Enforcement Administration at the time the theft is discovered. The local police department and the state bureau of narcotics enforcement should also be notified (see Chapter 6).

SMOKE ALARMS AND FIRE EXTINGUISHERS

Smoke alarms are required in all new buildings and should be installed in every existing medical facility. Their functioning must be checked regularly to ensure effectiveness if they should be needed. There should be a fire extinguisher readily accessible to any part of the facility.

FIRE EXITS

Fire exits should be clearly marked and the staff instructed on evacuation procedures in case of fire.

CONTACT WITH SECURITY SYSTEM MANAGEMENT

If the physician's office is located in a multiple-unit building or medical complex, know whom to contact if a security emergency should occur. Have the telephone number handy for local fire and police departments (i.e., 911 in many areas).

ROUTINE OFFICE SECURITY

Within the office, all valuables should be kept out of sight. A frequent target of thieves is the medical assistant's handbag, which is often left under a desk or table, where it can be easily spotted by an intruder.

It is important to secure all entrances, windows as well as doors. Have good double locks installed by a reliable locksmith. It may be well worth the cost to consult a professional security service and follow its advice. Making an office burglar proof is impossible, but entry can be made difficult; and this, in itself, usually discourages the amateur.

Outside sensor lights with unbreakable shields are extremely helpful. Leaving a light burning and a radio playing inside the office are additional deterrents. Tell the local police or the building security force which lights will always be left on.

Alarms can be helpful if they are reliable and are not easily disconnected by an expert. Loud local alarms are usually sufficient to frighten off a prowler. It is possible, if greater security is needed, to install an alarm system that will ring in the local police station or at a special security office.

Police departments urge that all valuables be protected by etching them with personal identification, such as the owner's name or Social Security number. This is easily done with an electric engraving tool that cuts into the equipment, and the marking is practically impossible to eradicate. Even if an attempt is made to scratch it off, a sufficient impression will be left so that police, with the aid of a special chemical, can bring the engraved characters up again (Fig. 23–7).

The most effective step in protecting your premises against break-ins is to remember to check carefully at the end of every day to make certain that all doors and windows are double locked.

WARNING

WE HAVE JOINED
OPERATION IDENTIFICATION
ALL ITEMS OF VALUE
ON THESE PREMISES
HAVE BEEN INDELIBLY MARKED
FOR READY IDENTIFICATION
BY LAW ENFORCEMENT AGENCIES

FIGURE 23–7 Warning sign indicating that valuables have been marked for the purpose of identification.

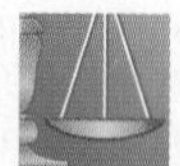

LEGAL AND ETHICAL ISSUES

The physician can be the victim of a lawsuit if a patient is injured on the premises. The medical assistant should report or eliminate any hazard observed.

Patients are entitled to confidentiality. Be aware of sound control and visual privacy.

Keep current and abide by OSHA regulations.

CRITICAL THINKING

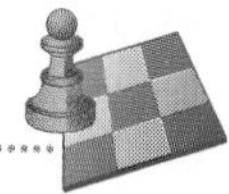

1 When you are visiting a professional office, observe the physical arrangements and try to think of ways the office could be made more efficient or more user-friendly.

2 Become informed on security procedures by examining your own living quarters. How might security be improved?

HOW DID I DO? Answers to Memory Joggers

1. Answers will vary but should include room temperature, lighting, and sound control.
2. Good housekeeping: saves time, conserves property, and eliminates incorrect use of materials. Poor housekeeping: could create physical danger for all occupants.
3. Exposure control plan.
4. Start at the top so that any drippings or dust will not fall on clean areas.
5. The inventory is valuable in preparing income tax reports and for reimbursement in case of loss and should include capital purchases, expendable equipment, and usable supplies.
6. *a.* Place in storage area until time to open packages.
   b. Compare items in packages with original purchase order.
   c. Check for correct items, sizes, and styles.
7. Replace entire bottle and solution for safety purposes.

REFERENCES

American Medical Association: Managing the Medical Practice. Norcross, GA, Coker Publishing Company, 1996.

Andress A: Manual of Medical Office Management. Philadelphia, WB Saunders, 1996.

Management Responsibilities

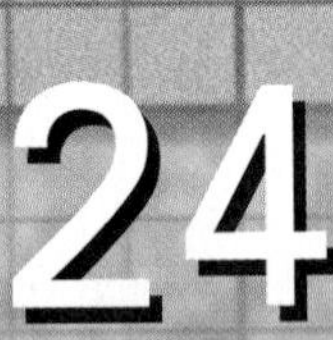

OUTLINE

LEARNING OBJECTIVES

Cognitive: On successful completion of this chapter you should be able to:

1. Define and spell the terms listed in the Vocabulary.
2. State the purpose and goals of medical office management.
3. Discuss the desirable qualities of an office manager and their importance in the selection of a supervisor.
4. Identify the goals of an office policy manual and how they may be achieved.
5. Explain how a procedure manual differs from a policy manual.
6. Discuss the steps in the hiring and dismissal of employees.
7. List five kinds of staff meetings.
8. Discuss the concept of practice development and its importance.
9. List at least 10 features of a patient information folder.
10. State two advantages of patient instruction sheets.
11. Discuss the supervisor's role in financial management.
12. Identify the source of reference for information on employer taxes and deposit requirements.

Performance: On successful completion of this chapter you should be able to:

1. Interview an applicant for a position, utilizing the guidelines in this chapter.
2. Prepare an outline of contents for a basic office policy manual.
3. Write a procedure sheet for a specific task.
4. Outline a patient information folder.
5. Outline a financial policies folder.
6. Write a patient instruction sheet.

VOCABULARY

ancillary Subordinate; auxiliary

appraisal Setting a value on or judging as to quality

candid Frank; straightforward

circumvention Going around or avoidance

discrimination A distinction based on race, religion, sex, or some other factor, especially one resulting in unfair or injurious treatment of an individual belonging to a specific group

disseminate To broadcast or spread over a considerable area

insubordination Refusing to submit to authority

meticulous Extremely careful of small details

motivation The process of inciting a person to some action or behavior

orientation The determination or adjustment of one's intellectual or emotional position with reference to circumstances

philosophy The general laws that furnish the rational explanation of anything

probationary Pertaining to a trial period to ascertain fitness for a job

recruitment The supplying of new members or employees.

Purpose of Management

The purpose of management in a medical practice is to provide a quiet, functional environment in which the physician or physicians can see and treat patients, provide competent medical care, safely store health information, and bill and collect for services to continue practicing medicine. We have learned that the daily functioning of a medical facility involves a multitude of details and that good management does not just happen.

Memory Jogger

What are the three basic purposes of medical office management?

WHO'S IN CHARGE?

If there is only one medical assistant, that person must be able to assume many of the management responsibilities with cooperation from the physician. When there are two medical assistants, one administrative and one clinical, it is often the administrative medical assistant who is expected to assume the management duties. In the office with a larger staff, a line of authority must be established.

A facility with three or more employees should have one person designated as supervisor or office manager. This individual should have management skills and the ability to deal with personnel matters. Other employees answer to the supervisor, the supervisor answers to the physician or physicians. This sets up an orderly way for

- The office staff to consult with the physician regarding administrative or clinical problems, complaints, or grievances
- The physician to check on the operation of the office, **disseminate** information on policy changes, and correct errors or grievances

The career of medical assisting becomes more challenging with the passing years. On the plus side, it also offers more opportunities for advancement than ever before. The recently graduated medical assistant whose first position possibly was as a receptionist may systematically be given more responsibilities and eventually become the office manager of a large staff. The single most critical short supply in health manpower is executive level personnel, specifically, individuals competent to develop and operate a health maintenance organization or prepaid group practice.

AVOIDING MANAGEMENT PROBLEMS

Management problems can often be avoided by carefully defining the areas of authority and responsibility of each employee. Many physicians say that friction between workers is their most common personnel problem. A definite chain of command must be established, and the physician must not undermine the supervisor's authority by **circumvention.** When employees know what is expected of them, they can plan both their daily and long-term work more effectively.

Qualities of a Supervisor

The selection of the right person to supervise the employees is critical. The supervisor may come from within the ranks or may be selected as a new member of the staff. Some employees do not wish to assume management responsibilities; others may not have the necessary qualifications.

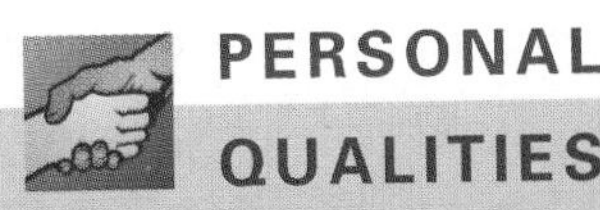

PERSONAL QUALITIES

SUPERVISORY QUALITIES

- Leadership ability
- Good judgment
- Good health
- Ability to organize
- Ability to learn and improve
- Original ideas
- A sense of fairness
- Strength to stand firm on policy, but enough flexibility to recognize when an exception should be made

The management aspect of a medical practice is becoming more complex every year. Practice management consultants frequently conduct seminars for medical office personnel. These are often arranged through a chapter of the American Association of Medical Assistants or the local medical society.

Management Duties

Medical office administrative procedures fall into three broad categories: patient scheduling, health information management, and practice management. We have dealt in detail with the first two categories in previous chapters. It is the third category—practice management process—that concerns us here.

The practice manager's duties vary with the practice but may include any or all of the responsibilities listed under Personnel Management.

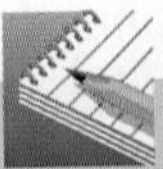

SKILLS AND RESPONSIBILITIES

PERSONNEL MANAGEMENT

- Prepare and update policy and procedure manuals and job descriptions
- Recruitment
- Orientation and training
- Performance and salary review
- Dismissal
- Plan staff meetings
- Maintain staff harmony
- Establish work flow guidelines
- Improve office efficiency
- Supervise purchase and care of equipment
- Patient education
- Eliminate time-wasting tasks for the physician
- Practice marketing

FINANCIAL MANAGEMENT

- Supervise cash transactions
- Maintain payroll records
- Manage employee benefits

OFFICE POLICY AND PROCEDURES MANUALS

Personnel management can best be accomplished with the backup of a well-designed policy manual and a detailed procedure manual.

A policy manual is informational, tells "what to do," and often has an opening statement of the philosophy of the practice, for example:

> The patient is the most important person in this office.
> The patient is the purpose of our being here.
> The patient shall receive our most courteous and attentive treatment at all times.

A procedure manual supplements the policy manual by telling "how to do it." Sometimes the two manuals are combined. The procedure manual will contain a job description for each position in the practice and detailed steps for carrying out each task.

Memory Jogger

Briefly state the difference between a policy manual and a procedure manual.

Office Policy Manual

The policy manual must be designed for a specific facility with its important goals and considerations outlined. It must be

- Comprehensive but flexible
- Easy to read
- Conform with professional ethics
- Reviewed frequently and kept up-to-date as changes occur

A well-designed policy manual will accomplish several results reflecting the expectations of the office:

- Solidifying what may have been vague thoughts into definite statements of policy
- Communicating these statements in exactly the same way to every employee
- Providing a permanent record of these policies

The manual may well be the office manager's best friend by serving as a clear and concise guide for policy information. It can serve as

- An informational guide for the new employee
- A ready reference for a temporary employee
- A reminder of policies for the regular employee
- A back-up for expectations when or if a controversy occurs

Development of the Policy Manual

Begin with the opening statement of the philosophy of the practice. Follow the opening statement with a staff chart that shows the line of authority and states who has authority to enforce the policies. Continue with professional information for each physician on the staff, including education and specialty board achievements, hospital staff memberships, memberships in professional societies, state license number, and narcotic registry number.

What are the expectations regarding the personal appearance of employees? Guidelines regarding appropriate dress, use of makeup, nail polish, perfume, cleanliness, grooming, and hygiene are difficult to discuss on a personal basis but can be matter-of-fact in an office manual.

Describe the work week, listing the daily office hours and any days off, the daily appointment schedule, and where the physician can be reached with messages or emergencies. Specify the time allowed each day for lunch and breaks and whether they must be taken at specific times.

Discuss the provisions for sick leave, emergency leave, and any other absences. Are medical services provided by the professional staff free to employees? Are they discounted? When is the employee eligible for benefits?

Describe the vacation policy, including how much vacation time the employee is allowed in terms of number of working days, who authorizes it, and whether there are any restrictions as to when vacation time may be taken. List the holidays observed.

Are there other benefits for employees, such as payment of professional dues, health insurance, uniform allowances, pension plan, profit sharing, and free parking?

Is time off given for education courses or for attending professional organization conventions or seminars? If so, is this time counted as paid time or as vacation time?

Does the office pay for courses, professional memberships, and expenses incurred at professional conventions?

When is payday? What is the policy on overtime? Are there annual bonuses? If so, how are they determined? What is the policy for performance reviews, salary reviews, and merit increases (Fig. 24–1)?

How much notice is expected if an employee wishes to quit? Can the employee who resigns receive severance pay? What are the grounds for immediate dismissal? How are complaints and grievances handled?

Office Procedure Manual

The office procedure manual supplements the office policy manual. It will contain a job description for each position in the practice and procedure sheets for carrying out each task.

Job Description

A job description is a detailed account of the duties and the qualifications for a specific position. In some cases it should state both primary and secondary responsibilities, emphasizing that the employee must be flexible. Job descriptions may change with personnel changes. No two people have the same capabilities and interests, and there is no need to try to mold a person to a job description when a simple shift in duties may accomplish a happier result. For instance, an administrative assistant might normally be expected to complete the computer sheets at the end of the day; but if a clinical assistant has special aptitude for this and really enjoys the task, there is no reason that this change in responsibility should not be made. Note it on the job description so that there is no confusion about who is responsible (Fig. 24–2). Following the list of duties, there should be a procedure sheet for each task.

Name ______________________ Soc. Sec. No. ______________

Job classification ______________________

Employment date ______________________ Starting salary ______________

Salary checks are issued every (week) (two weeks) (semi-monthly) (month) on ______________ (day or date).

Increase-in-pay review will be conducted six months after the completion of three-month probationary period and each six months thereafter.

Date of first pay review ______________________

Current maximum salary for this job classification $ ______________

Revised ______________ $ ______________

Revised ______________ $ ______________

SALARY SCHEDULE

Date	Amount of increase	Total salary

FIGURE 24–1 Example of page from an office policy manual.

JOB DESCRIPTION **OFFICE MANAGER**

The office manager is responsible for the coordination of all office activities, including recruitment and training of personnel, practice management, and financial procedures.

QUALIFICATIONS: CMA or degree in business administration
Previous medical office experience
Supervisory experience helpful

REPORTS TO: Physician

SPECIFIC TASKS:
1. Prepare annual budget
2. Prepare monthly profit and loss statement
3. Approve all expenditures
4. Review and dispose of delinquent accounts
5. Approve all write-offs
6. Maintain liaison with accountant
7. Recruit, hire, and fire
8. Conduct performance appraisals and report to physician
9. Arrange personnel vacations and keep records of leave days
10. Assist in improving work flow and office efficiencies
11. Supervise purchase and repair of equipment
12. Purchase and supervise storage of supplies
13. Arrange for practice insurance
14. Conduct regular staff meetings
15. Maintain current office policy and procedure manuals
16. Prepare patient education materials as needed

SUPERVISES: Administrative and Clinical Assistants
Service Personnel

Date of Revision: ____________

FIGURE 24–2 Example of job description.

Procedure Sheets

A procedure sheet is a verbal flow chart that lists step-by-step the logical sequence of activities involved in a given task. An employee should be able to perform the task by following the written instructions (Fig. 24–3). Procedure writing is sometimes difficult because, once we become proficient, we tend to take for granted many of the simpler steps involved in performing a task. After a task has been learned, it is unnecessary to refer to the procedure sheet for instructions, but the detailed procedure sheet is invaluable in training the new recruit and in assisting the temporary employee.

Memory Jogger

3 *What are the two categories of information that are included in an office procedure manual?*

PROCEDURE SHEET **PROCESS INCOMING MAIL**

1. Assemble all necessary tools and supplies: letter opener, paper clips, stapler, mending tape, date stamp.
2. Open all mail except letters marked personal.
3. Check to be sure writer's address is on letter before destroying envelope. Staple envelope to letter if address is missing.
4. Paper clip enclosures to letter (or note their absence if they are not enclosed).
5. Date stamp the letter or piece of mail.
6. Set aside cash receipts for processing.
7. Route insurance claim forms and inquiries to insurance clerk.
8. Arrange mail with second and third class on bottom, then first class, with any personal mail on top.
9. Place entire stack in mail tray on right side of physician's desk.

FIGURE 24–3 Example of procedure sheet.

Benefits and Subject Matter

Job descriptions and procedure sheets help the employee achieve expectations. Practice management specialists say that the most common remark from a discharged employee is "I didn't know I was supposed to. . . ." A written job description may also help avoid legal problems with an employee who is dismissed for not meeting performance standards.

A great deal of instruction can be incorporated into a procedure manual. Preferred performance procedures, both administrative and clinical, should be spelled out in detail, including the following information:

- A checklist of daily, weekly, monthly, quarterly, and yearly duties
- How much time is allotted for new patients? Established patients? Postoperative patients?
- How are records prepared and filed? A description of the filing system may save the day if a temporary employee needs to find something in the file during the regular medical assistant's absence.
- How is the telephone to be answered? Which calls are put through to the physician immediately, and which may the medical assistant handle? Include a list of the names and telephone numbers of persons who are called frequently—for example, consulting physicians, hospitals, laboratories, and the physician's spouse.
- Billing and collection procedures. Is billing done weekly, twice monthly, monthly? Are the statements prepared in the office? By what method? Is a collection agency used? Which one? What procedure is used for copays? What is the procedure for referrals?
- Completed samples of forms that need to be filled out and samples of correspondence (these provide excellent visual instruction)
- What kind of setup does the physician prefer for office surgeries or treatments? Is there a card index showing these setups? If so, where is it kept?
- Where and how are supplies ordered and stored? Include the name, address, and telephone number of every supplier. Also include an inventory of major equipment with serial numbers, where and when the equipment was purchased, and a telephone number for servicing.
- Any special duties the physician expects of the medical assistant, such as organizational activities or making travel arrangements

Management studies indicate that, in the multiple-employee facility, it is good practice to have an understudy for each position who can substitute in an emergency. A well-documented procedure manual that is kept current ensures continuity when one employee must, on occasion, fill in for or assist another.

Development of a procedure manual is a good discussion item for staff meetings; the cooperation of the staff is essential if the project is to be successful. Keep it simple to update by using a three-ring binder. Include date of revision. Be sure to destroy old pages when revisions are made. One complete master copy should remain in the custody of the office manager and one with the physician. Each employee should have a copy of the portion that pertains to his or her specific job.

RECRUITMENT

The office manager can be expected to initiate the recruitment and screening of prospective employees. Careful judgment and objectivity must be used in the search for an employee who is suitable for the practice. When possible, have the prospective employee complete an application form (Fig. 24–4) and screen it well before the initial interview.

Preliminary Steps

Before interviewing any applicant, the interviewer needs to know

- What personal qualities and abilities the applicant must have
- The responsibilities of the position
- Salary range
- How soon the position will be open

Add any other specifications for the position. Then, after reviewing the policy manual, prepare an outline for guidance in selecting prospective applicants.

EXAMPLE OF GUIDELINES IN SELECTING PROSPECTIVE APPLICANTS

- Do the applicant's appearance and personal grooming meet the standards set forth in the policy manual?
- Has the applicant been previously employed? What duties were performed?
- If previously employed, how long was the applicant in the last position? Why did the applicant leave?
- What are the applicant's skills? Do these meet the requirements for the position as set forth in the office procedure manual? Does the applicant seem to accept and enjoy responsibility?
- What is the applicant's formal education? Certified Medical Assistant? If not certified, is the applicant interested in taking the certifying examination? Is the applicant a member of a professional organization? Does he or she attend meetings?

APPLICATION FOR POSITION / Medical or Dental Office
AN EQUAL OPPORTUNITY EMPLOYER

(In answering questions, use extra blank sheet if necessary)

No employee, applicant, or candidate for promotion, training or other advantage shall be discriminated against (or given preference) because of race, color, religion, sex, age, physical handicap, veteran status, or national origin.

PLEASE READ CAREFULLY AND WRITE OR PRINT ANSWERS TO ALL QUESTIONS. DO NOT TYPE.

Date of Application

A. PERSONAL INFORMATION

Name - Last | First | Middle | Social Security No. | Area Code/Phone No. ( )

Present Address: - Street | (Apt #) | City | State | Zip | How Long At This Address?:

Previous Address: - Street | City | State | Zip | From: | To:

Person to notify in case of Emergency or Accident - Name: | Address: | Telephone:

B. EMPLOYMENT INFORMATION

For What Position Are You Applying?: | ☐ Full-Time ☐ Part-Time ☐ Either | Date Available For Employment?: | Wage/Salary Expectations:

List Hrs./Days You Prefer To Work | List Any Hrs./Days You Are Not Available: (Except for times required for religious practices or observances) | Can You Work Overtime, If Necessary? ☐ Yes ☐ No

Are You Employed Now?: ☐ Yes ☐ No | If So, May We Inquire Of Your Present Employer?: ☐ No ☐ Yes, If Yes: Name Of Employer: Phone Number: ( )

Have You Ever Been Bonded? ☐ Yes ☐ No | If Required For Position, Are You Bondable? ☐ Yes ☐ No ☐ Uncertain | Have You Applied For A Position With This Office Before? ☐ No ☐ Yes If Yes, When?:

Referred By / Or Where Did You Learn Of This Job?:

Can You, Upon Employment, Submit Verification Of Your Legal Right To Work In The United States?: ☐ Yes ☐ No
Submit Proof That You Meet Legal Age Requirement For Employment? ☐ Yes ☐ No

Language(s) Applicant Speaks or Writes (If Use Of A Language Other Than English is Relevant To The Job For Which The Applicant Is Applying:

C. EDUCATIONAL HISTORY

	Name & Address Of Schools Attended (Include Current)	Dates From	Dates Thru	Highest Grade/Level Completed	Diploma/Degree(s) Obtained/Areas of Study
High School					
College					Degree/Major
Post Graduate					Degree/Major
Other					Course/Diploma/License/Certificate

Specific Training, Education, Or Experiences Which Will Assist You In The Job For Which You Have Applied.

Future Educational Plans

D. SPECIAL SKILLS

CHECK BELOW THE KINDS OF WORK YOU HAVE DONE:

		☐ MEDICAL INSURANCE FORMS	☐ RECEPTIONIST
☐ BLOOD COUNTS	☐ DENTAL ASSISTANT	☐ MEDICAL TERMINOLOGY	☐ TELEPHONES
☐ BOOKKEEPING	☐ DENTAL HYGIENIST	☐ MEDICAL TRANSCRIPTION	☐ TYPING
☐ COLLECTIONS	☐ FILING	☐ NURSING	☐ STENOGRAPHY
☐ COMPOSING LETTERS	☐ INJECTIONS	☐ PHLEBOTOMY (Draw Blood)	☐ URINALYSIS
☐ COMPUTER INPUT	☐ INSTRUMENT STERILIZATION	☐ POSTING	☐ X-RAY
OFFICE EQUIPMENT USED: ☐ COMPUTER	☐ DICTATING EQUIPMENT	☐ WORD PROCESSOR	☐ OTHER:

Other Kinds Of Tasks Performed Or Skills That May Be Applicable To Position: | Typing Speed | Shorthand Speed

ORDER # 72-110 • © 1976 BIBBERO SYSTEMS, INC. • PETALUMA, CA. • (REV. 1/95)
TO REORDER CALL TOLL FREE: (800) BIBBERO (800-242-2376) OR FAX (800) 242-9330 MFG IN U.S.A.

(PLEASE COMPLETE OTHER SIDE)

FIGURE 24–4 Application for position in medical office. (Courtesy of Bibbero Systems, Inc., Petaluma, California (800) 242-2376, Fax (800) 242-9330.)

Illustration continued on following page

E. EMPLOYMENT RECORD

LIST MOST RECENT EMPLOYMENT FIRST | **May We Contact Your Previous Employer(s) For A Reference?** ☐ Yes ☐ No

1) Employer		Work Performed. Be Specific:
Address Street City State Zip Code		
Phone Number ( )		
Type of Business	Dates Mo. Yr. From Mo. Yr. To	
Your Position	Hourly Rate/Salary Starting Final	
Supervisor's Name		
Reason For Leaving		

2) Employer		Worked Performed. Be Specific:
Address Street City State Zip Code		
Phone Number ( )		
Type of Business	Dates Mo. Yr. From Mo. Yr. To	
Your Position	Hourly Rate/Salary Starting Final	
Supervisor's Name		
Reason For Leaving		

3) Employer		Worked Performed. Be Specific:
Address Street City State Zip Code		
Phone Number ( )		
Type of Business	Dates Mo. Yr. From Mo. Yr. To	
Your Position	Hourly Rate/Salary Starting Final	
Supervisor's Name		
Reason For Leaving		

F. REFERENCES — FRIENDS / ACQUAINTANCES NON-RELATED

(1) ____

Name Address Telephone Number (☐ Work ☐ Home) Occupation Years Acquainted

(1) ____

Name Address Telephone Number (☐ Work ☐ Home) Occupation Years Acquainted

Please Feel Free To Add Any Information Which You Feel Will Help Us Consider You For Employment

READ THE FOLLOWING CAREFULLY, THEN SIGN AND DATE THE APPLICATION

"I certify that all answers given by me on this application are true, correct and complete to the best of my knowledge. I acknowledge notice that the information contained in this application is subject to check. I agree that, if hired, my continued employment may be contingent upon the accuracy of that information. If employed, I further agree to comply with Company/Office rules and regulations."

Signature: ______________________________ Date: ______________

FIGURE 24–4 *continued*

ARRANGING THE PERSONAL INTERVIEW

If the applicant sent a letter asking for an interview, note whether the letter was correctly typed, included the essential information, and provided a personal data sheet (see Chapter 2). Forget the applicant who sends a letter handwritten in pencil. By telephoning the applicant, you will have an opportunity to judge the telephone voice. If it is poor, you may not wish to consider the applicant further.

Set a time for the personal interview when you most likely will be able to give the applicant your undivided attention. However, an applicant who is being considered for employment should have an opportunity to see your office when there is a fairly normal amount of activity. The prospective employee who is interviewed in a peaceful, quiet office on the physician's day out may not be prepared for the activity on a normal working day.

Before interviewing any applicant, make certain that you are thoroughly familiar with the federal, state, and local fair-employment practice laws affecting hiring practices. Both men and women are receiving protection from on-the-job discrimination, sexual harassment, mandatory lie detector tests, and unfair discharge.

Illegal questions are sometimes asked on preprinted employment applications or during interviews. Title VII of the Civil Rights Act of 1964, as amended by the Equal Employment Opportunity Act of 1972, prohibits inquiries into an applicant's race, color, sex, religion, and national origin. Inquiries regarding medical history, arrest records, or former drug use are also illegal. Most states have laws designed to protect the rights of job applicants, and these laws may impose additional restrictions.

Either send the applicant an application form to be completed and brought in at the time of the interview or allow ample time for its completion on the day of the interview. The application form can serve as a check of the applicant's penmanship and thoroughness as well as a permanent record for your files. If you wish it to be completed in the applicant's own handwriting, be sure to state this on the instructions. The applicant should be meticulous about following instructions and filling in all the blanks.

Memory Jogger

List five items of personal information that are prohibited from being requested under the Equal Employment Opportunity Act.

The Interview

First, make certain that the applicant feels at ease. You might shake his or her hand and ask a few social questions before starting the interview. In general, follow good manners and see that the person to be interviewed is comfortable.

Begin with a few open-ended questions that cannot be answered with a simple "yes" or "no," such as "What did you do in your last employment?" When interviewing a recent graduate who does not have experience, you might ask, "What was your favorite class?"

As you speak with the applicant, make a mental note of whether the applicant displays essential personal qualities.

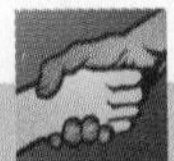

PERSONAL QUALITIES

APPEALING PERSONAL QUALITIES IN AN APPLICANT

- Converses easily
- Is a good listener
- Is free of annoying mannerisms
- Has a ready smile
- Is interested enough to ask as well as to answer questions
- Appears interested in the office and in the physician's specialty

Avoid questions that involve the applicant's privacy. Your questions should be related to the available position and the applicant's ability to do the job. An interview should be a two-way exchange of information between the applicant and the interviewer.

If the applicant appears to be one who will receive serious consideration, you have the responsibility of explaining what will be expected in the way of duties; office policies regarding appearance, working hours, overtime, time off, and vacations; what initial salary is offered and any fringe benefits; and the office policy on increases. If you fail to mention these items, the applicant may be hesitant to inquire.

If your employer is a member of a credit bureau, it may be advisable to request the applicant's permission to check his or her credit rating, especially if handling office finances will be one of the responsibilities. It can safely be assumed that one who is unable to handle personal financial affairs will be a poor risk in handling office finances.

Interview for Placement ______________________________
(position)

Name ______________________ **Date** __________ **Time** __________

	Superior	Above Average	Average	Poor	Remarks
Appearance/Grooming					
General Health					
Voice and Diction					
Mannerisms					
Poise					
Friendliness					
Interest in Work					
Did Applicant Ask Questions?					
Overall Impression					

FIGURE 24–5 Form for applicant rating after interview.

Review the job description for the position being filled. This is essential if you are to be certain that the person being interviewed understands the required duties and responsibilities. Ask if the applicant has any questions, and close the interview on a positive note.

During the hiring proceedings, you may wish to invite the prospective employee to lunch with the staff or for coffee in the more relaxed atmosphere of the employee lounge. This presents an opportunity to discover whether the applicant's personality will mesh with the atmosphere of the office.

Follow-Up Activities

When the interview is over, take a few moments immediately to rate the applicant on your checklist. Jot down some notes to refresh your memory when you refer this applicant to the physician for the final interview. Do not trust your impressions to memory, especially if several applicants will be interviewed. Figure 24–5 is a suggested checklist that may be modified to suit your own circumstances.

Checking References

It is always advisable to carefully check all references and to follow through on any leads for information. It is best to use the telephone in checking references because people are sometimes less than candid in a letter; furthermore, letter writing is time consuming and you may not get a reply.

Prepare a checklist before you place the call. When you talk with the person called, be sure to "listen between the lines." Note the tone of the replies to your questions. Do not ask questions that might incriminate the person answering them. You might ask the following questions as an introduction:

1. When did (the applicant) work for you?
2. How long?
3. What were the duties and responsibilities?
4. Did the employee assume responsibility well?

Hiring

When a decision has been reached to hire someone, notify the applicant of the decision and state when the applicant will be expected to report for work. Remember to notify all others who have applied. They may have hesitated to accept other interviews in the hope of hearing from you. It is unfair to keep individuals who are seeking employment "on the string." Good etiquette requires that you drop them a note or call by telephone and say that the position is filled. Thank the individual for applying, and say that you will keep his or her application on file.

ORIENTATION AND TRAINING

Recruitment does not end with the hiring. Some preliminary orientation and training will help new employees to understand what is expected and to develop their full potential. Acquaint the new employee with such aspects of the office as:

- Staff
- Physical environment
- Nature of the practice and specialty. Explain

what types of patients are dealt with and how the staff is expected to interact with them.
- Office policies. Have the employee read the policy manual and then discuss it.
- Long-range expectations

PERFORMANCE AND SALARY REVIEW

A new employee should be granted a probationary period. Sixty to 90 days has been traditional, but many employers believe that 2 weeks is sufficient to determine whether the employee will be able to learn and adapt to the position.

A definite date for a performance review at the end of the probationary period should be set at the time of employment. This review should not be squeezed in between patient visits or be given a token few minutes at the end of a day. There should be ample time to relax and talk. At this time, the new employee is told how well expectations have been met and whether there are any deficiencies. Then give the employee an opportunity to ask questions. Sometimes an employee fails to perform because of never having been told what was expected.

The performance **appraisal** includes a judgment of both the quality and quantity of work, personal appearance, attitudes and team spirit, dependability, self-discipline, **motivation,** attendance, and any other qualities essential to satisfactory performance of the job in question.

Although the probationary period does not always allow time to fully train an individual for a specific position, it is fair to assume that the potential for being a satisfactory employee can be judged at this time. Now is the time to talk out any problems and make suggestions for improvement.

The supervisor is responsible for ongoing performance appraisals of all employees, complimenting whenever possible and appropriate and offering helpful criticism when necessary. A formal performance appraisal at the end of the probationary period and at regular 6-month intervals thereafter, with a report to the physician employer, is helpful in the employee's salary review (Fig. 24–6).

DISMISSAL

The necessity for dismissing an employee is unpleasant at best, but if the ground rules are decided on in advance, written into the policy manual, and explained to all employees, the problem is partially solved. The policies must be applied equally and impartially to all. The final decision for dismissal will probably be made by the physician but may be based on the recommendation of the office manager/supervisor. The person who does the hiring should do the firing.

The probationary employee who does not prove satisfactory should be dismissed at the end of the probationary period, with tact and a full explanation of the reasons for dismissal. In all fairness, an individual should be told why the employment is ended and not be given weak excuses or untruths that do not help to correct deficiencies. If you are not straightforward in telling an employee the reason for dismissal, you are not helping that person to grow (Fig. 24–7).

An employee who has been in service for some time and is offering unsatisfactory performance should be warned and given an explanation of the specific improvements expected. If a second chance does not produce improvement in performance or attitude, then dismissal must follow. It should be done privately, with tact and consideration.

Most practice consultants believe that firing should come close to the end of the day, after all other employees have left, and that the break should be clean and immediate. If the office policy provides for 2 weeks' notice, give 2 weeks' pay. A dismissed employee should not be allowed to train or influence a replacement.

The exit meeting should be planned just as carefully as the employment interview. Be honest with the employee. Discuss the employee's assets as well as liabilities and give the reasons for the termination before you announce the dismissal. There is no need to dwell on the employee's deficiencies. These should have been thoroughly discussed at the warning interview, and the employee need only be told that the necessary improvements have not been made. Do listen to the employee's feedback. This may reveal some important administrative problems that need correction (Fig. 24–8).

After you dismiss an employee, do not leave that person in the office unattended. Request and get the office keys before giving a dismissed employee the final paycheck. And do not offer to give the employee a good reference unless you can do it sincerely.

Certain breaches of conduct, such as embezzlement and blatant insubordination or violation of patient confidentiality, are grounds for immediate dismissal without warning.

Occasionally, an employee voluntarily terminates a job without giving a valid reason. The physician or office manager may wish to follow up with a letter to the former employee to seek out any problem that may have prompted the resignation (Fig. 24–9).

Memory Jogger

What courtesy should be extended to a long-term employee whose performance is unsatisfactory?

Text continued on page 379

PERFORMANCE EVALUATION AND DEVELOPMENT PLAN
(OFFICE AND CLERICAL)

NAME: ______________________ DATE OF EVALUATION: ______________________

DATE OF HIRE: ______________________ DEPARTMENT: ______________________

JOB TITLE: ______________________ SUPERVISOR: ______________________

DATE APPOINTED THIS JOB: ______________________ MANAGER: ______________________

LAST REVIEW DATE: ______________________ LAST REVIEW RATING: ______________________

NEXT REVIEW DATE: ______________________ CURRENT REVIEW RATING: ______________________

PURPOSE

The purpose of this evaluation is to:

1. SET GOALS WITHIN SCOPE OF PRESENT JOB.
2. COMMUNICATE OPENLY ABOUT PERFORMANCE.
3. EVALUATE PAST PERFORMANCE.
4. DISCUSS FUTURE DEVELOPMENT PLANS FOR GROWTH.

INSTRUCTIONS

1. Supervisor to review form prior to completion. If specific items are not applicable they should be left blank.
2. Supervisor and employee to review job description prior to review.
3. In "COMMENTS" section supervisor may indicate which factors should be more heavily weighted in this particular evaluation.
4. Comments should be specific and job-related. All appropriate evaluation factors should be commented on to some degree.

I. POSITION OBJECTIVES AND MAJOR RESPONSIBILITIES. Summarize specific responsibilities of the job.

____

____

____

II. ACCOMPLISHMENTS AND/OR IMPROVEMENTS. What specific accomplishments and/or improvements has employee made since last review with respect to set goals?

____

____

____

PLEASE CONSIDER THE EMPLOYEE'S DEMONSTRATED PERFORMANCE AND MARK THE CIRCLE WHICH MOST CLOSELY DESCRIBES THAT PERFORMANCE.

4 - Performance consistently far exceeds expectations and requirements.
3 - Performance consistently exceeds normal expectations and job requirements.
2 - Performance consistently meets expectations and job requirements
1 - Performance usually meets expectations and minimum job requirements.
0 - Performance does not meet job requirements.

– CONTINUED, NEXT PAGE –

FORM # 72-119 © 1987 BIBBERO SYSTEMS, INC. PETALUMA, CA

TO REORDER CALL TOLL FREE: 800-BIBBERO /(800 242-2376) OR FAX: (800) 242-9330 MFG IN U.S.A.

FIGURE 24–6 Performance evaluation and development plan. (Courtesy of Bibbero Systems, Inc., Petaluma, California (800) 242-2376, Fax (800) 242-9330.)

7. **DEPENDABILITY:** CONSIDER ATTENDANCE, PUNCTUALITY, IDLE TIME AND RELIANCE WHICH CAN BE PLACED ON EMPLOYEE TO PERSEVERE AND CARRY THROUGH TO COMPLETION ALL ASSIGNED TASKS

○ 0 ○ 1 ○ 2 ○ 3 ○ 4

8. **COMPLIANCE WITH COMPANY POLICIES:** DOES THE EMPLOYEE COMPLY WITH RULES AND REGULATIONS WHICH APPLY TO SAFETY, FAIR EMPLOYMENT PRACTICES AND GENERAL ADMINISTRATIVE PROCEDURE.

○ 0 ○ 1 ○ 2 ○ 3 ○ 4

9. SPECIFIC PERFORMANCE	1	2	3	4	COMMENTS
A. Ability to handle scheduling:					
B. Willingness to work OT when necessary:					
C. Handling of calls and follow-up:					
D. Maintenance of equipment:					
E. Ability to handle patient complaints:					
F. Tact in dealing with patients:					
G. Speed (in specific technical procedures):					
H. Secretarial accuracy:					
I. Professional terminology:					
J. Assisting procedures:					
K. Laboratory techniques:					
L. X-ray techniques:					
M. Physical therapy:					
N. Collections:					
O. Medical Insurance:					
P. Bookkeeping:					

10. PERSONAL	1	2	3	4	COMMENTS
A. Grooming:					
B. Professional conduct:					
C. Energy, enthusiasm:					
D. Ability to handle stress:					

ADDITIONAL COMMENTS:

FORM # 72-119 © 1987 BIBBERO SYSTEMS, INC. PETALUMA, CA

FIGURE 24–6 *continued*

TERMINATION / REHIRE EVALUATION FORM

Employee Name____________________ Social Security No.__________

Department ____________________ Title __________

Termination Date __________

Reason for Termination: ________Resigned ______Laid Off________Retired

Evaluation of Job Performance	Excellent	Very Good	Average	Poor	Unacceptable
Quality (accuracy, etc.)	☐	☐	☐	☐	☐
Quantity (productivity, consistency, etc.)	☐	☐	☐	☐	☐
Knowledge of Duties	☐	☐	☐	☐	☐
Reliability (absenteeism)	☐	☐	☐	☐	☐
Punctuality	☐	☐	☐	☐	☐
Ability to Cooperate with Co-workers	☐	☐	☐	☐	☐
Relationship with Patients	☐	☐	☐	☐	☐
Overall Attitude (willingness and commitment)	☐	☐	☐	☐	☐
Initiative	☐	☐	☐	☐	☐
Judgment	☐	☐	☐	☐	☐

Recommendation for Rehiring: ____________________

____

____

Comments:____________________

____

____

____

____

____

____

____________________ Date __________

Supervisor's Signature

FORM # 72-123 PERSONNEL RECORDS ORGANIZING SYSTEMS • © 1987 BIBBERO SYSTEMS, INC. • PETALUMA, CA.
TO REORDER CALL TOLL FREE: (800) BIBBERO (800-242-2376) OR FAX (800) 242-9330 MFG IN U.S.A.

FIGURE 24–7 Termination/rehire evaluation form at end of probationary period. (Courtesy of Bibbero Systems, Inc., Petaluma, California (800) 242-2376, Fax (800) 242-9330.)

EXIT INTERVIEW QUESTIONNAIRE

Employee Name (Optional) ______________________ Date ________

Job Title ________________ Department ________________

Immediate Supervisor ________________ Dates of Employment ________________

SSN# ________________ EMP. ID# ________________

I. Please rate the following conditions.	**Excellent**	**Very Good**	**Average**	**Poor**	**Unacceptable**
Employer in General	☐	☐	☐	☐	☐
Administration	☐	☐	☐	☐	☐
Policies and Procedures	☐	☐	☐	☐	☐
New Employee Orientation	☐	☐	☐	☐	☐
Wages	☐	☐	☐	☐	☐
Vacation	☐	☐	☐	☐	☐
Holidays	☐	☐	☐	☐	☐
Sick Leave	☐	☐	☐	☐	☐
Other Benefits	☐	☐	☐	☐	☐
Immediate Supervisor	☐	☐	☐	☐	☐
Management	☐	☐	☐	☐	☐
Challenge of Position	☐	☐	☐	☐	☐
Satisfaction of Position	☐	☐	☐	☐	☐
Advancement	☐	☐	☐	☐	☐
Training Programs	☐	☐	☐	☐	☐
Co-workers	☐	☐	☐	☐	☐
Professional Staff	☐	☐	☐	☐	☐
Working Conditions (Physical)	☐	☐	☐	☐	☐
Hours	☐	☐	☐	☐	☐
Days	☐	☐	☐	☐	☐
Work Load	☐	☐	☐	☐	☐
Pressures / Stress	☐	☐	☐	☐	☐
Morale of Staff	☐	☐	☐	☐	☐

Specific comments on any of the above factors: ________________

II. Please rate the following conditions in your department.

	Excellent	**Very Good**	**Average**	**Poor**	**Unacceptable**
Orientation Program	☐	☐	☐	☐	☐
Intra-departmental Communication	☐	☐	☐	☐	☐
Inter-departmental Cooperation	☐	☐	☐	☐	☐
Opportunities for Training and Development	☐	☐	☐	☐	☐
Morale of Co-workers	☐	☐	☐	☐	☐

Specific comments on any of the above factors: ________________

ORDER # 72-122 PERSONNEL RECORD SYSTEM • © 1984 BIBBERO SYSTEMS, INC. • PETALUMA, CA.
TO REORDER CALL TOLL FREE: (800) BIBBERO (800-242-2376) OR FAX (800) 242-9330 (Rev. 5/96) MFG IN U.S.A.

FIGURE 24–8 Exit interview questionnaire after voluntary termination of employment. (Courtesy of Bibbero Systems, Inc., Petaluma, California (800) 242-2376, Fax (800) 242-9330.)

Illustration continued on following page

III. Please rate your immediate supervisor.	Excellent	Very Good	Average	Poor	Unacceptable
Follows Policies & Procedures	☐	☐	☐	☐	☐
Follows Regulations of Department	☐	☐	☐	☐	☐
Fair & Equal to Employees	☐	☐	☐	☐	☐
Assigns Work Fairly	☐	☐	☐	☐	☐
Provides Adequate Training	☐	☐	☐	☐	☐
Open to Suggestions	☐	☐	☐	☐	☐
Encourages and Praises Staff	☐	☐	☐	☐	☐
Encourages Team Effort and Cooperation	☐	☐	☐	☐	☐
Resolves Complaints & Problems	☐	☐	☐	☐	☐
Encourages Advancement	☐	☐	☐	☐	☐
Assigns Responsibility Equally	☐	☐	☐	☐	☐
Demands Realistic Standards	☐	☐	☐	☐	☐

Specific comments on any of the above factors: ____________________

____

____

IV. Please answer following general questions.

a. Why were you interested in working here? ____________________

____

b. Were you satisfied with your job here? ____________________

____

c. Positive conditions of work here? ____________________

____

d. Would you recommend employment here? ________Yes ________No

Why? ____________________

____

e. Please specify your reasons for leaving?

Moving to another location ____________________

Work schedule ____________________

Personal (family) ____________________

Supervision ____________________

Opportunity for Advancement ____________________

Transportation ____________________

Marriage ____________________

Pregnancy ____________________

Attend School ____________________

Retirement (voluntary) ____________________

Dissatisfied ____________________

Another Position ____________________

Other (Specify) ____________________

Conditions or benefits of new employment that you have found more appealing: ____________________

____

____

f. Suggestions for general improvements here or specifically within your department: ____________________

____

ORDER # 72-122 PERSONNEL RECORD SYSTEM • © 1984 BIBBERO SYSTEMS, INC. • PETALUMA, CA.
TO REORDER CALL TOLL FREE: (800) BIBBERO (800-242-2376) OR FAX (800) 242-9330 (Rev. 5/96) MFG IN U.S.A.

FIGURE 24–8 *continued*

Dear ____________________

Since your decision to leave our employ a few weeks ago, I have been concerned about your reasons for doing so. There may have been more than one reason—and one of them may have been dissatisfaction with the working conditions.

If there was in fact some reason for dissatisfaction that influenced your decision to leave our employ, I would appreciate your passing it along to me, so that I may avoid losing other valuable employees in the future.

Please drop me a note, telephone, or come in if you wish. I assure you that any comments you care to make will be treated with respect and appreciation.

Cordially yours,

FIGURE 24–9 Example of letter from physician to employee who resigned suddenly.

Business Management

STAFF MEETINGS

There must be some formal mechanism for keeping the office manager and other key employees current on the daily business affairs of the practice. One of the most common complaints from office personnel is that of being unable to discuss problems with the physician. The solution to this problem may be to hold regular staff meetings, which may be scheduled as frequently as weekly but should be no less often than quarterly. Some of the best ideas on improvement come from the office staff, and expressing ideas should be encouraged.

The simplest technique is to set aside a specific time for regular meetings at an hour when the most people can attend with the least disruption. The meetings need not be long or overly formal, but to be effective they must be planned and organized. There must be a leader, and a secretary should be appointed to take notes. The effectiveness of the leader, a person who can balance firmness with fairness, is an important aspect of the meeting. This is usually either the physician or the office manager/supervisor. All members of the staff should be encouraged to submit ideas for discussion.

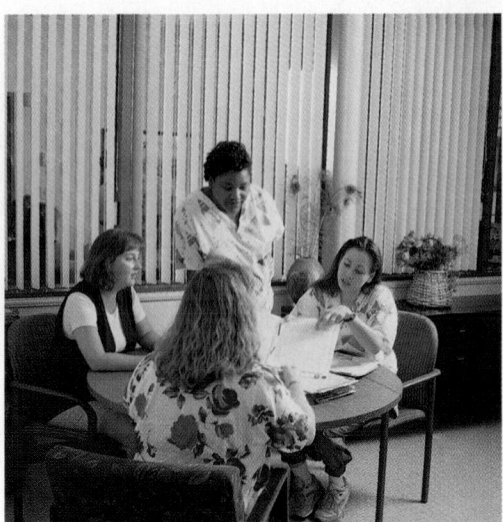

FIGURE 24–10 Staff meeting.

Draw up a simple outline of the issues you want to discuss and prepare any supporting data needed for the meeting. There are many kinds of staff meetings. They may be purely informational, or problem solving, or brainstorming; they may be work sessions for updating manuals, training seminars, or whatever is necessary to that individual practice. The staff should meet to discuss new ideas and any changes in office procedures and to resolve any problems. The staff meeting must not be allowed to deteriorate into a gripe session. Individual complaints should be handled privately.

The meeting must have a set agenda, with time for topics that need discussion on a regular basis, as well as time to handle any current problems. The agenda might be similar to that of any business meeting:

1. Reading of the last meeting's minutes
2. Discussion of any unfinished business
3. Discussion of any problems in the clinical area
4. Discussion of any problems in the administrative area
5. Discussion of any problems in common areas
6. Adjournment

Some physicians like to combine the staff meeting with a breakfast or lunch. The time or place is not important as long as it is "neutral" and suits the practice and the meetings are conducted regularly, democratically, and without interruption (Fig. 24–10). There must be follow-up to the items discussed; otherwise, the only result will be frustration and a reluctance to discuss problems at future meetings.

Memory Jogger

Why is it important to have an agenda for a staff meeting?

PRACTICE DEVELOPMENT

The business manager will play a large role in practice development, or "practice marketing" as it is often referred to. Practice development techniques are the outcome of a conscious need to improve the professional image, to increase exposure to the public, and to attract and keep patients. With the expansion of managed care in the health care industry, the average physician receives less income, has increased costs, and works a more competitive practice environment. In many instances it has become necessary to make slight changes in office hours to accommodate the patient population, including, in some cases, providing for evening and weekend hours or even house calls.

The medical assistant with management responsibilities can encourage the physician to participate in community affairs. For example, the practice might offer to give mass inoculations when needed, serve as a consultant in area health fairs, or speak on health topics to civic and professional groups. Some physicians gain public exposure by writing articles or a question-and-answer column for an area newspaper. Local events may suggest other ways of promoting the practice.

Communication with the patient is essential. The medical practice with a computer and word processing software can easily generate a newsletter several times a year containing information pertaining to the practice specialty or advances in health care in general. A letter to the patient and one to the patient's referring physician after a consultation are greatly appreciated by both and are easily and quickly accomplished with electronic equipment. Holiday and birthday remembrances are another easy way of keeping the patient aware of the practice and conveying your concern.

The first, last, and most important rule of marketing a medical practice, of course, is to treat the patients well, because the best source of patients consists of referrals from existing satisfied patients.

Memory Jogger

 *Memorize the most important rule of marketing a medical practice.*

PATIENT EDUCATION

Patients have many common concerns about the physician's policies, such as office hours, what is included in his or her specialty, directions for reaching the office, parking facilities, emergency services, answering service, cancellations, house calls, prescription renewals, and payment of fees. You can satisfy the patients' concerns and save your own time by putting these policies in writing and giving a copy to every patient.

Many management experts recommend that two separate folders or pamphlets be prepared—one devoted to general office information and another to financial policies.

Patient Information Folder

Only a very small percentage of practices have a booklet that explains the information basic to the operational and service aspects of the practice. Yet, a patient information folder can easily be compiled by the physician and staff cooperatively in a staff meeting. Experience has shown that if such a folder is given to every new patient, the number of incoming phone calls can be reduced by an average of 20% to 30%. It can also reduce misunderstanding and forgotten instructions. The folder must of necessity be tailored to the specific practice.

The patient information folder should be an introduction to the practice and, if possible, mailed to a new patient before the first visit. A supply may also be left with referring physicians' offices to be given to patients coming to your office. It should be designed to easily fit into a No. 10 business envelope.

The cover should show the name of the practice, its location, and the practice logo, if there is one. Consider using a photo of the medical building for easy identification by the new patient.

A statement of philosophy is frequently included in the introduction, followed by a description of the practice.

> The doctors and staff would like to welcome you to our office. We work as a team with the goal of providing prompt and thorough care of your problems. We are always working to improve our care and service in any way possible.
>
> Our practice is limited exclusively to the musculoskeletal system and its disorders. Therefore, it is important for each patient to have a primary care physician such as a pediatrician, family physician, or internist to oversee the primary medical care for the entire patient. Our role is most effective as a consultant to your primary care physician.

Describe the office policy regarding appointments and cancellations, telephone calls, and the function of the answering service. If a separate "business only" telephone line is available, be sure to include this information.

> This office has two receptionists available to answer phone calls during regular office hours. The office is very busy, and you will occasionally be asked to hold for a brief period. Please be patient with this. If you wish to speak to a doctor, your call will usually be returned during the next available break period or at the end of the office day. We receive many calls during the day, and it is unfair to the patients who have scheduled appointments to continually interrupt the doctor for telephone calls. Therefore, the receptionist will usually take a message and your call will be returned as soon as possible. Please inform the receptionist if your problem is urgent and she will let the doctor know this.

Describe any **ancillary** or laboratory services provided, how test results are reported, and your policy on prescription renewals.

Patients need to know the provisions for emergency procedures: What hospitals does the practice use regularly? What is the night and weekend coverage? Hospitalization procedures and postoperative care and follow-up may also be included.

> One of the doctors in the group is always on call for emergency situations. You may reach him by calling our office phone number (714) 333–2323, and the answering service will put you in touch with the doctor on call at that time. Our doctors are on staff at St. Joseph Hospital (714-222-3333) and, for children, Children's Hospital of Orange County, 714-222-4444. In case of emergency, call 911.

List all physicians in the practice; state their educational backgrounds, training, and board certifications; and define their specialties. List the names of key clinical and administrative staff members, such as registered nurses and nurse practitioners, medical assistants, the office manager, and the business manager. Provide the practice address, a map of how to get there, and information about the parking facilities.

Don't just stack these folders in the reception room for patients to pick up. Have the receptionist write the patient's name on the folder and hand it to the patient when he or she registers for the first appointment and suggest that the patient keep it for future reference.

Memory Jogger

In what ways does a patient information folder improve medical care?

Financial Policy Folder

A separate small folder of information covering the financial policies of the office can eliminate many questions and possible misunderstandings. Tailor the financial policy folder to your specific practice. Keep it small enough to fit into the billing envelope, and send it out with the first monthly statement. If the practice sends out a "welcome" package before the patient's first visit, include the financial policy folder. Otherwise, present one at the first visit.

Spell out policies regarding billing and collection procedures, and make it clear that patients are responsible for the uninsured portion of the fees. If you expect payment at the time of service, put this in the folder. Keep the language simple and straightforward so that the message is clear.

> FINANCIAL POLICY
>
> We ask that our services be paid for at the time they are rendered. You will be provided with a superbill so that you may bill your insurance company and be reimbursed for services paid at the time of your visit. Simply attach the superbill to your insurance form and mail it to the insurance company. The appropriate diagnoses and charges will be on the superbill. There is usually a greater charge for the initial visit because this involves more time than follow-up visits. If you are sent to an outside office for laboratory testing or special x-rays, you will be billed separately from that office. We will be available to help if special circumstances arise involving difficulty with forms or receiving reimbursement. We will bill your insurance if you have a special situation such as surgery, prepaid health plans, Medicaid, CCS, or Senior Savers. We will complete disability papers as promptly as possible. However, you must obtain the necessary forms from your employer or the disability office.

The financial policy folder should also clearly state that the ultimate responsibility for payment lies with the patient.

Patient Instruction Sheets

In most medical offices there are patient procedures that occur over and over again. Instead of attempting to orally instruct a patient each time, why not develop clearly stated instruction sheets that you can review with the patient and then give the patient the written instructions to take home?

> EXAMPLES OF PROCEDURES TO BE LISTED IN INSTRUCTION SHEETS
>
> - Preparation for x-ray or laboratory tests
> - Preoperative and postoperative instructions
> - Diet sheets
> - Performing an enema
> - Dressing a wound
> - Taking medications
> - Using a cane, crutches, walker, or wheelchair
> - Care of casts
> - Exercise therapy

Financial Management

A physician in a solo practice or small partnership may prefer to handle most financial aspects of the practice personally or may place that responsibility in the hands of a certified public accountant or management consultant. In this situation, the medical assistant's involvement may be limited to the billing and bookkeeping activities discussed in previous chapters.

The medical assistant who is able to handle more responsibility will probably have the opportunity to do so. This could be the most challenging part of the position and may include any or all of the following activities:

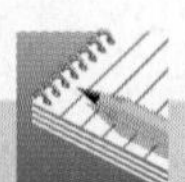

SKILLS AND RESPONSIBILITIES

ADVANCED RESPONSIBILITIES

- Supervising cash receipts:
  Banking
  Billing
  Collections
- Preparing periodic profit and loss statements
- Computing collection ratios
- Making provision for
  Practice insurance
  Professional liability
  Workers' compensation
  Employee's health benefits
  Disability insurance
  Unemployment insurance
- Writing payroll checks
- Paying bills
- Preparing reports for governmental agencies
- Serving as liaison with the accountant

PAYROLL RECORDS

Handling payroll records, whether for one employee or dozens of employees, involves frequent reporting activities. If it were necessary only to write a check to each employee for the agreed-upon salary for a given pay period, no discussion of payroll records would be necessary. But government regulations require the withholding of taxes from employees and payment of certain taxes due from both employees and employers.

To comply with government regulations, complete records must be kept for every employee. You must keep all records of employment taxes for at least 4 years. These should be available for review by the Internal Revenue Service (IRS). Such records include the following:

- Social Security number of the employee
- Number of withholding allowances claimed
- Amount of gross salary
- All deductions for Social Security and Medicare taxes; federal, state, and city or other subdivision withholding taxes; state disability insurance; and state unemployment tax, where applicable

Memory Jogger

How long must employee financial records be kept?

PAYROLL REPORTING FORMS

Each employee and each employer must have a tax identification number. The Social Security number is the employee's tax identification number. Any person who does not have a Social Security number should apply for one, using Form SS-5 available from any Social Security Administration office.

The employer applies for a number for federal tax accounting purposes using Form SS-4, available at Social Security Administration offices or by calling 1-800-TAX-FORM. In states that require employer reports, a state employer number must also be obtained.

Before the end of the first pay period, the employee should complete an Employee's Withholding Allowance Certificate (Form W-4) showing the number of withholding allowances claimed (Fig. 24–11). Otherwise, the employer must indicate withholding on the basis of a single person with no exemptions.

The employee should complete a new form when changes occur in marital status or in the number of allowances claimed. Each employee is entitled to one personal allowance and one for each qualified dependent. The employee may elect to take fewer or no allowances, in which case the tax withheld will be greater and a refund may be due when the employee's annual tax report is filed. If an employee claims more than 10 withholding allowances or an exemption from withholding and his or her wages would normally be more than $200 per week, the employer is required to send to the IRS copies of these W-4 forms.

A supply of all the necessary forms for filing federal returns, preprinted with the employer's name, will be furnished to an employer who has applied for an employer identification number. Extra forms may be obtained from the IRS office.

INCOME TAX WITHHOLDING

Employers are required by law to withhold certain amounts from employees' earnings and to report and forward these amounts to be applied toward payment of income tax. The amount to be withheld is based on the following:

- Total earnings of the employee
- Number of withholding allowances claimed

- Marital status of the employee
- Length of the pay period involved

The *Federal Employer's Tax Guide* includes tables to be used in determining the amount to be withheld. Sample pages are shown in Figure 24–12. There is one table for single persons and unmarried heads of households and one for married persons. The tables cover monthly, semimonthly, biweekly, weekly, and daily or miscellaneous periods.

Memory Jogger

What four items determine the amount of income tax withholding for each employee?

EMPLOYER'S INCOME TAX

The physician who is practicing as an individual is not subject to withholding tax but is expected to make an estimated tax payment four times a year. The accountant prepares four copies of Form 1040-S, Declaration of Estimated Tax for Individuals, for the ensuing year when the annual income tax return is prepared. The first form and the quarterly estimated tax for the next year is filed at the same time as the tax return. The remaining three forms, with the estimated tax due, must be filed on June 15, September 15, and January 15. It may be the business manager's responsibility to see that these returns are filed when due. The employer also contributes to Social Security and Medicare in the form of a self-employment tax.

SOCIAL SECURITY, MEDICARE, AND INCOME TAX WITHHOLDING

The Federal Insurance Contributions Act (FICA) provides for a federal system of old-age, survivors, disability, and hospital insurance. The tax rate is reviewed frequently and is subject to change by Congress. In 1998, the wage base for Social Security tax is $68,400 and the tax rate is 6.2% each for employers and employees. All wages (no ceiling) are subject to the Medicare tax at a rate of 1.45% each for both employees and employers.

QUARTERLY RETURNS

Each quarter of the year, all employers who are subject to income tax withholding (including withholding on sick pay and supplemental unemployment benefits) of Social Security and Medicare taxes must file an Employer's Quarterly Federal Tax Return on or before the last day of the first month after the end of the quarter (Fig. 24–13). Due dates for this return and full payment of the tax are April 30, July 31, October 31, and January 31. If deposits equaling full payment of taxes due have been made, the due date for the return is extended 10 days.

ANNUAL RETURNS

The employer is required to furnish two copies of Form W-2 Wage and Tax Statement to each employee from whom income tax or Social Security tax has been withheld or from whom income tax would have been withheld if the employee had claimed no more than one withholding allowance. The forms should be given to employees by January 31.

If employment ends before December 31, the employer may give the W-2 form to the terminated employee any time after employment ends. If the employee asks for Form W-2, the employer should give the employee the completed copies within 30 days of the request or the final wage payment, whichever is later.

Employers must file Form W-3, Transmittal of Income and Tax Statement, annually, to transmit wage and income tax withheld statements (Forms W-2) to the Social Security Administration. These forms are processed by the Social Security Administration, which then furnishes the IRS with the income tax data that it needs from those forms. Form W-3 and its attachments must be filed separately from Form 941 on or before the last day of February after the calendar year for which the W-2 forms are prepared.

HOW TO DEPOSIT

In general, the employer must deposit income tax withheld and both the employer and employee Social Security and Medicare taxes by mailing or delivering a check, money order, or cash to an authorized financial institution or Federal Reserve bank, using Form 8109, Federal Tax Deposit (FTD) Coupon. However, some taxpayers are required to deposit by electronic funds transfer. If the total deposits of Social Security, Medicare, railroad retirement, and withheld income taxes were more than $50,000 in 1996, then all depository tax liabilities that occur after 1997 must be made by electronic deposits. The Electronic Federal Tax Payment System (EFTPS) must be used to make electronic deposits. Failure to do so may result in being subject to a 10% penalty.

FEDERAL UNEMPLOYMENT TAX

Employers also contribute under the Federal Unemployment Tax Act (FUTA). Generally, credit can be taken against the FUTA tax for amounts paid into a state unemployment fund up to a certain percentage. Employers are responsible for paying the FUTA

Text continued on page 391

Personal Allowances Worksheet

A Enter "1" for **yourself** if no one else can claim you as a dependent . . . . A ______

B Enter "1" if: { • You are single and have only one job; or • You are married, have only one job, and your spouse does not work; or • Your wages from a second job or your spouse's wages (or the total of both) are $1,000 or less. } . . B ______

C Enter "1" for your **spouse.** But, you may choose to enter -0- if you are married and have either a working spouse or more than one job. (This may help you avoid having too little tax withheld.). . . . . C ______

D Enter number of **dependents** (other than your spouse or yourself) you will claim on your tax return . . . . D ______

E Enter "1" if you will file as **head of household** on your tax return (see conditions under **Head of household** above) . E ______

F Enter "1" if you have at least $1,500 of **child or dependent care expenses** for which you plan to claim a credit . . F ______

G **New—Child Tax Credit:** • If your total income will be between $16,500 and $47,000 ($21,000 and $60,000 if married), enter "1" for each eligible child. • If your total income will be between $47,000 and $80,000 ($60,000 and $115,000 if married), enter "1" if you have two or three eligible children, or enter "2" if you have four or more . . . . G ______

H Add lines A through G and enter total here. **Note:** This amount may be different from the number of exemptions you claim on your return. ▶ H ______

For accuracy, complete all worksheets that apply.
- If you plan to **itemize or claim adjustments to income** and want to reduce your withholding, see the Deductions and Adjustments Worksheet on page 2.
- If you are **single,** have **more than one job,** and your combined earnings from all jobs exceed $32,000 OR if you are **married** and have a **working spouse or more than one job,** and the combined earnings from all jobs exceed $55,000, see the Two-Earner/Two-Job Worksheet on page 2 to avoid having too little tax withheld.
- If **neither** of the above situations applies, **stop here** and enter the number from line H on line 5 of Form W-4 below.

Cut here and give the certificate to your employer. Keep the top part for your records.

Form **W-4** Department of the Treasury Internal Revenue Service

Employee's Withholding Allowance Certificate

▶ **For Privacy Act and Paperwork Reduction Act Notice, see page 2.**

OMB No. 1545-0010 **1998**

1 Type or print your first name and middle initial | Last name | 2 Your social security number

Home address (number and street or rural route) | 3 ☐ Single ☐ Married ☐ Married, but withhold at higher Single rate. **Note:** *If married, but legally separated, or spouse is a nonresident alien, check the Single box.*

City or town, state, and ZIP code | 4 If your last name differs from that on your social security card, check here and call 1-800-772-1213 for a new card . . . . . ▶ ☐

5 Total number of allowances you are claiming (from line H above or from the worksheets on page 2 if they apply) . | 5 |

6 Additional amount, if any, you want withheld from each paycheck . . . . | 6 | $

7 I claim exemption from withholding for 1998, and I certify that I meet **BOTH** of the following conditions for exemption:
- Last year I had a right to a refund of **ALL** Federal income tax withheld because I had **NO** tax liability **AND**
- This year I expect a refund of **ALL** Federal income tax withheld because I expect to have **NO** tax liability.

If you meet both conditions, enter "EXEMPT" here . . . . ▶ | 7 |

Under penalties of perjury, I certify that I am entitled to the number of withholding allowances claimed on this certificate or entitled to claim exempt status.

Employee's signature ▶ **Date ▶** , 19

8 Employer's name and address (Employer: Complete 8 and 10 only if sending to the IRS) | 9 Office code (optional) | 10 Employer identification number

Cat. No. 10220Q

FIGURE 24–11 Form W-4: Employee's Withholding Allowance Certificate.

Form W-4 (1998) Page 2

Deductions and Adjustments Worksheet

Note: *Use this worksheet only if you plan to itemize deductions or claim adjustments to income on your 1998 tax return.*

1 Enter an estimate of your 1998 itemized deductions. These include qualifying home mortgage interest, charitable contributions, state and local taxes (but not sales taxes), medical expenses in excess of 7.5% of your income, and miscellaneous deductions. (For 1998, you may have to reduce your itemized deductions if your income is over $124,500 ($62,250 if married filing separately). Get Pub. 919 for details.) . . . 1 $______

2 Enter: { $7,100 if married filing jointly or qualifying widow(er); $6,250 if head of household; $4,250 if single; $3,550 if married filing separately } . . . 2 $______

3 **Subtract** line 2 from line 1. If line 2 is greater than line 1, enter -0- . . . 3 $______

4 Enter an estimate of your 1998 adjustments to income, including alimony, deductible IRA contributions, and education loan interest . . . 4 $______

5 **Add** lines 3 and 4 and enter the total . . . 5 $______

6 Enter an estimate of your 1998 nonwage income (such as dividends or interest) . . . 6 $______

7 **Subtract** line 6 from line 5. Enter the result, but not less than -0- . . . 7 $______

8 **Divide** the amount on line 7 by $2,500 and enter the result here. Drop any fraction . . . 8 ______

9 Enter the number from Personal Allowances Worksheet, line H, on page 1 . . . 9 ______

10 **Add** lines 8 and 9 and enter the total here. If you plan to use the Two-Earner/Two-Job Worksheet, also enter this total on line 1 below. Otherwise, **stop here** and enter this total on Form W-4, line 5, on page 1 . . . 10 ______

Two-Earner/Two-Job Worksheet

Note: *Use this worksheet only if the instructions for line H on page 1 direct you here.*

1 Enter the number from line H on page 1 (or from line 10 above if you used the Deductions and Adjustments Worksheet) 1 ______

2 Find the number in **Table 1** below that applies to the **LOWEST** paying job and enter it here . . . 2 ______

3 If line 1 is **GREATER THAN OR EQUAL TO** line 2, subtract line 2 from line 1. Enter the result here (if zero, enter -0-) and on Form W-4, line 5, on page 1. **DO NOT** use the rest of this worksheet . . . 3 ______

Note: *If line 1 is **LESS THAN** line 2, enter -0- on Form W-4, line 5, on page 1. Complete lines 4–9 to calculate the additional withholding amount necessary to avoid a year end tax bill.*

4 Enter the number from line 2 of this worksheet . . . 4 ______

5 Enter the number from line 1 of this worksheet . . . 5 ______

6 **Subtract** line 5 from line 4 . . . 6 ______

7 Find the amount in **Table 2** below that applies to the **HIGHEST** paying job and enter it here . . . 7 $______

8 **Multiply** line 7 by line 6 and enter the result here. This is the additional annual withholding amount needed 8 $______

9 Divide line 8 by the number of pay periods remaining in 1998. (For example, divide by 26 if you are paid every other week and you complete this form in December 1997.) Enter the result here and on Form W-4, line 6, page 1. This is the additional amount to be withheld from each paycheck . . . 9 $______

Table 1: Two-Earner/Two-Job Worksheet

Married Filing Jointly				All Others			
If wages from **LOWEST** paying job are—	Enter on line 2 above	If wages from **LOWEST** paying job are—	Enter on line 2 above	If wages from **LOWEST** paying job are—	Enter on line 2 above	If wages from **LOWEST** paying job are—	Enter on line 2 above
0 - $4,000	0	38,001 - 43,000	8	0 - $5,000	0	70,001 - 85,000	8
4,001 - 7,000	1	43,001 - 54,000	9	5,001 - 11,000	1	85,001 - 100,000	9
7,001 - 12,000	2	54,001 - 62,000	10	11,001 - 16,000	2	100,001 and over	10
12,001 - 18,000	3	62,001 - 70,000	11	16,001 - 21,000	3		
18,001 - 24,000	4	70,001 - 85,000	12	21,001 - 25,000	4		
24,001 - 28,000	5	85,001 - 100,000	13	25,001 - 42,000	5		
28,001 - 33,000	6	100,001 - 110,000	14	42,001 - 55,000	6		
33,001 - 38,000	7	110,001 and over	15	55,001 - 70,000	7		

Table 2: Two-Earner/Two-Job Worksheet

Married Filing Jointly		All Others	
If wages from **HIGHEST** paying job are—	Enter on line 7 above	If wages from **HIGHEST** paying job are—	Enter on line 7 above
0 - $50,000	$400	0 - $30,000	$400
50,001 - 100,000	760	30,001 - 60,000	760
100,001 - 130,000	840	60,001 - 120,000	840
130,001 - 240,000	970	120,001 - 250,000	970
240,001 and over	1,070	250,001 and over	1,070

Privacy Act and Paperwork Reduction Act Notice. We ask for the information on this form to carry out the Internal Revenue laws of the United States. The Internal Revenue Code requires this information under sections 3402(f)(2)(A) and 6109 and their regulations. Failure to provide a completed form will result in your being treated as a single person who claims no withholding allowances. Routine uses of this information include giving it to the Department of Justice for civil and criminal litigation and to cities, states, and the District of Columbia for use in administering their tax laws.

You are not required to provide the information requested on a form that is subject to the Paperwork Reduction Act unless the form displays a valid OMB control number. Books or records relating to a form or its instructions must be retained as long as their contents may become material in the administration of any Internal Revenue law. Generally, tax returns and return information are confidential, as required by Code section 6103.

The time needed to complete this form will vary depending on individual circumstances. The estimated average time is: **Recordkeeping** 46 min., **Learning about the law or the form** 10 min., **Preparing the form** 1 hr., 10 min. If you have comments concerning the accuracy of these time estimates or suggestions for making this form simpler, we would be happy to hear from you. You can write to the Tax Forms Committee, Western Area Distribution Center, Rancho Cordova, CA 95743-0001. **DO NOT** send the tax form to this address. Instead, give it to your employer.

 ***Printed on recycled paper***

GPO: 1997-419-121

FIGURE 24–11 *continued*

SINGLE Persons—**MONTHLY** Payroll Period

(For Wages Paid in 1998)

If the wages are–		And the number of withholding allowances claimed is—										
At least	But less than	0	1	2	3	4	5	6	7	8	9	10
		The amount of income tax to be withheld is—										
$2,440	**$2,480**	364	302	268	235	201	167	133	100	66	32	0
2,480	**2,520**	375	312	274	241	207	173	139	106	72	38	4
2,520	**2,560**	387	324	280	247	213	179	145	112	78	44	10
2,560	**2,600**	398	335	286	253	219	185	151	118	84	50	16
2,600	**2,640**	409	346	292	259	225	191	157	124	90	56	22
2,640	**2,680**	420	357	298	265	231	197	163	130	96	62	28
2,680	**2,720**	431	368	305	271	237	203	169	136	102	68	34
2,720	**2,760**	443	380	317	277	243	209	175	142	108	74	40
2,760	**2,800**	454	391	328	283	249	215	181	148	114	80	46
2,800	**2,840**	465	402	339	289	255	221	187	154	120	86	52
2,840	**2,880**	476	413	350	295	261	227	193	160	126	92	58
2,880	**2,920**	487	424	361	301	267	233	199	166	132	98	64
2,920	**2,960**	499	436	373	310	273	239	205	172	138	104	70
2,960	**3,000**	510	447	384	321	279	245	211	178	144	110	76
3,000	**3,040**	521	458	395	332	285	251	217	184	150	116	82
3,040	**3,080**	532	469	406	343	291	257	223	190	156	122	88
3,080	**3,120**	543	480	417	354	297	263	229	196	162	128	94
3,120	**3,160**	555	492	429	366	303	269	235	202	168	134	100
3,160	**3,200**	566	503	440	377	314	275	241	208	174	140	106
3,200	**3,240**	577	514	451	388	325	281	247	214	180	146	112
3,240	**3,280**	588	525	462	399	336	287	253	220	186	152	118
3,280	**3,320**	599	536	473	410	347	293	259	226	192	158	124
3,320	**3,360**	611	548	485	422	359	299	265	232	198	164	130
3,360	**3,400**	622	559	496	433	370	307	271	238	204	170	136
3,400	**3,440**	633	570	507	444	381	318	277	244	210	176	142
3,440	**3,480**	644	581	518	455	392	329	283	250	216	182	148
3,480	**3,520**	655	592	529	466	403	340	289	256	222	188	154
3,520	**3,560**	667	604	541	478	415	352	295	262	228	194	160
3,560	**3,600**	678	615	552	489	426	363	301	268	234	200	166
3,600	**3,640**	689	626	563	500	437	374	311	274	240	206	172
3,640	**3,680**	700	637	574	511	448	385	322	280	246	212	178
3,680	**3,720**	711	648	585	522	459	396	333	286	252	218	184
3,720	**3,760**	723	660	597	534	471	408	345	292	258	224	190
3,760	**3,800**	734	671	608	545	482	419	356	298	264	230	196
3,800	**3,840**	745	682	619	556	493	430	367	304	270	236	202
3,840	**3,880**	756	693	630	567	504	441	378	315	276	242	208
3,880	**3,920**	767	704	641	578	515	452	389	326	282	248	214
3,920	**3,960**	779	716	653	590	527	464	401	338	288	254	220
3,960	**4,000**	790	727	664	601	538	475	412	349	294	260	226
4,000	**4,040**	801	738	675	612	549	486	423	360	300	266	232
4,040	**4,080**	812	749	686	623	560	497	434	371	308	272	238
4,080	**4,120**	823	760	697	634	571	508	445	382	319	278	244
4,120	**4,160**	835	772	709	646	583	520	457	394	331	284	250
4,160	**4,200**	846	783	720	657	594	531	468	405	342	290	256
4,200	**4,240**	857	794	731	668	605	542	479	416	353	296	262
4,240	**4,280**	868	805	742	679	616	553	490	427	364	302	268
4,280	**4,320**	879	816	753	690	627	564	501	438	375	312	274
4,320	**4,360**	891	828	765	702	639	576	513	450	387	324	280
4,360	**4,400**	902	839	776	713	650	587	524	461	398	335	286
4,400	**4,440**	913	850	787	724	661	598	535	472	409	346	292
4,440	**4,480**	924	861	798	735	672	609	546	483	420	357	298
4,480	**4,520**	935	872	809	746	683	620	557	494	431	368	305
4,520	**4,560**	947	884	821	758	695	632	569	506	443	380	317
4,560	**4,600**	958	895	832	769	706	643	580	517	454	391	328
4,600	**4,640**	969	906	843	780	717	654	591	528	465	402	339
4,640	**4,680**	980	917	854	791	728	665	602	539	476	413	350
4,680	**4,720**	991	928	865	802	739	676	613	550	487	424	361
4,720	**4,760**	1,003	940	877	814	751	688	625	562	499	436	373
4,760	**4,800**	1,014	951	888	825	762	699	636	573	510	447	384
4,800	**4,840**	1,026	962	899	836	773	710	647	584	521	458	395
4,840	**4,880**	1,038	973	910	847	784	721	658	595	532	469	406
4,880	**4,920**	1,051	984	921	858	795	732	669	606	543	480	417
4,920	**4,960**	1,063	996	933	870	807	744	681	618	555	492	429
4,960	**5,000**	1,076	1,007	944	881	818	755	692	629	566	503	440
5,000	**5,040**	1,088	1,018	955	892	829	766	703	640	577	514	451
$5,040 and over		Use Table 4(a) for a **SINGLE person** on page 34. Also see the instructions on page 32.										

FIGURE 24–12 Pages from 1998 Withholding Tax Table.

MARRIED Persons—**MONTHLY** Payroll Period

(For Wages Paid in 1998)

If the wages are–		And the number of withholding allowances claimed is—										
At least	But less than	0	1	2	3	4	5	6	7	8	9	10
		The amount of income tax to be withheld is—										
$0	$540	0	0	0	0	0	0	0	0	0	0	0
540	560	2	0	0	0	0	0	0	0	0	0	0
560	580	5	0	0	0	0	0	0	0	0	0	0
580	600	8	0	0	0	0	0	0	0	0	0	0
600	640	12	0	0	0	0	0	0	0	0	0	0
640	680	18	0	0	0	0	0	0	0	0	0	0
680	720	24	0	0	0	0	0	0	0	0	0	0
720	760	30	0	0	0	0	0	0	0	0	0	0
760	800	36	3	0	0	0	0	0	0	0	0	0
800	840	42	9	0	0	0	0	0	0	0	0	0
840	880	48	15	0	0	0	0	0	0	0	0	0
880	920	54	21	0	0	0	0	0	0	0	0	0
920	960	60	27	0	0	0	0	0	0	0	0	0
960	1,000	66	33	0	0	0	0	0	0	0	0	0
1,000	1,040	72	39	5	0	0	0	0	0	0	0	0
1,040	1,080	78	45	11	0	0	0	0	0	0	0	0
1,080	1,120	84	51	17	0	0	0	0	0	0	0	0
1,120	1,160	90	57	23	0	0	0	0	0	0	0	0
1,160	1,200	96	63	29	0	0	0	0	0	0	0	0
1,200	1,240	102	69	35	1	0	0	0	0	0	0	0
1,240	1,280	108	75	41	7	0	0	0	0	0	0	0
1,280	1,320	114	81	47	13	0	0	0	0	0	0	0
1,320	1,360	120	87	53	19	0	0	0	0	0	0	0
1,360	1,400	126	93	59	25	0	0	0	0	0	0	0
1,400	1,440	132	99	65	31	0	0	0	0	0	0	0
1,440	1,480	138	105	71	37	3	0	0	0	0	0	0
1,480	1,520	144	111	77	43	9	0	0	0	0	0	0
1,520	1,560	150	117	83	49	15	0	0	0	0	0	0
1,560	1,600	156	123	89	55	21	0	0	0	0	0	0
1,600	1,640	162	129	95	61	27	0	0	0	0	0	0
1,640	1,680	168	135	101	67	33	0	0	0	0	0	0
1,680	1,720	174	141	107	73	39	6	0	0	0	0	0
1,720	1,760	180	147	113	79	45	12	0	0	0	0	0
1,760	1,800	186	153	119	85	51	18	0	0	0	0	0
1,800	1,840	192	159	125	91	57	24	0	0	0	0	0
1,840	1,880	198	165	131	97	63	30	0	0	0	0	0
1,880	1,920	204	171	137	103	69	36	2	0	0	0	0
1,920	1,960	210	177	143	109	75	42	8	0	0	0	0
1,960	2,000	216	183	149	115	81	48	14	0	0	0	0
2,000	2,040	222	189	155	121	87	54	20	0	0	0	0
2,040	2,080	228	195	161	127	93	60	26	0	0	0	0
2,080	2,120	234	201	167	133	99	66	32	0	0	0	0
2,120	2,160	240	207	173	139	105	72	38	4	0	0	0
2,160	2,200	246	213	179	145	111	78	44	10	0	0	0
2,200	2,240	252	219	185	151	117	84	50	16	0	0	0
2,240	2,280	258	225	191	157	123	90	56	22	0	0	0
2,280	2,320	264	231	197	163	129	96	62	28	0	0	0
2,320	2,360	270	237	203	169	135	102	68	34	0	0	0
2,360	2,400	276	243	209	175	141	108	74	40	6	0	0
2,400	2,440	282	249	215	181	147	114	80	46	12	0	0
2,440	2,480	288	255	221	187	153	120	86	52	18	0	0
2,480	2,520	294	261	227	193	159	126	92	58	24	0	0
2,520	2,560	300	267	233	199	165	132	98	64	30	0	0
2,560	2,600	306	273	239	205	171	138	104	70	36	3	0
2,600	2,640	312	279	245	211	177	144	110	76	42	9	0
2,640	2,680	318	285	251	217	183	150	116	82	48	15	0
2,680	2,720	324	291	257	223	189	156	122	88	54	21	0
2,720	2,760	330	297	263	229	195	162	128	94	60	27	0
2,760	2,800	336	303	269	235	201	168	134	100	66	33	0
2,800	2,840	342	309	275	241	207	174	140	106	72	39	5
2,840	2,880	348	315	281	247	213	180	146	112	78	45	11
2,880	2,920	354	321	287	253	219	186	152	118	84	51	17
2,920	2,960	360	327	293	259	225	192	158	124	90	57	23
2,960	3,000	366	333	299	265	231	198	164	130	96	63	29
3,000	3,040	372	339	305	271	237	204	170	136	102	69	35
3,040	3,080	378	345	311	277	243	210	176	142	108	75	41
3,080	3,120	384	351	317	283	249	216	182	148	114	81	47
3,120	3,160	390	357	323	289	255	222	188	154	120	87	53
3,160	3,200	396	363	329	295	261	228	194	160	126	93	59
3,200	3,240	402	369	335	301	267	234	200	166	132	99	65

FIGURE 24–12 *continued*

Form **941** (Rev. January 1998) Department of the Treasury Internal Revenue Service (O)

Employer's Quarterly Federal Tax Return

▶ **See separate instructions for information on completing this return.**

Please type or print.

Enter state code for state in which deposits were made ONLY if different from state in address to the right ▶ (see page 3 of instructions).

Name (as distinguished from trade name) | Date quarter ended

Trade name, if any | Employer identification number

Address (number and street) | City, state, and ZIP code

OMB No. 1545-0029

T
FF
FD
FP
I
T

If address is different from prior return, check here ▶ ☐ IRS Use

1 1 1 1 1 1 1 1 1 1 2 3 3 3 3 3 3 3 3 4 4 4 5 5 5

6 7 8 8 8 8 8 8 8 8 9 9 9 9 9 10 10 10 10 10 10 10 10 10 10

If you do not have to file returns in the future, check here ▶ ☐ and enter date final wages paid ▶

If you are a seasonal employer, see **Seasonal employers** on page 1 of the instructions and check here ▶ ☐

1	Number of employees in the pay period that includes March 12th . ▶ 1	
2	Total wages and tips, plus other compensation . . .	2
3	Total income tax withheld from wages, tips, and sick pay . . .	3
4	Adjustment of withheld income tax for preceding quarters of calendar year . . .	4
5	Adjusted total of income tax withheld (line 3 as adjusted by line 4—see instructions) . . .	5
6	Taxable social security wages . . . 6a ____ × 12.4% (.124) =	6b
	Taxable social security tips . . . 6c ____ × 12.4% (.124) =	6d
7	Taxable Medicare wages and tips . . . 7a ____ × 2.9% (.029) =	7b
8	Total social security and Medicare taxes (add lines 6b, 6d, and 7b). Check here if wages are not subject to social security and/or Medicare tax . . . ▶ ☐	8
9	Adjustment of social security and Medicare taxes (see instructions for required explanation) Sick Pay $ ____ ± Fractions of Cents $ ____ ± Other $ ____ =	9
10	Adjusted total of social security and Medicare taxes (line 8 as adjusted by line 9—see instructions) . . .	10
11	**Total taxes** (add lines 5 and 10) . . .	11
12	Advance earned income credit (EIC) payments made to employees . . .	12
13	Net taxes (subtract line 12 from line 11). **This should equal line 17, column (d) below (or line D of Schedule B (Form 941))** . . .	13
14	Total deposits for quarter, including overpayment applied from a prior quarter . . .	14
15	**Balance due** (subtract line 14 from line 13). See instructions . . .	15

16 **Overpayment,** if line 14 is more than line 13, enter excess here ▶ $ ____
and check if to be: ☐ Applied to next return **OR** ☐ Refunded.

- **All filers:** If line 13 is less than $500, you need not complete line 17 or Schedule B (Form 941).
- **Semiweekly schedule depositors:** Complete Schedule B (Form 941) and check here . . . ▶ ☐
- **Monthly schedule depositors:** Complete line 17, columns (a) through (d), and check here . . . ▶ ☐

17 Monthly Summary of Federal Tax Liability. Do not complete if you were a semiweekly schedule depositor.

(a) First month liability	**(b)** Second month liability	**(c)** Third month liability	**(d)** Total liability for quarter

Sign Here Under penalties of perjury, I declare that I have examined this return, including accompanying schedules and statements, and to the best of my knowledge and belief, it is true, correct, and complete.

Signature ▶ **Print Your Name and Title ▶** **Date ▶**

For Privacy Act and Paperwork Reduction Act Notice, see page 4 of separate instructions. Cat. No. 17001Z Form **941** (Rev. 1-98)

FIGURE 24–13 Employer's Quarterly Federal Tax Return.

Form 941
Payment Voucher

Purpose of Form

Complete Form 941-V if you are making a payment with **Form 941,** Employer's Quarterly Federal Tax Return. We will use the completed voucher to credit your payment more promptly and accurately, and to improve our service to you.

If you have your return prepared by a third party and make a payment with that return, please provide this payment voucher to the return preparer.

Making Payments With Form 941

Make payments with Form 941 only if:

1. Your net taxes for the quarter (line 13 on Form 941) are less than $500 or

2. You are a monthly schedule depositor making a payment in accordance with the **accuracy of deposits** rule. (See section 11 of **Circular E,** Employer's Tax Guide, for details.) This amount may be $500 or more.

Otherwise, you must deposit the amount at an authorized financial institution or by electronic funds transfer. (See section 11 of Circular E for deposit instructions.) Do not use the Form 941-V payment voucher to make Federal tax deposits.

Caution: *If you pay amounts with Form 941 that should have been deposited, you may be subject to a penalty. See Circular E.*

*U.S. Government Printing Office: 1998 - 432-190/60347

Specific Instructions

Box 1—Amount paid. Enter the amount paid with Form 941.

Box 2. Enter the first four characters of your name as follows:

- **Individuals (sole proprietors, estates).** Use the first four letters of your last name (as shown in box 5).
- **Corporations.** Use the first four characters (letters or numbers) of your business name (as shown in box 5). Omit "The" if followed by more than one word.
- **Partnerships.** Use the first four characters of your trade name. If no trade name, enter the first four letters of the last name of the first listed partner.

Box 3—Employer identification number (EIN). If you do not have an EIN, apply for one on **Form SS-4,** Application for Employer Identification Number, and write "Applied for" and the date you applied in this entry space.

Box 4—Tax period. Darken the capsule identifying the quarter for which the payment is made. Darken only one capsule.

Box 5—Name and address. Enter your name and address as shown on Form 941.

- Make your check or money order payable to the Internal Revenue Service. Be sure to enter your EIN, "Form 941," and the tax period on your check or money order. Do not send cash. Please do not staple your payment to the voucher or the return.
- Detach the completed voucher and send it with your payment and Form 941 to the address provided in the separate **Instructions for Form 941.**

Printed on recycled paper

(Detach here)

Form 941-V
Department of the Treasury
Internal Revenue Service

Form 941 Payment Voucher

▶ Use this voucher when making a payment with your return.

OMB No. 1545-0029

1998

1 Enter the amount of the payment you are making ▶ $	2 Enter the first four letters of your last name (business name if corporation or partnership)	3 Enter your employer identification number

4 Tax period		5 Enter your business name (individual name if sole proprietor)
○ 1st Quarter	○ 3rd Quarter	Enter your address
○ 2nd Quarter	○ 4th Quarter	Enter your city, state, and ZIP code

For Privacy Act and Paperwork Reduction Act Notice, see Instructions for Form 941.

FIGURE 24–13 *continued*

Form **940** Department of the Treasury Internal Revenue Service (O)

Employer's Annual Federal Unemployment (FUTA) Tax Return

▶ For Paperwork Reduction Act Notice, see separate instructions.

OMB No. 1545-0028

1997

Name (as distinguished from trade name) Calendar year

Trade name, if any

Address and ZIP code Employer identification number

T	
FF	
FD	
FP	
I	
T	

A Are you required to pay unemployment contributions to only one state? (If "No," skip questions B and C.) . ☐ **Yes** ☐ **No**

B Did you pay all state unemployment contributions by February 2, 1998? ((1) If you deposited your total FUTA tax when due, check "Yes" if you paid all state unemployment contributions by February 10. (2) If a 0% experience rate is granted, check "Yes." (3) If "No," skip question C.) . . . . ☐ **Yes** ☐ **No**

C Were all wages that were taxable for FUTA tax also taxable for your state's unemployment tax? . . . . . ☐ **Yes** ☐ **No**

If you answered "No" to any of these questions, you must file Form 940. If you answered "Yes" to all the questions, you may file Form 940-EZ, which is a simplified version of Form 940. (Successor employers see **Special credit for successor employers** in the **Instructions for Form 940.**) You can get Form 940-EZ by calling 1-800-TAX-FORM (1-800-829-3676).

If you will not have to file returns in the future, check here, and complete and sign the return . . . . ▶ ☐
If this is an Amended Return, check here . . . . ▶ ☐

Part I **Computation of Taxable Wages**

		Amount paid		
1	Total payments (including payments shown on lines 2 and 3) during the calendar year for services of employees		1	
2	Exempt payments. (Explain all exempt payments, attaching additional sheets if necessary.) ▶	2		
3	Payments for services of more than $7,000. Enter only amounts over the first $7,000 paid to each employee. Do not include any exempt payments from line 2. The $7,000 amount is the Federal wage base. Your state wage base may be different. **Do not use your state wage limitation** .	3		
4	Total exempt payments (add lines 2 and 3)		4	
5	**Total taxable wages** (subtract line 4 from line 1) . . . . ▶		5	

Be sure to complete both sides of this return, and sign in the space provided on the back. Cat. No. 11234O Form **940** (1997)

DETACH HERE

Form **940-V** Department of the Treasury Internal Revenue Service

Form 940 Payment Voucher

Use this voucher only when making a payment with your return.

OMB No. 1545-0028

1997

Complete boxes 1, 2, 3, and 4. Do not send cash, and do not staple your payment to this voucher. Make your check or money order payable to the **Internal Revenue Service.** Be sure to enter your employer identification number, "Form 940," and "1997" on your payment.

1 Enter the amount of the payment you are making ▶ $	2 Enter the first four letters of your last name (business name if partnership or corporation)	3 Enter your employer identification number

Instructions for Box 2

—Individuals (sole proprietors, trusts, and estates)—Enter the first four letters of your last name.

—Corporations and partnerships—Enter the first four characters of your business name (omit "The" if followed by more than one word).

4 Enter your business name (individual name for sole proprietors)

Enter your address

Enter your city, state, and ZIP code

FIGURE 24–14 Employer's Annual Federal Unemployment Tax (FUTA) Return.

Form 940 (1997) Page **2**

Part II **Tax Due or Refund**

1	Gross FUTA tax. Multiply the wages in Part I, line 5, by .062	1	
2	Maximum credit. Multiply the wages in Part I, line 5, by .054 . . . | 2 |		
3	**Computation of tentative credit (Note:** *All taxpayers must complete the applicable columns.)*		

(a) Name of state	(b) State reporting number(s) as shown on employer's state contribution returns	(c) Taxable payroll (as defined in state act)	(d) State experience rate period From	(d) To	(e) State experience rate	(f) Contributions if rate had been 5.4% (col. (c) x .054)	(g) Contributions payable at experience rate (col. (c) x col. (e))	(h) Additional credit (col. (f) minus col.(g)). If 0 or less, enter -0-.	(i) Contributions actually paid to state
3a	Totals . . . ▶								

3b	**Total tentative credit** (add line 3a, columns (h) and (i) only—see instructions for limitations on late payments) ▶		
4			
5			
6	**Credit:** Enter the smaller of the amount in Part II, line 2 or line 3b	6	
7	**Total FUTA tax** (subtract line 6 from line 1)	7	
8	Total FUTA tax deposited for the year, including any overpayment applied from a prior year . .	8	
9	**Balance due** (subtract line 8 from line 7). This should be $100 or less. Pay to the Internal Revenue Service. See page 4 of the **Instructions for Form 940** for details . . . . ▶	9	
10	**Overpayment** (subtract line 7 from line 8). Check if it is to be: ☐ **Applied to next return** or ☐ **Refunded** . . . . ▶	10	

Part III **Record of Quarterly Federal Unemployment Tax Liability** *(Do not include state liability.)* Complete only if line 7 is over $100.

Quarter	First (Jan. 1–Mar. 31)	Second (Apr. 1–June 30)	Third (July 1–Sept. 30)	Fourth (Oct. 1–Dec. 31)	Total for year
Liability for quarter					

Under penalties of perjury, I declare that I have examined this return, including accompanying schedules and statements, and to the best of my knowledge and belief, it is true, correct, and complete, and that no part of any payment made to a state unemployment fund claimed as a credit was, or is to be, deducted from the payments to employees.

Signature ▶ **Title (Owner, etc.) ▶** **Date ▶**

FIGURE 24–14 *continued*

tax; it must not be deducted from employees' wages. For 1998 the FUTA tax was 6.2% of the first $7,000 in wages paid to each employee during the calendar year.

For deposit purposes, the FUTA tax is figured quarterly, and any amount due must be paid by the last day of the first month after the quarter ends. The formula for determining the amount due is set forth in the Federal Employer's Tax Guide.

An annual FUTA return must be filed on Form 940 on or before January 31 following the close of the calendar year for which the tax is due. Any tax still due is payable with the return. Form 940 may be filed on or before February 10 following the close of the year, if all required deposits were made on time and if full payment of the tax due is deposited on or before January 31 (Fig. 24–14).

Memory Jogger

11 *Who is responsible for the payment of FUTA tax?*

STATE UNEMPLOYMENT TAXES

All of the states and the District of Columbia have unemployment compensation laws. In most states, the tax is imposed only on the employer, but a few states require employers to withhold a percentage of wages for unemployment compensation benefits.

An employer may be subject to federal unemployment tax and not subject to state unemployment tax. In some states, for instance, the employer with fewer than four employees is not subject to the state unemployment tax. The regulations for a specific state should be checked.

STATE DISABILITY INSURANCE

Some states require that employees be covered by disability or sick-pay insurance. The employer may be required to withhold a certain amount from the employee's salary to pay for this insurance.

Special Duties

Before closing the chapter, we should mention certain events that do not occur with regularity but that may confront the office manager at some time.

MOVING A PRACTICE

The thought of moving into a shiny new spacious office can be exciting. However, unless the move is planned in advance, moving day and the weeks that follow can be a nightmare.

Planning the New Quarters

Do some careful measuring to see how the furniture and equipment you plan to move will fit into the new quarters. If possible, draw the rooms to scale and show where each item is to be placed by the mover. Include the location of available electrical outlets in your floor plan. If new furniture, carpets, or equipment is needed, try to have them in place before moving day. Don't expect to have the new carpet installed the day of your move.

Establishing a Moving Date

Decide what day you will move and whether you will close the office for 1 day or several. Select a mover and confirm the date. Patients must be notified of the move. As soon as the moving date is established, post a notice in the office and draw the patients' attention to it. You may want to send announcement cards to the active patients. Many physicians place a notice in the local newspapers.

Notifying Utilities and Mailers

At least 60 days in advance of the move, start a change-of-address notification campaign. Notify publishers of journals and suppliers of catalogs. (Cards for changes of address are available from the post office.) Six weeks' notice is generally required on all subscriptions, and postage due on forwarded journals can be very expensive. Notify the telephone company and utility companies well in advance so that there will no break in service. File a change of address card with the local post office. Order stationery and business cards with the new address.

Packing

The moving company will supply packing cartons for you to use. Have each employee be responsible for packing and labeling the items from his or her own work area. Tag each carton with a number and keep a master list of what is in each numbered carton. This will help you find items that you need. Also, if a carton should be lost or mislaid, you will have a record of what was in it. If time allows, just before moving is a good time to cull material from the files and discard old journals, supply catalogs, and any obsolete supplies or equipment.

Moving Day Strategy

Prepare a written outline of the moving day strategy, indicating each person's responsibility, and give each member of the office staff a copy. It may be wise to work in shifts to avoid confusion, but have one person stationed at the new address to direct the movers when they arrive.

Follow-Up

After the move, be sure to mention the new address when patients call for appointments. This is often neglected, especially after a few months have passed, and is very upsetting to the patient who tries to check in at the former address.

CLOSING A PRACTICE

A medical practice may be closed because of retirement, death, a change in geographic location, or a change in profession. If the closing is unexpected, as in the case of sudden death of the physician, much of the burden falls on the staff. If the closing is voluntary and planned for, the physician may wish to consult an attorney or the local medical society for guidelines. The following information is useful in either event.

Advance Notice to Patients

The physician who anticipates retirement can begin cutting back the practice months in advance. Patients can be notified as they come in that the practice will be closing on a specified date and asked to begin arrangements for care from another physician. The physician can also ask that patients pay at the time of service, to minimize accounts receivable at the time of retirement.

Avoiding Abandonment Charge

To avoid a charge of abandonment, the physician should notify active patients by letter that the practice is being discontinued. The letter should be sent out at least 3 months in advance, if possible. If a patient has been discharged or has not been given care by the physician for at least 6 years, there is no obligation to send the notice.

Public Announcement

About 1 month after the physician begins telling patients of the closing, an announcement should be placed in a local newspaper, giving the closing date of the office, explaining any arrangements made for continuing care and thanking patients for their support in prior years.

Other Notices

Hospital affiliations should be informed early, particularly if the physician will be leaving the community. If the office space is being rented, be sure to notify the landlord in observance of the rental contract if there is one. Insurance carriers must be advised of the change. The state medical licensure board should be contacted. If the practice is incorporated, an attorney should be consulted about disincorporation.

Patient Transfer and Patient Records

If another physician is taking over the practice, tell the patient about the new physician. However, be sure to explain that the patient's records will be transferred to any physician the patient chooses and that the request for transfer of records must be in writing. For convenience, the physician can have a form available that needs only the patient's signature.

Although the records belong to the physician, they can legally be transferred to another physician only with the consent of the patient. Any records not transferred should be stored, either in bulk or on microfilm or disk, until the statutes of limitations for malpractice and abandonment have run out.

Memory Jogger

12 *What action is required before transferring a patient's records to another physician?*

Financial Concerns

Income tax returns and supporting documents should be kept for at least 3 years after the tax return was filed. Appoint someone to take care of any remaining outstanding accounts receivable.

Disposition of Controlled Substances

Check with the Drug Enforcement Administration (DEA) for current regulations on disposal of controlled substances and the physician's certificate of registration. Do not simply toss them out. The certificate will have to be sent to the DEA for cancellation, and then it will be returned. It may be necessary to produce an inventory of all controlled substances on hand when the practice is terminated, along with duplicate copies of the official order forms that were used to obtain them. Return any unused forms to the DEA. Do not use leftover prescription blanks for note pads. Burn or shred them to avoid misuse.

Professional Liability Insurance

The physician who is discontinuing active medical practice can safely drop the professional liability insurance. However, do not destroy any of the previous policies. Most professional liability claims are covered by the policy that was in effect at the time the alleged act of negligence took place. The suit may be filed many years later, and it is important that the old policy be available.

Furnishings and Equipment

Unfortunately, used office furniture and equipment do not bring much in the marketplace. If another physician is taking over the practice, the value of the furnishings and equipment can be negotiated. Many physicians donate their libraries to the local hospital and declare the gift as a deduction from their income tax. This is an item to check with the accountant.

A physician may reward loyal employees with severance pay. On average, this equals at least 1 month's salary plus prorated compensation for any unused vacation time. A letter of reference is usually offered.

There are many details to take care of in closing a medical practice. Contact the local medical society for further guidance.

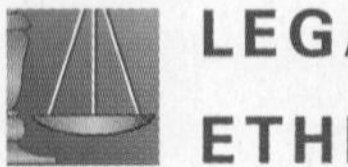

LEGAL AND ETHICAL ISSUES

The areas of authority and responsibility must be clearly defined to avoid management problems. Authority and responsibility are defined in the policy and procedures manual. This information must be available to every employee and updated on a regular basis.

The person in charge of hiring must be familiar with the Civil Rights Act of 1964, as amended by the Equal Opportunity Act of 1972 (available from EEOC, 2401 E Street, N.W., Washington, DC 20507).

A long-term employee whose performance declines should be counseled and given a chance to improve to attain specific practice goals.

CRITICAL THINKING

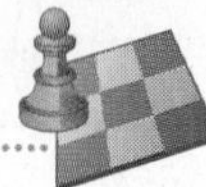

1 Practice your interviewing skills with another student, exchanging roles of interviewer and applicant.

2 Prepare a procedure sheet for a position that you would expect to seek.

3 Discuss with a colleague the ways in which a medical assistant could affect the success of the practice.

HOW DID I DO? Answers to Memory Joggers

1. The purpose of medical office management is to provide appropriate environment, safely store health information, and bill and collect for services.
2. The policy manual tells "what to do"; the procedures manual describes "how to do it."
3. Job descriptions and procedure sheets
4. Race, sex, religion, national origin
5. A warning and a full explanation of specific improvement expected
6. There should be an agenda for the staff meeting to prevent it from becoming a forum for individual complaints, which should be handled privately
7. The most important rule of marketing a medical practice is to "treat the patients well."
8. The patient information folder explains the philosophy and policies of practice and reduces misunderstanding and forgotten instructions.
9. At least 4 years
10. Total earnings, number of withholding allowances claimed, marital status, and length of pay period
11. Only the employer is responsible—not deducted from wages
12. Consent of the patient

REFERENCES

American Medical Association: Personnel Management in the Medical Practice. Norcross, GA, Coker Publishing, 1996.

U.S. Department of the Treasury, Internal Revenue Service: Circular E, 1998.

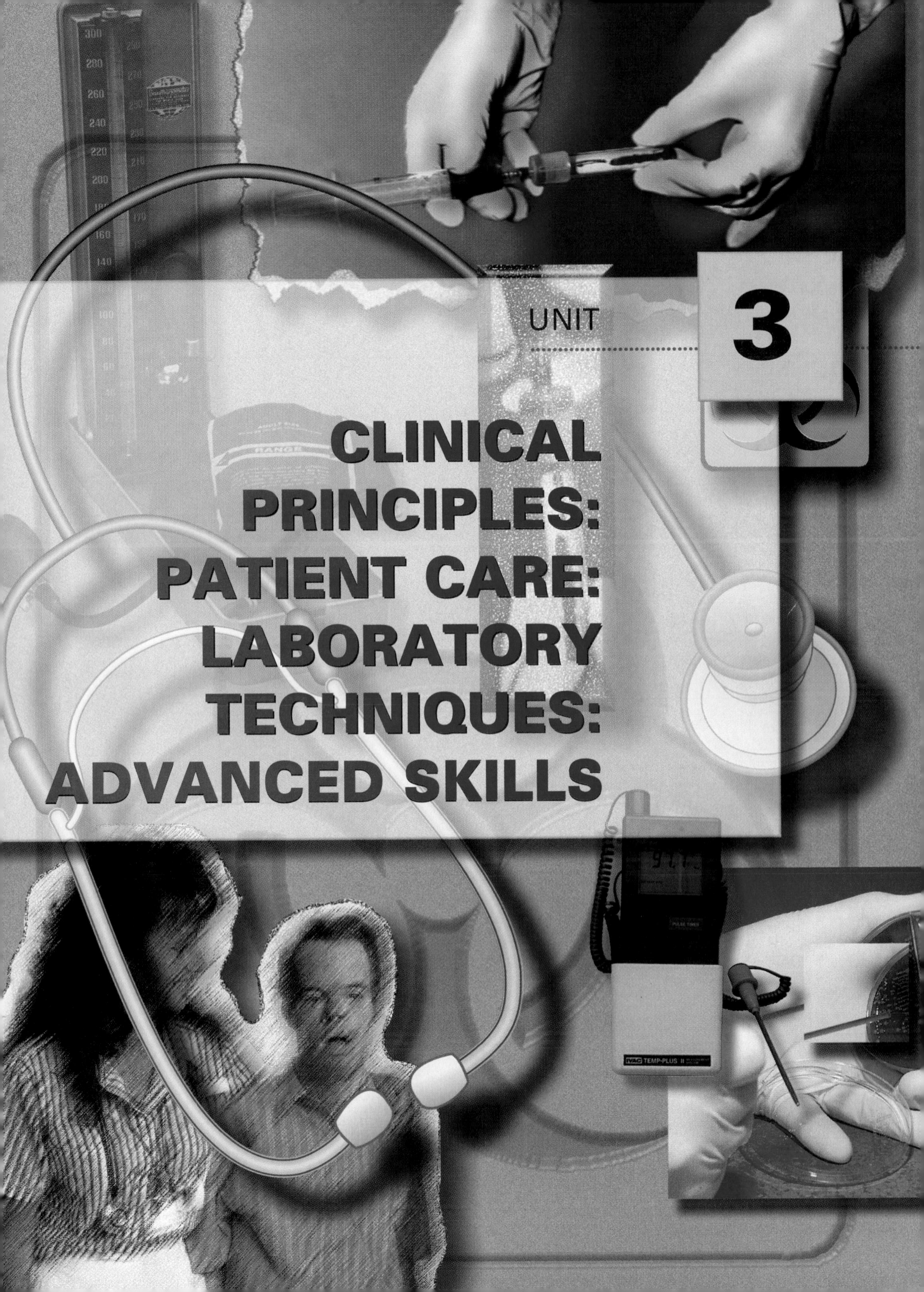
UNIT
3
CLINICAL
PRINCIPLES:
PATIENT CARE:
LABORATORY
TECHNIQUES:
ADVANCED SKILLS
TEMP-PLUS II

SECTION 7

Fundamental Principles of Patient Care

CURRICULUM CONTENT/COMPETENCIES

Chapter 25: Patient Assessment
- *Project a professional manner and image*
- *Adhere to ethical principles*
- *Manage time effectively*
- *Treat all patients with compassion and empathy*
- *Adapt communications to individual's ability to understand*

Chapter 26: Aseptic Concepts and Infection Control
- *Apply principles of aseptic technique and infection control*
- *Comply with quality assurance practices*
- *Follow federal, state, and local legal guidelines*
- *Comply with established risk management and safety procedures*
- *Evaluate and recommend equipment and supplies*

Chapter 27: Vital Signs and Anthropometric Measurement
- *Apply principles of aseptic technique and infection control*
- *Perform diagnostic tests*
- *Obtain patient history and vital signs*
- *Prepare and maintain examination and treatment areas*
- *Maintain confidentiality*
- *Document accurately*
- *Teach methods of health promotion and disease prevention.*

Patient Assessment

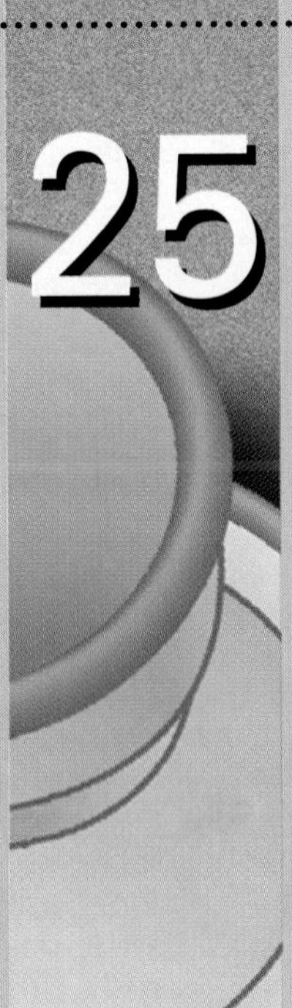

OUTLINE

LEARNING OBJECTIVES

Cognitive: On successful completion of this chapter you should be able to:

1. Define and spell the terms listed in the Vocabulary.
2. State the purpose of the medical history and how personal anxieties can affect the process.
3. List the three types of body language that can indicate your interest in the patient.
4. List the components of the medical history and explain the importance of each one.
5. Identify and explain the internal factors of communicating.
6. List and give an example of the external factors of communicating.
7. State when you should use open-ended questions.
8. Describe the purpose and usage of direct questions.
9. State the meaning of *interviewing restraints.*
10. Describe the medical assistant's role during the *system review.*
11. Differentiate between a sign and a symptom.
12. List the three medical record systems used in physicians' offices.

Performance: On successful completion of this chapter you should be able to:

1. Distinguish between verbal and nonverbal communication.
2. Provide examples of interviewing restraints.
3. Discuss the terminology used in the assessment process.
4. State your legal responsibilities in handling the patient's medical record.

VOCABULARY

biophysical Pertaining to the science dealing with the application of physical methods and theories to biologic problems

chief complaint Reason for patient seeking medical care

cognitive Pertaining to the operation of the mind process by which we become aware of perceiving, thinking, and remembering

diagnosis Concise technical description of the cause, nature, or manifestations of a condition or problem. *Initial:* Physician's temporary impression, sometimes called a *working diagnosis. Final:* Conclusion physician reaches after evaluating all findings, including laboratory and other testing results

familial Occurring in or affecting members of a family more than would be expected by chance

hereditary Transmitted from parent to offspring; genetically determined

present illness Amplification of the chief complaint, usually written in chronologic sequence with dates of onset

psychosocial Pertaining to or involving both psychic (behavior) and communal activity

rapport Relationship of harmony and accord between patient and physician

Assessment is the collection of data about an individual's health state. Not just physical data but **cognitive, psychosocial,** and behavioral data are significant for the analysis of a patient's health state. Assessment factors are a list of **biophysical** signs and symptoms. The patient is certified as healthy when these signs and symptoms of illness have been eliminated. When disease exists, medical **diagnosis** is worded to identify and explain the cause of disease.

This usually begins with the physician's working diagnosis, which he or she has determined through the patient's history and examination. Now the physician will order laboratory tests, possibly medications, and/or a referral visit to another physician to substantiate or refute the working diagnosis. Once all the facts are in, the clinical diagnosis is established. The patient is then treated and after a period of time will be reevaluated to see if the clinical diagnosis has changed. If it has, the new diagnosis is called the differentiated diagnosis.

Memory Jogger

 *What are the assessment factors?*

Patient care does not start with the physical examination; it begins when the patient makes first contact with the office. Even before the examination, you have the opportunity to interact with and react to the patient to ensure that he or she feels comfortable during the process and that all the necessary information is obtained.

Interviewing patients, assisting with examinations, and charting findings are important responsibilities for every medical assistant in every physician's practice. You must know the components and techniques for securing a medical history that will help the physician in the diagnosis and treatment of the patient. The more complete the medical history, the more efficient the physician's care and treatment will be.

Medical History

More than ever, medicine emphasizes the importance of communicating with the patient and providing a warm and caring environment. Positive reactions and interactions with the patient are essential to providing good patient care. As the patient progresses through the various stages of health care, all members of the medical team must exercise a variety of special skills to enhance the process. These skills are not all technical and medical; many involve the art of caring for the patient as a human being. Because medical care is of an extremely personal nature, the medical assistant must always remember that each patient is an individual with certain anxieties. These anxieties often cause people to act and react in different ways, and effective verbal and nonverbal communication with each patient is essential.

You can do much to put a patient at ease through the tone of your voice. Facial expression and the ease and confidence of your movements demonstrate to the patient a sincere interest. Give the patient your undivided attention, and let your body language inform each patient that you are interested in his or her medical problems (Fig. 25–1).

Memory Jogger

 *How can you put a patient at ease?*

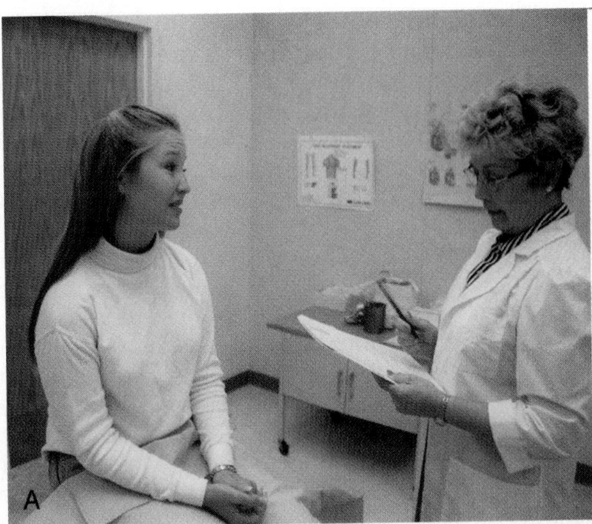

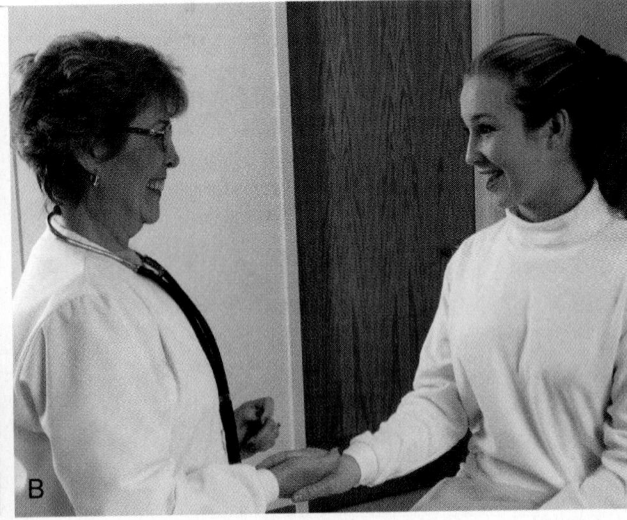

FIGURE 25–1 Right and wrong body language.

The patient is not concerned with the problems of the office staff, nor are you there to impress the patient with your medical knowledge. You are there for one purpose, to give each patient the best possible care.

COLLECTING THE HISTORY INFORMATION

When a new patient calls or comes in for an appointment, some medical offices ask him or her to complete a special self-history form. Besides being useful for diagnosing and treating the patient, the self-history allows the patient more participation in the process. The form may be mailed to the patient's home a week before the appointment or may be completed in the office during the first visit.

If you are responsible for taking a portion of the medical history, do it in an area free from outside interference and beyond the hearing range of other patients. Patients will not talk freely where they may be overheard or interrupted. The room should be physically comfortable and conducive to confidential communications. Legally and ethically, the patient has the right to privacy, and the access to the patient's medical record is only allowed to those individuals directly involved in this patient's care. Listen to the patient. Do not express surprise or displeasure at any of the patient's statements. Remember, you are there not to pass judgment but to gather medical data. Your responses should show interest and concern and should not be judgmental. Report the information gained to the physician in an organized manner, exactly as given by the patient, without opinion or interpretation.

In some medical offices, the physician takes the medical history, during the patient's initial interview. The physician will correlate the physical findings with the information in the history. The complete medical history and the physical examination form the foundation and starting point for all medical patient–physician contracts.

COMPONENTS OF THE MEDICAL HISTORY

Medical history forms may vary from office to office depending on the physician's preference and the practice speciality. The most utilized medical history method includes these components:

- *Database*—Record of the patient's name, address, date of birth, insurance information, personal data, history, physical examination, and initial laboratory findings. As new information is added, it becomes a part of this database. Check the name on the record and be certain that the information you are charting is recorded on the correct form on the correct patient's chart.
- *Past history (PH) or past medical history (PMH)*—Summary of the patient's previous health. It covers the dates and questions regarding the patient's usual childhood diseases (UCD or UCHD), major illnesses and surgeries, allergies, accidents, and immunization.
- *Family history (FH)*—Details regarding the patient's mother and father, their health, and, if deceased, the cause and age of death. **Hereditary** and/or **familial** diseases and disorders are recorded here and may include information about siblings and offspring. This information is important because certain diseases and disorders have familial and/or hereditary tendencies.
- *Social history (SH)*—Information regarding the patient's lifestyle, hobbies, entertainment preferences, education, occupation, use of tobacco and alcohol, sleeping habits, methods of exercise,

and sex life are noted in this section. This information assists the physician in planning treatment for the patient.

- *Systems review (SR) or review of systems (ROS)*—Guide to general health; tends to detect conditions other than those covered in the present illness. Often a patient may think certain health problems irrelevant and fail to mention them. These problems may help the physician in determining the cause of the disorder being presently explored. A system review is obtained by a logical sequence of questions, beginning with the head and proceeding downward.

Memory Jogger

What are the most utilized medical history components?

Interviewing Strategies

The interview is the first and the most important part of data collection. The medical history is important in beginning to identify the patient's health strengths and problems and as a bridge to the next step in data collection, the physical examination. At this point the individual knows everything about his or her own health state and you know nothing. Your skill in interviewing will glean all the necessary information as well as build **rapport** for a successful working relationship.

Consider the interview similar to forming a *contract* between you and your patient. A contract consists of spoken and unspoken language and concerns what the patient needs and expects from health care.

Memory Jogger

Name the most important part of data collection.

THE PROCESS OF COMMUNICATION

Communication is the vehicle that carries you and your patient through the interview. Communication is simply the exchanging of information so that each person clearly understands the other. Understanding is the difficult part. If you do not understand each other, you have not conveyed meaning; thus, there is no communication. Most of us believe that because we can talk and hear, we can communicate, but there is much more involved than just talking and hearing. Communication is all behavior, conscious and unconscious, verbal and nonverbal. *All behavior has meaning.*

Verbal communication consists of the words you speak, the tone of your voice, even the manner in which you speak. Nonverbal communication occurs through posture, gestures, facial expression, eye contact, touch, even where you place your chair. Because nonverbal communication is under less conscious control than verbal, it is probably more reflective of your true feelings.

You must be aware that the messages you send are only part of the process. Your words and gestures are merely symbols. They must be interpreted by the receiver (patient) to have meaning. You have a specific context in mind when you send your words, but the receiver puts his or her own interpretation on them. The receiver attaches meaning determined by his or her past experiences, culture, and self-concept, as well as current physical and emotional state. Sometimes these messages and interpretations do not coincide. It takes mutual understanding by both the interviewer and the person being interviewed to have successful communication. To maximize your communicating skill, first you need to be aware of internal and external factors and how they influence the interviewing process.

Memory Jogger

List five methods of nonverbal communication.

INTERNAL FACTORS

Internal factors are the feelings, interpretations, past experiences, culture, and your emotional state that you carry inside you and are what you bring to the interview. As a medical assistant you need to cultivate the three inner factors of liking others, empathy, and the ability to listen.

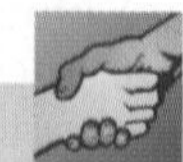

PERSONAL QUALITIES

DEFINING INNER FACTORS OF COMMUNICATION

- *Liking others* means a generally optimistic view of people. It is creating an atmosphere of warmth and caring so that the patient feels that he or she is accepted unconditionally.
- *Empathy* means recognizing and accepting the other person's feelings without criticism. It does not mean you become lost in the other person at the expense of your own self.
- *The ability to listen* requires your complete attention. To have empathy you need to listen. Listening is not a passive role in the communication process; it is active and demanding. You cannot be preoccupied with your own

TABLE 25-1 Types of Nonverbal Communication Observations

Area Observed	Hearing	Seeing	Perception
Breathing patterns	Prolonged respirations, sighing	Shallow thoracic breathing	Abdominal breathing
Eye movement		Side-to-side, down at hands	No eye contact
Hand movement	Tapping fingers, cracking of knuckles	Continuous movement	Wet/sweaty palms
Arm placement		Folded across the chest	Appears withdrawn
Leg placement	Tapping	Continuous movement	Tense, not relaxed

needs or the needs of others or you will miss something important. For the time of this interview, no one is more important than this patient. Listen to the way things are said, the tone of the patient's voice, and even to what the patient is not saying out loud.

Memory Jogger

6 *Identify three inner factors you must cultivate.*

Listening is probably the most effective communication technique available. It requires the medical assistant's complete attention and a great deal of energy. The nonverbal message the patient receives by the medical assistant's listening behavior is "You are a person of worth and I am interested in you as a unique person."

While listening to the patient try to attempt to determine what the patient's words mean to that individual. Many words in English have multiple meanings. For example: Consider the word "love" in the following three sentences. I love him very much. I love little dogs. I just love your new haircut. Does the word have the same meaning in all three sentences? Through careful listening, you should be able to understand the patient's message.

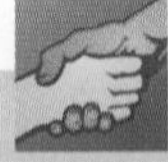

PERSONAL QUALITIES

RULES THAT WILL HELP YOU IN LEARNING TO LISTEN

- Relax while listening.
- Be patient and nonjudgmental.
- Don't interrupt.
- Never intimidate your patient.

OBSERVATION

The purpose of observing nonverbal communication is to become sensitive to, or aware of, the feelings of others as conveyed by small bits of behavior, rather than words. This sensitivity enables you to adapt your behavior to these feelings, to consciously select your response, either verbal or nonverbal, and thereby have a favorable effect on others. The favorable effect may consist of providing emotional support, conveying that you care, defusing the other's fear or anger, or providing an invitation to release pent-up feelings by talking about the situation that aroused the feelings. A message of need is most likely sent nonverbally (Table 25-1).

EXTERNAL FACTORS

Before you meet with the patient, prepare the physical setting. The setting may be an examination room, the staff lounge, or an office. In any location, optimal conditions are important to have a smooth, productive interview (Figure 25-2).

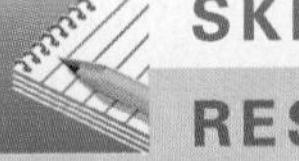

SKILLS AND RESPONSIBILITIES

PREPARING THE APPROPRIATE ENVIRONMENT

- *Ensure privacy.* Make sure the room you are using is unoccupied for the entire time allowed for the interview. The patient needs to

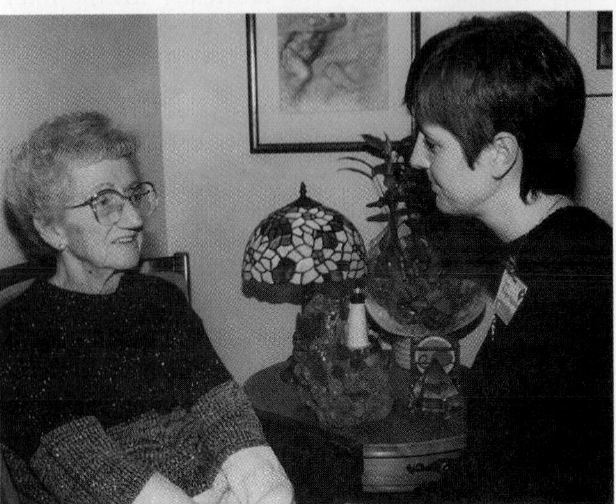

FIGURE 25-2 Comfortable interview area.

feel sure that no one can overhear the conversation or interrupt.

- *Refuse interruptions.* Inform your coworkers of the interview and ask them not to interrupt you during this time. You need to concentrate and to establish rapport. An interruption can destroy in seconds what you have spent many minutes building up.
- *Prepare comfortable surroundings.* This reduces patient anxiety. Keep the interviewing room at a comfortable temperature, and avoid facing the patient directly when there is a lighted window behind you. Keep the distance between you and the patient at 4 to 5 feet. Arrange chairs so both you and the patient are comfortably seated at eye level and the desk or table does not look like a barrier between you.
- *Take judicious notes.* Note taking should be kept to a minimum while you try to focus your attention on the person. Note taking during the interview has disadvantages such as breaking eye contact and shifting your attention away from the patient, which diminishes the patient's sense of importance. It is important to always write down pertinent details as you are interviewing because you may forget important facts if you do not note them at the time of the discussion. With experience, you will develop a personal type of shorthand that you will use during the interview process. In the beginning, your notes will be more involved.

Interviewing the Patient

INTRODUCTIONS

The patient is here and you are ready for the interview. If you are nervous about how to begin, remember to keep it short. The patient is probably nervous, too, and is anxious to get started. Address the patient, using his or her surname, and introduce yourself. If you are gathering a complete history, give the reason for the interview:

> Mr. Coleman, welcome to Dr Yang's family of patients. For us to become aware of your needs and concerns, I would like to take this time to talk to you. Would you mind sharing this information with me?

After this brief introduction, ask an open-ended question (see later) and then let the patient proceed with the conversation. You do not need friendly small talk to build rapport. This is not a social visit. You will build rapport best by letting the patient discuss his or her concerns early.

OPEN-ENDED QUESTIONS

An open-ended question asks for general information. It states the topic to be discussed but only in general terms. Use it to begin the interview, to introduce a new section of questions, and whenever the person introduces a new topic.

> What brings you to the doctor?
> Give me the reason you have come to see the doctor today.
> How have you been getting along?
> You mentioned having dizzy spells. Tell me more about that.

This type of question encourages the patient to respond in a manner that is comfortable for him or her. It allows the patient to express himself or herself fully.

DIRECT QUESTIONS

Direct questions ask for specific information. This form of questioning limits the answer to one or two words, a yes or no in many cases. Use this form of question when you need specific facts, such as when asking about past health problems (e.g., Have you ever broken a bone?) (Table 25–2).

Memory Jogger

What type of questions encourage the patient to talk?

TABLE 25–2 Therapeutic Communication Techniques

Technique	Value
Open-ended questions	Encourages patient to respond in a comfortable manner
Direct questions	Ask for specific information. Usually reply is a yes or no answer
Listening	Nonverbally communicates your interest in the patient
Silence	Nonverbally communicates your acceptance of the patient
Establishing guidelines	Helps the patient to know what is expected
Acknowledgment	Shows the importance of the patient's role
Restating	Checks your interpretation of the patient's message for validation
Reflecting	Shows the patient the importance of his or her feelings
Summarizing	Helps patient to separate relevant from irrelevant material

Interviewing Restraints

The verbal skills discussed to this point have all been positive and designed to enhance the interview. Now, let's consider nonproductive, defeating verbal messages that may be misleading or restrict the patient's response. This type of question can be an obstacle to obtaining complete data and to establishing rapport.

PROVIDING UNWARRANTED ASSURANCE

Mrs. Miller says to you "I know this lump is going to turn out to be cancer." The reply is almost automatic. "Don't worry, I'm sure everything will be all right." This type of answer makes her anxiety insignificant and denies her any further talk about it. Instead you could have said "You are really worried about the lump, aren't you?" This response acknowledges the feeling and opens the door to further communication.

GIVING ADVICE

Mrs. Thompson has just finished talking to the doctor and she looks at you and says, "Dr. Rowe says I must have surgery to get rid of these gallstones. I just don't know. What would you do?" If you give her an answer, you have shifted the accountability for decision making from her to you and she has not worked out her own solution. Does this woman really want to know what you would do? Probably not. Although it is quicker to give advice, medical assistants should never give advice. You may want to respond to her question with "Would you like to discuss these concerns with the doctor?"

USING PROFESSIONAL TERMS

You must adjust your vocabulary to the patient. The more the patient understands about what is happening and what the management of the problem will be, the better the outcome will be. Misinterpreted communication is the most frequent error encountered in patient care.

LEADING QUESTIONS

During the interview, you ask the patient, "You don't smoke, do you?" The patient knows that you want a yes answer and if he or she wants to please you the answer must be affirmative. To tell you that he or she does smoke would surely meet with your disapproval. Keep your questions positive. A better way of asking would be to say. "Have you ever smoked?" or "Do you use tobacco?"

TALKING TOO MUCH

Some medical assistants associate helpfulness with verbal overload. The patient lets the interviewer talk at the expense of his or her own need to express himself or herself. For example, the patient is telling you about having a problem of voiding whenever she coughs or sneezes and she tells you how embarrassing this is. You want to put her at ease so you answer, "I know just what your talking about, last week I was at a party and I had had a glass of wine, which of course made the situation worse, well, I started to cough and you can guess what happened, well, there I stood and. . . ." This type of conversation only delays the completion of your assigned task and can cause the time that the physician has with the patient to be reduced. Always remember, when interviewing a patient listen more than you talk.

Memory Jogger

 *Identify five obstacles to obtaining complete data.*

The time that we can spend with the patient has changed, and in many offices there is no longer time set aside for the interview process. If you are employed in one of the fast-paced offices, the health history forms are mailed to the new patient and before the patient arrives the forms have been returned and you have flagged any areas that might constitute a health problem. This means that the time you will have with the patient will be limited and you may find that most of your communication is done during the obtaining of the vital signs and while preparing the patient for the examination. If this happens, pick your questions carefully and let the patient do the talking (Fig. 25–3, p. 405).

Assessing the Patient

After the completion of the interview, the patient is escorted to an examination room and prepared for the physical examination, which is done by the physician. During this examination, the physician will methodically check all the body systems. As this examination is done, the physician is mentally comparing the patient's system with the established norms for that system. When something deviates from the accepted normal range, it is documented in the patient's chart. Table 25–3 (p. 406) lists the systems of the body and the signs and symptoms that would be evaluated for each system. The usual examination begins with the top of the head and progresses to the feet. Depending on the speciality of the physician, the order may vary.

PROCEDURE 25-1

Obtaining a Medical History

This procedure is to be done on another student. To make the experience more realistic, choose a student whom you know very little about.

GOAL

To obtain an acceptable written background from the patient to help the physician determine the cause and effects of the present illness. This includes the chief complaint, present illness, past history, family history, and social history.

SUPPLIES AND EQUIPMENT

A history form
Two pens, with red and black ink
A quiet, private area

PROCEDURAL STEPS

1 Greet and identify the patient in a pleasant manner. Introduce yourself and explain your role.
PURPOSE: To make the patient feel at ease.

2 Find a quiet, private area for the interview, and explain to the patient the need for the requested information.
PURPOSE: An informed patient is more cooperative and, thus, more likely to contribute useful information.

3 Complete the history form by asking appropriate questions. A self-history may have been mailed to the patient before the visit. If so, review the self-history for completeness.
PURPOSE: The self-history is designed to save time and to involve the patient in the process.

4 Speak in a pleasant, distinct manner, remembering to keep eye contact with your patient.
PURPOSE: Positive nonverbal behavior creates a friendly atmosphere.

5 Record the following statistical information on the patient information form:

Patient's full name, including middle initial
Address, including apartment number and ZIP code
Marital status
Sex (gender)
Age and date of birth
Telephone number
Employer's name, address, telephone number

6 Record the following medical history on the patient history form:

Chief complaint
Present illness
Past history
Family history
Social history

PURPOSE: This is information that the physician needs to know to make an accurate assessment and diagnosis. The physician usually completes the review of systems during the preexamination interview.

7 Ask about allergies to drugs and any other substances, and record any allergies in red ink on every page of the history form.
PURPOSE: The presence of an allergy may alter medication and treatment procedures.

8 Record all information legibly and neatly, and spell words correctly. Print rather than write in longhand. Do not erase; if you make an error, draw a single line through the error and initial the correction.
PURPOSE: To maintain a medical record that is understandable and defensible in a court of law.

9 Check for accuracy by repeating back to the patient the spelling of the name and the address, ZIP code, and phone number.

Continued

10 Thank the patient for cooperating, and direct him or her back to the reception area.

11 Review the record for errors before you hand it to the physician.

12 Use the information on the record to complete the patient's chart as directed by the physician. Keep the information confidential.
PURPOSE: All facts and information concerning the patient must remain in the office. This information may be legally and ethically discussed with only the physician.

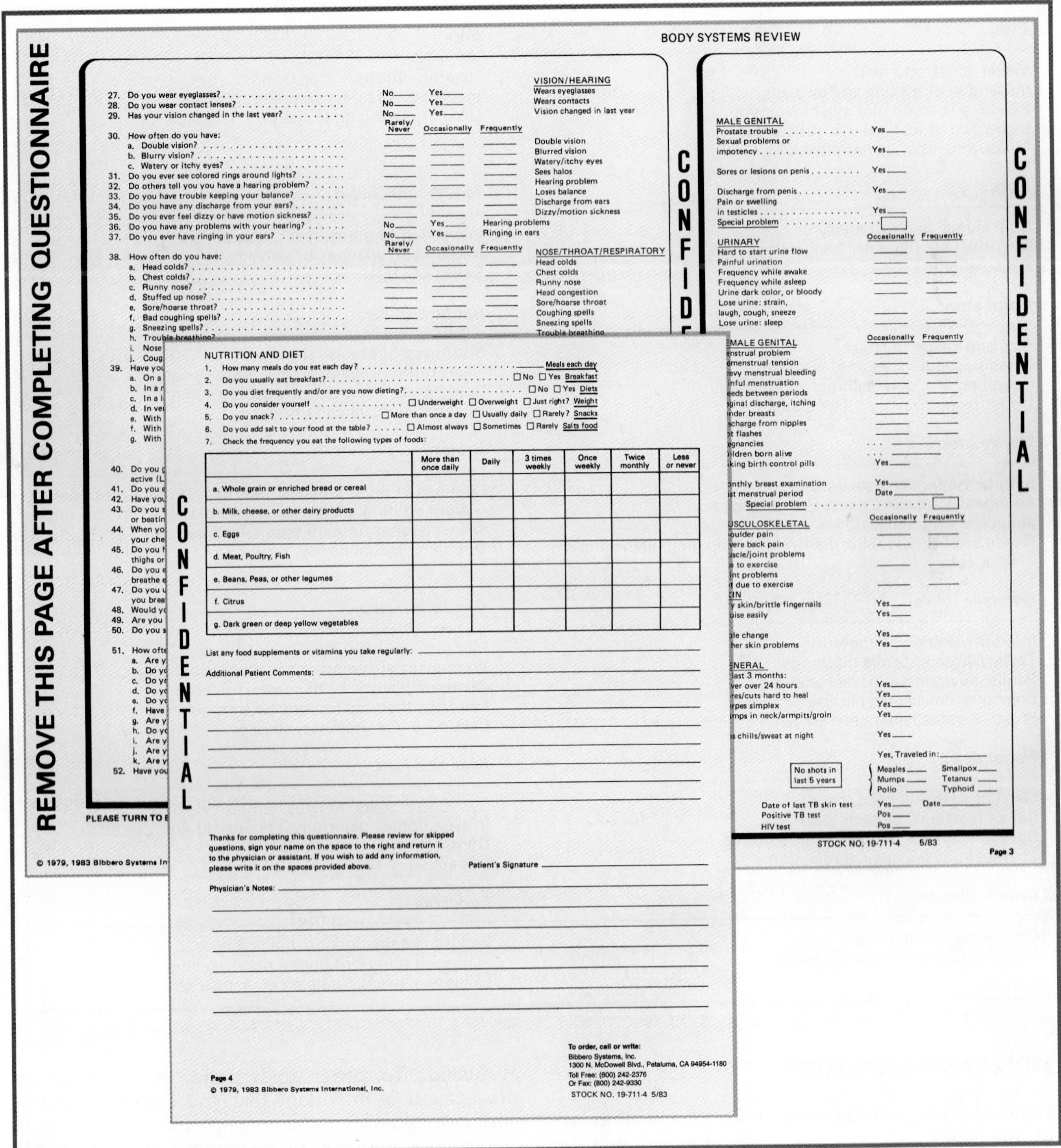

REMOVE THIS PAGE AFTER COMPLETING QUESTIONNAIRE

BODY SYSTEMS REVIEW

27. Do you wear eyeglasses? . . . . No___ Yes___ — VISION/HEARING: Wears eyeglasses
28. Do you wear contact lenses? . . . . No___ Yes___ — Wears contacts
29. Has your vision changed in the last year? . . . . No___ Yes___ — Vision changed in last year

	Rarely/Never	Occasionally	Frequently	
30. How often do you have:				
a. Double vision?				Double vision
b. Blurry vision?				Blurred vision
c. Watery or itchy eyes?				Watery/itchy eyes
31. Do you ever see colored rings around lights?				Sees halos
32. Do others tell you you have a hearing problem?				Hearing problem
33. Do you have trouble keeping your balance?				Loses balance
34. Do you have any discharge from your ears?				Discharge from ears
35. Do you ever feel dizzy or have motion sickness?				Dizzy/motion sickness

36. Do you have any problems with your hearing? . . . . No___ Yes___ Hearing problems
37. Do you ever have ringing in your ears? . . . . No___ Yes___ Ringing in ears

	Rarely/Never	Occasionally	Frequently	NOSE/THROAT/RESPIRATORY
38. How often do you have:				
a. Head colds?				Head colds
b. Chest colds?				Chest colds
c. Runny nose?				Runny nose
d. Stuffed up nose?				Head congestion
e. Sore/hoarse throat?				Sore/hoarse throat
f. Bad coughing spells?				Coughing spells
g. Sneezing spells?				Sneezing spells
h. Trouble breathing?				Trouble breathing

i. Nose
j. Coug
39. Have you
a. On a
b. In a r
c. In a l
d. In ve
e. With
f. With
g. With
40. Do you g active (L
41. Do you e
42. Have you
43. Do you s or beatin
44. When yo your che
45. Do you h thighs or
46. Do you e breathe e
47. Do you u you brea
48. Would y
49. Are you
50. Do you s
51. How ofte
a. Are y
b. Do y
c. Do y
d. Do y
e. Do y
f. Have
g. Are y
h. Do y
i. Are y
j. Are y
k. Are y
52. Have you

PLEASE TURN TO B

© 1979, 1983 Bibbero Systems In

CONFIDENTIAL

MALE GENITAL
Prostate trouble . . . . Yes___
Sexual problems or impotency . . . . Yes___
Sores or lesions on penis . . . . Yes___
Discharge from penis . . . . Yes___
Pain or swelling in testicles . . . . Yes___
Special problem . . . . ☐

URINARY	Occasionally	Frequently
Hard to start urine flow		
Painful urination		
Frequency while awake		
Frequency while asleep		
Urine dark color, or bloody		
Lose urine: strain, laugh, cough, sneeze		
Lose urine: sleep		

EMALE GENITAL	Occasionally	Frequently
enstrual problem		
emenstrual tension		
avy menstrual bleeding		
inful menstruation		
eeds between periods		
ginal discharge, itching		
nder breasts		
scharge from nipples		
t flashes		

egnancies . . . ___
ildren born alive . . . ___
king birth control pills Yes___
nthly breast examination Yes___
st menstrual period Date___
Special problem . . . . ☐

USCULOSKELETAL	Occasionally	Frequently
oulder pain		
vere back pain		
scle/joint problems		
e to exercise		
nt problems		
t due to exercise		

IN
y skin/brittle fingernails Yes___
uise easily Yes___
le change Yes___
her skin problems Yes___

ENERAL
last 3 months:
ver over 24 hours Yes___
res/cuts hard to heal Yes___
rpes simplex Yes___
mps in neck/armpits/groin Yes___
s chills/sweat at night Yes___
Yes, Traveled in:___

No shots in last 5 years — Measles___ Mumps___ Polio___ Smallpox___ Tetanus___ Typhoid___

Date of last TB skin test Yes___ Date___
Positive TB test Pos___
HIV test Pos___

STOCK NO. 19-711-4 5/83

Page 3

CONFIDENTIAL

NUTRITION AND DIET
1. How many meals do you eat each day? . . . . ___ Meals each day
2. Do you usually eat breakfast? . . . . ☐ No ☐ Yes Breakfast
3. Do you diet frequently and/or are you now dieting? . . . . ☐ No ☐ Yes Diets
4. Do you consider yourself . . . . ☐ Underweight ☐ Overweight ☐ Just right? Weight
5. Do you snack? . . . . ☐ More than once a day ☐ Usually daily ☐ Rarely? Snacks
6. Do you add salt to your food at the table? . . . . . ☐ Almost always ☐ Sometimes ☐ Rarely Salts food
7. Check the frequency you eat the following types of foods:

	More than once daily	Daily	3 times weekly	Once weekly	Twice monthly	Less or never
a. Whole grain or enriched bread or cereal						
b. Milk, cheese, or other dairy products						
c. Eggs						
d. Meat, Poultry, Fish						
e. Beans, Peas, or other legumes						
f. Citrus						
g. Dark green or deep yellow vegetables						

List any food supplements or vitamins you take regularly: ___

Additional Patient Comments: ___

Thanks for completing this questionnaire. Please review for skipped questions, sign your name on the space to the right and return it to the physician or assistant. If you wish to add any information, please write it on the spaces provided above.

Patient's Signature ___

Physician's Notes: ___

Page 4

© 1979, 1983 Bibbero Systems International, Inc.

To order, call or write:
Bibbero Systems, Inc.
1300 N. McDowell Blvd., Petaluma, CA 94954-1180
Toll Free: (800) 242-2376
Or Fax: (800) 242-9330
STOCK NO. 19-711-4 5/83

FIGURE 25–3 Comprehensive health history questionnaire.

TABLE 25–3 Body System Assessment

Appearance	Skin
Body build, posture, and gait Height and weight fluctuation Hygiene and grooming Emotional state and mood	Color, turgor, and tone Lesions or scars Temperature, rashes, itching Moles, sores, lumps, acne
Head and Neck	***Arms and Legs***
Size, shape, and contour of head Hair and scalp Palpation of neck, thyroid, trachea Difficulty in swallowing Change in voice, hoarseness	General appearance and symmetry Palpation of arm muscles Limitation of movement Inspection of fingernails Deformities, joint stiffness
Eyes	***Ears***
Visual acuity and field Inspection of eyelids and eyeballs Pupillary reaction and eye movement Inspection of internal eye structures Measurement of ocular pressure	Hearing deficits Inspection of size, symmetry, placement Discharge, ringing in the ears, infection
Nose	***Mouth and Throat***
Size, shape, and symmetry Deviated septum, nasal congestion Sense of smell	Inspection of gums, teeth, tongue, pharynx Bad breath, changes in salivation Sense of taste
Respiratory	***Cardiovascular***
Size and shape of chest Phlegm, cough, sneezing, wheezing Coughing of blood, asthma, emphysema Upper respiratory tract infections	Shortness of breath, chest pain Heart murmur, palpitations, night sweats Cold hands, leg cramps, varicose veins Hypertension, valvular disease
Gastrointestinal	***Urinary***
Symmetry, tenderness, pain Changes in appetite, nausea, vomiting Jaundice, ulcers, gallstones Change in bowel habits: diarrhea, constipation, hemorrhoids, stool color	Changes in urinary habits: hesitancy, urgency, frequency, night voiding, pain when voiding, loss of stream force Kidney stones, urinary tract infections Dribbling, incontinence
Genitalia (Male)	***Genitalia (Female)***
Infertility, sterility, impotency Testicular pain, penile discharge Penile enlargement or discomfort Erections, emissions, hernias Prostate or testicular enlargement	Menses regularity, flow, pain, duration Premenstrual symptoms, menopause Obstetric history, birth control method Estrogen therapy, reproductive surgeries Pain during intercourse, sterility
Neurologic	***Legs and Feet***
Level of consciousness, headaches Reflex reactions, general weakness Speech changes, memory loss, seizures Change in balance, incoordination	Symmetry, scars, bruises, lumps, swelling Broken bones, deformity, sprains, strains Gout, arthritis, osteoporosis Inspection of toenails
Lymph Glands	***Endocrine***
Enlargement, tenderness Female breasts: symmetry, lumps	Weight change, fatigue, bulging eyes Increased thirst or hunger, neck swelling Excessive sweating, heat/cold intolerance

SIGNS AND SYMPTOMS

When the physician completes the examination, all of the signs and symptoms documented will be evaluated. To better understand the examination processes it is important that you know the difference between a sign and a symptom.

Subjective findings, or symptoms, are perceptible

only to the patient; they are what the patient feels. An ache, pain, or dizziness is felt only by the patient, and only the patient can tell you it exists. The patient tells the physician about these symptoms, and the physician records them as subjective findings or symptoms. Symptoms of the greatest significance in identifying a disease are called *cardinal symptoms*.

Objective findings, or signs, are perceptible to a person other than the patient, specifically the physician and the medical assistant. They are the signs that a physician detects when examining a patient. The physician feels, sees, or hears the signs that are often associated with a certain disease or abnormal condition. Objective findings depend on another person's senses. A mass that a physician feels in the patient's abdomen is an objective finding and a sign of an abnormal condition. The medical assistant obtains the patient's vital signs, which are objective signs. Other terms that require understanding are the words *functional* and *physical* (organic). When a condition or disease is functional, it is without organic cause; that is, the organ appears normal but its function is not normal. A functional disease is any disease that alters the body functions but is not associated with any apparent organic, or physical, reason. An example of a functional problem would be if the patient has had repeated bouts of increased urinary albumin but all tests on the kidney show a normal healthy organ. A physical, or organic, disease or condition is one in which the abnormality can be seen or felt.

Memory Jogger

What is the difference between a subjective finding and an objective finding?

Charting

Charting may vary from office to office depending on the physician's preference. Regardless of the method used in the office, certain procedures have been standardized to meet the necessary legalities of maintaining medical records in an accurate and concise manner.

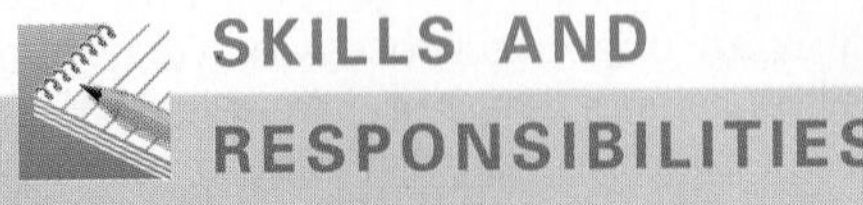

CORRECT METHOD OF CHARTING

- Check the name on the record and be certain that the information you are charting is recorded on the correct form on the correct patient's chart.
- All charting is done in black or blue ink. *Do not use pencil.*
- Write in a clear, legible manner.
- When you enter information on a patient's chart, you must sign the entry using your first initial and last name. The month, day, and year must precede the entry.
- All unusual complaints, symptoms, or reactions are noted in detail. If patient comments are entered in the patient's own words, then enclose them in quotation marks.
- Learn to be observant and to note anything that seems to be pertinent.
- Spelling, abbreviations, symbols, and terminology used must be accurate.
- Never scribble, erase, or white-out an error.
- Correct the error by drawing one line through it. Write the date and your initials next to the lined-out error (Fig. 25–4).

Professional Medical Offices
1722 E. North Avenue Suite 109
Aloha, Hawaii 99751

Patient Name Gestrin, Elenora C. (Last First MI) Date of Birth 8/15/40 Chart # 3361

Date	Subjective	Objective	Assess	Plan	Eval	Page------
7-4-98	~~T=99 P=72 R=61~~					7-4-98 S. Watkins CMA
7-4-98	T=99	P=72	R=16			S. Watkins CMA

FIGURE 25–4 Chart correction.

Memory Jogger

How do you correct a charting error?

TERMINOLOGY

Medical terminology differs from our ordinary language. Whenever an unfamiliar word is used, you must learn its meaning, how to spell it correctly, its pronunciation, and its proper usage. Learning medical terminology is an ongoing process of vocabulary building. Consistent use of a good medical dictionary is essential. To aid you in learning, a terminology glossary has been provided in the back of this textbook. It is your responsibility to make each new term a working part of your overall medical knowledge.

There are numerous terms that you will hear used; and when you hear an unfamiliar term, it will be your responsibility to make note of the term and, when the time is convenient, look the term up in a medical dictionary and discover the meaning of the word. Words and terms that may be seen on the history forms are listed for you at the beginning of the chapter, such as chief complaint, diagnosis, and present illness.

METHODS

Problem-Oriented Medical Record (POMR)

This method of medical record keeping introduced a logical sequence to recording the information obtained from the patient. It is based on the scientific method and was designed to solve a problem. The medical history and physical examination fit into a special format designed to clarify each patient's problem. The format includes supporting data that aid in solving the patient's problem. Because the POMR is universally organized, it is clear to anyone who reads the record. It leads to better audit of the medical record. The POMR is said to be the tool that revolutionized communication among the members of the health care team caring for the patient. The system is designed for and easily adapted to computerized medical records systems. The POMR system includes four basic parts:

- *Database*—Patient's personal information (previously discussed)
- *Problem list*—A list of the identified patient problems kept in the front of the patient's chart. It is the table of contents or the index of the chart. Each problem entered here is numerically listed and dated and is supported by the database. If the problem is resolved, the date of problem resolution is entered next to the problem.
- *Initial plan*—A written plan for each problem identified on the problem list, outlining further studies, treatments, and patient education (Fig. 25–5).
- *Progress notes*—Structured notes that correspond to each problem on the problem list, including (1) subjective data, (2) objective data, (3) assessment of the problem, (4) plans (diagnostic studies, treatments, and patient education), and (5) evaluation of the patient's understanding of the treatment and ability to comply to the treatment plan and diagnostics ordered.

The first letter of each part of the progress note adds up to SOAPE; therefore, this portion of the POMR system is called the SOAP notes, or SOAPE notes when evaluation is included (Fig. 25–6).

Source-Oriented Medical Records (SOMR)

This form of record keeping is still traditionally used by primary care physicians, especially those in sole practice. The notes are usually handwritten in chronologic order with the last on the top sheet. A handwritten chart has several disadvantages, which

PROGRESS SHEET

Date	Patient name: Fiddleman, Fred D. Allergies Iodine
9-9-98	c/o Fever for past two days. Productive cough
	Difficulty in breathing. Possible pneumonia
	Order Chest x-ray
	Rx: Keflex 500 mg #24 Cap i bid
	Phenergan Syrup ℥iv Sig: ʒii prn cough
	Return in one week

FIGURE 25–5 Initial plan for POMR progress notes.

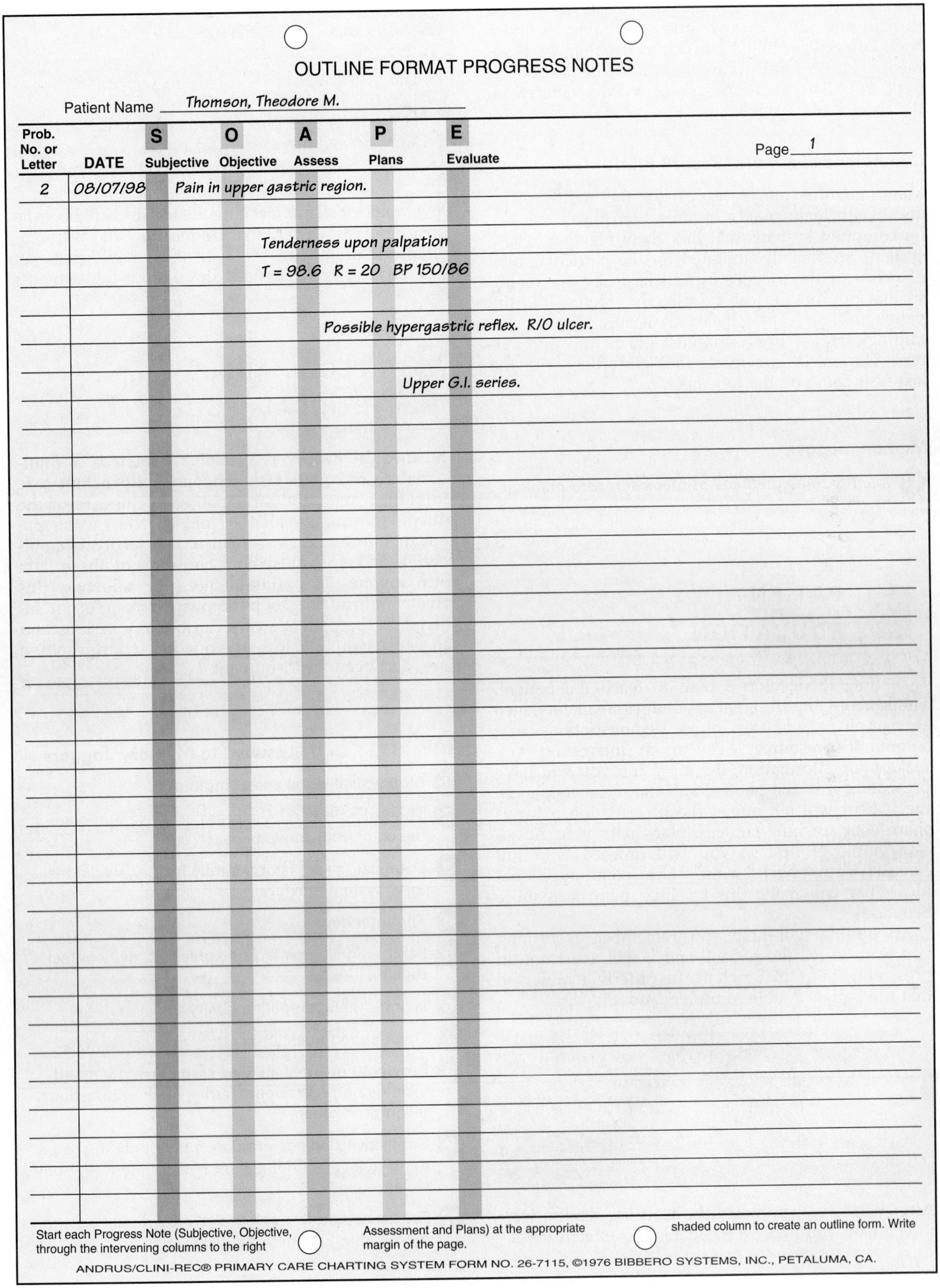

OUTLINE FORMAT PROGRESS NOTES

Patient Name Thomson, Theodore M.

Page 1

Prob. No. or Letter	DATE	S Subjective	O Objective	A Assess	P Plans	E Evaluate
2	08/07/98	Pain in upper gastric region.				
			Tenderness upon palpation			
			T = 98.6 R = 20 BP 150/86			
				Possible hypergastric reflex. R/O ulcer.		
					Upper G.I. series.	

Start each Progress Note (Subjective, Objective, Assessment and Plans) at the appropriate shaded column to create an outline form. Write through the intervening columns to the right margin of the page.

ANDRUS/CLINI-REC® PRIMARY CARE CHARTING SYSTEM FORM NO. 26-7115, ©1976 BIBBERO SYSTEMS, INC., PETALUMA, CA.

FIGURE 25–6 Structured notes for POMR system.

are primarily (1) handwritten entries are often hard to read and (2) it is very time consuming to find a back entry regarding a particular problem or treatment. The physical examination and medication orders would be in the chronologic order entered on the date of the service.

Computerized Medical Record (CMR)

Many medical offices, especially the multipractice and health maintenance organization physicians, are on computer systems that link them together. These systems are usually designed for the particular type of needs of the practice but all basically are set up so that information can be directly entered into the patient's chart. The physician usually dictates the findings, and a transcriptionist enters the information. The entries are in chronologic order, with the last visit being on the top sheet.

Memory Jogger

Identify three methods of medical record management.

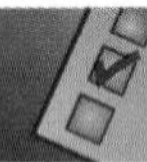

PATIENT EDUCATION

Take time to develop a plan to teach the patient. Think about the different modalities available, such as pamphlets, pictures, films, demonstrations, and community resources. The more interesting you make your information, the more fun you will have presenting it to the patient, and the more enjoyment the patient will get out of the presentation. Always share your teaching strategy plans with your physician/employer first so you will proceed with full consent. Your physician may have some additional ideas that will make this teaching plan even more beneficial.

An outline will help you remember everything you want to tell the patient, and it will assist you in presenting your material in an orderly manner so that the patient is able to understand and learn.

EXAMPLE OF A POSSIBLE OUTLINE

- Goal (what do you want to accomplish)
- Intervention (how do you plan to accomplish your goal)
- Evaluation (how will you know that the teaching was successful)

After you have completed the teaching session with the patient, you need to evaluate your effectiveness.

ANALYSIS OF TEACHING SESSION

- Did you cover all the items on your plan?
- Did the patient learn?
- How do you feel about your performance?
- Are you willing to try it again?
- How did the patient receive the information?

Developing patient teaching materials can be time consuming. However, sharing meaningful and helpful information with the patient is a gift that can have positive repercussions throughout the patient's life.

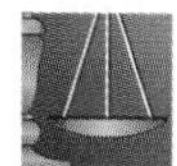

LEGAL AND ETHICAL ISSUES

The medical history record of a patient is a confidential record that is shared only with health care individuals who are participating in the care of the patient. Information that is told to you by the patient or information you read in this record is confidential, and you must not share any of these data with anyone. The consequences for allowing this private information to be known to people not involved in the patient's care can be very serious and can cause you the loss of your job, court-imposed fines, and even imprisonment.

HOW DID I DO? Answers to Memory Joggers

1. Biophysical signs and symptoms
2. Tone of voice, facial expression, ease and confidence of your movement
3. Database, past history, family history, social history, systems review
4. The interview
5. Posture, gestures, facial expression, eye contact, touch
6. Liking others, empathy, ability to listen
7. Open-ended questions
8. Providing unsubstantiated assurance, giving advice, using professional terms, leading questions, talking too much
9. Subjective findings are perceptible only to the patient; objective findings are perceptible to the physician.
10. Draw one line through the error, write error, and date and initial lined-out error.

11 Problem-oriented medical record, Source-oriented medical record, Computerized medical record

CRITICAL THINKING

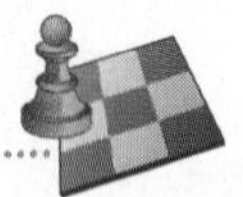

1 How would you handle a patient who is hesitant to talk to you?

2 Why is establishing rapport with the patient so important?

3 How might you cultivate the art of listening to others?

4 How do you think past experiences influence your nonverbal communication?

5 Identify your strong points and your weak points in doing patient interviews.

Aseptic Concepts and Infection Control

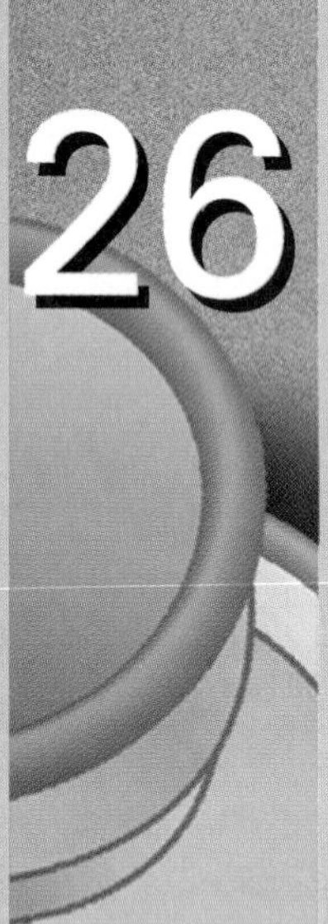
26

OUTLINE

LEARNING OBJECTIVES

Cognitive: On successful completion of this chapter you should be able to:

1. Define and spell the terms in the Vocabulary.
2. Explain the five links in the chain of infection.
3. Identify the eight specific reactions the body initiates as the inflammatory response.
4. Differentiate among the four types of infections.
5. Compare virus and bacteria cell invasion.
6. List the infectious materials covered in the Standard Precautions.
7. Identify the four major areas included in the OSHA Compliance Guidelines.
8. Differentiate between medical and surgical asepsis.
9. Differentiate among sanitization, disinfection, and sterilization.
10. Explain the types and uses of indicators.
11. Discuss the legal and ethical concerns regarding medical asepsis and infection control.
12. List possible methods of patient education.

Performance: On successful completion of this chapter you should be able to:

1. Demonstrate the proper hand washing technique for medical asepsis.
2. Clean and wrap instruments and equipment for autoclaving.
3. Load, run, and unload the autoclave with accuracy.

VOCABULARY

acute Having a rapid onset and severe symptoms; usually subsiding within a relatively short period of time

antiseptic Pertaining to substance that renders microorganisms harmless

asepsis Condition of being free from infection or infectious materials

carrier Unaffected person who can transmit infection to another person

chronic Persisting for a long period of time

coagulable Capable of being formed into clots

contamination Becoming soiled through contact with nonsterile material

disease Pathologic process having a descriptive set of signs and symptoms

disinfection Destruction of pathogenic organisms by chemical or physical means

edema Swelling between the layers of tissues

germicides Agents that destroy pathogenic organisms

infection Invasion and multiplication of microorganisms in body tissues causing injury and damage to the tissues

latent Describing the seemingly inactive time between the exposure of tissue to an injurious agent and the time that response signs and symptoms begin to appear

microorganisms Microscopic living parasites (also called *microbes*)

pathogens Disease-causing microorganisms

permeable To pass or soak through

pyemia The presence of pus-forming organisms in the blood

sanitization Reducing the number of microorganisms to a level that is relatively safe

septicemia Presence of pathogenic microorganisms in the blood

spores Thick walled reproductive cells formed within bacteria and capable of withstanding unfavorable environmental conditions

sterilization Complete destruction of all forms of microbial life

The concepts of disease transmission and the body's response to infection form the basis for understanding the importance of the first line of defense in preventing disease. Before we can assist in the prevention of disease, we have to look at methods we can use to minimize the chances of being a carrier of disease. One of the simplest ways of preventing the spread of disease is by washing your hands. As you continue through the remainder of this textbook, you will need to refer to the fundamental concepts of this chapter. Because of the need for infection control, every procedure begins with hand washing. The concepts in this chapter are basic to all clinical practice, and following them can lessen the transmission of disease, reduce the severity of disease, and might save the life of a patient or a co-worker or your own life.

Disease

Disease may be defined as any sustained, harmful alteration of the normal structure, function, or metabolism of an organism or cell. This pathologic condition of the body presents a group of clinical signs, symptoms, and laboratory findings that set it apart as an abnormal entity, differing from other normal and pathologic conditions. We recognize and categorize many different types of diseases: hereditary (genetic), drug-induced, autoimmune, degenerative, communicable, and infectious, to name only a few. Sometimes, a specific disease may fit two or more categories.

Any disease caused by growth of pathogenic microorganisms in the body falls into the category labeled *infectious diseases* (Tables 26–1 through 26–3). The entrance of a living microbe into the body is not disease, because until the infected cell or organism shows a harmful alteration of its structure, physiology, or biochemistry, disease is either not detected or not considered present. In fact, a living microbe may be ingested, injected, or inhaled and never cause disease in that person. An unaffected person, however, could still transmit the **infection** to another person. In this case, we call the unaffected person a **carrier.**

Microorganisms are almost everywhere. We carry them on our skin, in our bodies, and on our clothing. They are in ice, boiling water, the soil, and the air. The only places that are free of microorganisms are the insides of sterilized containers and in certain internal body organs and tissues. Organs and tissues that do not connect with the outside by means of

TABLE 26–1 Diseases Caused by Protozoa and Other Parasites

Disease	Organism	Transmission	Symptoms	Tests/Specimens
Malaria	*Plasmodium* species (protozoa)	Bite of the *Anopheles* mosquito	Chills, fever (cyclic)	Blood: examination of stained film for parasites
Toxoplasmosis	*Toxoplasma gondii* (protozoa)	Fecal contamination (cat litter); congenitally	Febrile illness, rash; congenital: jaundice, enlarged liver and spleen, brain abnormalities	Skin test
Amebic dysentery	*Entamoeba histolytica* (protozoa)	Fecal contamination of food and water	Bloody diarrhea, cramping, fever	Stool for O & P
Giardiasis	*Giardia lamblia* (protozoa)	Common in intestinal tract opportunist; contaminated surface water	Asymptomatic to severe diarrhea and abdominal discomfort	Stool for O & P; intestinal biopsy; string test
Interstitial plasma cell pneumonia	*Pneumocystis carinii*	Widely prevalent in animals. Occurs in debilitated persons, immunosuppressed; commonly associated with acquired immunodeficiency syndrome	Pneumonia-like	Biopsy
Trichinosis	*Trichinella spiralis* (roundworm)	Ingestion of undercooked pork, bear meat	Nausea, fever, diarrhea, muscle pain and swelling, edema of face	Biopsy; blood tests
Tapeworm	*Taenia* species	Undercooked meats (beef and pork)	Abdominal discomfort, diarrhea, weight loss	Stool for O & P
	Diphyllobothrium latum	Undercooked fish; common among Norwegians, Japanese	As above; may become anemic	Stool for O & P
Pinworm	*Enterobius vermicularis* (roundworm)	Fecal-oral	Severe rectal itching, restlessness, insomnia	Scotch tape applied to perianal region for ova
Scabies	*Sarcoptes scabiei* (itch mite)	Direct contact; clothing, bedding	Nocturnal itching; skin burrows	Skin scrapings for parasites
Lice	*Pediculus humanus; Phthirus pubis* (crab)	Direct contact; clothing, bedding, furniture (can transmit other diseases via bite)	Intense itching; skin lesions	Finding adult lice or eggs (nits) on body or hair

O & P, ova and parasites.

TABLE 26–2 Selected Fungal Diseases

Disease	Organism	Predisposing Conditions and Transmission	Symptoms	Tests/Specimens
Thrush (oral yeast); *Candida* (vaginal yeast)	*Candida* species (yeast)	Oral: during birth; other: following antibiotic therapy, oral birth control, severe diabetes	White, cheesy growth	Swab for KOH prep, culture
Athlete's foot, jock itch, ringworm (tinea)	Several species of dermatophytes (skin fungi)	Opportunist; direct contact; clothing; prolonged exposure to moist environment	Hair loss, thickening of skin, nails; itching; red, scaly patches	Skin scraping for KOH prep; skin, hair for culture
Histoplasmosis	*Histoplasma capsulatum*	Inhalation of dust contaminated with bird or bat droppings	Mild, flu-like to systemic	Serologic
Cryptococcosis	*Cryptococcus neoformans*	Contact with poultry droppings	Cough, fever, malaise; can become systemic	Sputum culture
Sporotrichosis	*Sporothrix schenckii*	Farmers, florists, people exposed to soil	Skin lesions that spread along lymphatics; can become systemic	Cerebrospinal fluid culture, India ink direct examination, scrapings; serologic

KOH, potassium hydroxide.

TABLE 26–3 Common Diseases Caused by Cocci

Disease	Organism	Description	Transmission	Symptoms	Specimens	Tests
Pneumonia	*Streptococcus pneumoniae*	Gram-positive cocci in pairs	Direct contact, droplets	Productive cough, fever, chest pain	Sputum; bronchoscopy secretions	Culture, Gram's stain
Strep throat	*Streptococcus pyogenes* (group A strep)	Gram-positive cocci in chains	Direct contact, droplets, fomites	Severe sore throat, fever, malaise	Direct swab	Direct agglutination; culture, white blood cell count and differential
Wound infection, abscesses, boils	*Staphylococcus aureus*	Gram-positive cocci in clusters	Direct contact, fomites, carriers; poor hand washing	Area red, warm, swollen; pus; pain; ulceration or sinus formation	Deep swab; aspirate of drainage	Culture and sensitivity (aerobic and anaerobic)
Staphylococcal food poisoning	*Staphylococcus aureus*	Gram-positive cocci in clusters	Poor hygiene and improper refrigeration of foods	Vomiting, abdominal cramps, diarrhea	Suspected food, stool	Culture
Toxic shock	*Staphylococcus aureus*	Gram-positive cocci in clusters	Use of absorbent packing materials (e.g., tampons, nasal packs)	Fever, headache, nausea, vomiting, delirium, low blood pressure	Swab, blood	Culture and serology
Gonorrhea	*Neisseria gonorrhoeae*	Gram-negative cocci in pairs; intracellular in white blood cells	Sexually transmitted	*Females:* pelvic pain, discharge. May be asymptomatic *Males:* urethral drip, pain on urination	Swab of cervix, urethra; rectal and pharyngeal swabs in homosexuals	Gram's stain; culture
Meningococcal meningitis	*Neisseria meningitidis*	Gram-negative diplococci	Respiratory tract secretions	High fever, headache, projectile vomiting, delirium, neck and back rigidity, convulsions, petechial rash	Nasopharyngeal swabs, cerebrospinal fluid, blood	Gram's stain; culture; cell counts and chemistries

mucus-lined membranes are, in the normal state, free from all living microorganisms. For example, the lungs, the heart, and the brain are all free of microorganisms.

Memory Jogger

Where on our bodies do we carry microorganisms?

THE CHAIN OF INFECTION

The life and growth of **pathogens** is a cycle, or chain. Break the chain, and you break the infectious process (Fig. 26–1).

The chain of infection starts at the *reservoir host.* A reservoir host may be an insect, animal, or human. Most pathogens must gain entrance into a host or else they will die. The reservoir host supplies nutrition to the organism, allowing it to multiply. The pathogen either causes infection in the host or exits from the host in great enough numbers to allow it to survive in the atmosphere, as it transfers to another host.

The chain of infection continues with the *means of exit.* This is how the organism escapes. Exits include the mouth, nose, eyes, ears, intestines, urinary tract, reproductive tract, and open wounds.

After exiting the reservoir host, organisms spread by *transmission* (see Table 26–1). Transmission is either direct or indirect. *Direct transmission* occurs from contact with an infected person or with the

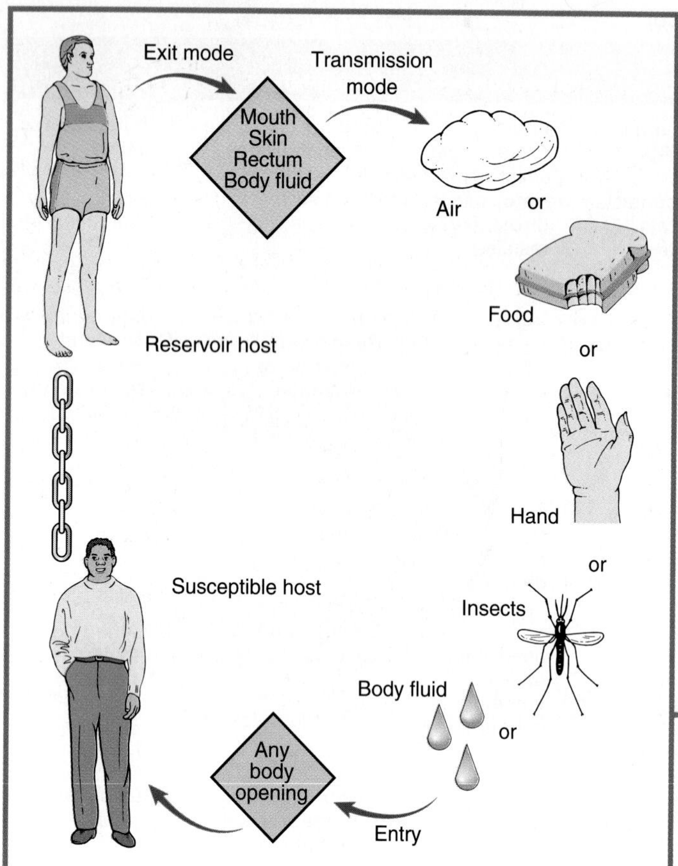

FIGURE 26–1 Chain of infection. (From Stepp CA, Woods MA: Laboratory Procedures for Medical Office Personnel. Philadelphia, WB Saunders, 1998.)

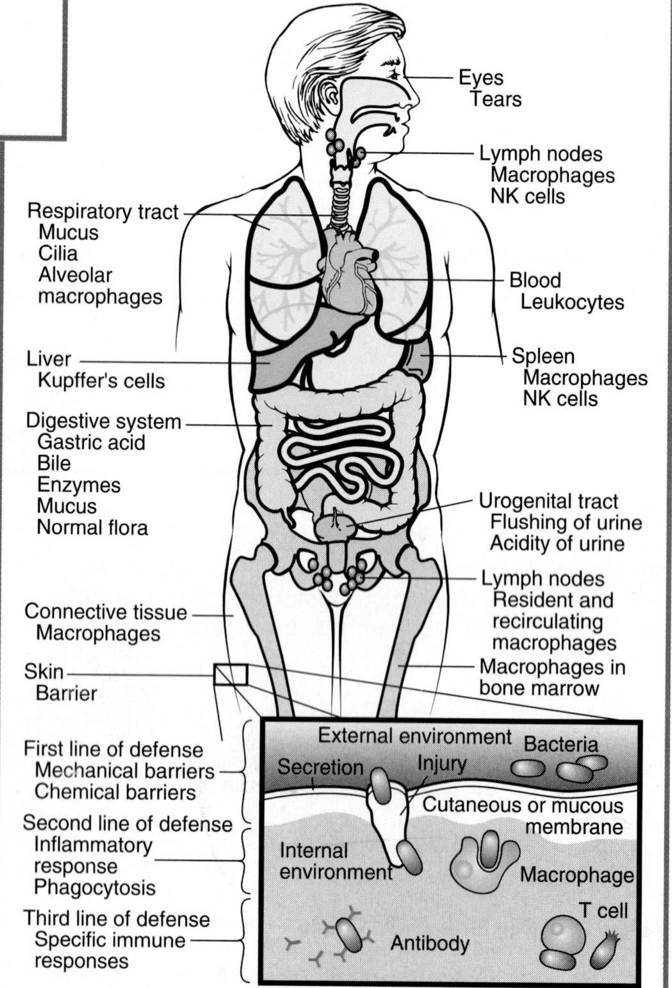

FIGURE 26–2 Natural protective mechanisms of the human body. (From Damjanov I: Pathology for the Health-Related Professions. Philadelphia, WB Saunders, 1996.)

discharges of an infected person, such as the feces or urine. *Indirect transmission* occurs from *droplets* in the air expelled from coughing, speaking, or sneezing; insects (called *vectors*) that harbor pathogens; contaminated food or drink; and contaminated objects (called *fomites*).

The next step is the *means of entry*. Now the transmitted organism will gain entry into a new host. The means of entry, like the means of exit, may be the mouth, nose, eyes, intestines, urinary tract, reproductive tract, or an open wound.

If the host is a *susceptible host,* that is, one that is capable of supporting the growth of the infecting organism, the organism will multiply. Factors affecting susceptibility include the location of entry, the dose of organisms, and the condition of the individual. If the conditions are right, the organisms reach infectious levels, the susceptible host becomes a *reservoir host,* and the cycle begins again (Fig. 26–2).

Memory Jogger

Trace the chain of infection.

THE INFLAMMATORY RESPONSE

When trauma occurs to our body, it alerts our protective mechanisms and our body responds in a predictable manner, called *inflammation* (Fig. 26–3). To defend itself, the body initiates specific responses that destroy and remove pathogenic organisms and their by-products or, if this is not possible, limit the extent of damage caused by pathogenic organisms and their by-products. This process characterizes the four classic symptoms of inflammation: redness, swelling, pain, and heat.

RESPONSES OF THE BODY TO PATHOGENIC ORGANISMS

- The blood vessels at the site of injury or invasion dilate, and the number of white blood cells in the area increases, causing redness.
- The white blood cells overpower and consume the pathogenic microorganisms in a process called phagocytosis.

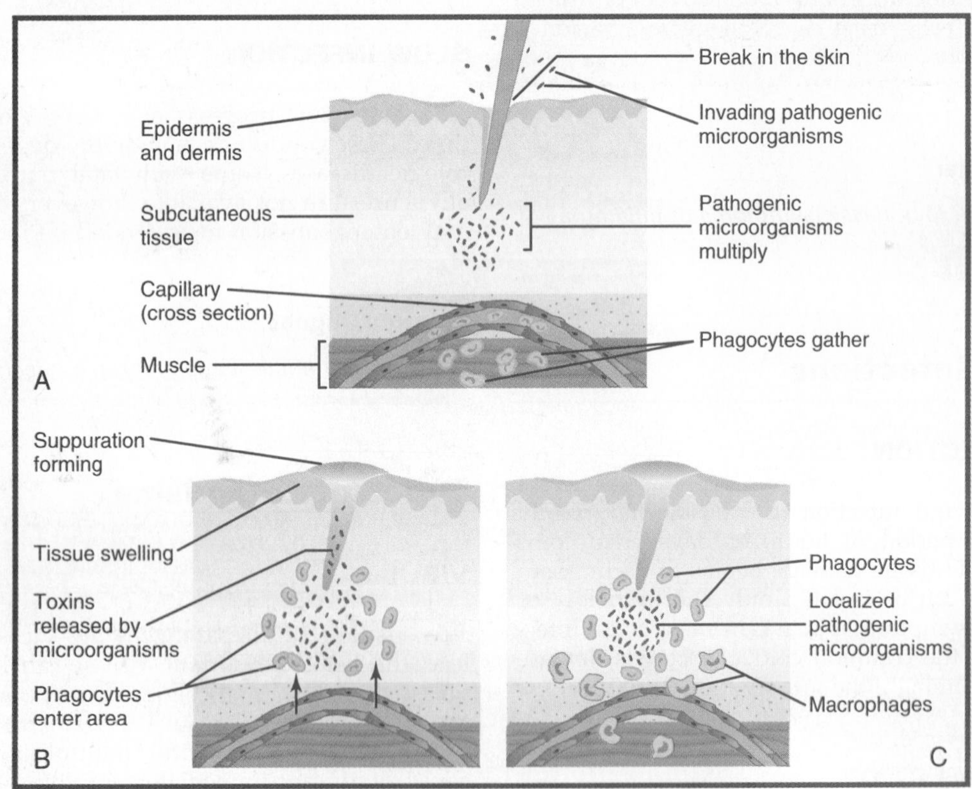

FIGURE 26–3 How the body defends itself against infection. *A,* Infection stage. A break in the skin allows pathogenic microorganisms to enter and multiply within the tissues. As a defense, the body prepares to send phagocytes (white blood cells) to fight the invading pathogenic microorganisms. *B,* Inflammation stage. As the pathogenic microorganisms multiply and die, toxins are released that destroy human tissue. Phagocytes have entered the infected area. Suppuration (liquefied dead tissue, pathogenic microorganisms, and phagocytes, also called pus) causes swelling and pain. *C,* Phagocytosis. Phagocytes engulf and ingest the invading microorganisms, localizing the infection. Macrophages (specialized phagocytes) now enter the area to ingest and clean up all the dead tissue debris. When all the debris has been enveloped and digested, swelling and pain subside, and the wound closes and heals.

- Fluids in the tissues increase, creating edema, which puts pressure on the nerves and causes pain.
- An increased blood supply to the area produces heat.

If the process is not reversed, it will continue through its course:

- Destroyed pathogens, cells, and white blood cells collect in the area and form a thick, white substance called pus.
- If the pathogenic invasion is too great for the white blood cells to control, the infection may collect in the body's lymph nodes, where more white blood cells are present to help fight the battle. This causes swollen glands.
- If the body is too weak or the number of pathogens is too great, the infection may spread to the bloodstream. This causes a systemic condition that could ultimately affect the entire body, called *septicemia* or blood poisoning.

When the entire body is invaded, the condition is called general **septicemia,** or **pyemia.** Without appropriate medical intervention, death can occur. Antibiotics must be used to help the white blood cells bring the pathogenic invasion under control.

Memory Jogger

 *Identify the four classic symptoms of inflammation.*

Types of Infections

ACUTE INFECTION

In the **acute** viral infection, the host cell typically dies within a period of hours or days. Symptoms appear after the tissue damage begins to occur. Usually, the virus can be isolated only shortly before or after the first symptom appears. In most acute infections, such as the common cold, the body's defense mechanisms eliminate the virus within 2 to 3 weeks.

CHRONIC INFECTION

Persistent viral infections are those in which the virus is present for a long period of time; some may persist for life. The person may be asymptomatic and the virus undetectable; or, as in **chronic** viral *hepatitis B,* the patient is asymptomatic but the virus may be detected and transmissible. Hepatitis B, or *serum hepatitis,* may be transmitted by blood or blood products and is a hazard to health care personnel. At one time hepatitis B could not be prevented, but now blood tests can determine the presence of certain antigens that identify a person as a carrier of hepatitis B, and thus the infection can be treated. A vaccine is also available to individuals for protection against the disease, and in many states, it is given as part of the well-baby immunizations.

LATENT INFECTION

A **latent** infection is a persistent infection in which the symptoms and the virus come and go. *Cold sores (oral herpes simplex)* and *genital herpes* are latent viral infections. The virus first enters the body and causes the original lesion. It then lies dormant, away from the surface, in a nerve cell, until certain provocation (illness with fever, sunburn, or stress) causes the virus to leave the nerve cell and seek the surface again. Once the virus reaches the superficial tissues it becomes detectable for a short time and causes another outbreak at that site. Another herpesvirus, *herpes zoster,* causes *chickenpox.* This virus then may lie dormant and later erupt as the painful disease shingles.

SLOW INFECTION

Slow infections progress over very long periods of time. These conditions include the degenerative neurologic diseases, some with fatal outcomes. Generally, cures are not available; however, these diseases may enter remission for extended periods.

Memory Jogger

 *Contrast a latent and a chronic infection.*

Types of Organisms

VIRUSES

The smallest of all pathogens are viruses, and they lead the list of important disease-causing agents. A virus enters a normal cell and incorporates itself into the cell's DNA or RNA. This growth may not appear right away, or viral multiplication may not cause significant immediate symptoms. Host cells infected with viruses may produce a substance called *interferon,* which protects nearby cells from invasion. Antibiotics are unable to destroy invaders that enter a normal cell and multiply within the cell. To counteract and destroy the virus invaders, interferon and the antiviral agents acyclovir and zidovudine (previously known as azidothymidine [AZT]) are widely prescribed.

BACTERIA

Bacteria are tiny, primitive cells that produce disease in a variety of ways. They can secrete toxic substances that damage human tissues, they may become parasites inside human cells, or they may form colonies in the body that disrupt normal human functions. Some bacteria can produce resistant forms called spores that make treatment difficult. When bacteria invade the body there are several ways to treat the patient. The most common approach is the use of antibiotics to destroy or inhibit the growth of the invader.

Memory Jogger

 *Why won't antibiotics destroy viruses?*

Prevention of Disease Transmission

For a pathogen to survive and multiply, it must be capable of getting all of its needs met. This means it must have an environment suitable for it to live, eat, and dispose of its waste products. After establishing this fact, the best way then to stop the growth and transmission of pathogens is to interfere with its environmental needs, thus breaking the chain of infection. For example, if pathogens thrive at 98.6° F, raise the temperature and most of them will die. If pathogens thrive in the dark, expose them to light.

Many **germicides** kill pathogens, provided the pathogens are exposed to the chemicals for a sufficient period of time. Spores are very resistant to germicides, but some can even kill spores after 10 hours or more of exposure. Temperatures of 250° F (121° C) maintained for 20 minutes with at least 15 pounds of pressurized steam kill all life forms, including spores. This is the basis of the autoclave method of sterilization. Meticulous sanitization, housekeeping controls, Occupational Safety and Health Administration (OSHA) Pathogen Standards, disinfection, and sterilization are necessary to control and break the chain of infection in the medical office.

STAYING HEALTHY WITH LIFESTYLE CHOICES

Avoidance of the infection is the best approach. This includes staying away from public areas during the flu season and isolating patients known to be infected with a virus. Patients must be vaccinated against polio (Sabin vaccine), German measles (rubella vaccine), measles (rubeola vaccine), and mumps (epidemic parotitis vaccine) (see Chapter 38). High-risk patients can be vaccinated against some other viruses, such as influenza, pneumonia, and hepatitis. This is especially important for the elderly and the chronically ill (see Chapter 39).

Memory Jogger

 *Identify three ways to avoid infections.*

OSHA Bloodborne Pathogen Standards

In July 1992, OSHA began enforcing work practice controls regarding bloodborne pathogens, which are defined as pathogenic microorganisms present in human blood and capable of causing disease. These controls include mandatory employee education on bloodborne disease transmission and exposure controls. In addition, employers must formally record all occupational injuries and be responsible for the labeling of all hazardous material located in the workplace. Failure to comply with the OSHA Standard by employees could result in a maximum penalty of $7,000 for the first violation and up to $70,000 for repeated violations.

NEW FUNDAMENTALS

OSHA has determined that employees face a significant health risk as the result of occupational exposure to blood and other potentially infectious materials because these materials may contain bloodborne pathogens, including hepatitis B virus and human immunodeficiency virus (HIV). OSHA concluded that exposure can be minimized or eliminated by a combination of engineering and work practice controls, the use of personal protective clothing and equipment, training, medical surveillance, hepatitis B virus vaccination, and the use of warning signs and labels.

The best way to reduce occupational risk of infection is to follow the Pathogen Standards. Health care workers must take adequate nondiscriminatory precautions to protect themselves. Standards apply to the handling of all potentially infectious body fluids and tissues.

POTENTIALLY INFECTIOUS FLUIDS

- Cerebrospinal, synovial, pleural, pericardial, peritoneal, mucous, and amniotic fluids
- Vaginal and seminal secretions
- Body fluid visibly contaminated with blood
- Unknown body fluid
- Human tissue including tissue culture, cells, or exudates

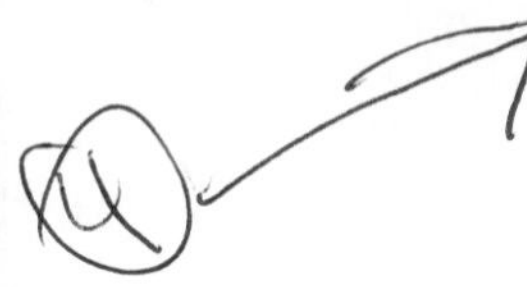

OSHA STANDARD PRECAUTION HIGHLIGHTS

* Wash Your Hands:
  After touching blood, body fluids, secretions, excretions, and contaminated items whether you have worn gloves or not.
  Immediately after you remove gloves
  Between patient contacts
  When necessary to prevent transfer of microorganisms
* Use plain soap for routine handwashing and an antimicrobial or antiseptic agent for specified situations.
* Wear clean, nonsterile gloves when touching blood, body fluids, secretions, excretions, mucous membranes, nonintact skin, and contaminated items.
* Change gloves between procedures on the same patient after exposure to potentially infective material.
* Remove gloves immediately after patient contact and wash your hands.
* Wear protective barrier equipment (e.g., mask, goggles, face shield, gown) to protect the mucous membranes of your eyes, nose, and mouth, and to avoid soiling your clothing when performing procedures that may generate splashes or sprays of blood, body fluids, secretions, or excretions.
* Care of linens and equipment that are contaminated with blood, body fluids, secretions, or excretions in a way that avoids skin and mucous membrane exposures, clothing contamination, and microorganism transfer to other patients and environments. Dispose of single-use items appropriately.
* Take precautions to avoid injuries before, during, and after any procedures using needles, scalpels, or other sharp instruments.
* Ensure that used needles are not recapped, purposely bent, broken, removed from disposable syringes, or otherwise manipulated by hand. Never direct the point of a needle toward any part of your body; instead use a one-handed "scoop" technique or a device designed for holding the needle sheath.
* Place used disposable syringes and needles, scalpel blades, and other used sharps in a puncture-resistant container that is located as close as possible to the area of use.
* Use barrier devices (e.g., mouthpieces, resuscitation bags) as alternatives to mouth-to-mouth resuscitation.

FIGURE 26–4 OSHA standard precaution highlights. (From Centers for Disease Control and Prevention and the Hospital Infection Control Practices Advisory Committee, January 1997.)

To ensure compliance, a state-designated agency is required to inspect all biohazardous wastes and all waste generators. (For interactive training support, call 1-[800]-547-0308.)

The Pathogen Standards are designed to reduce the risk of cross-infection of *any* infective agent in *any* body substance in *any* patient. The result is greater protection for health care workers and patients (Fig. 26–4).

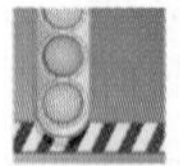

Safety Alert: Treat every patient as if he or she is infected with a bloodborne pathogen.

Memory Jogger

7 *List the body fluids considered to be potentially infectious.*

COMPLIANCE GUIDELINES

Because the Pathogen Standards are written to cover employees working in all health fields, it is obvious that only some of the regulations apply to the medical office. Safety and infection control fundamentals go beyond hand washing and disease cycle. The information presented here is as it applies to the medical assistant profession.

Barrier Protection

Medical assistants should routinely use appropriate barrier precautions when contact with blood or other body fluids is anticipated. Barrier protection is clothing or equipment such as gloves, face masks, face shields, protective glasses, laboratory coats, and barrier gowns (Fig. 26–5) that protect you from potentially infectious substances.

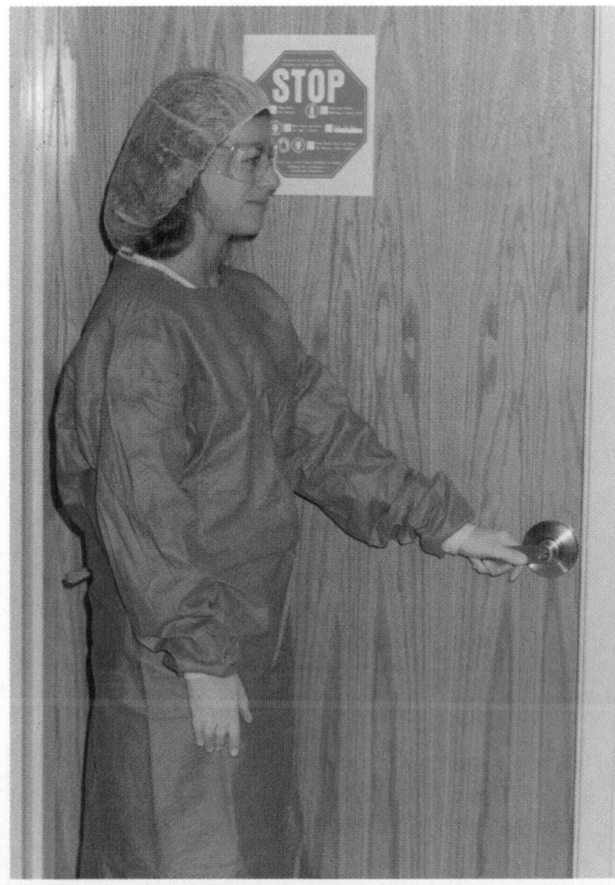

FIGURE 26–5 Barrier protection.

Protective equipment must be used if there is any chance that you will be involved in any of the following activities:

- Touching a patient's blood and body fluids, mucous membranes, or skin that is not intact
- Handling items and surfaces contaminated with blood and body fluids
- Performing venipuncture, finger punctures, injections, and other vascular access procedures
- Assisting with any surgical procedure. If a glove is torn or an injury occurs, the glove is removed and replaced with a new glove as soon as safety permits. The instrument involved in the incident is removed from the sterile field.
- Handling, processing, and disposing of all specimens of blood and body fluids
- Cleaning and decontaminating spills of blood or other body fluids

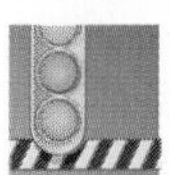

Safety Alert: *Gloves and gowns* contaminated with body fluid of any nature must be removed and placed in a designated area or container, and hands must be washed. *Protective eyewear* must be made of safety glass and have side shields. Standard prescriptive eyeglasses are not considered effective. All face shields, goggles, or glasses with side shields are acceptable. All personal protective equipment must be removed before leaving the medical facility.

Memory Jogger

What items of clothing are considered barrier protection?

Environment Protection

This section of the compliance guidelines covers controls to minimize the risk of occupational injury by isolating or removing any physical or mechanical health hazard in the medical workplace. Every medical assistant must adhere to these safety rules.

- Observe warning labels on biohazard containers and equipment (Fig. 26–6).
- Minimize splashing, spraying, and spattering of drops of potentially infectious materials.
- Remove contaminated gloves using proper technique and wash your hands.
- Bandage any breaks or lesions on your hands before gloving.
- If exposed skin surface comes in contact with potentially infectious body fluid, flush with wa-

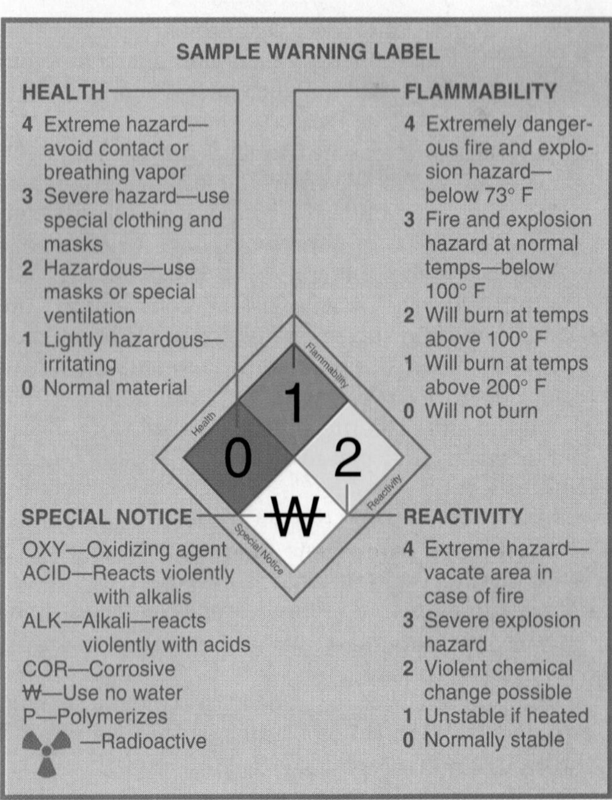

FIGURE 26–6 Sample warning label.

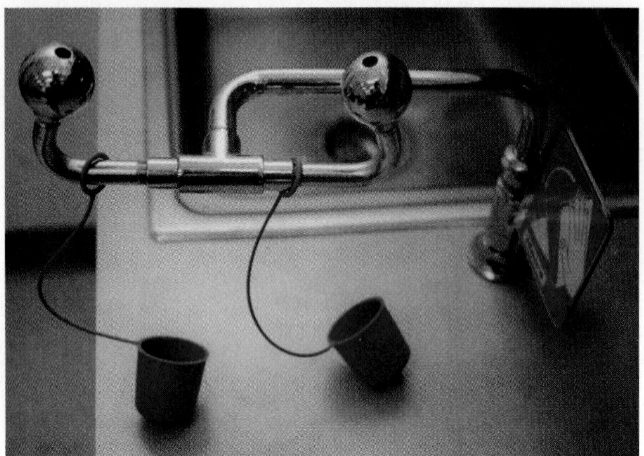

FIGURE 26–7 Eye washing unit.

ter and/or scrub with soap and water as soon as possible (Fig. 26–7).

- Do not recap used needles unless no other alternative is possible. If recapping must be done, use the scoop technique (Fig. 26–8). Sterile needles may be recapped after withdrawing medication from a vial.
- Do not bend, cut, break, or separate contaminated needles and syringes.
- Do not remove used scalpel blades from handles by hand. Use a hemostat to remove the blade.
- Immediately after use, dispose of syringes and needles, scalpel blades, and other sharp items in a puncture-resistant biohazard container. The container must be located as close as possible to the area where the instruments are used.
- Place all specimens in well-constructed containers with secure lids. Place this in a second container, such as an impervious bag, for transport. Check the bag for cracks or leaks. Avoid contaminating the outside of the container or the label with the specimen substance. If the outside is contaminated, the container should be disinfected, for example, with 1:10 dilution of 5.25% sodium hypochlorite (household chlorine bleach and water) and placed in an impervious bag for transport.
- Mouth pipetting or the sucking of blood through tubing is not to be done.
- Contaminated test materials should be decontaminated before reprocessing or should be placed in impervious bags and disposed of according to policy.
- Equipment that has been contaminated with blood or body fluids should be decontaminated before being repaired in the office or transported to the manufacturer.

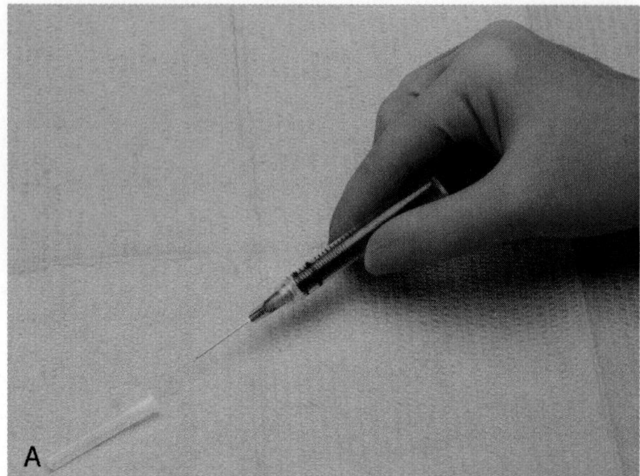

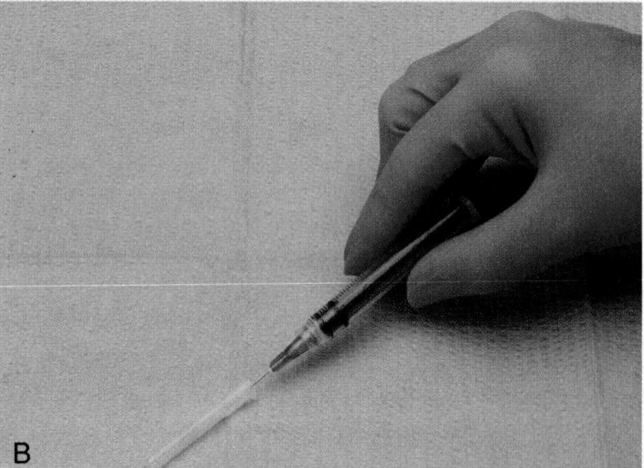

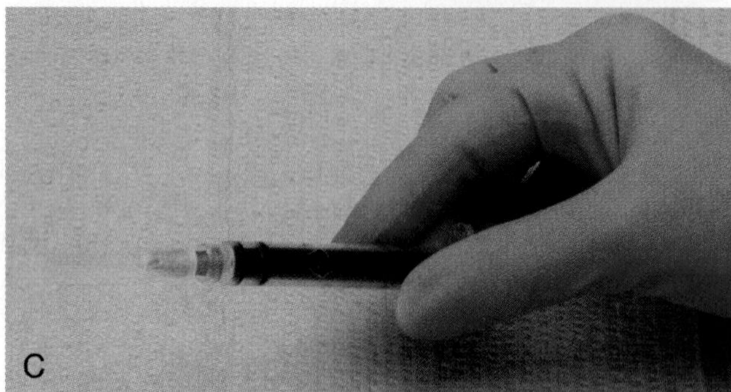

FIGURE 26–8 *A* through *C*, Scoop recapping method.

Memory Jogger

How would you make 100 mL of disinfectant using household bleach?

Housekeeping Controls

The OSHA Standard specifies certain housekeeping measures be followed to promote a work area that is clean and sanitary. Part of these guidelines includes that a documented schedule be maintained for cleaning and decontaminating each particular area where possible exposure occurs. This documentation must be specific and include the surface cleaned, the type of waste encountered, and procedures that are done in the designated area.

- Work surfaces must be immediately decontaminated with a disinfectant (such as sodium hypochlorite) after accidental spills of blood or body fluids and at the end of each procedure.
- Cleaning, removing soil, and decontaminating all reusable containers must be done on a routine basis.
- Sharps containers are to be maintained in an upright position to keep waste inside and as close as possible to the work usage area. Never attempt to reach inside a sharps container and do not overfill them. Replace containers on a routine basis and be certain that the lid is closed securely before placing it in the disposal waste.
- No attempt should be made to pick up spilled material or broken glassware with hands. Brooms, brushes, dustpans, and pickup tongs or forceps are to be used, and material should be immediately placed into an impervious bag at the spill site (Fig. 26–9). Use an absorbent professional biohazard spill preparation. If it is a large spill, call (HAZMAT) for decontamination and clean up.
- Handle soiled linen as little as possible. Linens soiled with blood or body fluids should be double bagged and transported in bags that will not leak.
- Contaminated materials and/or infective waste are to be handled with extreme caution to prevent exposure. Biohazardous waste must be collected in impermeable red polyethylene or poly-

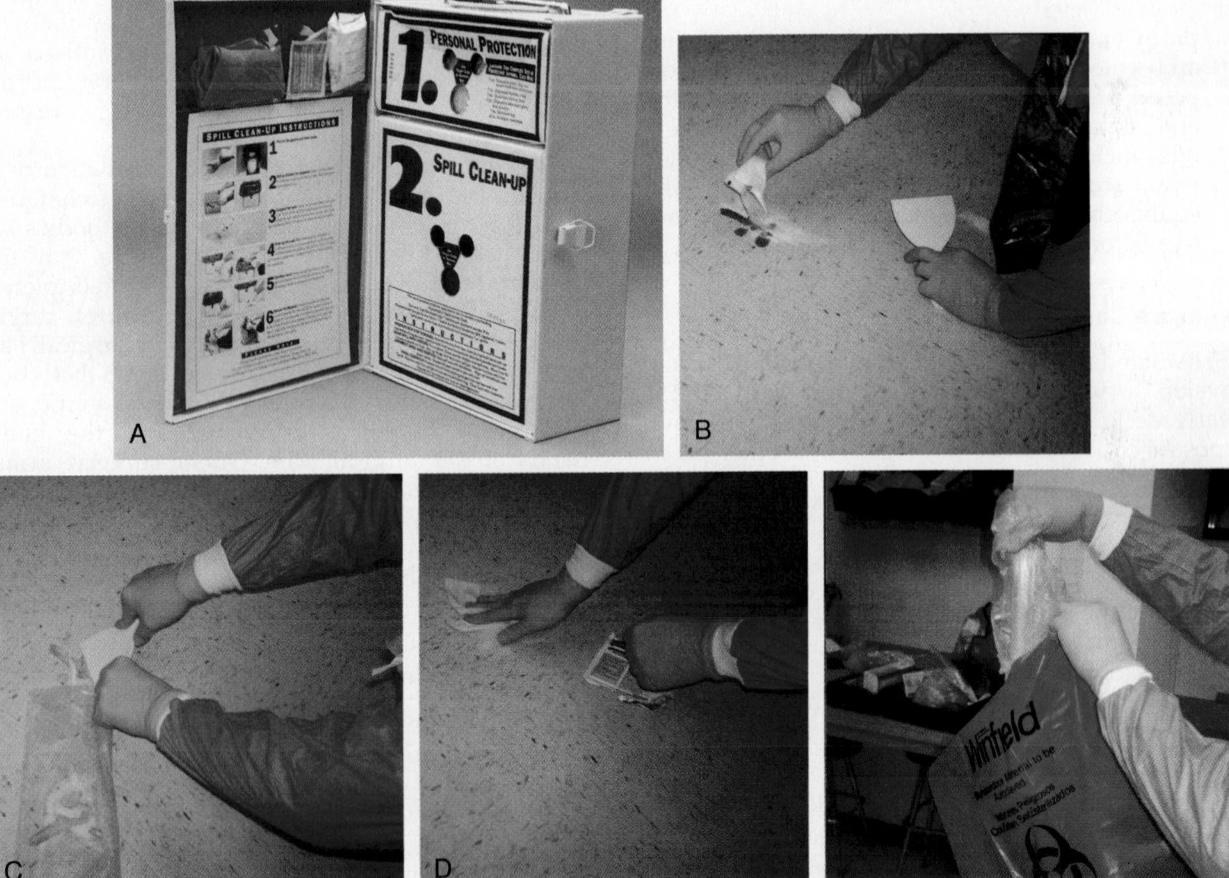

FIGURE 26–9 Cleaning spilled material. *A*, Clean-up kit with printed instructions. *B*, Sprinkle congealing powder over the spill. *C*, Scoop up spill and place in bag. *D*, Wipe area thoroughly with germicide. *E*, Place *all* contaminated items in biohazard bag.

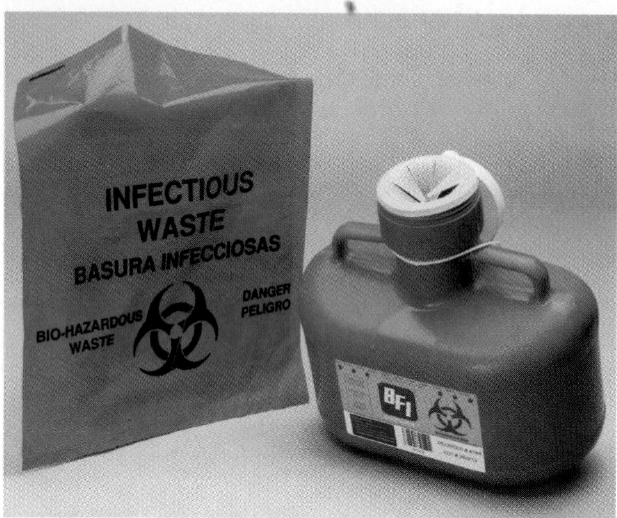

FIGURE 26–10 Biohazard bag and biohazard sharps container.

propylene biohazard-labeled bags or containers and sealed (Fig. 26–10). This waste must be disposed of in accordance with all applicable federal, state, and local regulations. Disposal methods include treatment by heat, incineration, steam sterilization, chemical treatment, or other equivalent methods that render the waste inactive before it can be placed in a landfill.

Exposure Control Plan

OSHA standards require that every medical facility develop a written exposure control plan that is clearly designed to eliminate or minimize employee exposure to bloodborne pathogens and other potentially infectious materials. This plan must be immediately available for review by all medical staff and must be updated on a regular basis, at least once a year.

- Exposure determination: tasks and the employment areas are listed in which occupational exposure would be likely.
- Method of compliance: specific health and safety measures are detailed that are taken to minimize the risk of exposure.
- Postexposure evaluation and follow-up: an incident report is filed and a confidential medical evaluation is provided to the injured employee.
- Information provided to the health care professional: employer must send the treating health care professional an incident report.
- Health care professional's written opinion: employer must give injured employee a copy of the health care provider's opinion within 15 days of the completion of the evaluation.
- Medical recordkeeping: medical records must be kept by Pathogen Standards guidelines.

A complete unabridged copy of the Occupational Exposure to Bloodborne Pathogens may be obtained from OSHA.

Memory Jogger

10 *Identify the six areas that must be included in the exposure control plan.*

Asepsis

Asepsis means freedom from infection or infectious material. *Medical asepsis* is defined as the destruction of organisms *after they leave the body.* When we practice the principles of medical asepsis, we are directing our efforts at preventing reinfection of the patient or cross-infection of other patients or ourselves. The goal is to isolate microorganisms by following Universal Blood and Body Fluid Precautions and disinfecting or sterilizing objects as soon as possible after they have been contaminated. This creates a nonsterile but clean environment.

Surgical asepsis is defined as the destruction of organisms *before they enter the body.* This technique is used for any procedure that invades the body's skin or tissues, such as surgery or injections. Any time the skin or mucous membrane is punctured, pierced, or incised (or will be during a procedure), surgical aseptic techniques are practiced. The surgical hand wash (scrub) must be used. Everything that comes into contact with the patient should be sterile, such as gowns, drapes, instruments, and the gloved hands of the surgical team. Minor surgery, urinary catheterizations, injections, and some specimen collections, such as blood and biopsies, are performed using surgical aseptic technique. This technique is presented in Chapter 50.

Memory Jogger

11 *What is the difference between medical and surgical asepsis?*

Because it is not possible to sterilize your hands, the goal of hand washing is to reduce skin bacteria by the use of mechanical friction, special soaps, and running water. Normally, there are two types of bacteria on your skin: *transient bacteria,* which are surface bacteria that are introduced by fomites and remain with you a short time, and *resident bacteria,* found under fingernails, in hair follicles, in the openings of the sebaceous glands, and in the deeper layers of the skin.

Resident bacteria in the deeper skin layers come to the surface with perspiration, which is why sterile gloves are used in addition to the surgical hand scrub in surgery.

The most effective barrier against infection is the unbroken skin. If the skin and mucous membranes are intact, medical asepsis can be practiced for most noninvasive (not penetrating through human tissues) procedures, such as pelvic and proctologic examinations. Instruments and objects not breaking the skin must be sterilized before being used on another patient, but then they may be stored and used under clean, nonsterile conditions. Gowns and masks may be used, but they are not presterilized; they are worn to protect you more than the patient. Hands are washed according to the principles of the medical aseptic hand wash.

Hand Washing

Hands must be washed, using the correct technique, before and after each patient is examined or treated. It is not necessary to do an extended scrub each time, but the first scrub in the morning should be extensive. Subsequent hand washing may be brief unless your hands become excessively contaminated. A good surgical soap with chlorhexidine, such as Hibiclens, which has antiseptic residual action that will last several hours, should be used. Each office sink should be equipped with a liquid soap dispenser. A water-soluble lotion may be rubbed into your hands after washing and drying them. Remember, dry, cracked skin can be a source of contamination.

Proper hand washing depends on two factors: running water and friction. Water should be warm; water that is too hot or too cold will cause the skin to become chapped. Friction means the firm rubbing of all surfaces of the hands and wrists. Remember that your fingers have four sides and fingernails have two sides. For the medical hand wash, all jewelry except a plain wedding band is removed. A wristwatch may be left on if it can be moved up on the forearm out of the wrist area. Your hands are washed under running water, with the fingertips pointing downward. Soap and friction are applied only to the hands and wrists. Allow the water to wash away debris from the wrists over the fingertips.

This procedure is used when you are performing medical procedures with patients. Your goal is to prevent cross-contamination of microorganisms from one patient to another. Use this procedure after you finish with one patient and before you attend to another patient; after you finish handling one specimen and before you handle another specimen; before and after you use toilet facilities; whenever you touch something that causes your hands to become contaminated; and on arrival to work and before you leave the office, before and after lunch, and at the end of the day.

Sanitization

Instruments and other items used in office surgery, examination, or treatment must be carefully cleaned *before* proceeding with the steps of disinfection or sterilization. **Sanitization** is the cleansing process that puts the number of microorganisms into a safe level as dictated in public health guidelines. This cleansing process removes debris such as blood and other body fluids from the instrument or equipment. Blood and debris must be removed so that later disinfection with chemicals or sterilization with steam, heat, or gases can penetrate to all the instrument's surfaces.

The medical assistant should always wear gloves while performing sanitization to prevent possible personal contamination of potentially infectious body fluids that may be present on the articles being cleaned.

When the procedure is completed, remove all used instruments to a separate work room or area to avoid cross-contamination with clean instruments and equipment. Instruments and equipment should be sanitized immediately after use. If this is not possible, rinse the used items under cold water and then place them in a low-sudsing, rust-inhibiting, enzyme-containing, detergent solution. Never allow blood or other **coagulable** substances to dry on an instrument. Be careful not to cut or puncture your skin when handling sharp instruments because this makes invasion of pathogenic organisms possible. When you are ready to sanitize instruments, drain off the soak solution and rinse each instrument in cold, running water. Separate the sharp instruments from the others; other metal instruments may damage the cutting edges and the sharp instruments may injure the other instruments or you. Clean all the sharp instruments at one time, when you can concentrate on avoiding the dangers of injury to yourself. Open all hinges, and scrub serrations and ratchets with a small scrub brush or toothbrush. Rinse the instruments in hot water, then check carefully for proper working order. The items are hand dried with a towel to prevent spotting. Sanitization is a very important step, and it cannot be overlooked or done carelessly.

It is not possible to know whether every patient is free of infectious pathogens; thus, extreme care must be taken when handling any item that has penetrated a patient's tissues. The use of *disposable* instruments, needles, and syringes when working with human blood or giving injections minimizes the need for sanitation and sterilization. Many disposable instruments are available.

Memory Jogger

Define sanitization.

PROCEDURE 26–1

Hand Washing for Assisting with Medical Procedures

GOAL

To minimize the number of pathogens on your hands, thus reducing the risk of pathogenic transmission.

EQUIPMENT AND SUPPLIES

Sink with running water
Liquid soap in a dispenser (bar soap is not acceptable)
Water-based antimicrobial lotion
Nail brush or orange stick
Paper towels in a dispenser

PROCEDURAL STEPS

1. Remove all jewelry except your wristwatch and a plain gold ring.
   PURPOSE: Jewelry is capable of concealing microorganisms.
2. Turn on the faucet and regulate the water temperature to lukewarm.
   PURPOSE: Water that is too hot can cause skin to become dry and chapped.
3. Allow your hands to become wet, apply soap, and lather using a circular motion with friction while holding your fingertips downward. Rub well between your fingers (Figure 1).
   PURPOSE: Friction removes soil and contaminants from your hands and wrists.
   If this is the first hand washing of the day, use a nail brush or an orange stick and thoroughly inspect and clean under every fingernail during step 3.
4. Rinse well, holding your hands so that the water flows from your wrists downward to your fingertips (Figure 2).
   PURPOSE: Soil and contaminants will wash off you and down the drain.

Continued

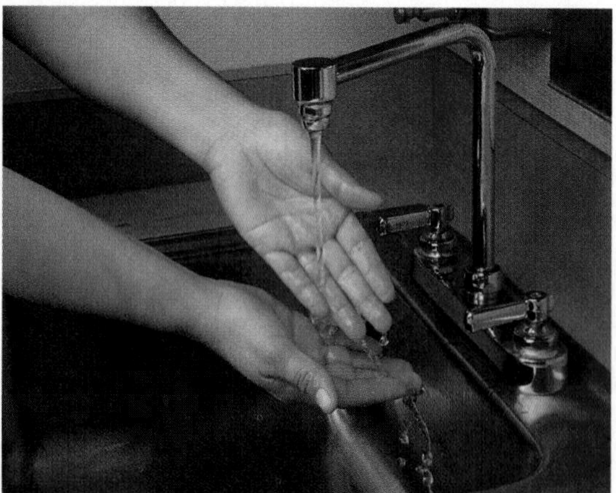

FIGURE 1

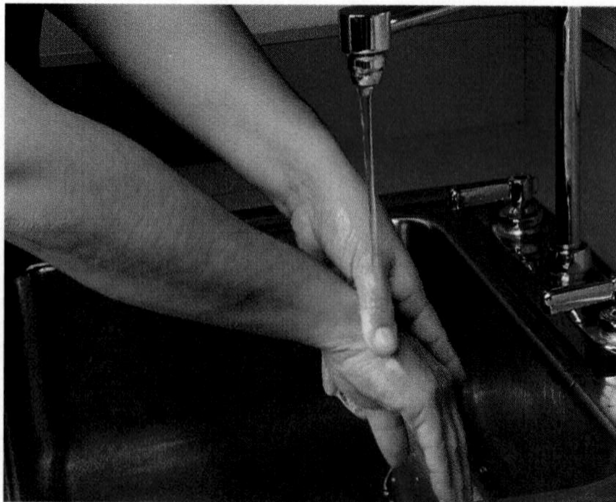

FIGURE 2

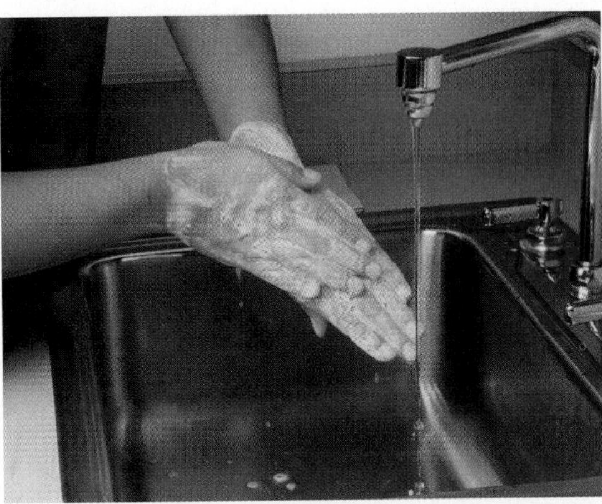
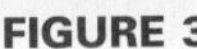

FIGURE 3

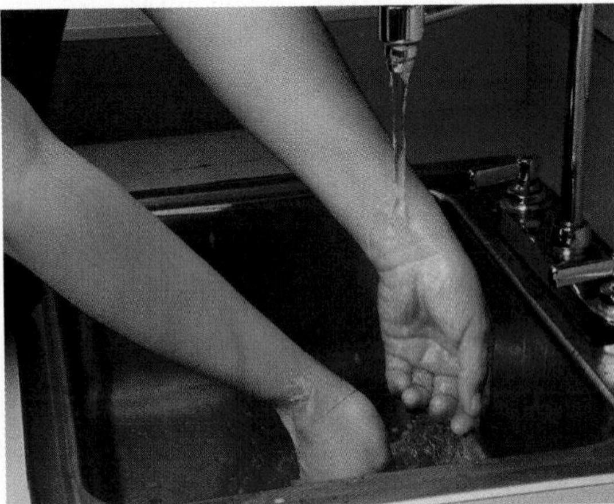

FIGURE 4

5. Wet your hands again and repeat the scrubbing procedure using vigorous, circular motion over wrists and hands for at least 1 full minute (Figure 3).
   PURPOSE: Time is required for friction and motion to eliminate all possible soil and contaminants.
6. Rinse your hands a second time, keeping fingers lower than your wrists, and take time to inspect them (Figure 4).
   PURPOSE: To ensure that the hands are really clean.
7. Dry your hands with paper towels. Do not touch the paper towel dispenser as you are obtaining towels (Figure 5).
   PURPOSE: Touching the dispenser contaminates your hands and you will need to start over.
8. If faucets are not foot operated, turn off the water faucet with the paper towel (Figure 6).
   PURPOSE: The faucet is dirty and will contaminate your clean hands.
9. After completion of drying your hands and turning off faucets (if necessary) place used towels into waste container.
   PURPOSE: Always discard contaminated waste immediately.
10. Apply a water-based antibacterial hand lotion to prevent chapped or dry skin.

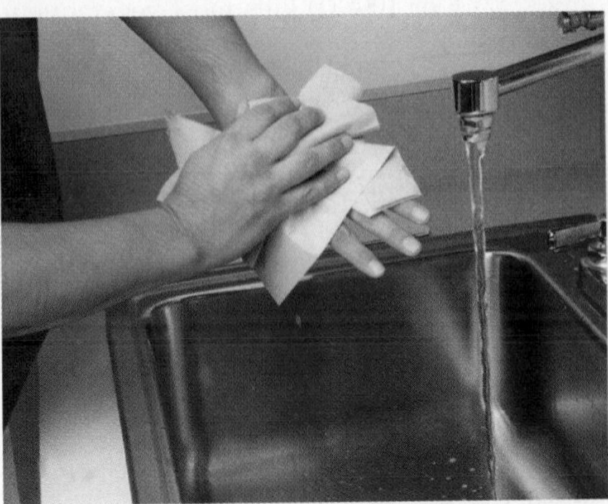

FIGURE 5

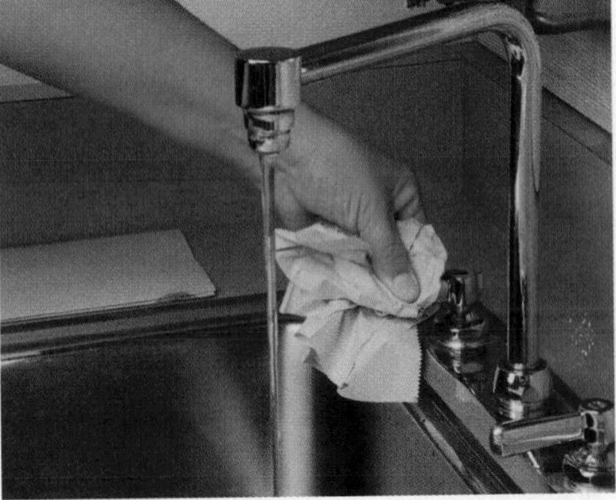

FIGURE 6

ULTRASONICS

Sound waves can be used for sanitization of instruments by placing the instruments in a bath of ultrasonic cleaner and water and then passing ultrasonic waves through the bath. The sound vibrates and causes bubbling, which loosens the materials attached to the instruments. Ultrasonic cleaners do not damage even the most delicate instruments.

Disinfection

Disinfection is the freeing of an item from infectious materials. It is not always effective against spores, the tubercle bacilli, and certain viruses. In the medical office, the term usually refers to disinfecting instruments with chemicals. Chemicals may kill microbes within a short time but are usually very hard on the instruments. Some chemicals are effective enough to kill all organisms, but the usual immersion time for these sterilants is 10 or more hours. There are various methods of disinfection with varying degrees of effectiveness. It is important to know how to properly use each method, as well as its advantages, disadvantages, and the possible sources of error.

Disinfectants are commonly applied to inanimate objects, because they are too strong to be used on human tissues. Items that will enter human tissue, the circulatory system, or a sterile body cavity may be disinfected or chemically sterilized but then are thoroughly rinsed with sterile water.

Disinfection is very difficult to verify, because there are no convenient indicators to ensure destruction of the organisms. Even when the manufacturer's directions for chemical strength and immersion times are followed, the following six common errors can cause chemicals to lose their effectiveness:

1. Instruments are not thoroughly sanitized, and attached organic matter inhibits or prevents the action of the disinfectant. No chemical can kill unless it reaches the instrument's surfaces; therefore, complete sanitization is absolutely necessary.
2. Sanitized instruments are not dried. The moisture on the instruments dilutes the solution beyond the effective concentration.
3. A solution is left in an open container, and evaporation changes its concentration.
4. Solutions are not changed after the recommended period for use has expired.
5. The solutions are not prepared properly or not mixed properly before using.
6. The recommended manufacturer's temperature for use and storage is not maintained.

Memory Jogger

List six common errors that cause chemicals to lose their effectiveness.

ALCOHOL

Alcohol is the most widely used **antiseptic,** but recent studies indicate that it is a poor antiseptic. Ethyl alcohol had been widely used in the past, but isopropyl alcohol has become more frequently used. It exhibits slightly greater germicidal action than does ethyl alcohol. It is an excellent fat solvent and, therefore, good for cleansing the skin, but continued use is hard on the hands. Iodine and other chemicals are sometimes added to alcohol to increase its lethal powers.

ALKALI

A popular product that is used frequently today is plain household bleach. When mixed with water to form a 10% solution, it is an effective and noncaustic disinfectant. It is used to wipe laboratory countertops where human blood and other body-fluid samples are handled. It can be used for soaking reusable rubber goods before sanitizing. Bleach is used to disinfect dialysis equipment and is an effective disinfectant for surfaces that have come into contact with viruses, including the HIV. It does "bleach out" clothing that comes in contact with it and is difficult to rinse off.

DISINFECTION BY BOILING (MOIST HEAT)

Boiling (212° F or 100° C) kills most vegetative forms of pathogenic bacteria, but bacterial spores and some viruses associated with infectious hepatitis are resistant to temperatures of 212° F and less. No matter how much heat is applied or how vigorous the boil, water will reach only 212° F at sea level. The higher the elevation, the lower the temperature required to obtain a boil (e.g., in Denver, Colorado, water boils at 202° F). This temperature is not high enough to kill spores and the virus that causes hepatitis. Because of these limitations, *boiling does not sterilize* and is used for disinfection only. Boiling can be used to disinfect instruments, such as nasal or ear specula, that do not penetrate body tissues. An article must be boiled at a rolling (not vigorous) boil for at least 15 minutes.

PROCEDURE 26-2

Sanitization of Instrumentations

GOAL

To remove all contaminated matter from instruments in preparation for sterilization.

EQUIPMENT AND SUPPLIES

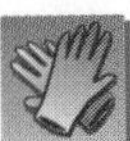

Sink or ultrasonic cleaner
Sanitizing agent or low-sudsing soap with enzymatic action
Gloves
Assorted instruments
Brush
Towels
Appropriate waste container

PROCEDURAL STEPS

1. Put on gloves.
   PURPOSE: To provide personal protection against potentially infectious matter.
2. Separate sharp instruments from other instruments to be sanitized.
   PURPOSE: To prevent possible self-injury (Figure 1).
3. Rinse the instruments under cold running water.
   PURPOSE: To help remove debris and makes sanitation easier.
4. Open hinged instruments and scrub all grooves, crevices, and serrations with a brush (Figure 2).
   PURPOSE: Microorganisms can hide under contaminants and not be destroyed by the disinfection process.
5. Rinse well with hot water.
   PURPOSE: Hot water removes all soap residue and promotes drying.
6. Towel dry all instruments thoroughly.
   PURPOSE: Wet instruments can rust or become dull.
7. Place sanitized instruments in designated area for sterilization.
   PURPOSE: Sanitized instruments are always removed from cleaning area to prevent possible cross-contamination.

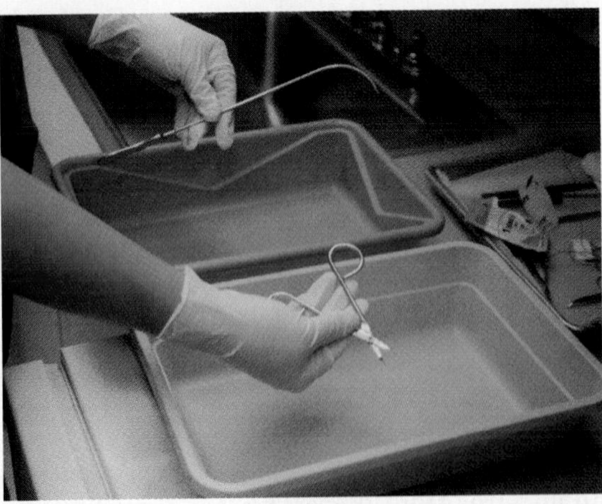

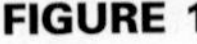

FIGURE 1

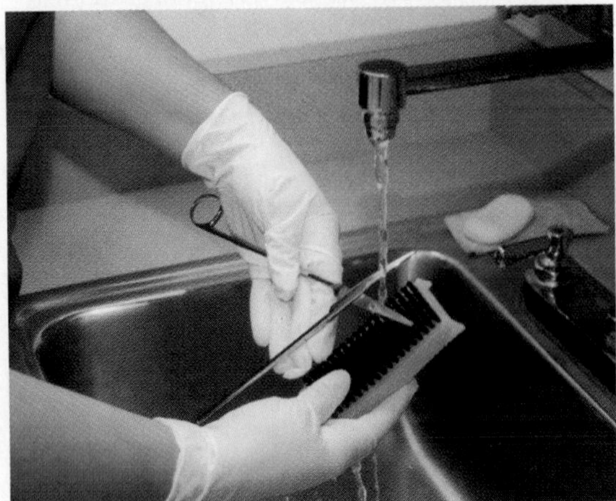

FIGURE 2

Sterilization

Sterilization reduces the perpetual threat of **contamination** to patients, to the physician, and to the medical assistant. To ensure proper sterilization for aseptic procedures, an area should be set aside in each office for just this purpose. The area should be divided into two sections. One section is used for receiving contaminated materials. This area should have a sink as well as receiving basins, proper cleaning agents, brushes, sterilizer wrapping paper, sterilizer envelopes and tape, sterilizer indicators, and disposable gloves. The other section should be reserved for receiving the sterile items after they are removed from the sterilizer. Clear, clean plastic bags in which to store sterile packs may be kept in the sterile area. Both areas should be spotlessly clean and well organized. Designated waste containers are needed for gloves worn when handling contaminated items.

Sterilization can be achieved by dry heat, as in a gas autoclave, and by steam heat, which is the most commonly used device in the medical office.

MOIST HEAT STERILIZATION

Steam under pressure is the best and most accepted method of sterilization because it kills all pathogens and spores. It is the principal operation of the *autoclave* (Fig. 26–11). Steam under pressure is fast, convenient, and dependable. The pressure allows for heat higher than the boiling point; and when combined with moisture, these two factors create a very effective mechanism for killing all microorganisms. When steam is admitted into the autoclave chamber, it simultaneously heats and wets the object, coagulating the proteins present in all living organisms.

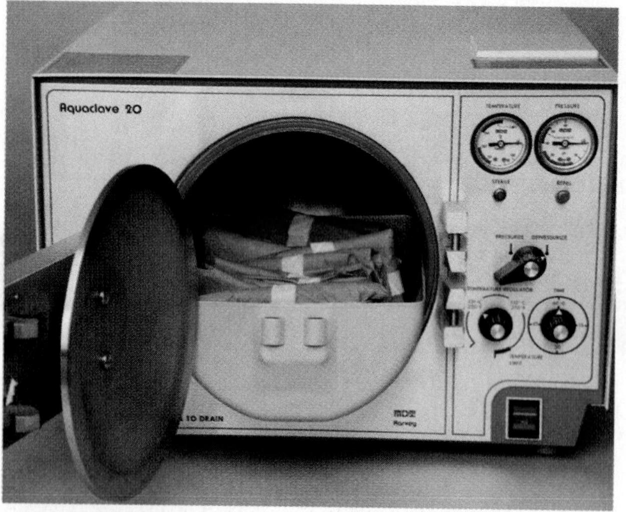

FIGURE 26–11 Autoclave. (Courtesy of Aquaclave by MDT.)

When the cycle is complete and the chamber cooled, the steam condenses and explodes the cells of microorganisms, thus destroying them. To be effective, all surfaces must be contacted by the moisture. Steam under pressure is capable of much faster penetration of fabrics and textiles than is dry heat, but it has definite limitations if the proper techniques are not followed.

Memory Jogger

14 *Why is steam the most accepted method of sterilization?*

The recommended temperature for sterilization in an autoclave is 250° F to 255° F. Unwrapped items should be sterilized for 20 minutes, small wrapped items for 30 minutes, and large or tightly wrapped items for 40 minutes.

Incorrect operation of an autoclave may result in *superheated* steam. If steam is brought to too high a temperature, it is literally dried out, and the advantage of a higher heat is diminished. *Wet* steam is another cause of incomplete sterilization. Wet steam results from failing to preheat the chamber, which results in excessive condensation in the interior of the chamber. Condensation is necessary, but too much prevents the sterilization process from coming to a proper completion. It can be compared to taking a hot shower in a cold bathroom, which results in heavily steamed mirrors, tile walls, and towels. If fabric packs become too saturated to dry during the drying cycle, the packs will pick up and absorb bacteria from the air or any surface they are placed on (Table 26–2). Cold instruments placed in a hot chamber also increase condensation. Other causes of wet steam include opening the door too wide during the drying cycle or allowing a rush of cold air into the chamber. Also, overfilling the water reservoir may produce this same effect.

The main cause of incomplete sterilization in the autoclave is the presence of residual air. Without the complete elimination of air, an adequately high temperature cannot be reached. Air and steam do not mix. Because air is heavier than steam, it will pool wherever possible. One tenth of 1% residual air trapped around an instrument will prevent complete sterilization. This is especially dangerous in older autoclaves that do not have a chamber thermometer separate from the pressure gauge. Chamber pressure does not guarantee a proper chamber temperature. All release valves and discharge lines must be kept clean and free from dirt and lint.

WRAPPING MATERIALS

The maintenance of sterility is completely dependent on the wrapper and its porosity as well as on the

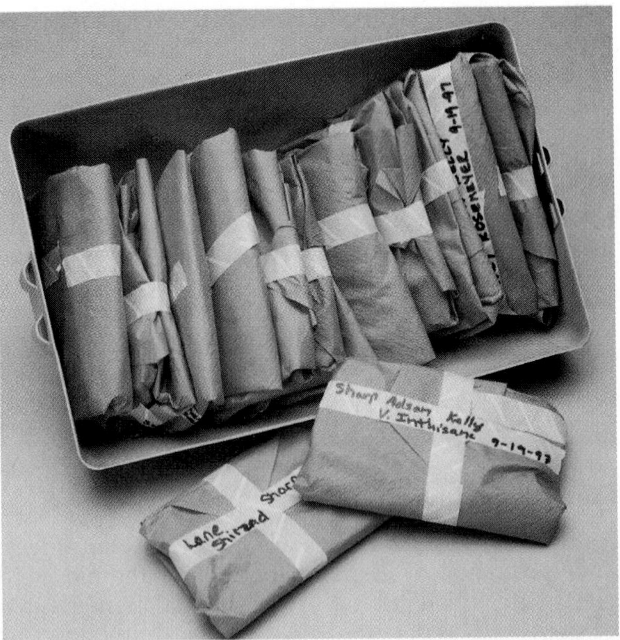

FIGURE 26–12 Autoclave paper wrap. Note chemical lines in tape.

method of wrapping. The wrapping material must be **permeable** to steam but impervious to contaminants such as dust and insects. A double thickness of material should be used.

Acceptable wrapping materials for autoclaving should be made of a substance that allows the steam to penetrate while preventing pathogens from entering during storage and handling. A wrapper should not be used if it is torn or has a hole in it. Clean muslin and disposable autoclave paper are examples of autoclave instrument wrap (Fig. 26–12).

WRAPPING INSTRUMENTS

The method used to wrap instruments for autoclave sterilization must allow the pack to be opened without becoming contaminated. To protect the package contents, the following rules are helpful:

1. Hinged instruments are wrapped in the open position to allow steam penetration.
2. Place a gauze sponge between the tips of sharp instruments to prevent the instrument from piercing through the wrap.
3. If a number of instruments are to be placed on a nonpermeable tray for wrapping, place a double-folded towel between the tray and the instruments to protect the instruments and absorb moisture.
4. When using sterilizing bags, insert the jaws of the instrument first to ensure that the grasping end of the instrument can be reached easily when the bag is opened.
5. Indicate on the wrapper what is in the package or prepare a list of what is in the package and store the list with the sterile package.
6. Label by identifying the contents, the date sterilized, and your initials. Use an indelible ink pen, *never* a ball-point pen because it may smear.

You may need to wrap several items into one wrapper; the procedure remains the same. Be sure to remember to pick a wrapper that will adequately cover the items to be sterilized.

INDICATORS

Sterilization is achieved only when steam reaches an optimum temperature for a designated length of time and has penetrated to the center of the articles. To eliminate the constant doubt of complete sterilization, *indicators* are used. These indicators show, by melting or by changing color, that a certain temperature for a given period of time has been reached, irrespective of pressure. There are several types of indicators. Some of the commonly used types are discussed here.

Autoclave Tape

This tape contains a chemical dye that will change color when exposed to steam (Fig. 26–13). It is not to be a sterilizing indicator independent of all other types. The tape does not make certain that proper sterilization time and temperature has been maintained, it just indicates that a high temperature has been reached while the article was in the autoclave. Its primary purpose is to give immediate verification that the package has been autoclaved.

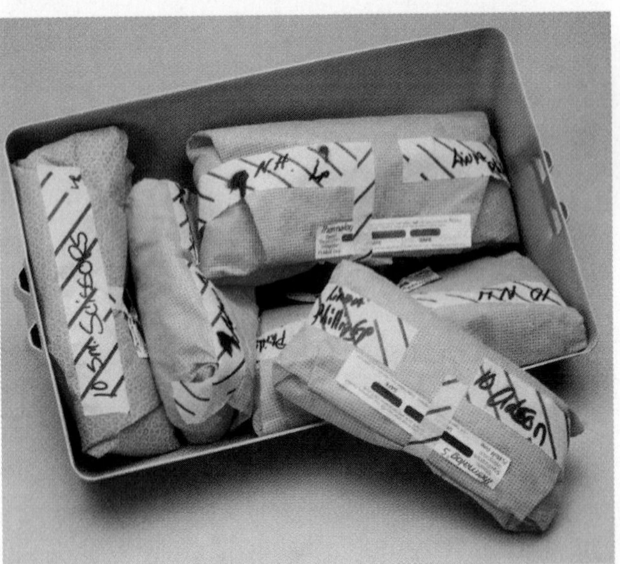

FIGURE 26–13 Autoclave wrapped instruments. Note strip indicators on packages.

Sterilization Indicator Strips

A popular strip indicator that is easy to use is one that contains a thermolabile (temperature-sensitive) dye that changes from white to black when the proper combination of steam, temperature, and time has been achieved. This type of indicator should be placed with each load in one of the following places:

- Buried deep in packs
- In constriction tubes
- In the bottom of containers that cannot be turned on their sides
- In places that might be inaccessible to the flow of steam

Culture Tube Test

Most types of sterilization indicators indicate effective sterilization by color changes. An example of an excellent system for testing the effectiveness of your office autoclave is the culture test. It is a bioindicator that consists of a double-walled tube that, when broken, releases a microorganism into a culture medium. If the sterilization cycle is defective and the microorganism still lives, growth should occur within 24 hours. It can be cultured in an office water bath or a dry block incubator. Another method for determining the efficiency of sterilization processes is the indicator that contains dried bacterial spores of established, heat-resistant organisms. These bacterial spore strips are available commercially from reliable suppliers, but the indicators are not always practical for a physician's office because the strip, after autoclaving, must be sent to a bacteriology laboratory for sterility testing.

When a culture tube is used in the sterilizing process, the tube should be clearly visible when looking into the autoclave. This tube is handled with care until the report comes back from the laboratory indicating that all spores are dead within the tube.

Every office will have the protocols to follow when doing a quality assurance evaluation of the autoclave. This is done at specific intervals of time depending on the volume of use that the autoclave undergoes. A record must be kept of the type of control test done, when it was done, and the testing results. If the testing results indicate that the sterilization was inadequate, a report indicating the method used to correct the problem will be completed and filed.

Sterilization Indicator Bags

Sterilization indicator bags are also very convenient. They are made of disposable paper or thermostable plastic, in which tubing and many other items can be sterilized and stored. The paper or transparent material is permeable to steam and provides a barrier against airborne bacteria during storage. Each bag has an indicator printed on it, similar to the sterilizer tape, which shows that the bag has been autoclaved but does not prove that its contents are sterile.

Memory Jogger

15 *What system is the most effective for testing the accuracy of the autoclave? Why?*

PROCEDURE 26-3

Wrapping Instruments and Supplies for Steam Sterilization

GOAL

To place dry, checked, sanitized supplies and instruments inside appropriate wrapping materials for sterilization and storage without contamination.

EQUIPMENT AND SUPPLIES

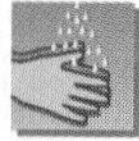

- Dry, checked, sanitized items
- Assorted wrapping materials
- Autoclave tape
- Indicator tape
- A waterproof felt-tipped pen

PROCEDURAL STEPS

1. Collect and assemble items to be wrapped.
2. Place the wrapper to be used on a clean flat surface.

Continued

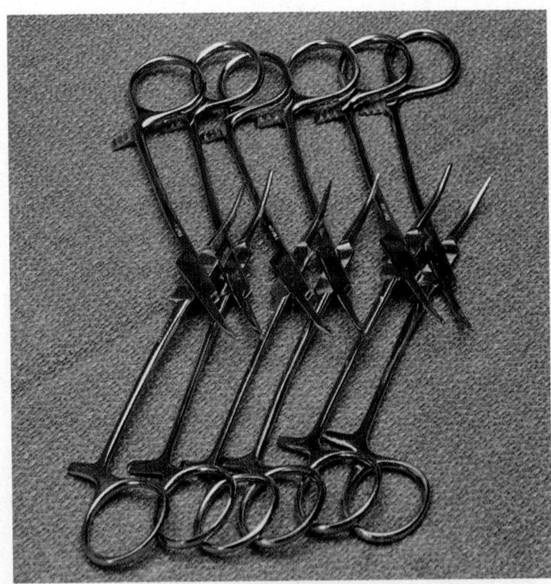

FIGURE 1

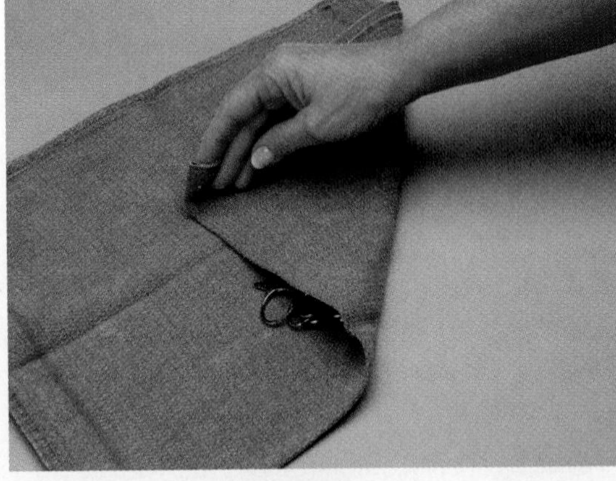

FIGURE 2

3. Place the item(s) diagonally at the approximate center of the wrapping material. Make sure the size of the square is large enough for the items (Figure 1).
   PURPOSE: Each of the four corners must fold over and completely cover the item(s), with a few extra inches of overlap for folding back a flap.
4. With the squares that are cloth fabric, use two pieces if the cloth is single layered, or follow the manufacturer's recommendation when using commercial autoclave wrapping paper.
   PURPOSE: To ensure sterility until the sterile item is needed for use.
5. Open slightly any hinged instruments. If the instrument is sharp, its teeth or tip should be shielded with cotton or gauze.
   PURPOSE: To prevent puncture of the package or the operator.
6. If the package is to contain several items, place a commercial sterilization indicator inside the package at the approximate center.
   PURPOSE: To ensure that the autoclave is reaching effective levels of heat and pressure.
7. Bring up the bottom corner of the wrap, and fold back a portion of it.
   PURPOSE: This folded-back flap is the only part of each wrapper corner that can be touched when opening a sterile package (Figure 2).
8. Fold over the right corner, and turn back a portion of it (Figure 3). Fold over the left corner, and turn back a portion of it (Figure 4).

Continued

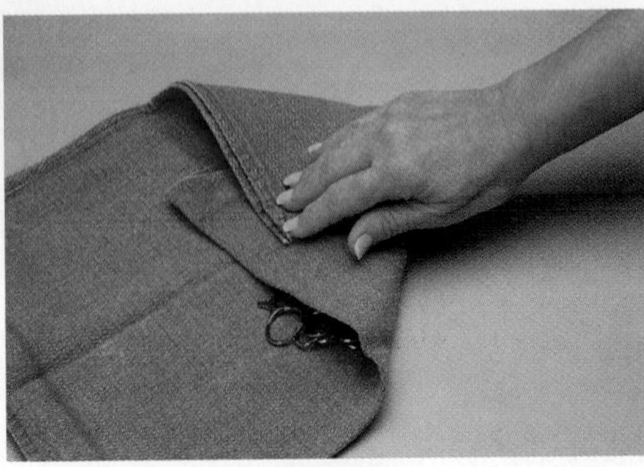

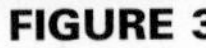

FIGURE 3

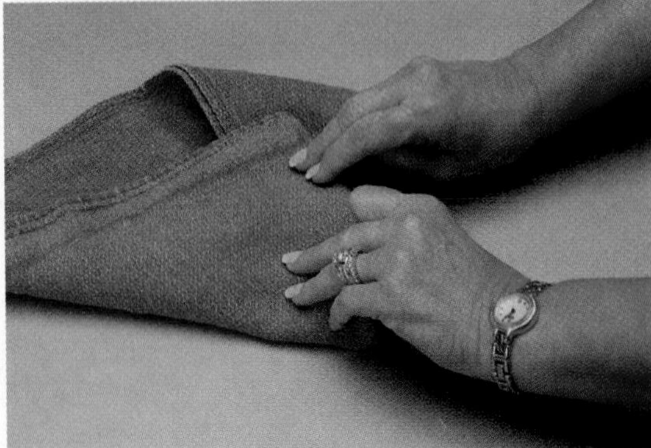

FIGURE 4

PROCEDURE 26-3 (CONTINUED)

Wrapping Instruments and Supplies for Steam Sterilization

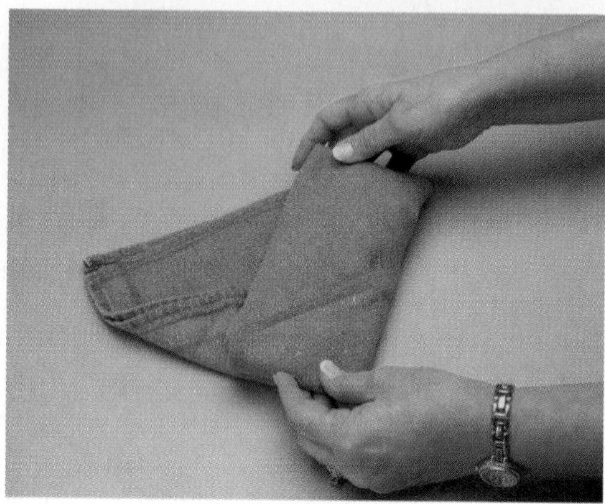

FIGURE 5

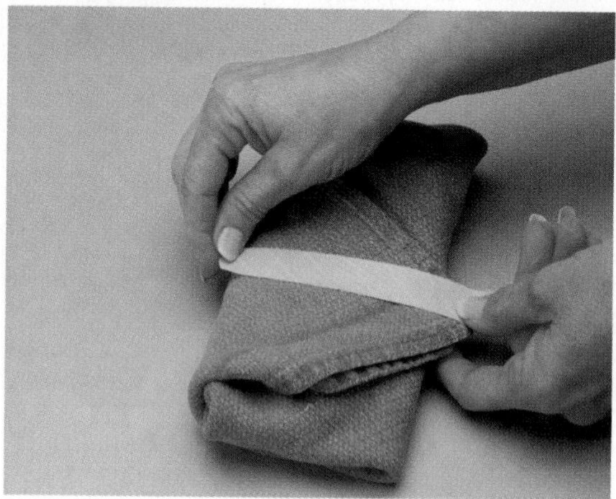

FIGURE 6

9. Fold the last flap over (Figure 5).
10. Secure with autoclave tape (Figure 6).
11. Secure with autoclave tape and label package with the date including year, contents, and your initials (Figure 7).
    PURPOSE: To know what is in the pack at a later date, whether or not the shelf life has expired (expiration date), and who performed the task. As a general rule, most office autoclaved packs are considered sterile (usable) for 30 days.

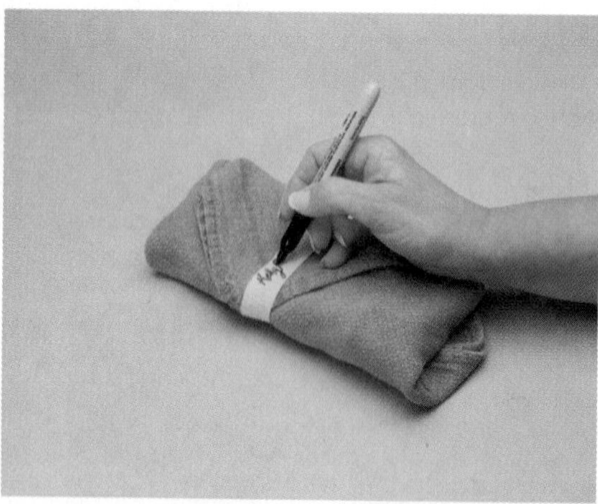

FIGURE 7

The Steam Autoclave

The office autoclave is similar to the home pressure cooker. It operates on the principle of steam under pressure. Water in an outer chamber, or jacket, is heated to produce steam. The pressure in this outer jacket builds and forces steam into the inner chamber. As steam is forced in, air is forced out. Visualize the air flowing out of the chamber as water flowing down a sink drain. Read the manufacturer's instructions carefully. An autoclave usually has three gauges: (1) the jacket pressure gauge, which indicates the steam pressure in the outer chamber; (2) the chamber pressure gauge, which indicates the steam pressure in the inner chamber; and (3) the temperature gauge, which indicates the temperature in the inner chamber, where the items are sterilized. When the temperature gauge reaches 250° F (121° C) and the pressure gauge indicates 15 pounds of steam pressure, the load of articles to be sterilized can be timed for the recommended length of time (Table 26–4).

TABLE 26–4 Sterilization Chart

Article	Method	Temperature	Time
Gauze, small, loosely packed	Autoclave	250° F	30 min
Gauze, large, loosely packed	Autoclave	270° F	30 min
Gauze, small, tightly packed	Autoclave	250° F	40 min
Gauze, large, tightly packed	Autoclave	270° F	40 min
Gauze, tightly packed	Dry heat	320° F	3 h
Gauze, loosely packed	Dry heat	320° F	2 h
Glass syringes in tubes	Autoclave	250° F	30 min
Glass syringe in muslin	Dry heat	320° F	1 h
Instruments on tray, muslin under and over	Dry heat	320° F	1 h
Instruments on tray, muslin under and over	Autoclave	250° F	15 min
Solutions in flasks with gauze plug	Autoclave	250° F	30 min
Glassware unwrapped	Dry heat	320° F	1 h
Glassware wrapped	Autoclave	250° F	30 min
Petroleum jelly, 1-oz jar	Dry heat	340° F	1 h
Petroleum jelly, 1-oz jar	Dry heat	320° F	2 h
Petroleum gauze in instrument tray	Dry heat	320° F	150 min
Powder, 1-oz jar	Dry heat	320° F	2 h
Powder, small glove packs	Autoclave	250° F	15 min

Remember to always place an indicator in areas where there is doubt that the steam will penetrate.

Do not measure by chamber pounds. A thermometer and indicator are the reliable methods of judging a killing temperature.

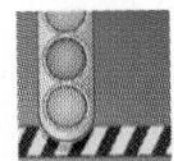

Safety Alert: The manufacturer's recommended time and/or pressure required for autoclaving must never be shortened because items will not be sterile when cycle is completed.

CLEANING AND MAINTENANCE

The autoclave chamber must be cleaned after each load. If the load contained containers filled with solutions, check for possible overflow of some of the solution into the autoclave. If there has been boiling over of solutions, the water reservoir must be drained and thoroughly cleaned and rinsed. Check the manufacturer's instructions carefully and do not use a commercial cleaner unless advised by the manufacturer. A mild detergent may be used in the chamber, but make certain the chamber is very thoroughly rinsed after any type of cleaner has been used.

The trays must also be kept clean and free of lint. Be sure to replace the bottom (chamber) tray after cleaning; it must be in place for proper steam circulation. Periodically check the rubber gasket in the door for cracks or tears because this will interfere with the sealing of the door when it is closed. The air exhaust valve is one of the most important parts of the autoclave and must be clean and free of lint, otherwise the air will not exhaust from the chamber. Unless proper care is taken of the autoclave, the dressings and instruments will have been *well heated but not sterilized.* Table 26–5 provides tips to improve autoclaving techniques.

LOADING THE AUTOCLAVE

Prepare all packs and arrange the load in such a manner to allow maximum circulation of steam and heat. Articles should be placed so that they rest on their edges, to permit proper permeation of the materials with moisture and heat (Fig. 26–14). Under no conditions should you permit the crowding of packs into tight masses.

Jars, bottles, and trays must be wrapped and placed on their sides if they are to be used to store sterile items. Covers on jars and containers should be put to one side or left ajar to allow steam to circulate. Extreme care must be taken not to contaminate the jars when replacing the lids after autoclaving is complete.

Instruments may be autoclaved unwrapped if they are to be used immediately or do not need to be sterile when used later. Perforated trays are used for sterilizing unwrapped instruments. Place a lint-free towel under and over the instruments to facilitate

TABLE 26–5 Tips for Improving Autoclaving Techniques

Problem	Causes	How to Correct
Damp linens	Clogged chamber drain	Remove strainer; free openings of lint.
	Goods removed from chamber too soon after cycle	Allow goods to remain in sterilizer an additional 15 min with door slightly open.
	Improper loading	Place packs on edge; arrange for least possible resistance to flow of steam and air.
Stained linens	Dirty chamber	Clean chamber with Calgonite solution; never use strong abrasives, such as steel wool; rinse thoroughly after cleaning.
Corroded instruments	Poor cleaning; residual soil	Improve cleaning; do not allow soil to dry on instruments; sanitize first.
	Exposure to hard chemicals (e.g., iodine, salt, and acids)	Do not expose instruments to these chemicals; if exposure occurs, rinse immediately.
	Inferior instruments	Use only top-quality instruments.
Spotted or stained instruments	Mineral deposits on instruments	Wash with soft soap and detergent with good wetting properties.
	Residual detergents from cleaning	Rinse instruments thoroughly.
	Mineral deposits from tap water	Rinse with distilled water.
Instruments that have soft hinges or joints	Corrosion or soil in joint	Clean with warm, weak acid solutions (10% nitric acid solution); rinse thoroughly.
	Jaws and shanks out of alignment	Have realignment done by qualified instrument repair professional.
Ebullition, or caps that blow off solutions	Exhausting chamber too rapidly	Use slow exhaust, cool liquids, or turn autoclave off and let cool on its own; that is, let the pressure decrease at its own rate.
Steam leakage	Worn gasket	Replace.
	Door closes improperly	Reopen door and shut carefully; have serviced if unable to close door properly.
Chamber door does not open	Vacuum in chamber (check chamber pressure gauge)	Turn on controls to starting steam pressure; wait until equalized, then vent and open door.

drying and to prevent contamination when removing them from the autoclave.

UNLOADING THE AUTOCLAVE

When the sterilization cycle is complete, release the pressure with the control setting. Once the pressure gauge reads "0" stand back from the door and, with oven mitts, open the door about a fourth of an inch. Allow the load to dry for at least 15 minutes (this will vary according to the type of autoclave and the size of the load). *Capillary attraction* is the term describing the force that draws moisture through surfaces of materials. Materials act like a sponge. Any moisture outside the pack contains microorganisms, which, in turn, are drawn into the pack with the moisture. Touching a wet pack will allow the microorganisms on your hands to penetrate the wrappings and to render the contents nonsterile. Dry, wrapped packs may be removed with clean, dry hands, but it is safer to wear oven mitts to reduce the possibility of burns from the hot instruments inside the packs. If possible, allow all packs to cool in the autoclave with the door open. Place the packs on a dry, dust-free surface, inside an enclosed cupboard or drawer for storage. Avoid cold surfaces, because the hot packs may cause condensation and moisture will contaminate the contents.

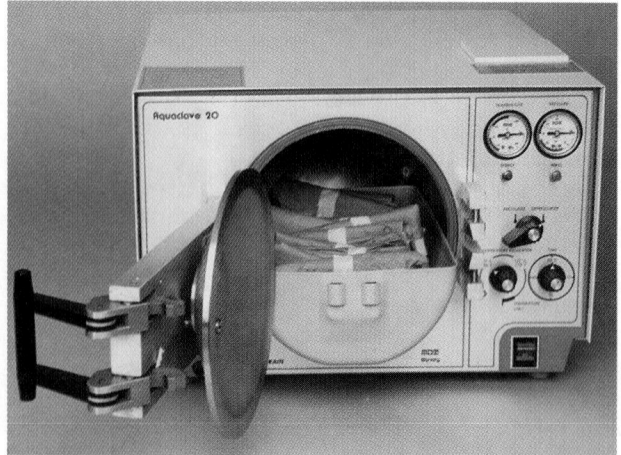

FIGURE 26–14 Articles placed so that they rest on their edges to permit proper permeation.

Memory Jogger

Why does touching a wet package render the contents nonsterile?

STORAGE OF WRAPPED SUPPLIES

Although experts do not agree on the length of time that wrapped supplies remain sterile, shelf-life rules are fairly standard.

PROCEDURE 26-4
Using the Steam Autoclave

GOAL
To sterilize properly prepared supplies and instruments, using the autoclave.

EQUIPMENT AND SUPPLIES
An autoclave
Wrapped items ready to be sterilized

PROCEDURAL STEPS
1. Check the water level in the reservoir and add distilled water as necessary.
   PURPOSE: Too much or too little water may alter the effectiveness of the equipment. Tap water will leave lime deposits in the chamber.
2. Turn the control to "fill" to allow water to flow into the chamber. The water will flow until you turn the control to its next position. Do not let the water overflow.
3. Load the chamber with wrapped items, then space them for maximum circulation and penetration.
   PURPOSE: Ensure sterilization of all items.
4. Close and seal the door.
   PURPOSE: The door must be closed or the heated water in the chamber will evaporate.
5. Turn the control setting to "on" or "autoclave" to start the cycle.
6. Watch the gauges until the temperature gauge reaches at least 250° F (121° C) and the pressure gauge reaches 15 pounds of pressure.
   PURPOSE: Proper temperature and pressure must be reached before sterilization can begin.
7. Set the timer for the desired time.
8. At the end of the timed cycle, turn the control setting to vent.
   PURPOSE: This releases the steam and pressure. The water at the bottom of the chamber will drain back into the reservoir.
9. Wait for the pressure gauge to reach zero.
10. Open the chamber door a fourth of an inch.
    PURPOSE: To allow steam to escape faster.
11. Leave the autoclave control at vent to continue producing heat.
    PURPOSE: To dry the items faster.
12. Allow complete drying of all articles.
13. Using heat-resistant gloves or pads, remove the items from the chamber and place the sterilized packages on dry, covered shelves or open door and allow items to cool.
14. Turn the control knob to "off," and keep the door slightly ajar.
    PURPOSE: Allows the inside of the autoclave to dry completely.

STANDARD SHELF-LIFE RULES TO MAINTAIN STERILE SUPPLIES

- Double-wrapped muslin and double-wrapped paper packs are considered sterile up to 28 days from the date of sterilization.
- Nonpermeable plastic-wrapped packs are considered sterile up to 6 months from the date of sterilization. (Most medical offices do not have the equipment to sterilize supplies in nonpermeable packages. Purchased nonpermeable packs will have expiration dates printed on the outside.)
- All supplies should be stored on dry, dust-free, covered shelves or in drawers. Fabric wrappers must be relaundered. A damaged pack or a broken seal renders the package nonsterile. Spills of any fluid onto a package render the pack nonsterile. When a pack is no longer sterile because of a broken seal or an expiration date that has passed, the contents must be reprocessed starting with the sanitization process.

Gas Sterilization

There are considerable differences among the various gas sterilizers on the market, and each manufacturer has its own set of conditions necessary to achieve sterilization. The major disadvantages with the use of gas sterilization are time and the general hazards connected with using gas. The length of exposure time is usually 1½ to 2 hours, although exposure times sometimes can be lessened by slightly increasing the temperature. Another disadvantage is the time required for aeration after sterilization. Sterilizers must be properly vented to reduce human exposure to the gas. In August 1984, standards were issued by OSHA. If you work with ethylene oxide gas, you should have a copy of these standards on the premises. The human hazards of gas sterilization include the possibility of damage to the reproductive organs of the operator as well as the development of cancer from prolonged exposure to high concentrations of ethylene oxide, making gas sterilization unrealistic for use in the physician's office.

The Medical Assistant's Role in Asepsis

Medical asepsis is one of the very few procedures that directly affect the health of the patient, physician, and office staff. The spread of pathogens in the office can be controlled only through effective sterilization of all reusable equipment.

The medical assistant must develop an inner sense for aseptic procedures. It is important that these techniques be done on such a routine basis that they become an unbreakable habit. Conscientious attention must be given to sterilizing *all* items at *all* times. Frequent rechecking of the solutions and techniques helps to ensure that the procedures employed are effective. The use of disposable items is highly recommended in the control of the infection process, and these items have become commonplace in many offices. However, when disposable equipment is used, the assistant must be conscious of disposal guidelines and provide the office and the environment with continuous protection.

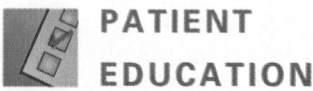

PATIENT EDUCATION

The best time to instruct your patients in aseptic techniques that they can use at home is while you are performing the aseptic procedure. For example:

- While hand washing explain to the patient that this routine is part of daily hygiene and is particularly important for patients who are very young or old or who seem to get sick frequently. Discuss with the patient that hands should be washed before and after meals; after sneezing, coughing, or nose blowing; after using the bathroom; before and after changing a bandage; and after changing an infant's diaper.
- Explain to the patient how using disposable tissues to cover the nose and mouth when coughing or sneezing decreases the possibility of transmitting illness between household members.
- Discuss proper ways for disposing of used tissues, especially when one member of the household is suspected of having a communicable disease.
- Instruct the patient regarding the differences between sterile and clean dressings and bandages. Show him or her step by step how to change a dressing properly and then how to dispose of the contaminated items.

There are many ways that the medical assistant can help the patient. Thinking up creative ideas for patient education might be a project for the office staff. Here are a few more suggestions to educate and inform the patient about asepsis and infection control:

1. Set up an information table in the waiting room with take-home pamphlets and literature.
2. Mail a periodical newsletter to patients.
3. Demonstrate and explain aseptic procedures to patients, inviting them to participate.

Sometimes in the course of a general conversation, the medical assistant can pick up hints of concerns that the patient has and can direct the conversation into a discussion of these concerns.

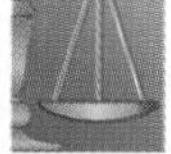

LEGAL AND ETHICAL RESPONSIBILITIES

A number of legal and ethical concerns are related to medical asepsis and infection control in the medical office. Personal discipline is the primary concern in medical asepsis. Often, the assistant is alone when performing a medical aseptic procedure; if contamination occurs, no one may know except the medical assistant. It is the medical assistant's responsibility to begin the procedure again with clean supplies if it is believed that contamination has occurred. One of the medical assistant's main responsibilities is to carry out sterilization and disinfection procedures with precision and with total effectiveness. There is no room for compromise. Patients should have absolute assurance that they are being taken care of in an aseptic atmosphere and under aseptic conditions. This assurance is just as important for the protection of the physician and staff as it is for the patient.

Allowing the physician to assume that the correct aseptic techniques have been employed in the preparation of equipment and allowing him or her to use contaminated equipment on a patient can result in claims of malpractice. Honesty on the part of the assistant builds self-respect and contributes to professional achievement.

To have a good understanding of the subject, you must become familiar with the various techniques of sterilization and disinfection. Ignorance or carelessness can be dangerous and is inexcusable before the law.

Memory Jogger

17 *Describe your responsibilities in medical asepsis and infection control.*

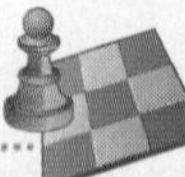

CRITICAL THINKING

1 How would you handle a fellow employee who continuously comes to work with a runny nose and cough?

2 A patient becomes upset when you put on gloves. How might you explain your actions?

3 You drop and break a glass container of supplies. How would you proceed to clean it up?

4 Last night you cut your finger at home. What must you do to protect yourself against potential infection today at work?

5 You need to sterilize the gauze and applicator containers in the exam rooms. How would you do this?

6 In obtaining the scissors requested by the physician, you drop the instrument on the floor. Now what?

HOW DID I DO? Answers to Memory Joggers

1 We carry microorganisms
a. On our skin
b. In our bodies
c. On our clothing

2 The chain of infection starts at the reservoir host → means of exit → means of transmission → susceptible host → who now becomes a reservoir host.

3 The four classic symptoms of inflammation are
a. Redness
b. Swelling
c. Pain
d. Heat

4 A latent infection is a persistent infection with symptoms that come and go. A chronic infection is a persistent infection in which the virus is present for long periods of time.

5 Antibiotics will not destroy viruses because viruses incorporate themselves into the DNA and RNA inside the invaded cell.

6 Three ways to avoid infections are
a. Avoid infected places
b. Get vaccinated
c. Isolate people who are infected

7 Body fluids that are considered potentially dangerous are
a. Blood
b. Cerebrospinal
c. Pleural
d. Pericardial
e. Peritoneal
f. Amniotic
g. Vaginal
h. Seminal
i. Unknown

8 Items of clothing considered barrier protection include
a. Gloves
b. Face masks
c. Face shields
d. Protective eye wear
e. Laboratory coats
f. Barrier gowns

9 90 mL of water + 10 mL of bleach = 100 ml of 10% disinfectant solution

10 An exposure control plan includes
a. Exposure determination
b. Method of compliance
c. Postexposure evaluation and follow-up
d. Information to health care provider
e. Health care provider's written opinion
f. Medical record keeping

11 Medical asepsis is freedom from infection or infectious materials. Surgical asepsis is destruction of organisms before possible entry into the body.

12 Sanitation is reducing the number of microorganisms to a level that is relatively safe.

13 Chemicals can lose their effectiveness if
a. Instruments are not left in solution long enough.
b. Sanitized instruments are not dried.
c. The solution is left to evaporate.
d. Solutions have expired.
e. Solutions are mixed improperly.
f. Recommended temperatures are not maintained.

14 The most accepted method of sterilization is the steam autoclave.

15 The most accurate system for determining autoclave accuracy is the culture tube test.

16 Capillary attraction will render the contents nonsterile.

17 Your responsibility in medical asepsis and infection control is to ensure asepsis and infection control in every procedure.

Vital Signs and Anthropometric Measurements

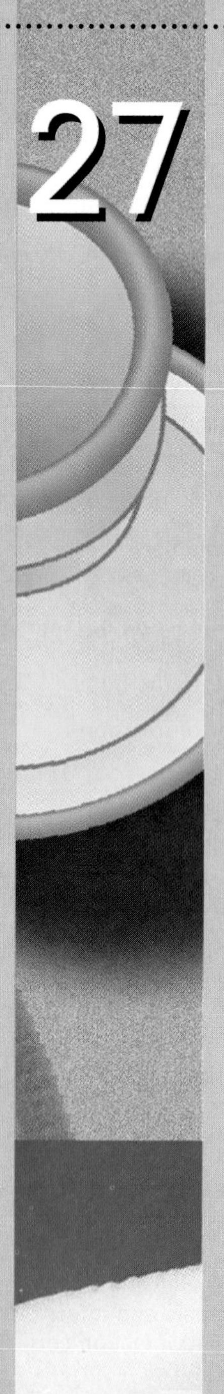

OUTLINE

LEARNING OBJECTIVES

Cognitive: On successful completion of this chapter you should be able to:

1. Define and spell the words in the Vocabulary.
2. Cite the average values of body temperatures, pulse rates, respiratory rates, and blood pressure.
3. Describe how emotional and physical factors cause body temperature to increase or decrease.
4. Identify the 24-hour patterns for three types of fevers.
5. List six methods for obtaining a patient's temperature.
6. Describe pulse rate, volume, and rhythm.
7. List four important characteristics to note when taking a pulse.
8. List six respiratory rate variations.
9. Describe the best way to obtain accurate respiration counts.

10 List four physiologic factors affecting blood pressure.
11 Differentiate between essential and secondary hypertension.
12 Describe the methods for obtaining weight and height of a patient.
13 Identify patient education possibilities.
14 Describe legal and ethical responsibilities in obtaining vital signs.

Performance: On successful completion of this chapter you should be able to:
1 Locate eight pulse sites.
2 Identify the different Korotkoff phases.
3 Convert kilograms to pounds and pounds to kilograms.
4 Complete all chapter procedures at the satisfactory level determined by your instructor.

VOCABULARY

apnea Absence or cessation of breathing
arrhythmia Irregular heart rhythm
bounding pulse Pulse characterized by increased tension
bradycardia A slow heartbeat; a pulse below 60 beats per minute
bradypnea Respirations that are regular in rhythm but slower than normal in rate
cerumen A waxy secretion in the ear canal; commonly called *ear wax*
dyspnea Difficult or painful breathing
elastic pulse Pulse with regular alterations of weak and strong beats without changes in cycle
essential hypertension Elevated blood pressure of unknown cause that develops for no apparent reason; sometimes called *primary hypertension*
homeostasis Internal adaptation and change in response to environmental factors
hyperpnea Increased rate of respiration
hypertension High blood pressure (systolic pressure consistently above 160 mm Hg and diastolic pressure above 90 mm Hg)
hyperventilation Abnormally prolonged and deep breathing usually associated with acute anxiety or emotional tension
hypotension Blood pressure that is below normal (systolic pressure below 90 mm Hg and diastolic pressure below 50 mm Hg)
intermittent pulse Pulse in which beats are occasionally skipped
irregular pulse Pulse that varies in force and frequency
otitis media Inflammation of the middle ear
orthopnea Breathing in an upright position
orthostatic (postural) hypotension Temporary fall in blood pressure when a person rapidly changes from a recumbent position to a standing position
pulse deficit Difference between the apical pulse and the radial pulse
pulse pressure Difference between the systolic and the diastolic blood pressures (less than 30 points or more than 50 points is considered normal)
rales Abnormal or crackling chest sounds during breathing
remittent fever Fever in which temperature fluctuates greatly but never falls to the normal level
rhonchi Rattling noises in the throat that may resemble snoring
secondary hypertension Elevated blood pressure due to another condition
sinus arrhythmia Irregular heartbeat originating in the sinoatrial node (pacemaker)
stertorous Describing a deep snoring sound that occurs with each inspiration
tachypnea Respirations that are regular in rhythm but faster than normal in rate
thready pulse Pulse that is scarcely perceptible
unequal pulses Difference felt between right and left radial and/or femoral pulse counts

The measurement of vital signs is an important aspect of almost every visit a patient makes to the medical office. These signs are the human body's indicators of internal **homeostasis** and represent the general state of health of the patient. Because the medical assistant is chiefly responsible for obtaining these measurements, it is imperative for you to have confidence in both their theoretical and practical applications. When the principles of and the reasons for these measurements are understood, you will become a valuable asset to any medical office.

Accuracy is essential. A change in one or more of the patient's vital signs may indicate a change in general health. Variations may indicate the presence or disappearance of a disease process and, therefore, a change in the treatment plan. Although you will obtain vital signs routinely, it is not a routine task. These findings are crucial to a correct diagnosis, and you should never perform them with indifference or casualness. In addition to accurate measurement, you must use care when charting your findings on the patient's medical record.

The vital signs are the patient's temperature, pulse, respiration, and blood pressure. These four signs are abbreviated *TPR* and *BP* and may be referred to as *cardinal signs.* It is the medical assistant's duty to understand the significance of the vital signs and to accurately measure and record them. Anthropometric measurements are not considered vital signs but are usually obtained at the same time as the vital signs. These measurements include height, weight, and other body measurements, such as fat composition and head and chest circumference.

Memory Jogger

 *What are vital signs?*

Factors That May Influence Vital Signs

The vital signs are influenced by many factors, both physical and emotional. A patient may have consumed a hot or cold beverage just before the examination or may be angry or afraid of what the doctor may find. For example, your patient has been asked to return to have a repeat Papanicolaou test because the first one showed the presence of unidentifiable cells. You take her blood pressure and find it to be markedly elevated when compared with previous readings. It may be possible, even probable, that this individual is suffering from anxiety and is apprehensive about the test results. What type of a temperature reading would you expect on a patient who couldn't find a parking place and had to walk four blocks to the office and knew he would be late for his appointment? If you said it would be elevated, you are right. Certainly this patient would have an increase in his metabolism because of the physical exercise, and, as a result, his temperature would be elevated along with his pulse and probably his respirations. Most patients, for one reason or another, are apprehensive during an office visit. These emotions may alter the vital signs, and it is necessary for the medical assistant to help the patient relax before taking any readings. It sometimes is necessary to obtain some measurements a second time, after the patient is calmer or more comfortable. To obtain a better picture of the patient's vital signs, you may be asked to record the vital signs twice: at the beginning of the visit and just before the patient leaves the office.

Temperature

PHYSIOLOGY

Body temperature is defined as the balance between the heat lost and the heat produced by the body. It is measured in degrees. The process of chemical and physical change within our bodies that produces heat is called *metabolism.* Body temperature is a result of this process. Examples of the factors that may elevate body temperature include respiration, muscle activity, emotional changes, and reproductive activities. Temperature elevation may also be caused by external factors, such as the temperature of the environment. A healthy person's temperature varies slightly during the day, depending on both internal and external stimuli.

In illness, the individual's metabolic activity is increased; this causes internal heat production to increase, which, in turn, increases body temperature. The increase in body temperature is thought to be the body's defensive reaction, because heat is believed to inhibit the growth of some bacteria and viruses.

When a fever is present, superficial blood vessels near the surface of the skin constrict. The small papillary muscles at the bases of hair follicles also constrict and cause goosebumps. Chills and shivering follow, causing internal heat to be produced. As this process repeats itself, more heat is produced, and body temperature becomes elevated or increases above normal levels. When more heat is lost than is produced, the opposite effect occurs and body temperature drops below normal levels.

A variation from the patient's average range of body temperature may be the first warning of an illness or change in the patient's present condition.

Average body temperature varies from person to person and is at different levels at different times in each person. The daily average oral temperature of a healthy person may vary from 97.6° F to 99° F (36.4° C to 37.3° C), with the average daily temperature being 98.6° F. The lowest body temperature occurs in the early morning (from 2 AM to 6 AM). The highest body temperature occurs in the evening (from 5 PM to 8 PM). Body temperature may vary to a greater degree and is generally higher in an infant or young child than in an adult.

Memory Jogger

A variation from the patient's average range of body temperature may indicate ________?

FEVER

Fever usually accompanies infection and many other disease processes. If the average temperature of the healthy patient is 98.6° F (37° C), a fever is present when the oral temperature is 99.2° F (37.3° C) or higher. Temperatures of 104° F (40° C) or higher indicate a possible serious illness.

Fevers are classified according to the 24-hour pattern they follow. The three most commonly seen patterns are illustrated in Figure 27–1. As you look at the temperature charts you notice the following:

1. Continuous fever rises and falls only slightly during the 24-hour period. It remains above the patient's average normal range and is called continuous because that is exactly what the pattern shows.
2. Intermittent fever comes and goes, or it spikes and then returns into average range. Notice the pattern: around 10 AM it begins to elevate, it reaches its maximum at about 3 PM and by 12 AM it is back into average range; thus it is an intermittent fever.
3. Remittent fever has great fluctuation but never gets back into the average range. It is a constant fever with fluctuating levels and thus is remittent.

Memory Jogger

Describe the difference between an intermittent and a remittent fever.

TEMPERATURE READINGS

A clinical thermometer is used to measure body temperature and is calibrated in either the Fahrenheit or the Celsius scale. The Fahrenheit (F) scale has been used most frequently in the United States to measure body temperature, but hospitals often use the Celsius scale (Table 27–1). The thermometer is placed under the tongue, in the rectum, in the ear, or in the axilla because large blood vessels are near the surface at these points. The average temperature

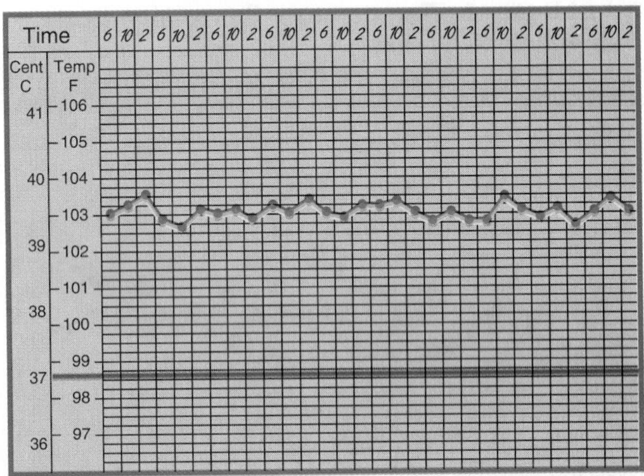

A

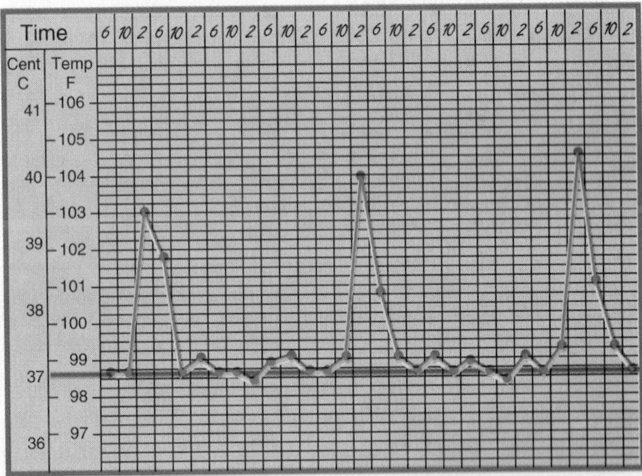

B

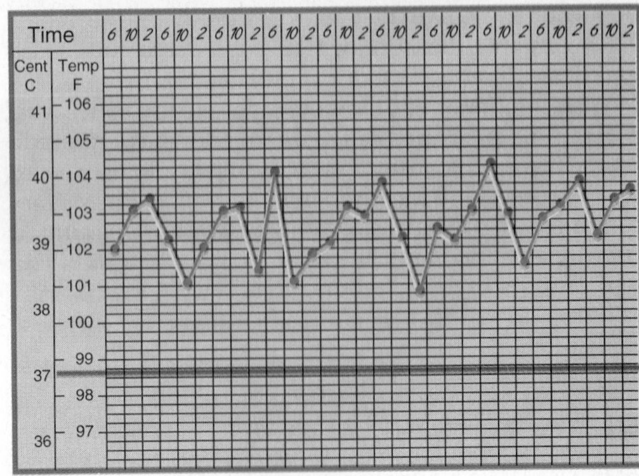

C

FIGURE 27–1 Common temperature patterns. *A*, Continuous fever. *B*, Intermittent fever. *C*, Remittent fever.

values for these four sites, based on statistical survey, are shown in Table 27–2.

Rectal temperatures, when taken accurately, are approximately 1° F or 0.6° C higher than oral readings. Axillary temperatures are approximately 1° F or 0.6° C lower than accurate oral readings. Tym-

TABLE 27–1 Temperature Conversion Scale: Fahrenheit to Celsius*

F	C	F	C	F	C
95.0	35.0	100.2	37.9	105.4	40.8
95.2	35.1	100.4	38.0	105.6	40.9
95.4	35.2	100.6	38.1	105.8	41.0
95.6	35.3	100.8	38.2	106.0	41.1
95.8	35.4	101.0	38.3	106.2	41.2
96.0	35.5	101.2	38.4	106.4	41.3
96.2	35.6	101.4	38.5	106.6	41.4
96.4	35.7	101.6	38.6	106.8	41.5
96.6	35.9	101.8	38.7	107.0	41.6
96.8	36.0	102.0	38.8	107.2	41.8
97.0	36.1	102.2	39.0	107.4	41.9
97.2	36.2	102.4	39.2	107.6	42.0
97.4	36.3	102.6	39.3	107.8	42.1
97.6	36.4	102.8	39.4	108.0	42.2
97.8	36.5	103.0	39.5	108.2	42.3
98.0	36.6	103.2	39.6	108.4	42.4
98.2	36.8	103.4	39.7	108.6	42.5
98.4	36.9	103.6	39.8	108.8	42.6
98.6	37.0	103.8	39.9	109.0	42.7
98.8	37.1	104.0	40.0	109.2	42.9
99.0	37.2	104.2	40.1	109.4	43.0
99.2	37.3	104.4	40.2	109.6	43.1
99.4	37.4	104.6	40.3	109.8	43.2
99.6	37.5	104.8	40.4	110.0	43.3
99.8	37.6	105.0	40.5		
100.0	37.7	105.2	40.6		

*To convert degrees F to degrees C, subtract 32, then multiply by 5/9. To convert degrees C to degrees F, multiply by 9/5, then add 32.

panic temperature is measured the same as oral temperature. Rectal temperature measurements are considered the most accurate because the mucous membrane lining with which the thermometer comes in contact is not exposed to the air; thus, it does not vary like that of the mouth or the axilla. The tympanic measurement is considered the fastest and easiest method.

When obtaining temperatures using the oral method of measurement, you do not have to indicate it when recording the reading. You do record an R for rectal, T for tympanic, and an A for axillary readings. In pediatrics, the temperature reading is usually obtained by the rectal or tympanic method, and an O is used for an oral reading.

Memory Jogger

4 *Identify the four body sites used for obtaining temperature readings. Give the average normal value for each site.*

TABLE 27–2 Average Temperature Values

Site	Fahrenheit Scale	Celsius Scale
Oral	98.6°	37°
Rectal	99.6°	37.6°
Axillary	97.6°	36.4°
Tympanic	98.6°	37°

Types of Thermometers and Their Usage

GLASS

A glass thermometer has a short, blunt mercury bulb that allows surface contact with tissues when it is placed in the mouth under the tongue, in the axilla, or during rectal insertion. The upper tips are usually colored for identification. Red is used for rectal measurement, clear is used for axillary measurement, and blue is used for oral measurement (Fig. 27–2).

The mercury in the bulb of the glass thermometer expands on contact with warm body tissue. In 3 minutes, the mercury registers its highest reading and no longer expands. The reading is obtained by viewing the calibration scale on the thermometer and noting the highest point reached by the mercury. Because the glass thermometer measures heat, it will not cool down or decrease in reading, unless shaken.

The longest lines on all glass thermometers represent 1 degree of temperature. On the Fahrenheit scale, the shorter lines represent 0.2-degree increments; and on the Celsius scale, the lines represent 0.1-degree increments (Fig. 27–3).

Because of the risk of cross-contamination of body fluids, the glass thermometer has been replaced in many offices and hospitals by disposable thermome-

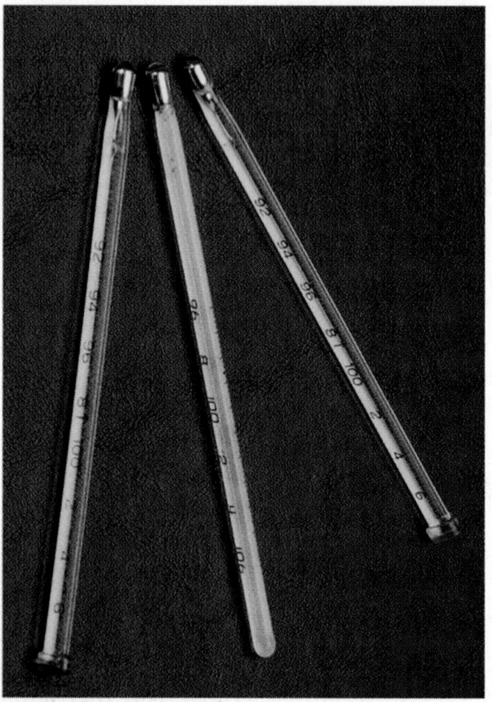

FIGURE 27–2 Glass thermometer. Note the red and blue tips indicating oral and rectal, respectively. The middle thermometer is universal but not used for rectal readings.

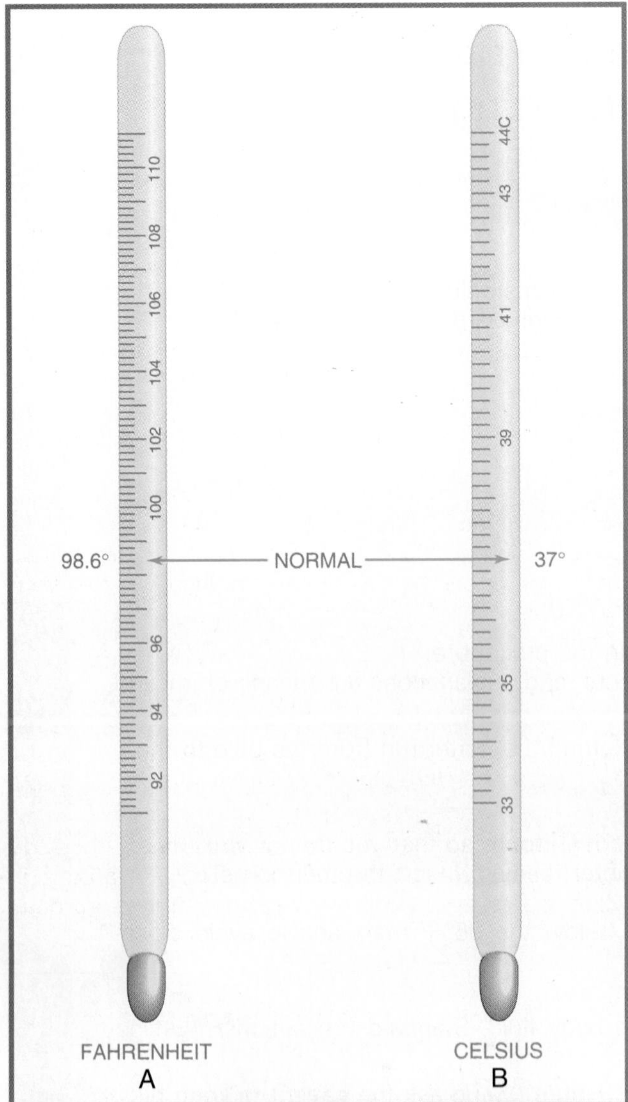

FIGURE 27–3 Comparing Fahrenheit (*A*) and Celsius (*B*) scales. Normal body temperature is about 98.6° F or 37° C when measured orally.

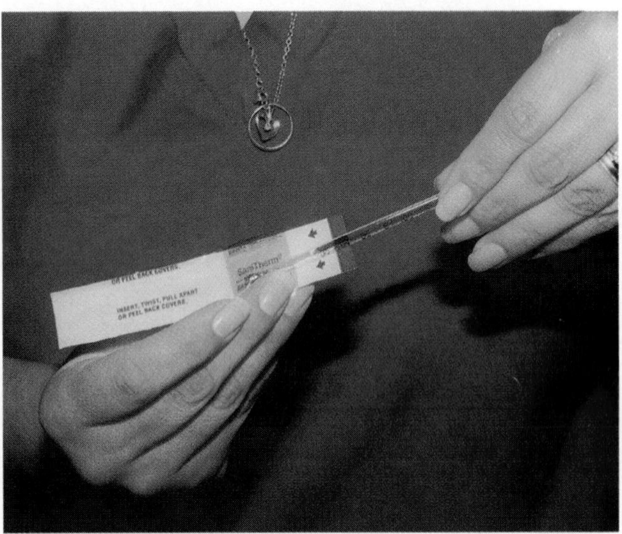

FIGURE 27–4 Thermometer with disposable sheath.

ters or a tympanic or an electronic device. If a glass thermometer is used, a disposable plastic sheath should be placed over it to ensure cleanliness (Fig. 27–4) (see Procedure 27–1).

Always rinse the thermometer clean before placing it in the plastic sheath. Lower the mercury column to below 95° F (35° C) by shaking the thermometer with a snap of the wrist. Be sure to hold the thermometer tightly between your thumb and forefinger at the end opposite the bulb. Be careful not to strike the thermometer against a hard object, because the glass will break and the mercury will spill. Such spills require special handling because mercury is a poisonous substance.

ELECTRONIC

Electronic thermometers have become increasingly popular and are available in both Fahrenheit and Celsius scales. They are battery operated and can be

PROCEDURE 27–1

Obtaining an Oral Temperature Using a Glass Thermometer

GOAL

To accurately determine and record a patient's temperature as part of the patient assessment using a glass thermometer.

Continued

PROCEDURE 27-1 (CONTINUED)
Obtaining an Oral Temperature Using a Glass Thermometer

EQUIPMENT AND SUPPLIES

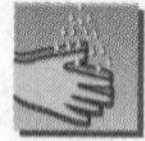
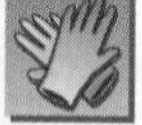
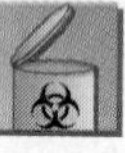

Oral Fahrenheit thermometer
Thermometer sheaths
A supply of tissues
Nonsterile gloves
Biohazard waste container

PROCEDURAL STEPS

1 Read the physician's order.
2 Wash your hands.
PURPOSE: Infection control.
3 Gather equipment and supplies.
4 Introduce yourself, identify your patient, and explain the procedure.
PURPOSE: Identification of the patient prevents errors, and explanations are means of implied consent.
5 Rinse the thermometer under cool running water, letting the water run from the bulb to the tip (Figure 1).
PURPOSE: To remove antiseptic solution.
6 Shake down the thermometer, allowing yourself enough room so that you do not strike it against an object and break it. Check the thermometer reading. Insert the thermometer mercury end first into a disposable sheath (Figure 2).
PURPOSE: To force the column of mercury to fall below the 95° F mark and to avoid cross-contamination.
7 Put on gloves.
PURPOSE: When there is a possible exposure to a body fluid, Standard Precautions must be followed.
8 Place the thermometer under the patient's tongue (Figure 3) and ask the patient to keep his or her lips firmly closed and to breathe through the nose. Caution the patient not to bite the thermometer (Figure 4).
PURPOSE: Air seeping into the mouth interferes with an accurate body temperature reading, and biting may cause it to break.

Continued

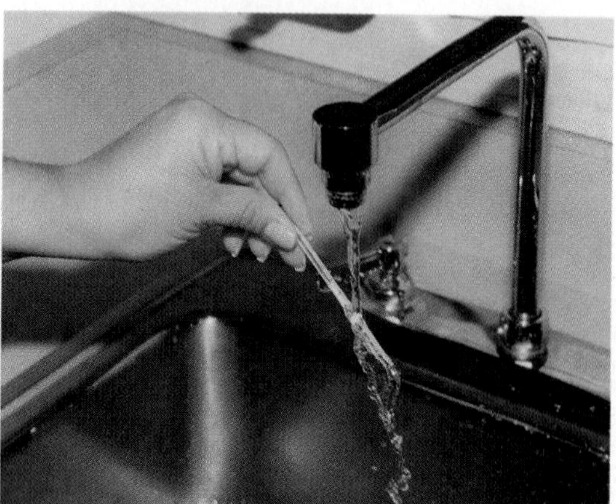

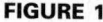

FIGURE 1

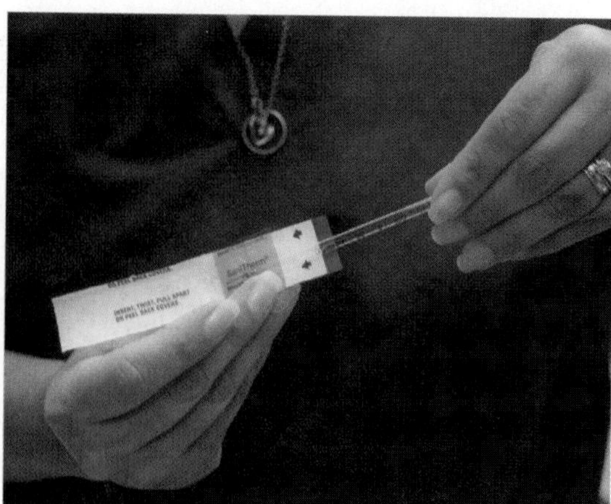

FIGURE 2

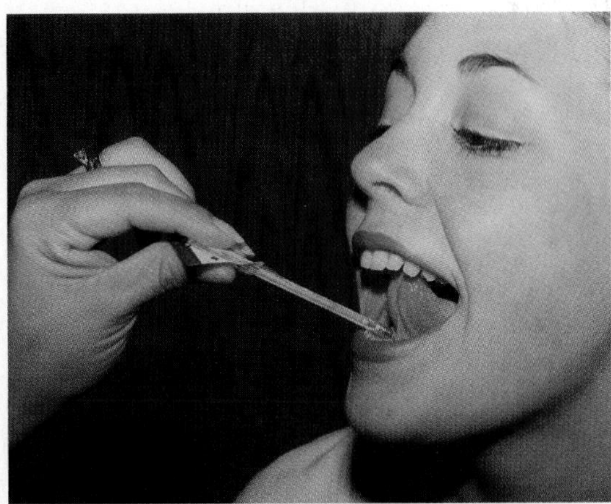

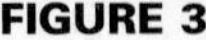

FIGURE 3

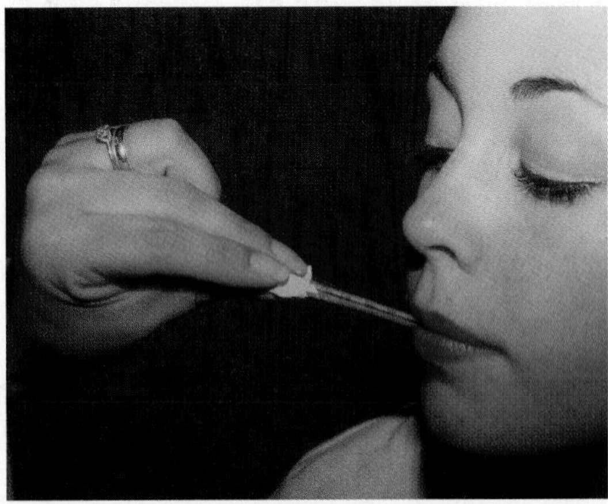

FIGURE 4

9 Advise the patient that the thermometer needs to be held in place for at least 3 minutes.
PURPOSE: This is the required time to obtain an accurate oral reading.

10 Remove the thermometer, peel off the protective sheath, and discard the sheath in the appropriate waste container (Figure 5).
PURPOSE: Makes the mercury column easier to read and reduces the risk of cross-contamination.

11 Read the thermometer, making certain that you hold it at eye level. Look for the silver column of mercury, and follow it until it ends. Align the end of the column to the scale marked in degrees (Figure 6).
PURPOSE: Holding the thermometer at eye level facilitates an easier and more accurate reading.

12 Shake down the mercury column to below the 95° F mark.

13 Wash the thermometer with soap and cool water, rinse, and dry. Place it into the designated disinfectant for the recommended length of time.
PURPOSE: Thermometers must be thoroughly washed, dried, and disinfected before being returned to their containers for use with another patient.

14 Remove gloves, discard in appropriate container, and wash your hands.

15 Record the temperature reading on the patient's medical record. Record it as T = 98.6°
PURPOSE: Procedures that are not recorded are considered not done.

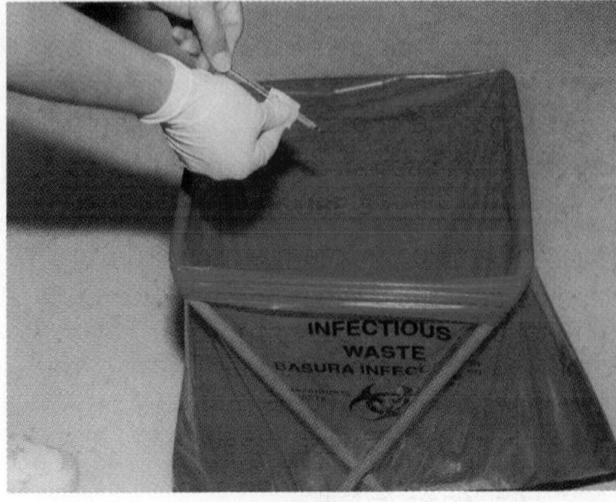

FIGURE 5

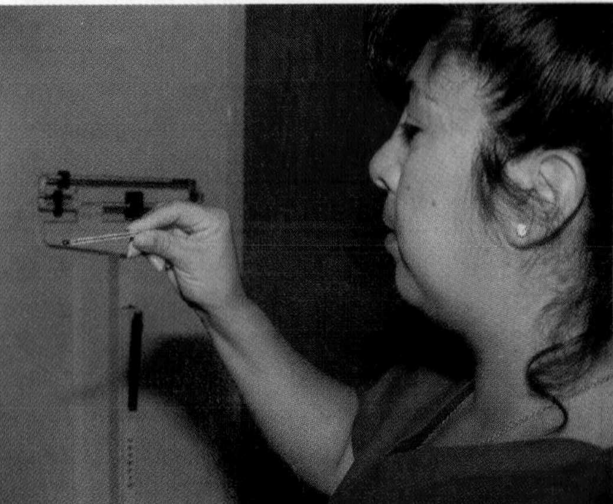

FIGURE 6

PROCEDURE 27-2

Obtaining an Oral Temperature Using an Electronic Thermometer

GOAL

To accurately determine and record a patient's temperature using an electronic thermometer.

EQUIPMENT AND SUPPLIES

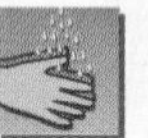
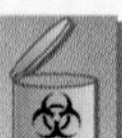

Electronic thermometer
Probe covers
Biohazard waste container

PROCEDURAL STEPS

1 Wash your hands and assemble equipment and supplies.
PURPOSE: Infection control.

2 Identify your patient and explain the procedure.
PURPOSE: Identification of the patient prevents errors, and explanations are means of implied consent.

Continued

held in your hand for convenient use. The unit is equipped with two probes: a blue one for oral use and a red one for rectal use only. A disposable cover fits snugly over the probe and is easily and quickly removed by pushing in the colored end of the probe (see Procedure 27–2). The instrument sounds an audible "beep" when the process is complete (between 10 and 60 seconds), and the reading appears on a digital screen located on the face of the instrument. Because the only part of the instrument that comes in contact with the patient is the probe, and that is sheathed, the risk of cross-infection is greatly reduced (Fig. 27–5).

TYMPANIC

The tympanic membrane of the ear can also be used for the quick, accurate, and safe assessment of a patient's temperature. It shares the blood supply that reaches the hypothalamus, which is the brain's temperature regulatory control. Because the ear canal is lined with skin rather than mucous membrane, the risk of spreading communicable diseases during temperature measurement is greatly reduced.

The tympanic measurement system consists of a hand-held processor unit equipped with a tympanic probe that is covered with a disposable speculum when being used (Fig. 27–6). When the probe is

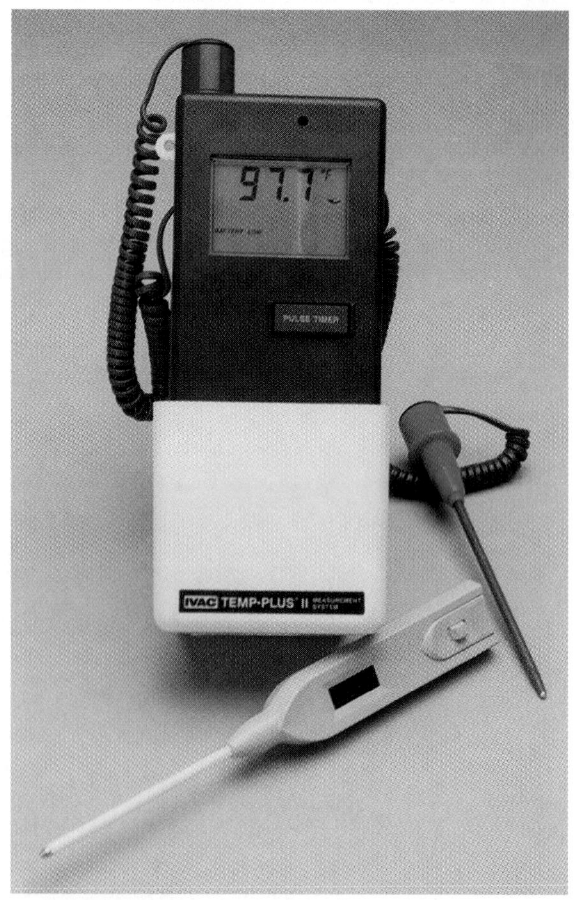

FIGURE 27–5 Electronic thermometers.

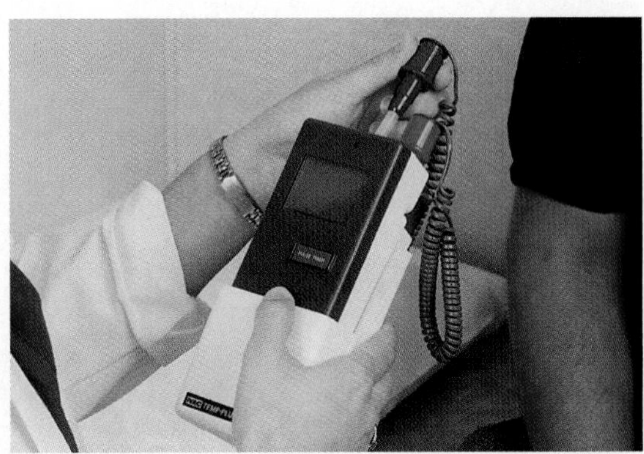

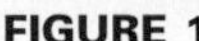

FIGURE 1

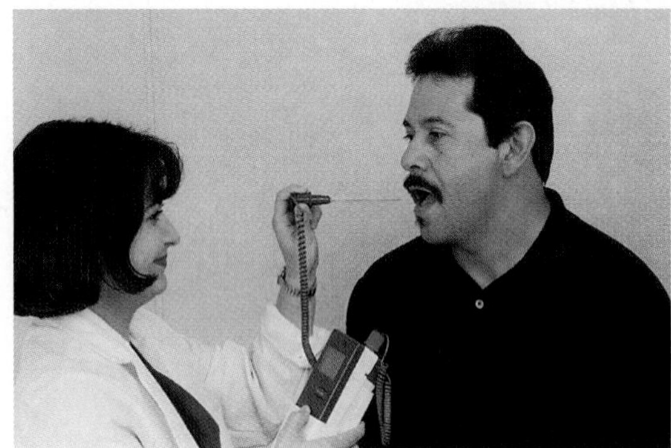

FIGURE 2

3 Prepare the probe for use as described in the "directions for usage" (Figure 1).

4 Place the probe under the patient's tongue (Figure 2), and instruct the patient to close the mouth tightly (Figure 3). Assist the patient by holding the probe end.
PURPOSE: Air seeping into the mouth interferes with an accurate body temperature reading. Probe is heavier than glass and hard to hold tightly.

5 When the "beep" is heard, remove the probe from the patient's mouth and immediately eject the probe cover into the appropriate waste container.
PURPOSE: Probe cover will be contaminated.

6 Note the reading in the LED window of the processing unit you are holding (Figure 4).

7 Record the reading on the patient's medical record as T = 97.7°.
PURPOSE: Procedures that are not recorded are considered not done.

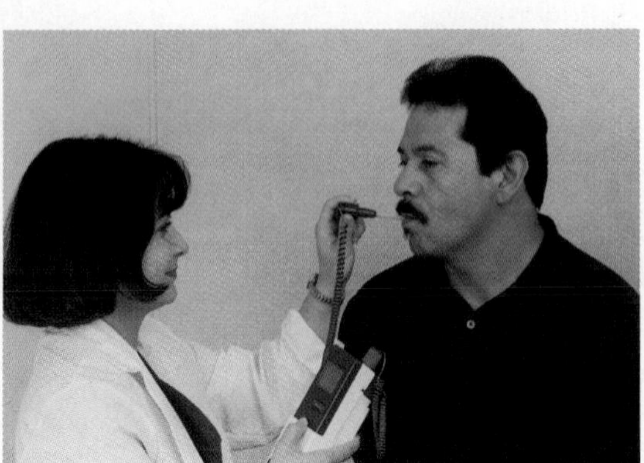

FIGURE 3

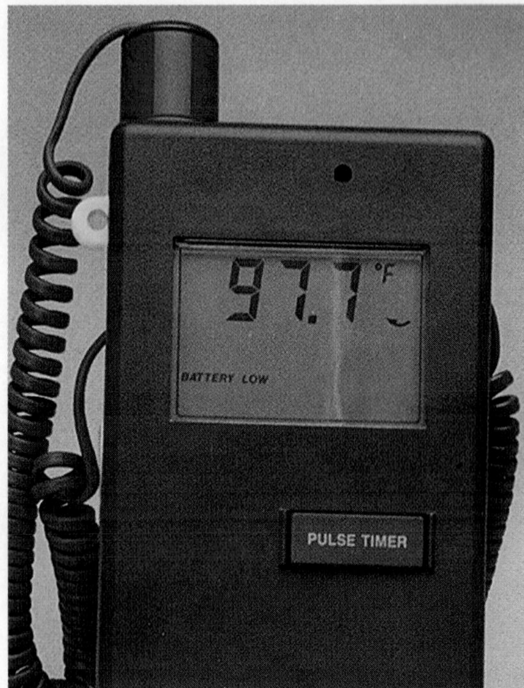

FIGURE 4

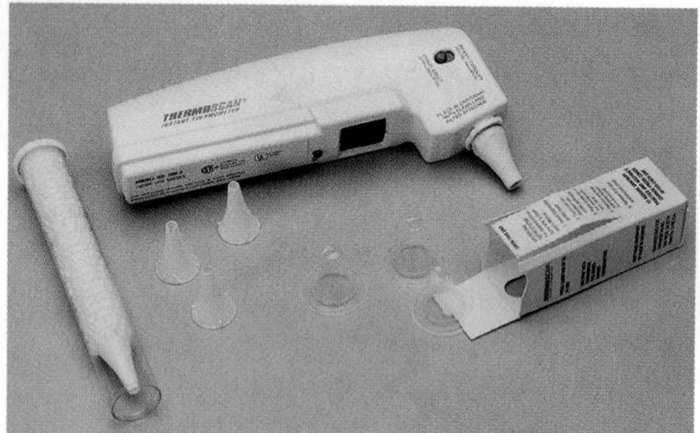

FIGURE 27–6 Tympanic thermometer.

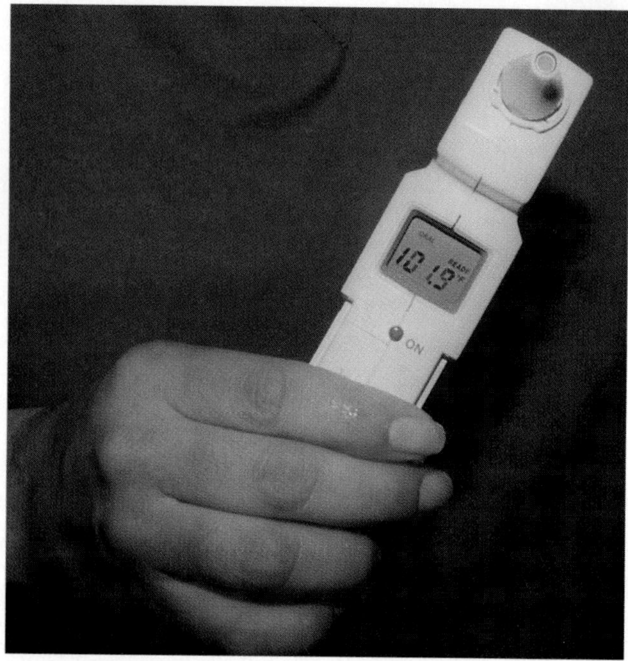

FIGURE 27–7 LED read-out on tympanic thermometer.

placed into the ear canal, it gently seals the external opening of the ear canal and the infrared energy emitted by the tympanic membrane is gathered. This signal is then digitalized by the processor unit and shown on the display screen (Fig. 27–7). Accurate readings are obtained in approximately 2 seconds (see Procedure 27–3). The speed and patient comfort have greatly influenced the popularity of the tympanic thermometer. This unit should not be used if the patient has **otitis media** or impacted **cerumen** or is in an increased emotional state. Physicians have found the readings to be occasionally inaccurate in such situations.

Memory Jogger

 *Why are tympanic thermometers so popular?*

PROCEDURE 27–3

Obtaining an Aural Temperature Using the Tympanic System

GOAL

To accurately determine and record a patient's temperature using the tympanic membrane.

EQUIPMENT AND SUPPLIES

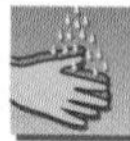 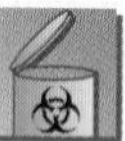

Tympanic thermometer
Disposable probe covers
Biohazard waste container

PROCEDURAL STEPS

1 Wash your hands.
PURPOSE: Infection control.

2 Gather the necessary equipment and supplies.

3 Identify your patient and explain the procedure.
PURPOSE: Identification of the patient prevents errors, and explanations are means of implied consent.

Continued

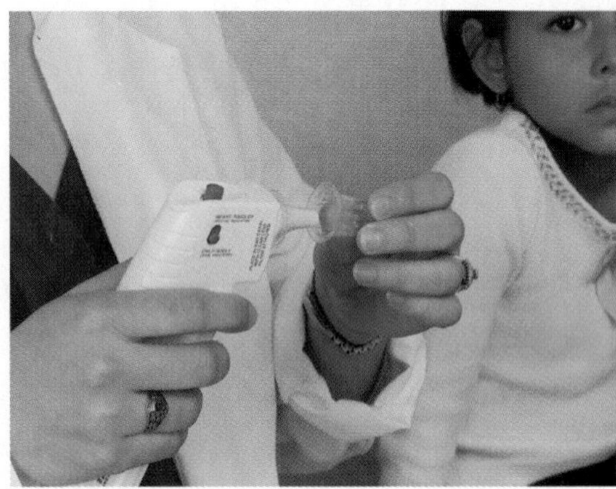

FIGURE 1

4 Place disposable probe cover on probe, avoiding sharp edges (Figure 1).
PURPOSE: To ensure a clean surface and prevent cross-contamination.

5 Engage the thermometer by pressing the "start" indicator.

6 Insert the probe into the ear canal far enough to seal the opening. Do not apply pressure (Figure 2).
PURPOSE: Air seeping around the probe interferes with an accurate body temperature reading.

7 Press the "temp" button on the probe. The temperature will be on the display screen in 1 to 2 seconds.

8 Remove the probe, note the reading (Figure 3), and discard the probe cover.
PURPOSE: The probe cover will be contaminated and must be disposed of in a biohazard waste container.

9 Wash your hands.
PURPOSE: Infection control.

10 Record temperature results as T = 98.6° (T) on the patient's medical record.
PURPOSE: Procedures that are not recorded are considered not done.

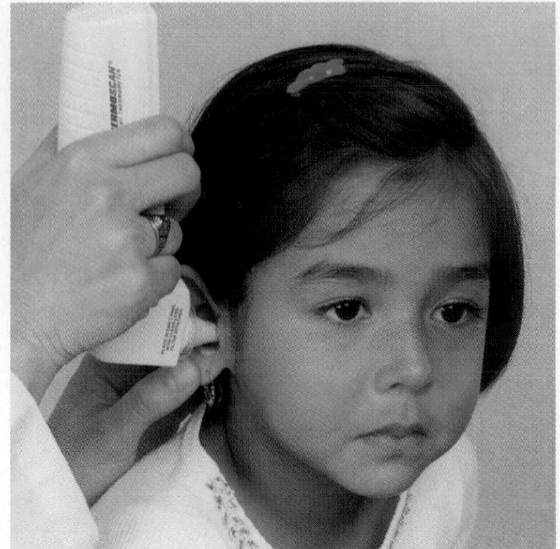

FIGURE 2

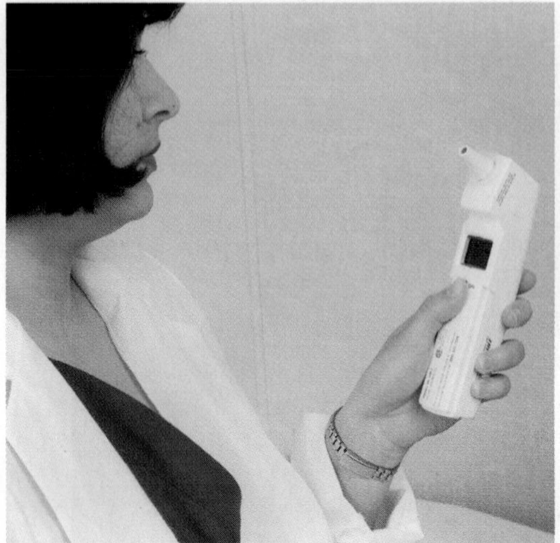

FIGURE 3

PROCEDURE 27-4

Obtaining Temperature Using a Disposable Thermometer

GOAL

To accurately determine and record a patient's body temperature using a disposable thermometer.

EQUIPMENT AND SUPPLIES

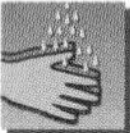

Forehead thermometer
Tissue
Watch with sweep second hand

PROCEDURAL STEPS

1 Wash your hands.
PURPOSE: Infection control.

2 Gather needed supplies.

3 Identify your patient and explain the procedure. Be sure that the patient has not eaten, drunk fluids, or exercised for 30 minutes before taking the temperature.
PURPOSE: Temperature will be inaccurate if food or fluids have been ingested or exercise has been done within 30 minutes.

4 Peel off the disposable thermometer's protective tape, exposing the adhesive.

5 Center the thermometer strip on clean dry forehead just above the eyebrow level.
PURPOSE: Forehead must be dry for adhesive to stick to the skin.

6 Press the thermometer strip firmly to the forehead (Figure 1).

7 Leave strip in place until colors stop changing; approximately 20 seconds.

8 Green indicates the correct temperature; if green does not appear, your temperature will be midway between that indicated by the tan and blue (Figure 2).

9 Remove the strip, and wipe any excess adhesive from the patient's forehead.

10 Record the temperature results on the patient's medical record.
PURPOSE: Procedures that are not recorded are considered not done.

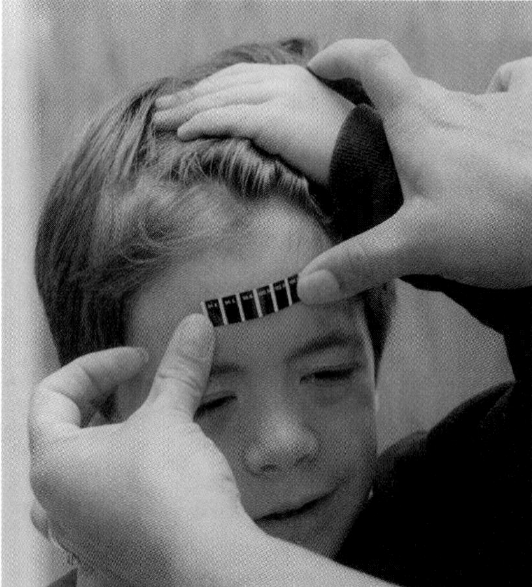

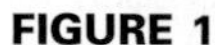

FIGURE 1

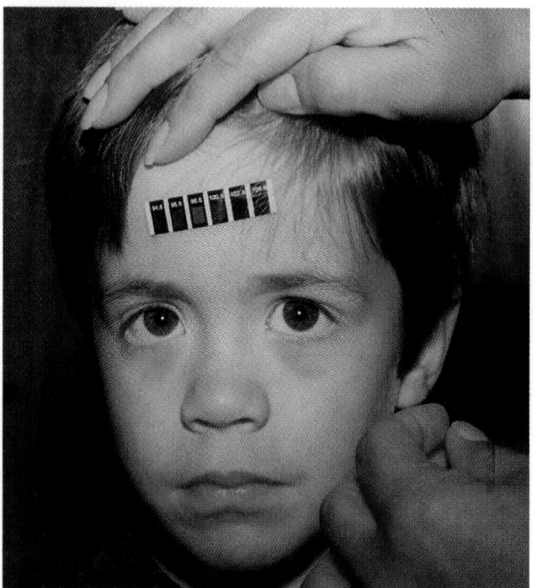

FIGURE 2

DISPOSABLE

Disposable thermometers (those that are used only once) are also available for obtaining body temperatures. They are frequently used in the home on small children. The reading is obtained by a heat-sensitive material that changes color according to the elevation of body temperature (see Procedure 27–4). There are two types of disposable thermometers that are frequently used by parents of young children. One type is placed on the child's forehead (Fig. 27–8*A*), and the other is placed under the tongue (Fig. 27–8*B*). Both methods are fairly reliable, but both carry expiration dates, which often are overlooked. These methods are considered good screening methods but not as accurate as the electronic or the tympanic thermometers.

RECTAL

The rectal method is usually required for the very young patient, patients with breathing difficulties, patients who are uncooperative or unconscious, or when the axillary method cannot be used. The procedure is the same as for the oral method, except the bulb or probe (sheath) must be lubricated with a water-soluble jelly (see Procedure 27–5). The patient's temperature will register on the glass thermometer within 3 minutes and on the electronic probe in 10 to 60 seconds. Stay with the patient. Adults should be kept in the prone or Sims' position, with their toes pointed inward, until the thermometer is removed. Place an infant in the supine position. Hold the legs straight up with one hand, and hold the thermometer in place with the other. Alternatively, restrain the small child in the prone position with one hand at the buttocks, and hold the thermometer in place with the other (Fig. 27–9). You must *never* leave the thermometer in an infant or child without you or the parent holding onto the thermometer and the child's feet.

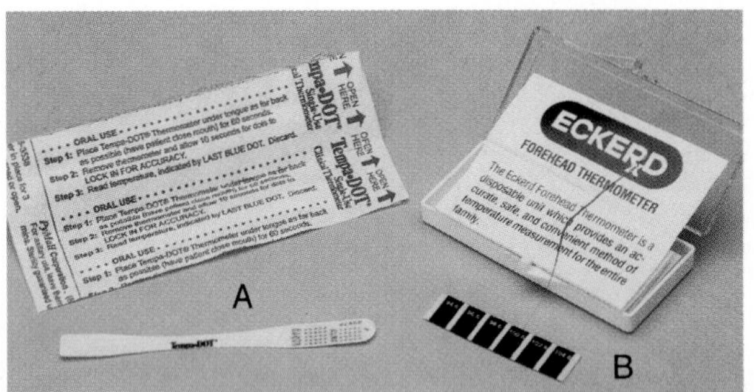

FIGURE 27–8 *A*, Tempa-Dot disposable oral strip thermometer. (Courtesy of Tempa-Dot, Sommerville, NJ.) *B*, Eckerd forehead disposable thermometer. (Courtesy of Eckerd, San Jose, CA.)

Memory Jogger

When might it be necessary to take a rectal temperature?

AXILLARY

Recent studies reveal that the axillary temperature is very accurate when performed correctly. Axillary temperatures take more time to register the correct body temperature, but the method is safe, simple, and easily accessible (see Procedure 27–6). It may be the method of choice when obtaining temperatures on patients who have had facial or oral surgery or are mouth breathers, patients using oxygen, and/or patients who have recently ingested hot or cold liquids. When taking an axillary temperature using the electronic thermometer use the oral (blue) probe and prepare it in the same manner as you did for the oral thermometer. When using a glass thermometer, the use of a sheath is not required but it is a healthy practice to follow.

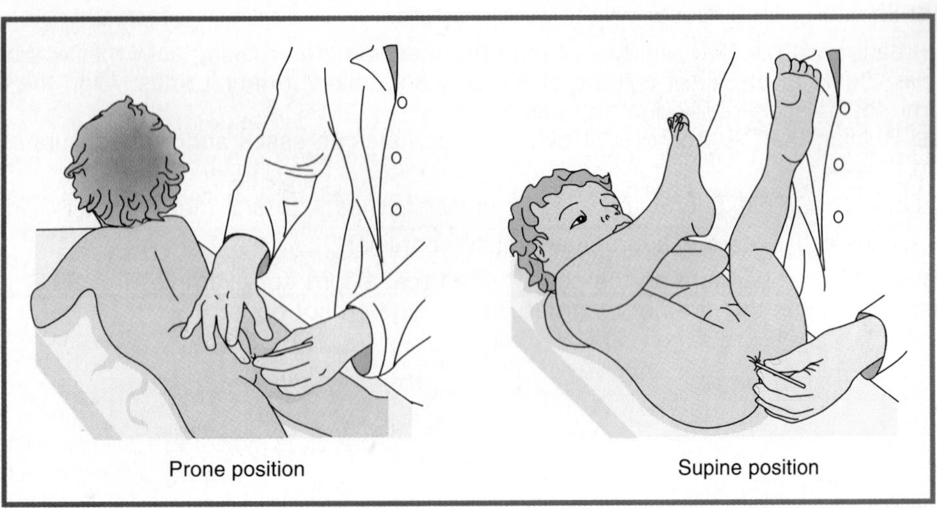

FIGURE 27–9 Rectal temperature taken with child prone or supine with legs elevated.

PROCEDURE 27-5

Obtaining Temperature Using the Rectal Method

GOAL

To accurately determine and record a patient's temperature using the rectal method.

EQUIPMENT AND SUPPLIES

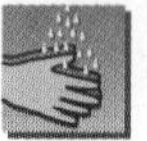

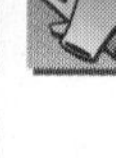

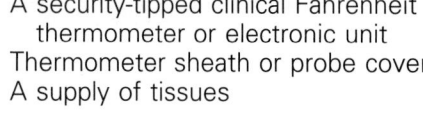

- A security-tipped clinical Fahrenheit thermometer or electronic unit
- Thermometer sheath or probe cover
- A supply of tissues
- Alcohol sponge
- Nonsterile gloves
- Biohazard waste container

PROCEDURAL STEPS

1 Wash your hands.
PURPOSE: Infection control.

2 Gather equipment and supplies.

3 Introduce yourself, identify your patient, and explain the procedure.
PURPOSE: Identification of the patient prevents errors, and explanations are means of implied consent.

4 Prepare thermometer using a lubricated sheath or electronic unit in the same manner as done for oral usage.
PURPOSE: Covering prevents cross-contamination.

5 Put on gloves.
PURPOSE: When there is a possible exposure to body fluid, Standard Precautions must be followed.

6 Place adult patient in Sims' position.
PURPOSE: This position will make the insertion of the probe easier and more comfortable to the patient.

7 Hold the glass thermometer in place for 3 minutes or the electronic probe until it "beeps."
PURPOSE: Due to normal peristaltic movement, the probe will not stay in place unless it is held.

8 Remove the thermometer, remove the sheath, and discard the sheath in waste container. Or remove the probe and immediately eject the used probe into the appropriate waste container.
PURPOSE: Sheath or probe cover will be contaminated.

9 Note the reading on the LED window or read the thermometer, making sure that you hold it at eye level. Look for the silver column of mercury and follow it until it ends. Align the end of the column to the scale marked in degrees.
PURPOSE: Holding the thermometer at eye level facilitates an easier and more accurate reading.

10 If glass thermometer has been used, clean and disinfect as with oral thermometer.

11 Remove gloves and discard in appropriate waste container.

12 Record the rectal temperature on the patient's medical record; for example, T = 99.6° (R).
PURPOSE: Procedures that are not recorded are considered not done.

PROCEDURE 27-6

Obtaining an Axillary Temperature

GOAL

To accurately determine and record a patient's temperature using the axillary method.

EQUIPMENT AND SUPPLIES

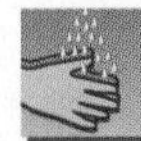
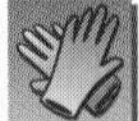
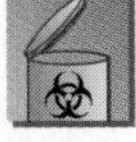
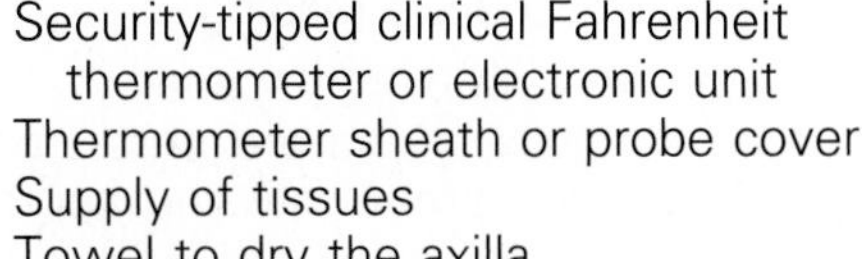

- Security-tipped clinical Fahrenheit thermometer or electronic unit
- Thermometer sheath or probe cover
- Supply of tissues
- Towel to dry the axilla
- Alcohol sponge
- Nonsterile gloves
- Biohazard waste container

PROCEDURAL STEPS

1 Wash your hands.
PURPOSE: Infection control.

2 Gather equipment and supplies.

3 Introduce yourself, identify your patient, and explain the procedure.
PURPOSE: Identification of the patient prevents errors, and explanations are means of implied consent.

4 Prepare thermometer or electronic unit in same manner as done for oral usage.

5 Put on gloves.
PURPOSE: When there is a possible exposure to body fluids, Standard Precautions must be followed.

6 Pat the patient's axillary area dry with a towel.
PURPOSE: To ensure an accurate reading. Do not rub area, because this may cause an elevated reading (Figure 1).

7 Place the bulb of the thermometer or the tip of the probe into the center of the armpit, pointing the stem to the upper chest, making sure the thermometer is touching only skin, not clothing (Figure 2).
PURPOSE: Location offers the most accurate reading, and contact with clothing will alter reading.

Continued

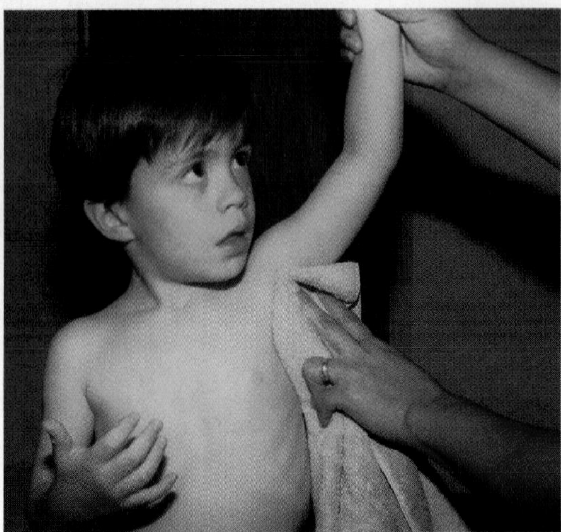

FIGURE 1

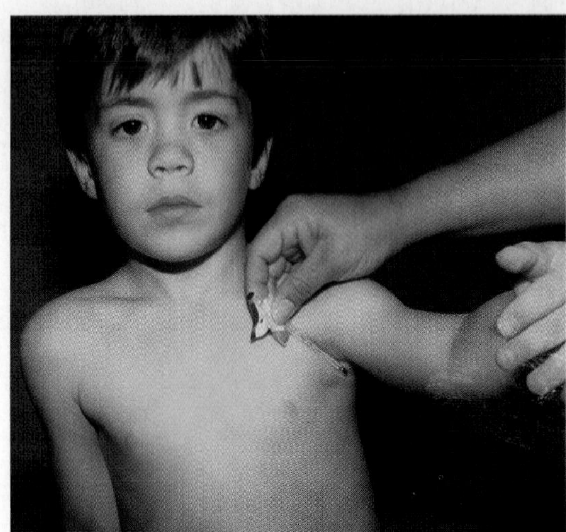

FIGURE 2

PROCEDURE 27-6 (CONTINUED)

Obtaining an Axillary Temperature

8 Instruct the patient to hold the arm snugly against the ribs with the other hand (Figure 3).
PURPOSE: Prevents air from leaking in and interfering with closed environment.

9 Inform the patient that the thermometer needs to be held in place for at least 10 minutes (glass) or until unit "beeps."
PURPOSE: Time needed must be extended to obtain an accurate reading.

10 Remove the thermometer and wipe it dry from stem to bulb with a tissue.
PURPOSE: Wiping with a tissue cleans the surface for visibility and prevents cross-contamination. Or remove probe and immediately eject the used probe into the appropriate waste container (Figure 4).
PURPOSE: Probe cover will be contaminated.

11 Note the reading on the LED window *or* read the thermometer, making sure that you hold it at eye level. Look for the silver column of mercury and follow it until it ends. Align the end of the column to the scale marked in degrees.
PURPOSE: Holding the thermometer at eye level facilitates an easier and more accurate reading.

12 If glass thermometer has been used, clean and disinfect it like an oral thermometer.

13 Remove gloves and discard in appropriate waste container.

14 Read and record the axillary temperature on the patient's medical record, for example, T = 97.6° (A)
PURPOSE: Procedures that are not recorded are considered not done.

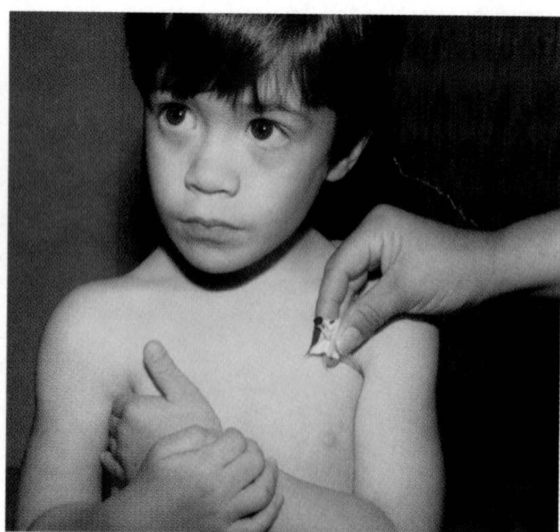

FIGURE 3

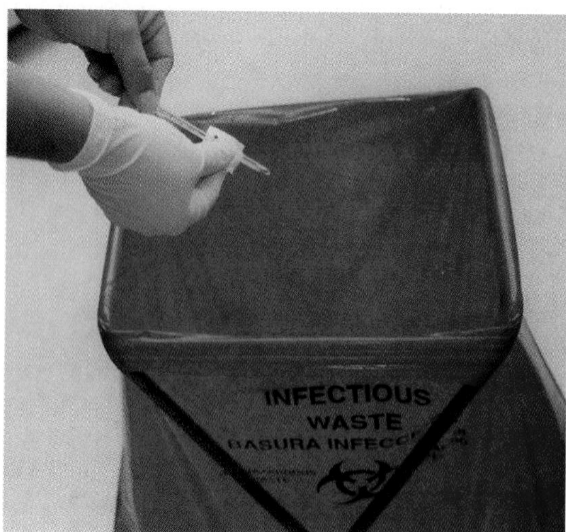

FIGURE 4

Cleaning Thermometers

GLASS

After use, the thermometer is never returned to its storage container until it is sanitized and disinfected. Sanitize it by cleaning the thermometer with soap and cool water, and then rinse and dry the instrument. The choice of a disinfecting solution should be based on its effectiveness and safety for human use. Soak the thermometer in the disinfectant for 30 to 60 minutes depending on the manufacturer's directions.

Memory Jogger

 *List the steps in cleaning a glass thermometer.*

ELECTRONIC

The electronic unit needs to be wiped off at the end of every day when all other environmental cleaning is done. Care needs to be taken when you eject the probe shield so as not to contaminate the probe or the processing unit. If there is a chance that patient body fluid got onto the unit, wipe it with disinfectant before returning it to its storage area.

TYMPANIC

Cleaning the tympanic unit follows the same guidelines as for the electronic unit. When using it on a small child, be conscious of what the child touches. If the processing unit is touched, be sure to clean it after use.

DISPOSABLE

When using a disposable thermometer, always discard it into the appropriate waste container immediately after use to avoid the possibility of contamination and spreading of the pathogen to others. If you are instructing the parent in using a disposable thermometer at home, be sure to emphasize that it should be discarded immediately. A used disposable thermometer is not something that other children can touch and "play" with.

RECTAL

The thermometer that is used to obtain a rectal temperature is handled the same as the oral thermometer. The major consideration is to never mix the two. Always keep them separated. This means washing, rinsing, drying, and disinfecting them separately. Never use the same container for both types, even after they are cleaned. Keep the rectal thermometers in a clearly labeled separate container.

AXILLARY

In most offices, an axillary thermometer is cleaned in the same manner as the rectal thermometer. Put it through the same cleaning and disinfecting process and store it in a container labeled "axillary." Remember that the axillary thermometer has a clear tip and can be distinguished in this manner from a rectal thermometer.

TIPS FOR OBTAINING ACCURATE TEMPERATURE READINGS

- Do not take an oral temperature within 30 minutes after the patient has ingested food or fluids or smoked.
- Label containers to differentiate thermometers that are contaminated or soaking from those that are clean.
- Label rectal thermometers carefully. If you are not using the different bulb types for identification, mark the stem ends of the rectal thermometers with red nail polish.
- Keep rectal thermometers in clearly labeled solutions separate from the oral and axillary thermometers.
- Use security-tipped bulbs for obtaining axillary temperatures.
- Place disposable covers on all thermometers, except disposable ones, before use.

Pulse

Pulse reflects the palpable beat of the arteries as they expand with the beat of the heart. With every beat, the heart pumps an amount of blood, known as the *stroke volume,* into the aorta. Every artery throughout our entire body has a pulse beat, but it is impossible for us to measure all of them. When pulse is measured, an artery that is close to the body surface that can be pushed against a bone is used. Palpating the peripheral pulse gives the rate and rhythm of the heartbeat, as well as local data on the condition of the artery. Determining the pulse is such a routine part of the physical examination that it is often taken in a mechanical way and some of the finer aspects are neglected.

PULSE SITES

A pulse rate may be counted any place where an artery is near the surface of the body and the vessel can be pressed against a bone. The most common sites that are used to feel this rhythmic throbbing are at the following arteries: temporal, carotid, apical, brachial, radial, femoral, popliteal, and dorsalis pedis.

The *temporal* pulse is located at the temple area of the skull, parallel and lateral to the eyes (Fig. 27–10*A*). It is seldom used as a pulse site but may be used as a pressure point to assist in controlling bleeding from a head injury.

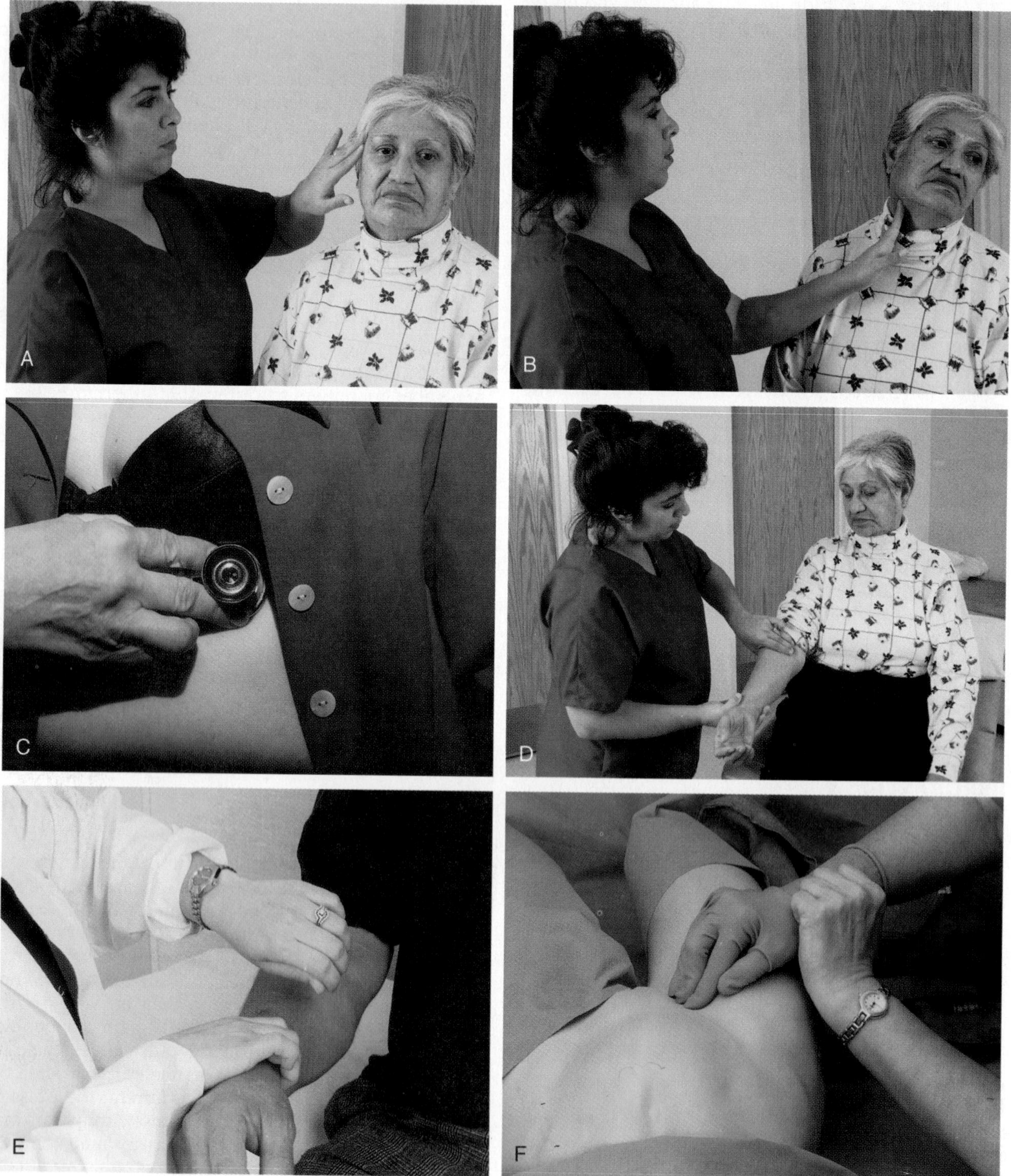

FIGURE 27–10 Pulse sites. *A*, Temporal. *B*, Carotid. *C*, Apical. *D*, Brachial. *E*, Radial. *F*, Femoral.

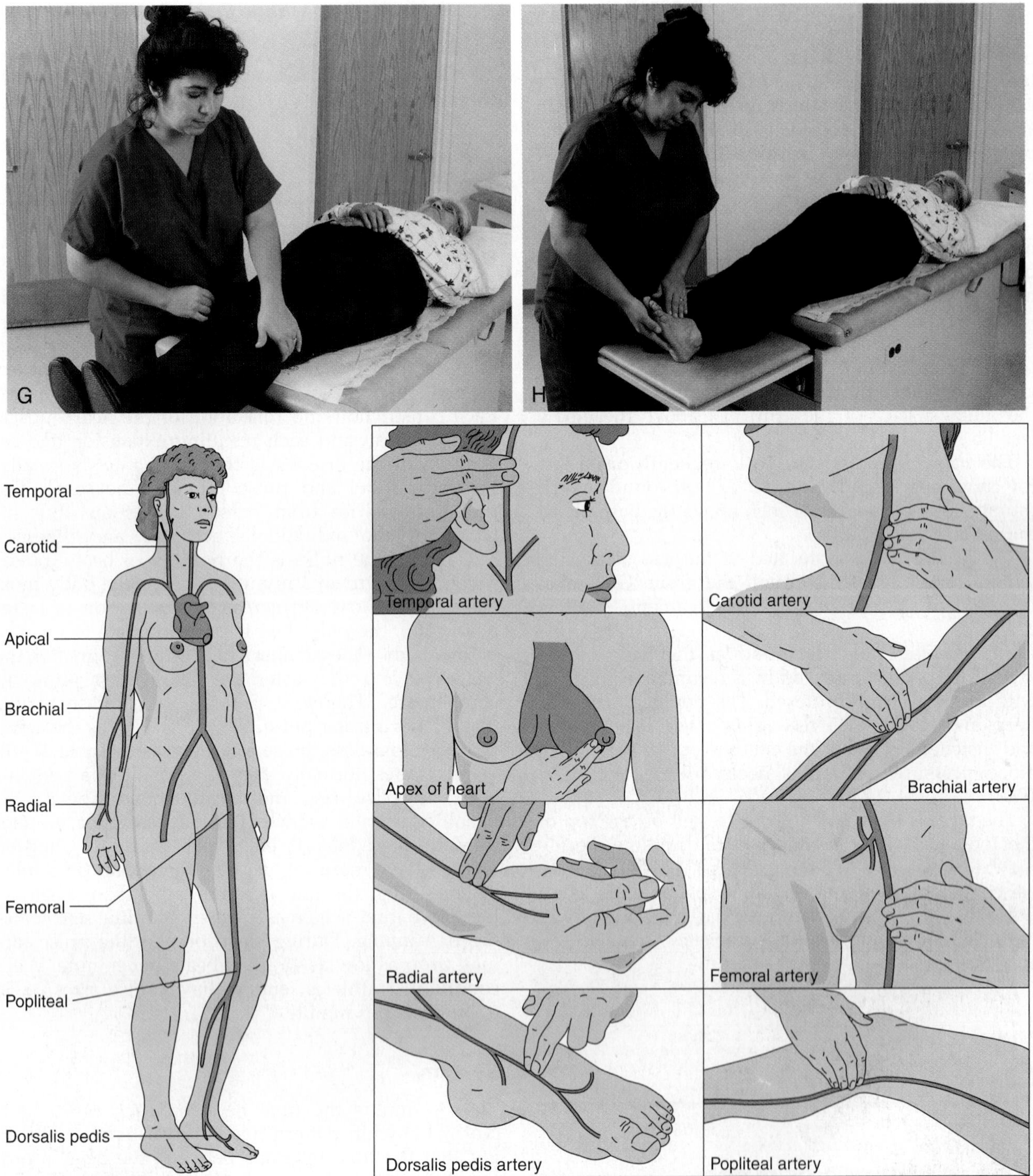

FIGURE 27–10 *Continued.* *G,* Popliteal. *H,* Dorsalis pedis. Although the radial artery is the most frequently used, it is important for the medical assistant to be able to obtain a pulse rate from alternative sites.

The *carotid* artery is located between the larynx and the sternocleidomastoid muscle in the front and to the side of the neck (see Fig. 27–10*B*). It is most frequently used in emergencies and during cardiopulmonary resuscitation. It can be felt by pushing the muscle to the side and pressing against the larynx.

The *apical* heart rate, or the heartbeat at the apex of the heart, is heard with a stethoscope. It is often used for infants and young children or in adults if the radial pulse is difficult to feel. An apical count may be requested if the patient is taking cardiac drugs or has **bradycardia** (slow heartbeat) or a rapid, irregular pulse at one of the other pulse sites.

The physician may listen to the apical beat while you count the pulse at another site. This is to determine equal pulse between the heartbeat and the artery. The difference between the apical rate and the pulse rate at another site is called the **pulse deficit.** The stethoscope is placed just below the left nipple between the fifth and sixth ribs. Count for 1 minute, and note the method by placing an "AP" beside the recorded count.

The apex of the heart is located in the left fifth intercostal space on the midclavicular line, that is, between the fifth and sixth ribs on a line with the midpoint of the left clavicle. (see Fig. 27–10C).

The *brachial* pulse is felt at the inner (antecubital) aspect of the elbow. It is the artery heard and felt when taking a blood pressure. It is also felt in the groove between the biceps and triceps muscles on the inner surface of the arm, just above the elbow (see Fig. 27–10*D*).

The *radial* artery is the most frequently used site for counting the pulse rate. It is best found on the thumb side of the wrist, 1 inch above the base of the thumb (see Fig. 27–10*E*).

The *femoral* pulse is located at the site where the femoral artery passes through the groin. One must press deeply below the inguinal ligament (see Fig. 27–10*F*).

The *popliteal* pulse is found at the back of the knee. The patient must be in a recumbent position, with the knee slightly flexed. The popliteal artery is deep and difficult to feel. This artery is palpated and listened to with the stethoscope when a leg blood pressure reading is necessary (see Fig. 27–10*G*).

The *dorsalis pedis (pedal)* artery is felt on the top of the foot, just slightly lateral to the midline, beside the extensor tendon of the great toe. This pulse may be congenitally absent in some patients. A good pulse rate at this site is an indicator of normal lower limb circulation and arterial sufficiency (see Fig. 27–10*H*).

Memory Jogger

 *Locate the eight pulse sites.*

CHARACTERISTICS OF PULSE

When you are taking a pulse, there are four important characteristics to note: (1) rate, (2) rhythm, (3) volume of the pulse, and (4) condition of the arterial wall. These characteristics depend on the size and elasticity of the artery, the strength of the contraction of the heart, and the tissues surrounding the artery. A patient's pulse may reveal valuable information regarding abnormalities of the circulation of the heart.

TABLE 27–3 Average Pulse Rates

Age	Average	Normal Limits (beats per minute)
At birth	120	70–190
Children 1–4 years	120	80–120
Children 6–12 years	90	70–110
Children 12–16 years	75–90	60–100
Adults	60–80	60–100

Rate

The pulse rate is a method of counting the heartbeat by feeling the pulsing of an artery. When the heart contracts, pressure throughout the arteries increases and the arteries expand. When the heart relaxes, arterial pressure decreases and the arteries relax. Each constriction and relaxation of the heart muscle is a heartbeat, and each resulting expansion and relaxation of the arteries is the pulse rate. Normally, heartbeat (rate) and pulse rate are the same. The pulse rate varies from person to person. It is affected by the individual's activities and illnesses. The rate of the pulse is the number of beats (pulsations) that occur in 1 minute. Because the body must balance heat loss by increasing circulation (a faster heart rate), the pulse rate is proportionate to the size of the body. The smaller the body, the greater the heat loss and the faster the heart must pump to compensate. Therefore, infants and children normally have a faster pulse than do adults; as the aging process progresses, pulse rate decreases (Table 27–3).

Pulse rates normally vary as a result of a person's age, body size, sex, and health status. The rate is usually faster in women (70–80 beats per minute) than in men (60–70 beats per minute). Children tend to have more rapid pulse rates than do adults. When sitting, the rate is more rapid than when lying down, and it increases when standing and walking or running. During sleep or rest, the pulse rate may drop as low as 45 to 50 beats per minute. Well-conditioned athletes tend to have pulse rates of 50 to 60 beats per minute.

Rhythm

The rhythm is the time between each pulse beat. Normal rhythm pattern has an even tempo, indicating that the time intervals between the beats are of equal duration. Abnormal rhythm is described according to the rhythm pattern you detect with your hand. Skipping an occasional beat (intermittent pulse) occurs in all normal individuals and may be more noticeable during exercise or after drinking a beverage containing caffeine. One irregularity that is commonly found in children and young adults is **sinus arrhythmia.** Here the heart rate varies with the respiratory cycle, speeding up at the peak of inspiration and slowing to normal with expiration. If there are frequently skipped beats or if the beats are markedly irregular, the physician should be advised, because this may indicate heart disease. It is sometimes helpful to count the radial pulse for 1 minute and then count the apical pulse for 1 minute. Record both readings. The difference between the two is called the pulse deficit.

Volume

The volume or force of the pulse refers to the strength of the beat and is described as full, strong, feeble, thready, weak, hard, or soft. The force of the heartbeat and the condition of the arterial walls influence the volume. It is possible for the pulse to vary only in intensity and otherwise be perfectly regular. This condition can also indicate heart disease. The pulse force is recorded using a three-point scale.

THREE-POINT SCALE

- 3 + = full, bounding
- 2 + = normal pulse
- 1 + = weak, thready
- 0 = no pulse detected

Vessel Elasticity

As you palpate the pulse through the skin, you must also evaluate the condition of the arterial wall. Normally, the wall would be described as being springy, resilient, and elastic. Abnormal findings include hard, ropelike, knotty, or wiry-feeling vessels, or any combination of these.

DETERMINING PULSE RATE

Radial, Brachial, and Apical

The patient should be in a comfortable position, with the artery to be used at the same level as or lower than the heart (see Procedure 27–7). The limb should be well supported and relaxed. The patient may be lying down or sitting. As with all pulse readings, the pads of your first three fingers are placed over the artery. Push until you feel the strongest pulsation.

As you begin the counting process, start with "zero" for the first pulse felt, the second pulse beat felt is "one," and so on. The pulse is counted for 1 full minute. The 15- or 30-second interval is found to be less accurate than the longer interval. Using shorter intervals invites error because you often will be unable to evaluate the quality of the pulse rhythm.

Variations from the normal quality, such as an **arrhythmia** or a pulse that is **thready, elastic, intermittent, irregular, bounding,** or **unequal,** are noted and recorded. Some pulses are more difficult to feel than are others, and the correct pressures to be used for each patient and site require practice and experience.

Both you and your patient should be in relaxed positions. The sensitivity in your counting fingers is greatly reduced if you are in an awkward position. Too much pressure obliterates the patient's pulse, and too little pressure prevents detection of irregularities or of all of the beats. Record the number of beats in 1 minute. Assess the pulse, including rate, rhythm, volume, and elasticity. If the pulse rate is counted at any site other than the radial, the site should be recorded along with a notation of the site used.

Femoral, Popliteal, and Pedal

Pulses in the lower extremities may be difficult to find and equally difficult to hear. The Doppler unit, which is an ultrasound unit that magnifies the pulsation, may be used to locate and count these pulses accurately (Fig. 27–11). This unit is battery operated and can be attached to your stethoscope so only you hear the beat, or it can be set so that both you and your patient can hear the pulsations.

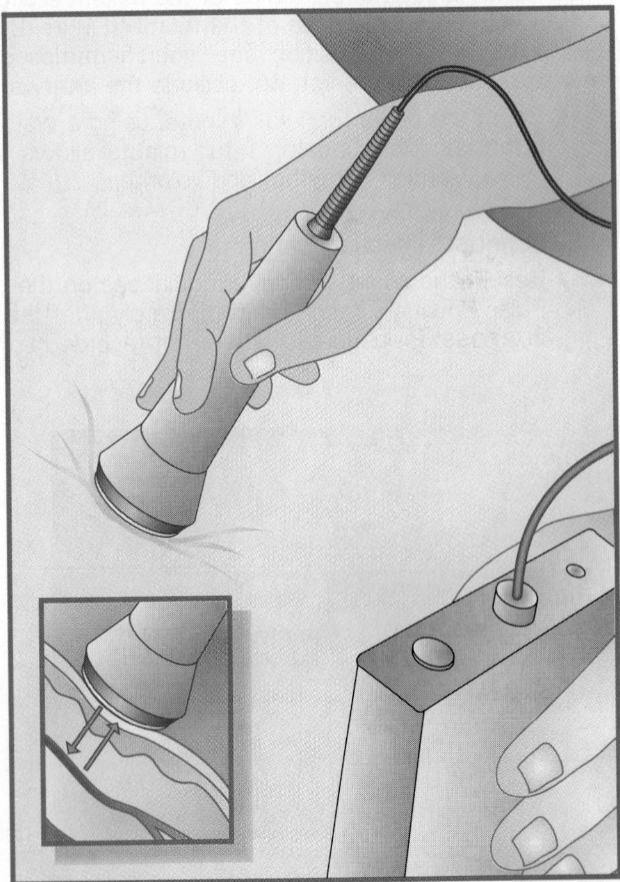

FIGURE 27–11 Doppler ultrasound unit for measuring pulses of lower extremities.

PROCEDURE 27-7

Assessing the Patient's Pulse

GOAL

To determine and record a patient's pulse rate, rhythm, volume, and elasticity. (*Note:* When TPR measurements are ordered, count the patient's pulse while the glass thermometer is in his or her mouth.)

EQUIPMENT AND SUPPLIES

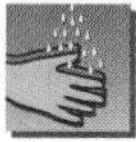

A watch with a second hand

PROCEDURAL STEPS

1 Wash your hands.
PURPOSE: Infection control.

2 Introduce yourself, identify your patient, and explain the procedure.
PURPOSE: Identification of the patient prevents errors, and explanations are means of implied consent.

3 Place the patient's arm in a relaxed position, palm downward.
PURPOSE: The patient's radial artery is more easily palpated when the patient is relaxed and in this position.

4 Gently grasp the palm side of the patient's wrist with your first three fingertips approximately 1 inch above the base of the thumb (Figure 1).
PURPOSE: This position puts your fingertips directly over the artery. Press firmly, but if you press too hard, you will occlude the artery and feel nothing.

5 Count the beats for 1 full minute, using a watch with a second hand.
PURPOSE: Counting for 1 full minute allows you to obtain an accurate count, including any irregularities in rhythm and volume.

6 Wash your hands.
PURPOSE: Infection control.

7 Record the count and any irregularities on the patient's medical record. Record as P = 72. Pulse is usually recorded immediately after the temperature.
PURPOSE: Procedures that are not recorded are considered not done.

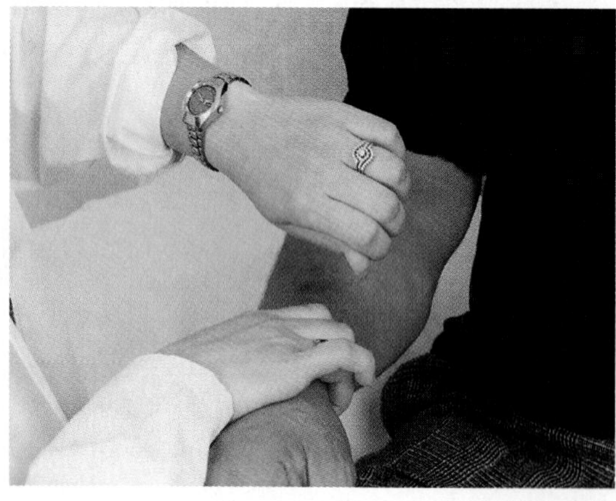

FIGURE 1

Respiration

PHYSIOLOGY

The purpose of respiration is to provide for the exchange of oxygen and carbon dioxide between the atmosphere, the blood, and the body cells. Oxygen is taken into the body to be used for life-sustaining body processes, and carbon dioxide is released as a waste product.

One complete inspiration and expiration is called a *respiration.* During the inspiration phase, the diaphragm contracts, causing the lungs to expand and fill with air. Then, during the expiration phase, the diaphragm returns to its normal, elevated position, causing the lungs to expel the waste air back into the atmosphere.

Respiration is both internal and external. *External respiration* refers to the exchange of oxygen and carbon dioxide in the lungs. *Internal respiration* occurs at the cellular level, when the oxygen in the bloodstream is utilized and the cells release carbon dioxide as a waste product to be transported back to the lungs for exhalation.

When there is build-up of carbon dioxide in the blood, a message is sent to the medulla oblongata, which is located in the brain between the top of the spine and the brain stem. This control center sends a message to trigger respiration.

Respiration is controlled by the involuntary nervous system; this means we breathe automatically. Because a person can control respiration to a certain extent, it is also a voluntary body function. Breathing is ultimately under the control of the medulla oblongata, which is why we can hold our breath only for a given length of time. Once the blood carbon dioxide level increases to the point at which cells become oxygen starved, a stimulus is sent and breathing begins involuntarily.

CHARACTERISTICS OF RESPIRATIONS

Normally, a person's breathing is relaxed, automatic, and silent. When determining the respiratory rate of a patient, three important characteristics must be noted: (1) rate, (2) rhythm, and (3) depth.

Rate

The rate of respiration refers to the number of respirations per minute. It is described as *normal, rapid,* or *slow.* Variations occur in the respiratory rate (fast or slow), volume (deep or shallow), and rhythm (regular or irregular) (Fig. 27–12). **Dyspnea,** meaning difficult breathing, occurs in patients with pneumonia or asthma. It also occurs after physical exertion or at very high altitudes. Other alterations in

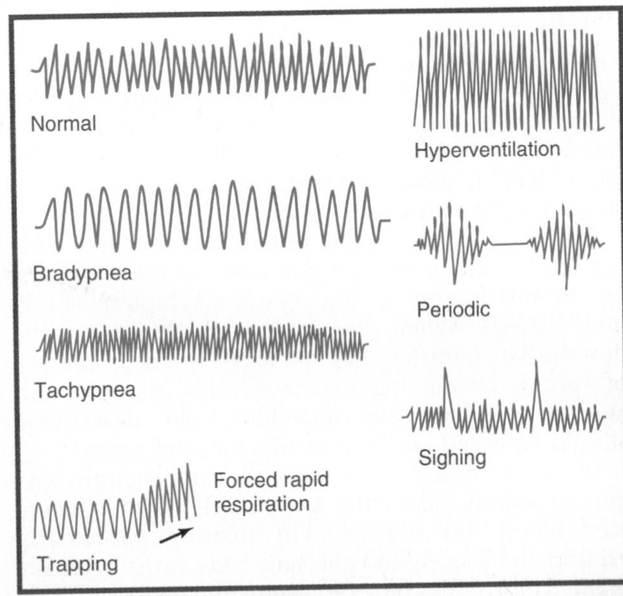

FIGURE 27–12 Respiration rate patterns called spirograms, which are recorded using a spirometer.

breathing are **bradypnea** (abnormally slow respiration), **apnea** (temporary cessation of respiration), **tachypnea** (excessively rapid breathing), and **hyperpnea** (increased rate of breathing). Hyperpnea is usually accompanied by **hyperventilation** and is frequently found in emotional conditions. **Orthopnea** is difficulty in breathing while lying down, as found in patients with congestive heart failure. See Table 27–4 for normal respiratory rates according to age.

A fairly constant ratio of four pulse beats to one respiration exists. As a general rule, both pulse and respiration rates normally respond to exercise or emotional upsets.

Rhythm

The rhythm refers to the breathing pattern. A regular breathing pattern is normal in adults; however, the breathing pattern for infants is irregular. Automatic interruptions, such as sighing, are also considered normal.

TABLE 27–4 Respiratory Rates

Age	Breaths per Minute
Newborn	30–40
1 year	20–40
2 years	25–32
4 years	23–30
6 years	21–26
8 years	20–26
12 years	18–22
16 years	16–20
18 years	18–20
Adult	14–20

Depth

The depth of respiration refers to the amount of air being inhaled and exhaled. When a patient is at rest, normal respirations have a consistent depth, which can be noted as you watch the rise and fall of the chest. Rapid, shallow breathing at rest occurs in some disease states.

Normally, no noticeable breath sounds occur during the breathing process; the one exception is snoring. Noticeable breath sounds are a symptom of certain diseases. When referring to breath sounds, the descriptive characteristics are represented by the use of specific terminology, such as **rales, rhonchi,** and **stertorous.** The term matching the description should be noted on the patient's medical record.

When an individual cannot inspire enough oxygen to supply all of the body's cells with oxygenated blood, the normal skin coloring particularly around the mouth and the nail beds turns a bluish, dusky color. This color represents the increased level of carbon dioxide that is present in the blood and is termed *cyanosis*.

COUNTING RESPIRATIONS

Because most people are unaware of their breathing, do not mention that you will be counting the respirations (see Procedure 27–8). Sudden awareness may alter the normal breathing pattern. Respiration rate is easily controlled and patients self-consciously alter their breathing rates when they are being watched. It is best to count the respirations while appearing to count the pulse. Keep your eyes alternately on the patient's chest and your watch while you are counting the pulse rate, and, then, without removing your fingers from the pulse site, determine the respiration rate. It may be easier to count the respirations first, because that number is not as hard to remember. If the patient is lying down, the arm may be crossed over the chest so the respirations can be felt with the rise and fall of the chest. Count the respirations for 30 seconds and multiply the number by 2. Avoid the 15-second interval because this can vary by a factor of +4 or −4, which is significant when dealing with such a small num-

PROCEDURE 27-8
Determining Respirations

GOAL

To determine and record a patient's respirations. (Remember that the respiration count may be altered if the patient is aware that you are counting his or her breaths.)

EQUIPMENT AND SUPPLIES

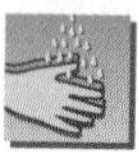

A watch with a second hand

PROCEDURAL STEPS

1 Wash your hands.
PURPOSE: Infection control.

2 Identify your patient.
PURPOSE: Identification of the patient prevents errors, and explanations are means of implied consent.

3 Place the patient's arm in the same position as it was when you were counting the pulse.
PURPOSE: This position allows you to feel the rise and fall of the chest wall.

4 Count the respirations for 30 seconds, using a watch with a second hand, and multiply by 2.
PURPOSE: Counting for 30 seconds allows you to obtain an accurate count and determine any irregularities in rhythm or depth or unusual breathing patterns, such as apnea or dyspnea.

5 Release the patient's wrist.

6 Wash your hands.
PURPOSE: Infection control.

7 Record the respirations on the patient's medical record after the pulse recording. Record as R = 18.
PURPOSE: Procedures that are not recorded are considered not done.

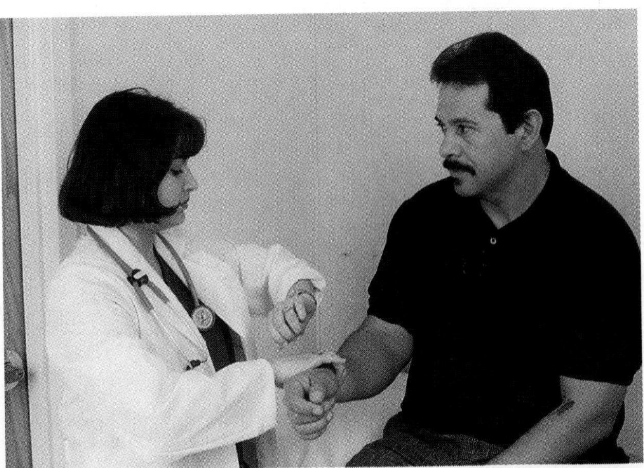

FIGURE 27–13 Hand position when counting respirations. Hands should be left in place as if still counting the patient's pulse.

ber. Note any variation or irregularity in the rate. Record the respiration count on the medical record.

If a glass thermometer is used for the temperature reading, the pulse and respiration rates are usually counted while an oral temperature is being obtained. Doing the three procedures together is very efficient, and the patient cannot distract you with conversation. After recording the pulse and respiration counts, remove the thermometer and record that reading.

If the electronic or tympanic methods are employed, count the respirations when you count the pulse. Leave your hands in place as if to be still counting the pulse (Fig. 27–13).

Memory Jogger

9 *How would you tell someone that you are going to count his or her respirations?*

Blood Pressure

Blood pressure is a reflection of the pressure of the blood against the walls of the arteries. Each time the ventricles contract, blood is pushed out of the heart and into the aorta and pulmonary artery, exerting pressure on the walls of the arteries. There are actually two blood pressure readings: the systolic pressure is the highest pressure level that occurs when the heart is contracting and the pulse beat is felt, and the diastolic pressure is the lowest pressure level when the heart is relaxed and no pulse beat is felt. Systole (heart contraction) and diastole (heart relaxation) together make up the cardiac cycle. The difference between the systolic and diastolic pressures reflects the volume of circulating blood and is called the **pulse pressure.**

Blood pressure is read in millimeters of mercury, abbreviated mm Hg. However, the abbreviations are not necessary when recording the reading on the patient's medical record. Blood pressure is recorded as a fraction, with the systolic reading the numerator (top) and the diastolic reading the denominator (bottom), for example, 130/80.

FACTORS AFFECTING BLOOD PRESSURE

The physiologic factors that determine the blood pressure include blood volume, peripheral resistance created by blood viscosity, vessel elasticity, and the condition of the heart muscle and the arterial walls.

Volume is the amount of blood in the arteries. An increased blood volume increases the blood pressure, and a decreased blood volume decreases blood pressure. If a hemorrhage occurs, the blood volume drops, and so does the pressure.

Peripheral resistance of blood vessels refers to the relationship of the lumen of the vessel and the amount of blood flowing through it. The smaller the lumen, the greater the resistance to the blood flow. Blood pressure is high with a small lumen and low with a large lumen. Vessels affected by fatty cholesterol deposits result in increased blood pressure owing to the narrowing of their diameters or lumina.

Vessel elasticity refers to a vessel's capability to expand and contract to supply the body with a steady flow of blood. With age, vessel elasticity lessens, and the arterial walls become resistant; as a result, blood pressure increases.

Heart muscle condition is of primary importance to the volume of blood flowing through the body. A strong, forceful pump works efficiently and tends to keep blood pressure within normal limits. If the muscle becomes weak, blood pressure begins to increase in an attempt to maintain the necessary level of oxygen and nutrients needed by the body.

Memory Jogger

10 *Identify the five physiologic factors that determine the blood pressure.*

As previously stated in this chapter, pulse pressure is the difference between the systolic and diastolic pressures and is an important measurement in diseases and trauma of the nervous system, especially of the spinal cord and brain. The average pulse pressure is 40 mm Hg. If the blood pressure is 120/80, then the pulse pressure is 40 (resulting in a 3:1 ratio). Conditions such as brain tumors and cerebrovascular accident (stroke) greatly increase pulse pressure.

Memory Jogger

11 *Clarify the difference between pulse deficit and pulse pressure.*

EVALUATING BLOOD PRESSURE

When tracking a patient's blood pressure, frequent readings should be taken about the same time of day and by the same person. A person is said to have **hypertension** (elevated blood pressure) if the pressure is persistently above normal, which means the systolic pressure remains above 160 mm Hg and diastolic pressure is greater than 90 mm Hg. Hypertension may have no known cause (**essential hypertension**), or it may be associated with some other disease (**secondary hypertension**). Essential hypertension is common among Americans. Secondary hypertension often accompanies renal diseases, pregnancy, endocrine imbalances, obesity, arteriosclerosis, atherosclerosis, and brain injuries. Temporary hypertension may occur with stress, pain, exercise, and exhaustion.

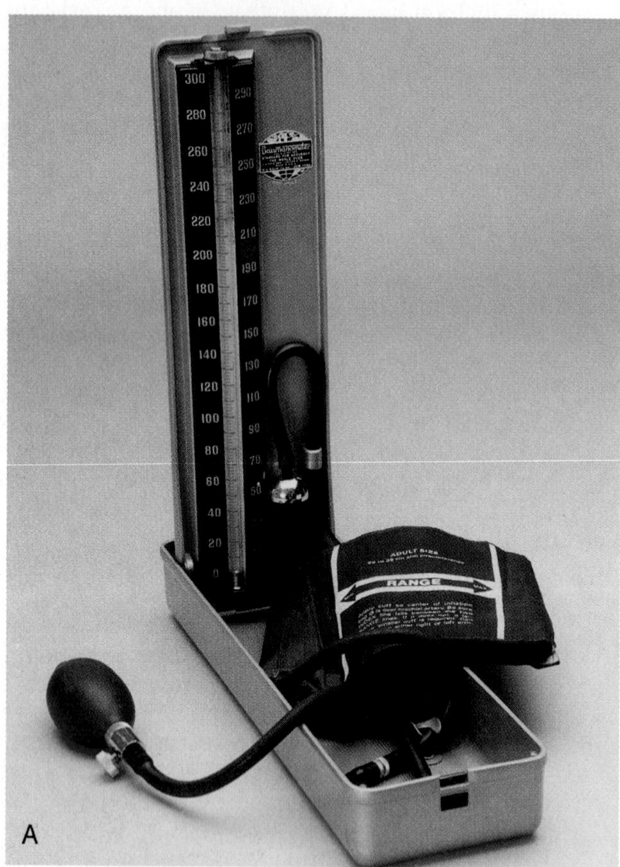

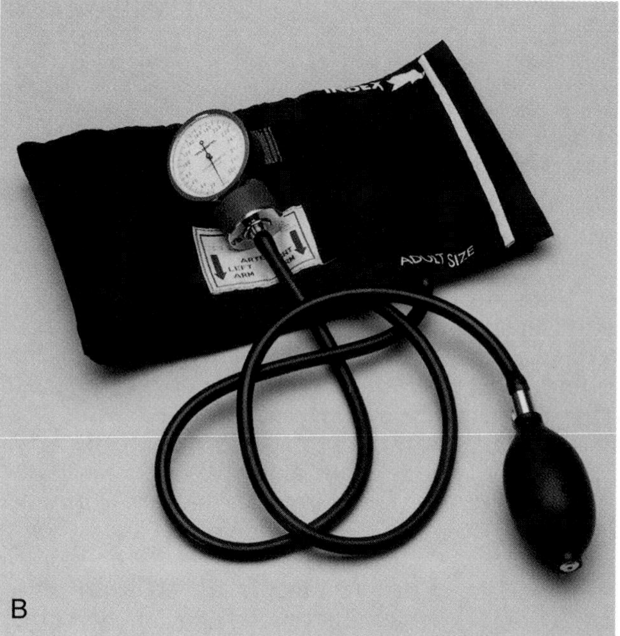

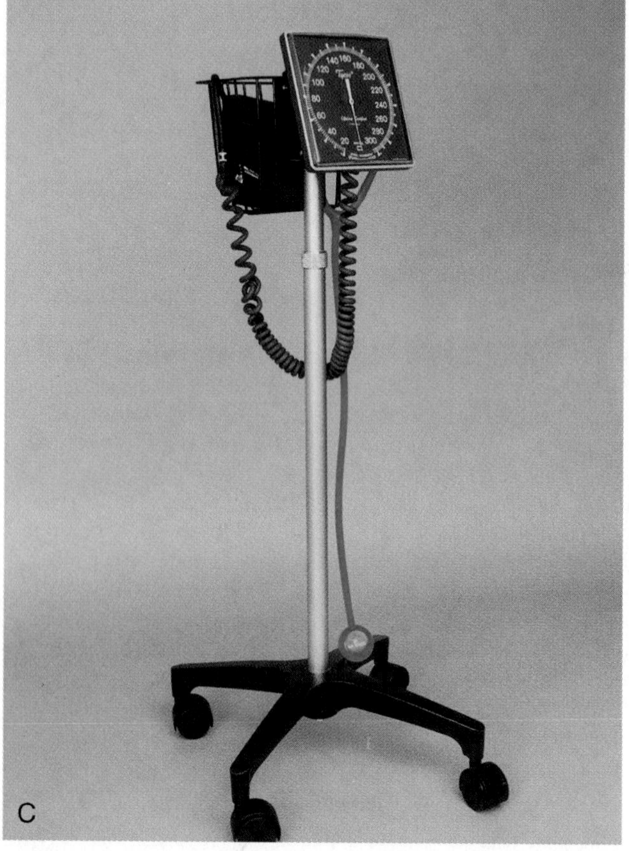

FIGURE 27–14 *A*, Blood pressure mercury column pressure gauge system. *B*, Aneroid dial system. *C*, Aneroid floor model with large slanted face.

Hypertension has been called the silent disease because it has no symptoms, and persons may go for long periods of time without knowing that they have a problem. Often, hypertension is discovered by accident during the medical or dental treatment of another problem. Long-term, untreated hypertension is suspected to be a major cause of strokes.

Hypotension is abnormally low blood pressure and may be caused by shock, both emotional and traumatic; hemorrhage; central nervous system disorders; and chronic wasting diseases. Persistent readings of 90/60 mm Hg or below are usually considered hypotensive. **Orthostatic (postural) hypotension** is the temporary fall in blood pressure that occurs when a person rapidly changes from a recumbent position to a standing position or when a person stands motionless in a fixed position, such as standing at attention. Some medications can cause orthostatic hypotension. The patient may feel suddenly dizzy and have blurred vision or may actually faint.

Memory Jogger

Compare and contrast hypertension and hypotension.

MEASURING BLOOD PRESSURE

The instrument used to measure blood pressure is called the sphygmomanometer. The term *manometer* refers to an instrument used to measure the pressure of a liquid or a gas. *Sphygmo* means pulse. Thus, sphygmomanometer means an instrument used for measuring blood pressure in the arteries. The instrument consists of an inflatable cuff, an inflation bulb with a control valve, and a pressure gauge. There are two common types of pressure gauges: the mercury column (Fig. 27–14*A*) and the aneroid dial (see Fig. 27–14*B*). The aneroid dial also comes in a floor model with a large angled face (see Fig. 27–14*C*). Sphygmomanometers are delicately calibrated instruments and must be handled carefully. They should be recalibrated regularly and checked for accuracy, either by you or a medical supply dealer. The recording needle on the aneroid dial sphygmomanometer should rest within the small square or circle at the bottom of the dial. The meniscus of mercury on the mercury column sphygmomanometer should rest at zero (0).

The sphygmomanometer must be used with a stethoscope. The objective of the procedure is to use the inflatable cuff to obliterate (cause to disappear) circulation through an artery, similar to when using a tourniquet. The stethoscope is placed over the artery just below the cuff, and then the cuff is slowly deflated to allow the blood to flow again. As blood flow is resumed, the cardiac cycle sounds may be heard again through the stethoscope, and gauge readings are taken when the first and last sounds are heard (see Procedure 27–9).

Blood pressure cuffs and stethoscopes are available in drug stores and retail stores for patients to use to measure their own blood pressure at home. These units can be aneroid, electronic or computerized sphygmomanometers (Fig. 27–15). If you have

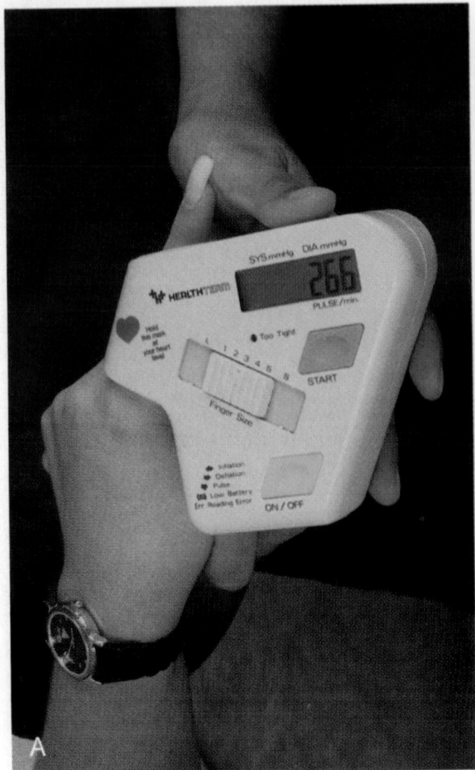

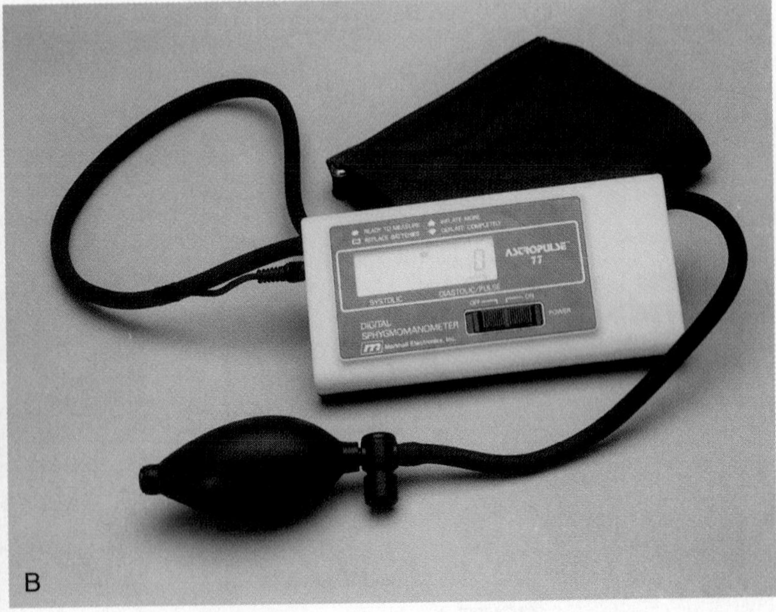

FIGURE 27–15 Personal blood pressure systems. *A*, Home system finger cuff. *B*, Digital blood pressure home system arm cuff.

PROCEDURE 27-9

Determining a Patient's Blood Pressure

GOAL

To perform a blood pressure measurement that is correct in technique and accurate and comfortable to the patient.

EQUIPMENT AND SUPPLIES

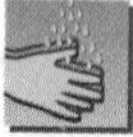

Sphygmomanometer
Stethoscope
Antiseptic wipes

PROCEDURAL STEPS

1 Wash your hands.
PURPOSE: Infection control.

2 Assemble the equipment and supplies needed.

3 Introduce yourself, identify the patient, and explain the procedure.
PURPOSE: Identification of the patient prevents errors, and explanations are a means of implied consent.

4 Seat the patient in a comfortable position with legs uncrossed.
PURPOSE: To promote relaxation and aid you in obtaining a true reading.

5 Determine the correct cuff size (Figure 1).
PURPOSE: An incorrect cuff size prevents accurate measurement of blood pressure.

6 Roll up the sleeve to about 5 inches above the elbow, or have the patient remove his or her arm from the sleeve.
PURPOSE: Tight clothing interferes with an accurate reading.

7 Palpate the brachial artery in both arms. If one arm has a stronger pulse, use that arm; if the pulses are equal, select the right arm (Figure 2).
PURPOSE: A stronger pulse is easier to measure; the right arm is the universal arm of choice.

8 Support the patient's arm at heart level or slightly lower.
PURPOSE: If the upper arm is higher than the heart, the reading will be inaccurate.

Continued

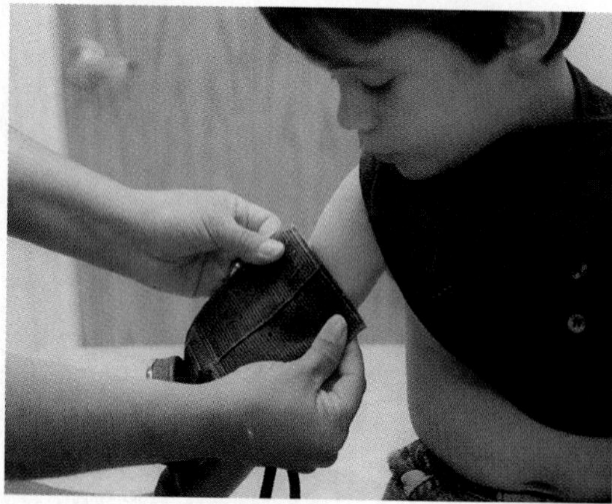

FIGURE 1

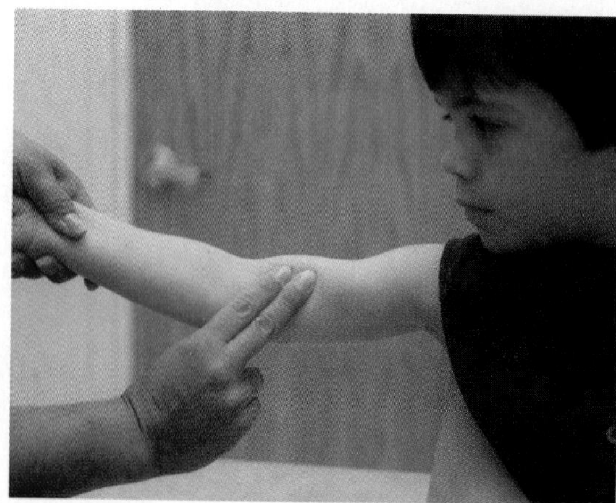

FIGURE 2

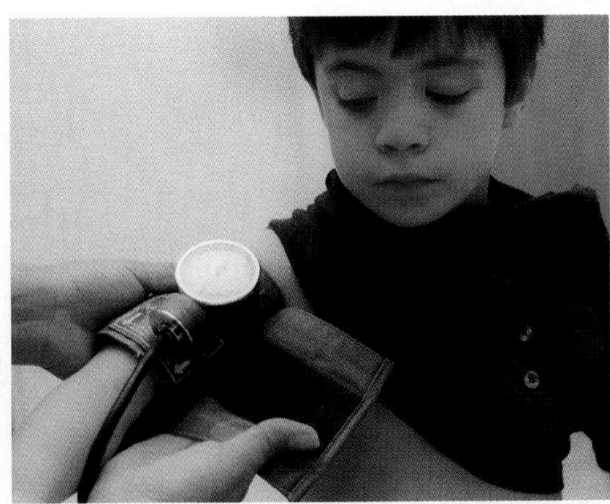

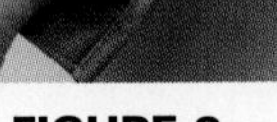

FIGURE 3

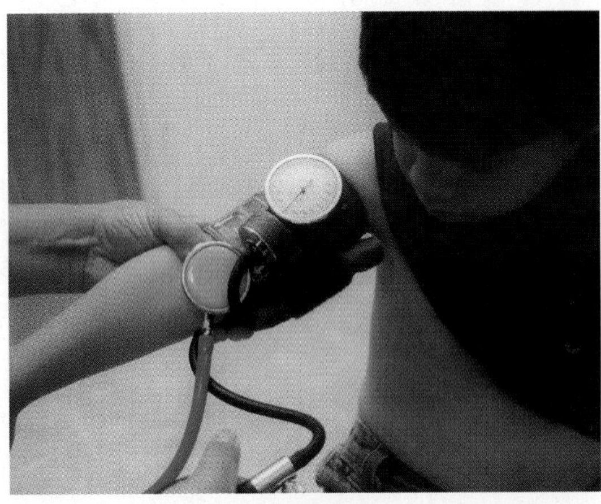

FIGURE 4

9 Center the cuff bladder over the brachial artery, with the connecting tube away from the patient's body and the tube to the bulb close to the body (Figure 3).
PURPOSE: Pressure must be applied directly over the artery for an accurate reading.

10 Place the lower edge of the cuff about 1 inch above the palpable brachial pulse, normally located in the natural crease of the inner elbow, and wrap it snugly and smoothly.
PURPOSE: This helps ensure an accurate reading.

11 Position the gauge of the sphygmomanometer so that it is at eye level.
PURPOSE: The dial is calibrated to be read in this position.

12 Take the patient's brachial pulse, and mentally add 40 mm to the reading.
PURPOSE: This is to determine the inflation level needed to find phase I of the Korotkoff sounds.

13 Insert the earpieces of the stethoscope turned down and forward into your ears.
PURPOSE: With the ear pieces in this position, the openings follow the anatomic line of the ear canal and blood pressure will be accurately heard.

14 Place the stethoscope bell over the palpated brachial artery firmly enough to obtain a seal but not so tightly that you constrict the artery (Figure 4).
PURPOSE: The bell magnifies the low pitch sounds better than the diaphragm and also forms a better seal.

15 Close the valve, and squeeze the bulb to inflate the cuff at a rapid but smooth rate to 20 mm above the palpated pulse level that was previously determined in step 12 (Figure 5).

Continued

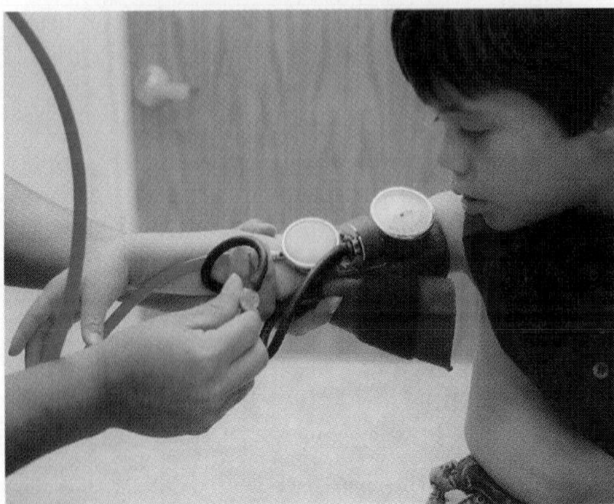

FIGURE 5

PROCEDURE 27-9 (CONTINUED)

Determining a Patient's Blood Pressure

16 Open the valve slightly and deflate the cuff at the constant rate of 2 mm Hg per second.
PURPOSE: Careful, slow release allows you to listen to all of the sounds.

17 Listen throughout the entire deflation until the sounds have stopped for at least 10 mm Hg.

18 Remove the stethoscope from your ears, and record the systolic and diastolic readings as BP systolic/diastolic (e.g., BP 120/80).

19 If you are uncertain of your reading, release the air from the cuff, wait 1 to 2 minutes, then repeat the process. It is advisable to have the patient gently wiggle his or her fingers during the waiting period.
PURPOSE: This waiting time allows circulatory congestion to dissipate.

20 Remove the cuff from the patient's arm and return it to its proper storage area. Clean the earpieces of the stethoscope with alcohol and return it to storage.

21 Wash your hands.
PURPOSE: Infection control.

patients who are monitoring their pressures at home, be sure that they understand the mechanics of accurately obtaining a reading. It is a wise idea to have them bring their equipment to the office and demonstrate how they use it. While the patient is showing you his or her home equipment, you will have an ideal time to check the calibration and answer any questions the patient might have regarding the usage of their equipment.

HEART SOUNDS

There are two basic heart sounds produced by the functioning of the heart during the cardiac cycle. The first sound produced at systole (contraction) is dull, firm, and prolonged and is heard as a lubb sound. The second sound, produced at diastole (relaxation) when the heart valves close, is shorter and sharper and is heard as a dupp sound. The lubb-dupp is the sound of one heartbeat.

The Korotkoff sounds are the sounds heard during the measurement of blood pressure. These sounds are thought to be produced by the vibrations of the arterial wall as the wall suddenly distends when compressed by the blood pressure cuff. However, it has not been determined whether the sounds come from within the wall itself or from the blood passing through the vessel. The sounds were first discovered and classified into five distinct phases by Nicolai Sergevich Korotkoff, a Russian neurologist.

PHASE I This is the first sound heard as the cuff deflates. The blood is resurging into the patient's artery and can be heard quite clearly as a sharp, tapping sound. Note the gauge reading when this first sound is heard. Record this as the systolic pressure.

PHASE II As the cuff deflates, even more blood flows through the artery. The movement of the blood makes a swishing sound. If proper procedure is not followed in inflating the cuff, these sounds may not be heard because of their soft quality. Occasionally, blood pressure sounds completely disappear during this phase. The loss of the sounds and their reappearance later is called the auscultatory gap. The silence may continue as the needle or the column of mercury falls another 30 mm Hg. Auscultatory gaps occur particularly in hypertension and certain heart diseases. So, if you notice such a gap, be certain to report it to the physician.

PHASE III A great deal of blood is now pushing down into the artery. The distinct, sharp tapping sounds return and continue rhythmically. If you do not inflate the cuff enough, you will miss the first two phases completely and you will incorrectly interpret the beginning of phase III as the systolic blood pressure (phase I).

PHASE IV At this point, the blood is flowing easily. The sound changes to a soft tapping, which becomes muffled and begins to grow fainter. Occasionally, these sounds continue to zero. This may occur in children, after exercise, with a fever, or in pregnancy if anemia is present. The American Heart Association recommends that the beginning of phase IV be recorded as the diastolic reading for a child. Some physicians call the change at phase IV the fading sound and want it recorded between the systolic and the diastolic recordings (for example, 120/84/70, with the 84 representing the gauge reading when the sounds of phase III have ended and those of phase IV are beginning. Other physicians consider phase IV the true diastolic pressure.

PHASE V All sounds disappear in this phase. Note the gauge reading when the last sound is heard. Record this as the diastolic *pressure.*

Memory Jogger

 *Describe the different sounds you hear in each of the Korotkoff phases.*

Palpatory Method

The systolic pressure may be checked by feeling the radial pulse rather than hearing (auscultatory method) it with the stethoscope. Place the cuff in the usual position and palpate the radial pulse, noting the rate and rhythm. Now inflate the cuff until the pulse disappears, and then add 30 mm more of inflation to get above the systolic pressure. Do not remove your fingers from the pulse or change the pressure of your fingers. Now, slowly release the pressure in the cuff and wait for the pulse to be felt again. Note the reading on the gauge, and record the first pulse felt as the systolic pressure. The diastolic and the Korotkoff phases cannot be determined by this method, and its use, other than in combination with the auscultatory method, is not recommended.

COMMON CAUSES OF ERRORS IN BLOOD PRESSURE READINGS

1 The limb being used is not at the same level as the heart. (It is not necessary for the manometer to be at the same level as the heart.)
2 The rubber bladder in the cuff has not been completely deflated before starting or retaking a reading.
3 The mercury column is allowed to drop too rapidly, resulting in an inaccurate reading.
4 The patient is nervous, uncomfortable, or too anxious, which may cause a reading higher than the patient's actual blood pressure.
5 The cuff is improperly applied.
6 The cuff is too large or too small.
7 The cuff is not placed around the arm smoothly.
8 The cuff is too loose or too tight.
9 The bladder is not centered over the artery.
10 The rubber bladder bulges out from the cover.
11 Failing to wait 1 to 2 minutes between measurements.
12 Defective instruments:
  a Air leaks in the valve.
  b Air leaks in the bladder.
  c Dirty mercury column.
  d Mercury column or aneroid needle that is not calibrated to zero

Anthropometric Measurement

Anthropometry is the science that deals with the measurement of the size, weight, and proportions of the human body. These measurements are often included in the initial measurement of the vital signs. Because they are indicators of the state of health and well-being of the patient, the measurements of height and weight are discussed as part of the vital signs. Other measurements are discussed when pertinent in the speciality chapters.

MEASURING HEIGHT AND WEIGHT

The patient's height and weight are often helpful in diagnosis, and the medical assistant must determine these readings with accuracy and empathy (see Procedure 27–10). Weight and height measurements are often routinely done in many medical settings as the patient is being escorted to the examination room. If this is the first visit for this patient, the anthropometric measurements will be written in the baseline information and used as reference data in future visits when or as needed.

There are certain medical specialties and specific medical problems that may require continuous monitoring of weight. Hormone disorders (e.g., diabetes), growth patterns (seen in children), and eating disorders (e.g., obesity and bulimia) necessitate accurate weight checks as part of every medical visit. In addition, maternity patients and heart patients with fluid retention difficulties also need weight monitoring. Some scales are calibrated in kilograms, whereas others are in pounds. When it is necessary to convert a weight, use the formulas under Conversion Formulas.

CONVERSION FORMULAS

TO CONVERT KILOGRAMS TO POUNDS

1 kilogram = 2.2 pounds
Multiply the number of kilograms by 2.2.
Example: If a patient weighs 68 kilograms, multiply 68 by 2.2 = 149.6 pounds.

TO CONVERT POUNDS TO KILOGRAMS

1 pound = 0.45 kilogram
Multiply the number of pounds by 0.45.
Example: If a patient weighs 120 pounds, multiply 120 by 0.45 = 54 kilograms.

Memory Jogger

 *Patient D weighs 87 kilograms; how many pounds does he weigh?*

PROCEDURE 27-10

Measuring a Patient's Height and Weight

GOAL

To accurately weigh and measure a patient as part of the physical assessment procedure.

EQUIPMENT AND SUPPLIES

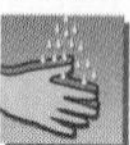

A balance scale with a measuring bar

PROCEDURAL STEPS

1 Wash your hands.
PURPOSE: Infection control.

2 Identify your patient and explain the procedure.
PURPOSE: Identification of the patient prevents errors, and explanations are means of implied consent.

3 If the patient is to remove his or her shoes for weighing, place a paper towel on the scale platform. The patient may be given disposable slippers to wear.

4 Check to see that the balance bar pointer floats in the middle of the balance frame when all weights are at zero.
PURPOSE: A floating pointer indicates that the scale is properly adjusted and in balance.

5 Help the patient onto the scale. Be sure that the female patient is not holding a purse and that the male patient has removed any heavy objects from pockets.

6 Move the large weight into the groove closest to the estimated weight of the patient. The grooves are calibrated in 50-lb increments. If you choose a groove that is more than the patient's weight, the pointer will immediately tilt to the bottom of the balance frame. You then must move it back one groove (Figure 1).

Continued

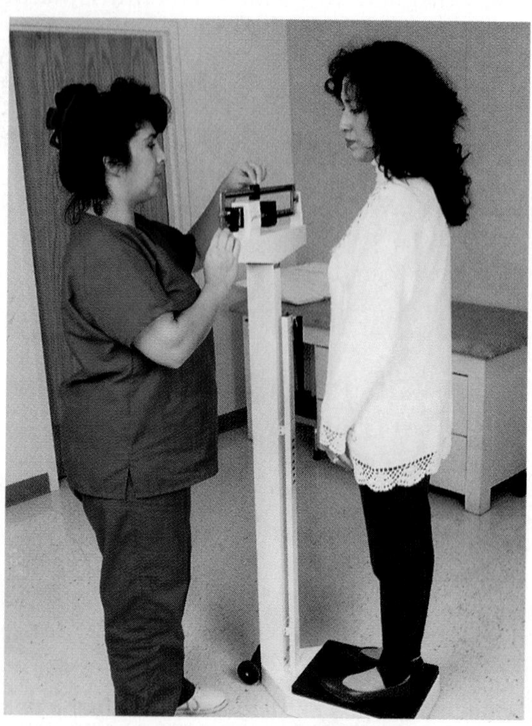

FIGURE 1

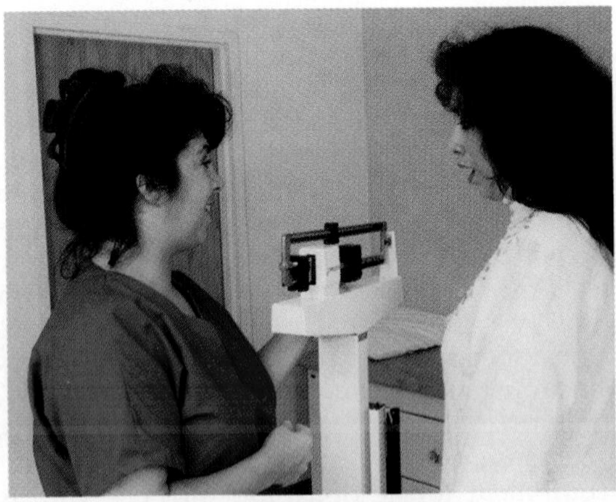
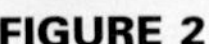

FIGURE 2

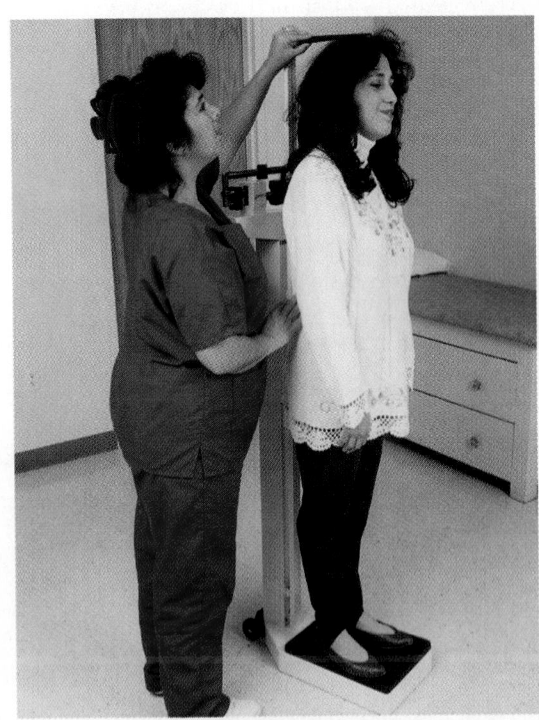

FIGURE 3

7 While the patient is standing still, slide the small upper weight to the right along the ¼-pound markers until the pointer balances in the middle of the balance frame (Figure 2).
PURPOSE: The pointer will float between the bottom and the top of the frame when both lower and upper weights together balance the scale with the patient's weight.

8 *Leave the weights in place.*

9 Ask the patient to stand up straight and to look straight ahead.

10 Adjust the height bar so that it just touches the top of the patient's head (Figure 3).

11 Leave the elevation bar set but fold down the horizontal bar.
PURPOSE: Patient safety.

12 Assist the patient off the scale. Be sure all items removed for weighing are given back to the patient.

13 Read the weight scale. Add the numbers at the markers of the large and the small weights and record the total to the nearest ¼ pound on the patient's medical record (e.g., Wt: 122½).

14 Record the height. Read the marker at the movable point of the ruler, and record the measurement to the nearest quarter inch on the patient's medical record (e.g., Ht: 64½).

15 Return the weights and the measuring bar to zero.

16 Record the results on the patient's medical record.
PURPOSE: Procedures that are not recorded are considered not done.

Weight

Some patients are sensitive or secretive about their body weight, so placement of the scale in the office should offer privacy from staff and other patients who might be in the office area. Your manner and approach are very important in keeping patients from feeling embarrassed or shy. Whether your patients are obese or petite persons who do not want their weight known to others or who are handicapped with appliances that must be removed, make certain that the scale is placed in an area of privacy.

It is not necessary to remove shoes and clothing if patients are consistently weighed and measured with them on. Although the exact weight and height may not be determined, changes in the patient's weight and height can be detected and analyzed

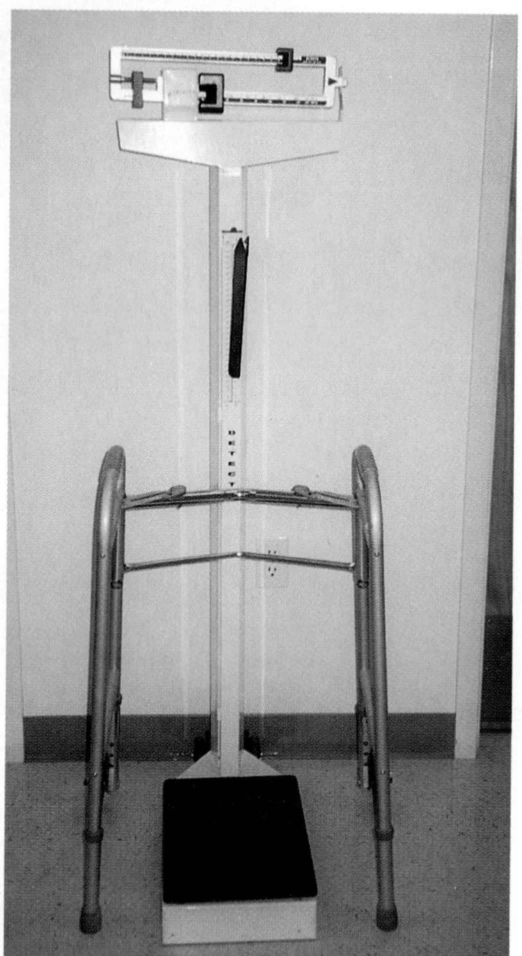

FIGURE 27–16 Walker over scale to aid patient in balancing.

(see Chapter 47). If patients are unstable, assist them onto the scale and to balance themselves. A walker can be placed over the scale for the patient to use as hand support when getting on or off or to balance on the scale (Fig. 27–16).

Do not comment on a patient's weight or his or her progress in a weight program; this is the physician's or counselor's responsibility. When the physician prescribes weight measurement at home, make certain that the patient understands the importance of weighing himself or herself each day at the same time in clothing of similar weight. Body weight may vary considerably from early morning to late afternoon. Teach the patient how to record the weight on a graphic record and how to make any other important notations.

Height

Height can be measured in inches or in centimeters. It is easily accomplished by moving the parallel bar attached to the ruler on the scale. Height measurements used in pediatrics are discussed in Chapter 34 and those in elder care in Chapter 39.

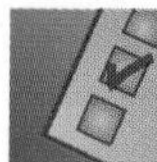

PATIENT EDUCATION

All patients should know how to use a thermometer safely and how to read a thermometer accurately. Because many types of temperature reading equipment are sold, ask the patient what type of equipment he or she uses at home to obtain temperature readings. By talking with the patient, you will be able to determine whether the patient understands how to use a thermometer. You might have the patient actually read the thermometer.

When instructing a patient in methods of pulse assessment, it is important to familiarize him or her with counting the beats and also in how to determine the rate, rhythm, and regularity of the beat. Have the patient take your pulse to assess accuracy.

If a patient is to keep track of his or her own respirations, he or she will need assistance in counting; however, the patient can be taught self-assessment of impending complications as well as preventive breathing exercises.

Monitoring blood pressure at home has become very common. Suggest to the patient to bring his or her equipment to the office and practice with it. In this way, you can be sure that the patient is using the equipment correctly and is hearing the diastolic and systolic beats using his or her own stethoscope and sphygmomanometer and recording the results accurately in a record book. One of the most common problems in hearing blood pressure accurately is in the placement of the earpieces in the ears. Patients frequently have the earpieces pointing backward instead of forward. This simple correction may eliminate the patient's problem in using home equipment.

Weight management can be a trying and emotional experience for a patient. Understanding how weight is affected by the time of day, by a particular activity, or by the type of scale used can help the patient to maintain a positive attitude. Have an assortment of weight management literature available for the patient to take home.

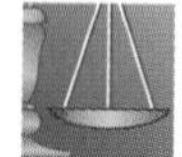

LEGAL AND ETHICAL ISSUES

The medical assistant must always remember that, as the physician's agent, he or she plays an important role in preventing legal claims against the physician and the medical office. The medical assistant always functions within the legal boundaries of the profession. When obtaining vital signs, carefully select your response to a patient who asks about the results. Patients should be told the results *only* when the physician has given the assistant consent to do so. Even when the physician has given consent, remember that you are *never* to diagnose; that is, you are never to evaluate or give an opinion of what the results may mean. For example: The patient asks "Is my blood pressure better?" You might reply, "My reading is 160/90." You have not said that it is worse, the same, or better.

Always be very accurate in the transcribing of the results onto the patient's medical record. If the results are incorrectly recorded, there is a chance that the patient will be incorrectly diagnosed or treated. This can result in legal action that may implicate you. A careless attitude toward the assessment of vital signs and toward documentation can lead to possible legal entanglement. In every procedure you did in this chapter there was a reminder to record the test results. If there is no entry, the assumption is that it was not done. Cultivate a sensitivity toward proper conduct and performance so that you can protect yourself and your physician employer.

Memory Jogger

15 *Why can't you tell a patient that his or her blood pressure has improved?*

CRITICAL THINKING

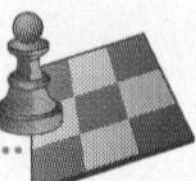

1 How would you handle a patient who is continuously talking with the thermometer in his or her mouth?

2 Your patient has a documented thready, soft pulse. What would be the best site at which to take the pulse and how would you expect it to feel?

3 Your patient is wearing a heavy knit sweater and you need to get a respiration count. How would you handle the situation?

4 The medical record of Mr. Black states "severe orthostatic hypotension." What would be the position(s) of choice to get a blood pressure reading?

5 Mrs. Johnson has come for her first visit. In what order would you take her vital signs and her anthropometric measurements? Why?

HOW DID I DO? Answers to Memory Joggers

1 Vital signs are temperature, pulse, respiration, and blood pressure.

2 A variation from the patient's average range of body temperature may be the *first warning of an illness or change in present condition.*

3 An intermittent fever spikes and then returns to normal. A remittent fever has great fluctuation but never gets to normal.

4 The body sites used to obtain a temperature are
a. Oral: Average normal value = 98.6° F
b. Rectal: Average normal value = 99.6° F
c. Axillary: Average normal value = 97.6° F
d. Tympanic: Average normal value = 98.6° F

5 Tympanic thermometer units are popular because of speed and patient comfort.

6 A rectal temperature might be used if a patient is unconscious, is uncooperative, has breathing difficulties, has had oral surgery, or is very young.

7 Steps in cleaning a glass thermometer:
a. Wash with soap and cool water.
b. Rinse and dry.
c. Soak in disinfecting solution 30 to 60 minutes.

8 The eight pulse sites are temporal, carotid, apical, brachial, radial, femoral, popliteal, and pedal.

9 You never tell someone that you are going to count his or her respirations because when one is conscious of breathing the rate frequently changes. Tell the patient you want to take his or her pulse, then hold the wrist and count the respirations.

10 Physiologic factors determining blood pressure are volume, peripheral resistance of blood vessels, vessel elasticity, and condition of the heart muscle.

11 Clarify the difference:
a. Pulse deficit is the difference between the apical and the radial pulses.
b. Pulse pressure is the difference between the systolic and diastolic blood pressures.

12 Hypertension is pressure persistently above normal, and hypotension is pressure of 90/60 or below.

13 Describe Korotkoff sounds:
a. Phase I = sharp, tapping sound
b. Phase II = swishing sound
c. Phase III = distinct, sharp rhythmically tapping
d. Phase IV = soft muffled tapping sound growing fainter
e. Phase V = last sound is heard, sound disappears

14 87 kilograms = 191.4 pounds

15 Medical assistants are not allowed to diagnose. A lower reading may not indicate improvement.

SECTION 8

The Protocols of Patient Care

CURRICULUM CONTENT/COMPETENCIES

Chapters 28–38: Assisting in Specialty Practices

- *Prepare the patient for examinations, procedures, and treatments*
- *Assist with examinations, procedures, and treatments*
- *Perform diagnostic tests*
- *Project a professional manner and image*
- *Recognize and respond to verbal and nonverbal communication*
- *Adapt communications to individual's ability to understand*
- *Document accurately*
- *Screen and follow up patient test results*

Chapter 39: Assisting With the Elder Client

- *Prepare the patient for examinations, procedures, and treatments*
- *Assist with examinations, procedures, and treatments*
- *Project a professional image*
- *Adhere to ethical principles*
- *Treat all patients with compassion and empathy*
- *Adapt communications to the individual's ability to understand*
- *Recognize and respond to verbal and nonverbal communication*
- *Explain procedures*

Chapter 40: Assisting With Office Emergency Procedures

- *Recognize and respond to emergencies*
- *Adhere to established triage procedures*
- *Perform diagnostic tests*
- *Maintain confidentiality*
- *Practice within the scope of education, training, and personal capabilities*
- *Document accurately*

Assisting with the Primary Physical Examination

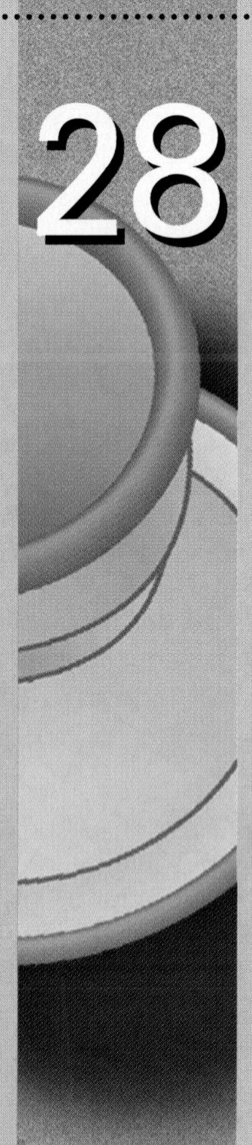

OUTLINE

LEARNING OBJECTIVES

Cognitive: On successful completion of this chapter you should be able to:

1. Define and spell the words in the Vocabulary.
2. Describe the structural development of the human body.
3. Identify the 11 body systems and the major organs or units in each.
4. List 10 instruments that may be used during a physical examination.
5. Describe the six methods of examination and give an example for each.
6. Outline the basic principles of properly draping a patient for examination.
7. List eight positions that may be used in examinations.
8. Outline the sequence of a routine physical examination.
9. Identify the medical speciality for each body system.
10. Discuss the legal and ethical implications of the physical examination.

Performance: On successful completion of this chapter you should be able to:

1. Prepare the examination room and instruments for a physical examination.
2. Position and drape a patient in six different examining positions with ease while mindful of patient modesty.
3. Assist in the physical examination of a patient, correctly completing each step of the procedure in the proper sequence.

VOCABULARY

bruit Abnormal sound or murmur heard on auscultation of an organ, vessel, or gland

emphysema Pathologic accumulation of air in the tissues or organs; in the lungs, the bronchioles become plugged with mucus and lose elasticity

manipulation Moving or exercising a body part by an externally applied force

murmur Abnormal sound heard when auscultating the heart that may or may not be pathologic

nodule Small lump, lesion, or swelling felt when palpating the skin

sclera White part of the eye that forms the orb

transillumination Inspection of a cavity or organ by passing light through its walls

trauma Physical injury or wound caused by an external force or violence

uremia Toxic renal condition characterized by an excess of urea, creatinine, and other nitrogenous end-products in the blood

The human body is a creation that can never be duplicated. Imagine billions of microscopic parts, each with its own functioning identity yet all working together in a systematic organizational manner for the perfect harmony of the entire creation. There has always been an intense interest in understanding how and why the body functions and what happens when parts become diseased or wear out. The only way any health care professional can help in the repair or maintenance of the human body is by understanding how the body is put together, what role each part plays, and how each part functions.

Anatomy and Physiology

The study of how the body is shaped and structured is *anatomy*. It encompasses a wide range of subjects, including (1) structural development, (2) levels of organization, (3) relationships between microscopic parts, and (4) interrelationship of structure and function.

The study of body functions is *physiology*. This field is also subdivided into areas of study, and some physiologists spend their entire lives studying only one function, such as how cells work or how a single organ such as the small intestine is interrelated in function with the stomach and the large intestine.

It is almost impossible to separate these two sciences because one continuously influences the other. Function affects structure, and structure affects function; for example, an infant has the ability to suck effortlessly because of the lack of teeth in its mouth. Once teeth appear, sucking becomes more tiresome and the child now begins to chew and bite. Phenomena in structure and function affect the interrelationship of the entire gastrointestinal system, which is responsible for providing nourishment to the entire body.

Memory Jogger

Why is it important to understand how the body functions?

STRUCTURAL DEVELOPMENT

Cells

The basic unit of life is the cell, and it determines the functional and structural characteristics of the entire body. Cells come in a variety of shapes and sizes and provide a vast array of functions. It is estimated that the human body is composed of about 100 trillion living, functioning cells.

Tissue

When cells with similar structure and function are placed together, they form tissues. All of the body tissues are grouped into four types: epithelial, connective, muscle, and nervous. Every tissue in our body is classified as one of these types of tissues.

Memory Jogger

What type of tissue do you think blood is?

Organs

An *organ* is composed of two or more types of tissue bound together to form a more complex structure for a common purpose or function. An organ may have one or many functions and may be considered a unit in one or several systems.

Systems

A body *system* is composed of several organs and their associated structures. These structures work to-

TABLE 28–1 Body System Organization

Body System	Systems, Organs, and Structures
Integumentary	Skin, sweat glands, sebaceous glands, ceruminous glands, hair, and nails
Musculoskeletal	Bones, joints, muscles, tendons, ligaments, and cartilage
Nervous	Brain, spinal cord, nerves
Special senses	Eye and ear
Gastrointestinal	Mouth, pharynx, esophagus, stomach, small intestine, large intestine, liver, gallbladder, pancreas, anus
Cardiovascular	Heart, arteries, veins
Respiratory	Nose, pharynx, larynx, trachea, lungs
Endocrine	Pituitary, pineal, thyroid, thymus, pancreas, adrenal, parathyroid, ovaries, testes
Lymphatic and hematic	Lymph, spleen, tonsils, thymus, white blood cells, red blood cells, platelets, plasma
Urinary	Kidneys, ureters, bladder, urethra
Reproductive	Ovaries, fallopian tubes, uterus, vagina, mammary glands, testes, vas deferens, prostate gland, penis

gether to accomplish a definite assignment or purpose. There are 11 systems in the human body; each system has specific units within it, and each performs specific functions. Put these eleven systems all together and we have a human being (Table 28–1).

Memory Jogger

List the 11 systems of the human body.

Medical Specialties

As the knowledge and understanding regarding the anatomy and physiology of the human body increased, the medical profession realized it was becoming impossible for one physician to be an expert in all systems. To solve this, physicians began to specialize in one system to master the problems and treatments of the body functions controlled by that system. Some systems are so interrelated that they remain combined under one specialty whereas others are so large they have become divided into subspecialties (Table 28–2).

FAMILY PRACTICE PHYSICIAN

Family practice physicians treat all the members of the family for broad ranges of different diseases and complaints. This physician is qualified to provide continuing health care for the entire family, from birth to old age, regardless of sex, age, or type of problem.

Although the field of medicine has become highly specialized, the need for a physician who will treat the entire family has never diminished. Within the health care system of today, many health insurance programs have gone to the primary care referral system. This means that everyone must have a primary care physician as their gatekeeper in personal health care. A family practice physician serves as the physician of first contact and means of entry into the health care system. The physician can evaluate the patient's total health care needs, can provide personal medical care within one or more fields of medicine, and can arrange for their patient to receive further care with a specialist when an advanced or serious condition warrants additional expertise. In 1969, family practice became a board-certified specialty and is now one of the fastest growing medical specialties because it incorporates the family as a unit.

The medical assistant's clinical responsibilities in the family practice office encompass assisting with patients and procedures on all age groups with problems in all systems. When a practice becomes so diversified, the physician and the medical assistant must work as an efficient team to utilize their time and still provide for the needs of the patients served. The medical assistant can ease the roles of both the physician and the patient by following the physician's instructions quickly, accurately, and confidentially.

TABLE 28–2 Medical Specialties

Speciality	Speciality Area
Allergist	Respiratory system
Cardiologist	Cardiovascular system
Dermatologist	Integumentary system
Endocrinologist	Endocrine system
Family Practice Physician	All systems
Gastroenterologist	Gastrointestinal system
Geriatrics	Elder care
Gynecologist	Female reproductive system
Internist	Cardiovascular, endocrine, respiratory, gastrointestinal, lymphatic, and hematic
Nephrologist	Kidneys
Neurologist	Brain and nervous system
Obstetrician	Pregnancy and birth
Oncology	Tumors and masses (cancer)
Ophthalmologist	Eyes
Orthopedist	Muscloskeletal system
Otorhinolaryngologist	Ears, nose, and throat
Pediatrician	Infants and children
Physical Medicine	Muscles and joints
Proctologist	Large intestine (colon) and anus
Psychiatrist	Brain and nervous system
Pulmonary Medicine	Chest and lungs
Urologist	Urinary system, male reproductive system

Physical Examination

The purpose of the physical examination is to determine the overall state of well-being of the patient. All major organs and all body systems are checked during a physical examination. As the physician examines the entire body, the findings are interpreted, and by the time the examination is completed, the physician has formed an initial diagnosis regarding the patient's condition. Frequently, laboratory and other diagnostic tests are ordered to supplement the physician's initial diagnosis. The results of these tests are often used to aid the physician in planning a treatment for the patient, in maintaining drug therapy, or in evaluating the patient's progress.

PREPARING FOR THE PHYSICAL EXAMINATION

The Medical Assistant's Role in the Physical Examination

The examination begins when the patient first makes contact with the office. Before the examination, you have the opportunity to interact with and react to the patient to ensure that he or she feels comfortable during the examination process and that all the necessary information is obtained.

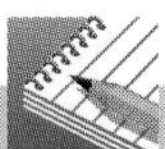

SKILLS AND RESPONSIBILITIES

The medical assistant's duties can be divided into three areas

1 Preparation of the room and equipment
2 Preparation of the patient
3 Assisting the physician

Room preparation includes stocking and checking the room to be sure that it is aesthetically ready and assures patient privacy and comfort. Drapes, gowns, and gloves should be arranged and ready for use. The instruments and equipment that will be used are prepared and properly covered.

Patient preparation includes checking the medical record for completeness and making sure that any needed consent forms are signed; obtaining any specimens such as urine and blood; performing an electrocardiogram; determining height, weight, and vital signs; and helping the patient physically prepare (removing clothing and gowning). Throughout this entire sequence of events, the medical assistant offers explanations of what he or she is doing to the patient.

Assisting the physician includes handing the physician the instruments and equipment requested, positioning and draping the patient during the different phases of the examination, writing down any pertinent information, and acting as an advocate for the patient.

Memory Jogger

Identify three duty areas that the medical assistant is responsible for.

Instruments and Equipment Needed for Physical Examination

The instruments most frequently used for the physical examination are described in the following paragraphs. These instruments enable the physician to see, feel, and listen to parts of the body. All the equipment and supplies needed should be ready for the physician's use during the examination.

- *Nasal speculum*—stainless-steel instrument used to inspect the lining of the nose, nasal membranes, and internal septum (Fig. 28–1*A*). By squeezing the handles of the nasal speculum, the tips spread apart to dilate the nostrils, allowing the physician to visualize the internal aspects (see Fig. 28–1*B*). An otoscope with a special attachment may be used for nasal visualization.
- *Ophthalmoscope*—instrument used to inspect the inner structures of the eye (Fig. 28–2*A*). It has a stainless-steel handle containing batteries, onto which a head is attached. The head is equipped with a light and magnifying lenses and an opening through which the eye is viewed (see Fig. 28–2*B*).
- *Otoscope*—instrument used to examine the ear canal and tympanic membrane. It has a stainless steel handle containing batteries, onto which a head is fastened (Fig. 28–3*A*). The head contains a light that is focused through a magnifying lens and ear speculum. The specula are long, narrow, and numbered according to the size of the lumen. Some offices prefer to use a disposable speculum (Fig. 28–3*B*).

The previously described three instruments may all work off a common handle unit, and only the examination head is changed for each part of the examination. Some offices use handles equipped with rechargeable batteries that must be placed in a charger when not in use, or the exam room may contain a wall-mounted electrical unit to which the scopes are attached and batteries are not needed (Fig. 28–4).

Memory Jogger

Spell the names of the three instruments that may work off one handle.

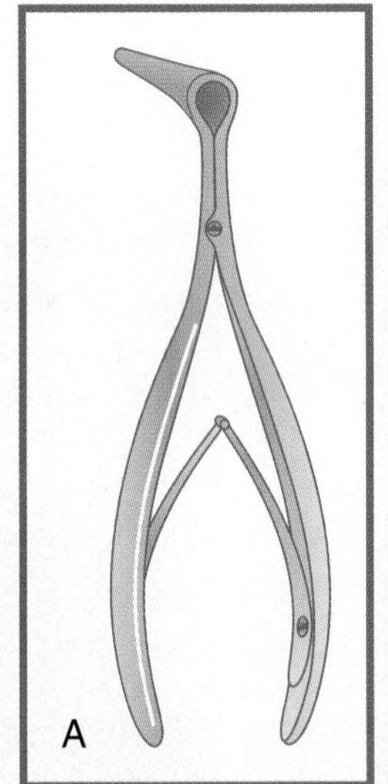

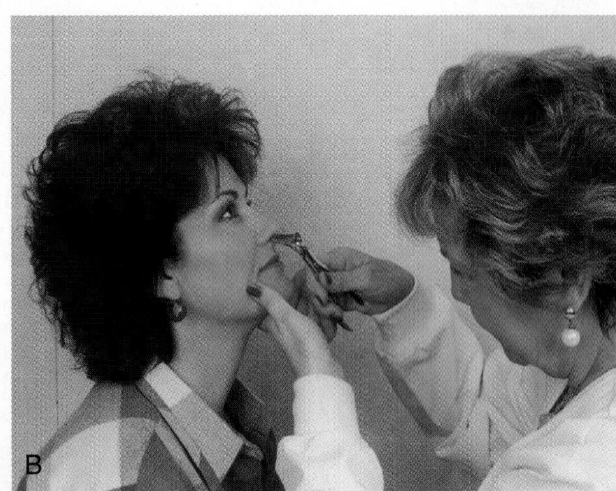

FIGURE 28–1 *A,* Nasal speculum. *B,* Nasal examination.

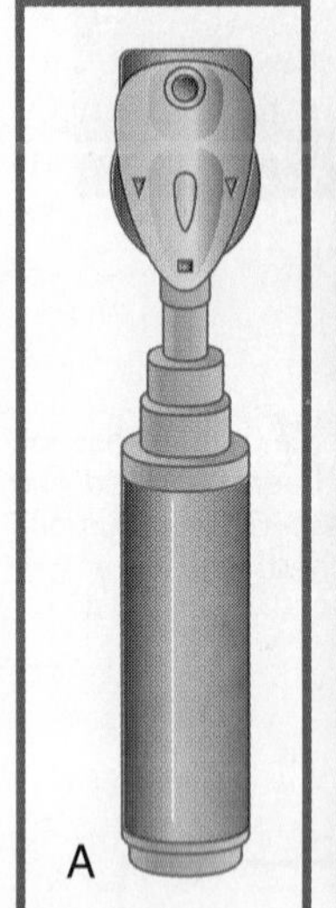

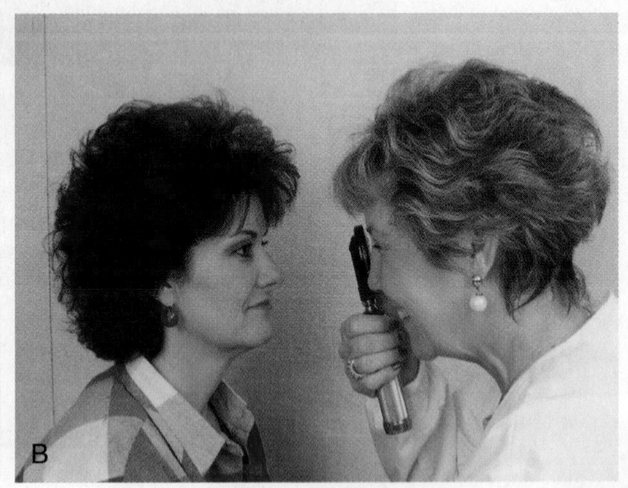

FIGURE 28–2 *A,* Ophthalmoscope. *B,* Eye examination.

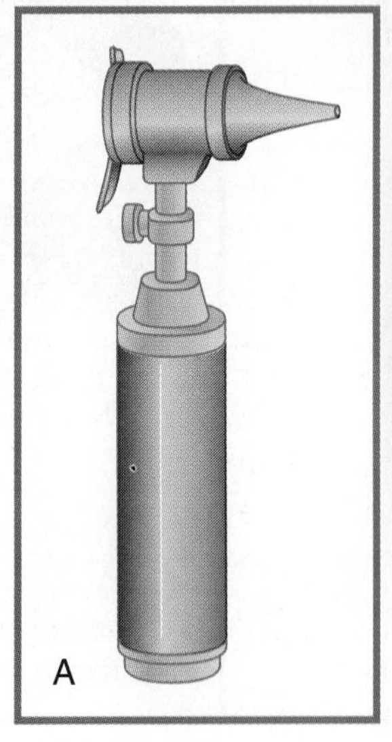

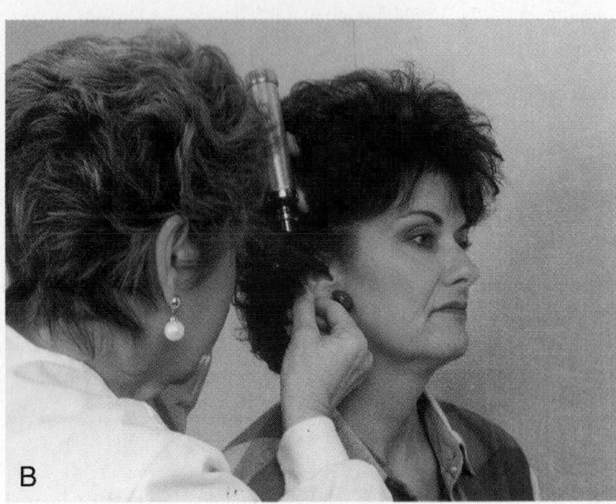

FIGURE 28–3 *A,* Otoscope. *B,* Ear examination.

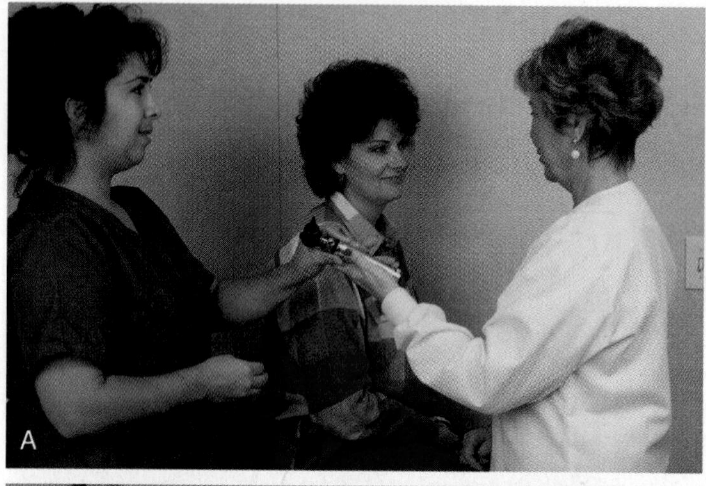

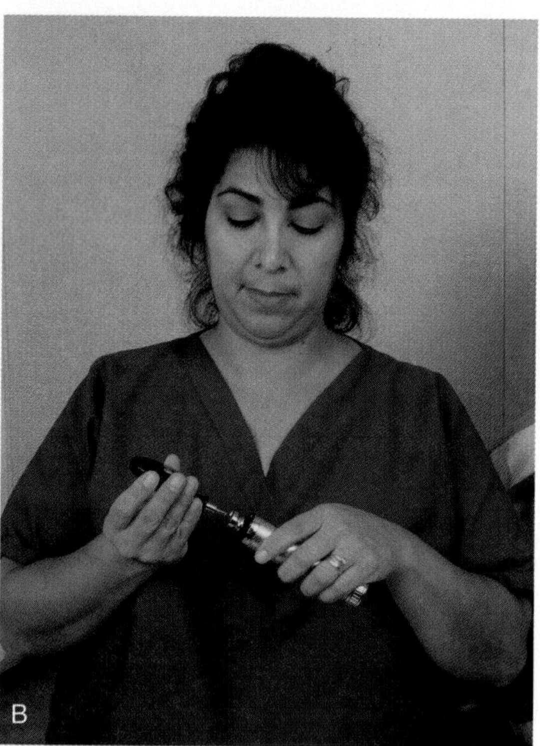

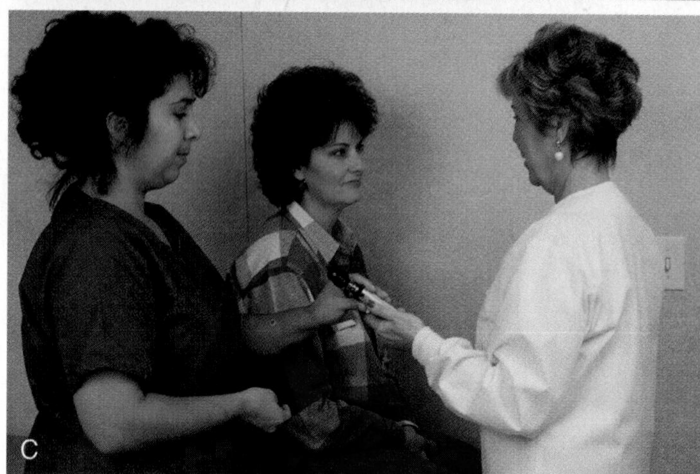

FIGURE 28-4 *A,* Multipurpose handle with otoscope head attached. *B,* Otoscope head has been removed and ophthalmoscope head is being attached. *C,* Multipurpose handle with ophthalmoscope head attached.

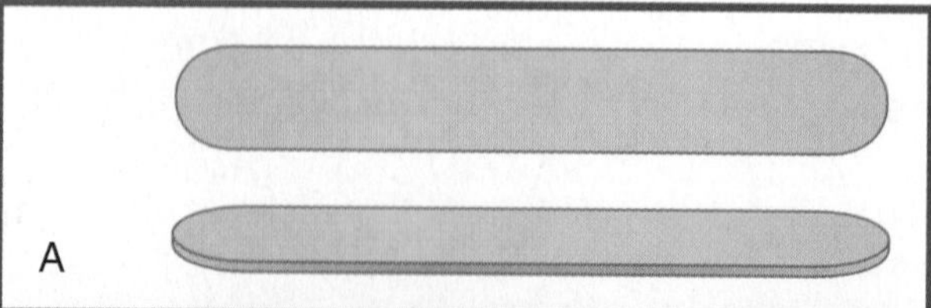

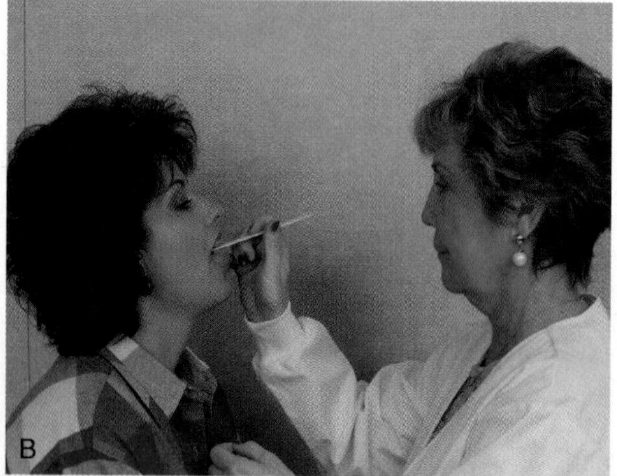

FIGURE 28-5 *A,* Tongue depressor. *B,* Pharyngeal examination.

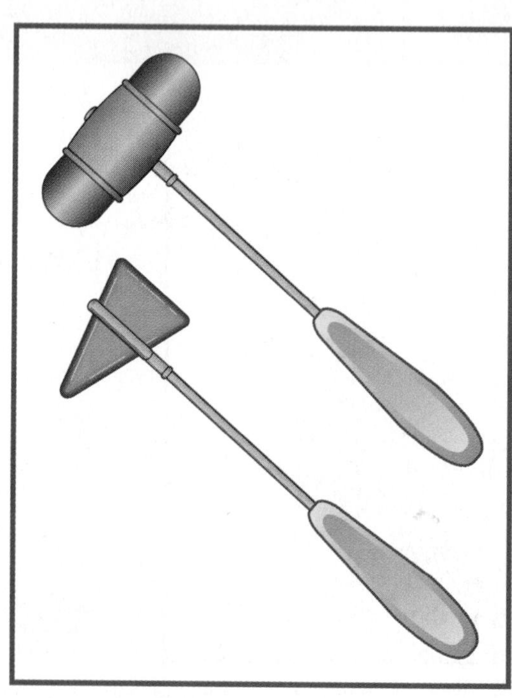

FIGURE 28-6 Reflex hammers.

- *Tongue depressor*—flat, wooden blade used to hold down the tongue when examining the throat (Fig. 28–5).
- *Reflex hammer*—sometimes referred to as a percussion hammer. This stainless steel instrument has a hard rubber head used to test neurologic reflexes of the knee and elbow by striking the tendons (Fig. 28–6).
- *Tuning fork*—The forks come in different sizes, and each size produces a different pitch level (Fig. 28–7*A*). The tuning fork is used to check a patient's auditory acuity and to test bone vibra-

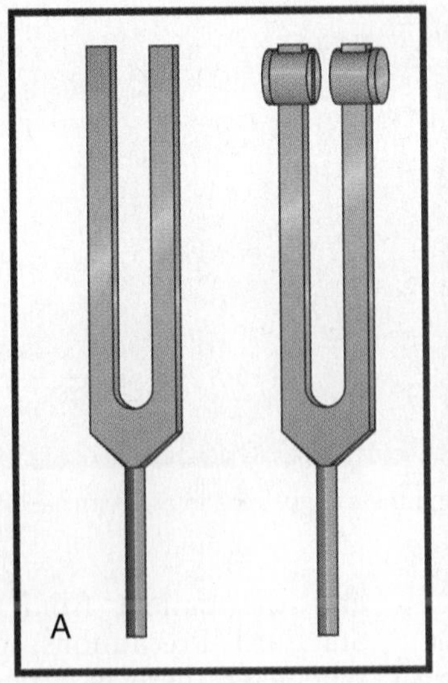

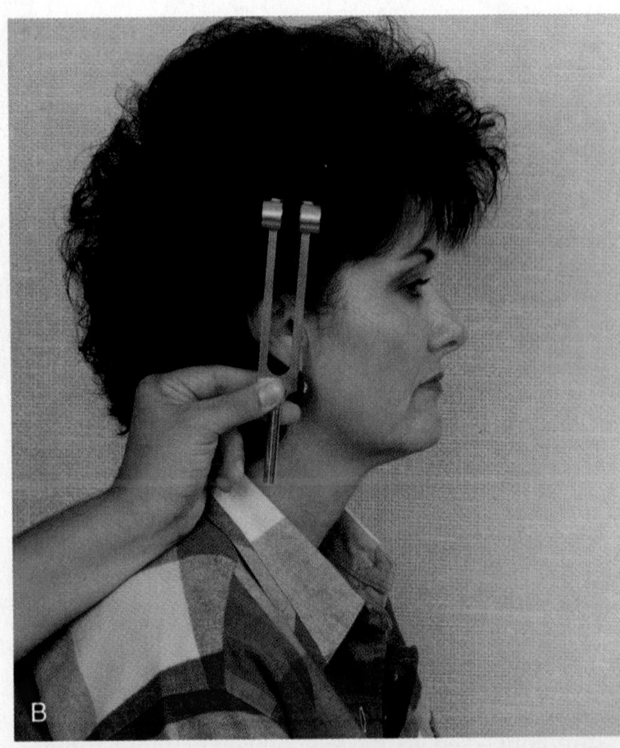

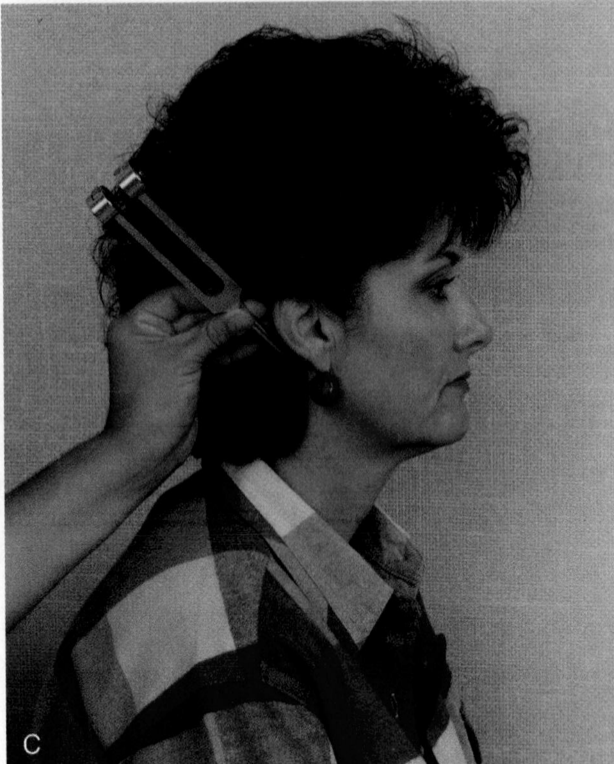

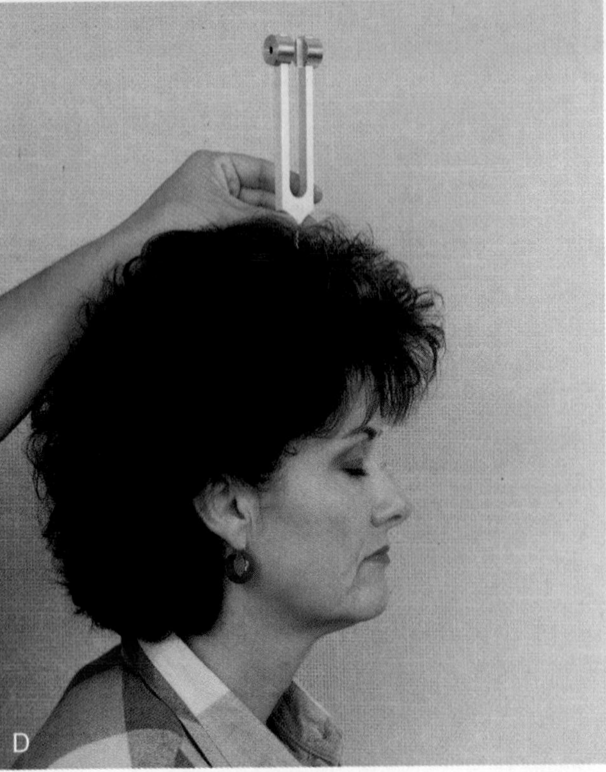

FIGURE 28–7 *A,* Tuning fork. *B,* Auditory acuity testing. *C,* Bone vibration testing, using mastoid process. *D,* Bone vibration testing using parietal suture line.

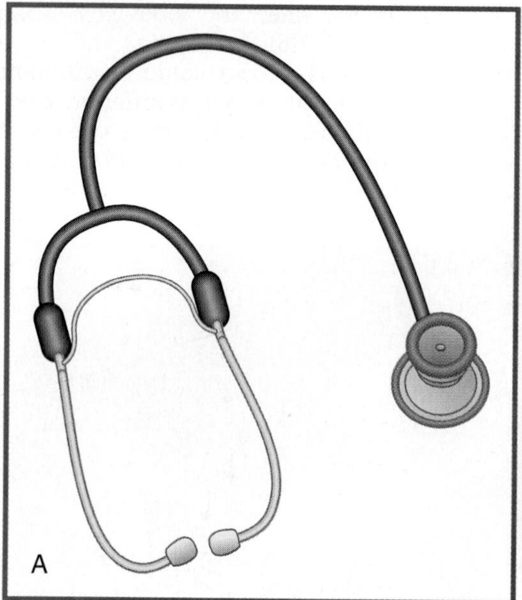
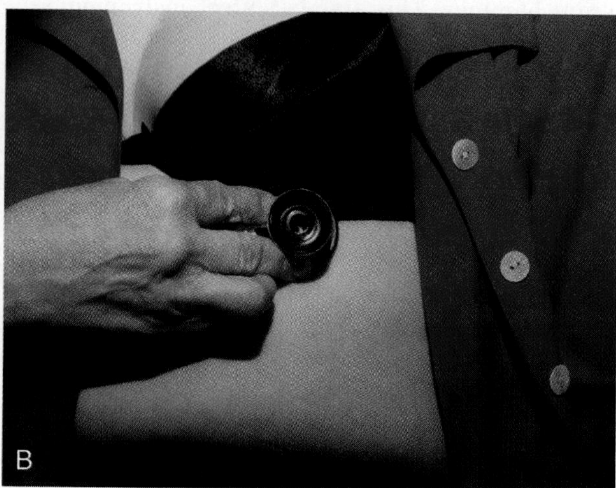

FIGURE 28–8 *A,* Stethoscope. *B,* Using the stethoscope in an examination.

tion. This stainless steel instrument consists of a handle and two prongs that produce a humming sound when the physician strikes the prongs against his or her hand (see Fig. 28–7*B* through *D*).

- *Stethoscope*—listening device used when auscultating certain areas of the body, particularly the heart and lungs. This instrument comes in many shapes and sizes. All have two ear pieces that are connected to flexible rubber or vinyl tubing (Fig. 28–8*A*). At the distal end of the tubing is a diaphragm or bell (many have both) that when placed securely on the patient's skin enables the physician to hear internal body sounds (see Fig. 28–8*B*).
- *Gloves*—disposable gloves protect the physician and the patient from microorganisms. Under Standard Precautions, gloves are to be worn whenever there is a possibility of contact with body fluids and contaminated items.
- *Tape measure*—Flexible ribbon ruler usually printed in inches and feet on one side and in centimeters and meters on the opposite side (Fig. 28–9). Measurement is used to assess developmental progress or determine the size of an abnormality found during an examination.
- *Headmirror and penlight*—used if additional light is needed for **transillumination**. Lights may be battery operated or electrical (Fig. 28–10). The medical assistant must always check the light to be sure that it works correctly before placing it with the examination equipment.
- *Additional supplies*—gauze squares, cotton balls, glass slides, cotton-tipped applicators, and laboratory request forms should be easily accessible for use during the examination.

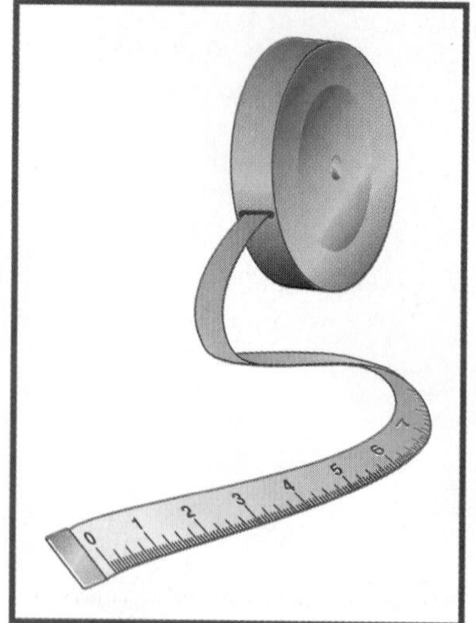

FIGURE 28–9 Tape measure.

Memory Jogger

6 *Explain the difference between visualization and transillumination.*

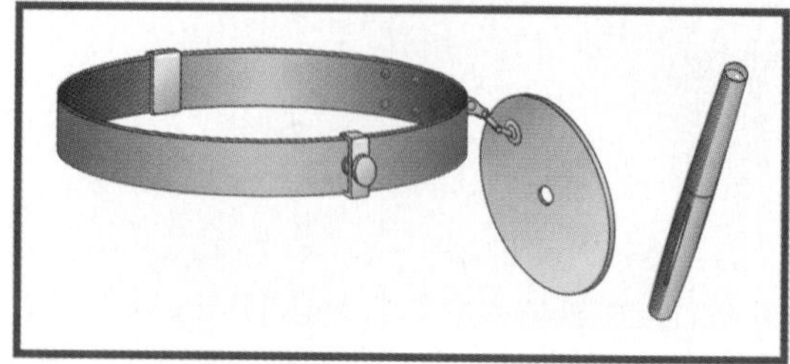

FIGURE 28–10 Headmirror and penlight.

ASSISTING WITH THE PHYSICAL EXAMINATION

Methods of Examination

Examinations are performed as both a routine confirmation of the absence of illness and a means of diagnosing disease. There are six methods of examining the human body that are used by the physician. All six methods are part of a complete physical examination.

INSPECTION Inspection is the art of observation that involves the ability to detect significant physical features. The focus of this method of examination ranges from the patient's general appearance (the general state of health, including posture, mannerisms, grooming) to the more detailed observations, including body contour, symmetry, visible injuries and deformities, tremors, rashes, and color changes.

PALPATION Palpation uses the sense of touch (Fig. 28–11*A*). A part of the body is felt with the hand

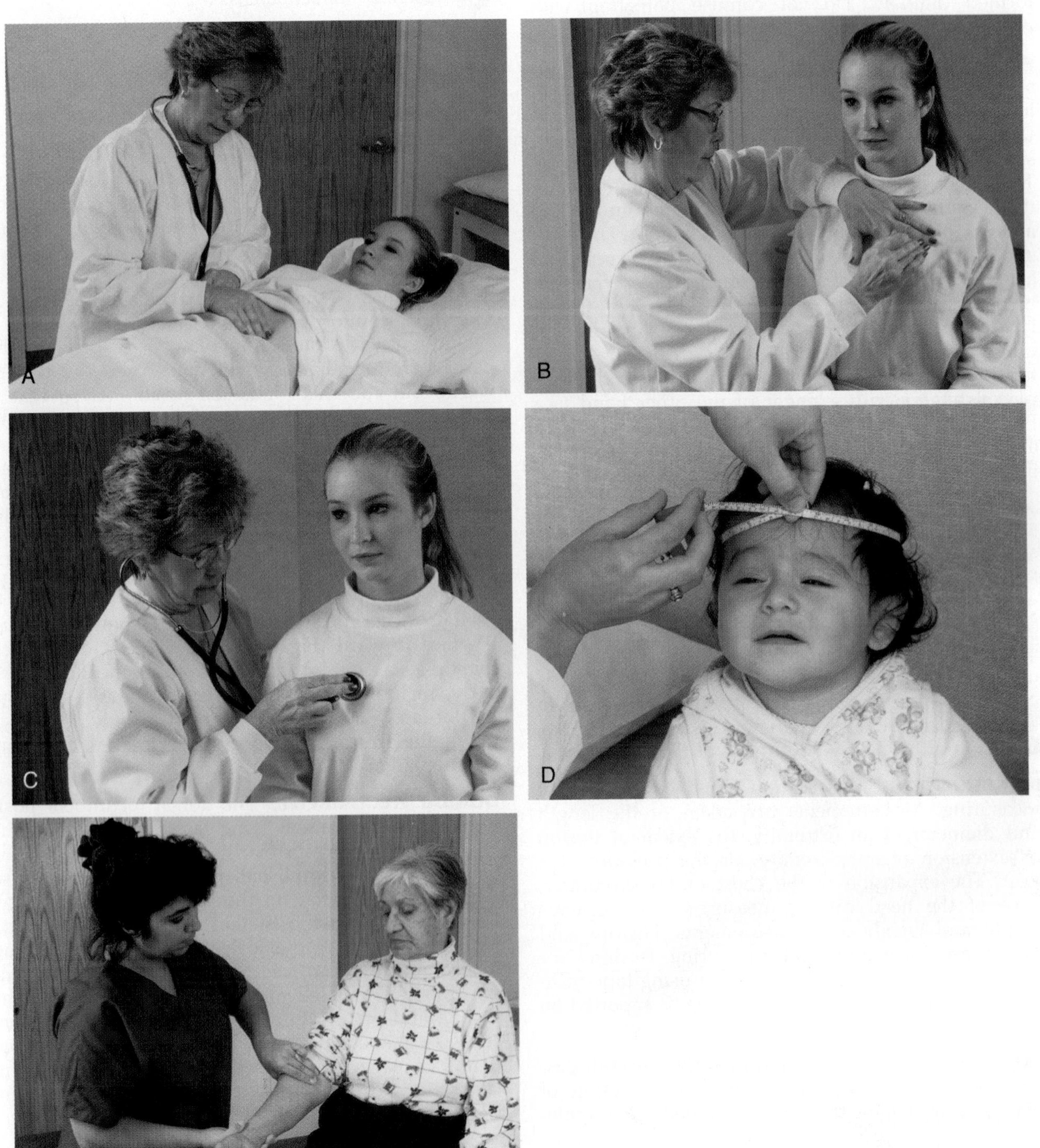

FIGURE 28–11 *A*, Demonstration of palpation. *B*, Demonstration of percussion. *C*, Demonstration of auscultation. *D*, Demonstration of mensuration. *E*, Demonstration of manipulation.

for the purpose of determining its condition or that of an underlying organ. Palpation may include touching the skin or the more firm feeling of the abdomen for underlying masses. This technique involves a wide range of perceptions: temperature, vibrations, consistency, form, size, rigidity, elasticity, moisture, texture, position, and contour. Palpation is performed with one hand, both hands (bimanual), one finger (digital), the fingertips, or the palmar aspect of the hand. A pelvic examination is done bimanually, whereas an anal examination is performed digitally. Do not confuse palpation with *palpitation*, which is a throbbing pulsation.

PERCUSSION Percussion is the art of tapping or striking the body, usually with the fingers or a small hammer, to elicit sounds or vibratory sensations. Percussion aids in the determination of the position, size, and density of an underlying organ or cavity. The effect of percussion is both heard and felt by the examiner. It is helpful in determining the amount of air or solid matter in an underlying organ or cavity. The two basic methods of percussion are *direct* and *indirect*. Direct (immediate) percussion is performed by striking the body with a finger. Indirect (mediate) percussion is used more frequently and is done by the physician placing his or her own fingers on the area and then striking the placed fingers with a finger of the other hand (see Fig. 28–11*B*). Both a sound and a sense of vibration are evident here. The examiner will speak of sounds in terms of pitch, quality, duration, and resonance.

AUSCULTATION Auscultation is the process of listening to sounds arising from the body (not the sound produced by the physician as in percussion but sounds that originate within the patient's body). Auscultation is a difficult method of examination because the physician must distinguish between a normal and an abnormal sound. A stethoscope is used to amplify the sounds (see Fig. 28–11*C*). It is particularly useful in appraising sounds arising from the lungs, heart, and abdomen such as **murmurs, bruits,** and the clicks and gurgles of the intestine.

MENSURATION Mensuration is the process of measuring. Measurements are taken of the length and diameter of an extremity, the extent of flexion or extension of an extremity, or the pressure of a grip. The expansion of the chest or the circumference of the head can be measured. The patient's height and weight are measurements. Hearing and vision are measured, and measuring is done for pregnancy. Measurements are taken using tape measures or small rulers and are usually reported in centimeters (see Fig. 28–11*D*).

MANIPULATION **Manipulation** is the forceful, passive movement of a joint to determine the range of extension or flexion of a part of the body. Manipulation may or may not be grouped with palpation. It is usually considered separate from the four standard methods of examination (inspection, palpation, percussion, and auscultation) and is grouped with mensuration, especially by the orthopedist and the neurologist. Insurance and industrial reports often request this information in detail (see Fig. 28–11*E*).

Memory Jogger

Describe indirect percussion.

Positioning and Draping for Physical Examinations

There are various positions in which a patient may be placed to facilitate a physical examination. The medical assistant instructs the patient about, and assists the patient into, these positions with as much ease and modesty as possible and helps the patient to maintain a position during the examination with as little discomfort as possible.

Draping with an examination sheet protects the patient from embarrassment and keeps the patient warm, but the sheet must be positioned so that it allows complete visibility for the examiner and does not interfere with the examination. During the general examination, each part of the body is exposed one portion at a time. For gynecologic and rectal examinations, the sheet may be positioned on the diagonal across the patient. The following positions are used for medical examinations.

SUPINE (HORIZONTAL RECUMBENT) Supine is used to describe the patient who is lying flat with the face upward (Fig. 28–12). This position is used for the examination of the frontal portion of the body, including the heart, breasts, and the abdominal organs. The patient's gown should be open down the front, and the drape is placed over any exposed area that is not being examined.

DORSAL RECUMBENT The dorsal recumbent position places the patient lying face upward, with the weight distributed primarily to the surface of the back. This is accomplished by flexing the knees so that the feet are flat on the table. This position relieves muscle tension in the abdomen and is used for examination of the lower extremities, including inspecting the rectal, vaginal, and perineal area. This position can be used for digital examinations of the vagina and rectum but is not used if an instrument such as a speculum is needed. To ensure the patient's privacy, it is important to keep the patient completely draped until the physician is present (Fig. 28–13).

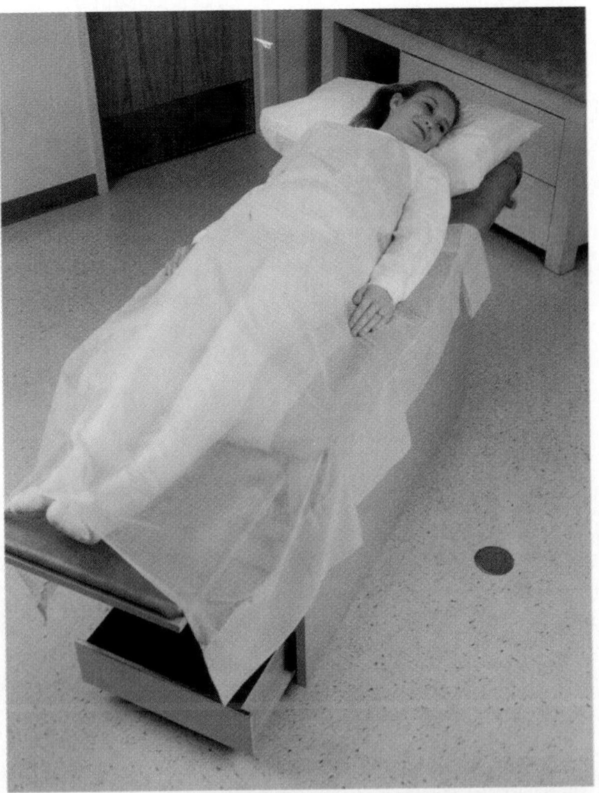

FIGURE 28–12 Patient in supine position.

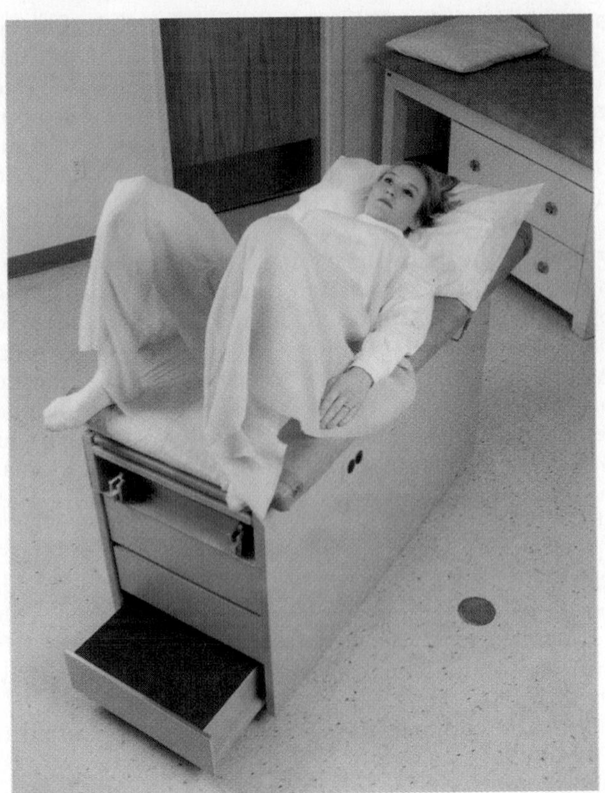

FIGURE 28–13 Patient in dorsal recumbent position.

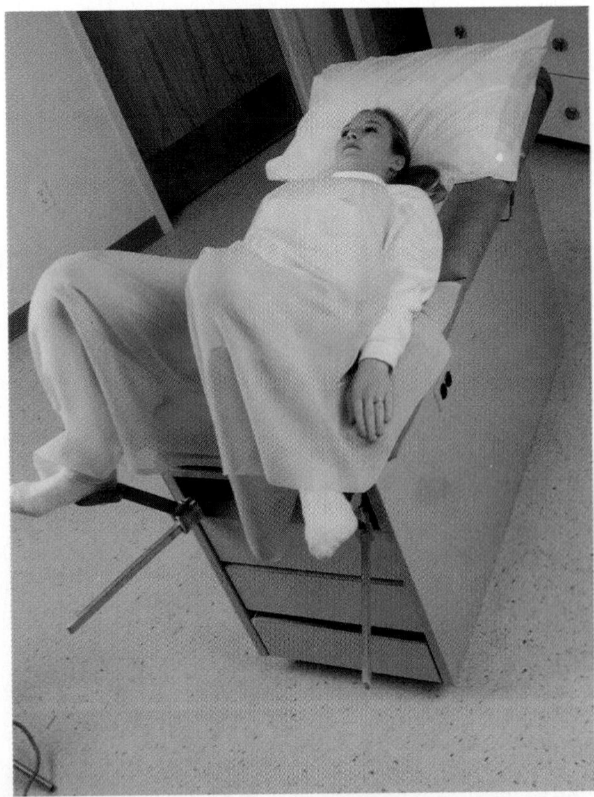

FIGURE 28–14 Patient in lithotomy position.

LITHOTOMY The patient is placed on the back, with the knees sharply flexed, the arms placed at the sides or folded over the chest, and the buttocks to the edge of the table. The feet are supported in table stirrups. The stirrups should be placed wide apart and somewhat away from the table. If the heels are too close to the buttocks, the possibility of leg cramps is increased, and it is more difficult for the patient to relax the abdominal muscles. Make sure that the stirrups are locked in place. A towel is placed under the patient's buttocks, and a drape is placed over the patient's abdomen and knees. The drape should be large enough to cover the breasts if the patient is not wearing a gown. The drape must be long enough to cover the knees and touch the ankles and wide enough to prevent the sides of the thighs from being exposed. The physician will push the drape away from the pubic area when the examination begins (Fig. 28–14).

FOWLER'S The patient is sitting on the examination table with the head elevated. The head usually is raised to a level of about 90 degrees. This position is useful for examinations and treatments of the head, neck, and chest. The drape will vary according to the exposure of the patient, but the female breasts should be covered by the gown or the drape (Fig. 28–15).

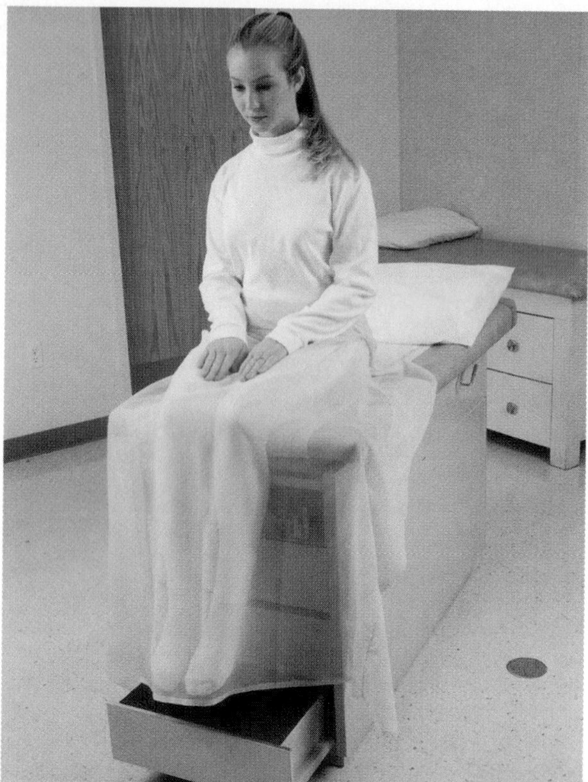

FIGURE 28–15 Patient in Fowler's position.

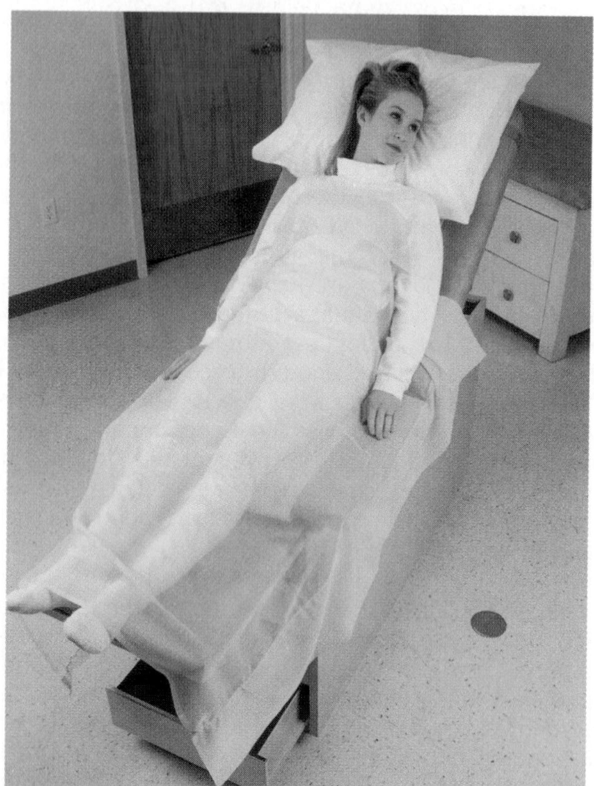

FIGURE 28–16 Patient in semi-Fowler's position.

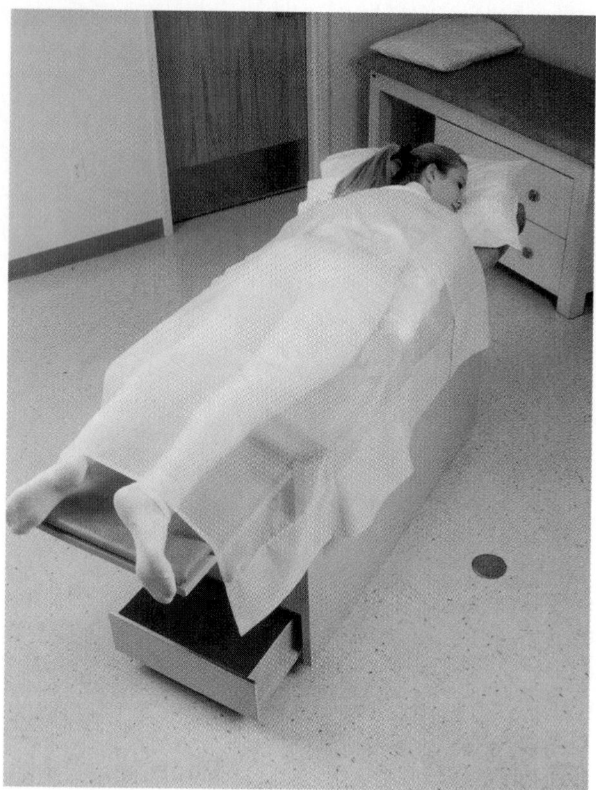

FIGURE 28–17 Patient in prone position.

SEMI-FOWLER'S This position is a modification of Fowler's position. Instead of the head at a full 90-degree angle the head is lowered to a 45-degree angle. This position is useful for postsurgical examinations and when the patient has an elevated temperature or is suffering from head trauma or pain (Fig. 28–16).

PRONE The patient is lying face down on the table, on the ventral surface of the body. This is the opposite of the supine position and is another one of the recumbent positions. The patient is covered with a drape large enough to cover from the middle of the back to below the knees. The drape on the female patient should extend high enough to cover her breasts if she is to be turned over to the dorsal recumbent position during the examination (Fig. 28–17).

SIMS' This position is sometimes called the *lateral* position. The patient is placed on the left side, with a towel or small pillow under the left cheek. The left arm and shoulder are drawn back behind the body so that the body's weight is predominantly on the chest. The right arm is flexed upward for support. The left leg is slightly flexed, and the buttocks are pulled to the edge of the table. The right leg is sharply flexed upward. A towel is placed on the

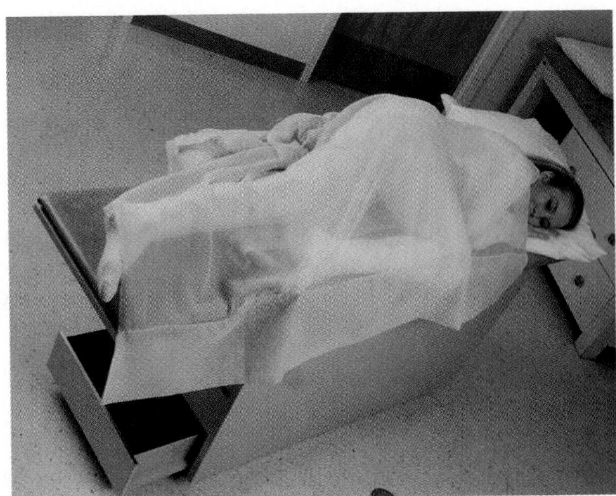

FIGURE 28–18 Patient in Sims' position.

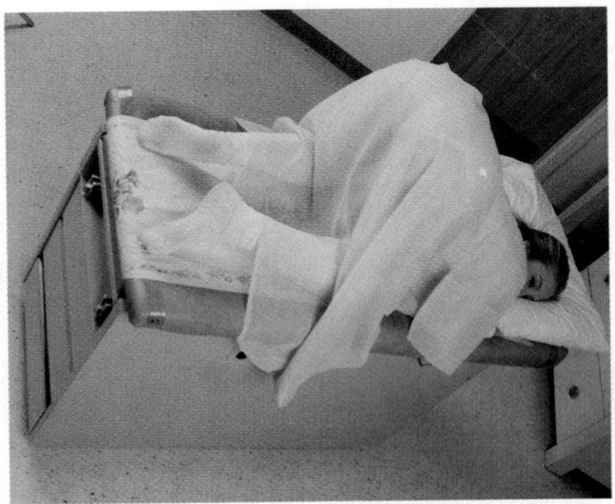

FIGURE 28–19 Patient in knee-chest position.

upper left thigh, just below the perineal area. A sheet is placed over the patient, extending from under the arms to below the knees. The physician will raise a small portion of the sheet from the back of the patient to sufficiently expose the rectum. The remaining portion of the sheet will cover the patient's chest area and thighs. This position is used for rectal examinations, because the rectal ampulla is dropped down into the abdominal cavity; this facilitates entrance to and examination of the rectum. Sims' position is also used for perineal and some pelvic examinations (Fig. 28–18).

KNEE-CHEST The patient rests on the knees and the chest. The head is turned to one side, with one arm flexed under the abdomen and the other hanging over the side of the table or both arms extended along the sides of the body. The thighs are perpendicular to the table and are slightly separated. The patient's back should not be rounded but curved inward somewhat to an anterior convexity. The patient will need assistance to obtain this position correctly. It is a difficult position for most patients to maintain, and you must remain with the patient for assistance and support the entire time that this position is needed. If the correct knee-chest position cannot be obtained, the patient may have to be placed in a knee-elbow position. This position puts less strain on the patient and is easier to maintain. These positions are used for protologic examinations and sigmoid, rectal, and occasional vaginal examinations. A fenestrated (opening) drape is used, or a single sheet may be draped over the patient's back at the sacral area. Two smaller sheets may be used, with one sheet over the patient's back and the other from the curve of the buttocks down over the thighs. It will be necessary to join the two sheets together on each side of the examination area with towel clamps (Fig. 28–19).

TRENDELENBURG'S The patient is supine on a table that has been raised at the lower end about 45 degrees. This places the patient's head lower than the legs. The patient's legs are then flexed over the end. This position is sometimes used in cases of shock or low blood pressure. Recent studies in emergency care question the value of lowering the patient's head, and experts are suggesting that this position is no longer necessary for shock victims. It is also a position for abdominal surgery because the abdominal viscera gravitate upward and out of the way of the surgical procedure. A sheet is placed over the patient, covering from the underarms to below the knees. Never cover the neck, the head, or the hands.

Memory Jogger

Into what position would you place the patient for a rectal examination?

EXAMINATION SEQUENCE

The physical examination sequence is fairly standard; however, variations may occur depending on the physician's speciality, the medical necessity, and the physician's preference. There is much the medical assistant can do to facilitate the quality of patient care and the physician's schedule. The successful medical assistant orchestrates a routine that is organized yet flexible enough to adjust to the individual problems that may arise.

Give your patient a brief explanation of the type of examination to be done. Patients are more cooperative and less anxious if they understand what is expected of them. Assemble all the instruments that

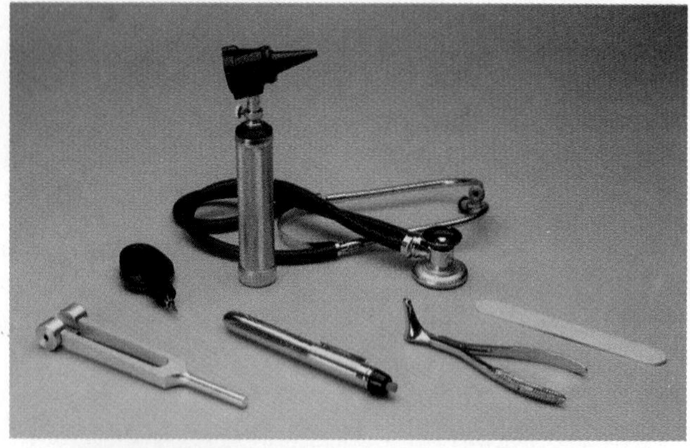

FIGURE 28–20 Physical examination instruments.

will be used during the examination (Fig. 28–20). As the physician proceeds with the examination, make sure the patient remains unexposed by adjusting the drapes as needed. In every examination, you have the responsibility to assist the physician by handing him or her the correct instruments and supplies needed. For legal reasons, if the physician is male, a female medical assistant must remain with the female patient throughout the examination unless the physician excuses you from the room. A female assistant in the room during the examination of the female patient can avert potential lawsuits.

As soon as the physician begins the examination, keep your conversation to a minimum and remain inconspicuous. The examination usually starts with the patient seated on the examining table. If the physician uses reflected light, then the light source should be behind the patient's right shoulder. If illuminated instruments are used, then the standard overhead lights are sufficient. Be careful not to shine a light directly into the patient's eyes. Turn on lights while they are directed away from the patient, and then carefully move the light toward the area to be examined.

Memory Jogger

How can potential lawsuits be averted during the examination?

Presenting Appearance (General Appearance)

The physical examination starts as the patient appears before the physician. Either of the terms *presenting appearance* and *general appearance* may be used on the medical record. These terms note whether the patient appears well and in good health. The patient may appear disoriented or in distress. The patient's responses to the opening remarks or questions may show an alertness or dullness.

The patient's gait, that is, the manner or style of walking, will often give some information. The patient may limp, walk with the feet wide apart, or have difficulty in maintaining his or her balance. In addition to gait, the patient's entire body movement is observed for possible muscle movement that the physician would deem out of average range. A patient's posture may indicate an area of pain. A rigid posture may indicate a fixed spine, and an altered posture may result from an extremity with limited motion.

Nutrition and Stature

The patient's height is measured. The physician notes the body build and proportions. Any gross (immediately obvious; taking no account of details, or minutiae) deformities are recorded. Sometimes, abnormalities in height or body proportion may be due to hormonal imbalances. Charts are published containing what is considered average healthy weight for the age and height of an individual (see Chapter 47). Being overweight or underweight is considered as being above or below the designated average healthy range.

Speech

Speech may reveal a pathologic condition. Some basic speech defects are *aphonia,* the inability to speak because of a loss of the voice, commonly seen with severe laryngitis or overuse of the voice; *aphasia,* the loss of the power of expression through speech, writing, or sign due to injury or disease of the brain centers; and *dysphasia,* a lack of coordination and failure to arrange words in proper order, usually due to a brain lesion. Other comments concerning speech may include the terms *incoherent, jumbled,* or *slurred.*

Breath Odors

Breath odors may or may not be diagnostic, although they are often associated with poor oral hygiene or dental care. Acidosis will give the strong odor of acetone, which is sweet and fruity, and may result from diabetes mellitus, starvation, or renal disease. A musty odor is usually associated with liver disease, and the odor of ammonia may be found in cases of uremia.

Skin

Comments on the skin are included as a part of the general appearance, unless the chief complaint involves a condition related to the skin. If so, then the skin is listed as a separate category. Skin texture refers to smoothness, roughness, and scaling. Loss of elasticity is when the skin does not return immediately to normal when it has been pulled or stretched. This can occur as an inherited condition or from prolonged injury, such as excessive exposure to the sun.

Fingernails and toenails often give some indication of a person's health. Brittle, grooved, or lined nails may indicate either local infection or systemic disease. *Clubbing* of the fingertips is associated with some congenital heart or lung diseases. *Spooning* of the nail is seen in some patients with severe *iron-deficiency anemias. Beau's lines* appear after an acute illness but will grow out and disappear.

Skin disorders have become very common. When the primary care physician believes that the patient has a definite skin problem, the patient will be referred to a dermatologist for diagnosis and treatment.

Reflexes

The patient's reflexes are checked with the patient in the sitting and supine positions. While the patient is sitting, the biceps are checked with the patient's arm flexed and supported by the examiner. The knee jerk (patellar reflex) and the ankle jerk (Achilles reflex) are checked using tapotement (a tapping or percussing movement) with either the fingers or the reflex hammer. The plantar reflexes (Babinski and Chaddock reflexes) are tested with the patient in either the sitting or the lying position.

Head

The patient's head and face are usually the starting place for the examination. The face reflects the patient's state and tells the physician a great deal about how the patient handles stress and illness. The skull, scalp, and face are palpated for size, shape, and symmetry. The distribution or the lack of hair and the hair texture may indicate hormonal changes. Excessive hair, especially facial hair in the female, indicates some bodily change. As the head is examined, the physician watches for possible **nodules,** masses, or signs of **trauma.**

Neck

The neck is examined for *range of motion* (ROM) by having the patient move the head in various directions. The thyroid gland is given special attention for symmetry, size, and texture. The physician manually palpates the thyroid area, and the patient is asked to swallow several times. The medical assistant may help by giving the patient a small amount of water in a paper cup. The physician palpates the thyroid gland both anteriorly and posteriorly. The carotid artery is palpated and auscultated for possible bruit. The lymph nodes are palpated. Swollen lymph nodes usually are present when there is infection in the face, head, or neck.

Eyes

Eyes are checked for reaction while shining a light into the pupils. This is known as *light and accommodation* (L&A). The **sclera** is checked for color, which ranges from white to pale yellow. The movements of the eyes are tested by having the patient follow the physician's finger. If the movement is within average range it is written as extraocular movement (EOM) intact. The physician uses the ophthalmoscope to examine the interior of the eye, including the retina and the intraocular vessels.

Ears

The ears are examined using the otoscope. The external ear is first checked for redness of the ear canal or the presence of ear wax (cerumen). The tympanic membrane (ear drum) may be seen in most patients and appears pearly gray. Scars appearing on the eardrum are frequently the result of earlier, chronic ear infections or perforations. The color of the eardrum is important to the diagnosis because it may indicate fluids such as blood or pus behind the eardrum in the middle ear. The patient may be asked to swallow several times to observe movement of the tympanic membrane, which occurs on pressure changes in the eustachian tube. The eustachian tube equalizes air pressure between the middle ear and the throat.

Mouth and Throat

The mouth, or oral cavity, is usually thought of in terms of oral hygiene and dental care. Dental hygiene includes the condition of the teeth, how the patient cares for the teeth and gums, and whether the teeth of the upper and lower jaws meet properly (occlude) for chewing. Healthy gums are pale pink, glossy, and smooth and do not bleed when pressure from a tongue depressor is applied. The palatine tonsils are usually visible. The physician may use a tongue depressor and a piece of gauze to grasp the tongue for careful examination of it. The floor of the mouth is examined by both inspection and palpation for enlarged lymph nodes, salivary gland function, and ulcerations. The insides of the cheeks are also examined for any abnormal marks or color.

Nose and Sinuses

The nasal cavity basically requires an examination of the color and texture of the mucosa. The sinus meatus cannot be seen, but the frontal and maxillary sinuses may be examined by the application of pressure over the area and transillumination.

When disorders in the eyes, ears, nose, and throat are observed, and the physician believes that the condition warrants the attention of a specialist, the patient will be referred to an ophthalmologist or an otorhinolaryngologist (ear, nose, and throat specialist). These specialities are discussed in Chapter 31.

Chest

While the patient is still in the sitting position, the chest, heart, lungs, and breasts are examined. The chest is examined for symmetric expansion. A tape measure may be used, especially if there is a variation between the upper and lower chest expansion. A patient with a history of **emphysema** may display a chest that is barrel-like.

With the stethoscope to the patient's back, the examiner listens to the lung sounds. The patient is asked to take deep and regular breaths during this examination. This may produce a slight dizziness, which is acceptable; the patient may be assured that it is only the result of the deep respirations and will rapidly pass. The types of respiration are noted. Some common variations in respiration can be found in Chapter 27.

Because it takes considerable concentration to interpret the heart sounds, it is necessary to have complete silence when the physician is listening to the patient's heart. The heart is examined using a stethoscope from both the anterior and posterior approaches to the patient. Further examination may include auscultation on the left, lateral side. In cases of heart disease, the physician may spend an extended period of time listening to the heart sounds.

When the examining physician finds chest or heart abnormalities, the next step will be blood tests, x-rays, and usually a resting electrocardiogram. Once all these results are analyzed, the physician may refer the patient to a specialist such as a cardiologist for the heart or a pulmonary specialist/respiratory care for the breathing disorder.

Breasts

A careful breast examination is part of the examination of every female, whether or not the patient is symptomatic. The patient is usually examined in the sitting position but may be examined later in the supine position. Breast cancer is the most common malignancy occurring in women, and early detection is the key to successful treatment (see Chapter 33 for more detailed examination procedures).

Abdomen

The patient is lowered to the dorsal recumbent position, and the drape is lowered to the pubic hair line. The gown is raised to just under the breasts. A towel should be placed over the female breasts if a gown is not worn. The physician stands to the patient's right side if at all possible. The patient's arms may be placed at the side, or the hands may be crossed over the chest. If the table is narrow and the patient cannot relax completely, it may help to have the patient tuck the thumbs under the buttocks to relax the shoulders. Relaxation of the abdominal muscles is absolutely essential for the abdominal examination. It sometimes helps to place a small pillow under the patient's head or the knees. If the patient exhibits ticklishness, it is best to disregard it and try to continue the examination by changing the routine.

To complete the abdominal examination, the patient may be placed in the knee-elbow position to better determine the presence of free abdominal fluid. The Sims position may also be used for this purpose.

Rectum

The rectal examination usually follows the abdominal examination or may be part of the examination of the male and female genitalia. The patient's comfort and dignity are vital. The examination is limited to an area of within 6 to 8 cm (2.5 to 3.5 inches). For this part of the examination, the physician needs one to two fingercots or an examining glove and lubricating jelly. Some physicians prefer to use an anoscope. The examination light must be directed at the perineal area during the examination.

Hemoccult test specimens are often collected at the time of the digital rectal examination. If this is a procedure that the physician does, be sure to include the necessary collection folder with the examination equipment.

The speciality area for disorders and diseases of the stomach and small intestine is gastroenterology. Proctology is the speciality of the large intestine and rectum. These specialities are discussed in Chapter 32. The examinations of the female and male reproductive systems are covered in Chapters 33 and 38, respectively.

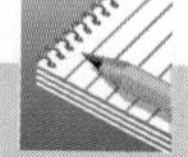

SKILLS AND RESPONSIBILITIES

EACH PATIENT'S NEEDS ARE SPECIAL

The physical examination establishes a baseline from which a patient's health care can be determined. This examination should not be considered routine. Every examination is unique, just as is every patient physically and emotionally. Each patient's needs are special, and the medical assistant must learn to foresee the patient's needs and be prepared to assist when needed.

Memory Jogger

10 *List the systems examined in a physical examination.*

PROCEDURE 28–1
Assisting with a Physical Examination

GOAL

To help the physician examine patients by preparing the necessary equipment and ensuring patient safety and comfort during the examination.

EQUIPMENT AND SUPPLIES

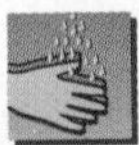

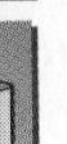
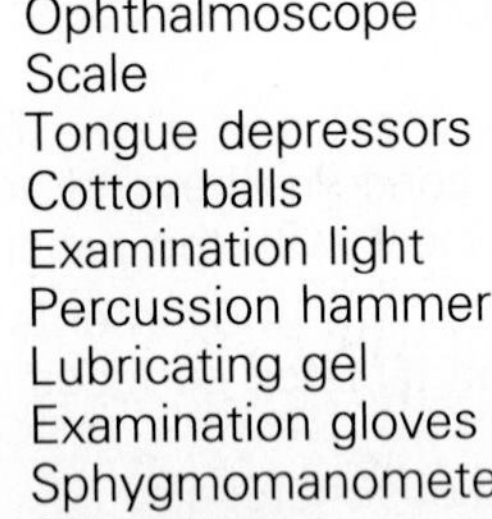

Stethoscope
Ophthalmoscope
Scale
Tongue depressors
Cotton balls
Examination light
Percussion hammer
Lubricating gel
Examination gloves
Sphygmomanometer
Otoscope
Tape measure
Gauze sponges
Head mirror
Pen light
Nasal speculum
Tuning fork
Biohazard container
Laboratory request forms
Specimen bottles/glass slides
Patient gown
Drape
Thermometer
Fingercots or gloves
Cotton-tipped applicators

PROCEDURAL STEPS

1. Prepare the examining room according to acceptable medical aseptic rules.
   PURPOSE: Room must be aseptically clean.
2. Wash your hands.
   PURPOSE: Infection control.
3. Locate the instruments for the procedure. Set them out in sequence.
   PURPOSE: Promotes time management and ensures that all needed equipment and supplies are ready.
4. Identify the patient, and determine whether the patient understands the procedure. If the patient does not understand, explain what you and the physician will be doing.
   PURPOSE: To increase patient cooperation during the examination.
5. Review the medical history with the patient.
   PURPOSE: Verifies that all information is current and complete.
6. Measure and record the patient's vital signs, height, and weight.
   PURPOSE: To gather data needed before the examination begins.
7. Instruct the patient on how to collect the urine specimen, and hand the patient the properly labeled specimen container (see Chapter 43). Obtain any blood samples that are required (see Chapter 44). Obtain resting electrocardiogram if ordered (see Chapter 29).
   PURPOSE: To obtain all specimens and tests that have been ordered by physician.
8. Hand the patient a gown and sheet. Instruct the patient on how to put the gown on. Help patient with undressing as needed; however, most patients prefer to undress in privacy.
   PURPOSE: To assist the patient in preparing for the examination.
9. Assist the patient in sitting on the narrow end of the examination table; place the drape over the patient's lap and legs. If the patient is elderly, confused, or feeling faint or dizzy, DO NOT leave him or her alone.
   PURPOSE: To provide for the patient's warmth and modesty and to prevent a fall and injury.
10. Advise the physician that the patient is ready.
11. Assist during the examination by handing the physician each instrument as it is needed and by positioning and draping the patient.

Continued

PROCEDURE 28–1 (CONTINUED)

Assisting with a Physical Examination

12. When the physician has completed the examination, allow the patient to rest for a moment, then help the patient from the table. Assist with dressing, if necessary.
    PURPOSE: Ensure patient's stability.
13. Record the necessary notes on the patient's chart and forward it to the physician for further notations.
14. Return to the patient and ask him or her if there are any questions. Give the patient any final instructions, and schedule the next appointment if that is appropriate. Escort patient from the room.
    PURPOSE: To clarify directions, eliminate any misunderstandings, and allow the patient to discuss any concerns. If there are misunderstandings or concerns beyond your scope of experience or skill, you must arrange for the physician to speak with the patient again.
15. Put on gloves and dispose of used supplies and linens with minimal movements to prevent stirring the dust and air in designated waste containers. Clean tabletop surfaces with disinfectant.
    PURPOSE: Prevent cross-contamination of any potential infectious materials.
16. Remove gloves and discard them in the biohazard waste container and wash your hands.
    PURPOSE: Infection control.

Now it is time to practice the procedures learned. Once you feel confident, demonstrate your skills and knowledge to your instructor by accurately preparing for and assisting with the routine physical examination (Procedure 28–1).

PATIENT EDUCATION

To improve the overall health status of individuals and to enlist the patient as an ally in the examination process, the medical assistant may educate the patient in many different ways. Patient education is an important function of the profession, the procedure process, and the concepts of holistic health.

The physical examination process is an excellent time for the medical assistant to assess the need for patient education. This assessment should be performed to identify the best way to meet the needs of the patient. When identifying these needs, consider the following:

- The information that the patient needs to know.
- How to convey the information so that the patient will understand.
- How the patient will use the information once he or she has it.

Develop a plan to teach the patient. Think about the different modalities available, such as pamphlets, pictures, films, demonstrations, and community resources. The more interesting you make your information, the more fun you will have presenting it to the patient, and the more enjoyment the patient will get out of learning. Always share your teaching strategy plans with your physician/employer so you will proceed with full consent. Your physician may have some additional ideas that will make this teaching plan even more exciting.

An outline will help you remember everything you want to tell the patient, and it will assist you to present material in an orderly manner so that the patient is able to understand and learn. An outline might contain the following subdivisions:

A. Goal (what do you want to accomplish?)
B. Intervention (how do you plan to accomplish this?)
C. Evaluation (how will you know that the teaching was successful?)

After you have completed the teaching session with the patient, you need to evaluate your effectiveness.

- Did you cover all the items on your plan?
- Did the patient learn?
- How do you feel about your performance?
- Are you willing to try it again?
- How did the patient receive the information?

Developing patient teaching materials can be time consuming. However, sharing meaningful and helpful information with the patient is a gift that can have positive repercussions throughout the patient's life.

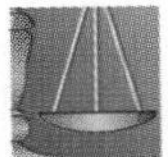

LEGAL AND ETHICAL ISSUES

The medical assistant must recognize that a legal and ethical contract exists between the patient and the physician. As the physician's employee, you also become part of that contract. You must remember that information gained during the physical examination is confidential and must remain that way. You have a responsibility to the patient, to the physician, to yourself, and to society to uphold the ethical responsibilities as written in the AAMA Code of Ethics: to render service, respect confidential information, and uphold the honor and high principles of the profession.

Memory Jogger

11 *Why is information obtained during the physical examination confidential?*

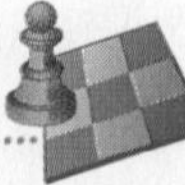

CRITICAL THINKING

1 Why should everyone have a physical examination every 1 or 2 years even if he or she is not "sick"?

2 Why are people afraid to have a physical examination?

3 How would you recognize anxiety or fear in a patient? What would you do about it?

4 Have you had a physical examination in the past 2 years? Why?

HOW DID I DO? Answers to Memory Joggers

1 The only way we can help in the repair and maintenance of the human body is by understanding how the body is put together, what role each part plays, and how each part functions.

2 Blood is connective tissue.

3 The 11 systems of the body are
a. Musculoskeletal
b. Endocrine
c. Nervous
d. Integumentary
e. Cardiovascular
f. Respiratory
g. Lymphatic and hematic
h. Gastrointestinal
i. Urinary
j. Reproductive
k. Special senses

4 The medical assistant's three duty areas are
a. Preparation of the room and equipment
b. Preparation of the patient
c. Assisting the physician

5 The otoscope, ophthalmoscope, and nasal speculum can all work off of the same handle.

6 Visualization is inspection by physically looking at a structure. Transillumination is inspection of a cavity or organ by passing light through its walls.

7 Indirect percussion is done by placing your fingers on the area and then striking the placed fingers with a finger of the other hand.

8 Sims' position is used for rectal examination.

9 When a male doctor is examining a female patient, the female medical assistant remains in the examination room to avert possible lawsuits.

10 All 11 systems are examined during a physical examination.

11 Information is confidential because it involves the personal life and welfare of the patient.

Assisting in Cardiovascular Medicine

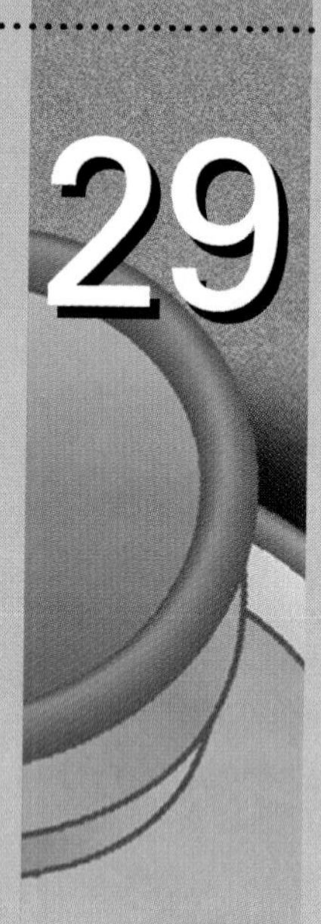

29

OUTLINE

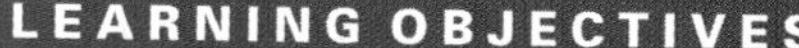

LEARNING OBJECTIVES

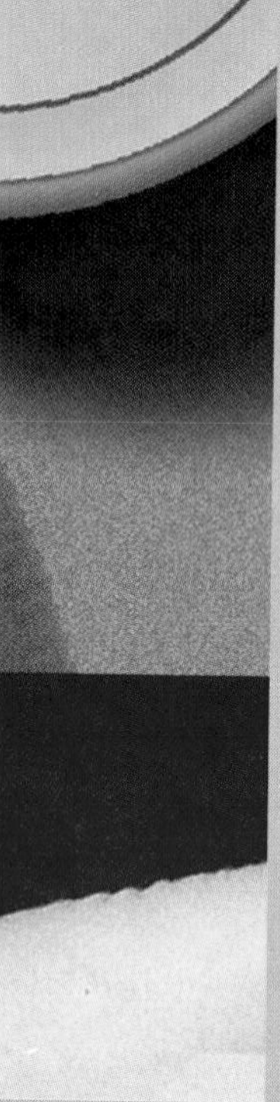

Cognitive: On successful completion of this chapter you should be able to:

1 Define and spell the terms in the Vocabulary.
2 Anatomically and physiologically describe the heart and its significant structures.
3 Identify the important presenting symptoms of cardiovascular disease.
4 List the signs, symptoms, and diagnostic and therapeutic procedures employed with coronary artery disease and hypertension.
5 Anatomically and physiologically describe the circulatory vessels.
6 List the most frequently diagnosed vascular conditions.
7 Trace the electrical conduction system through the heart.
8 State the meaning of the horizontal and vertical lines on the ECG paper.
9 List four types of artifacts commonly seen and explain the probable cause for each.
10 Discuss the process of obtaining the ECG.
11 Recognize the differences between patient preparation of the basic ECG and the stress test.

Performance: On successful completion of this chapter you should be able to:

1 Match the contractions of the heart with the deflections on the ECG tracing.
2 Point out the 12 leads recorded on an ECG, state the electrical activity of each, and identify the coding used for each.
3 Obtain a 12-lead ECG tracing.
4 Obtain a multichannel ECG tracing.
5 Apply and connect the Holter monitor.

VOCABULARY

angina pectoris Acute pain in the chest, resulting from decreased blood supply to the heart muscle

arrhythmia Abnormality or irregularity in heart rhythm

arteriosclerosis Hardening and thickening of the walls of the arterioles

asymptomatic Showing no symptoms

atherosclerosis Common type of arteriosclerosis in which deposits of yellow plaques form on the interior walls of the arterioles

atrioventricular (AV) node Part of the conductive system located between the atria and the ventricles near the septum that receives the impulses from the sinoatrial node and sends them down the bundles of His and the bundle branches

atria Upper chambers of the heart

bifurcates Divides into two branches

bradycardia Slow heartbeat

bruit Abnormal sound or murmur heard on auscultation of an organ, vessel, or gland

bundle of His Atrioventricular bundle of impulse-conducting fibers in the myocardium

cardiac arrest Total cessation of a functional heartbeat

cardiomyopathy Disease of the myocardium that is caused by a primary disease of the heart muscle

defibrillator Apparatus used to produce a brief electroshock to the heart through electrodes placed on the chest wall

diaphoresis Profuse perspiration

dyspnea Difficult or painful breathing

edema Intracellular accumulation of excess fluid

epistaxis Nosebleed

erythema Redness of the skin caused by congestion of the capillaries in the skin layers

erythrocytes Red blood cells

hypertension High blood pressure in which the systolic reading is consistently above 160 mm Hg and the diastolic pressure is above 90 mm Hg

infarction Area of tissue that has died because of lack of blood supply

insidious Diseases that come on in a symptomatic manner; of gradual and subtle development

ischemic Refers to a temporary deficiency of blood supply to a tissue or organ

mediastinal Pertaining to the space in the center of the chest under the sternum, containing the heart, great vessels, esophagus, and trachea

myocardial Pertaining to the middle layer of the walls of the heart muscle

orthopneic Pertaining to difficult breathing except in an upright or straight position

pericardium Sac that surrounds the heart

pleural Pertaining to a two-layer serous membrane that encapsulates the lungs

sinoatrial (SA) node Pacemaker of the heart located in the right atrium

stent Device used to prevent the lumen of the vessel from closing after angioplasty

syncope Brief loss of consciousness; fainting

symptoms Any indication of disease felt by the patient

tachycardia Fast heartbeat

thallium scan Intravenous administration of a radioisotope that localizes calcium in the myocardium in areas referred to as "cold spots," thus pinpointing the site of occlusions of coronary arteries

triglyceride Neutral fat that is the usual storage form of lipids in the human body

ventricles Lower chambers of the heart

vertigo Sensation of rotation or movement; dizziness

In the past, heart disorders were problems seen in men but seldom in women. That has changed, and today the most frequent cause of illness and death, regardless of gender, is cardiovascular disease. Medical assistants in all specialties often care for patients with heart disorders. Seldom does the cardiologist discover the heart problem. Most patients who see this specialist have already been given a diagnosis of a suspected heart disorder and have been referred to the cardiologist for verification and treatment.

Due to the overwhelming number of people with cardiovascular problems, all medical assistants need to understand this system, be able to recognize early symptoms of potential disorders, perform basic screening tests when ordered by the physician, and assist the physician in the examination of the heart and vessels.

Anatomy of the Heart

The heart is a hollow, muscular organ situated in the thoracic cavity in the **mediastinal** region, between the right and left **pleural** spaces. It weighs approximately 9 ounces and is about 9 × 12 cm or the size of a closed fist, and approximately two thirds of it is located to the left of the sternum (Fig. 29–1). The heart is a muscular pump that provides the force needed to push blood through all the arteries of the body, thus circulating a continuous supply of oxygen and nutrients to the cells and picking up the metabolic waste products from them. At the same time, the heart also pushes the deoxygenated blood through the pulmonary artery to the lungs for oxygen saturation and then back through the pulmonary veins into the left side of the heart. Deprived of these vital functions, the cells will die. The heart is the organ that keeps the blood moving through the arteries. The average adult heart pumps about 5 L of blood every minute (which is equal to two and one-half 2-L drink containers) throughout your life time. If the heart loses its pumping action for even a few brief minutes, death may occur or permanent damage may result.

The heart is really a double pump. On the right side, one pump receives blood that has just come from the body after delivering nutrients and oxygen to the tissues. The right side pumps deoxygenated blood to the lungs, where the carbon dioxide is exchanged for a fresh supply of oxygen. The pump on the left side of the heart receives this fresh oxygenated blood from the lungs and pumps it out through the aorta, to be distributed to all parts of the body.

Memory Jogger

How much blood passes through the heart in 1 minute?

LAYERS OF THE HEART

The heart is enclosed in a sac called the **pericardium.** The outer layer of the pericardial sac is a tough protective layer, the middle layer is a serous layer, and the inside layer forms the epicardium (outside layer) of the heart itself. The heart also possesses three more layers: the outer epicardium, the middle myocardium, and the inner endocardium (Fig. 29–2). The epicardium is a thin, protective

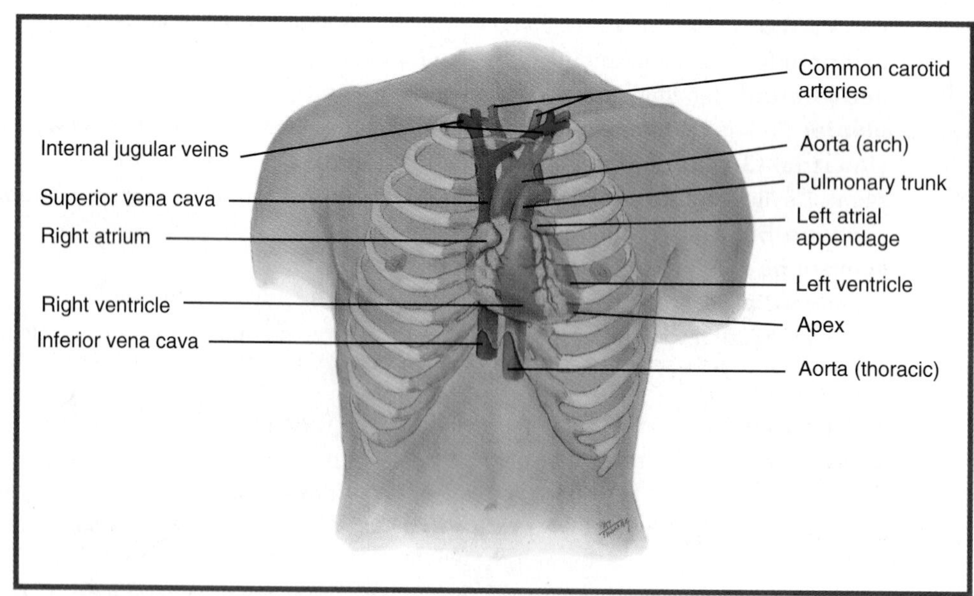

FIGURE 29–1 Location of the heart in the thoracic cavity. (From Applegate EJ: The Anatomy and Physiology Learning System. Philadelphia, WB Saunders, 1995.)

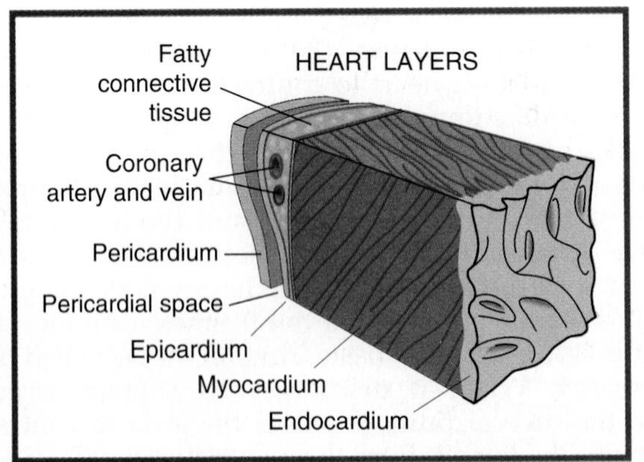

FIGURE 29–2 Layers of the heart. (From Danjanov I: Pathology for the Health-Related Professions. Philadelphia, WB Saunders, 1995.)

layer of connective tissue that is firmly attached to pericardial muscle tissue within the center of the chest. Blood vessels that nourish the heart wall are located in the epicardium.

The middle layer of the heart is the myocardium, which is the muscle layer that composes the largest percentage of the heart wall. It is the contractions of this muscle layer that force the blood from the heart into the vessels.

The smooth inner layer of the heart is the endocardium. The endocardial layer forms a smooth lining that allows the blood to flow effortlessly through the heart and into the arteries. The endocardium also forms the hearts valves and the lining of the blood vessels.

Memory Jogger

 *Identify the four layers of the heart.*

HEART CHAMBERS AND VALVES

The heart is divided into four cavities (Fig. 29–3). The **atria,** the top chambers, receive blood, and the **ventricles,** the bottom chambers, pump the blood out. The right atrium receives the deoxygenated

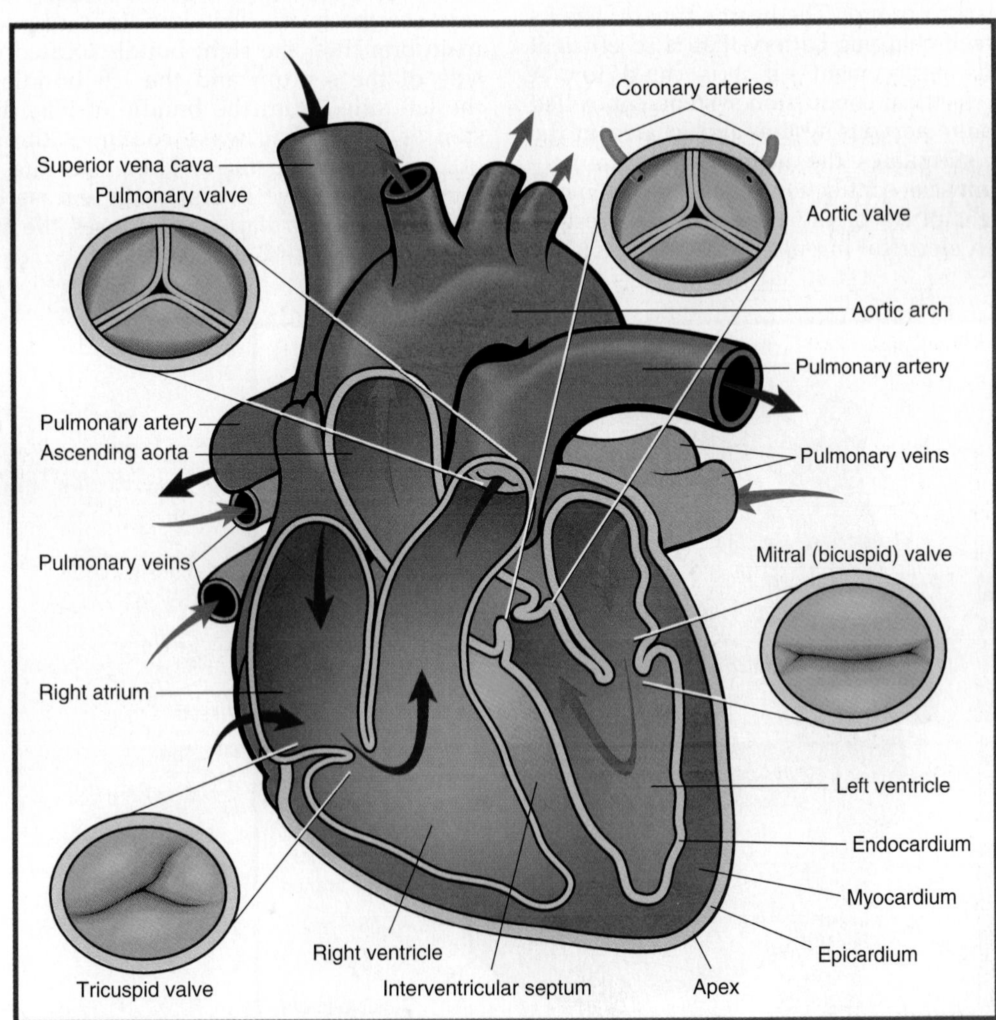

FIGURE 29–3 Chambers of the heart. (From Danjanov I: Pathology for the Health-Related Professions. Philadelphia, WB Saunders, 1995.)

blood from the body, and the left atrium receives the oxygenated blood from the lungs. The left ventricle sends the deoxygenated blood to the lungs, and the right ventricle pumps the blood out to the entire body system.

To keep the blood flowing in one direction, the chambers need valves. These little valves open and close to ensure the correct flow of the blood as it passes through the heart. There are four valves within the heart; two are located between the atria and the ventricles and two where the blood enters the arteries when leaving the heart (see Fig. 29–3).

Memory Jogger

3 *Identify the chamber that pumps blood into the entire body.*

HEART CONDUCTION

Because no other organ in our body has pumping ability, how is the heart capable of performing this pumping action every second of our life? What causes the heart to pump? The heart's muscle has its own built-in, self-charging battery that is so efficient it never needs replacement—if it is cared for. A sophisticated electrical conduction system, controlled by the autonomic nervous system and located in the myocardium, stimulates the heart muscle contractions. These muscle contractions make blood move through the chambers of the heart and the rest of the body. Each electrical impulse moves through the heart muscle in a twisting, spiral motion. These rhythmic waves cause the cardiac cells to beat, which causes the heart to contract.

The cardiac impulse originates in specialized muscle tissue called the **sinoatrial (SA) node.** The SA node is located in the right atrium, just at the junction of the superior vena cava and the atrium. This wave spreads in concentric circles over the atrial walls, and the atria contract. The SA node rhythmically initiates impulses 70 to 80 times a minute; because it creates the basic rhythm, it is called the *pacemaker*. When it discharges its rhythm pattern into the myocardium, it causes the atria to contract, forcing the blood into the ventricles of the heart. The wave then passes through a second area of specialized muscle tissue between the right atrium and right ventricle, called the **atrioventricular (AV) node.** The AV node holds the impulse for a fraction of a second to prevent inappropriately high atrial rates as well as to allow for atrial dumping. The chordae tendineae, at this moment, close the valves between the atria and the ventricles tightly. Then the AV node releases the charge, sending it down through a bundle of nerve tissue **(bundle of His)** located in the septum between the right and left sides of the heart. This bundle is divided into two main branches, the right bundle located on the right side of the septum and the left bundle located on the left side. From the bundle of His, the transmission of the cardiac wave continues through a mass of cardiac muscle fibers known as the Purkinje fibers. The Purkinje fibers totally encase both ventricles, and the cardiac wave causes the ventricles to contract (Fig. 29–4).

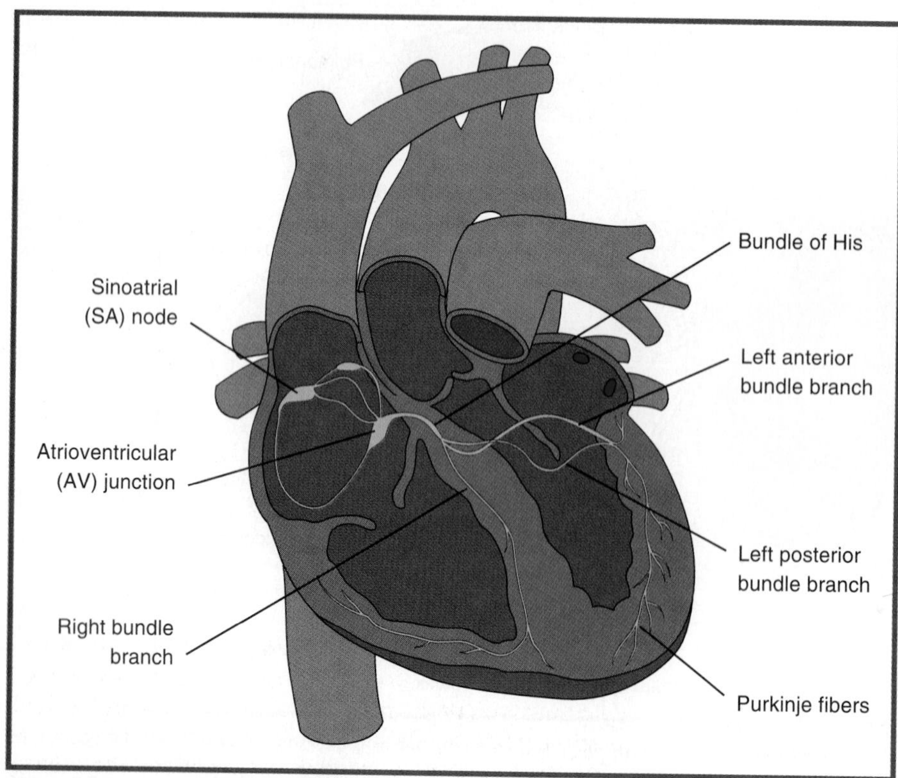

FIGURE 29–4 Cardiac conduction system.

The transmission of the cardiac impulse from the SA node to the muscles in the ventricles is called *depolarization.* A period of electric *recovery,* called *repolarization,* then occurs. The heart returns to resting (*polarization*), and the entire cycle begins again. The normal cardiac cycle consists of atrial contraction, ventricular contraction, and then recovery and heart rest. This cycle maintains the average range of 60 to 100 beats per minute and a normal heart rhythm. It is this electrical force that is traced and evaluated when an electrocardiogram is done.

Memory Jogger

4 *Trace the heart's conduction system.*

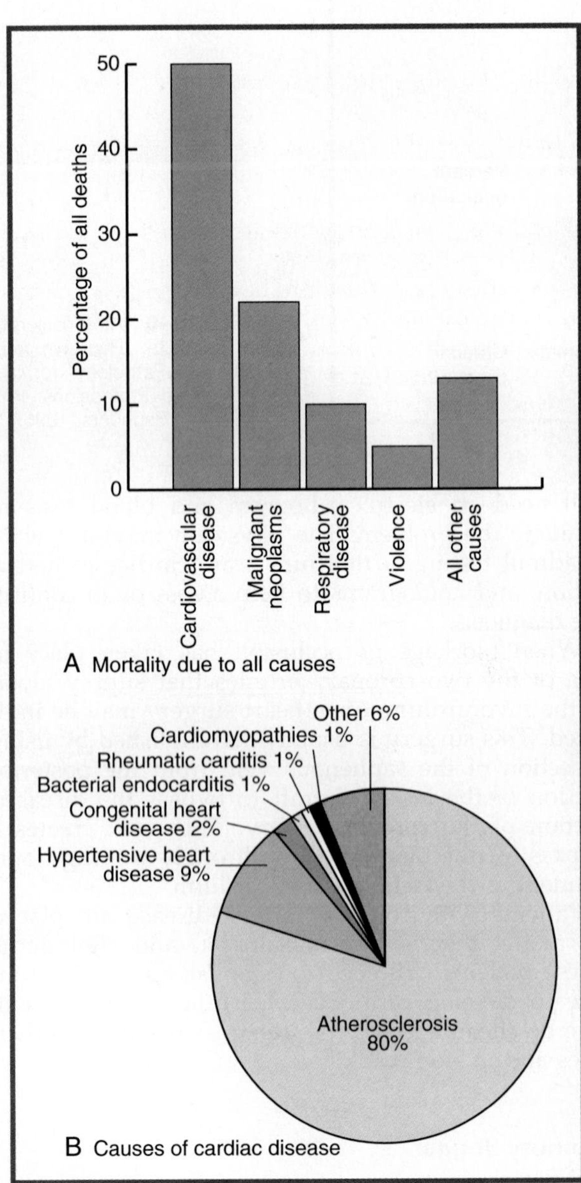

FIGURE 29–5 Incidence of cardiovascular diseases. (From Damjanov I: Pathology for the Health-Related Professions. Philadelphia, WB Saunders, 1995.)

Diseases and Disorders of the Heart

There are many diseases and disorders of the heart and blood vessels. In some disorders, the rhythm of the heartbeats becomes irregular **(arrhythmia),** too fast **(tachycardia),** or too slow **(bradycardia)** (Fig. 29–5). About one third of all cardiovascular deaths are due to coronary artery disease and hypertension. The lifestyles of Americans along with the diets in this country have been definitely linked to the increase in premature death by cardiovascular causes.

PRESENTING (OFTEN RECURRENT) SYMPTOMS OF CARDIOVASCULAR DISEASE

- Chest pain
- **Dyspnea** (difficulty in breathing) on exertion
- Tachypnea (rapid breathing)
- Palpitations (rapid beating of the heart)
- Cyanosis (bluish tinge to the skin)
- **Edema**
- Fatigue
- **Syncope** (fainting)
- **Diaphoresis**

CORONARY ARTERY DISEASE

In coronary artery disease the arteries supplying the myocardium become narrowed by atherosclerotic deposits. These deposits of plaque narrow the opening (lumen) of the arteries and inhibit the normal flow of blood through the arteries, thus depriving the heart of an adequate nutritious blood supply (Fig. 29–6).

PERSONS AT HIGHER RISK OF CORONARY ARTERY DISEASE

- Those with genetic predisposition and familial history
- Those older than 40 years
- Smokers or those living in areas with poor air quality
- Persons with hypertension, diabetes, or obesity
- Persons with a history of elevated cholesterol
- Persons living a sedentary lifestyle
- Persons with excessive stress

Signs and Symptoms

Patients may be without symptoms, or **asymptomatic,** until the disease becomes fully developed. The first symptom may be pain in the chest called **angina pectoris,** followed by pressure or fullness in the chest, syncope, edema, unexplained coughing

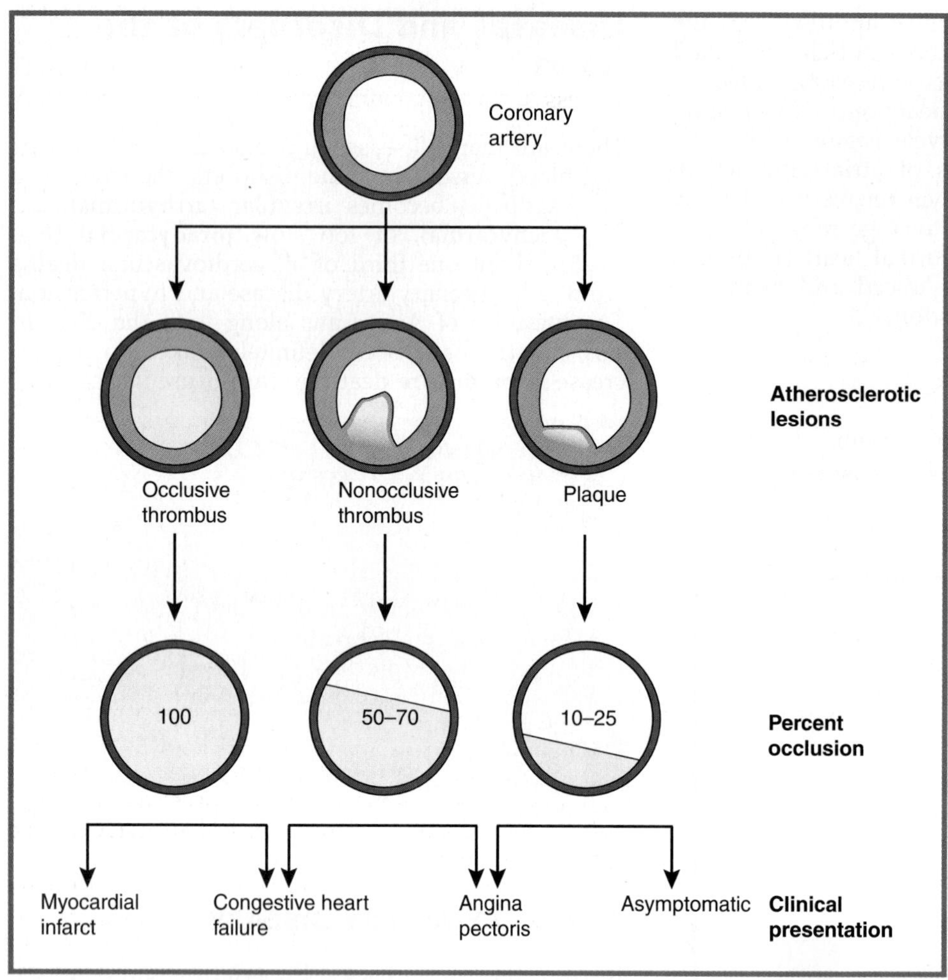

FIGURE 29–6 Atherosclerotic vessel deposits. (Redrawn from Danjanov I: Pathology for the Health-Related Professions. Philadelphia, WB Saunders, 1995.)

spells, and unexplainable fatigue. When a patient tells you he or she is experiencing any of these symptoms, the individual should be seen by the physician immediately.

The major concern in heart disease is the lack of blood to the heart muscle, which occurs when a vessel becomes totally blocked. Death of a portion of the heart muscle is **myocardial infarction** (MI), commonly called a heart attack. Symptoms of myocardial infarction are very similar to those of angina, but myocardial infarction is identified by pain lasting longer than 30 minutes and is unrelieved by rest or nitroglycerin tablets. A myocardial infarction is life threatening, and intervention must begin within the first hour or death usually occurs.

Memory Jogger

5 *What is the correct terminology for a heart attack?*

Diagnostic and Therapeutic Procedures

The treatment objective consists of restoring adequate blood flow to the myocardium. The patient will need an electrocardiogram and blood tests to evaluate the problem. The physician may also want treadmill testing, a **thallium scan,** cardiac catheterization, and angiograms to help assess or to confirm the diagnosis.

When blockage or occlusion has taken place in one of the two coronary arteries that supply blood to the myocardium, open-heart surgery may be indicated. This surgery is usually accomplished by using a section of the saphenous vein from the posterior section of the leg as a graft to bypass the diseased section of the coronary artery. This graft creates a bypass for the blood to flow through to bring nourishment to the **ischemic** myocardium.

Patients with coronary artery disease are placed on a diet that is low in salt, fat, and cholesterol. These patients will need to establish an exercise routine to develop cardiovascular fitness. Patients will also be encouraged to reduce stress reactions in their lives and to stop smoking.

Memory Jogger

6 *What can be done to bring nourishment to the ischemic section of the myocardium?*

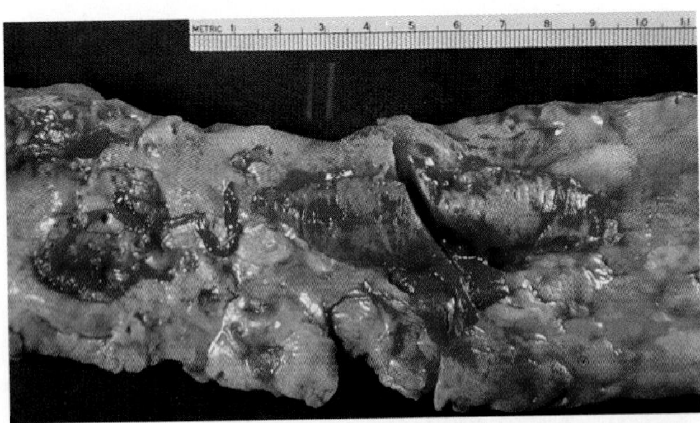

FIGURE 29–7 Atherosclerotic vessel. (From Danjanov I: Pathology for the Health-Related Professions. Philadelphia, WB Saunders, 1995.)

HYPERTENSIVE HEART DISEASE

Hypertensive heart disease results from chronic elevated blood pressure and is the major cause of stroke and renal failure. Hypertension is frequently familial, but it can be caused by **atherosclerosis, arteriosclerosis,** renal disorders, or any condition that causes the heart to work harder as it pumps against increased resistance (Fig. 29–7).

Signs and Symptoms

The two types of hypertension are primary and secondary. Primary hypertension has an insidious onset, with the patient showing few, if any, symptoms until permanent damage is done. The individual may have excessive headaches, **epistaxis,** lightheadedness, bouts of nausea, and/or syncope. Secondary hypertension is sometimes called malignant hypertension because it is a severe form of the disease and is life threatening. Its cause may be unknown, or it may be the effect of another condition present in the body.

Both forms of hypertensive heart disease result from unknown causes, although many factors are thought to contribute to the condition. Stress is believed to be a major factor in hypertension. In addition, age, heredity, smoking, obesity, and type A personality are all possible contributing factors.

Diagnostic and Therapeutic Procedures

One of the symptoms will usually cause the patient to seek medical attention, and the hypertension is generally detected when blood pressure is taken during the examination or screening process. This is the primary purpose for taking the patient's blood pressure accurately during every visit. Patients with a resting systolic blood pressure higher than 140 mm Hg and a diastolic pressure of greater than 90 mm Hg are said to be hypertensive. The diagnosis is based on a series of blood pressure readings, with elevated values being obtained repeatedly (Fig. 29–8).

In secondary hypertension, marked blood pressure elevation is present with the systolic pressure above

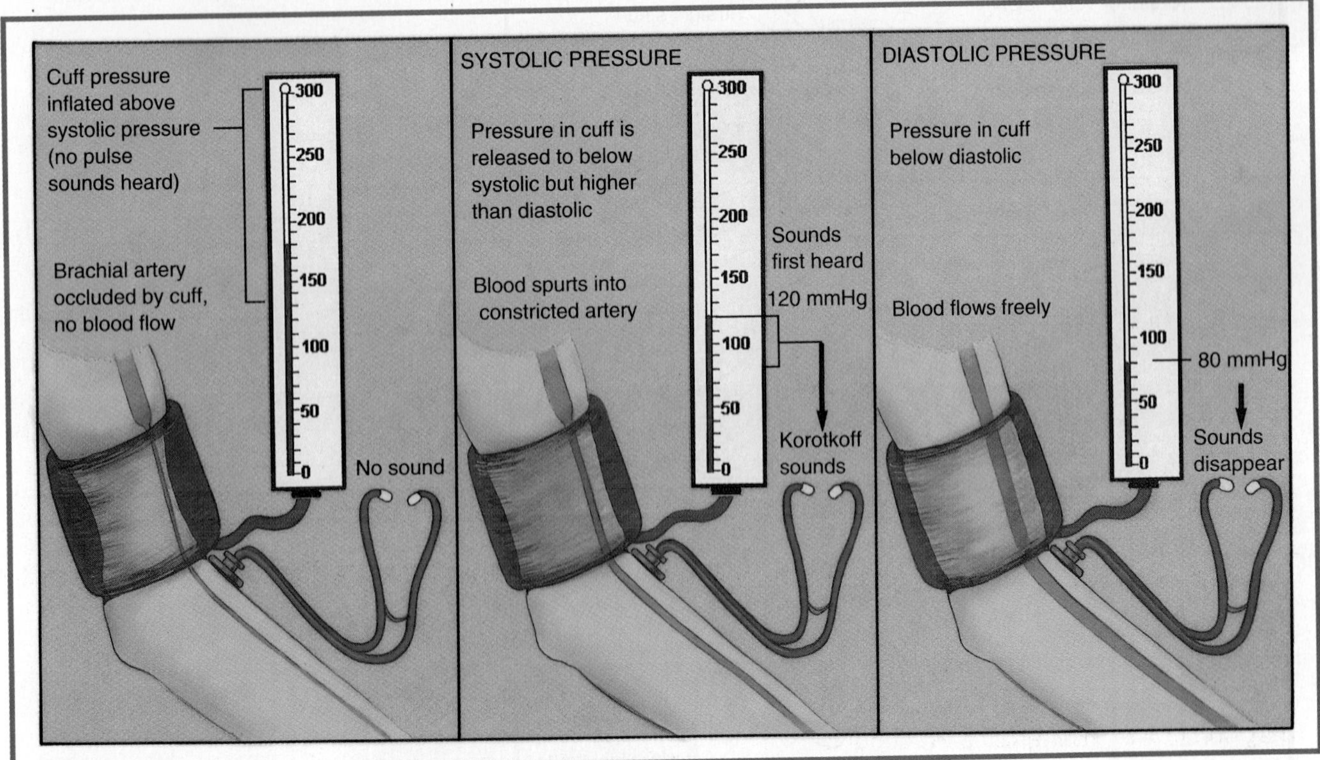

FIGURE 29–8 Measurement of blood pressure. (From Applegate EJ: The Anatomy and Physiology Learning System. Philadelphia, WB Saunders, 1995.)

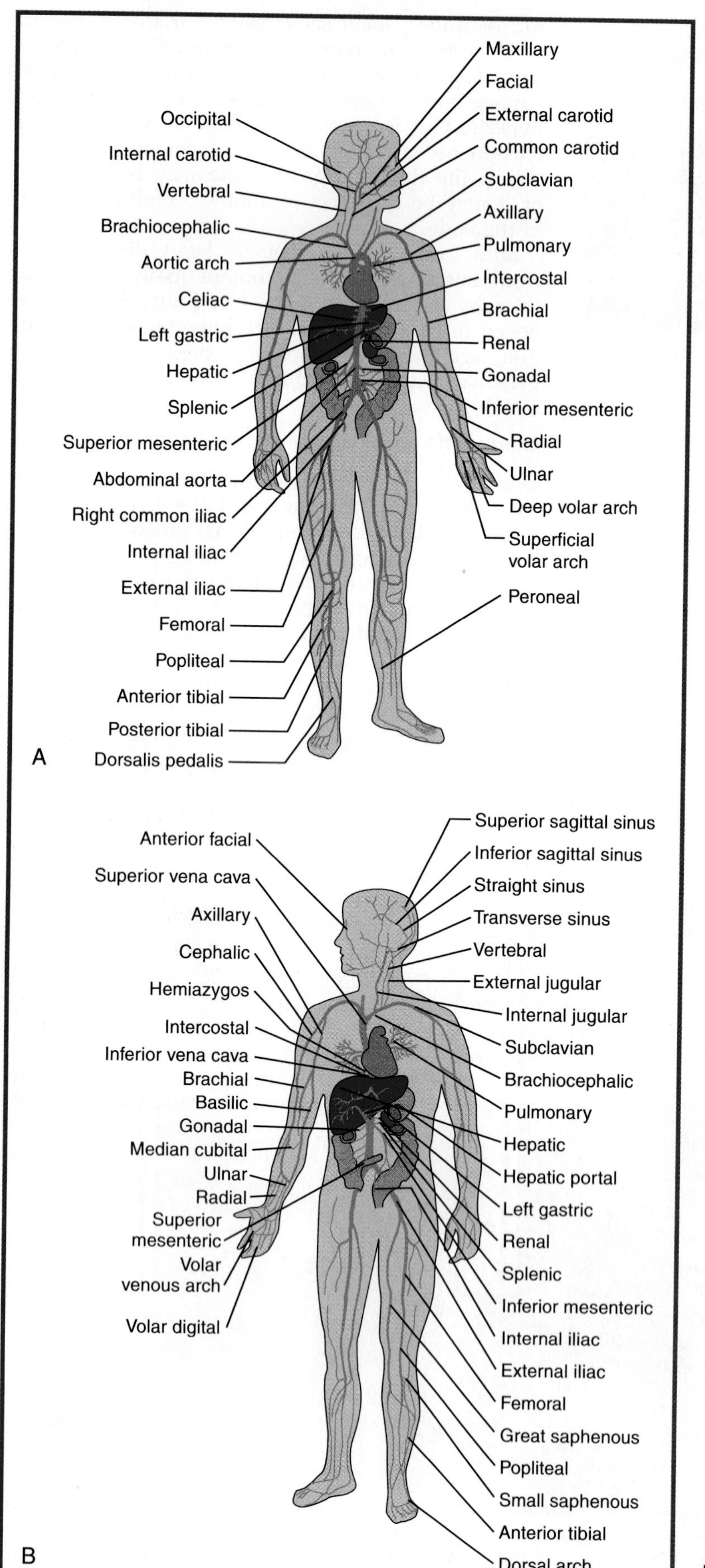

FIGURE 29–9 *A,* Systemic arteries. *B,* Systemic veins.

200 mm Hg. These patients are at risk for a cerebrovascular accident, or stroke, and irreversible renal damage.

A program of drug therapy is commonly used in the treatment of hypertension. The drug therapy program is designed to fit each patient's needs and response. In additional to the medications, the patient is encouraged to limit salt intake, follow a diet regimen, reduce stress, and exercise. The medical assistant can be an interactive part of this therapy in teaching the patient how to take his or her own blood pressure, providing literature that reinforces the necessity of monitoring the blood pressure, and helping the patient to understand that this condition is not cured, but can be controlled, for the rest of his or her life.

Memory Jogger

Would a patient with continuous blood pressure readings of 170/90 mm Hg be considered to have hypertensive heart disease? Why or why not?

Blood Vessels

The blood vessels are the pipes through which the blood travels to all parts of our body. These vessels are divided into two systems that begin and end with the heart (Fig. 29–9). The *pulmonary system* carries blood from the right ventricle to the lungs and then back to the left atrium. The *systemic system* carries blood from the left ventricle throughout the entire body and back to the right atrium. The vessels are classified according to their structure and function as arteries, which carry the blood away from the heart; capillaries, the microscopic vessels that are responsible for the exchange of oxygen and carbon dioxide in the tissue; and veins, the vessels that carry blood back to the heart.

ARTERIES

All arteries carry blood from the heart but not all arteries carry oxygenated blood. Pulmonary arteries transport the deoxygenated blood from the right ventricle to the lungs for reoxygenation. Systemic arteries carry the oxygenated blood away from the heart to all the cells of the body. The largest of these vessels is the aorta, which starts at the left ventricle and travels through the center of the body into the lower abdomen, where it **bifurcates** into the right and left femoral arteries and continues down to the feet. As the aorta passes through the body, the blood leaves the large aorta and enters smaller arteries that branch into smaller and smaller arteries until the branching becomes microscopic. These vessels are referred to as *arterioles* and terminate into *capillaries,* which are the smallest and most plentiful of the blood vessels. In these very tiny vessels, **erythrocytes** must travel in single file and every cell is nourished and cared for. When the blood leaves the capillary bed, the oxygen supply has been depleted and it now begins the return portion of the blood cycle.

VEINS

As the blood leaves the capillary beds, it enters the smallest veins, called *venules.* From this point on, the blood will flow into larger and larger veins until it reaches the largest vein in the body, the *vena cava.* The vena cava deposits the blood into the right atrium, where the blood again begins its trip through the heart, into the pulmonary arteries to the lungs, and then through the pulmonary veins, which will bring the extremely rich oxygenated blood back from the lungs to the left atrium.

The walls of veins are thinner than those of the arteries and have valves to prevent backflow of blood. These venous valves are especially important in the arms and legs because they prevent pooling of blood due to the pull of gravity.

Memory Jogger

All arteries carry oxygenated blood from the heart, and all veins carry deoxygenated blood to the heart. True or False.

Vascular Disorders

Through every moment of our lives the vascular system is busy supplying blood containing oxygen and nutrients to all of our tissues and picking up the metabolic waste from the tissue. For our tissues to receive an adequate amount of oxygen and nutrients, the arterial vessel must maintain its elasticity and the lining has to remain smooth to allow decreased friction of the blood flow. Constriction or dilation of the vessel walls causes alterations in blood pressure that, in turn, cause heart disease.

COMMON VASCULAR CONDITIONS

- Emboli and thrombi
- Arteriosclerosis
- Aneurysms
- Phlebitis and varicose veins

EMBOLUS AND THROMBUS

An embolus is a mass of undissolved material moving in a blood or lymphatic vessel. Emboli may be

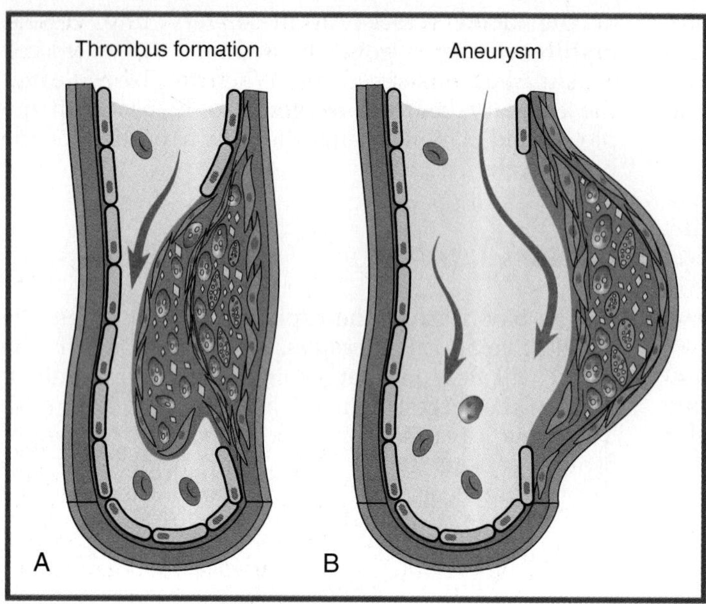

FIGURE 29–10 *A*, Thrombus nesting in vessel and curbing the flow of blood. *B*, Aneurysmal dilation of vessel caused by weakening of the vessel wall. (From Danjanov I: Pathology for the Health-Related Professions. Philadelphia, WB Saunders, 1995.)

solid, liquid, or gaseous. This undissolved material may be fat, air, bits of tissue, clumps of bacteria, or foreign matter. Emboli may be created within the body or may gain entrance from the outside. Occlusion of a vessel from emboli usually results from the development of a thrombus.

A thrombus is a blood embolus that obstructs a blood vessel or a cavity of the heart (Fig. 29–10). Thrombi nest in a blood vessel and curb the flow of blood. They are a life-threatening event because the clot can occlude a vessel and stop the blood supply to an organ or a part of an organ. The thrombus, if detached and moving, becomes an embolus and may occlude a vessel at a distance from the original nesting site. For example, a clot may begin in the leg, break free from the vessel in the leg, and begin moving and continue traveling through the circulation until it causes a pulmonary occlusion or pulmonary thrombosis.

Signs and Symptoms

Symptoms depend on the location of the vessel that has the clot. The patient may feel agitated or restless. If the embolus is in the chest, the symptoms can include difficult unequal breathing, cyanosis, and a drop in blood pressure. The initial symptom is usually pain in the area of the thrombus if it is stationary. When a large artery is involved, the individual may experience nausea, vomiting, syncope, and eventually shock.

Diagnosis and Treatment

Diagnosis is usually based on the clinical picture and a history of inactivity or heart disease. The treatment is immediate to prevent death of the tissue that relies on the blocked vessel for its nourishment. Blood flow is reestablished to the affected part by lowering the appendage below the heart. The patient is placed in full Fowler's orthopneic or another comfortable position to improve ventilation. Prescribed pharmaceutical agents such as heparin, warfarin (Coumadin), corticosteroids, and diazepam may be given. If this treatment does not work, surgical intervention may be necessary to remove the obstruction.

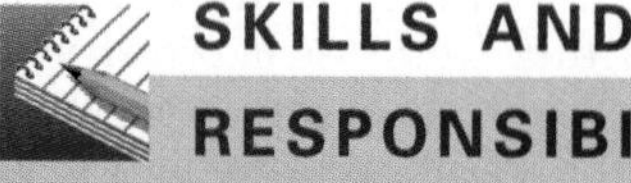

SKILLS AND RESPONSIBILITIES

ENCOURAGING AND SUPPORTING A PATIENT

Frequent, sometimes daily, blood tests may be ordered by the physician to manage and control vessel disorders. The medical assistant can assist the physician by helping the patient to understand the need for these tests and why these tests play a vital role in vessel disorder management. Listening to the patient and offering encouragement and support may be a vital part in recovery.

Memory Jogger

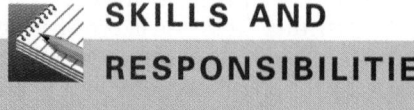

9 *Explain the difference between an embolus and a thrombus.*

ATHEROSCLEROSIS AND ARTERIOSCLEROSIS

Hardening of the arteries has two general forms. One is called atherosclerosis, in which the hardening is caused by a buildup of plaque of cholesterol and lipids along the inside vessel wall. It is responsible for the majority of myocardial infarctions. The second form is arteriosclerosis, in which there is a thickening of the walls of the arteries with loss of elasticity and contractibility.

Diagnosis and Treatment

Diagnosis is usually made during a routine physical examination or screening process. Blood tests frequently show an elevation in cholesterol, **triglyceride,** and lipid levels. Hypertension may be present, and Doppler auscultation of the major vessels shows reduced blood flow. Doppler auscultation is explained in Chapter 33.

Treatment consists of dietary reductions in saturated fats and foods high in cholesterol. Patients are encouraged to stop smoking. Drugs such as lovastatin (Mevacor) and simvastatin (Zocor) may be used to reverse the plaque buildup. The medical assistant can help in the treatment with encouragement and by educating the patient about risk factors and alterations in lifestyle.

Memory Jogger

10 *Differentiate between atherosclerosis and arteriosclerosis.*

ANEURYSM

An aneurysm is a ballooning or dilation of the wall of a vessel caused by a weakening of the vessel wall. A common cause is the buildup of plaque, which weakens the vessel wall. The two most common points for this to occur are in the abdominal aorta and in the cerebral arteries. In either case, the patient seldom has any signs or symptoms. Occasionally, the patient may describe a pounding or pulsating pain in the area of the aneurysm.

Diagnosis and Treatment

When the physician auscultates the vessel over the area of the aneurysm, a **bruit** will usually be heard. Radiologic studies, ultrasonography, and tomography all help to confirm the diagnosis. The treatment sometimes is to watch and wait. Surgical repair is recommended for all aneurysms 6 cm or greater, but smaller ones can also rupture. If an aneurysm is tender and known to be enlarging rapidly, no matter what the size, surgery is essential. If a rupture occurs, immediate lifesaving intervention must be done.

The medical assistant may aid the physician by observing the patient for signs of pain, mental changes, and changes in pulse and respirations. If any of these signs are observed, the physician must be notified immediately. As with any serious condition, the patient is going to exhibit a high level of anxiety and the medical assitant's strongest role is to support the patient and the family.

Memory Jogger

11 *Describe an aneurysm.*

PHLEBITIS AND VARICOSE VEINS

Phlebitis is an inflammation of the veins most commonly seen in the lower legs. The disorder may appear for no apparent reason. It is believed that obesity and vascular injury, both internal and external, may be possible causes. Varicose veins are swollen, knotted veins that can result from repeated bouts of phlebitis, prolonged standing, and pregnancy. Advanced varicosities cause a brownish discoloration of the skin around the affected area (Fig. 29–11).

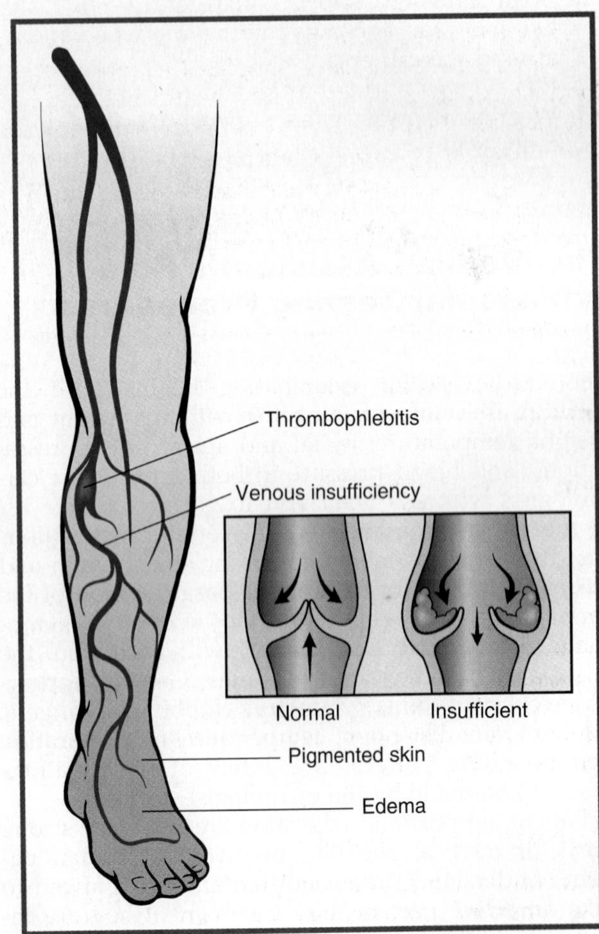

FIGURE 29–11 Varicose veins of the calf. (From Danjanov I: Pathology for the Health-Related Professions. Philadelphia, WB Saunders, 1995.)

Diagnosis and Treatment

Inspection of the extremities along with the symptoms is usually sufficient to make a definite diagnosis for both phlebitis and varicosities. Treatment includes rest periods during which the feet are elevated above the heart. Support stockings may be recommended for individuals who must stand for long periods of time. Varicose veins may need surgical intervention consisting of laser treatments, saline injections, or surgical ligation and stripping.

The medical assistant can assist in the prevention of phlebitis and varicosities by discussing methods of prevention with the patient. Help the patient to understand that weight gain, standing in one position for long periods of time, and lack of exercise to assist in maintaining good circulation all put added pressure and stress on the body and circulation.

SUGGESTIONS TO PREVENT PHLEBITIS AND VARICOSE VEINS

- Join a weight-control group.
- Use shoes with different heel heights during the workday.
- Wear full-length support stockings.
- Do not wear stockings that have elastic bands around the calf area.
- Elevate legs during breaks and rest periods.
- Wear shoes with good support when taking daily walks.

The Medical Assistant's Role in Vascular Testing Procedures

The cardiovascular examination begins with the medical assistant obtaining the patient's height and weight, temperature, radial and apical pulses, respirations, and blood pressure in both arms. Most cardiologists will also want you to get a complete list of the prescription and over-the-counter medications that the patient is taking, including the strength and frequency of use for each one. A large portion of the examination will center around subjective symptoms. The actual examination will focus on the chest, heart, and vascular systems. General appearance, color of skin, symmetry, clubbing of fingers, jugular vein distention, temperature of extremities, and breathing patterns are a few of the notations that will be made by the cardiologist.

Patient support and education are two very strong areas of medical assisting involvement. When patients understand their condition and are allowed to take an active part in their treatments, they are inclined to follow and/or comply with the physician's orders in a more precise and orderly fashion.

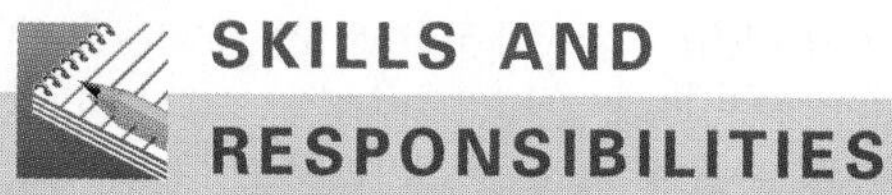

SKILLS AND RESPONSIBILITIES

THE MEDICAL ASSISTANT'S CLINICAL RESPONSIBILITIES

1 Prepares patient for exam by obtaining thorough drug history and preliminary exam procedures.
2 Explains and clarifies any direction or information that has been said that the patient is having difficulty understanding.
3 Performs the testing procedures that will assist the cardiologist or physician in diagnosing the disorder. Among these tests are the 12-lead electrocardiogram, application of the Holter monitor, assisting with a treadmill, and preparing the patient for radiologic procedures.

Electrocardiography

Electrocardiography is a painless and safe procedure that is frequently used in the diagnosis of heart disease. To perform electrocardiography, wires with electrodes are attached to the patient. The machine, called an *electrocardiograph,* amplifies many times the natural electrical currents generated by the electrical impulses of the heart. A pattern of the heart impulses is traced on heat-sensitive graph paper with a balanced tracing pen, or heated stylus. This tracing, called an *electrocardiogram* (ECG or EKG), is an exact graphic representation of the heart's electrical activity. The tracing is then mounted in a predesigned folder or on mounting paper for the physician to read, evaluate, and keep as a permanent record.

For the ECG recording to depict the true cardiac activity, the medical assistant must have an understanding of normal cardiac function and its relationship to the ECG markings. It is the medical assistant's responsibility to ensure that the patient has been prepared mentally and physically and that the equipment is set up properly. When performing the test, the medical assistant must be able to recognize electrical interferences and make appropriate corrections or adjustments. The validity of the test depends on the accuracy and skill of the technician.

CARDIAC CYCLE

The term *cardiac cycle* refers to one complete heartbeat, which consists of depolarization (contraction), repolarization (recovery), and polarization (relaxation). The cardiac impulse can be transferred to the electrocardiograph, which records the intensity and the time factor of this natural electrical activity. This

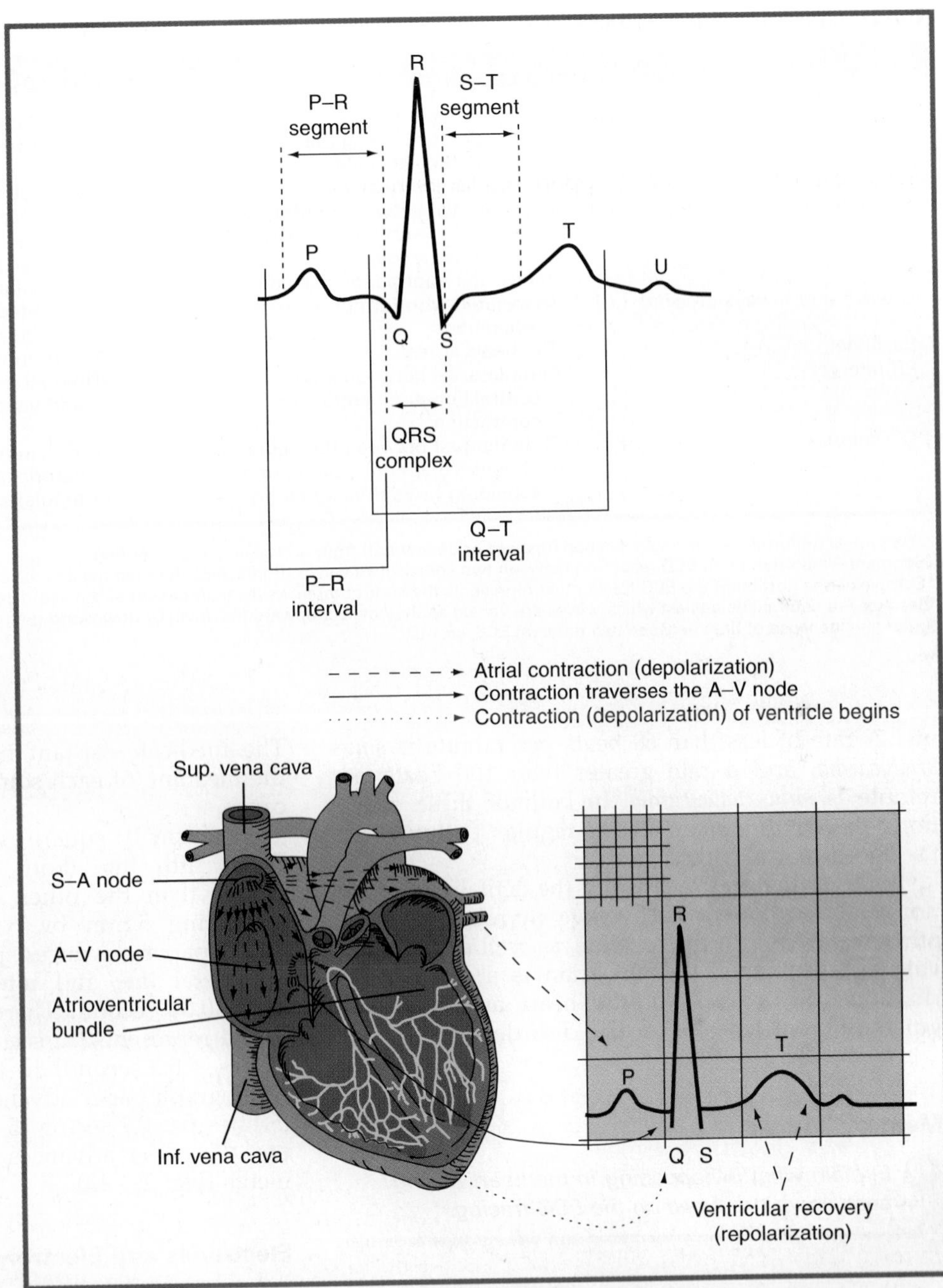

FIGURE 29–12 Cardiac cycle.

is the physiologic basis of electrocardiography. The ECG measures the normal conductive mechanism of the heart muscle and detects any disturbances or disruptions of heart rhythm (Fig. 29–12).

The ECG records a series of waves, or deflections, above or below a baseline. Each deflection corresponds to a particular part of the cardiac cycle (Table 29–1). The normal ECG cycle consists of waveforms that have been arbitrarily labeled the P wave, the Q wave, the R wave, the S wave, and the T wave. The Q, R, and S waves are frequently identified as the QRS complex. The *P wave* reflects contraction of the atria (beginning depolarization). The *PR interval* reflects the time it takes from the beginning of the atrial contraction to the beginning of the ventricular contraction. The *QRS complex* reflects the contraction of the ventricles (depolarization of both ventricles). The *ST segment* reflects the time interval from the end of the ventricular contraction to the beginning of ventricular recovery. The *T wave* reflects ventricular recovery (repolarization of the ventricles). After the T wave, there is a period of heart rest (polarization); and the tracing shows a straight line, indicating the resting state of the heart. This flat horizontal line is called the *baseline.* Occasionally, after the T wave, another small *U wave* is seen. It may appear in patients who have a low serum potassium level and other metabolic disturbances. *Normal sinus rhythm* refers to an ECG that is within the average limit range of 60 to 100 beats per min-

TABLE 29–1 The Cardiac Cycle

Stage	Heart Activity	Electric Current
P wave*	Atrial contraction	Atrial depolarization
PR segment†	Contraction traversing the atrioventricular node	Depolarization traversing the atrioventricular node
QRS complex‡	Ventricular contraction	Ventricular depolarization
ST segment	Time interval between ventricular contraction and the beginning of ventricular recovery	Time interval between ventricular depolarization and ventricular repolarization
T wave	Ventricular contraction subsides	Ventricular repolarization (electric recovery)
U wave (not always present)	Associated with further ventricular relaxation	Associated with further ventricular repolarization
Baseline§	The heart at rest	Polarization
PR interval‖	Time interval between atrial contraction and ventricular contraction	Time interval between atrial depolarization and ventricular depolarization
QT interval	Time interval between the beginning of ventricular contraction and the subsiding of ventricular contraction	Time interval between the beginning of ventricular depolarization and ventricular repolarization (electric recovery)

*Wave—a uniformly advancing deflection (upward or downward) from a baseline on a recording.
†Segment—a portion of an ECG recording between two consecutive waves. Represents the time needed for an electric current to move on.
‡Complex—the portion of the ECG tracing that represents the sum of three waves (contraction of the ventricles).
§Baseline—a neutral line against which waves are valued as they deflect upward (positive) or downward (negative) from the line.
‖Interval—the lapse of time between two different ECG events.

ute. A rate of less than 60 beats per minute is *sinus bradycardia,* and a rate greater than 100 beats per minute is *sinus tachycardia.* In both of these conditions the rhythm maintains a regular pattern; it is the speed that is pathologic.

By observing and measuring the actual configuration and location of each wave in relation to the other waves and to the baseline, as well as the intervals and segments, the physician is able to detect rhythmic disturbances of the heart and to distinguish different types of cardiac disorders.

Memory Jogger

Explain what is happening in the heart during each wave produced on the ECG tracing.

THE ELECTROCARDIOGRAM

Electrocardiograph Paper

Electrocardiograph paper is heat sensitive and pressure sensitive. The recording or writing device of the electrocardiograph is called a *stylus.* When the machine is on, the heated stylus moves along a horizontal line and burns the paper. Because the paper is also pressure sensitive, it must be handled carefully to avoid any markings that would blemish the tracing.

Electrocardiograph paper is graph paper with internationally accepted increments for measuring the cardiac cycle. These universal measurements allow physicians anywhere, anytime, to interpret the significance of each person's ECG in the same manner. The medical assistant needs to know the size and the meaning of each square to understand its significance.

Each small square measures 1 mm by 1 mm. Every fifth line (both vertical and horizontal) is darker than the other lines and defines a square measuring 5 mm by 5 mm. As the electrocardiograph paper advances, the stylus moves along one horizontal line and intersects with a vertical line every 0.04 second. Therefore, every fifth line intersected represents 0.2 second (0.04 second per line for 5 lines = 0.2 second) in time. Routinely, the electrocardiograph paper advances at a speed of 25 mm/sec (5 lines per 0.2 sec or 25 lines = 1 second). In 1 minute, the paper advances three hundred 5-mm increments (Fig. 29–13).

Electrodes and Electrolytes

Sensors or *electrodes* are placed on the patient's limbs and chest to pick up the electrical activity of the heart. The cardiac impulses are transmitted to the electrocardiograph by the metal tips and wires that are attached to the sensors or electrodes (Fig. 29–14). Most offices prefer to use disposable electrodes, which are permeated with the needed electrolyte and can be used to secure all 12 leads.

The standard 12-lead electrocardiograph may have 5 or 10 electrodes. Two electrodes are attached to the fleshy part of the arms and 2 to the fleshy part of the legs. If the machine has 5 electrodes, the fifth electrode is moved to six different positions on the chest. If there are 6 or 10, these are placed in the positions recommended by the manufacturer and moved only if indicated in the instruction procedure. The electrodes are coded to ensure accurate placement of each (Fig. 29–15*A*).

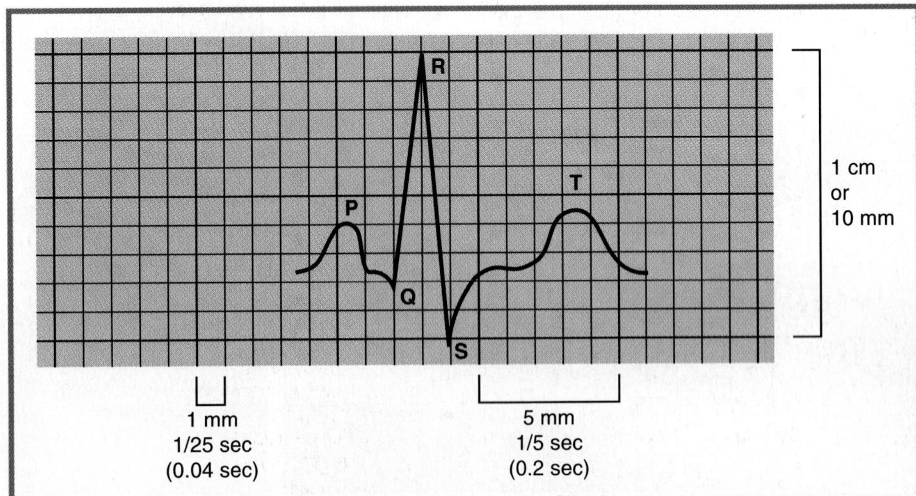

FIGURE 29–13 ECG paper measurement.

The skin is a poor conductor of electricity. To aid in the conduction of this electrical current, an *electrolyte* is applied to each electrode. Electrolyte products are available in the form of pastes, gels, pads saturated with electrolyte solution, or self-stick disposable electrode pads.

The cardiac impulses travel from the electrodes and wires to an amplifier, where they are magnified. The amplified impulses are then converted into mechanical action by a *galvanometer* or into electrical action fed into a computer and then are recorded on the electrocardiograph paper by the stylus or computer-produced recording (Fig. 29–15*B*).

Leads

The standard ECG consists of 12 separate *leads*, or recordings, of the electrical activity of the heart, from different angles. Each lead must be marked, or

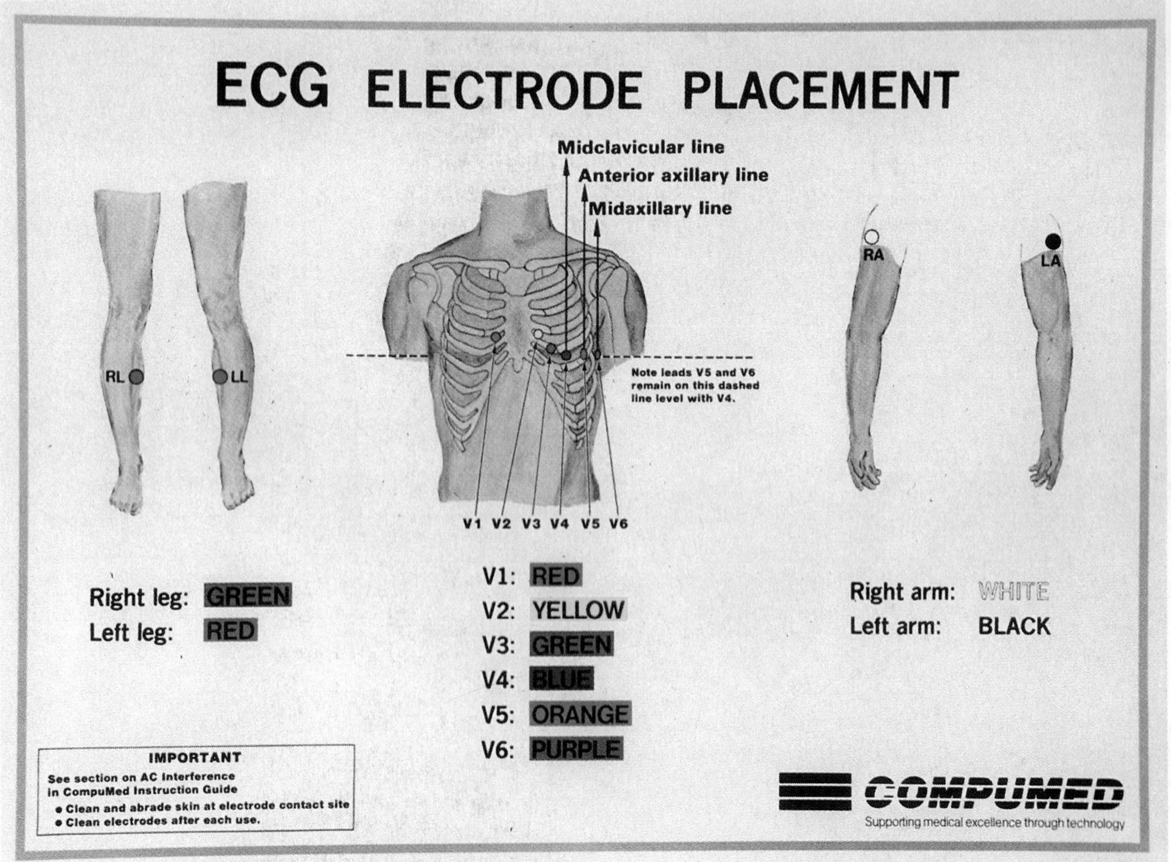

FIGURE 29–14 ECG electrode placement. (Courtesy of Compumed, San Diego, CA.)

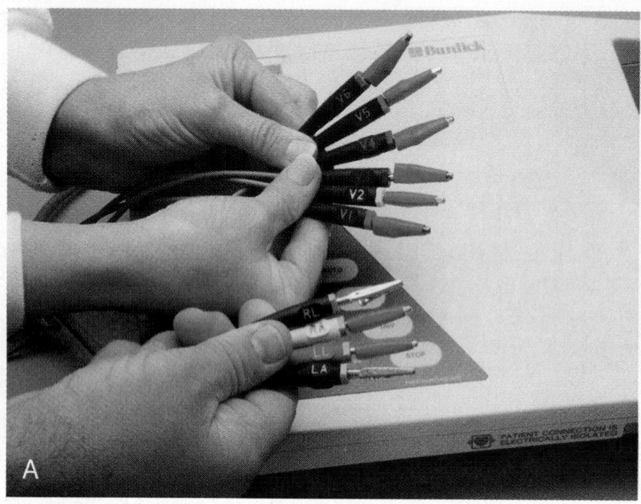

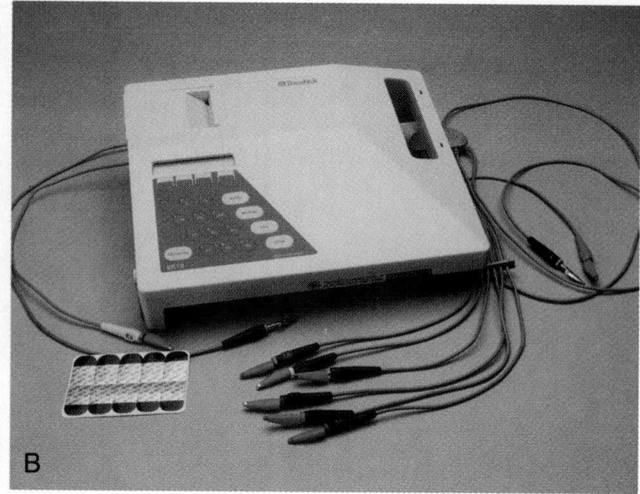

FIGURE 29–15 *A*, ECG electrode identification. Note code on terminal end. *B*, ECG machine with electrodes and wires attached to base. (Courtesy of Burdick Corporation, Melton, WI.)

coded, for the physician to know the angle recorded. Most machines being used automatically mark the 12 leads as the *lead selector switch* is turned. However, there may be times when the assistant will be required to mark or code each lead manually. A certain coding system is used to identify each lead recorded. Codes consist of a series of dots and dashes. One standard marking code is illustrated in Table 29–2.

Standard, or Bipolar, Leads

The first three leads recorded are called the standard, or *bipolar,* leads. They are referred to as bipo-

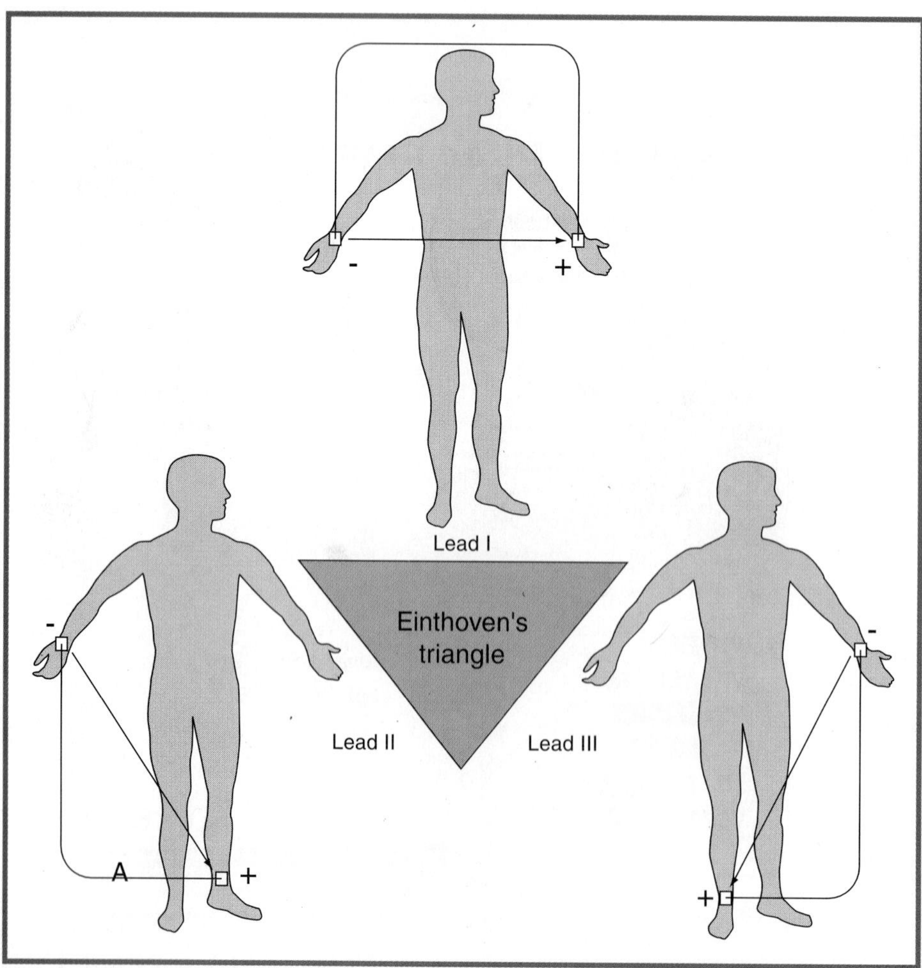

FIGURE 29–16 Bipolar leads and axes.

TABLE 29–2 The Standard Marking Codes

	Electrodes Connected	Marking Code
Standard or Bipolar Limb Leads		
Lead 1	LL & RA	•
Lead 2	LL & RA	••
Lead 3	LL & LA	•••
Augmented Unipolar Limb Leads		
aVR	RA & (LA-LL)	—
aVL	LA & (RA-LL)	——
aVF	LL & (RA-LA)	———
Chest or Precordial Leads		
V	C & (LA-RA-LL)	V1—• V2—•• V3—••• V4—•••• V5—••••• V6—••••••

(Courtesy of The Burdick Corporation, Milton, WI.)

lar because they each use two limb electrodes to record the electrical activity. Roman numerals are used to designate these leads (Fig. 29–16).

- Lead I records the electrical activity between the right arm and the left arm.
- Lead II records the electrical activity between the right arm and the left leg.
- Lead III records the electrical activity between the left arm and the left leg.

Augmented Leads

The next three leads recorded are the augmented or combined leads. They are aVR, aVL, and aVF. The aV stands for augmented voltage, the R for right arm, the L for left arm, and the F for the left leg. The right leg electrode acts as the grounding electrode. These leads are unipolar (Fig. 29–17).

- *Lead aVR* records the electrical activity from the midpoint between the left arm and the left leg to the right arm.
- *Lead aVL* records the electrical activity from the midpoint between the right arm and the left leg to the left arm.
- *Lead aVF* records the electrical activity from the midpoint between the right arm and the left arm to the left leg.

Chest, or Precordial, Leads

The last six leads are the chest, or *precordial,* leads. These leads are unipolar and are designated V_1, V_2,

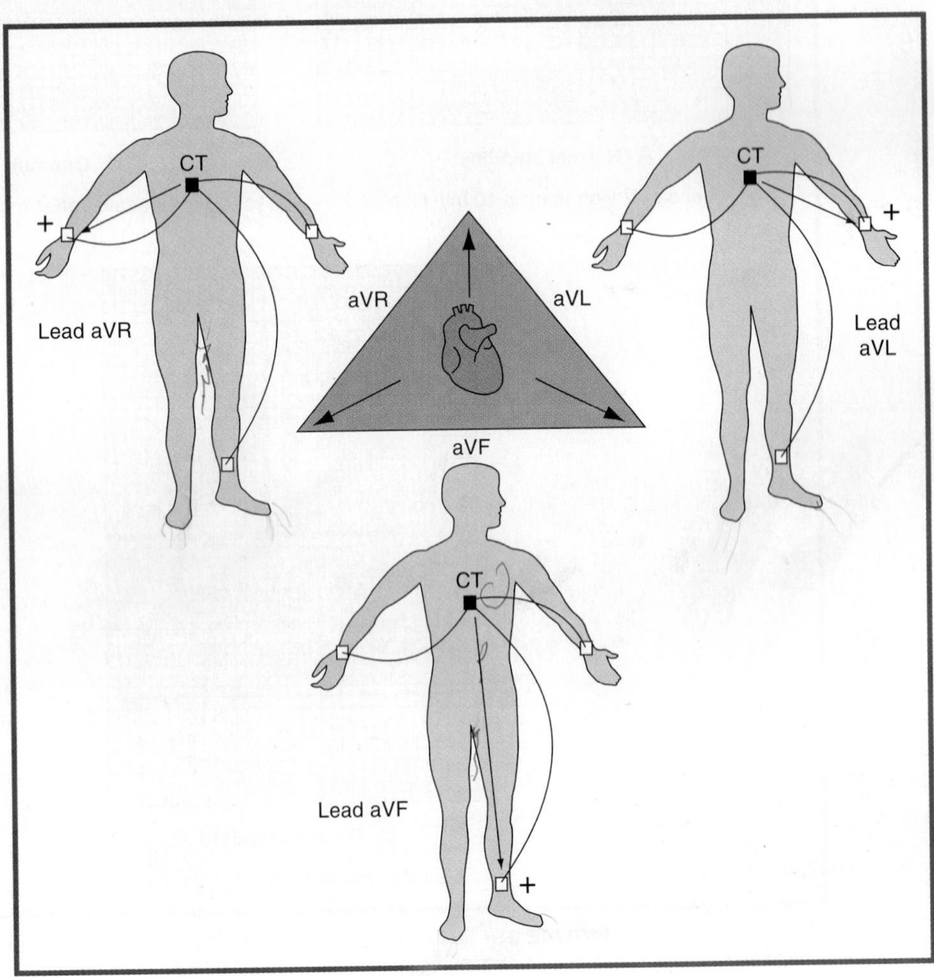

FIGURE 29–17 Augmented leads and precordial leads.

V_3, V_4, V_5, and V_6. Each number signifies the position of the electrode on the chest. Leads V_1 through V_6 record the electrical activity between six points on the chest wall and a point within the heart (see Fig. 29–15*A*).

Memory Jogger

13 *How many different leads make up an ECG tracing?*

Standardization and Sensitivity

Standardization has been determined by an international agreement to ensure that an ECG can be interpreted anywhere in the world. It assumes that the electrocardiograph used has been calibrated according to universal measurements. Before recording a patient's tracing, you must make certain that the machine is correctly standardized.

When a machine is in standard (1 STD), 1 millivolt (mV) of electricity causes the stylus to move vertically 10 mm. Thus, it is possible to calculate

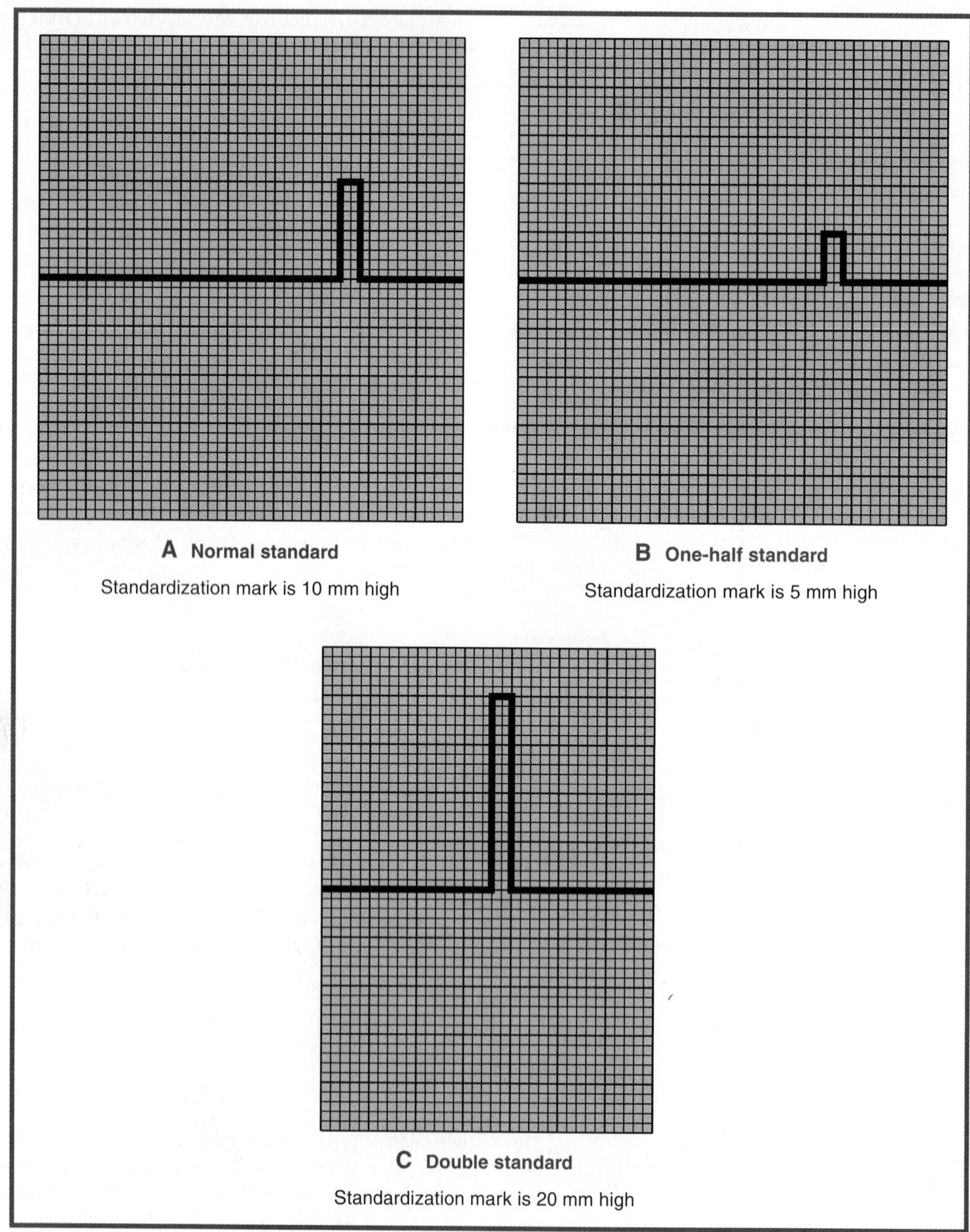

FIGURE 29–18 *A* through *C*, Standardization sensitivity controls.

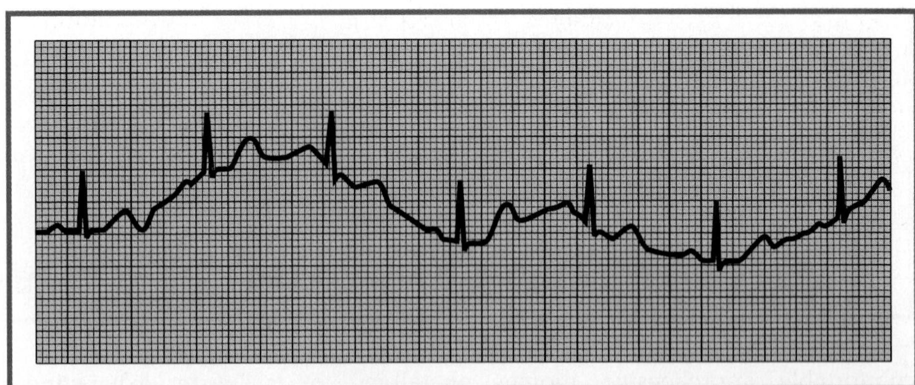

FIGURE 29–19 Wandering baseline.

electric voltages by the vertical movement of the stylus on the paper. The stylus should deflect exactly 10 mm when the *standardization button* is depressed with a quick pecking motion. The standardization should be 2 mm wide and rectangular. Each manufacturer's manual explains the method of adjustment to obtain a perfect standardization.

Standardization is usually performed at the beginning of the first lead recording, although some physicians require a standardization within each of the 12-lead recordings.

Most machines have three sensitivity (STD) positions that may be used. They are ½ STD, 1 STD, and 2 STD. When recording ½ STD, 1 mV causes the stylus to deflect 5 mm. If the amplitude (height) of the QRS complex is too high and is causing the stylus to move off the paper, the machine should be put on ½ STD. If the amplitude of the QRS complex is too small, the machine should be put on 2 STD, causing the stylus to deflect 20 mm. Figure 29–18 shows the three sensitivity positions. Make note of any variation from the normal 1 STD.

As mentioned, the standard speed for recording an ECG is at 25 mm/sec. If the patient's heart rate is very rapid or if certain parts of the complex are too close together, it may be necessary to adjust the paper run to 50 mm/sec. This will double the speed of the paper run and extend the recording to twice its normal length (see Fig. 29–18). Again, make certain that this is noted on the tracing.

Memory Jogger

14 *What are the three sensitivity settings on the ECG machine?*

TRACING ERRORS IN THE PLACEMENT OF THE LIMB LEADS

- If there is interference in limb leads I and II, check the electrode connection on the patient's right arm.
- If there is interference in limb leads I and III, check the electrode connection on the patient's left arm.
- If there is interference in limb leads II and III, check the electrode connection on the patient's left leg.

Artifacts

An artifact is unwanted movement of the stylus on the paper produced by outside electrical interference. The electrocardiograph is extremely sensitive to any kind of electrical activity. Artifacts on the tracing make the interpretation of the recording difficult. The medical assistant should have a thorough understanding of the causes and remedies of these artifacts. The types of artifacts include wandering baseline, somatic tremor, alternating current, and baseline interruption.

Wandering Baseline

This artifact is a gradual shifting of the stylus away from the center of the paper, usually resulting from unnoticed movement of the patient (Fig. 29–19). If this occurs, remind the patient to remain still. Other causes include metal electrodes that are corroded or dirty or have been applied too loosely or too tightly; tension on the electrode from a dangling cable; poor-quality electrolyte paste, or too little applied to the electrode; and improper preparation of the patient's skin before applying the electrolyte.

Somatic Tremor

Somatic tremor means muscle movement. Natural electrical voltage from muscle movement causes additional stylus movement across the paper. This results in a recording with jagged peaks of irregular height and spacing and a shifting baseline (Fig. 29–20). Usually, this is because the patient is un-

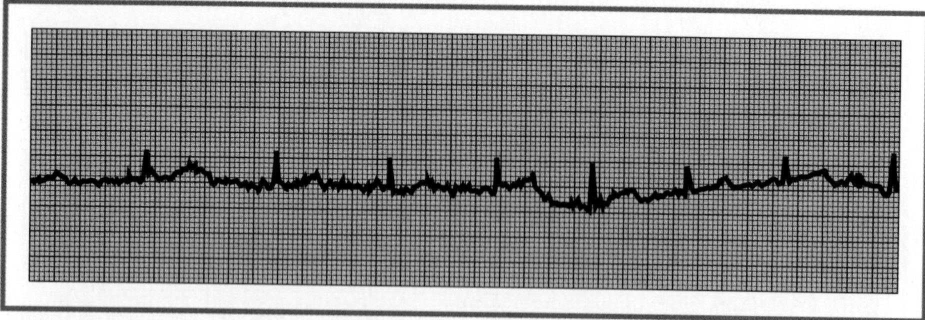

FIGURE 29–20 Somatic tremor.

comfortable, apprehensive, moving or talking, or suffering from a disorder that causes body tremors. Explaining the procedure beforehand alleviates apprehension and relaxes the patient. Reposition the patient comfortably, or offer the patient a pillow. Sometimes it helps to place the patient's hands under the buttocks or to ask the patient to take slow, deep breaths. Chills cause somatic tremor; check the room temperature and offer the patient a blanket. If the patient is having great difficulty in relaxing or is trembling, cover him or her with a blanket and consult the physician regarding a possible intervention.

Alternating Current Interference

Alternating current (AC) interference appears as a series of uniform small spiked lines on the paper (Fig. 29–21). Alternating current present in nearby equipment or wires can radiate small amounts of energy into the room where the ECG is being performed. Some of this energy can be detected by the sensitive electrocardiograph. If there is AC interference, check the machine for proper grounding. You may need to use an external ground wire provided with the machine. Be certain to follow the manufacturer's directions. Check to see that the lead wires are not crossed. Also check that the electrodes are clean. If the interference is still present, unplug other electrical appliances in the room. Move the patient table to another area of the room, or turn the table around. Move the table away from the wall, because the interference may be in the electrical wiring in the wall or in an adjoining room. Make certain that your patient is not touching anything on the patient table. If necessary, turn off the overhead fluorescent lights.

After exhausting all of the probable causes, try using a different location, such as a different examination room in a totally different area of the facility. The last step is to call the manufacturer or your local service representative.

Baseline Interruption

Baseline interruption occurs when the electric connection has been interrupted. The stylus moves onto the margin of the paper (Fig. 29–22). The stylus moves violently up and down, or it may record a straight line across the top or the bottom of the paper. Most baseline interruption is caused by noticeable patient movement jarring the electrodes. Other causes can be a broken wire in the patient cable or cable tips that are attached too loosely to the electrodes.

Memory Jogger

Name four types of artifacts and what may cause each of them.

Pathological Tracings

The medical assistant working in the cardiovascular practice needs to be able to recognize rhythm abnormalities that may appear on the tracing. Alerting the physician to the presence of an arrhythmia while the patient is still connected to the machine may allow the physician the opportunity to observe the patient while the machine is running or institute some type of intervention immediately.

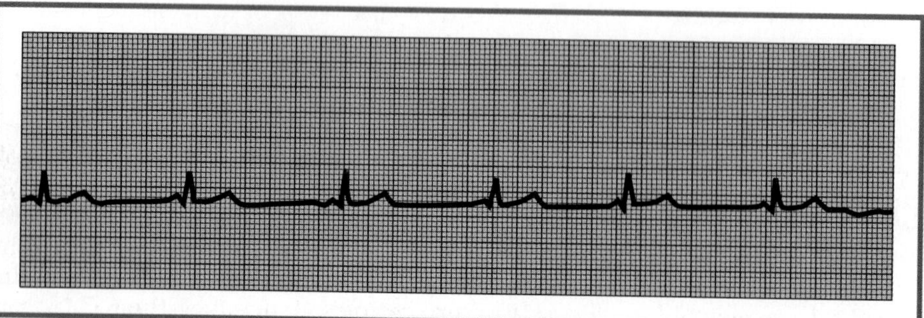

FIGURE 29–21 AC interference.

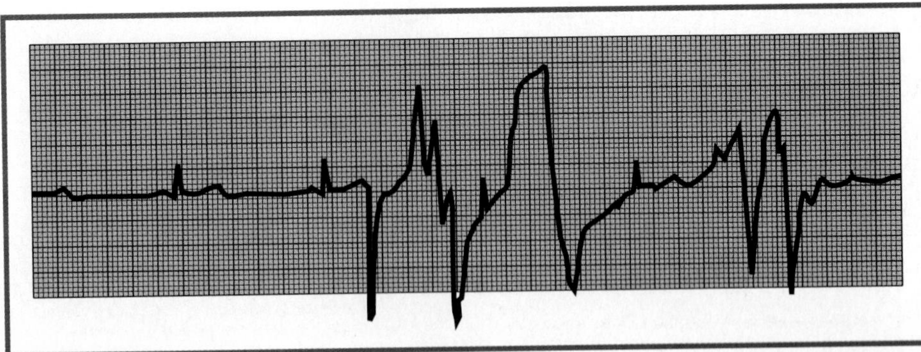

FIGURE 29–22 Baseline interruption.

OBTAINING THE ELECTROCARDIOGRAM

Preparing the Room and the Patient

The room should be free from interruptions, and the machine should be as far away from other electrical equipment as possible. This includes x-ray machines, diathermy equipment, centrifuges, fans, refrigerators, and air conditioners. The room should be quiet and warm.

The treatment table should be comfortable and wide enough for the patient to be fully supported to avoid excess muscle movement. It should be wood or have some form of insulation between metal legs or surfaces. Position the table so that you are working from the patient's left or right side. Try both positions to determine which way is more comfortable for you. If you work from the patient's left side, you will be connecting the electrodes moving toward you. If you work from the right you will be moving away from you or to the left for V_5 and V_6. As long as the electrodes are placed in the proper position, the positioning is up to you.

Small pillows are helpful in relaxing the patient. One pillow may be used under the patient's head, but it should not be elevating the patient's shoulders. A small pillow placed under the patient's knees may also help relax the muscles of the abdomen and the lower extremities.

The patient must disrobe to the waist and expose the lower legs. A patient gown may be put on with the opening in the front (female), or a drape may be placed over the exposed chest (male). Pantyhose or stockings must be removed to expose bare skin and all tight clothing loosened.

Place the patient in the supine position, with arms at the sides and the legs not touching one another. If the patient is **orthopneic,** semi-Fowler's position may be used or the patient can be seated on a wooden chair. Check with the physician before obtaining the ECG tracing in an alternate position. In the sitting position, the patient's feet should be on the floor on a rubber mat or on a wooden footstool or on a stack of books. The legs must not hang free, nor should there be any pressure on the back of the lower thighs. If the patient is in a sitting or semi-Fowler's position, *note this on the patient's recording.*

It is advisable to have the patient rest for at least 10 minutes before the recording. Check to determine whether the patient was able to follow the instructions given (Fig. 29–23). Note on the patient's record that all vital signs and medications taken have been recorded.

Explain to the patient the nature and purpose of the ECG. Chat with the patient while preparing for the procedure. Stress the importance of not moving during the entire procedure, and assure the patient that there is no danger. When you tell patients to lie still, make sure their breathing remains normal. Frequently, when you tell patients to lie still they tend to hold their breath. Allow time for the patient to ask questions or to express any concerns before you begin obtaining the tracing.

Memory Jogger

 *Describe a patient with orthopnea.*

Applying the Electrodes and Lead Wires

There are many types of electrocardiograph equipment. Each machine has a slightly different method for attaching the electrodes and lead wires. The age of the machine also can determine the method of attachment. It is always necessary to become familiar with the equipment that you will be using. Read the manufacturer's directions and practice doing an ECG with the equipment before performing the procedure on a patient.

Before beginning, plug in the machine and turn the power switch on to allow the machine to warm up. Make certain that the patient cable is pushed in all the way into the patient cable jack on the machine. Expose the patient's arms and legs. If you are using the electrodes with lead connectors, attach an electrode strap to each electrode, then place a small amount of electrolyte or an electrolyte pad on each electrode. Make certain that you have the same amount on each electrode. With the electrode, rub the electrolyte into the skin on the fleshy part of the arms and legs. *Avoid the muscle and bone area.* Rub the skin's surface until a slight **erythema** appears.

INSTRUCTIONS FOR PATIENT BEFORE AN ELECTROCARDIOGRAM

Name: ______________________________

Your cardiogram appointment is ______________ , ____________________ at ________ AM/PM
Day Date Time

These instructions are simple, but it is important that you follow them. Please call us if you are unable to follow these instructions or keep your appointment so we may make another appointment.

1. There is no discomfort or sensation in having an electrocardiogram. No electricity is put into the patient in any way. Small metal plates are placed on the calf of each leg and on each arm and at different places on the chest. The minute impulse generated by your heart is simply picked up by these plates and recorded by the machine.
2. You will be asked to lie down on a comfortable table while the test is being performed by the technician.
3. For your convenience, it is best to wear loose clothing. You will be asked to disrobe to your waist to expose the chest. It will also be necessary to expose your lower legs from the knees down and the upper arms just below the shoulders.
4. The actual test only takes about 5 minutes, but you will be asked to rest for about one-half hour before the test. It is best you do not have a heavy meal for about 2 hours before the test. You should not consume any cold drinks or ice cream or smoke just before the test. It is also advisable to refrain from excessive exercise just before the test. Do not take any medications without the physician's usual instructions and knowledge.
5. During the test, you will be asked to lie absolutely still and relax, because the slightest movement interferes with an accurate tracing. Do not talk.
6. The skin on the legs, arms, and chest must be free from skin ointments, oils, and medications.
7. The technician taking the test is specially trained to perform the test but is unable to tell you the results of the test, because he or she is neither trained nor authorized to make any interpretations of the cardiogram. This is the task of the physician.

FIGURE 29–23 ECG patient instructions.

Wipe off any excess electrolyte. Do not allow your hands to carry the electrolyte from the patient to the equipment. Unequal amounts of electrolyte or the spreading of it to the wires and equipment may cause artifacts.

Position the electrodes with the lead connectors pointing toward the center of the body. Place the electrodes on the prepared skin areas. Place each strap around the limb until the hole just meets the hook. Then move the strap one hole tighter and fasten it. This should provide the correct tension. Avoid having the lead connectors cross over the plates. An accurate tracing cannot be made if the straps are too loose or too tight.

Place the disc-shaped chest electrode in the first chest lead position (V_1). Depending on the type of machine being used, the chest electrode may be moved to the other chest points, one lead at a time, during the procedure. A *Welch electrode* is one type of bulb-shaped electrode that may be used for the chest leads. Some multichanneled ECGs use sensors or electrodes, which are all connected at the same time. These sensors consist of a rubber bulb with a metal suction cup. Locate each of the chest lead sites. Squeeze a dab of electrolyte on each electrode site, pinch the bulb slightly, and secure the metal cup over the selected site. Take care that the bulbs do not touch each other.

Insert the tips of the lead cords into the lead connector holes of the leg and arm electrodes. Check to make certain that you have connected the correct lead terminal into the corresponding electrode. As you attach the electrodes consciously think of what you are doing, for example, "right arm electrode into right arm terminal." The lead cords are color coded, but it is still easy to confuse the patient's right and left sides. Make sure all wires lie on the patient's body because this will reduce interference and prevent drag on the cable, which can cause an improper electrode connection. Check that each lead cord terminal is snug.

If you are using the disposable sensor tabs, the placement remains the same and the small alligator clips are fastened to the tab on the sensor pads.

Recording the Electrocardiogram

Check the manufacturer's instructions for the specific amount of warm-up time needed. Set the *lead selector control* to STD. Turn the *recorder control* to "on" and then to "run." Using the *position control knob,* center the *stylus* on the baseline. Check the standardization by pressing the *standardization button:* the stylus should move to a height of 10 mm when the sensitivity is at "1."

After obtaining a proper standardization, turn the *lead selector control* to "automatic." The machine will code each part of the tracing and run the appropriate length needed for mounting.

Before removing the equipment from the patient, show the tracing to the physician for his or her approval. Then you can remove the equipment and assist the patient to a sitting position. The patient should remain on the table for a few moments to rest and then be assisted off the table and with dressing, if needed.

Caring for the Equipment

Remove the tips of the lead wires from the electrodes, unfasten the rubber straps, and remove the electrodes from the patient. Clean the electrode sites with a warm, wet paper towel, and dry them. If sensors were used, remove the alligator clips and then remove the disposable sensors, discarding them in the acceptable manner. Change the table paper, and discard any used disposable materials.

Clean the rubber straps with a mild detergent, and dry them. The electrodes must be cleaned with a mild detergent first, then polished with a fine grade of scouring powder. Do not use steel wool or any metal-based polish because it will interfere with the tracing and cause artifacts. Always rinse the electrodes well and let them dry before storing them. Use an applicator to clean the connecting holes and the inside of the suction-type chest electrode.

MULTICHANNEL/AUTOMATIC ELECTROCARDIOGRAPH

Most physicians are now using an electrocardiograph with a three-channel or six-channel capability that can simultaneously record three or six different leads. For these machines, there are six chest electrodes and all are placed into position before the test is run. Once started, some machines run through all 12 leads automatically and mark each lead with its identifying letters instead of the dot-dash coding seen on the single-channel tracing. These tracings are shorter when they are produced and need no special mounting when placed into the patient's chart.

PROCEDURE 29–1
Performing a Multichannel ECG

GOAL

To obtain an accurate, artifact-free recording of the electrical activity of the heart.

EQUIPMENT AND SUPPLIES

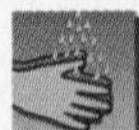

- Multichannel ECG machine, loaded with paper
- 10 disposable self-adhesive electrodes
- Patient cables
- Patient gown and drape
- Gauze squares
- Pencil and paper
- Mounting board

PROCEDURAL STEPS

1 Wash hands.
PURPOSE: Infection control.

2 Explain the procedure to the patient.
PURPOSE: To gain patient cooperation and alleviate apprehension.

3 Ask the patient to disrobe to the waist and remove socks, stockings, or pantyhose.
PURPOSE: Electrodes must be applied to bare skin.

4 Position the patient on the ECG table and drape appropriately.
PURPOSE: To ensure safety, modesty, and comfort of the patient.

Continued

PROCEDURE 29–1 (CONTINUED)

Performing a Multichannel ECG

5 Turn on the machine to warm the stylus (Figure 1).
PURPOSE: Ensure machine performance.

6 Label the beginning of the tracing paper with patient's name, date, and time of test (Figure 2).
PURPOSE: Proper identification of test results.

7 Apply self-adhesive electrodes to dry fleshy areas on the limbs. Make sure that the points of the electrotabs point toward the feet (Figure 3).
PURPOSE: Position ensures a better connection and places less stress on the electrodes.

8 Palpate the chest for the location sites of the chest electrodes and secure all tabs with points facing downward.

9 Connect lead wires using the alligator clips at the end of each wire (Figure 4).

10 Press the AUTO button on the machine and run the ECG tracing (Figure 5). The machine will automatically place the standardization at the beginning, and then the 12 leads will follow in the three-channel matrix.

11 Watch for artifacts (Figure 6).

12 Remove the electrode tapes from the patient, disconnect the lead wires, and place used electrodes in the waste container.

13 Assist the patient in dressing as needed.

14 Clean and return equipment to its storage area.

15 Mount ECG or give the physician the unmounted tape as directed (Figure 7).

16 Wash hands.

17 Document procedure in the patient's medical record.
PURPOSE: Procedures that are not recorded are considered not done.

Continued

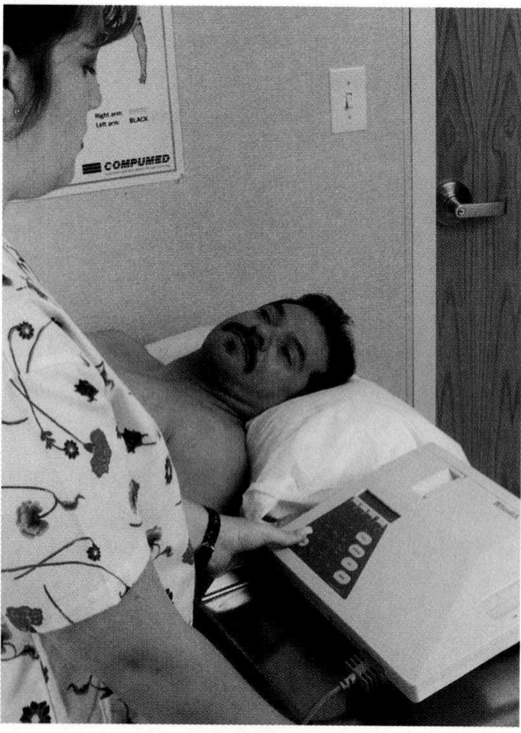

FIGURE 1

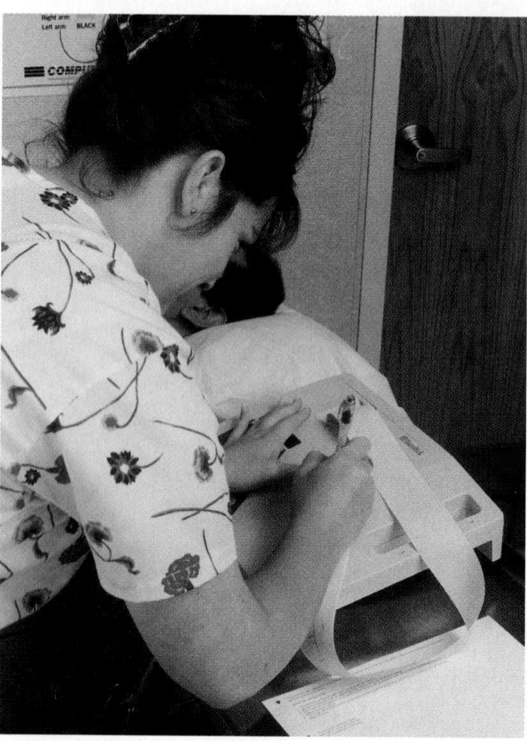

FIGURE 2

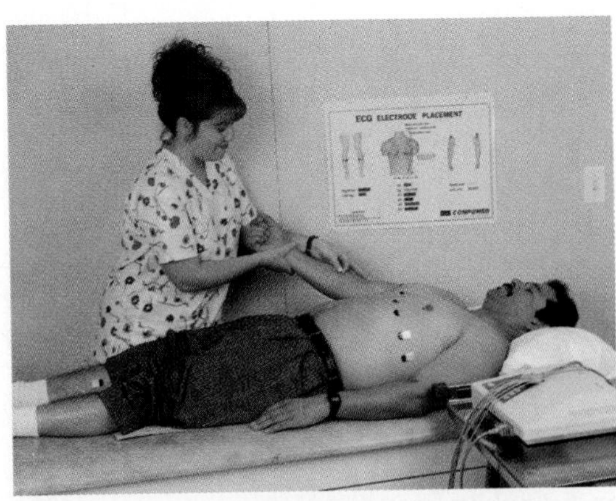

FIGURE 3

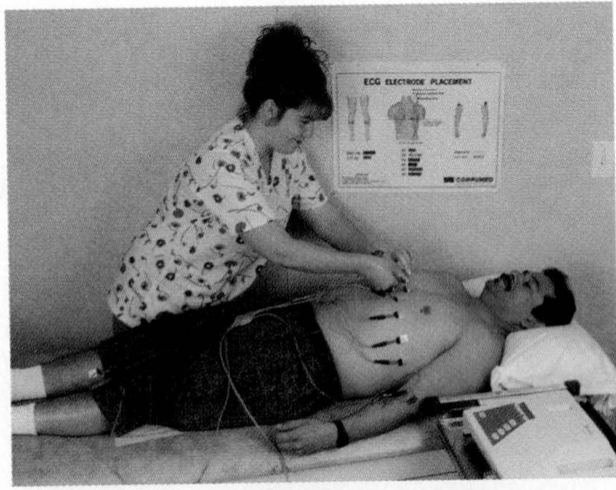

FIGURE 4

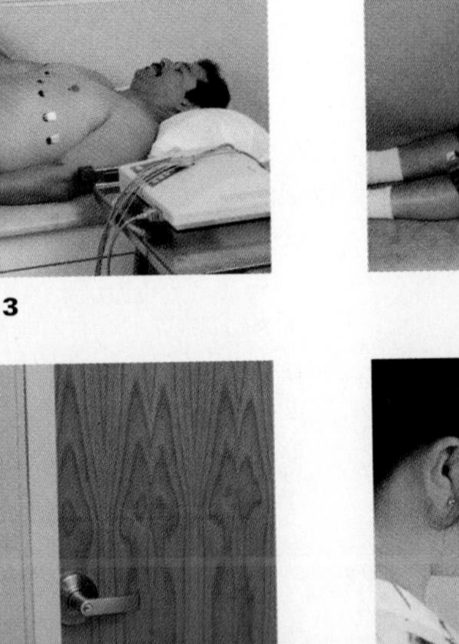

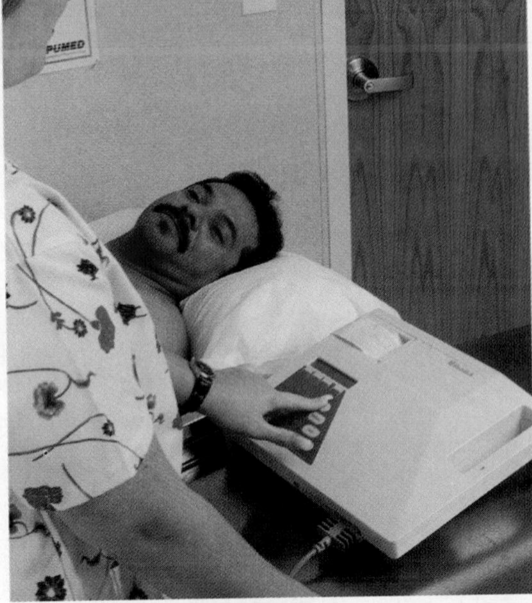

FIGURE 5

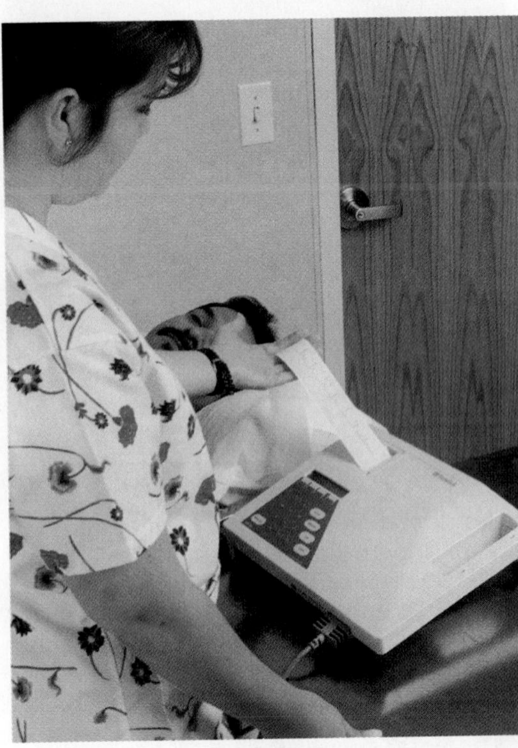

FIGURE 6

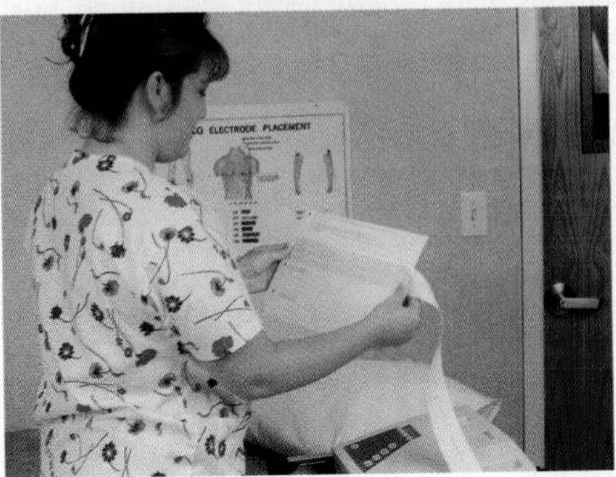

FIGURE 7

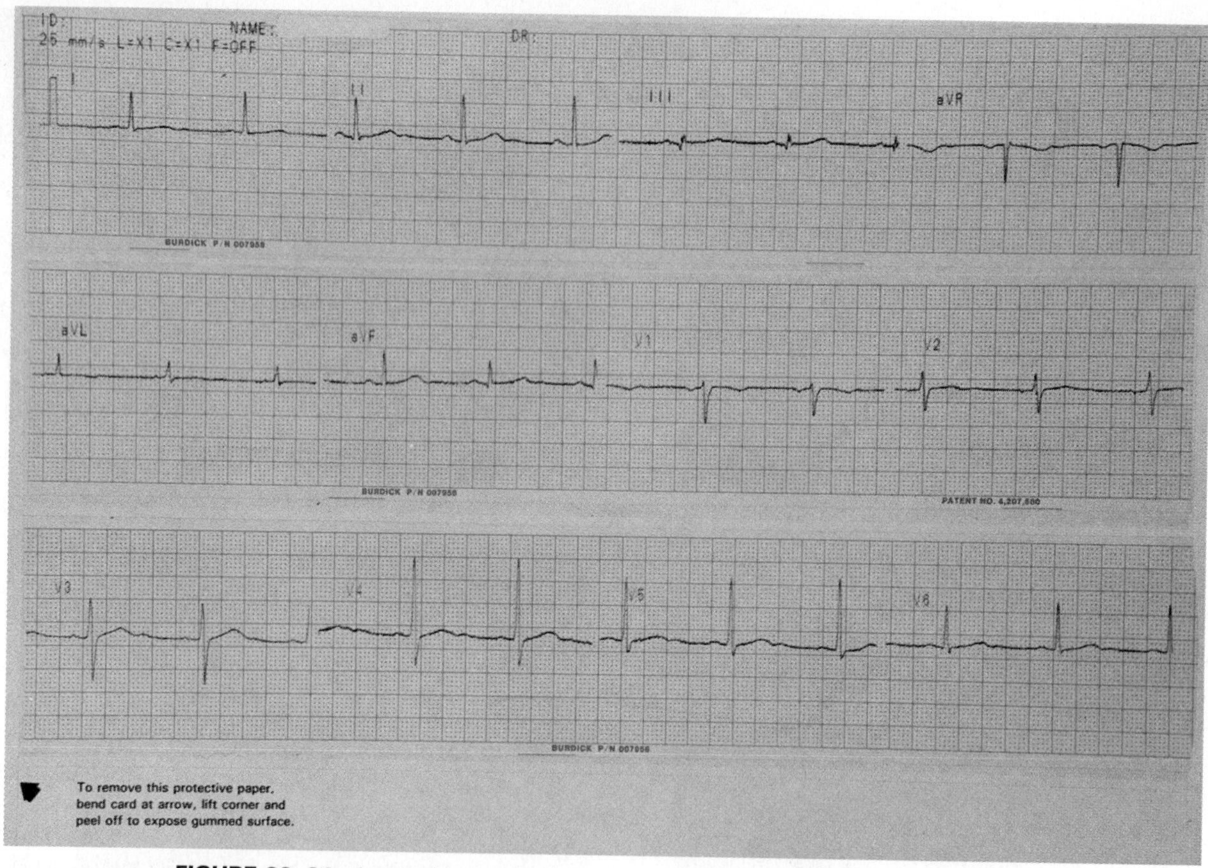

FIGURE 29–24 Accurately mounted ECG. (Courtesy of Burdick Corporation, Melton, WI.)

MOUNTING AN ECG TRACING

There are many different types of ECG mounts. An office selects the mount that is best adapted to the types of ECG equipment used in the office. It is advisable to select a mount that can be easily read in its entirety on one surface. The most commonly used mounts are self-adhesive mounting pages that are designed so that an entire test is placed on a single-sided page (Fig. 29–24). Tracings are usually a series of records over a period of years; a mount must last for a considerable length of time.

Paper clips and staples are not used because they will scratch a tracing. Clear tape can be used, but some tape becomes sticky or yellow with time. Copy machines can be used to make a single-sheet copy of the tracing without damaging the original record. Photocopies take up less filing space.

Regardless of the style of mount used, each ECG should be neatly and carefully mounted, with complete information recorded on each one.

INFORMATION THAT MUST APPEAR ON THE MOUNT

- Patient's full name
- Sex
- Age
- Date and time of ECG
- Medications
- Variations from normal sensitivity and variation from a machine speed of 25 mm/sec

A notation is made of any variation from the routine, such as a very nervous patient, a different position of the patient, lack of rest before the test, or smoking immediately before the test. If the lead placements were different from the routine, this also should be noted.

Care is taken when mounting an ECG. If you are using a trimmer, do not allow your desk to become cluttered with tracing trimmings. Discard the trimmings into a waste container as you trim them off. Most tracings are easily scratched, so be careful not to damage the tracing with finger rings or sleeve buttons. Do not stack other items on top of the open-faced type of mount.

If trimming the strip is required, do not cut off the lead coding until you are ready to mount that particular lead. Double-check each lead code with the mount placement. Some mounts place the precordial leads horizontally whereas others place them vertically. Take great care not to mount a lead upside down. If you have been requested to show the

STD in a lead, be sure to include it. Do not cover the tips of the QRS complexes with the sides of the slotted-type mount. Place the mounted ECG tracing on the physician's desk for evaluation with the patient's medical record and any previous ECG tracings.

Some physicians will want to see the entire strip before it is mounted and will decide which sections to keep. In this case, mount the ECG sections according to the decisions made by the physician.

Memory Jogger

What information should be included on the mounted ECG tracing?

INTERPRETATION OF THE ECG

The physician can determine two important heart functions when interpreting the ECG. These two functions are heart rate and heart rhythm.

On the ECG tracing, each cycle consists of a P wave, a QRS complex, and a T wave. When the rhythm is regular, it is possible to calculate heart rate by counting the number of 5-mm boxes between two R waves. Divide this number into 300. Your answer will be the beats per minute.

Heart rhythm is determined to be either regular or irregular. The horizontal distance between the P waves is measured first. If the distance is the same, atrial rhythm is regular; and if not, it is irregular. Next, measure the horizontal distance between the R waves. If the distance is the same, ventricular rhythm is regular; if it is not, it is irregular.

Memory Jogger

If there are four 5-mm boxes between two R waves, what is the heart rate?

AUTOMATIC LEAD CONTROL SWITCH

Both single-channel and multiple-channel electrocardiographs may be equipped with automatic sequencing ability. This connects the correct electrode combinations so the technician does not have to advance a control. In the single-channel machine, the 12 leads automatically record one at a time until all 12 are recorded; in the multichannel machines, 3 or 6 leads record one at a time until all leads have been recorded. A standardization mark is also automatically recorded on the tracing. Most of these machines also have a manual recording capability that can be used when longer tracings are required for interpretations. If the machine has a copy capability, it can produce an accurate copy of the last ECG recorded.

TELEPHONE TRANSMISSION

An electrocardiograph with telephone transmission capabilities can transmit a recording over the telephone line to an ECG data interpretation center. The machine is equipped with a direct ECG fax transmitter. The recording is interpreted by a computer at the data center and verified by the cardiologist, and a printout with the computer-assisted interpretations is returned to the sender by fax or mail. Patient information that may be important to the interpretation, such as age, sex, height, weight, blood pressure, and medications, may also be relayed to the center. In some cases, the physician may want an expert comparison of two ECG tracings done on different visits by a patient. Both the old and new tracings may be sent, and the center will do the comparison and send them back immediately. This type of reporting often can allow the physician to begin treatment with the initial visit and save a return visit for the patient.

INTERPRETIVE ELECTROCARDIOGRAPHS

Interpretive electrocardiographs are equipped with a built-in computer, which analyzes the recording as it is being run. With this capability, immediate information on the heart's activity is available and can help in earlier diagnosis and treatment. It is necessary to enter patient baseline data into the computer *before* the tracing is taken. The computer analysis of the ECG and the reason for each interpretation is printed on the top of the recording.

Do not tell or allow the patient to read this interpretation. Give this to the physician immediately and allow him or her to decide what the patient is to be told.

Memory Jogger

What is the primary advantage of an ECG data interpretation center?

Cardiac Stress Testing

Cardiac stress testing is conducted to observe and record the patient's cardiovascular response to measured exercise challenges. Stress testing is performed to diagnose cardiac disease that cannot be detected by the standard resting ECG, to determine an individual's energy performance capacity, or to prescribe a specially designed exercise plan. The stress test is done while the patient is exercising on either a bicycle or a treadmill and under careful supervision.

Cardiac Stress Test

Cardiac stress testing (also known as an exercise tolerance test or treadmill test) is a means of observing, evaluating, and recording your heart's response during a measured exercise test. This test determines your capacity to adapt to physical stress.

There are various reasons that your physician may suggest this test for you:

1. To aid in determining the presence of suspected coronary heart disease.
2. To aid in the selection of therapy.
   a. For angina pectoris (tightness or pain in the chest).
   b. Following a myocardial infarction (heart attack).
   c. Following coronary bypass surgery (open heart surgery).
3. To determine your physical work capacity.
4. To authorize participation in a physical exercise program.

Preparation for the Test

1. Avoid eating a heavy meal within 2 hours of your appointment.
2. Take your medications as you usually do, unless your doctor advises you not to take them.
3. Wear a shirt or blouse that buttons down the front with slacks, a skirt, jogging pants, or shorts.
4. Do not wear one-piece undergarments, jumpsuits, or dresses.
5. Tennis shoes are ideal if you have them. Otherwise, wear comfortable flat or low-heeled shoes. Do not wear clogs, sling-backs, crepe soles, boots, or high heels, as they make walking on the treadmill more difficult.

The Procedure

When you arrive in the Cardiology Department, areas of your chest may be shaved (men only) to allow the electrodes to adhere tightly to your chest. A blood pressure cuff will be wrapped around your arm, and an electrocardiogram (ECG) is taken while you are at rest. The technician will then demonstrate how to walk on the treadmill and will answer any questions you may have.

You will then perform a graded exercise test on a motor-driven treadmill. You will begin walking very gradually at a rate you can easily accomplish.

Progressively throughout the test, the speed and grade of the treadmill will be increased, and you will be walking at a faster pace up a slight incline. At no time will you be asked to jog or run, nor will you be asked to exercise beyond your capabilities.

At all times during the test, trained personnel are in the room with you, monitoring your heart rate and blood pressure and observing you for signs of fatigue or discomfort. We do not wish to exercise you to a level that is medically unsafe or physically distressing.

An ECG is taken again when you finish walking. Your cardiologist will immediately interpret the results of the test and explain his or her findings to you. If necessary, medications or treatment will be discussed. A letter with the results of the stress test will be sent to your referring physician.

The entire procedure will take 1 to 1 1/2 hours. If you have any questions regarding the cardiac stress test or any problems with your appointment, please contact us.

FIGURE 29–25 Patient information for stress test.

After you have carefully recorded a patient's history, inform the patient of the details of the procedure. The purpose of the test is to increase physical exertion until a *target heart rate* is reached or signs of deficiency of blood supply to the heart appear. The patient must read and sign a consent form. Some offices publish information booklets for their patients (Fig. 29–25).

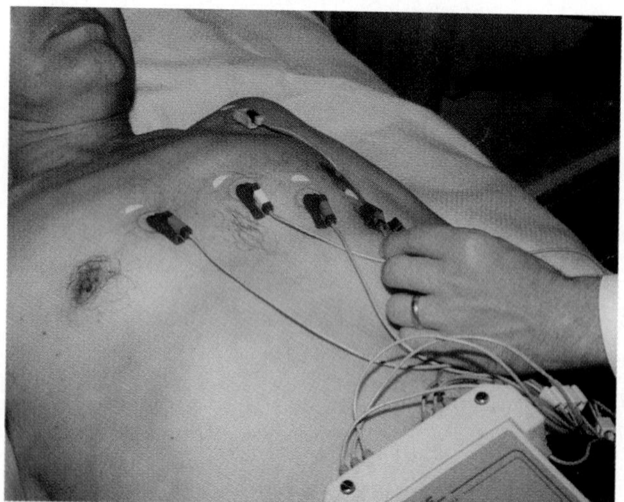

FIGURE 29–26 Stress test chest electrodes.

The chest electrodes are placed on the patient and are connected to the cable wires (Fig. 29–26). One team member demonstrates how to walk on the treadmill. The patient's blood pressure and heart rate are recorded resting before the test begins. When the physician is present, the treadmill is turned on, and a continuous ECG is run during the exercise (Fig. 29–27). The patient's blood pressure and heart rate are also monitored. Immediately after the termination of the test, the blood pressure and heart rate are again recorded with the patient lying down. A post-resting ECG is then run on the monitor for 5 minutes before the patient is discharged.

Stress testing can cause **cardiac arrest.** The medical assistant must be able to recognize symptoms of dyspnea, **vertigo,** extreme fatigue, severe arrhythmia, and other abnormal ECG readings that may develop during the stress test or during the rest period immediately after the exercise.

All members of a cardiac stress testing team must be prepared to terminate testing immediately if the patient is unable to continue or when abnormalities appear on the monitor. Therefore, cardiac stress testing team members need to be trained in cardiopul-

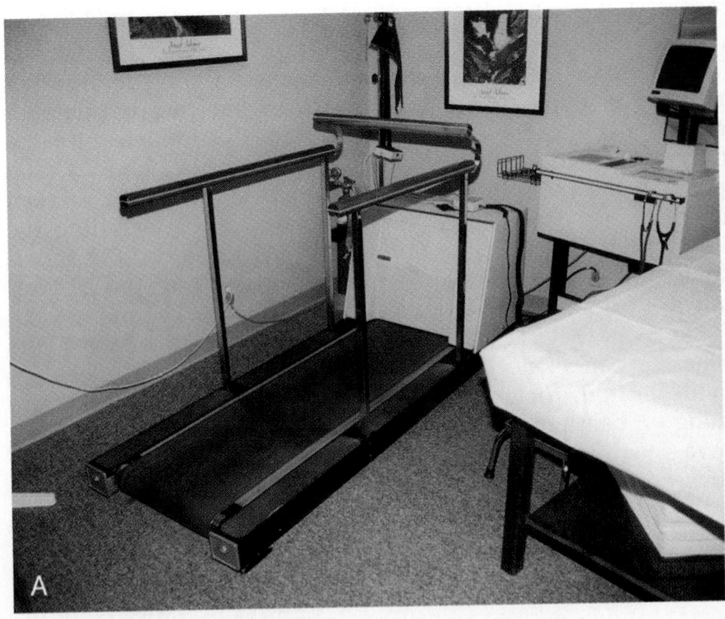

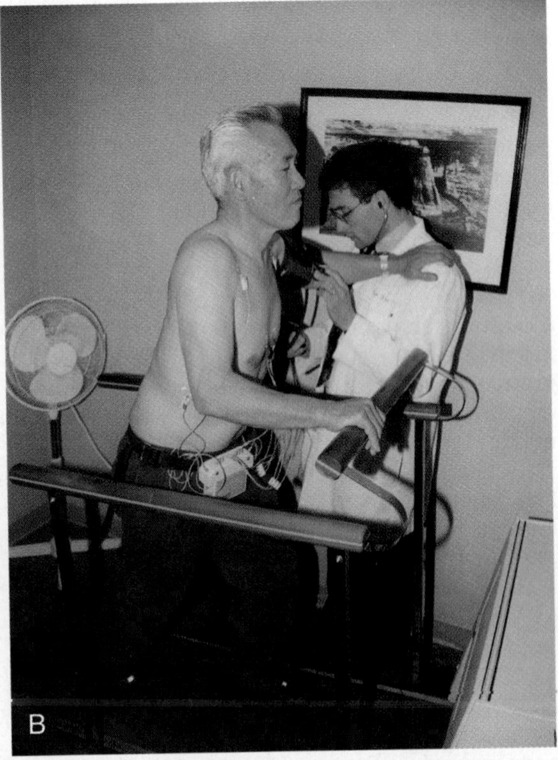

FIGURE 29–27 *A,* Treadmill prepared for test. *B,* Physician is monitoring patient's blood pressure during test. (*A,* courtesy of Dr. Sam Borno, Fresno, CA.)

monary resuscitation and emergency intervention. The physician must be present during this procedure. Besides the monitoring equipment, oxygen, a **defibrillator** (Fig. 29–28), and emergency cardiac medications are to be available in case of cardiac crisis.

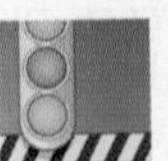

Safety Alert: The medical assistant will need additional training before performing the following tests. Be sure to check with your state scope of practice regarding requirements in your area.

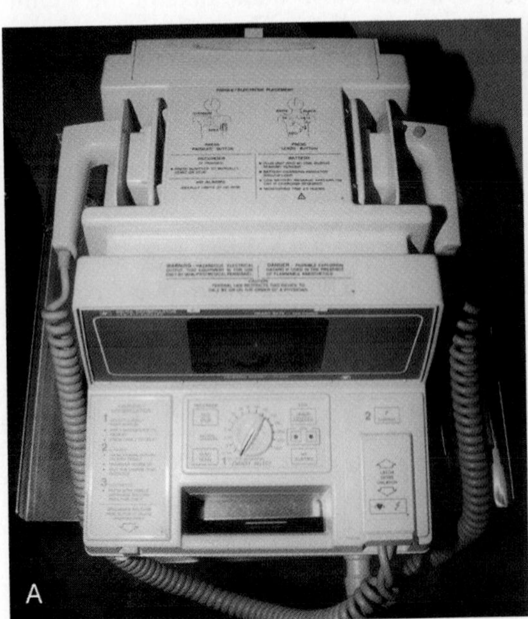

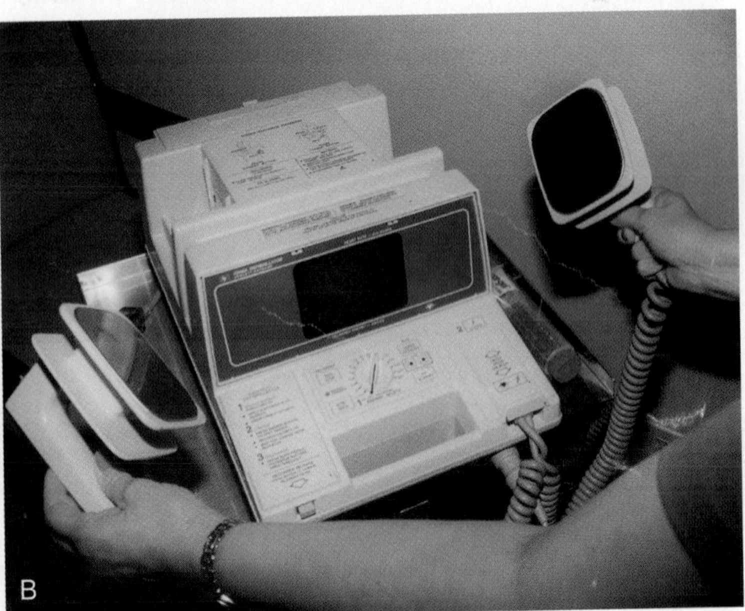

FIGURE 29–28 *A,* Cardiac defibrillator. *B,* Defibrillator paddles to be placed on the chest by the physician.

Echocardiography

Echocardiography makes use of ultrasound to measure the structure and movement of the various parts of the heart. It can be done in two or three dimensions. The patient is placed in a supine position, and the transducer is held against the chest wall. The sound waves are sent out and echoed back through the transducer into the machine, where they are converted into a picture that shows the exact size and movement of the parts of the heart that are being measured. The use of the echogram is convenient; it has the advantage of providing immediate visualization of what is happening inside the heart without the complication of an invasive heart catheterization procedure. It is particularly helpful in diagnosing valvular disease, the level of heart failure, and **cardiomyopathy.**

Holter Monitor Cardiography

A Holter monitor is a portable monitoring system for recording cardiac activity of a patient over a 24-hour period or longer (Fig. 29–29). This machine is lightweight so the patient can wear it while doing usual daily activities. The Holter monitor can be programmed to take a continuous recording for the 24-hour period or only at certain points of the time span. It can also be set to record when activated by the patient when symptoms occur or during periods of stress.

It is very important that the patient keep a written diary of all activities during the day that cause stress, such as driving in rush hour traffic, bowel movements, intercourse, stair climbing, and other symptoms associated with possible heart problems. This diary should be explained completely to the patient so that proper entries can be made during the monitoring period, along with the time of each entry. Some machines are capable of recording the patient's voice while he or she describes the activities and symptoms experienced during the 24-hour monitoring. Although the majority of the monitoring periods last 24 hours, there are instances when the patient needs to wear the monitor for a longer period, for example, when only certain symptoms are being monitored by a patient activating the machine.

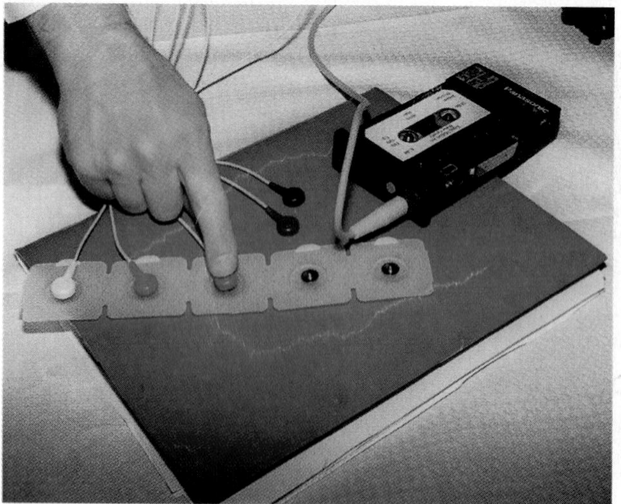

FIGURE 29–29 Holter monitor equipment. (Courtesy of Panasonic, Los Angeles, CA.)

Many cardiologists have Holter monitors in their offices. The medical assistant may be responsible for preparing the patient, applying and removing the equipment, and instructing the patient in the guidelines of the procedure. The number of electrodes and leads varies with the number of channels on the machine. The electrode positions may not be any of the standard locations, but the assistant should always check with the physician regarding placement before attaching the electrodes. Because electrodes must be firmly placed, it may be necessary to shave the sites for secure placement. The lead wires are run from the electrodes to the monitor, which is usually attached to a belt that is worn diagonally over the shoulder or around the waist. The patient is taught how to use the monitor. If the monitor is equipped with an event marker, the patient is shown how to use this in case a significant symptom is experienced. This marker alerts the technician when the tape is being interpreted. If the marker is used, the patient must also make note of the significant symptom in the diary. The patient may be allowed to take only sponge baths during the test period because the equipment must not get wet. Sometimes the cardiologist will direct the patient to remove the monitor while taking a shower. Be certain that the patient has a full understanding of the physician's orders.

At the end of the monitoring time, the patient returns to the office, and the machine is disconnected and removed. The tape and diary covering the testing period are placed into a Holter scanner or computer by a trained technician, who analyzes the results. Any portion of the tape can be printed for further study.

Memory Jogger

How does a Holter monitor test differ from a stress test?

PROCEDURE 29–2
Applying the Holter Monitor

GOAL
To establish possible correlation between coronary disorders and daily activity.

EQUIPMENT AND SUPPLIES
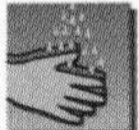

Holter monitor and blank magnetic recording tape
Disposable electrodes
Razor
Tape
Activity diary
Carrying case with belt or shoulder strap
Gauze 4 × 4-inch pads
Alcohol swabs
Nonallergenic tape

PROCEDURAL STEPS
1 Wash your hands.
PURPOSE: Infection control.

2 Assemble equipment needed.

3 Install new battery in the monitor or insert fully charged rechargeable battery (Figure 1).
PURPOSE: A new or fully charged battery ensures accurate monitor function for the 24-hour period.

4 Greet the patient and explain the procedure.
PURPOSE: An informed patient helps ensure testing accuracy.

5 Ask the patient to disrobe to the waist and sit at the end of the examination table or on an elevated stool.
PURPOSE: Places patient at a better working level and provides a degree of patient comfort.

6 If the patient has a hairy chest, dry shave the patient's chest at each of the electrode sites.
PURPOSE: Skin must be hairless to provide adherence of electrodes.

7 Using alcohol swabs, rub each shaved site and then allow these sites to air dry.
PURPOSE: To remove all surface skin oil and residue.

Continued

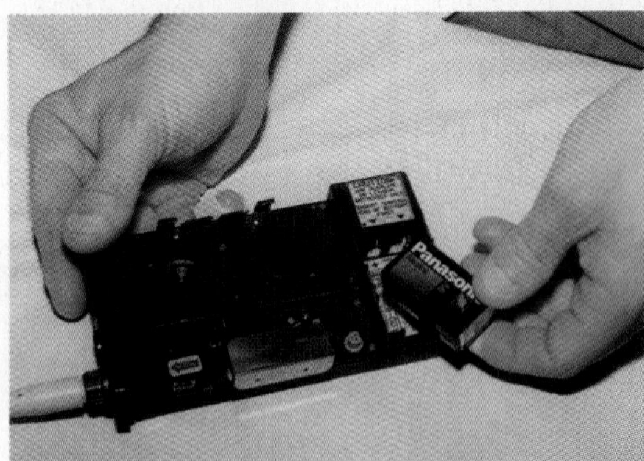

FIGURE 1

PROCEDURE 29-2 (CONTINUED)
Applying the Holter Monitor

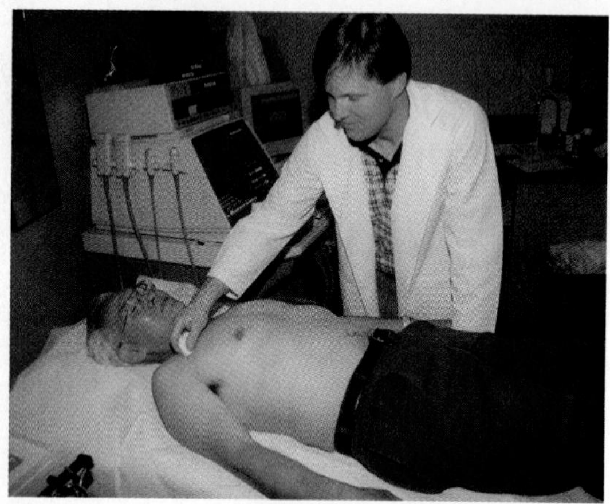
FIGURE 2

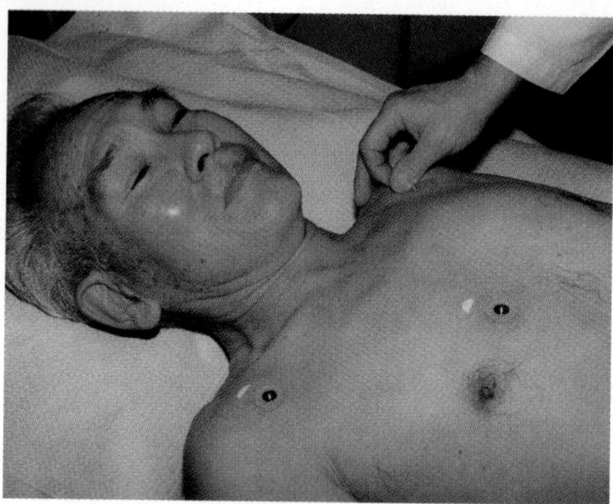
FIGURE 3

8 Fold a gauze pad over your index finger and briskly rub the sites (Figure 2).
PURPOSE: Will make removal of the electrodes less painful in 24 hours.

9 Peel backing from electrodes and apply to the appropriate skin sites by firmly pressing the center of the electrode and then move pressure outward until entire electrode is securely pressed into place. As an added measure, rub the edges of each electrode a second time to make doubly certain that the electrode will stay in place. Note that the electrodes will be damp (Figure 3).
PURPOSE: Secure attachment of the electrodes is absolutely necessary to produce an accurate tracing.

10 Attach the lead wires to the electrodes and connect the end terminal to the patient cable (Figure 4).

11 Place a strip of nonallergenic tape over each electrode.
PURPOSE: Aids in securing electrode placement if there would be any pulling of the wires during the testing period.

Continued

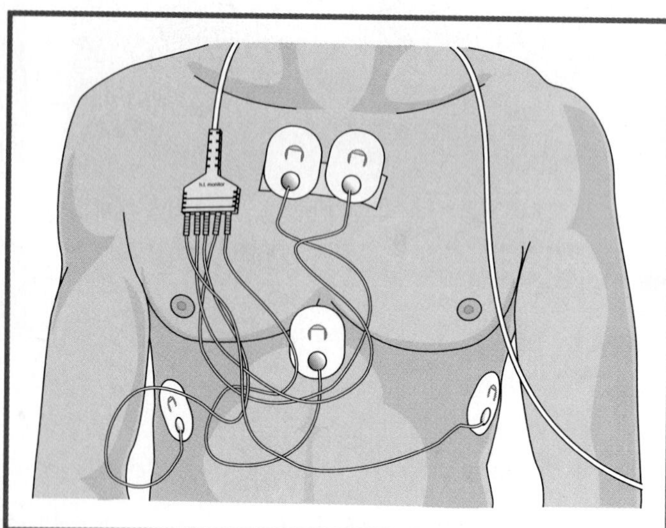
FIGURE 4

12 Attach the *test cable* to the monitor and plug it into the electrocardiograph. Run a baseline test tracing (Figure 5).
PURPOSE: Ensures proper connections of the electrodes and running of the monitor.

13 Help the patient put on a shirt or bra and blouse over the connected electrodes. Be certain that the cable extends through the buttoned front or out the bottom of the shirt or blouse.

14 Place the monitor in the carrying case (Figure 6), and attach it to the patient's belt or place it over the shoulder (Figure 7). Check to ensure that the wires are not taut or bent in half.
PURPOSE: Taut or badly crimped wires may loosen or malfunction.

15 Plug the electrode cable into the monitor.

16 Record the patient's name, date of birth, and starting time in the patient's activity diary.
PURPOSE: Establish starting time of test and cardiac activity.

17 Give the patient the activity diary and advise him or her to begin by writing in his or her present activity state.
PURPOSE: Diary must correlate patient's activity with cardiac activity.

18 Give patient appointment for returning in 24 hours.

19 Wash hands.
PURPOSE: Infection control.

20 Enter procedure information in the patient's record.
PURPOSE: A procedure is not done until it is entered into the patient's record.

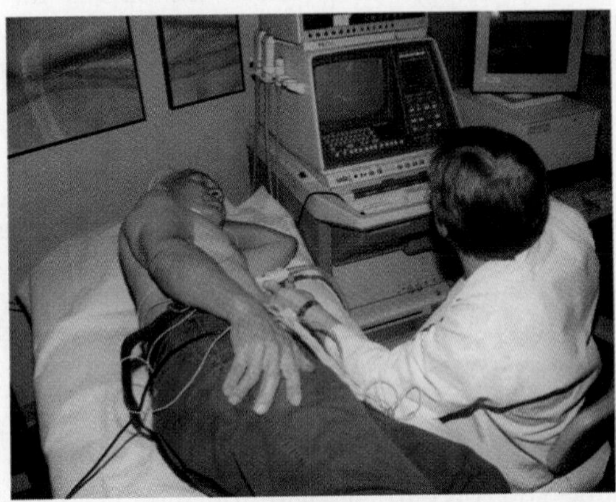

FIGURE 5

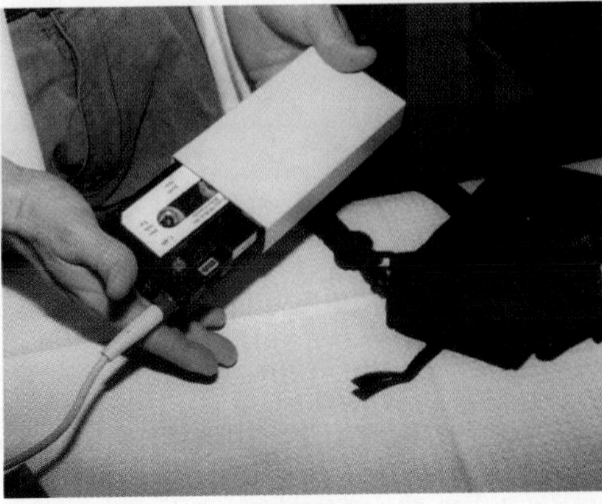

FIGURE 6

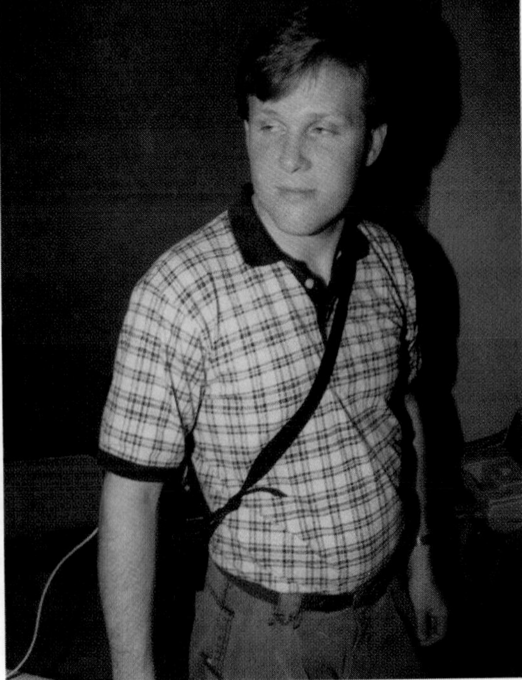

FIGURE 7

Heart Catheterization and Angioplasty

These procedures are not done in the cardiologist's office and are included for information only. These two techniques are not part of the scope of practice of the medical assistant.

Heart or cardiac catheterization is used to diagnose or evaluate a variety of heart disorders. Patients complaining of chronic shortness of breath, dizziness or syncope, chest pain, heart palpitations, and noticeable changes in heart rhythm patterns, and who also have abnormal stress test or echocardiography results, are all considered likely candidates for a heart catheterization procedure.

In this procedure, the cardiologist makes an incision into a blood vessel, in the arm or groin, and inserts a small soft catheter into the vessel. The catheter is then carefully threaded in the vessel toward the heart. Once it is in position, a contrast medium is injected. This medium allows the heart's chambers, valves, great vessels, and coronary arteries to be viewed on a fluoroscopic monitor as the procedure is done (Fig. 29–30). The cardiologist can evaluate the condition of these structures, and any deviation from normal can be noted.

During this procedure, if the physician notes deposits of atherosclerotic material in one of the coronary vessels, percutaneous transluminal coronary angioplasty may be performed. When the plaque area is found, a balloon that surrounds the upper portion of the catheter is inflated and the atherosclerotic material is pressed against the vessel walls, relieving the obstruction. Lasers may also be used, or a **stent** may be inserted and left in place within the vessel to keep the vessel open.

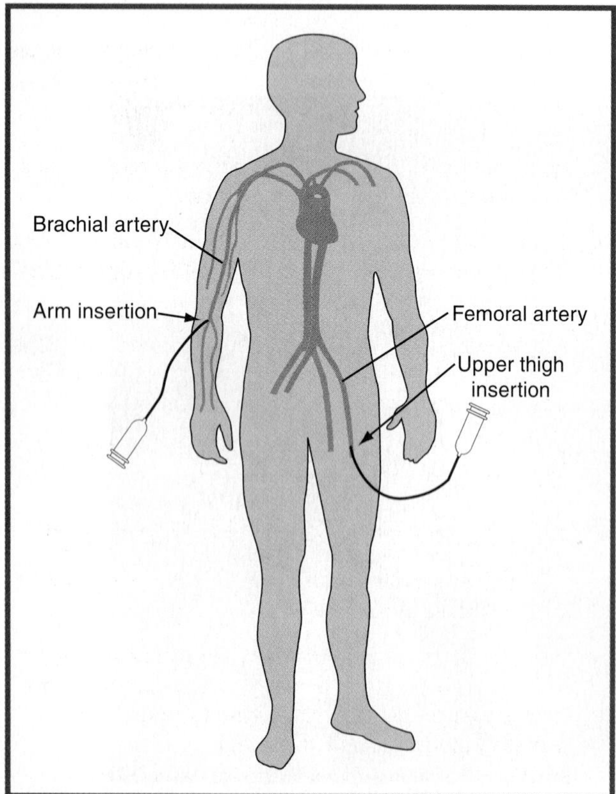

FIGURE 29–30 Cardiac catheterization.

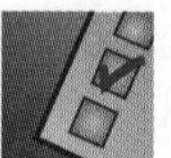

PATIENT EDUCATION

Heart disease and stroke account for more than one third of all deaths. Familial genetics, predisposition, and lifestyle habits such as smoking, lack of exercise, and diet play a significant role in the acquisition of heart disease. There is a constant need for communication skills in your relationship with the patient and with the physician. Talk to the patient about factors that could be changed or modified.

Before you can successfully counsel a patient in changing a habit, you will need to obtain background knowledge in possible techniques to use. Places to obtain information to prepare yourself include the American Heart Association, the public library, and the Internet.

Patients like visual aids in learning, and having pictures, brochures, and pamphlets to give them is a marvelous way to generate learning and questions. Make a note in the chart that you gave them certain educational items so that on a return visit you can ask if the information helped, if they tried any of the modifications, what the results were, and if they have any suggestions to help another patient with the same problem. You may be surprised to learn that patients are inclined to try something new if it has more than one purpose. If they feel that they are helping you prepare a plan for modification and you need their input, they may be willing to try.

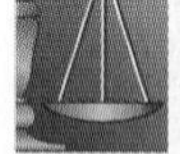

LEGAL AND ETHICAL ISSUES

Electrocardiography is a valuable diagnostic tool. It is one of the primary procedures used in the diagnosis of the patient with a possible heart problem. The cardiologist compares and measures the patient's heart activity with known values by using the ECG tracing. He or she can also note changes in the patient's heart condition by comparing previous ECGs with current tracings. For the doctor to be able to interpret the ECG tracing and establish its value in diagnosing the patient's problem, the medical assistant has the ethical obligation to complete the task as accurately and properly as possible.

Diagnostic procedure can have a marked effect on the patient's treatment. When you are entrusted with performing testing procedures, you are assuming the responsibility for accuracy and performing the testing precisely. This is a very important role, and the results you submit as accurate could strongly influence the therapeutic plan of treatment. Never assume that this test is just routine.

CRITICAL THINKING

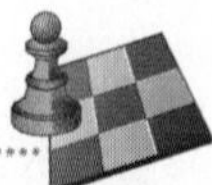

1 How would you handle a telephone call from a patient who complains of nausea, has difficulty taking a deep breath, and thinks he or she is going to faint? What questions would you ask to substantiate the seriousness of the problem?

2 What could you do to help patients with primary hypertension? Think of informational materials, possible take-home VCR tapes or audio cassette tapes, office show-and-tell programs, and group therapy sessions.

3 You are doing an ECG and the QRS complex is swinging the entire width of the recording paper. What do you have to do to ensure a readable tracing?

HOW DID I DO? Answers to Memory Joggers

1 Five liters of blood passes through your heart every minute.

2 The four layers of the heart are the pericardium, epicardium, myocardium, and endocardium.

3 The left ventricle pumps blood into the aorta that carries blood through the system.

4 The heart's conduction begins in the sinoatrial node located in the sinus of the right atrium. The conduction then travels to the atrioventricular node, down the bundle of His, and then to the Purkinje fibers.

5 Myocardial infarction is the medical term for a heart attack.

6 An ischemic myocardium can be corrected by coronary bypass surgery.

7 Yes, because constant blood pressure readings are above 140/90 mm Hg.

8 False. All arteries except the pulmonary artery carry oxygenated blood from the heart and all veins except the pulmonary vein carry deoxygenated blood to the heart.

9 Emboli are moving clots of foreign material. If a clot is blood and nested in a vessel and may be causing occlusion, it is called a thrombus.

10 Atherosclerosis is artery hardening caused by a buildup of plaques of cholesterol or lipids along the inside vessel wall. Arteriosclerosis is a thickening and hardening of the arterial walls that causes loss of elasticity and contractibility.

11 An aneurysm is a ballooning or dilation of the wall of a vessel caused by a weakening of the vessel wall.

12 During the ECG tracing the following occurs:
P wave = contraction of the atria
Q wave = excitement of the ventricles
R wave = beginning of the ventricle contraction
S wave = completion of the ventricle contraction
T wave = resting and repolarization of the myocardium

13 In a standard ECG tracing, there are 12 different tracings: L1, L2, L3, aVR, aVL, aVF, V_1, V_2, V_3, V_4, V_5, and V_6.

14 Three sensitivity deflections are on an ECG machine:
1/2 STD = 5-mm deflection
1 STD = 10-mm deflection
2 STD = 20-mm deflection

15 There are four types of artifacts:
a. Wandering baseline is a gradual shifting of the stylus away from the baseline.
b. Somatic tremor results in jagged peaks of irregular height and spacing.
c. Alternating current appears as a series of uniform, small spiked lines.
d. Baseline interruption appears as a straight line or violent movements up and down.

16 An orthopneic patient has breathing difficulty in any position except standing or sitting upright.

17 Information that is written on the ECG tracing includes the patient's name, sex, age, date and time of ECG, medications, and any variation from normal STD and variation of speed.

18 If there are four 5-mm boxes between R waves, the heart rate is 75 beats per minute.

19 An ECG interpretive center analyzes the recording immediately and gives immediate information on the heart's activity. Diagnosis and treatment can be instituted much sooner.

20 The Holter monitor test traces heart activity during a 24-hour period of normal physical activity. The stress test measures heart activity under controlled induced physical activity.

Assisting in Pulmonary Medicine

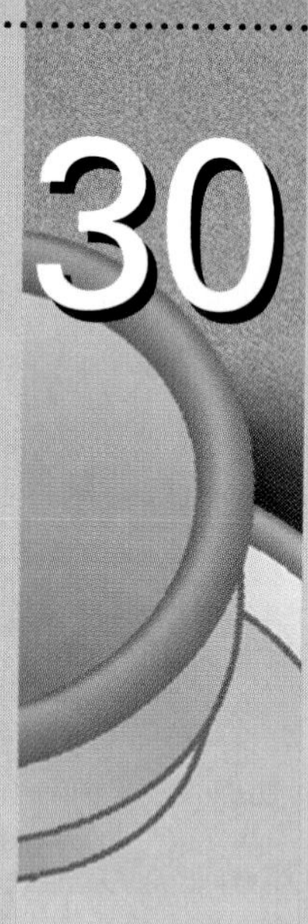

OUTLINE

LEARNING OBJECTIVES

Cognitive: On successful completion of this chapter you should be able to:

1 Name and locate the structures of the respiratory system.
2 Describe the functioning purpose of each respiratory structure.
3 Demonstrate understanding of ventilation.
4 Identify the major categories of respiratory diseases.
5 Differentiate the signs and symptoms and the diagnosis and treatment for the diseases discussed in this chapter.
6 Be able to assist the pulmonary care physician in the examination of the chest and lungs.
7 Spell and define the terms in the vocabulary.

Performance: On successful completion of this chapter you should be able to:

1 Accurately administer a Mantoux tuberculin skin test.
2 Prepare a patient for pulmonary function testing.
3 Obtain an accurate volume capacity spirometric test.
4 Prepare a patient for throat culture.
5 Collect a specimen by swab for throat culture.
6 Demonstrate the standard safety precautions used when handling a sputum sample.
7 Prepare the patient and obtain a sputum sample for culture.

VOCABULARY

anoxia Severe hypoxia; absence of oxygen in inspired gases or in arterial blood

atelectasis Collapsed or airless state of the lung

bifurcates Divides into two branches

bronchiectasis Dilation of the bronchi and bronchioles associated with secondary infection or ciliary dysfunction

catheter Thin flexible tube inserted into the body to permit introduction or withdrawal of fluid

chronic bronchitis Recurrent inflammation of the membranes lining the bronchial tubes

cilia Hairlike projections from the surface of a cell; provide locomotion in free unicellular organisms

cyanosis Bluish discoloration of the skin, extremities, and mucous membranes caused by a decreased level of oxygen transported to cells

cytology Biologic science devoted to the study of cell morphology

emphysema Pathologic accumulation of air in the tissues or organs; in the lungs, the bronchioles become plugged with mucus and lose elasticity

eosinophil Granular leukocyte that increases in number in allergic conditions

eradicated Wiped out or cancelled

exudate Fluid with a high concentration of protein and cellular debris that has escaped from blood vessels and has been deposited in tissues or on tissue surfaces

glomerulonephritis Disease that interferes with the basic functions of the kidneys

homeostasis Ability of the body systems to maintain relatively constant conditions in the internal environment

malaise Feeling of uneasiness or indisposition

metabolic Referring to the processes concerned with the disposition of nutrients absorbed into the blood after digestion

nebulization Treatment by a spray

neoplasm Abnormal new mass of tissue that serves no purpose; often cancerous

phlegm Expectorated matter; saliva mixed with discharges from the respiratory tract

pulmonary consolidation Process of the lungs becoming solidified as they fill with exudates in pneumonia

purulent Consisting of or containing pus

rales Abnormal or crackling chest sounds that occur during the inspiration portion of ventilation

rheumatic endocarditis Disease associated with hemolytic streptococci in the inside lining of the heart, valves, and great vessels

rheumatic fever Delayed sequela of an upper respiratory tract infection caused by the group A hemolytic *Streptococcus.*

rhonchi Rattling noises in the throat that may resemble snoring

saliva Liquid substance secreted into the mouth by the salivary gland; moistens the mouth and starts the digestion of starches

tachypnea Respirations that are regular in rhythm but faster than normal in rate

tenacious Stubbornly unyielding; sticking together

virulent Exceedingly pathogenic, noxious, or deadly

Have you ever stopped to think about how often you breathe? We all know that we cannot live without breathing, but it is a life-sustaining phenomenon that we seldom think about as long as everything is working according to plan. Respiration, or ventilation, is the exchange of oxygen and carbon dioxide between the atmosphere and the lungs.

PRECONDITIONS FOR NORMAL RESPIRATION

- An open airway leading to the lungs
- Ability of the lungs to expand rhythmically

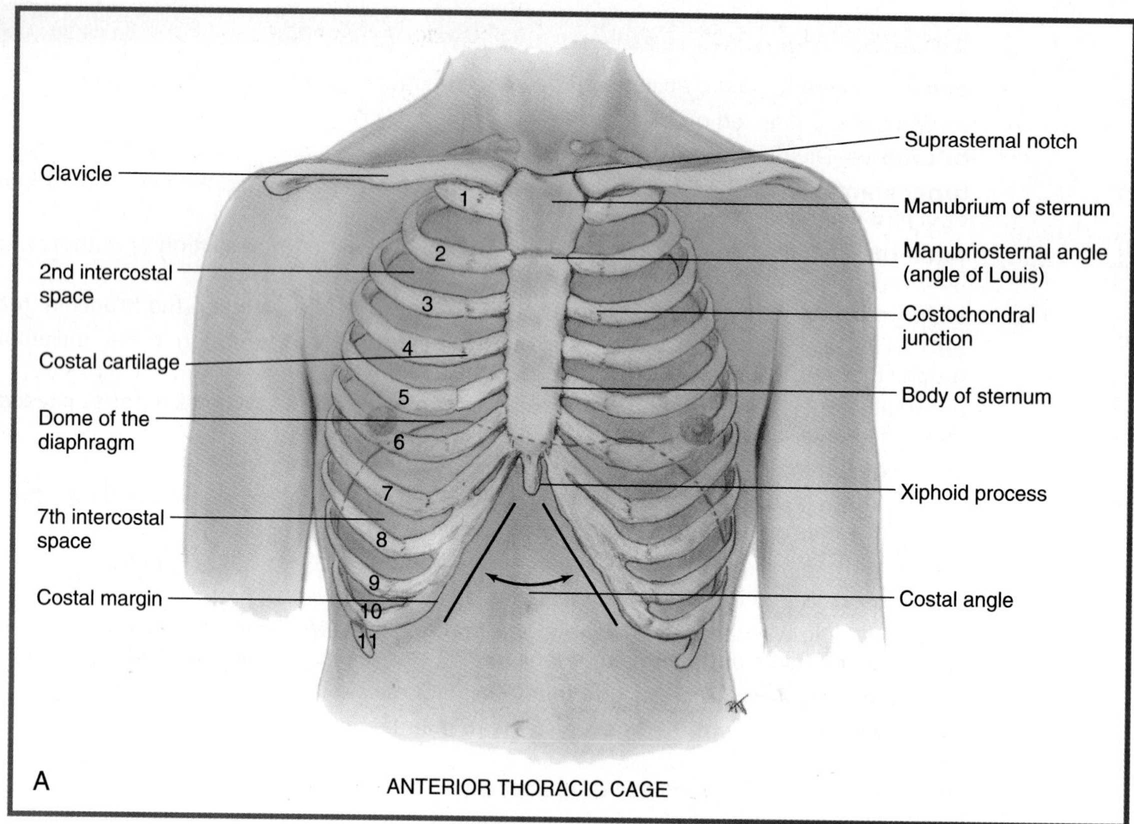

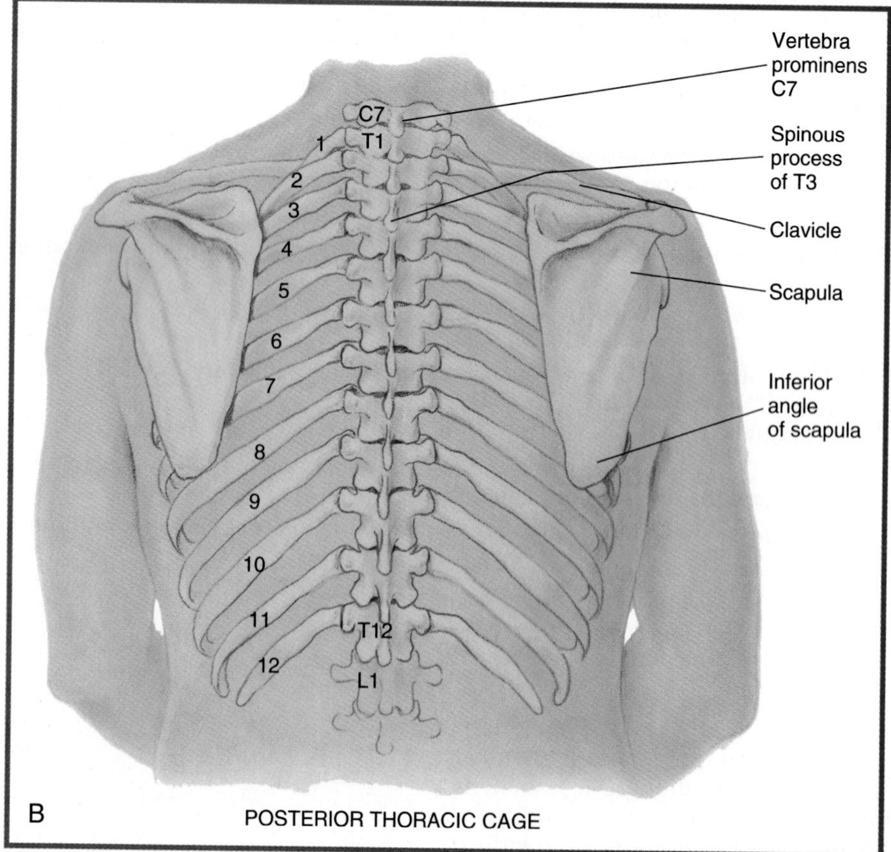

FIGURE 30–1 *A,* Anterior thoracic cage. *B,* Posterior thoracic cage. (From Jarvis C: Physical Examination and Health Assessment, 2nd ed. Philadelphia, WB Saunders, 1996.)

- Alveolar membranes must be intact
- Coordination of the intercostal muscles and the diaphragm
- Proper action of the central nervous system's control center

The major metabolic function of the lungs is maintaining the acid-base balance within the body. Failure of this function may result in respiratory acidosis or alkalosis. The respiratory system and the circulatory system work together to supply the body cells with oxygen and to remove the **metabolic** wastes. Failure in the ability of these systems to work together can lead to changes in the kidney or gastrointestinal tract such as lactic acidosis secondary to diabetes mellitus.

Respiratory System

The thoracic cage, sometimes referred to as the rib cage, is a bony structure that is narrower at the top and wider at the base. It is held in place by the thoracic vertebrae of the spine in the center of the back and the sternum in the center of the frontal aspect of the body. The first seven ribs attach directly to the sternum and are referred to as the true ribs; ribs 8, 9, and 10, fasten one to another, forming the false ribs; and ribs 11 and 12 are the "floating" ribs or half ribs because their only attachment is to the thoracic vertebrae. At the base or floor of the rib cage is the diaphragm, a musculotendinous membrane that divides the thoracic cavity and the abdominal cavity (Fig. 30–1).

These surface thoracic landmarks are guideposts for the underlying respiratory structures. Knowledge of these landmarks will help you in communicating a possible finding to the physician.

Memory Jogger

Identify the surface landmarks and use your fingers to palpate the location on your thoracic cage.

In the center section of the thoracic cavity is the mediastinum. In this region is the esophagus, trachea, heart, and great vessels, as discussed in Chapter 29. On either side of the mediastinum are the right and left pleural sacs containing the lungs. Disorders of the respiratory system are usually divided into two major groups: upper respiratory and lower respiratory.

UPPER RESPIRATORY TRACT

The upper respiratory tract includes the nose, pharynx, or throat, and larynx (Fig. 30–2). As air enters

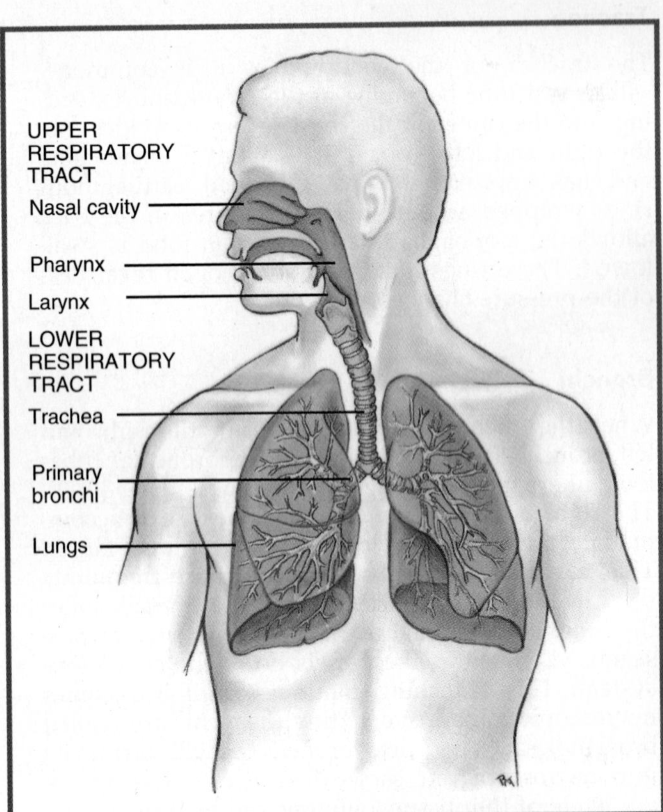

FIGURE 30–2 Upper and lower respiratory tract. (From Applegate EJ: The Anatomy and Physiology Learning System. Philadelphia, WB Saunders, 1995.)

the nasal cavity, it is cleaned by the **cilia,** warmed by the capillary blood vessels, and moistened by the mucous membranes. The air is moved through the pharynx past the tonsils, which function in immunity and help defend the body from potential pathogens. As the air continues toward the lungs, it passes through the larynx, which is the voice box. Once the air leaves the larynx, it enters the lower respiratory tract.

LOWER RESPIRATORY TRACT

The lower respiratory tract consists of the trachea, bronchial tubes, and the lungs (see Fig. 30–2). These structures are also lined with mucous tissue that is covered with cilia. The collection of dust and foreign particles on the cilia should initiate the coughing reflex, aiding us in expectorating mucus that may contain possible pathogens. Without these defense mechanisms, these pathogens would remain in our lungs, which could cause disease. Cigarette smoke and other air pollutants can slow down or paralyze the cleansing action of the cilia in the trachea.

Memory Jogger

Name the structures located in the upper respiratory tract and in the lower respiratory tract.

Trachea

The trachea, or the windpipe as it is commonly called, is a tube beginning at the larynx and extending into the center of the chest where it divides into the right and left bronchi. It is about 5 inches long and has approximately 18 C-shaped cartilaginous rings wrapped around it. The open area in the back allows the esophagus to enlarge when food is swallowed. These rings hold the trachea open regardless of the pressure changes exerted.

Bronchi

When the trachea **bifurcates,** it forms the right and left bronchi. It is often said that the bronchial tubes look like a tree hanging in your chest (Fig. 30–3). The right bronchus is wider than the left to accommodate the right lung lobes, which are also larger. This means foreign substances are more frequently seen in the right bronchus. Once the bronchi enter the lungs, they branch into smaller and smaller passageways, much as the vessels do in the circulatory system. This branching continues until it becomes microscopic. These very tiny bronchi are called bronchioles. Every tiny bronchiole will terminate into microscopic air sacs called *alveoli.* The alveoli are made of thin tissue, only one cell wall thick, that allows the exchange of oxygen and carbon dioxide through the cell wall.

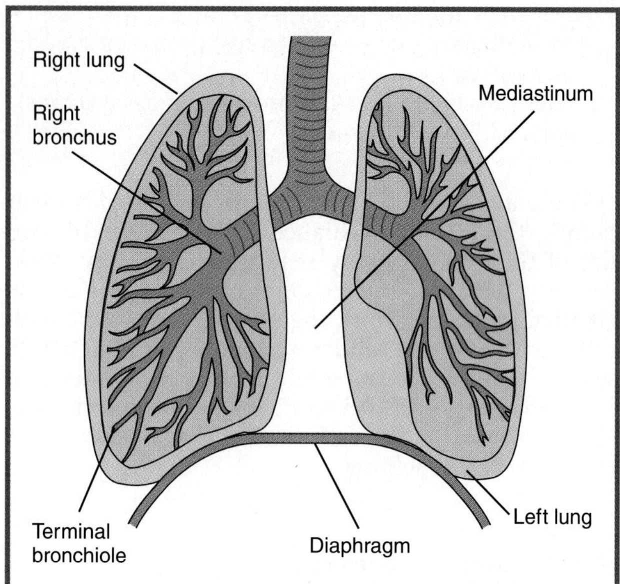

FIGURE 30–3 Bronchial tree.

Lungs

The bronchial tree and the alveoli are the major structures housed within the right and left lungs. Lungs are soft and spongy masses, owing to the air sacs that compose a great percent of their mass. They hang in the right and left sides of the chest, separated by the pericardial sac containing the heart.

The right lung is divided into three lobes and has a greater volume capacity than the left lung. Each

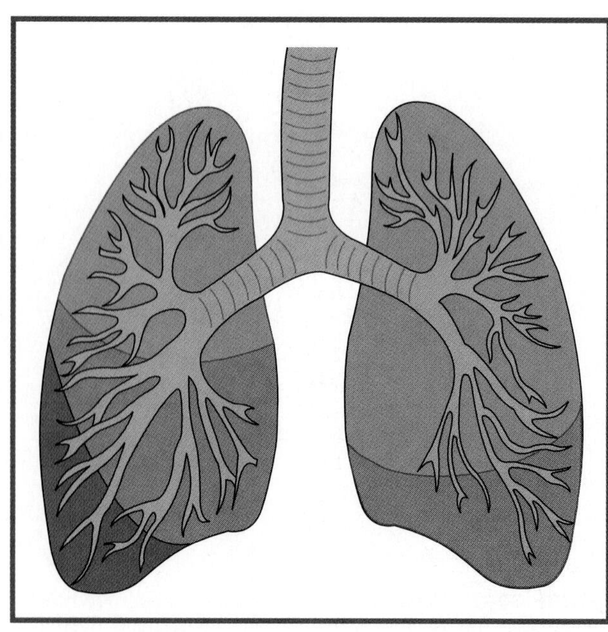

FIGURE 30–4 Lobes of the lungs.

lobe has its own bronchus and blood supply and is really an independently functioning organ. This independent structure makes it possible for a person to have one lobe removed, and the rest of the lung sustains little, if any, damage.

The left lung is longer and narrower and has a distinct indentation in the center of it known as the *cardiac notch.* This is the location for the left ventricle of the heart. It is also the spot where you would obtain an apical pulse. The left lung has only two lobes, an upper and lower (Fig. 30–4).

As you remember, the heart is encased in a sac called the pericardium, and each lung is encased in a sac called the pleural sac. These double-layered membranes aid the lung in its function and protect the very fragile lung tissue from harm and abuse.

Ventilation

In the very delicate lung tissue, the bronchioles deposit the oxygenated air into the grapelike structures called the alveoli. Surrounding each alveolus is a network of pulmonary capillaries filled with waste air. The oxygenated air moves through the single-celled walls of the alveoli and through the single-celled walls of these capillaries (Fig. 30–5). As this is happening, the waste air is forced out of the capillaries back into the alveoli and then into the bronchioles. Air exchange has taken place, and the capillaries carry the oxygenated air back to the heart and the waste gases are being exhaled. This exchange is referred to as *ventilation.* The movement of oxygen from the atmosphere into the alveoli is called *inspiration,* and the movement of the waste gases from the alveoli back into the atmosphere is called *expiration.*

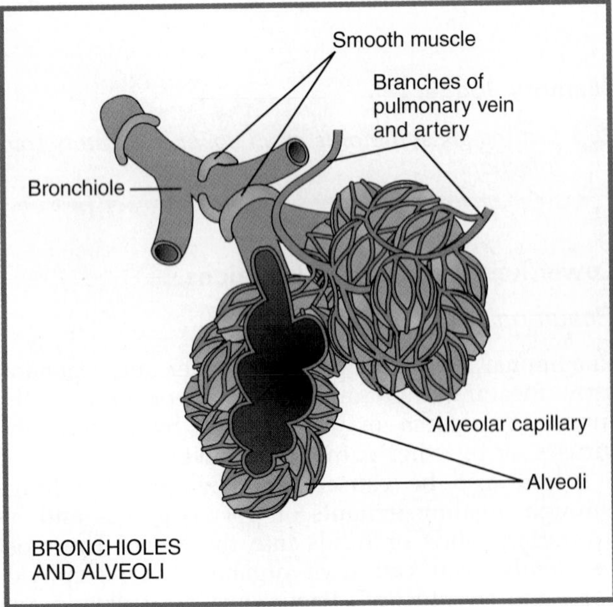

FIGURE 30–5 Alveoli with capillary network.

INSPIRATION

Inspiration begins with a signal from the medulla oblongata in the brain stem. This signal is carried by the phrenic nerve to the major muscle of inspiration, the diaphragm. When the diaphragm receives the signal, it flattens out and pulls downward. At the same moment, the intercostal muscles located between the ribs contract, causing the ribs to move outward and the chest cavity to enlarge. This movement causes the lungs to expand and increase their volume. The more these muscles are contracted, the deeper the inhalation is and the greater the air volume becomes. When an individual is unable to move enough air using the diaphragm and intercostal muscles to meet the body's needs, the individual will be diagnosed with a respiratory disease.

EXPIRATION

The second half of ventilation is expiration. Once inspiration is completed the diaphragm and intercostal muscles relax, causing the chest to move inward and the lungs to decrease in volume. This movement forces the waste air out of the lungs and back into the atmosphere. This phase of ventilation needs very little energy and takes place with minimal effort by the body. In asthma and/or emphysema, the individual has difficulty in getting the air out of the lungs, and accessory muscles in the chest will need to assist the intercostal and diaphragm muscles to accomplish exhalation.

Respiratory System Defenses

Every part of the respiratory system has a defense mechanism. In the upper respiratory tract, the mucus-covered ciliated surface of the mucous membrane traps particles; through the continuous flow of the mucus back toward the nasopharynx, the particles are swallowed.

The lower respiratory tract is sterile, which is a phenomenal feat considering that each day these airways are exposed to approximately 10,000 L of air containing an endless number of bacteria and foreign material. It is the ever-changing air flow, inspiration to expiration, that creates a turbulence that makes it very difficult for these invading substances to remain in the bronchi. This, combined with coughing, sneezing, and our functioning immune system, protects the respiratory tract and helps the body maintain **homeostasis.** Disease occurs when something happens to upset the normal homeostatic chain of events.

Major Diseases of the Respiratory System

Many diseases affect this system; however, the major diseases can be divided into four categories:

- Infectious diseases
- Immune diseases
- Environmental diseases
- Tumors

INFECTIOUS DISEASES

Respiratory tract infections are in two groups. Diseases of the nose and upper respiratory tracts (URIs) are more common, and diseases of the lower respiratory tract (e.g., pneumonia) are less common. Respiratory tract infections account for approximately 75% of all human infections diagnosed clinically. Only about 5% of these infections involve the lungs. Most lung infections are seen in hospitalized patients, the elderly, drug addicts, alcoholics, and patients with the acquired immunodeficiency syndrome (AIDS). Even if we eliminate patients with AIDS, most of whom die of lung infection, pneumonia is listed as the cause of death of approximately 30,000 people every year in the United States.

Memory Jogger

Name the groups of society in which most lung infections are seen.

Upper Respiratory Tract Infections

An upper respiratory tract infection, also known as the common cold, is an acute inflammatory process affecting the mucous membranes that line the nose, pharynx, larynx, and bronchus. Usually the term *cold* is used when only the membrane of the nose and pharynx are affected; however, the same virus can affect the larynx and the lungs. The common cold is a group of minor illnesses that can be caused by approximately 200 different viruses. The viral invasion can be followed by bacterial infections of the pharynx and middle ear.

SIGNS AND SYMPTOMS Nasal congestion and discharge (rhinorrhea), sneezing, watery eyes, sore throat (pharyngitis), hoarseness (laryngitis), and coughing are the frequently seen signs of an upper respiratory tract infection. The symptoms can vary depending on the invading virus. The nasal discharge is usually clear and watery in the early stage but can become greenish yellow and **tenacious** as the virus becomes more virulent or when bacteria invade. The patient usually complains of headache, feeling slightly feverish, having chills, and having no appetite.

DIAGNOSIS AND TREATMENT The physician usually makes the diagnosis from the symptoms present. If there is a possibility of a more serious problem, a culture of the nasal discharge and sputum and a complete blood cell count will be ordered. If these tests confirm a bacterial infection in the respiratory tract, a more active treatment will be prescribed.

CHIEF COMPLAINTS INDICATING RESPIRATORY TRACT DISORDERS

- Chest pain or feeling of heaviness in the chest
- Difficulty in breathing, increasing in supine position
- Cough, either productive or nonproductive
- Sore throat or hoarseness
- Chills and sweats
- Fever
- Generalized malaise

Colds usually clear in 3 to 5 days, but the nasal discharge may continue for a much longer period of time. There is no cure for the common cold, and the best way to treat it is by getting plenty of rest and drinking fluids. Taking an over-the-counter cold remedy, cough syrups, and acetaminophen may lessen the discomfort. Echinacea, an herbal remedy, has been found to enhance immunologic activity and may be taken to improve the immune system or complement other cold medications. Antibiotics are of little value in a viral disorder and are only prescribed if the physician wants to protect the bronchi from possible bacterial invasion or a secondary bacterial infection.

Memory Jogger

List the six symptoms of an upper respiratory tract infection.

Lower Respiratory Tract Infections

Pneumonia

Pneumonia is both a specific disorder and a general term meaning inflammation of all or part of the lungs. Pneumonia may be caused by bacteria, by viruses, or by other pathogens (Table 30–1).

It can also be caused by damaging the lungs through inhaling irritants or poisonous gas and by aspirating solids or fluids into the lungs. The most frequently seen causative organisms are staphylococci and streptococci. Pneumonia can occur in any

TABLE 30–1 Pathogens Causing Pneumonia

Pathogen	Type of Infection
Bacteria	*Streptococcus pneumoniae* *Haemophilus influenzae* *Staphylococcus aureus* Mycobacteria
Virus	Influenza virus
Fungi	*Aspergillus fumigatus* *Candida albicans* *Mycoplasma pneumoniae*
Parasite	*Pneumocystis carinii* (opportunistic infection, seen in immunosuppressed, debilitated, or terminally ill patients)

age group but most often affects preschool age children and the elderly (older than 65). Other risk factors include smoking, alcoholism, and immunosuppression caused by diseases or treatment. Pneumonia is a common component of AIDS. Pneumonia can range from a mild complication to an upper respiratory tract infection to a life-threatening illness and is the fifth leading cause of death in the United States.

SIGNS AND SYMPTOMS The patient usually comes to the office with symptoms of high fever, chills, and total **malaise.** Signs of the illness include the appearance of great distress, shortness of breath (dyspnea), increased rate of respiration (tachypnea), chest pain during inspiration, and a relentless cough with expectoration of blood-tinged, "rusty," sputum.

Memory Jogger

What is the fifth leading cause of death in the United States?

DIAGNOSIS AND TREATMENT The physician will use the signs and symptoms and the patient's history to begin a preliminary diagnosis. Auscultation of the chest with a stethoscope usually reveals **rales, rhonchi,** and other signs of **pulmonary consolidation.** The preliminary diagnosis must be confirmed by additional studies such as a chest radiograph to assess the pulmonary consolidation; bacteriologic studies of the sputum to identify the invading organism; and white blood cell count including a differential count to determine whether the pneumonia is viral or bacterial. If the pneumonia is viral, there will be no increase in the number of white cells; but if it is bacterial, the greater the invasion, the higher the white cell count will be and the differential count will indicate an elevation in the neutrophil and monocyte levels.

The treatment is based on destroying the invading organism. If the organism is bacterial, the treatment of choice is with antibiotic therapy and lung function therapy until the patient has recovered.

Memory Jogger

Name three tests that might be ordered to confirm diagnosis of pneumonia.

Tuberculosis

For more than 50 years, the incidence of tuberculosis steadily declined, but since the late 1980s it has shown a serious increase in the United States. This increase is believed to be due to the number of illegal immigrants who originated in countries where tuberculosis was prevalent, to AIDS patients with little resistance to disease, and to the overwhelming appearance of drug-resistant bacteria.

Mycobacterium tuberculosis is the bacterium that causes tuberculosis. This organism is covered with a waxy substance that makes it possible for it to survive outside a living host for a long period of time. Infected droplets of sputum that are expectorated into the environment dry up, but the organisms remain as dust particles. This "infective" dust can be inhaled by a healthy host; in the presence of the warm, moist respiratory tract, these organisms again become active. This person can cough or sneeze in the presence of others, and the airborne infected droplets are inhaled by the individuals present, infecting them and now making them all hosts of the disease. Although tuberculosis is primarily a lung disease, it can spread to the bones, brain, and kidneys (Fig. 30–6). Tuberculosis seems to be spreading most quickly in large cities, in the elderly, nonwhites, alcoholics, and among AIDS patients. All tuberculin-negative health care workers should undergo a skin test annually. In tuberculin-positive cases, a chest radiograph should be obtained annually.

Memory Jogger

In what groups of people is tuberculosis spreading most quickly?

SIGNS AND SYMPTOMS Symptoms of the primary infection include an intermittent fever peaking in the afternoon, night sweats, weight loss, and general malaise. As the infection becomes **virulent** within the host, there will be a productive cough with thick, dark, frequently blood-tinged mucus being expectorated.

DIAGNOSIS AND TREATMENT The primary diagnosis of tuberculosis is established through the signs and symptoms accompanied by the auscultation of the chest for evaluation of the lungs. The infection is confirmed by culturing expectorated **exudate** or **phlegm** and by a radiologic workup of the chest. Once the diagnosis is confirmed, the patient will be

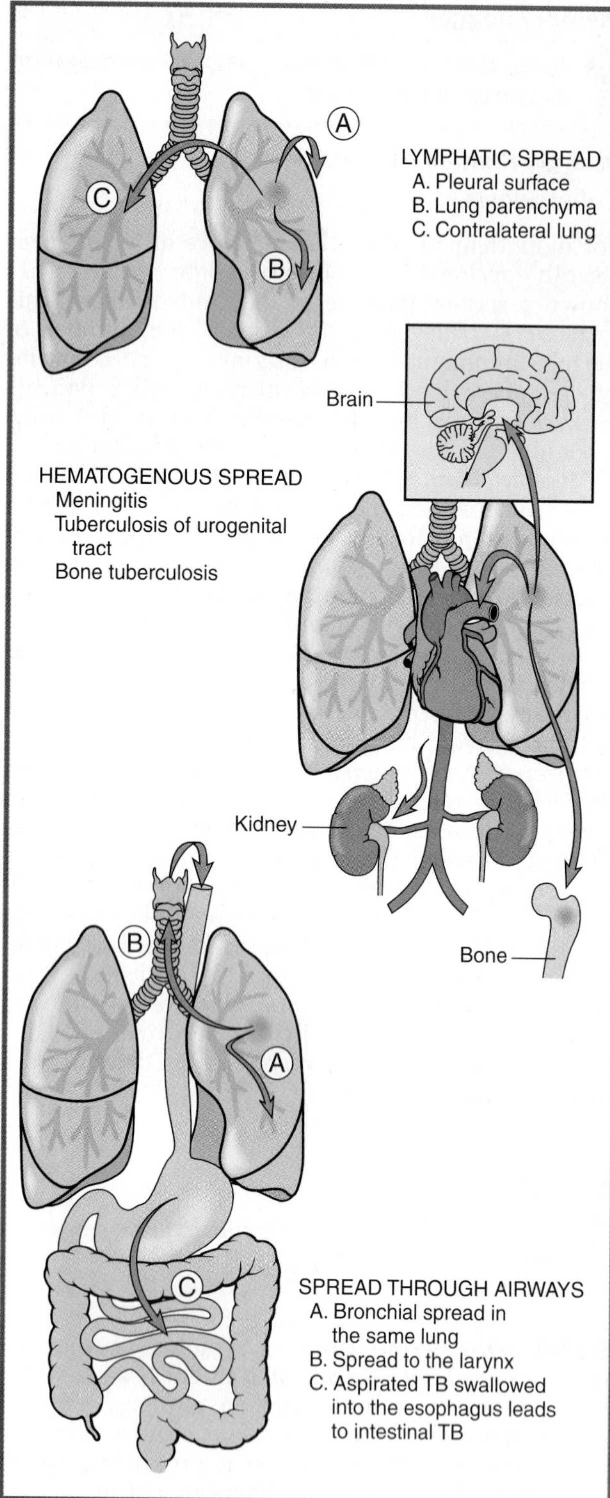

FIGURE 30–6 Spread of tuberculosis. (From Damjanov I: Pathology for the Health-Related Professions. Philadelphia, WB Saunders, 1996.)

given isoniazid, 300 mg, an antituberculous medication, taken daily for 6 months, after which the testing is repeated. Occasionally, these medications are unable to control the progression of the disease and the diseased portion of the lung must be removed surgically.

Memory Jogger

What are the common symptoms of tuberculosis?

Chronic Obstructive Pulmonary Disease

Chronic obstructive pulmonary disease (COPD) is a group of diseases with the common characteristic of chronic airway obstruction. Among the diseases included in this group are **chronic bronchitis, bronchiectasis,** and **emphysema.** Although the mechanism of the obstruction may vary, the patient with COPD is unable to ventilate the lungs freely, resulting in an ineffective exchange of respiratory gases. This will cause the patient increased difficulty in eliminating the carbon dioxide from the lungs during expiration.

SIGNS AND SYMPTOMS The symptoms of COPD vary depending on the amount of tissue infected with the disease. Patients with bronchitis exhibit prolonged bouts of coughing, expectoration of thick, **purulent** mucus, and difficulty in breathing. Patients with emphysema have no bronchial obstructions and thus will not have the cough. Instead they exhibit **tachypnea, anoxia, cyanosis,** and an overexpanded chest (barrel chest), and they often hunch forward and hyperventilate to oxygenate the blood (Fig. 30–7).

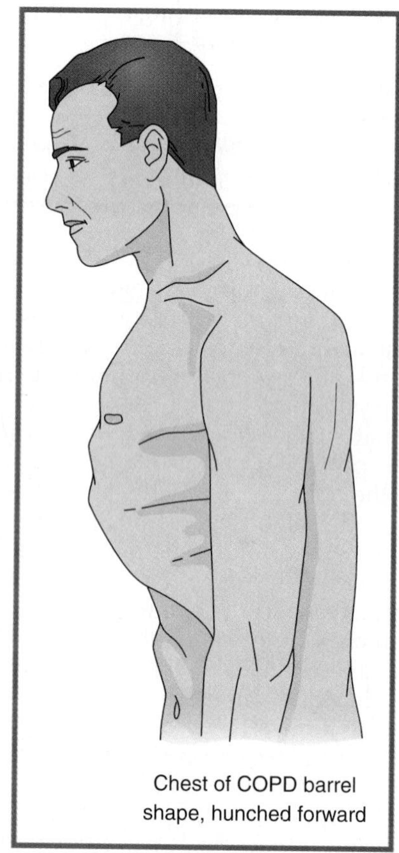

FIGURE 30–7 Barrel chest in a patient with chronic obstructive pulmonary disease.

DIAGNOSIS AND TREATMENT Diagnosis is made on the signs and symptoms and confirmed with chest radiographs that will show the abnormal markings in the chest, heart, and lungs of COPD. The physician will then begin a symptomatic treatment regimen based on supportive measures. Even if the patient now quits smoking, the symptoms will still persist but it is hoped will not worsen.

Memory Jogger

 *Recall three forms of COPD.*

IMMUNE DISEASES

Many immune diseases affect the respiratory tract. A significant group of immune diseases are associated with the environment and employment. The two immune problems that are most frequently seen in the physician's office are asthma and allergic rhinitis (hay fever).

Asthma

Asthma is a chronic disease characterized by increased activity or sensitivity of the bronchial tubes, resulting in spasm. The spasm can be related to external factors, such as environmental irritants, poor air quality, and other allergies, or to internal factors, such as stress, exercise, infection, and allergen inhalation. Asthma also has a strong hereditary factor.

SIGNS AND SYMPTOMS Asthma attacks can be mild to severe and can last minutes to days. They can be severe enough to constitute a medical emergency. The asthmatic patient has a nonproductive cough accompanied by a wheezing expiration. The breathing is rapid and shallow. Because of this difficult breathing, the pulse becomes rapid and there is generalized pallor with profuse perspiration. When you speak to the patient, the reply will be only a few words and then the patient may need to stop to regulate his or her air intake.

DIAGNOSIS AND TREATMENT When the chest is auscultated, the physician hears diminished breath sounds with wheezes and rhonchi in the lungs. The spasm in the bronchi has trapped air and thick mucus in the lungs. The best way to evaluate the lungs' ability to function is with a pulmonary function test during the attack. This test may be normal between attacks so timing is very important. Chest radiographs may also show changes in the lungs owing to the mucous obstructions. Blood tests include a complete blood cell count with a differential count to reveal the elevation of the **eosinophil** count and elevated serum immunoglobulin.

The treatment consists of a regimen of medications to expand the bronchi and aid in the expectoration of the mucus. Immunotherapy through allergy evaluation and allergy shots is often beneficial. If the attack is severe, it may require injections of epinephrine, corticosteroids, and inhalation therapy. This treatment is only given under direct supervision of the physician.

Allergic Rhinitis (Hay Fever)

Allergic rhinitis affects millions of people every year. It is caused by a reaction of the nasal mucosa to an environmental allergen. The most frequent allergen is plant pollen, and this is where the term *hay fever* originated. The sneezing can be controlled with antihistamines and nasal sprays. The list of possible allergens is extensive. When this condition is seen in the respiratory practice, the patient will be referred to the allergist for testing and a desensitizing treatment regimen.

Memory Jogger

 *Name two immune diseases that may be helped through allergy injections.*

ENVIRONMENTAL DISEASES

Environmental causes of respiratory diseases are the result of inhalation of dusts, fumes, and various kinds of organic or inorganic matter. A majority of these diseases are occupational, which means these diseases are the consequence of long-term exposure to unsafe air in the workplace. These air pollutants include

- Car exhaust
- Smoke
- Tobacco
- Paint spray propellant
- Building insulation
- Laboratory fumes
- Smog
- Mining dust
- Stone cutting
- Artificial nail resins and sanding dust

The symptoms are usually nonspecific and follow the same symptomatic characteristics as COPD. As the diseases become more advanced, breathing becomes increasingly difficult and the final result is death by respiratory failure.

Memory Jogger

 *List 10 air pollutants.*

TUMORS

The most prevalent **neoplasms** of the respiratory system are lung cancer and carcinoma of the larynx (Fig. 30–8).

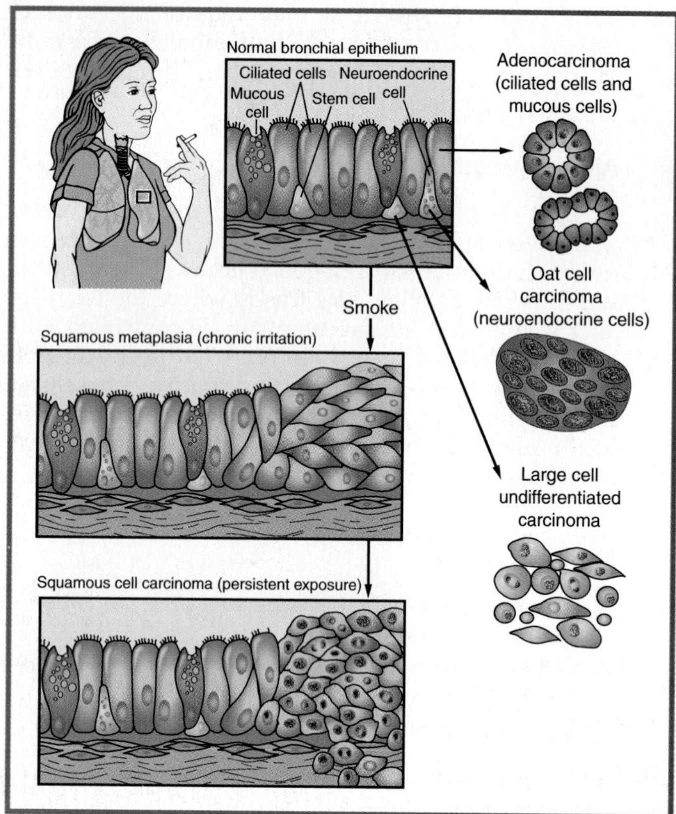

FIGURE 30–8 Classification of lung cancer. (From Damjanov I: Pathology for the Health-Related Professions. Philadelphia, WB Saunders, 1996.)

Lung Cancer

Lung cancer is the leading cause of death in the United States. It is estimated that more than 150,000 people die of lung cancer every year. In most cases, the most prominent cause of lung cancer is cigarette smoking. There is no definite proof to support this statement, but it is a fact that better than 90% of patients with lung cancer are smokers. Lung cancer usually appears after the age of 40 in both men and women, and then the incidence increases as age increases.

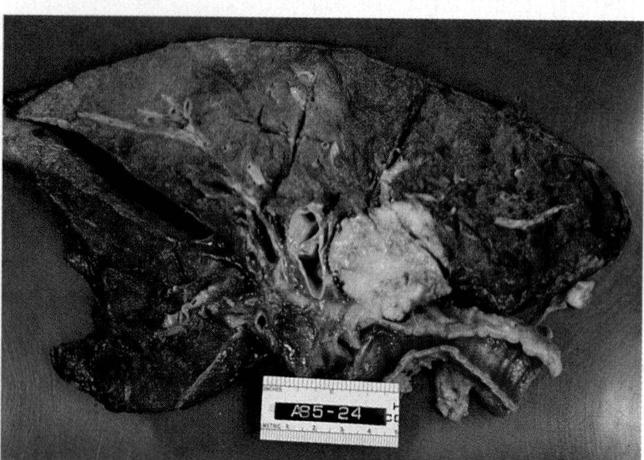

FIGURE 30–9 Lung cancer. (From Damjanov I: Pathology for the Health-Related Professions. Philadelphia, WB Saunders, 1996.)

About 15% of patients with lung cancer display no obvious symptoms, and the tumor is discovered incidentally during routine chest radiography. The ones that do show symptoms usually display local effects of a tumor in the chest such as bronchial obstruction and **atelectasis.**

Lung cancer is essentially incurable. Treatment consists of surgery, radiation therapy, and chemotherapy. The 5-year survival rate is about 12%. The tumors that are successfully **eradicated** are the ones that are found by chance and are in the very infant stages of development (Fig. 30–9).

Carcinoma of the Larynx

Less than 2% of all human cancers are carcinoma of the larynx. This type of cancer is pathologically linked to smoking and chronic alcohol consumption. Men are affected seven times more frequently than women. The incidence of this cancer is also seen in people older than 40 and then increases as age increases. Patients show early signs of hoarseness and loss of voice; occasionally, respiration becomes impaired. Owing to these early symptoms, most laryngeal tumors are discovered in their early stages and can be removed with a very good prognosis. About 75% of people who have had the tumor removed and then received radiation therapy have survived to live a normal life span.

Memory Jogger

What are four types of lung diseases that are directly linked to smoking?

Medical Assistant's Role in Pulmonary Procedures

ASSISTING WITH THE EXAMINATION

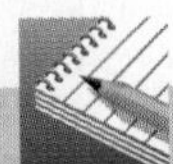

SKILL AND RESPONSIBILITIES

MEDICAL ASSISTANT'S CLINICAL RESPONSIBILITIES

1 Prepare patient for examination
2 Support patient by helping to position and drape patient
3 Administer various tests if qualified

Ask the patient to disrobe to the waist. If the patient is female, give her an examination gown and tell her to put it on with the opening in the front. Then invite the patient to sit upright on the end of the examination table. The examination begins just after the palpation of the thyroid gland, with the physician standing in front of the patient. When the physician is ready to begin this portion of the examination, lift up the gown of a female patient and drape it on her shoulders rather than completely removing it. This draping procedure gives a woman the feeling of being somewhat covered and will aid in maintaining patient privacy.

The examination will be done using inspection, palpation, percussion, and auscultation on the anterior thorax and then will be repeated on the posterior and lateral thorax.

ADMINISTRATION OF THE MANTOUX TUBERCULIN SKIN TEST

The Mantoux test is used for routine screening and in the diagnosis of tuberculosis. The test uses a purified protein derivative (PPD) from a live tuberculin bacillus culture to test for the presence of tuberculin antibodies.

The preferred site for the PPD test is the upper third of the anterior forearm. Avoid areas with excessive hair, scarring, or any other abnormality of the skin surface. Alcohol, acetone, or ether may be used to cleanse the skin. The area must be thoroughly dry before the intradermal injection.

The results should be read at 48 to 72 hours after the test is given. Vesiculation or the extent of induration is the determining factor in reading the results: redness without induration is of no significance. The reading should be made in good light, with the forearm slightly flexed. The size of the induration is determined in millimeters by inspection, measuring, and palpation. The tests come with cards for measuring and reading (Fig. 30–10). A positive Mantoux reaction is indicated when the induration is greater than 10 mm and indicates the possibility of active or dormant tuberculosis or exposure to the disease. Further testing by sputum culture and radiographs is required for a definitive diagnosis. Ad-

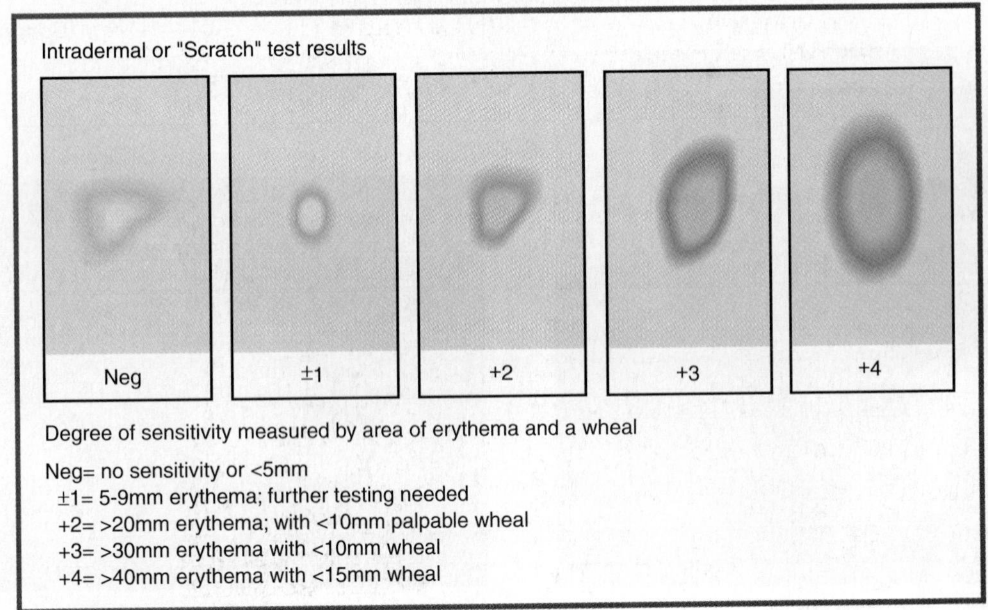

FIGURE 30–10 Positive indurations (TB test). (From Stepp CA, Woods MA: Laboratory Procedures for Medical Office Personnel. Philadelphia, WB Saunders, 1998.)

PROCEDURE 30–1

Administering the Mantoux Tuberculin Skin Test

GOAL

To accurately administer the Mantoux TB test.

EQUIPMENT AND SUPPLIES

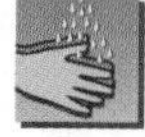

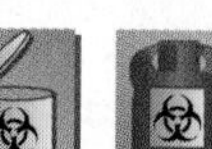

Alcohol preps
Nonsterile gloves
Tuberculin syringe with 3/8 to 1/2-inch, 26- or 27-gauge needle containing 0.1 mL purified protein derivative (PPD)
Patient instruction leaflet with millimeter ruler
Biohazard waste and sharps container

PROCEDURAL STEPS

1 Wash your hands.
PURPOSE: Infection control.

2 Identify your patient and explain the procedure.
PURPOSE: Eliminate possible administration to the wrong patient.

3 Check the patient's arm and select an appropriate site to administer the test. The anterior surface of the forearm halfway between the antecubital space and the wrist is recommended. Hairy or traumatized areas are to be avoided (Figure 1).
PURPOSE: The use of skin areas that are hairy or traumatized makes it difficult to read the results.

4 Prepare the site by cleansing the area with alcohol or other appropriate cleansing agent.
PURPOSE: The skin surface should be made as free from organisms as possible.

5 Put on gloves.
PURPOSE: Gloves provide barrier protection.

6 Grasp the forearm where the test is to be given and stretch the skin tightly to make it easier to puncture the skin (Figure 2).
PURPOSE: Stretching the skin allows for easier insertion of the needle.

Continued

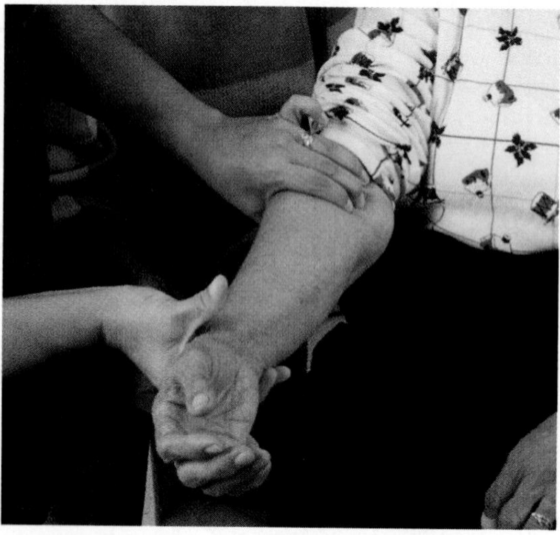

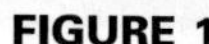

FIGURE 1

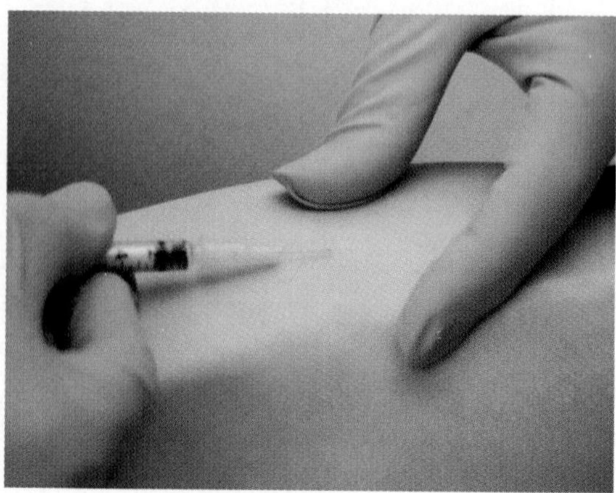

FIGURE 2

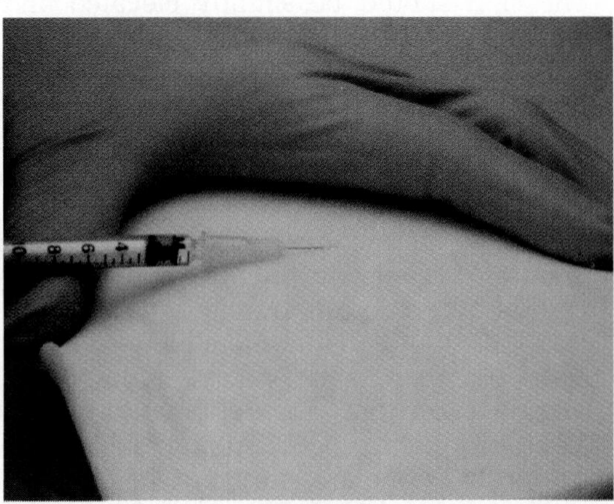
FIGURE 3

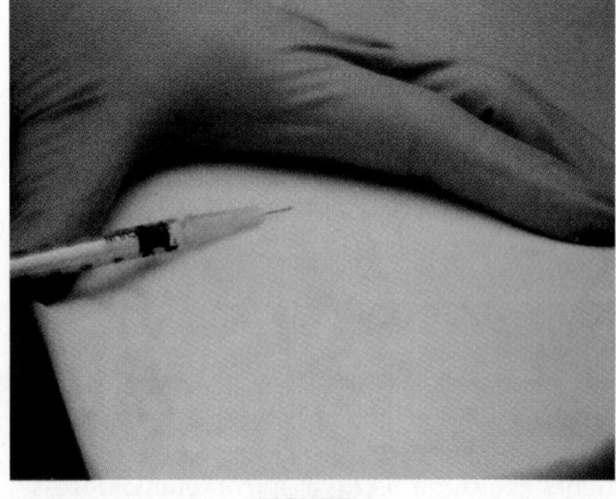
FIGURE 4

7 With the bevel of the needle facing up, insert the needle at a 10- to 15-degree angle into the upper layer of the skin. The needle will be slightly visible below the skin (Figure 3).
PURPOSE: The needle should be inserted almost parallel to the skin to ensure that penetration occurs within the dermal layer.

8 DO NOT ASPIRATE. Hold the needle steady in position and inject the medication slowly by depressing the plunger (Figure 4). A wheal will form as the medication enters the dermis (Figure 5).
PURPOSE: Moving the needle once it has penetrated the skin will cause patient discomfort. If the needle is turned so that the bevel faces downward, no wheal will form and the medication will be absorbed into the tissue.

9 Remove the needle from the skin at exactly the same angle it was inserted. Do not massage or press on the site.
PURPOSE: Pressure on the wheal may cause the medication to enter the tissue.

10 Dispose of the uncapped needle into the biohazard sharps container.
PURPOSE: Reduce the risk of an accidental needle stick.

11 Advise the patient to return to have the test read in 48 to 72 hours, or instruct the patient in assessing the test at home and calling in the results.
PURPOSE: Optimal results occur within 48 to 72 hours. The test *must* be read during that time span for clinically acceptable results to be obtained.

12 Record the test given and the administration site on the patient's medical record. Include the date and time if not previously recorded. Initial or sign the entry.
PURPOSE: Procedures that are not recorded are considered not done.

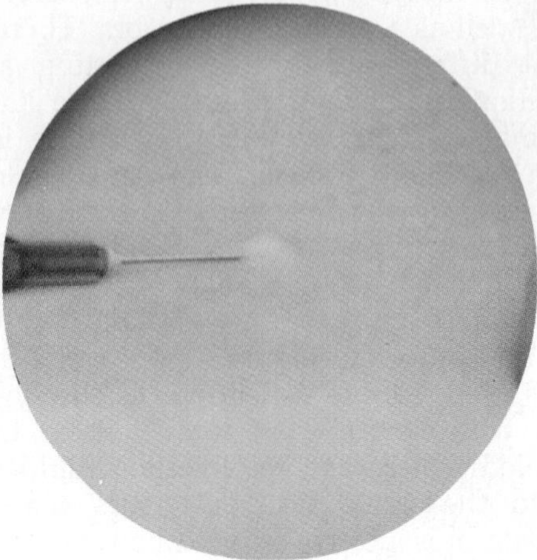
FIGURE 5

verse reactions include pain, itching, and discomfort at the test site. Rarely, bleeding may occur at the puncture site, but it is of no significance.

Memory Jogger

 *Where is the preferred site for the Mantoux test?*

PULMONARY FUNCTION TESTS

Pulmonary function tests are done to measure the amount of air a patient can inhale and exhale and the speed at which he or she can process it. The measurements are done using a spirometer. Successful spirometry requires the application of a consistent technique for preparing the patient, explaining and performing the procedure, and determining the results.

Patient preparation begins when the procedure is scheduled. At that time the patient should be instructed on which medications should be withheld (if any), whether he or she should stop smoking for a specific time period, and possibly other factors. You may need written orders from the physician regarding precisely what each patient should do to prepare for this test.

Patient Preparation

When the patient arrives for testing, the assistant should explain the purpose of the test, determine if there are any contraindications to performing the test, obtain the patient's vital signs, position the patient, and explain the actual maneuver. Explain spirometry in simple terms, and be brief. One statement that works well is "I am going to have you blow into a machine to see how big your lungs are and how fast the air comes out. It doesn't hurt, but it does require your cooperation and lots of effort."

The next step is to get the patient comfortable and in the proper position. Have the patient loosen any tight clothing such as a necktie, belt, or bra. There is no significant difference between the sitting and standing positions, but many people become lightheaded and may faint or stumble; thus, sitting is a safer position for them to be in. The patient's legs should be uncrossed, and both feet should be on the floor.

Explain the actual maneuver next. Show the patient the mouthpiece and noseclips. Explain how the mouthpiece fits into the mouth. If a cardboard mouthpiece is used, tell the patient not to bite down because this will obstruct the tubing hole. Lips should be sealed tightly, and the tongue should not stick out into the mouthpiece. Dentures that fit poorly may be a nuisance and should be removed if you think they will interfere.

Show the patient the proper chin and neck position. The chin should be slightly elevated and the neck slightly extended. This position should be maintained throughout the forced expiratory procedure. Don't let the patient bend the chin to the chest. Bending at the waist is common and acceptable, but discourage the patient from bending all the way over.

Give specific instructions in simple, direct terms. For example, "I want you to take the deepest breath possible, put the mouthpiece in your mouth and seal your lips tightly, and then blow all your air into the tube as hard and as fast as you can in one long, complete breath." For spirometers that allow the patient to already be breathing on the mouthpiece, the instructions are simpler. One analogy that is sometimes helpful to further explain the maneuver is, "It's like blowing out the candles on a birthday cake and they all don't go out, so you need to keep blowing in the same breath until they do."

Next, demonstrate the maneuver. Many patients will forget some or all of the instructions they just received, so the demonstration reinforces exactly what they are to do. Show the patient proper chin and neck position, how to get the mouthpiece in at the right time, and how to blow the air out and continue to blow.

When the demonstration is done, remind the patient of the following points:

- Take as deep a breath as possible.
- Blow air out hard.
- Don't stop blowing until you are told to stop.

Use good active and forceful coaching while the patient is performing the maneuver. You may need to raise your voice with some urgency, using such phrases as "blow, blow, blow!" "Keep blowing, keep blowing!" and "Don't stop blowing!" Coaching improves the performance of most effort-dependent activities, which include spirometry. After the maneuver, give the patient some feedback on the quality of the test and describe what improvements could be made. Continue to repeat efforts until *three acceptable maneuvers* are obtained. If, after eight trials, no acceptable curves are obtained, stop and report this to the physician.

Memory Jogger

 *What are three reminder points you need to tell the patient before spirometric testing?*

ACCEPTABLE MANEUVERS

Acceptability consists of five characteristics:

1 No coughing
2 Good start of test

3 No early termination
4 No variable flows
5 Consistency

Memory Jogger

15 *List the five acceptable characteristics of a spirometric test.*

Infection Control

After a spirometric test is completed, the medical assistant must clean the equipment thoroughly. Microorganisms reportedly have been collected from pulmonary function devices. The transmission of the microorganisms to other patients has also been reported. There is a risk of cross-contamination when using pulmonary function equipment. It would seem safe to speculate that this risk is in proportion to the frequency of cleaning or changing equipment parts. The use of filters to trap microorganisms might reduce this risk; however, these filters are costly and may interfere with the accuracy of the test. The National Association of Respiratory Care Therapists has made recommendations to aid in avoiding cross-contamination.

AIDS IN PREVENTING CROSS-CONTAMINATION

1 Use disposable mouthpieces and discard them after each patient's use. If rubber mouthpieces are used, clean with high-level disinfectant and rinse well between every patient.
2 Change external spirometer tubing between patients. Give the contaminated tubing high-level disinfection; rinse and dry the tubing before reuse.
3 Change noseclips between patients, and discard or clean with high-level disinfectant.
4 Change water in water-sealed spirometers as indicated by the volume of patient use.
5 Do not spend a great amount of time and effort cleaning the surfaces inside the spirometers.
6 Wash hands thoroughly, using proper handwashing technique, before and after performing testing maneuvers, whether or not gloves are worn.

Memory Jogger

16 *How many acceptable maneuvers must you obtain to complete the test procedure?*

Test Results

Place the results of the maneuvers with the patient's chart on the physician's desk when the tests are completed. Many physicians rely on the assistant to include comments pertinent to the testing with these results. If there are any questions regarding the quality of the results, you should ask the patient to wait while you check with the physician. Never allow the patient to leave the office before the physician gives you approval to do so. If the patient has delayed taking medication, check with the physician as to when the patient should resume taking it.

PROCEDURE 30-2
Performing Volume Capacity Spirometric Test

GOAL

To perform volume capacity testing.

EQUIPMENT AND SUPPLIES

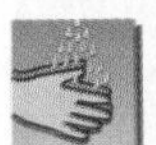

Balance scale with measuring device
Volume capacity spirometer with recording paper in place
External spirometric tubing
Disposable mouth piece
Noseclip
Biohazard waste container

Continued

PROCEDURE 30-2 (CONTINUED)

Performing Volume Capacity Spirometric Test

PROCEDURAL STEPS

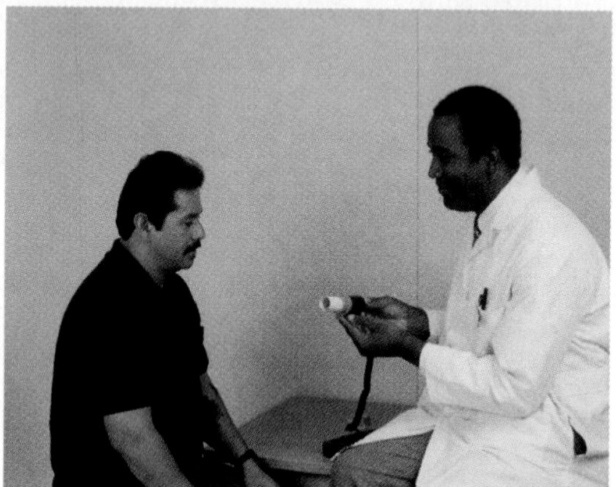

FIGURE 1

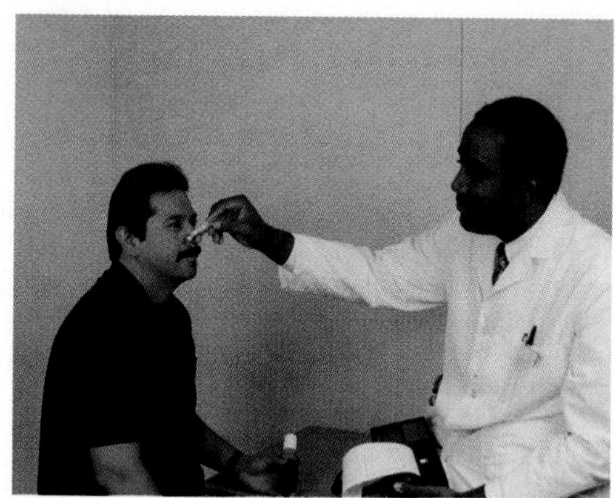

FIGURE 2

1 Introduce yourself and confirm the identity of the patient. Ascertain if any special preparation was needed by this patient and if it was followed.
PURPOSE: If special procedures were not followed, the test may have to be rescheduled.

2 Explain the purpose of the test
PURPOSE: To help reassure the patient.

3 Obtain the patient's vital signs.

4 Explain the actual maneuver (Figure 1). Demonstrate the use of the noseclips (Figure 2).
PURPOSE: The patient needs to understand the maneuver so he or she can cooperate fully to obtain best testing results.

5 Be certain the patient is comfortable and in proper sitting or standing position (Figure 3).
PURPOSE: Proper positioning is necessary to ensure accurate test results.

6 Loosen any tight clothing, such as necktie, belt, or bra.
PURPOSE: Tight clothing may restrict breathing capacity.

7 Show the patient the proper chin and neck position (Figure 4).

Continued

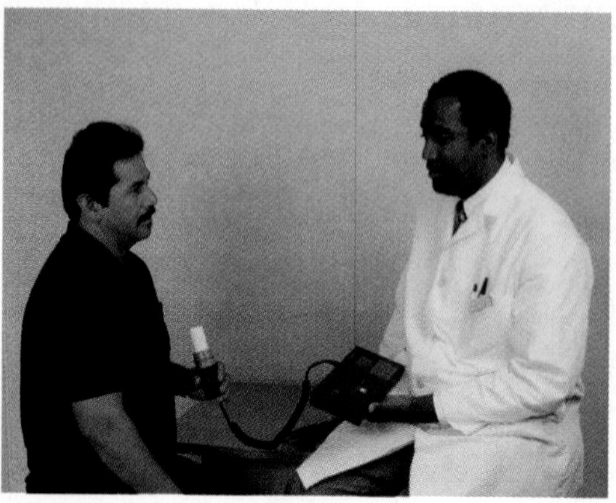

FIGURE 3

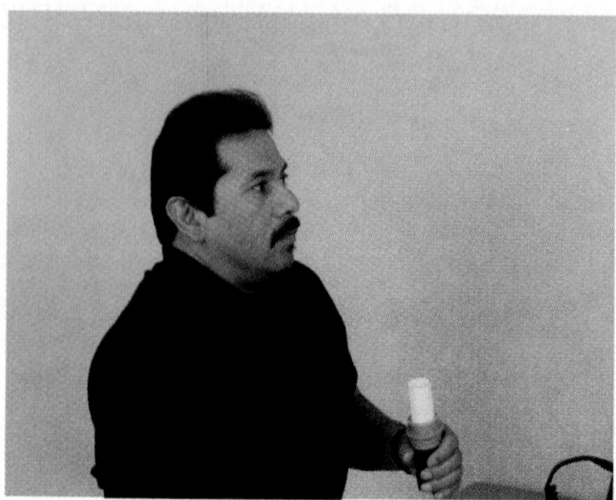

FIGURE 4

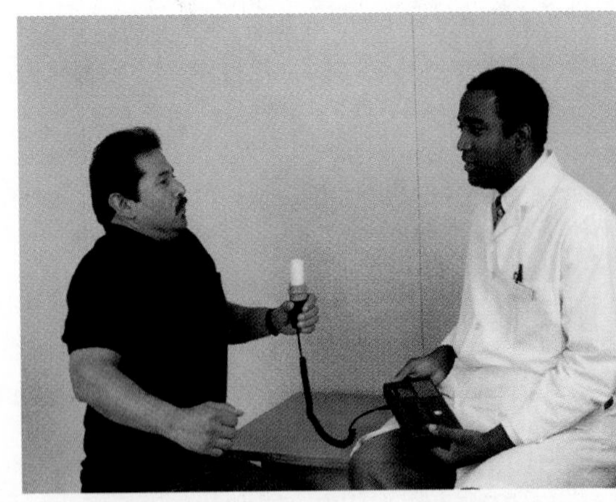

FIGURE 5

8 Practice the maneuver with the patient and tell patient "Inhale" (Figure 5).
PURPOSE: To relieve apprehension and enhance understanding.

9 Use active, forceful coaching during testing. Begin by saying "Blow" (Figures 6 through 8). Then say "Blow out hard." Then say "Keep blowing, keep blowing." Then say "Don't stop—blow harder."
PURPOSE: Coaching improves performance.

Continued

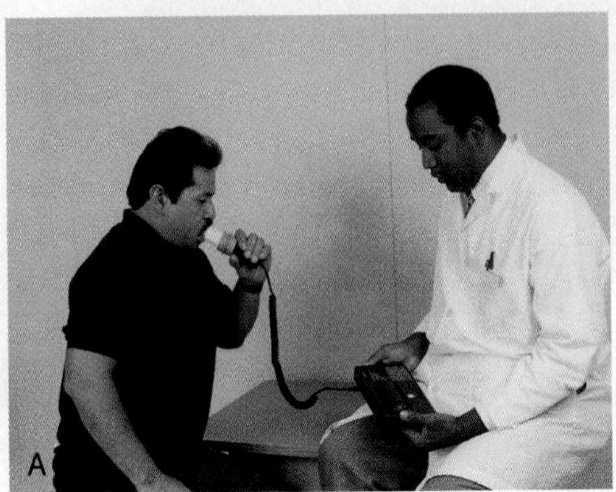

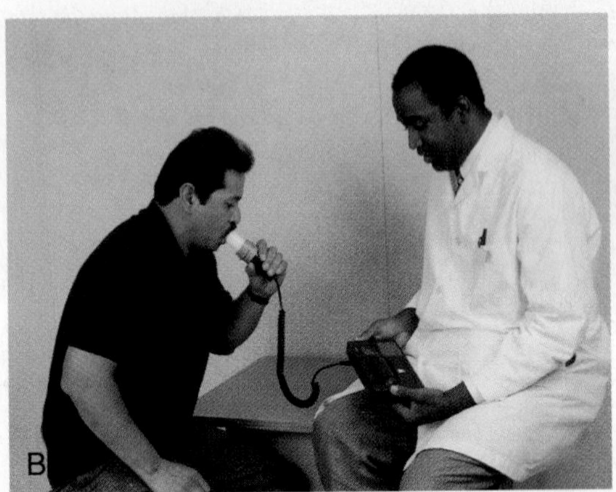

FIGURE 6

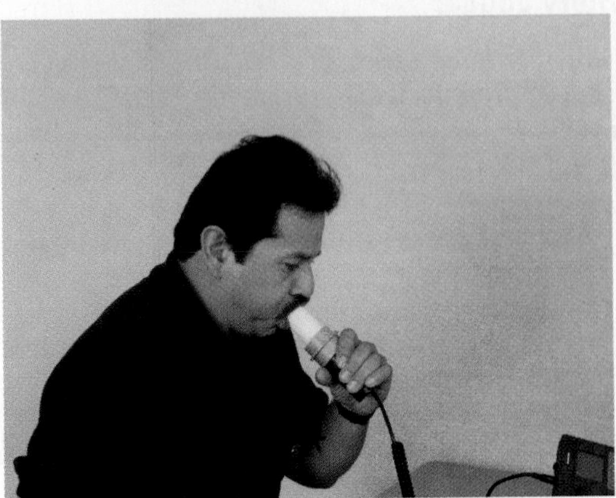

FIGURE 7

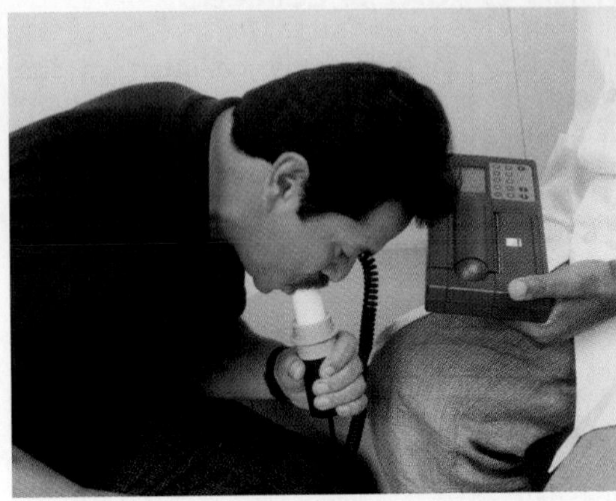

FIGURE 8

PROCEDURE 30-2 (CONTINUED)
Performing Volume Capacity Spirometric Test

10 Give the patient feedback after the maneuver is completed (Figure 9).
PURPOSE: Compliments and explanations of mistakes in the maneuver will help improve patient compliance.

11 Continue testing until three acceptable maneuvers have been obtained (Figure 10).

12 Dismiss the patient only if results are satisfactory.

13 Clean and disinfect the equipment. Discard waste in a biohazard waste container.

14 Wash hands.
PURPOSE: Infection control.

15 Record testing information on the patient's chart and place the chart with the test results on the physician's desk for interpretation.
PURPOSE: Procedures that are not recorded are considered not done.

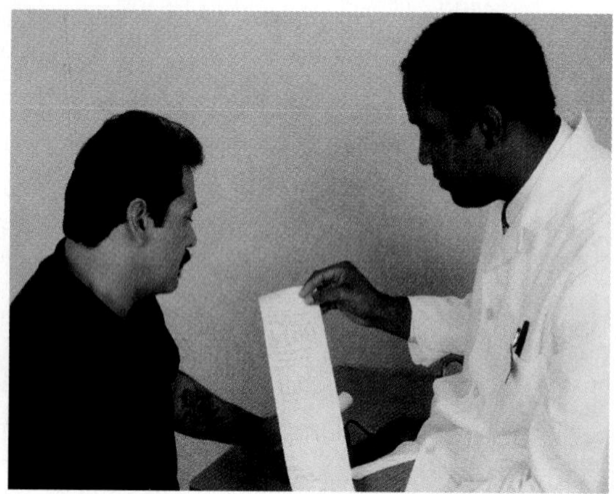

FIGURE 9

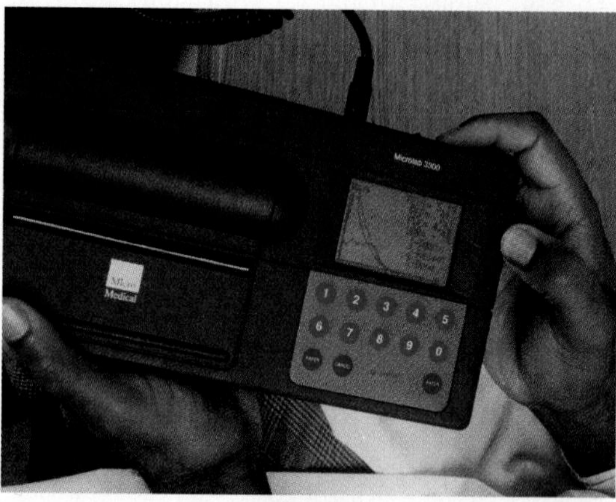

FIGURE 10

COLLECTING THROAT SPECIMENS

Throat specimens are frequently collected in the physician's office to assist in the diagnosis of strep throat infections. Strep throat (type A) is caused by the bacteria called *Streptococcus* and, if left untreated, can cause serious complications such as **rheumatic fever, rheumatic endocarditis,** and **glomerulonephritis.**

Throat cultures are collected by gently swabbing the back of the throat and the surfaces of the tonsils with a sterile swab. The mouth and tongue should be avoided to prevent contamination of the swab with the normal flora of the mouth. Throat cultures are best obtained by depressing the tongue and instructing the patient to say "ah."

Memory Jogger

Identify three serious complications that may occur if strep throat is untreated.

OBTAINING SPUTUM FOR CULTURE

Sputum culture is requested when there are signs and symptoms accompanied by physical evidence of pneumonia, tuberculosis, or other infectious diseases of the lower respiratory tract. The sample is sent to a laboratory that is equipped to handle bacteriologic samples that are potentially infectious. Once the sample arrives at the laboratory, it will be cultured

PROCEDURE 30-3

Collecting a Specimen by Swab for Throat Culture

GOAL

To collect a throat culture, using sterile technique, for either immediate testing or transportation to the laboratory.

EQUIPMENT AND SUPPLIES

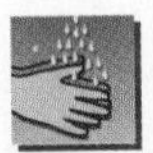

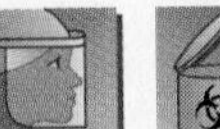

Nonsterile gloves and face protection barrier
Sterile swab
Sterile tongue depressor
Transport medium
Biohazard waste container

PROCEDURAL STEPS

1 Wash and dry your hands.
PURPOSE: Infection control.

2 Gather the materials needed.

3 Don gloves and face protection (Figure 1).
PURPOSE: Standard Precautions.

4 Position the patient so that the light shines into the mouth.
PURPOSE: Visualization of the area to be swabbed.

5 Remove the sterile swab from the sterile wrap with your dominant hand, and grasp the sterile tongue depressor with your nondominant hand (Figure 2).
PURPOSE: Better control of the swabbing process.

Continued

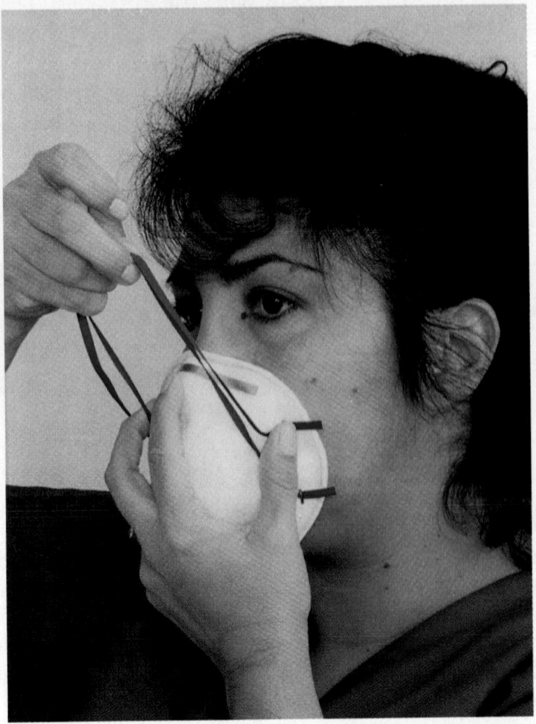

FIGURE 1

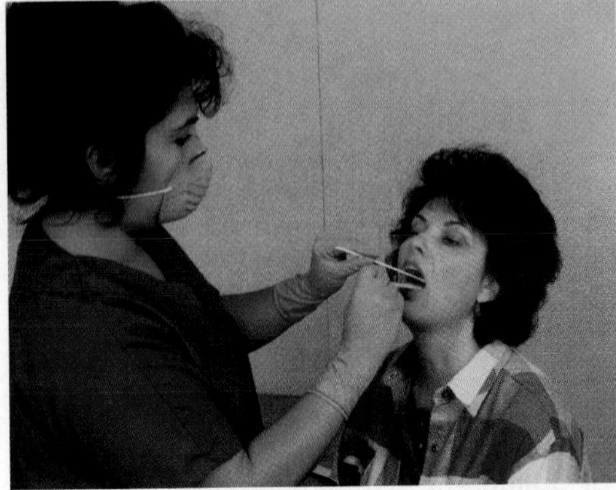

FIGURE 2

PROCEDURE 30-3 (CONTINUED)
Collecting a Specimen by Swab for Throat Culture

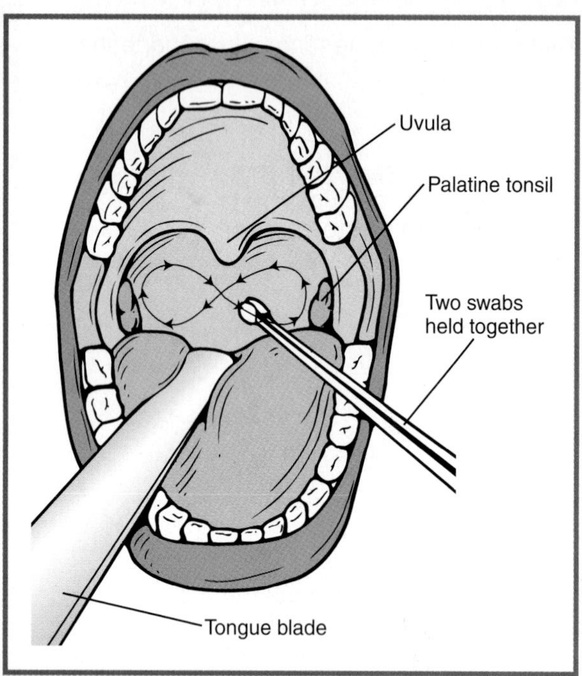

FIGURE 3

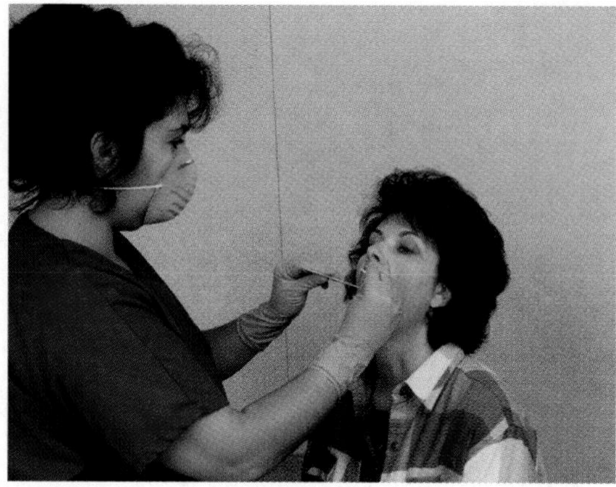

FIGURE 4

6 Instruct the patient to open the mouth and to say "ah." Depress the tongue with the depressor (Figure 3*).
PURPOSE: Saying "ah" helps elevate the uvula and reduces the tendency to gag. The tongue is depressed so that you can see the back of the throat.

7 Swab the back of the throat between the tonsillar pillars and especially the reddened, patchy areas of the throat, white pus pockets, purulent areas, and the tonsils (Figure 4*).
PURPOSE: Pathogenic organisms are found in the back of the throat and on the tonsils.

Continued

* Figures 3 and 4 from Stepp CA, Woods MA: Laboratory Procedures for Medical Office Personnel. Philadelphia, WB Saunders, 1998.

and incubated. The pathogenic organism grown in the culture media will then be identified. The sample may also be sent to laboratory **cytology** for analysis that might suggest a cancerous condition of the lungs or bronchi.

Methods of Collection

There are three methods of collection: expectoration, tracheal suctioning, and bronchoscopy. If the sample is to be collected by expectoration, encourage the patient to drink fluids the night before the collection to help increase sputum production. The patient also needs to understand that he or she is not to brush the teeth or use mouthwash before the test. (If this is done, the tests results will be unreliable.) It is acceptable to rinse the mouth with water. On the morning of the test, instruct the patient how to expectorate by taking three deep breaths and forcing a deep cough. It is important to remember that spu-

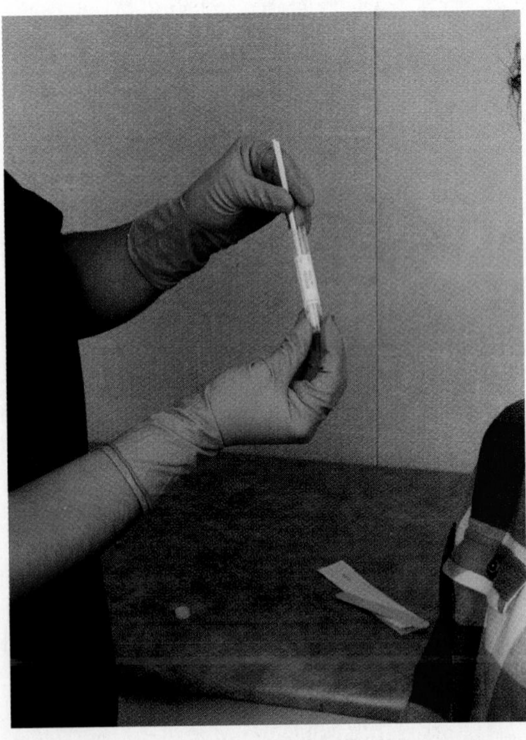

FIGURE 5

8 Place the swab into the transport medium, label it, and send it to the laboratory. If direct slide testing is requested, return the labeled swab to the laboratory (Figure 5).
PURPOSE: Transport media prevent the swab from drying. Labeling immediately after collection prevents mixing up specimens.

9 Dispose of contaminated supplies in biohazard waste container.
PURPOSE: Prevents the spread of infection.

10 Disinfect the work area.

11 Remove gloves; place in biohazard waste container.

12 Wash your hands.
PURPOSE: Infection control.

13 Record procedure in the patient's record.
PURPOSE: Procedures that are not recorded are considered not done.

tum is not the same as **saliva,** which is unacceptable for culturing. The sputum is to be spit directly into the laboratory container. If the cough does not produce sputum, chest physiotherapy or **nebulization** (a heated aerosol spray) may be ordered by the physician to induce it. Sputum collection may be required for three consecutive mornings.

If the specimen is to be collected by tracheal suctioning, a **catheter** is passed through the nostril into the trachea, then suction is used for up to 15 seconds. This method is not used if the patient has abnormalities in the esophagus or has heart disease.

In a specimen collected by bronchoscopy, the patient must fast for 6 hours before the procedure. A local anesthetic is sprayed into the patient's throat immediately before the physician inserts the bronchoscope into the throat and into the bronchus. Secretions are collected with a bronchial brush or aspirated through the inner channel of the scope.

Test results are usually available in 48 to 72 hours. However, cultures for tuberculosis take up to 2 months. The diagnosis of this disorder is generally based on the patient's symptoms and on results of an acid-fast bacilli test, chest radiograph, and a skin test.

Memory Jogger

18 *Why are standard safety precautions so carefully followed when collecting and handling sputum samples?*

PROCEDURE 30–4

Obtaining a Sputum Sample for Culture

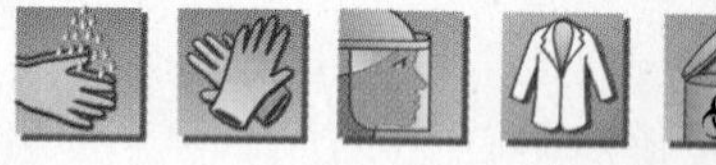

GOAL

To collect a sputum sample while observing standard precautions.

EQUIPMENT AND SUPPLIES

Sterile laboratory specimen cup, accurately labeled
Plastic laboratory specimen bag
Biohazard waste container

PROCEDURAL STEPS

1 Assemble the equipment.

2 Greet patient and explain the procedure.
PURPOSE: An informed patient is more cooperative.

3 Wash hands and put on gloves, faceshield, and gown.
PURPOSE: Standard precautions must be followed when collecting potentially infectious materials.

4 Have the patient rinse the mouth with water.
PURPOSE: Any food particles in the mouth will contaminate the specimen.

5 Instruct the patient to take three deep breaths and then cough deeply to bring up secretions from the lower respiratory tract.
PURPOSE: The organisms for culture must be from the lung fields in the lower respiratory tract.

6 Tell the patient to spit directly into the specimen container and to avoid getting any sputum on the sides of the container.
PURPOSE: Sputum on the sides of the container is considered hazardous.

7 Place the lid on the container securely and then place the container into the plastic specimen bag.
PURPOSE: Minimize the possibility of spreading the potentially hazardous specimen.

8 Offer the patient a glass of water or ginger ale.
PURPOSE: The patient may have a bad taste in the mouth after the test, which may cause nausea.

9 If another test is ordered for tomorrow morning, instruct the patient when to come and remind him or her to follow the same instructions for preparation.

10 Clean the work area and properly dispose of all supplies.
PURPOSE: Observe standard precautions.

11 Wash your hands.
PURPOSE: Infection control.

12 Process the specimen immediately to ensure optimal test results.
PURPOSE: Microorganisms may propagate or die, creating an elevated or false-negative result.

13 Record the procedure in the patient's record.
PURPOSE: Procedures that are not recorded are considered not done.

Overview

The respiratory system provides the body with oxygen, which is the primary substance needed for cell metabolism. Cells soon stop functioning and die when they are deprived of oxygen. In addition to supplying oxygen, the respiratory system assists the body in eliminating carbon dioxide, which if not eliminated will cause the acid-base balance to change, causing acidosis. The respiratory system is exposed to the atmosphere and is susceptible to airborne infections, contaminants, and irritant injury. The medical assistant can play an important role in assisting the patient to maintain a health respiratory system and in helping the physician in diagnosing and treating respiratory diseases.

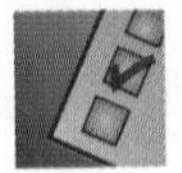

PATIENT EDUCATION

It is often said that the greatest fear a person ever has is the fear of the unknown. Often the patient worries and fears the tests that the physician orders. The imagination can create all types of frightening scenarios with even more alarming outcomes.

You can help the patient by explaining any diagnostic testing procedure and making sure that the patient understands what will be expected of him or her during the testing procedure. Make sure that you have literature explaining the test ordered to give to the patient to read at his or her leisure before the testing time. Answer all of the patient's questions; if a concern is voiced that you cannot answer, consult with the physician regarding this concern before the patient leaves the office.

As medical assistants, we need to be aware of opportunities to give advice and help by answering questions and alerting the physician to possible symptoms that we noticed in preparing the patient. Sometimes the most insignificant comment makes the greatest difference. Of course, above all, we must set an example, and basically that means practice what you preach.

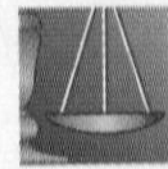

LEGAL AND ETHICAL ISSUES

When the respiratory system is mentioned, people generally think of breathing, but this is only one of the activities of the respiratory system. Our body cells need a continuous supply of oxygen to maintain life. The respiratory system works together with the circulatory system to supply this oxygen and to remove the waste products of metabolism. Too often people take breathing for granted and assume that nothing could possibly happen to their ability to breathe. Sadly, respiratory diseases are the leading cause of death, and that means there are people we know and love who will suffer and die of some of the diseases discussed in this chapter.

If the pulmonary test ordered is an invasive test such as bronchoscopy, be certain that a written consent form is obtained from the patient and is in the patient's chart. If the patient is to see another specialist, a consent form must be signed to give permission to copy and forward patient information to the consultant. If it is your responsibility to copy and forward this information to the consultant, be sure you do so as quickly as possible. The consultant may need time to review the information before seeing the patient.

CRITICAL THINKING

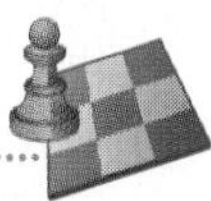

1 Sometimes patients with respiratory diseases or patients who have had a lung removed have a deformed chest. What could you do to protect these patients' dignity and assist them through the examination?

2 What type of a spirometric test would you have if you had the patient follow written instructions rather than verbal coaching? How would you handle the patient who refuses to follow your instructions?

3 You are a cigarette smoker and you work in a pulmonary medicine clinic. Do you think you can hide your habit from the patients? How convincing will you be as an advocate of respiratory care? What could you do to be more convincing?

HOW DID I DO? Answers to Memory Joggers

1. The surface landmarks of the respiratory system are
   a. rib cage
   b. vertebrae
   c. sternum
   d. diaphragm
2. Upper respiratory structures include the nose, pharynx, and larynx. The lower respiratory tract includes the trachea, bronchus, and the lungs.
3. The groups of society in which most lung infections are seen include hospitalized patients, the elderly, drug addicts, alcoholics, and patients with AIDS.
4. The six symptoms of an upper respiratory tract infection include rhinorrhea, sneezing, watery eyes, pharyngitis, laryngitis, and coughing.
5. The fifth leading cause of death in the United States is pneumonia.
6. Three tests that confirm pneumonia are chest radiography, sputum studies, and blood leukocyte analysis.
7. Tuberculosis is spreading quickly in crowded city areas and in the elderly, nonwhites, alcoholics, and people with AIDS.
8. Common symptoms of tuberculosis include afternoon fever, night sweats, weight loss, general malaise, and a productive cough.
9. Three diseases included under COPD include chronic bronchitis, bronchiectasis, and emphysema.

10 Two immune diseases that may be helped through allergy desensitizing injections are asthma and hay fever.

11 The ten air pollutants include car exhaust, smoke, tobacco, paint spray propellant, building insulation, laboratory fumes, smog, mining dust, stone cutting dust, and artificial nail resins and sanding.

12 Four lung diseases linked to smoking include chronic bronchitis, emphysema, lung cancer, and carcinoma of the larynx.

13 The preferred site for the Mantoux tuberculin skin test is the upper one third of the anterior forearm.

14 When doing spirometric testing, three points you need to tell the patient are

a. Take as deep a breath as possible.
b. Blast air out hard.
c. Don't stop blowing until you are told to stop.

15 Five acceptable characteristics of acceptable spirometric testing include

a. No coughing
b. Good start of test
c. No early termination
d. No variable flows
e. Consistency

16 You need three acceptable maneuvers to complete the testing procedure.

17 The serious complications that untreated strep throat can lead to include rheumatic fever, rheumatic endocarditis, and glomerulonephritis.

18 You must carefully follow standard safety precautions when collecting and handling sputum samples owing to their high degree of potentially hazardous contents.

Assisting with Ophthalmology and Otorhinolaryngology Procedures

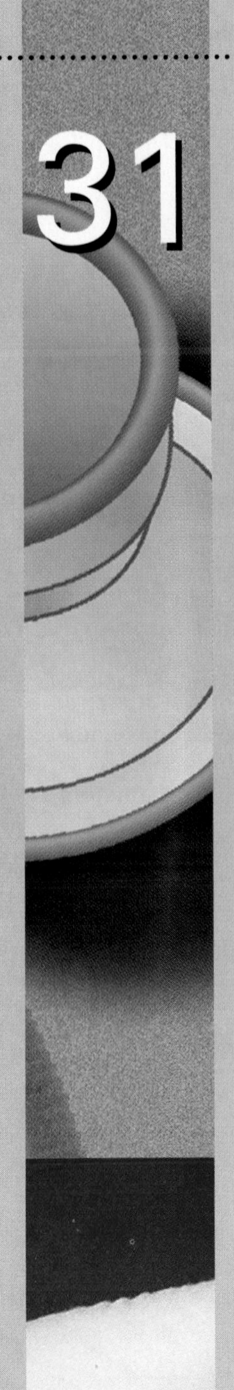

OUTLINE

LEARNING OBJECTIVES

Cognitive: On successful completion of this chapter you should be able to:

1 Explain the differences among an ophthalmologist, optometrist, and optician.
2 Identify the anatomic structures of the eye.
3 Describe how vision occurs.
4 Differentiate among the four major types of refractive errors.
5 Be able to give four reasons each for eye irrigation and instillation of medication.
6 Identify the structures and explain the functions of the external, middle, and internal ear.
7 List disorders that can cause hearing losses.
8 Differentiate between conductive and sensory losses.
9 Describe four methods used to assess hearing acuity.
10 State three reasons for ear irrigations and/or instilling ear medication.
11 State reasons for ensuring aseptic technique in both eye and ear procedures.
12 Spell and define terms in the vocabulary.

Performance: On successful completion of this chapter you should be able to:

1 Correctly label the results of a Snellen vision test.
2 Accurately measure distance visual acuity.
3 Assess color acuity.
4 Properly irrigate a patient's eyes.
5 Accurately instill eye medication.
6 Assist with the removal of a foreign object from an eye.
7 Properly irrigate a patient's ears.
8 Accurately instill otic drops.

VOCABULARY

accommodation Adjustment of the eye for seeing various sizes of objects at different distances

amblyopia Reduction or dimness of vision with no apparent organic cause; often referred to as lazy eye syndrome

analgesics Drugs that relieve pain without loss of consciousness

audiologist An allied health care professional specializing in evaluation of hearing function, detection of hearing impairment, and determination of the anatomic site of impairment

auditory ossicles Three small bones of the middle ear responsible for converting air conduction to bone conduction

blepharitis Inflammation of the glands and lash follicles along the margin of the eyelids

ceruminous Pertaining to the waxy secretion of the glands of the external auditory canal known as cerumen (commonly called ear wax)

chalazion A small eyelid mass resulting from inflammation of a meibomian gland

choroid Middle, vascular layer of the eye containing many blood vessels and brown pigment that serves to reduce reflection when it falls on the retina

chronic Persisting for a long period of time and showing little change

cones Structures found in the retina that make the perception of color possible

conjunctiva Delicate membrane lining of the eyelids and covering of the eyeball

conjunctivitis Inflammation of the conjunctiva

cornea Clear, transparent anterior covering of the eye

diplopia Double vision

eustachian tube Narrow tube leading from the middle ear to the pharynx

exophthalmia Pertaining to an abnormal protrusion of the eyes

exophthalmometer Instrument used to measure the pressure in the central retinal artery

fovea centralis A small pit in the center of the retina that is considered the center of clearest vision

hertz (Hz) Unit of frequency equal to one cycle per second

hordeolum Inflammation of one or more sebaceous glands of the eyelid; often called a stye

iris Circular pigmented membrane behind the cornea, perforated by the pupil

keratitis Inflammation of the cornea of the eye

lacrimal sac Sac located over the upper, outer corner of the eye that secretes tears

lens Transparent, biconvex body separating the posterior chamber and the vitreous body of the eye

masking To obscure or diminish a sound with the presence of another sound of different frequency

opaque Impervious to light rays; neither translucent nor transparent

ophthalmologist Physician specializing in the diagnosis and treatment of disorders of the eye

optic disc Region at the back of the eye where the optic nerve meets the retina; considered the blind spot of the eye because it contains only nerve fibers and no rods or cones and thus is insensitive to light

optic nerve Second cranial nerve that carries impulses for the sense of sight

optician One who can translate, fill, and adapt ophthalmic prescriptions, products, and accessories and who does not need to be licensed

optometrist Professional trained to examine the eyes and prescribe eyeglasses to correct irregularities in vision

orbit Bony cavity containing the eyeball and its associated structures

organ of Corti Located within the cochlear duct; contains special sensory receptors for hearing

otalgia Pain in the ear; an earache

otosclerosis Formation of spongy bone in the labyrinth of the ear, often causing the auditory ossicles to become fixed and unable to vibrate when sound enters the ears

prenatal Period of time between conception and birth

psoriasis Usually chronic, recurrent skin disease marked by bright red patches covered with silvery scales

ptosis Drooping of the upper eyelid

purulent Consisting of or containing pus

refraction Deviation of light produced by the eye and resulting in the focusing of images upon the retina

retina Innermost layer of the eye composed of light-sensitive neurons

rods Structures located in the retina of the eye and forming the light-sensitive elements

sclera Tough, white, outer layer of the eyeball, covering about five sixths of its surface

seborrhea Excessive discharge of sebum from the sebaceous glands forming greasy scales or cheesy plugs on the body

tinnitus Ringing in the ears; a symptom of labyrinthitis, eighth cranial nerve damage, or cerebral arteriosclerosis

vascular Pertaining to blood vessels or indicative of a copious blood supply

vitreous Glasslike or hyaline fluid found inside the eye

As a medical assistant you may be responsible for performing a wide variety of procedures in an ophthalmologic or otologic specialty. You must have an understanding of the anatomy and physiology of these sensory organs. It is through this understanding that you will be able to master the skills needed to be a valuable asset to the physician.

Many disorders of the eyes and the ears are not covered in this chapter. The conditions covered are the ones that are seen most often. Knowing the fundamental procedures will give you the knowledge on which to build the advanced techniques that you will be called on to learn if you choose to concentrate your expertise in these areas. There are many subspecialty areas for medical assistants to enter within the eye and ear medical practice arena.

Examination of the Eye

Ophthalmology is the science that is concerned with the eye and its disorders and diseases. The physician who specializes in the diagnosis and treatment of the disorders and diseases of the eye is an **ophthalmologist.** An **optometrist** is trained and licensed to examine the eyes and treat visual defects through corrective lenses and eye exercises. The **optician** receives training in filling prescriptions for corrective lenses, grinding the lenses, and fitting the eyewear. The optometrist and the optician are not medical physicians.

ANATOMY AND PHYSIOLOGY OF THE EYE

The eyes are two of the smallest yet most detailed and complex organs of your body. They are located within a bony **orbit** in the skull. This bony orbit provides protection and support to the eye. Only about one sixth of the eye lies outside this orbit. The eyelid assists in protecting the eye from physical trauma. The eyebrows help to keep perspiration, which is an irritant, out of the eyes. The eyelashes line the margin of the eyelid and help trap foreign particles.

The **conjunctiva** is a thin mucous membrane that lines the eyelid and covers the outside of the eyeball except for the centralmost portion, which is covered by the **cornea.** The mucus secreted from the conjunctiva helps to keep the eye moist. An inflammation of the conjunctiva is called **conjunctivitis.** It can be caused by irritation, allergy, or bacteria.

The eye blinks every 2 to 3 seconds. Blinking causes the lacrimal gland, which is located in the upper outer portion of the upper eyelid, to secrete tears. These tears move across the eyes, cleansing and moistening the eye, and then drain into the **lacrimal sac,** which opens into the nasal cavity. Thus, when you cry, the excess tears fill the lacrimal sac, which empties into your nose and produces a watery nasal discharge.

Memory Jogger

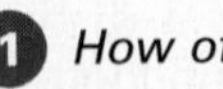

1 *How often do you blink and why?*

Eyeball

The eyeball consists of three layers. The outermost layer is the white **opaque sclera** and the transparent cornea. The sclera protects all of the eyeball lying within the orbit, and the transparent cornea covers the exposed one sixth that serves as a clear window that lets light enter your eye (Fig. 31–1). The cornea was one of the first organs to be transplanted, and now corneal transplants are a common procedure. Long-term success after corneal implant surgery is excellent.

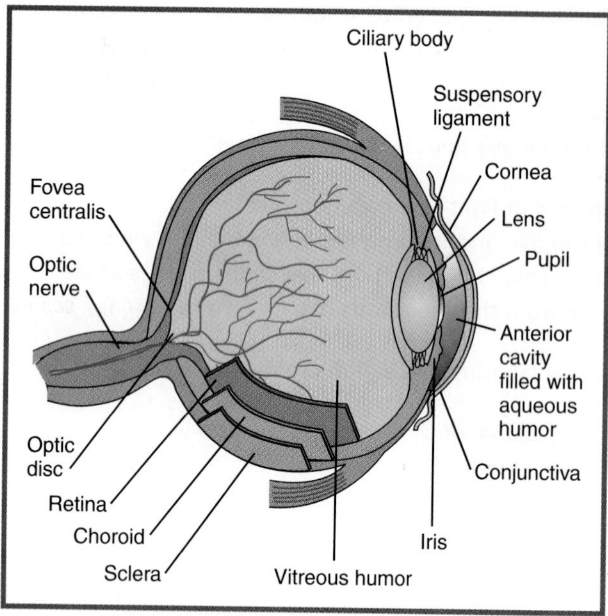

FIGURE 31–1 Anatomical eye.

TABLE 31–1 Functions of the Major Parts of the Eye

Structure	Function
Sclera	External protection
Cornea	Light refraction
Choroid	Blood supply
Iris	Light absorption and regulation of pupillary width
Ciliary body	Secretion of vitreous fluid; changes the shape of the lens
Lens	Light refraction
Retinal layer	Light receptor that transforms optic signals into nerve impulses
Rods	Means of distinguishing light from dark and of perceiving shape and movement
Cones	Color vision
Central fovea	Area of sharpest vision
Macula lutea	Blind spot
External ocular muscles	Movement of the globe
Optical nerve (cranial nerve II)	Transmission of visual information to the brain
Lacrimal glands	Secretion of tears
Eyelid	Eye protection

Modified from Damjanov I: Pathology for the Health-Related Professions. Philadelphia, WB Saunders, 1996.

The middle layer includes the **choroid** within the orbit and the **iris** covering the exposed one sixth. This layer is very **vascular.** The choroid contains brown pigment that absorbs excess light rays that could interfere with vision. The iris is the colored portion of the eye. It is doughnut shaped with the opening of the pupil in the center. The iris regulates the size of the pupil according to the intensity of the light, becoming smaller in bright light and opening wider in dim light.

The inner layer comprises the **retina** in the posterior portion and the **lens** in the anterior portion. It is in the retina where the **rods** and **cones,** the **optic nerve,** the **optic disc,** and the **fovea centralis** are located. The delicate tissue of the retina converts light into impulses. These impulses travel to the brain by means of the optic nerve, and the brain converts them into what you see. The lens helps focus light after it passes through the cornea. The **vitreous** is a clear gel-like substance that fills the back of the eye. Each part of the eye has a distinct function, and every part must be able to function for vision to occur (Table 31–1).

Memory Jogger

 *Name the layers of the eye.*

Vision

Vision requires light and depends on the proper functioning of all parts of the eye. A visual impulse begins with the triggering of our 100 million **rods** and 3 million **cones,** which are the photoreceptor cells, and ends with interpretation in the visual cortex of the occipital lobe of the brain. Vision also depends on the shape of the orbit, the cornea, and the lens. When all of these structures are formed correctly, we still must have muscles that will accommodate, contract, and dilate the respective parts of the eye when they are stimulated. The most common visual problems are in visual acuity, which involves the acuteness or sharpness of vision. An individual with average visual acuity can see clearly and is able to distinguish fine details both at a reasonable distance and up close.

DISORDERS OF THE EYE

Refractive Errors

Four major types of refractive error result when the eye is unable to focus light effectively on the retina. **Refraction** refers to the ability of the lens of the eye to bend parallel light rays coming into the eye so the ray can focus on the retina. An error of refraction means that the light rays are not being refracted or bent properly and thus do not focus correctly on the retina. Defects in the shape of the eyeball may cause a refractive error. Most refractive errors can be corrected by wearing corrective lenses (Fig. 31–2).

Hyperopia (Farsightedness)

When light enters the eye and focuses behind the retina, the person has hyperopia. This disorder is caused by an eyeball that is too short from the ante-

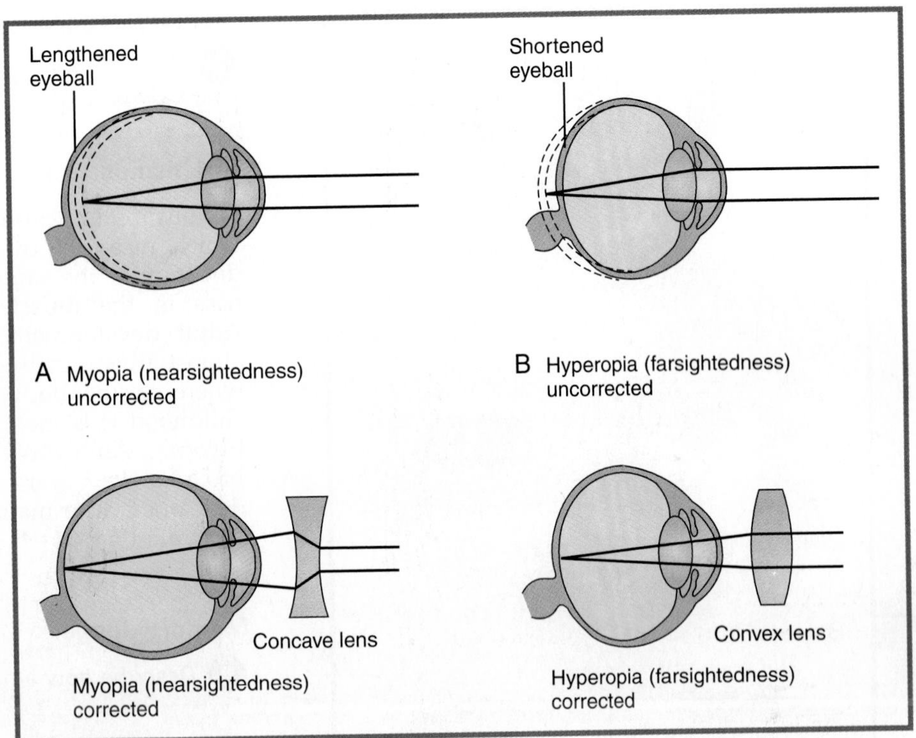

FIGURE 31–2 Errors in refraction. *A*, Myopia. *B*, Hyperopia.

rior to posterior wall. A hyperopic person has difficulty seeing objects close up, at reading or working level. A convex-shaped corrective lens aids the eye's internal lens to place objects on the retina to secure a sharp, detailed image.

Myopia (Nearsightedness)

Myopia occurs when light rays entering the eye focus in front of the retina, causing objects at a distance to appear blurry and dull. Objects viewed at reading or working level can be seen clearly. In this disorder the eyeball is elongated from the anterior to the posterior walls and the image cannot be sharpened by the internal lens of the eye. A concave corrective lens is used to focus the light rays on the retina.

Presbyopia

As people age, most experience a decrease in the elasticity of the internal lens of the eye. This often causes vision changes after 40 years of age. The condition is characterized by a decrease in the ability to see at reading level and then again at a distance. A combination corrective lens, known as a bifocal lens correction, is used to focus both distal and proximal objects directly on the retina.

Astigmatism

Astigmatism is an irregular focusing of the light rays entering the eye. This is usually caused by the cornea or the lens not being a smooth sphere but instead having an irregular shape or having wavy lines in it. This causes the light rays to be unevenly or diffusely focused on the retina, and images appear clear in the center but blurry around the perimeter. It is like attempting to focus on objects seen through a wavy piece of window glass (Fig. 31–3).

SIGNS AND SYMPTOMS Refractive errors in vision can lead to squinting, frequent rubbing of the eyes, and headaches. The individual begins noticing blurring of vision and/or fading of words at reading level. A strong clue is when the individual cannot read numbers correctly in the phone book or is unable to recognize friends, by their appearance only, at a distance.

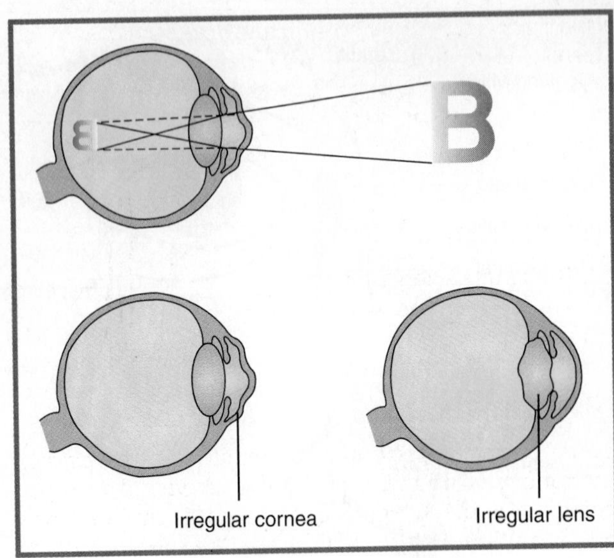

FIGURE 31–3 Astigmatism.

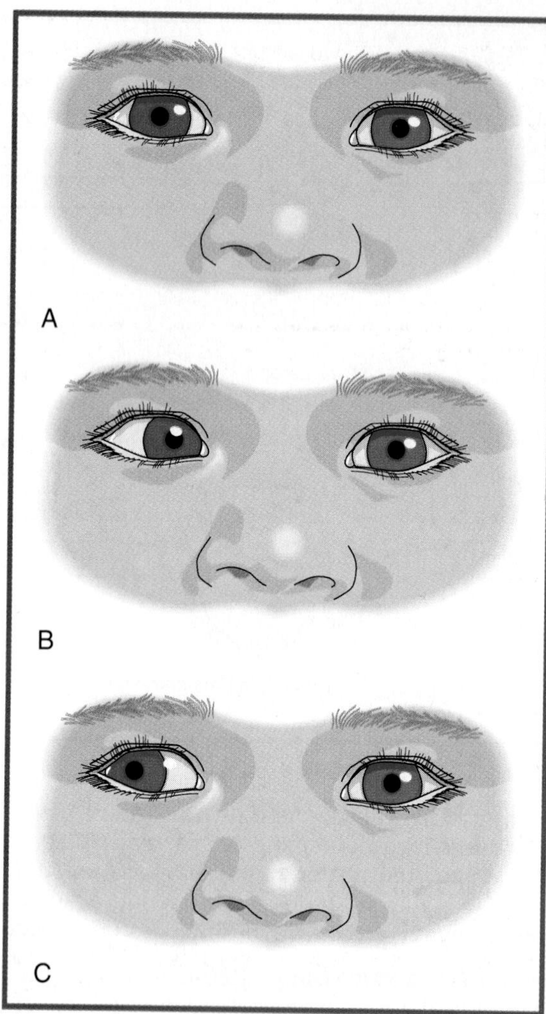

FIGURE 31–4 Strabismus. *A*, Normal. *B*, Right esotropia. *C*, Right exotropia.

Memory Jogger

 *State the four major types of refractive error.*

Strabismus

Strabismus is failure of the eyes to track together, which means both eyes do not look in the same direction at the same time. This is caused by weakness in the muscles that control eye movement. Adult development of any form of strabismus is almost always caused by a condition or disease elsewhere in the body. If this appears in infancy or childhood it is most commonly associated with **amblyopia.** Amblyopia is often correctable until approximately 7 years of age or until the retina is fully developed. The main symptom in all age groups is **diplopia** (Fig. 31–4).

Memory Jogger

 *Describe how amblyopia differs from diplopia.*

Disorders of the Orbit

There are many simple acute disorders of the eyelid that are frequently seen in the ophthalmology office. These include a **hordeolum** (stye), a **chalazion** (cyst), **keratitis, blepharitis,** and **conjunctivitis.** The treatment of these disorders depends on the causative agents. The commonly used treatments include combinations of warm compresses, antibiotic eye drops, and/or a minor office surgical procedure for removal or drainage of cysts (Fig. 31–5).

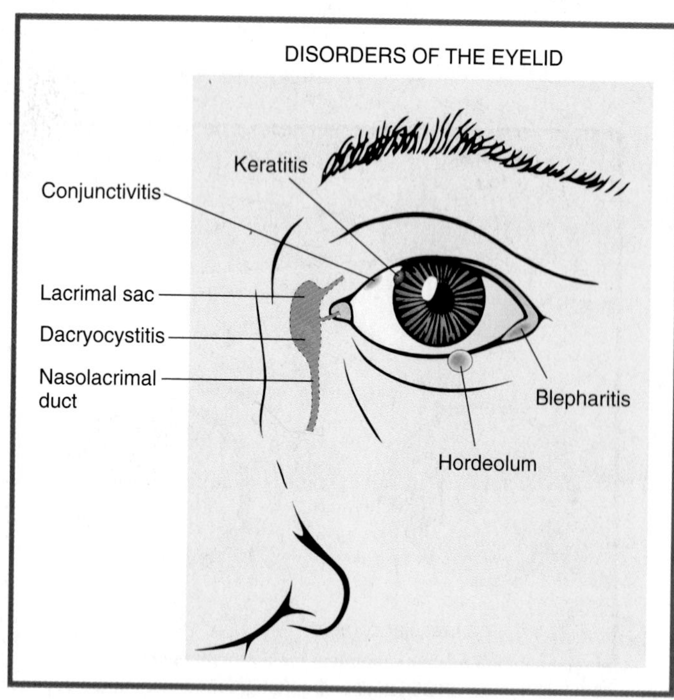

FIGURE 31–5 Disorders of the eyelid. (From Damjanov I: Pathology for the Health-Related Professions. Philadelphia, WB Saunders, 1996.)

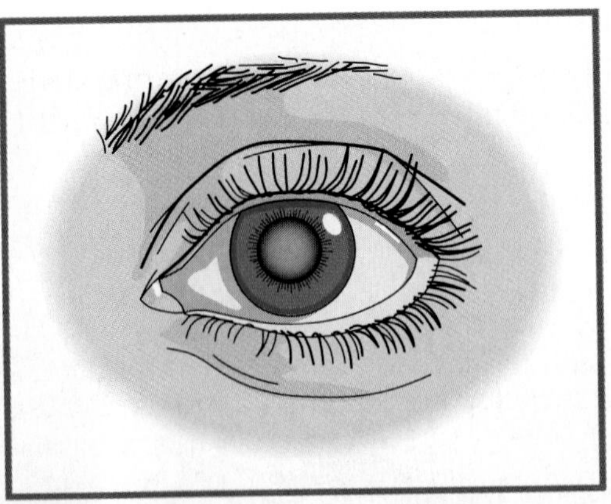

FIGURE 31–6 Cataract. Lens appears gray or cloudy.

Disorders of the Eyeball

Cataract

A cataract is a cloudy or opaque area in the normally clear lens of the eye. This condition may result from injury to the eye, exposure to extreme heat or radiation, or inherited factors. The majority of cataracts result from the natural aging deterioration of the lens of the eye (Fig. 31–6).

SIGNS AND SYMPTOMS Blurred and dimmed vision is often the first symptom of a cataract. The patient may need a brighter reading light or must hold objects closer to the eyes for better viewing. The continued clouding of the lens may cause double vision. Often the patient will need frequent changes of eyeglasses.

DIAGNOSIS AND TREATMENT When the patient's vision becomes distorted or appears to be deteriorating, the ophthalmologist performs a simple penlight or slit lamp examination (Fig. 31–7) to confirm the diagnosis. The only known effective treatment is surgical removal of the lens. This is often done as an outpatient procedure within the ophthalmologist's office. After the eye is anesthetized, the inner portions of the lens, the nucleus and cortex, are removed. The capsule is retained, and an artificial lens is slipped into place. The incision is then closed with tiny sutures, and the eye is bandaged for 24 to 48 hours. When the bandage is removed the person enjoys healthy restored vision. This procedure may be done through several methods, including freezing (cryoextraction), with a laser, and phacoemulsification (ultrasound).

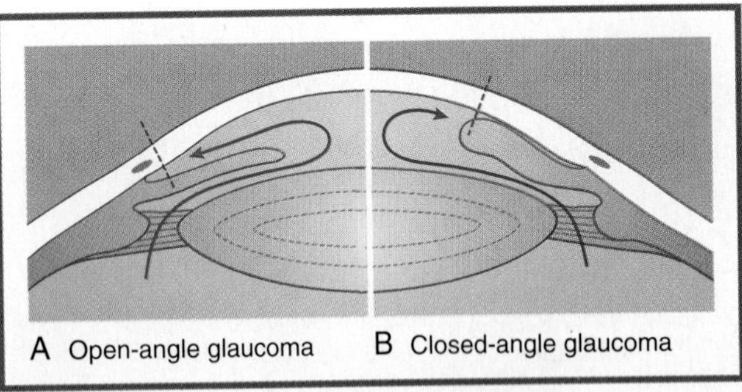

FIGURE 31–8 Glaucoma. (From Damjanov I: Pathology for the Health-Related Professions. Philadelphia, WB Saunders, 1996.)

Memory Jogger

What is a cataract?

Glaucoma

One of the most common and severe ocular disorders is a group of diseases known as glaucoma. It is characterized by increased intraocular pressure, resulting in pathologic changes in the optic disc that will eventually cause blindness if not treated. It rarely occurs in people younger than 40 and usually is seen in people older than 60. The cause is unknown, but there is a hereditary tendency toward the development of the most common forms. Glaucoma is responsible for about 12% of all cases of blindness and strikes about 2% of all persons older than 40 in the United States.

The normal eye is filled with fluid in an amount carefully regulated to maintain the shape of the eyeball. In glaucoma, fluid is formed more rapidly than it can leave the eye and pressure builds up. The increased pressure damages the retina and will eventually damage the optic nerve, interrupting the flow of impulses and causing blindness (Fig. 31–8).

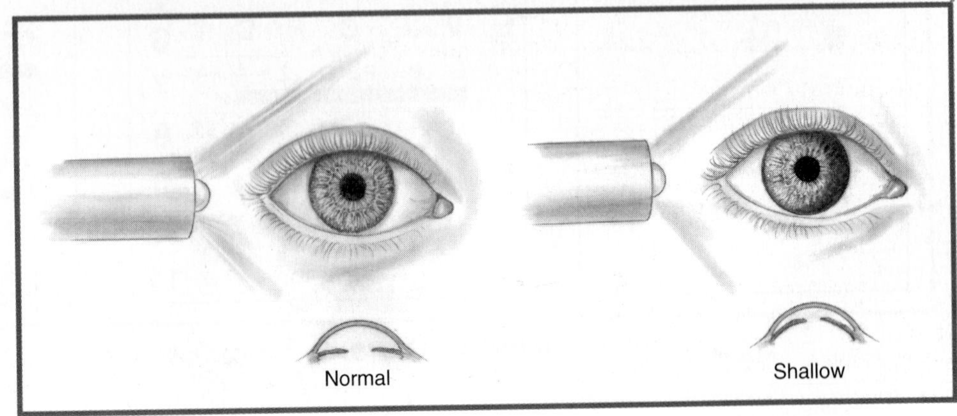

FIGURE 31–7 Light reaction/chamber abnormalities. (From Jarvis C: Physical Examination and Health Assessment, 2nd ed. Philadelphia, WB Saunders, 1996.)

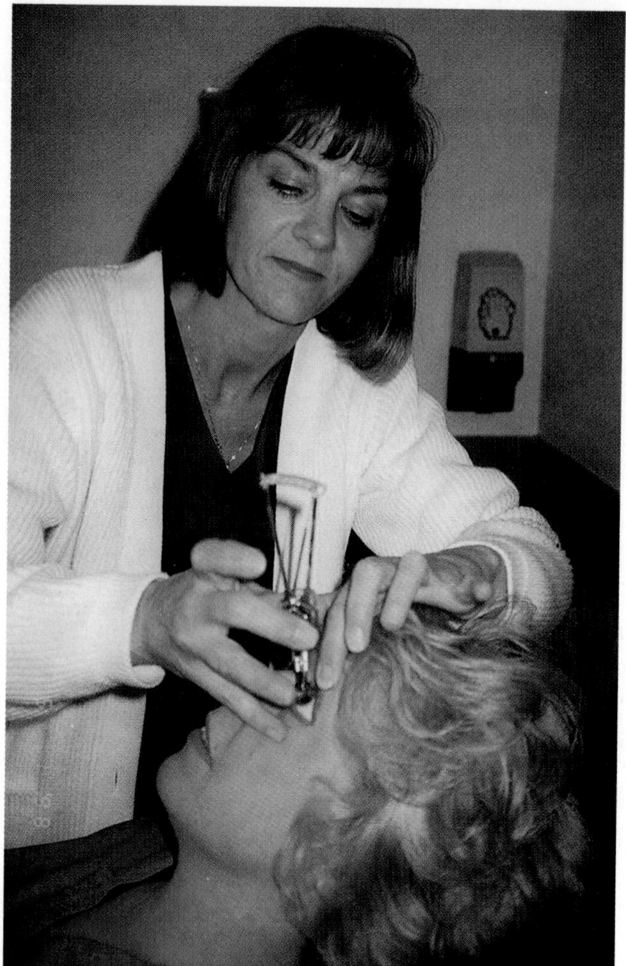

FIGURE 31–9 Tonometer.

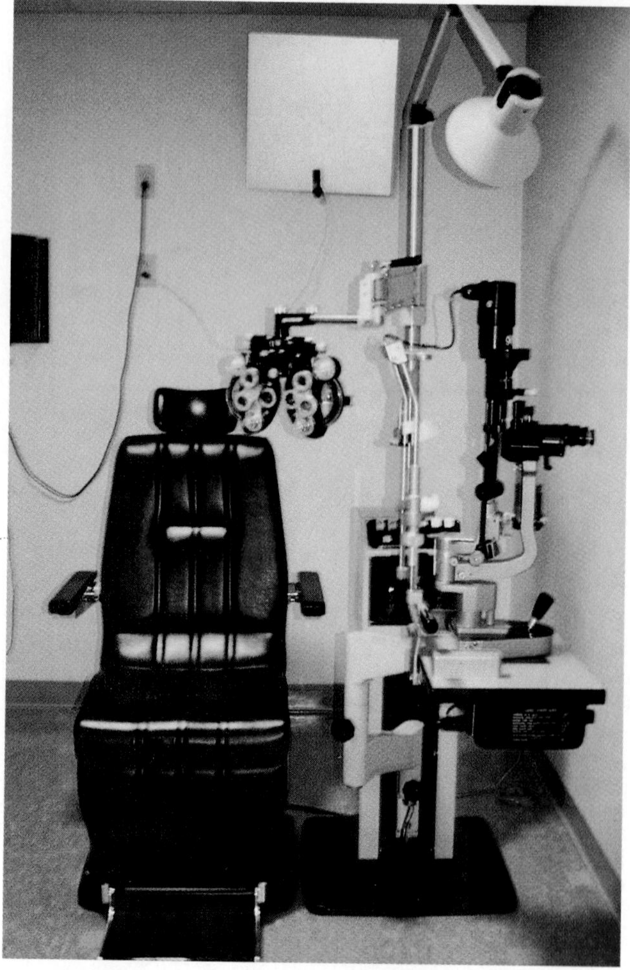

FIGURE 31–10 Ophthalmology examination room.

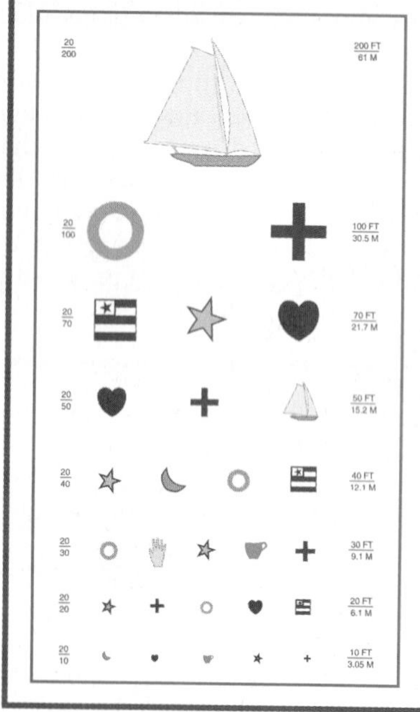

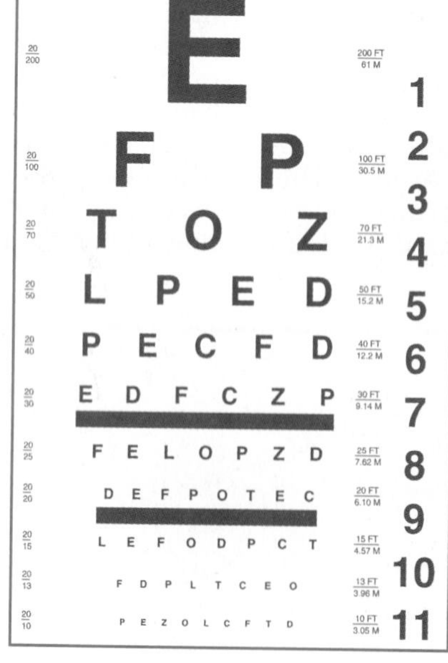

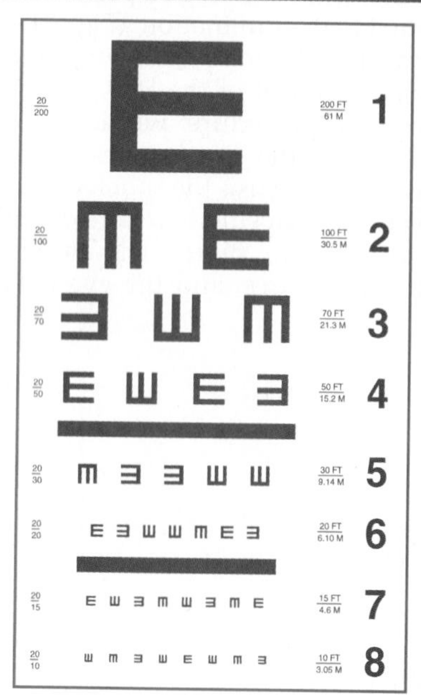

FIGURE 31–11 Different types of Snellen charts.

SIGNS AND SYMPTOMS Glaucoma may not cause symptoms. It is usually detected by an abnormal intraocular pressure measurement. The frequent need to change eyeglass prescriptions, vague visual disturbances, mild headaches, and impaired dark adaptation may also be present. If the patient has mild aching in the eyes, has loss of peripheral vision, sees halos around lights, and complains of reduced visual acuity especially at night, the ophthalmologist may suspect open-angle glaucoma, which is an ophthalmic emergency.

DIAGNOSIS AND TREATMENT Intraocular pressure is checked using the tonometer in most individuals older than age 35. The patient is placed in a reclining position or sits with the head resting back on a support. A topical anesthetic is instilled in each eye. After 1 minute, the patient is instructed to fix his or her vision on a spot in the machine. The physician then touches the sterile footplate of the tonometer to the cornea of the eye (Fig. 31–9).

When pressure increases, it can be relieved through eye drop medications. The combinations of drugs used to treat glaucoma can vary considerably. It is imperative that prescribed eye drops and oral medications be taken on an uninterrupted basis. The treatment for glaucoma must not be neglected. Occasionally, laser surgery may be used to seal off or destroy the diseased tissue. This is a relatively simple procedure that can stop or slow the progression of glaucoma.

Memory Jogger

Identify the risk group for glaucoma.

THE MEDICAL ASSISTANT'S ROLE IN OPHTHALMOLOGIC PROCEDURES

A complete examination of the eye is technical and requires expensive equipment and the expertise of an ophthalmologist (Fig. 31–10). The family practitioner does offer some basic examinations and treatments of the eye. The use of the ophthalmoscope to examine the retina of the eye is an essential part of every complete physical examination. The eye often reflects an individual's general health or may be involved in a systemic disease or injury. Reactions to a systemic medication the patient is taking may also be evident in the eye.

The most routine eye test, other than the use of the ophthalmoscope, is the distance acuity test, which is usually given with the *Snellen chart* (Fig. 31–11). This test may be administered by the medical assistant, who may also check the patient's near vision with the *near-vision acuity chart* (Fig. 31–12). This is especially done on the patient older than 40 years of age for possible presbyopia.

60

Nothing can take the place of "the only pair of eyes you will ever have." That is why you are exercising such good judgment in taking care of them as you are now doing.

50

For this reason, you will welcome the suggestion about lenses which are designed and made to give you "greater comfort and better appearance." In man's earliest days he had little use for glasses. He used his eyes chiefly for long distance.

40

He worked by daylight and at tasks with little detail. But now, you use your eyes for much close work—reading, writing, sewing and many other uses which the eyes of primitive man did not know. Now your eyes meet all sorts of lighting conditions, artificial and natural.

30

Many of these conditions produce "overbrightness" or glare. Sometimes it is the direct or reflected glare of sunlight; often it is direct or reflected from artificial light. And very often this glare is uncomfortable—impairs your efficiency. But special lenses, developed by America's leading optical scientists, combat this glare.

25

These lenses give you more comfortable vision and blend harmoniously with your complexion. These lenses are less conspicuous. We are glad to recommend them because they will give you greater comfort and better appearance. Thousands of satisfied wearers testify to their real benefits.

20

You are wise in taking good care of "the only pair of eyes you will ever have." You know how valuable they are, that you can never have another pair. For this reason, you will welcome the suggestion about lenses which are designed and made to give you "greater comfort and better appearance." In man's earliest days he had little use for glasses.

The above letters subtend the visual angle of 5' at the designated distance in inches.

FIGURE 31–12 Near vision acuity chart.

Testing a patient's color vision is important, especially if the patient is in certain occupations. By the age of 5, all children should be checked with color vision (e.g., Ishihara) charts (Fig. 31–13).

The eyelids are examined for edema, which may be the result of nephrosis, heart failure, allergy, or thyroid deficiency. **Ptosis** of the eyelid may be caused by a disorder of the third cranial nerve.

The pupils of the eyes are normally round and equal. Normal pupils constrict rapidly in response to light and during **accommodation.** This is demonstrated by shining a bright pinpoint light into one eye from the side of the patient's head. The pupil of the illuminated eye constricts, and the pupil of the other eye constricts equally. This test is called *light and accommodation (L&A).* An older patient's eyes do not accommodate as well as a younger person's.

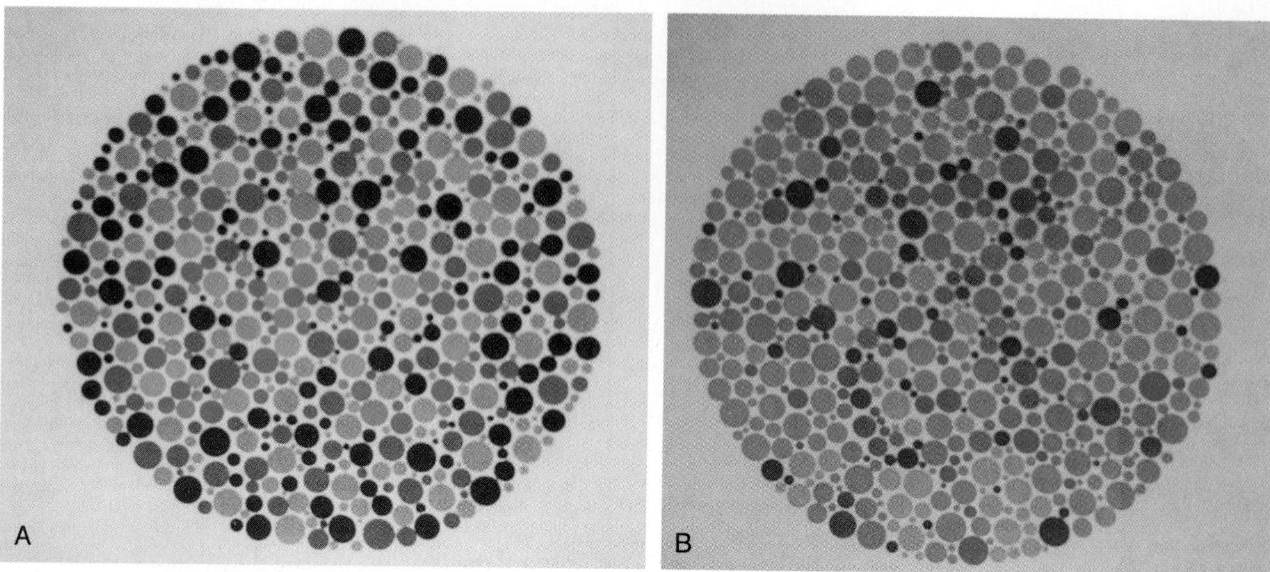

FIGURE 31–13 *A* and *B*, Ishihara color plates.

Each eye is checked this way. Then the patient is asked to look at the physician's finger as it is moved directly toward the patient's nose to check for eye coordination. If the pupils are equal, regular, respond normally to light, and adjust and focus on objects at different distance in a reasonable length of time, the physician will chart "PERRLA."

PERRLA

P = PUPILS
E = EQUAL
R = REGULAR
R = REACTIVE
L = LIGHT
A = ACCOMMODATION

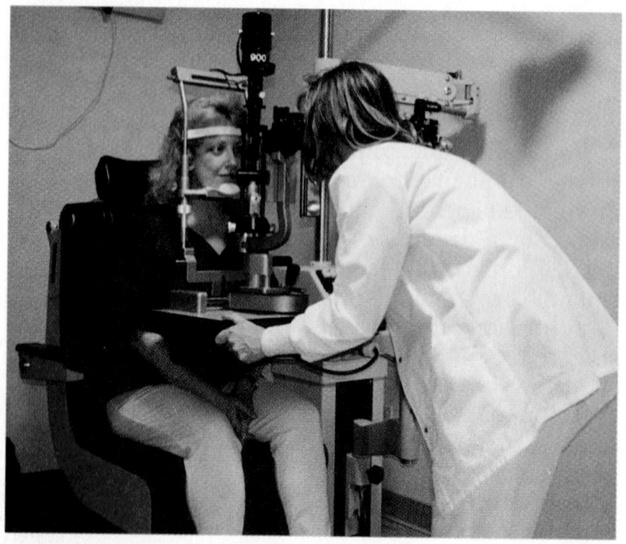

FIGURE 31–14 Slit lamp.

The ophthalmoscope is used for examining the interior of the eye. It projects a bright narrow beam of light that permits the physician to examine the interior parts of the eye and retina through the lens of the eye. It is helpful in detecting disorders of the eyes as well as disorders of other organs, the conditions of which are reflected in the condition of the eyes.

Special techniques employed in the ophthalmologist's office include the use of a slit-lamp biomicroscope (Fig. 31–14). This device is used to view the fine details in the anterior segments of the eye. It may be used to view a foreign body because it gives a well-illuminated and highly magnified view of the area. The patient with **exophthalmia** (abnormal protrusion of the eye due possibly to an overactive thyroid or to a tumor behind the eyeball) is checked with the **exophthalmometer.** This instrument is designed to measure the pressure of the central retinal artery. It is helpful in patients with circulatory disease because it measures the blood pressure in the retinal artery.

Memory Jogger

 *Name the instrument designed to measure the pressure of the central retinal artery.*

Distance Visual Acuity

Distance visual acuity is frequently part of a complete physical examination (see Procedure 31–1). It is widely used in schools and industry. It is the best single test available for visual screening. Many cases of myopia, astigmatism, or hyperopia have been detected by this routine test. The most common chart used is the Snellen alphabetical chart. This chart has various letters of the alphabet and is for general use. Patients with limited knowledge of the English alphabet can be tested with the E chart (see Fig. 31–11). In addition, there is a chart available that uses pictures as symbols (see Fig. 31–11). This chart is also used for preschool patients, slow learners, or mentally retarded children who have not yet learned the English alphabet. The symbol on the top line of the chart can be read by persons of normal vision at 200 feet. In each of the succeeding rows, from the top down, the size of the symbols is reduced so that a person with normal vision can see them at distances of 100, 70, 50, 40, 30, and 20 feet.

The patient must not be allowed to study the chart before the test. The room or hall should be long enough so that the 20-foot distance can be marked off accurately. The chart should be hung at eye level and illuminated with maximum light, without glare on the chart. The patient may be standing or sitting with the chart at eye level.

Most adults do not need the chart explained, but the assistant must have the patient's cooperation. With the E chart, for example, an explanation must be given as to how the Es are to be read. The patient may point up or down or right or left. The patient may prefer to hold three fingers in the same direction that the letter is facing. Use the same routine each time the patient is tested, by starting with the right eye. If the patient is wearing glasses, the physician may want the eyes tested first with the glasses on and then without them. Indicate on the patient's record "with" or "without." Test one eye at a time. Both eyes are to be kept open during the test, but the eye not being tested is to be covered with a paper cup or a piece of cardboard (Fig. 31–15). If there is no occluder available, the paper cup is best because it does not touch the eye. Under no circumstances should the patient use fingers to hold the eye closed because any applied pressure will interfere with visual acuity.

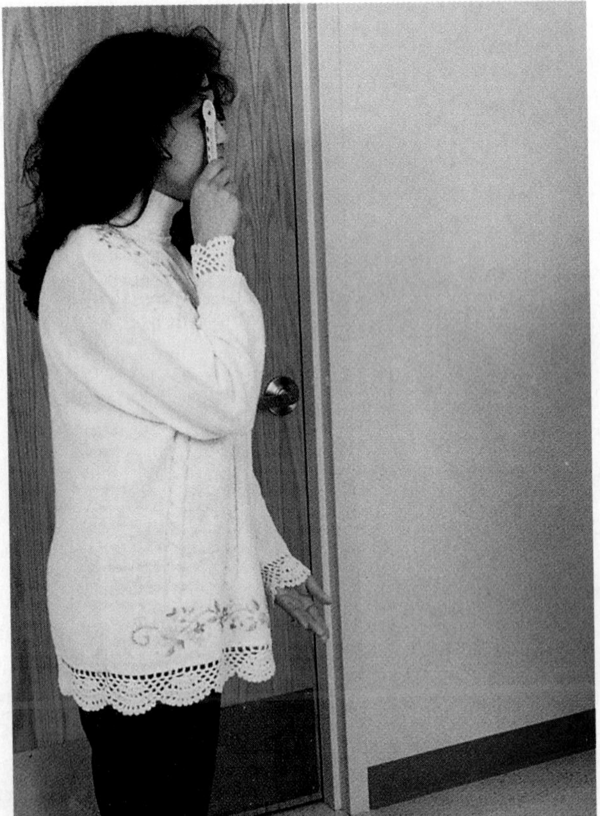

FIGURE 31–15 Using the occluder to block the eye not being tested.

Allow a moment between changing eyes. The medical assistant should stand beside the chart and point to the line to be read. Start with the line having the larger symbols, and then proceed to the lower lines. Record the smallest line that the patient can read without a mistake, and also record any behavioral observations such as squinting, straining, tearing, or turning of the head. Record the responses of each eye separately. The response is recorded as a fraction. The numerator (top number) is the distance of the patient from the chart, the denominator (bottom number) is the lowest line read satisfactorily by the patient. For example, if the patient reads the 20 line at 20 feet, the fraction 20/20 is recorded for that eye. Make certain the record reads "right eye" (OD), "left eye" (OS), and both eyes (OU).

Memory Jogger

 *When recording the Snellen test results, does the numerator reflect distance or acuity?*

PROCEDURE 31-1

Measuring Distance Visual Acuity Using the Snellen Chart

GOAL

To determine the patient's degree of visual clarity at a measured distance, using the Snellen chart.

EQUIPMENT AND SUPPLIES

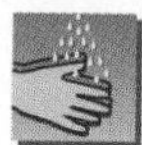

Snellen eye chart
Eye cover
Pen or pencil and paper

PROCEDURAL STEPS

1 Wash your hands.
PURPOSE: Infection control.

2 Prepare the examination room. Make sure that (a) the room is well lighted, (b) a distance marker is 20 feet from the chart, and (c) the chart is placed at eye level.

3 Identify the patient, and explain the procedure.
PURPOSE: Explanations help gain patient cooperation and alleviate apprehension.

4 Position the patient in a standing or sitting position at the 20-foot marker (Figure 1).
PURPOSE: Twenty feet is the standard testing distance.

5 Position the Snellen chart at eye level to the patient. If the patient is seated, have the patient's eyes even with the 20″ line on the chart.

6 Cover the patient's left eye (Figure 2).
PURPOSE: The right eye is traditionally tested first.

Continued

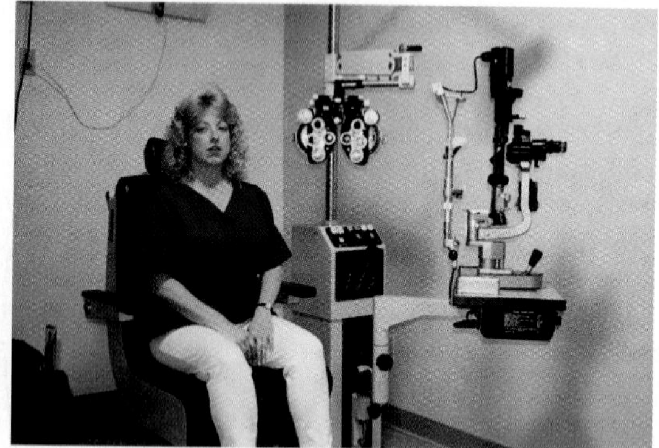

FIGURE 1

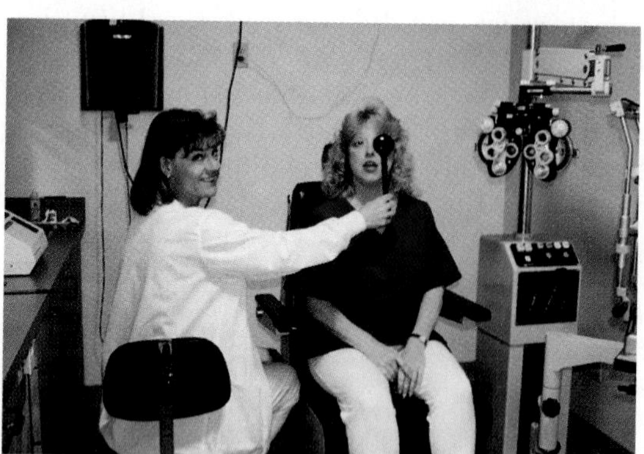

FIGURE 2

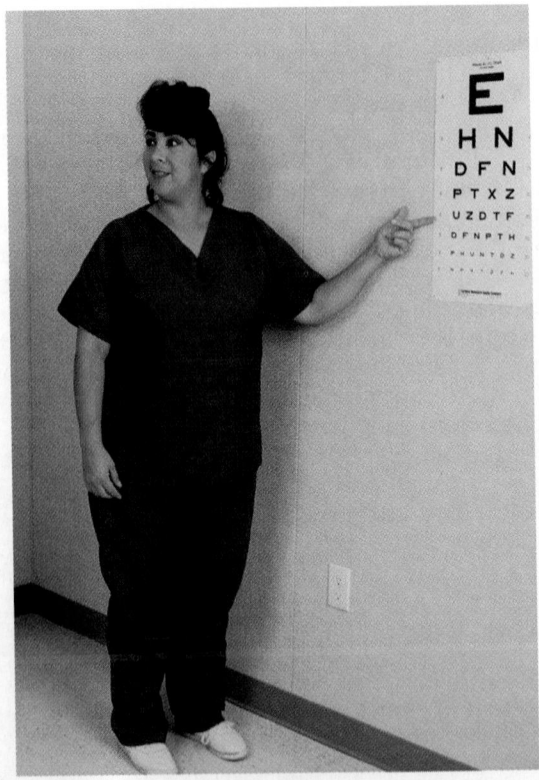

FIGURE 3

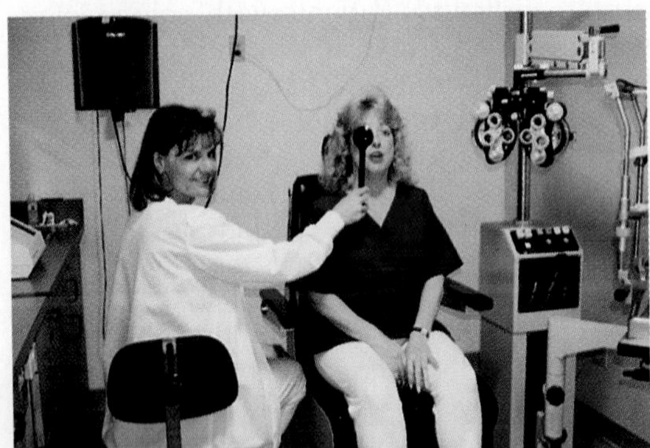

FIGURE 4

7 Stand beside the chart, and point to each row as the patient orally reads down the chart, starting with the 20/200 row (Figure 3).
PURPOSE: Starting with larger letters allows the patient to gain confidence and allows accommodation of vision.

8 Record any patient reactions in reading the chart.
PURPOSE: Reactions such as squinting, leaning, tearing, or blinking may indicate that the patient is experiencing difficulty with the test.

9 Record the smallest line that the patient can read without making a mistake.

10 Repeat the procedure on the other eye (Figure 4).

11 Enter the procedure and the results on the patient's record.
PURPOSE: Procedures that are not recorded are considered not done.

The Ishihara Color Vision Test

Defects in color vision are classified as either congenital or acquired. Congenital defects are the most common and are found in 8% of men and 5% of women. The Ishihara test is a simple, convenient, and accurate procedure that detects total colorblindness as well as the red-green blindness that is prevalent in congenital blindness (see Procedure 31–2). The test assesses the perception of primary color as well as shades of colors.

The test booklet contains polychromatic plates made up of colored dots in numerical patterns. The numbers are one color, and the background dots are a different color. Patients with average visual acuity will be able to read the numbers within the dot matrix without difficulty. Patients with color vision defects will not be able to read the number or will see a totally different number. There is also a section of plates that contain colored line trails through a background of dots. These plates are designed to be used on children or adults who are not able to read numbers. In this situation, the patient is asked to take his or her finger and follow the dotted trail through the picture.

When you are asked to perform this test, it is important that you do so in a quiet room that is well illuminated by sunlight and not artificial lighting. If this is not possible, create the best situation possible. If there is a quiet outside patio area, use it or try to set the electric lights to create an artificial sunlight effect. The test uses 14 color plates. The basic test consists of plates 1 through 11. Plates 12 through 14 are used if the patient appears to be having difficulty with the red-green differentiations, and it is not necessary to use plates 12 and 14. If the patient appears to have average-range color perception. The medical assistant records the number of plates that were read correctly. If the results are 10 or greater, the patient is within the average range. If the score is 7 or less, the patient is suspected of having a color deficiency and the ophthalmologist will perform additional assessment tests using more precise color vision testing equipment.

The test booklet is designed in such a way that it is very unusual for the final score to be 8 or 9. The patient with a color vision deficit generally does not read 8 or 9 plates correctly.

Memory Jogger

State two classifications of color vision defects.

PROCEDURE 31-2
Assessment of Color Acuity

GOAL

To correctly assess a patient's color acuity and record the results.

EQUIPMENT AND SUPPLIES

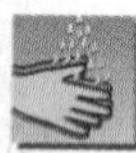

- Appropriate room area with natural light
- Ishihara Color Plate book
- Pen, pencil, and paper
- Watch with a second hand

PROCEDURAL STEPS

1 Assemble the necessary equipment and prepare the room for testing. The room should be quiet and illuminated with natural light.

PURPOSE: For testing colors to be seen correctly, natural light is needed.

2 Identify the patient and explain the procedure. Use a practice card during the explanation and be sure that the patient understands that he or she has 3 seconds to identify each plate.

PURPOSE: An informed patient is a cooperative patient. The first plate is a practice plate and is designed to be read correctly.

Continued

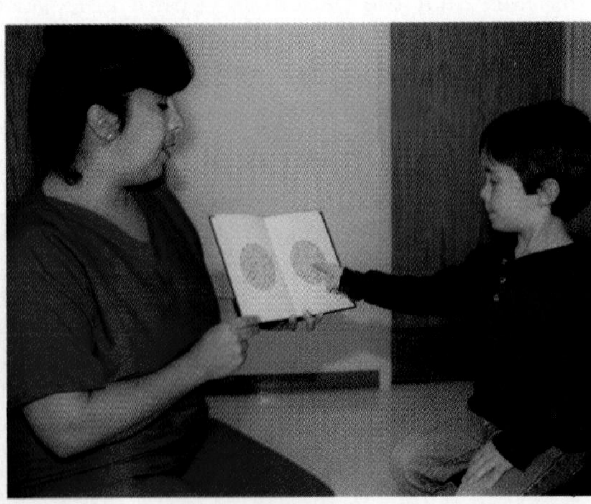

FIGURE 1

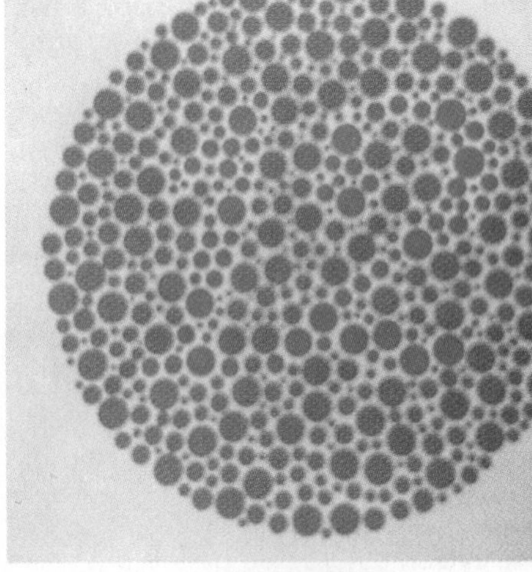

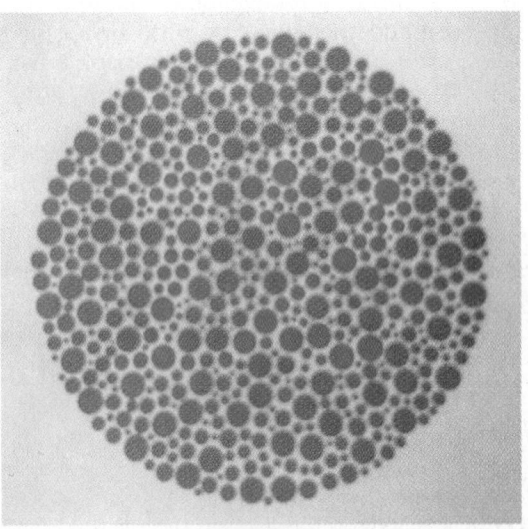

FIGURE 2

3 Hold up the first plate at a right angle to the patient's line of vision and 30 inches from the patient. Be sure both eyes are kept open during the test (Figure 1).

4 Ask the patient to tell you what number is on the plate and record the plate number and the patient's answer (Figure 2).

5 Continue this sequence until all 11 plates have been read. If the patient cannot identify the number on the plate, place an X in the record for that plate number. Your record should look like this:
Plate 1 = pass, Plate: 2 = pass, Plate: 3 = x, Plate 4 = pass, and so on.

6 Include any unusual symptoms in your record, such as eye rubbing, squinting, or excessive blinking (Figure 3).

7 Place the book back into its cardboard sleeve and return the book to its storage space. The Ishihara color plates need to be stored in a closed position away from external light to protect the colors.

8 Record the procedure and the testing results in the patient's record.
PURPOSE: Procedures that are not recorded are considered not done.

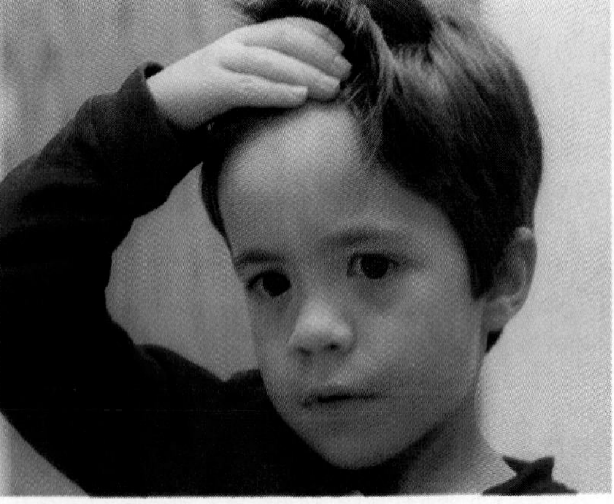

FIGURE 3

Eye Irrigation

The eye is irrigated to relieve inflammation, remove drainage, dilute chemicals, or wash away foreign bodies. Sterile technique and equipment must be used to avoid contamination (see Procedure 31–3).

When an eye irrigation is ordered by the physician, the assistant may perform the procedure, provided that he or she has completed proper training and is competent in the application of the technique. The solution should be warmed to body temperature (98.6° F). Follow the procedure as prescribed, making sure that the patient is comfortable. Always record the treatment on the patient's record immediately after completing it. Remember if it is not recorded, it has not been done.

PROCEDURE 31–3
Irrigating a Patient's Eyes

GOAL

To cleanse the eye(s), as ordered by the physician.

EQUIPMENT AND SUPPLIES

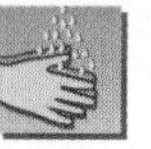
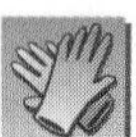
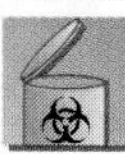

Prescribed sterile irrigation solution
Sterile irrigating bulb syringe
Sterile basin for solution
Basin for drainage
Sterile gauze squares
Disposable drape
Towel
Nonsterile gloves
Biohazard waste container

PROCEDURAL STEPS

1 Wash your hands. Put on gloves.
PURPOSE: Infection control.

2 Check the physician's orders to determine which eye (or both) requires irrigation.
PURPOSE: To check the abbreviations: OD (right eye), OS (left eye), OU (both eyes).

3 Assemble the materials needed.

4 Read the label of the solution three times.
PURPOSE: To follow the rules for administering medications.

5 Identify the patient, and explain the procedure.
PURPOSE: Explanations help gain patient cooperation and alleviate apprehension.

6 Assist the patient into a sitting or supine position, making certain that the head is turned toward the side of the affected eye. Place the disposable drape over the patient's neck and shoulder.
PURPOSE: This position causes the solution to flow away from the unaffected eye so as to reduce the chances for cross-contamination of the healthy eye.

7 Place or have the patient hold a drainage basin next to the affected eye to receive the solution from the eye. Place a polylined drape under the basin to avoid getting the solution on the patient.

8 Moisten a gauze square with solution and cleanse the eyelid and lashes. Start at the inner canthus (near nose) to the outer canthus (farthest from nose) and dispose of the gauze square (Figure 1).
PURPOSE: Debris on the lids or lashes must be cleansed away before exposing the conjunctiva.

Continued

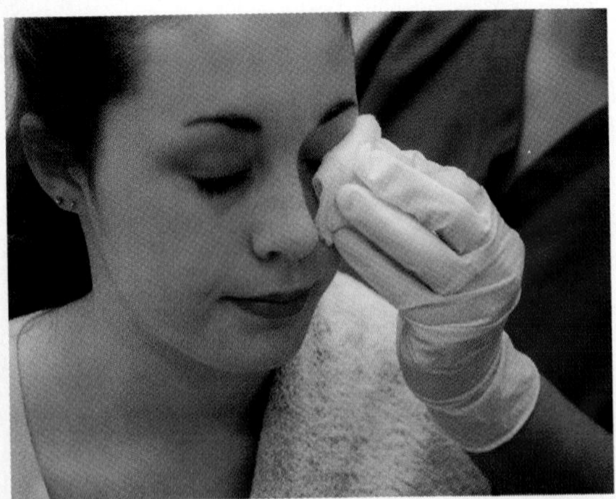
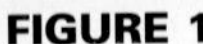

FIGURE 1

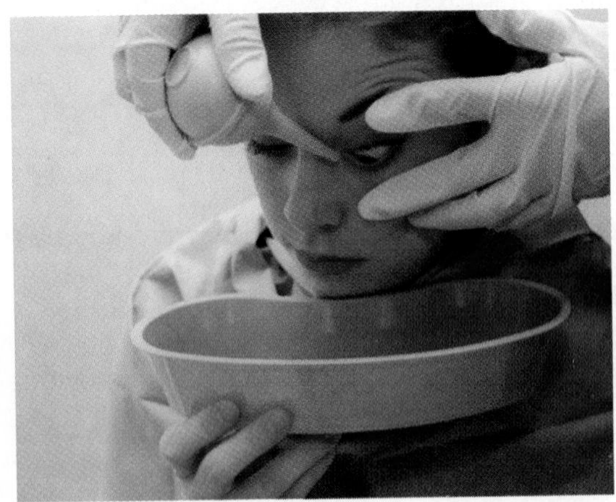

FIGURE 2

9 Pour the required volume of body-temperature irrigating solution into the basin and withdraw solution into the bulb syringe.
PURPOSE: Cold solution will cause the patient pain and discomfort.

10 Separate and hold eyelids with the index finger and thumb of one hand. With the other hand, place the syringe on the bridge of the nose parallel to the eye.
PURPOSE: To support and steady the syringe.

11 Squeeze the bulb, directing the solution toward the inner contour of the eye and allowing the solution to flow steadily and slowly. Do not allow the syringe to touch the eye or eyelids (Figure 2).
PURPOSE: Prevents possible injury to the eye.

12 Dry the eyelid with sterile gauze. Do not use cotton balls because fibers might remain in the eye.

13 Clean the work area.

14 Remove gloves and wash your hands.
PURPOSE: Infection control.

15 Record the procedure and the results in the patient's record.
PURPOSE: Procedures that are not recorded are considered not done.

Instillation of Medication

Medication may be instilled into the eye for treatment of an infection, to soothe an eye irritation, to anesthesize the eye, or to dilate the pupils before examination or treatment (see Procedure 31–4). Ophthalmic medications come in several forms. Liquid drops are usually in small squeeze bottles with tips that allow one drop at a time to be dispensed, or the bottle may contain a dropper with a small rubber attachment used to dispense the medication by drops. Eye ointments are dispensed in small metal or plastic tubes with an ophthalmic tip that allows you to dispense a small stream of ointment directly into the eye.

Safety Alert: Whatever the medication, the container is never to touch the eye while the prescribed amount of medication is dispensed.

Memory Jogger

List four reasons for the instillation of eye medications.

PROCEDURE 31-4

Instilling Eye Medication

GOAL

To apply medication to the eye(s), as ordered by the physician.

EQUIPMENT AND SUPPLIES

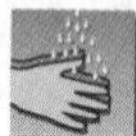
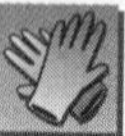

Sterile medication with sterile eye dropper or ophthalmic ointment
Disposable drape
Gauze squares
Nonsterile gloves

PROCEDURAL STEPS

1 Wash your hands.
PURPOSE: Infection control.

2 Check the physician's order to determine which eye(s) require medication and the name and strength of the medication you will be using.
PURPOSE: To prevent possible drug error.

3 Assemble equipment and supplies.

4 Read the label of the medication three times.
PURPOSE: To follow the rules for administering medications.

5 Identify the patient, and explain the procedure.
PURPOSE: Explanations help gain patient cooperation and alleviate apprehension.

6 Put on nonsterile gloves and rinse your gloved hands under warm water to remove all powder from gloves (Figure 1).
PURPOSE: Gloves assist you in holding the eye open and protect against the possibility of your hand slipping or your nail poking the patient's eye.

7 Assist the patient into a sitting or supine position. Ask the patient to tilt the head backward and look up.
PURPOSE: Looking up helps to prevent touching the cornea with the tip of the dropper. It also helps keep the patient from blinking as the medication is instilled.

8 Pull the lower conjuctival sac downward (Figure 2).
PURPOSE: Create a pocket for the medication.

Continued

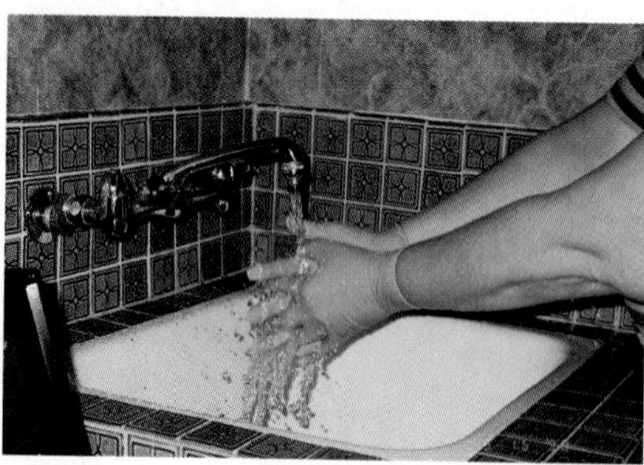

FIGURE 1

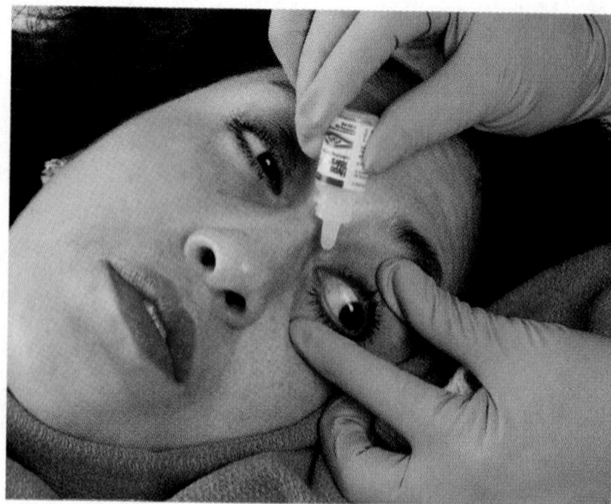

FIGURE 2

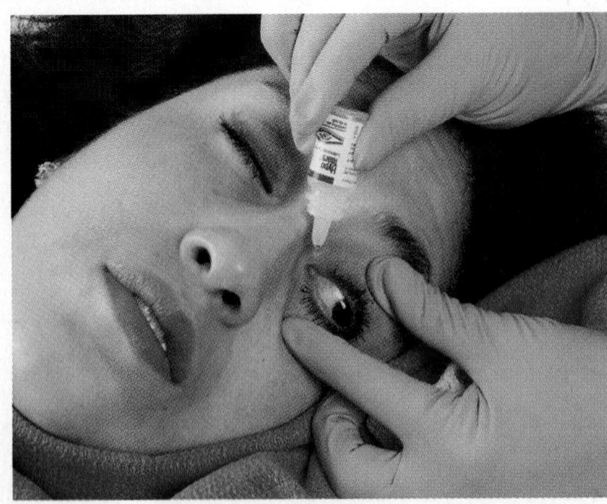

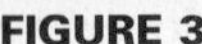

FIGURE 3

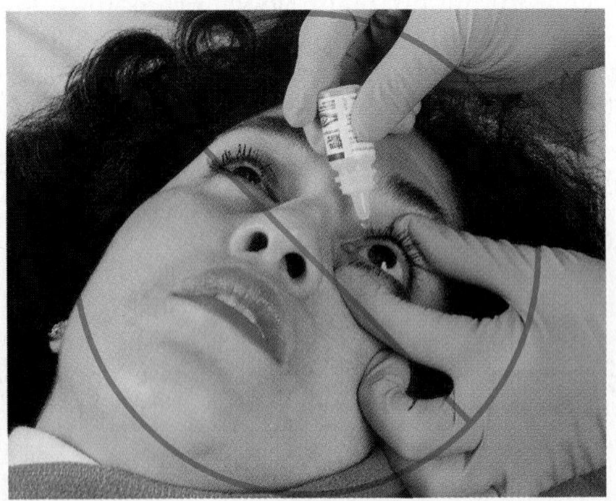

FIGURE 4

9 Insert the prescribed number of drops or amount of ointment into the eye, directly over the center of the lower conjunctival sac while holding the dropper parallel to the eye and ½ inch away (Figure 3).
PURPOSE: Never point the dropper toward the pupil of the eye or touch the eye with the dropper (Figure 4).

10 Instruct the patient to close the eye immediately and to rotate the eyeball.
PURPOSE: Rotating the eyeball distributes the medication (Figure 5).

11 Dry any excess drainage.

12 Clean the procedure area.

13 Remove your gloves and wash your hands.
PURPOSE: Infection control.

14 Record the procedure on the patient's chart.
PURPOSE: Procedures that are not recorded are considered not done.

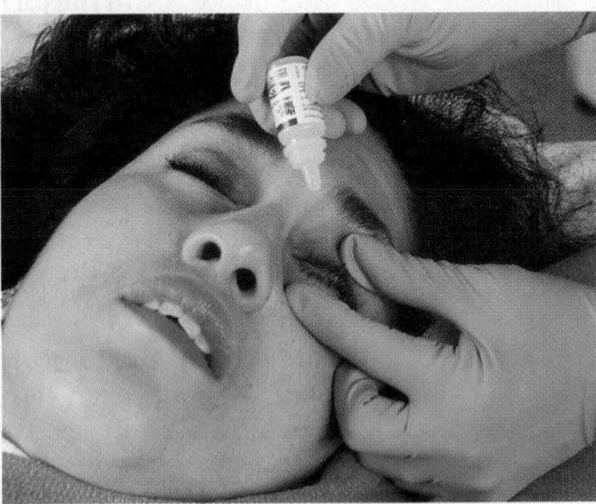

FIGURE 5

Aseptic Procedures in Ophthalmology

A major concern in ophthalmologic procedures is the careless use of eye ointment and the careless handling of the medicine dropper. The use of stock eye irrigation solutions has been discouraged because of the dangers of the solution's becoming contaminated with pathogenic bacteria. Eye ointments present a similar problem. The sterility of all eye medications is critical for good patient care. Newly opened sterile solutions must be used if there is a laceration or ulceration of the eye. All instruments used for the removal of a foreign body should be sterile. If possible, label and reserve a medication for the patient for whom it is prescribed and do not use it on other patients.

Foreign Bodies

Foreign bodies are very irritating and may cause considerable pain. They may be noticed on the eyeball itself, on the lower eyelid, or under the upper eyelid. If the foreign body is under the upper lid, the patient usually feels it when blinking. Most foreign bodies are superficial and can be easily removed. Occasionally, foreign particles may be deeply embedded and require eye surgery.

When a patient comes into the office and has something in his or her eye, notify the physician immediately. The first objective of the physician's examination will be inspection. The lower lid and most of the eyeball are easily visualized. The patient may be asked to look to either side and up and down so that the anterior surface can inspected. For the physician to fully inspect under the upper lid, the patient must cooperate by looking downward while the physician everts the upper lid using a cotton-tipped applicator. While maintaining the lid everted, any foreign materials may be rinsed away with sterile water or saline. Contact lenses may need to be removed to properly care for the eye.

If the physician gives the order for you to remove the foreign body, do so through irrigation only. If this technique is unsuccessful, cover both eyes with a gauze dressing and notify your supervisor immediately.

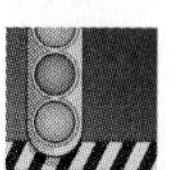

Safety Alert: Never attempt to anesthesize the eye or remove a foreign body from the cornea using an applicator, as scratches to the cornea may result, causing scar formation and impairment of vision.

Memory Jogger

11 *List the steps followed when looking for a foreign body in the eye.*

Examination of the Ear

Otorhinolaryngology is the medical specialty that deals with the ear, nose, and throat. It is frequently referred to as otolaryngology or even as a single specialty of otology or laryngology. Usually, the specialty otorhinolaryngology is referred to simply as ear, nose, and throat (ENT) (see Chapter 30).

ANATOMY AND PHYSIOLOGY OF THE EAR

The ears are only a small portion of the actual organ of hearing. Most of this structure lies hidden in the temporal bone. Anatomically, the organ of hearing is divided into three sections: the outer ear, the middle ear, and the inner ear (Fig. 31–16).

Outer or External Ear

The outer ear consists of the auricle or pinna, the fleshy part of the ear that you see on the side of the head, and the external auditory canal, the tube that extends from the auricle to the tympanic membrane (ear drum). The auricle collects the sound waves and sends them down the auditory canal.

The skin that lines the auditory canal contains numerous hair follicles, many nerve endings, and **ceruminous** glands that secrete cerumen (commonly called ear wax), which lubricates the canal. Both the hair and the waxy cerumen help prevent foreign objects from reaching the ear drum. The canal has a slight S shape to it and is approximately 2.5 cm long.

Middle Ear

The middle ear, which is sometimes referred to as the tympanic cavity, is an air-filled cavity that begins with the ear drum and terminates at the round and oval windows. It contains the **auditory ossicles** or bones—the malleus, incus, and stapes—and the opening into the **eustachian tube.** The oval window is closed by the stapes. The round window is closed by a membrane.

The ear drum, or tympanic membrane, is a thin disc-shaped membrane that totally seals off the outer ear from the middle ear. Sound waves hit this membrane and cause it to vibrate. These vibrations are picked up by the three ossicles and changed from air-conducted sound waves to bone-conducted sound waves.

The eustachian tube connects the middle ear with the throat. External atmospheric pressure and the pressure in the middle ear are equalized through this tube. This equalized pressure makes hearing possible. Throat infections may spread to the middle

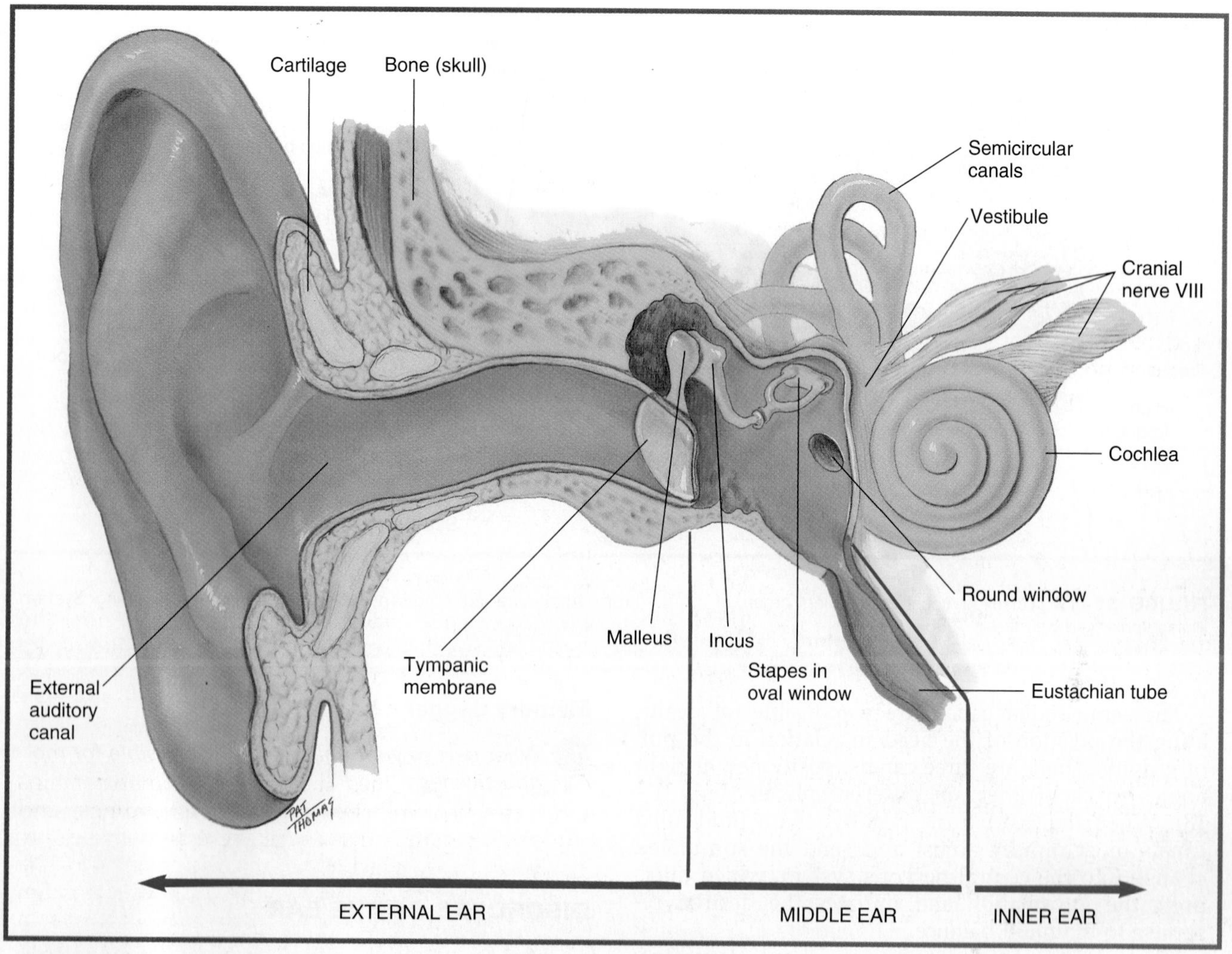

FIGURE 31–16 Anatomy of the ear. (Adapted from Jarvis C: Physical Examination and Health Assessment, 2nd ed. Philadelphia, WB Saunders, 1996.)

ear through the eustachian tube. This type of exposure is very common in young children.

The auditory ossicles are three tiny bones that are linked together through minute ligaments to form a bridge across the space of the tympanic cavity. As the tympanic membrane vibrates, the ossicles transmit the sound as bone-conducted sound waves through the middle ear to the oval window. Here these sound waves are moved into the fluids of the inner ear. This fluid motion excites the receptors, changing the bone-conducted sound into sensory-neural impulses.

Inner Ear

The inner ear is divided into the vestibule, semicircular canals, and cochlea. The vestibule and the semicircular canals function in the sense of equilibrium, and the cochlea functions in the sense of hearing.

The **organ of Corti** contains the receptors for sound and is located within the cochlea. These hair-like sensory cells are surrounded by sensory nerve fibers that form the cochlear branch of the eighth cranial nerve. Sound impulses cause the hairs to bend and rub against the nerve fibers, which initiate impulses to travel through the cochlear nerve (Fig. 31–17).

The eighth cranial nerve transmits auditory impulses to the medulla oblongata. Then impulses travel to the thalamus and then to the auditory cortex of the temporal lobe of the brain, where they are interpreted into audible sound and speech patterns.

Memory Jogger

12 *Trace sound from the atmosphere to the auditory cortex of the temporal lobe.*

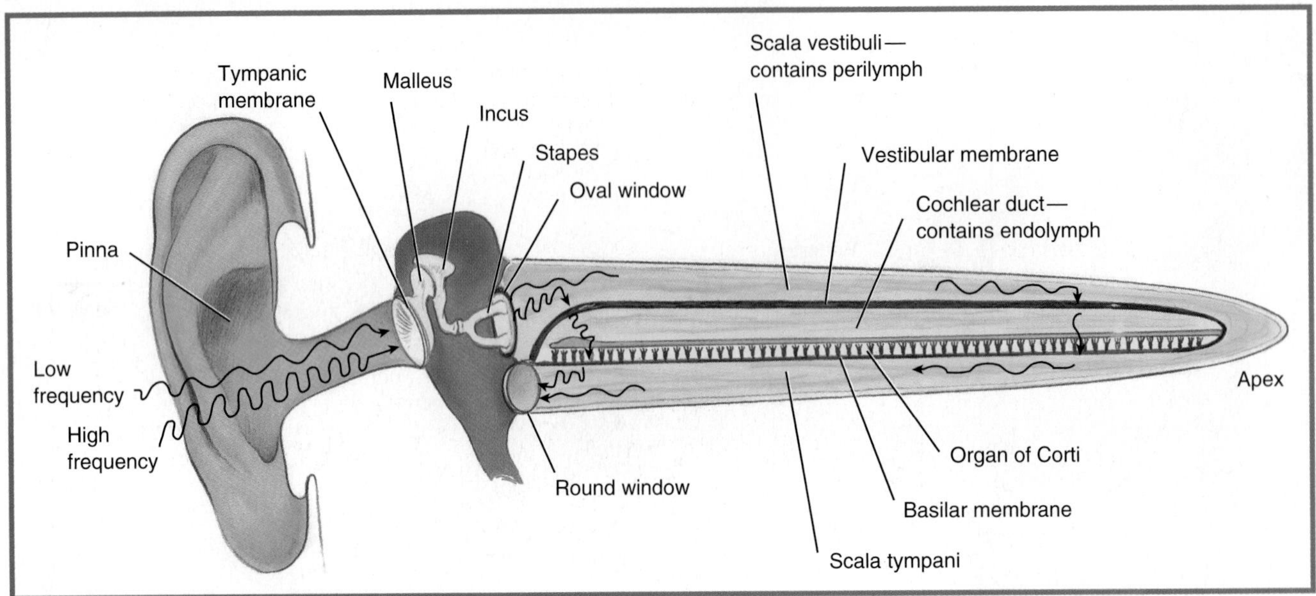

FIGURE 31–17 Uncoiled cochlea showing organ of Corti. (From Applegate EJ: The Anatomy and Physiology Learning System. Philadelphia, WB Saunders, 1995.)

The semicircular canals are responsible for evaluating the position of the head in relation to the pull of gravity. There are three canals, positioned at right angles to each other, on different planes (Fig. 31–18). When the head turns rapidly, these fluid-filled canals must rapidly adjust and send the stimulated change into the central nervous system, which interprets the information and initiates the desired response to maintain balance.

Through this interpretation, you can accurately judge objects around you when you are standing, lying down, or hanging upside-down. When there is repetitive and/or excessive stimulation to the equilibrium receptors, some people become nauseated and may vomit. This condition is known as motion sensitivity or motion sickness.

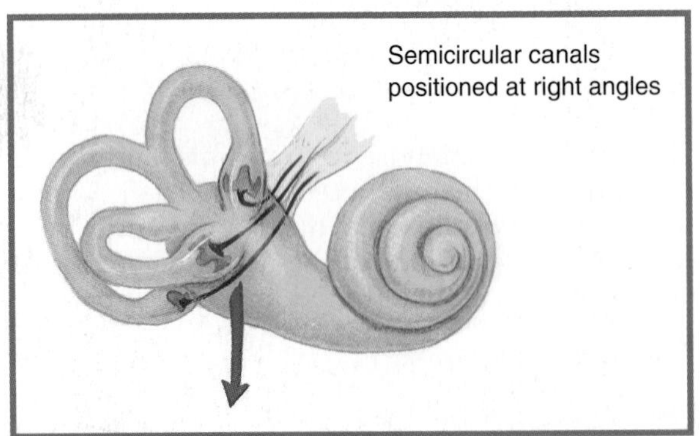

FIGURE 31–18 Semicircular canals. (From Applegate EJ: The Anatomy and Physiology Learning System. Philadelphia, WB Saunders, 1995.)

Memory Jogger

13 *What part of your anatomy is responsible for motion sickness?*

DISORDERS OF THE EAR

Deafness

There are almost 30 million people in the United States who have some form of hearing loss, and over 2 million of these are totally deaf. Deafness is classified into three types: conductive, sensory, and mixed.

A conductive loss is caused by a problem that originates in the external or middle ear. Some of the common causative factors include impacted cerumen, trauma to the tympanic membrane, hemorrhage in the middle ear, **otosclerosis, prenatal** complications, and recurrent chronic ear infections. It is the patient with conductive hearing loss who receives the greatest benefit from a hearing aid.

A sensory loss results from damage to the inner ear and especially affects the cochlea. Trauma from noise is often the causative factor. This trauma can be from pitch, such as a repeating noise in the workplace, or from intensity, such as listening to music with the volume increased to damaging levels. Presbycusis, the hearing loss of unknown etiology that affects elderly people, is also classified as a sensory loss (Fig. 31–19).

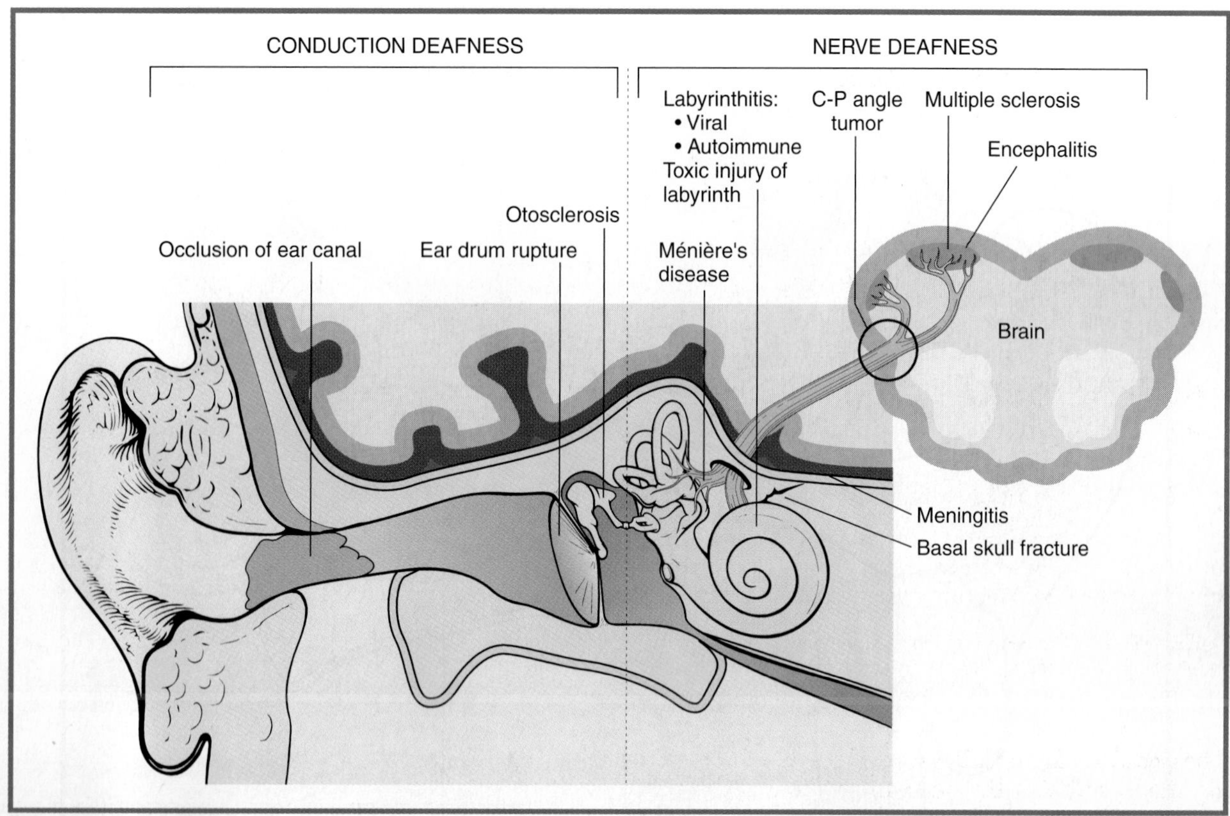

FIGURE 31–19 Causes of deafness. (From Damjanov I: Pathology for the Health-Related Professions. Philadelphia, WB Saunders, 1996.)

A mixed hearing loss is the combination of conductive and sensory deafness. This type of loss can result from tumors, toxic levels of certain medications, hereditary factors, and stroke.

Memory Jogger

14 *Identify three types of hearing loss.*

Otitis

There are two common types of otitis that are seen in patients in an otologic practice. The first affects the external ear canal and is called otitis externa, or swimmer's ear. Otitis externa may be caused by **seborrhea, psoriasis,** trauma to the canal, or through the continuous use of ear plugs. Swimmers frequently have otitis externa because water collects in the ears. The water may carry pathogens that can mix with the cerumen and form an ideal culture medium for bacteria and fungus to grow in. Rubbing can cause additional trauma to the canal and may worsen the condition (Fig. 31–20).

Otitis media is an inflammation of the normally air-filled middle ear, which means there is a collection of fluid behind the ear drum. In otitis media the cause is often associated with an upper respiratory tract infection that has spread through the eus-

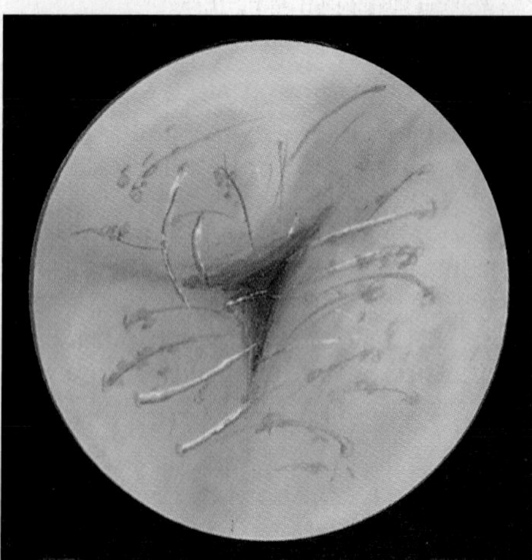

FIGURE 31–20 Otitis externa. (From Jarvis C: Physical Examination and Health Assessment, 2nd ed. Philadelphia, WB Saunders, 1996.)

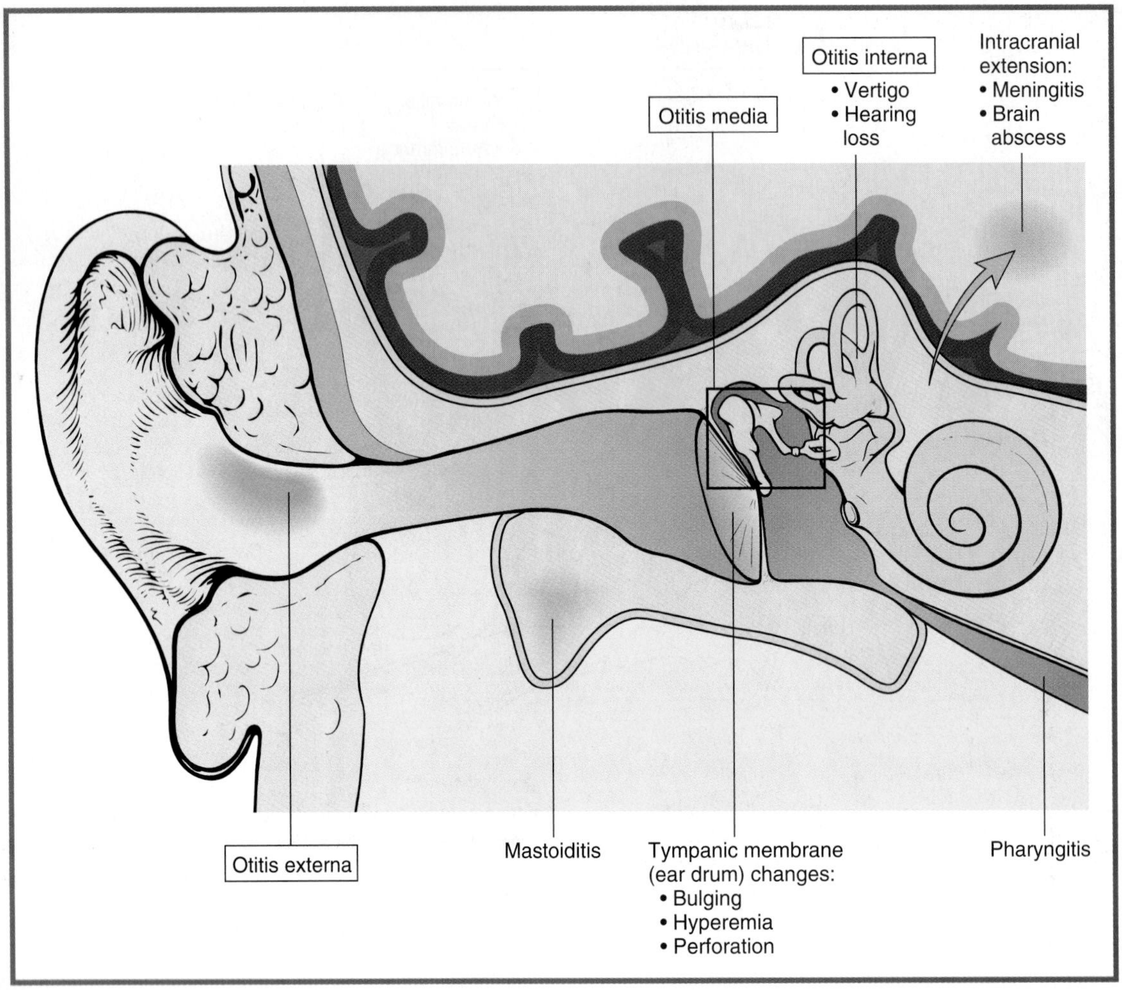

Otitis interna
• Vertigo
• Hearing loss
Intracranial extension:
• Meningitis
• Brain abscess
Otitis media
Otitis externa
Mastoiditis
Tympanic membrane (ear drum) changes:
• Bulging
• Hyperemia
• Perforation
Pharyngitis

FIGURE 31–21 Otitis media. (From Damjanov I: Pathology for the Health-Related Professions. Philadelphia, WB Saunders, 1996.)

tachian tube into the middle ear or as a result of an allergic reaction (Fig. 31–21).

SIGNS AND SYMPTOMS When an inflammation occurs in either the external ear canal or the middle ear cavity, it can cause severe pain. The canal becomes red, swollen, and tender to touch. The individual often experiences a fever, hearing loss, and a **purulent** discharge. The patient may also complain of the sensation of itching within the ear. Individuals with swimmer's ear will often use a cotton applicator to rub the inside of the ear canal to relieve the itching sensation. Individuals with otitis media often describe a sensation of fullness or pressure within the ear.

DIAGNOSIS AND TREATMENT Otoscopy shows the normally pearly gray ear drum to be inflamed and swollen, sometimes referred to as bulging. In otitis externa or if the ear drum has ruptured, fluid may be present in the canal, which can be cultured to determine the causative pathogen. The individual may be given antibiotics, **analgesics,** and often a decongestant to promote drainage. If this condition becomes **chronic,** the physician may recommend a myringotomy with the insertion of a tympanostomy tube (Fig. 31–22).

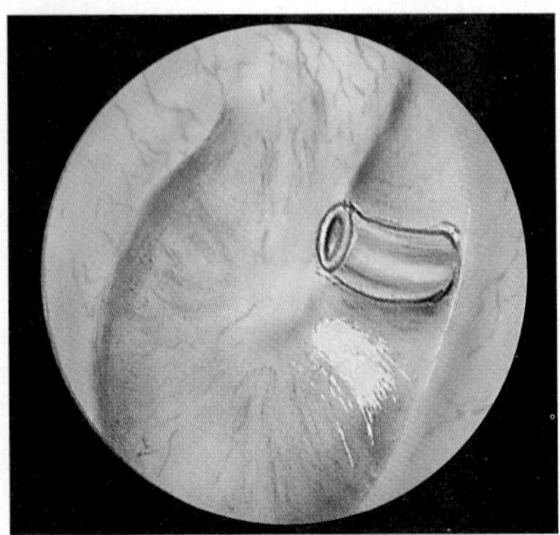

FIGURE 31–22 Insertion of tympanostomy tubes. (From Jarvis C: Physical Examination and Health Assessment, 2nd ed. Philadelphia, WB Saunders, 1996.)

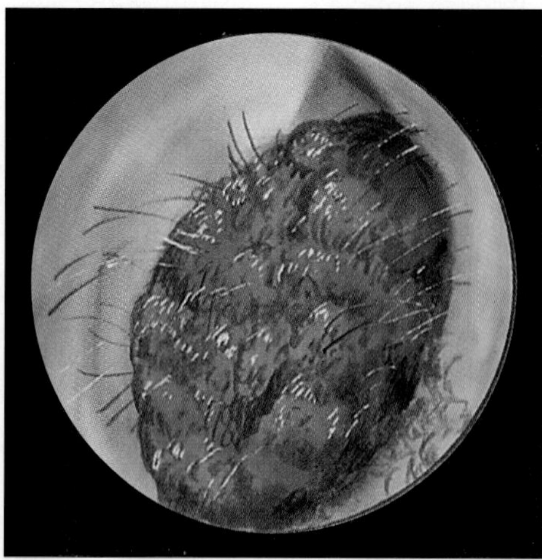

FIGURE 31–23 Cerumen impaction. (From Jarvis C: Physical Examination and Health Assessment, 2nd ed. Philadelphia, WB Saunders, 1996.)

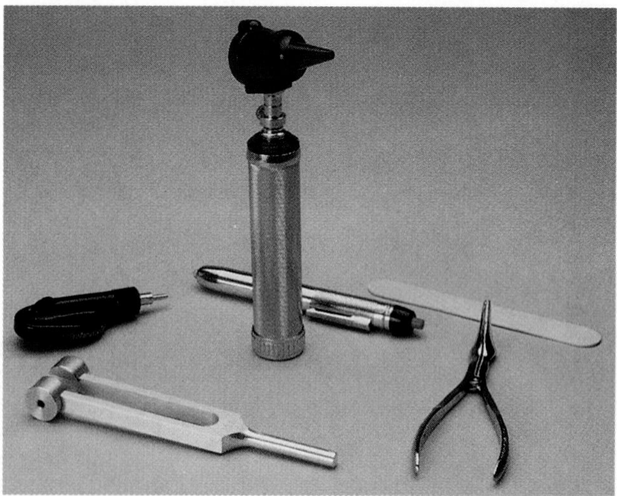

FIGURE 31–24 Otoscopy examination instruments.

Cerumen Impaction

Cerumen is normally a soft, yellowish waxy substance lubricating the external ear canal. An excessive secretion of cerumen can gradually cause hearing loss, **tinnitus,** and **otalgia.** Surprisingly, impacted cerumen that has pushed tightly up against the ear drum is a frequent cause of conductive hearing loss (Fig. 31–23). Individuals with abnormally narrow ear canals or who have an excessive amount of hair growing within the ear canal are more prone to this condition.

DIAGNOSIS AND TREATMENT A simple otoscopic examination quickly reveals this problem. If impacted cerumen is found, it must be removed. This can be done by softening the wax with oily drops such as carbamide peroxide (Debrox) and then irrigating the ear with warm water until the plug is removed. Because this condition can recur, the patient needs to have a schedule of periodic examinations. A hearing deficit diagnosis is always based on clinical data plus documented audiologic techniques and testing.

THE MEDICAL ASSISTANT'S ROLE IN OTOLOGIC PROCEDURES

The anatomic point at which the ear examination begins varies with the physician (Fig. 31–24). The external auditory canal is viewed with an otoscope or a light and an ear speculum (Fig. 31–25). The normal external canal contains a small amount of cerumen. Normally the ear drum is pearly gray and concave, but infection may cause discoloration, and fluids from behind the ear drum may cause the membrane to bulge. In addition to the otoscopic examination, the physician will palpate the area around the pinna for abnormalities or sensations.

There are a number of tests used to assess hearing acuity, ranging from simple tuning fork tests to quantitative and qualitative audiometric testing.

During the examination, the physician may perform a simple screening qualitative test by asking the patient to repeat a series of numbers or words that the physician recites in a quiet voice approximately 2 feet from the ear. The physician evaluates the patient's response for accuracy, speed, and fluency of response. When a hearing loss is suspected, the next test is usually done with a tuning fork.

Tuning Fork Testing

Tuning fork tests measure hearing by air conduction and bone conduction. In bone conduction the sound vibrates through the cranial bones to the inner ear. There are different-sized tuning forks, each with a different frequency. The most commonly used fork is the "c," which has a frequency of 1024 hertz, because this frequency reflects the level of normal speech patterns. To activate the fork, the physician

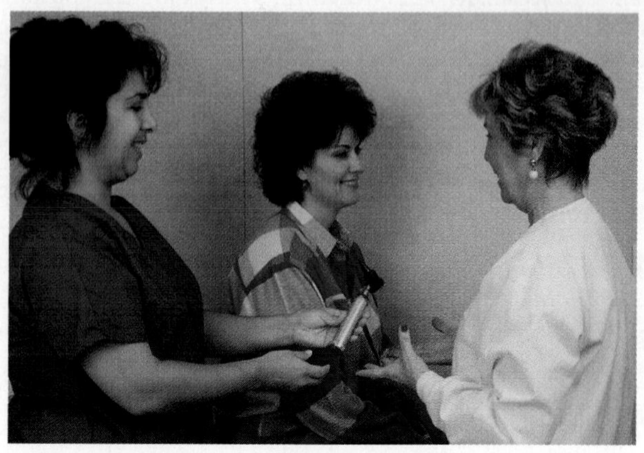

FIGURE 31–25 Examination with otoscope.

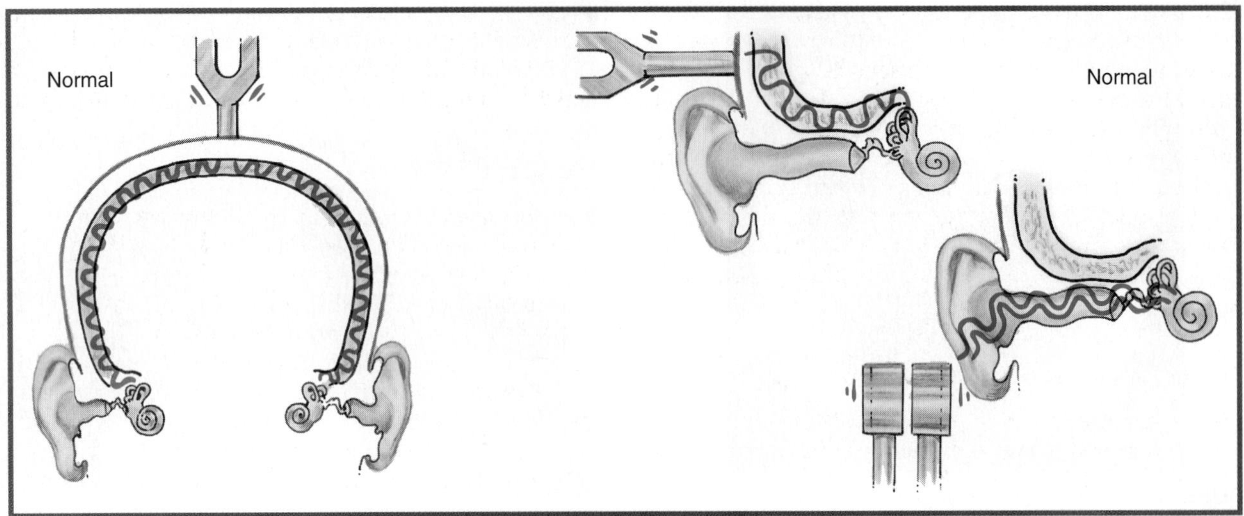

FIGURE 31–26 Tuning fork tests. (From Jarvis C: Physical Examination and Health Assessment, 2nd ed. Philadelphia, WB Saunders, 1996.)

holds it by the stem and strikes the tines softly on the palm of the hand. Striking the tines too forcefully will create a tone that is too loud for diagnostic use. The two testing evaluations that are used to evaluate hearing are the Weber and the Rinne tests. Both of these procedures are commonly used to evaluate conductive and sensory losses (Fig. 31–26).

The *Weber test* is used if the patient states that hearing is better in one ear than the other. The vibrating fork is placed in the center of the top of the head, and the patient is asked in which ear the tone is louder or if the tone is the same in both ears. Because the patient is hearing the tone by bone conduction through the head, the sound should be equal in both ears.

The *Rinne test* is designed to compare air conduction sound with bone conduction sound. In this test the stem of the vibrating fork is placed on the patient's mastoid process and the patient is advised to raise his or her hand when the sound disappears. The fork is quickly inverted so that the vibrating tines are approximately 1 inch in front of the external ear canal. If the hearing is normal, the patient should still hear a sound. In normal hearing the sound is heard twice as long by air conduction as by bone conduction. The normal response would be that air conduction is greater than bone conduction.

Memory Jogger

15 *State the value of the results from the Weber and Rinne tests.*

Audiometric Testing

A simple audiometric test may be done in the otologic office; and if the medical assistant has received additional training in audiometric testing, this test may be done by the assistant. It consists of hearing different levels of tones at different intensity levels and it is commonly done in elementary schools to evaluate the hearing levels of young children (Fig. 31–27.)

After the physician completes the screening test procedures, the patient may be given an appointment to see an **audiologist** for audiometric testing and evaluation. This testing consists of a battery of tests that evaluate the level of hearing impairment and provide valuable information as to how the patient may be helped. The testing is conducted in a quiet area that has no distracting noise. The first tests are usually to evaluate speech comprehension and to assess the patient's ability to follow instructions. Once this evaluation is completed, the patient is placed in a sound-proof booth and earphones are placed over the ears. From this point on, the audiologist will speak to the patient and conduct all testing through the earphones. The testing battery will

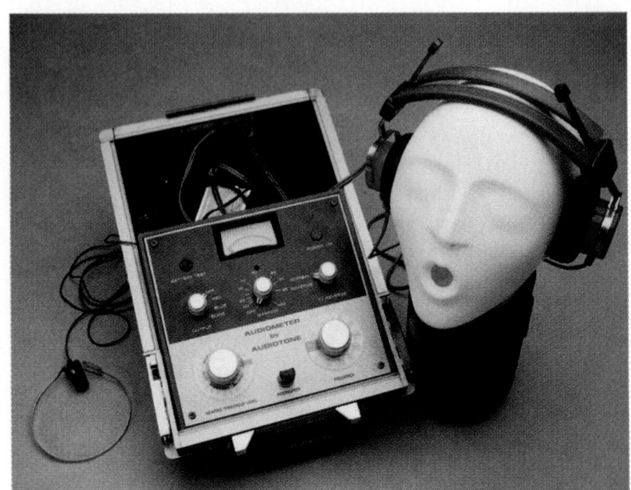

FIGURE 31–27 Audiometric testing equipment.

include testing the frequency, intensity, and audibility of sound. The testing usually takes approximately an hour. The patient receives no medication and will experience no discomfort. Most of the time, patients find the testing a pleasant experience.

Whatever type of testing is being done, it is important to remember that only one ear can be tested at a time because a hearing loss level must be determined for each ear. Frequently, the ear not being tested will be blocked with an ear plug or by **masking.**

Aseptic Procedures in Otology

Routine examination instruments are sterilized after each use and stored in a clean area. Surgical asepsis must be practiced when changing dressings, placing packs, and performing minor surgery. Dressing forceps must be sterilized after their use with each patient. Medications, such as ear and nose drops, must be handled carefully to avoid contamination.

Ear Irrigation

Ear irrigation is performed to remove excessive or impacted cerumen (see Procedure 31–5). When an ear irrigation is ordered by the physician, the assistant may perform the procedure provided that proper training has been completed and that the assistant is competent in the technique. The solution should be warmed to average body temperature (98.6° F). Follow the procedure as prescribed, making sure that the patient is comfortable. Always chart the treatment immediately after completing it.

PROCEDURE 31–5
Irrigating a Patient's Ear

GOAL

To remove excessive or impacted cerumen from a patient's ear(s).

EQUIPMENT AND SUPPLIES

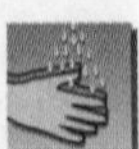

- Irrigating solution
- Basin for irrigating solution
- Bulb syringe or an approved otic irrigating device
- Gauze squares
- Otoscope
- Drainage basin
- Disposable drape with polylined barrier
- Cotton-tipped applicators

PROCEDURAL STEPS

1 Wash your hands.
PURPOSE: Infection control.

2 Check the physician's order and assemble the materials needed (Figure 1).

3 Check the label of the solution three times: (a) when you remove it from the shelf, (b) when you pour it, and (c) when you return it to the shelf.
PURPOSE: Prevent possible medication error.

Continued

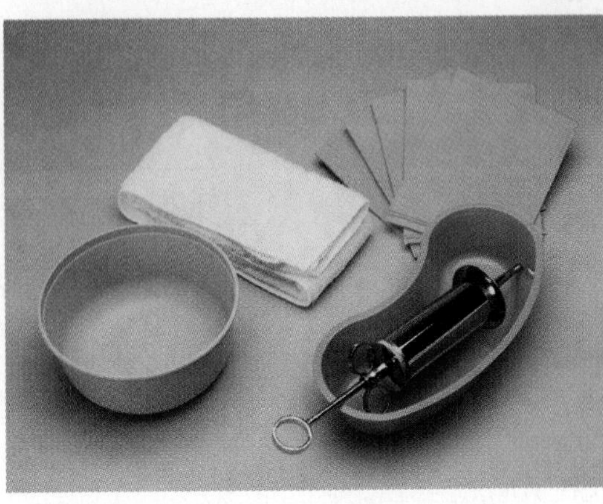

FIGURE 1

PROCEDURE 31-5 (CONTINUED)
Irrigating a Patient's Ear

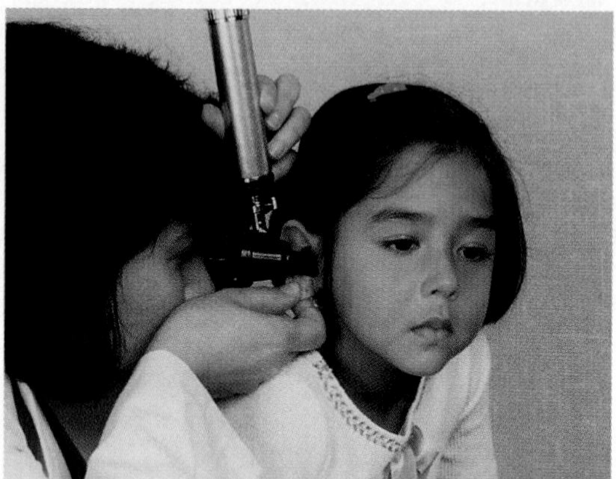
FIGURE 2

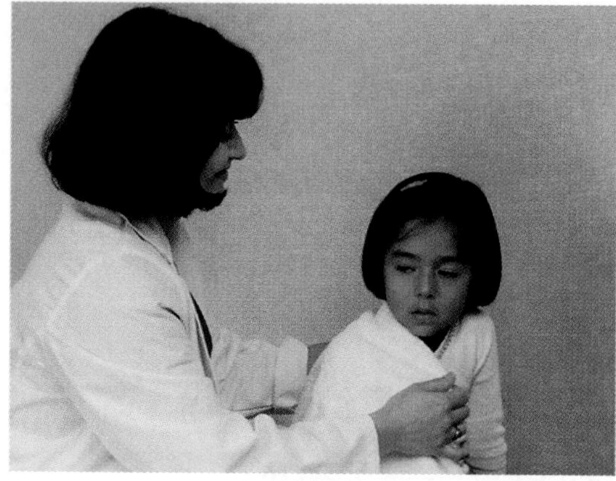
FIGURE 3

4 Prepare the solution as ordered. The solution temperature should be at body temperature (98.6° F to 100° F) to help loosen the cerumen.
PURPOSE: Solutions at 100° F are most comfortable to the patient. Ask the patient if the solution temperature is comfortable.

5 Identify the patient, and explain the procedure.

6 View the affected ear with an otoscope to locate impaction or a foreign object (Figure 2).

7 Place the patient in a sitting position with the head tilted toward the affected ear. A water-absorbent towel is placed over a polylined barrier on the patient's shoulder (Figure 3), and the collecting basin is placed on the towel flush against the base of the ear. The patient may be asked to assist you by holding the collecting basin in place (Figure 4).
PURPOSE: This technique will minimize the risk of getting the patient's clothing wet and will aid the water flow into the collecting basin.

8 Wipe any particles from the outside of the ear with gauze squares.
PURPOSE: This prevents the introduction of foreign materials into the ear canal.

9 Fill the syringe and flush warm solution through the irrigating syringe or apparatus and test to be certain that the solution is warm when it leaves the syringe (Figure 5).

Continued

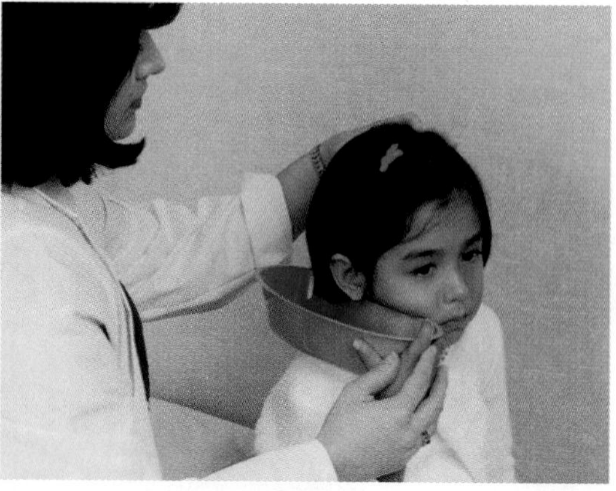
FIGURE 4

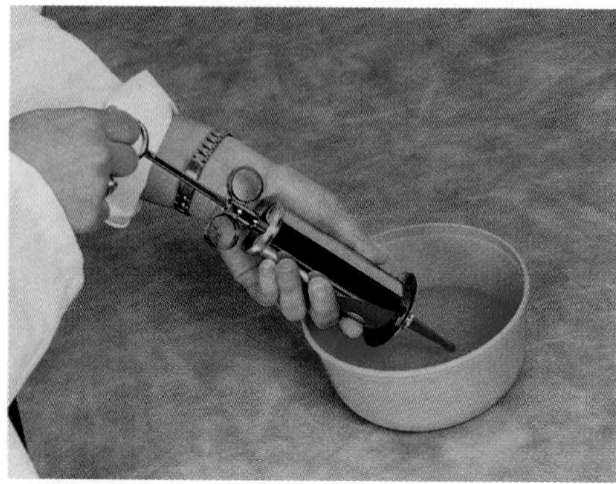
FIGURE 5

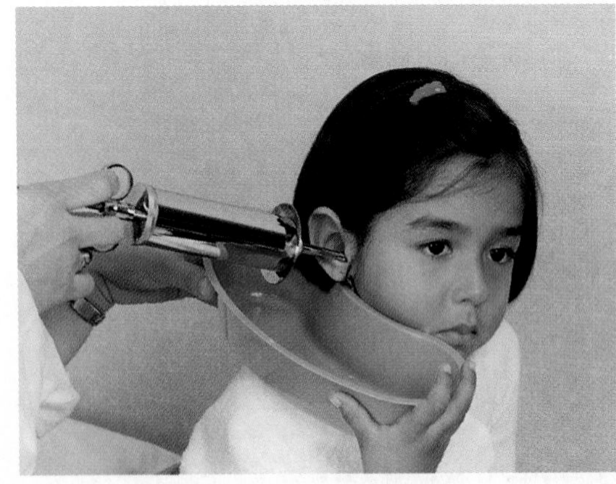

FIGURE 6

10 Place the tip of the syringe into the meatus of the ear.

11 Gently direct the flow of the solution (Figure 6).
PURPOSE: This will help to prevent injury to the tympanic membrane and will aid in the removal of the imbedded material.

12 Refill the syringe with warm solution and continue until the material has been removed. Note the particles in the collecting basin to evaluate when the material has been successfully removed.

13 Dry the patient's external ear with gauze squares and the visible ear canal gently with cotton-tipped applicators.
PURPOSE: Inserting the applicator into the canal may cause serious trauma.

14 Inspect the ear with an otoscope to determine the results.

15 Place a clean, absorbent towel against the freshly irrigated ear and allow the patient to rest quietly while you wait for the physician to return to check the affected ear.

16 Clean the work area, and return all equipment after it has been properly disinfected. Wash your hands.
PURPOSE: Infection control.

17 Record the procedure and the results in the patient's record. Be certain to include which ear was irrigated and the results of that irrigation.
PURPOSE: Procedures that are not recorded are considered not done.

Instilling Otic Medications

Medication that is to be instilled into the ear generally is given to soften impacted cerumen or to relieve pain or is an antibiotic drop needed to fight an infectious pathogen (see Procedure 31–6). The patient may be apprehensive and in considerable pain. Often he or she is hoping that these drops will provide immediate relief or at least lessen the level of discomfort.

PERSONAL QUALITIES

INSTILLING MEDICATION

You will get the best results when instilling medication if your voice remains calm and distinct and if your instructions are simple and direct.

Often the patient may be experiencing difficulty hearing, which makes this a poor time for conversation to evaluate the patient's understanding of his or her illness. Wait until after the procedure is completed or on a follow-up visit, depending on the condition of the patient.

Memory Jogger

16 *Identify three reasons for instilling medication in the ear.*

PROCEDURE 31-6

Instilling Medicated Otic Drops

GOAL

To instill the correct medication in the accurate dosage directly into the external auditory canal.

EQUIPMENT AND SUPPLIES

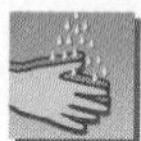

Prescribed otic drops
Disposable sterile dropper
Cotton balls

PROCEDURAL STEPS

1 Wash your hands and gather the needed equipment and supplies.
PURPOSE: Infection control and to reduce procedure time.

2 Check the medication order three times: (a) when you remove it from the shelf, (b) when you prepare it, and (c) when you return it to the shelf.
PURPOSE: To avoid possible medication error.

3 Identify your patient and explain the procedure.

4 Have the patient lie down on the side with the affected ear upward.
PURPOSE: Ensures patient comfort and encourages patient relaxation (Figure 1).

5 Check the temperature of the medication bottle. If it feels cold, gently roll the bottle back and forth between your hands to warm the drops. When the bottle feels at body temperature, open and withdraw the prescribed amount into the sterile disposable dropper (Figure 2).
PURPOSE: Cold medication may increase the pain level or cause symptoms of nausea and vertigo.

6 Hold the dropper firmly in your dominant hand. With the other hand, gently pull the pinna up and back if the patient is an adult or down and back if patient is younger than 3 years old (Figure 3).
PURPOSE: To straighten the ear canal and make it easier for the medication to reach its designated position.

7 Place the tip of the dropper in the ear canal meatus and instill the medication drops along the side of the canal (Figure 4).

Continued

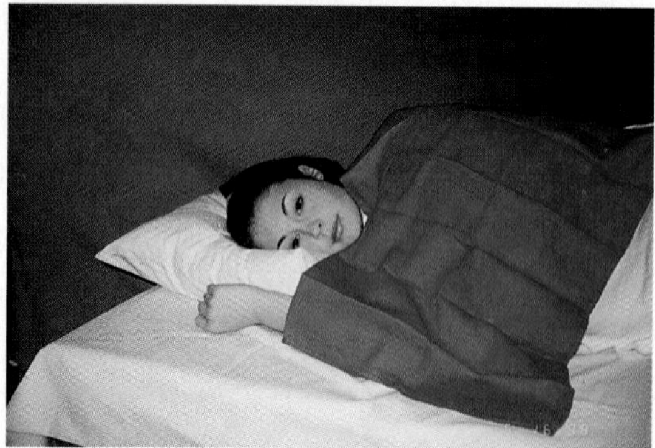

FIGURE 1

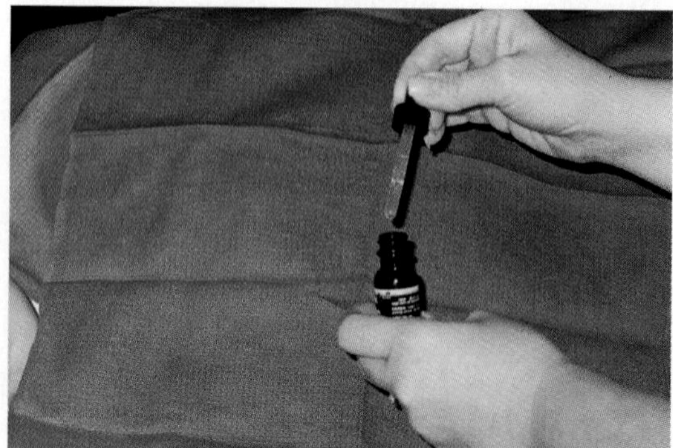

FIGURE 2

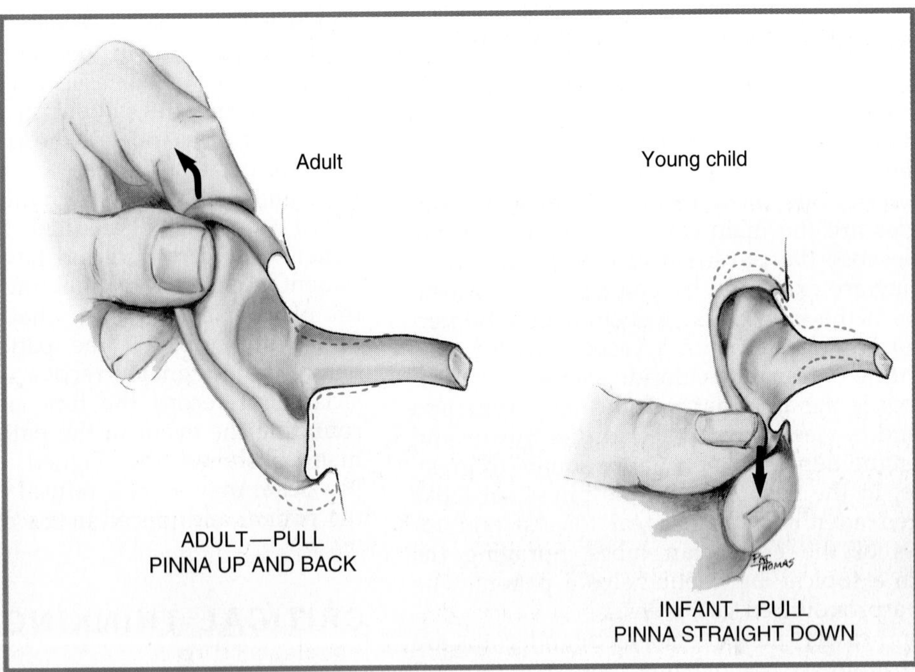

FIGURE 3*

8 Instruct the patient to remain in this position for about 3 minutes.
PURPOSE: This time will allow the medication to reach the base of the canal and will prevent it from running out of the ear (Figure 5).

9 If instructed by the physician, place a moistened cotton ball into the ear canal. The cotton ball is moistened with the physician's designated fluid.
PURPOSE: Protects the ear canal and inhibits medication from leaking back out of the ear.

10 Clean the work area and wash your hands.
PURPOSE: Infection control.

11 Record the procedure, including which ear, the medication, and the amount instilled, in the patient's record.
PURPOSE: Procedures that are not recorded are considered not done.

*From Jarvis C: Physical Examination and Health Assessment, 2nd ed. Philadelphia, WB Saunders, 1996.

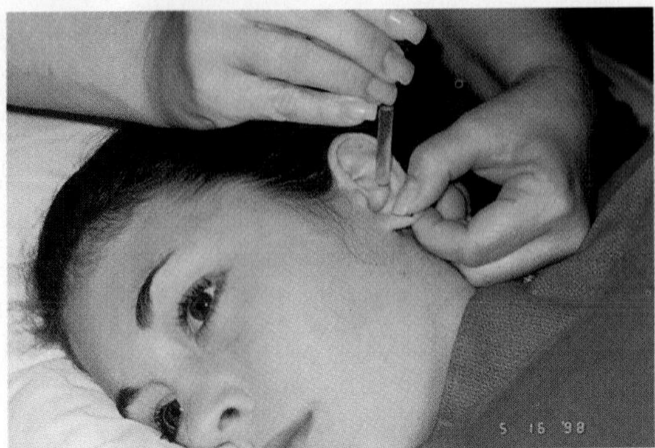

FIGURE 4

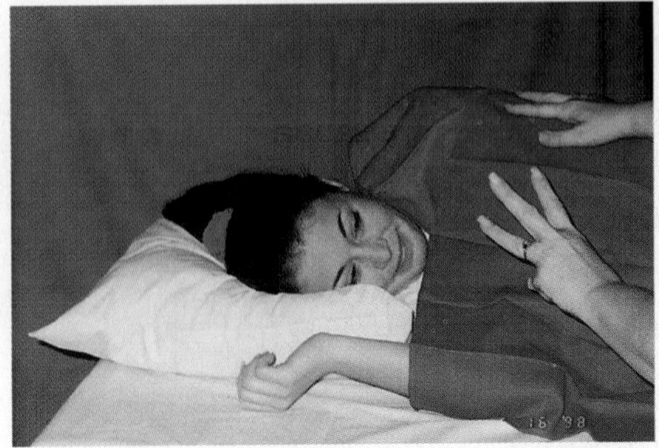

FIGURE 5

Examination of the Nose and Throat

If you are working in an ENT speciality office, you will also be assisting in the examination of the nasal cavity and the throat (see also Chapter 30).

Examination of the nasal cavity is mainly inspection of the mucous membrane. The common cold and allergies are the main causes of changes in the mucosa. Because the physician cannot see the nasal sinuses, they are examined by palpation and transillumination. If the mucosa is swollen, it may be necessary to spray the area with a vasoconstrictor such as epinephrine (adrenaline chloride solution).

The throat is the area that includes the larynx and pharynx and is viewed with the aid of a mirror and either a tongue depressor or a gauze square to grasp the tongue. In the nasopharynx, the physician looks for enlarged adenoids (pharyngeal tonsils) and for the orifices of the eustachian tubes. Spraying the throat with a topical anesthetic helps a patient who may have a pronounced gag reflex.

In the oral cavity, the patient's teeth and gums are carefully examined. The palatine tonsils (if present) are checked for size and the presence of crypts. The lingual tonsils are also checked. The salivary glands are palpated.

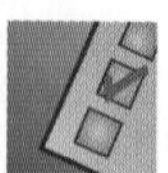

PATIENT EDUCATION

Unless you have personally experienced an eye or ear disorder that has rendered you with a temporary sight or hearing disorder, you can only attempt to imagine this very helpless feeling. Many patients do not want to talk or listen to someone explain why this problem occurred or how it could have been prevented. At this particular time, the primary thought is "get me through this and make me well." This is the time for good listening skills and accurate action. Of course, whenever a patient comes in sick, you need to be a good listener and take accurate action; but when the special senses are involved, you need to be even more aware of the nonverbal communication that can be implemented to show the patient that you do care. Try a touch or holding the patient's hand. Sometimes just being there, without saying a word, is comforting. Try to put yourself in the patient's shoes and practice empathy.

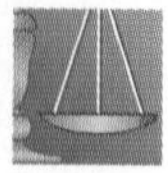

LEGAL AND ETHICAL ISSUES

Diminished sight and/or hearing may render the patient seriously impaired. To avoid possible accidents and office injuries, always ask the sight- or hearing-impaired patient how you can assist them and listen to what is asked of you. Follow the patient's requests, as in this case, the patient definitely knows what type of assistance he or she will need. When placing the patient in an examination room, offer your arm and tell the patient the approximate distance that you will be walking. If the patient is to have an examination that will involve local anesthesia or eye drops that dilate the pupil, be sure the patient has recovered and have someone to take the patient home before allowing him or her to leave the office. Never assume that the patient is capable of leaving alone. If the patient insists on leaving before the designated recovery time, inform the physician and record the time and circumstances surrounding the event in the patient's chart. This information should be signed and witnessed. The physician may want a refusal of care form signed by the patient and placed in the chart.

CRITICAL THINKING

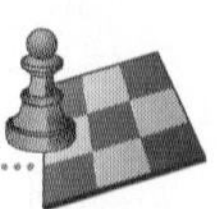

1 Myopia can be corrected through an outpatient surgical/laser procedure. Why won't this same procedure work for hyperopia?

2 Can you justify the reasons people consider ear wax to be a sign of poor hygiene and believe that it must be removed from the ears?

3 Considering all the advancements in medicine, what could be a reason for deafness to be constantly increasing?

4 Using outside sources, determine the number of years of school required to become an optometrist, an audiologist, and an optician. Did this information surprise you? Why?

HOW DID I DO? Answers to Memory Joggers

1. When you blink, the lacrimal gland secretes tears that move across the eye cleansing and moistening it. You blink approximately every 2 to 3 seconds.
2. The layers of the eye are outside = sclera and cornea, middle = choroid and iris, and inner = retina and lens.
3. The four major types of refractive error are (a) hyperopia, (b) myopia, (c) presbyopia, and (d) astigmatism.
4. Amblyopia is correctable up to the age of 7 or until the retina is fully developed. A symptom of strabismus occurring at any age is diplopia.
5. A cataract is a cloudy or opaque area in a healthy clear lens.

6 The group that is at the highest risk for glaucoma includes people older than age 60 years.

7 The exophthalmometer is used to measure the pressure of the central retinal artery.

8 In the results of a Snellen vision test, the numerator reflects the distance from the chart and the denominator is the lowest line that is correctly read.

9 Congenital and acquired are the two classifications of color defects.

10 Four reasons to instill medications into the eye are (a) to treat an infection, (b) to soothe an eye irritation, (c) to dilate pupils for eye examination, and (d) to anesthesize the eyes for treatment.

11 When looking for a foreign body in the eye, first inspect the eye; second, have the patient look to each side and then up and down; third, inspect under the lower lid; and fourth, inspect under the upper lid.

12 Sound waves travel into the external ear by air conduction and hit the tympanic membrane; the ossicles of the middle ear pick up the vibrations and turn them into bone conduction impulses; when the bone conduction reaches the oval/round window, the sound is moved into the inner ear; and the organ of Corti receives the impulses and converts them into nerve conduction frequencies, which travel up the otic nerve into the temporal lobe of the brain where they are translated into sound patterns.

13 Motion sickness is caused by a disorder in the semicircular canals in the inner ear.

14 Three types of hearing deficits are conductive, sensory, and mixed.

15 The Weber test is valuable in determining with which ear the patient can hear best. The Rinne test compares air-conduction hearing with bone-conduction hearing levels.

16 The reasons for instilling otic drops are to soften impacted cerumen, to relieve pain, and to instill an antibiotic drop to fight an infectious pathogen.

Assisting in Gastroenterology and Proctology

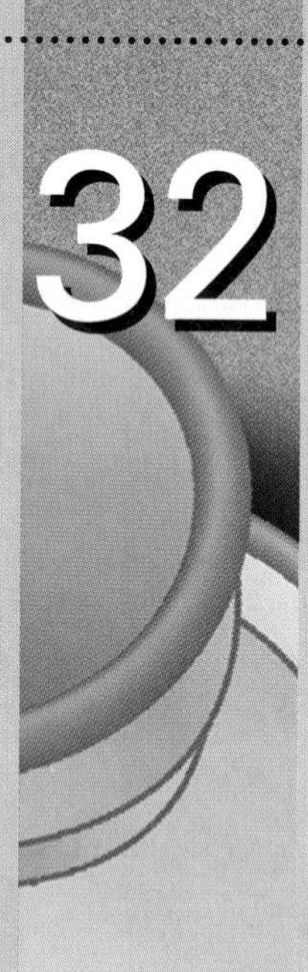

OUTLINE

LEARNING OBJECTIVES

Cognitive: On successful completion of this chapter you should be able to:

1. Describe the three primary functions of the gastrointestinal system.
2. Identify the major functions of the system and describe the physiology of each phase.
3. Name the six fundamental aspects of the gastrointestinal system.
4. List eight diseases or disorders of the gastrointestinal system and the signs, symptoms, methods of diagnosis, and treatment for each.
5. Describe the significance of the gastrointestinal system and its relationship with other body systems.
6. Define hepatitis and describe the similarities and differences of the five types.
7. Identify the methods used to diagnose gallstones.
8. Identify the types of disorders that might be referred to a proctologist.
9. List 10 possible laboratory procedures that could be ordered to assist the physician in obtaining a diagnosis.
10. Explain the indication of a positive occult blood screening.
11. List the types of laboratory samples that can be obtained during an endoscopic procedure.
12. Spell and define the terms in the vocabulary.

Performance: On successful completion of this chapter you should be able to:

1. Demonstrate the medical assistant's role during the physical examination of the gastrointestinal area.
2. Demonstrate the preparation of a patient for a colorectal procedure.
3. Assist with a colon examination.
4. Accurately obtain a stool specimen collection.
5. Demonstrate the points that need to be explained to the patient who will be receiving a suppository or rectal ointment.
6. Properly insert a rectal suppository.

VOCABULARY

abscesses Localized collections of pus that may be located under the skin or deep within the body and causes tissue destruction

absorption Passage of the products of digestion from the gastrointestinal tract into the blood and lymphatic vessels and the tissue cells

anorexia Lack or loss of appetite for food

anus Opening of the rectum on the body surface

asymptomatic Showing no symptoms

biopsy Excision of a small sample of living tissue from the body for diagnostic or therapeutic purposes

bolus The mass of food, made ready by mastication, that enters the esophagus as one swallows

cholangiogram Film obtained by x-ray examination of the bile ducts, using a radiopaque dye as a contrast medium

cholecystogram Film obtained by x-ray examination of the gallbladder, using a radiopaque dye as a contrast medium

cirrhosis Disease of the liver that causes impairment in the metabolism of nutrients and the detoxification of poisons absorbed from the intestines

colostomy Artificial opening (stoma) created in the large intestine and brought to the surface of the abdomen for the purpose of evacuating the bowels

cryosurgery Destruction of tissue by application of extreme cold

cytology Study of cells, their origin, structure, function, and pathology

defecation Elimination of wastes and undigested food, as feces, from the rectum

digestion Process of converting food into chemical substances that can be used by the body

dysphagia Difficult or painful swallowing

electrolyte Chemical substance that when dissolved dissociates into electrically charged particles and is capable of conducting an electric current and is essential to the normal function of all cells through involvement in metabolic activity

elimination Discharge from the body of indigestible materials and of waste products of body metabolism

epigastric Medial area of the abdominal cavity located between the umbilical area and the diaphragm

feces Body waste discharged from the intestine; also called stool or excreta

fissures Narrow slits or clefts in the abdominal wall

fistulas Abnormal, tubelike passages within the body tissue, usually between two internal organs

flatus Gas expelled through the anus

gangrene Death of body tissue due to loss of nutritive supply and followed by bacteria invasion and putrefaction

guarding Act of physically protecting a specific part of the body from another person's touch

Helicobacter pylori Gram-negative spiral bacterium that causes gastritis and pyloric ulcers in humans

hematocrit Volume percentage of erythrocytes in whole blood

hemoglobin Protein found in erythrocytes that transports molecular oxygen in the blood

hypogastric Medial area of the abdominal cavity located below the umbilical area and above the pubic bone

ileocecal valve Valve guarding the opening between the ileum and cecum; also called the ileocolic valve.

ingestion Taking of food, drugs, and other substances into the body by mouth

jaundice Yellowness of the skin and mucous membranes caused by deposition of bile pigment that is not a disease but a symptom of a number of diseases, especially liver disorders

ligation Process of tying off something to close it, usually a blood vessel during surgery, with a tie called a ligature

malaise Feeling of uneasiness or indisposition

mastication Act of chewing

necrosis Morphologic changes indicative of cell death caused by enzymatic degradation

NSAIDS Nonsteroidal antiinflammatory drugs; nonnarcotic analgesics that do not belong to the steroid group of drugs; drugs that have antiinflammatory, antipyretic, and analgesic effects

obturator Disk or plate that closes an opening

peristalsis Wavelike movement by which the gastrointestinal tract moves food downward

polyps Tumors on stems frequently found in the mucosal lining of the colon

reabsorption Act or process of absorbing again, as the absorption in the colon of the fluids already secreted into the gastrointestinal tract

rectum Distal portion of the large intestine located between the sigmoid colon and the anus

sclerotherapy Injection of sclerosing solutions in the treatment of hemorrhoids, varicose veins, or esophageal varices

truss Elastic, canvas, or metallic device for retaining a reduced hernia within the abdominal cavity

ulcer Lesion on the surface of an organ or tissue, produced by sloughing of necrotic inflammatory tissue

Valsalva's maneuver Occurs when one strains to defecate and urinate, uses the arms and upper trunk muscles to move up in bed, or strains during laughing, coughing, or vomiting; causes a trapping of blood in the great veins, preventing it from entering the chest and right atrium and may cause heart attack and death.

Internal medicine is a nonsurgical specialty with several subspecialties. Gastroenterology is one of these subspecialties and covers an extremely wide area known as the gastrointestinal system or the alimentary canal. Gastroenterologists are concerned with the diseases and disorders involving the stomach, small intestine, large intestine (colon), appendix, and the accessory organs of the liver, gallbladder, and pancreas. Proctology is concerned with disorders of the rectum and **anus.** The major purpose of the gastrointestinal system is to prepare, digest, and absorb the necessary nutrients to keep the body in homeostasis and to excrete the end-products that the body cannot use.

The primary functions of the gastrointestinal organs are threefold. When food is taken in through the mouth, it is broken down, enzymes are added to it, and it is mechanically and chemically changed. This process is called **digestion.** The second function begins when the food enters the small intestine. Here, the digested food must be absorbed into the bloodstream by passing through the walls of the small intestine. By the time this **bolus** of food reaches the terminal end of the small intestine, every nutrient that your body needs at this particular time should have been absorbed. What is left is copious amounts of fluids containing by-products and waste nutrients. This mass enters the colon or large intestine, where the order of business is **reabsorption** of the excess fluid, to prevent dehydration of the body tissues. Once the fluid has been reabsorbed, the remaining solid waste materials, called **feces,** are moved into the sigmoid colon and **rectum** and, thus, **elimination** occurs through the anus.

Anatomy and Physiology

The gastrointestinal system is basically a long hollow tube that has essentially the same structural organization from its beginning to its termination (Fig. 32–1). It is closely governed by the autonomic nervous system, which gives the entire system its unique ability to move slowly in some locations and to increase the movement in other sections. This also ensures that food will be prepared in one section, absorbed in another, and eliminated in the terminal section. The gastrointestinal tract is rich in lymphatic tissue, which is very important for the absorption of nutrients from the ingested food. Unfortunately, the lymphatic vessels are also the main route for the spread of cancers.

The major functions of the gastrointestinal tract are the digestion of food and the elimination of the excretory products of metabolism. These functions can be divided into the following specific phases.

Food is selected and manually prepared for consumption. It is then placed into the mouth and the process begins. This is called **ingestion.**

When food is taken in through the mouth, it must be broken down, saliva-containing enzymes are added to it, and it is mechanically and chemically prepared. This process is called **mastication.** The primary structures in this phase of preparation are the teeth and the tongue, which do the ripping, mincing, and mixing. Now this mass, called a bolus, is swallowed and the food enters the esophagus. Contractions of the smooth muscles are activated, and the food is now moved by **peristalsis.** The sec-

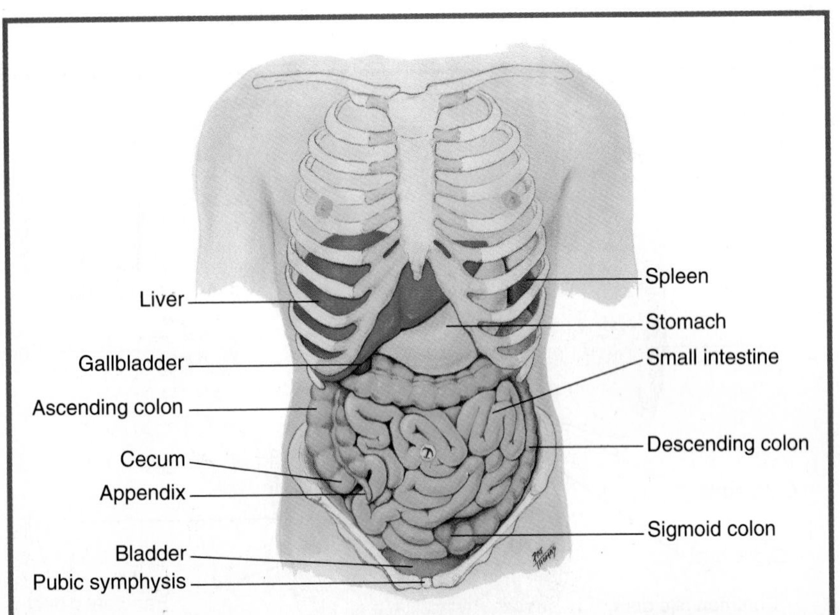

FIGURE 32–1 Gastrointestinal system. (From Jarvis C: Physical Examination and Health Assessment, 2nd ed. Philadelphia, WB Saunders, 1996.)

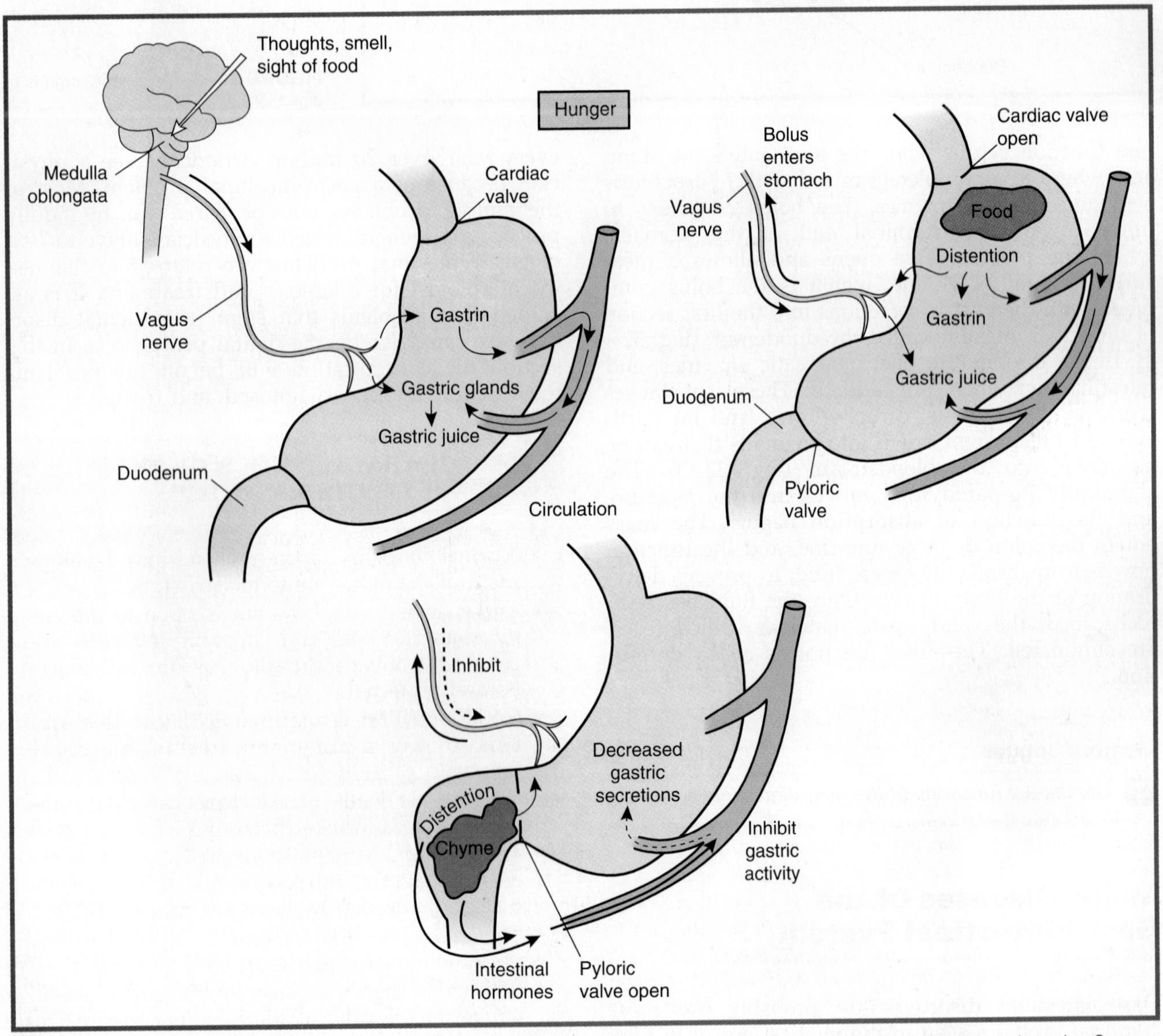

FIGURE 32–2 Regulation of food through the stomach. (Modified from Applegate EJ: The Anatomy and Physiology Learning System. Philadelphia, WB Saunders, 1995.)

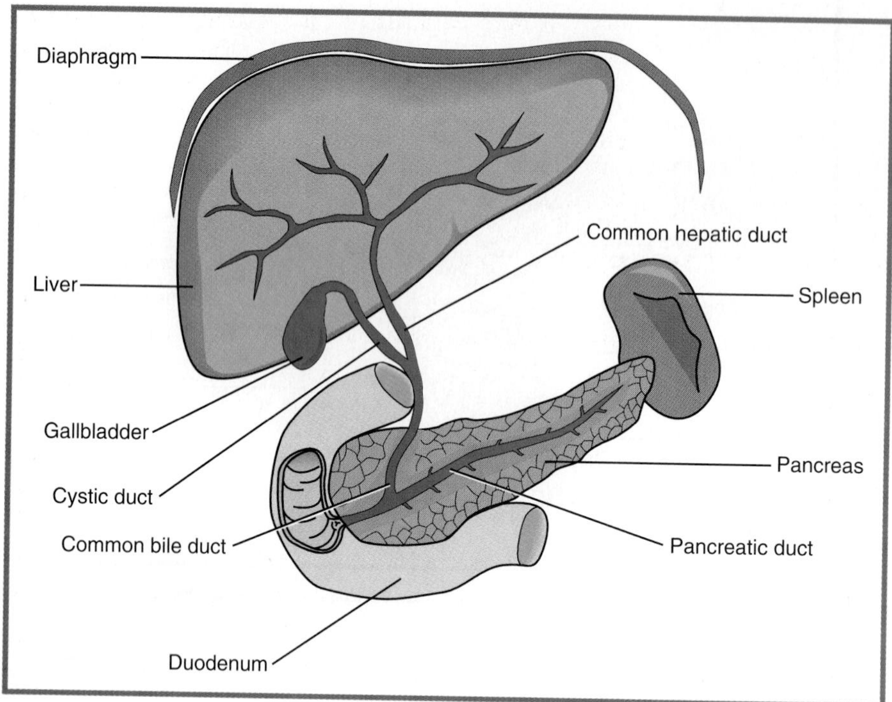

FIGURE 32–3 Accessory organs of digestion.

ond function begins when the food enters the stomach, where it is completely mixed with hydrochloric acid and gastric enzymes. The bolus continues to move toward the terminal end of the stomach, where the pyloric valve opens and allows a measured amount of chyme, which is the bolus combined with the gastric secretions into the first section of the small intestine called the duodenum (Fig. 32–2). In the duodenum, bile, pancreatic enzymes, and intestinal enzymes are added. These substances work on the proteins, carbohydrates, and fat particles and break them down into elements that can be absorbed into the bloodstream (Fig. 32–3). The chemically prepared food moves into the jejunum, and the function of **absorption** begins. The mass enters the colon or large intestine, and the function now is to reabsorb the excess fluid, to prevent dehydration of the body tissues. Once the fluid has been reabsorbed, the solid waste materials, called feces, are eliminated. This final function is called **defecation.**

Memory Jogger

 *List the six functions of the gastrointestinal system.*

Major Diseases of the Gastrointestinal System

Gastrointestinal disorders are probably the most common problem seen in the medical office. In fact, every year over 20 million Americans see a physician because of a gastrointestinal problem. Most of the simple problems will be cared for by family practice and general practice physicians. Five to 10% of gastrointestinal problems are referred to the gastroenterologist for diagnosis and treatment. It is assumed that problems that stem from dental disorders are cared for by the dental professions. In this section the concentration will be on the problems most frequently seen, diagnosed, and treated.

SOME CHARACTERISTICS OF THE GASTROINTESTINAL SYSTEM

- Normal function depends on normal development of the entire anatomic structure.
- The gastrointestinal system is open to the environment at both ends, making it readily accessible to invading pathogens but amazingly is rarely infected.
- Good nutrition is required to allow this system to stay healthy and free of functional damage.
- The muscle walls of this tube can dilate abnormally and/or obstruct.
- The gastrointestinal system provides the nutrients for all the other systems; if it becomes diseased, all other systems are affected.
- The gastrointestinal system is exposed to environmental carcinogens in food and water.
- Pathogens ingested through the gastrointestinal system readily invade the bloodstream.

Memory Jogger

Why is the gastrointestinal system readily accessible to invading bacteria?

A patient with a gastrointestinal problem may complain of such things as nausea, **anorexia,** and abdominal pain, as well as numerous other symptoms. It may be difficult for the medical assistant to organize a patient's complaints when a patient first contacts the office by telephone for an appointment. The patient may say he or she has a stomachache when the discomfort is really not in the stomach area but rather in the transverse portion of the colon. Or, the patient may say he or she has a stomachache when the discomfort is in the **hypogastric** area and not in the **epigastric** area (Fig. 32–4).

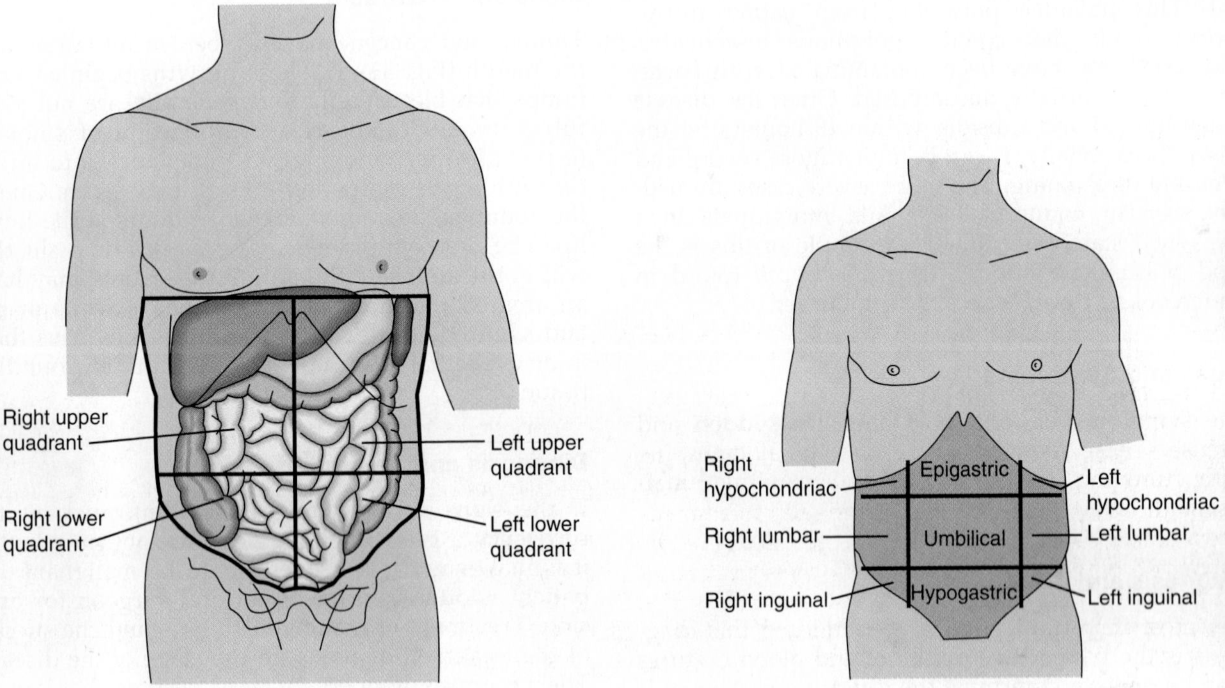

Right upper quadrant
Left upper quadrant
Right lower quadrant
Left lower quadrant

Right hypochondriac
Epigastric
Left hypochondriac
Right lumbar
Umbilical
Left lumbar
Right inguinal
Hypogastric
Left inguinal

RIGHT UPPER QUADRANT (RUQ)

Liver
Gallbladder
Duodenum
Head of pancreas
Right kidney and adrenal
Hepatic flexure of colon
Part of ascending and transverse colon

LEFT UPPER QUADRANT (LUQ)

Stomach
Spleen
Left lobe of liver
Body of pancreas
Left kidney and adrenal
Splenic flexure of colon
Part of transverse and descending colon

RIGHT LOWER QUADRANT (RLQ)

Cecum
Appendix
Right ovary and tube
Right ureter
Right spermatic cord

LEFT LOWER QUADRANT (LLQ)

Part of descending colon
Sigmoid colon
Left ovary and tube
Left ureter
Left spermatic cord

MIDLINE

Aorta
Uterus (if enlarged)
Bladder (if distended)

FIGURE 32–4 Abdominal areas and quadrants and the organs located in each.

When discussing the abdominal pain with the patient, ask the patient to point to or touch the area where the pain is located. This is one way of making sure that the correct area is identified and prepared for the physician to examine. Record the area or region of the pain.

FOOD POISONING

Food poisoning is a disorder resulting from the ingestion of food that contains bacterial or toxic material. This includes poisoning from eating mushrooms, foods that contain poisonous insecticides, and foods that have been contaminated with bacteria or have partially decomposed. Often the disease is self-limited and subsides within 48 hours after the onset. Occasionally, it can be much more severe and even life threatening. The more severe cases are usually seen in young children and individuals in a weakened state of health. An example of this is the food poisoning caused by *Escherichia coli* found in undercooked meat, especially hamburger.

Signs and Symptoms

The symptoms of food poisoning are sudden and intense. These include severe abdominal cramping with rumbling noises, nausea and vomiting, **malaise,** and fever.

Diagnosis and Treatment

The most important point in determining this diagnosis is the patient history. Stool and blood cultures may be done to determine the causative pathogen. If the patient has a remaining portion of the suspected ingested food, this will be sent to the laboratory for analysis. The physician may order an endoscopic examination of the gastrointestinal system in severe cases to determine the extent of the damaged or the condition of the mucosal lining of the system.

The treatment of choice is to treat the symptoms. The important aspect is to minimize dehydration and maintain **electrolyte** balance. Medications are used to control the vomiting and the diarrhea. These are often given in a suppository form. If the diarrhea and vomiting cannot be corrected within a reasonable length of time (determined by age, body size, and health condition), the patient may be hospitalized so that intravenous fluid replacement can be given.

Memory Jogger

How long before food poisoning usually subsides without medication?

ORAL TUMORS AND CANCER

Causes for oral tumors of any kind are unknown. It is well known that the use of tobacco and chronic alcoholism are definite risk factors. Oral tumors and cancers occur more frequently in men older than 50. Simple, benign tumors develop slowly, over a period of years and remain non–life threatening whereas cancerous tumors develop rapidly and metastasize within a few months.

Signs and Treatment

Tumors and cancers may be seen in all surfaces of the mouth (Fig. 32–5). These growths begin as small lumps that bleed easily and generally are not painful. A mouth tumor is a complication of smoking (especially pipe smoking) and may turn into an ulcer with a soft center and a hard, raised rim. One of the common sites for malignant tumors is the lower lip. The first symptom may be a sore or a slit that will not heal. Inside the mouth the patient may have an area on the mucosal surface that is white or red and slightly elevated. The patient usually says there is an area that does not look like the surrounding tissue.

Diagnosis and Treatment

If the signs and symptoms are confirmed by the physician, a **biopsy** will be done to confirm whether it is malignant. If it proves not to be malignant, the patient is often referred to an oral surgeon for excision. Treatment of malignant tumors and the success of the treatment depends on the stage of the disease. The prognosis is good for early lesions that can be surgically removed and/or treated with radiation therapy. Unfortunately, many patients do not seek medical attention for these growths because there is

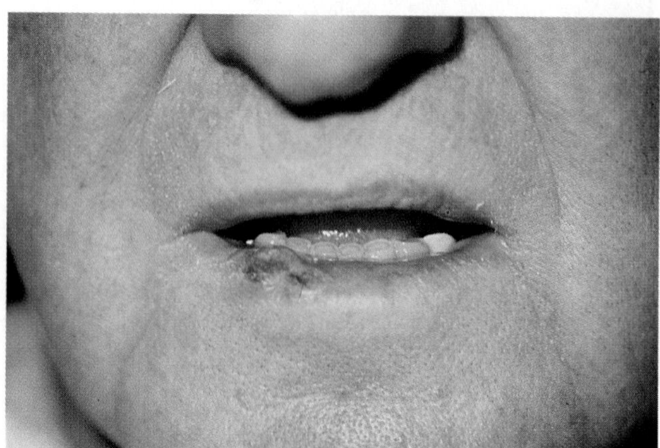

FIGURE 32–5 Cancer of the lip. On gross examination the tumor appears to be ulcerated. (From Damjanov I: Pathology for the Health-Related Professions. Philadelphia, WB Saunders, 1996.)

rarely any pain in the early stages. Thus, when medical attention is sought, the growth is advanced cancer and the overall 5-year survival rate is only 25%.

Memory Jogger

 What causes oral tumors?

HERPES SIMPLEX (COLD SORES)

Cold sores, sometimes referred to as fever blisters, are caused by herpes simplex virus type 1. They appear around the lips and in the mouth (Fig. 32–6). After the initial infection, the virus remains dormant in a cutaneous nerve until it is activated by stress, fever, or ultraviolet radiation. Exposure to sunshine, wind, or the common cold may also reactivate the virus.

Signs and Symptoms

Herpes simplex lesions are small fluid-filled blisters that itch and are painful. Besides the usual sites, these ulcers may also be seen on the gums as tender, red, swollen areas. Tingling and numbness around the mouth may precede or follow the appearance of the ulcer.

Diagnosis and Treatment

An oral examination usually can confirm the diagnosis. No treatment is advised if the infection is mild and localized. Herpes simplex virus seldom causes any risk to the patient's general health. Occasionally, if the patient rubs his or her eyes after touching the moist area of the blister, a herpetic corneal ulcer may form. In an immunocompromised patient, such as someone with the acquired immunodeficiency syndrome, this virus can cause serious complications. The treatment prescribed usually consists of rest, analgesics, and a topical cream that will dry and heal the affected area.

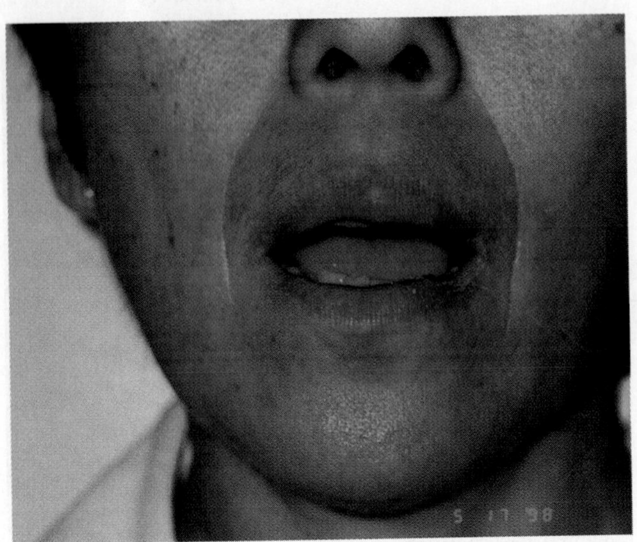

FIGURE 32–6 Herpes simplex.

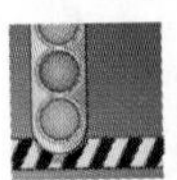

Safety Alert: Avoid contamination through direct contact.

Memory Jogger

 Name the usual sites for herpes simplex lesions.

GASTRIC AND DUODENAL ULCERS

Gastric and duodenal ulcers usually do not appear; but when they do, it is usually in the midlife years. Ulcers can, however, be seen in all ages, even young children. Ulcers can appear under a variety of predisposing circumstances, including the use of alcohol, aspirin, and nonsteroidal antiinflammatory drugs (NSAIDs); psychological anxiety or emotional stress; erosion and/or breakdown of the mucosal lining; ***Helicobacter pylori*** infection in the stomach or duodenum; and genetic predisposition. Duodenal ulcers are seen more frequently than gastric ulcers, but both are characterized by an area of breakdown of mucosal membrane that leads to ulceration of the epithelial lining of the stomach or intestine (Fig. 32–7).

Signs and Symptoms

The most inclusive symptom is intense pain in the area of the ulcer occurring about 2 hours after the ingestion of food and at night. Gastric ulcers may cause loss of weight, and duodenal lesions often produce nausea and vomiting. Some patients state that eating very small amounts frequently relieves the intensity of the pain. If the ulcerative area is bleeding internally, the patient may find blood in vomit and/or the feces. The blood may be digested and appear as coffee-ground and/or "tarry" black stools. Often, blood in the stool is occult or "hidden" blood.

Diagnosis and Treatment

The description of the patient's pain gives the physician a clear suspicion of the disorder. The examination often shows the patient to have a guarding of

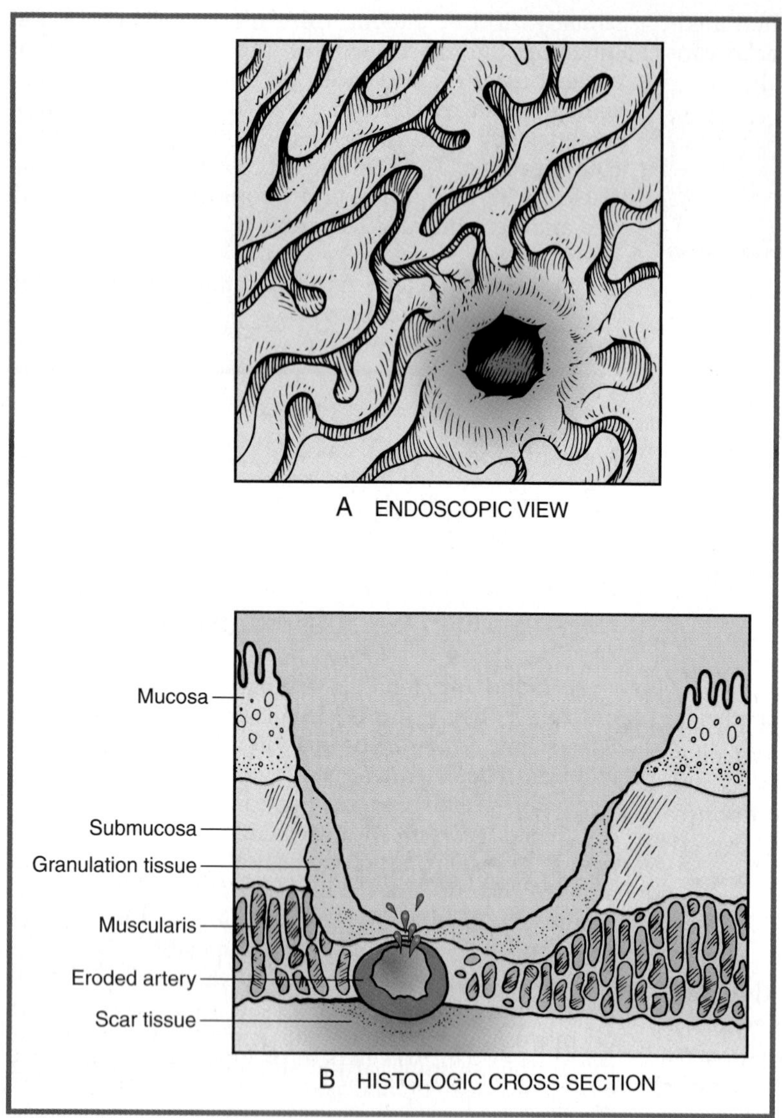

FIGURE 32–7 *A* and *B*, Peptic ulcer.

the painful area, which is characterized by clutching of the upper abdominal area and keeping the knees drawn up toward the chest. A definitive diagnosis is based on an upper gastrointestinal series (x-ray), or endoscopy (visualization) of the upper gastrointestinal tract is ordered (Fig. 32–8). A biopsy of the affected area may be taken during the endoscopy to rule out possible cancer. A sampling of the gastric contents may be collected to establish the level of acidity or presence of blood, and/or a culture may be ordered to rule out bacteria. A stool test may be ordered to check for the presence of occult blood. Blood tests will also be ordered to establish **hemoglobin** and **hematocrit** levels. Treatment involves rest, medications (e.g., histamine-2 blockers), possibly diet modification, and changes in lifestyle. If the causative agent is *Helicobacter pylori,* the treatment will involve antibiotics. In most cases, ulcers will heal with medical treatment but patients will need to observe preventive measures to prevent the condition from recurring. In severe cases, surgery may

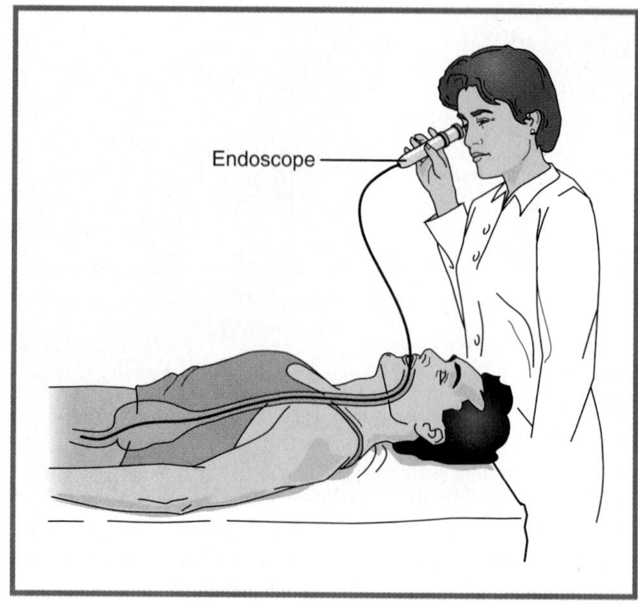

FIGURE 32–8 Endoscopy.

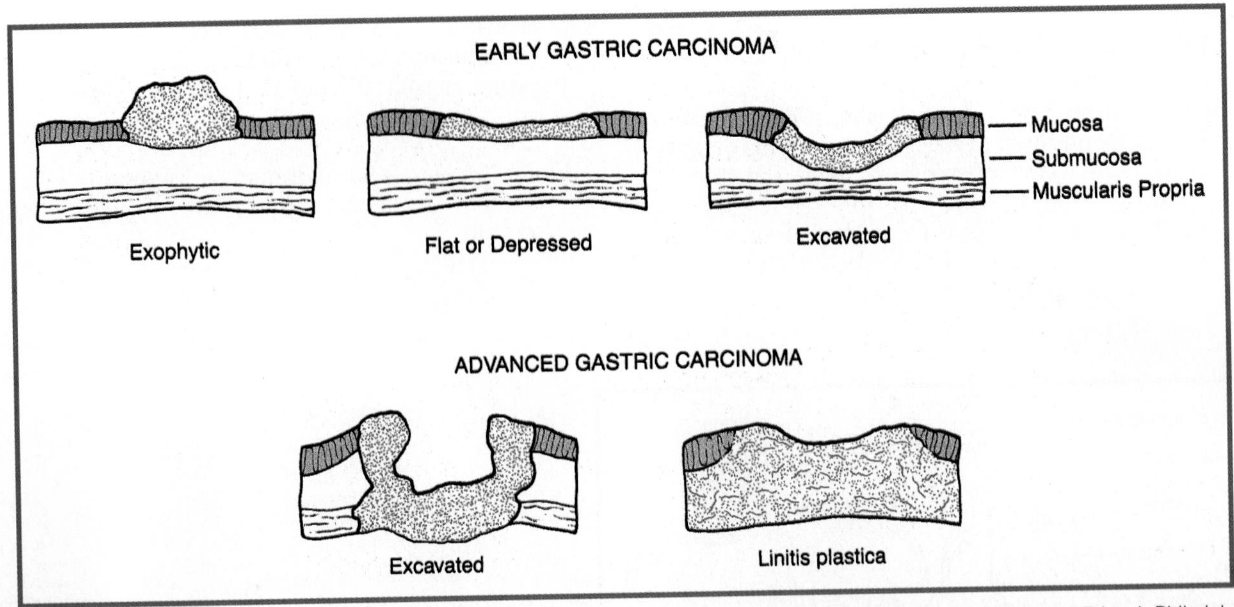

FIGURE 32–9 Gastric cancer. (From Cotran RS, Kumar V, Robbins SL [eds]: Robbins Pathologic Basis of Disease, 5th ed. Philadelphia, WB Saunders, 1994.)

be indicated. Any nonhealing ulcer will be periodically reevaluated through endoscopy to rule out cancer.

Memory Jogger

6 *What two tests may be ordered to assist in the diagnosis of ulcers?*

GASTRIC CANCER

Stomach cancer is most often seen as a complication of gastric ulcer. The reason why some ulcers end up as cancer is unknown, but diet is suspected as a possible contributing factor (Fig. 32–9). In the United States, the incidence of gastric cancer has markedly decreased in the past several decades; yet it still causes approximately 14,000 deaths a year. This research substantiates the suspicion that carcinogens are present in the foods ingested or are in the environment. This has not been definitely identified, but it is known that this decrease has been the result of limiting the use of carcinogenic agents in agriculture and in food processing techniques.

Signs and Symptoms

The signs and symptoms of gastric cancer are nonspecific, and patients seldom seek medical attention early. By the time a diagnosis is made, the lesions are often inoperable, owing to the advanced stage. The patient's early signs are weight loss, **dysphagia,** malaise, generalized weakness, and anemia. As the tumor advances, symptoms include severe pain in the upper abdomen, marked weight loss, frequent vomiting, bloody bowel movements, and bloody emesis.

Diagnosis and Treatment

The signs and symptoms of stomach cancers are a strong indication of the diseases or disorder. The physician will order an upper gastrointestinal series and endoscopy with tissue biopsy of the stomach. Gastric secretion analysis may also be used. Treatment consists of partial or total removal of the stomach followed by radiation therapy. If the situation is inoperable, chemotherapy may be recommended. Gastric carcinoma has a very poor prognosis and only about 12% survive the 5-year period.

Memory Jogger

7 *What is believed to be a contributing factor for gastric cancer?*

HERNIAS (HIATAL, ABDOMINAL, INGUINAL)

A hernia is the abnormal protrusion of part of an organ or tissue through the structures normally containing it. These protrusions can develop in various parts of the body but most frequently are seen in the abdominal region. Causes of herniation include congenital weakness of the structures, trauma, relaxation of ligaments and skeletal muscles, or increased upward pressure from the abdomen. It is most often found in middle-aged or older individuals. The location of the hernia determines the term by which the protrusion is identified.

TYPES OF HERNIAS

Hiatal hernia: upper part of the stomach protrudes through the esophageal opening of the diaphragm. This opening is called the hiatal sphincter (Fig. 32–10).

Abdominal hernia: an organ or part of an organ protrudes through a weakened area in the abdominal muscle wall (Fig. 32–11).

Inguinal hernia: a loop of the bowel protrudes into the inguinal canal of the male (Fig. 32–12).

Other types of herniations: fat, femoral, incarcerated, incisional, umbilical, vaginal, and scrotal.

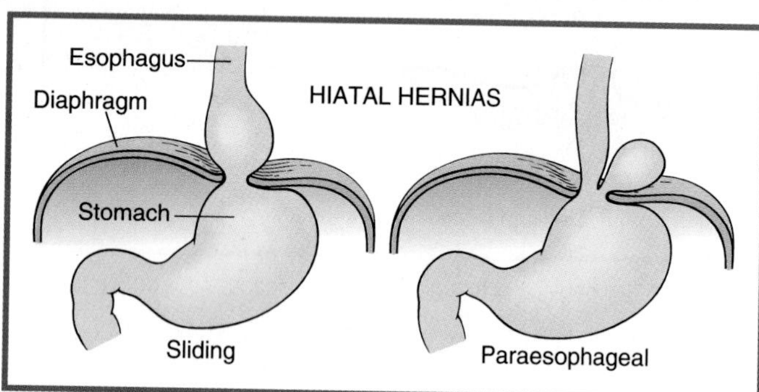

FIGURE 32–10 Hiatal hernia. (From Damjanov I: Pathology for the Health-Related Professions. Philadelphia, WB Saunders, 1996.)

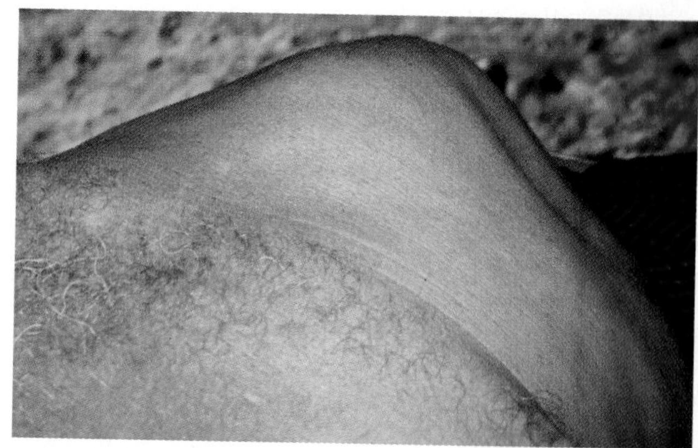

FIGURE 32–11 Epigastric abdominal hernia.

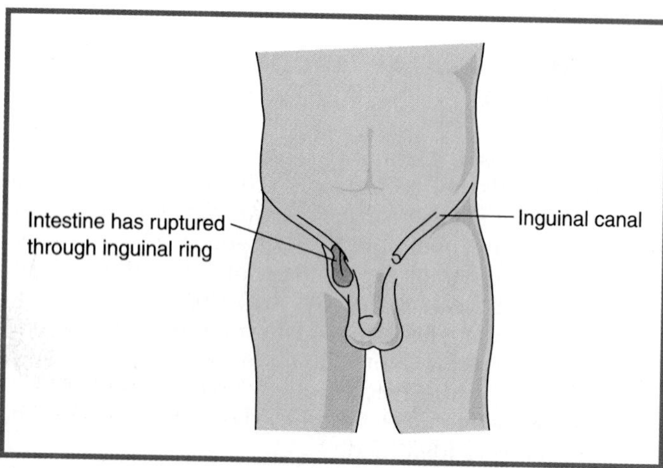

FIGURE 32–12 Herniated inguinal canal.

Signs and Symptoms

The usual sign of an abdominal hernia is an abnormal lump or bulge that the patient finds while bathing. This bulge is tender, but the pain is mild. The patient may also discover that the bulge can be pushed back into the abdomen and it will stay that way until there is some type of moving activity and then it reappears. If there is severe pain, the hernia may be trapped or strangulated if blood flow has been compromised; and if immediate medical intervention is not performed, the tissue may die and **gangrene** may set in.

The hiatal hernia usually produces chronic pain related to regurgitation of acidic gastric contents accompanied by facial grimacing. The hiatal hernia patient may verbally discuss with the medical assistant vivid accounts of "burping up dinner." This patient may also talk about having difficulties in lying down too soon after eating because the stomach contents come "back up" or after eating a full meal the abdominal pain becomes intense and may even cause breathing difficulties.

Diagnosis and Treatment

The physician can palpate a visible abdominal or inguinal hernia for size and inspect the area with the patient standing and lying down. An inguinal hernia can be detected in the male by performing **Valsalva's maneuver.** The medical assessment may also include x-rays and an upper gastrointestinal series (hiatal), and in severe cases computed tomography or magnetic resonance imaging may be ordered. The most frequent treatment is surgical repair in the form of a herniorraphy or hernioplasty. If the person is in poor health, the physician may have the patient fitted with a device known as a **truss.**

The patient with the diagnosis of a hiatal hernia is usually treated with medications, such as antacids (aluminum hydroxide [Amphojel]), anticholinergics (propantheline bromide [Pro-Banthine]), and histamine-2 antagonists (ranitidine [Zantac]). The treatment may also include diet modification and changes in lifestyle.

Depending on the patient's diagnosis, the medical assistant may want to discuss the medications and expectations. If the drug may produce constipation, the patient may need to increase the daily intake of fiber. Antacids need to be well shaken before the prescribed dose is poured. They should also be taken before drinking milk or water. Histamine-2 antagonists may cause a dry mouth and may be ordered to be taken at bedtime. If the patient understands the rationale, it is likely that the treatment regimen will be followed.

Memory Jogger

8 *When do most patients discover abdominal hernia?*

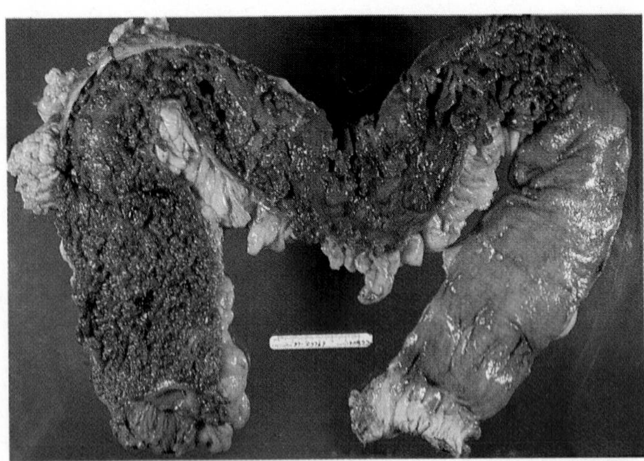

FIGURE 32–13 Ulcerative colitis. (From Damjanov I: Pathology for the Health-Related Professions. Philadelphia, WB Saunders, 1996.)

ULCERATIVE COLITIS

Ulcerative colitis is a chronic inflammatory disease of the lining of the colon. The cause is not definitely known, but it may be an abnormal gastrointestinal immune reaction to foods or certain microorganisms. Ulcerative colitis can occur at any age, but it is most frequent in women in their 30s and 40s. It is characterized by extensive ulcerations along the lining of the bowel, which leads to bloody diarrhea and as many as 20 bowel movements a day (Fig. 32–13).

Signs and Symptoms

The patient seeks medical attention due to the frequent episodes of bloody diarrhea, abdominal cramping, and the continuous urge to have a bowel movement. He or she may also describe loose, light-colored, and/or mucus in the bowel movement, rectal bleeding, and continuous thirst, which is due to fluid loss.

Diagnosis and Treatment

When a patient sees the physician with the signs and symptoms discussed, the clinical picture is fairly conclusive that the problem is ulcerative colitis. The physician will order laboratory tests including a stool analysis and culture, hemoglobin and white blood cell analysis, and radiographs of the abdomen. Occasionally a lower gastrointestinal series and/or colonoscopy will be done. Treatment will consist of removing any irritating food from the diet. Medications to quiet gastrointestinal activity (antacids) and control the diarrhea (antiemetics) are often prescribed. In severe cases, surgical removal of the bowel, and the creation of a **colostomy,** may be the treatment of choice. The patient with ulcerative colitis is at increased risk of developing colon cancer and needs to undergo frequent examinations to monitor any colon changes.

Memory Jogger

What kind of allergies contribute to ulcerative colitis?

HEMORRHOIDS

Hemorrhoids are varicose veins of the anus and rectum and affect about 5% of all adults. There is a familial, hereditary predisposition to the disorder, and it is common in persons with varicose veins of the lower extremities and inguinal hernias. The cause is related to increased pressure in the rectum often caused by constipation. If the swollen veins are within the rectal wall, they are considered to be internal hemorrhoids; and if they are firm, protruding, and can be felt and/or seen, they are external.

Signs and Symptoms

These tumor-like masses may have a variety of symptoms. Some patients experience no pain whereas other patients experience definite rectal pain. Frequently, anal itching and burning discomfort immediately after a bowel movement is reported. If the patient must strain to defecate, bleeding and a protrusion of the swollen mass can occur. Often patients will state that it is necessary to bathe the anal area with warm water or even soak in warm water to get relief from the itching and pain after every bowel movement.

Diagnosis and Treatment

A proctologic examination and inspection of the anal area will reveal external hemorrhoids. Proctoscopy is done to visualize internal hemorrhoids of the rectum. A hemoglobin level and red blood cell count may be ordered to determine if there has been any significant blood loss. Hemorrhoids are treated with stool softeners, a diet high in whole grains or bulking agents, vegetables, and fruits, and an analgesic ointment applied locally or a suppository to relieve swelling. If these measures do not correct the problem, the next step may be **sclerotherapy** injections, **cryosurgery**, or **ligation.**

Memory Jogger

10 *Hemorrhoids are more common in persons with __________ and __________.*

Diseases of the Accessory Organs

VIRAL HEPATITIS

Acute viral hepatitis is an inflammatory process and infection of the liver. There are several forms of this virus, known as hepatitis A, B, C, D, and E. It is the most prevalent liver disease in the world. In the United States about 1 person in every 500 will be affected yearly. Hepatitis A is frequently **asymptomatic,** which helps us to understand why 40% of all Americans have antibodies to hepatitis A virus and approximately 10% have antibodies to hepatitis B virus, even though most of these individuals cannot identify a time when they had hepatitis. The main features of hepatitis are listed in Table 32–1. Vaccines are given for hepatitis A virus (HAV) and hepatitis B virus (HBV). Immunization of persons who are at increased risk is highly recommended. All health care personnel are included in this group because they are at increased risk of infection through exposure to blood or blood products and body fluids.

Hepatitis is spread from person to person through body fluid contact. As a health care professional, the medical assistant cares for sick people on a daily basis who may be carriers of the hepatitis virus.

TABLE 32–1 Features of Known Human Hepatitis (A, B, C, D, and E) Viruses

Feature	HAV	HBV	HCV	HDV	HEV
Family	Picoma	Hepadna	Flavi	Viroid	Calici
Genome	RNA	DNA	RNA	RNA	RNA
Size	27 nm	42 nm	30–60 nm	35 nm	32 nm
Viremia	Brief	Long	Long	Like HBV	Brief
Transmission	F/O	Par/sex	Par/sex	Par/sex	F/O
Incubation (days)	15–45	14–180	15–150	30–50	14–60
Fulminant hepatitis risk (%)	0.1	1	0.1	10	1–2 (if pregnant, 20)
Chronicity	No	10%	50%	10%	No
HCC association	No	Yes	Yes	No	No
Chronic carrier state	No	Yes	Yes	Yes	No
Vaccine available	Yes	Yes	No	No	No

F/O, fecal/oral; Par/sex, parenteral/sexual; HCC, hepatocellular carcinoma.
From Damjanov I: Pathology for the Health-Related Professions. Philadelphia, WB Saunders, 1996.

Inhaling droplets released by a cough, holding a patient's hand that was just used to cover the mouth, and discarding a wet baby diaper are all possible ways that exposure can occur. If you have washed your hands 50 times already today, that's okay, wash them again.

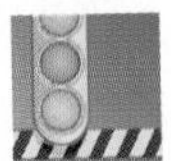

Safety Alert: The best preventive measure is WASH YOUR HANDS.

Signs and Symptoms

Hepatitis A symptoms usually develop within 3 to 4 weeks after exposure. The infection is characterized by fever, vomiting, loss of appetite, and **jaundice** (Fig. 32–14). Recovery is within a week, and there are seldom any long-term complications. Transition to chronic hepatitis or liver **cirrhosis** never occurs.

Symptoms and signs of hepatitis B are the same as those of hepatitis A except the intensity is more severe. They include fever, chills, headache, generalized body aches and pains, anorexia, nausea, vomiting, dark yellowish brown urine, diarrhea, enlarged and tender liver, pale, clay-colored stools, and jaundice.

The features of hepatitis C (HCV) are difficult to distinguish from those of hepatitis B, but the disease is usually less severe. Before the antibody test to HCV became available, it was believed that over 90% of all patients with HCV had posttransfusion hepatitis or had had intimate contact with an infected partner. This has proven to be inaccurate, and today it is not known how these patients became infected. What is known is that 50% of affected individuals progress to chronic hepatitis and develop cirrhosis and that many of these will then develop cancer.

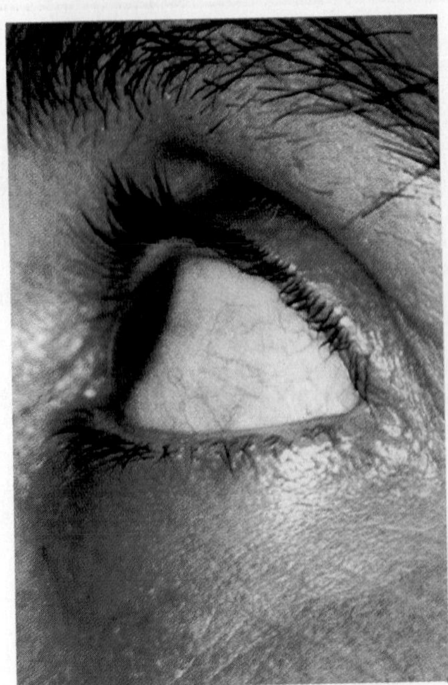

FIGURE 32–14 Jaundice of the sclera. (From Damjanov I: Pathology for the Health-Related Professions. Philadelphia, WB Saunders, 1996.)

Hepatitis D virus (HDV) requires HBV to be present before it can replicate within an individual's body. The fact that this exists as a co-infection means the symptoms are the same as those of hepatitis B. A superinfection of HBV may activate this disease. The progression to cirrhosis will accelerate, and it is also likely that the patient's liver will become necrotic as the chronic hepatitis continues.

Hepatitis E (HEV) is not seen in the United States. This virus is endemic in parts of Asia, Africa, and South America. It is spread through waterborne epidemics; and although the infection is mild, it heals with serious complications, including liver **necrosis.**

Diagnosis and Treatment

Diagnosis of hepatitis A, B, and C is based on identifying the virus or the antibodies to the virus in the blood. Another test that is very useful is a liver biopsy for tissue examination. The treatment generally consists of bed rest and a high-protein diet.

The best form of treatment for hepatitis B is prevention by being vaccinated against the disease. The vaccine is given in three doses. The first two are given 30 days apart, and the third is given 6 months later. Before beginning employment in a health care facility, you may be required to show proof of vaccination or submit to the vaccination procedure, which is provided by the employer. Today many states require the hepatitis vaccine be given as part of the preschool well-baby immunizations. This is covered in Chapter 38.

Memory Jogger

11 *What type(s) of hepatitis are health care providers at risk of contracting?*

CIRRHOSIS

Cirrhosis is a chronic liver disease in which the structure of the liver deteriorates and the function becomes decreasingly impaired. Cirrhosis is an irreversible disease; the only cure is liver transplantation. The disease is often a complication of chronic alcoholism and substance abuse. It is the fourth most common cause of death in men between the ages of 40 and 60. In approximately 30% of cirrhosis cases, the cause cannot be positively established (Fig. 32–15).

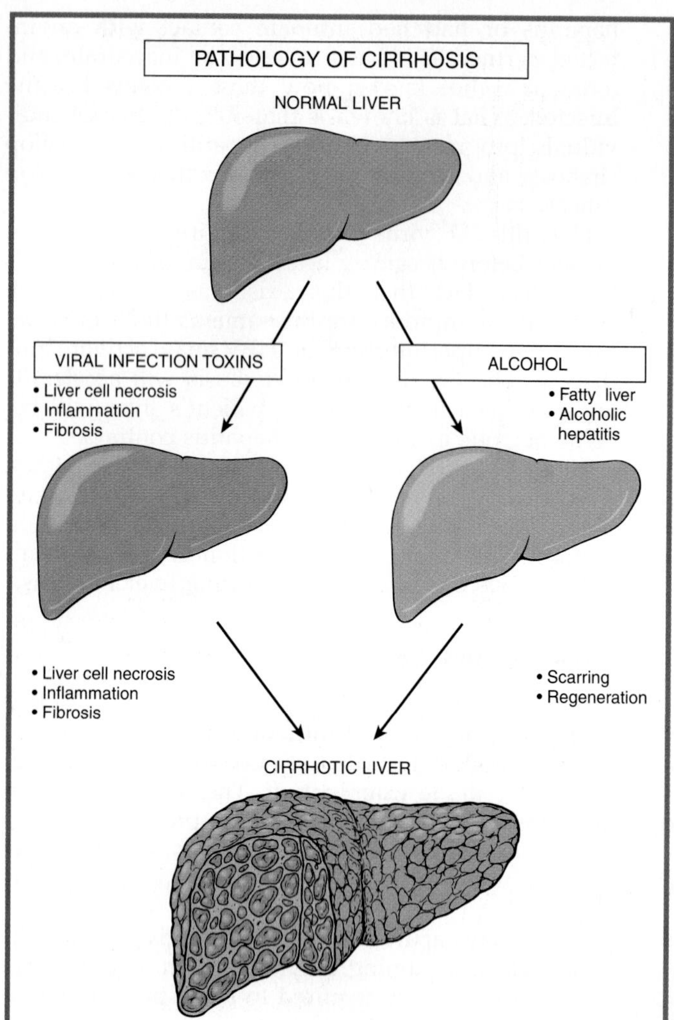

FIGURE 32–15 Pathology of cirrhosis. (From Damjanov I: Pathology for the Health-Related Professions. Philadelphia, WB Saunders, 1996.)

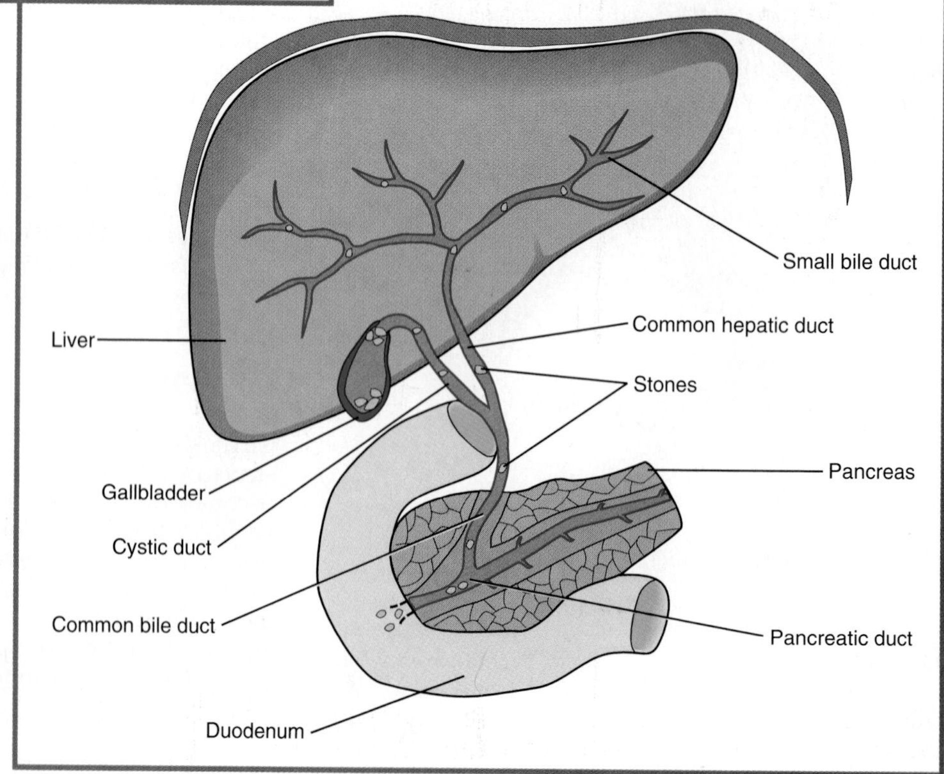

FIGURE 32–16 Gallstones.

CHOLELITHIASIS (GALLSTONES)

About 500,000 people in the United States undergo surgery for gallstones every year. It is estimated that 20% of people older than age 65 years have gallstones and women are three times more at risk than men. There used to be a saying that if the patient had upper right quadrant pain radiating into the back and was female, fat, fair, and over 40, it was gallstones. Of course, this is no longer true, but whites still develop gallstones at a higher frequency than races of color. Gallstones form in the gallbladder from insoluble cholesterol and bile salt and vary in size and number. The reasons for formation are not always clear, although occurrence is more frequent with a high-calorie, high-cholesterol diet and is associated with obesity (Fig. 32–16).

Signs and Symptoms

Most gallstones are asymptomatic and are incidentally discovered during a routine radiograph. Pain usually occurs when the stones move to and obstruct the biliary duct. The pain is in the epigastric and right upper quadrant region, often radiating into the right upper back area. Nausea and vomiting may accompany the pain. The pain hits in a wavelike pattern and is referred to as colicky pain or biliary colic. If the obstruction is not corrected, jaundice may appear.

Diagnosis and Treatment

The physician will base the preliminary diagnosis on the signs and symptoms noted on palpation of the upper right quadrant. To confirm the diagnosis, ultrasonography of the gallbladder and the biliary duct is ordered or radioisotope scan, an oral **cholecystogram,** and a **cholangiogram** may be requested. In a blood chemistry analysis, the serum bilirubin level is elevated.

Treatment is removal of the gallbladder (cholecystectomy), which can be accomplished through the traditional incision along the base of the ribs or may be done by laparoscopy.

Memory Jogger

12 *Describe the pain associated with biliary duct obstruction.*

The Medical Assistant's Role in the Gastrointestinal Examination

Emotional factors play an important part in many gastrointestinal problems, often making the separation of functional disorders and organic disorders difficult. You may be faced with making the determination of whether the abdominal pain may be classified as chronic or acute. The chronic abdomen, or chronic pain, may or may not be abdominal in origin. It may originate in the thoracic cavity or musculoskeletal system. The acute abdomen may demand immediate attention, as in acute appendicitis or acute gastritis with possible hemorrhage. Both may demand surgical therapy. Careful questioning will guide the patient to a more precise description of the symptoms and will give you the information needed by the physician. Your role as the liaison between the patient and the physician may strongly help the physician in making the diagnosis and getting the patient the treatment needed.

There are many abdominal symptoms that are commonly associated with changes in bowel patterns (Table 32–2). Abdominal symptoms that a patient may report during the history include *dyspepsia* (indigestion), *dysphagia* (difficulty in swallowing), a sensation of burning starting just below the sternum and radiating upward into the neck, a change in bowel habits including constipation and/or diarrhea, excessive *flatulence* (gas), nausea, and vomiting. General abdominal discomfort (colic) is common, because abdominal pain is frequently referred pain (Fig. 32–17), that is, pain that is felt in the abdomen but is actually being generated from an organ elsewhere.

TABLE 32–2 Gastrointestinal Symptoms and Related Disorders

Symptom	Related Disorder
Constipation	Inadequate bulk in the diet Neuromuscular or musculoskeletal impairment Pain on defecation Pregnancy, aging, medication, stress Inadequate physical activity Chronic use of laxatives and enemas Gastrointestinal growths and lesions
Diarrhea	Effects of medications, radiation, surgery Dietary alterations, food intolerance Allergies

REFERRED PAIN

When a person sees the physician and repeatedly describes abdominal pain, the pain's location may not be directly over the involved organ or over the point of the disorder. The reason for this is that the human brain has no way of determining the felt image for internal organs. However hard to imagine, the pain is referred to a site where the organ was located in fetal development. Even though the organ moves during fetal development, its nerves persist in referring sensations from its primitive or primary location.

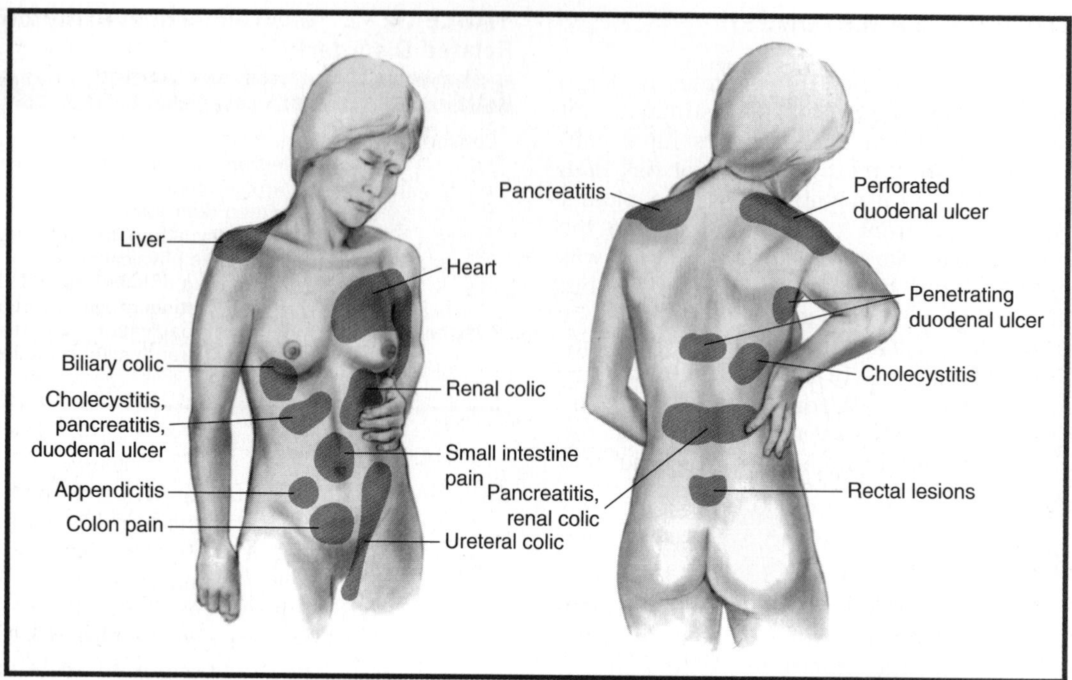

FIGURE 32–17 Common site of referred abdominal pain. (From Jarvis C: Physical Examination and Health Assessment, 2nd ed. Philadelphia, WB Saunders, 1996.)

The accessory organs of the digestive system also play an important role. These are the liver, the gallbladder, and the pancreas. The diseases and disorders for just these three structures number more than 100.

EXAMPLES OF ACCESSORY ORGAN DISEASES AND DISORDERS

- Jaundice as a sign of liver disease, or obstructive jaundice due to *choledocholithiasis* (a calculus in the common bile duct)
- *Acute pancreatitis,* which produces diffuse pain and tenderness in the epigastrium
- Carcinoma, which can invade and cripple all or any one of the accessory organs

ASSISTING WITH THE EXAMINATION

When the patient describes and points to the location of the pain being felt, it is important to know the topography of the abdomen and the underlying organs. Mentally divide the abdomen into quadrants (see Fig. 32–4). The vertical line extends from the xiphoid process of the sternum to the symphysis pubis; the horizontal line crosses the abdomen at the level of the umbilicus (navel). Another method of dividing the abdomen is by regions, or sections (see Fig. 32–4). Note that the right and left hypochondriac regions are composed almost entirely of the costal margins. This is because the abdomen extends up under the rib cage to the dome of the diaphragm. The liver and spleen are located in these two regions. Record the quadrant in which the pain is located, such as "pain in LLQ." Now the physician can move directly into this location when the examination begins. This saves time and also builds patient rapport and confidence as the patient knows that the information you were told was important to the physician.

The inspection of the abdomen begins with noting any change in skin color such as jaundice. *Striae* (silver stretch marks), *petechiae* (small purple hemorrhagic spots), cutaneous *angiomas* (spider nevi), scars, and visible masses may be observed. The contour of the abdomen may be flat, rounded, or bulging in localized areas. A bulging in the right and left lumbar regions (the flanks) may be the result of the presence of free abdominal fluid *(ascites).* Abdominal hernias are examined with the patient in the supine and standing positions.

The physician will use palpation and percussion to evaluate the entire abdominal area. As this is done, your responsibility is to remove the drape from the area to be examined and to re-drape the patient once the physician has completed the examination segment. In addition, the physician may want you to make notations of findings as the examination is being done. Be sure to have pencil and paper ready to complete this task. When the physician wishes to examine the anal area, have the patient turn onto his or her left side and assist the patient into Sims' position. As this is done, be sure the patient remains draped or covered. After the position is achieved, position the drape so that it can be easily lifted for the final segment of the examination.

Memory Jogger

 *During the physical examination, what is your primary role?*

PROCTOLOGIC EXAMINATION

Proctology is the branch of internal medicine concerned with the diseases and disorders of the colon, rectum, and anus. The examination of the anal area is done with a 3-inch anoscope or a proctoscope that permits the detection of hemorrhoids, **polyps, fissures, fistulas,** and **abscesses.** The rectum and the sigmoid colon are examined with either a rigid or flexable sigmoidoscope, and the examination of the descending, transverse, and ascending colon sections or the entire colon is done with a colonoscope.

Many individuals are apprehensive about colorectal examinations. The patient may suffer from anxiety from the moment he or she enters the examining room. It is important for the medical assistant to create an atmosphere of confidence and relaxation.

Memory Jogger

 *Identify five abnormalities that can be detected with a proctoscope.*

Patient Preparation

In an attempt to alleviate apprehension, the patient needs to understand exactly what to do before the examination and may need to be reminded as the procedure is being done. Let the patient know that some discomfort such as cramping can be experienced. Furthermore, the sensations of expelling **flatus** or of an impending bowel movement may be felt. These sensations are caused by the instrument and the procedure.

Depending on the type and purpose of the colorectal procedure and the physician's preference, the patient may be required to prepare the colon for the examination. The patient may be asked to eat a light, low-residue meal the evening before the test is scheduled or may be restricted to only clear liquids. An evening laxative and/or a sodium phosphate (Fleet) enema may be ordered. On the morning of the procedure, some physicians may allow a light breakfast followed by a cleansing enema whereas other physicians may insist that the patient have nothing by mouth until after the procedure is completed. The object of this preparation is to remove all fecal material so that the bowel mucosa can be readily observed. Other physicians prefer to view the lining of the colon in its normal state and feel that the bowel prep may change the appearance of the intestinal mucosa, thus making the diagnosis difficult or altered. The medical assistant must always check the office procedure manual and confirm that this is the protocol that the physician desires for this particular patient. Be certain of the preferred preparation.

Patient Positioning on a Proctologic Table

This position requires an examining table that can be elevated and tilted in the center and lowered at the head and legs. The patient's head and legs are at an angle lower than the buttocks (Fig. 32–18). It must be understood that the patient's body is flexed at the hip joint and not at the waist. If this flexion is not correct, the patient will experience considerable discomfort, and the bowel will not be displaced forward. A single sheet is draped in and around the anal area. Do not bind the patient's legs together with the drape because it may be necessary to separate the legs during the examination. This position is often used for a sigmoidoscopic examination because it straightens the rectosigmoidal area and displaces the lower bowel. It is a convenient position for examining the perineal area, the anus, and hemorrhoids. If the protologist uses a flexible scope, the patient will be placed in the Sims position for the procedure.

Sigmoidoscopy and Colonoscopy Examinations

Sigmoidoscopy provides direct visualization of the sigmoid colon and the rectum. Colonoscopy is more extensive and includes the rectum, the sigmoid, the descending, transverse, and ascending colon, or all structures up to the ileocecal valve.

Sigmoidoscopy may be done with a rigid scope that is 10 to 12 inches long. This hard metal or disposable plastic instrument is calibrated in centimeters (Fig. 32–19). At the insertion end is an **obturator,** which allows the physician to introduce the instrument into the anus and rectum with only minimal discomfort. At the external end is the handle containing the light source and a magnifying lens that assists the physician in viewing the lining of the colon. The lens can be moved aside to allow for laboratory samples to be obtained. The scope is equipped with a air device that enables the physician to expand the walls of the sigmoid colon, making it easier to diagnose hemorrhoids, polyps, and disorders of the diverticula.

A more widely used sigmoidoscope is the flexible fiberoptic sigmoidoscope. This scope allows the physician to complete this examination with very little discomfort to the patient. The entire examination can be done with the patient in the Sims position, which is less traumatic for the patient to maintain than the proctologic position needed when the rigid scope is used. This scope is very thin and bendable so that it can be maneuvered around the curves and

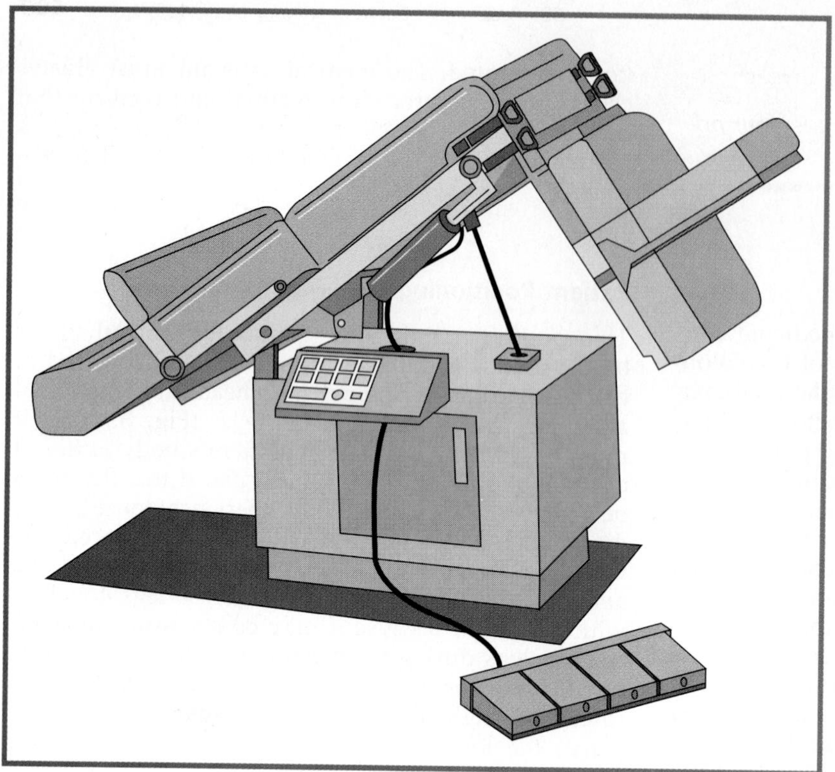

FIGURE 32–18 Proctologic examination table.

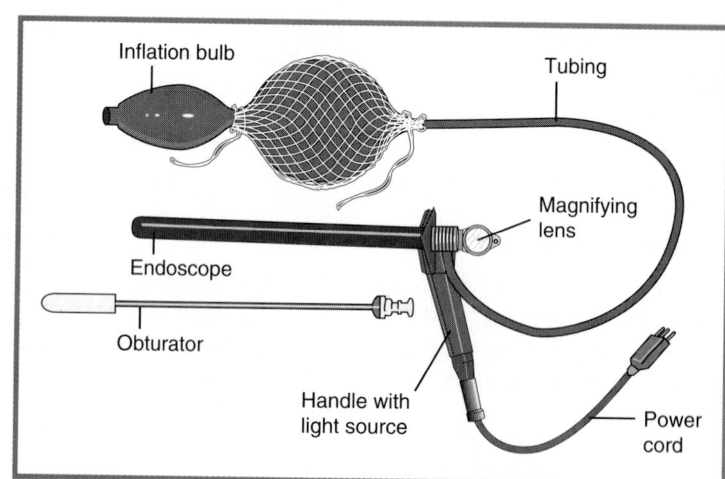

FIGURE 32–19 Rigid sigmoidoscope. (Redrawn from Bonewit-West K: Clinical Procedures for Medical Assistants, 4th ed. Philadelphia, WB Saunders, 1995.)

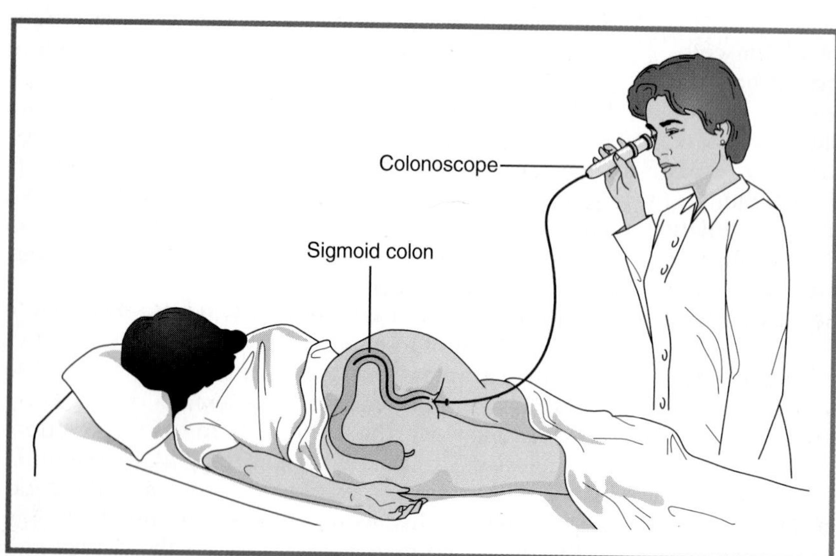

FIGURE 32–20 Flexible colonoscope.

bends of the sigmoid colon (Fig. 32–20). Because the flexible sigmoidoscope is easier to insert and move, the entire sigmoid colon can be examined. To examine beyond the sigmoid section of the colon, the colonoscope is used (see Procedure 32–1).

Memory Jogger

15 *Describe the primary difference between an examination with an anoscope, a rigid and flexible sigmoidoscope, and a colonoscope.*

PROCEDURE 32-1

Assisting with a Colon Examination

GOAL

To assist the physician with the examination, to prepare collected specimens as requested, and to promote patient comfort and safety.

EQUIPMENT AND SUPPLIES

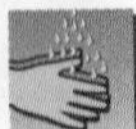

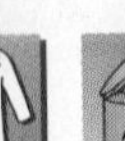
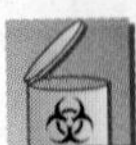

Gloves (for physician)
Appropriate instrument:
  sigmoidoscope, anoscope, or proctoscope
Water-soluble lubricant
Drape and patient gown
Long cotton-tipped swabs
Suction source
Biopsy forceps
Specimen containers with appropriate preservative added
Tissue wipes
Biohazard container

PROCEDURAL STEPS

1 Wash your hands and assemble all needed equipment and supplies.
PURPOSE: Infection control.

2 Identify the patient and explain the procedure.
PURPOSE: Helps to alleviate patient apprehension.

3 Ask the patient to empty his or her bladder.
PURPOSE: Aids in patient comfort during the examination.

4 Give the patient an examination gown and instruct him or her to remove all clothing below the waist and put on the gown with the operating to the back.

5 Obtain and record the patient's vital signs.
PURPOSE: Baseline vital signs allow detection of variations that might occur during the examination.

6 Assist the patient onto the table. When the physician is ready, place the patient in the appropriate position for the type of examination ordered.

7 Drape the patient so that only the anus is exposed. A fenestrated drape (drape with a circular opening placed over the anus) may be used in place of the rectangular drape.

8 Put on gloves and assist the physician as requested during the examination. This includes
- Lubricating the physician's gloved index finger for the digital examination
- Lubricating the obturator tip of the instrument before insertion
- Plugging in the scope's light source when the physician is ready
- Handing the needed supplies to the physician
- Collecting specimens by holding the container to accept the sample
- Labeling specimens immediately because several specimens may be taken from different areas
- Disposing of contaminated supplies as you are given them by the physician

9 Throughout the examination, observe the patient for any undue reactions. Encourage the patient to breath slowly through pursed lips to facilitate relaxation.

Continued

PROCEDURE 30–1 (CONTINUED)

Assisting with a Colon Examination

10 On completion of the examination, cleanse the patient's anal area with tissue wipes. Remove gloves and assist the patient into a resting position and allow the patient time to recover from the procedure.
PURPOSE: A drop in blood pressure often occurs after an invasive procedure, and this may cause fainting.

11 Assist patient off of table and instruct him or her to get dressed. Show the patient where the sink, towels, and tissues are, and provide assistance if needed.

12 Complete all laboratory request forms and specimen container labels, and place specimens in appropriate location for laboratory pick up.

13 Clean work area and all equipment used.
PURPOSE: Infection control.

14 Record procedure and any pertinent information on the patient's record.
PURPOSE: Procedures that are not recorded are considered not done.

LABORATORY TESTS

Many of the diagnostic tests for gastrointestinal symptoms are noninvasive. The patient may be asked to have various radiographs taken of the digestive system. These include a barium swallow, an upper gastrointestinal series, and a barium enema. The gallbladder is viewed by cholecystography. Liver function is checked by various blood tests, such as the "liver function studies" (aspartate aminotransferase, alanine aminotransferase). The urine is tested for bilirubin and urinary amylase levels. The stool is tested for occult blood, intestinal ova and parasites, fat excretion, and color.

Occult Blood Screening

Most family practitioners and internists routinely screen all patients older than 50 years of age for occult blood. This test may be performed on younger patients if a familial history indicates a need. Fecal examination is one means of evaluating patients with gastrointestinal bleeding, obstruction, parasites, dysentery, colitis, or increased fat excretion. This is a screening test (qualitative) and will not diagnose the exact problem but rather gives a positive indication that additional testing is desirable.

Blood is not found in the stool of healthy individuals. If the person is experiencing bleeding of the intestinal wall, the blood is likely to be occult or hidden. This means it cannot be seen with the naked eye. This condition may remain relatively asymptomatic for some time and is why the American Cancer Society recommends an occult blood stool screening test be done as part of the routine physical examination of adults.

A number of easy-to-perform testing kits are available for the detection of occult blood. Most of these kits consist of a test card containing paper squares coated with guaiac, which reacts with the hemoglobin in blood when in the presence of hydrogen peroxide. This reaction produces a blue color on the paper squares of the test card. Two commonly used testing kits are ColoScreen (Helena Laboratories) and Hemoccult II (SmithKline Diagnostics). (See Procedure 32–2.)

Memory Jogger

16 *Why can't occult blood tests be mailed back to the physician's office?*

PROCEDURE 32-2
Stool Specimen Collection

GOAL

Possible detection of the presence of occult blood in a fecal specimen as a screening test for colorectal bleeding disorders.

EQUIPMENT AND SUPPLIES

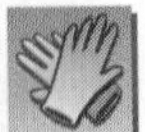 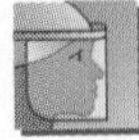

Hemoccult II testing kit
Hemoccult developer
Gloves and face protection
Quality control color strip

PROCEDURAL STEPS

Instructions according to the physician's guidelines are to be given to the patient. The following is a sample of what might be given:

1 For the next 2 days, eat a high-fiber diet. This diet may consist of
   - Well-cooked poultry and fish
   - Cooked fruits and vegetables
   - Bran breads
   - Raw lettuce, carrots, and celery
   - Moderate amounts of peanuts and popcorn

   Avoid
   - Red and partially cooked meats
   - Turnips, cauliflower, broccoli, parsnips, and melons (especially cantaloupe)
   - Alcohol, aspirin, and supplemental vitamin C, and products that contain these elements

2 On the days of the collection, write your name, age, date, and address on the front of the card (Figure 1).

3 After a bowel movement, open the front of one of the cards and using one of the wooden applicators, collect a small sample of feces from the toilet bowl and spread a very thin smear in box A (Figure 2).

Continued

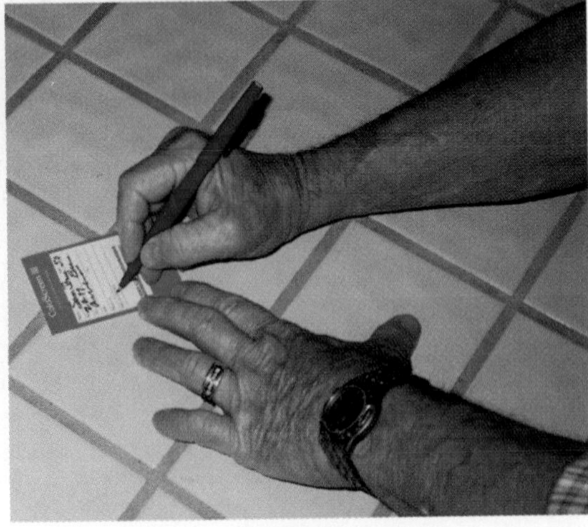

FIGURE 1

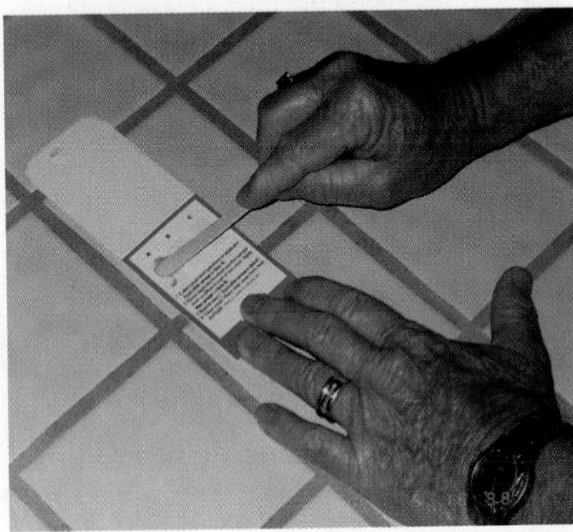

FIGURE 2

PROCEDURE 32-2 (CONTINUED)
Stool Specimen Collection

4 Using the same wooden applicator, collect a second sample from a different part of the stool and spread this sample in box B.

5 Discard the wooden applicator into a trash container. Do not throw this into toilet because it may cause a plumbing problem.

6 Reseal the cover of the specimen card and complete the information requested on the outside of the cover of the card. Wash your hands as usual.

7 Repeat steps 3 to 6 for each of your next two bowel movements.

8 Place all three cards containing samples in the envelope provided and transport it to your doctor or laboratory immediately. Do not attempt to mail the cards to the physician because this material is considered potentially hazardous and is unlawful to mail in a plain envelope.

9 When the slides arrive at the office, confirm that all the necessary information is written on the slide covers.
PURPOSE: Proper identification saves time and possible errors.

10 Wash your hands and put on gloves and face protection.
PURPOSE: Infection control.

11 Open the back sides of all three cards.

12 Follow the manufacturer's directions. The following procedure follows one manufacturer's protocols: place two drops of the developer on each specimen square (Figure 3).

13 Wait 30 seconds and then read the results within 2 minutes. Any blue color visible around the fecal smears indicates a positive result (Figure 4).

Continued

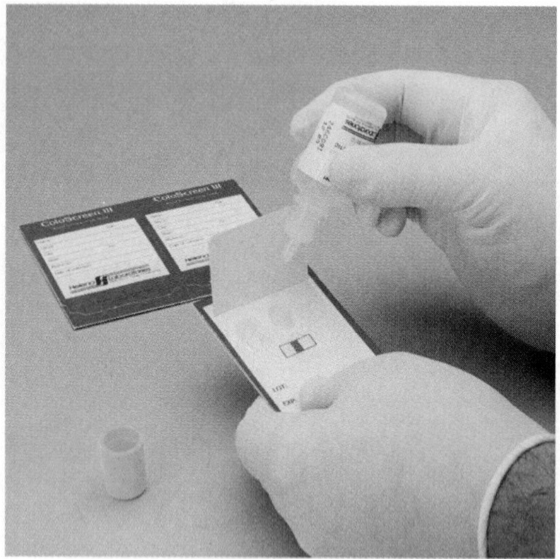

FIGURE 3

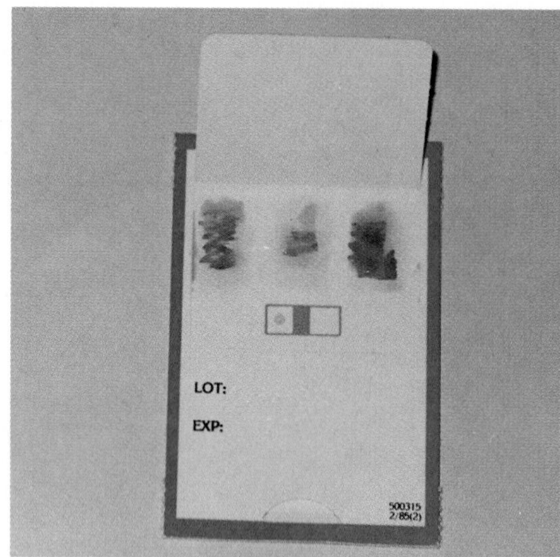

FIGURE 4

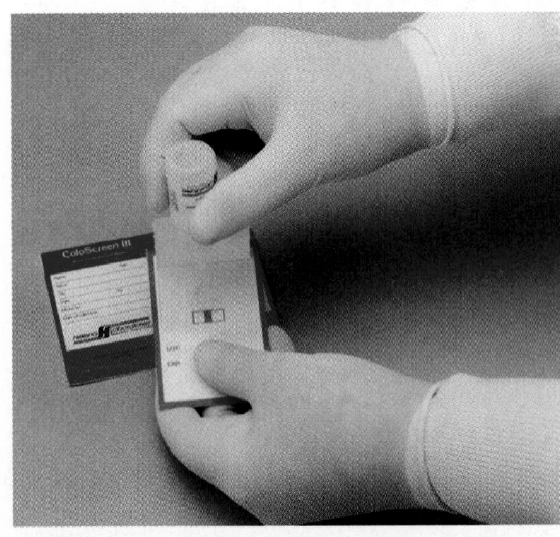

FIGURE 5

14 To develop the test monitor, place one drop of developer between the boxes (Figure 5).

15 Wait 30 seconds and then read the results within 2 minutes.

16 Compare your results with the color photo strip located in the informational folder included in the test pack.
PURPOSE: Quality test control.

17 Discard contaminated supplies, clean work area, remove gloves, and wash hands.
PURPOSE: Infection control.

18 Record test and the results in the patient's record.
PURPOSE: Procedures that are not recorded are considered not done.

ENDOSCOPIC OBSERVATIONS

The unequivocal test for the organs of the entire gastrointestinal system is an endoscopic analysis. The upper gastrointestinal system is examined by passing a soft, flexible tube down the esophagus into the stomach and small intestine up to the **ileocecal valve.** The colon is examined through an ascending technique with entrance through the anus. This fiberoptic technology allows for photographs, filming, and laboratory samples such as tissue biopsy samples, gastric fluid, pathogens, bile crystals, and cytology samples to be obtained during the procedure with only minor discomfort to the patient.

Endoscopic procedures can be used to observe the functioning gallbladder, biliary ducts, and the pancreatic ducts by injecting a dye directly into the vessel ducts of the gallbladder and the pancreas. The examination can then render definitive results regarding patency and function of the organs.

Rectal Suppository Medication

The rectal mucosa provides a rapid absorption due to the high vascularity of the membranes. Drugs are absorbed directly into the bloodstream, without being altered as they would be by the digestive processes and without irritation to the patient's gastric mucosa. Rectal medications are useful if the patient is nauseated, vomiting, or unconscious. Manufacturers supply rectal medications in the form of gelatin or cocoa butter–based suppositories, which melt in the warmth of the rectum and release the medication (see Procedure 32–3), or in the form of enemas. Suppositories and enemas are also used for their local effect, that is, to treat constipation. Rectal suppositories are used to soften the stool or stimulate evacuation of the bowel; enemas are used to cleanse and evacuate.

The best time to administer a rectal drug intended for a systemic effect is after a bowel movement or enema. The patient should be cautioned to remain lying down for 20 to 30 minutes to prevent accidental evacuation of the drug by a bowel movement or elimination of the enema. Suppositories intended to treat constipation, of course, are administered to bring about bowel evacuation. The patient should be instructed to insert the suppository about 2 inches above the rectal sphincter muscles; a little mineral oil or vegetable oil may be used as lubrication. If suppositories are individually wrapped in foil, make sure the patient knows that the foil is the wrapper and is not part of the treatment.

PROCEDURE 32-3
Inserting a Rectal Suppository

GOAL
To insert the prescribed medication accurately into the rectal mucosa.

EQUIPMENT AND SUPPLIES
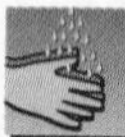  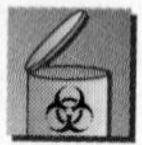

Prescribed suppository medication

Biohazard waste container

PROCEDURAL STEPS
1 Wash your hands, read order, and obtain the necessary supplies.

2 Identify the patient and explain the procedure.
PURPOSE: Proper identification saves time and avoids possible errors.

3 Ask patient to remove clothing covering the anal area.

4 Assist patient into a Sims position and drape exposed area (Figure 1).

5 Put on gloves.
PURPOSE: Infection control.

6 Remove covering from the suppository and smooth any rough edges on the suppository.
PURPOSE: Eliminate any possible trauma to the rectal mucosa.

Continued

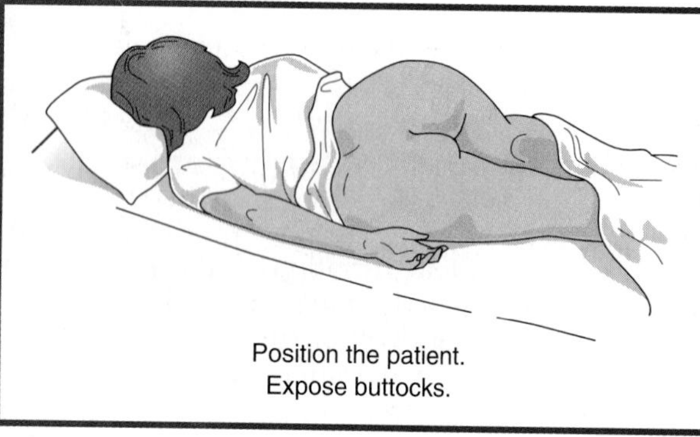
Position the patient.
Expose buttocks.

FIGURE 1

Memory Jogger

 *Why must the individual remain lying down for 20 to 30 minutes after the insertion of a suppository?*

INSTILLING OF OINTMENT

If you are to instill ointment into the rectum using a tube with a rectal applicator attached, review the preceding technique. To lubricate the applicator, remove its protective cover and squeeze the tube. This will push the ointment through the small openings on the applicator and facilitate its insertion into the rectum. Insert the applicator gently to avoid injury to the rectal canal or to hemorrhoids. Squeeze the prescribed amount of ointment into the rectum. Remove the applicator and clean the rectal area with tissues.

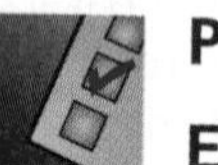

PATIENT EDUCATION

The gastrointestinal system is responsible for the nutrition of the entire body. Digestion is broken into several components: ingestion, digestion, absorption, reabsorption, and elimination. It is through this proc-

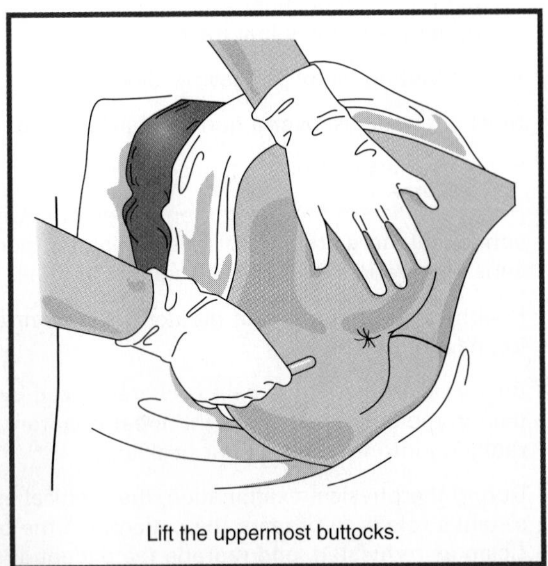
Lift the uppermost buttocks.

FIGURE 2

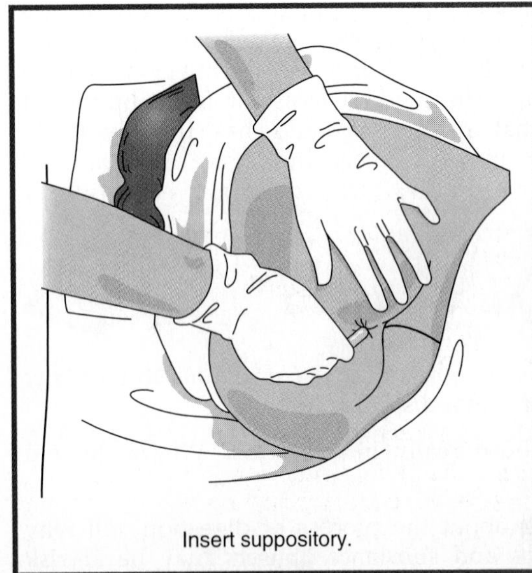
Insert suppository.

FIGURE 3

7 Generously lubricate the suppository with a water-soluble lubricant.
PURPOSE: Promotes ease of insertion.

8 With your free hand, gently lift the uppermost buttock (Figure 2).

9 With your index finger, guide the suppository into the anus, directing it along the rectal wall and away from any fecal masses (Figure 3).

10 To prevent immediate expulsion, be sure to insert the suppository beyond the internal sphincter.

11 Use tissue to gently press on the anus for a few minutes to help the patient retain the rectal medication. Then with the same tissue, wipe any excess lubricant from the rectal area. Dispose of used tissue in a biohazards waste container.

12 Allow patient to rest for a short time before getting up and leaving the office.
PURPOSE: Medication retention.

13 Clean up area, remove gloves, and wash hands.
PURPOSE: Infection control.

14 Record procedure and any pertinent information on the patient's record.
PURPOSE: Procedures that are not recorded are considered not done.

ess of metabolism that nutrients are converted into usable energy units that make it possible for every cell in our body to receive the necessary nutrients to keep it in good health. When disease interferes with this process, the entire body may become disabled and illness can lead to marked pathologic disorders. Listen for a patient's concerns that may indicate a possible problem within this system and its accessory organs. Report these concerns to the physician or note them on the patient's medical record for the physician to read. If the office has information that may assist the patient in dealing with a particular problem, lay out the information for the physician to give to the patient; or with the physician's authorization, talk to the patient and offer suggestions that might help in dealing with a particular concern. Learning to perform and assist with diagnostic procedures can aid the physician in the diagnostic sequence and assist the patient in maintaining a healthy gastrointestinal system, which in turn assists the entire body in homeostasis.

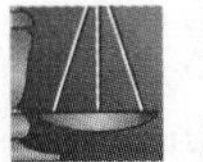

LEGAL AND ETHICAL ISSUES

Legally and ethically the medical assistant's responsibility is to assist the physician and act as the patient's advocate. All information that is discussed between the patient and the physician as well as all testing procedures ordered and done continue to fall under the umbrella of confidentiality. Confidentiality and trust are very closely linked, and these two issues form the basis for a sound patient–physician relationship. The medical assistant is an important part of that relationship and has the ability to strengthen it when practicing ethical professional conduct.

CRITICAL THINKING

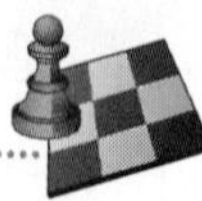

1 Give reasons why alcohol contributes to so many gastrointestinal disorders.

2 Is heartburn really in the heart? Where do you think it is?

3 Thinking about the process of digestion, tell why alcoholics and substance abusers may be at risk for cirrhosis.

4 What are ways you can create a confident and relaxed atmosphere for the apprehensive patient?

HOW DID I DO? Answers to Memory Joggers

1 The six functions of the gastrointestinal system are ingestion, mastication, digestion, absorption, reabsorption, and elimination.

2 The gastrointestinal system is readily accessible to invading bacteria because it is open at both ends.

3 It usually takes about 48 hours to recover from food poisoning.

4 The cause of oral tumors is unknown, but use of tobacco products and chronic alcoholism are definite risk factors.

5 The usual sites for herpes simplex are the lips, mouth, and gums.

6 Two tests that assist in the diagnosis of ulcers are an upper gastrointestinal series and endoscopy of the upper gastrointestinal tract.

7 A contributing factor for gastric cancer is diet.

8 Most patients discover a hernia while bathing.

9 Food allergies contribute to ulcerative colitis.

10 Hemorrhoids are more common in persons with a congenital, hereditary predisposition and in persons with varicose veins and inguinal hernias.

11 Health care workers are at greater risk in contracting hepatitis B.

12 Biliary duct obstruction pain is characterized by pain in the epigastric and right upper quadrant radiating into the right upper back area.

13 During the physical examination, the medical assistant's role is to prepare the patient, aid the physician as requested, and redrape the patient as the examination is completed. When the examination is done, assist the patient in redressing and clean the examination area.

14 The proctoscope may be used to detect hemorrhoids, polyps, fissures, fistulas, and abscesses.

15 An anoscope examination extends 3 inches into the anus. The sigmoidoscope extends approximately 10 inches or through the anus, rectum, and sigmoid colon; and the colonoscope extends from the anus up to the ileocecal valve, which is the entire length of the colon.

16 The occult blood test cards cannot be mailed back to the office because it is potentially a biohazard test and it is unlawful to mail such material unless it is in a designated carton and labeled as biohazard material.

17 The individual remains in a lying position for 20 to 30 minutes after receiving a suppository to prevent accidental evacuation of the drug.

Assisting in Gynecology and Obstetrics

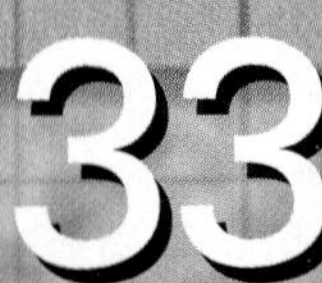

33

OUTLINE

LEARNING OBJECTIVES

Cognitive: On successful completion of this chapter you should be able to:

1 Identify the major organs of the female reproductive system and explain the primary function of each.
2 Trace the ovum through the three phases of menstruation.
3 Explain the physiology of pregnancy from conception through the three trimesters and parturition.
4 Identify the three types of pregnancy complications.
5 List and explain the diseases and disorders that may affect the female.
6 Name and describe seven sexually transmitted diseases.
7 Outline the medical assistant's role in the reproductive examination.
8 Compare and contrast the yearly physical examination with the initial pregnancy examination.
9 Name and describe the medical assistant's role in seven diagnostic tests that may be done in evaluating the female reproductive system.
10 Define family planning and the three classifications of birth control that are used.
11 Spell and define terms in the vocabulary.

Performance: On successful completion of this chapter you should be able to:

1 Prepare the instruments and equipment for a female examination including a Papanicolaou test.
2 Teach the patient how to perform a breast self-examination.
3 Describe cryosurgery preparation to a patient.
4 Determine the estimated day of delivery when given the date of the last menstrual period.

VOCABULARY

adhesions Fibrous scar tissue that clings to the surface of adjoining tissue sometimes forming an unwanted union of two surfaces

anomalies Marked deviations from normal as the result of faulty development of the fetus

atrophy Wasting away; decrease in size from normal

cervical spatula Wooden instrument designed to remove cervical secretions from the cervical os and from the cervical cuff; used to obtain secretions for the Papanicolaou test

cervix The narrow lower end of the uterus, sometimes called the *neck of the uterus*

chancre Primary lesion of syphilis occurring at the site of entry of the infection

clitoris Small, elongated erectile body situated above the urinary meatus at the superior point of the labia minora

coitus Sexual union between male and female; also known as intercourse

colostrum Thin, yellow, milky fluid secreted by the mammary glands a few days before and after delivery

dysmenorrhea Painful menstruation

dysuria Difficult or painful urination

estrogen Female sex hormone secreted primarily by the ovaries

fallopian tubes Extensions from the uterus that capture the expelled ova and transport them to the uterus; usual location of fertilization; also called the *oviducts*

fimbriae Fringelike border found on the distal part of the fallopian tube

fixative Agent used in preserving a histologic or pathologic specimen to maintain its normal structure

fundus Part of the uterus between the junctions of the fallopian tubes

gestation Period of development from fertilization until birth

hemoptysis Coughing and spitting of blood as a result of bleeding in the respiratory tract

human chorionic gonadotropin (hCG) Hormone secreted by the female when pregnant

hysterectomy Surgical removal of the uterus

in vitro Created in an artificial environment, such as a test tube or a petri dish

labia majora Two folds of adipose tissue that extend from the mons pubis to the perineum in the female

labia minora Two thin folds of epithelial tissue between the labia majora and the opening of the vagina

lubricant Water-soluble substance used on the glove when the rectum or vaginal cavity is examined

malaise Feeling of uneasiness

mammary glands Milk-producing glands in the breasts

menarche Onset of the menstrual cycle

menopause Biologic end of the reproductive cycle of the female; also called *climacteric*

menstruation Cyclic shedding of the lining (endometrium) of the uterus

mons pubis Fat pad that covers the symphysis pubis

multiparous Pertaining to women who have had two or more pregnancies

ovaries Pair of almond-shaped organs located at the distal end of the fallopian tubes that are responsible for the production and release of ova and a large percentage of the female hormones

parturition Act or process of giving birth to a child

placenta Vascular structure that develops within the uterus during pregnancy and through which the fetus receives nourishment

progesterone Female hormone that plays a major part in the menstrual cycle

umbilicus Depressed scar on the abdomen marking the site of entry of the umbilical cord; also called the navel

urethral meatus External opening to the urinary system

uterus Pear-shaped organ located in the pelvic cavity between the bladder and the rectum and ending in the cervix; holds the fetus during pregnancy

vagina Collapsible muscular tube extending from the vaginal opening to the cervix

vaginal speculum Instrument used to expand the vaginal orifice and allow the physician to examine the vagina and cervix or to obtain a cytologic specimen for the Papanicolaou test

viability State or quality of being capable to live after birth

void To urinate

vulva The external female genitalia, which begins at the mons pubis and terminates at the anus

zygote Cell resulting from the union of the male and female sex cells

The branch of medicine that deals with pregnancy, labor, and the postnatal period is known as *obstetrics,* and the branch of medicine that deals with diseases of the genital tract in women is called *gynecology.* Frequently, a physician practices both specialties and is known as an OB/GYN physician. The assessment of the female reproductive system is an important part of health care. Often, patients are hesitant and uncomfortable with talking about sexual matters and wait until symptoms are intolerable or disease is advanced before seeking medical care. In addition to the signs and symptoms of disease, the medical assistant must be aware of signs of the patient's emotional state and give support when needed.

Anatomy and Physiology

THE FEMALE REPRODUCTIVE SYSTEM

The female reproductive system contains both internal and external organs. The internal organs are located within the pelvis and cannot be seen without special instrumentation such as a vaginal speculum or a laparoscope. The external organs can be seen visually during the physical examination.

The primary parts of the female reproductive system are the **vulva, vagina, uterus, fallopian tubes,** and the **ovaries** (Fig. 33–1). The vulva includes the **clitoris,** the **urethral meatus,** and the vaginal orifice. These structures are covered by two sets of lips of tissue. The **labia minora** is a thin layer of skin extending from the top of the clitoris to the base of the vaginal opening. The external set is known as the **labia majora,** and these, along with the **mons pubis,** are covered with hair in the adult.

The vagina is the structure that connects the internal and external organs. This tubelike structure is constructed to easily receive the penis during **coitus.** It is lubricated by its mucous membrane and has tremendous elasticity, as noted in its expansion during delivery. At the upper end of the vagina is the **cervix,** often called the neck of the uterus. This muscle controls the opening to the uterus.

The uterus is a pear-shaped muscular organ with the sole purpose of housing and nourishing the fetus from implantation shortly after conception until **parturition.** The uterine walls have three layers. The inner layer is the endometrium, which is rich in blood and will change in consistency during the menstrual cycle. The middle layer is the myometrium. This is the powerful muscular layer that contracts to make the delivery of the fetus possible. The outer layer is the perimetrium, which protects the

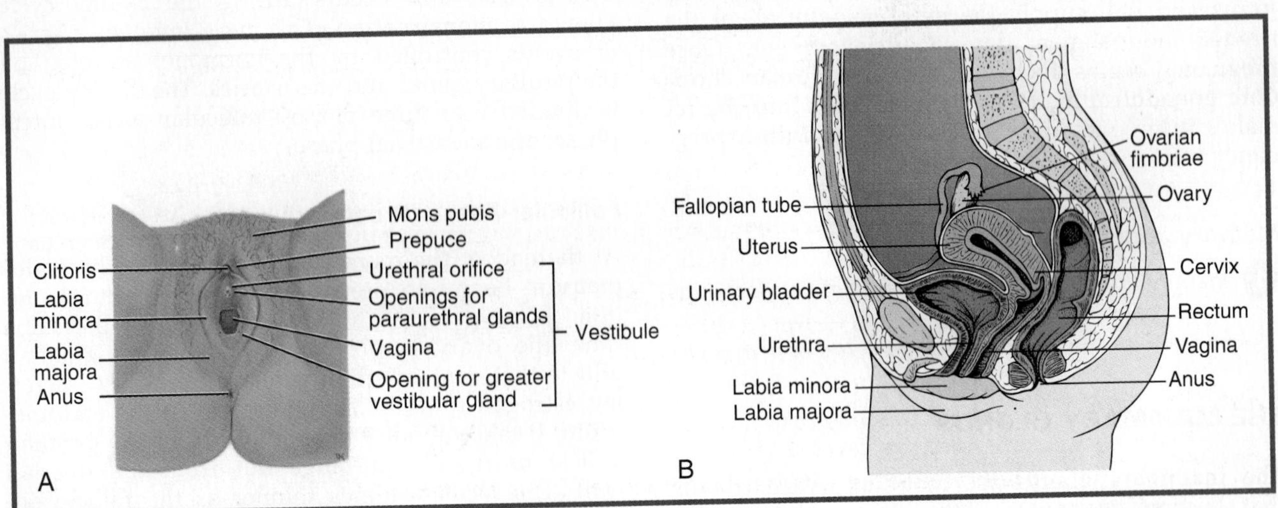

FIGURE 33–1 *A,* Female external genitalia. *B,* Normal female reproductive system. (*A,* from Applegate EJ: The Anatomy and Physiology Learning System. Philadelphia, WB Saunders, 1995; *B,* from Frazier MS, Drzymkowski JA, Doty SJ: Essentials of Human Diseases and Conditions. Philadelphia, WB Saunders, 1996.)

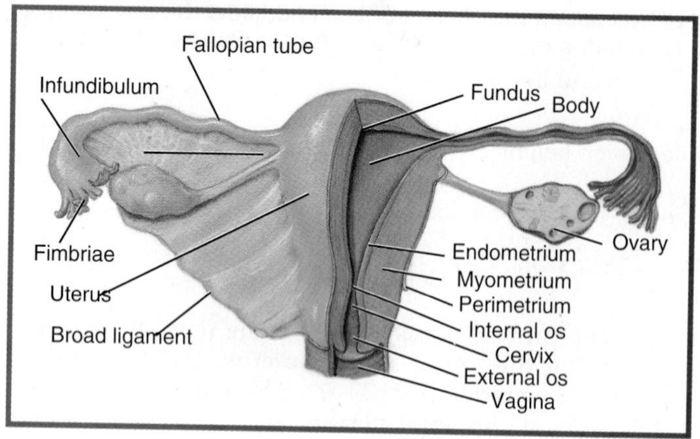

FIGURE 33–2 Uterus and fallopian tubes. (Adapted from Applegate EJ: The Anatomy and Physiology Learning System. Philadelphia, WB Saunders, 1995.)

structure and attaches to ligaments that support and hold the uterus in place (Fig. 33–2).

On either side of the **fundus** of the uterus are the fallopian tubes, which are also called the oviducts. These tubes extend from the uterus to the ovaries but do not attach to the ovaries. The distal end of the tube opens freely into the abdominopelvic cavity and acts as the passageway for the ovum to the uterus and for the sperm as they search for the ovum. At the superior end of the tubes are hairlike fingers called **fimbriae.** The fimbriae move in a wavelike pattern to draw the ovum into the tube.

The ovaries are almond-shaped organs that produce and release the egg and hormones necessary for the development of secondary sex characteristics and the maintenance of a pregnancy. The hormones progesterone and estrogen secreted by the ovaries regulate the reproductive function. The vagina receives the sperm from the male, and fertilization takes place in the lower portion of the fallopian tube. The tiny fertilized ovum, now called a **zygote,** leaves the tube and implants itself into the wall of the uterus. After implantation occurs, the **placenta** forms and will supply the new life with all of the needed nourishment for its development. Once pregnancy begins, the serum levels of **human chorionic gonadotropin** (hCG) rise and spill into the female's urine, where it can be detected with a pregnancy test.

Memory Jogger

1 *Identify the internal and external female reproductive organs.*

THE MAMMARY GLANDS

The **mammary glands** are modified sweat glands that become the organs of milk production. The glands are located in the breast tissue of both sexes but usually function only in the female.

In the center of each breast there is a raised area known as the nipple, which is surrounded by a pigmented region called the areola. Inside the breast are lobules of granular tissue that are separated by connective support tissue and surrounded by adipose tissue. The amount and distribution of the adipose tissue determines the size and shape of the breast (Fig. 33–3).

There are four hormones that control the mammary glands. Estrogen is responsible for the increase in size, progesterone stimulates the development of the duct system, prolactin stimulates the production of milk, and oxytocin causes the ejection of the milk from the glands.

MENSTRUATION

When a young girl enters puberty, one of the many changes that will occur is **menarche,** or the beginning of the menstrual cycle. This is a normal body process that occurs in every female and is the physiologic way of ridding her body of the thickened uterine wall that occurs during the 28-day cycle known as **menstruation.** This cycle involves a series of events controlled by the hormones secreted by the pituitary gland and the ovaries. The 28-day cycle is divided into three phases: follicular phase, luteal phase, and menstrual phase.

Follicular Phase (Proliferative Phase)

At the end of the menstrual flow (day 5), the endometrium begins to prepare for a possible implantation of a zygote by rapidly enlarging. At the same time, the ovary is producing one mature graafian follicle that contains the ovum, and it is also secreting **estrogen** to assist in the growth of the endometrium. It takes about 9 days (day 14) for the graafian follicle to ripen and bulge out from the ovarian wall. This wall becomes thinner as the follicle enlarges until it bursts, allowing the ovum to be liberated into the abdominal cavity. Now the fimbriae begin their wavelike motion to fan the ovum into the fallopian tube. The rupture spot on the ovary,

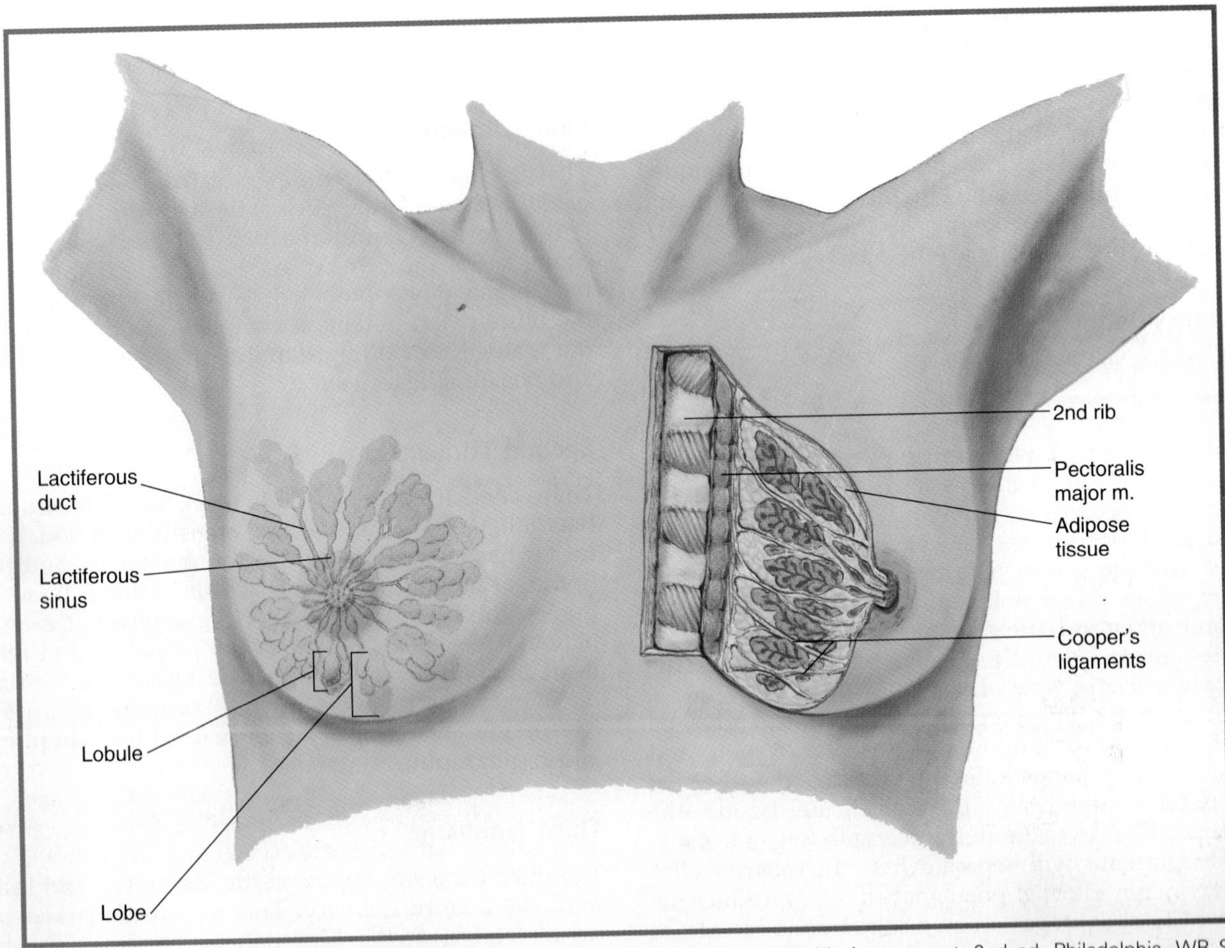

FIGURE 33–3 Normal female breast. (From Jarvis C: Physical Examination and Health Assessment, 2nd ed. Philadelphia, WB Saunders, 1996.)

now called the corpus luteum, begins to secrete **progesterone.** All of this activity causes an increase in body temperature, and some women experience cramping and tenderness in the lower abdominal area at this time.

Luteal Phase (Secretory Phase)

Once ovulation is complete, the luteal phase begins (day 15). During this phase, progesterone secreted from the corpus luteum causes extensive growth of the endometrium as it prepares for the possible pregnancy. If conception occurs, the corpus luteum will continue to secrete progesterone until the placenta is well established and can take over the secreting function of progesterone and hCG.

If conception does not occur, the hCG secretion will be absent and the corpus luteum will **atrophy.** With these hormones missing, the endometrium begins to break down the buildup of implantation tissue.

Menstrual Phase

On day 28, menstruation begins. This discharge is made up of dead endometrial tissue, mucus, and the blood that was in the endometrial engorgement. As the uterus contracts to shed the excess tissue, a woman may experience cramping pain and irritability. This phase usually lasts about 5 days and then the follicular phase begins again.

When conception has taken place, the menstrual cycle is interrupted and will not appear until after the termination of the pregnancy.

Memory Jogger

In what phase does pregnancy occur?

PREGNANCY

If fertilization does occur in the fallopian tube, the fertilized egg, now called a zygote, is formed. This zygote begins with the 23 chromosomes of the ovum uniting with the 23 chromosomes of the sperm to form the first complete cell. This cell begins to grow and multiply immediately. The zygote will reach the uterus in 5 to 6 days and implants in the uterine endometrium. Enzymes are secreted by the zygote to aid in the implantation process.

The placenta forms within the uterine wall. It is derived from maternal endometrium and partly from the chorion, the outermost membrane that surrounds the developing zygote. The amnion is the innermost layer of the membranes, and it holds the fetus suspended in an amniotic cavity surrounded by a fluid called the amniotic fluid. The amnion and fluid are sometimes known as the "bag of water." When this breaks it signals the onset of labor.

Memory Jogger

Where does fertilization occur?

After the first 2 weeks of the pregnancy are completed, and the zygote is well established in the uterus, it becomes an embryo. It will remain an embryo until close to the end of the first trimester (12 weeks) of pregnancy. During the embryonic period, every cell in this new life will be formed. During the second and third trimester periods, the embryo becomes a fetus. During these periods, the cells develop and begin their primary functions.

Throughout the pregnancy, maternal and fetal blood never mix. Important nutrients, oxygen, and wastes are exchanged through the blood vessels of the fetus's umbilical cord, which lie beside the mother's blood vessels in the placenta (Fig. 33–4).

The placenta will separate from the uterus after delivery, but during pregnancy it will produce its own hCG and progesterone. Progesterone maintains the development of the placenta, and low levels of progesterone can lead to spontaneous abortion in pregnant women and menstrual irregularities in nonpregnant women. The average **gestation** is calculated at 9 calendar months, 10 lunar months, or 266 to 280 days and is divided into first, second, and third trimesters.

First Trimester

The first trimester is the period from the beginning of the last menstrual period through the 14th week. It is a period of multiple physical and psychologic changes for the female and is a crucial period of fetal organ development. It is during this time that the obstetrician obtains a complete health history of the patient, including family, medical, menstrual, and obstetric histories.

Second Trimester

The second trimester extends from the 15th through the 28th weeks after the last menstrual period. The uterus has enlarged to above the **umbilicus,** and the first fetal movements are felt by the patient. In addition to the basic health history and physical examination, assessment by abdominal palpation and fetal heart monitoring is conducted. Diagnostic testing during this period may include amniocentesis (Fig. 33–5), ultrasonography, chorionic villus sampling, and radiography.

Third Trimester

The third trimester begins at the 28th week and lasts until the time of delivery. This period is marked by rapid fetal growth. The patient continues to be closely monitored. Childbirth preparation classes usually begin during this time. The patient experiences noticeable breast enlargement and may experience occasional discharge from the nipples of the clear sticky fluid **colostrum.**

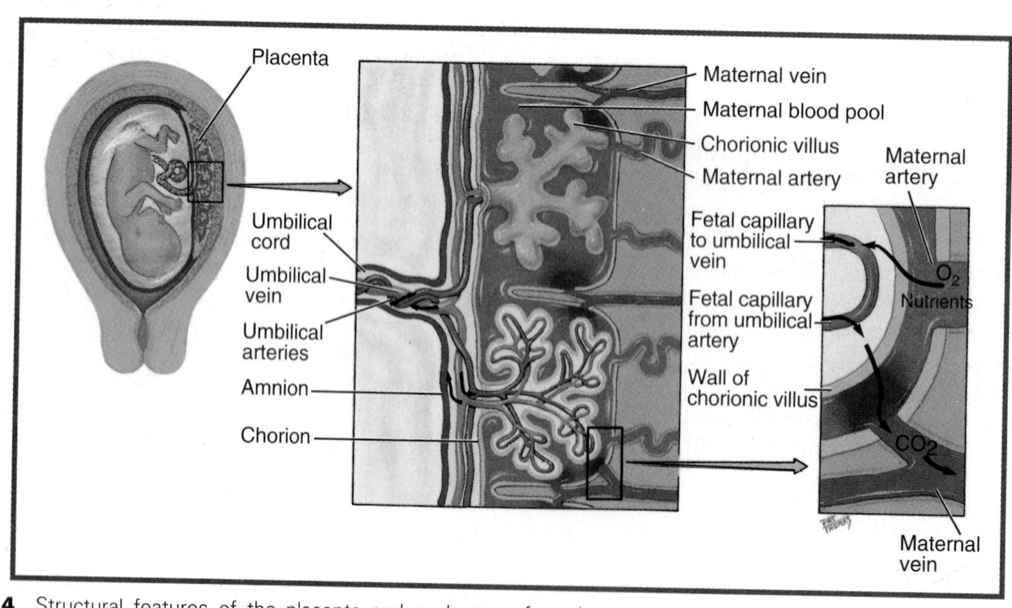

FIGURE 33–4 Structural features of the placenta and exchange of nutrients and wastes between maternal and fetal blood. (From Applegate EJ: The Anatomy and Physiology Learning System. Philadelphia, WB Saunders, 1995.)

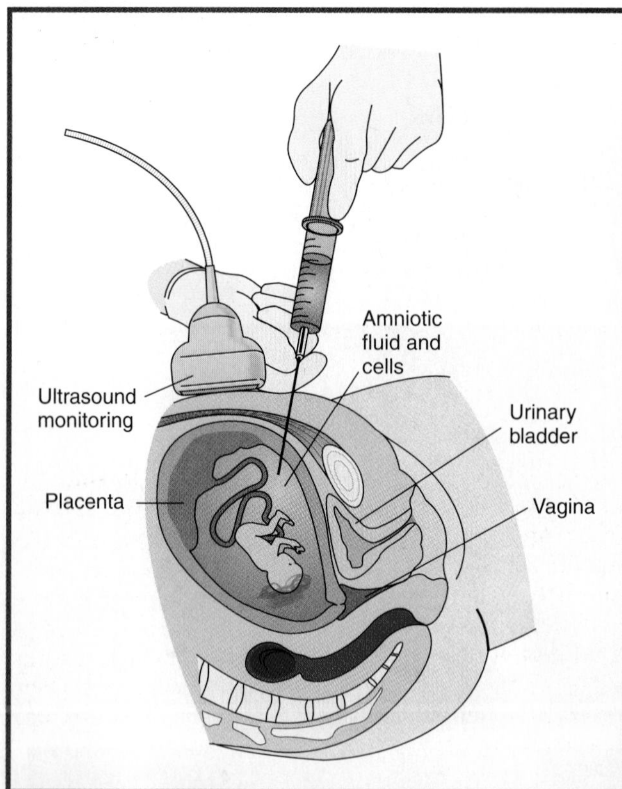

FIGURE 33–5 Amniocentesis.

Memory Jogger

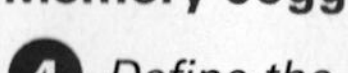

Define the terms zygote, embryo, and fetus.

Parturition

Labor is the physiologic process by which the uterus expels the fetus and the placenta (Fig. 33–6*A*). It is divided into three stages:

- Stage I: From onset of labor through complete dilation and effacement of the cervix (see Fig. 33–6*B*)
- Stage II: From complete dilation and effacement of the cervix through the birth of the fetus (see Fig. 33–6C).
- Stage III: From the birth of the fetus through the expulsion of the placenta and the membranes (see Fig. 33–6*D*).

Pregnancy Complications

Pregnancy complications can occur at several points in time and are classified into three areas: abnormal fertilization, improper implantation, and interruption of pregnancy.

Abnormal Fertilization

Some couples are unable to have a child because of the inability of the sperm and ovum to unite. Ovarian factors are not totally understood; however, it is known that some women have "healthier" ova than others. The ova in women older than 40 are generally of inferior quality, but mature, apparently healthy ova of young women do not fertilize in 20% of cases.

Improper Implantation

Ectopic pregnancy refers to a pregnancy that occurs outside the uterus. This can occur in the ovary, fallopian tube, or even the abdominal cavity, but about 90% of the time, it occurs in the fallopian tube. When the cells of the forming placenta erode the muscle layer of the tube, it causes bleeding and can destroy the tube's muscle layer and rupture the tube. Rupture of the fallopian tube containing an ectopic pregnancy is a very serious event and requires immediate surgical intervention to prevent fatal hemorrhage.

A placenta that is implanted in the lower portion of the uterus is referred to as placenta previa. When this happens, symptoms may not appear until the seventh or eighth month of pregnancy. At that time slight hemorrhage, recurring with greater severity and accompanied by a gradual anemia, pallor, rapid weak pulse, air hunger, and low blood pressure, occurs. The prognosis depends on control of hemorrhage and prevention of uterine infection, and a cesarean delivery is usually performed as soon as possible.

Interruption of Pregnancy

An interruption of pregnancy before the term of fetal **viability** is called an abortion.

TYPES OF ABORTIONS

- *Spontaneous*—abortions that do not have an identifiable cause
- *Complete*—complete expulsion of both fetus and placenta without any medical intervention
- *Incomplete*—expulsion of only parts of the fetus and placenta. A dilation and curettage (D&C) must be done to remove the remaining pieces.
- *Missed*—the fetus dies in utero and must be evacuated surgically.
- *Threatened*—cervical bleeding but no dilation occurs, and the pregnancy continues uninterrupted.
- *Induced*—evacuation of the uterus at the request of the mother of the fetus

It is estimated that one in three pregnancies will terminate by abortion, and in most cases the causes are not clear. Chromosomal **anomalies** are fre-

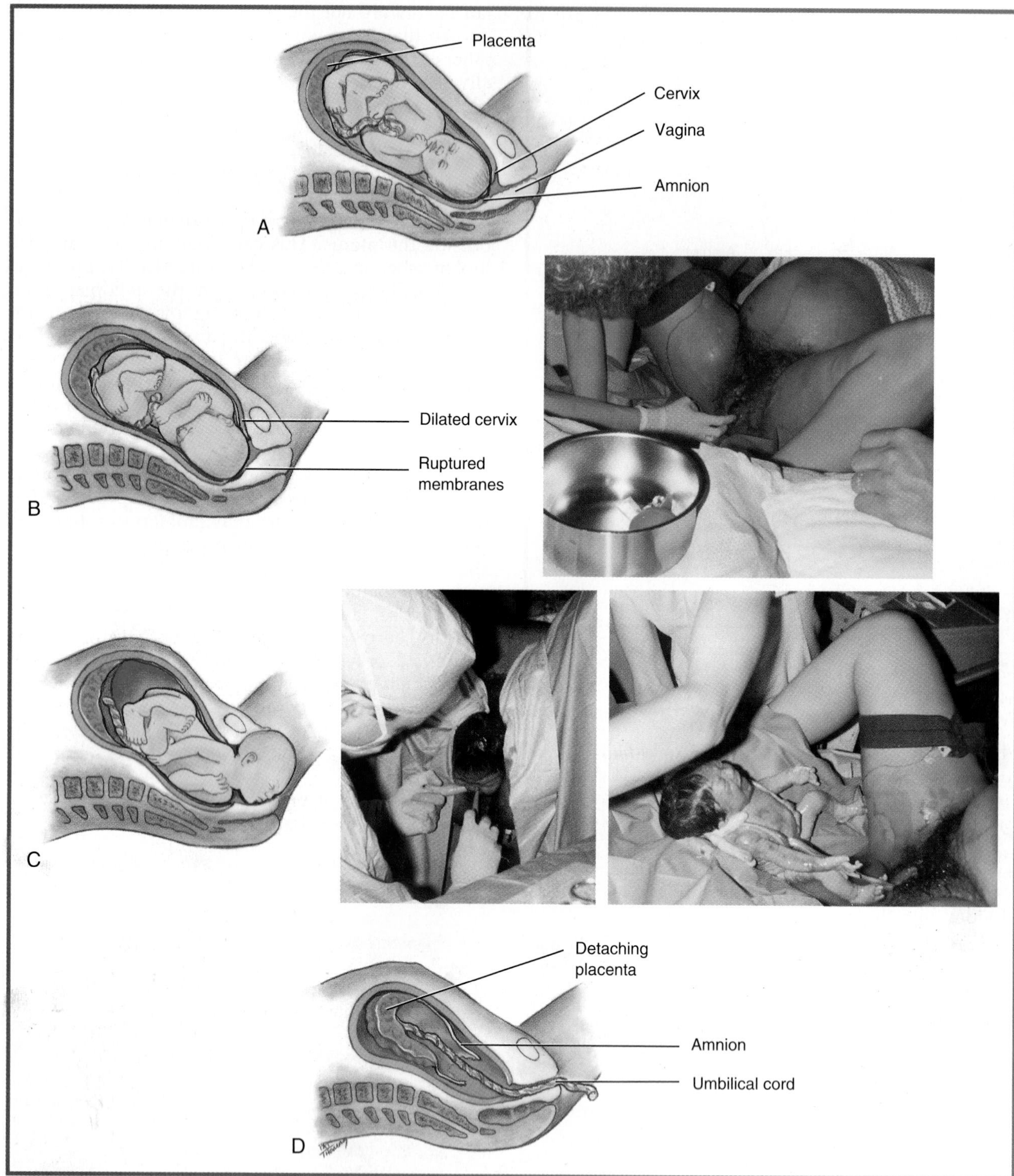

FIGURE 33–6 Three stages of labor. *A*, Before labor begins. *B*, Dilation stage. *C*, Expulsion stage. *D*, Placental stage. (From Applegate EJ: The Anatomy and Physiology Learning System. Philadelphia, WB Saunders, 1995.)

quently detected in an aborted fetus and/or placenta.

Spontaneous abortion (miscarriage) is the loss of a pregnancy before the 20th week of fetal development. Common causes are defective development of the embryo, abnormalities of the placenta, endocrine disorders, malnutrition, infection, drug reaction, blood group incompatibilities, severe trauma, and shock. Symptoms include vaginal bleeding of varying degrees of severity and lower abdominal cramping progressing to cervical dilation with rupture of membranes and complete expulsion of the products of conception.

Memory Jogger

Name three classifications of pregnancy complications.

Disease and Disorders

CERVICITIS

Cervicitis is an inflammation of the cervix caused by an invading organism. The main symptom is a thick, purulent, whitish discharge with an acrid odor. Dysuria may also be present. Cervicitis is common after vaginal delivery, resulting from infection of cervical lacerations. Treatment consists primarily of antibiotics, although cauterization, or electrocoagulation, may be indicated when cervical erosion exists.

CERVICAL POLYPS

Polyps are the second most common lesion of the cervix. They are most prevalent during the reproductive years. The most common symptom is genital bleeding after intercourse, douching, or tampon insertion. Treatment consists of surgical removal of the polyps in the office.

CYSTOCELE

A cystocele is a protrusion of the bladder into the vagina. A diagnosis can be made by requesting the patient to bear down as the vaginal opening is examined. A cystocele may result from injury during childbirth, obesity, heavy lifting, chronic coughing, and poor musculature due to aging (Fig. 33–7).

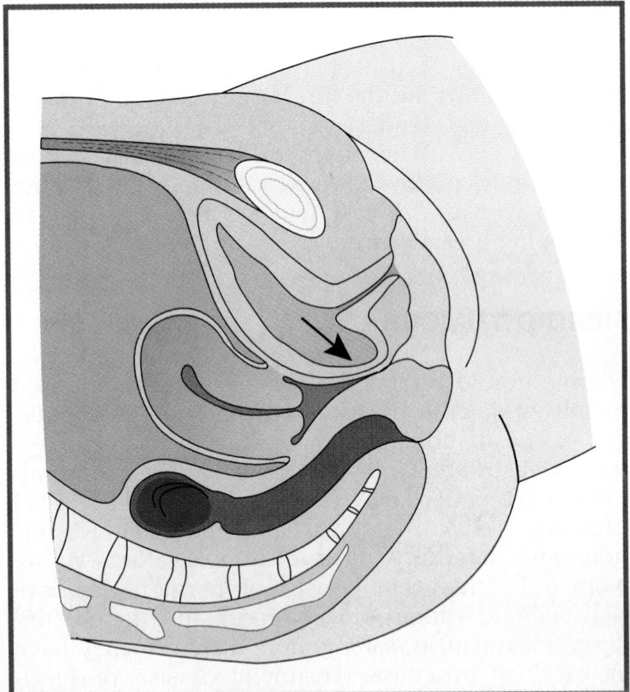

FIGURE 33–7 Cystocele.

ENDOMETRIOSIS

Endometriosis is characterized by the presence of endometrial tissue outside the uterus. It is commonly found in the pelvic area attached to the vulva, urinary bladder, uterus, fallopian tubes, ovaries, intestines, and peritoneum. The cause is unknown, but the use of tampons has been suggested as a possible cause. **Dysmenorrhea** and contact pain in the lower abdomen, pelvis, vagina, and back beginning 7 days before menses and lasting 3 days after onset characterize this condition. Other symptoms can include profuse menses, hematuria, rectal bleeding, nausea, vomiting, and abdominal cramps. Conservative treatment through the use of hormones is used when the woman wants to have children. Treatment may consist of a laparoscopy to remove the ectopic endometrial tissue. In severe cases, a total **hysterectomy** may be indicated. There is no cure, but pregnancy, nursing an infant, or natural menopause frequently causes remission (Fig. 33–8).

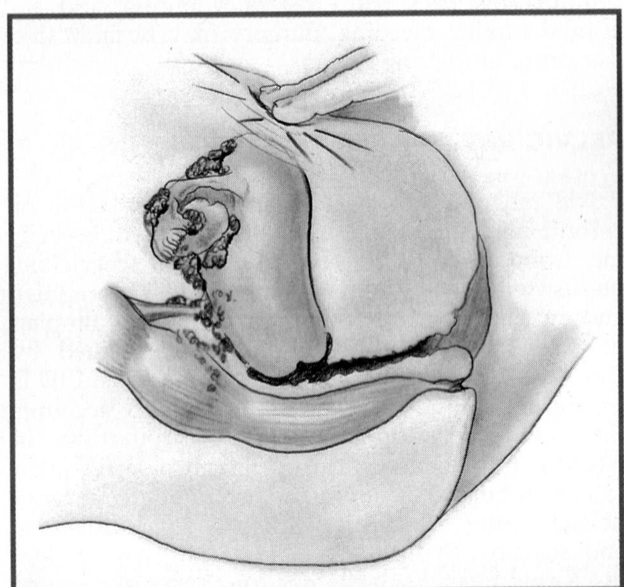

FIGURE 33–8 Endometriosis showing nodular masses on uterus, ovaries, and sigmoid colon. Ovaries are often enlarged. (Redrawn from Jarvis C: Physical Examination and Health Assessment, 2nd ed. Philadelphia, WB Saunders, 1996.)

FIBROCYSTIC BREAST DISEASE

Fibrocystic breast disease is the presence of multiple palpable lumps in the **breasts,** usually associated with pain and tenderness that fluctuate with the menstrual cycle. The lumps may be fibrous tumors that have degenerated or sacs filled with fluid. Women with the disease may be at greater risk of developing breast cancer.

FIBROID TUMORS

Uterine fibroid tumors are benign tumors composed mainly of smooth muscle and some fibrous connective tissue of unknown cause. Menorrhagia (excessive menstruation) is the primary symptom, although the patient may experience bladder or rectal pressure, pelvic pressure, pain, abdominal distortion, and infertility. Fibroid tumors affect young women because they consist of hormone-sensitive cells. Fibroid tumors do not recur and do not undergo malignant transformation; therefore, they have an excellent prognosis. Treatment consists of surgical removal of the mass, but a hysterectomy may be indicated when there is greater involvement (Fig. 33–9).

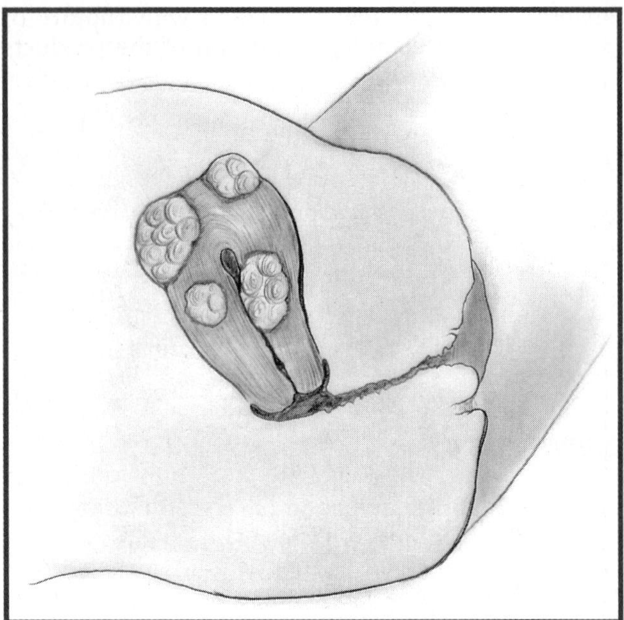

FIGURE 33–9 Uterine fibroid tumors are composed of hormone-sensitive cells, and treatment consists of surgical removal. (Redrawn from Jarvis C: Physical Examination and Health Assessment, 2nd ed. Philadelphia, WB Saunders, 1996.)

OVARIAN CYSTS

Ovarian cysts are sacs of fluid or semisolid material located on the ovary. Most cysts are nonmalignant, small, and asymptomatic, and the underlying cause is unknown. They can occur in the follicle or the corpus luteum at any time between puberty and **menopause.** Large or multiple cysts may cause discomfort, low back pain, nausea, vomiting, and abnormal uterine bleeding. Surgery may be indicated if rupture of the cyst occurs.

PELVIC INFLAMMATORY DISEASE

Pelvic inflammatory disease (PID) is any acute or chronic infection of the reproductive system ascending from the vagina (vaginitis), cervix (cervicitis), uterus (endometritis), fallopian tubes (salpingitis), and ovaries (oophoritis). In these cases, the fallopian tubes may contain pus or may be deformed by chronic attacks of inflammation or **adhesions.** PID is frequently caused by gonorrhea and also accounts for a large percentage of cases of infertility in women. In women with PID, **in vitro** fertilization can often be successfully done. Uterine infection can develop after pelvic surgery, tubal examinations, and abortion. Symptoms include a purulent vaginal discharge, fever, **malaise, dysuria,** lower abdominal pain, bleeding, and nausea and vomiting. PID treatment may include antibiotics, analgesics, and bed rest.

RECTOCELE

A rectocele is a protrusion of the rectum into the vagina. Diagnosis can be made by requesting the patient to bear down as the vaginal opening is examined. Rectocele is most often seen in postmenopausal women. A rectocele may result from pregnancy, difficult delivery, prolonged labor, obesity, chronic coughing, and lifting heavy objects.

MALIGNANCY

The majority of the problems encountered with the female reproductive organs are related to abnormal cell growth. Early screening and preventive intervention are essential. Most malignant tumors require surgical removal. Radiation, chemotherapy, and hormone therapy may be alternative treatment choices. Uterine cancer is the most common reproductive organ cancer, usually affecting women between the ages of 50 and 60 years. The first signs of uterine cancer include uterine enlargement and unusual bleeding. The only reliable diagnostic procedure is a biopsy. Cervical cancer is asymptomatic until the malignancy has penetrated through the membranes and spread (Fig. 33–10). The earliest symptoms include abnormal vaginal bleeding, persistent discharge, and bleeding and pain during intercourse. Cervical cancer can be detected early by a Papanicolaou (Pap) smear (Fig. 33–11). The American Cancer Society recommends that all sexually active women have annual Pap smears.

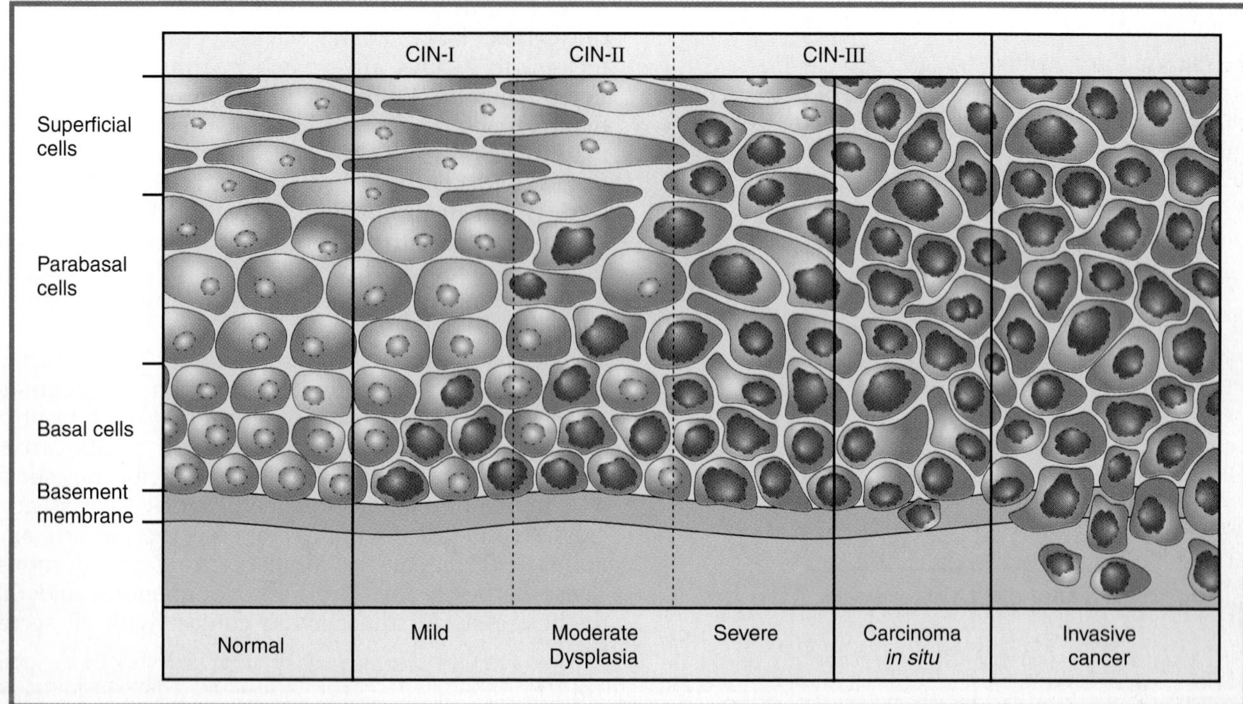

FIGURE 33–10 Carcinoma of the cervix. (From Damjanov I: Pathology for the Health-Related Professions. Philadelphia, WB Saunders, 1996.)

Ovarian Cancer

Ovarian neoplasms represent the most important pathologic disorder of the ovaries. Ovarian cancer is the second most common gynecologic cancer but is ranked first in gynecologic cancer deaths. In fact, it causes more deaths than all other tumors of the reproductive system. Approximately 19,000 new cases are reported annually, and 12,000 women die of ovarian cancer every year.

Very little is known about how or why ovarian cancer occurs, but it is known that ovarian cancer is linked to ovulation. Women who do not ovulate do not develop ovarian cancer. Oral contraceptives suppress ovulation and reduce the risk of ovarian cancer. Ovarian tumors are classified on the basis of their biologic features. About 20% of all ovarian tumors are cancerous, and the recovery rate is linked to the location, stage of the tumor development, and age of the patient.

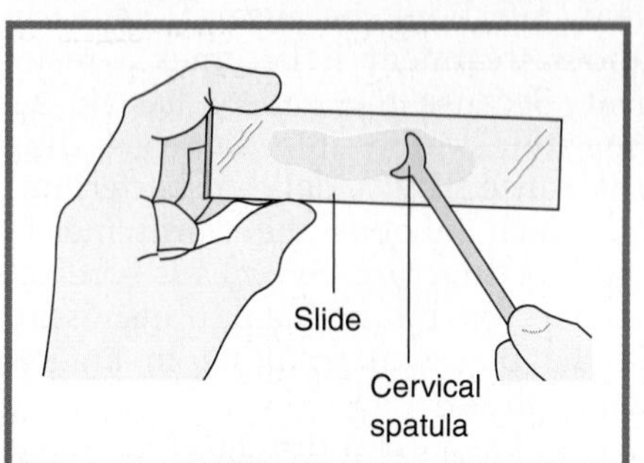

FIGURE 33–11 Preparation of slide for Papanicolaou smear.

Breast Cancer

Breast cancer is the leading cause of death among women between 35 and 55 years of age. Although the cause is unknown, predisposing factors include family history of breast cancer, early menarche and late menopause, first pregnancy after the age of 35 years or no pregnancy, high socioeconomic status, obesity, stress, high-fat diet, extensive use of oral contraceptives, and other cancers. The American Cancer Society recommends monthly breast self-examination and a baseline mammogram before age 40. After age 40, it should be part of the yearly physical examination.

Breast cancer appears most commonly in the upper outer quadrant of the left breast. It spreads through the lymphatic and circulatory systems to other parts of the body. Specific signs include

- A lump in the breast (Fig. 33–12)
- Changes in breast shape and size
- Change in the appearance of the skin
- Change in skin temperature
- Drainage or discharge
- Change in the nipple

Diagnosis is made through routine monthly breast self-examinations, mammography, ultrasonography, needle aspiration, and surgical biopsy.

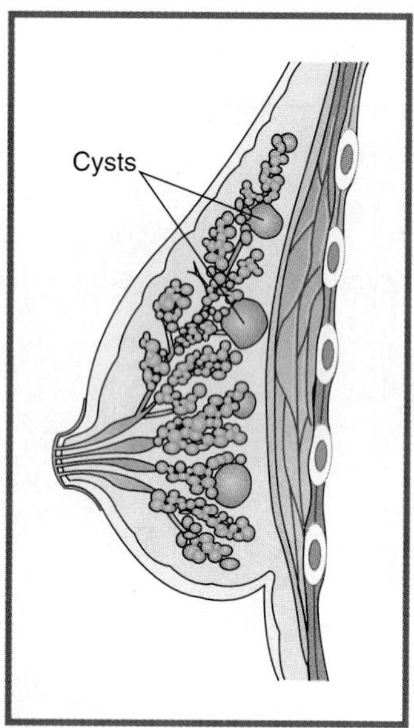

FIGURE 33–12 Breast cysts.

TREATMENT OF BREAST CANCER

- A lumpectomy (removal of tumor only)
- Simple mastectomy (removal of breast only)
- Modified radical mastectomy (removal of breast and axillary nodes)
- Radical mastectomy (removal of breast, axillary nodes, and muscle of chest wall)

Memory Jogger

Name three gynecologic diseases with unknown causes.

SEXUALLY TRANSMITTED DISEASES

The list of infectious diseases spread by sexual contact continues to grow. These diseases are considered to be the most common contagious diseases in the United States. All sexually transmitted diseases are transmitted from one person to another through body fluids such as blood, semen, and vaginal secretions during vaginal, anal, or oral sex (Fig. 33–13).

Herpes Simplex Virus Infection

Herpes simplex virus (HSV) infection is spread by direct skin-to-skin contact with another lesion. There are two strains of the virus: HSV-1 and HSV-2. HSV-1 causes the typical cold sore on the lip or edge of the nose, whereas HSV-2 is the more frequent cause of an infection of the skin in the genital area. Painful genital blister-like lesions appear on the cervix, labia, vulva, vagina, perineum, or buttocks 3 to 7 days after contact with infected secretions. After the lesions heal, the virus becomes dormant but hides in the nervous system: thus attacks may recur throughout life. Newborns can be infected with herpes through active lesions in the birth canal during vaginal deliveries. Brain damage, blindness, or death of the newborn may occur. Most physicians choose to perform a cesarean section when a woman has active lesions at the time of birth.

Diagnosis is made by observation of the characteristic vesicles, from patient history, and from tissue culture techniques. The Centers for Disease Control and Prevention states that one in six adults carries the highly contagious HSV-2. Treatment consists of a combination of antiviral medications such as acyclovir, sulfa-based creams to ease discomfort, and antibacterial agents to combat secondary infections. These herpes lesions are highly contagious, and the medical assistant must avoid contact with all secretions.

Gonorrhea

Gonorrhea is a common sexually transmitted infection of the genitourinary tract. It is widespread throughout the world. The causative organism of gonorrhea is the bacterium *Neisseria gonorrhoeae,* which is quite fragile and can survive only in a moist, dark, warm area of the body. The most common sites are the vagina, penis, rectum, mouth, and throat. The disease is spread only through direct sexual contact. Infants can become infected during birth if the mother has the disease. Women may develop a greenish yellow discharge from the cervix and experience dysuria. Preliminary diagnosis may be made by microscopic examination using Gram's stain and viewing intracellular or extracellular gram-negative diplococci. To confirm the diagnosis, the gonococci from the discharge are cultured. Antibiotic therapy is the recommended treatment. With early treatment the recovery rate is high.

Syphilis

Syphilis is of unique importance among the sexually transmitted infections because if its early lesions heal without treatment it becomes a major risk to the patient. Because the patient has no symptoms, he or she thinks the infection has disappeared. Syphilis is caused by a delicate bacterium called a *spirochete,* which inhabits the warm moist areas of the genitalia and rectum. Syphilis is spread by direct sexual contact or by prenatal transmission to the fetus via the placenta, resulting in an infant with congenital syphilis.

The disease progresses through four stages. Symptoms vary according to the stage of involvement.

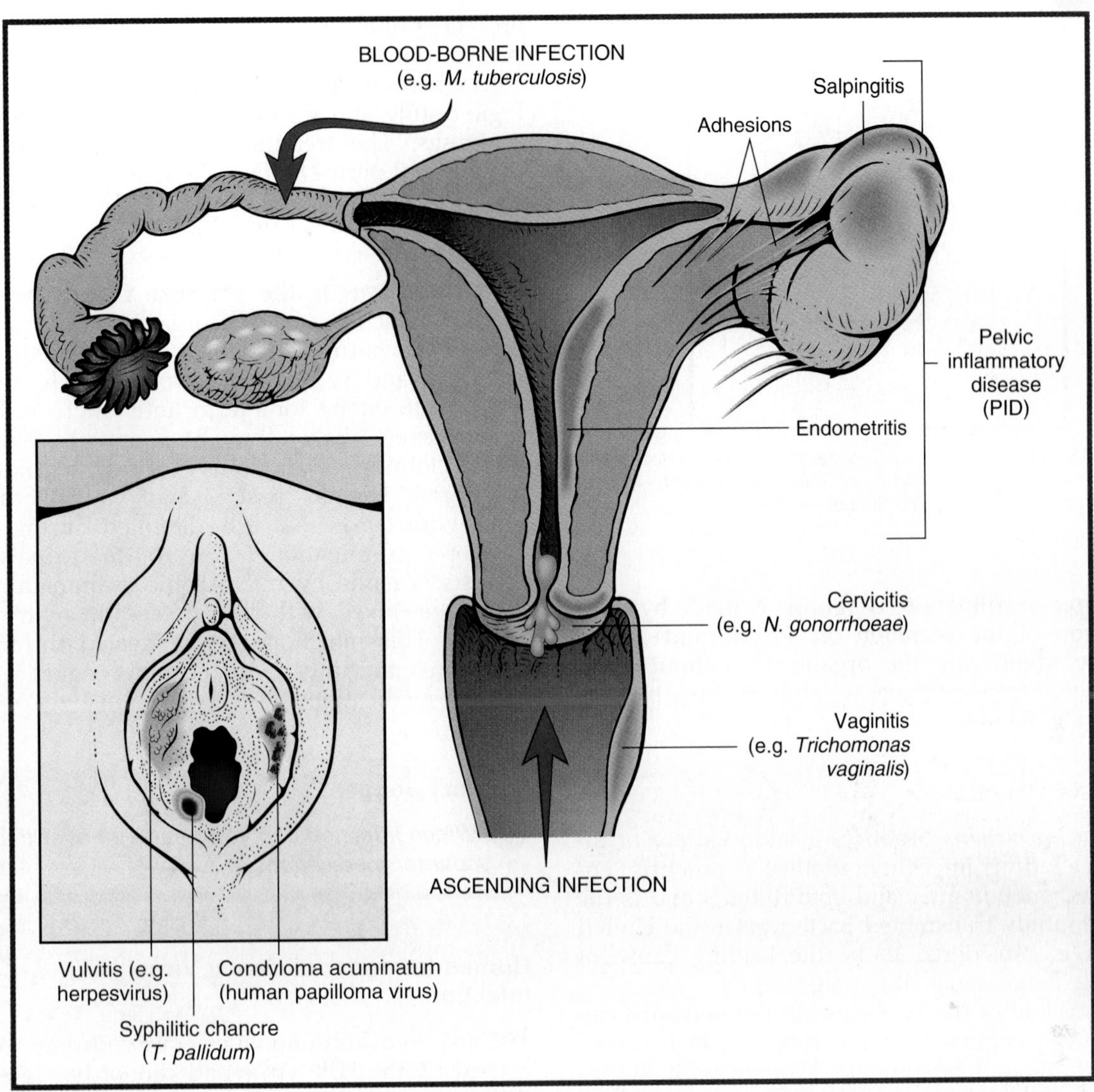

FIGURE 33–13 Ascending infections of the female genital organs are usually caused by sexual contact, pregnancy, or instrumentation. Descending infections usually begin in the blood or lymph fluids. (From Damjanov I: Pathology for the Health-Related Professions. Philadelphia, WB Saunders, 1996.)

The primary stage (first stage) begins with the organism entering the mucous membranes or the genitalia as a result of sexual contact with an infected person. Three or four weeks later, a lesion called a **chancre** appears at the site of the organism's entrance. Secondary syphilis (second stage) develops 6 to 8 weeks after the chancre. Skin, mucous membranes, and lymph nodes are involved. This stage is characterized by a generalized, painless, nonitching rash. Systemic manifestations include loss of appetite, hair, and weight; fever; sore throat; headache; nausea; constipation; and bone, muscle, and joint pain. Without treatment, the disease becomes asymptomatic in 2 to 6 weeks. Early latent syphilis (third stage) is asymptomatic and may last for years. The organism is invading the blood vessels, brain, spinal cord, and bones. After 1 year, the disease is no longer infectious. Late latent syphilis (fourth stage) is characterized according to the type of involvement, such as internal organs, heart and major blood vessels, and brain and spinal cord.

Syphilis is diagnosed by darkfield microscopic examination of the spirochete or by a blood test called the VDRL (Venereal Disease Research Laboratory). Diagnosis is confirmed with the fluorescent treponemal antibody-absorption test or the *Treponema pallidum* hemagglutination test. Penicillin is the treatment of choice for syphilis.

Trichomoniasis

Trichomonas vaginalis is a protozoon that infects the lower genitourinary tract. The infection can be passed back and forth between sexual partners; therefore, both persons must be treated. The prime and discriminating symptom is a foul, profuse, yellowish, frothy discharge that may be identified by visual examination or during routine urinalysis or

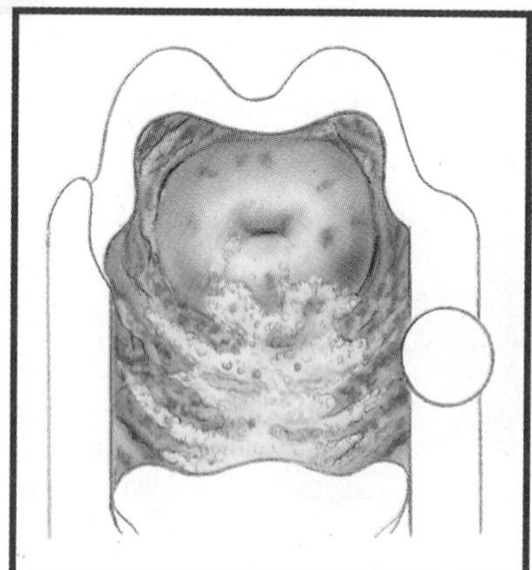

FIGURE 33–14 Trichomoniasis is passed between sexual partners. (From Jarvis C: Physical Examination and Health Assessment, 2nd ed. Philadelphia, WB Saunders, 1996.)

microscopic examination. Diagnosis is made by placing a drop of the secretion on a slide and microscopically identifying the organism. Without treatment the infection remains and it can become chronic (Fig. 33–14).

Chlamydia

Chlamydia trachomatis produces a wide variety of illnesses, including infertility, urethritis, proctitis, endometritis, pneumonitis, and epididymitis and is the most commonly transmitted bacterium in the United States. It is considered to be the leading cause of PID and a major cause of female sterility.

Transmission of the bacterium to the newborn can occur during vaginal delivery, resulting in neonatal eye infections and pneumonia. Women with the infection may be asymptomatic. Some experience a vaginal discharge, dysuria, urinary frequency, and soreness in the affected area. In men, the symptoms are the same except that the discharge is usually present only in the morning after waking.

Diagnosis is made through antigen-specific serologic testing and through specialized staining of cell scrapings. The treatment is antibiotic therapy for both sexual partners (Fig. 33–15).

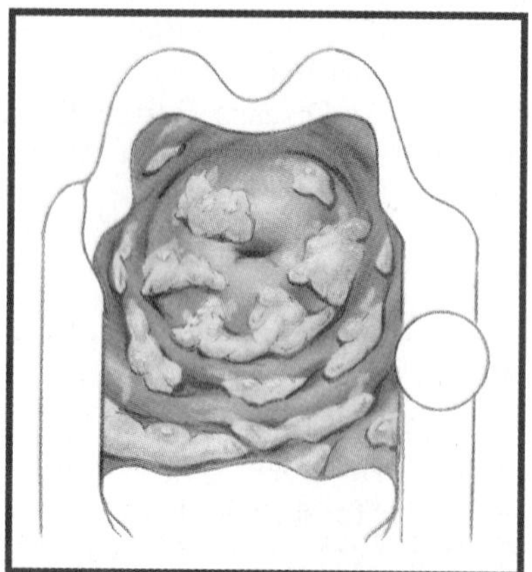

FIGURE 33–15 Candidiasis is a yeastlike fungal infection often found in the vagina. (From Jarvis C: Physical Examination and Health Assessment, 2nd ed. Philadelphia, WB Saunders, 1996.)

Candidiasis

Candida albicans is the yeastlike fungus responsible for this infection. *Candida* organisms are commonly part of the normal flora of the mouth, skin, intestinal tract, and vagina. Overgrowth of the organism can be caused by long-term antibiotic use, high estrogen levels, diabetes mellitus, and the wearing of tight clothing. Symptoms include itching; dry, bright-red vaginal tissue; and vaginal discharge thick with curds that are identified during the microscopic examination of the routine urinalysis. Diagnosis is made by microscopic examination of the discharge mixed with 10% potassium hydroxide on a slide. This infection can be treated through prescription antifungal medications and over-the-counter medications.

Memory Jogger

Which infection can you treat with over-the-counter medications?

Human Immunodeficiency Virus (HIV) Infection

The acquired immunodeficiency syndrome (AIDS) is caused by the HIV virus and cannot be classified as a disease with a definite cause and treatment (Fig. 33–16). Instead, AIDS is a syndrome of clinical conditions in which the body's immune response is compromised and eventually destroyed. It is transmitted by sexual intercourse, by injection-drug use, by transfusion or transmission of virus-contaminated blood or blood products, and by mother to infant either before or at the time of birth or breast feeding.

Signs and symptoms of HIV infection vary but may begin with patients complaining of burning, numb, or itching feet or with respiratory problems such as cough, shortness of breath, or dyspnea on exertion, pleuritic chest pain, or **hemoptysis.** The brain is the only organ that shows HIV-specific changes that are linked to lesions caused by opportunistic infections causing meningitis and encephalitis.

There are many ways of diagnosing HIV, including skin scrapings cultures, shave or punch biopsies, and radioimmunoprecipitation assay. HIV culture can be performed using blood of the suspected infected individual.

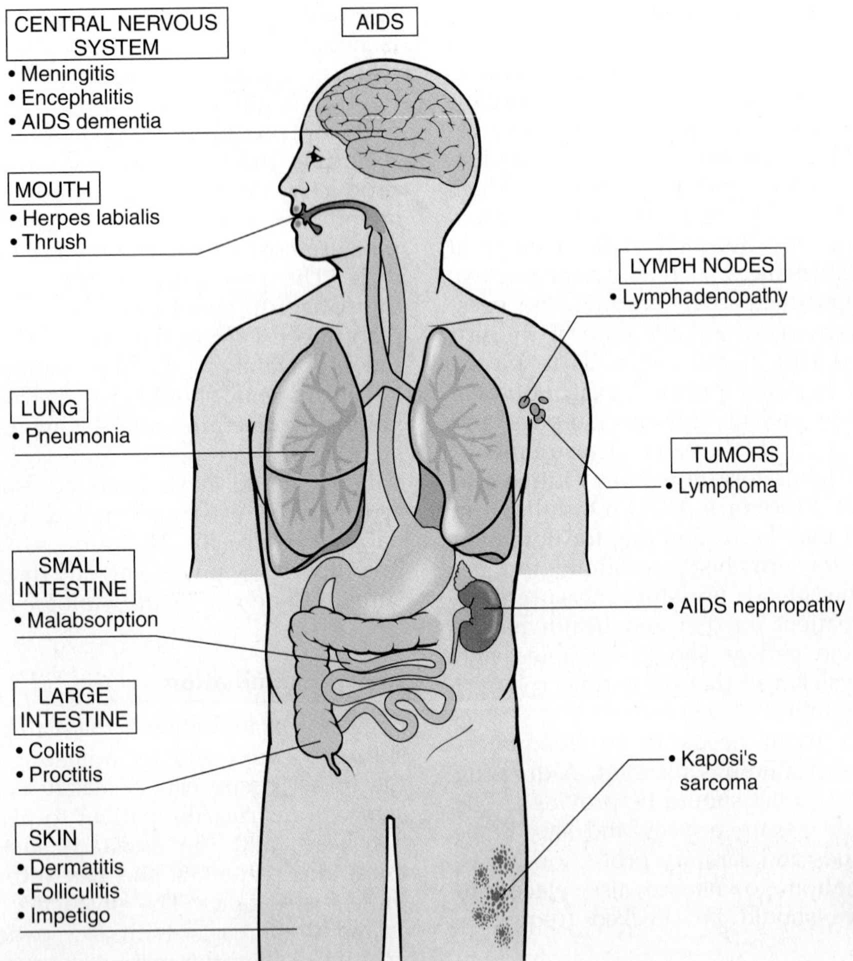

FIGURE 33–16 Pathologic changes associated with the acquired immunodeficiency syndrome. (Redrawn from Damjanov I: Pathology for the Health-Related Professions. Philadelphia, WB Saunders, 1996.)

Treatment may be done with antiviral drugs used in series. For example, drugs such as acyclovir (Zovirax), didanosine (Videx), ganciclovir (Cytovene), zalcitabine (HIVID), and zidovudine (formerly azidothymidine [AZT]) may be given in tablet form or intravenously. Patients receiving antiviral drugs for HIV infections may continue to develop opportunistic infections and other complications of HIV infection. All patients must be closely monitored for signs of infection such as fever (even a low-grade one), malaise, sore throat, or lethargy and should call the physician immediately if experiencing numbness, tingling, or pain in the feet or hands.

Memory Jogger

8 *Identify the five methods through which AIDS is transmitted.*

The Medical Assistant's Role in Gynecologic and Obstetric Procedures

As the female travels from menarche, through the child-bearing years, and then through menopause her medical concerns change and the focal point of the physical examination may also change. Even though this is true, the overall concentration of the medical office is to keep her physically and mentally healthy and productive. Being able to assist the physician in identifying possible problems before the problem becomes a threat to the patient's health is a major priority in her care. The best way to accomplish this is by listening to your patient. The patient isn't interested in your health, but you must be alert to the signs that give clues to their concerns. Remember, to the patient there is no such thing as a routine examination.

EXAMINATION PREPARATION

Examination of the female reproductive system is done to assure normality of the reproductive organs or to diagnose and treat abnormalities of these organs. Before the physician begins the examination, you will need to obtain a gynecologic history, which includes age at menarche, regularity of the menstrual cycle, amount and duration of the menstrual flow, menstrual disturbances such as dysmenorrhea, intermenstrual or postmenstrual bleeding, the presence of vaginal discharges, and the date of the last menstrual period (LMP). If the patient is to be examined as part of her first prenatal visit, you will need to prepare the patient and the supplies and equipment necessary to obtain pelvic measurements, serologic tests, and laboratory tests both routine and state mandated (see Procedure 33–1). On follow-up prenatal visits, you may be responsible for obtaining a urine specimen for urinalysis, weighing the patient, obtaining the blood pressure measurement, and advising the patient on diet and health habits. Any concerns of the patient should be noted and reported to the physician so that these concerns may be alleviated at this time.

The examination room needs to be adequately equipped and the surroundings pleasant. A dressing area with an adjacent toilet should be provided. The dressing area should assure privacy and should be equipped with tissues and sanitary protection items. Disposable examination gowns are also placed in this room. Supplies should be checked frequently throughout the day.

Memory Jogger

9 *What is usually included in a follow-up prenatal visit?*

ASSISTING WITH THE EXAMINATION

This is probably the most emotionally charged medical experience the average female undergoes. Even women with relatively sophisticated attitudes toward their bodies and sexuality may be mortified by the casual impersonal approach of the medical team during this procedure. Many women may have a fear of the physician's findings, which one does not encounter when treating the common cold. These anxieties and fears may be eased by the knowledge of what will be occurring during the examination. Anxieties and fears are best handled through explanations and showing a genuine interest in the patient's concerns.

If the physician is male, the female medical assistant should be in attendance while the patient is exposed during the examination. The only exception to this rule is if the patient requests that the medical assistant leave the room; if this is done, the request is noted on the patient's medical record. The male medical assistant is usually not in the room during the examination except when it is necessary to assist with a procedure. The physician makes the decision regarding the male assistant's role in the female reproductive system examination. When you are in attendance, it is your responsibility to support the patient and to assist the physician during the procedure. The procedure should be fully explained to the patient to avoid unnecessary embarrassment and discomfort. During the explanation, the assistant has the opportunity to do some patient teaching.

The patient should be instructed to void and empty her rectum, completely disrobe, and put on an examination gown. Unless contraindicated, the patient should have been advised at the time the appointment was made not to douche or have sexual intercourse for 24 hours before the examination to properly evaluate vaginal discharges and to ensure accurate results of cytologic studies.

Breast Examination

Begin the examination by assisting the patient into a sitting position and by adjusting the gown so that the breast tissue can be easily exposed. The physician will instruct the patient to place her arms above her head, and the assistant should be present to assist the patient if she has difficulty in following these instructions. The physician may prefer to examine the breasts with the patient in the supine position. When the patient is instructed to assume a supine position, you help the patient and adjust the gown and drape as needed for the physician and for the patient's comfort. A small pillow may be placed under the patient's head for comfort. When the examination is completed, the gown is readjusted to cover the breast tissue. The physician may choose to discuss breast self-examination with the patient at this time or may inform the patient that you will be explaining the technique at the end of the exam (Procedure 33-2).

Abdominal Examination

After the examination of the patient's breasts, cover her breasts and position the drape to allow the physician to palpate the abdomen to confirm normal symmetry and the presence of possible masses. In the case of pregnancy, the uterine enlargement is also evaluated. For this examination, the patient's arms should be placed at her sides to achieve better relaxation of the abdominal muscles.

Pelvic Examination

The medical assistant should remain in the examination room to provide reassurance to the patient as well as offer legal protection to the male physician

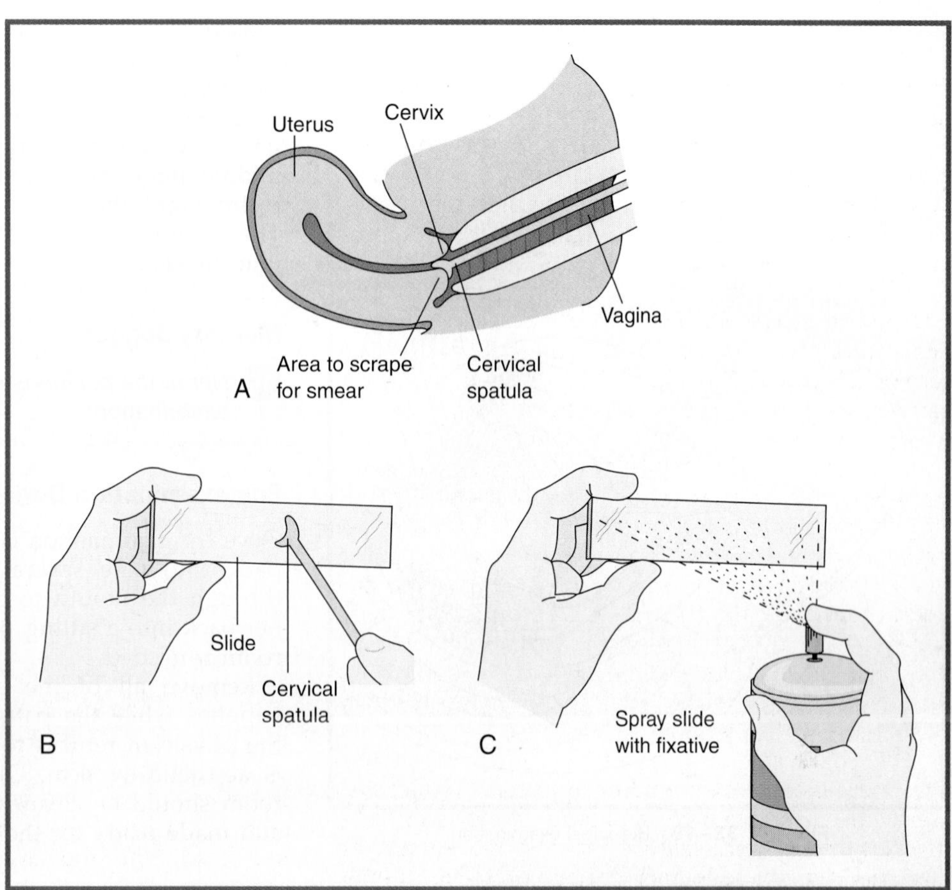

FIGURE 33–17 *A* through *C*, Procedure to obtain a Papanicolaou smear.

while the patient's vagina and perineal areas are being examined. Furthermore, the patient should be offered assistance in getting on and off the table. The lithotomy position is very awkward to get into unassisted and may be embarrassing to the patient. Never position the patient in the lithotomy position until the physician is ready to begin the examination. When you assist the patient into the lithotomy position, always keep the patient totally covered.

The best place for you to stand during the pelvic examination is at the patient's side. In that position, you will be able to observe the patient and also be able to move quickly if you are needed by the physician.

First, the physician inspects the external genitalia and palpates the perineal body, Bartholin's and Skene's glands, and the urethral meatus. The patient may be asked to bear down to show any muscular weaknesses that may be the result of lacerations of the perineal body during childbirth. A third-degree laceration may have involved the rectal sphincter and may cause rectal incontinence.

Next, the **vaginal speculum,** without lubrication, is inserted for examination of the cervix and the vaginal canal and for obtaining the Pap smear (Fig. 33–17). You may want to warn the patient that this instrument may feel cool and have her take some deep breaths to help relax the abdominal muscles. The normal cervix points posteriorly and has smooth, pink squamous epithelium. The abnormalities most frequently seen are ulcerations (erosions), Bartholin cysts, and cervical polyps. Because erosions cannot be palpated, inspection is the only method of knowing their presence. Healed lacerations resulting from childbirth are common in the **multiparous** patient. Pregnancy increases the size of the cervix, and hormone deficiency causes it to atrophy. The vaginal wall is reddish pink and has a corrugated appearance. Vaginal infections change the appearance of the vaginal mucosa. When the Pap specimen is obtained, you may be responsible for applying the **fixative** to the glass slide, labeling the slide(s), and preparing the specimen for transport to the cytology laboratory. Be sure to follow the laboratory instructions in the preparation to avoid possibly repeating the examination to obtain another specimen.

After the vaginal speculum has been removed, the physician does a bimanual examination; that is, the second and third gloved fingers are lubricated with a water-soluble jelly (**lubricant**) and inserted into the vaginal canal, and the other hand palpates the abdomen over the pelvic organs and the mons pubis (Fig. 33–18). The uterus is examined for shape, size, and consistency. The position of the uterus is noted. The normal uterus is freely movable with limited discomfort. A laterally displaced uterus is usually the result of pelvic adhesions or displacement

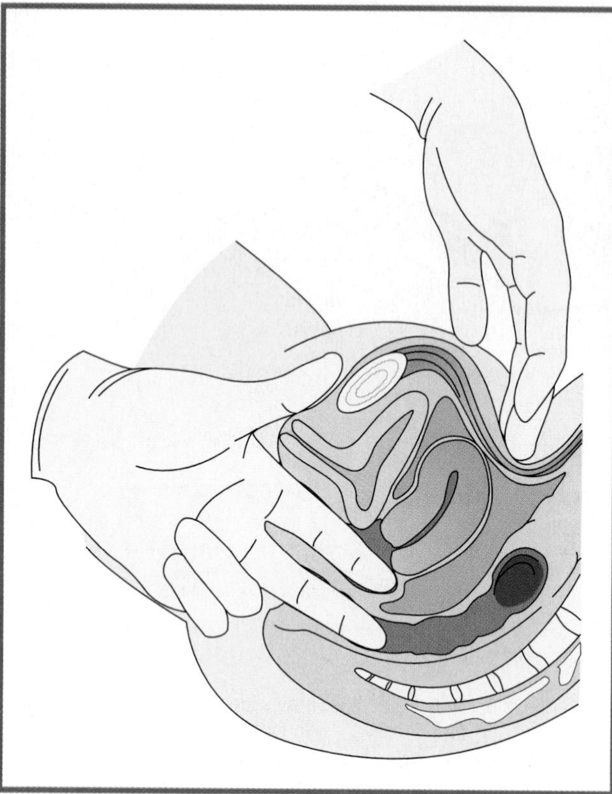

FIGURE 33–18 Bimanual examination.

caused by a pelvic tumor. The fallopian tubes and ovaries are evaluated. The normal tubes and ovaries are difficult to palpate. The physician may now complete the examination by performing a rectovaginal abdominal examination. This is done with the middle finger of the minor hand inserted into the rectum and the index finger in the vaginal canal. The rectum is checked by the index finger inserted into the rectum.

Memory Jogger

Name the positions used for the female physical examination.

Postexamination Duties

Once the examination is concluded, you may ask the patient to take several deep, even breaths slowly through the mouth to help her to relax. Then help her back into a sitting position and into the dressing room if needed.

Remove all of the examination equipment and supplies while the patient is dressing so that when the physician returns to talk to the patient the room is aesthetically neat. Once the patient has left, the room should be cleaned and restocked as necessary and made ready for the next patient.

PROCEDURE 33-1
Assisting with Examination of the Female Patient

GOAL

To assist the physician in examination of a female patient.

EQUIPMENT AND SUPPLIES

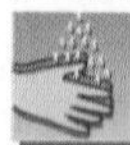 

- Patient gown
- Lubricant
- 4 × 4-inch gauze flats
- Laboratory slips
- Drape sheet
- Examination light
- Cervical spatula
- Microscopic slides
- Vaginal speculum
- Uterine sponge forceps
- Disposable gloves
- Fixative for Pap smear

PROCEDURAL STEPS

1 Assemble the materials needed, and prepare the room. Prepare the equipment and supplies needed for the Pap smear (Figure 1).
PURPOSE: Efficiency.

Continued

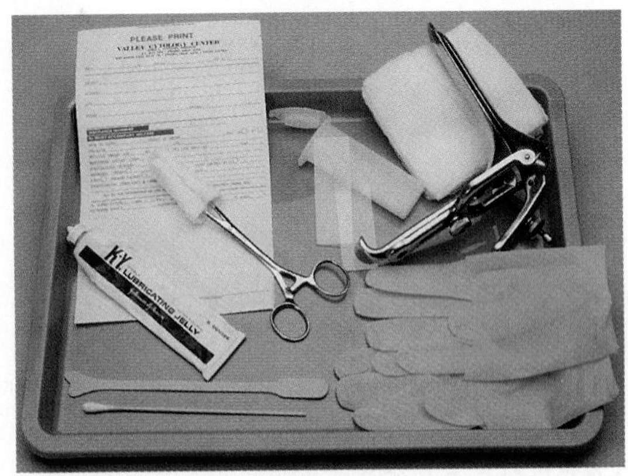

FIGURE 1

2 Wash your hands. Follow Standard Precautions. Don gloves.
PURPOSE: Infection control.

3 Identify the patient, and briefly explain the procedure.
PURPOSE: Explanations gain patient cooperation and alleviate apprehension.

4 Instruct the patient to empty the bladder and collect a urine specimen if needed.
PURPOSE: Organ palpations are performed on an empty bladder.

5 Instruct the patient to disrobe completely and to put on a gown. Explain proper gown opening (front or back).

6 Assist the patient into a sitting position at the end of the examination table. Drape the patient and assist the physician with the examination. Provide reassurance to the patient as needed.

7 When the physician is ready to examine the breasts and the abdomen in the supine position, assist the patient into the supine position and drape as needed.
PURPOSE: To avoid exposing the patient unnecessarily.

8 When the physician is ready to begin the vaginal examination, assist the patient into the lithotomy position. Remember to always position the patient underneath the drape.

9 Direct the light source into the vaginal speculum.
PURPOSE: Facilitates better viewing of the cervix.

10 Pass the proper instruments to the physician in proper sequence.
PURPOSE: Teamwork enhances efficiency.

11 Assist the physician with preparation of the smear, its labeling, and its transportation to the laboratory.

12 Apply the water-soluble lubricant to the physician's fingers.
PURPOSE: Facilitates the bimanual examination.

13 Place the soiled instruments in a basin.
PURPOSE: Helps produce better aesthetic surroundings.

14 Instruct the patient to breathe deeply through the mouth with hands crossed over the chest.
PURPOSE: Helps relax muscles.

15 Assist the patient off the table and with dressing if needed.

16 While patient is in the dressing room, clean the room, removing used equipment.

17 Remove gloves and wash your hands.
PURPOSE: Infection control.

18 Label the slides and prepare the Pap smear for transportation to the laboratory.

19 Record all procedures that you did on the patient's medical record.
PURPOSE: A procedure is not done until it is entered into the patient's record.

PROCEDURE 33-2
Teaching the Patient Breast Self-Examination

GOAL
Teach the patient how to palpate her breast for possible abnormalities.

EQUIPMENT AND SUPPLIES
Instruction pamphlet
Teaching model (to use to demonstrate the technique before a return demonstration by patient)

PROCEDURAL STEPS
1 Assemble equipment.

2 Tell patient to always examine breast while bathing or showering in warm water. The best time to perform this examination is immediately after the menstrual period is completed because at this time there is minimal breast engorgement.
PURPOSE: Fingers will move more smoothly over wet tissue.

3 Have patient raise one arm. With her fingers flat, she should press gently in small circles, starting at the outermost top edge of the breast and spiraling in toward the nipple. Touch every part of each breast, gently feeling for a lump or thickening. Use the right hand to examine the left breast and the left hand for the right breast (Figure 1).

4 After the bath/shower is completed, the patient should continue the examination in front of a mirror with arms at the sides. Then with arms raised above the head, look carefully for changes in the size, shape, and contour of each breast. Look for puckering, dimpling, or changes in skin texture (Figure 2).

Continued

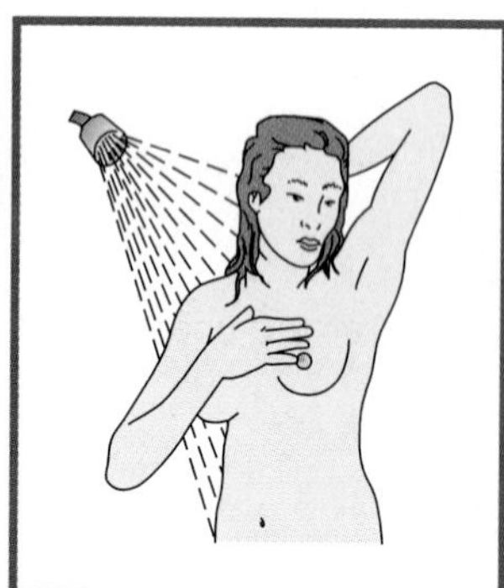

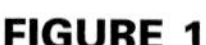

FIGURE 1

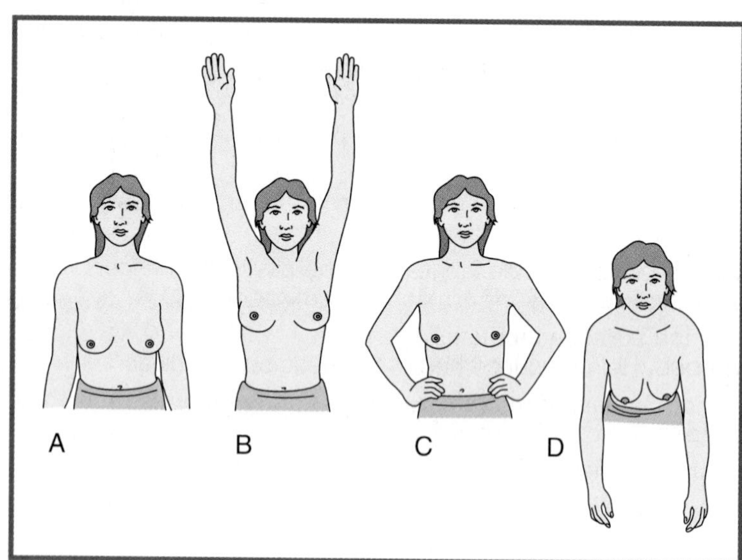

FIGURE 2

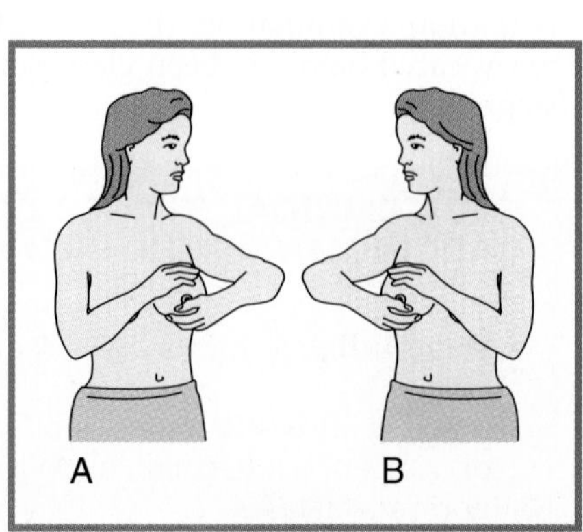

FIGURE 3

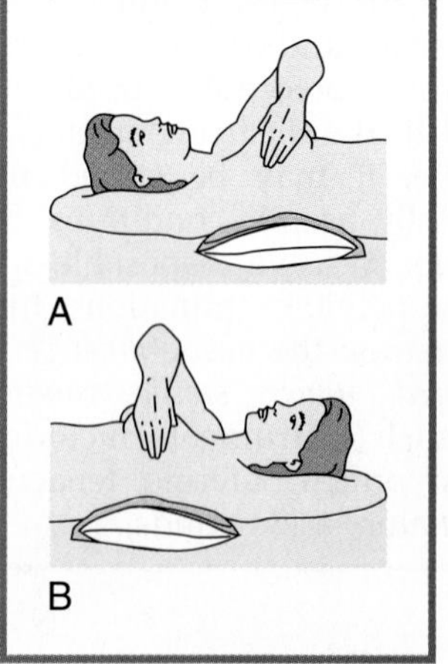

FIGURE 4

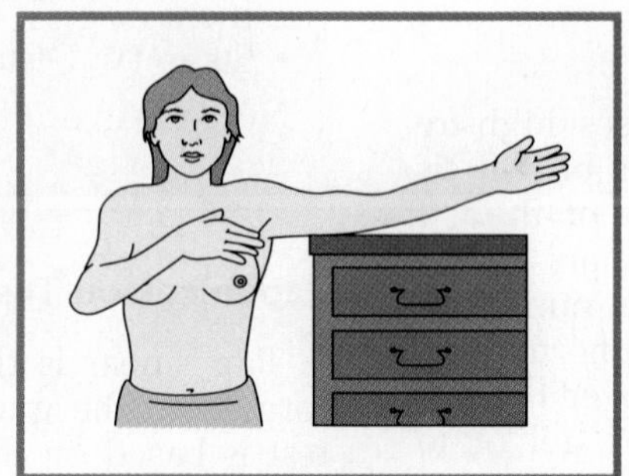

FIGURE 5

5 Gently squeeze both nipples and look for discharge (Figure 3).

6 Before dressing, lie on a bed. Place a towel or pillow under the right shoulder and the right hand behind the head. Examine the right breast using the left hand. Press gently in small circles, starting at the outermost top edge and spiraling in toward the nipple. Repeat with left breast (Figure 4).

7 In a standing position, with the arm resting on a firm surface such as a chest or dresser, use the same circular motion to examine the underarm area.
PURPOSE: This area is also breast tissue (Figure 5).

8 Give the patient the instruction pamphlet to use at home. If you have given her the shower card to follow, show her how it will hang inside the shower on a faucet or the shower nozzle and be a quick reference for her.

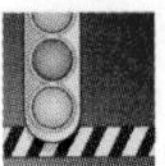

Safety Alert: Any instrument that comes in contact with a patient should be sterilized in an autoclave for 15 to 20 minutes at 15 pounds of pressure and at 250° F or with a germicide chemical before it is used for another patient. If the instrument does not penetrate tissue, it may be stored under clean or medically aseptic conditions. Some physicians prefer to use a disposable speculum for routine pelvic examinations. Instruments that penetrate the tissue *must be sterilized and stored under sterile conditions.* Examples of such instruments include the uterine biopsy punch, uterine tenaculum, and cervical dilators and sounds.

DIAGNOSTIC TESTING

Ultrasonography

Ultrasonography is a technique that uses high-frequency sound waves to produce images of soft tissues of the body and of accumulations of fluid. It can distinguish between cysts and tumors and is used during pregnancy to determine the number of fetuses, age and sex of the fetus, fetal abnormalities, and position of the placenta. The skin over the area being studied is coated with conductive gel or lotion, and the transducer is pressed lightly against the skin. Once the sound waves reach the underlying body structure, they bounce back to the transducer that converts the returning sound waves into electrical impulses.

Ultrasound technology is divided into two methods. The gray scale image converts soundwave echoes into graphs or dots that form pictures of organ and blood vessels (Fig. 33–19). The Doppler method converts the ultrasound into audible sounds that are heard as pulsations (Fig. 33–20). Color-coded Doppler signals, three-dimensional imaging, and contrast medium enhancement of ultrasound image provide more accurate images and data related to organ structure and function.

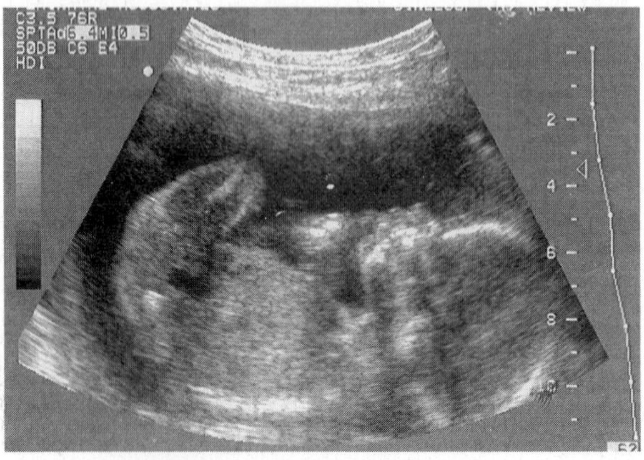

FIGURE 33–19 Ultrasound of fetus.

Mammography

Mammography provides an x-ray image of the breast tissue performed to identify abnormal masses that would otherwise go undetected under a breast palpation examination (Fig. 33–21). Invasive mammary carcinoma has been classified into four clinical stages.

FOUR CLINICAL STAGES OF CARCINOMA OF THE BREAST

- Stage I: Breast tumors less than 2 cm in diameter
- Stage II: Breast tumors 2 to 5 cm in diameter, or cancers with small, mobile axillary lymph node metastases
- Stage III: Breast tumors over 5 cm in diameter with lymph node metastases or skin involvement
- Stage IV: Distant metastases

Noninvasive mammary carcinomas are classified as stage TIS (tumor in situ).

Papanicolaou Test

A Pap smear is the single most important test performed in the gynecology and obstetrics office. The test is based on the premise that normal and abnormal cervical cells fall from the lining of the cervix and pass into the cervical and vaginal secretions. A smear is the removal of secretions from the cervix and upper vagina. The secretions are scraped from the cervix with a **cervical spatula,** spread on a slide, prepared according to the directions of the cytology laboratory, and sent to the laboratory for analysis. In the laboratory the secretions are examined and any abnormalities can be identified before symptoms become apparent. The abnormal changes of the cervical epithelium are graded from mild, to moderate, to severe, to carcinoma in situ as follows:

CLASSIFICATION OF CARCINOMA OF THE CERVIX

The grades of cervical intraepithelial neoplasia (CIN) are

CIN I = mild dysplasia
CIN II = moderate dysplasia
CIN III = severe dysplasia to carcinoma in situ

When the carcinoma progresses to carcinoma of the cervix, the cancer can be classified by the following stages:

Stage 0 = carcinoma in situ
Stage I = carcinoma of the cervix with no adnexal involvement
Stage II = carcinoma of the cervix with minimal adnexal invasion

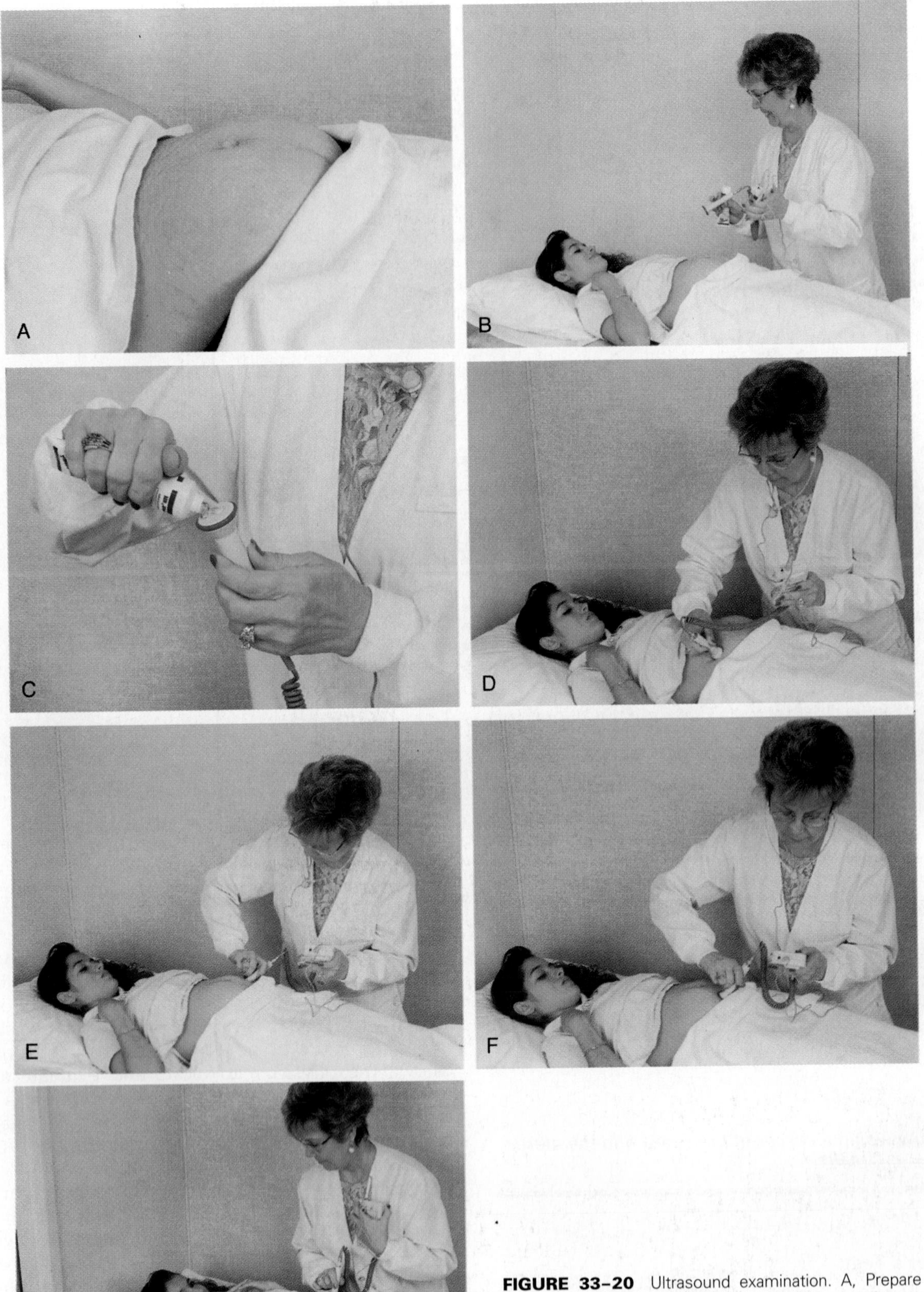

FIGURE 33–20 Ultrasound examination. A, Prepare the patient for Doppler reading. B, Explain procedure to the patient. C, Place conductive gel on skin or transducer. D, Place listening device into ears and begin to sound the abdominal area for fetal heart sounds. E, Sound from patient's right to left until fetal sounds are audible. F, When sounds are audible, note rate and intensity. G, Allow patient to share in the experience.

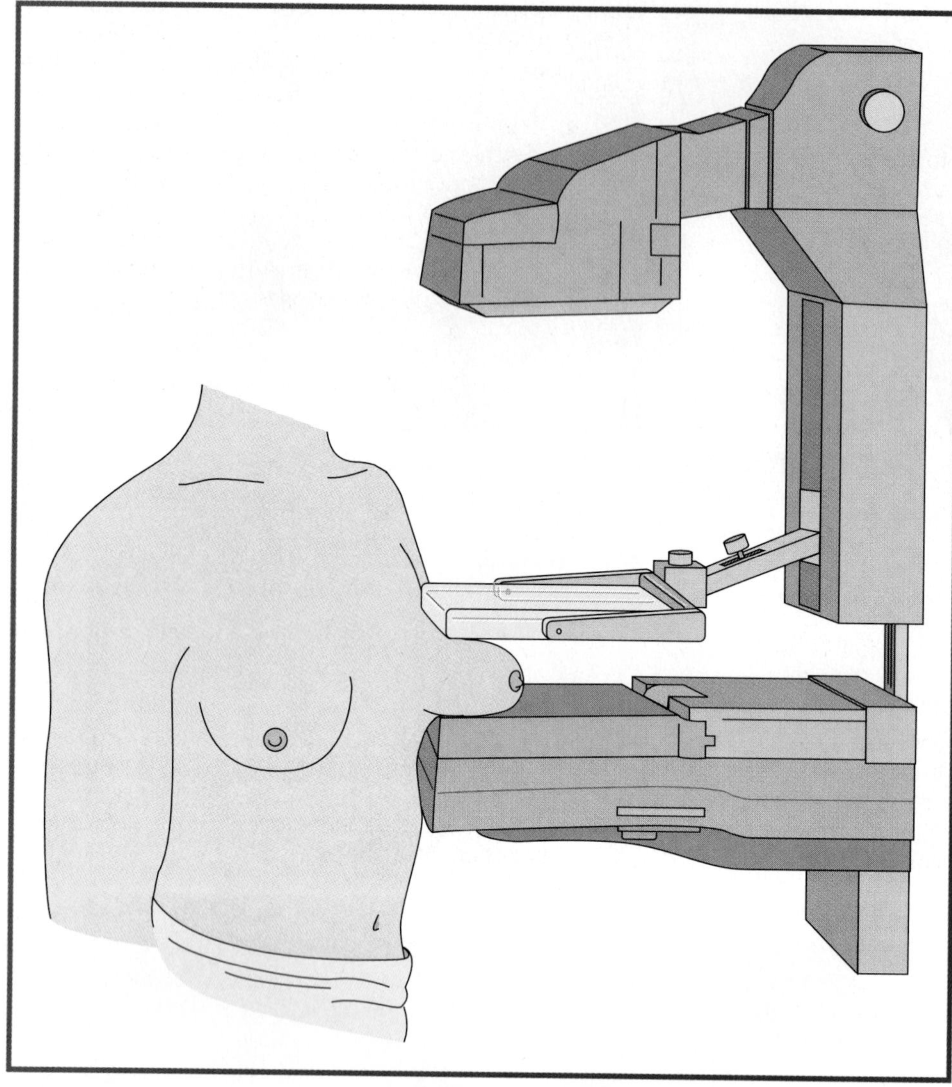

FIGURE 33–21 Proper position of breast for mammogram.

Stage III = carcinoma of the cervix with involvement to the pelvic area
Stage IV = carcinoma of the cervix with involvement of structures outside the pelvic area.

Memory Jogger

 *How would a cancer of the cervix and the uterus be classified?*

Schiller's Test

Schiller's test can be used during the pelvic examination by the physician as a means to diagnose cervical and vaginal neoplasia. An iodine stain is painted onto the mucous membrane. Cancerous cells are easily identified because they do not absorb the stain. Noncancerous cells absorb the stain and turn a brownish color.

Colposcopy

Colposcopy is the visual examination of the vagina and the cervical surfaces through the use of a colposcope. The colposcope is a stereoscopic microscope that is fitted with a camera, making it possible to photograph the tissue being examined. Colposcopy allows the physician to locate and evaluate abnormal cells and detect cancer of the cervix in its early stages, examine tissue from which an abnormal Pap smear has been obtained, and monitor areas of the cervix from which malignant lesions have been removed. A cervical biopsy may be performed in junction with a colposcopy.

Colposcopy may also be used to monitor women who are at risk for developing cervical cancer because their mothers were given diethylstilbestrol (DES) during their pregnancy. Colposcopy may also be used to examine male genitalia when sexually transmitted diseases are suspected.

The colposcope is not inserted into the vaginal cavity; thus, colposcopy is a relatively safe and painless procedure. Discomfort may occur when the speculum is inserted into the vagina to improve visualization of the tissue. Discomfort and bleeding can occur when tissue is taken for biopsy.

Cryosurgery

This procedure is often done to treat chronic cervicitis and cervical erosion problems through the use of freezing temperatures. The freezing causes the cells it contacts to die, and in about 1 month these dead, discarded cells are replaced with healthy cells.

The procedure involves placing a probe against the problem area on the cervix and then allowing liquid nitrogen to flow over the area for about 3 or 4 minutes or until the area is frozen (see Procedure 33–3). The patient may experience some pain for about 30 minutes after the procedure and a slight watery discharge for up to a week. If there are any signs of infection, foul discharge, or pain, the patient should call the physician's office. She is advised not to engage in sexual intercourse for 1 month and to expect a heavier than usual menstrual flow for the first period after the procedure.

PROCEDURE 33-3
Preparing the Patient for Cryosurgery

GOAL

To prepare the patient and assist the physician in cryosurgery.

EQUIPMENT AND SUPPLIES

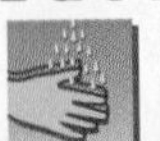
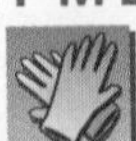

- Cryosurgery machine equipped with liquid nitrogen canister
- Cryoprobe
- Cervical tenaculum
- Cervical ring forceps or disposable cervical swabs
- Vaginal speculum
- 4 × 4-inch gauze squares
- Gloves
- Gowns and face protection
- Specimen containers
- Cytology request forms

PROCEDURAL STEPS

1 Assemble equipment
PURPOSE: Expedite procedure.

2 Wash hands and don gloves.
PURPOSE: Infection control.

3 Obtain the patient's temperature and blood pressure and record them on the patient's record.
PURPOSE: To establish an average base range.

4 Drape and assist the patient into the lithotomy position. Don gloves.

5 Assist the physician with the procedure by handing the equipment needed.

6 Encourage the patient to take deep breaths to promote relaxation of the pelvic muscles during the procedure. Observe patient for any sign of distress.
PURPOSE: Patient safety.

7 When the procedure is completed, place the patient in a supine position and allow her to rest while you tidy the room and remove the used supplies. Retake temperature and blood pressure.
PURPOSE: Ensure that vital signs and blood pressure return to average range.

8 Help patient sit up and assist her in dressing if needed.
PURPOSE: Patient safety.

8 Remove gloves and wash hands.
PURPOSE: Infection control.

9 Return equipment to the proper storage area.

10 Record procedure and final vital sign measurements on the patient's record.
PURPOSE: A procedure is not done until it is recorded.

Pregnancy Testing

Most pregnancy tests are designed to detect hCG, normally found in the serum and urine of pregnant women about 1 week after the first missed menses. In the physician's office, urine testing and blood testing are commonly performed. The urine test should be conducted on the first-voided urine specimen in the morning, because the hormone is most concentrated at this time. (Pregnancy testing is covered in Chapter 45.) The patient undergoes a complete medical and obstetric examination, which includes a number of laboratory tests (Table 33–1).

When it is determined that the patient is definitely pregnant, her estimated day of delivery (EDD) will need to be determined (see Procedure 33–4). The EDD is frequently called her expected due date. The due date can be determined by several methods, including Nägele's rule, lunar method, or the commercially prepared gestational wheel. Regardless of the method, the date determined will only be an educated guess, and most obstetricians rely on quickening, the enlargement of the uterus, and the sonogram for more reliable data.

TABLE 33–1 Diagnostic Pregnancy Testing

Complete blood cell count
Blood type and Rh factor
Serologic test for syphilis
Rubella titer
Sickle cell trait or disease (for black patients)
Blood glucose (for high-risk patients)
Papanicolaou smear
Smears for infections (when indicated)
Urinalysis
Pregnancy test

Family Planning

Family planning refers to the process of deciding whether to have children, how many to have, and when to have them. Choices of whether to use a contraceptive method, which to use, and how to use it may be influenced by many external factors and internal feelings.

When it has been decided that a method of birth

PROCEDURE 33–4

Establishing the EDD Using Nägele's Rule and Lunar Method

GOAL

To establish the patient's due date.

EQUIPMENT AND SUPPLIES

Calendar for present and following year
Paper and pencil
Commercial EDD wheel (optional)

PROCEDURAL STEPS

1 Ask patient for the date of the onset of the last menstrual period. Be sure that this is the date of the onset and not the date of the termination of the menses.

2 Patient informs you that her LMP was June 7, 1998.

3 Calculate her EDD using Nägele's method.

4 Using Nägele's method: Begin with the date of the first day of her last menstrual period (LMP). Count back 3 months and add 1 year plus 7 days.
Example: LMP = June 7, 1998, May, April, March 7, 1998. Add 1 year and 7 days = March 14, 1999. Thus her EDD is March 14, 1999.

6 Using the same LMP, Calculate her EDD using the lunar rule.

7 Using lunar rule:
Example: LMP = June 7, 1998 + 9 months = March 7, 1999 + 7 days = March 14, 1999

8 Compare the results for accuracy. Did you obtain the same EDD using both methods?

control is to be employed, the next step is to determine the type of intervention that is the best for each individual patient. There are three methods of control used: hormonal, barrier, and permanent.

The hormonal methods include the birth control pill, injection, and implants. The barrier method includes the use of the condom (male or female), the diaphragm, and the vaginal sponge. Permanent methods of contraception include the surgical procedures of vasectomy for the male and tubal ligation for the female. Every method has advantages and disadvantages.

When the physician prescribes the method and type of control to be used, the assistant usually gives the patient the literature explaining this intervention and should be able to answer any questions that the patient asks. Remember one answer is, "I am not sure, but I will have the doctor answer that question for you."

Tubal ligation is a surgical procedure in which the fallopian tubes are occluded to prevent the passage of future ova. It can be performed using several different surgical techniques, each of which produces the same result.

A woman needs to be fully informed about sterilization before she gives consent for the procedure. The U.S. Department of Health and Human Services has set up the following guidelines for federally funded sterilizations to make sure that a woman fully understands the procedure; the risks, benefits, and alternatives of the procedure must be explained.

- A statement that describes sterilization as a permanent and irreversible method of birth control is given to the patient.
- A 30-day waiting period is required between the time of consent and the surgery.
- The consent forms must be in the woman's native language, or provisions for an interpreter must be provided.

Sterilization does not stop the normal menstrual cycle, nor does it cause any changes in physiologic or sexual responses.

There are many effective methods of contraception available to the couple who wants to plan a family. Table 33–2 provides information on the most commonly used methods of temporary contraception used in family planning.

Memory Jogger

Name three methods of birth control used by the female.

TABLE 33–2 Effective Method Suggestions of Family Planning

Method	Description	Patient Education
Condom		Prevents sperm from entering the vagina
Male	Sheath applied over the erect penis	may tear or slip; STD barrier
Female	Sheath held in the vagina by rings	Expensive; must be put in place prior to intercourse; STD barrier
Diaphragm	Rubber cervical cap	Female must be measured for correct size and taught how to insert; limited STD protection; must be in place before intercourse
Spermicide	Chemical preparations that kill sperm	Best used in combination with sheath or cervical cap; may cause irritation, rash, or allergic reactions; very limited STD protection
Birth control pill	Female hormones taken orally to prevent ovulation	Highly effective if taken as prescribed; alters natural hormonal secretions; may produce numerous side effects; no STD protection
Birth control injection	Injection of synthetic progesterone that prevents ovulation	Highly effective; lasts 3 to 4 months; alters hormonal physiology; may produce side effects including menses irregularity; no STD protection.
Vasectomy	Cutting and tying of the vas deferens	99.9% effective; permanent sterilization; surgical reversal may be done but is very expensive and not guaranteed; no STD protection
Tubal ligation	Cutting and tying of the fallopian tubes	99.9% effective; involves outpatient surgery; reversal can be done but is very expensive and there is no guarantee; no STD protection
Rhythm method	Abstinence during the female's monthly fertile period	Requires continuous careful menstrual cycle record keeping; high incidence of failure

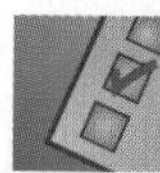

PATIENT EDUCATION

The medical assistant can assist the physician by providing information for the patient that promotes sexual health, safe sex behaviors, and safe pregnancies and that prevents sexual dysfunctions that are related to illness and injury throughout the life of the patient.

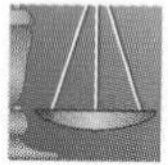

LEGAL AND ETHICAL ISSUES

Every time the physician sees this patient, the patient is there for a definite reason, and listening to her is a primary point in identifying the symptoms that can lead to that very important diagnosis.

Many ethical and legal issues arise as a result of missed communication. Listen to what every patient is telling you and write down any information that will assist the physician in treating the patient. The issue may appear to be an insignificant problem to you, but to the patient it may be a major concern. Let the physician be the judge of whether the problem is relevant. As the patient's advocate and the physician's assistant, you play an important role in assisting in the establishment of good communication as a vital link in patient care.

CRITICAL THINKING

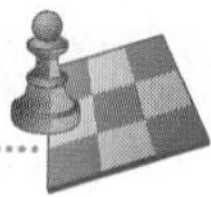

1 Identify possible signs of emotional distress that you may observe in a gynecologic patient.

2 What patient-expressed signs and symptoms would give you clues indicating that you should prepare the instruments and supplies needed to obtain a gynecologic smear for possible infectious organisms?

3 Justify the 30-day waiting period between consent and a sterilization surgical procedure.

HOW DID I DO? Answers to Memory Joggers

1 Internal = vagina (connecting organ), cervix, uterus, fallopian tube, and ovary.
External = vulva (clitoris, urethral meatus, and vaginal meatus), labia minora, labia majora, and mons pubis.

2 Pregnancy occurs in the luteal, or secretory, phase.

3 Fertilization occurs in the fallopian tube.

4 Zygote = union of sex cells until formation of placenta; first 2 weeks
Embryo = balance of first trimester
Fetus = second and third trimester

5 Abnormal fertilization; improper implantation; abortion

6 Endometriosis, ovarian cysts, and breast cancer

7 Candidiasis

8 Sexual intercourse, injection-drug use, transfusion of virus-contaminated blood or blood products, mother to child during pregnancy and/or birth, and breast feeding

9 Follow-up includes urinalysis, weight, blood pressure check, and advice on diet and health habits.

10 Sitting, Fowler's, supine, lithotomy

11 CIN III stage III

12 Hormonal, barrier, permanent

Assisting in Pediatrics

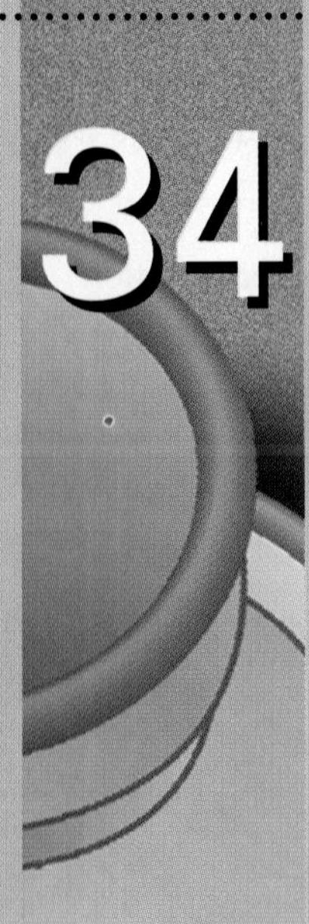

OUTLINE

LEARNING OBJECTIVES

Cognitive: On successful completion of this chapter you should be able to:

1. Compare the different growth and development patterns.
2. Name and briefly explain the major diseases discussed in the chapter.
3. Understand how vaccines are made.
4. List the AAP-approved immunizations and the appropriate age at which each is given.
5. Compare and contrast the well-child and the sick-child examinations.
6. Understand the medical assistant's role in the pediatric examination.
7. Be able to obtain accurate pediatric measurements.
8. Accurately obtain pediatric vital signs.
9. Understand when and how to apply restraints.
10. Show knowledge in handling child abuse.
11. Spell and define the terms in the Vocabulary.

Performance: On successful completion of this chapter you should be able to:

1. Properly obtain head measurement.
2. Obtain accurate height and weight measurements and plot growth pattern.
3. Accurately obtain pediatric vital signs.
4. Apply pediatric restraints.
5. Correctly obtain a pediatric urine sample.
6. Demonstrate methods for giving pediatric medications.

VOCABULARY

anomaly A marked deviation from normal: a congenital deformity

attenuated Weakened, or change in, virulence of a pathogenic microorganism

congenital Present at and existing from birth

electrolyte Chemical substance that when dissolved dissociates into electrically charged particles and is capable of conducting an electric current; essential to the normal function of cells

excoriation Scratch or similar abrasion to the skin

hydrocephaly Enlargement of the cranium caused by abnormal accumulation of cerebrospinal fluid within the cerebral system

laryngoscopy Visual examination of the voice box area through a endoscope equipped with a light and mirrors for illumination

maturation Physical and mental development process from beginning to maximum growth

microcephaly Small size of the head in relationship to the rest of the body

myringotomy Surgical process performed to relieve pressure and allow fluid drainage from the middle ear

purulent Containing or forming pus

rhonchi Continuous dry rattling in the throat or bronchial tube due to partial obstruction

serous Thin, watery, serum-like drainage

stridor Shrill, harsh respiratory sound heard during inhalation in laryngeal obstruction

suppurative Formation and/or discharge of pus

Pediatrics deals with the development and care of children and with the treatment of childhood diseases. The age range of the pediatric patient is from birth to puberty. Some practices continue to see the child until he or she is 14 to 16 years of age. Occasionally, children will continue to see the pediatrician until high school graduation. There are subspecialties within pediatrics such as surgery, cardiology, and psychiatry. About 50% of the patients in the pediatric office are well-baby or well-child care patients. The role of the pediatrician and the medical office staff is to supervise and help maintain the health of these patients. An increasing number of auxiliary health care personnel are being involved in the health services provided to young patients. Parents of these young patients must be involved with their care and development. The medical assistant can help a great deal in the communications between the patient, the parents, and the medical staff. The confidence a child develops in the care and the consideration received in the physician's office is the basis of good medical care.

Pediatric care actually starts before the child is born, with the promotion of the mother's good general health before conception and during pregnancy. The confidence and enthusiasm of the parents also affect the infant's physical and emotional well-being.

Normal Growth and Development

During the examination of a pediatric patient, the pediatrician looks for any sign of growth abnormality by comparing a child's physical, intellectual, and social signs to national average data charts. This comparison will indicate if the child is in the appropriate stage of growth and development for his or her chronologic age.

GROWTH PATTERNS

Physical growth is one of the most visible changes in childhood. By the time the child is 6 months old, the birth weight has doubled. The growth slows down slightly so that at 1 year, birth weight has tripled and height has increased 10 to 12 inches. Between ages 1 and 2, the child will gain approximately ½ pound per month and grow 3½ to 5 inches. From age 2 to age 3, the weight gain will average 3 to 5 pounds and height will increase 2 to 2½ inches. Most children slim down during this period; by the time their third birthday arrives, the potbellied toddler has become the characteristic preschooler.

During the preschool period, ages 3 to 6 years, weight increases 3 to 5 pounds a year and height increases at a slower but steady rate of 1½ to 2½ inches per year. By age 4, the child usually doubles his or her birth length. During this time the legs are the fastest growing part and fatty connective tissue continues to increase slowly until about age 7. This same growth rate continues through the school-age period, 6 to 12 years; and as this period of development terminates, the child usually is into a growth spurt that indicates impending puberty.

The growth spurt continues for approximately 2

years, and now the child is into adolescence, ages 12 to 18 years. During this period, the adolescent gains almost half of his or her adult weight and the skeleton and organs double in size. These changes are more noticeable in boys than in girls. Weight will increase in girls by 20 to 25 pounds and in boys by 15 to 20 pounds. Girls will grow 5 to 6 inches, and boys will grow 4 to 5 inches. Growth in height is fairly well complete by age 18.

As the growth spurt is completed, the teenager reaches sexual maturity. In the female, sexual maturity is known by the onset of the menstrual cycle; and in the male, maturity is determined by the presence of sperm in the semen. Timing of sexual maturity in both sexes varies greatly.

Completion of skeletal growth occurs in girls between 15 and 16 years of age and in boys between ages 17 and 18. Skeletal growth completion is established when the growth plates of the long bones of the extremities have completely fused.

Memory Jogger

At what age does the average child double in length?

DENVER II DEVELOPMENTAL SCREENING TEST

Each child develops individually and will display differences in attaining developmental plateaus. There are many theories concerned with stages of development common to all children as they mature. The Denver II Developmental Screening Test is given to children between the ages of 1 month and 6 years to assess normal development and identify possible developmental delays (Figs. 34–1 and 34–2). This assessment focuses on four developmental areas:

- Gross motor skills: Evaluation of the child's ability to control the body's large muscle groups. *Examples:* standing, kicking, running, and balance.
- Language: Evaluation of the child's verbal comprehension. *Examples:* word comprehension, following simple commands, use of subjects, and counting.
- Fine motor–adaptive skills: Evaluation of the child's coordination of the fine motor muscles. *Examples:* reaching, grasping, piling blocks, and drawing.
- Personal skills: Evaluation of child's self confidence and socialization. *Examples:* Playing games, using fork and spoon, dressing, and brushing teeth.

Once the test is completed, the results are analyzed and then determined to be normal, suspect, or untestable. When the results are not normal, the child may be retested with other developmental tests either by the pediatrician or by a professional pediatric testing agency.

DEVELOPMENTAL PATTERNS

General patterns of child development occur rapidly during the first year of life as the infant progresses from reflex activities such as grasping fingers and sucking to learning to manipulate simple objects such as pulling open drawers or throwing toys out of the crib. In addition to these motor skills, the child also learns verbal patterns, progressing from cooing and crying for attention to speaking first words.

By age 3, the child is showing increased autonomy. Now the child can walk, is toilet trained, sits at the table and eats with the family, can make simple sentences, understands the word "no," and even imitates the parent by using verbal gestures that he or she has seen used. The vocabulary consists of more than 500 words.

During the preschool stage, the child becomes increasingly independent and now initiates activities. Preschoolers have mastered many gross motor skills and are perfecting their fine motor development. Verbal communication has increased to full simple and even complex sentences but remains quite literal. For example, if you tell a preschool child that you are going to fly to visit Aunt Sue, the child would think you are going to flap your arms and fly. Nonverbal communication skills are also being mastered. The vocabulary now includes more than 2000 words. During this period, children need to develop social skills, such as sharing and taking part in peer-group activities.

The school-age child has perfected fine motor skills and can paint, draw, and play an instrument: enjoys team activities; and expands reading and writing skills. His or her intellectual skills are developing, and social skills are going through refinement as a sense of self-achievement and self-worth is developed. It is during this time that the child learns and tests the rules for socializing outside the immediate family as an independent individual.

The adolescent, or transition, stage is when the individual attempts to establish an adult identity. This is usually done through trial and error by experimenting with adult roles and behavior patterns. Traditional values learned in childhood may be questioned and peer relationships take on new importance. It is in this time frame that the teenager must develop the emotional maturity and motivation to make beneficial decisions. The family is looked to for encouragement and guidance in making decisions that will help the adolescent develop self-confidence and to become patient and less impulsive and self-centered.

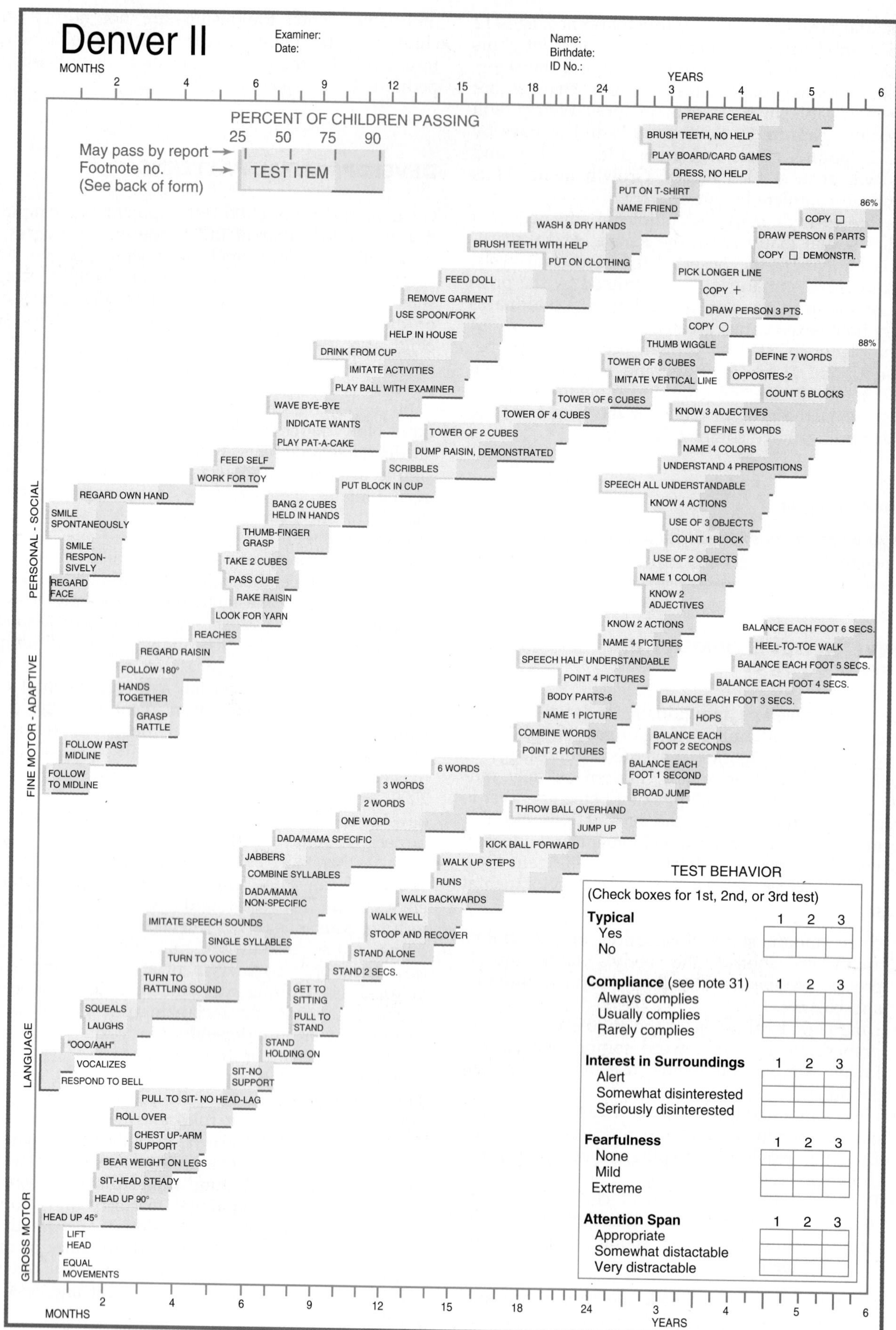

FIGURE 34–1 Denver II Developmental Screening Test (DDST). (Copyright 1990 by W.K. Frankenburg and J.B. Dodds.)

DIRECTIONS FOR ADMINISTRATION

1. Try to get child to smile by smiling, talking or waving. Do not touch him/her.
2. Child must stare at hand several seconds.
3. Parent may help guide toothbrush and put toothpaste on brush.
4. Child does not have to be able to tie shoes or button/zip in the back.
5. Move yarn slowly in an arc from one side to the other, about 8" above child's face.
6. Pass if child grasps rattle when it is touched to the backs or tips of fingers.
7. Pass if child tries to see where yarn went. Yarn should be dropped quickly from sight from tester's hand without arm movement.
8. Child must transfer cube from hand to hand without help of body, mouth, or table.
9. Pass if child picks up raisin with any part of thumb and finger.
10. Line can vary only 30 degrees or less from tester's line.
11. Make a fist with thumb pointing upward and wiggle only the thumb. Pass if child imitates and does not move any fingers other than the thumb.

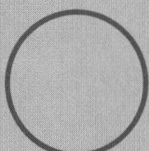

12. Pass any enclosed form. Fail continuous round motions.

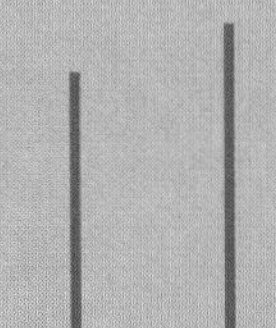

13. Which line is longer? (Not bigger.) Turn paper upside down and repeat. (pass 3 of 3 or 5 of 6)

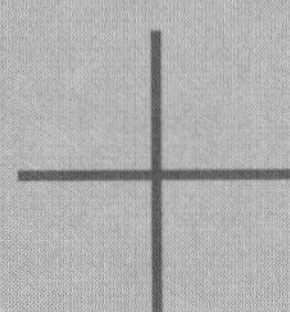

14. Pass any lines crossing near midpoint.

15. Have child copy first. If failed, demonstrate.

When giving items 12, 14, and 15, do not name the forms. Do not demonstrate 12 and 14.

16. When scoring, each pair (2 arms, 2 legs, etc.) counts as one part.
17. Place one cube in cup and shake gently near child's ear, but out of sight. Repeat for other ear.
18. Point to picture and have child name it. (No credit is given for sounds only.) If less than 4 pictures are named correctly, have child point to picture as each is named by tester.

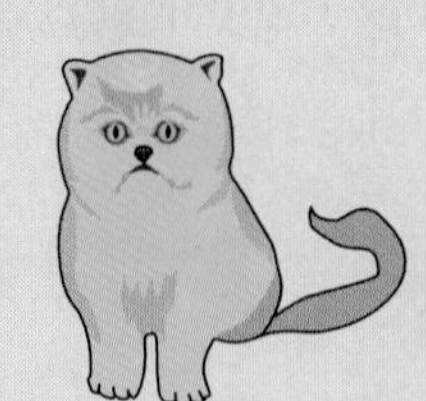
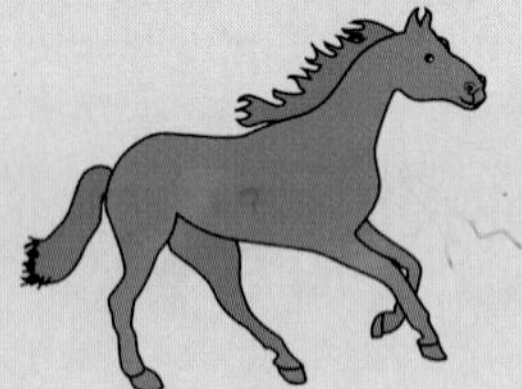
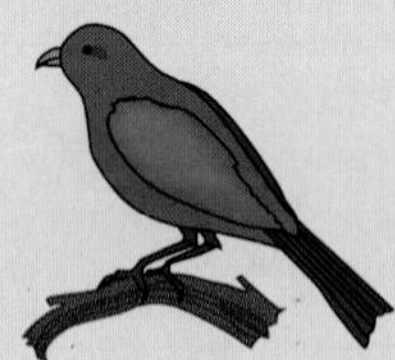
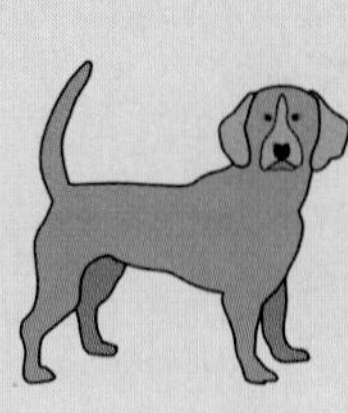
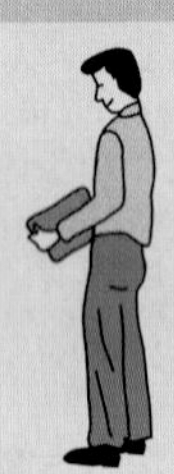

19. Using doll, tell child: Show me the nose, eyes, ears, mouth, hands, feet, tummy, hair. Pass 6 of 8.
20. Using pictures, ask child: Which one flies? . . . says meow? . . . talks? . . . barks? . . . gallops? Pass 2 of 5, 4 of 5.
21. Ask child: What do you do when you are cold? . . . tired? . . . hungry? Pass 2 of 3, 3 of 3.
22. Ask child: What do you do with a cup? What is a chair used for? What is a pencil used for? Action words must be included in answers.
23. Pass if child correctly places and says how many blocks are on paper. (1, 5).
24. Tell child: Put block **on** table; **under** table; **in front of** me, **behind** me. Pass 4 of 4. (Do not help child by pointing, moving head or eyes.)
25. Ask child: What is a ball? . . . lake? . . . desk? . . . house? . . . banana? . . . curtain? . . . fence? . . . ceiling? Pass if defined in terms of use, shape, what it is made of, or general category (such as banana is fruit, not just yellow). Pass 5 of 8, 7 of 8.
26. Ask child: If a horse is big, a mouse is __? If fire is hot, ice is __? If the sun shines during the day, the moon shines during the __? Pass 2 of 3.
27. Child may use wall or rail only, not person. May not crawl.
28. Child must throw ball overhand 3 feet to within arm's reach of tester.
29. Child must perform standing broad jump over width of test sheet (8 1/2 inches).
30. Tell child to walk forward, ⊂⊃⊂⊃⊂⊃⊂⊃ → heel within 1 inch of toe. Tester may demonstrate. Child must walk 4 consecutive steps.
31. In the second year, half of normal children are non-compliant.

OBSERVATIONS:

FIGURE 34–2 Instructions for DDST. (Copyright 1990 by W.K. Frankenburg and J.B. Dodds.)

Memory Jogger

A vocabulary of over 2000 words is expected in what age stage?

Diseases and Disorders

The process of illness in the pediatric patient poses special problems as children are constantly changing physically and functionally. When **maturation** moves along through a normal process, the child's natural immune system expands and, with the aid of routine prophylactic immunization, the child is fortified with long-term protection. Rapid advances in preventive medicine combined with advances in treatment have brought about the control of many serious infectious diseases that only a decade ago often resulted in death.

Various diseases still frequently affect the child, some of which are discussed next.

COLIC

Colic is usually seen in the newborn period or in early infancy. The problem is intermittent. During an attack, the infant draws up the legs, clenches the fists, and has a painful cry. This abdominal distress usually occurs in the late afternoon and evening. The cause is unknown, but it is thought that improper feeding techniques, overeating, swallowing excessive air while eating, and an allergy to cow's milk are all possible causes. Whatever is the cause, the infant is extremely uncomfortable and painfully cries throughout the attack.

The treatment consists of finding out what the possible cause could be. Often the child will outgrow the condition before the causative agent can be determined. The usual time for colic is from birth until 4 months of age. In severe cases, the infant may be given a gastric antispasmodic agent and the parent may need counseling and assistance in developing coping techniques.

Memory Jogger

Describe the signs expressed by an infant with colic.

DIARRHEA

Diarrhea is diagnosed when the child has two or more watery or apparently abnormal stools within a 24-hour period. The child may or may not show other signs of illness. If the diarrhea continues for more than 2 days, it needs medical intervention because it can cause rapid dehydration and **electrolyte** imbalance when fluid loss becomes excessive. Diaper rash along with **excoriation** of the anus can produce painful stool elimination.

Treatment consists of observation of the stools both physically and with laboratory analysis for color, consistency, odor, and amount. Oral intake may be restricted to rest the intestinal tract, or a special diet may be advised. Antibiotics may be prescribed if the causative agent is infectious. The child may require hospitalization to maintain electrolyte and fluid levels.

Memory Jogger

What is the importance of an electrolyte?

CROUP

Croup is a viral disorder that affects primarily the larynx with edema and spasm to the vocal cords. This varying degree of obstruction to the cords produces hoarseness, a high-pitched raspy cough, and **stridor** during inhalation. The episodes usually occur at night, and all symptoms may be gone by morning. If the child becomes frightened or anxious during the height of the episode, the symptoms can worsen. If the problem becomes chronic or continues for a period of time, it may become necessary to do a **laryngoscopy** or obtain throat cultures to determine the underlying cause.

COMMON COLD

A cold is a common viral occurrence in every family and frequently happens when there is a decided

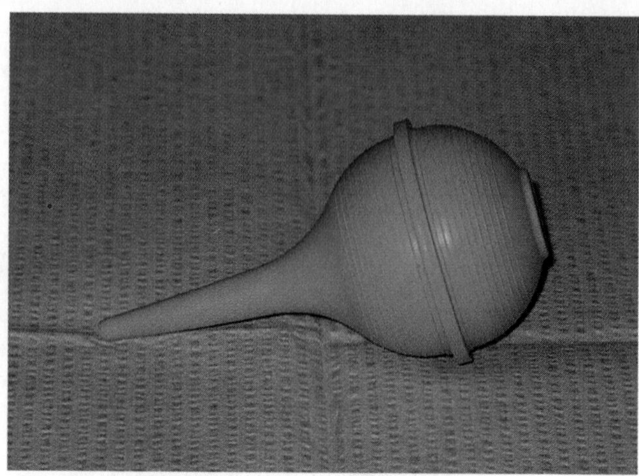

FIGURE 34–3 Nasal bulb syringe.

change in environmental temperature. Most colds are self-limiting and run their course in about a week. In infants and young children, the primary concern is nasal congestion and loss of appetite. The parent may need to be shown how to use a nasal bulb-syringe to suction the nose (Fig. 34–3). The possibility of a secondary infection in the lower respiratory tract or in the middle ear is a potentially dangerous side effect.

Memory Jogger

 *List the dangers of the common cold.*

CHICKENPOX (VARICELLA)

Chickenpox is caused by a member of the herpesvirus group and is transmitted by direct or indirect droplet from the respiratory tract of an infected person. The incubation period is 14 to 21 days. The child usually runs a slight fever for up to 3 days before the skin eruptions occur and is contagious at this time. The skin lesions tend to be more abundant on covered parts of the body. These lesions continue to erupt for 3 to 4 days and cause intense itching. The infection lasts for about 2 weeks and, in most cases, leaves the child with lifetime immunity. A varicella virus vaccine, Varivax, is now available for protection against chickenpox.

Memory Jogger

 *How long is the incubation period for chickenpox?*

INFLUENZA

Influenza is an acute, highly contagious viral infection of the respiratory tract. Its highest incidence is in schoolchildren, but it is most severe in infants and toddlers. It is transmitted by direct contact with moist secretions. Children tend to have high fevers with influenza and are susceptible to pulmonary complications. There is a broad range in the severity of flu cases from very mild to life threatening. The virus can destroy the respiratory epithelium, which is one of the body's strong defense mechanisms against bacterial invasion. With the loss of this protective mechanism, bacteria can invade any part of the respiratory tract and cause pneumonia.

There is no medication that cures influenza. Sometimes antibiotics are prescribed to prevent a secondary bacterial infection. The usual treatment consists of bed rest, increased fluids, and a nonaspirin analgesic to reduce fever. Flu vaccines are available but are only beneficial if obtained before the onset of the disease, and this immunization does not give immunity for all strains of the flu virus.

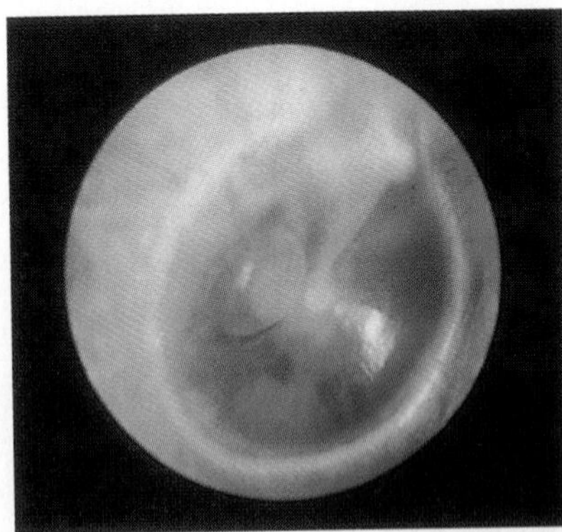

FIGURE 34–4 Serous otitis media. (From Swartz MH: Textbook of Physical Diagnosis, 3rd ed. Philadelphia, WB Saunders, 1997.)

OTITIS MEDIA

Infection in the middle ear is usually a side effect of a cold or other upper respiratory tract disorder, but it can also be the result of allergy. It is classified as either **serous** (Fig. 34–4) or **suppurative** or **purulent** (Fig. 34–5), depending on the composition of the accumulating fluid. Symptoms vary according to the type, but generally all types cause dizziness and pain.

The treatment usually consists of analgesics, decongestants, and antibiotics. For cases that become chronic and/or do not respond to conventional treatment, **myringotomy** may be needed (Fig. 34–6).

Memory Jogger

 *Identify the three types of otitis media.*

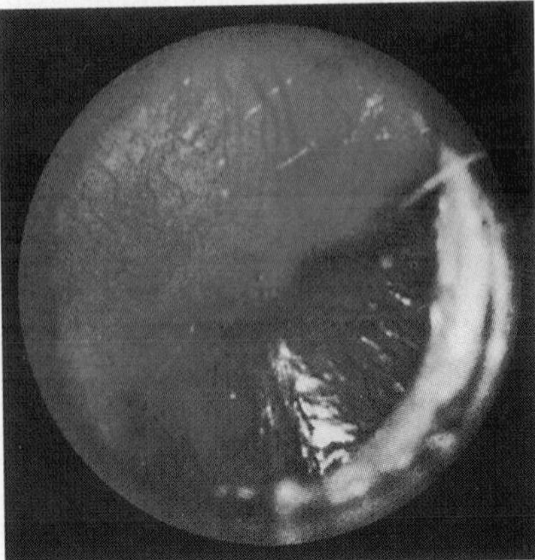

FIGURE 34–5 Purulent otitis media. (Courtesy of Dr. Richard A. Buckingham and Dr. George E. Shambaugh, Jr.)

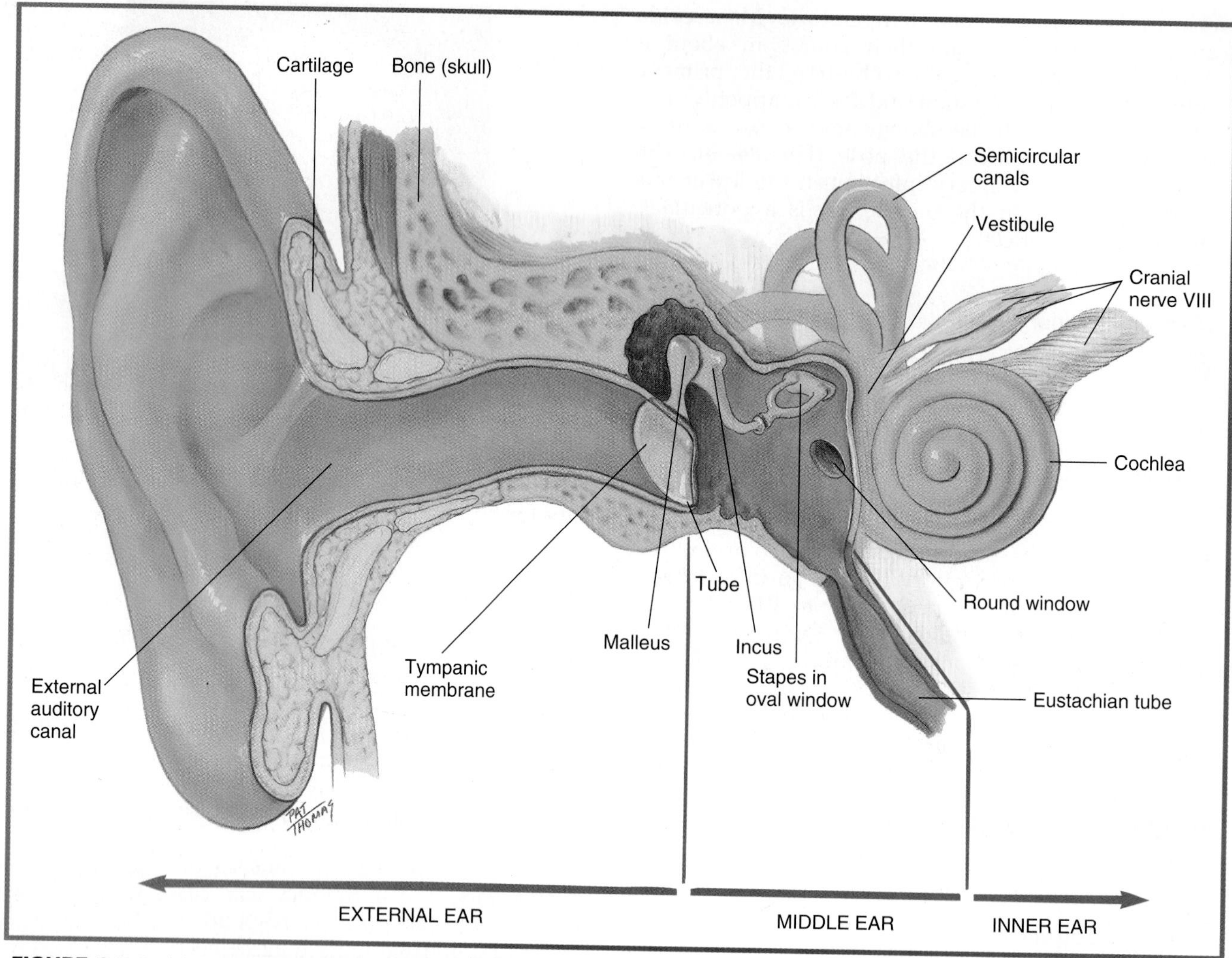

FIGURE 34–6 Myringotomy procedure. Tube is inserted into a small opening in the ear drum to allow drainage and air to pass from and into the middle ear. (Adapted from Jarvis C: Physical Examination and Health Assessment, 2nd ed. Philadelphia, WB Saunders, 1996.)

TONSILLITIS

Tonsillitis is caused by many infectious agents, but the most frequent is beta-hemolytic *Streptococcus.* The onset is sudden and can become intensely painful in a brief time period. The tonsils appear red and infected, and a culture is done to determine the causative organism. The treatment usually consists of bed rest, liquid to soft diet, gargling with salt water, and oral antibiotics. The danger is in the secondary problems that can occur, which include rheumatic heart disease and kidney disease.

ASTHMA

Asthma is the result of hypersensitive bronchial tubes that trigger bronchial spasms. These spasms trap air and thick mucus in the lungs and can be brought on by allergy, stress, infection, strenuous activity, and inhalation of innocuous fumes. The disease has a strong hereditary factor and is a leading cause of absenteeism from school. The child usually has a nonproductive cough accompanied by an expiratory wheeze and shallow respirations. The shallow breathing will increase the pulse rate and make it difficult for the child to speak more than a few words at a time. The child complains of a tight chest, and the physician will hear **rhonchi** when the chest is auscultated. An asthmatic attack can last minutes to days and/or can be a medical emergency. Each child and each attack needs to be evaluated independently.

Treatment requires medical management by a specialist. Many pediatricians will refer asthmatic patients to an ear, nose, and throat or allergy specialist who specializes in asthmatic disorders. Specialists may order intradermal skin testing to identify the causative inhalant or allergy substance. Pulmonary function testing and respiratory therapy may also be employed.

HEPATITIS B

Hepatitis B virus (HBV) infection can lead to serious and chronic infection of the liver. The virus can be transmitted across the placenta or during the birth process if the mother is infected. HBV can also be transmitted sexually, by blood transfusion, or by direct contact. A child can carry the virus for years and only later develop liver failure or liver cancer as a result. Many states now include immunizations for HBV in the recommended immunization schedule. This immunization may be begun between 2 and 3 months of age.

REYE'S SYNDROME

The cause of Reye's syndrome is unknown, but it has been linked to the use of aspirin during illness. It is an acute and sometimes fatal illness that is characterized by fatty invasion of the inner organs, especially the liver, and swelling of the brain. It is most often seen in children between infancy through puberty (age 16). The syndrome moves through five stages (Table 34–1).

Prevention is the best treatment, which means give children no aspirin. Use nonsalicylate analgesics and antipyretics such as ibuprofen and acetaminophen. Early recognition, hospitalization, and treatment have greatly reduced the mortality rate.

Memory Jogger

8 *Reye's syndrome is linked to the use of _____?*

TABLE 34–1 Five Stages of Reye's Syndrome

Stage	Signs and Symptoms
1	Restlessness, vomiting, liver malfunction
2	Elevated respiratory rate, hyperactive reflexes, increased liver dysfunction
3	Internal organ tissue changes, coma
4	Loss of brain function, deepening coma
5	Seizures, respiratory arrest, death

Immunizations

Over the years immunization has helped dramatically reduce potentially lethal childhood infections. According to the Centers for Disease Control and Prevention the record is impressive:

- Measles: Cases of this acute viral affliction plunged from 481,000 in 1962 to 277 in 1997.
- Whooping cough (pertussis): Cases of this sometimes deadly illness dropped from 74,700 in 1948 to less than 5000 in 1997.
- Polio: This paralyzing disease fell from 18,000 cases in 1954 to 2 in 1993 and none in 1997.
- Diphtheria: Cases of this occasionally lethal bacterial "sore throat" plummeted from nearly 9,500 in 1948 to none in 1993 through 1997.
- Tetanus: This potentially fatal bacterial infection declined from 600 cases in 1948 to 42 in 1997.

Because any of these diseases could rebound in a newer, more deadly form, the CDC recommends immunization against infectious diseases for all children except those for whom a particular vaccination would pose a risk. The American Academy of Pediatrics (AAP) has developed an immunization schedule outlining vaccines recommended for all children before entering school (Fig. 34–7). Each individual state develops its own immunization program and a method for enforcement. Periodically, this schedule is updated as new vaccines become available and/or research indicates a better method in giving the vaccine.

Immunizations are a vaccine suspension of dead or **attenuated** organisms given to stimulate an active immune response to increase the permanent resistance to specific pathogenic viruses and organisms (Table 34–2). Booster doses are usually equivalent to one single dose of the initial immunization and are prescribed at designated intervals to ensure maintenance of the immune levels.

Vaccine manufacturers have trade names for each product and have established protocols to ensure potency and stability. All vaccines are tested for safety and effectiveness. In every package of vaccine is an insert that fully describes the vaccine, its use, and route of administration and also describes adverse reactions and symptoms that the parent might observe after immunization that would indicate a potential problem. Untoward responses include high

TABLE 34–2 Suggested Immunizations

Vaccine	Vaccination for	Contraindications
TOPV or OPV	Polio	Acute illness, immunosuppression
DPT	Diphtheria, pertussis, tetanus	Fever, history of neurologic disorders
DT	Diphtheria, tetanus	
MMR	Measles, mumps, rubella	Allergy to eggs, fever untreated tuberculosis
Hib	*Haemophilus influenzae* type b	Acute illness
Hepatitis B	Hepatitis B	Allergy to yeast, active infection, cardiovascular disease
Varivax	Chickenpox	Fever, previously had disease
PPD	Skin test for tuberculosis	Previous positive test

RECOMMENDED CHILDHOOD IMMUNIZATION SCHEDULE UNITED STATES, JANUARY – JUNE 1996

[1]**Infants born to HBsAg-negative mothers** should receive 2.5 μg of Merck vaccine (Recombivax HB) or 10 μg of SmithKline Beecham (SB) vaccine (Engerix-B). The second dose should be administered ≥1 mo after the first dose.

Infants born to HBsAg-positive mothers should receive 0.5 mL Hepatitis B Immune Globulin (HBIG) within 12 hr of birth, and either 5 μg of Merck vaccine (Recombivax HB) or 10 μg of SB vaccine (Engerix-B) at a separate site. The second dose is recommended at 1–2 mos of age and the third dose at 6 mos of age.

Infants born to mothers whose HBsAg status is unknown should receive either 5 μg of Merck vaccine (Recombivax HB) or 10 μg of SB vaccine (Engerix-B) within 12 hr of birth. The second dose of vaccine is recommended at 1 mo of age and the third dose at 6 mos of age.

[2]Adolescents who have not previously received 3 doses of hepatitis B vaccine should initiate or complete the series at the 11–12 year-old visit. The second dose should be administered at least 1 mo after the first dose, and the third dose should be administered at least 4 mos after the first dose and at least 2 mos after the second dose.

[3]DTP4 may be administered at 12 mos of age, if at least 6 mos have elapsed since DTP3. DTaP (diphtheria and tetanus toxoids and acellular pertussis vaccine) is licensed for the fourth and/or fifth vaccine dose(s) for children ≥15 mos and may be preferred for these doses in this age group. Td (tetanus and diphtheria toxoids, absorbed, for adult use) is recommended at 11–12 years of age if at least 5 years have elapsed since the last dose of DTP, DTaP, or DT.

[4]Three *H. influenzae* type b (Hib) conjugate vaccines are licensed for infant use. If PRP-OMP (PedvaxHIB [Merck]) is administered at 2 and 4 mos of age, a dose at 6 mos is not required. After completing the primary series, any Hib conjugate vaccine may be used as a booster.

[5]Oral poliovirus vaccine (OPV) is recommended for routine infant vaccination. Inactivated poliovirus vaccine (IPV) is recommended for persons with a congenital or acquired immune deficiency disease or an altered immune status as a result of disease or immunosuppressive therapy, as well as their household contacts, and is an acceptable alternative for other persons. The primary 3-dose series for IPV should be given with a minimum interval of 4 wks between the first and second doses and 6 mos between the second and third doses.

[6]The second dose of MMR is routinely recommended at 4–6 yrs of age or at 11–12 yrs of age, but may be administered at any visit, provided at least 1 mo has elapsed since receipt of the first dose.

[7]Varicella zoster virus vaccine (Var) can be administered to susceptible children any time after 12 months of age. Unvaccinated children who lack a reliable history of chicken pox should be vaccinated at the 11–12 year-old visit.

Vaccines are listed under the routinely recommended ages. Bars *indicate range of acceptable ages for vaccination.* Shaded bars *indicate* catch-up vaccination: *at 11–12 years of age, hepatitis B vaccine should be administered to children not previously vaccinated, and varicella zoster virus vaccine should be administered to children not previously vaccinated who lack a reliable history of chicken pox.*

Age ▶ / Vaccine ▼	Birth	1 mo	2 mos	4 mos	6 mos	12 mos	15 mos	18 mos	4–6 yrs	11–12 yrs	14–16 yrs
Hepatitis B[1,2]	Hep B-1 (Birth–2 mos)										
		Hep B-2 (1–4 mos)			Hep B-3 (6–18 mos)					Hep B[2]	
Diphtheria, Tetanus, Pertussis[3]			DTP	DTP	DTP	DTP[3] (DTaP at 15+ m) (12–18 mos)			DTP or DTaP	Td (11–16 yrs)	
H. influenzae type b[4]			Hib	Hib	Hib[4]	Hib[4] (12–15 mos)					
Polio[5]			OPV[5]	OPV	OPV (6–18 mos)				OPV		
Measles, Mumps, Rubella[6]						MMR (12–15 mos)			MMR[6] or	MMR[6]	
Varicella Zoster Virus Vaccine[7]						Var (12–18 mos)				Var[7]	

Approved by the Advisory Committee on Immunization Practices (ACIP), the American Academy of Pediatrics (AAP), and the American Academy of Family Physicians (AAFP).

FIGURE 34–7 Immunization schedule.

fever, swelling at the site of the injection, breathing difficulties, severe headache, and convulsions. Any of these should be reported to the physician immediately.

Some vaccines are grown in bird eggs or on media made from animal organs or are weakened with chemicals. The child is screened for certain allergies or previous reactions to vaccine or the growth media. It is the responsibility of the medical assistant to know these effects and to be certain that the parent is informed. Informed consent must be signed and attached to the child's health record before immunizations are given.

Memory Jogger

List the ages at which the DPT immunization is given.

The Pediatric Patient

The newborn's first physical assessment comes at the time of delivery, when the pediatrician assesses the newborn's ability to thrive outside the uterus. The Apgar score is a system of scoring the infant's physical condition at 1 and 5 minutes after birth (Table 34–3). The heart rate, respiration, muscle tone, response to stimuli, and color of the infant are each rated 0, 1, or 2. The maximum total score is 10. Those infants with low scores must be given immediate attention.

WELL-CHILD VISITS

The frequency of the well-child visits varies with the physician and the community. It may follow this pattern: 2 weeks, 7 weeks, 4 months, 1 year, 2 years, 5 years, 10 years, and 15 years. These visits focus on maintaining the health of the child through basic system examinations, immunizations, and upgrading of the child's medical history record.

The decision of whether the child is to be seen alone or with the parent depends on the pediatrician and on the age of the child. Often the child will look to the parent for approval before answering or performing a skill; and for this reason, the physician may want the child alone. If this is the case, explain to the parent that the physician wants to evaluate the child's independent abilities and that as soon as the testing is completed, you will return so that the physician can relate the results of the testing protocols.

The medical history is an essential guide to the pediatric examination. With the infant, the physician is dependent on the parent for the history, but as the child gets older some history may be obtained from the child and clarified or amplified by the parent. Generally, the child is extremely honest regarding the facts of the illness. Close observation also gives the physician considerable information. A wince may indicate tenderness, and the facial expression associated with nausea should alert the physician and the staff.

SICK-CHILD VISITS

The sick-child visits occur whenever needed and usually on short notice. For this reason, most pediatric offices keep open appointments in the scheduling to accommodate the sick child. The length and frequency of this type of visit depend entirely on the child and the illness.

Memory Jogger

What are the three focus points in the well-child examination?

The Medical Assistant's Role in Pediatric Procedures

When assisting in the pediatric office, in addition to assisting the pediatrician with examinations through upgrading the patient history, performing the or-

TABLE 34–3 The Apgar Scoring System*

Clinical Sign	Assigned Score		
	0	*1*	*2*
Heart rate	Absent	Under 100	Over 100
Respiratory effort	Absent	Slow and irregular	Good and crying
Muscle tone	Limp	Some flexion of the arms and legs	Active movement
Reflex irritability	No response	Grimace	Coughing and sneezing
Color	Blue and pale	Body pink and extremities blue	Pink all over

*The readings are taken by the pediatrician at 1-minute and 5-minute intervals after birth. At *1 minute,* if the score is 7 or less, some nervous system problems are suspected. If the score is below 4, resuscitation is usually necessary. At *5 minutes,* if the score is at least 8, the pediatrician can conduct a complete examination. The child is probably reacting normally.

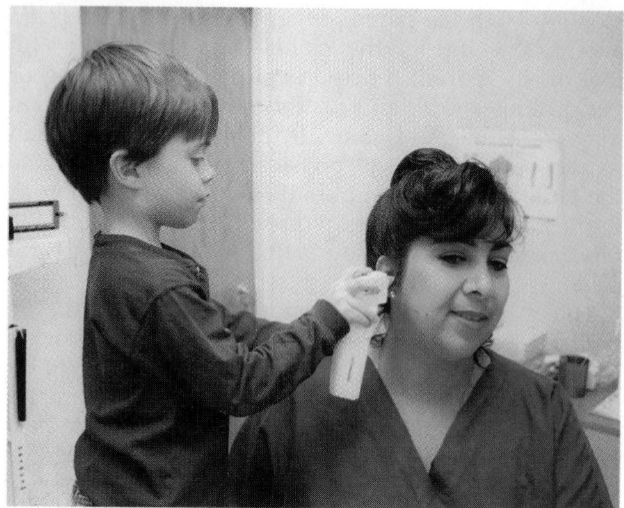

FIGURE 34–8 Making a game out of a procedure.

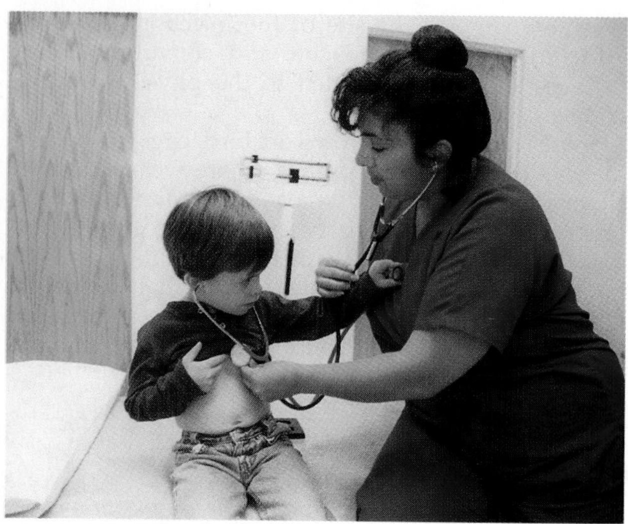

FIGURE 34–9 Explaining a procedure.

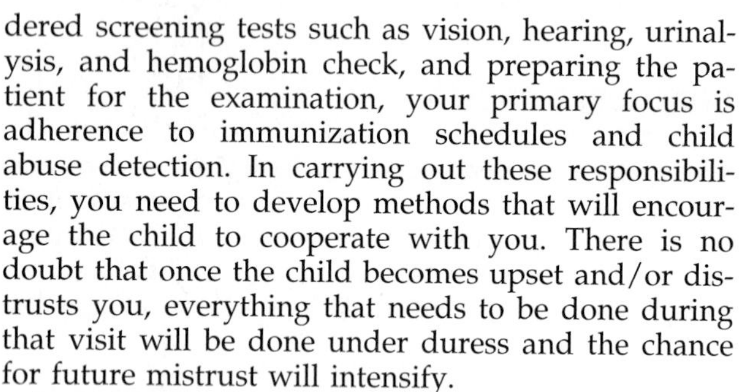

dered screening tests such as vision, hearing, urinalysis, and hemoglobin check, and preparing the patient for the examination, your primary focus is adherence to immunization schedules and child abuse detection. In carrying out these responsibilities, you need to develop methods that will encourage the child to cooperate with you. There is no doubt that once the child becomes upset and/or distrusts you, everything that needs to be done during that visit will be done under duress and the chance for future mistrust will intensify.

Interacting with children requires special techniques, depending on the age of the child. If you gain the child's trust and confidence, the child tends to be more cooperative during the examination. Children younger than 2 feel better when the parent is holding them or remains very close. Between the ages of 2 and 4, children enjoy making a game out of the situation (Fig. 34–8). Your duties may be to weigh and measure the infant, to record this information on the patient's chart, and to check whether immunizations are due.

The sequence of the examination varies and is frequently adapted to the cooperation of the child. The pediatrician may leave until last the areas to which the patient may object the most and in which the patient may be the least cooperative. Sometimes, a tongue depressor in each little hand keeps an infant from grabbing the stethoscope. Explaining what is to be done and showing the child the instruments to be used often contribute to his or her cooperation (Fig. 34–9). The instruments and the examiner's hands should be warm.

The physician is concerned with the patient's growth and development. The child's alertness and responses tell the physician a considerable amount. In infancy and in the young child of preschool age, the parent is closely questioned about the child's eating, sleeping, and elimination habits. The school-age child is usually a little more cooperative during an examination and can answer most questions without parental assistance. Adolescent patients are usually sensitive, are easily embarrassed, and are concerned about their health and appearance. Adolescent medicine is now a subspeciality in pediatrics.

MEASUREMENT

Examination of the child during routine well-child care includes the measurement of the circumference of the infant's head (see Procedure 34–1). The head of the infant is measured to determine normal growth and development (Fig. 34–10). If the circumference of the head deviates greatly from normal measurements, **hydrocephaly** or **microcephaly** may be suspected. It is important to discover any **congenital** problem as early as possible so that appropriate treatment measures can be initiated. Measurement of head circumference should be performed during routine office visits until the child is 36 months old (Fig. 34–11). You will measure the head

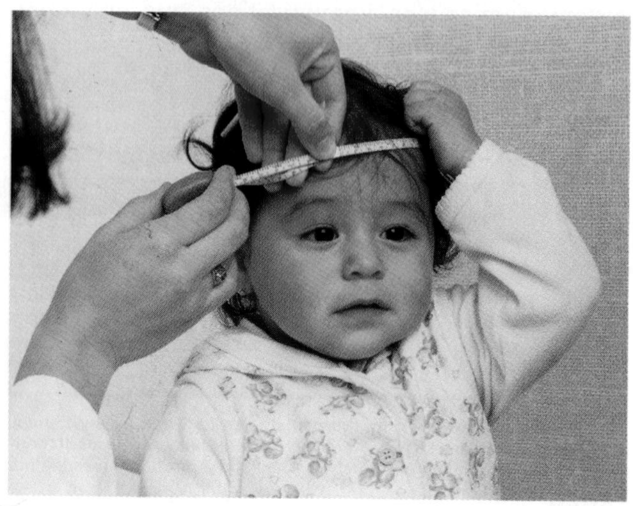

FIGURE 34–10 Head circumference.

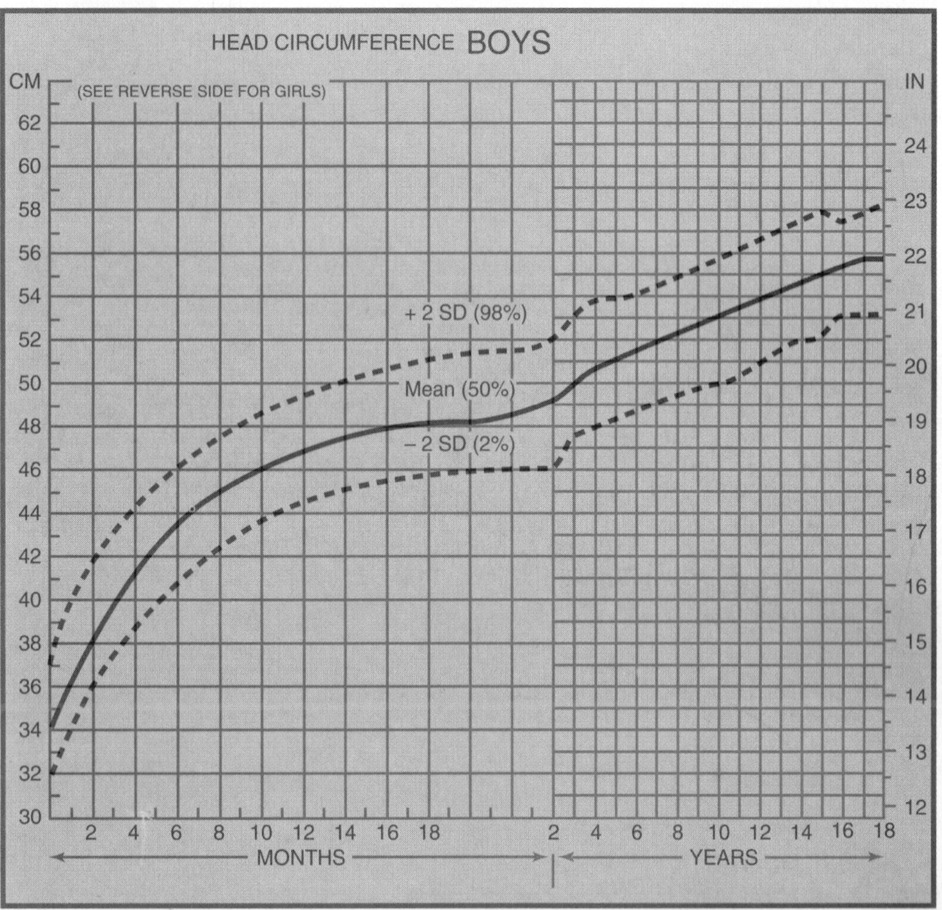

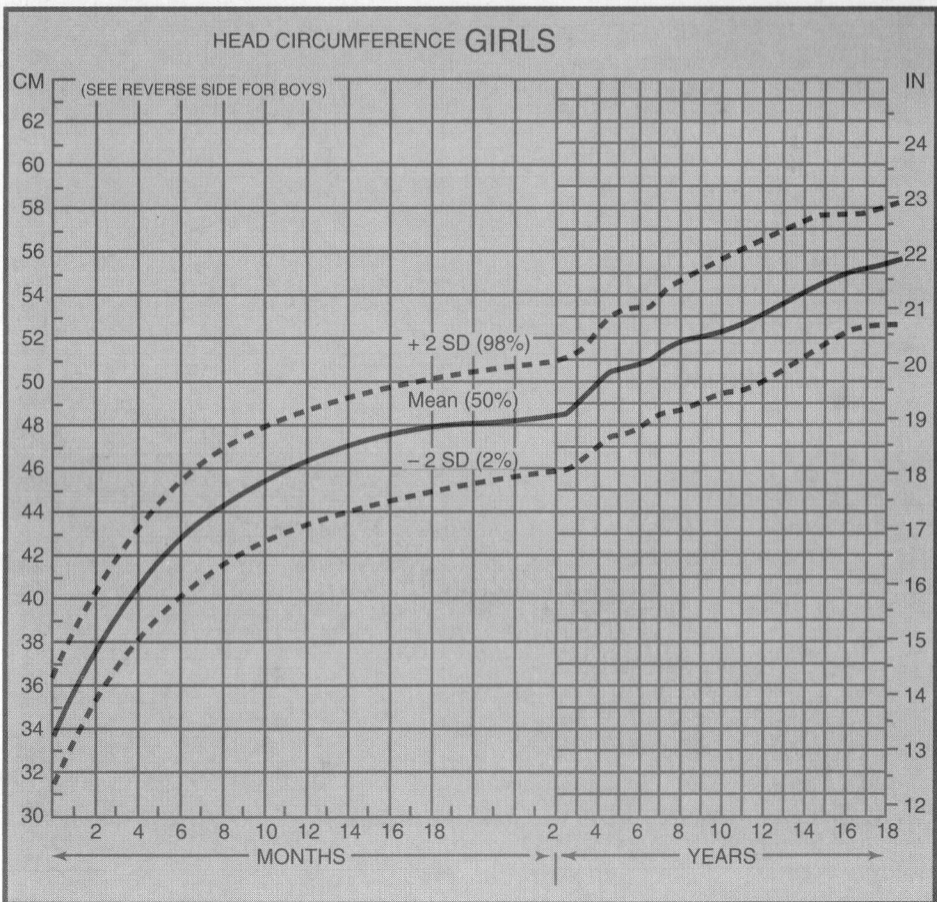

FIGURE 34–11 Head circumference chart. (From National Center for Health Statistics.)

HEIGHT AND WEIGHT MEASUREMENTS FOR GIRLS

	Height by Percentiles						Weight by Percentiles					
	5		50		95		5		50		95	
Age*	cm	Inches	cm	Inches	cm	Inches	kg	lb	kg	lb	kg	lb
Birth	45.4	17 3/4	49.9	19 3/4	52.9	20 3/4	2.36	5 1/4	3.23	7	3.81	8 1/2
3 months	55.4	21 3/4	59.5	23 1/2	63.4	25	4.18	9 1/4	5.4	12	6.74	14 3/4
6 months	61.8	24 1/4	65.9	26	70.2	27 3/4	5.79	12 3/4	7.21	16	8.73	19 1/4
9 months	66.1	26	70.4	27 3/4	75.0	29 1/2	7.0	15 1/2	8.56	18 3/4	10.17	22 1/2
1	69.8	27 1/2	74.3	29 1/4	79.1	31 1/4	7.84	17 1/4	9.53	21	11.24	24 3/4
1 1/2	76.0	30	80.9	31 3/4	86.1	34	8.92	19 3/4	10.82	23 3/4	12.76	28 1/4
2†	81.6	32 1/4	86.8	34 1/4	93.6	36 3/4	9.95	22	11.8	26	14.15	31 1/4
2 1/2†	84.6	33 1/4	90.0	35 1/2	96.6	38	10.8	23 3/4	13.03	28 3/4	15.76	34 3/4
3	88.3	34 3/4	94.1	37	100.6	39 1/2	11.61	25 1/2	14.1	31	17.22	38
3 1/2	91.7	36	97.9	38 1/2	104.5	41 1/4	12.37	27 1/4	15.07	33 1/4	18.59	41
4	95.0	37 1/2	101.6	40	108.3	42 3/4	13.11	29	15.96	35 1/4	19.91	44
4 1/2	98.1	38 1/2	105.0	41 1/4	112.0	44	13.83	30 1/2	16.81	37	21.24	46 3/4
5	101.1	39 3/4	108.4	42 3/4	115.6	45 1/2	14.55	32	17.66	39	22.62	49 3/4
6	106.6	42	114.6	45	122.7	48 1/4	16.05	35 1/2	19.52	43	25.75	56 3/4
7	111.8	44	120.6	47 1/2	129.5	51	17.71	39	21.84	48 1/4	29.68	65 1/2
8	116.9	46	126.4	49 3/4	136.2	53 1/2	19.62	43 1/4	24.84	54 3/4	34.71	76 1/2
9	122.1	48	132.2	52	142.9	56 1/4	21.82	48	28.46	62 3/4	40.64	89 1/2
10	127.5	50 1/4	138.3	54 1/2	149.5	58 3/4	24.36	53 3/4	32.55	71 3/4	47.17	104
11	133.5	52 1/2	144.8	57	156.2	61 1/2	27.24	60	36.95	81 1/2	54.0	119
12	139.8	55	151.5	59 3/4	162.7	64	30.52	67 1/4	41.53	91 1/2	60.81	134
13	145.2	57 1/4	157.1	61 3/4	168.1	66 1/4	34.14	75 1/4	46.1	101 3/4	67.3	148 1/4
14	148.7	58 1/2	160.4	63 1/4	171.3	67 1/2	37.76	83 1/4	50.28	110 3/4	73.08	161
15	150.5	59 1/4	161.8	63 3/4	172.8	68	40.99	90 1/4	53.68	118 1/4	77.78	171 1/2
16	151.6	59 3/4	162.4	64	173.3	68 1/4	43.41	95 3/4	55.89	123 1/4	80.99	178 1/2
17	152.7	60	163.1	64 1/4	173.5	68 1/4	44.74	98 3/4	56.69	125	82.46	181 3/4
18	153.6	60 1/2	163.7	64 1/2	173.6	68 1/4	45.26	99 3/4	56.62	124 3/4	82.47	181 3/4

HEIGHT AND WEIGHT MEASUREMENTS FOR BOYS

	Height by Percentiles						Weight by Percentiles					
	5		50		95		5		50		95	
Age*	cm	Inches	cm	Inches	cm	Inches	kg	lb	kg	lb	kg	lb
Birth	46.4	18 1/4	50.5	20	54.4	21 1/2	2.54	5 1/2	3.27	7 1/4	4.15	9 1/4
3 months	56.7	22 1/4	61.1	24	65.4	25 3/4	4.43	9 3/4	5.98	13 1/4	7.37	16 1/4
6 months	63.4	25	67.8	26 3/4	72.3	28 1/2	6.20	13 3/4	7.85	17 1/4	9.46	20 3/4
9 months	68.0	26 3/4	72.3	28 1/2	77.1	30 1/4	7.52	16 1/2	9.18	20 1/4	10.93	24
1	71.7	28 1/4	76.1	30	81.2	32	8.43	18 1/2	10.15	22 1/2	11.99	26 1/2
1 1/2	77.5	30 1/2	82.4	32 1/2	88.1	34 3/4	9.59	21 1/4	11.47	25 1/4	13.44	29 1/2
2†	82.5	32 1/2	86.8	34 1/4	94.4	37 1/4	10.49	23 1/4	12.34	27 1/4	15.50	34 1/4
2 1/2†	85.4	33 1/2	90.4	35 1/2	97.8	38 1/2	11.27	24 3/4	13.52	29 3/4	16.61	36 1/2
3	89.0	35	94.9	37 1/4	102.0	40 1/4	12.05	26 1/2	14.62	32 1/4	17.77	39 1/4
3 1/2	92.5	36 1/2	99.1	39	106.1	41 3/4	12.84	28 1/4	15.68	34 1/2	18.98	41 3/4
4	95.8	37 3/4	102.9	40 1/2	109.9	43 1/4	13.64	30	16.69	36 3/4	20.27	44 3/4
4 1/2	98.9	39	106.6	42	113.5	44 3/4	14.45	31 3/4	17.69	39	21.63	47 3/4
5	102.0	40 1/2	109.9	43 1/4	117.0	46	15.27	33 3/4	18.67	41 1/4	23.09	51
6	107.7	42 1/2	116.1	45 3/4	123.5	48 1/2	16.93	37 1/4	20.69	45 1/2	26.34	58
7	113.0	44 1/2	121.7	48	129.7	51	18.64	41	22.85	50 1/4	30.12	66 1/2
8	118.1	46 1/2	127.0	50	135.7	53 1/2	20.40	45	25.30	55 3/4	34.51	76
9	122.9	48 1/2	132.2	52	141.8	55 3/4	22.25	49	28.13	62	39.58	87 1/4
10	127.7	50 1/4	137.5	54 1/4	148.1	58 1/4	24.33	53 3/4	31.44	69 1/4	45.27	99 3/4
11	132.6	52 1/4	143.3	56 1/2	154.9	61	26.80	59	35.30	77 3/4	51.47	113 1/2
12	137.6	54 1/4	149.7	59	162.3	64	29.85	65 3/4	39.78	87 3/4	58.09	128
13	142.9	56 1/4	156.5	61 1/2	169.8	66 3/4	33.64	74 1/4	44.95	99	65.02	143 1/4
14	148.8	58 1/2	163.1	64 1/4	176.7	69 1/2	38.22	84 1/4	50.77	112	72.13	159
15	155.2	61	169.0	66 1/2	181.9	71 1/2	43.11	95	56.71	125	79.12	174 1/2
16	161.1	63 1/2	173.5	68 1/4	185.4	73	47.74	105 1/4	62.10	137	85.62	188 3/4
17	164.9	65	176.2	69 1/4	187.3	73 3/4	51.50	113 1/2	66.31	146 1/4	91.31	201 1/4
18	165.7	65 1/4	176.8	69 1/2	187.6	73 3/4	53.97	119	68.88	151 3/4	95.76	211

Modified from National Center for Health Statistics (NCHS), Health Resources Administration, Department of Health, Education and Welfare, Hyattsville, MD. Conversion of metric data to approximate inches and pounds by Ross Laboratories.

*Years unless otherwise indicated.

†Height data include some recumbent length measurements, which make values slightly higher than if all measurements had been of stature (standing height).

FIGURE 34–12 Height and weight chart.

at the time that the weight and height measurements are determined (Fig. 34–12).

Growth charts using the National Center for Health Statistics (NCHS) system for evaluating and comparing young children's growth rates with those of similar children of similar ages are used by most pediatricians. Slowed growth patterns and nutritional variances are easily detected. Because boys and girls differ in normal growth rates, separate charts are used. There are charts for two age groups: birth to 36 months (Figs. 34–13 and 34–14) and ages 2 to 18 years (Figs. 34–15 and 34–16). Frequently, medical assistants are asked to plot a growth pattern.

Memory Jogger

At what age is the head circumference no longer measured?

Text continued on page 664

PROCEDURE 34–1
Measuring the Circumference of an Infant's Head

GOAL

to obtain an accurate measurement of the circumference of an infant's head.

EQUIPMENT AND SUPPLIES

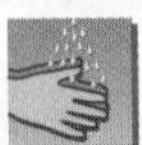

Flexible tape measure
Growth chart
Patient's chart
Pen or pencil

PROCEDURAL STEPS

1 Wash your hands
PURPOSE: Infection control.

2 Identify the patient and gain infant cooperation through conversation.
PURPOSE: Alleviate anxiety and gain child's trust.

3 Place the infant in the supine position; an older child may sit on the examination table; alternatively, the infant may be held by the parent.

4 Hold the tape measure with the zero mark against the infant's forehead, above the eyebrows.

5 Bring the tape measure around the head, just above the ears, to meet at the mid forehead (Figure 1).

6 Read to the nearest 0.01 cm or ¼ inch.

7 Record the measurement on the growth chart and the patient's chart.
PURPOSE: A procedure is not done until it is recorded.

8 Clean the work area.

9 Wash your hands.
PURPOSE: Infection control.

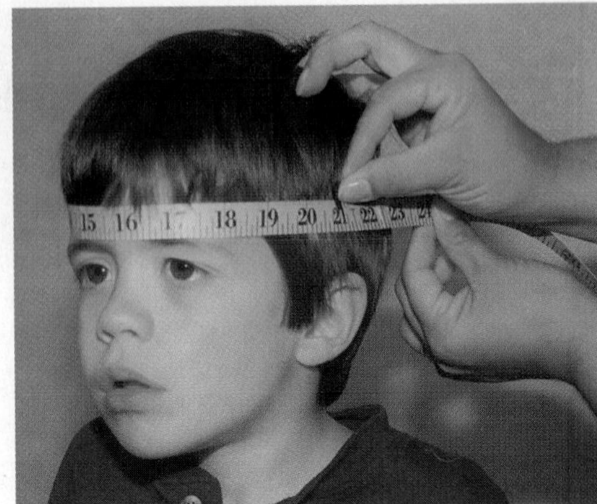

FIGURE 1

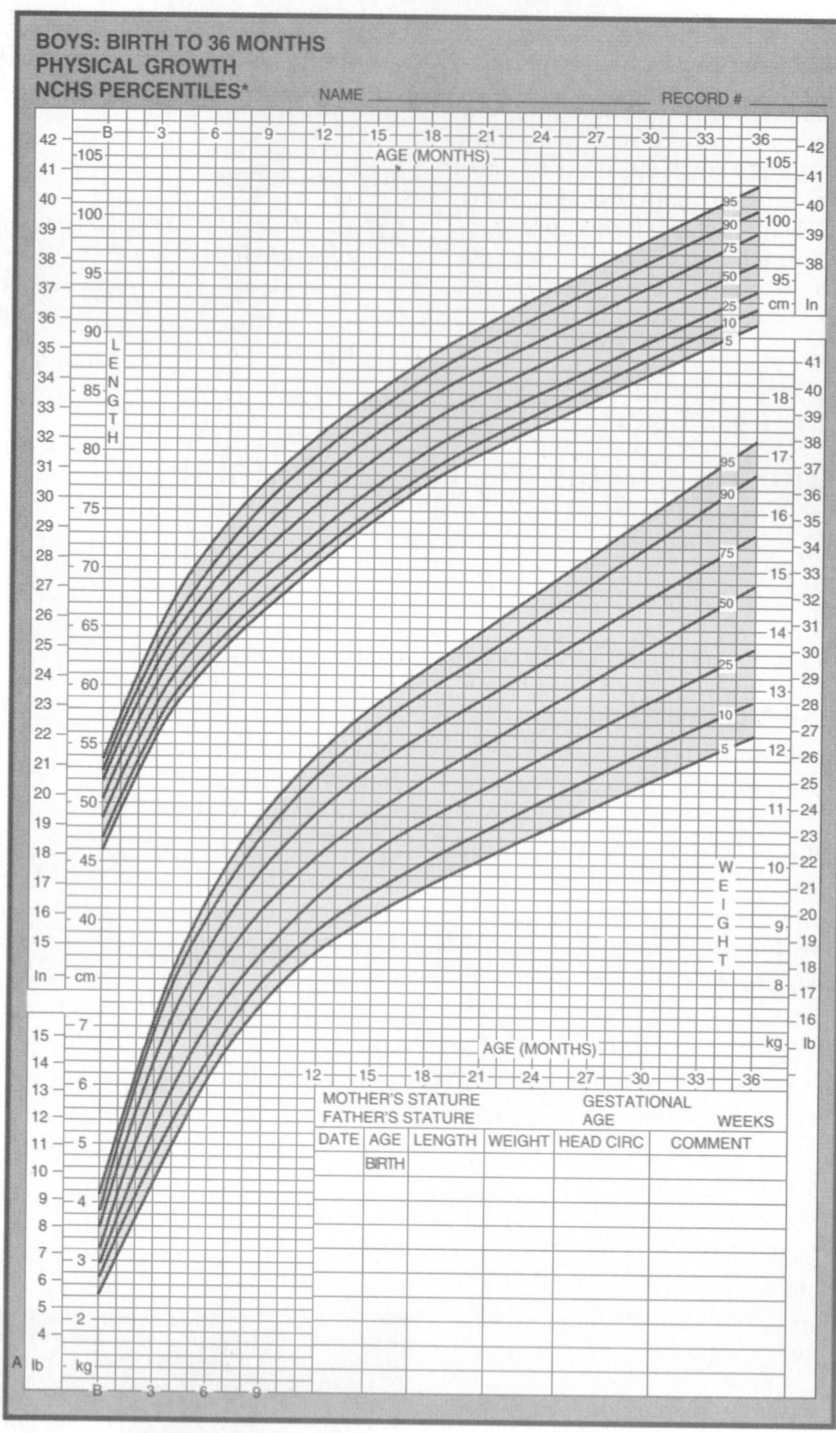

FIGURE 34–13 Growth rate graph: males (0–36 months).

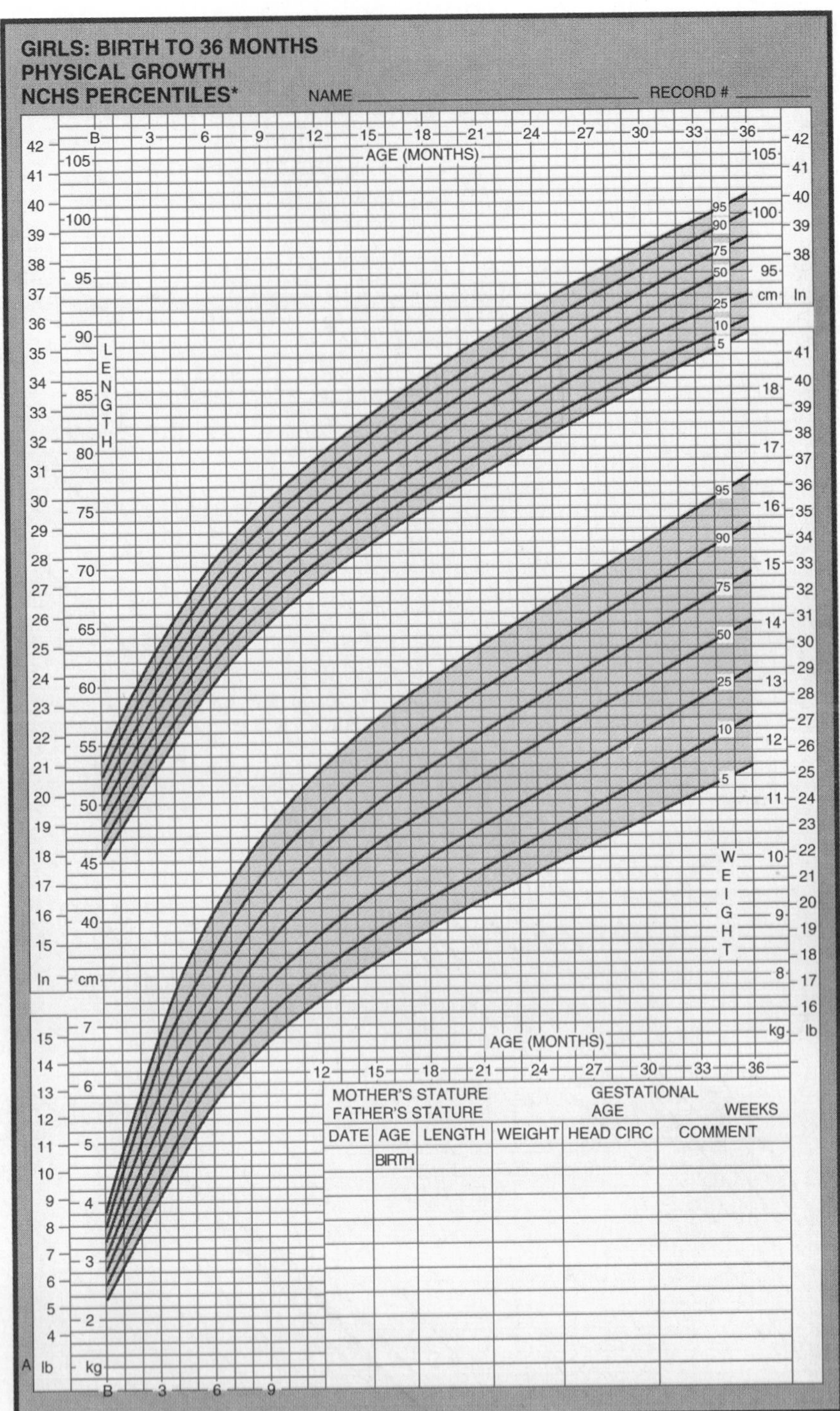

FIGURE 34–14 Growth rate graph: females (0–36 months).

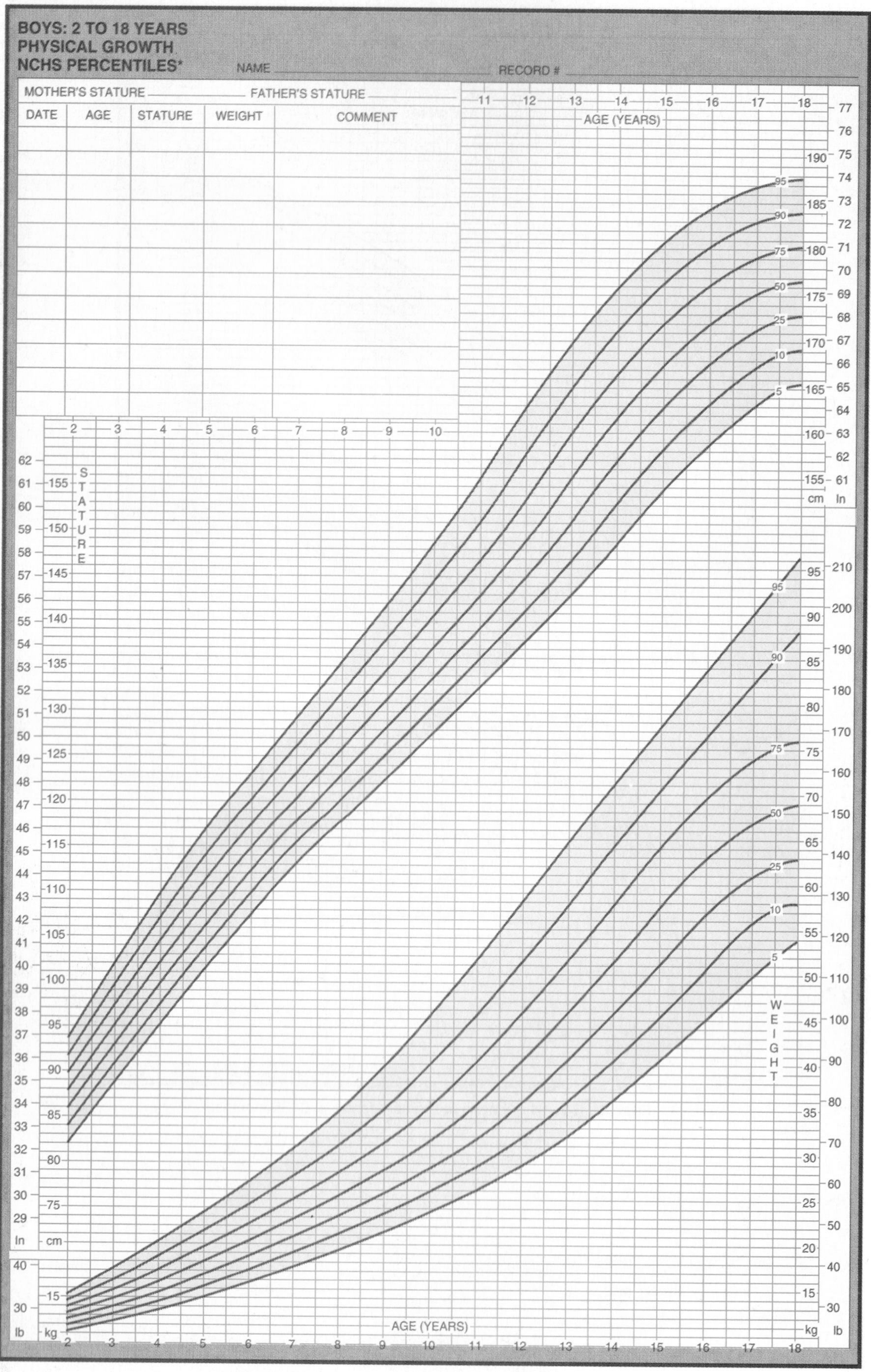

FIGURE 34–15 Growth rate graph: males (2–18 years).

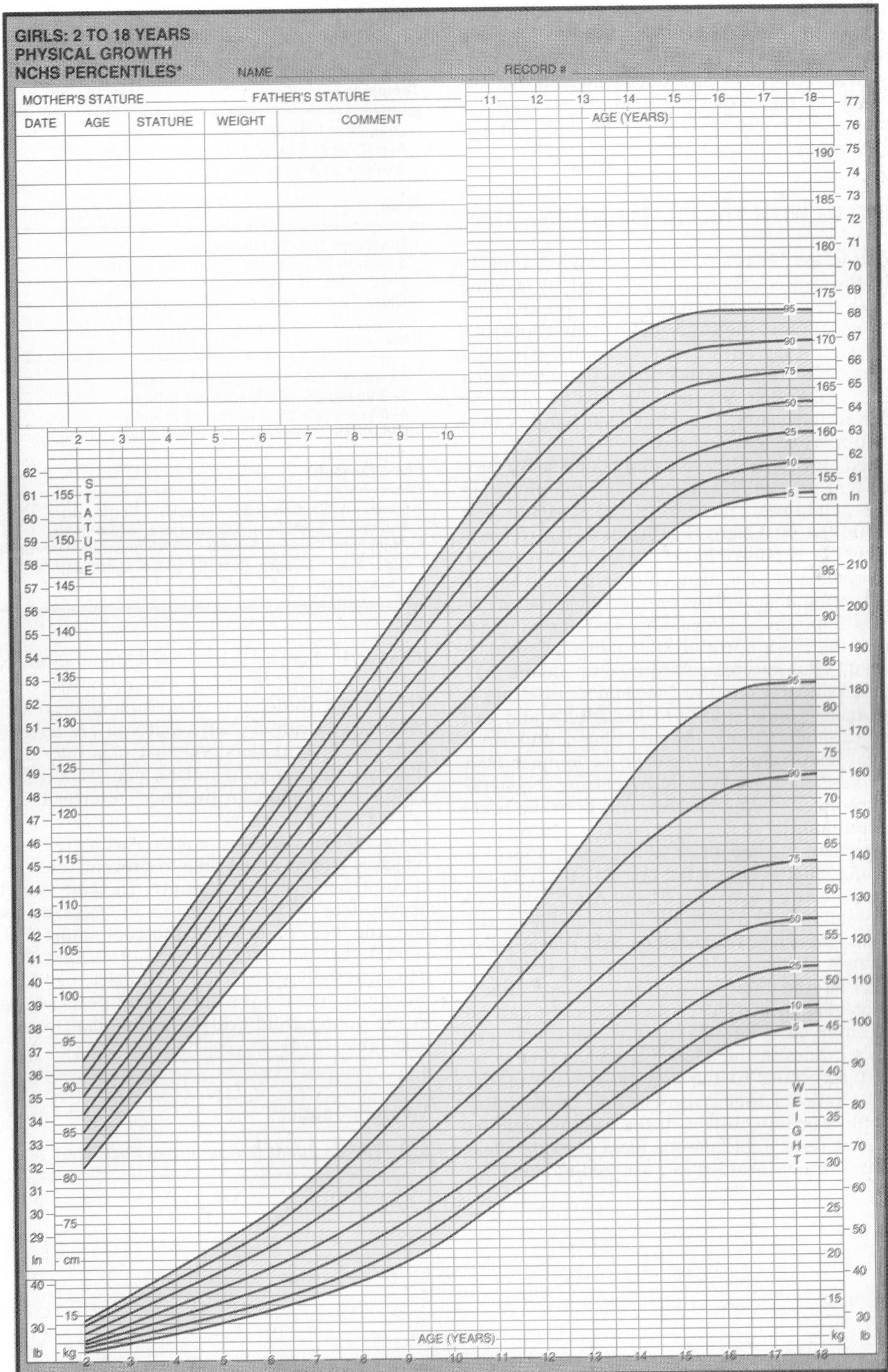

FIGURE 34–16 Growth rate graph: females (2–18 years).

Many medical offices evaluate young children's rates of growth and development with the Denver II Developmental Screening Test. This test helps detect delays in development and documents normal development in the preschool child. It is a simple screening test and is easy to use. It does not test intelligence.

ASSISTING WITH THE EXAMINATION

For routine examinations, begin by taking time to explain the procedure to the child and by gaining his or her confidence. If you maintain a positive and reassuring attitude, the child will usually cooperate. A small child may be held on an adult's lap, with the child's right arm tucked under the adult's left arm. The child's left arm may be held in place by the adult's right hand. The adult's left hand is then free to support the child's head.

The pediatrician will have a designated set of procedures that you will complete before the physician sees the child (see Procedure 34–2). Usually you will obtain the vital signs first (Table 34–4). *Temperature* may be obtained by axillary, rectal, oral, or tympanic method. The temperature is most easily obtained using the axillary or the tympanic methods. It is important to remember that the younger the child, the more immature the ability to regulate body heat. Thus the temperature of an infant may fluctuate easily and rapidly. The child's pulse rate is affected in a fashion similar to the adult's and can increase through activity, anxiety, illness, and environmental temperature. If the child is younger than 2, the *pulse* is measure apically by placing the stethoscope medial to the nipple. Always count the beats for 1 full minute.

An alternate method of obtaining the pulse of a very young child is to use the brachial artery in the upper arm at heart level (Fig. 34–9). After 2 years of age, the child's pulse may be taken at the radial pulse site. Anticipate a higher than adult level pulse rate because the younger the child, the faster the pulse will be (see Table 34–4). The *respiratory rate* is easily obtained in a child because the chest can be readily observed. The rate of the child will not change as it does in the adult. Expect the rate to be increased according to the age and health of the child. The ratio of four pulse beats to one respiration should remain constant in the healthy child as in the adult (see Table 34–4). *Blood pressure* measurements are not included in most pediatric examinations. If there is a heart or kidney **anomaly,** you may be required to obtain a blood pressure reading. This is not difficult in the child older than age 2 because you can explain what you are about to do, and once it is understood that it is only a balloon that you are going to inflate, you usually have the child's cooperation. In the child younger than 2, obtaining blood pressure can be quite a feat. The two obstacles that you must contend with are movement, which is almost impossible to prevent, and the small circumference of the extremity. The cuff must be the appropriate width to obtain an accurate reading, and the bell of your stethoscope must be small enough to seal over the site. It is best to use a pediatric stethoscope with a pediatric bell when obtaining an infant's pressure. Blood pressure readings in the young child will be lower than in the adult (see Table 34–4).

TABLE 34–4 Reference Ranges for Pediatric Vital Signs

Temperature
Oral: 98.6° F or 37° C
Rectal: 99.6° F or 37.6° C
Axillary: 97.6° F or 36.4° C
Pulse
Newborn: 100–180 beats per minute
3 months–2 years: 80–150 beats per minute
2–10 years: 65–130 beats per minute
Older than 9 years: 60–100 beats per minute
Respiratory
Newborn: 30–35 breaths per minute
1–2 years: 25–30 breaths per minute
4–6 years: 23–25 breaths per minute
Older than 7 years: 16–20 breaths per minute
Blood Pressure
Newborn: Systolic <90; diastolic <70 mm Hg
1–5 years: Systolic <100; diastolic <70 mm Hg
Older than 9 years: Systolic <120; diastolic <84 mm Hg
Older than 13 years: Systolic 100 + age; diastolic 30–40 beats less

Memory Jogger

 *Why do infant temperatures fluctuate?*

PROCEDURE 34-2

Obtaining Pediatric Vital Signs and Vision Screening

GOAL

To accurately obtain vital signs and vision on a pediatric patient.

EQUIPMENT AND SUPPLIES

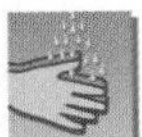

Tympanic thermometer
Pediatric blood pressure cuff
Wristwatch with sweep second-hand
Weight scale
Stethoscope
Pencil and paper

PROCEDURAL STEPS

1 Gather equipment.
PURPOSE: Efficiency.

2 Wash hands.
PURPOSE: Infection control.

3 Explain the procedure to the parent and if you want the parent to help by holding the child, explain the technique you want him or her to employ.
PURPOSE: Explanations ahead of time save time and enhance cooperation.

4 Help child stand in the center of the scale and weigh the child (Figure 1). Ask child to turn around and obtain the child's height (Figure 2). Record your findings.

Continued

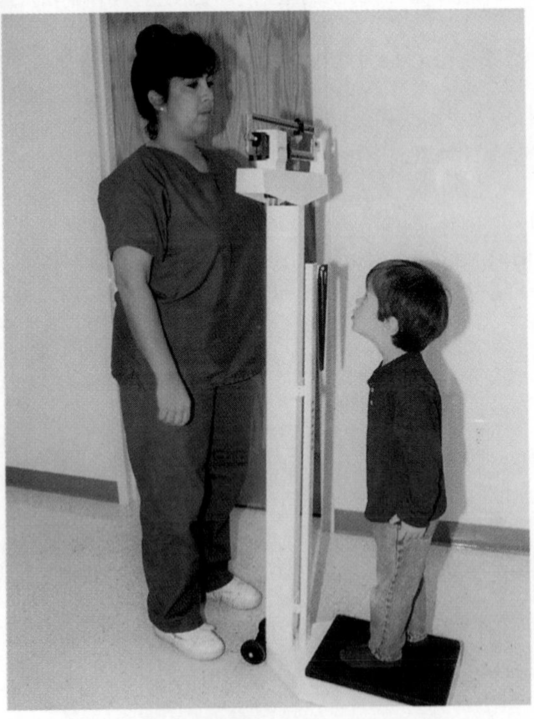

FIGURE 1

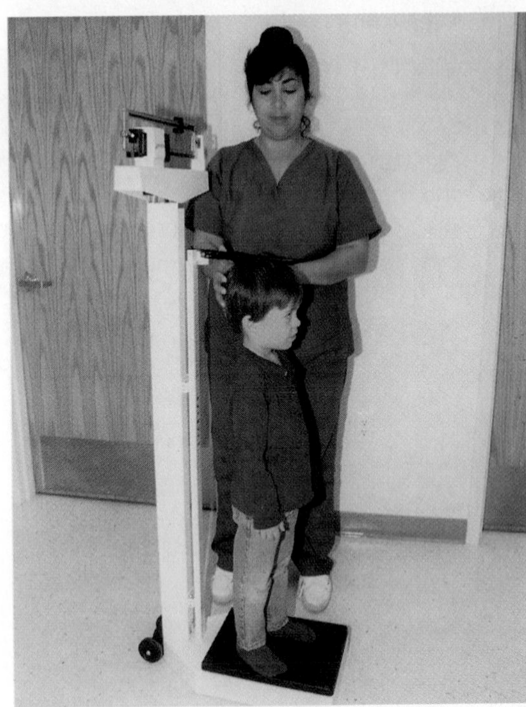

FIGURE 2

PROCEDURE 34-2 (CONTINUED)

Obtaining Pediatric Vital Signs and Vision Screening

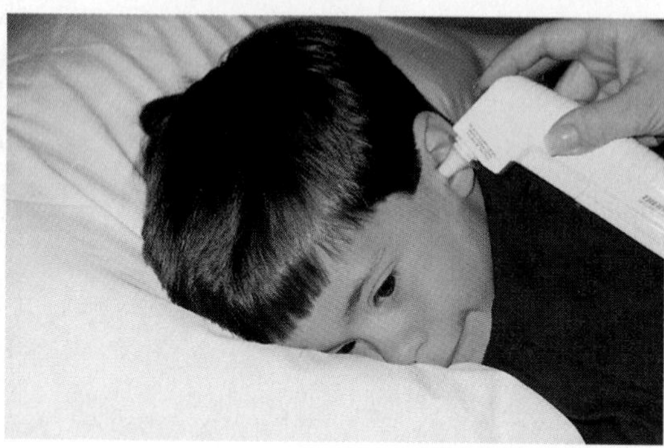

FIGURE 3

5 Obtain tympanic or axillary temperature using the procedure explained in Chapter 27 (Figure 3).

6 Record temperature. Indicate the method used: A = axillary; R = rectal.
PURPOSE: A procedure is not done until it is recorded on the patient's record.

7 Place stethoscope on child's chest at the mid-point between the sternum and the left nipple and listen for the apical beat (Figure 4).

8 Count the apical beat for 1 full minute.

9 Record the apical pulse. Be sure to place an (A) behind the rate to indicate that this is an apical pulse reading.
PURPOSE: A procedure is not done until it is recorded on the patient's record.

10 Place your flat hand on the child's chest and count the respirations for 1 full minute.

11 Record the respiration rate.
PURPOSE: A procedure is not done until it is recorded on the patient's record.

12 Check to be sure that you have the correct-size blood pressure cuff and then proceed with taking the blood pressure. Follow procedure in Chapter 27 (Figure 5).

13 Record the blood pressure.
PURPOSE: A procedure is not done until it is recorded on the patient's record.

Continued

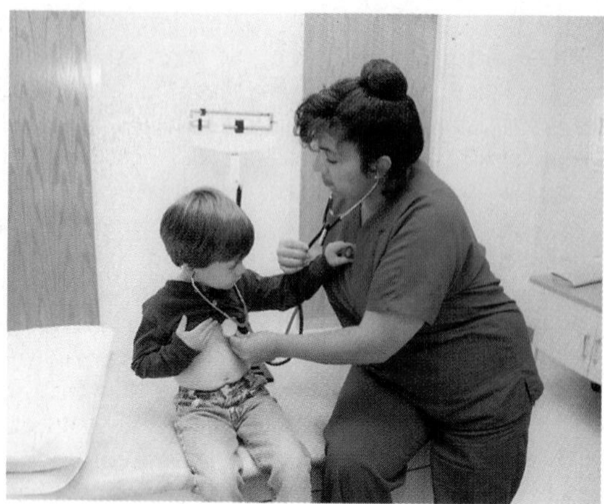

FIGURE 4

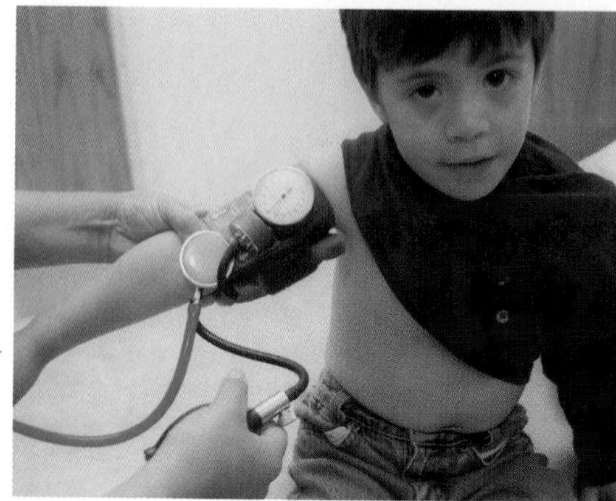

FIGURE 5

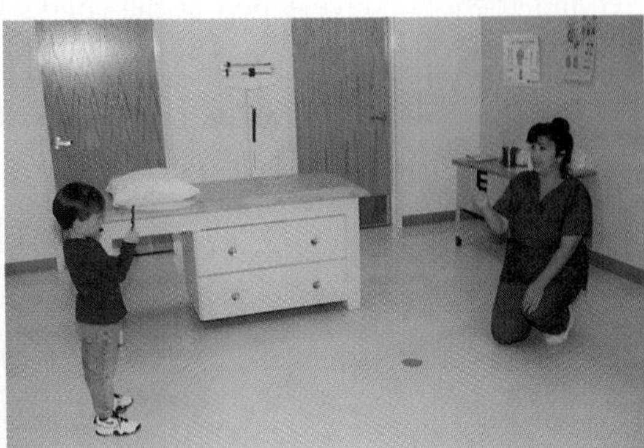

FIGURE 6

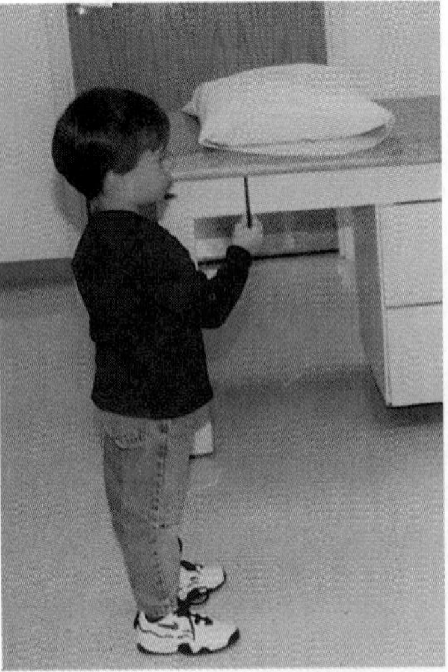

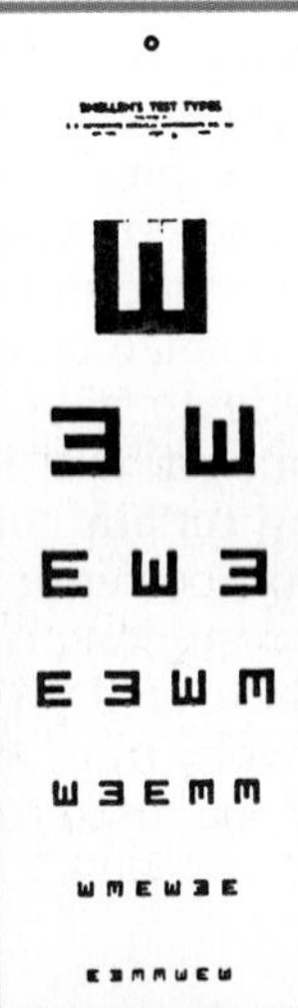

FIGURE 7

14 If vision screening is to be done, familiarize the child with the E by asking him or her to make an E point the same way as your E is pointing (Figure 6). Then position the child in front of the pediatric E Snellen chart (Figure 7) and have him or her match the E using his or her hands with the one that you are pointing to.

15 Record the vision results: OD = right eye, OS = left eye, OU = both eyes.
PURPOSE: A procedure is not done until it is recorded on the patient's record.

16 Compliment the child on his or her performance, and if the parent is present, share the praise with the parent.
PURPOSE: Builds rapport and encourages self-confidence in the child.

17 Wash your hands.
PURPOSE: Infection control.

18 Return all equipment used to proper storage area.

When the pediatrician wishes to examine and/or treat the ears, eyes, nose, or throat, place the child on the examination table. You will need to immobilize the head as gently as possible. Try to gain the child's cooperation. Ask the parent to assist. The parent can frequently help hold the child. A familiar face and voice can help to calm children's anxieties and fears.

The examination of the pediatric patient follows the same pattern as that for the adult, with the exception that the examination is altered to focus on normal growth and development. Because the child is continuously growing and changing, the physiologic and psychologic growth patterns must be carefully noted and recorded. Depending on the age of the child, the physician may make changes in the routine examination procedure. You will need to be flexible and ready to adapt to changes to assist the physician and the patient. It is important that you be knowledgeable of the major problems that affect children in different age groups and develop the skills needed to identify possible areas of concern.

PREVENTIVE WRAPPING OF CHILDREN

When wrapping a crying child (see Procedure 34–3), check your own position and that of the child. Sometimes a child cries from the pain of too tight a hold rather than from the pain of the examination. For example, when holding an infant's legs to expose the buttocks, place your index finger between the ankles to reduce pressure.

When more extensive examinations are necessary, place the child on a large sheet that has been folded into a triangle, keeping the long side of the sheet even with the shoulders and the triangular point just below the feet. Leave a greater portion of the sheet on the left side of the child. Now bring this longer side back over the left arm and under the body and right arm. Next, bring the sheet back over the right arm and under the body again. The two arms will be completely wrapped, leaving the abdomen exposed. When wrapping the entire body, bring the right portion of the sheet over the abdomen, and tuck it securely under the entire back and out again on the right side.

This wrap can be quickly and easily made and can be used to leave either arm exposed while securing the opposite arm as well as the legs and body. It may be pinned if necessary. Elbow restriction may be made by using a blood pressure cuff or a towel wrapped around the elbow several times.

To prevent a small child or infant from rolling the head from side to side, stand at the head of the table and support the child's head between your hands, making certain not to press on the ears or on the anterior or posterior fontanelle. The reverse of this may be restricting a child with your body by taking the place of the physician and allowing the physician to work from above the child's head. This position may be used for an examination of the child's eyes. A small infant may be placed crosswise on the table that has both the head and base raised slightly, forming a large V in the table. This prevents the infant from rolling, as might happen on a flat surface.

It is not necessary to drape an infant, but the older child's modesty should be respected. Sincere respect and friendly conversation at the child's level accomplish a great deal. Always be patient with children. Be certain that they understand what is expected. Always involve the parents as much as possible.

Memory Jogger

When might preventive wrapping be used?

PROCEDURE 34-3
Preventive Wrapping of a Child

GOAL

To prevent possible injury of a child by wrapping the child.

EQUIPMENT AND SUPPLIES

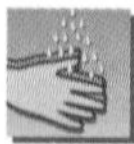

Large sheet

PROCEDURAL STEPS

1 Wash your hands.
PURPOSE: Infection control.

2 Fold the sheet into a triangle, and place it on the examining table. The distance from the fold to the lower corner of the sheet should be twice the length of the child.
PURPOSE: Prepare the wrap before taking the child from the parent.

3 Place the child on the sheet, with the fold slightly above the shoulders. Bring the lower corner of the sheet up over the child's body (Figure 1).

Continued

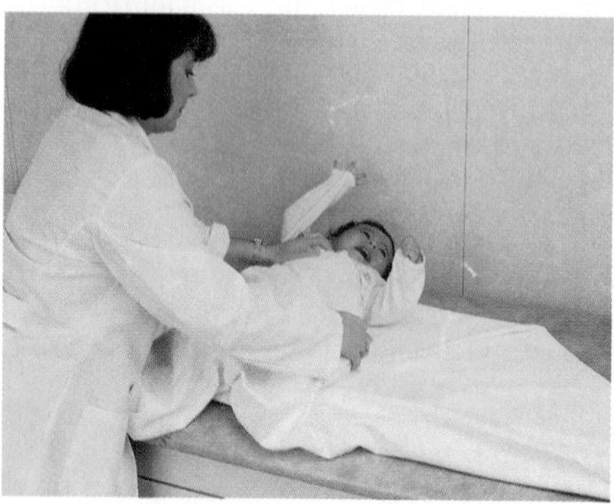

FIGURE 1

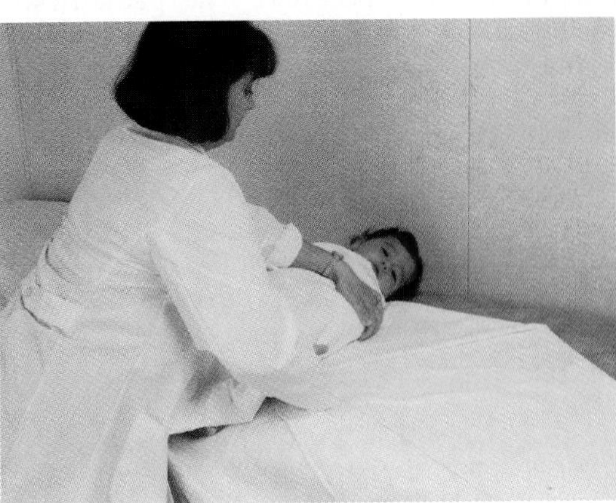

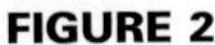

FIGURE 2

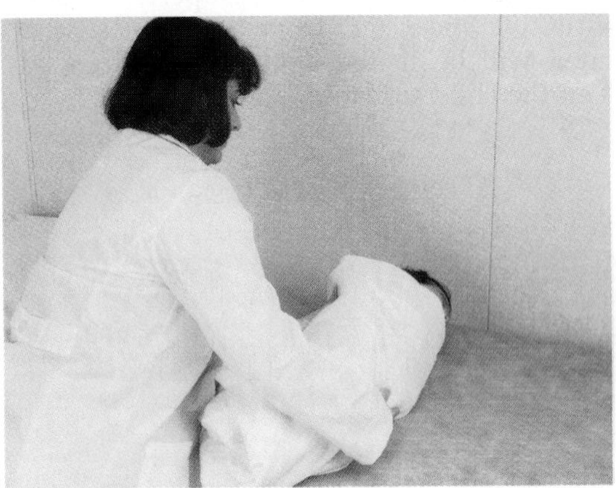

FIGURE 3

4 Loosen tight clothing and straighten the child's arms and legs. The right corner is brought over the body and tucked under the body snugly (Figure 2).

5 Bring the left corner over the child and under and around the child's body. (Figure 3).

6 Never leave the child alone once the wrap is in place (Figure 4).
PURPOSE: Child safety.

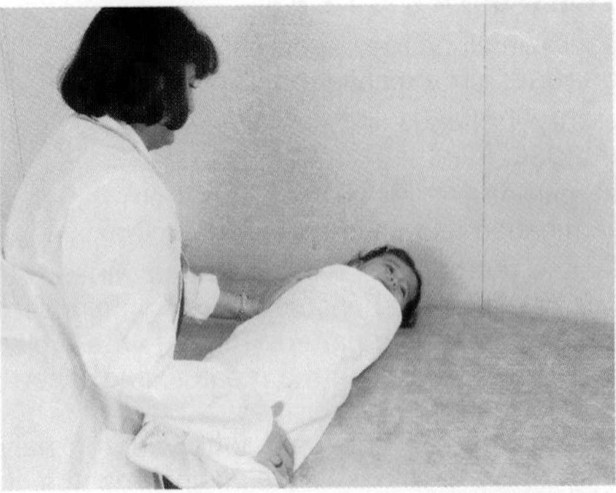

FIGURE 4

OBTAINING A URINE SAMPLE

The easiest way to obtain a urine sample on a child older than 2 and toilet trained is to give the parent the container and instructions ahead of time. Then when the child appears at the office for the examination, you have the sample to be tested. If you need to obtain the sample while the child is at the office, consult with the parent for the best method to use. No one knows the child's habits better than the parent, and to prevent a lot of frustration, consult the "expert." If the child is younger than 2 years old, you will need to apply a pediatric urine collection device (Fig. 34–17; see Procedure 34–4). Place this device on the child as soon as the child appears in the office, so that you increase your chances of obtaining the needed sample before the child leaves.

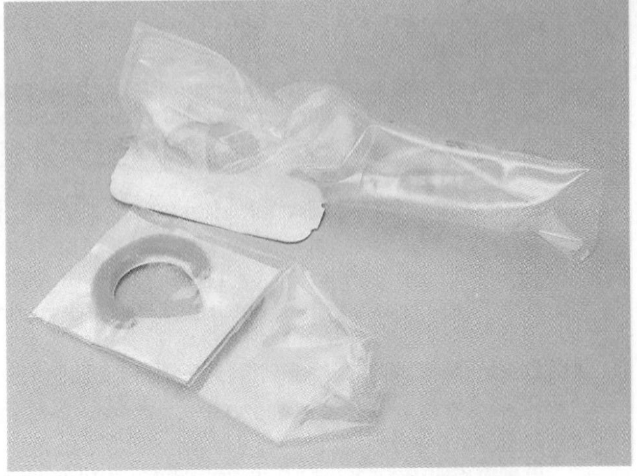

FIGURE 34–17 Urine collection devices.

Once the device is in place, the child can be diapered to aid in holding the device properly. Be sure that the adhesive sticks tightly to the child so that the specimen will be in the device and not in the diaper when the child urinates.

In some cases the child may need to be catheterized to obtain the specimen. The pediatrician will order the catheterization and may ask you to prepare the equipment needed. There are pediatric cath-kits available that contain all the supplies

PROCEDURE 34-4
Applying a Urinary Collection Device

GOAL

To properly apply a pediatric urinary collection device.

EQUIPMENT AND SUPPLIES

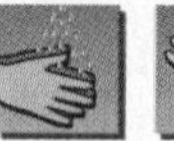
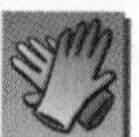
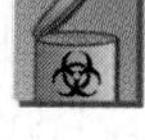
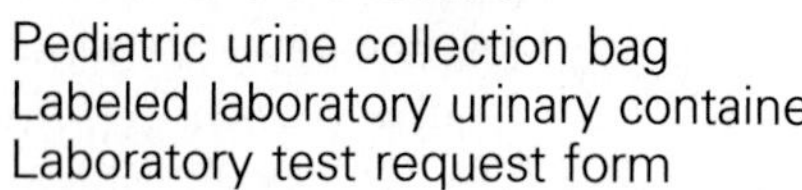

Pediatric urine collection bag
Labeled laboratory urinary container
Laboratory test request form
Antiseptic wipes
Biohazard waste container
Gloves

PROCEDURAL STEPS

1 Assemble all needed supplies.
PURPOSE: Time management.

2 Wash your hands and don gloves.
PURPOSE: Infection control.

3 Ask parent to remove the diaper from the child or lay the child in a supine position on the examination table and remove the diaper.

4 Cleanse the genitalia with antiseptic wipes.
Male: Cleanse the urinary meatus in a circular motion starting directly on the meatus and work in an outward pattern. Repeat with a clean wipe. If the child is not circumcised, retract the foreskin to expose the meatus, and when you have completed cleansing, return the foreskin to its natural position.
Female: Hold the labia open with your left hand and with your right hand, cleanse the inner labia, from the clitoris to the vaginal meatus, in a superior to inferior pattern. Discard the first wipe and repeat with a clean wipe.

5 Unfold the collection device and remove the paper from the upper portion and place this portion over the mons pubis and press it securely into place. Make sure the area is dry and then continue by removing the lower portion of the paper and securing this portion against the perineum. Be sure that the device is attached smoothly and that you have not taped it to part of the infant's thigh.

6 Rediaper the infant, or if the parent is helping, the parent may rediaper the infant at this time. The diaper will help hold the bag in place.

7 Suggest that the parent give the child liquids if allowed and to check the bag for urine at frequent intervals.
PURPOSE: Increased intake helps increase output.

8 When there is a noticeable amount of urine in the bag, remove the device, cleanse the skin area that was attached to the device, and rediaper the child.

9 Pour the urine carefully into the laboratory urine container and handle the sample in a routine manner.

10 Dispose of all used equipment in a biohazard waste container.

11 Remove your gloves, dispose of them in a biohazard container, and wash hands.

12 Record the procedure in the patient's record.
PURPOSE: A procedure is not done until it is recorded.

needed for this procedure. In getting this kit ready for the pediatrician's use, always remember that this is a sterile procedure. The pediatrician will usually ask the parent to hold the infant's legs apart, and you will be responsible for handling the specimen, labeling it, and preparing it for the laboratory. You will not do a pediatric catheterization unless you have received special training and have been authorized by the pediatrician to perform the procedure.

On a newborn or small infant, the pediatrician may simply wipe povidone-iodine (Betadine) on the suprapubic area, insert a needle with syringe, and aspirate urine from the bladder. Your responsibility would remain the same.

ADMINISTERING MEDICATIONS

Giving young children medications orally and by injection may be difficult and can require participation by both the parent and medical assistant to accomplish. The methods to use are discussed in Chapter 49.

Child Abuse

The Federal Child Abuse Prevention and Treatment Act states that all threats to a child's physical and/or mental welfare must be reported. This means that every teacher, health care worker, and social worker, in fact every citizen who suspects that a child is being neglected or abused, must report this to the proper authority. When this is reported, the agency must record the report and after three similar reports, the agency must investigate.

When you call in a suspected abuse, you are required to give your name, but this is considered confidential information and your name will not be given to the child's parent or guardian, nor is it given to the investigating officer. You are also protected under law from any liability for reporting your suspicions. Figure 34–18 lists the signs of abuse you need to learn.

If you suspect that the child that you are caring for in the office is a victim of abuse, consult with the pediatrician immediately, before the patient is seen. In this manner, you can discreetly work as a team member to substantiate or rebuff the suspected injuries. In most states, both you and the physician can make separate reports to the authority. State laws do vary, and the state and local reporting protocols should be outlined in your office procedure manual.

You have the ethical and moral obligation to file this report. You do not have the right to share this suspicion with another party.

SIGNS OF ABUSE

Obvious Signals

Previously filed reports of physical or sexual abuse of child
Documented abuse of other family members
Different stories of how an accident happened between parents and child
Stories of incident and injuries found are suspicious
The cause of the injuries are blamed on other family members
Repeated visits to the emergency room for injuries

Findings on Examination

Trauma to the nervous system
Internal abdominal pain
Discolorations/bruising to the buttocks, back and abdomen
Elbow, wrist, and shoulder dislocations

Changes in Behavior

Too eager to please the parent
Overly passive and too compliant
Aggressive and demanding
Parenting the parent—role reversal
Delays in the normal growth and development patterns
Erratic school attendance

Physical Indicators

Poor hygiene
Malnutrition
Obvious dental neglect
Neglected well-baby procedures such as immunizations

FIGURE 34–18 Signs of abuse.

Memory Jogger

14 *How many incident reports must be on file before the child welfare agency is forced to investigate?*

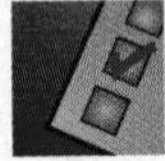

PATIENT EDUCATION

In pediatrics, the child is usually joined by one or both parents during visits to the physician. The health of the child is the concern of both parents and may be confronted with the parents' questions and comments concerning their child. Parents need to have reinforcement, praise, and understanding in dealing with the health and welfare of their child, and they expect to receive such support from the pediatrician and the office staff. Provide parents with information to help them understand their children's behavior and improve their parenting skills. Understanding the normal behavior characteristics of a particular developmental stage may increase the parents' confidence and reinforce their expectations for their child (Fig. 34–19).

When you are attending the child, a good rule to remember is that a child is just a small adult and

PARENT EDUCATION TOPICS

Normal growth and development
Child safety
Pediatric nutrition needs
Alternative feeding habits
Immunizations
Sexual curiosity
Answering "sex" questions
Toilet training
Adolescent behavior
Adolescent trust vs mistrust
Common health problems

FIGURE 34–19 Parent education topics.

needs the same love, compassion, and understanding. Children need to be talked to, not talked at.

If the pediatrician has pamphlets available for parents that offer advice and assistance in caring for their child, you should discuss them with the parents. You need to answer questions whenever possible or alert the physician so that questions can be answered during the office visit. It is important that you make the most of every opportunity to teach parents about sound health care.

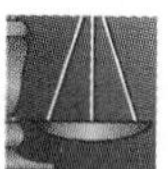

LEGAL AND ETHICAL ISSUES

In the United States children are considered individuals who are growing and developing physically, emotionally, and mentally. Our laws view children as a distinct group, and there are laws and customs dealing with the protection of children's rights. Occasionally in the pediatric office, legal and ethical issues arise and the entire office staff may be faced with an ethical situation. If this type of situation occurs, the first option is to talk it over with the pediatrician. It may be necessary to have a office staff meeting to identify the conflict, note pertinent laws and facts, consider possible options and the consequences of each, and decide on a course of action. Facing ethical issues confidently may reduce the risk of liability. You may find that the pediatrician feels differently than you do, and this might be a totally separate dilemma that you will have to deal with. Always remember that as your employer, the physician makes the final decision and as long as you work in that office, you are required to do things according to that decision.

If something happens that you cannot ethically support, seek the help of your local medical assistant organization. You may find that others have been in similar situations and that they can suggest possible methods to solve the problem.

CRITICAL THINKING

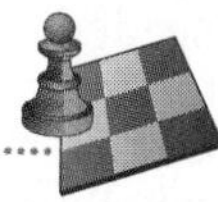

1 The physician wants you to do a Denver II Developmental Screening Test on a 3 year old, without the parent present. How would you explain this to the parent?

2 Why do parents need reinforcement and praise in dealing with a child's health and welfare? How could you assist with this?

3 You notice when you are measuring a 1-year old that there are bruises on the child's neck and when you touch the child's right shoulder, the child winces. What would you do? Explain your rationale step by step.

HOW DID I DO? Answers to Memory Joggers

1 A child doubles in length by age 4.

2 A 2000-word vocabulary is expected in the preschool stage.

3 The infant draws up the legs, clenches the fists, and has a painful cry.

4 Water dissolves electrolytes so that they can produce the electrically charged particles that are essential to cell activity. If the person becomes dehydrated, the lack of water will cause an electrolyte imbalance.

5 Dangers include a lower respiratory tract infection and middle ear infection.

6 Incubation period is 14 to 21 days.

7 Serous, suppurative, purulent

8 Linked to aspirin

9 DPT is given at 2 months, 4 months, and 6 months, with a booster at 4 to 6 years.

10 Well-baby examination focuses on maintaining the health of the child through basic system examinations, immunizations, and upgrading the medical history record.

11 Head circumference is taken until the child is 36 months old.

12 Fluctuation is due to immaturity of the heat-regulating body mechanisms.

13 Preventive wrapping may be used when a more extensive examination is necessary.

14 Three incident reports must be on file before there is an investigation.

Assisting in Neurology

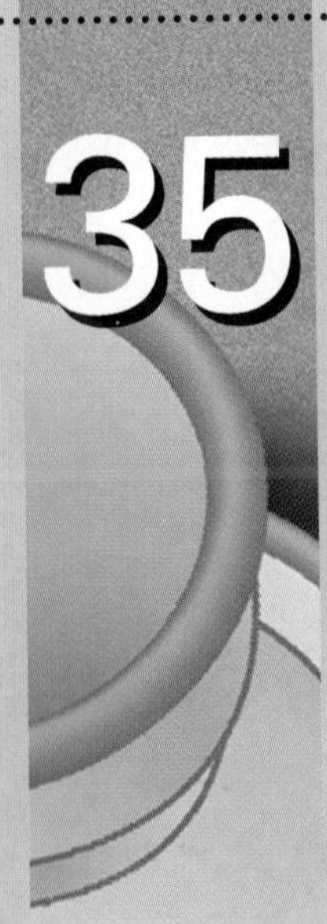

OUTLINE

LEARNING OBJECTIVES

Cognitive: On successful completion of this chapter you should be able to:

1. Identify the anatomic structures that compose the nervous system.
2. Explain the functions of the peripheral and central nervous systems.
3. Differentiate between the different layers of the brain's protective covering.
4. Define a synapse.
5. Name and describe the functions of the three major sections of the brain.
6. List the seven symptoms that suggest possible neurologic problems.
7. Identify three brain disorders that result from injury.
8. Name two disorders that could be work-related injuries.
9. Identify the frequently used diagnostic procedure for nerve disorders.
10. Define and spell vocabulary terms.

Performance: On successful completion of this chapter you should be able to:

1. Describe three tests that might be used during the neurologic examination.
2. Prepare a patient for a neurologic procedure.
3. Assist with the neurologic examination.

VOCABULARY

anomalies Deformities or deviations from normal as a result of faulty development of the fetus

anoxia Absence of oxygen in the tissues

ataxia Failure or irregularity of muscle actions and coordination

atrophy Decrease in the size of a normally developed organ

aura A peculiar sensation preceding the appearance of more definite disturbance

benign Not cancerous, not recurrent

collodion A preparation of cellulose nitrate that, when applied to the skin, dies to form a strong, thin, transparent film

coma An unconscious state from which the patient cannot be aroused

compression The state of being pressed together

convulsions A series of involuntary contractions of the voluntary muscles

delirium An acute, reversible organic mental syndrome characterized by reduced ability to maintain attention to external stimuli

diplopia Double vision

exacerbation Aggravation of symptoms or increased severity of a disease

gait The manner of walking

glioma A neoplasm of the supporting structure of nervous tissue in the brain

homeostasis To maintain constant internal environmental conditions

incontinence The inability to control excretory functions

malignant Cancerous

medulloblastoma A tumor composed of embryonic cells in the medulla oblongata

meningioma A hard vascular tumor invading the dura and skull

paresthesia An abnormal sensation of burning, prickling, or stinging

paroxysmal Pertaining to a sudden recurrent spasm of symptoms

remission A lessening in the severity of a disease or symptoms

sheath The covering surrounding the axon of the nerve cell that acts as an electrical insulator to speed the conduction of nerve impulses

stroke A sudden loss of consciousness and/or paralysis caused by extreme trauma or injury to an artery in the brain

syncope Fainting

transection A cross section; division by cutting transverse

The human brain weighs about 3 pounds, consumes the power equivalent to a 20-watt light bulb, stores over 100 trillion bits of information, and works better than any computer. The matter that makes up the brain is about 85% water; and when removed from the skull and placed on a dissection table, it slumps like a blob of gelatin. Early scientists believed that the brain's function was to cool the blood. Today's scientists have shown us that even though the brain does receive 20% of the body's blood supply, its function is much more complex than that of a cooling apparatus.

The physician who specializes in the diseases and disorders of the nervous system is the neurologist. Often this specialization is combined with psychiatry, which is the speciality that deals with the diseases and disorders of the brain. Because the brain is made up entirely of nervous tissue, it is a logical marriage of specialties.

Anatomy and Physiology

Functioning as an elaborate central processing unit, the brain constantly receives input in the form of billions of electrical and chemical impulses that keep it informed about the state of affairs both inside and outside the human body. The brain then analyzes this information and transmits messages to the body's various organs, glands, and muscles, enabling them to respond appropriately. Your brain, and specifically that portion termed the *cerebrum,* is also the source of consciousness, emotions, memory, language, creativity, and thought (Fig. 35–1).

Emerging from the base of the brain is a cable of nerve tissue termed the *spinal cord,* which extends about 17 inches from the brain stem to the lower part of the back. Together, your brain and spinal cord comprise the central nervous system. Both components are encased in bone for protection: the

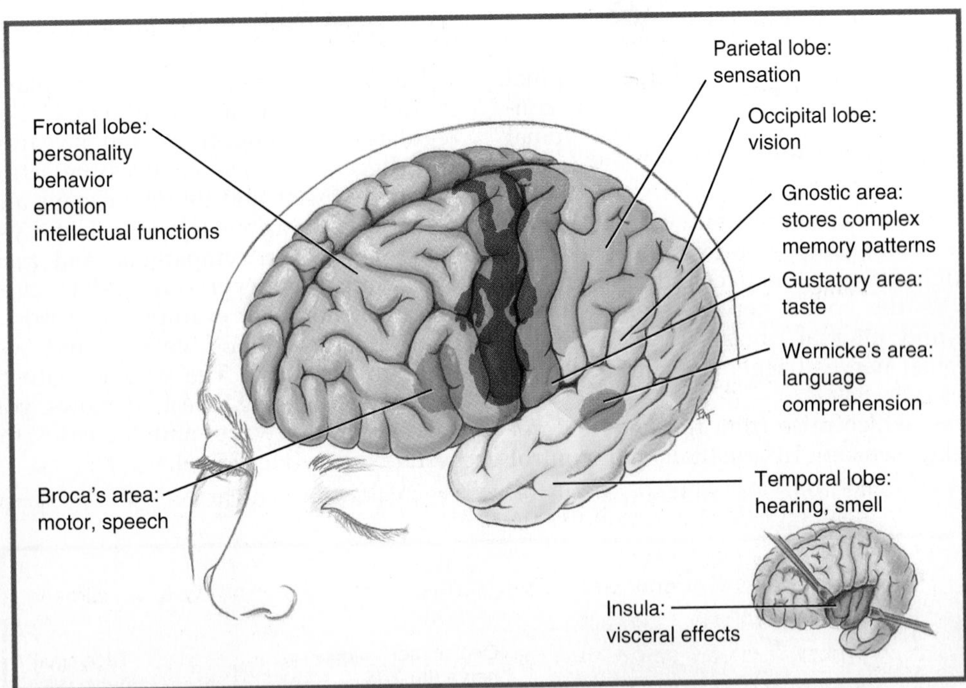

FIGURE 35–1 Functional areas of the cerebrum. (Modified from Applegate EJ: The Anatomy and Physiology Learning System. Philadelphia, WB Saunders, 1995.)

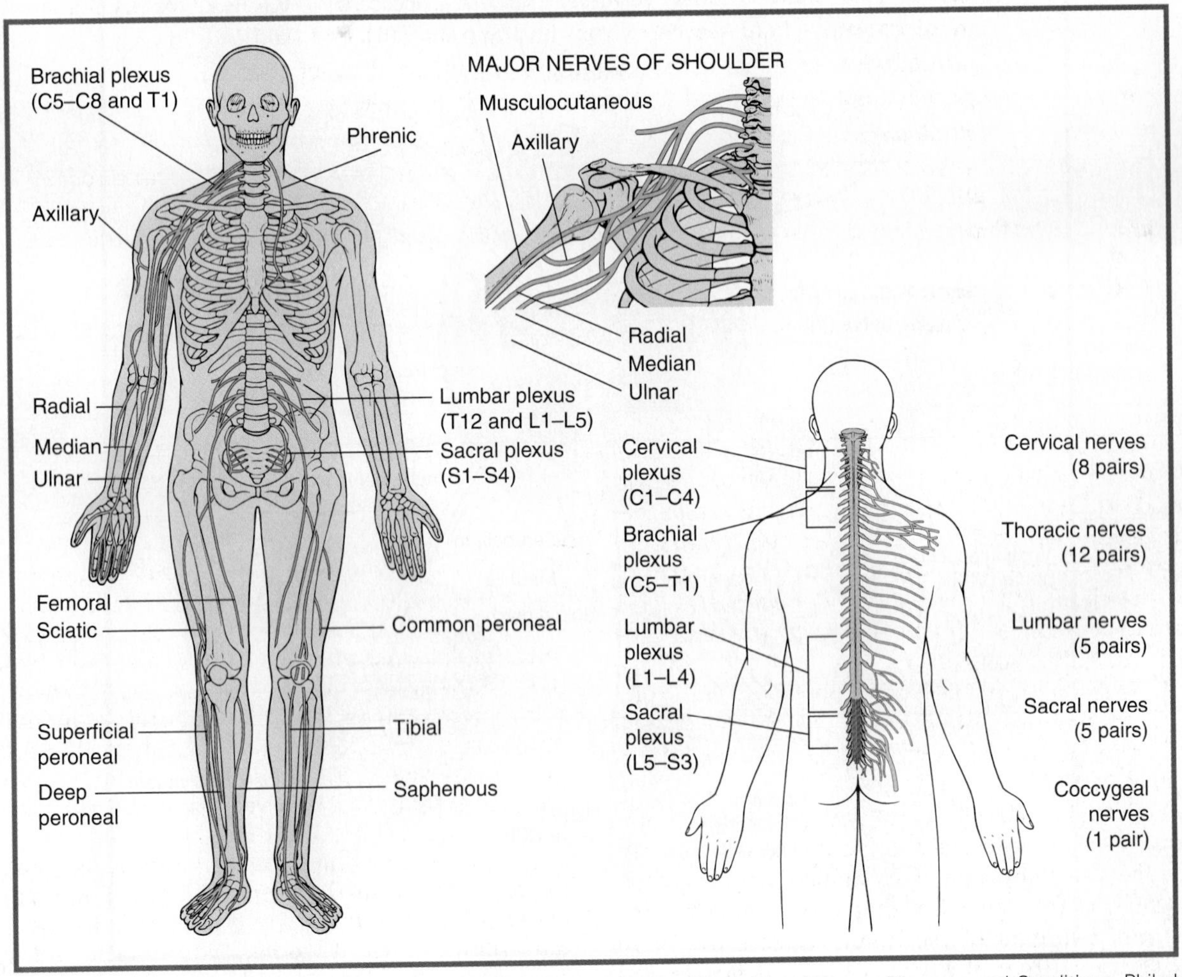

FIGURE 35–2 Spinal nerves. (From Frazier MS, Drzymkowski JA, Doty SJ: Essentials of Human Diseases and Conditions. Philadelphia, WB Saunders, 1996.)

skull encloses the brain, whereas the vertebral canal surrounds the spinal cord.

Extending outward from your brain and spinal cord is the peripheral nervous system, which consists of three main components: peripheral spinal nerves, cranial nerves, and the autonomic nervous system.

The spinal nerves, which transmit information to and from your brain, emerge from the spinal cord and exit through openings between the vertebrae. Sensory fibers in the spinal nerves receive stimuli from the skin and internal organs, whereas motor fibers in the spinal nerves trigger the contraction of skeletal muscles (Fig. 35–2).

Cranial nerves, which arise from the underside of your brain, relay sensory information and control muscles primarily in the head and neck region (Fig. 35–3).

The autonomic nervous system plays the key role in functions that are involuntary. For example, it regulates breathing, heart rate, sweating, circulation, and digestion. It also controls the actions of muscles in blood vessels and internal organs and governs the activities of various glands. This system has two components: the sympathetic and parasympathetic. The sympathetic nervous system prompts various body functions: for example, it speeds up your heart rate, constricts blood vessels, and widens the airways in the lungs. The parasympathetic system has a counterbalancing effect: it slows your heart rate, narrows the airways, and increases the flow of digestive juices (Fig. 35–4).

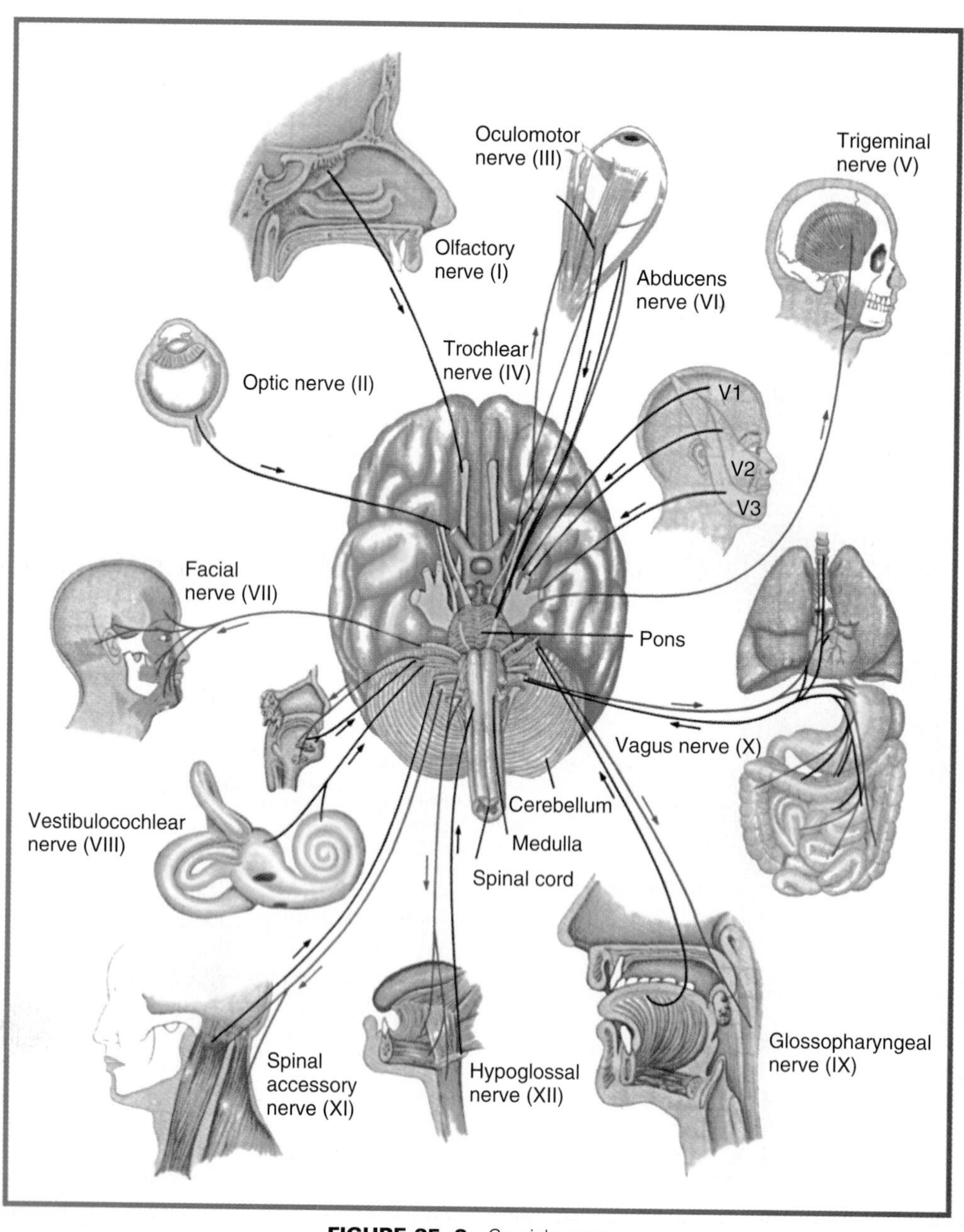

FIGURE 35–3 Cranial nerves.

The fundamental unit of the nervous system is the *neuron* or nerve cell. The brain contains billions of individual neurons. These connections begin to form in the last trimester before birth and continue to create a network until the age of 2. Each neuron consists of a cell body with a central nucleus, a major projection termed an *axon,* its covering, known as **sheaths,** and numerous smaller filaments called *dendrites* (Fig. 35–5). Axons, some of which are very long, reaching a length of more than 3 feet, conduct electrical impulses away from the cell body, while the dendrites receive electrical signals from other neurons. Each neuron makes contact with an adjacent nerve cell at a point termed the *synapse,* where it triggers the release of chemical neurotransmitters. These substances then bind to receptor sites on a target cell. Electrical and chemical impulses spirit from neuron to neuron in this fashion until the message reaches its destination and produces the desired effect.

Memory Jogger

How many neurons does a fully developed brain contain?

Although the brain probably accounts for only about 2% of your total body weight, it commands 20% of your heart's output of blood. To maintain stable brain function, a so-called blood–brain barrier exists that controls the flow of molecules to your brain. This barrier consists of a highly impermeable layer of cells in the brain capillaries surrounded by a layer of astrocytes (supporting nerve cells). Relatively small molecules such as oxygen, water, and glucose easily penetrate this barrier, but many drugs and chemicals are unable to do so. Brain inflammation can increase the permeability of many drugs that normally fail to penetrate the blood–brain barrier.

Memory Jogger

Which system contains the voluntary nerve cells?

BRAIN

The brain is divided into areas according to its function and location (Fig. 35–6). The *cerebrum* is the largest part of the brain and is the site of higher learning. It is divided into right and left hemispheres. Within the interior of the cerebrum are four hollow spaces called *ventricles.* In these ventricles is the cerebrospinal fluid, which lubricates and nourishes the brain and the spinal cord.

The *diencephalon* is made up of the thalamus and the hypothalamus. The thalamus acts as a relay station in which sensory neurons transfer stimuli to other sensory neurons. The hypothalamus helps regulate the autonomic nervous system by maintaining internal homeostasis.

The *brain stem* consists of the midbrain, the pons, and the medulla oblongata. The midbrain is involved with visual and auditory reflexes such as moving the eyes or turning the head to view or hear better. The pons serves as another sensory relay station. The medulla oblongata is the vital link for eyes, ears, respiratory, and circulatory activities. Specialty areas within this structure control waking and sleeping, heart rate, blood pressure, and respiration.

The *cerebellum,* which is located below the occipital lobe of the cerebrum, is important in maintaining balance, muscle coordination, and equilibrium. Any cerebellar disorder produces ataxia and loss of balance.

SPINAL CORD

The spinal cord begins at the termination point of the medulla oblongata and extends to approximately the second lumbar vertebra. Within the spinal cord are 31 pairs of spinal nerves. Each pair is responsible to one specific portion of the body (see Figs. 35–2 and 35–4). It is the spinal cord's responsibility to convey messages to the brain. All stimuli traveling to the brain travel through some portion of the spinal cord, and the same is true about motor responses.

Memory Jogger

Where is the vital link for eyes, ears, respiratory, and circulatory activities located?

PROTECTIVE COVERING OF THE BRAIN

Both the brain and the spinal cord are of critical importance to life, and for this reason both structures are well protected. Besides being totally surrounded by thick bone, these structures are also protected by three membranes called *meninges.* The cerebrospinal fluid is located beneath the middle layer (see Fig. 35–6).

The outer membrane is called the *dura mater,* and it is tough and thick. The middle layer is the *arachnoid.* This layer gets its name from its spider web appearance. The innermost layer is the *pia mater,* which contains many blood vessels and is the thinnest.

The cerebrospinal fluid is a clear fluid containing protein, chloride, and white blood cells. It is located just beneath the arachnoid membrane around the brain and in the canal within the spinal cord. It is

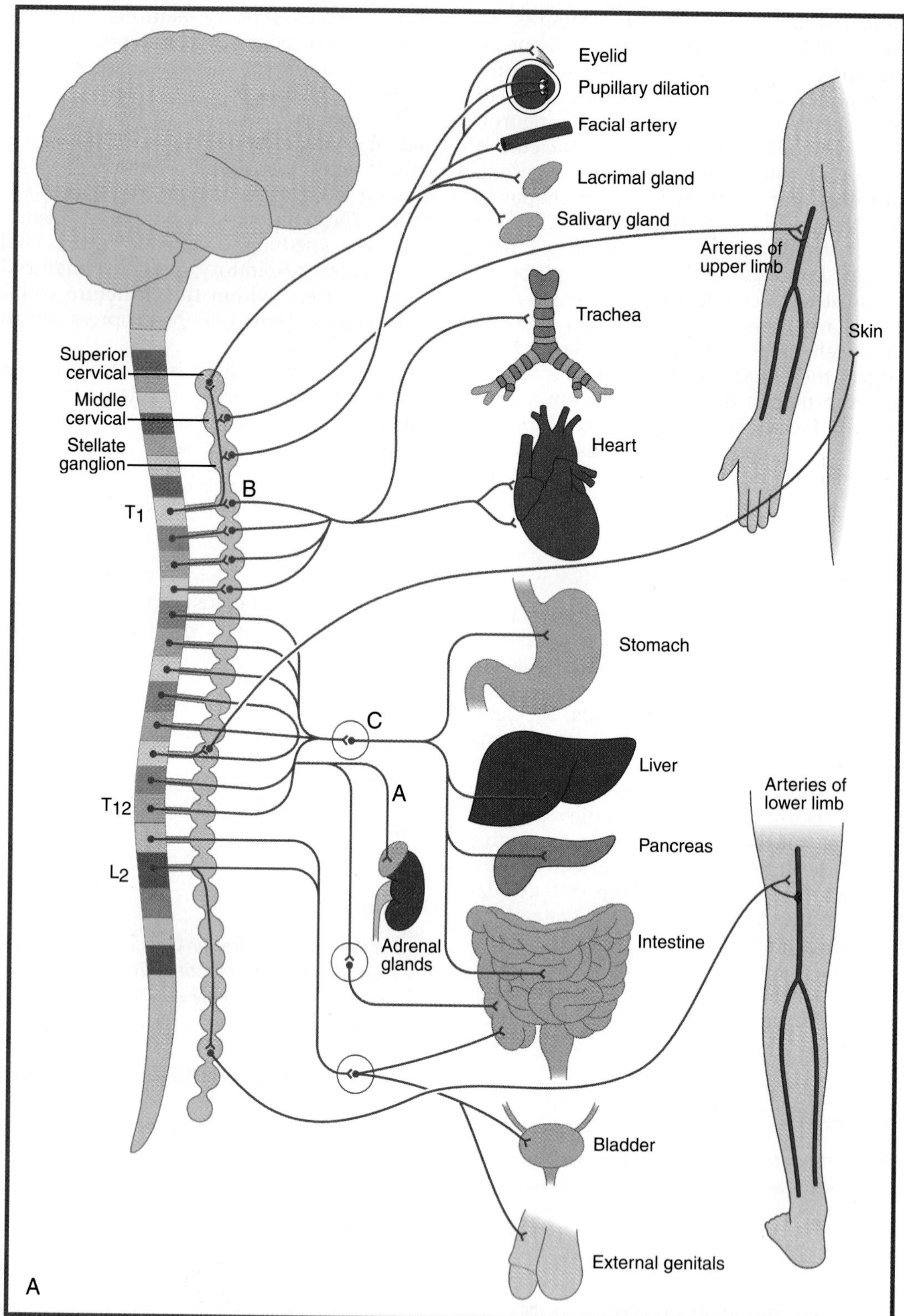

FIGURE 35-4 *A* and *B*, Sympathetic/parasympathetic nerves. (From Lundy-Ekman L: Neuroscience: Fundamentals of Rehabilitation. Philadelphia, WB Saunders, 1998.)

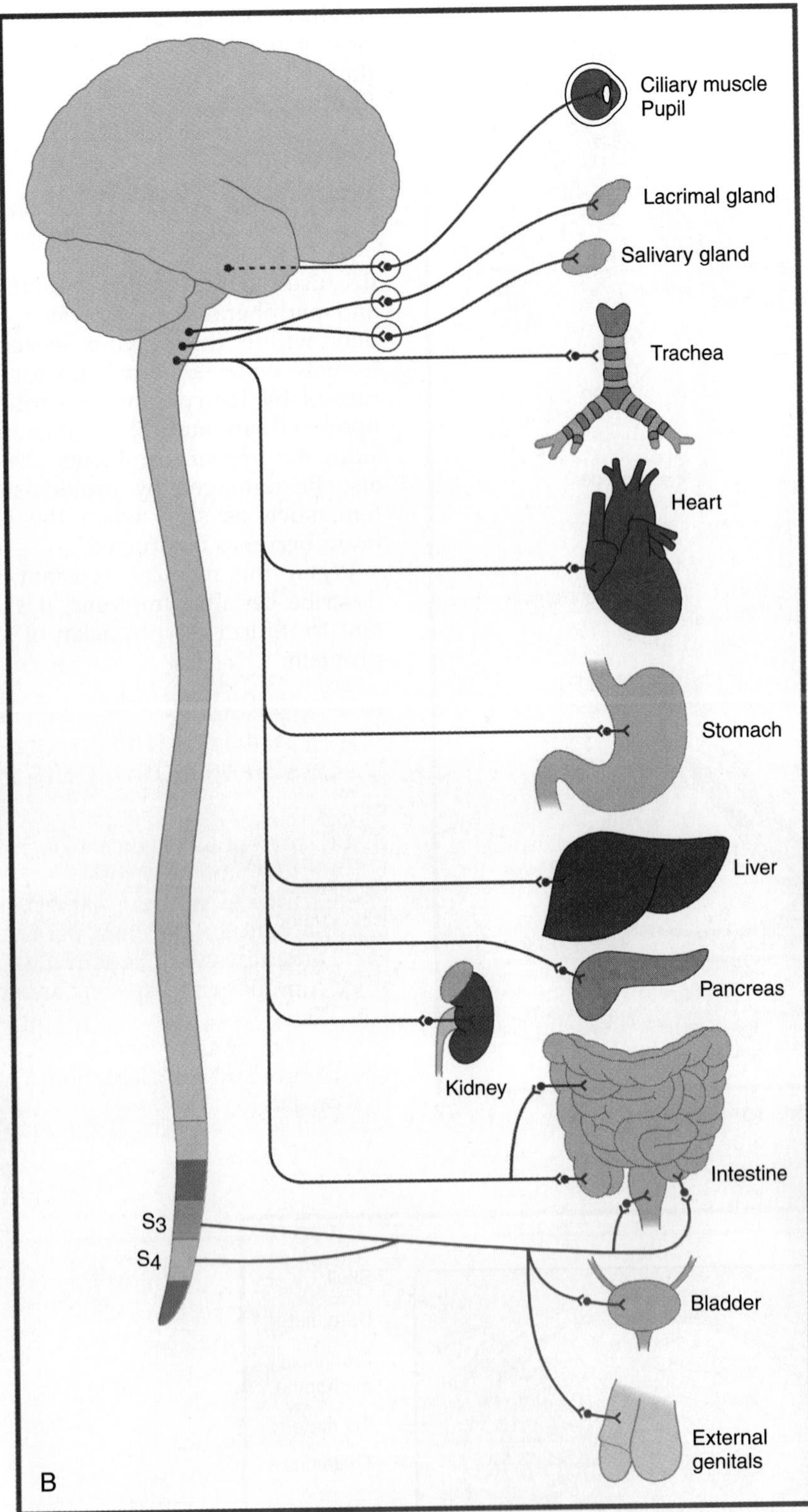

FIGURE 35–4 *Continued*

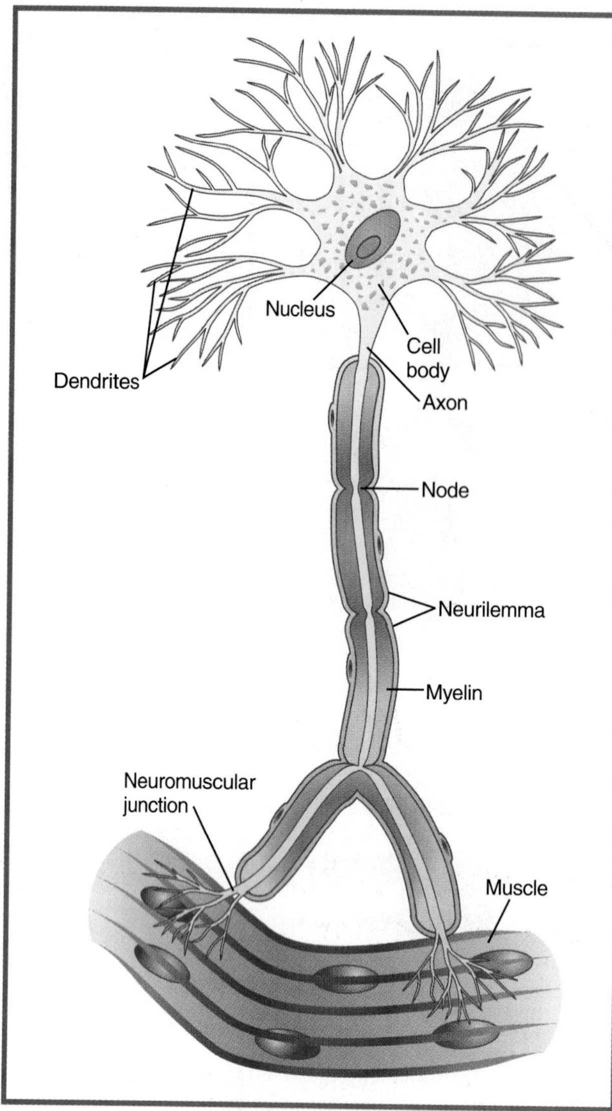

FIGURE 35–5 Neuron.

produced in specialized cells located in the ventricles of the brain. This fluid continuously circulates through the ventricles and spinal cord cleansing and filtering the tissue.

Diseases and Disorders

Because of the complex structure of both the central and peripheral nervous systems, diseases and disorders within the nervous system can cause an extremely wide range of damage. This damage can be caused by injury, infection, inherited defects, developmental **anomalies,** degeneration, or tumors. Besides the primary problems, the nervous system can also be damaged by problems within another system, such as seen when the blood supply to the brain becomes obstructed.

When the medical assistant listens to a patient describe certain symptoms, it should alert the assistant to inform the physician of a possible neurologic problem.

SYMPTOMS THAT SUGGEST POSSIBLE NEUROLOGIC PROBLEMS

- Recurrent localized headache
- Periodic memory loss
- Change in sleeping patterns
- Inability to hold onto items
- Difficulties with certain speech patterns
- Numbness in a specific area of the body
- Visual disturbances
- Loss of consciousness
- Confusion/disorientation to time, place, and/or date.

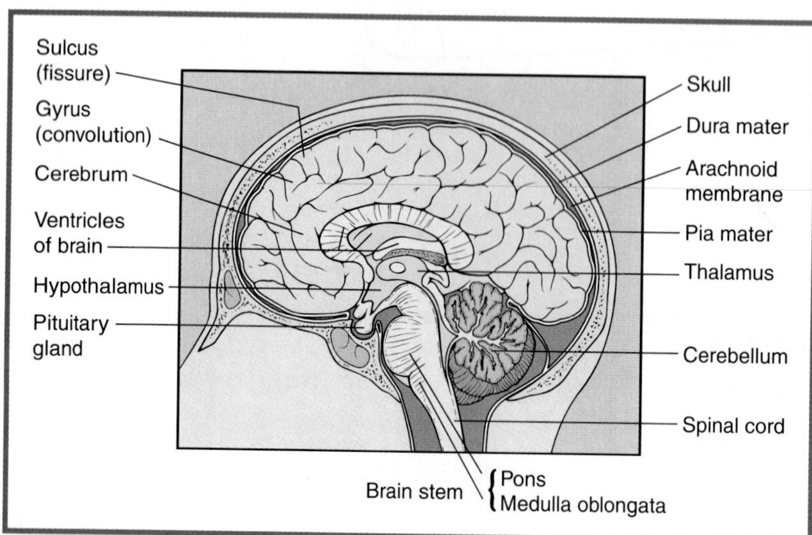

FIGURE 35–6 Normal brain. (From Frazier MS, Drzymkowski JA, Doty SJ: Essentials of Human Diseases and Conditions. Philadelphia, WB Saunders, 1996.)

CEREBROVASCULAR DISEASE

Cerebrovascular disease (CVD) is the third largest cause of death and the most frequently seen crippling disease in the United States. Generally, CVD is related to atherosclerosis of the cerebral arteries and most frequently occurs in older individuals. Important genetic factors include hypertension and blood clot disorders. Atherosclerosis may involve the major arteries or their branches. The narrowing of these arteries may be gradual, owing to fatty deposits or hardening of the vessel walls, or sudden, when a vessel becomes blocked by thrombi.

This disorder is usually diagnosed through cerebral angiography, which is done by injecting a dye into the vessel and doing a radiologic scan of the vessel (Fig. 35–7). Other confirming tests include magnetic resonance imaging (MRI), computed tomography (CT), and electroencephalography (EEG).

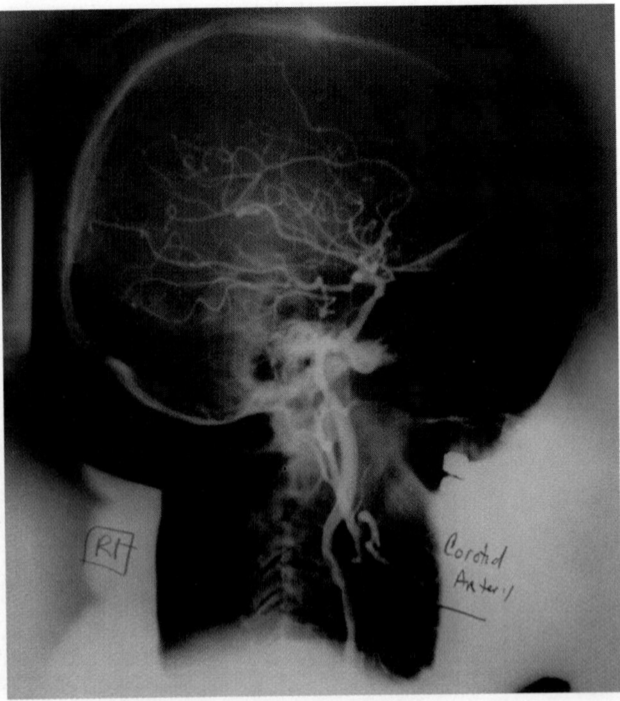

FIGURE 35–7 Angiogram of right carotid artery.

CEREBROVASCULAR ACCIDENT

The most important clinical manifestation of CVD is cerebrovascular accident (CVA), commonly referred to as **stroke.** This occurs when a vessel in an anatomic part of the brain ruptures or totally occludes as a result of CVD. Cerebral ruptures are most often caused by an occlusion of an atherosclerotic artery or the tearing of a weakened section of the artery. The rupture causes the surrounding brain tissue to become filled with blood, thereby destroying the affected tissue. In an occlusion, the embolus or thrombus becomes wedged in an artery and obstructs the flow of blood to an area of the brain (Fig. 35–8).

The symptoms largely depend on the site of the arterial occlusion. Some of the more common symptoms include slurred or inaudible speech, difficulty in swallowing, paralysis on one side of the body, loss of consciousness, dizziness, and double vision.

After a stroke, the treatment of an unconscious patient includes hospitalization, usually in the intensive-care unit. Brain edema, the most life-threatening problem, is usually treated with corticosteroids and diuretic agents that drain the water from the brain tissue. As the patient recovers, physical therapy is important.

CARPAL TUNNEL SYNDROME

Carpal tunnel syndrome occurs when there is **compression** or entrapment of the median nerve at the passageway for the median nerve and the flexor tendons of the forearm. Compression may occur spontaneously or may be due to repetitious overuse. One frequently reported cause is through the daily use of a typing/computer keyboard. The symptoms of compression are pain and **paresthesia** of the radial-palmar region of the hand.

Treatment consists of therapy designed to change the position of the hands at intervals through the use of some form of wrist support. In addition, carpal tunnel syndrome may be treated with nonsteroidal antiinflammatory drugs (NSAIDs), ice, supportive work devices such as wrist supports, and physical therapy. If this does not correct the problem, surgery may be required to relieve the pressure.

Memory Jogger

4 *Why do computer operators commonly suffer from carpal tunnel syndrome?*

MIGRAINE HEADACHE

Migraine headaches are **paroxysmal** attacks of headaches that may be completely incapacitating and are frequently associated with other symptoms such as nausea, vomiting, visual disturbances, and throbbing pain in one side of the head. This type of headache manifests differently from one individual to another (Fig. 35–9). Many describe an **aura** before the onset of the headache that often consists of some form of visual disturbance, such as dark lines across the visual field or spots within the visual field.

Medical research has yet to discover the reason why some individuals suffer from migraine. What is known is that this form of headache tends to be hereditary and often seems to be associated with

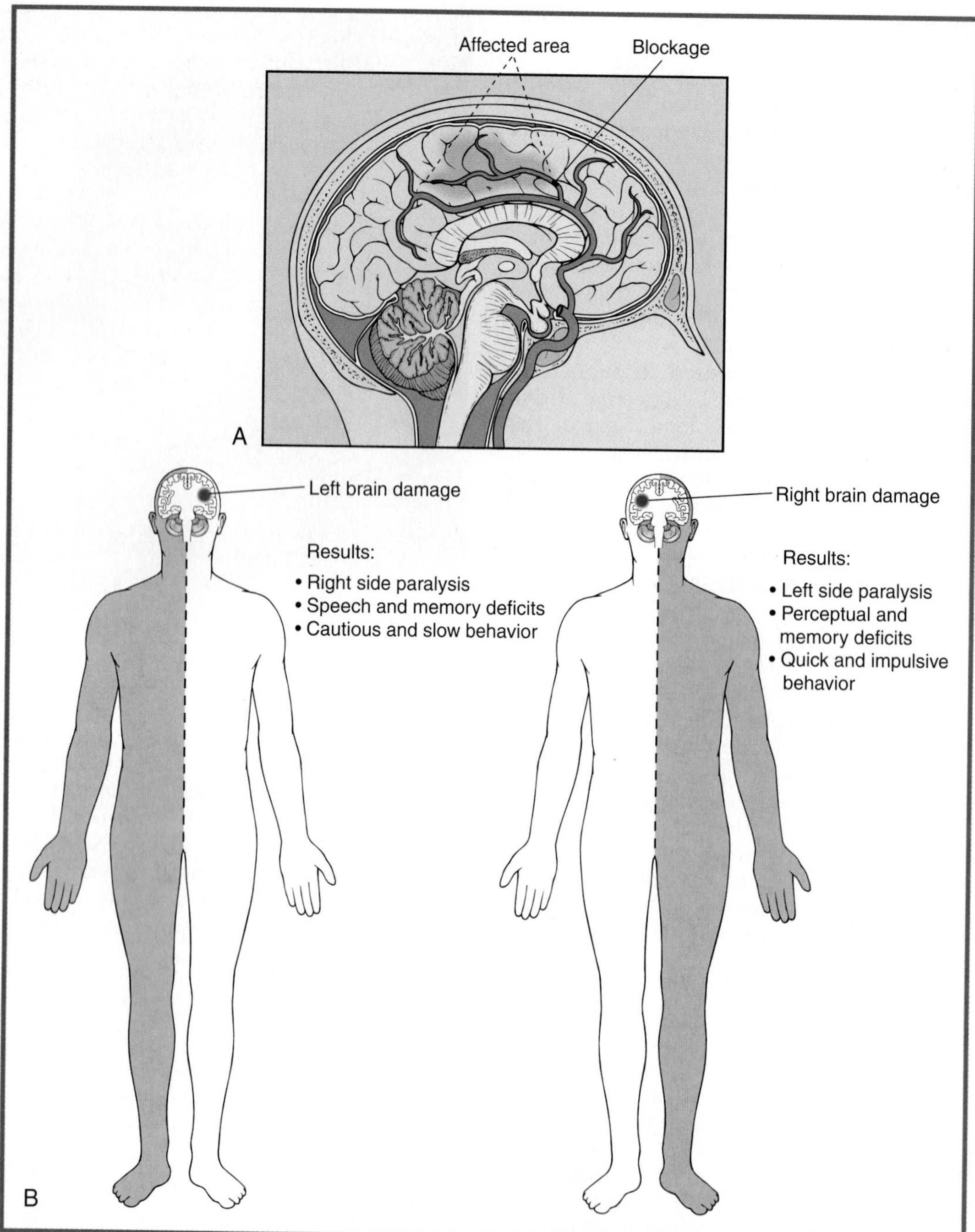

FIGURE 35–8 Cerebrovascular accident. (From Frazier MS, Drzymkowski JA, Doty SJ: Essentials of Human Diseases and Conditions. Philadelphia, WB Saunders, 1996.)

food allergies. There is evidence that a migraine is provoked by cerebrovascular constriction followed by dilation of these vessels. Migraine headaches are marked by severe, throbbing pain caused by an initial constriction of blood vessels surrounding the brain followed by the dilation of blood vessels in the scalp. Diagnosis is usually established through medical history, but physicians may order an EEG, MRI, or CT scan to rule out any organic disorder. Drugs used to prevent migraine, such as methysergide maleate, block the action of certain chemicals that provoke the initial blood vessel constriction leading to the migraine attack. Agents given to abort an acute attack, such as sumatriptan succinate, constrict the dilated blood vessels, thereby relieving the severe pain. Additional treatment may include biofeedback techniques to reduce stress levels and elimination diets.

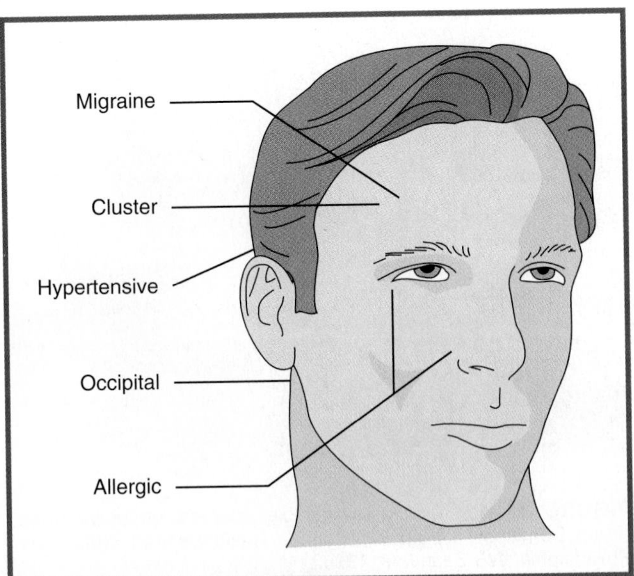

FIGURE 35–9 Types of headaches. (Redrawn from Ferguson GG: Pathophysiology: Mechanisms and Expressions. Philadelphia, WB Saunders, 1984.)

Memory Jogger

5 *Describe the visual aura that may precede a migraine headache.*

CEREBRAL CONCUSSION

Frequently referred to as being "knocked out," this is a traumatic injury resulting from impact with a blunt object. Loss of consciousness may last from a few seconds to several minutes, followed by a period of 12 to 24 hours of disorientation. The concussion causes a disruption in the normal electrical activity in the brain, but the brain is not usually injured. The brain tissue may sustain a contusion or bruised area (Fig. 35–10).

Symptoms may include headache, nausea, vomiting, vision disturbances, and sensitivity to light. On talking to the patient, there may be decreased levels of concentration, irritability, and/or difficulty in recall.

ENCEPHALITIS (SLEEPING SICKNESS)

Most cases of encephalitis are caused by viruses. Some of these are transmitted from animal to human and others from human to human. The symptoms range from mild to serious. In the mild form, the patient has headaches, muscle aches, malaise, and, in general, symptoms that are associated with influenza. The severe cases include fever, **delirium, convulsions, coma,** and even death.

A quiet and nonstimulating environment is necessary to avoid triggering convulsions and to relieve headache and promote rest. The patient may suffer from confusion and disorientation and other behavioral changes owing to the inflammation of nerve tissues. The family will need support and reassurance that these behavior changes are part of the disease and usually disappear as the patient's condition improves.

Management consists of treating the symptoms and is aimed at controlling the fever, electrolyte maintenance, and constant observance of respiratory and urinary functions. In the severe cases, with serious damage to the central nervous system, the convalescence is usually prolonged, and physical therapy is needed to overcome the neurologic and musculoskeletal complications.

Memory Jogger

Can you explain why encephalitis is also known as sleeping sickness?

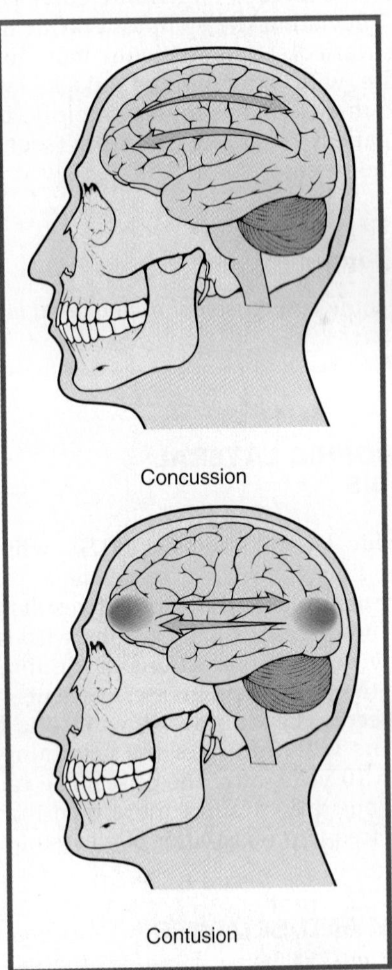

FIGURE 35–10 Concussion and contusion. (From Frazier MS, Drzymkowski JA, Doty SJ: Essentials of Human Diseases and Conditions. Philadelphia, WB Saunders, 1996.)

MULTIPLE SCLEROSIS

Around the nerve fibers in the peripheral system are protective sheaths called myelin. Multiple sclerosis (MS) occurs when the myelin sheaths become inflamed and deteriorate, leaving the nerve tissue unprotected. This then causes a variety of neurologic disorders, such as visual disturbances, urinary dysfunctions, emotional instability, muscle weakness, and degrees of paralysis. The common onset of this disease occurs in women in their early 30s. The cause remains unknown, although it is known that MS is more common in temperate climates and often associated with an autoimmune reaction. It remains difficult to diagnose, and the diagnosis may be made based on the **exacerbation** and **remission** characteristics of the disease. One of the tests that can assist in the diagnosis is lumbar puncture, which will show an increase in the gamma-globulin level in the cerebrospinal fluid when the disease is present. Another test is the MRI, which shows actual plaques on the nerve fibers (Fig. 35–11).

Great strides have been made toward a cure for MS, but as yet there is no definite cure. Treatment is aimed at alleviating the symptoms with the prognosis being varied. Some patients may live a quite normal life with only limited attacks, whereas in others the disease may progress rapidly, incapacitating the patient, resulting in death soon after the onset of the disease.

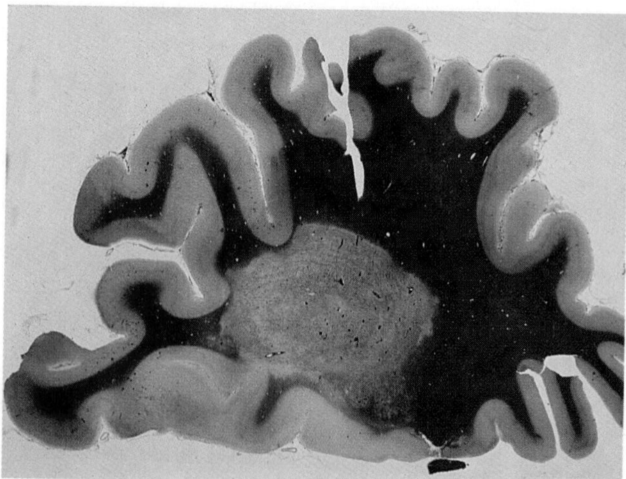

FIGURE 35–11 Plaque of multiple sclerosis on nerve fibers. (From Damjanov I: Pathology for the Health-Related Professions. Philadelphia, WB Saunders, 1996.)

Memory Jogger

7 *How is the cerebrospinal fluid altered in multiple sclerosis?*

AMYOTROPHIC LATERAL SCLEROSIS

Amyotrophic lateral sclerosis (ALS), which is also known as Lou Gehrig's disease, is a progressive, destructive neurologic disease that results in muscle **atrophy.** The disease usually begins with small local involuntary muscle contractions in the forearms and hands. As the disease progresses, patients have difficulty in speech, chewing, swallowing, and breathing. Death occurs with failure of the respiratory muscles within 6 to 10 years after the onset. The cause is still unknown, but it does affect more men than women, with most frequent onset after 50 years of age.

EPILEPSY AND SEIZURES

A seizure is characterized by abnormalities in levels of consciousness, sensory disturbances, and impaired motor function. These attacks of altered cerebral functions are due to uncoordinated and disorganized electrical impulses in the brain. In a majority of cases, the cause is unknown; however, possible causes include high fever, brain tumors, central nervous system infections, **anoxia,** and head injury.

There are several different types of seizures, each of which may be preceded by a significant aura, which acts as a warning signal indicating that a seizure is going to occur. A tonic-clonic seizure (grand-mal) is characterized by a sudden loss of consciousness, falling down, and then tonic contractions (stiffening of muscles) followed by clonic contractions (twitching and jerking movements of the limbs). Absence seizures (petit mal) are a minor form of seizure consisting of momentary clouding of consciousness and loss of contact with the environment. Diagnosis is made by the succession of seizures, and the test that is relied on the most for diagnosis is the EEG. Seizures can be effectively controlled but cannot be cured by drugs. Phenytoin (Dilantin), phenobarbital, and valproic acid are frequently prescribed.

Most seizures are not medical emergencies in an individual with epilepsy, but in someone who does not have epilepsy, the seizure could be a sign of serious illness (Fig. 35–12).

SPINAL CORD INJURIES

Spinal cord injuries are usually the result of an accident in which there has been severe trauma to the back and neck. These injuries are most common among 16- to 30-year-old individuals and associated with automobile and sport accidents. If the cord is completely severed, there will be no neurologic communication between the brain and any of the structures located below the injury. The higher the **transection** of the cord, the more serious the injury becomes. The paralysis that is sustained falls into three categories according to the location of the transection (Fig. 35–13).

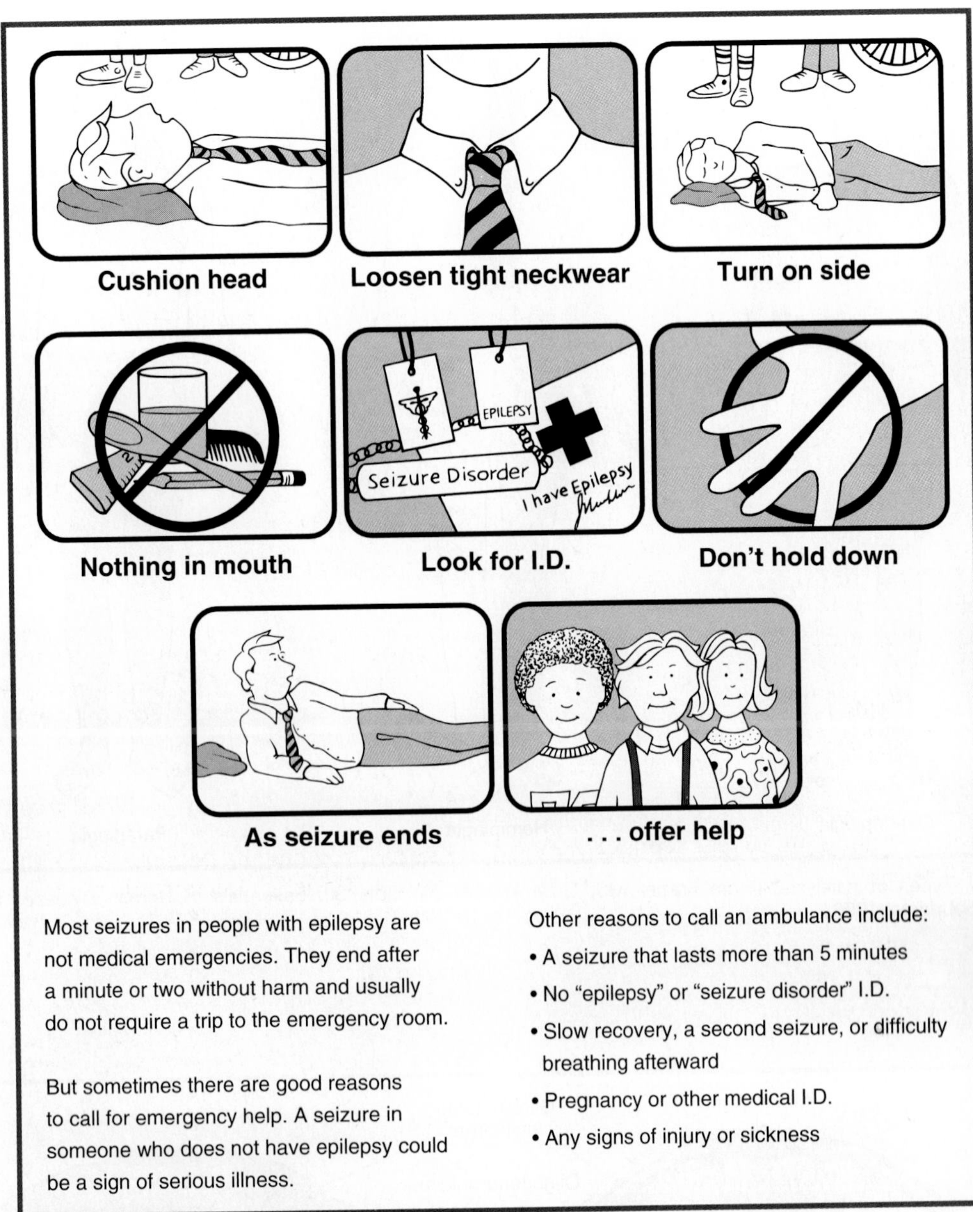

Cushion head
Loosen tight neckwear
Turn on side
EPILEPSY
Seizure Disorder
I have Epilepsy
Nothing in mouth
Look for I.D.
Don't hold down
As seizure ends
. . . offer help
Most seizures in people with epilepsy are not medical emergencies. They end after a minute or two without harm and usually do not require a trip to the emergency room.
But sometimes there are good reasons to call for emergency help. A seizure in someone who does not have epilepsy could be a sign of serious illness.
Other reasons to call an ambulance include:
• A seizure that lasts more than 5 minutes
• No "epilepsy" or "seizure disorder" I.D.
• Slow recovery, a second seizure, or difficulty breathing afterward
• Pregnancy or other medical I.D.
• Any signs of injury or sickness

FIGURE 35–12 First aid for seizures. (From Epilepsy Foundation of America, Landover, MD, 1990.)

THREE CATEGORIES OF TRANSECTION

Paraplegia: Transection occurs below the midpoint of the spinal cord, and the paralysis involves the lower two quadrants.

Quadriplegia: Transection occurs in the upper thoracic and cervical portions of the cord, causing paralysis of all four quadrants.

Hemiplegia: No cord involvement; instead this paralysis is caused by a cerebrovascular accident or brain tumor and affects one hemisphere of the body.

There is no treatment or surgery that can repair the cord. If the spinal cord is injured but not totally severed, the paralysis and neurologic ability of the patient will depend on the degree of injury. These patients usually respond well to physical therapy and their ability to recover motor function is good; however, there may always be some limitations in function.

Memory Jogger

8 *Why isn't hemiplegia caused by a severing of the spinal cord?*

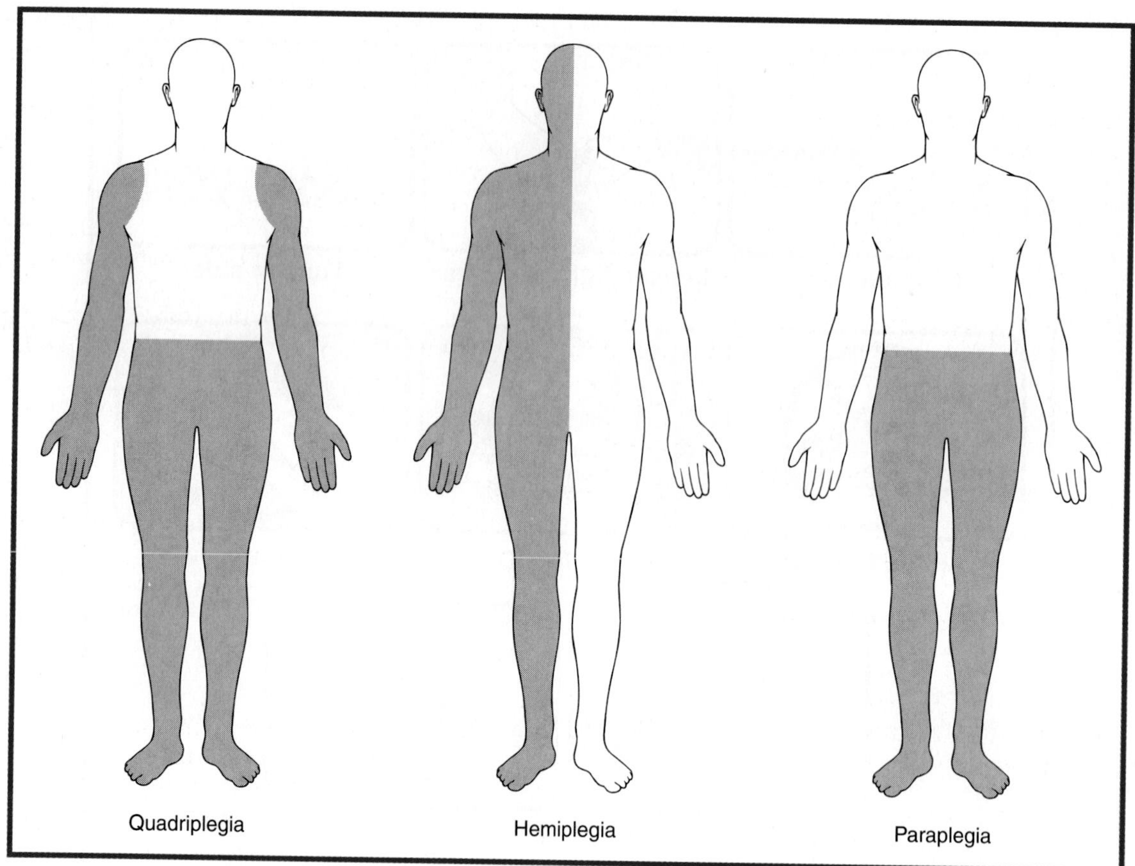

FIGURE 35–13 Types of paralysis. (From Frazier MS, Drzymkowski JA, Doty SJ: Essentials of Human Diseases and Conditions. Philadelphia, WB Saunders, 1996.)

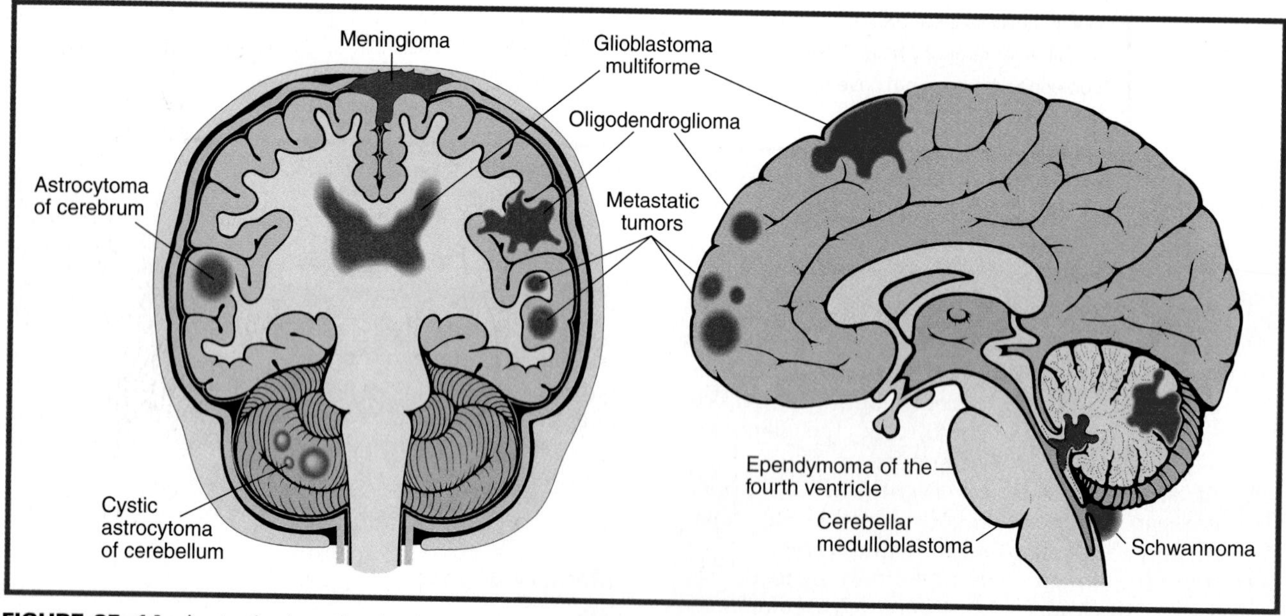

FIGURE 35–14 Anatomic sites of various brain tumors. (From Damjanov I: Pathology for the Health-Related Professions. Philadelphia, WB Saunders, 1996.)

BRAIN TUMORS

A tumor of the brain is probably one of the most feared medical problems. People will suffer with migraine headaches for years without seeking any medical help because of the fear of brain tumor. Modern medicine has taken great steps in the ability to diagnose a tumor and in the treatment of brain tumors. The type of treatment that will be followed greatly depends on whether the tumor is **malignant** or **benign** plus the determination of the tumor's primary site. Approximately 50% of all brain tumors represent metastases from a malignant tumor involving some other site within the body. Although any malignant tumor can metastasize to the brain, lung cancer, breast cancer, and melanoma have a special predilection for spreading to the brain.

Tumors originating from nerves collectively are called neuromas and are composed of cells encasing the axons. Three of the more frequently seen neurologic brain tumors are **glioma, meningioma,** and **medulloblastoma** (Fig. 35–14). Regardless of the type or location of the tumor, each can produce serious complications for the patient because of the limited space inside the skull.

The symptoms depend on the type and location of the tumor but generally the initial symptoms are headaches, vomiting, dizziness, double vision, and changes in muscle strength and coordination. Changes in personality and mental function, seizures, paralysis, loss of speech, and sensory disorders appear as the tumor enlarges Diagnosis is made through radiologic studies specifically the MRI and the CT and EEG. Lumbar puncture may reveal increased pressure in the fluid and the presence of tumor cells. Edema of the optic nerve may be observed with an ophthalmoscope. The treatment can be surgery, chemotherapy, and nuclear therapy, and often is a combination of all three.

Memory Jogger

Name the three most often seen brain tumors.

The Medical Assistant's Role in the Neurologic Examination

As in other physical examinations, a careful history provides the physician with valuable clues in diagnosing neurologic malfunctions. These may be seizures, **syncope, diplopia, incontinence,** and the subjective symptoms mentioned earlier in this chapter. The patient's general health often complicates a neurologic diagnosis. The purposes of a neurologic examination are to determine whether a nervous system malfunction is present, discover its location, and identify its type and extent. During the examination, the physician may determine the effect of the symptoms in relationship to the patient's emotional status, intellectual performance, cognitive ability, and general behavior. One method of evaluation may be evident in the patient's grooming and mannerisms. The patient's ability to communicate is also observed at this time. These include speech, language, and written skills. As you listen to the patient, listen for difficulty in putting words together, the slurring of speech, and whether what is being said makes sense. If you notice changes in the patient, note them on the patient's record for the physician's attention and evaluation.

The physician may grade the patient's mental status with the Glasgow Coma Scale, which is a standardized system for assessing the response to stimuli. Each cranial nerve is checked by the physician. You can assist by helping the patient assume the position needed for each test and by having the instruments that the physician will need ready for use. For example, the first cranial nerve, the *olfactory nerve,* is examined by determining the patient's ability to identify familiar odors, such as coffee, tobacco, or cloves. The fifth cranial nerve, the *trigeminal nerve,* is checked by the patient's differentiating between warm and cold objects held on his or her right and left cheeks.

The motor system is examined by observing the patient's muscular strength, **gait,** and movements. The diameters of the upper arms and the calves of the legs are measured for muscular atrophy. Motor functioning may be assessed through the use of the Romberg test, in which the patient will be asked to stand with the feet together, arms horizontal to the body, and the eyes closed. The sensory system is examined by noting the patient's ability to perceive superficial sensations, such as a wisp of cotton brushed on the skin, a light pinprick, or hot and cold touching certain areas. Several reflexes, such as the patellar and Achilles reflexes, are examined (Fig. 35–15). A stroke with a dull instrument on the lateral aspect of the sole of the foot may produce a positive Babinski reflex (Fig. 35–16), in which the great toe dorsiflexes whereas the smaller toes fan out. This may indicate a possible stroke or a brain lesion. In plantar reflex (Fig. 35–17) the great toe plantarflexes and the smaller toes contract.

Other tests may include skull radiographs, carotid angiograms, myelograms, and MRI and CT studies. An EEG also is performed.

Memory Jogger

What is one of the ways that you can help the physician in diagnosing a neurologic disorder?

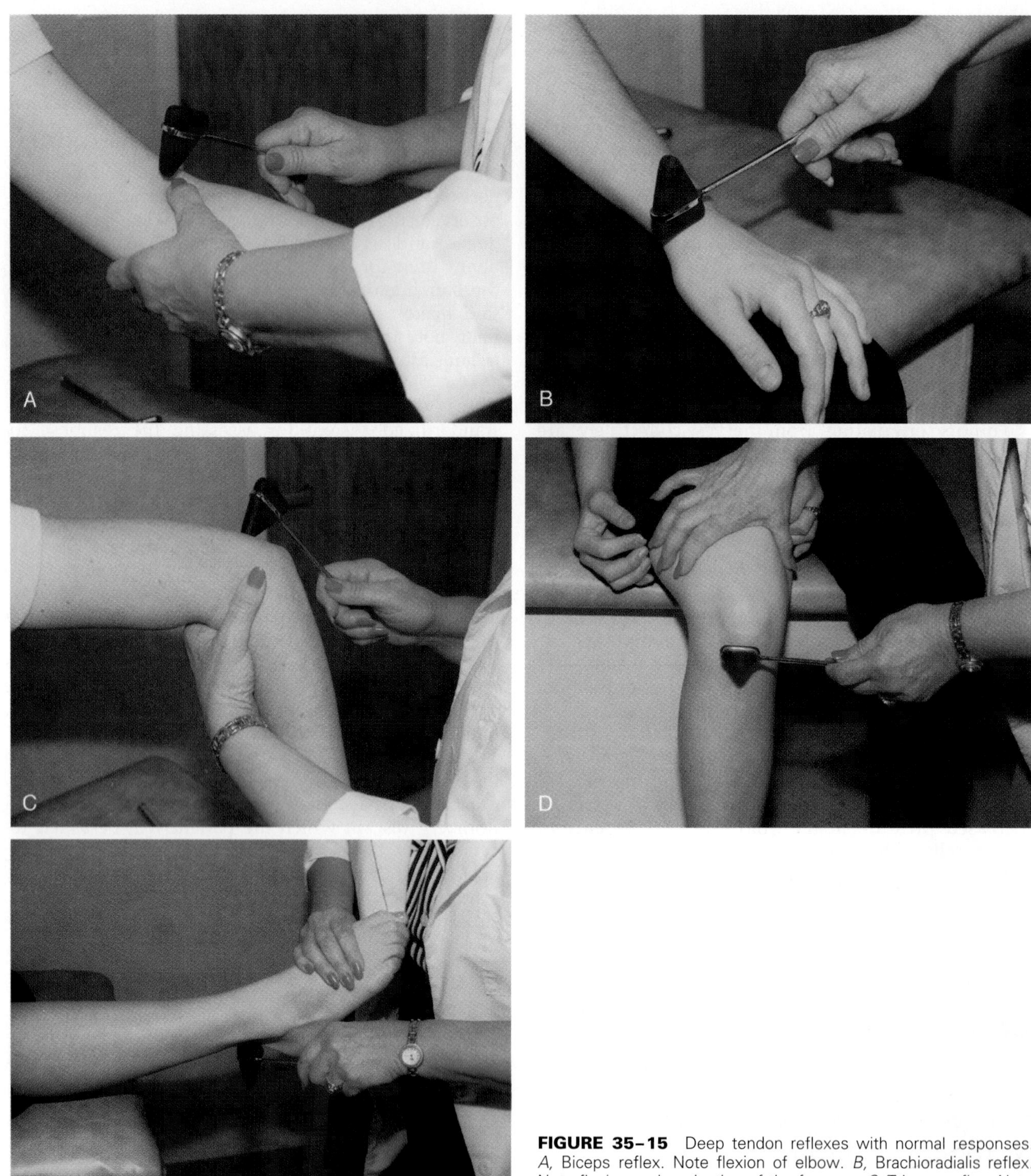

FIGURE 35–15 Deep tendon reflexes with normal responses. *A,* Biceps reflex. Note flexion of elbow. *B,* Brachioradialis reflex. Note flexion and supination of the forearm. *C,* Triceps reflex. Note extension of the arm. *D,* Patellar reflex. Note extension of the leg. *E,* Achilles reflex. Note plantar flexion of the foot.

Diagnostic Testing

ELECTROENCEPHALOGRAPHY

Electroencephalography is the recording of changes in the electrical impulses in various areas of the brain by means of electrodes placed on the scalp, on the brain surface, or within the brain itself. These electrodes are connected to an amplifier that amplifies the impulses more than a million times. Once magnified to this intensity, the impulses can move an electromagnetic pen that records the brain waves.

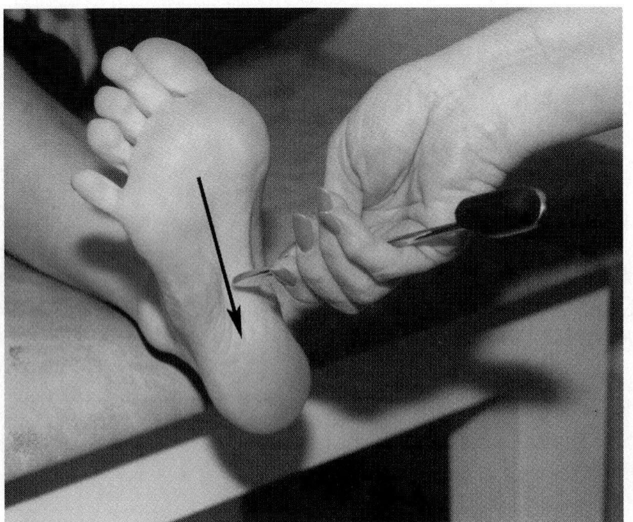

FIGURE 35–16 Babinski reflex. Toes abduct (fan out) and great toe dorsiflexes. Result is positive.

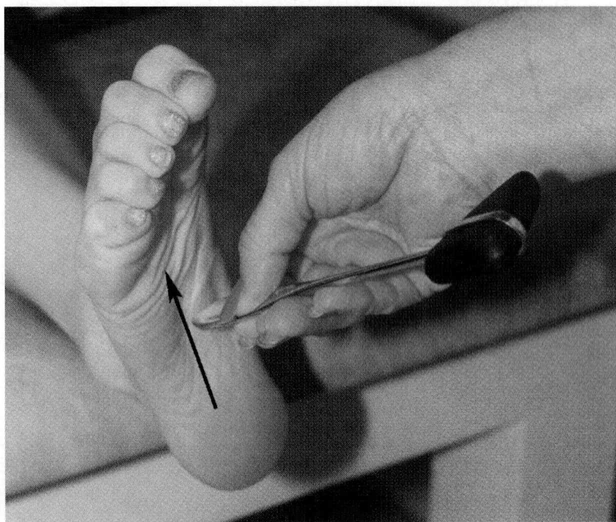

FIGURE 35–17 Plantar reflex. Great toe plantarflexes and toes contract. Result is negative.

The rate, height, and length of the waves vary in different parts of the brain, and every individual has a unique and characteristic pattern. In a healthy brain, most of the recorded waves are the occipital alpha waves, which are obtained from the back of the head. The beta waves, which are related to the sensory-motor parts of the brain, are obtained from the central and front parts of the head. Irregular slow waves are called delta waves and are normally found in deep sleep and in infants and young children. If the delta wave pattern is found in the awake adult, it is considered abnormal. Rhythmic slow waves are called theta waves and show a decrease in brain activity. Electrical silence indicates no evidence of brain activity and is one of the criteria of death.

Electroencephalography is widely used in studying brain functions and in tracing the connections between the parts of the central nervous system. EEG is particularly valuable in diagnosing epilepsy, brain tumor, and other diseases of and injury to the brain (see Procedure 35–1).

PROCEDURE 35–1
Preparing the Patient for an EEG

GOAL

To properly prepare a patient physically and psychologically to obtain an accurate and useful recording.

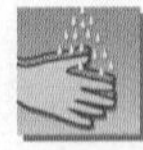

PROCEDURAL STEPS

1 Greet patient and introduce yourself. Explain to the patient that you want to go over the test step by step to ensure the best results.

2 Explain to the patient the purpose of the test, how the procedure will be carried out, and what will be expected of the patient during the testing period.

3 Tell the patient that the electrodes lead minute amounts of electrical charge from the body and that there is no danger of electric shock.

4 Explain that the test is painless because the electrodes are attached to the scalp with **collodion.**

Continued

PROCEDURE 35-1 (CONTINUED)

Preparing the Patient for an EEG

5 If this is to be a sleep recording, suggest that the patient stay up later than usual the night before so that it will be easier to fall asleep.
PURPOSE: Sleep medications are very seldom used because this may alter the wave pattern.

6 Go over the physical preparation, which includes the diet to be followed for 48 hours before the test. This usually requires no stimulants and no meal skipping.
PURPOSE: Meal skipping may cause hypoglycemia, which alters brain function.

7 Tell the patient that at the beginning of the test a baseline EEG will be taken and during this time the patient will be asked to avoid all movement, even eye and tongue movement.
PURPOSE: These activities can be very disruptive in the wave tracing.

8 Explain that the brain will be stimulated by a "photic" stimulator, which employs flickering lights to stimulate the brain.

9 Ask the patient if there are any questions; and, if there are, be certain that these questions are answered to the patient's satisfaction.
PURPOSE: Patients are more likely to be cooperative if they are informed so they will not be unduly apprehensive before and during the test.

LUMBAR PUNCTURE

When the physician suspects meningitis, a possible infection or inflammation in the central nervous system, it is common for a lumbar puncture to be requested. This procedure is done to obtain a small amount of the cerebrospinal fluid so that it can be tested for possible glucose, protein, bacteria, and blood and so the cells seen can be differentiated and counted. The fluid can also be used to evaluate intracranial pressure or an intracranial bleeding disorder.

When lumbar puncture is done in the physician's office, sterile technique is observed. The patient is placed on the side (usually left) in a fetal position, the area is anesthetized, and then fluid is obtained with the use of a special needle, which is inserted into the subarachnoid space, below the spinal cord, at the level of L4 and L5 (Fig. 35–18).

Because patients must remain flat in bed for approximately 8 hours after the procedure, some neurology practices have a specially equipped room in which special procedures are performed. If you are working in such an office, you may be expected to assist with a lumbar puncture and be responsible for the patient after the procedure. When assuming this responsibility, you will be expected to watch for side effects such as severe headaches, visual disturbances, and pain. You will also need to know the physician's protocols regarding the frequency in taking the patient's vital signs, measuring urinary output, fluid intake, and the presence of family members.

If the office does not have the space to conduct the procedure and post care, the lumbar puncture may be performed in outpatient clinics or surgical centers.

COMPUTED TOMOGRAPHY AND MAGNETIC RESONANCE IMAGING

These revolutionary radiologic imaging modalities use computer processing to generate an image of tissue density in a slice as thin as 1 to 10 mm in thickness through a person's body. When it is necessary to differentiate between different layers of soft tissue within the nervous system, a contrast medium or dye can be introduced into the area to produce a contrast in the radiograph and a CT scan is done (Fig. 35–19).

Using MRI, a hologram can be created to show tumor masses and help the surgeon study the approach into the skull to remove the tumor. Radiologists can also make a video from the MRI that peels away the skin, skull, and covering of the brain to allow the surgeon to view the tumor from all directions with three-dimensional glasses before going into the operating room to remove the real tumor (Fig. 35–20).

ALPHA-FETOPROTEIN TESTING

When a fetal neural abnormality is possible, the physician may order this blood test to be done to

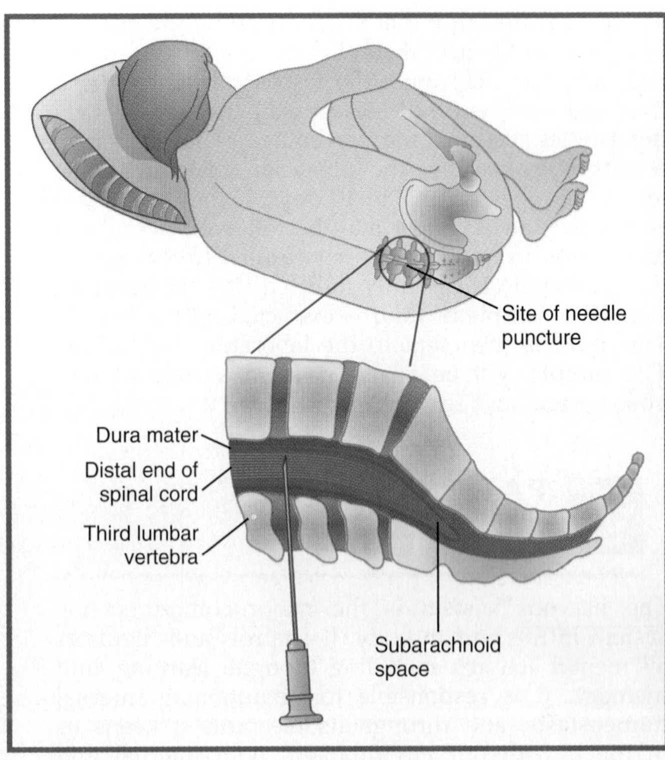

FIGURE 35–18 Lumbar puncture.

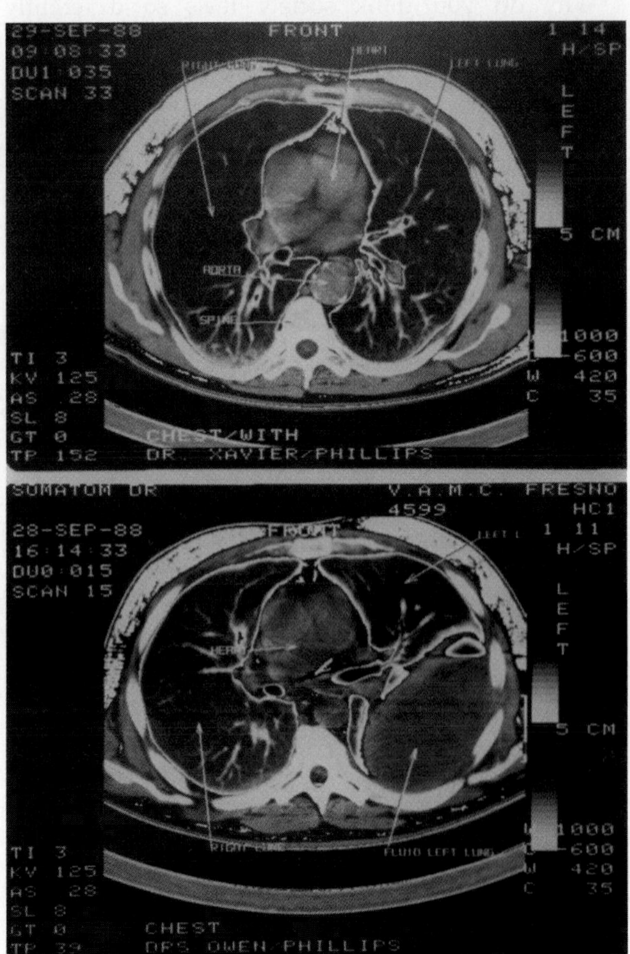

FIGURE 35–19 Computed tomogram of spine.

evaluate the development of the neural tube, which will eventually develop into the brain and spinal cord. The blood sample is obtained from the pregnant mother between 16 and 18 weeks of gestation. The blood is then tested for alpha-fetoprotein (AFP),

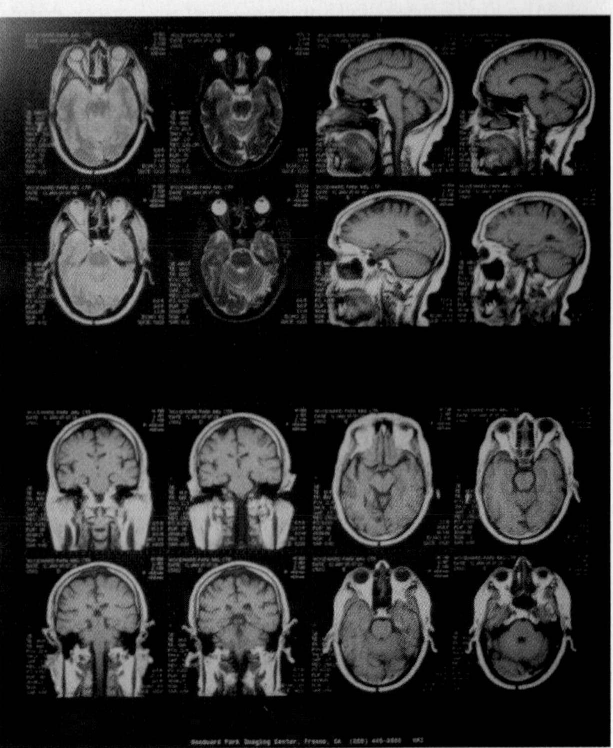

FIGURE 35–20 Magnetic resonance image of skull.

which is a substance that is produced by the embryo and in later development by the fetal liver. If the AFP levels are elevated, the test is considered positive, and this then indicates possible nervous system deformities. Because the percentage of false-positive results is noticeable, the physician may order the test to be repeated in 7 to 10 days. If the second test is positive, an AFP test may be followed by an amniocentesis to qualify the first results. In this procedure, a needle is carefully inserted into the amniotic sac and a sample of fluid is extracted into a syringe. This fluid is then sent to the laboratory for testing. The sample will be analyzed for a variety of nervous system and sex-linked disorders.

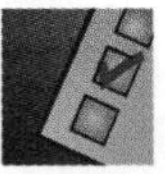

PATIENT EDUCATION

The nervous system is the major communication system in the human body. It controls and regulates all mental activity, including thought, learning, and memory. It is responsible for maintaining internal **homeostasis,** and through its receptors it keeps us in touch with our environment, both internal and external.

When this system becomes damaged or diseased, the signs and symptoms appear in every system. Motor activity becomes erratic, or the activity level decreases so that the person becomes unable to complete tasks that should be of no problem. Patients may seem to be always complaining about something, and no one seems to listen to them.

As the medical assistant in neurology, your prime responsibility will be to observe, list, and report any change you observe. Even things that may seem rather slight may give the physician that one last clue needed to put the puzzle together and get this person into the right treatment program. Neurology will not be the specialty that every medical assistant would like to be associated with, because there are very few exciting procedures. To enjoy this type of practice, you will need to have the ability to talk to people and, above all, listen to what the patients are telling you.

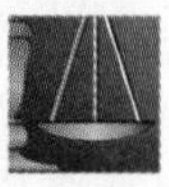

LEGAL AND ETHICAL ISSUES

In neurology, you will be faced with many degrees of behavior and personality changes that are all part of neurologic diseases. Often the patient is not aware of the changes and may feel that there is nothing wrong with him or her. Some are concerned that loved ones have turned against them and are treating them in an abusive manner. The patient's family may be experiencing emotional stress in coping with the patient's behavior. It is in this type of a situation that you must remember the medical assistant's code of ethics and the need for total confidentiality. Everything that is said or discussed in the examination room is not repeated to other staff members in the office and never discussed outside the office. Confidentiality must be strictly observed.

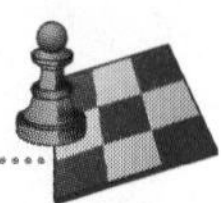

CRITICAL THINKING

1 The mother of a 10-year-old child calls the office and wants to bring the child to see the doctor today. She tells you that her son has had a bout of flu with fever and nasal congestion for the past 3 days. Today when she woke him to get up for school, he said he had a terrible headache and that everything in his room looked blurry. She also noticed that he had rigidity in his neck. What might be the cause of these symptoms? Would you give him a STAT appointment or the last appointment of the day or tell the mother to take him to the emergency department at the hospital? Why?

2 Have you ever noticed how people treat someone who has a gastrointestinal disorder compared with someone who has a neurologic disorder? Why do you think society feels so differently toward neurologic disorders?

HOW DID I DO? Answers to Memory Joggers

1. A fully formed human brain contains 100 billion neurons or nerve cells.
2. Voluntary nerves are part of the peripheral nervous system.
3. The medulla oblongata is the vital link.
4. Computer operators get carpal tunnel syndrome due to the repetition and positioning of the hands on the keyboard for extended periods of time.
5. The visual aura may be dark lines across the visual field or spots within the field.
6. Encephalitis is also called sleeping sickness because of the fever, delirium, and coma that are part of the severe symptoms.
7. The cerebrospinal fluid will show an increased level of gamma globulin if multiple sclerosis is present.
8. Hemiplegia is one-sided paralysis that is not possible when the spinal cord is severed.
9. The three most frequently reported brain tumors are glioma, meningioma, and medulloblastoma.
10. You can help the physician by listening carefully and observing the patient and then reporting to the physician any observations that appear to be out of context for this particular patient.

Assisting in Dermatology

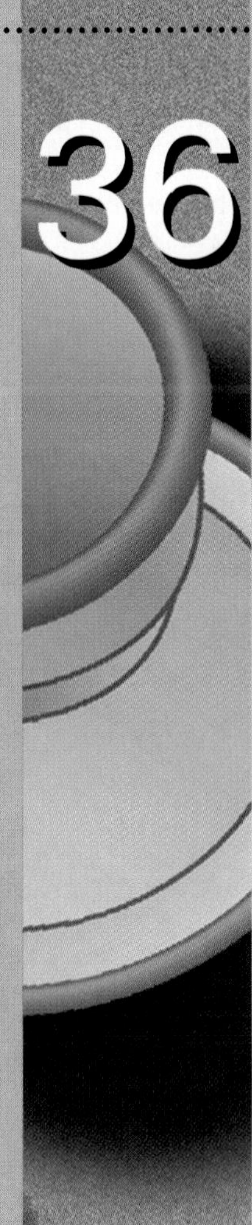

OUTLINE

LEARNING OBJECTIVES

Cognitive: On successful completion of this chapter you should be able to:

1. Identify the anatomic structures of the skin.
2. Explain the major functions of the skin.
3. Identify different lesions by name.
4. List and describe types of thermal skin injuries.
5. Name eight diseases or disorders of the skin.
6. Discuss your role in assisting with dermatologic testing.
7. Identify six forms of dermatologic medications.
8. Analyze your role in patient education.
9. Discuss legal issues in caring for the dermatologic patient.
10. Define and spell vocabulary terms.

Performance: On successful completion of this chapter you should be able to:

1. Assist the dermatologist with the examination of the skin.
2. Accurately obtain an exudate sample from a wound for laboratory analysis.
3. Assist with a skin biopsy.
4. Prepare a list of possible patient education skin issues.

VOCABULARY

adipose Pertaining to fatty tissue

allergens Substances that are capable of producing an allergic reaction

antipruritics Agents that prevent or relieve itching

aspirating To draw in by suction

bilirubin Orange-colored pigment in bile, which when it accumulates leads to jaundice

cancer Any cellular tumor or neoplastic disease in which there is a transformation of normal body cells into malignant cells

collagen Strong, fibrous, insoluble protein found in connective tissue

cryosurgery Technique of exposing tissue to extreme cold to produce a well-defined area of cell destruction

cyanosis Blue discoloration of the skin usually caused by depressed circulation

debridement Removal of foreign material and dead, damaged tissue from a wound

dermatophytes Fungal parasite that grows in or on the skin

ecchymosis Bluish-black skin discoloration produced by hemorrhagic areas

electrodesiccation Destructive drying of cells and tissue by means of short high-frequency electrical sparks

erythema Redness or inflammation of the skin

jaundice Yellow discoloration of the skin and mucous membranes

keratin Very hard, tough protein found in hair, nails, and epidermal tissue

keratinocytes Any one of the skin cells that synthesizes keratin

keratolytic Substance that causes the shedding of skin cells at regular intervals

leukoderma White patches on the skin

melanin Protein manufactured by the body that gives the skin its color and protects the body from ultraviolet light rays

neoplasm New growth of cells (used interchangeably with the term *cancer*)

nits Eggs of the louse

onychomycosis Fungus of the nail bed

opaque Not translucent or transparent

palliative Substance that alleviates or eases a painful situation without curing it

pallor Lack of color; pale skin

petechiae Small, purplish hemorrhagic spots on the skin

pruritus Itching

sebaceous glands Oil-secreting gland of the skin

sebum Fatty secretion of the sebaceous glands

vitiligo Loss of pigment in areas of the skin

wheal Localized area of edema on the skin that is usually accompanied by itching

The skin, the largest organ in the human body, covers a total area of about 20 square feet in an average-sized adult. Forming the outer boundary of your body, skin carries out several essential functions: it acts as a barrier to protect vital internal organs against infection and injury, it helps dissipate heat and regulate body temperature, and it synthesizes vitamin D when exposed to ultraviolet light. In addition, the various sensory receptors present throughout the skin enable it to respond to such sensations as heat, cold, pain, and pressure.

The specialization of dermatology deals with the skin, its accessory structures such as the hair and sweat glands, and the subcutaneous tissue that lies beneath the skin. The physician specializing in dermatology is called a dermatologist.

Anatomy and Physiology

Each square inch of the skin contains millions of cells, numerous specialized nerve endings, hair follicles, muscles, sweat glands to cool the body, and **sebaceous glands** that release oil to lubricate the skin. These diverse structures and glands are nour-

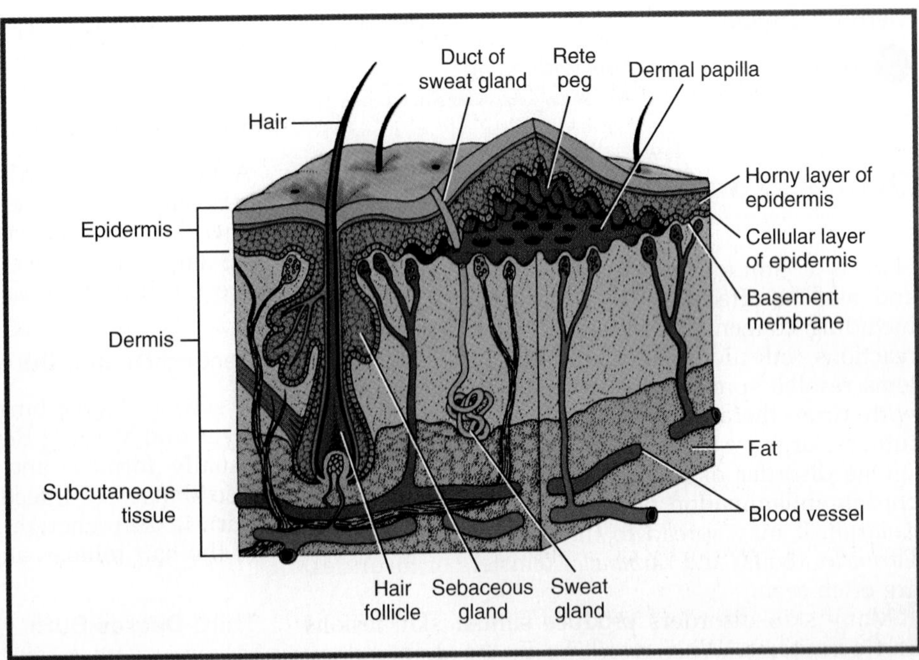

FIGURE 36–1 The three layers of the skin.

ished by a permeating, elaborate network of blood vessels. The thickness of human skin varies markedly on different parts of your body, ranging from fairly thin over protected areas, such as the eyelids, to very thick over areas subject to abrasion, such as the palms of the hands and the soles of the feet.

Skin is composed of three layers. The epidermis, which is the thin uppermost layer; the dermis, which is the thicker layer beneath, is often referred to as the true skin, and makes up about 90% of the skin mass; and the subcutaneous layer, which is composed primarily of fatty or **adipose** tissue (Fig. 36–1).

Memory Jogger

 *Where is the human skin relatively thin?*

EPIDERMIS

New skin cells called **keratinocytes** are found in the basal cell layer of the epidermis and migrate upward over a period of about 4 weeks. As the cells move toward the surface, they grow flatter and more scaly, eventually losing their nuclei and changing into dead skin cells that contain an inert protein called **keratin.** Keratin, which makes up the outermost layer of the epidermis, forms a protective barrier that helps control water loss from the body. Ultimately, the outermost keratin layer sloughs off as a result of washing and friction. Hair and nails, which are also composed of keratin, are products of the epidermis.

About 95% of the cells in the epidermis are keratinocytes. The other 5% of epidermal cells are pigmented cells, or melanocytes. **Melanin** is a protein manufactured in the body that gives coloring to the skin and also protects the body from ultraviolet light. Skin coloring is determined not by the total number of melanocytes, which is relatively constant for all races, but rather by the rate at which these cells produce melanin.

Memory Jogger

 *What is the function of keratin?*

DERMIS

The underlying dermis contains fibers such as **collagen** and elastin as well as water and jelly-like materials that make the skin compressible. The dermis consists of connective tissue through which are found collagen and elastin fibers. Collagen fibers help to prevent tearing of the skin, and elastin is a flexible fiber that makes the skin resilient. Distributed throughout the dermis are blood vessels, lymph vessels, nerve fibers, muscle cells, hair follicles, and sebaceous and sweat glands.

SUBCUTANEOUS LAYER

The subcutaneous layer, which manufactures fat, provides insulation and serves as a depository for reserve calories. Subcutaneous tissue is unevenly distributed; and as the human body ages, this layer thins considerably.

Memory Jogger

 *Which layer of skin thins with aging?*

Diseases and Disorders

Skin is continuously exposed to the environment and may be affected by a wide range of disorders, including congenital diseases, inflammation, allergic reactions, infections, and tumors. Many skin problems resolve spontaneously, others can be managed with drug therapy, and still others, such as skin tumors, large cysts, or moles, may require surgery.

One disorder of the skin is *seborrheic dermatitis,* a chronic inflammation of the scalp, commonly called *dandruff.* It may spread to the face, neck, and body. *Furuncles* (boils) and *carbuncles* (clusters of furuncles) are often seen.

Many skin disorders produce similar skin lesions and symptoms. When working in the dermatology office, it is important to learn and understand the terms used to describe skin lesions (Fig. 36–2). Being able to describe the lesion to the physician using the correct term is important and also professional, such as "Large, black nodule on right anterior forearm" or "Big black mole on the right arm below the elbow."

Disorders of the skin may be divided into primary and secondary lesions. *Primary lesions* are those that appear immediately. Macules, papules, plaques, nodules, cysts, wheals, and pustules are all primary lesions. *Secondary lesions* never appear originally but are the result of alterations in a primary lesion. Examples of secondary lesions are scales, crusts, fissures, erosions, ulcerations, and scars. A burn gives a blister. The blister is the primary lesion, the blister breaks and an ulceration forms, and then healing ends in a scar. The ulceration and the scar formation are secondary lesions.

Memory Jogger

 *Are acne cysts primary or secondary lesions?*

THERMAL INJURIES

Skin can be damaged and injured by exposure to moderately high or low temperatures over an extended time period. It also can be injured in a relatively short time period when exposed to very high or low temperatures. The most frequent thermal injury are burns, caused by heat and cold injuries such as frostbite. Other types include electrical, radiation, and sunburn injuries.

Heat burns are classified as first-degree, second-degree, or third-degree, depending on the depth of the wound (Fig. 36–3*A*).

First-Degree Burn

A first-degree burn shows **erythema** of the epidermis only. The tissue destruction is superficial, without blistering. The use of cold packs (see Chapter 41) on a first-degree burn until the pain stops may prevent it from becoming a second-degree burn.

Second-Degree Burn

A second-degree burn includes the entire epidermal layer and varying depths of the dermis. Blisters are usually formed, and there is some pain. There is also danger of infection in the blistered area. If the burn is deep enough, there may be some destruction of the hair follicles and the sebaceous glands.

Third-Degree Burn

A third-degree burn is the destruction of all the epithelium and may involve underlying muscle tissue. Destroyed skin sloughs, leaving a raw area. There is danger of infection. Third-degree burns do not cause pain because the nerve endings are destroyed.

Burns are also classified according to the percentage of body surface involved (see Fig. 36–3*B*). A method called the *rule of nines* has been developed to determine burn surface involvement.

In adults, the body surface area is divided into areas of 9% and 18%. Areas involving 9% of the body surface are the head, neck, and each arm. Areas involving 18% of the body surface are the front torso, the back torso, and each leg. The genitalia and each palm represent 1% each. The sum of all body percentages is 100%. In children, an adjustment is made because a child's head is relatively large compared with the body. The head is given 18%, and each lower limb is considered 14%.

Treatment depends on the source of the burns. Analgesics may be given to treat the pain. Minor burns may be treated with an antibacterial cream or ointment. Severe burns require specialized care, possible hospitalization in a burn unit, with possible surgical **debridement** of the burned tissue and skin grafting.

COLD INJURIES

Cold injuries are usually less severe than burns, but prolonged exposure can result in amputation and, in severe situations, death. Frostbite is caused by exposure to subfreezing temperatures. The damage occurs at the level of the small blood vessels, which, stunned by the cold, become permanently dilated and unable to regulate local blood flow. Venous

PRIMARY LESIONS

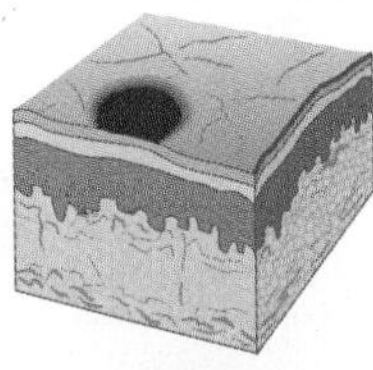

MACULE
Flat area of color change (no elevation or depression)

Example: Freckles

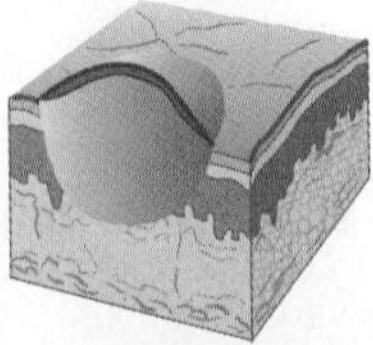

PAPULE
Solid elevation less than 0.5 cm in diameter

Example: Allergic eczema

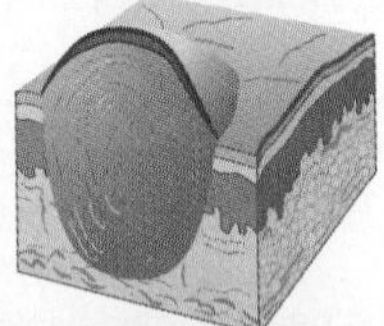

NODULE
Solid elevation 0.5 to 1 cm in diameter. Extends deeper into dermis than papule

Example: Mole

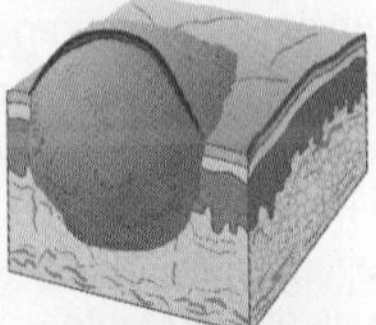

TUMOR
Solid mass—larger than 1 cm

Example: Squamous cell carcinoma

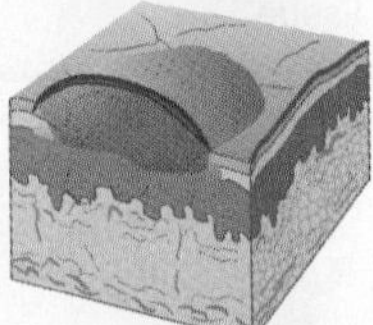

PLAQUE
Flat elevated surface found on skin or mucous membrane

Example: Thrush

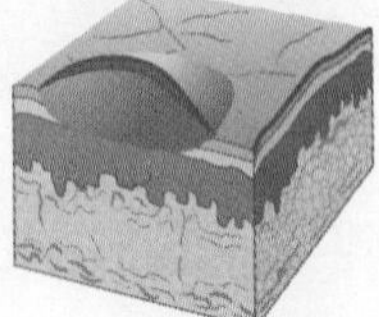

WHEAL
Type of plaque. Result is transient edema in dermis

Example: Intradermal skin test

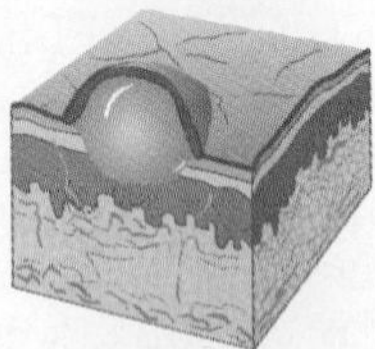

VESICLE
Small blister—fluid within or under epidermis

Example: Herpesvirus infection

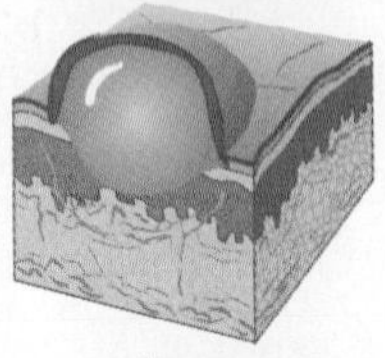

BULLA
Large blister (greater than 0.5 cm)

Example: Burn

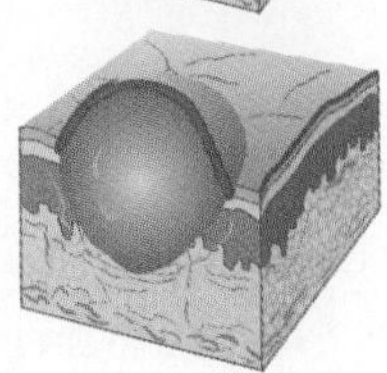

PUSTULE
Vesicle filled with pus

Example: Acne

SECONDARY LESIONS

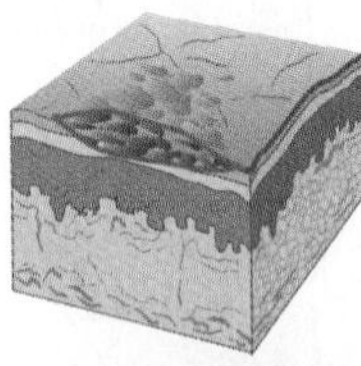

SCALES
Flakes of cornified skin layer

Example: Psoriasis

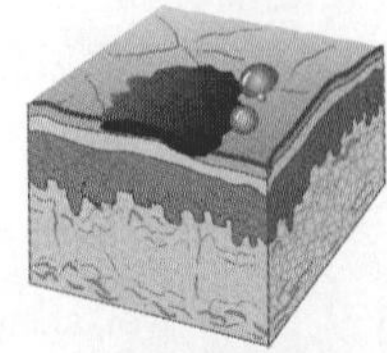

CRUST
Dried exudate on skin

Example: Impetigo

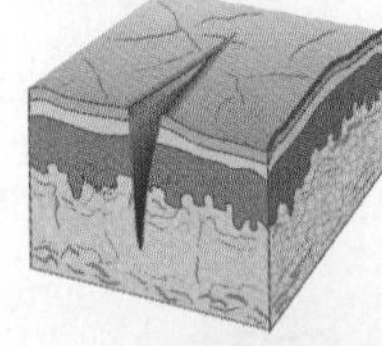

FISSURE
Cracks in skin

Example: Athlete's foot

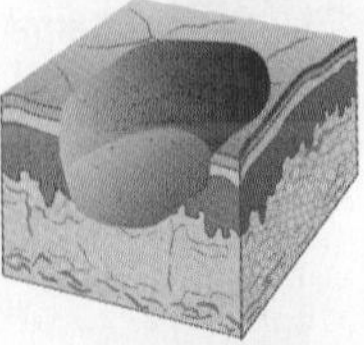

ULCER
Area of destruction of entire epidermis

Example: Decubitus (pressure sore)

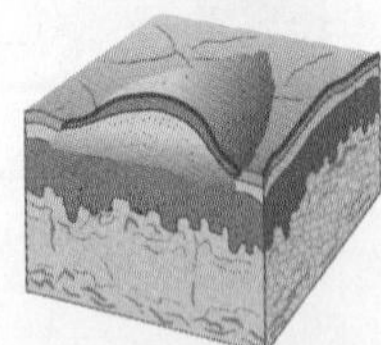

SCAR
Excess collagen production after injury

Example: Surgical healing

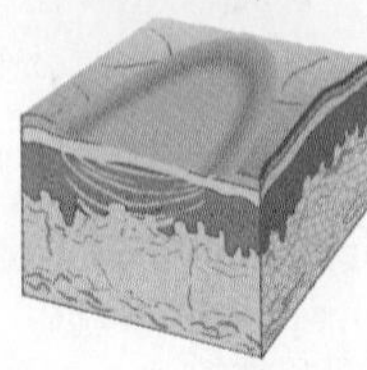

ATROPHY
Loss of some portion of the skin

Example: Paralysis

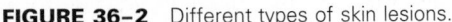

FIGURE 36–2 Different types of skin lesions.

EPIDERMIS
Sweat duct
Capillary
Sebaceous gland
Nerve endings
DERMIS
Hair follicle
Hair follicle
Sweat gland
Fat
Blood vessels
SUBCUTANEOUS TISSUE

A

	APPEARANCE	SENSATION	COURSE
SUPERFICIAL BURN	Mild to severe erythema; skin blanches with pressure Skin dry Small, thin-walled blisters	Painful Hyperesthetic Tingling Pain eased by cooling	Discomfort lasts about 48 hours Desquamation in 3–7 days
PARTIAL-THICKNESS BURN	Large thick-walled blisters covering extensive area (vesiculation) Edema; mottled red base; broken epidermis; wet, shiny, weeping surface	Painful Hyperesthetic Sensitive to cold air	Superficial partial-thickness burn heals in 10–14 days Deep partial-thickness burn requires 21–28 days for healing Healing rate varies with burn depth and presence or absence of infection
FULL-THICKNESS BURN	Variable, e.g., deep red, black, white, brown Dry surface Edema Tissue disrupted	Little pain Anesthetic	Full-thickness dead skin suppurates and liquefies after 2–3 weeks Spontaneous healing impossible Requires removal of eschar and skin grafting Scarring deformities and function loss Beneath eschar capillary tufts and fibroblasts organize into granulating tissue

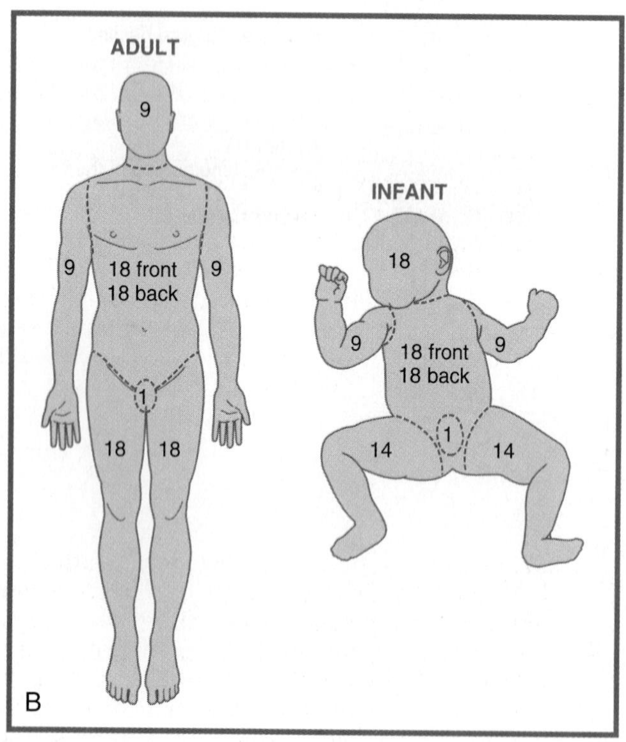

FIGURE 36–3 Rule of nines classification of burns.

stagnation occurs, and skin necrosis develops with formation of blisters and ulcers.

Diagnosis is made by visual examination and knowing the history of the exposure. Treatment consists of warming the area with an external source of low, even heat not above 105° F. The area should never be rubbed. Vital signs should be monitored, and the physician's orders should be explicitly followed.

Memory Jogger

5 *When warming a frostbitten area, the heat should not exceed ____.*

ACNE

Acne typically begins at puberty, probably under the influence of sex hormones (Fig. 36–4). Although acne is an infectious disease, it is thought that hereditary, hormonal factors, and general hygiene are important. Sebum reaches the skin surface through the hair follicles and stimulates the follicle walls, causing a more rapid shedding of the skin cells. This then causes the cells and sebum to stick together and form a plug that promotes the growth of bacteria in the follicles that forms blackheads, pimples and pustules, or larger abscesses. Scratching, picking, or pressing on these lesions predisposes the individual to secondary infections.

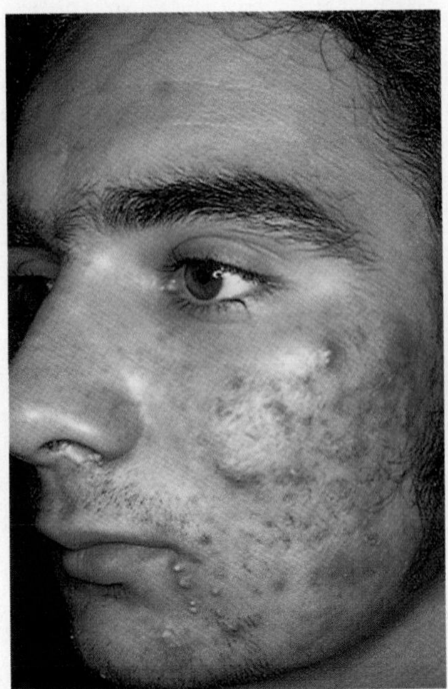

FIGURE 36–4 Acne. (From Hurwitz A: Clinical Pediatric Dermatology: A Textbook of Skin Disorders in Childhood and Adolescence, 2nd ed. Philadelphia, WB Saunders, 1993.)

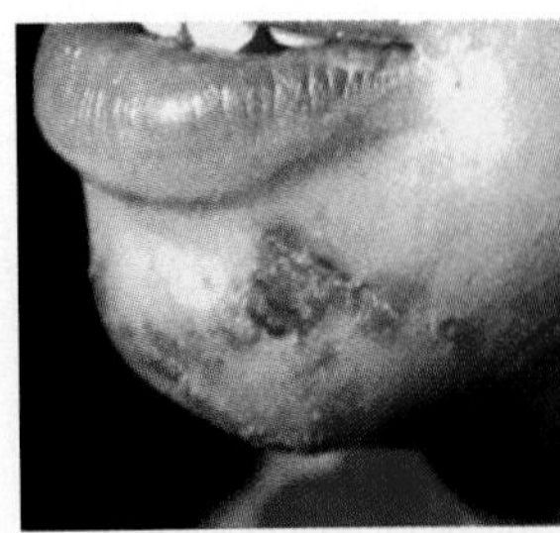

FIGURE 36–5 Impetigo. (From Lookingbill D, Marks J: Principles of Dermatology, 2nd ed. Philadelphia, WB Saunders, 1993.)

Treatment may include the use of topical and/or systemic antibiotics. Topically applied **keratolytic** agents may be appropriate for many acne problems. Ultraviolet light treatments and application of medications related to vitamin A such as tretinoin (Retin-A) may be used to reduce the skin's natural oils and promote drying and peeling of the acne lesions.

Memory Jogger

6 *Scratching or pressing on acne lesions can lead to ____.*

IMPETIGO

Impetigo is a common contagious superficial infection caused by streptococci or *Staphylococcus aureus*. It appears as vesicular or pustules found on the face of young children, around the nose and mouth (Fig. 36–5). The skin lesions are itchy and are spread through scratching the infected area. Affected children often spread the infection to other sites on their bodies or to other children through sharing toys and touching. Treatment consists of properly cleaning the infected areas and applying an antibiotic ointment three or four times a day. The infected areas will usually heal without any scars.

FUNGAL INFECTIONS (DERMATOPHYTOSES)

Fungal infections such as tinea pedis (athlete's foot) (Fig. 36–6*A*), tinea cruris (jock itch) (see Fig. 36–6*B*), and tinea corporis (ringworm) (see Fig. 36–6*C*) are extremely common. These pathogens tend to live in the "dead tissues" such as the surface keratin layer, hair, or nails and cause almost no inflammation in the underlying skin. These fungi species can invade the skin where the skin has been damaged. All of these lesions are characterized by an distinct border and are marked by scaling with a clear area in the center of the lesion.

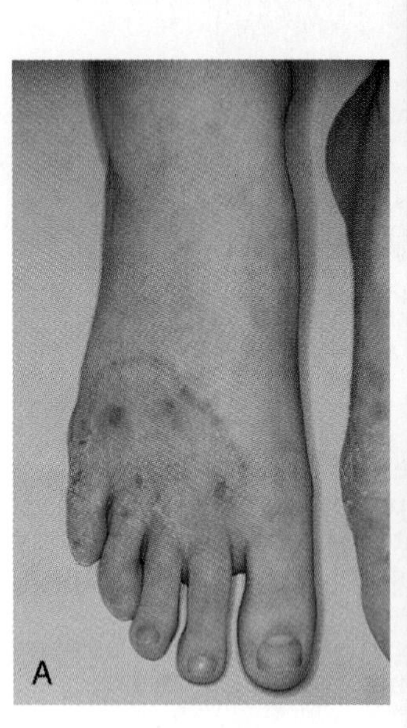

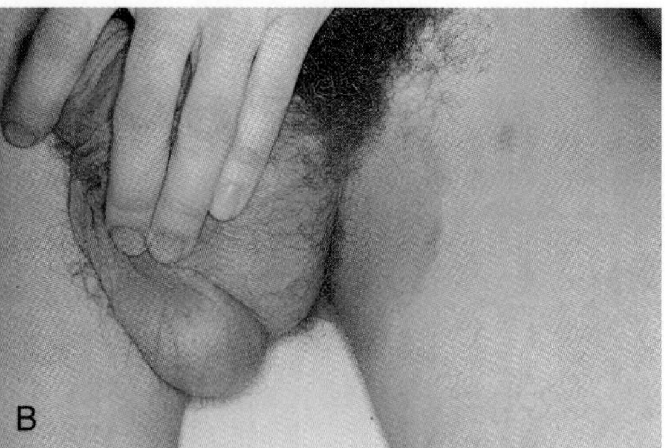

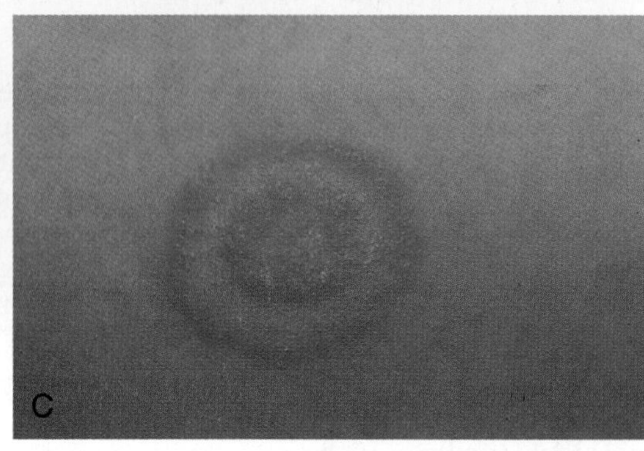

FIGURE 36–6 Fungal Infections. *A,* Tinea pedia. *B,* Tinea cruris. *C,* Tinea corporis. (From Callen J, Greer K, Hood A, et al: Color Atlas of Dermatology. Philadelphia, WB Saunders, 1993.)

Treatment may consist of topical and/or oral antibiotics depending on the severity of the infection. The patient needs to be advised to keep the area clean and dry and to wear loose clothing over the infected area if at all possible. All forms of dermatophytosis can be persistent and become chronic. You can help the patient by explaining how to clean and dry the affected area and why this is necessary to correct the condition.

Memory Jogger

 *Name three common forms of fungal infections.*

SCABIES AND PEDICULOSIS

Scabies (itch mite) and pediculosis (lice) are the two most common parasites to infest individuals. Scabies is a tiny organism, barely visible with the eye, that burrows into the epidermis (Fig. 36–7). Pediculosis consists of three species of lice: the head louse (Fig. 36–8*A*), the body louse, and the pubic louse (Fig. 36–8*B*). Both infestations are highly contagious. Diagnosis is done by looking for the infected skin area for scabies and looking for **nits** on the hair shafts when checking for lice. Patients describe symptoms of intense itching, possible body rash, and a sensation of something crawling on their skin.

Treatment consists of ridding the body of the parasite, controlling the itching, and disinfecting the home environment to prevent reinfestation. This may be done by using medicated shampoo, cream, and/or lotion. If a secondary infection has begun, antibiotics may also be prescribed. All family members and other individuals who have had direct personal contact with the infested person must also be treated.

You can assist the patient through explanations regarding the washing and/or dry-cleaning of all clothing and bedding. Washing must be done in hot water. If clothes worn by the infested person have been placed back into the closet, all items in the closet must be washed or dry-cleaned. Furniture and carpets will need to be washed or vacuumed; and, if possible, both should be sprayed with a surface-disinfecting cleaning agent.

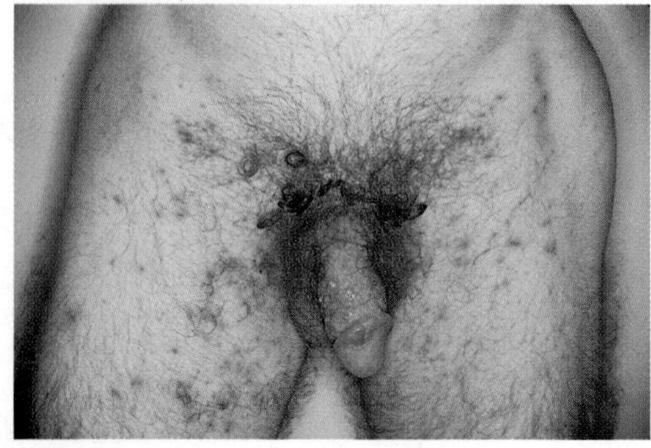

FIGURE 36–7 Scabies rash. (From Callen J, Greer K, Hood A, et al: Color Atlas of Dermatology. Philadelphia, WB Saunders, 1993.)

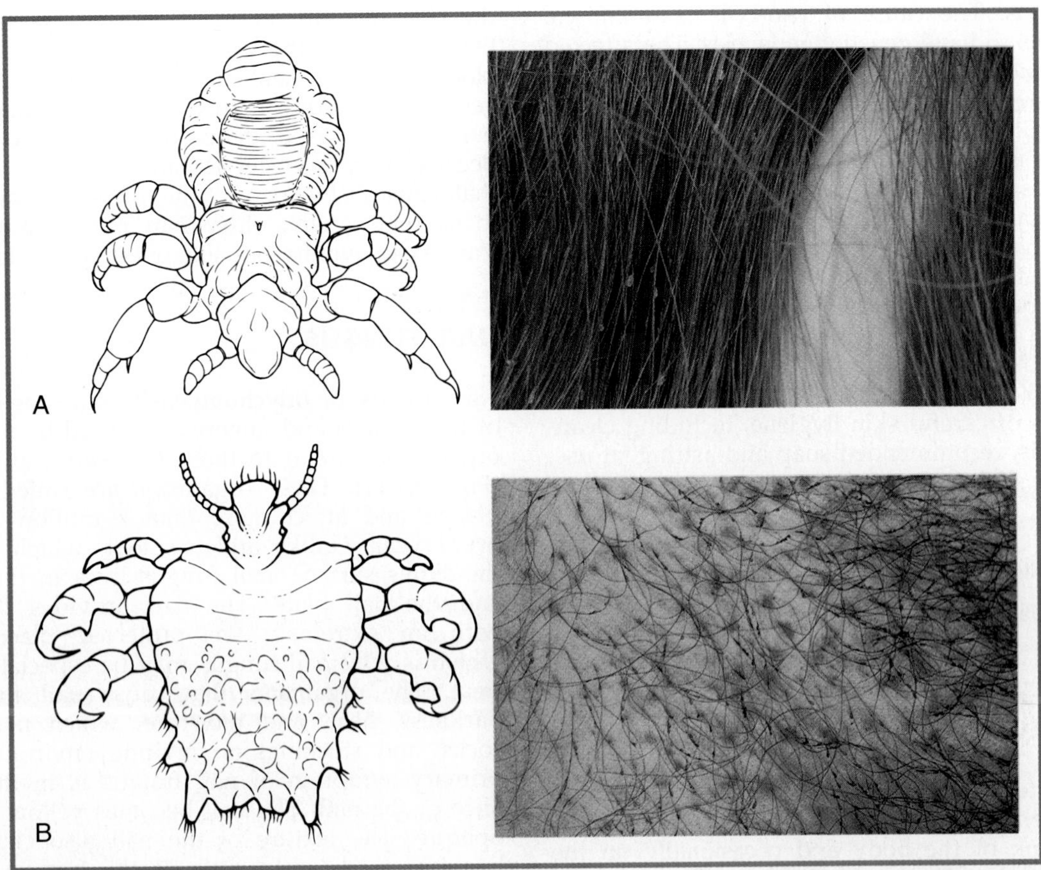

FIGURE 36–8 Pediculosis. *A, Pediculus humanus capitis* (head louse) and lice in hair. *B, Phthirus pubis* (pubic, or crab, louse) and pubic lice rash. (From Callen J, Greer K, Hood A, et al: Color Atlas of Dermatology. Philadelphia, WB Saunders, 1993.)

Memory Jogger

What is a nit?

ECZEMA

Eczema is a collection of different forms of inflammatory skin diseases. Eczema is characterized by chronic skin cell inflammation, blood vessel dilatation, and edema. Generally, eczema causes the patient to scratch the skin continuously, and this scratching causes scales, crusts, and oozing of the skin. Eczema can usually be traced to a specific irritant or allergen. Occasionally, a drug-induced systemic rash may also be diagnosed as eczema.

Because its cause may be different from one patient to another, the diagnosis is based on the signs and symptoms. The patient may be asked to make a list of all of the possible items that might be responsible. If you are working with the patient in making out this list, you might ask the patient to go through a daily routine from the moment the alarm goes off. Then with every activity, help the patient pinpoint a change. For example, has the patient used a different toothpaste, shower soap, makeup, shaving cream, or deodorant, different laundry products, new underwear, and so on. Finding out the causative agent can be a real problem.

PSORIASIS

Psoriasis is a chronic skin disease that produces discrete pink or red lesions covered with silvery scaling (Fig. 36–9). The disease may begin at any age and is

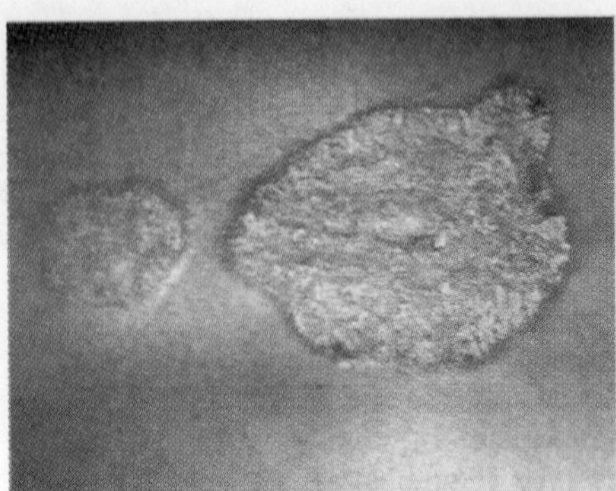

FIGURE 36–9 Psoriasis. (From Lookingbill D, Marks J: Principles of Dermatology, 2nd ed. Philadelphia, WB Saunders, 1993.)

noninfectious. The cause of psoriasis is unknown, but it seems to have genetic tendencies. The affected skin is typically dry, cracked, and encrusted. The lesions may appear on the scalp, chest, buttocks, and extremities.

Psoriasis is diagnosed by observations of the skin, a careful patient history, and/or a skin biopsy. The treatment can only be **palliative** because there is no cure for the disease. Exposure to ultraviolet light may retard the cell production, and coal tar preparations may be applied to the affected areas. The physician may also order corticosteroid creams, low-dosage antihistamines, oatmeal baths, and open, wet dressings. You may be asked to educate the patient in methods of careful skin hygiene, including cleaning methods, recommended soap and astringent use, and proper skin-drying techniques.

Memory Jogger

 *Is psoriasis an acute infectious disease?*

HERPES ZOSTER (SHINGLES)

Herpes zoster is an acute inflammatory disorder that is characterized by highly painful vesicle eruptions on the trunk of the body and occasionally on the face (Fig. 36–10). The lesions occur on the portion of the skin located above the nerve pathway that has been infected by the virus. Herpes zoster primarily affects adults older than 50 years of age.

The onset of the disorder is usually pain along the nerve pathway and then in approximately 3 days the lesions will appear. The lesions begin as a red rash, and in a short time period the vesicles appear. The site of these lesions is usually on one side of the truck of the body, and the area around the site may be intensely painful.

Diagnosis is through the characteristic pattern of painful lesions and may be confirmed by isolating the virus in cell cultures. It can also be detected by the presence of the varicella-zoster antibodies in the blood. The treatment may consist of sedatives, analgesics, and **antipruritics.** Antibiotics may also be used if there is evidence of a secondary infection. Because herpes zoster is caused by the same virus that causes chickenpox, the physician may recommend that patients older than 50 be vaccinated with Varivax to avoid a possible outbreak of shingles.

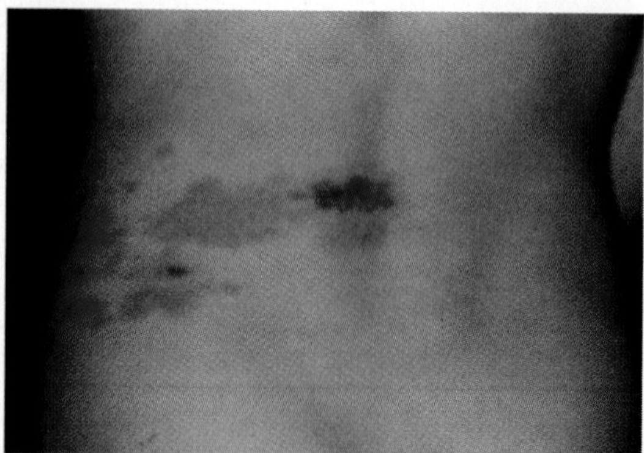

FIGURE 36–10 Herpes zoster (shingles). (From Callen J, Greer K, Hood A, et al: Color Atlas of Dermatology. Philadelphia, WB Saunders, 1993.)

NAIL FUNGUS

Nail fungus, or **onychomycosis,** is a fungal infection of the toenails and fingernails caused by microscopic organisms, similar to those that cause athlete's foot (Fig. 36–11). These organisms are called **dermatophytes** and affect more than 7 million Americans every year. Unlike athlete's foot, which occurs on the skin's surface, nail fungus lives in the nail bed and the nail plate. The nail provides the fungus with an extremely well-protected place to live, which is why nail fungus may be especially hard to treat. The organisms that cause nail fungus like darkness, heat, and moisture, which make shoes, socks, and stockings an inviting environment. The primary symptom of nail fungus is in the appearance of the nail. The nail becomes yellow, white, or **opaque.** The texture of the nail also changes and becomes thick and brittle. If the fungus has been present for a long time, the nail can even become twisted or distorted. Occasionally the patient will experience pain, but the psychological effects of unsightly nails are much greater.

Diagnosis is done by inspecting the nail for the classic symptoms described, but the physician may want to clip off a piece of the infected nail and send it to the laboratory for analysis and confirmation of the causative organism. The most effective way to treat nail fungus appears to be with new medications taken orally (e.g., terbinafine [Lamisil]). These medications attack the fungus from the inside out, which is something that no topical medication can do. Other treatments may include removing the affected nail with surgery, laser, or chemicals or ap-

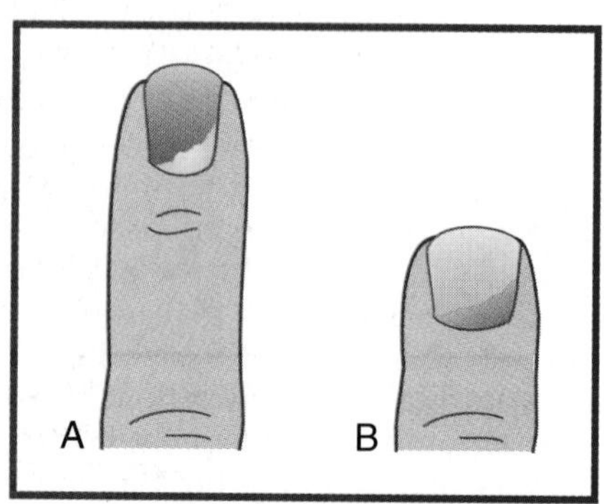

FIGURE 36–11 *A* and *B*, Nail fungus.

plying medications such as lotions or ointments directly to the affected nail.

Memory Jogger

10 *Describe the appearance of nail fungus.*

BENIGN AND MALIGNANT NEOPLASMS

A **neoplasm** is an abnormal growth characterized by uncontrolled cell multiplication. Neoplasms of the skin may be benign or malignant. Examples of benign tumors include birthmarks and moles. Occasionally, a tumor may be a benign tumor that is said to have a predisposition to **cancer,** which means it can go from the benign state to a cancerous one. Whenever a tumor-like mass is discovered, the physician may want to do a biopsy on the lesion to establish the type of cells involved.

The most common skin cancers are basal cell and squamous cell carcinomas. Malignant melanoma is a third type. It is not seen as frequently but is the most serious of the three types.

Basal cell carcinoma is most frequently seen in blond, fair-complected males and is the most frequently seen form of skin cancer. The most common sites are areas of the body that are exposed to the sun. It appears as a painless, smooth, small, waxy, translucent nodule (Fig. 36–12).

Squamous cell carcinoma is more serious because it has a tendency to metastasize. Like the basal cell, it is most frequently seen in fair-skinned, blond males. It appears as a firm, red nodule with visible scales and may ulcerate and form a crust (Fig. 36–13).

Malignant melanoma is composed of abnormal melanocytes. The incidence of malignant melanoma has doubled in the past 10 years and results in more deaths than all other skin diseases. It appears as a brown or black, flat lesion that will change in size and color with time. It tends to have irregular edges, be circular, and be slightly elevated (Fig. 36–14).

All skin cancers are diagnosed by their appearance, and confirmation is done through biopsy. The treatment depends on the type, level of invasion, and location. The physician may choose to remove the tumor or irradicate the tumor with **cryosurgery, electrodesiccation,** or through the application of chemotherapeutic agents.

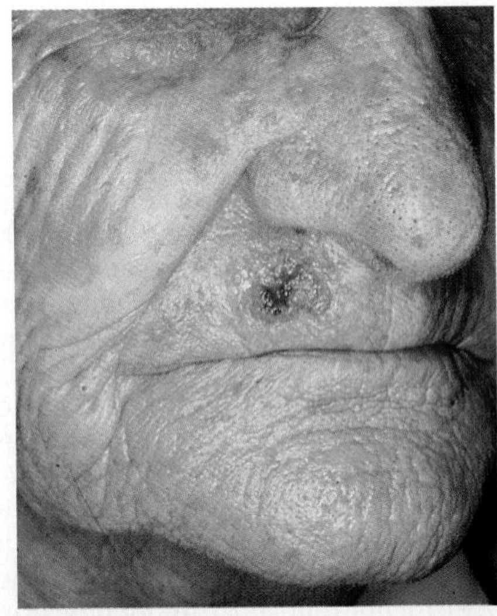

FIGURE 36–13 Squamous cell carcinoma. (Modified from Damjanov I: Pathology for the Health-Related Professions. Philadelphia, WB Saunders, 1996.)

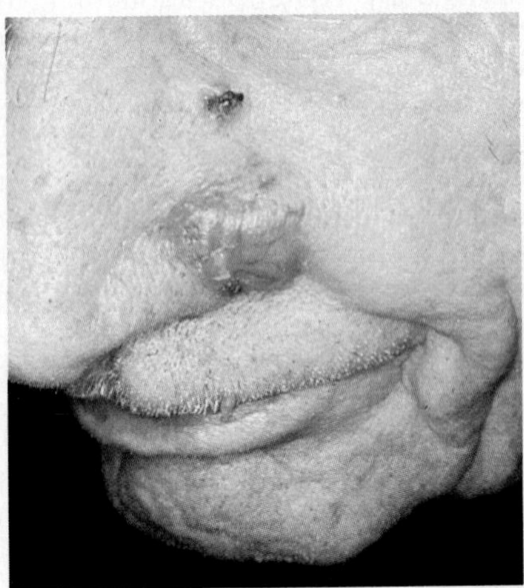

FIGURE 36–12 Basal cell carcinoma. (Modified from Damjanov I: Pathology for the Health-Related Professions. Philadelphia, WB Saunders, 1996.)

Memory Jogger

11 *What is the most common type of skin cancer?*

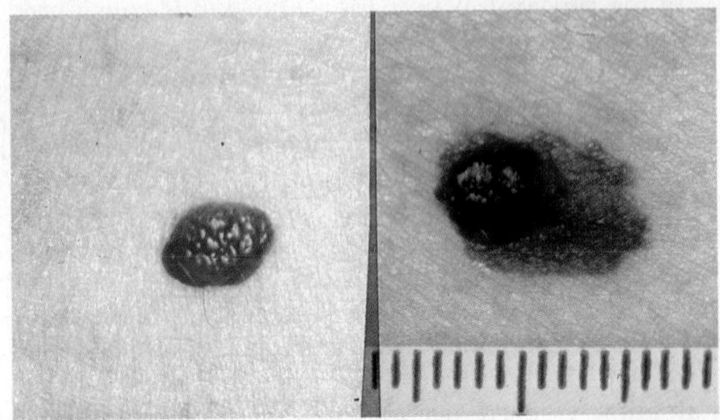

FIGURE 36–14 Pigmented skin lesions. *Left,* Benign pigmented nevus (mole). *Right,* Malignant melanoma. (Courtesy of the National Cancer Institute, Bethesda, MD.)

The Medical Assistant's Role in Dermatologic Procedures

The skin reflects both internal and external contact reactions. It also acts as a mirror reflecting aging changes that proceed in all of the organs of the body. Because the aging changes in the skin and hair can be viewed directly, these changes carry profound psychologic impact. For many people, self-esteem is linked to a youthful appearance. As you are preparing the patient for a dermatologic examination, allow the patient to express his or her anxieties. The skin holds information about the body's circulation, nutritional status, and signs of systemic diseases. Normality of the skin depends on the person's age, sex, and physical and emotional health.

The impairments that most frequently bring a patient to the dermatologist's office are the cosmetic disfigurements caused by a skin disease, pain and **pruritus,** and interference with sensations or movements. The possibility that a skin lesion is the result of a systemic condition is sometimes a major concern.

ASSISTING WITH THE EXAMINATION

The dermatologist will examine the visible top layer of skin of the entire body, beginning with the scalp and continuing through to the soles of the feet. This will also include the genital area. The skin assessment is basically accomplished through inspection followed with detailed examination by palpation, diascopy, and special tests. The *diascope* is a glass plate held against the skin to permit observation of changes produced in the underlying areas by the pressure. Inspection may include using a magnifying lens and a bright light to closely examine a suspicious lesion or growth. You may be instructed to take photographs of the affected area or to chart measurement results of the lesion to aid in determining future changes.

In the physical examination, the skin is considered a separate organ of the body. Concerns include abnormal coloring such as redness, **cyanosis, pallor,** erythema, **leukoderma,** or excessive brown patches. **Jaundice** may indicate an increase in the level of **bilirubin** in the blood. Decreased pigmentation is found in **vitiligo,** which is the acquired loss of melanin and is characterized by white patches. Lesions, ulcers, and bruises may be the result of pathologic conditions. Localized red or purple changes may be the result of vascular neoplasms, birthmarks, or subcutaneous hemorrhages (**petechiae** and **ecchymoses**). Palpation is used to confirm and amplify findings seen by inspection. Inspection and palpation are interrelated in confirming diagnoses. Palpatory findings may include texture, elasticity, or edema.

Draping a patient for a skin examination depends on the area to be examined. Remember to expose the area adequately but protect the patient's privacy. Try to make the patient as comfortable as possible and offer support when it is needed.

Memory Jogger

What equipment would you have available for the dermatologist for skin examination?

ASSISTING WITH TESTING PROCEDURES

Wood's Light Examination

One dermatology test performed in the dermatologist's office is the *Wood's light examination.* This is a visual examination of the skin made in a darkened room with the ultraviolet lamp (black light). The lamp is directed 4 to 5 inches from the patient's skin, and abnormalities in the skin and hair appear as fluorescent colors. Differences in the ultraviolet light absorption and fluorescence bring out characteristics of some mycologic skin diseases, such as *tinea capitis (ringworm).*

Allergy Skin Testing

Scratch Test

The scratch and puncture tests may be performed on any smooth surface of the skin, but the arm and back are most popular. The arm is safer (either the outer surface of the upper arm or the anterior surface of the lower arm), because a serious reaction may be limited by the application of a tourniquet above the site. However, the back is favored in infants and in young children because of the large area of skin available. It is also easier to immobilize the child in this position. The skin surface is labeled or numbered in rows 1½ to 2 inches apart. A short scratch is made with a needle or lancet, and a drop of various **allergens** is placed on each scratch or puncture. Fifty or more tests may be done at one time, and a certain pattern is followed so that the site of each allergen is identified (Fig. 36–15).

A reaction usually occurs within 10 to 30 minutes. If the reaction is positive, a **wheal** (hive) will be formed at the site of the scratch. The interpretation of the test should always be based on a comparison of this reaction with that of the control, which is a scratch with a plain base fluid free of any allergy-producing extract.

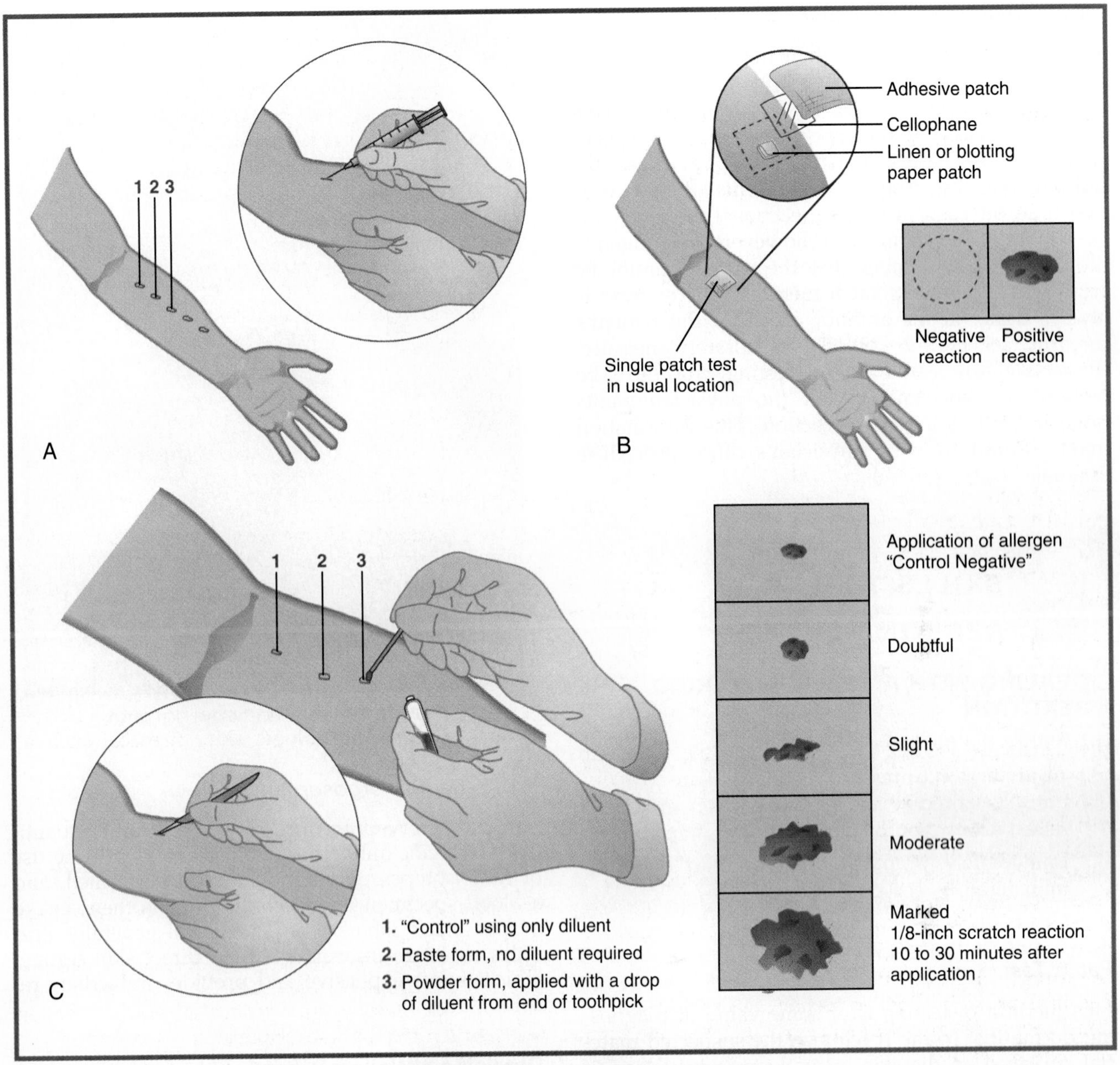

FIGURE 36–15 Allergy skin testing.

The interpretation, or reading, of the skin tests is performed by the physician or a trained technician. Reactions are commonly graded from 2 to 4. No precise definition of a reaction can be given, and indeed the intensity may vary among individuals. However, as a general rule, a 2 reaction implies a wheal that is definitely larger than that of the control. A larger wheal is interpreted as a 3, whereas the presence of pseudopods (finger-like extensions around the periphery of the wheal) may be read as a 4. Carefully wipe off the extract to stop the reaction when a strong reaction is occurring. Erythema, or reddening, around the wheal is usually disregarded in the interpretations. Frequently, the large or significant reactions are accompanied by local itching.

Memory Jogger

13 *What skin area(s) are usually used for the scratch test on an adult?*

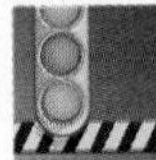

Safety Alert: Patients are to remain in the office for a minimum of 30 minutes after the completion of the allergy testing procedure in case of a delayed allergic reaction.

Intradermal (Intracutaneous) Test

This test is more accurate than the scratch test. Extracts are injected into the skin, with the usual sterile technique, in a dose of 0.1 to 0.2 mL. This method is used for the tuberculin (purified protein derivative [PPD]) test and the Valley Fever coccidioidomycosis test. Ten to 15 tests may be done at one time on each arm. The reaction time is identical to that of the scratch test; however, the antigen is more dilute. Remember that the extract cannot be wiped off as in the scratch method. This method is always done on the anterior aspect of the patient's forearm (see Fig. 36–15). This is a safety measure. If you are responsible for the testing procedure, be certain that you know what the physician wants done if there is a severe reaction. This information maybe found in your physician's office procedure manual.

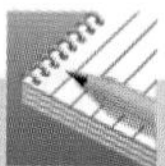

SKILLS AND RESPONSIBILITIES

DEALING WITH A SEVERE ALLERGIC REACTION

1 Notify the physician immediately.
2 Apply a blood pressure cuff and inflate to 100 mm Hg directly above the reaction area to retard absorption of the extract.
3 Immediately prepare epinephrine to be administered by the physician.

Patch Test

This method of testing is of some value in diagnosing dermatitis. In the patch test, the suspected material is placed on the skin (near the original lesion, if possible), covered with a small square of cellophane, and held down with strips of adhesive or transparent tape or even collodion (Fig. 36–16). Twenty to 30 tests may be done at one time. The reaction is read within 1 to 4 days.

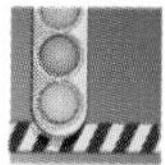

Safety Alert: Allergy skin testing is usually done by a technician trained in this procedure with a physician present in the facility. The possibility of anaphylactic shock must always be considered as a risk factor.

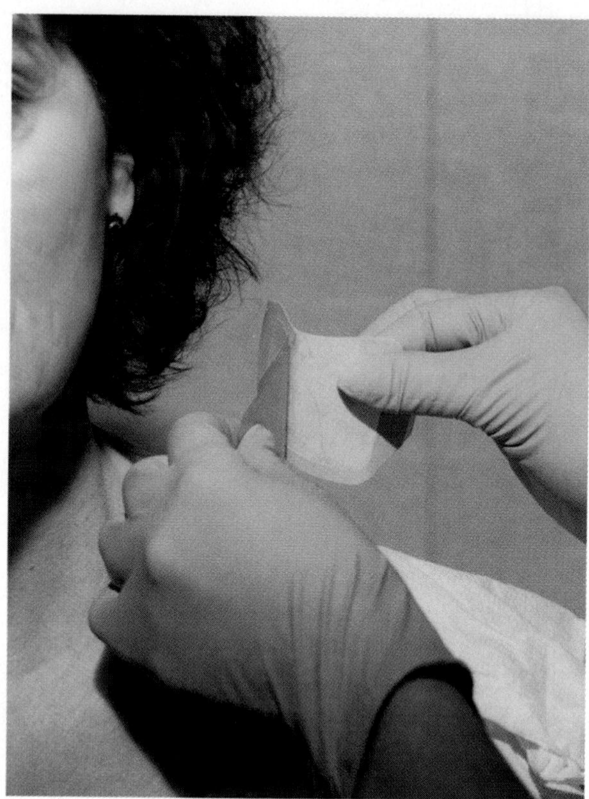

FIGURE 36–16 Transdermal skin patch.

RAST (Radioallergosorbent Test)

This laboratory procedure measures minute quantities of specific antibodies against foods with the use of radioisotopes. A venipuncture is performed, and a blood specimen is collected, which is then sent to a specialized laboratory. The RAST generally provides no more information than direct skin testing, which is less expensive and provides immediate results.

Obtaining a Wound Culture

A wound culture is obtained to diagnose bacterial or fungal pathogens, which are the causative agents (see Procedure 36–1). A sufficient sample of the organism must be collected to grow a representative culture. This is accomplished by either swabbing the wound with a sterile Dacron swab or **aspirating** the wound area with a syringe and needle.

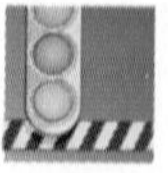

Safety Alert: Do not use cotton swabs because cotton may inhibit the growth of streptococcus.

PROCEDURE 36-1
Obtaining Wound Exudate for Culture

GOAL
To obtain an adequate, noncontaminated sample for culture.

EQUIPMENT AND SUPPLIES
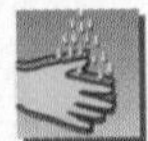

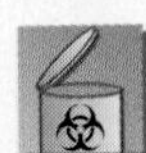
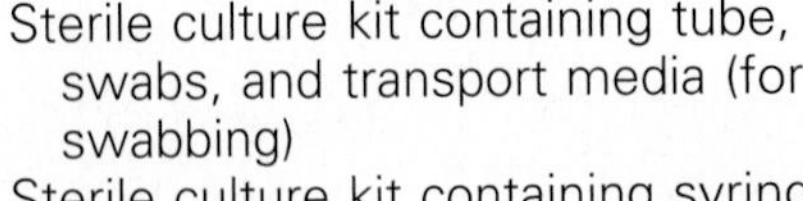

Sterile culture kit containing tube, swabs, and transport media (for swabbing)
Sterile culture kit containing syringe and transport media (for aspirating)
Gauze flats
Recommended wound cleansing solution
Clean sterile dressing

PROCEDURAL STEPS
1 Wash your hands, gather supplies (Figure 1), and don gloves and face protection.
PURPOSE: Infection control.

2 Remove dressing from the wound and dispose of it in biohazard waste container.
PURPOSE: Infection control.

3 Observe the wound and make note of the color, odor, and amount of exudate present.
PURPOSE: Information will be noted for the physician on the patient's record when procedure is completed.

4 Swabbing. Remove the swab from the culture kit, insert the swab into the wound, and saturate it with the exudate (Figure 2).

5 Aspirating. Remove the syringe from the kit, insert the tip into the wound exudate, and draw back the plunger, drawing the exudate up into the syringe.

Continued

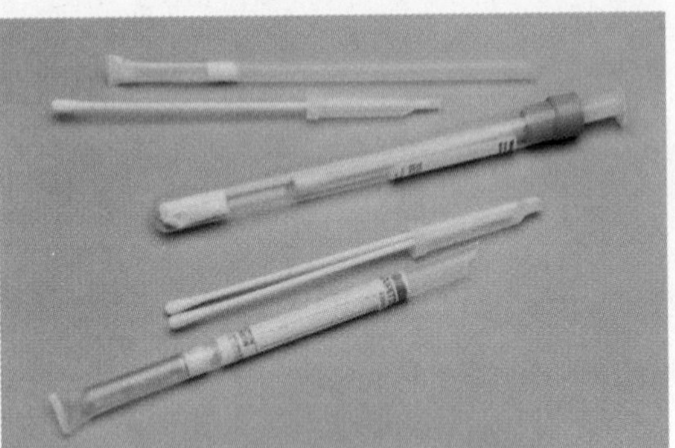
FIGURE 1

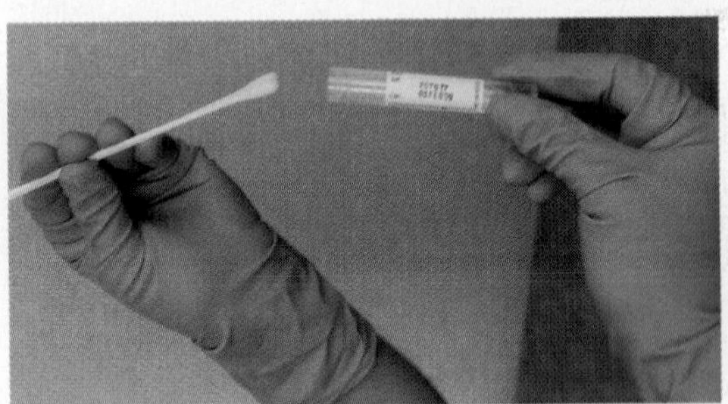
FIGURE 2

PROCEDURE 36-1 (CONTINUED)
Obtaining Wound Exudate for Culture

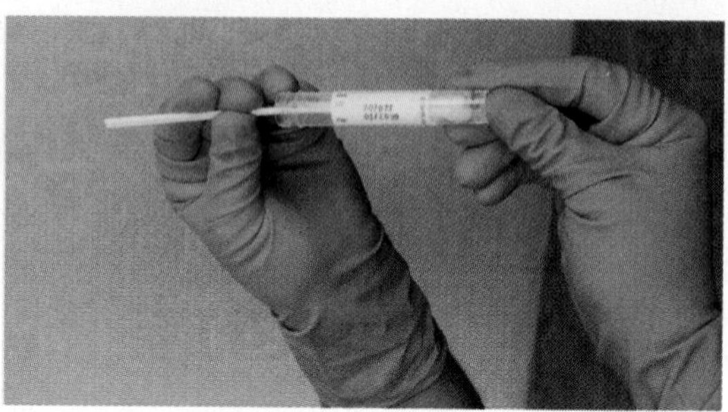

FIGURE 3

6 Place the swab into the culture tube and crush the transport media ampule, which is in the transport tube, by squeezing the walls of the transport tube slightly. Or place the exudate-filled syringe directly into the transport tube (Figure 3).
7 Label the culture tube accurately.
8 Clean the wound as ordered by the physician and apply a clean sterile dressing to the area. See Chapter 52 for dressing procedure.
9 Clean area, disposing of all waste materials in biohazard waste container. Remove gloves and wash your hands.
PURPOSE: Infection control.
10 Place culture tube in the laboratory collection area. Chart the procedure and all wound data on the patient's record.
PURPOSE: A procedure is considered not done until it is recorded.

Assisting with a Tissue Biopsy

There are three methods for obtaining a small piece of tissue to be examined under a microscope for differentiation and diagnosis. In an excision biopsy, the entire lesion may be removed for analysis such as in a wart or mole removal. A punch biopsy involves the removal of a small section from a designated location within the lesion, usually the center is the optimal site. This can be done with a punch instrument or a large-gauge needle such as in a breast biopsy. A shave biopsy is done with a scalpel by cutting or shaving off the growth or lesion just above the skin line. This may be used to biopsy a possible squamous cell carcinoma lesion.

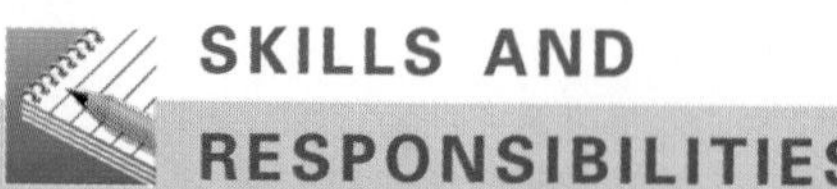

SKILLS AND RESPONSIBILITIES

ASSISTING WITH A TISSUE BIOPSY

1 Assemble all of the supplies needed for the procedure.
2 Prepare the patient by explaining the procedure.
3 Prepare the site of the biopsy according to office protocol.
4 Assist the physician as needed.
5 Label the sample container and prepare it for transport to the testing laboratory. Remember to include the laboratory request forms.
6 Clean the procedure area, properly disposing of all waste materials.

Memory Jogger

 14 *Name three types of skin biopsies.*

Administration of Dermatologic Medications

The skin is an important route of administration for drugs. Many topical drugs are applied to the skin as a cream, ointment, or liquid. Most do not significantly penetrate the skin layers, and thus tend to cause fewer side effects than systemic drugs (those taken orally or injected). Systemic drugs are taken up by the circulation and widely distributed through the body. Also available are transdermal skin patches, worn on the chest or behind the ear, for example, which release controlled amounts of drug (Fig. 36–16). Subcutaneous injections of certain drugs are given to deeper layers of skin, where they may be absorbed by the circulation. Finally, solid pellets containing hormones or other agents are sometimes implanted under the skin, where the drug is absorbed slowly over weeks or months. For information regarding the administering of medications see Chapter 49.

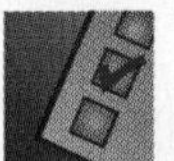

PATIENT EDUCATION

There are many areas of patient education within the dermatology field. If you enjoy patient teaching, you will be able to find a long list of topics regarding the care of the skin. Skin care products are advertised in the newspaper, on billboards, in magazines, and on television. People are willing to try almost anything to keep a youthful appearance. Consult the dermatologist you work for and get recommendations of skin care procedures that the office can recommend to the patients. Sometimes skin care companies will give you samples of their products if you write and tell them that your office recommends a certain product's use to patients. Patients enjoy receiving samples and encouragement to try a new skin care technique.

Another area of patient education is on the effects of sunlight on the skin. Some may be shocked to learn that sunburn constitutes first- and second-degree burns. Obtain literature showing how ultraviolet rays cause premature aging and may cause cancerous lesions later in life. You can explain the meaning of sun protective factor (SPF) on suntanning lotions. Most sunscreen products contain para-aminobenzoic acid, which causes allergy in many people. Tanning beds and sun lamps should be avoided, especially by those who have a skin disorder or by those who are on certain medications, owing to the ultraviolet light concentration.

If the patient needs help in meal planning due to food allergy, you can help by recommending a nutritional center or a dietetic service that may be of help, or for other types of allergy you could recommend other possible outside assistance and resource information centers.

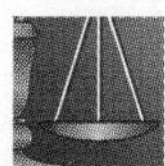

LEGAL AND ETHICAL ISSUES

When working in the dermatology office, you will hear many patients express concerns regarding a skin disorder. Expressing their concerns, knowing that you are listening, is always helpful, but be careful when offering encouragement about the course and outcome of their treatment. No treatment can restore youth. The improvement achieved may be slow and gradual. Keep your encouragement on a positive level. Compliment the patient on small improvements, but let the physician describe the possible course and outcome of the prescribed treatment.

CRITICAL THINKING

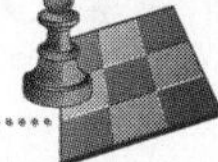

1 Why is it unwise to tell the patient that if the dermatologist's treatment is followed exactly as prescribed the patient's condition will be completely corrected?

2 What suggestions could you make to a parent who has a son with chronic bouts of athlete's foot?

3 A patient is in for a punch biopsy of the breast and is very apprehensive about the possible results. How might you assist the patient?

HOW DID I DO? Answers to Memory Joggers

1 The skin is fairly thin over protected areas such as the eyelids.

2 Keratin forms a protective barrier that helps control water loss from the body.

3 The subcutaneous layer thins with aging.

4 Acne cysts are primary lesions.

5 The maximum heat temperature is 105° F.

6 Scratching and pressing on acne lesions tends to cause infections.

7 Three common forms of fungal infections are athlete's foot, jock itch, and ringworm.

8 A nit is the egg of the louse.

9 Psoriasis is chronic and noninfectious.

10 Nail fungus causes the nail to become discolored or opaque, twisted, and/or distorted.

11 The most common type of skin cancer is basal cell carcinoma.

12 Equipment that the dermatologist may use in a skin inspection includes gloves, diascope, bright light, magnifying lens, camera, and tape measure or metric ruler.

13 Areas used for an adult scratch test are the outer surface of the upper arms and the anterior surface of the lower arms.

14 Three types of biopsies are the excision, punch, and shave.

Assisting in Orthopedic Medicine

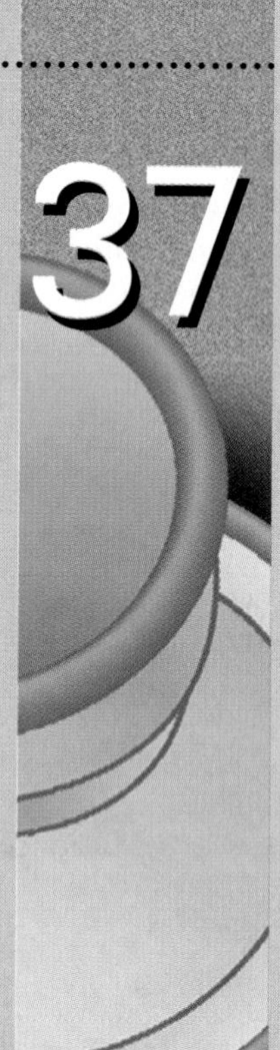

OUTLINE

LEARNING OBJECTIVES

Cognitive: On successful completion of this chapter you should be able to:

1. Describe the principal structures of the musculoskeletal system.
2. Identify five types of bones and give an example of each type.
3. Describe three forms of muscles.
4. Differentiate between tendons, bursae, and ligaments.
5. List and describe the major disorders of the system.
6. Describe the different types of fractures.
7. Explain types of diagnostic procedures used.
8. Describe four types of ambulatory devices.
9. Explain the uses for cold applications.
10. Define and spell vocabulary terms.

Performance: On successful completion of this chapter you should be able to:

1. Prepare and assist with cast application.
2. Accurately apply a sling to immobilize an injury.
3. Properly apply an ice bag.

VOCABULARY

crepitation Dry, crackling sound or sensation produced by the grating of the ends of a fractured bone

diaphysis Portion of the long bone between the ends enclosing the medullary cavity

epiphyses Ends of the long bone, which are wider than the shaft of the bone

gait Manner or style of walking

goniometer Instrument for measuring muscle angles

kyphosis Abnormally increased convex curve of the thoracic spine; also called *hunchback*

lordosis Forward curvature of the lumbar spine

luxation Total dislocation of the bone from the joint

malaise Feeling of uneasiness or indisposition

medullary cavity Inner portion of the bone that contains the bone marrow

reduction Correction of a fracture, dislocation, or hernia

scoliosis Lateral deviation in the normal vertical curve of the spine

subluxation Partial dislocation of the bone from the joint

synovial Pertaining to synovia, which is a clear fluid found in the joint cavities that facilitates smooth painless movement

The orthopedic specialist treats diseases and disorders of the musculoskeletal system but primarily deals with bone diseases and disorders. Rheumatologists are physicians who treat joint diseases and disorders. Osteopaths are doctors of osteopathic medicine and base their practice on the belief that the body is capable of healing itself when the body is healthy and bones are in proper position. Chiropractors are neither physicians nor osteopaths, and they use physical means to manipulate the spinal column, believing that disease is caused by pressure on nerves.

The musculoskeletal system consists of the body's bones, joints, muscles, and supportive connective tissue (cartilage, tendons, and ligaments). This system provides for

- Internal organ protection
- Support to stand erect
- Movement
- Production of the red blood cell in the bone marrow
- Mineral storage

Memory Jogger

What are the principal structures of the musculoskeletal system?

Anatomy and Physiology of the Musculoskeletal System

BONES

The body contains 206 bones, which make up about one tenth of the body weight. The bones provide a framework that encases and protects the body's vital internal organs. A bone's size is directly related to the mobility and weight-bearing function of that bone. In some cases, bone size and shape are also related to the protection of underlying internal organs and tissues. For example, ribs surround and protect the lungs, heart, liver, and kidneys, while the skull protects the delicate tissue of the brain. The 33 vertebrae of the spinal column shields the spinal cord and protects this pathway for nervous impulses to and from the brain. Bones in the pelvic girdle protect the bladder as well as the reproductive organs of the female (Fig. 37–1).

In the body are long, short, flat, rounded, and irregularly shaped bones. The long bone is a shaft **(diaphysis)** with two large ends **(epiphyses)** (Fig. 37–2). The epiphyses of one bone will join the epiphyses of another bone to form a joint. Cartilage covers each epiphysis to lesson the stress and friction on the bone ends during movement and weight bearing. The thickness of the cartilage layer varies, depending on the amount of stress placed on that particular joint. In the interior portion of the diaphysis is the **medullary cavity,** which contains the bone marrow.

Bones are usually perceived as solid and inert, but they are actually living, changing tissues that are constantly being remodeled. Bone also serves as a repository for vital minerals such as calcium and phosphate, whereas the bone marrow, a spongy core of tissue located in the center of the long and the flat bones, manufacturers new blood cells.

Memory Jogger

Identify the five primary bone shapes.

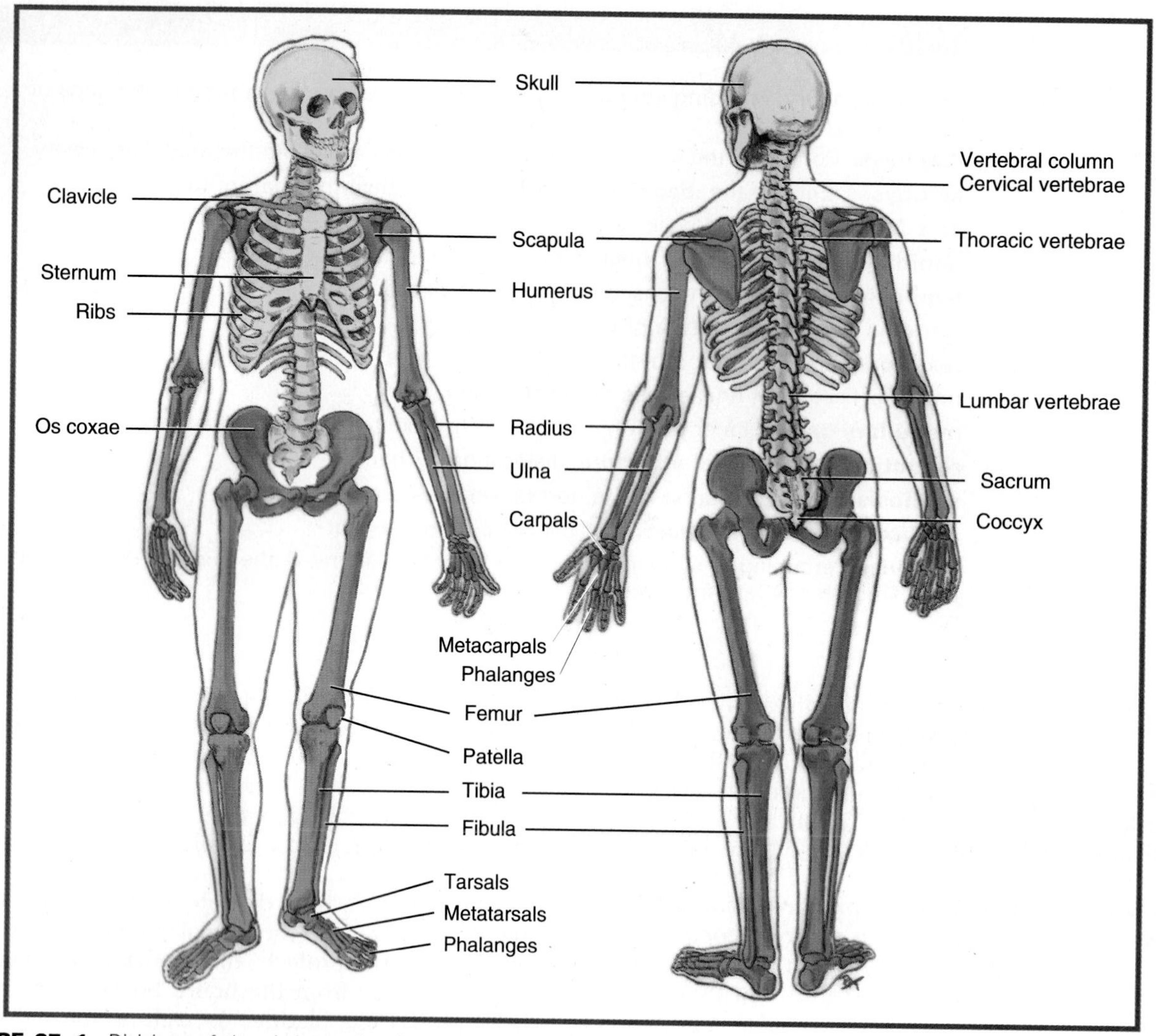

FIGURE 37–1 Divisions of the skeleton showing major bones. (From Applegate EJ: The Anatomy and Physiology Learning System. Philadelphia, WB Saunders, 1995.)

JOINTS

The bones of the body are connected to each other at junctions or joints. Joints can be nonsynovial or **synovial.** In nonsynovial joints, the bones are joined by fibrous cartilage and are immovable, such as the sutures of the skull, or only slightly movable, such as the vertebrae. Synovial joints are freely movable because the bones are separated from each other and are encased in a joint cavity that is filled with a lubricant called synovial fluid. Synovial joints, such as the elbow, are basically hinges that permit movement in only one plane. Other joints such as the hip and shoulder allow a much wider range of motion (Fig. 37–3).

MUSCLES

More than 600 muscles cover the bony skeleton, account for 40% to 50% of the body's weight, and give the human body its distinctive shape. There are three types of muscle: (1) smooth or involuntary muscle, which is found in such internal organs as the stomach, intestines, and bladder, and within the walls of the blood vessels; (2) cardiac muscle, which is found only in the heart; and (3) skeletal, or striated, muscle that controls voluntary movement and is connected to your bones by strong fibrous bands of tissue called tendons (Fig. 37–4). The elastic fibers in skeletal muscles can shorten and lengthen and thus produce movement at the joints. Only skeletal muscles are under voluntary control, which means that they are the only muscles in the body that can be consciously flexed and relaxed.

Memory Jogger

Name the three types of muscles found in the human body.

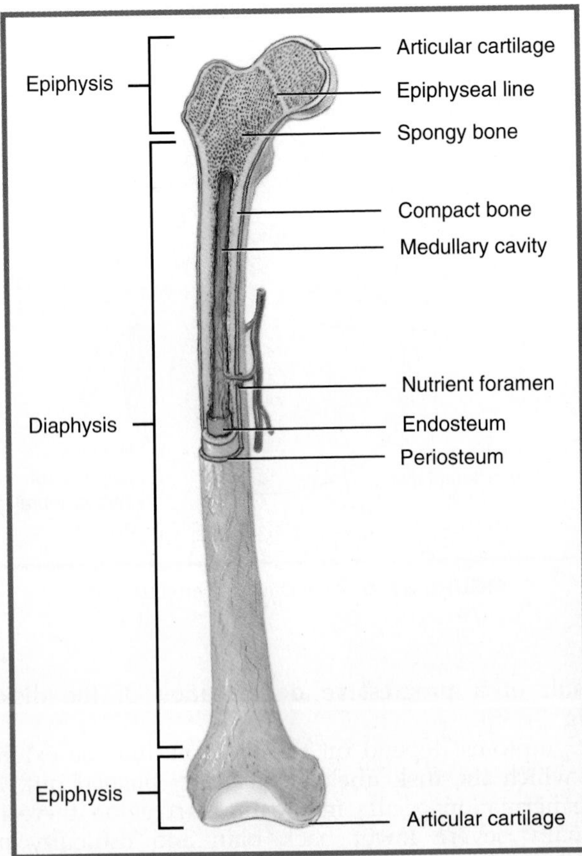

FIGURE 37-2 Cross section of a long bone. (From Applegate EJ: The Anatomy and Physiology Learning System. Philadelphia, WB Saunders, 1995.)

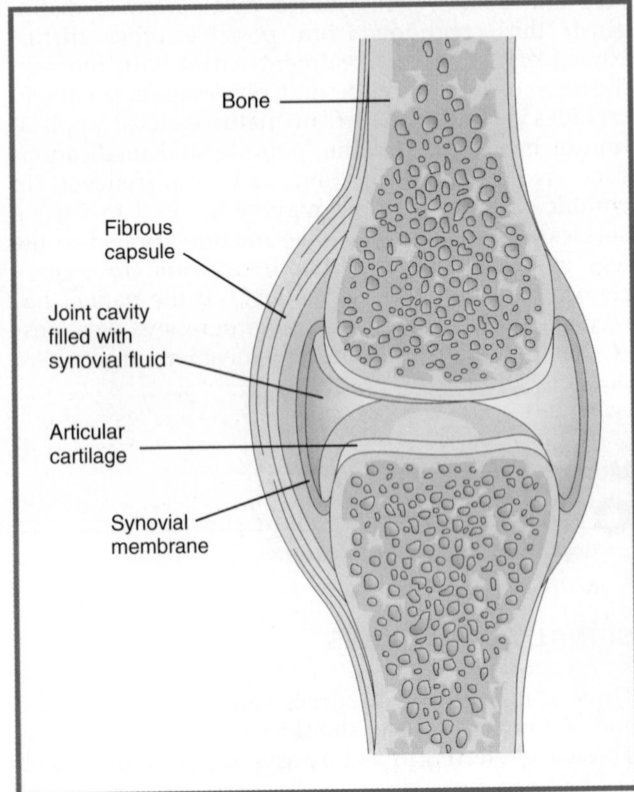

FIGURE 37-3 Synovial joint.

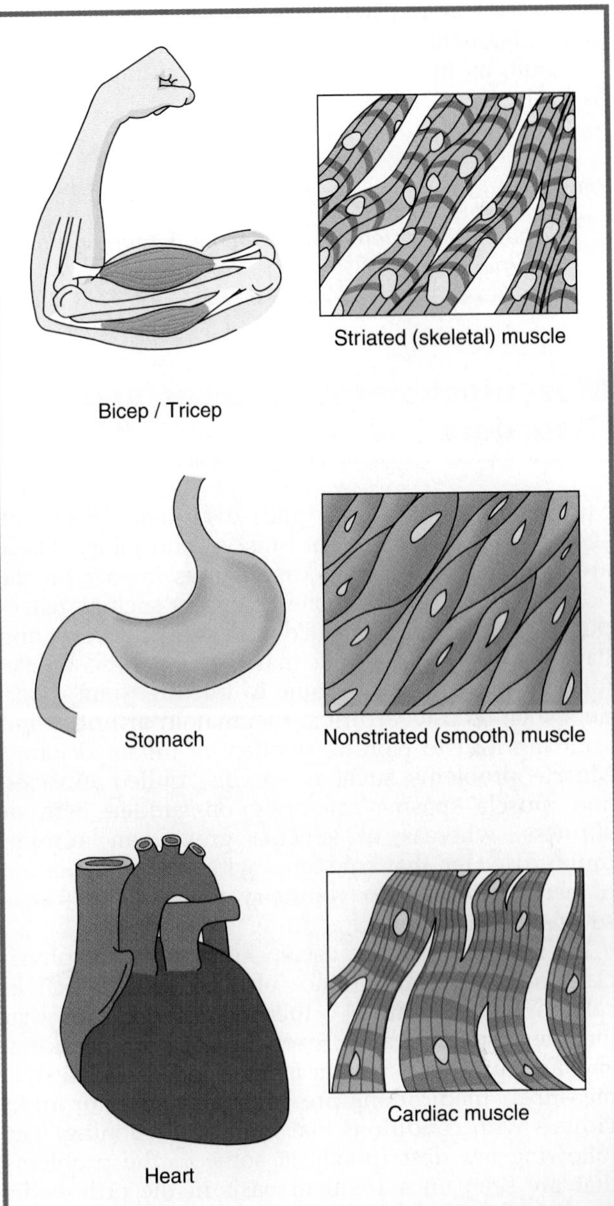

FIGURE 37-4 Types of muscle tissue.

TENDONS, BURSAE, AND LIGAMENTS

A *tendon* is a strong connective tissue sheath that attaches the muscle to a bone. Tendons begin within the muscles, surround the muscle mass, and then bind the whole mass to its accompanying bone. Tendons can be flat or round and can pass between muscles, between bones, or through specialized openings between bones.

Bursae are sacs filled with fluid and act as cushions between bone and tendon or tendon and ligament. The bursae reduce friction and help muscles and tendons glide smoothly over bone.

Ligaments are powerful, strong, fibrous connective tissue that connect bone to bone at the joint and encase the joint capsule. Ligaments support purposeful joint movement and prevent joint movement that would be detrimental to that particular type of joint. Ligaments are found oblique to or parallel to the joint, as in the knee, and surrounding the joint, as in the hip.

Memory Jogger

 *What is the difference between a tendon and a ligament?*

Musculoskeletal Diseases and Disorders

Musculoskeletal disease and disorders affect the skeleton and its system of muscles and joints. These are common and have a tremendous impact on the normal quality of life. Bone disorders such as osteoporosis, osteomalacia (called rickets in children), and Paget's disease are often marked by brittle or deformed bones that are prone to fracture. Joint disorders such as osteoarthritis, rheumatoid arthritis, and gout can lead to painful, swollen, or inflamed joints. Muscle problems such as sprains, pulled muscles, and muscle spasms can bring on sudden pain or stiffness, whereas myasthenia gravis, an autoimmune disorder that interferes with the transmission of nerve impulses to voluntary muscles, can cause severe muscle weakness.

To help maintain musculoskeletal health, physicians stress the importance of eating foods rich in calcium and vitamin D, following a program that includes weight-bearing exercises such as walking, and avoiding smoking. In addition to these lifestyle measures, medications are often required for individuals with conditions that impair functioning. The following are descriptions of some of the problems that are seen on a frequent basis in the orthopedic practice.

Memory Jogger

 *List three items stressed by physicians to help maintain musculoskeletal health.*

HERNIATED DISK

A herniated or ruptured disk occurs when the soft nucleus of an intervertebral disk protrudes through a tear or weakened area in the tough outer disk covering. The condition occurs most often in the lumbar or lower back, occasionally in the neck or cervical area and rarely in the thoracic vertebrae. Herniation of the disks may be caused by injury or by sudden straining with the spine in an unnatural position. The condition may come on gradually as a result of a progressive deterioration of the disks (Fig. 37–5).

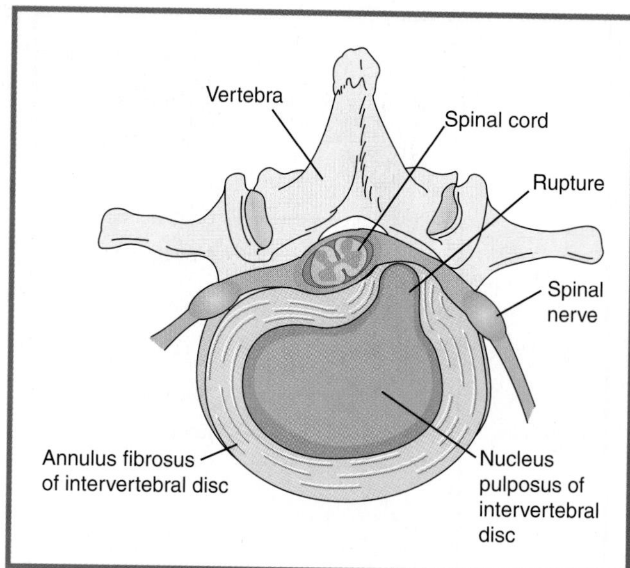

FIGURE 37–5 Herniation of vertebral disk.

Symptoms depend on the location and the extent to which the disk nucleus has been pushed out. If the herniation occurs in the lumbar region there is usually severe lower back pain and difficulty in walking. If a cervical disk is affected, the severe pain will be in the back of the neck radiating down the arms into the fingers.

The physician may want to carefully examine the area and usually will want a myelogram to distinguish this condition from possible other disturbances of the spine. Treatment varies with the seriousness of the herniation. Conservative treatment includes bed rest on a firm mattress, local application of heat for short time periods, and medications such as a muscle relaxant and pain reliever. In chronic cases, the patient may be advised to wear a surgical support and/or have traction applied to the legs and pelvis (for lumbar injury) and to wear a cervical collar (for cervical injury). If the patient has recurring pain, numbness, and progressive weakness of the area, the physician may consider surgery as a possible solution.

Memory Jogger

 *A herniated disk occurs most often in the _______.*

SPINAL CURVATURES

Three abnormal spinal curves can affect the posture and alignment of the shoulders and pelvic girdle. These are referred to as **lordosis** or swayback, which is identified by a deep lumbar curvature; **scoliosis,** which is a side-to-side or lateral curvature that is

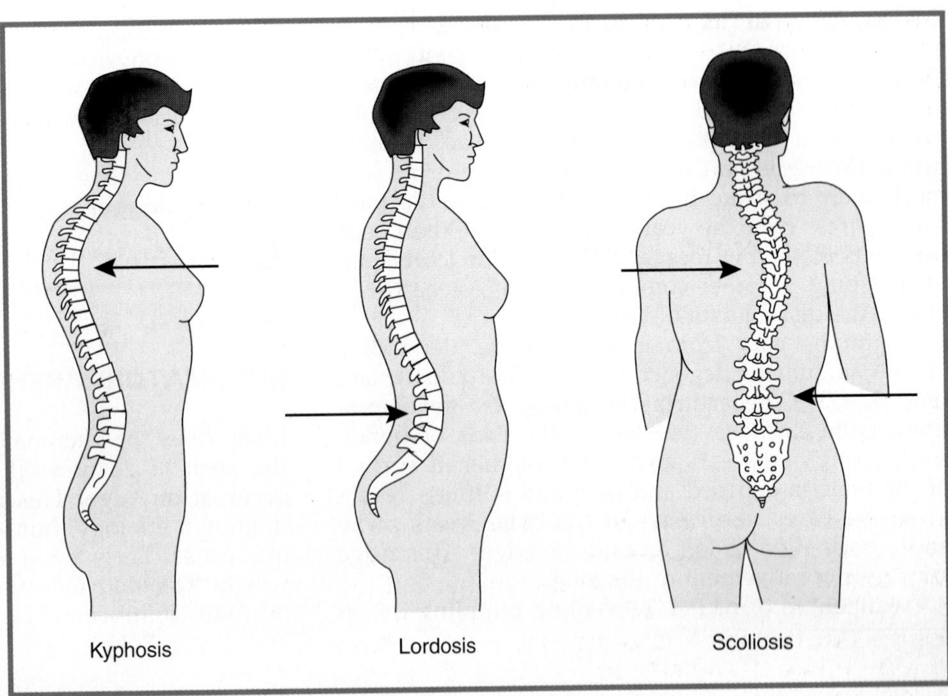

FIGURE 37–6 Spinal curve abnormalities.

most common in teenagers; and **kyphosis,** or hunched back, which is an abnormal curvature of the upper thoracic vertebrae. Diagnosis is done by inspection and palpation of the spine, which may be confirmed by radiography (Fig. 37–6).

Treatment involves the use of devices such as braces, shoe lifts, exercises, and electrical muscle stimulation. In severe cases, rigid casting may be used. Surgical intervention is indicated when the curve is so great that it is interfering with daily movement.

Memory Jogger

7 *Which form of spinal curvature is most common in teenagers?*

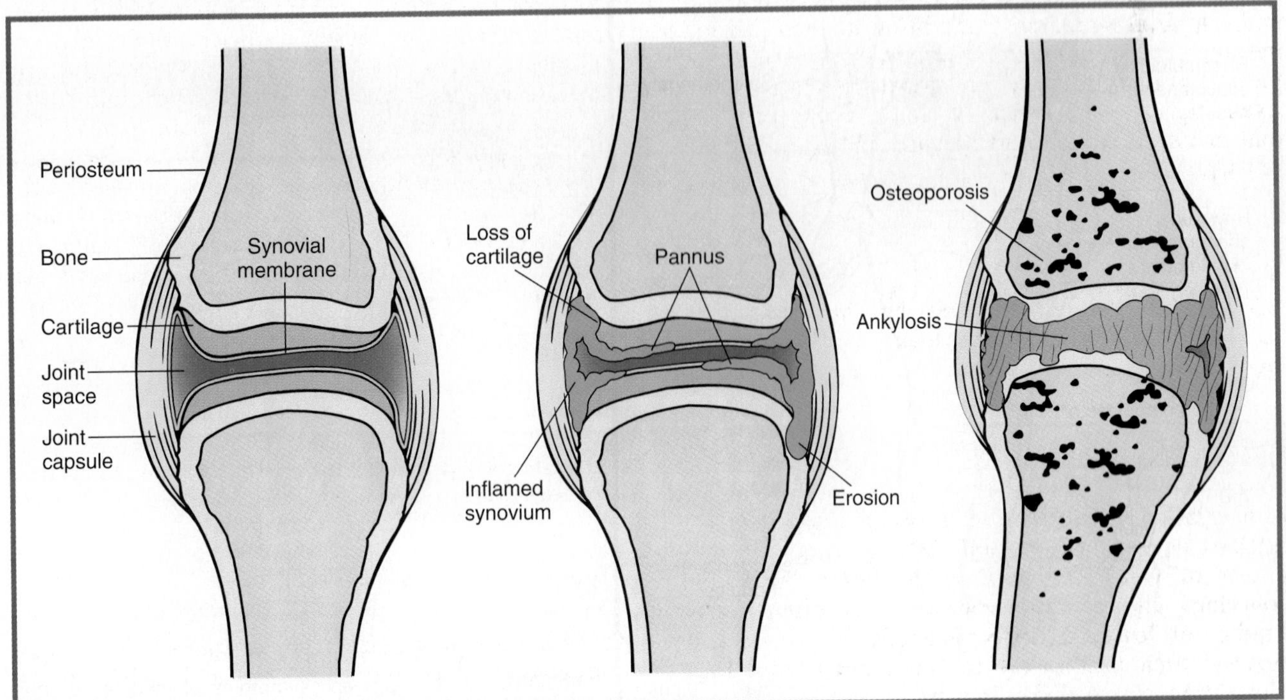

FIGURE 37–7 Pathologic changes in osteoarthritis. (From Damjanov I: Pathology for the Health-Related Professions. Philadelphia, WB Saunders, 1996.)

OSTEOARTHRITIS

Osteoarthritis is a noninflammatory degenerative joint disease marked by degeneration of the joint cartilage and changes in the synovial sac. Primary osteoarthritis, as part of the normal aging process, is most likely to strike the joints that receive the most use or stress over the years. These include the knees, the joints of the big toes, and those of the lower part of the spine. Another common form of osteoarthritis affects the distal joints of the fingers.

Symptoms vary from mild to severe, depending on the amount of degeneration that has taken place (Fig. 37–7). Osteoarthritis is caused by disintegration of the cartilage that covers the ends of bones. As the cartilage wears away, the roughened surface of the bone is exposed and pain and stiffness result. In severe cases, the center of the bone wears away and a bony ridge is left around the edges. This ridge may restrict movement of the joint.

Treatment is aimed at preventing crippling deformities, relieving pain, and maintaining motion of the joint. The physician may prescribe antiinflammatory medications, intraarticular corticosteroid injections, and the use of a walker or cane.

Memory Jogger

8 *What causes osteoarthritis?*

RHEUMATOID ARTHRITIS

Most cases of rheumatoid arthritis begin between the ages of 20 and 40; however, the disease may occur at any age. This autoimmune disease has an unknown etiology, but it is thought that there is no one cause. Early symptoms include **malaise,** fever, weight loss, and morning stiffness of the joints. One or more joints may become painful and inflamed

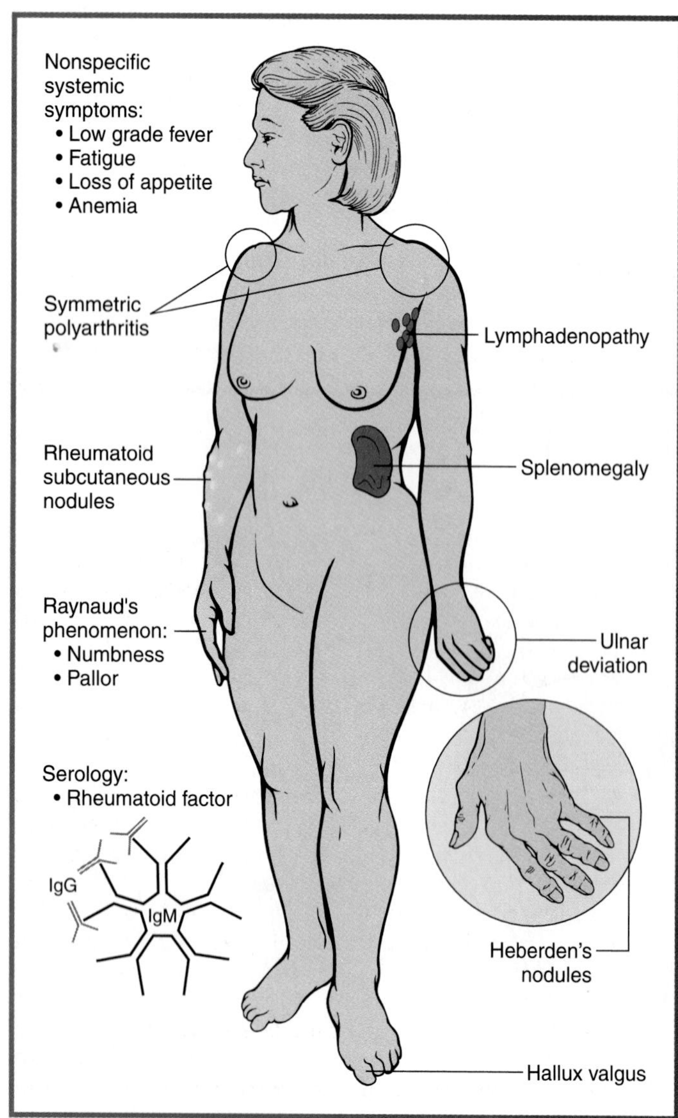

FIGURE 37–8 Signs and symptoms of rheumatoid arthritis. (From Damjanov I: Pathology for the Health-Related Professions. Philadelphia, WB Saunders, 1996.)

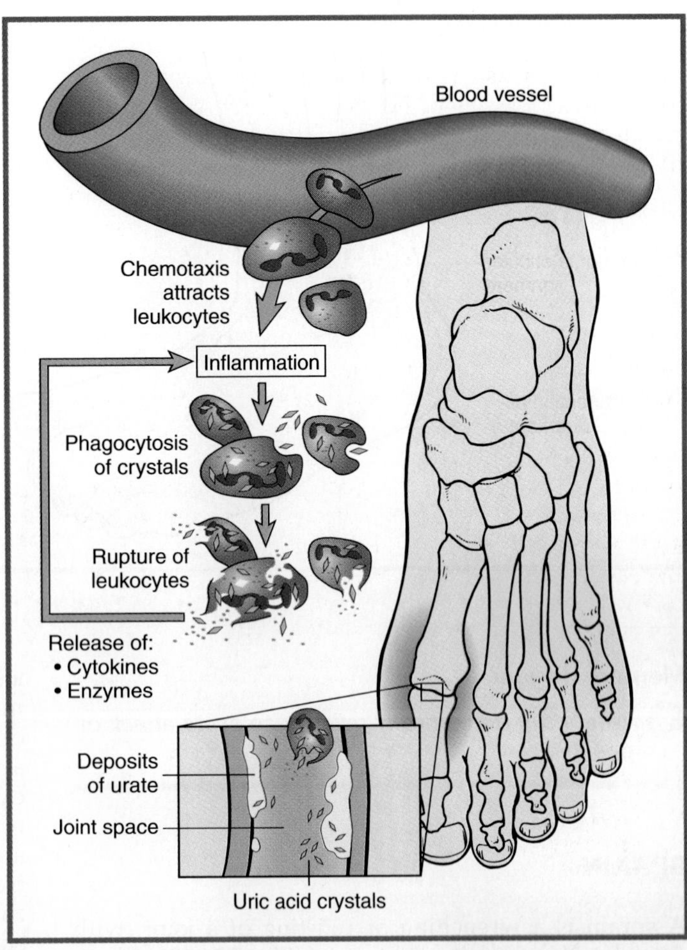

FIGURE 37–9 Gouty arthritis. Deposits of uric acid crystals in the connective tissue. The inflammation most often affects the joint of the big toe. (From Damjanov I: Pathology for the Health-Related Professions. Philadelphia, WB Saunders, 1996.)

(Fig. 37–8). Typically, arthritis attacks will increase in severity and frequency. As the severity increases, the joints become damaged and deformity occurs. Patients with rheumatoid arthritis may appear undernourished and chronically ill due to the formation of degenerative lesions occurring in the collagen in the lungs, heart, blood vessels, and pleura.

PATHOLOGIC STAGES OF RHEUMATOID ARTHRITIS

1 Increased inflammation of the synovial sac causing excretions that thicken the sac walls
2 Formation of granular tissue that causes destruction of the bone capsule
3 Fibrous stiffening of the joint
4 Fusion of the joint bone ends, causing fixation of the joint

Rest and exercise seem to be the key in the treatment of rheumatoid arthritis, as in osteoarthritis. Therapeutic exercises are designed to prevent and correct deformities, control pain, strengthen weakened muscles, and improve function. The most frequently prescribed antiinflammatory medications are still aspirin (acetylsalicylic acid) and nonsteroidal antiinflammatory drugs such as indomethacin (Indocin), sulindac (Clinoril), naproxen (Naprosyn), and ibuprofen (Motrin).

GOUT

Gout, sometimes called gouty arthritis, is a metabolic disease in which there is an overproduction of uric acid. Gout usually affects the big toe, which becomes inflamed, hot, and painful (Fig. 37–9). The disorder will have periods of remission and exacerbation, but the symptoms will continue to worsen if left untreated and may produce degeneration of the joints and deformity.

Treatment consists of dietary avoidance of all foods containing purine, such as liver, certain cold meats, and some forms of sausage. Alcohol-related products must also be avoided. The physician may administer the drug colchicine to confirm the diagnosis. If colchicine dramatically relieves an acute attack of joint pain, the disorder is almost certainly gouty arthritis. Precisely how colchicine works to ease the symptoms of gout is still unknown. Other medications include uricosuric drugs, which promote the excretion of uric acid. Drugs that reduce the level of uric acid production are also being used.

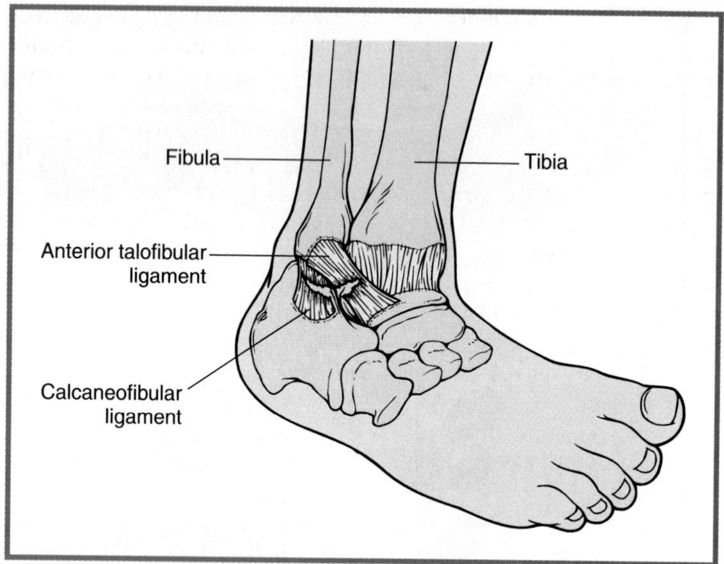

FIGURE 37–10 Ankle sprain. (From Frazier MS, Drzymkowski JA, Doty SJ: Essentials of Human Diseases and Conditions. Philadelphia, WB Saunders, 1996.)

Memory Jogger

What drug dramatically relieves an acute attack of gout?

SPRAIN

A sprain is a wrenching or twisting of a joint, with partial tearing of its ligaments (Fig. 37–10). There may be damage to the associated blood vessels, muscles, tendons, and nerves. A sprain is more serious than a muscle strain, which is simply the overstretching of a muscle, without swelling. Severe sprains are so painful that the joint cannot be used. There is much swelling, with reddish to blue discoloration owing to hemorrhage from ruptured blood vessels.

Treatment includes rest and elevation of the injured joint with no weight bearing to prevent further damage. The injured part should be elevated to decrease swelling. Applications of ice or cold compresses (not heat) to the injured part during the first 12 hours may help relieve pain and prevent swelling. If there is severe tearing or rupture of a ligament or tendon, total immobilization in a cast or surgical repair or both may be required.

DISLOCATION

Dislocation of a joint is called **luxation** when the end of the bone is displaced from the joint and joint structures and **subluxation** if the dislocation is only partial and the bone is pulled out of the joint but all joint structures remain in alignment. The most common dislocations involve a finger, thumb, or shoulder (Fig. 37–11). A dislocation is usually caused by a blow or fall. It is possible to have congenital dislocation, especially of the hip. Symptoms include loss of motion, temporary paralysis of the involved joint, and pain and swelling. A dislocation is usually treated as a fracture, with **reduction** and immobilization. Occasionally, surgery may be necessary to stabilize the joint.

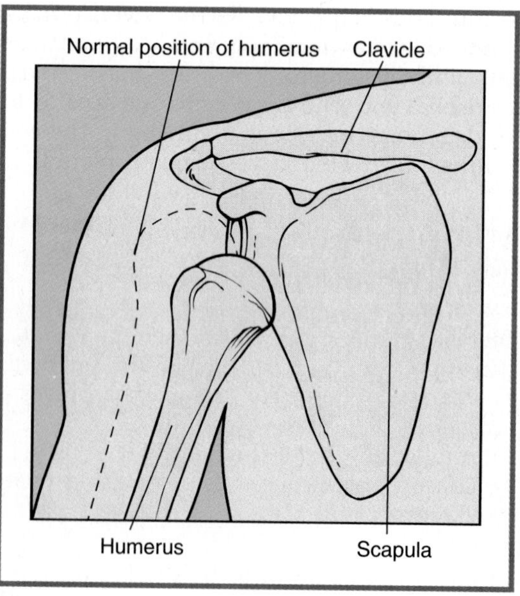

FIGURE 37–11 Dislocation of the shoulder. (From Frazier MS, Drzymkowski JA, Doty SJ: Essentials of Human Diseases and Conditions. Philadelphia, WB Saunders, 1996.)

TENDINITIS

Tendinitis is one of the most common causes of acute pain in the shoulder. Inflammation of tendons may be associated with a calcium deposit involving the bursa that is around or near the joint, causing bursitis. Diagnosis is determined by the shoulder pain becoming more profound when the affected arm is abducted between 50 and 130 degrees. The treatment includes relieving pain and decreasing inflammation so that exercise is possible and permanent immobility of the shoulder is avoided. Injections of long-acting corticosteroids may be given along with short-acting analgesics. Applications of ice are helpful in relieving the pain, and heat tends to aggravate the calcium tendinitis.

MUSCULAR DYSTROPHY

Muscular dystrophy is a hereditary disease that affects almost a quarter of a million Americans. In muscular dystrophy, the muscle suffers a vital loss of protein and muscle fibers are gradually replaced by fat until the voluntary muscle becomes virtually useless. The symptoms of childhood muscular dystrophy are noticeable about the second or third year of life. The child gradually finds it more difficult to play and get about. As the weakening process continues, the child will be wheelchair bound; and in many cases death comes before the age of 20. This type of muscular dystrophy is the most common type and is known as the Duchenne type. Other types will appear in teenagers and in young adults, but these forms progress more slowly than the childhood form. Treatment is activity. The more active the patient is, the better the physical and mental status remains. Obesity must be avoided. Splints, braces, and occasionally corrective orthopedic surgery may be needed.

The Muscular Dystrophy Associations of America (3561 East Sunrise Drive, Tucson, AZ 85718) are concerned with every aspect of the care and comfort of dystrophic patients and can offer many valuable suggestions to the patient and the family.

Memory Jogger

10 *Why do voluntary muscles become virtually useless in muscular dystrophy?*

MUSCLE SPASMS AND TICS

Involuntary muscle movements are frequently *tics,* which may be habit spasms (usually found around the eyes, neck, or face) or the result of various conditions. Tics are involuntary, rhythmic movements by a group of muscles that go into spasm at irregular intervals. A *tremor* is an involuntary trembling or quivering. A tremor may be the beating of the thumb against a flexing finger or a rhythmic oscillation of the head, as may occur in old age.

Torticollis (wryneck) may be present as a result of a spasm or the shortening of the neck and chest muscles.

FRACTURES

A fracture is a break or crack in a bone and can result from trauma or disease. There are many types of fractures, and each may have its own set of problems (Fig. 37–12). The one symptom that is shared by all patients with a bone fracture is pain. Other symptoms may include swelling, bleeding, lack of movement, malalignment of the bone, and discoloration of the area.

When a patient with a fracture is brought into the office, you should make the patient as comfortable as possible. Have the patient lie down in a position that does not place strain on the area. First aid includes preventing movement of the injured part; elevation of the affected extremity; application of ice; and control of bleeding, if present. Do not apply too much pressure on the bleeding area if there is a fracture beneath. Be gentle. Do not attempt to straighten the fracture or move it in any way. If the patient must be moved, give support to the fractured area before moving the patient. If possible, an x-ray film of the area should be ready when the physician arrives.

Treatment consists of putting the broken ends back into proper alignment. This procedure is called *reduction* and consists of two methods. The first is closed reduction, which involves bone alignment and then splinting, wrapping, taping, or casting of the fracture site including the immobilization of the joint above and the joint below the fracture. If it is not possible to achieve proper alignment by the closed reduction method, surgery is required and this procedure is called open reduction. When an open reduction is done, the surgeon may use pins, screws, and metal plates to fixate the bone ends into alignment. The internal fixation devices may remain in the bone until total healing is seen on the x-ray film. At that time the devices will be removed.

Memory Jogger

11 *One symptom shared by all bone fracture victims is ________.*

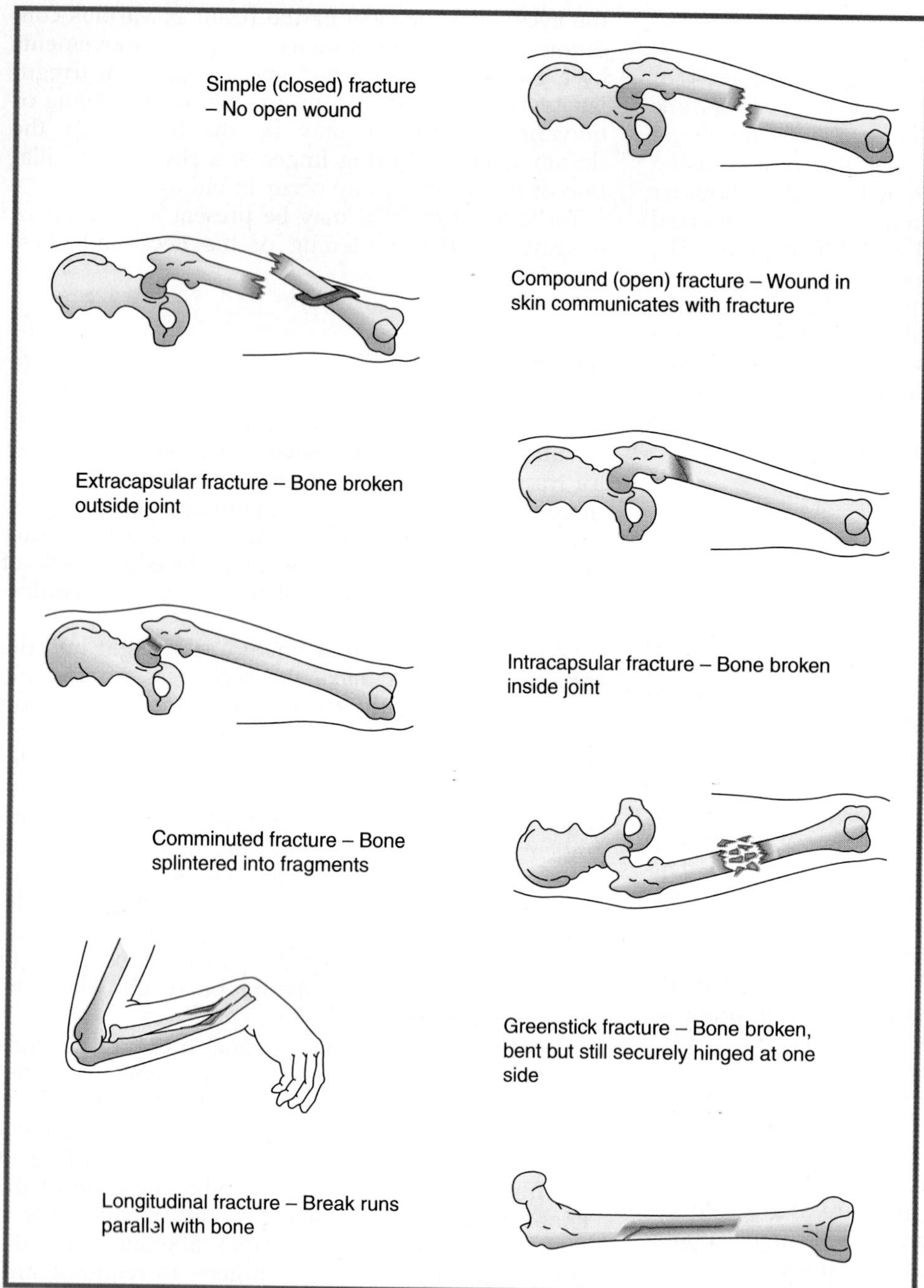

FIGURE 37–12 Various types of fractures.

The Medical Assistant's Role in Assisting with Orthopedic Procedures

The role of the medical assistant begins with an accurate recording of the patient's description of the circumstances surrounding the onset of the disability, what was done to alleviate the problem, and, by comparison, what the major concerns right now are. Where is the pain, and on a scale of 1 to 10 at what level would the patient put the pain? Be sure to include any medication that has been taken, and the amount and the time it was taken.

When taking the patient to an examination room, be sure to offer assistance. It may be necessary to use a wheelchair to transfer the patient from the reception area to the examination room. In the examination room, assist the patient to a comfortable position. Offer a pillow or folded blanket to support a painful body part. If necessary, provide assistance with disrobing because there may be limited mobility due to pain. Check with the patient to be certain that the room temperature is comfortable. Be clear

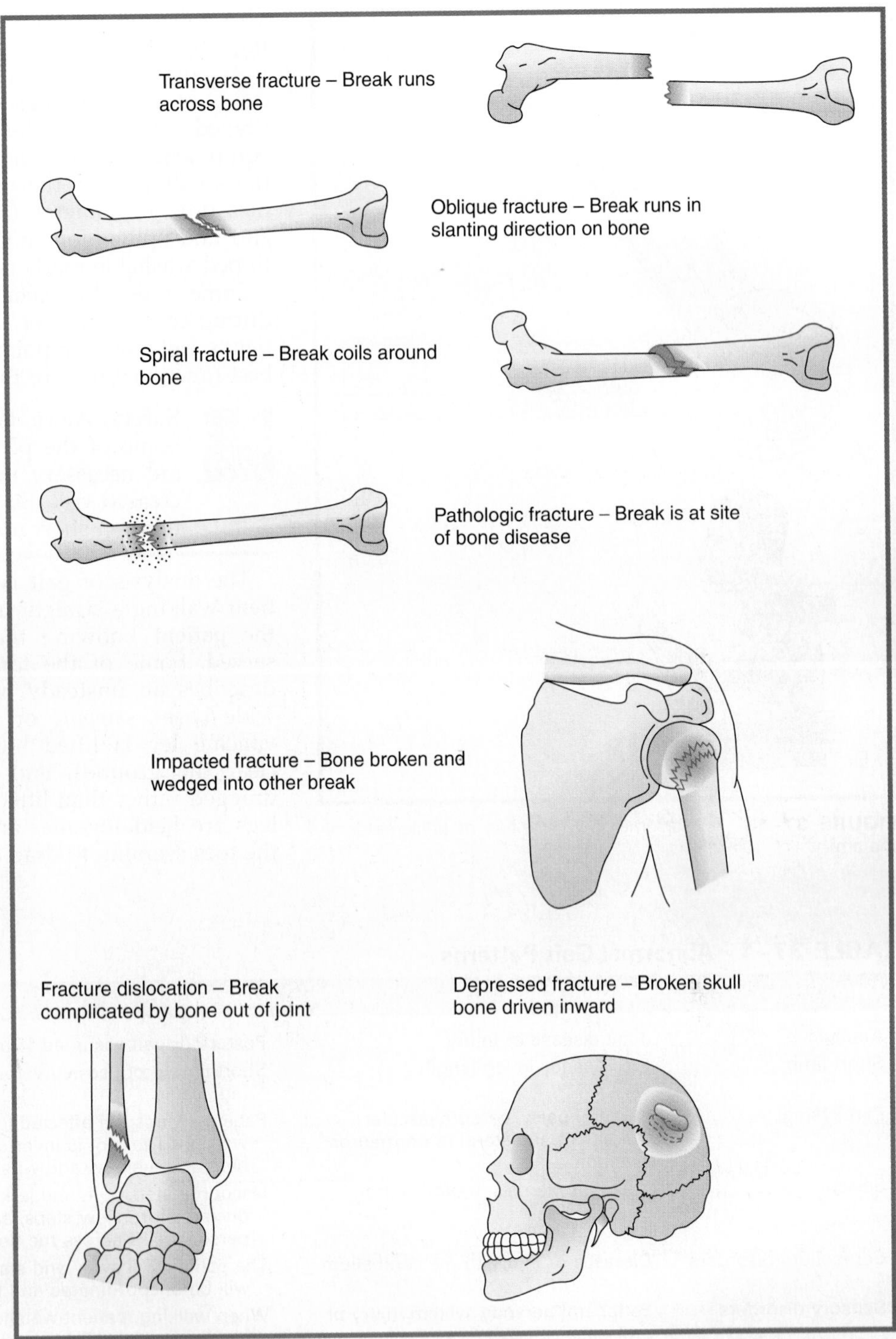

FIGURE 37–12 *Continued*

and concise in your explanations to the patient. Notify the physician as soon as the patient is prepared and ready for the physician's examination.

ASSISTING WITH THE EXAMINATION

The physician may use inspection, palpation, range of motion, and muscle testing as means of examining the major voluntary muscles and joints of the body. Much of the examination is done by comparing paired muscles and joints for size, position, and strength. When the patient is to be in a certain position, you may find it helpful to demonstrate the position or the movement desired. Watch the patient's nonverbal language for signs of changes in tolerance of the manipulative portion of the examination.

As a general rule, the physician will examine the unaffected side before examining the affected side.

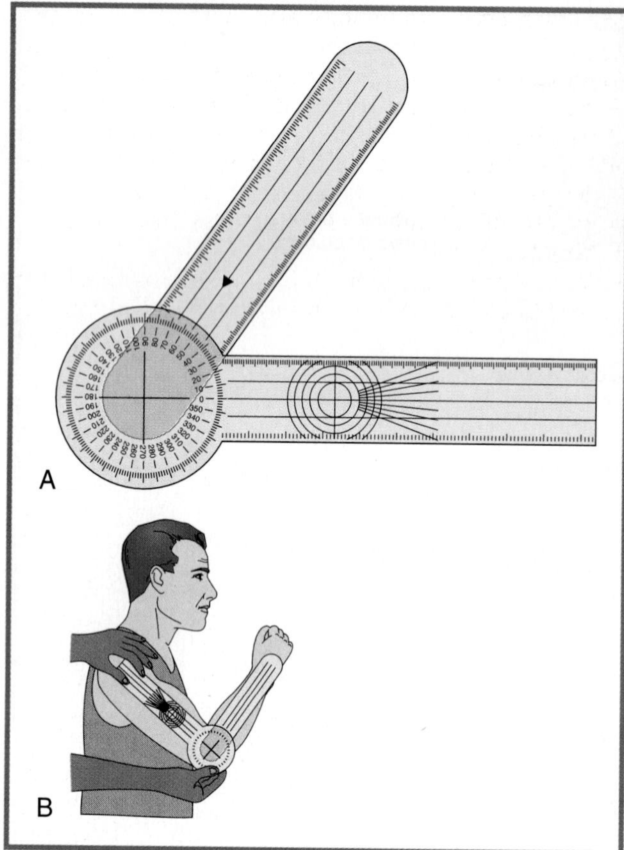

FIGURE 37–13 *A*, Goniometer. *B*, Position of goniometer on the arm.

This will give the physician a guideline for comparing the affected with the unaffected muscle. You may be responsible for making note of the physician's clinical findings. Keep the patient properly draped, and assist the physician by handing the equipment to him or her as needed. Most examinations will require the use of a nonstretchable tape measure, **goniometer** (Fig. 37–13), blood pressure cuff and sphygmomanometer, stethoscope, and felt-tipped washable markers.

Some musculoskeletal problems may be worse during certain parts of the day. Arrange for the patient's follow-up appointments during the patient's best functional time of the day.

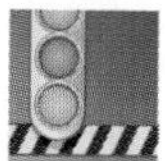

Safety Alert: Guard against patient falls. Some of the positions and movements that are necessary may place the patient at increased risk. Be prepared to support the patient on short notice to prevent a fall.

The analysis of **gait** is usually done with the patient walking a straight line or may be done without the patient knowing that he or she is being observed. Some of the terms used are *ataxic* (which describes an unsteady, uncoordinated walk over a wide base), *slapping* or *steppage* (in which the advancing leg is lifted high enough for the toes to clear the ground), *drag-to* (in which the feet are dragged rather than lifted), and *spastic* (in which the legs are held together and move in a stiff manner, the toes seeming to drag and catch (Table 37–1).

TABLE 37–1 Abnormal Gait Patterns

Type	Possible Cause	Description
Antalgic	Joint disease or injury	Posture or gait assumed to avoid or lessen pain.
Short limb	Discrepancy in leg length	Short limb produces curvature of spine and limp when walking.
Paroxysmal	Cerebral palsy, cerebrovascular accident, unilateral motor neuron tumor	Patient swings the affected leg in a wide semicircle when walking. The foot is inverted and planterflexed. The arm is bent at the elbow and wrist.
Scissor	Multiple sclerosis, motor neuron disease	Uncoordinated, stiff, and jerky gait. Knees are adducted, producing short, slow steps, and the foot may drag as the person walks across the floor.
Cerebellum disorders	Diseases or injury to the cerebellum	The patient will sway and stagger while walking. The gait will be uncoordinated and broad based.
Sensory disorders	Peripheral nervous system injury or disease	When walking, patient watches the floor to help in correctly placing the foot. The foot will be lifted exceptionally high and then slapped to the floor, heel first. The patient appears to be uncertain of spatial position.
Festination	Parkinson's disease	An involuntary tendency to take short accelerating steps when walking results in a shuffling gait with the feet barely leaving the floor. Body remains rigid, with knees slightly flexed when standing and walking.
Footdrop	Polio, paralysis of dorsiflexor muscles	The whole sole of the foot is slapped on the floor at once and the hip and knee is flexed to lift the foot off of the floor.
Bandy-legged	Alzheimer's disease or frontal lobe tumor	Patient appears "stuck" to the floor; once gait begins, it is slow and shuffling.
Waddling	Hip dysplasia or muscular dystrophy	When walking, the patient's pelvis on the unaffected side will drop as weight bearing is shifted to the affected side, producing a "hula" motion of both hips.

Memory Jogger

Four means of examining the major muscles and joints are ________.

ASSISTING WITH RANGE OF MOTION (ROM) EVALUATION

An orthopedist who specializes in industrial medicine and workers' compensation cases has a knowledge of special terminology and methods for recording and measuring muscle and joint movement. The American Academy of Orthopedic Surgeons has a published guide called "Joint Motion: Method of Measuring and Recording." When working in the orthopedic office, you will need to become familiar with the terms used (Fig. 37–14 illustrates upper extremity ROM and 37–15 illustrates lower extremity ROM).

When evaluating ROM the physician will ask the patient to move the joint through each of its various

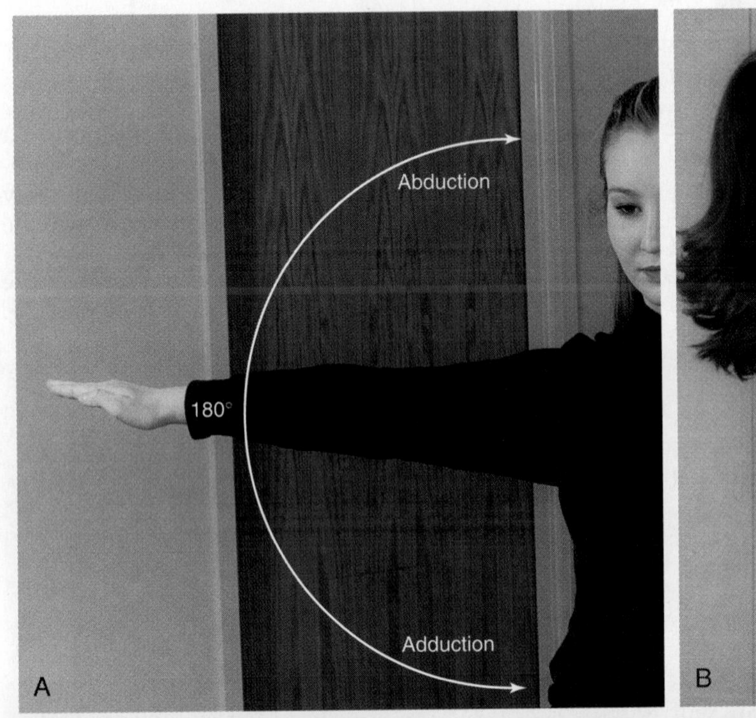

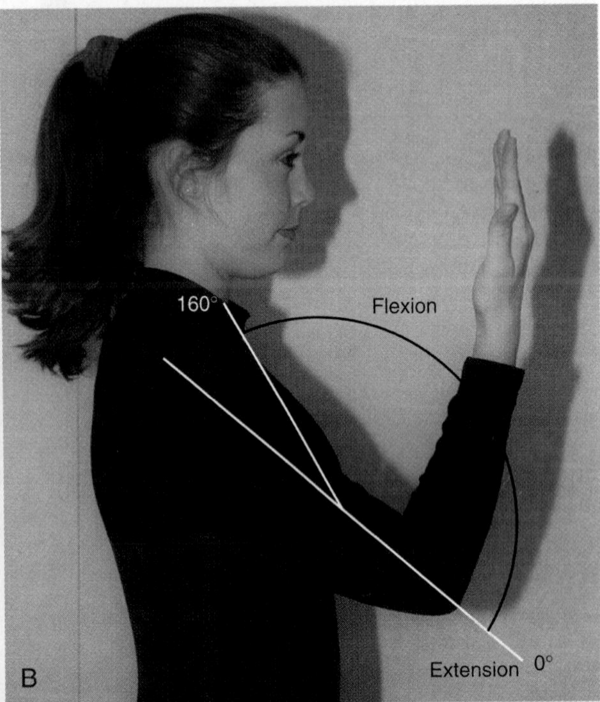

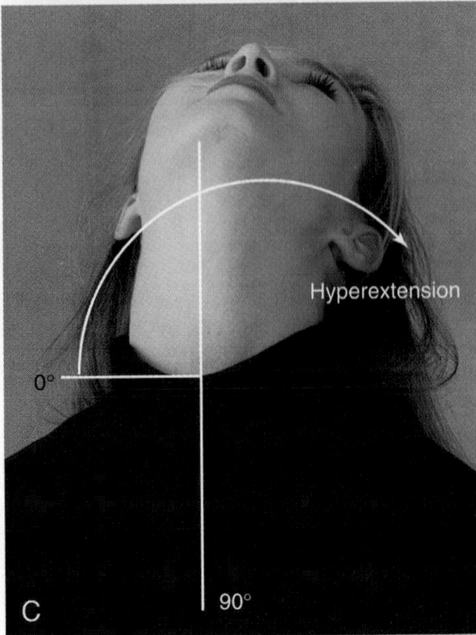

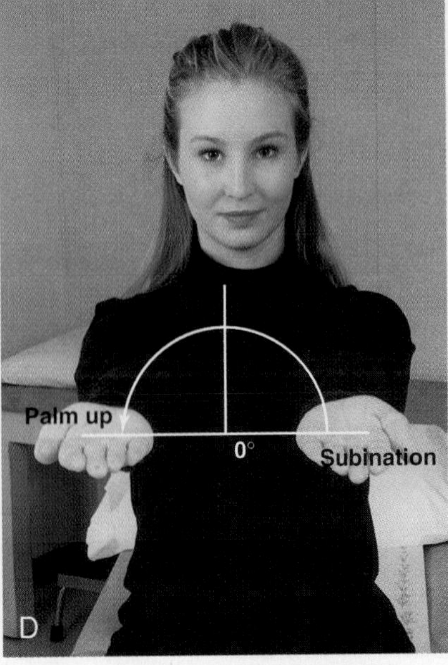

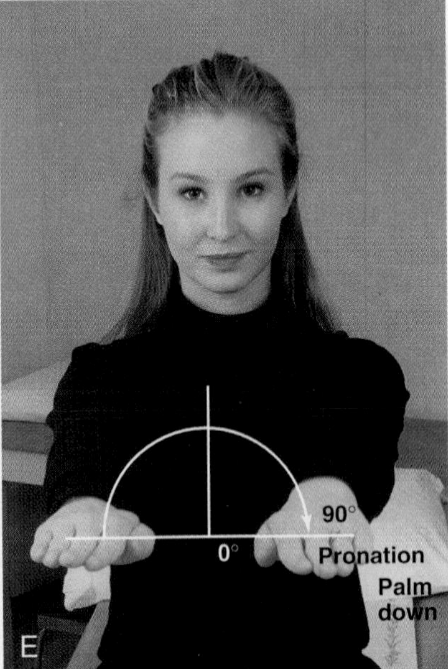

FIGURE 37–14 Range of motion exercises for upper extremities. *A*, Abduction/adduction. *B*, Flexion/extension. *C*, Hyperextension. *D*, Supination. *E*, Pronation.

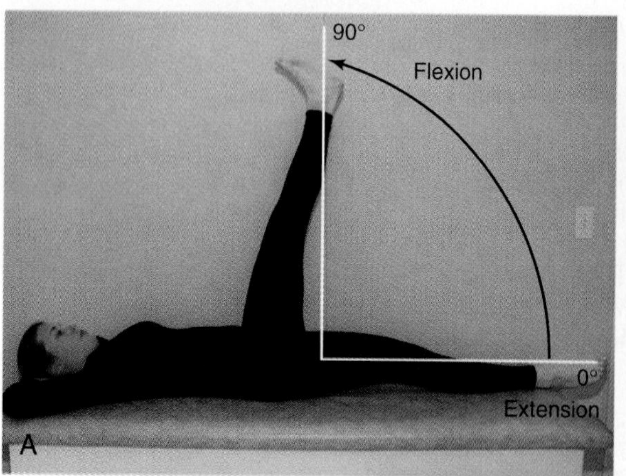

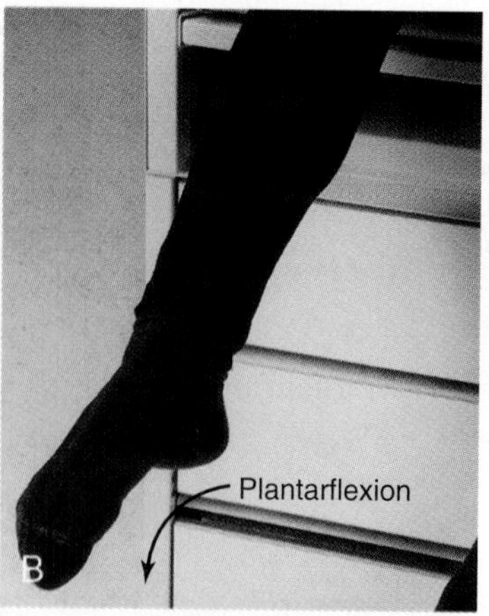

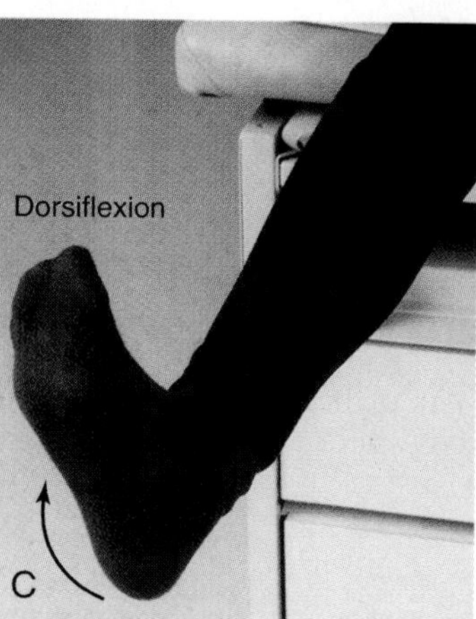

FIGURE 37–15 Range of motion exercises for lower extremities. *A*, Flexion/extension. *B*, Plantarflexion. *C*, Dorsiflexion.

ROM movements. If the patient can do this without assistance, the motion is recorded as active movement. You may be responsible for recording the angle of each movement, along with any pain, tenderness, or **crepitation** experienced by the patient. If the patient is unable to perform active ROM, the physician may attempt to put the joint through the desired movement range. When the movement is done in this fashion, it is recorded as passive ROM. No joint is forced to move beyond its normal anatomic angle.

Joint mobility is measured in degrees. In a hinged joint such as the knee, 180 degrees would be total ROM; and in a freely movable joint such as the hip, 360 degrees would illustrate total ROM.

ASSISTING WITH MUSCLE STRENGTH EVALUATION

During the evaluation of ROM, the physician will also assess each muscle group for strength. Normal muscle strength allows for complete voluntary ROM in the presence of resistance. This resistance can be gravity, such as in rising from a sitting position to a standing position, and/or physical, such as in pulling or lifting an object. Muscle strength is bilaterally equal in normal conditions. The evaluation will be conducted by comparing like muscles in each hemisphere of the body (e.g., comparing the grip of the right and left hand using a blood pressure cuff) (Fig. 37–16).

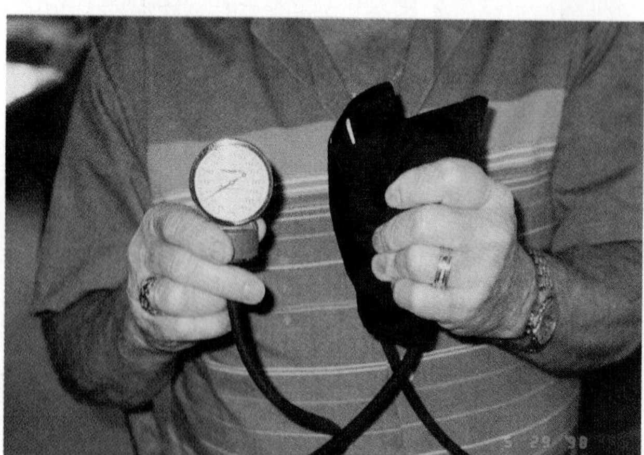

FIGURE 37–16 Assessing grip strength using a blood pressure cuff.

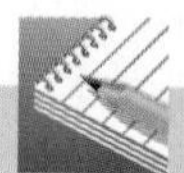

SKILLS AND RESPONSIBILITIES

ASSESSMENT OF STRENGTH USING A BLOOD PRESSURE CUFF

- Fold up an aneroid blood pressure cuff and ask the patient to grasp the rolled cuff.
- Inflate the cuff to 20 mm Hg.
- Ask the patient to squeeze the cuff as tightly as possible.
- Note the increase in millimeters of mercury on the aneroid dial. A normal grip will be above 150 mm Hg.
- Record the hand tested and the result of the test.
- Repeat the test on the opposite side.

You may be recording whether the tested muscle groups are strong and equal in strength, the level of muscle involvement, and the patient's response to the assessment. Muscle strength is graded on a 0 to 5 scale. If the strength was normal the grade would be a 5, about 50% of normal would be 2 to 3, and no visible contraction would be 0.

RADIOLOGY AND DIAGNOSTIC IMAGING

Diagnostic imaging and radiology are two detection interventions that are frequently used in orthopedic medicine. Many orthopedists have the ability to perform radiology procedures within their offices and may employ a full-time radiology technician. Radiography is used to diagnose fractures, dislocations, degenerative disorders, and diseases of bone and joints. In addition, x-ray films are used to evaluate the healing process and to determine when a cast can be removed or if a fracture needs to be repositioned and recasted. Arthrograms are used to visualize joints, myelograms check for vertebral disk disorders, and a bone scan evaluates bone growth, density, development, tumors, as well as other types of bone disease and disorder patterns.

If it is necessary to visualize soft tissue such as in tumors, masses, lesions, or ruptured or torn spine injuries, computed tomography will be requested.

In some disorders, the muscle does not get the stimulation from the nerve fibers and the physician will need to conduct tests that measure nerve conduction. These tests are electromyography and a nerve conduction velocity. These tests are designed to measure the nerve's ability to conduct impulses to the muscle fibers and measure muscle functional responses.

The goniometer was previously discussed as a method of measuring the amount of movement available in a joint.

As in other systems, the biopsy remains a valuable diagnostic tool. The biopsy of bone and/or muscle tissue allows for microscopic examination to determine the type of cell in the biopsy, if there is cell damage present, the presence of tumors and neoplasms, and the possible presence of other pathogens.

When one of these tests is to be done, you will need to explain the procedure, how it is done, where it will be done, and how long will it take to have it done. Besides these explanations, the most common question you will be asked is "will it hurt?" Tell the truth. If it is a painful procedure, let the patient know so that he or she will be prepared for it. Most painful procedures are done only after the patient has been given a mild sedative or analgesic. Discuss the testing procedure in a professional, yet empathetic manner. If the patient wishes to speak to the physician regarding the procedure, inform the physician so that the patient's request will be honored.

Memory Jogger

Name two tests designed to measure stimulation of nerve fibers.

ASSISTING WITH CASTING

When the physician orders a casting as the means of immobilization of a musculoskeletal injury, you will need to know what type of cast will be used. Casting material used includes plaster-of-Paris, fiberglass or plastic, synthetic material, or the air cast. Plaster-of-Paris is the oldest of the casting materials and is formed by soaking roller gauze that is impregnated with calcium sulfate in warm water and then rolling it over the fracture site, like a wet bandage, molding it to fit smoothly, and allowing it to dry (see Procedure 37–1). The plastic or fiberglass casting material has impregnated fiber or resin in the rollers and is applied is the same fashion. The advantage of this type of cast is that it is stronger, lighter in weight, and relatively waterproof. This cast allows the patient to get the cast wet without damaging the casting material. If the patient will need to wear the cast only when using the limb, the physician may use a synthetic cast that is a formed boot or sleeve that fits like a sandwich over the fracture and is held in place by Velcro tapes (Fig. 37–17). An air cast is a temporary cast and operates as an inflatable immobilizer. The type of cast to be used will depend on the location of the injury, the age and/or occupation of the patient, and the physician's preference.

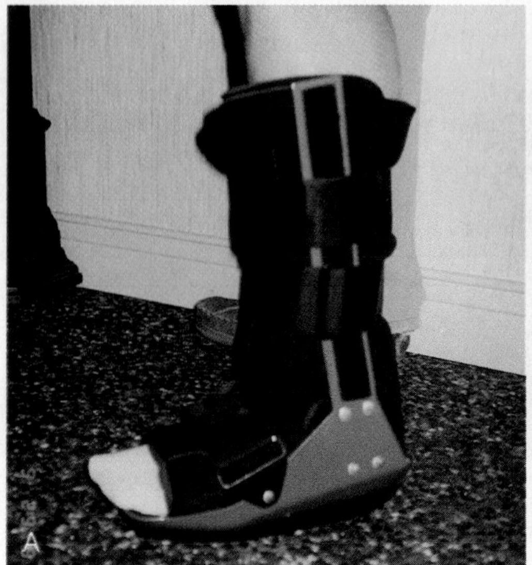

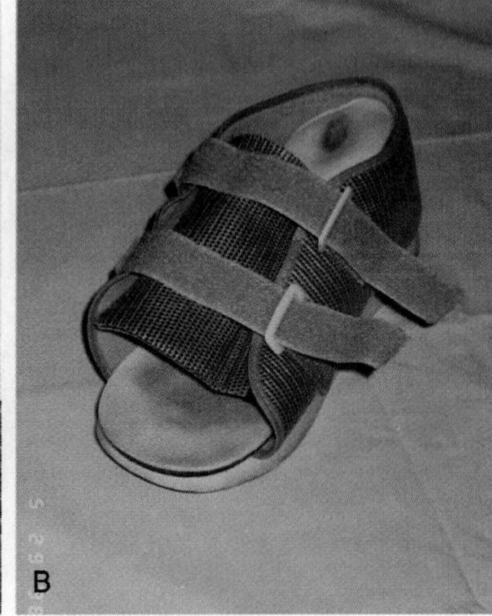

FIGURE 37–17 *A,* Synthetic boot cast. *B,* Synthetic foot immobilizer.

PROCEDURE 37-1

Assisting with Applying a Plaster-of-Paris Cast

GOAL

To assist the physician in applying a plaster cast.

EQUIPMENT AND SUPPLIES

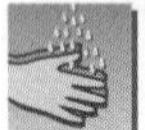

- Tubular stockinette, sized according to limb
- Sheet wadding or roller padding
- Roller plaster or other casting material
- Container of cool or room temperature water (a bucket is best)
- Cast knife or shears
- Heavy rubber gloves

PROCEDURAL STEPS

1. Assemble equipment and supplies. Be sure that the stockinette is adequate to fit comfortably over the fractured area.
   PURPOSE: To alleviate circulation difficulties.
2. Assist the physician in covering the injured limb with the stockinette leaving extra fabric above and below the proposed casting area (Figure 1).
   PURPOSE: This fabric will be used to encase the cast ends.
3. Hand the physician the sheet wadding and support the patient's limb as directed. The physician will apply a thick layer over the stockinette with extra padding layers over any bony prominence (Figure 2).
   PURPOSE: To prevent possible secondary pressure sores.
4. Place the roller plaster into the water to soak. When bubbles no longer appear around the ends of the roller, squeeze the rollers.
   PURPOSE: To be certain that the water has completely saturated the roller.
5. Press out the extra water and hand the physician the saturated rollers as requested (Figure 3).
   PURPOSE: Never wring or twist the rollers because it will damage the casting material.
6. When the physician has completed the cast plaster application, hand the physician the plaster knife or plaster shears and assist as needed in trimming the rough plaster edges (Figure 4).
7. After the edges are smooth, assist in folding the excess stockinette over the cast ends to form cuffs at each of the cast ends (Figure 5).
   PURPOSE: Patient comfort.

Continued

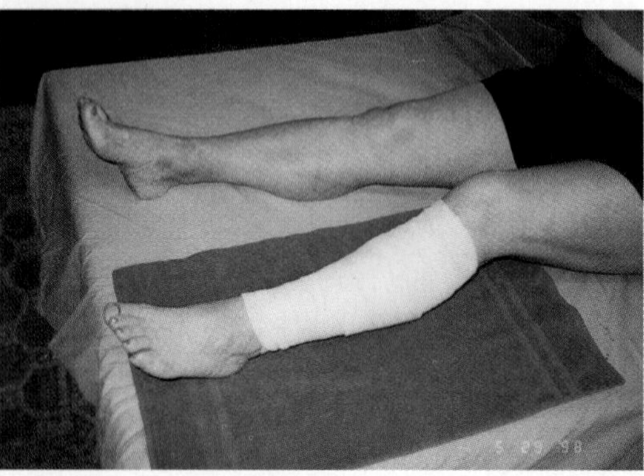

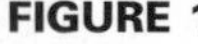

FIGURE 1

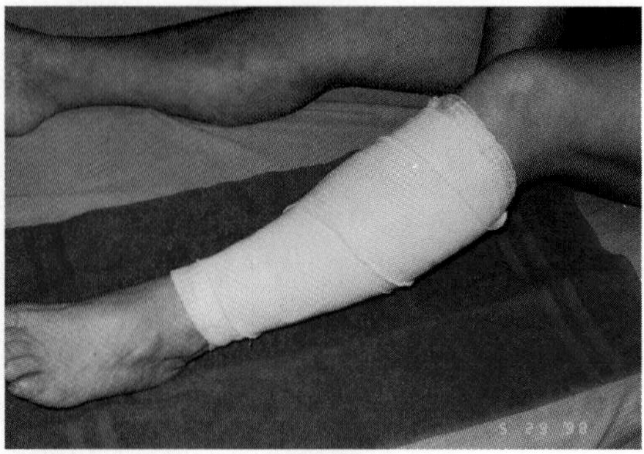

FIGURE 2

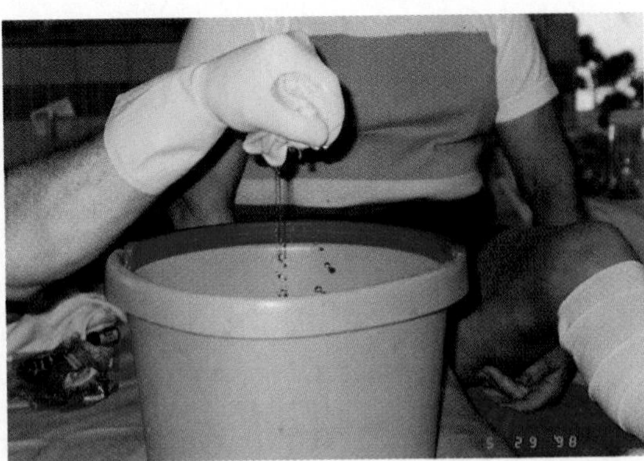

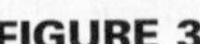

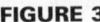

FIGURE 3

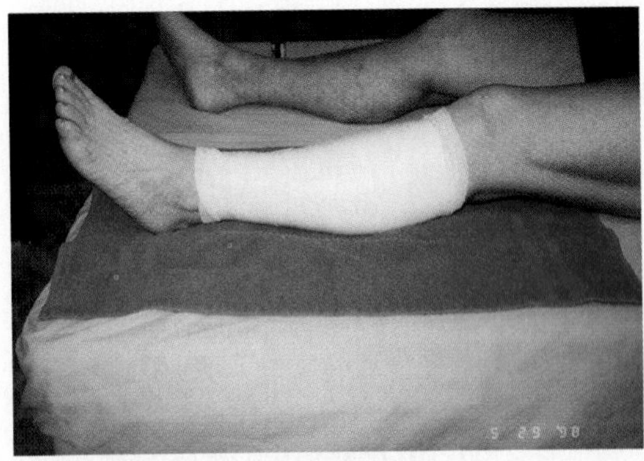

FIGURE 4

8 Place the casted limb carefully on a pillow to begin drying. Avoid squeezing the soft cast.
PURPOSE: Indentations in the cast may inhibit blood flow to the limb area underneath the indentation.

9 Clean the skin of all casting material.
PURPOSE: To avoid discomfort and create a hygienically appearing cast.

10 Instruct the patient to report odors, staining, undue warmth, changes in limb color, swelling, and numbness and to keep the limb elevated for at least the first 24 hours.
PURPOSE: Ensure against possible nerve or vascular damage.

11 Review cast care instructions with the patient and a family member if the cast was placed on a child. Give the patient a copy of the cast care instructions and if the physician has ordered a form of isometric exercises, be certain to demonstrate the exercise technique. Be sure to reinforce any precautions the physician has informed the patient about.
PURPOSE: Reviewing all of the physician's orders with the patient may help in avoiding complications to the circulatory system.

12 Discard water down the sink drain but keep all plaster residue out of the drain. Discard the used plaster bandage and plaster residue in designated container for disposal.
PURPOSE: Plaster will dry in the drain pipe and form an obstruction.

13 Check the limb in 20 to 30 minutes for color, swelling, numbness, and temperature. Advise the physician and chart your findings.
PURPOSE: Establish record of patient's status before discharge from office.

14 If arm has been casted, and the physician has ordered a sling, place the limb into a sling for support.
PURPOSE: Avoid undue stress and strain on the shoulder muscles. If a foot has been casted, and crutches are ordered, continue instructions with patient in the use of crutches.
PURPOSE: Patient cannot bear weight on the injured limb until cast is dry and/or physician gives permission.

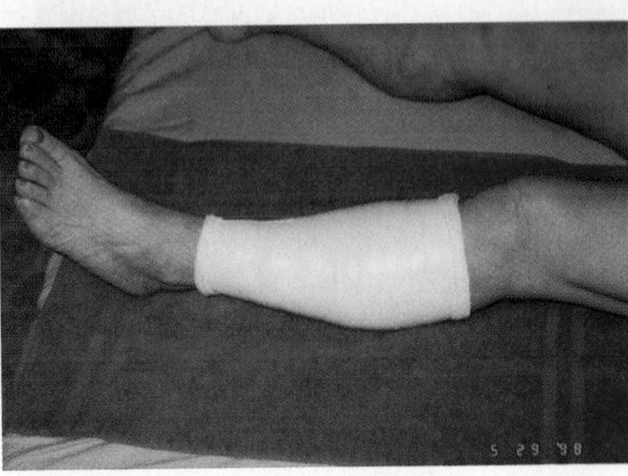

FIGURE 5

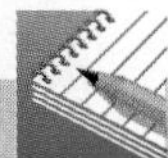

SKILLS AND RESPONSIBILITIES

INSTRUCTIONS TO THE PATIENT ON CAST CARE

- Keep cast uncovered for first 12 hours to allow casting material to dry completely.
- Avoid pressure indentations during the drying period because these may cause underlying tissue damage.
- Check the fingers or toes that are extending from the cast for color and temperature. Notify physician if there are any changes that might indicate that the cast is too tight.
- Elevate the limb as often as possible to help prevent swelling and help circulation.
- Do not pour, shake, or stick any creams, powders, or objects under the cast. This may cause tissue damage or injury.
- Do not get a plaster cast wet. Clean cast with a wet cloth and then dry completely.
- Use only water-soluble pens to decorate the cast. The cast must be allowed to breathe.

PLACING THE CASTED ARM IN A SLING

If an arm has been casted, the patient may need to place the cast into a sling to support the shoulder muscles. This sling may be a commercially designed sling (Fig. 37–18*A* and *B*) or a triangular-shaped piece of soft material (see Fig. 37–18C) (see Procedure 37–2). Slings may also be used if the arm did not have to be casted but must be immobilized to promote the healing process.

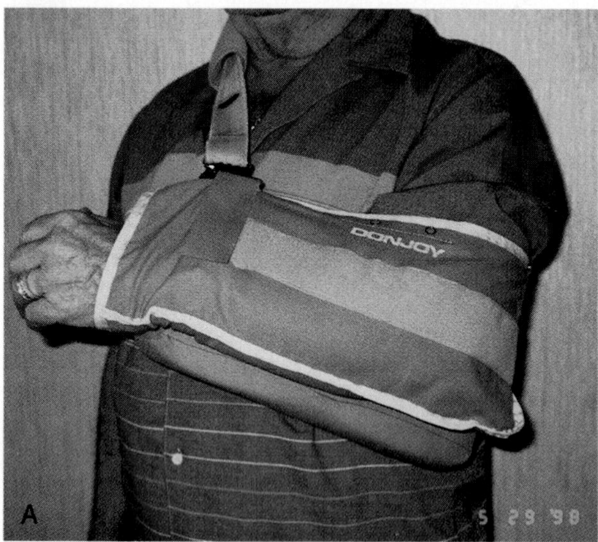

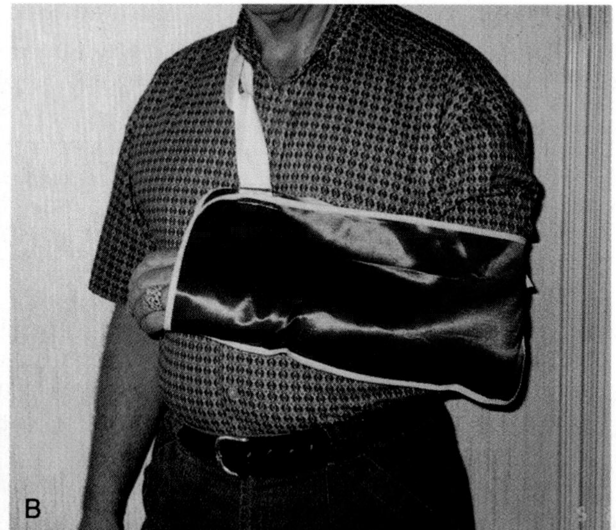

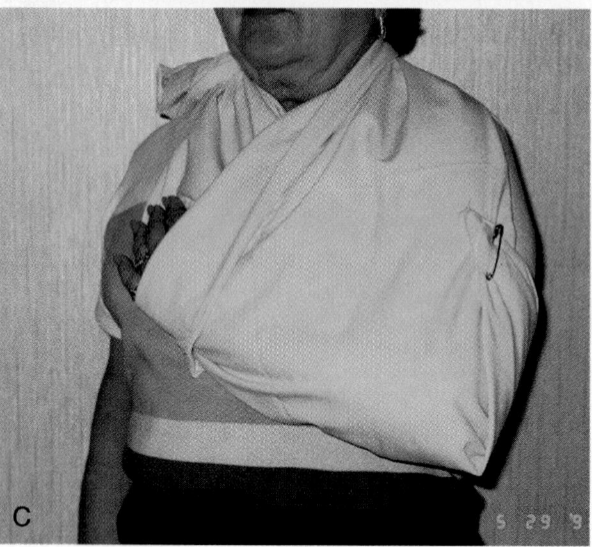

FIGURE 37–18 Types of slings. *A,* Commercial sling with foam wedge to maintain anterior angle. *B,* Commercial sling for simple immobilization or used with an arm cast. *C,* Soft material triangular sling.

PROCEDURE 37-2

Application of a Triangular Arm Sling

GOAL

To properly place a casted arm in a triangular sling.

EQUIPMENT AND SUPPLIES

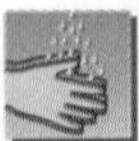

Triangular-shaped arm sling

PROCEDURAL STEPS

1 Check the physician's order to be certain that a triangular arm sling was requested.

2 Wash your hands and obtain the desired sling.

3 Explain the procedure to the patient.

4 Position the patient's injured arm across the chest at a 90-degree angle to the waist with the hand slightly elevated (Figure 1).
PURPOSE: This position helps to reduce swelling.

5 Carefully slide the triangular sling between the patient's chest and the affected arm (Figure 2).

Continued

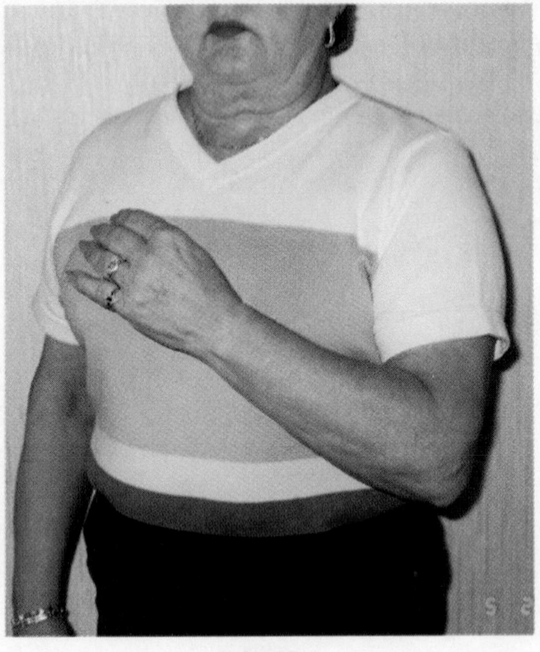

FIGURE 1

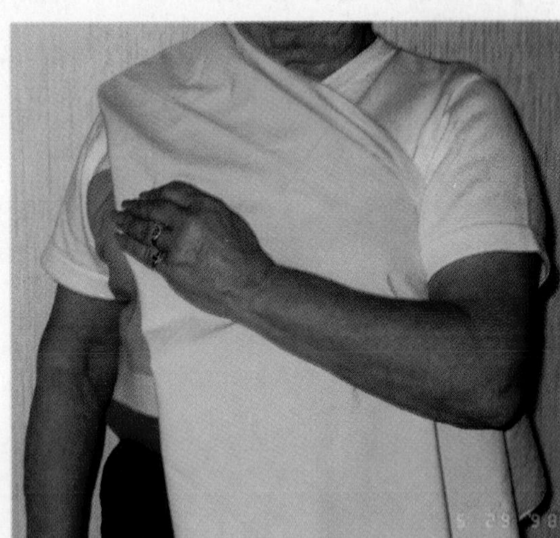

FIGURE 2

PROCEDURE 37-2 (CONTINUED)

Application of a Triangular Arm Sling

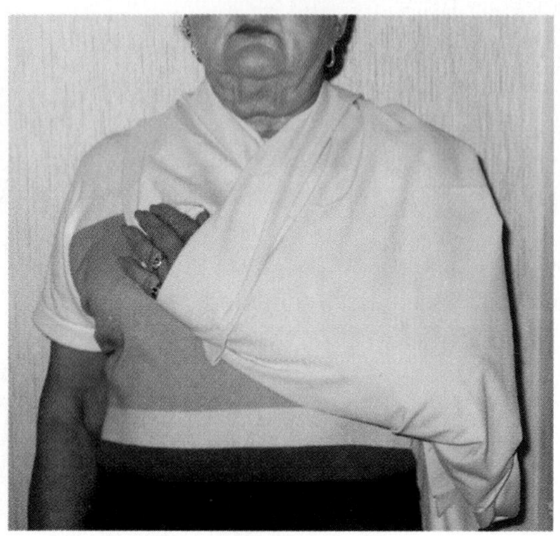

FIGURE 3

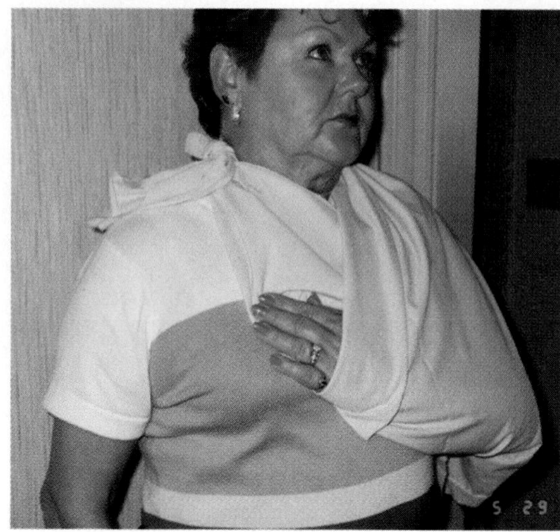

FIGURE 4

6 Bring the lower front corner up over the shoulder of the affected side to the neck (Figure 3).

7 Grab the opposite corner and tie or pin the ends together at the side of the neck (Figure 4).
PURPOSE: Never tie at the back of the neck because it may cause headache and muscle discomfort.

8 Fold in the tail and secure with a pin or adhesive tape to secure the elbow (Figure 5).

9 Fold the sling edge to form smooth edge along the wrist.
PURPOSE: Patient comfort.

10 Record the procedure in the patient's record.
PURPOSE: A procedure is considered not done until it is recorded.

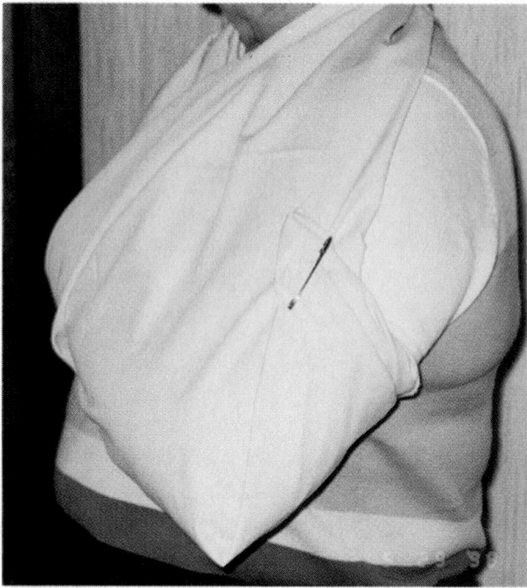

FIGURE 5

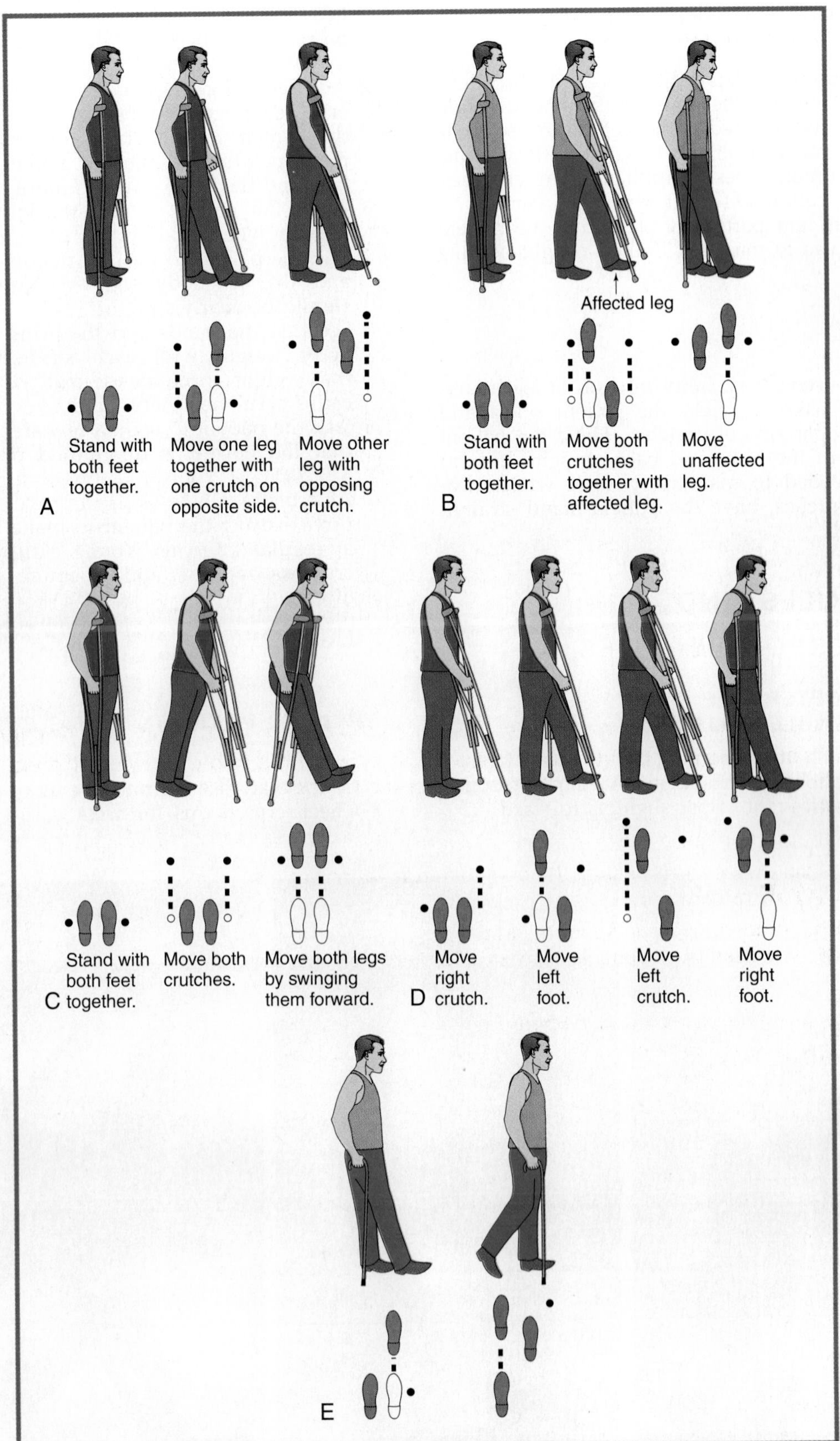

FIGURE 37–19 Crutch gait patterns. *A,* Two-point gait. *B,* Three-point gait. *C,* Four-point alternate crutch gait. *D,* Swing-through gait. *E,* Proper cane stance.

Ambulatory Appliances

In many musculoskeletal diseases and disorders, walking and mobility become painful and difficult. The patient may be faced with needing to use some type of ambulatory appliance to assist with walking. The most common types of appliances are crutches, walkers, and canes. Different types of injuries will indicate a different pattern of steps that the patient will need to use to maintain limited weight bearing (Fig. 37–19).

CRUTCHES

Crutches are used for mobility in cases of leg injury. You may be asked to help the patient select and adjust the proper size of crutches. Have the patient stand tall, with the head and back straight. If extra support is needed to maintain posture while measuring the crutches, have the patient stand straight against a wall.

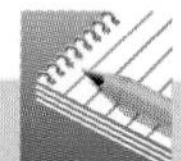

SKILLS AND RESPONSIBILITIES

HOW TO DETERMINE A COMFORTABLE CRUTCH FIT

1 Place crutch tips about 6 inches away from and parallel to the toes. (A thin person should move the tips slightly forward; a heavy person, with wide hips, should allow more space between the crutches and the toes.)
2 Adjust the length of the crutches so that two or three fingers fit between the armpit and the crutch top (about 2 inches). You may measure from the anterior axillary fold to the heel and then add 2 inches more.
3 Have the patient bend the elbow 20 to 30 degrees when holding the hand grip.
4 Ask the patient to push down on the crutches and lift the body slightly. Now the arms should be nearly straight.
5 See that the hands and the arms hold all the body weight with each stride. (Remember that weight borne by the axillary region may cause permanent nerve damage.)
6 Ask the patient to walk a few steps to be sure that the weight is distributed properly (Fig. 37–20).
7 As crutch-walking skills improve, so will posture. Instruct the patient to make adjustments at regular intervals. Young children outgrow crutches rapidly, and fit must be checked often.

TIPS FOR PATIENTS USING CRUTCHES

- Check that all wing nuts are tight.
- Check crutch tips for wear. Crutch tips may

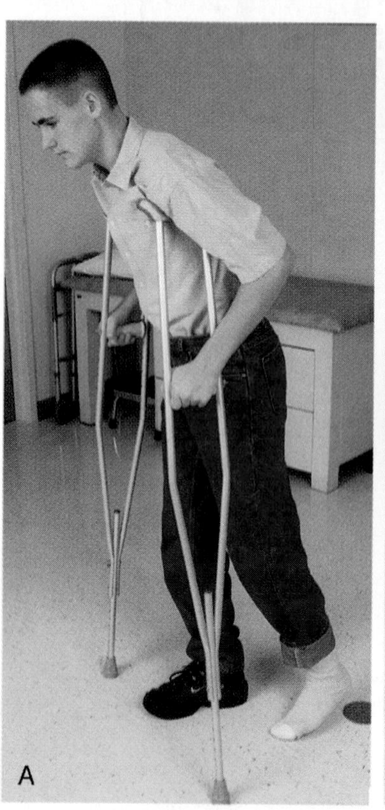

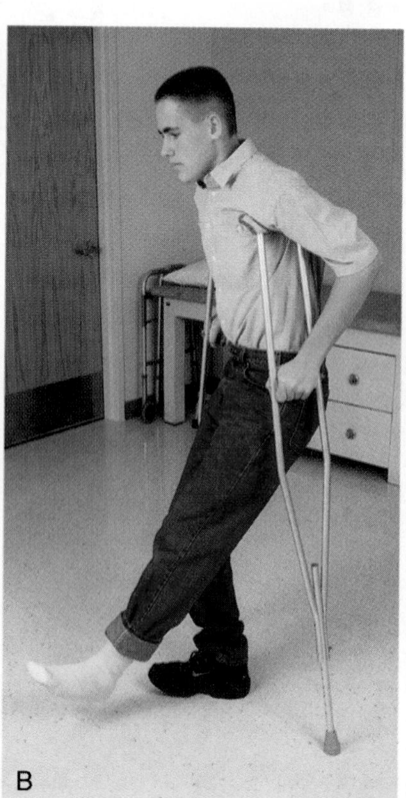

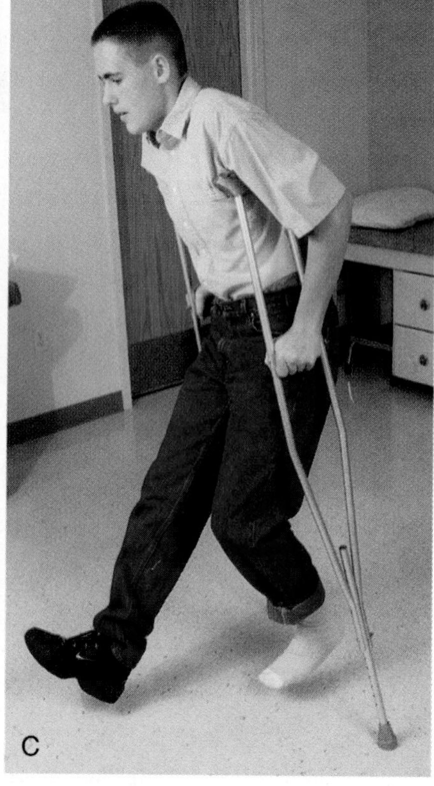

FIGURE 37–20 Three-point crutch walking. *A*, Both feet together. *B*, Move crutches with affected foot. *C*, Move unaffected foot.

be purchased at any drugstore or hardware store.
- Make sure foam pads at the armpits and around the hand grips are comfortable.
- Wear a sturdy low-heeled shoe on your unaffected foot.
- Keep the injured leg as relaxed as possible, and bend the knee to ensure that the leg clears the floor.
- Avoid scatter rugs, spills on the floor, extension cords, pets, and walking in the dark.

WALKERS

Walkers are usually made of aluminum and can be easily adjusted to fit the individual. Walkers are lightweight, can be folded for storage and traveling, and can be equipped with a front tray so that the user can carry items on it; it can also be fitted with a fold-down bench seat. The disadvantage to using a walker is the inability to use the walker on stairs and in small, tight areas such as a narrow hallway or bathroom.

If you are responsible for adjusting the height of a walker, ask the patient to stand. A chair or the examination table can be used to assist the patient in standing. The top of the walker should be just below the patient's waist, or at the same height as the top of the hip bone. Ask the patient to use the walker and observe the angle of the elbow. If the height is correct, the elbow should be bent at a 30-degree angle (Fig. 37–21).

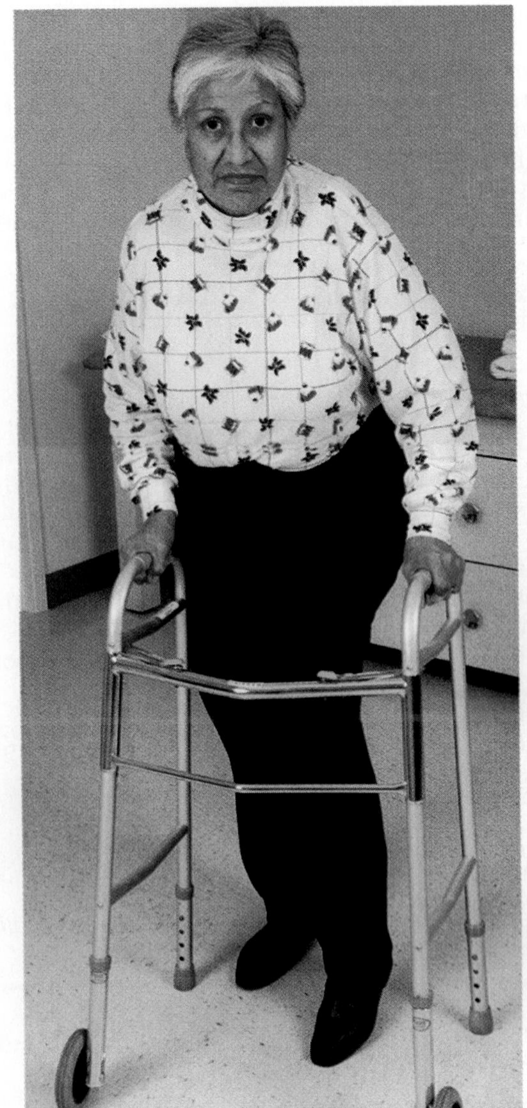

FIGURE 37–21 Using a walker. Note angle of arms and height of walker.

CANES

Canes come in two basic designs (Fig. 37–22). The first type is the conventional standard or single-tipped cane. It has a curved end that makes it easy to grip, and some have a hand grip built into the curved end. This type of cane is recommended for individuals who can ambulate with only minimal assistance.

The second type is the tripod (three legged) or the quad (four legged) cane. This type of device can stand alone if the patient needs to have his or her hands free. This cane is bulkier and heavier than the single-tipped cane and is recommended for patients who need greater support.

To measure the proper cane height, have the patient stand up straight. Adjust the cane so that the cane is level with the top of the patient's femur and the elbow should be bent at a 30-degree angle. Use Figure 37–19 to instruct the patient in the proper walking technique.

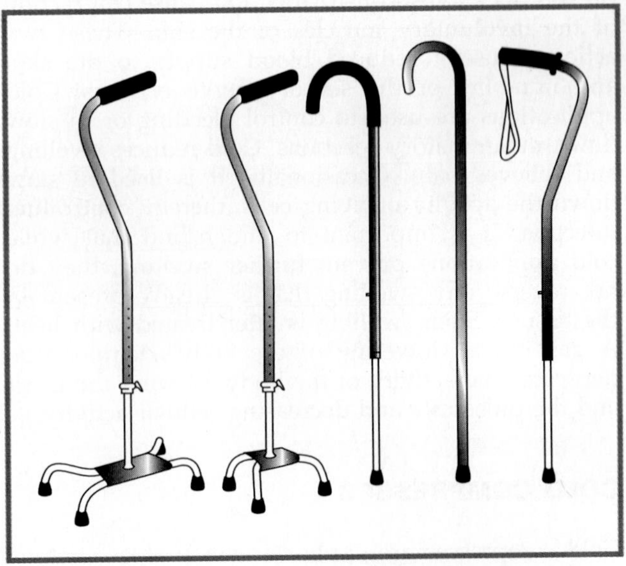

FIGURE 37–22 Types of standard canes.

WHEELCHAIRS

Wheelchairs provide mobility to patients who are paralyzed, have had an amputation, or have a crippling disease. A manual wheelchair uses arm muscles rather than leg muscles for mobility. Wheelchairs also come in motorized models that are controlled by the patient. The size of the chair depends on the size of the patient. The patient needing a wheelchair will need to be referred to a store that sells orthopedic prostheses to pick out the type of chair wanted and for fitting the chair to the patient.

TIPS FOR PATIENTS USING A WHEELCHAIR

- Lock the chair so that it cannot move.
- Fold back the foot rests.
- Back into the chair, and support yourself on the arm rests as you lower your body into the seat.
- To leave the chair, first lock the chair and then fold back the foot rests.
- Lift your body, supporting yourself on the arm rests.
- Place your unaffected foot flat on the floor, just slightly under the seat.
- Push into an upright position, using your thigh muscles along with your arm and shoulder muscles.

Memory Jogger

Name three common types of ambulatory appliances.

General Principles of Cold Application

Cold applications such as ice packs and cold compresses act as vasoconstrictors and cause contraction of the involuntary muscles of the skin. These two actions cause a reduced blood supply to the skin and numbing of the sensory nerve endings. Cold applications are used to control bleeding or to slow down inflammatory reactions. Cold reduces swelling and relieves pain. Occasionally, it is used to slow down the activity of living cells, thereby controlling infection. It is important to understand that while cold applications prevent further swelling, they do not reverse any swelling that is already present in the tissues. Such swelling is later treated with heat. A generalized lowering of the body's temperature depresses the activity of the body, slowing the heart and the pulse rate and decreasing cellular activity.

COLD COMPRESSES

Cold compresses are applied to small areas such as the face and the head. Gauze sponges or washcloths are most often used. The first cloth should be applied gently so that the patient gets used to the cold. Compresses should be changed every 3 minutes, and the total treatment is ordered usually for 20 minutes at a time. Advise patients to check the skin for signs of redness and swelling at the application site. Applications should be stopped if the cold causes pain.

ICE PACKS

Ice packs may be prescribed to control swelling and bleeding. The length of time for the ice pack to be used will depend on the injury and the purpose of the cold treatment. Always check the physician order to determine the area of the body that is to have the cold treatment and the length of time the ice pack is to remain on the area (see Procedure 37–3).

Usually, an ice pack is applied up to 1 hour or until the patient complains of pain from the cold or numbness, whichever occurs first. Ice packs should be covered with a cloth or towel to keep the patient dry. Ice packs without a covering may be too cold for the patient to tolerate.

Do not assume that a patient knows the correct technique of applying an ice pack. Instruct the patient on how to care for and apply ice packs at home. Ice packs may be made from items found in the home such as plastic bags and towels.

Commercially prepared chemical ice packs may be used and should be covered with a cloth before applying it to the injured area (Fig. 37–23). Because the chemical ice pack does not freeze and become solid, this form of ice pack is ideal for contouring to the body part being treated.

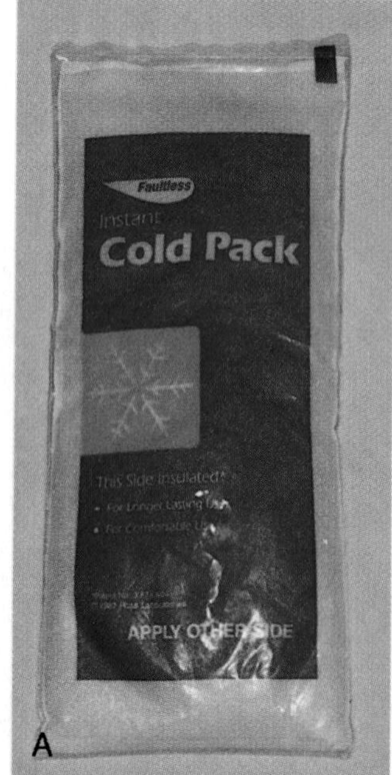

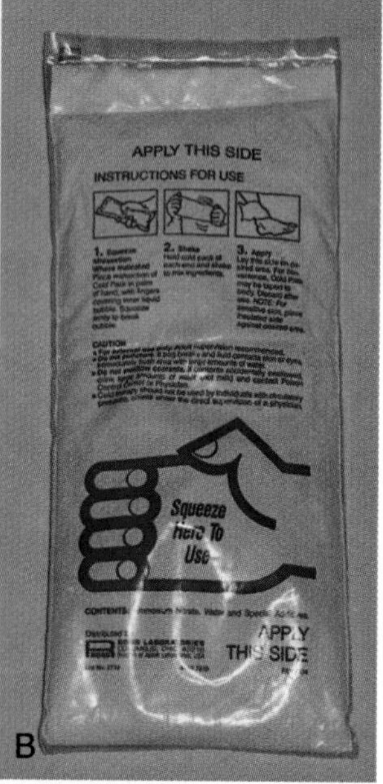

FIGURE 37–23 *A*, Commercial ice pack. *B*, Note instructions on back side.

PROCEDURE 37-3
Applying an Ice Bag

GOAL

To instruct a patient on how to apply dry cold to a body area to prevent swelling.

EQUIPMENT AND SUPPLIES

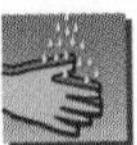

Ice bag
Small cubes or chips of ice
Towel

PROCEDURAL STEPS

1 Wash your hands.

2 Explain the procedure, and answer any questions that the patient may ask.

3 Check the bag for possible leaks.

4 Fill the bag with small cubes or chips of ice until it is about two-thirds full.
PURPOSE: Small chips conform better to the body part.

5 Push down on the top of the bag to expel excess air, and apply the cap.
PURPOSE: To remove air, which is a poor conductor of cold.

6 Dry and cover the bag.

7 Help the patient position the ice bag on the affected area.

8 Advise the patient to leave the ice bag in place for about 30 minutes or until the area feels numb.

9 Check the skin for color, feeling, and pain.
PURPOSE: If the area being treated becomes very painful, remains numb, or is pale or blue, the ice bag should be removed and the physician notified.

10 Record the procedure.
PURPOSE: A procedure is considered not done until it is recorded.

Memory Jogger

15 *Name two uses of cold application.*

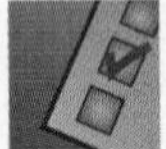

PATIENT EDUCATION

Musculoskeletal problems, particularly arthritis, are so widespread that its victims are easy prey for miracle drug promotions. It is important for you to recognize the need for patient education and work diligently with the patient and family encouraging participation in care programs that are effective.

Home care is an essential part of arthritic management. The Arthritis Foundation (1314 Spring Street NW, Atlanta, GA 30309) provides a number of pamphlets and other educational materials. The foundation also supports a broad program of research and education in the treatment of arthritis.

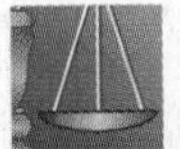

LEGAL AND ETHICAL ISSUES

Working with orthopedic patients may involve triage procedures, assisting with assessments, and performing procedures that directly involve the patient's recovery plan. Whenever you perform any independent technique, you are responsible for the procedure. To assist you in determining whether or not you are legally and ethically prepared to complete the task, ask yourself the following question:

1. Is there a written order for me to do the procedure?
2. Can I complete the procedure as it is ordered?
3. What am I to tell the patient regarding the reason for this procedure?
4. Do I know the instructions given to the patient by the physician?
5. Do I feel comfortable in doing the procedure?
6. If I am not comfortable, who can help me?

Always remember you are the assistant and this is the physician's patient and the physician is ultimately responsible for the patient's care. If you feel uncertain or unsure of an order that the physician has written, the time for clarification is before you proceed. Always stay within the ethical guidelines of the medical assistant profession.

CRITICAL THINKING

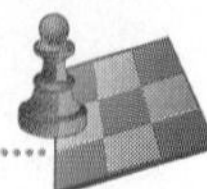

1 The father of a teenager comes into the office and says his son fell out of a tree and can't move his right leg. The father is quite sure that the leg is broken. The young man is in the car in the emergency parking area immediately in front of the office. Outline how you would handle the situation if the doctor is in the office. Would your plan change if the doctor was not in the office?

2 What methods would you use to teach a deaf, elderly patient to use crutches?

3 A patient has crippling arthritis and has broken the left ulna. What type of walking support would be the best for this patient? Where could you get advice to assist you in helping this patient (exclude your physician-employer)?

HOW DID I DO? Answers to Memory Joggers

1. Principal structures include bones, muscles, joints, cartilage, tendons, and ligaments.
2. Bone shapes include long, short, flat, rounded, and irregular.
3. Three types of muscle fibers are smooth, cardiac, and skeletal.
4. A tendon holds the muscle fibers to bone, and a ligament holds bone to bone.
5. To help maintain musculoskeletal health, physicians stress eating foods rich in calcium and vitamin D, exercising, and avoiding smoking.
6. Herniated disk most often occurs in the lumbar or lower back.
7. Scoliosis is most common in teenagers.
8. Osteoarthritis is caused by disintegration of the cartilage that covers the ends of bones.
9. Colchicine dramatically relieves gout pain.
10. Voluntary muscles become virtually useless because fat replaces the muscle fiber.
11. The symptom shared by all patients with a bone fracture is pain.
12. The physician may use inspection, palpation, range of motion, and muscle testing in an examination.
13. Two tests that measure nerve conduction are electromyography and nerve conduction velocity.
14. Three common types of appliances include crutches, canes, and walkers.
15. Two uses for cold application are to control bleeding or to slow down inflammatory reactions.

Assisting in Urology and Male Reproduction

38

Lance Granum, LVN, CHHA

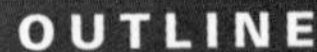

OUTLINE

Anatomy and Physiology of the Urinary System
- KIDNEY
- URETER
- URINARY BLADDER
- URETHRA

Disorders of the Urinary System
- URINARY INCONTINENCE
- GLOMERULONEPHRITIS
- RENAL FAILURE
- KIDNEY DIALYSIS
- PYELONEPHRITIS
- RENAL CARCINOMA
- RENAL CALCULI
- CYSTITIS
- HYDRONEPHROSIS
- POLYCYSTIC KIDNEYS
- URETHRITIS
- BLADDER CANCER

Pediatric Urologic Disorders
- ENURESIS
- URINE REFLUX DISORDER
- CRYPTORCHIDISM
- HYDROCELE

Diagnostic Testing
- RADIOLOGY OF KIDNEY, URETERS, AND BLADDER
- INTRAVENOUS PYELOGRAPHY/UROGRAPHY
- ANGIOGRAPHY
- COMPUTED TOMOGRAPHY
- CYSTOSCOPY
- RETROGRADE PYELOGRAPHY
- VOIDING CYSTOURETHROGRAPHY
- ULTRASONOGRAPHY

Anatomy and Physiology of the Male Reproductive System
- TESTES
- EPIDIDYMIS
- VAS DEFERENS
- PROSTATE GLAND
- PENIS
- HORMONE PRODUCTION

Disorders of the Male Reproductive Tract
- BENIGN PROSTATIC HYPERTROPHY
- PROSTATITIS
- PROSTATE CANCER
- EPIDIDYMITIS
- BALANITIS
- TESTICULAR CANCER
- IMPOTENCE
- INFERTILITY
- PEYRONIE'S DISEASE
- SEXUALLY TRANSMITTED DISEASES

The Medical Assistant's Role in the Urologic and the Male Reproductive Examinations
- CATHETERIZATION
  - *Procedure 38–1: Catheterization of the Female Patient*
  - *Procedure 38–2: Catheterization of the Male Patient*
- ASSISTING WITH THE UROLOGIC EXAMINATION
- ASSISTING WITH THE MALE REPRODUCTIVE EXAMINATION
- VASECTOMY
- DIAGNOSTIC TEST EXPLANATIONS
  - *Procedure 38–3: Teaching Testicular Self-Examination*
- PROSTATIC ACID PHOSPHATASE
- PROSTATE-SPECIFIC ANTIGEN
- TISSUE BIOPSY
- SEMEN TEST
- OTHER PROCEDURES

Patient Education

Legal and Ethical Issues

Critical Thinking

Answers to Memory Joggers

LEARNING OBJECTIVES

Cognitive: On successful completion of this chapter you should be able to:

1. List the organs of the urinary system and explain the function of each.
2. Explain the reason the urinary system has many opportunities for contracting diseases and disorders.
3. Compare and contrast the diseases and disorders of the urinary system.
4. Identify the primary signs and symptoms of urinary problems.
5. List the radiologic procedures used to diagnose urinary disorders.
6. List the organs included in male reproduction.
7. Trace sperm through the male reproductive tract.

8 Explain the cause and effects of prostate disorders.
9 Compare the effects of sexually transmitted diseases in the male with those in the female.
10 Understand and demonstrate the medical assistant's role in urology.
11 Define and spell vocabulary terms.

Performance: On successful completion of this chapter you should be able to:

1 Demonstrate with accuracy the catheterization of both the female and the male patient.
2 Accurately prepare a patient for a vasectomy.
3 Instruct a patient in performing self-testicular examination.
4 Explain to the patient reasons for a prostatic acid phosphatase (PAP) or prostate-specific antigen (PSA) test.
5 Prepare a patient for a tissue biopsy.

VOCABULARY

albumin Water-soluble, heat-coagulable protein

albuminuria Abnormal presence of albumin in the urine

anuria Complete suppression of urine formation by the kidney

casts Fibrous or protein material molded to the shape of the part in which it has accumulated and thrown off into the urine in kidney disease

catheter Thin, flexible tube inserted into the body to permit introduction or withdrawal of fluid

circumcision Surgical removal of the foreskin

copulation Sexual intercourse

creatinine Nitrogenous waste from muscle metabolism excreted in urine

dysuria Painful or difficult urination

edema Intracellular accumulation of excess fluid swelling between the layers of tissue

ejaculation Ejection of the seminal fluid from the male urethra

erythropoietin Substance released from the kidney and liver that promotes red blood cell formation

fenestrated drape Surgical drape or cover that has a prepared opening

frequency Excessive need to urinate

hematuria The presence of blood in the urine

hemodialysis Type of kidney dialysis in which an artificial kidney machine is used to cleanse the blood

incontinence Inability to control urination functions

invasive Procedure in which a body cavity is entered or tissue is pierced

irrigation Cleansing of the bladder or other body cavity with water or other fluids to treat inflammation or infection

malaise Feeling of discomfort or uneasiness

malignant Growing worse, resisting treatment, threatening to produce death; cancerous

micturition Urination; act of voiding

nitrogenous waste Product of metabolism that if left to accumulate may become toxic

nocturia Urination occurring during the night

oliguria Sudden drop in urine volume

peritoneal dialysis A type of dialysis in which fluid is injected through a catheter into the abdomen to remove waste products

pyuria Pus in the urine

reflux Return or backward flow

renin Enzyme produced in the kidney that helps in the regulation of blood pressure

residual Urine left in the bladder after urination

retention Inability to empty the bladder

semen Thick, whitish secretion containing spermatozoa

spermatozoa Mature male sex cells or germ cells

urea End product formed by protein metabolism after ammonia is broken down by the liver

urgency Sudden, compelling desire to urinate and the inability to control its release

vasectomy Male sterilization procedure

viable Able to sustain life

Urology is the study of the urinary tract in both male and female patients. The physician who specializes in the diseases and disorders of the urinary system is a urologist. The urologist also specializes in the diseases and disorders of the male reproductive system. There is a wide variety of medical treatments, from radiologic to surgical, available to the urologist to treat the diseases and disorders of the urinary system.

Anatomy and Physiology of the Urinary System

The urinary tract consists of two kidneys, two ureters, one urinary bladder, and one urethra (Fig. 38–1). The main function of the urinary system is to remove waste products from the body. A variety of wastes are produced as by-products of the body's metabolic processes and, if left to accumulate, can become toxic. The urinary system removes salts and **nitrogenous waste,** which is the product of protein breakdown, in the form of soluble urea from the blood and carries it outside the body through tube-like organs. The urinary system also helps to maintain the normal concentration of water and electrolytes, regulate pH and volume of fluid, and control red blood cell production and blood pressure.

KIDNEY

The kidneys are red-brown, bean-shaped glandular organs. They are retroperitoneal (behind the peritoneum) and against the muscles of the back, roughly between the T12 and L3 vertebrae. The left kidney is located approximately 2 cm higher than the right owing to the location of the liver.

The kidneys are responsible for removing unwanted substances from the blood and forming urine. They also help control the rate of red blood cell formation by secreting the hormone **erythropoietin,** help regulate blood pressure by the secretion of the enzyme **renin,** and encourage calcium ion absorption by activating vitamin D.

The kidneys receive a great deal of blood for their cleansing process, somewhere between 15% and 30%

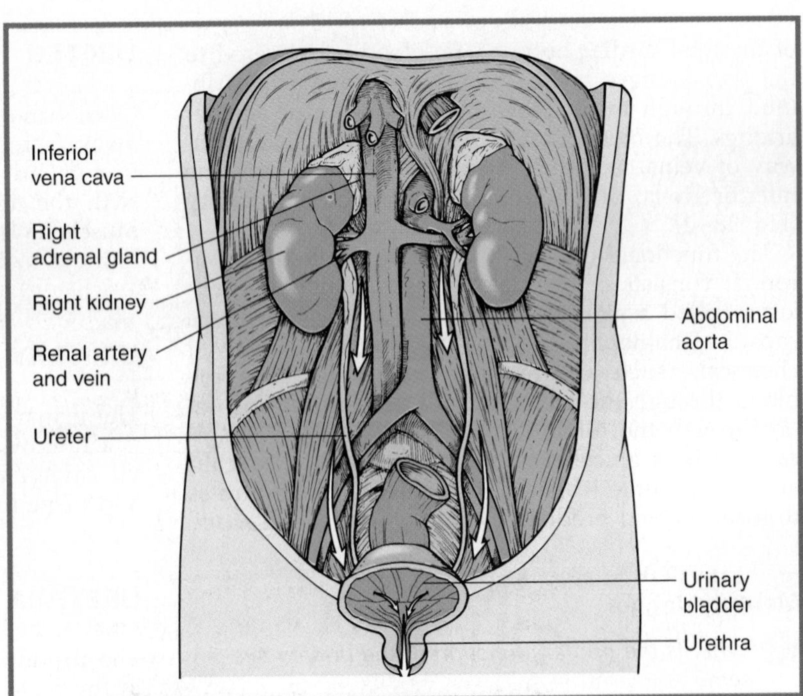

FIGURE 38–1 The urinary system. (From Frazier MS, Drzymkowski JA, Doty SJ: Essentials of Human Diseases and Conditions. Philadelphia, WB Saunders, 1996.)

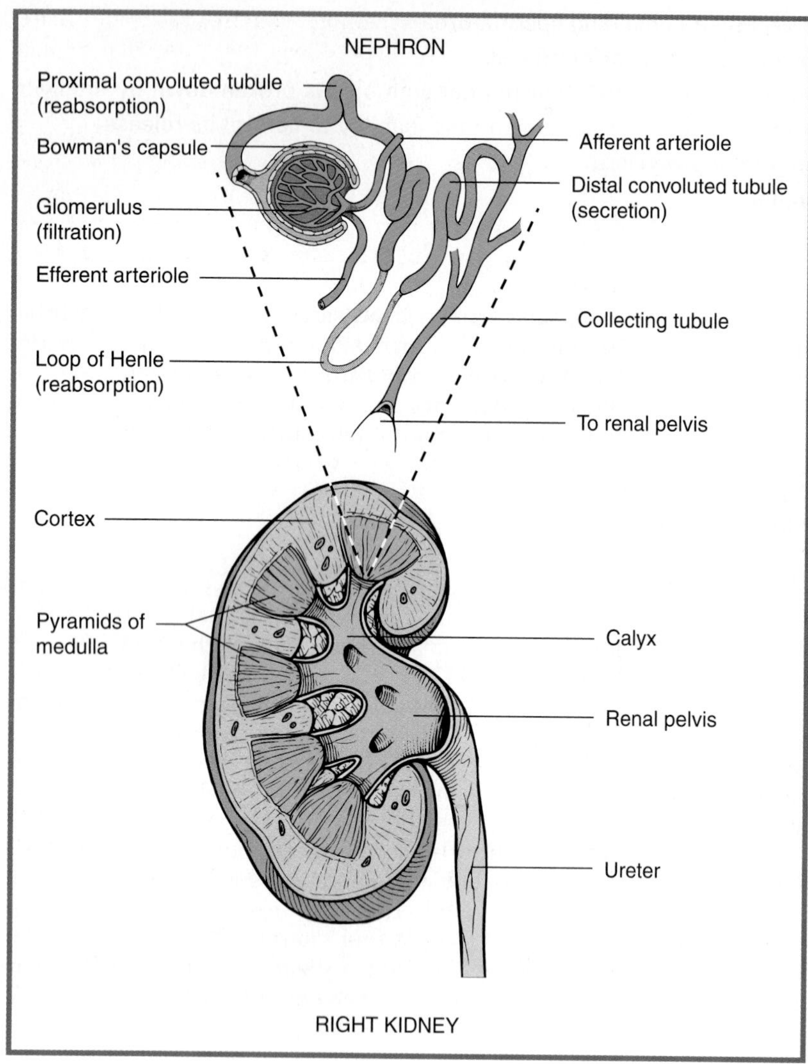

FIGURE 38–2 The kidney. (From Frazier MS, Drzymkowski JA, Doty SJ: Essentials of Human Diseases and Conditions. Philadelphia, WB Saunders, 1996.)

of the total cardiac output. The blood is delivered to the two kidneys by the renal artery and is distributed through the kidneys by a highway of smaller arteries. The blood is then returned through a pathway of veins, including the renal vein that joins the inferior vena cava through the abdominal cavity (Fig. 38–2).

The functional unit of the kidney is called a nephron. It consists of a tangled cluster of blood capillaries called a glomerulus surrounded by Bowman's capsule. The nephrons filter out water and dissolved chemicals, such as **urea** and **creatinine,** from the blood through the glomerulus. As the filtrate passes on through the tubules, it reabsorbs needed chemicals, such as glucose, and secretes excess chemicals; and by the time it reaches the calyx, it concentrates to form the end product, urine.

Memory Jogger

What is the primary function of the urinary system?

URETER

Once urine is produced, the job of transporting it away from the kidneys falls to the ureter. The two ureters are tubular organs about 25 cm long; and with the aid of peristaltic waves generated by the muscle layer, the ureters move the urine from the kidneys to the urinary bladder.

URINARY BLADDER

The urinary bladder is basically a urine reservoir. It is a hollow, muscular organ that lies within the pelvic cavity. When the bladder is full, sphincters open and urine flows into the urethra.

URETHRA

The urethra is lined with a mucous membrane and in the male functions as both urinary canal and passageway for cells and secretions from various reproductive organs. In the male, the urethra is divided into three sections: the prostatic urethra, the membranous urethra, and the penile urethra. The urethra conveys the urine from the bladder. It passes through the meatus and outside the body. The process of urinating urine through the urethra is known as voiding or **micturition.**

Memory Jogger

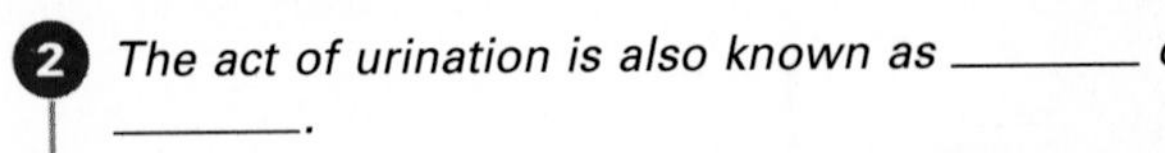

The act of urination is also known as ______ or ______.

Disorders of the Urinary System

The urinary tract has many opportunities for contracting diseases and disorders; and, as a result, there are a wide range of symptoms, with the most common involving changes in the frequency of urination. **Dysuria,** difficult or painful urination, **urgency,** and **incontinence** are all common symptoms. Abnormal functions of any part of the urinary tract can often be determined with urinalysis, which is the most common test, with blood urea nitrogen (BUN) levels, and with creatinine clearance. These tests are discussed in Chapter 43. Radiologic testing is also important to detect urinary tract diseases. Specialized radiographs such as from the radiography of the kidneys, ureters, and bladder (KUB) or intravenous pyelography/urography are important diagnostic tools for urologists.

Memory Jogger

Name three common symptoms involving changes in the frequency of urination.

URINARY INCONTINENCE

Urinary incontinence, the involuntary release of urine, can be the result of many conditions. Infections of the urinary tract, brain disorders, and tissue damage can all lead to urinary incontinence. This disorder can also be caused by straining or coughing in postsurgical patients and in patients with relaxed pelvic musculature. When caused in this manner it is termed stress incontinence.

Treatment methods for incontinence will depend on the causative factor. Retraining a patient to recognize the sensation of having to void can be successful in cases in which mental confusion is the basis for the incontinence. In cases in which relaxed musculature is at fault, teaching the patient to perform muscle-strengthening exercises, known as Kegel exercises, can help solve the problem. Special appliances have also been developed to aid incontinent patients. For the male patient, an external drainage apparatus may be applied. The incontinence urinal is a rubber device that resembles a jock strap with a collection bag strapped to the lower thigh. A catheter is inserted through the meatus and drains into the bag. The bag is drained by a tube at the bottom.

When all other treatments have failed, surgical intervention in the guise of an artificial bladder sphincter can be implemented. This hydraulically activated mechanism is placed around the urethra, or bladder neck, and is made to open and close by squeezing one of two bulbs implanted under the skin of the scrotum or labia.

GLOMERULONEPHRITIS

Many urinary tract diseases and disorders arise from bacterial infections. Glomerulonephritis, the degenerative inflammation of the kidney glomeruli, usually develops in children and young adults after a previous streptococcal infection such as strep throat or scarlet fever. Its symptoms usually include fever and chills, loss of appetite, and general **malaise. Edema** may be present in the face and ankles. A urinalysis will show the presence of blood and increased **albumin.** Prognosis is usually good for an attack of acute glomerulonephritis, but prolonged reinfection can lead to a chronic condition that can eventually cause the kidneys to fail.

Memory Jogger

In glomerulonephritis, urinalysis will show the presence of ______.

RENAL FAILURE

Chronic glomerulonephritis as well as other severe kidney diseases and certain toxic chemicals, or poisons, can also cause the kidneys to cease functioning. The end result is that the kidneys can no longer remove waste products from the blood and toxicity develops.

In an acute condition, there is usually **oliguria,** a sudden drop in urine volume, or a total absence of urine, known as **anuria.** The patient's symptoms can include gastrointestinal upset; deep, sighing respiration; a distinct urine smell of the breath; and drowsiness. When examined, the urine can also show **pyuria, hematuria, albuminuria,** and **casts.** If treated, acute renal failure has a good prognosis; however, chronic renal failure can develop, and this very serious disease can result in death. In these conditions, dialysis is usually done.

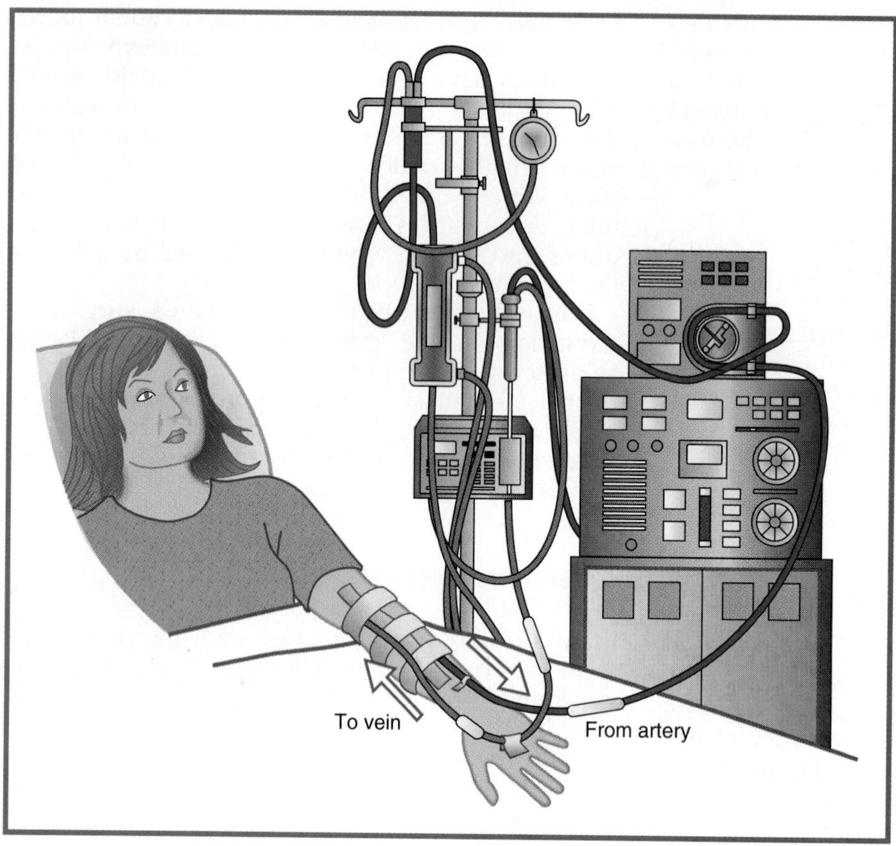

FIGURE 38–3 Hemodialysis.

KIDNEY DIALYSIS

Dialysis, or cleansing of the blood, can be done in two methods. The first, **hemodialysis,** is the removal of waste-filled blood from the body by a machine known as an artificial kidney. It filters out the waste products and returns the cleansed blood to the body (Fig. 38–3). **Peritoneal dialysis** is a blood-cleansing process by which dialyzing fluid is infused into a patient's abdomen with a peritoneal catheter. The fluid absorbs the waste products and then is released out of the body again through the catheter. This process can be controlled either by the aid of a machine or by the patient himself or herself.

Memory Jogger

5 *Name two forms of kidney dialysis.*

PYELONEPHRITIS

Pyelonephritis, inflammation of the kidney and renal pelvis, is another urinary disease caused by bacterial infection. It is a suppurative disease, which means that formation of pus is associated with it. The infection is usually caused by a bacteria, such as *Escherichia coli,* that originates in the lower gastrointestinal tract and spreads into the kidneys. It may also arise from a descending infection carried by the bloodstream. The symptoms of pyelonephritis include chills and fever, back pain, and dysuria. Urine examination will show pyuria and hematuria. The prognosis is good when antibiotics are employed.

RENAL CARCINOMA

One disease of the urinary tract that is not caused by bacteria is renal carcinoma. This tumor may not manifest itself right away and does metastasize to the lungs, liver, male urogenital system, bone, and brain. Roughly 2% of all cancers in adults are renal carcinomas. In children, a malignant form of the disease is known as Wilms' tumor. Symptoms of the disease include pain, loss of appetite, anemia, and an increased white blood cell count. Urinalysis will show hematuria. Surgical nephrectomy is the best treatment, and prognosis for the tumor has improved over the past few years.

Memory Jogger

6 *Identify the malignant form of renal carcinoma seen in children.*

RENAL CALCULI

Another nonbacterial disorder is renal calculi, or kidney stones. Kidney stones are created when salts in the urine collect in the kidney and grow. Small stones usually do not cause any difficulty until they grow large enough to lodge in the ureters or renal pelvis. These may pass spontaneously. The stones can be removed either with surgery or by lithotripsy (Fig. 38–4), which is the crushing of the stones by laser or shock waves. The patient will experience dysuria and back pain. A urine examination will show hematuria and leukocytes if the stones form in the bladder and cause cystitis. Ultrasonography and urography can both confirm the diagnosis.

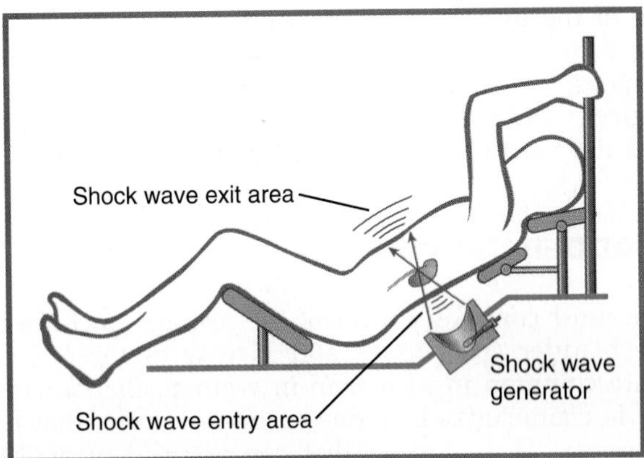

FIGURE 38–4 Lithotripsy.

CYSTITIS

Kidney stones are just one of the few causes of cystitis, or bladder infection. The condition tends to arise from an invading organism that ascends through the urethra. Cystitis occurs more frequently in women than men, owing to the shorter urethra in women. The symptoms of cystitis are usually **frequency** and urgency of urination as well as a stinging sensation when voiding. Urinalysis shows bacteria, pyuria, casts, and leukocytes. Antibiotics are used to cure the condition.

Memory Jogger

7 *Why is cystitis more frequently seen in women?*

HYDRONEPHROSIS

Kidney stones are also responsible for the condition known as hydronephrosis, the extreme dilation of the kidneys by water. An enlarged prostate or a tumor can also lead to this condition because either can close off the passage of urine. Hydronephrosis can occur bilaterally or unilaterally. Pain occurs that is directly related to the nature of the blockage. Urine testing will detect hematuria and, if infection develops from stagnant urine, pyuria. Removing the blockage will correct the condition (Fig. 38–5).

POLYCYSTIC KIDNEYS

Polycystic kidney is a congenital abnormality that consists of multiple cysts developing in one or both kidneys. Kidney tubules that do not open into the renal pelvis become enlarged, fuse, and then become infected. As the cysts enlarge, they compress the surrounding tissue and this eventually leads to uremia, the toxic condition resulting from kidney failure, and then to death.

URETHRITIS

Urethritis is the inflammation of the urethra and is more common in males. It results from a gonococcal infection or infection with other pathogenic bacteria, viruses, and chemicals. The symptoms include discharge of pus and an itching sensation at the open-

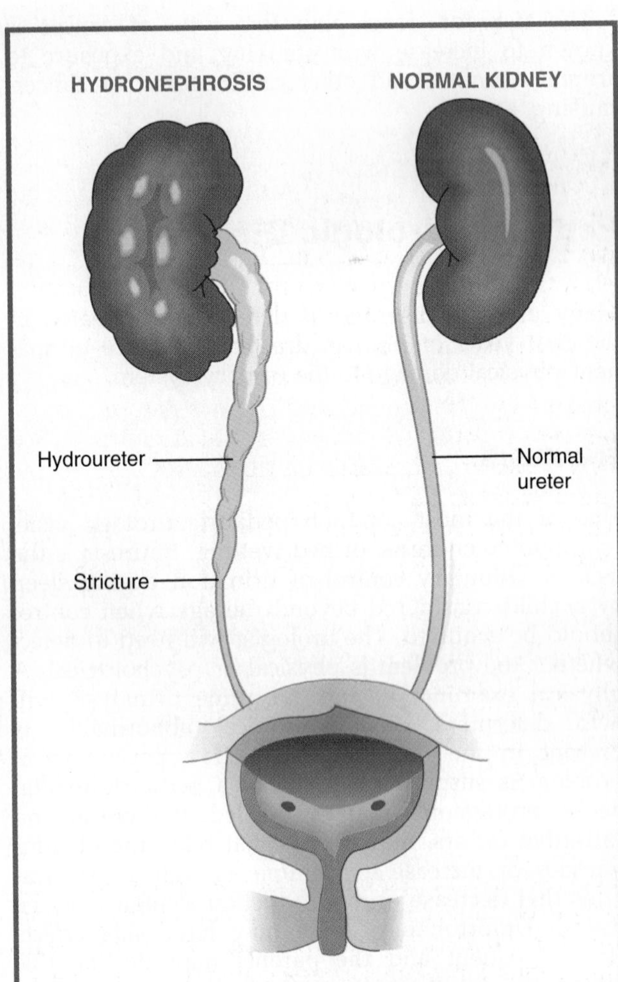

FIGURE 38–5 Hydronephrosis.

ing of the urethra. There is a burning sensation during urination, and it can accompany cystitis in females. Urinalysis may show hematuria as well as pyuria. Antibiotics are used to treat the condition, and the female partner should be treated as well.

BLADDER CANCER

The most common cancer of the urinary tract affects the bladder (Fig. 38–6) and is two to three times more common in men than in women. Bladder cancer is characterized by one or more tumors that can reappear. Thus, testing that can identify recurrence is extremely important. A urine test, known as NMP22, has been approved by the Food and Drug Administration for use in identifying a recurrence of the disease in the half million patients monitored every year. This test is twice as sensitive as urine cytology and is painless and inexpensive. It works by identifying the nuclear matrix protein present in the transitional cells of the bladder. Ninety percent of bladder cancers are attributed to these particular cells, called transitional cells, owing to their ability to be cubelike when the bladder is empty and flat when it is full.

The risk for developing this type of cancer is known to increase with smoking and exposure to aromatic amines and other carcinogenic, or cancer-causing, agents.

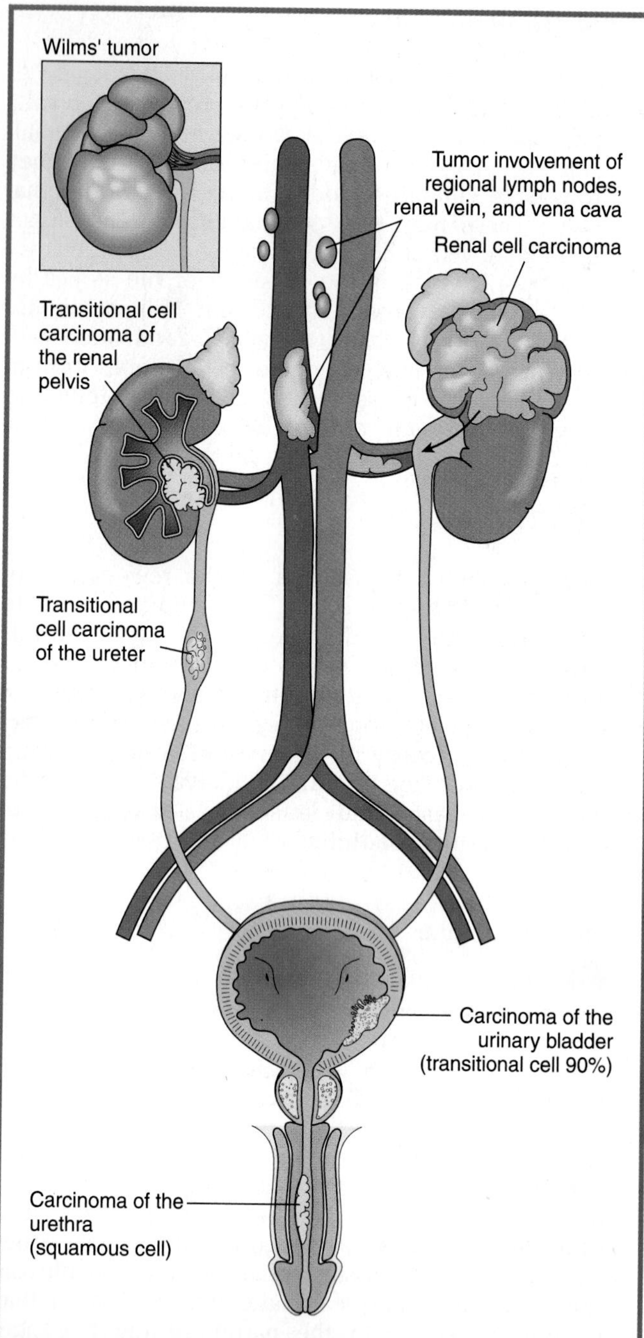

FIGURE 38–6 Neoplasms of the urinary tract. (From Damjanov I: Pathology for the Health-Related Professions. Philadelphia, WB Saunders, 1996.)

Pediatric Urologic Disorders

Many urologic disorders if detected and treated in the first years of life can drastically reduce permanent physical damage to the urinary system.

ENURESIS

One of the most common pediatric urology visits will involve enuresis, or bed wetting. Enuresis is the lack of voluntary control of urination during sleep by a child considered beyond the age when control should be acquired. The urologist will need to detect whether the problem is physical or psychological. A physical examination and a routine urinalysis will help determine if any physical abnormality is present in the urinary system. If a psychological problem is suspected, help from a pediatric mental health professional may be needed. If there are no causative factors, medications that relax the bladder muscles or increase its volume as well as medications that decrease urine production at night may be useful. Unfortunately, these may have side effects for the patient and the parents may decline this treatment. In these instances, conditioning with alarms may be an effective way to help treat the patient.

URINE REFLUX DISORDER

Another reason for pediatric urology referrals may be urine reflux disorders. Urine **reflux** is caused by the backward flow of urine in the ureters during voiding. This can be detected early in utero by ultrasonography or later with a voiding cystourethrogram (Fig. 38–7). This test involves the placing of a urinary catheter in the bladder and filling it with a dye or radioactive material that helps visualize the flow of urine. Although an uncomfortable proce-

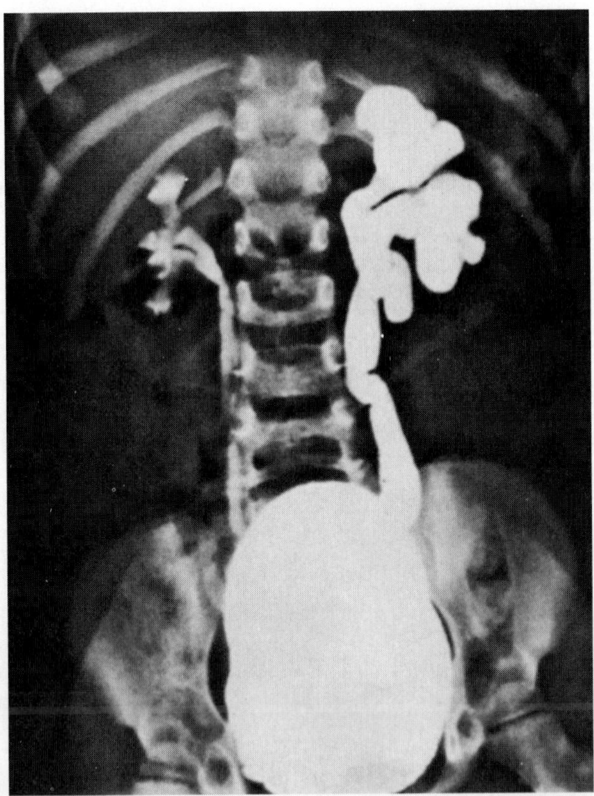

FIGURE 38–7 Voiding cystourethrogram. (From James AE Jr, Squire LF: Nuclear Radiology. Philadelphia, WB Saunders, 1973.)

dure, the benefit of early detection and decreased damage to the kidney makes the screening worthwhile.

Treatment of reflux is usually determined by grading severity on a 1 to 5 scale, with 5 being the highest. Prophylactic antibiotics are given in low doses daily to avoid damaging kidney infections, and this is usually sufficient for low-grade reflux, which can disappear on its own. However, with higher grade reflux that persists after 4 or 5 years or for patients who have breakthrough infections despite the antibiotics, surgical repair of the ureters is necessary. Patients and physicians may also opt for surgery because the procedure has a high success rate of 95% and poses little risk.

CRYPTORCHIDISM

A common disorder for young boys involves undescended testes, a condition known as cryptorchidism (Fig. 38–8). Normally, the testes develop in the abdominal cavity of the fetus and then descend into the scrotum near the end of the pregnancy. In some instances, however, the path is incomplete or incorrect. Most testes will come down within 3 to 4 months from birth, but persistent cryptorchidism should be treated. Infertility, owing to slightly warmer temperature effect on sperm, and increased chance of testicular cancer are two reasons for treatment.

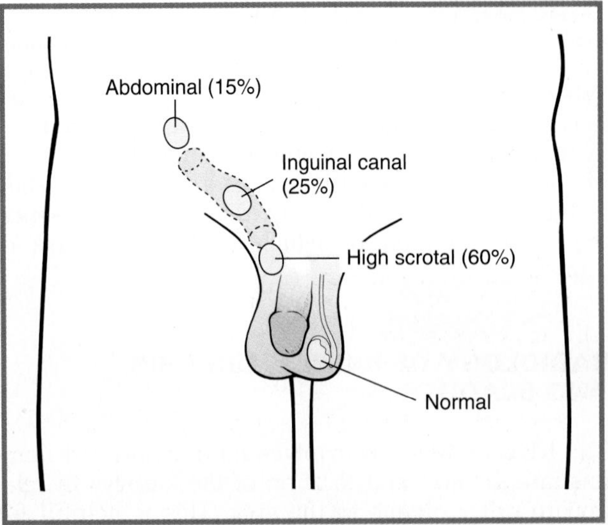

FIGURE 38–8 Cryptorchidism. (From Damjanov I: Pathology for the Health-Related Professions. Philadelphia, WB Saunders, 1996.)

Location of the errant testes will dictate the form of treatment. Testes that are palpable are usually treated with hormones or with an outpatient surgical procedure known as orchidopexy. If the testes is impalpable (cannot be felt), then a laparoscopy is necessary to locate it. This procedure includes inserting a telescope into the abdomen by way of a small incision near the navel. Once found, the testes is either moved into proper position or removed. Success rates decrease with testes that are placed higher.

HYDROCELE

During the descent of the testes, a small canal develops for them to pass through. If the canal does not close after birth, fluid from the peritoneal cavity may pass through and form in the scrotum. This is called a hydrocele and must be corrected surgically (Fig. 38–9). It is usually benign but may lead to scrotal swelling, which can be painful.

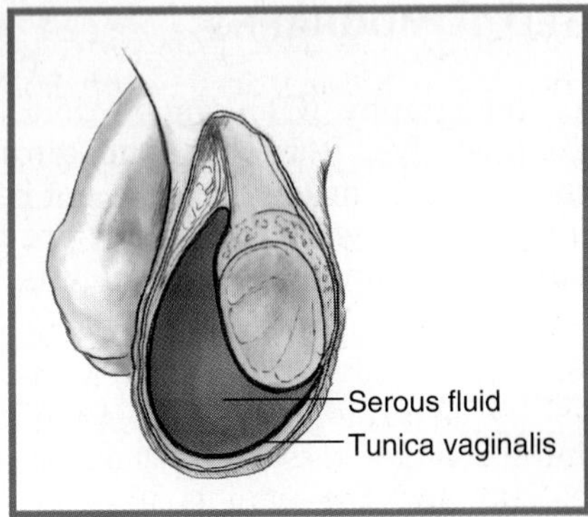

FIGURE 38–9 Hydrocele. (From Jarvis C: Physical Examination and Health Assessment, 2nd ed. Philadelphia, WB Saunders, 1996.)

Diagnostic Testing

When urinalysis detects an abnormality in the urinary tract, there are many new testing procedures available for in-depth diagnostic determinations. All of the previously mentioned disorders have certain testing procedures that help detect their presence, the most common of which involves the use of x-rays.

RADIOLOGY OF KIDNEY, URETERS, AND BLADDER

The KUB radiograph involves no dye and can demonstrate the size and location of the kidneys in relation to other organs in the area. This is helpful for spotting an enlarged or deteriorating kidney, such as can be found with hydronephrosis.

INTRAVENOUS PYELOGRAPHY/ UROGRAPHY

Intravenous pyelography (IVP), also known as urography, is another radiographic technique, but it involves the injection of dye into the veins. This contrast material travels to the urinary system, where it fills the kidneys, ureters, bladder, and urethra. The x-ray films taken provide an overall view of renal function as well as show the presence of cysts, tumors, infection, and calculi.

ANGIOGRAPHY

Another diagnostic examination using dye for visualization of the urinary system is renal angiography. The dye is injected into the circulation, filling arteries and veins of the kidney, and radiographs are taken. Vessel narrowing, cysts, blood clots, and tumors in the kidney can all be determined by this examination.

COMPUTED TOMOGRAPHY

Computed tomography (CT) can be done with or without contrast dye. It is not done during renal failure, when contrast material should not be administered. Transverse views of the kidney are taken by CT and can detect tumors, abscesses, cysts, and hydronephrosis.

CYSTOSCOPY

Cystoscopy is an examination that views the urinary bladder, not by injecting dyes and using radiographs but by inserting a cystoscope into the bladder (Fig. 38–10). The cystoscope is a hollow metal tube that is passed through the urethra and into the bladder. By using fiberoptic lights and reflections, the cystoscope allows the bladder mucosa to be observed for inflammation, calculi, and tumors. Sterile urine samples from the bladder can be removed for testing by inserting a catheter through the cystoscope. Cystoscopy is usually performed as an outpatient procedure in a surgical center.

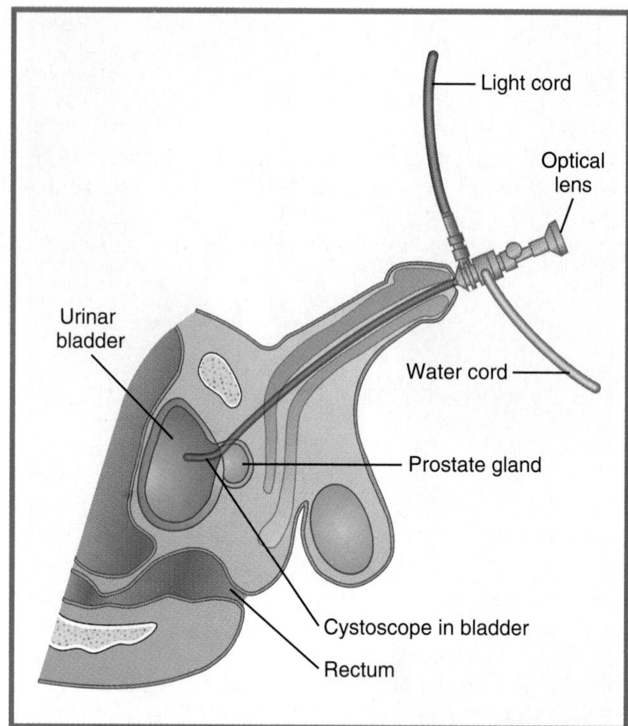

FIGURE 38–10 Cystoscopy.

RETROGRADE PYELOGRAPHY

Dye can be injected into the bladder, ureters, and kidney through a cystoscope in the same manner that the urine sample is gathered. This technique is used to detect stones and other obstructions. It is also used to replace an IVP for patients with renal failure, with physical blockages, or with allergies to the intravenous dye.

VOIDING CYSTOURETHROGRAPHY

In a voiding cystourethrogram (VCUG), dye is injected into the bladder after a straight catheter is inserted. The catheter is removed, and radiographs are taken while the patient is urinating. It can show reflux of urine, which is not a normally occurring phenomenon, and excessive urine retention. Obstructions and hydronephrosis can also be seen.

ULTRASONOGRAPHY

Ultrasonography, scans taken using sound waves, is a noninvasive examination that helps detect abnormalities in the urinary system. Kidney size can be examined; and disorders such as hydronephrosis, polycystic kidneys, and obstructions of the ureters and bladder can all be seen using ultrasonography. No renal function information can be determined.

Memory Jogger

Name eight radiologic tests that can be done to diagnose urinary disorders.

Anatomy and Physiology of the Male Reproductive System

The male reproductive system plays an important role in the continuation of the human species. Although not necessary for individual survival, the production, sustaining, and transport of male sex cells is vital to the creation of life.

The male reproductive system consists of both primary and secondary organs. The secondary organs are further broken down into external and internal organs (Fig. 38–11).

TESTES

The primary reproductive organs in the male are a pair of testes. Each testis is an oval structure 4 to 5 cm in length and 2.5 to 3 cm in diameter. Each is surrounded by a white, fibrous capsule, and they are contained together in the retractable saclike scrotum. The testes are primarily responsible for production of the male hormone testosterone and produce **spermatozoa,** the male sex cells. These cells contain 23 chromosomes, or half of the DNA chain needed to form a complete cell. When conception takes place, these 23 chromosomes plus the ovum's 23 chromosomes will unite to form a new complete cell.

The sperm cells are tadpole-like structures less than 0.1 mm long and, when mature, will be stored in the epididymis (Fig. 38–12).

EPIDIDYMIS

The epididymis is a long, coiled tube that rests on the top and lateral side of each testis. Each epididymis is approximately 6 meters long and connects

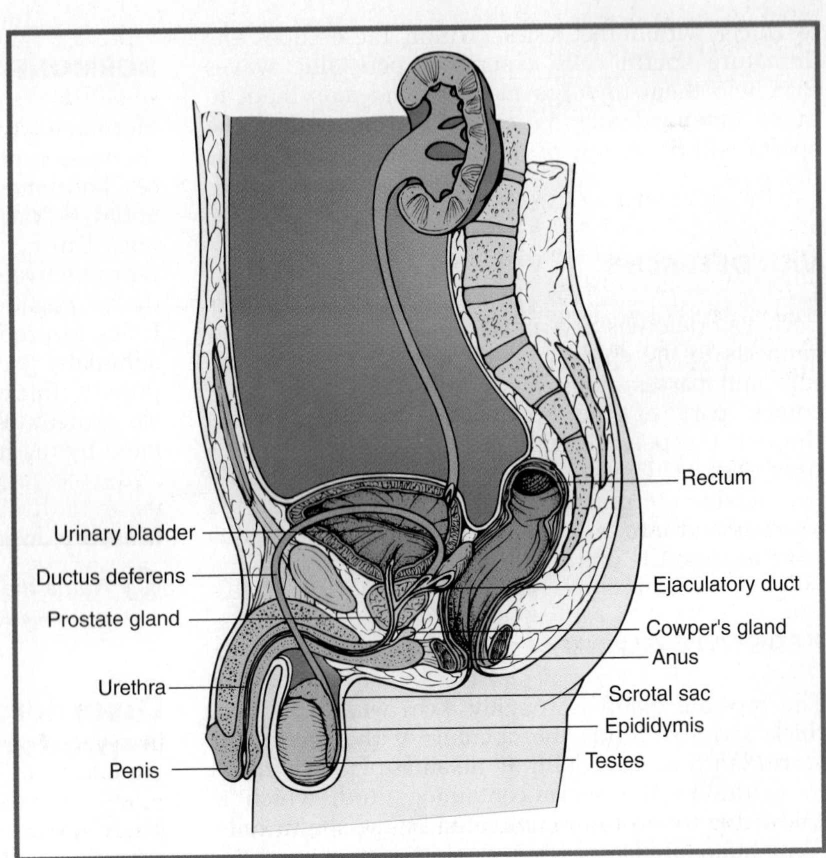

FIGURE 38–11 Male reproductive anatomy. (From Frazier MS, Drzymkowski JA, Doty SJ: Essentials of Human Diseases and Conditions. Philadelphia, WB Saunders, 1996.)

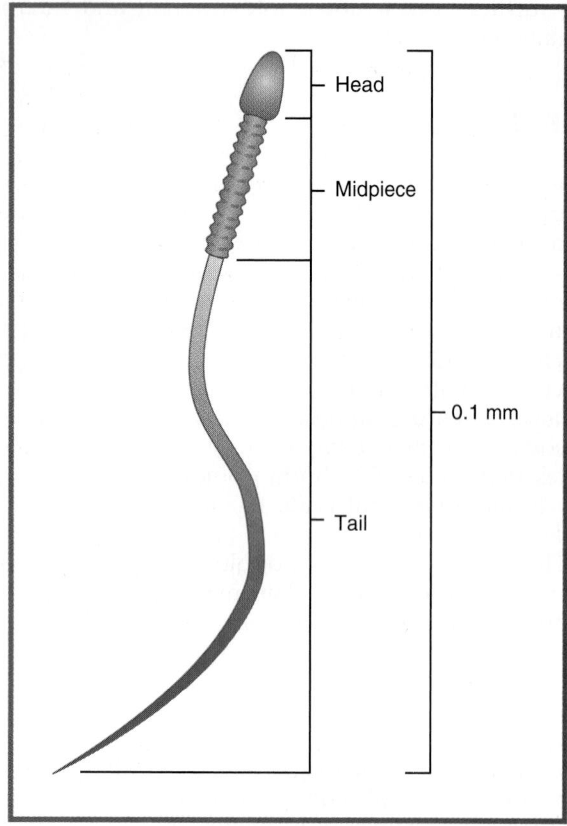

FIGURE 38–12 Sperm.

to ducts within the testes. Within these tubes the immature sperm cells experience peristaltic waves that help them undergo maturity and aids them to move independently. When **ejaculation** occurs, the sperm will move out of the epididymis into the vas deferens.

VAS DEFERENS

Each vas deferens is a muscular, 45-cm tunnel that connects to the epididymis at the base of the structure and passes along the side of the testes. It becomes part of the spermatic cord that passes through the pelvic cavity and ends behind the urinary bladder. Uniting there with the seminal vesicle just outside the prostate gland, it passes through the prostate and into an ejaculatory duct that empties its contents into the urethra.

PROSTATE GLAND

The prostate gland is roughly 4 cm wide and 3 cm thick and surrounds the opening of the urethra. It secretes a thin fluid with an alkaline pH. This helps to neutralize the sperm-containing fluid, which is acidic due to wastes accumulated by the sperm cells. This fluid can also neutralize acidic secretions of the vagina, thereby helping to sustain the sperm cells that enter the female reproductive tract, and, added to secretions from the vas deferens, seminal vesicles, and bulbourethral gland, makes up **semen.** The volume of semen in one ejaculate varies from 2 to 6 mL and averages roughly 120 million sperm per milliliter.

PENIS

The organ of male **copulation** is the penis. It is a cylindrical organ consisting of an elongated body with a slightly enlarged end, called the glans penis. Around the glans penis there is a fold of skin that begins just behind the glans and extends forward to cover it like a sheath. This is called the prepuce, or foreskin, and is sometimes removed in a surgical procedure known as **circumcision.** The penis is responsible for conveying urine and semen through the urethra and outside the body. When transmitting semen to the female tract, the penis must enlarge and stiffen for insertion. This is done when three columns of erectile tissue within the penis become stimulated. The arteries within the penis dilate and the veins compress. This compression of the veins allows a reduction of blood flow away from the penis, causing it to swell. Motor impulses are stimulated by the swelling of the urethra due to semen collection, and the contracting of the urethra causes the semen to be ejaculated through the penis.

HORMONE PRODUCTION

Hormone production is also an important aspect of the male reproductive system. As a group, the male sex hormones are called androgens. The most influential product of hormone production is testosterone. During pubescence, when the male becomes reproductively functional, the pituitary gland produces gonadotrophic hormones that stimulate the testes to produce testosterone. Testosterone, in turn, stimulates the testes to enlarge, increases body hair growth, thickens skin and bone, and increases muscle growth. The production of testosterone is regulated by the hypothalamus in the brain.

Memory Jogger

9 *Name the most influential male hormone.*

Disorders of the Male Reproductive Tract

There are many diseases and disorders of the male reproductive tract. The most common of these involve enlargement or inflammation of certain organs as well as **malignant** tumors. The prostate is the most widely affected organ.

BENIGN PROSTATIC HYPERTROPHY

For men older than 50 the occurrence of enlargement of the prostate is very common. Benign prostatic hyperplasia increases with age. The swelling of the prostate gland partially blocks the flow of urine, causing a medium for bacterial infection that can lead to cystitis. This blockage can also extend to the ureters and kidneys.

Benign prostatic hyperplasia is usually brought on by the decrease of testosterone production as the male ages. This condition is usually found during routine examination and is treated by hormone therapy, chemotherapy, or surgical removal (Fig. 38–13). Although the gland can be removed through an abdominal incision, the most common approach is through the urethra. This procedure is a transurethral resection of the prostate.

PROSTATITIS

The cause of inflammation of the prostate is not always known but usually develops in the presence of infection. The common symptoms are dysuria, tenderness of the prostate region, and secretion of pus from the tip of the penis. Treatment is usually with an antibiotic such as penicillin.

PROSTATE CANCER

Cancer of the prostate is common in older men. The American Cancer Society reports that 165,000 American men, most older than 65, contract the disease every year and approximately 30,000 die of this disease every year. These tumors can be small and asymptomatic and are usually found during a digital rectal examination. The patient may experience many symptoms. Urinary obstruction, increased bouts of urinary infection, and frequent **nocturia** (the need to void at night) are all symptoms of prostate cancer.

These malignant tumors spread rapidly to the bladder and rectum and often metastasize to the lymph nodes, bones, lungs, and brain. The prognosis for these cancers is rather poor unless the tumor is discovered in its early stages of development.

The extent of the prostate cancer will dictate treatment options. Hormone therapy is generally prescribed because estrogen will inhibit the production of testosterone and testosterone has been proven to increase tumor growth. The surgical removal of the testosterone-producing testes as well as of the tumor itself is also performed. This is a debilitating surgery that has side effects such as impotence and incontinence. An alternative procedure is radioactive seed implant, a variant of radiation therapy. In this procedure, tiny radioactive seeds are placed directly in the prostate gland through a precisely placed hollow needle. The radiation is quite strong but has a very short range, so that it destroys the tumor and minimizes damage to surrounding tissue.

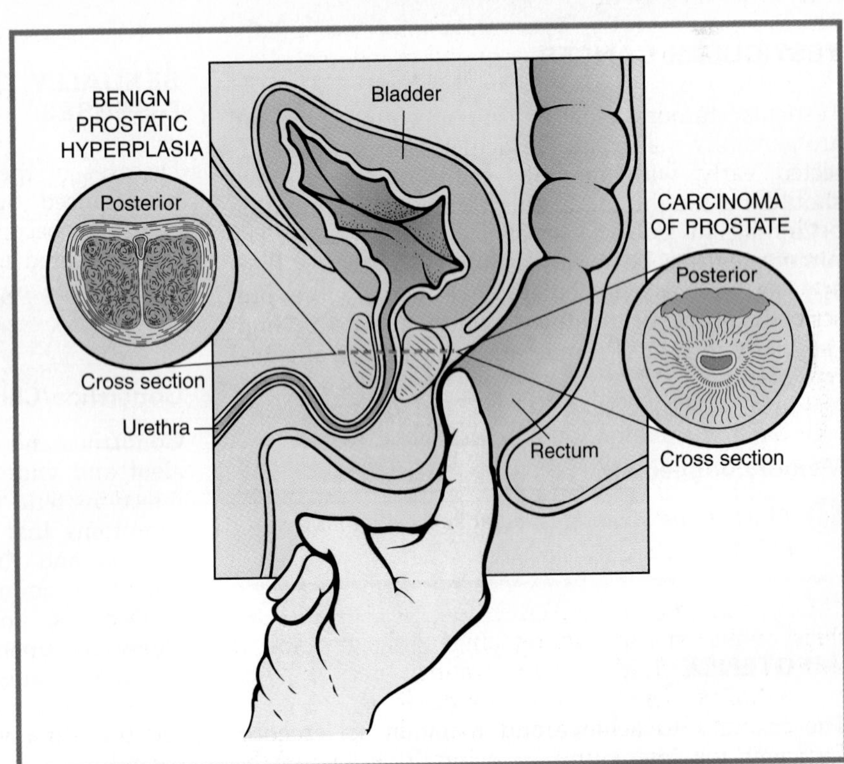

FIGURE 38–13 Benign prostatic hypertrophy. (From Damjanov I: Pathology for the Health-Related Professions. Philadelphia, WB Saunders, 1996.)

Memory Jogger

 *List the signs and symptoms of prostate enlargement.*

EPIDIDYMITIS

Epididymitis is the inflammation of the tubular epididymis. It is most often attributed to a urinary tract infection or an inflamed prostate. Patients experience severe low abdominal and testicular pain as well as swelling and tenderness of the scrotum. If abscesses form and produce scar tissue, sterility can occur if both sides are affected. Antibiotics are the usual treatment. Rest and implementing a diet that avoids irritants such as spicy food and alcohol also encourage healing.

BALANITIS

The inflammation of the glans is known as balanitis. It occurs most often in uncircumcised patients with narrow foreskins that do not retract easily and in diabetics. It has many causes, including allergic reaction to certain chemicals such as contraceptive foam, build-up of skin secretions, called smegma, as well as urinary tract and yeast infections. Treatment follows causative factors. Antibiotics are used for infections, and cleansing for build-up and avoidance of chemicals that cause reactions can help avoid the problem.

TESTICULAR CANCER

Testicular tumors usually occur in young men and are generally malignant. Testicular cancer can be detected early with monthly self-examination. Men should be taught to do this 3-minute examination beginning in puberty or at 15 years of age. The tumors tend to be radiosensitive, so radiation therapy, as well as chemotherapy, is usually the prescribed course of treatment. Survival rate is high especially in stage I seminoma, which has a survival rate of almost 95%.

Memory Jogger

 *At what age should testicular self-examinations begin?*

IMPOTENCE

The inability to achieve and maintain an erection sufficient for intercourse is a condition known as impotence. It has many causes, both psychologic and physiologic. Stress, anxiety, and fear of unsatisfactory performance as well as physical distresses such as arteriosclerosis, alcoholism, and diabetes mellitus can all lead to impotence . Certain medications also have impotency as a side effect. Treatment is centered toward the causative factor.

INFERTILITY

Fertility peaks in men at the age of 25. Although infertility is certainly present in female patients, 40% of infertile marriages are due to infertile males. In 10% to 20% of infertility cases there is no known cause. For the remaining cases, there can be many causative factors. Cryptorchidism, stricture, and varicoceles (dilated spermatic cord veins), low sperm count and motility, and obstruction of the vas deferens are all factors in infertility.

Examination of sperm samples can be helpful in making a diagnosis of infertility. These tests can determine the presence of sperm, the number of sperm in an ejaculation, as well as the health and motility of the sperm. The use of ultrasound is also helpful in detecting blockages of the vas deferens.

PEYRONIE'S DISEASE

Peyronie's disease is an incurable disorder that affects the erectile functioning of the penis. Scarring on one of two corpora cavernosa within the penis causes it to bend almost 90 degrees when erect.

SEXUALLY TRANSMITTED DISEASES

Diseases of the male reproductive system can also be acquired during sexual intercourse. These diseases can become quite serious and lead to death if left untreated (see Chapter 37). The discussion here explains the signs and symptoms experienced by the male.

Gonorrhea/Chlamydia

Gonorrhea and chlamydia are among the most prevalent and widespread venereal diseases. These two infections tend to coexist. The man tends to develop symptoms that include acute urethritis as well as dysuria and discharge of pus. Early detection is done by examining the discharge for the presence of gonococcus, and penicillin is effective treatment. However, superinfection has been known to develop and the organism can become resistant. Chlamydia is resistant to penicillin; thus, a regimen of antibiotics other than penicillin should be used if the patient has been diagnosed with both conditions.

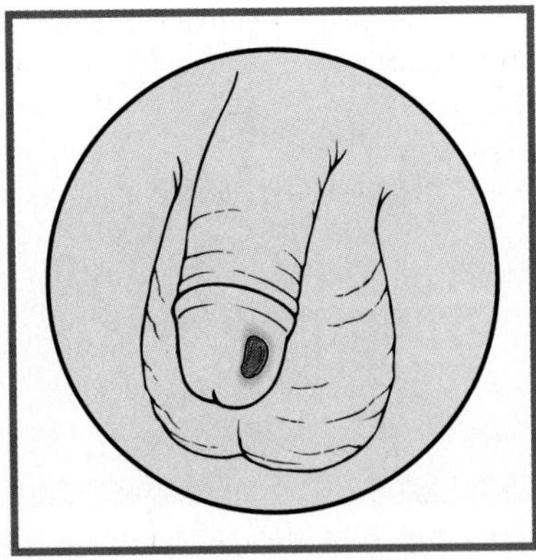

FIGURE 38–14 Syphilitic chancre. (From Frazier MS, Drzymkowski JA, Doty SJ: Essentials of Human Diseases and Conditions. Philadelphia, WB Saunders, 1996.)

Syphilis

A syphilitic lesion, called a chancre, develops on the male genitalia, usually the penis, within a few days to a few weeks after exposure (Fig. 38–14). It can be treated successfully with penicillin but can go unnoticed. Lack of treatment leads to a secondary phase indicated by a nonitching rash that can affect any part of the body. The patient is still infectious at this stage and yet is treatable with penicillin.

Syphilis can remain undetected or dormant for years. Symptoms that appear years after the primary infection lead to the most serious phase of the disease.

Herpes

Genital herpes, an extremely painful viral disease, has no cure. Symptoms of the disease include pain, a burning sensation, and multiple blisters that appear on the genitalia or surrounding area (Fig. 38–15). These usually appear within 2 to 3 weeks after exposure. The virus can remain dormant even after the lesions heal and recurrences may be either frequent or seldom. Although the disease does not yet have a **viable** cure, the lesions can be treated by keeping them clean and dry, using cold compresses, and taking medications such as acyclovir (Zovirax).

Acquired Immunodeficiency Syndrome

One of the most deadly diseases spread by sexual intercourse, acquired immunodeficiency syndrome (AIDS) is caused by a virus that comes into contact with mucous membranes of the reproductive tract. This causative virus is called the human immunodeficiency virus (HIV). It affects white blood cells and destroys their ability to fight infection.

Early symptoms include weight loss, enlarged lymph nodes, diarrhea, fever, and night sweats. There is a long latent period, (from 2 to 8 years) in which HIV infection leads to full-blown AIDS. The patient is considered to be HIV positive until such time as the T-cell count is below 200 mm^2. Then the patient is considered to have full-blown AIDS.

Research is very close to perfecting a vaccination against AIDS, and it is believed that by the year 2000 this dreaded disease will begin to be controlled.

The Medical Assistant's Role in the Urologic and the Male Reproductive Examinations

Much of the diagnosis of urinary dysfunction is dependent on the patient's history, which may include frequency or urgency of urination, dysuria, or incontinence.

A major part of the urologic examination is urinalysis. The medical assistant must be able to instruct the patient in how to obtain a clean-catch urine specimen (see Chapter 43). It is best to have the patient void in the physician's office so that the specimen can be examined immediately. The urologist may need to examine a catheterized specimen, which is collected using a sterile technique. A small **catheter** is introduced into the bladder, and the urine is collected in a sterile container.

CATHETERIZATION

Because of the possibility of introducing contagious agents, catheterization is not the ideal method for obtaining a urine sample. Many experts believe that a midstream urine catch is as dependable a speci-

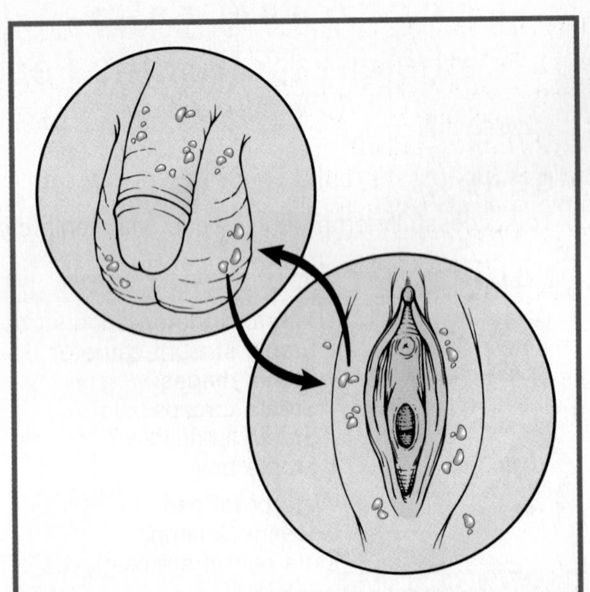

FIGURE 38–15 Genital herpes. (From Frazier MS, Drzymkowski JA, Doty SJ: Essentials of Human Diseases and Conditions. Philadelphia, WB Saunders, 1996.)

men as that obtained by an **invasive** catheterization. Often patients who have urine **retention** can void after the stimulus of hearing running water or submerging their hands in warm water.

REASONS FOR PERFORMING A CATHETERIZATION

- To relieve urinary retention
- To obtain a sterile urine sample from a female
- To measure the amount of **residual** urine in the bladder
- To obtain a urine sample when it cannot be obtained by any other method
- To empty the bladder before and/or during surgery or before specific diagnostic procedures

Catheters will vary in size, type, and construction material. When the procedure is done for the purpose of obtaining the contents that are present in the bladder, a straight or urethral No. 14 French is the most frequently used on female patients and the coudé with its slightly curved tip may be preferred for the male. The office will usually stock sizes 14 to 20 French for adults and sizes 8 to 10 French for pediatric use. In addition to the straight and coudé catheters there is also the Foley or indwelling type, which is designed to be left in the bladder for a period of time. The Foley catheter has a small inflatable balloon by its tip. When inflated, the balloon allows the catheter to remain in place within the bladder. To remove this type of catheter, the balloon must first be deflated (Fig. 38–16).

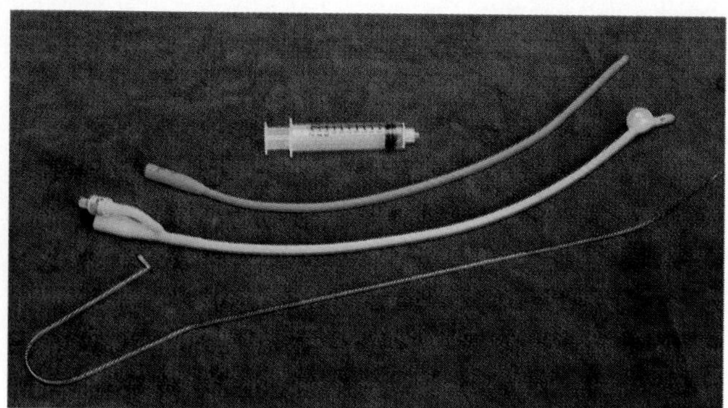

FIGURE 38–16 Types of catheters: straight and Foley with metal catheter guide. Syringe is used to inflate the balloon at the end of the Foley.

This procedure may be done by the physician or by the medical assistant if specially trained to do so.

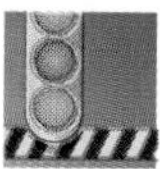

Safety Alert: This procedure should never be performed by a medical assistant who does not have the necessary training in the sterile technique or the knowledge of the responsibilities of catheterization.

Memory Jogger

12 *List five reasons for catheterization.*

Text continued on page 758

PROCEDURE 38–1

Catheterization of the Female Patient

GOAL

To successfully empty the bladder via sterile catheterization.

EQUIPMENT AND SUPPLIES

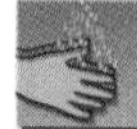 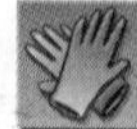

Urethral catheterization kit containing
- Sterile straight catheter
- Sterile drapes
- Sterile forceps
- Sterile lubricant
- Sterile tray
- Sterile gloves
- Sterile cotton balls or gauze flats
- Povidone-iodine (Betadine)
- Specimen container

Waterproof pad
Gooseneck lamp
Extra pair of sterile gloves

Continued

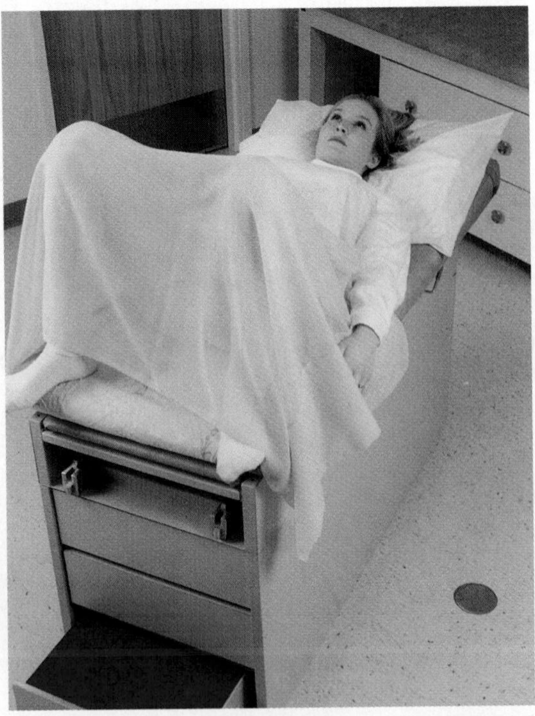
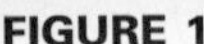

FIGURE 1

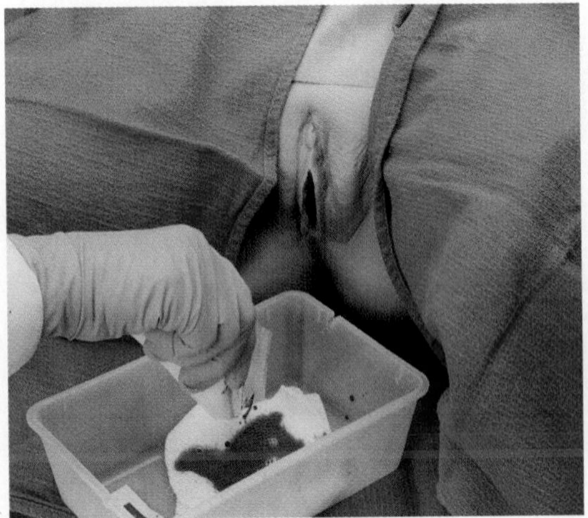

FIGURE 2

PROCEDURAL STEPS

(*A demonstration model has been used to illustrate this procedure.*)

1 Wash your hands and collect necessary supplies.
PURPOSE: Infection control.

2 Explain the procedure to the patient and have the patient remove necessary clothing.
PURPOSE: Knowledge leads to patient cooperation.

3 Place your patient in the dorsal recumbent position (Figure 1).

4 Drape the patient's upper body, leaving the genital area exposed.
PURPOSE: Drape provides a degree of dignity and comfort.

5 Position a gooseneck lamp on the genital area.
PURPOSE: The female urinary meatus may be difficult to identify.

6 Wash your hands and open the catheterization tray on a clean stable surface; often a Mayo stand is used.
PURPOSE: This is a sterile technique.

7 Open the sterile underpad drape and hold the underpad so that the undersurface of the two corners encircles your hands. Slide it under the patient while she is lifting her hips off the table. *Be careful not to touch the patient or the table with your hands.*

8 Open the sterile drape and place it over the patient's exposed genital area so that the vulvar area is exposed.

9 Place the insertion kit and any other supplies on the sterile drape between the patient's legs.

10 Put on gloves following sterile procedure (see Chapter 50). Open the povidone-iodine (Betadine) and pour it over cotton balls or gauze flats in the tray (Figure 2).

11 Open the sterile lubricant package and place it on the sterile field.

12 Open all other items, including the catheter. Stand the specimen container on the tray.

Continued

PROCEDURE 38-1 (CONTINUED)
Catheterization of the Female Patient

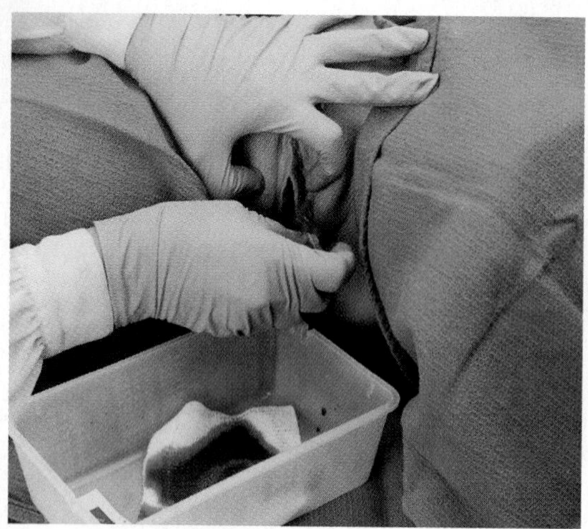
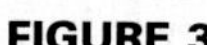
FIGURE 3

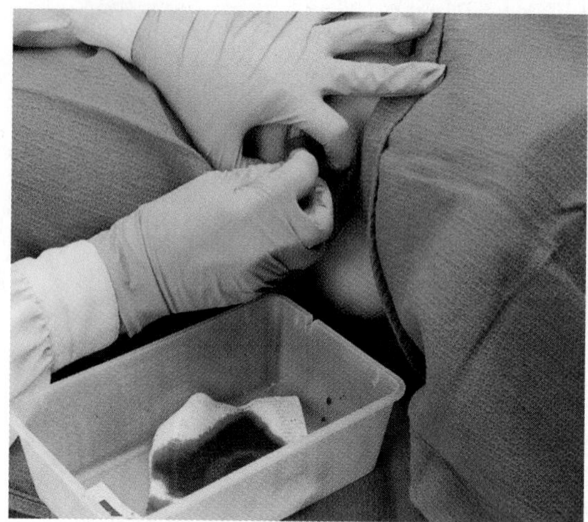
FIGURE 4

13 With the thumb and index finger of your nondominant hand, separate the patient's labia as widely as possible. *Your nondominant hand must maintain this position throughout the balance of the procedure.* With your dominant hand, pick up one of the povidone-iodine–soaked gauze flats and wipe from top to bottom on one side of the labia. Discard the used gauze flat (Figure 3).

14 Pick up another gauze flat and wipe from top to bottom on the other side of the labia. Discard the gauze flat.

15 Pick up another gauze flat and using a circular motion wipe over the urinary meatus from the inside outward (Figure 4). Discard the gauze flat.

16 With your dominant hand, pick up the catheter about 3 inches from the insertion end and dip the tip into the sterile lubricant. Position the other end of the catheter in the collection compartment of the kit tray.

17 Insert the lubricated tip into the urinary meatus and continue inserting the catheter 2 to 3 inches or until urine begins flowing out the catheter into the kit tray (Figure 5). *Never force the catheter.*

PURPOSE: Resistance may indicate a problem. Remove catheter and notify the physician.

Continued

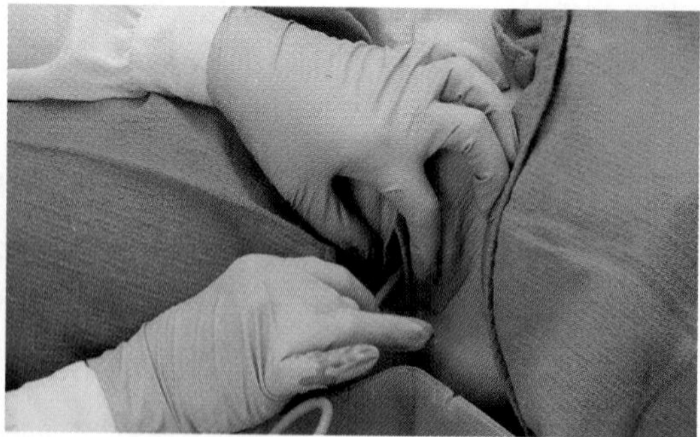
FIGURE 5

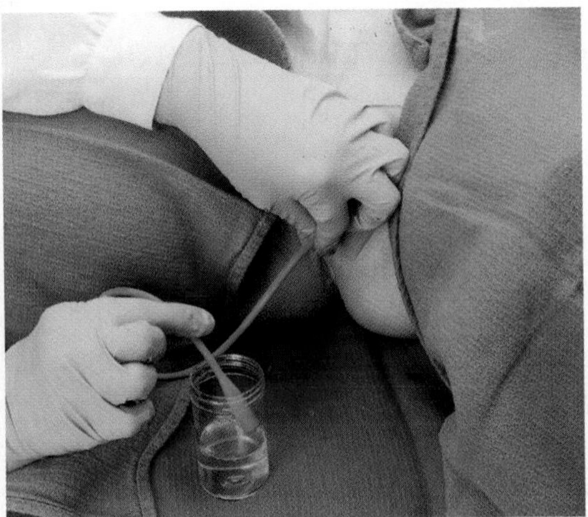

FIGURE 6

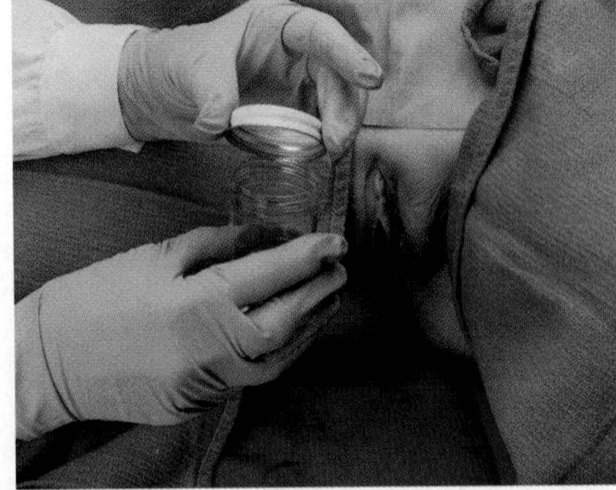

FIGURE 7

18 Let some of the urine flow and then place the specimen container over the end of the catheter and collect the specimen (Figure 6).

19 When the bladder is completely emptied, and the urine stops flowing, gently remove the catheter. If more than 500 mL of urine drains into the collection tray, clamp the catheter and wait 10 to 15 minutes, then reopen the catheter and allow the bladder to empty.
PURPOSE: A distended bladder that is emptied too quickly may cause bladder spasm.

20 Secure the lid to the urine specimen (Figure 7).
PURPOSE: Protect sterility of the specimen.

21 Remove all supplies and dispose of them according to Standard Precautions.

22 Assist patient off table and with dressing as needed.

23 Record the procedure, and include the number of milliliters of urine removed from the bladder.
PURPOSE: A procedure is considered not done until it is entered into the patient's record.

PROCEDURE 38-2

Catheterization of the Male Using a Straight Catheter

GOAL

To successfully obtain a urinary specimen through catheterization.

EQUIPMENT AND SUPPLIES

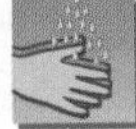 

Urethral catheterization kit containing
- Sterile straight catheter
- Sterile drapes
- Sterile forceps
- Sterile lubricant
- Sterile collection tray
- Sterile gloves
- Sterile cotton balls
- Povidone-iodine (Betadine)
- Specimen container

Waterproof pad
Extra pair of sterile gloves

Continued

PROCEDURE 38-2 (CONTINUED)

Catheterization of the Male Using a Straight Catheter

PROCEDURAL STEPS

1 Wash your hands and collect the necessary supplies.
PURPOSE: Infection control.

2 Explain the procedure to the patient and ask him to remove pants and underwear.
PURPOSE: Knowledge leads to patient cooperation.

3 Place the patient in the supine position.

4 Wash your hands and open the catheterization kit on a clean surface following sterile technique; often a Mayo stand is used.

5 Hold the sterile underpad so that the undersurface of the two corners encircles your hands. Position it over the patient's thighs under his penis.
PURPOSE: This is a sterile technique (Figure 1).

6 Put on sterile gloves.

7 Open the **fenestrated drape** and position it so the opening exposes the penis (Figure 2). Be careful not to touch the patient or the table.

8 Place the sterile kit on the table on top of the sterile drape and open all the supplies as in Procedure 38–1, steps 10 through 12.

9 Grasp the penis below the glans with your nondominant hand. In uncircumcised males, you must pull back the foreskin to see the meatus. You must do this and hold the penis upright with your nondominant hand *only*.

10 Using your dominant hand and forceps, pick up a povidone-iodine (Betadine)–soaked cotton ball and clean around the meatus in circular motions from the center outward. Repeat this a total of three times using a fresh soaked cotton ball each time (Figure 3).
PURPOSE: Ensures that the urinary meatus is properly cleaned.

11 After a thorough cleansing, wipe the glans with a dry cotton ball (Figure 4).

Continued

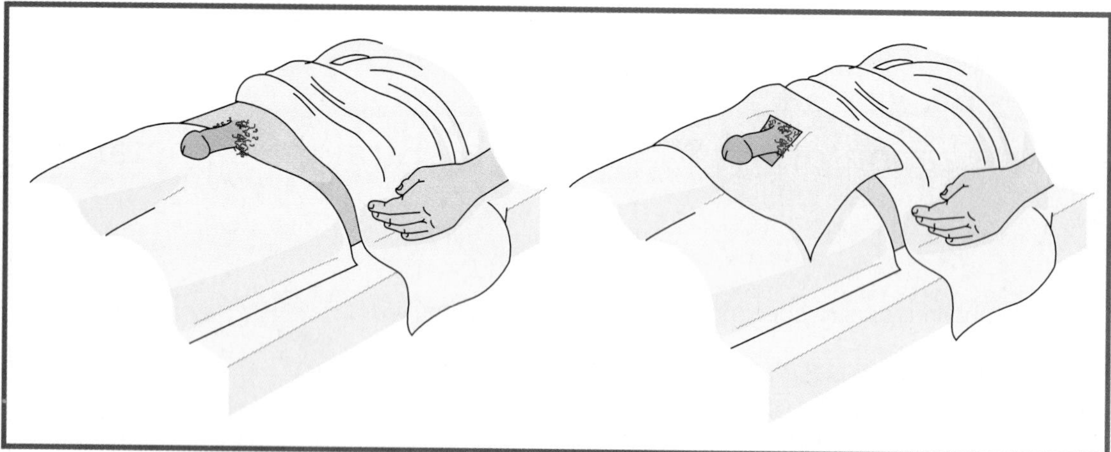

FIGURE 1 FIGURE 2

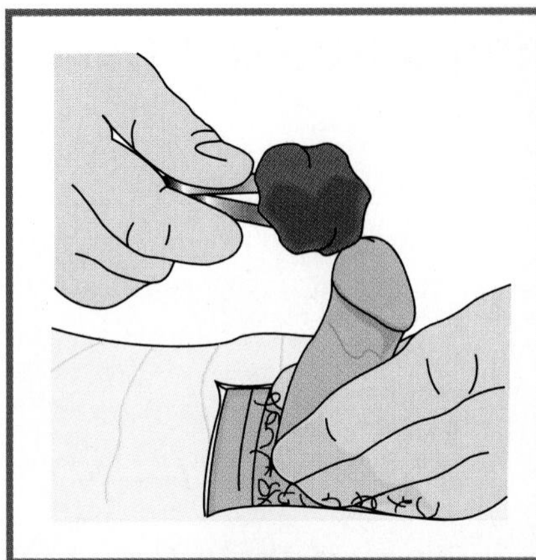

FIGURE 3

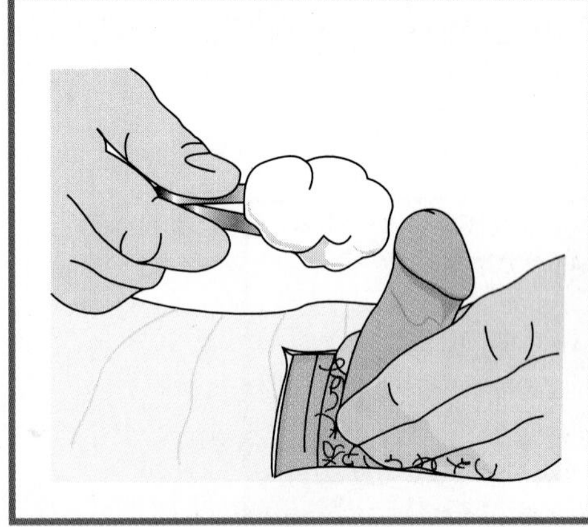

FIGURE 4

12 Hold the penis upright and straight with your nondominant hand. With your dominant hand, pick up the catheter approximately 3 inches from the insertion end and lubricate the tip of the catheter at least 7 inches; or if the catheterization kit contains a premeasured, lubricant-filled syringe, you can inject the lubricant directly into the urethra of an adult (Figure 5). Be sure to put the other end of the cathether into the collection compartment of the kit tray.
PURPOSE: Straight position keeps anatomic alignment of urethra for easier insertion.

13 Continue to hold the shaft of the penis at a 90-degree angle to the patient's abdomen. Apply gentle traction to straighten the urethra, and ask the patient to bear down as if to urinate. Gently insert the catheter tip into the urinary meatus 6 to 8 inches or until urine begins flowing out of the catheter (Figure 6). *Never force the catheter; if you meet resistance, remove the catheter and notify the physician.*

Continued

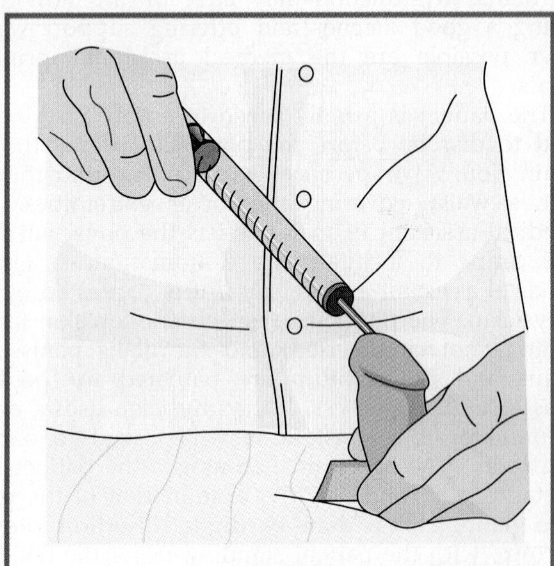

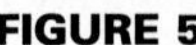

FIGURE 5

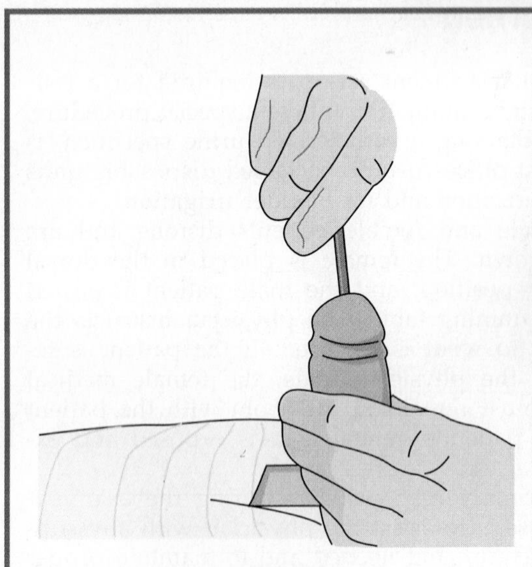

FIGURE 6

PROCEDURE 38-2 (CONTINUED)

Catheterization of the Male Using a Straight Catheter

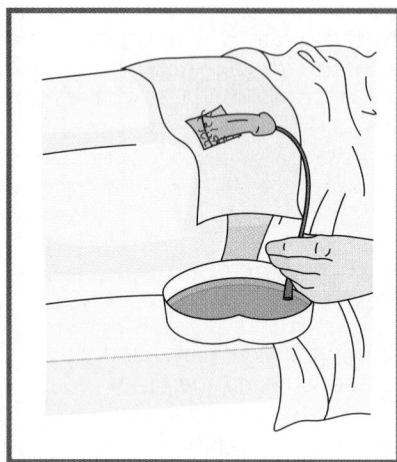

FIGURE 7

14 Obtain the specimen (Figure 7) and complete the procedure following steps 17 through 23 of the female catheterization procedure.

ASSISTING WITH THE UROLOGIC EXAMINATION

No special instrument set-up is required for a routine urologic examination unless a special procedure, such as obtaining a catheterized urine specimen, is done. Most offices use prepackaged disposable units for catheterization and for bladder **irrigation.**

Both male and female patients disrobe and are given a gown. The female is placed in the dorsal recumbent position, and the male patient is seated on the examining table. The physician instructs the patient as to what is required. If the patient is female and the physician male, the female medical assistant must remain in the room with the patient while the patient's genital area is exposed and examined.

Your primary responsibility during the examination process is to assist the physician with any supplies and equipment needed and to maintain proper draping of the patient.

ASSISTING WITH THE MALE REPRODUCTIVE EXAMINATION

The primary function of the medical assistant in the male reproductive system examination is to understand the male reproductive system and to be supportive. It is impossible to know what meaning a particular dysfunction may have on an individual. Being a good listener and offering support whenever possible are the medical assistant's primary goals.

The patient is usually asked to empty his bladder and to disrobe before the physician begins the examination. A drape sheet is placed around the patient's waist, covering the lower extremities. The medical assistant (if male) assists the physician with the drape to facilitate the examination. A female medical assistant assists *only* if it is requested by the physician. The physician inspects the foreskin (if patient is not circumcised) and the glans penis. The penis and the scrotum are palpated for possible masses and tenderness. If the physician uses a transilluminator, the assistant may be asked to darken the room. The assistant then assists the patient into a standing position for the examination of the prostate gland. This is done by digital insertion into the rectum, with the patient standing using the table for support (see Fig. 38–13). At this time, the physician may also check the patient for possible inguinal hernias (Fig. 38–17).

If the assistant is male, he may be needed to assist the physician with the examination and aid the patient with draping and positioning. The assistant should watch the patient for signs of discomfort and anxiety; if these signs are noted, he should notify the physician immediately. Answering the patient's questions and reinforcing understanding of the phy-

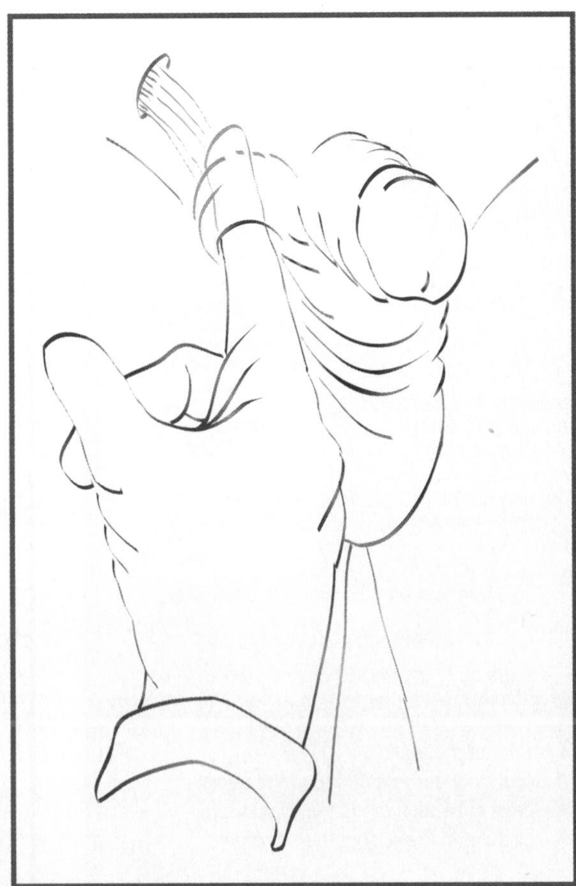

FIGURE 38–17 Hernia palpation.

sician's orders are among the assistant's responsibilities.

When the examination has been completed, the assistant aids the patient as needed.

VASECTOMY

The medical assistant may assist the physician with a **vasectomy.** A vasectomy is a surgical procedure for sterilizing the male patient (Fig. 38–18). It is performed by surgically removing a section of each vas deferens to stop sperm from reaching the prostate and mixing with semen. The sexual characteristics of the patient remain the same, and the ability to have an erection is entirely unchanged.

More than 500,000 of these procedures are done in doctors' offices with a local anesthetic agent such as lidocaine (Xylocaine). The conventional technique consists of the doctor making one or two small incisions with a scalpel to reach and clip the vasa and then closing them with sutures or stitches. A newer procedure, first introduced in the United States in 1988, uses a no-scalpel method. Rather than making incisions with a scalpel, a special instrument is used to pierce the skin of the scrotum and then gently stretch it to reach the tubes. The tubes are cut in the normal way, but no sutures are required to close the stratum and there is less loss of blood. The opening heals quickly, and there is little, if any, scarring. Recovery is complete in 3 to 5 days. Sperm checks are required 4 to 6 weeks apart to ensure the effectiveness of the procedure.

DIAGNOSTIC TEST EXPLANATIONS

The urinary system remains a very private, personal system. Patients often feel embarrassed to ask questions regarding how to obtain the requested urine or semen sample. Often the patient's foremost thought is "will this hurt?" These are the types of explanations that the medical assistant can assist the physician with.

The physician may ask you to give the patient the pamphlet and shower card on testicular self-examination (Fig. 38–19). There are two ways you can do this. One way is to take the information to the patient, tell him to follow the pictures, and if he has any questions to call for clarification. Will he call? Would you? The second way is to take the pamphlet in and go over the instructions with the patient. If it is possible for a male assistant to explain this procedure, the assistant can assist the patient in doing the examination for the first time to ensure that the patient knows how to do each step.

When the patient will be sent to another laboratory or to another area within your office for tests, always explain exactly what will be the procedure and how the sample must be obtained. Sometimes pictures and diagrams help in the explanations. It is best to never assume that the patient knows exactly what to do.

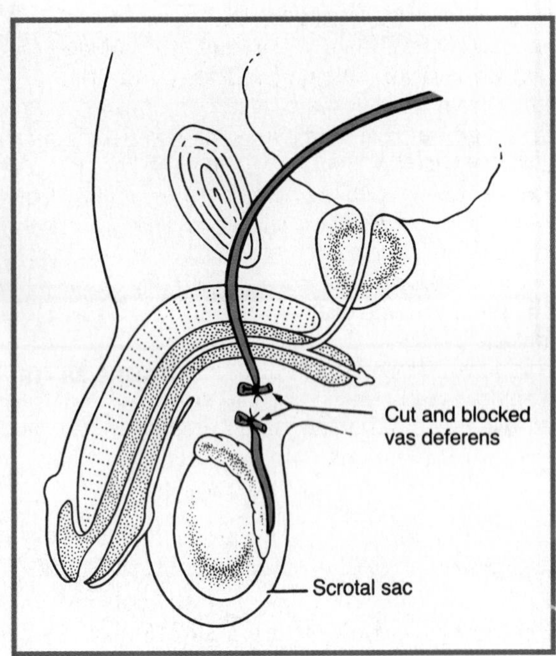

FIGURE 38–18 Vasectomy. (From Chabner DE: The Language of Medicine, 5th ed. Philadelphia, WB Saunders, 1996.)

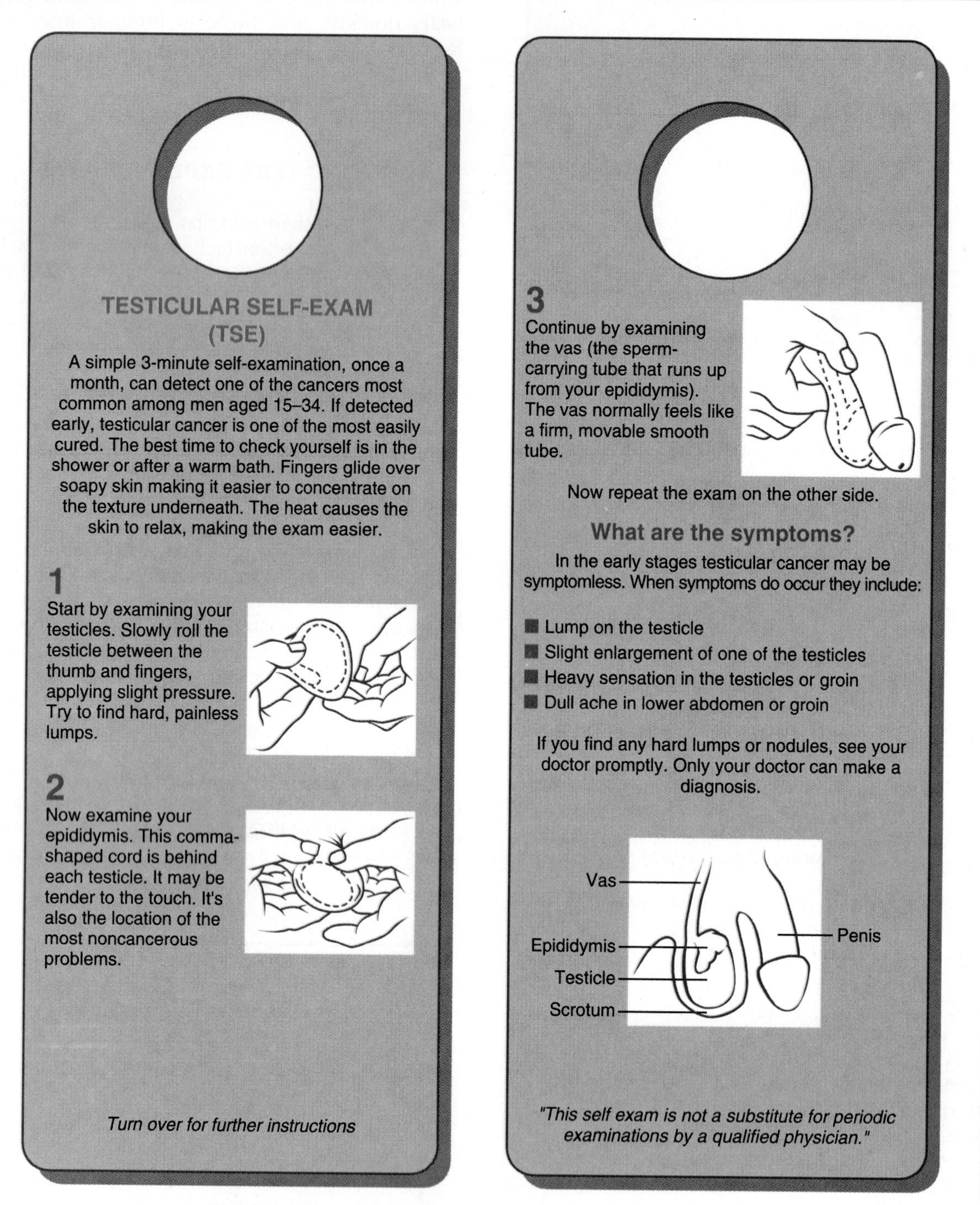

TESTICULAR SELF-EXAM
(TSE)
A simple 3-minute self-examination, once a month, can detect one of the cancers most common among men aged 15–34. If detected early, testicular cancer is one of the most easily cured. The best time to check yourself is in the shower or after a warm bath. Fingers glide over soapy skin making it easier to concentrate on the texture underneath. The heat causes the skin to relax, making the exam easier.
1
Start by examining your testicles. Slowly roll the testicle between the thumb and fingers, applying slight pressure. Try to find hard, painless lumps.
2
Now examine your epididymis. This comma-shaped cord is behind each testicle. It may be tender to the touch. It's also the location of the most noncancerous problems.
Turn over for further instructions
3
Continue by examining the vas (the sperm-carrying tube that runs up from your epididymis). The vas normally feels like a firm, movable smooth tube.
Now repeat the exam on the other side.
What are the symptoms?
In the early stages testicular cancer may be symptomless. When symptoms do occur they include:
Lump on the testicle
Slight enlargement of one of the testicles
Heavy sensation in the testicles or groin
Dull ache in lower abdomen or groin
If you find any hard lumps or nodules, see your doctor promptly. Only your doctor can make a diagnosis.
Vas
Epididymis
Testicle
Scrotum
Penis
"This self exam is not a substitute for periodic examinations by a qualified physician."

FIGURE 38–19 Self-examination shower card.

PROCEDURE 38-3

Teaching Testicular Self-Examination

GOAL

To instruct the patient in the steps of testicular self-examination.

EQUIPMENT AND SUPPLIES

Self-examination pamphlet and shower card
Demonstration model
Nonsterile gloves

PROCEDURAL STEPS

1 Wash your hands and collect needed supplies.
PURPOSE: Infection control.

2 Explain to the patient what you are going to do.
PURPOSE: Understanding helps with cooperation.

3 Begin by explaining to the patient that testicular cancer may produce no symptoms in early stages and that it is important to examine the testes once a month. This should begin at puberty or about 15 years of age. It is best to do the examination in the shower or in a warm bath. The total examination takes about 3 minutes.
PURPOSE: Heat causes the scrotal skin to relax, making the examination easier.

4 Examination of the testes: Start by holding the scrotum in the palms of the hands. Then feel one testicle. Apply a small amount of pressure. Slowly roll it between the fingers, and try to find hard, painless lumps (Figure 1).

5 Examination of the epididymis: This comma-shaped cord is found behind the testis. Its job is to store and transport sperm. Tender when touched, it is the location of most noncancerous problems. Check for hard spots and lumps (Figure 2).

6 Examination of the vas deferens: Continue by examining the sperm-carrying tube that runs up the epididymis. Normally, the vas feels like a firm, movable, smooth tube (Figure 3).

7 Now repeat the entire examination on the other side beginning with the opposite testis.

8 After completing the examination on the model, ask the patient to do a return-examination using the model. A male assistant can have the patient do a self–testicular examination.

9 Give the pamphlet to the patient along with the shower card with instructions regarding hanging it in the shower as a monthly reminder and guide.

10 Record the instructional transaction in the patient's medical record.
PURPOSE: If it is not recorded it was not done.

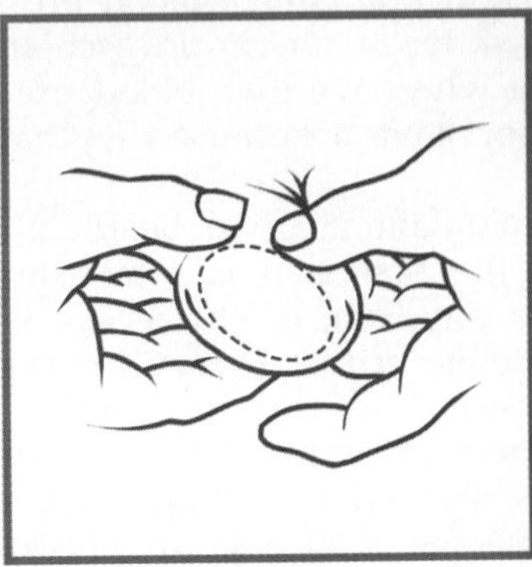

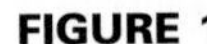

FIGURE 1

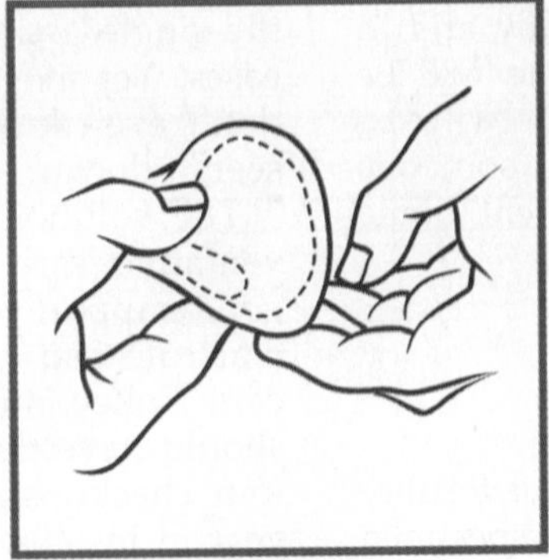

FIGURE 2

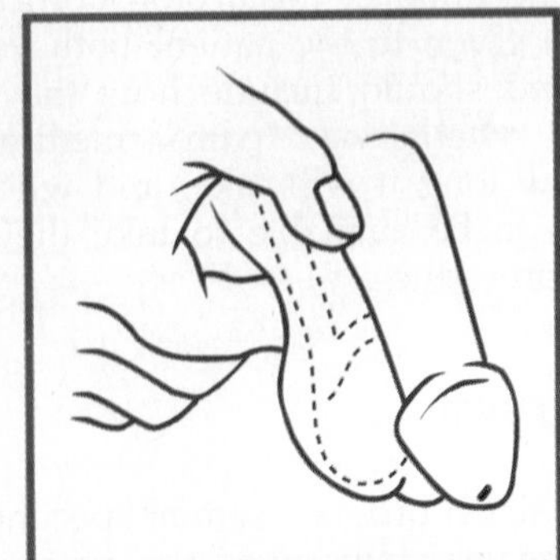

FIGURE 3

PROSTATIC ACID PHOSPHATASE

Acid phosphatases are enzymes that can be found in the kidney, spleen, liver, bone, red blood cells, and platelets. In the male prostate gland the activity of these enzymes is 100 times greater. This finding makes the prostatic acid phosphatase (PAP) test valuable in the diagnosis of metastatic cancer and in evaluating the prognosis of treatment. Acid phosphatase is also present in high concentration in seminal fluid, and the presence of this enzyme may be used to investigate rape.

Palpation of the prostatic gland and biopsy procedures before testing cause abnormal increases in the testing results. Therefore, when this test is ordered, the patient must be advised that there is to be *no* palpation of the prostate gland 2 to 3 days before testing. Drugs may cause increased and/or decreased results. Venous blood or seminal fluid may be used for this test.

PROSTATE-SPECIFIC ANTIGEN

The prostate-specific antigen (PSA) test differs from the prostatic acid phosphatase (PAP) test because this antigen is found in both normal prostatic epithelial cells and prostatic cancer cells. Because of this special finding, this test is believed to be the most reliable in monitoring recurrent prostatic carcinomas. The American Cancer Society recommends that the PSA test be used in conjunction with a digital rectal examination for the detection of prostatic cancer. The PSA test is also a valuable test in the follow-up prognosis of patients at high risk for prostatic cancers.

TISSUE BIOPSY

A tissue biopsy may be ordered if a mass is detected by the physician when the reproductive organs are palpated. Obtaining the biopsy specimen is usually done at the hospital on an outpatient basis but may be done in the urology office. Instructions should be given to the patient both verbally and in writing and should include how the tissue will be obtained, whether a "pain" medication will be given, how long it will take, and whether someone will need to be available to take the patient home after the procedure.

SEMEN TEST

If the physician orders a semen specimen for fertility testing, the assistant gives the patient a specimen container along with instructions on how to collect the specimen at home. The assistant also provides the patient with the laboratory forms to take along with the specimen to the testing center.

OTHER PROCEDURES

Other procedures may include drawing a blood sample, making microscopic smears on glass slides, or sending the patient to a laboratory with request forms for specific tests to be performed.

Memory Jogger

What blood test is recommended by the American Cancer Society for the detection of early prostate cancer?

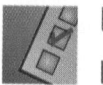

PATIENT EDUCATION

Most men under the age of 50 haven't seen a doctor in years. The most common excuses for this are "no time and no need, after all, I'm not sick." This "bulletproof mentality" also can keep men from gaining knowledge needed to maintain good health. It's no coincidence that women outlive men by an average of 7 years.

Medical studies reveal that attitude, not biology, has a lot to do with the difference between men's and women's life spans. Men's misconceptions about their invincibility make them more vulnerable to illnesses and death. Not only do men refuse to visit a physician, they typically lead higher risk lives than do women. Men drive faster and are twice as likely as women to die in an automobile accident. Men drink more alcohol, are more violent, and avoid danger less. For example, more men know how to swim, yet five times more men than women drown.

In 1997, more than 300,000 men will be diagnosed with prostate cancer, typically a slow-growing disease that has a high cure rate. Yet too many men with the disease will wait until it has reached an advanced state before seeking treatment.

Another common affliction is high blood pressure, the single greatest risk factor for cardiovascular diseases. Yet most men who have high blood pressure don't even know they have it because they haven't seen a doctor.

The solution to maintaining good health is preventative care and the first step is establishing a good rapport with a physician of choice. As a general rule and a guideline of the Agency for Healthcare Policy and Research, a man in good health should have three checkups in his 20s, from three to four checkups in his 30s, and a checkup every other year in his 40s. At the age of 50, a yearly checkup is recommended. In addition to testing for conditions like cancer, heart disease, stroke, and diabetes, four of the top male health problems, the entire medical team can empower male patients with the knowledge to make responsible decisions regarding good health.

There are many procedures required in a urology setting, and there is a strong need for patient education, especially of the male patient. The medical assistant should see this need as an opportunity to become a greater asset to the physician/employer, the patient, and the profession. The greater the interest taken in the needs and desires of the patients, the greater the personal reward.

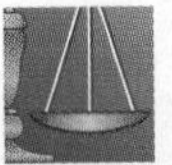

LEGAL AND ETHICAL ISSUES

When working in a urology office, the medical assistant must be very careful to ensure that patients have given informed consent for the procedures to be performed. When the patient refuses a procedure, the assistant needs to have the patient sign the appropriate informed refusal forms; these forms are then included in the medical record. All patient education should be done after the doctor has completed the explanation and has given the assistant instructions to do so. Never diagnose, prescribe, or offer comment about a patient's condition. Remember that as the physician's agent your comments can be considered as those of the physician.

Medical assistants who overstep their professional boundaries may place the doctor and themselves in legal jeopardy. Remember that the patient who is legally informed and satisfied with the care received is less likely to find the need to take legal action against the physician and the assistant.

CRITICAL THINKING

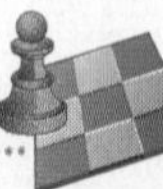

1 Examine the cultural reasons that are present in your community regarding discussing a problem in the urinary system.

2 You need to catheterize a 16-year-old. What special problems may arise? How could you attempt to solve them?

3 What suggestions could you make to a 70-year-old man who has an incontinence problem?

HOW DID I DO? Answers to Memory Joggers

1 The urinary system removes salts and nitrogenous wastes.

2 Urination is also known as voiding and micturition.

3 The common symptoms involving changes in the frequency of urination are dysuria, urgency, and incontinence.

4 The urinalysis of a patient with glomerulonephritis shows the presence of blood and increased albumin.

5 Two forms of kidney dialysis are hemodialysis and peritoneal dialysis.

6 In children, a malignant form of renal carcinoma is Wilms' tumor.

7 Cystitis occurs more frequently in women owing to the short urethra.

8 Radiologic tests include kidney-ureter-bladder films, intravenous pyelography, angiography, computed tomography, cystoscopy, retrograde pyelography, voiding cystourethrography, and ultrasonography.

9 The most influential male hormone is testosterone.

10 Signs and symptoms of prostate carcinoma include urinary obstruction, increased urinary infections, and frequent nocturia.

11 Testicular self-examination should begin at age 15.

12 Five reasons to catheterize are

a. To relieve urinary retention
b. To obtain a sterile urine sample from a female
c. To measure the amount of residual urine in the bladder.
d. To obtain a urine sample when it cannot be obtained by any other method
e. To empty the bladder before and/or during surgery or before specific diagnostic procedures.

13 The PSA blood test is recommended along with a digital rectal examination.

Assisting with the Older Patient

39

Myra M. DeWulf, MT (ASCP), BB MHA

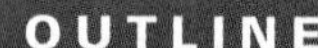

OUTLINE

LEARNING OBJECTIVES

Cognitive: On successful completion of this chapter you should be able to:

1 Identify the various impacts of an increasing aging population on society.
2 Explain the changes caused by aging in each of the body systems.
3 Identify the major disease and disorders faced by the elderly.
4 Explain why sleep disorders are a major concern of the elderly.
5 Differentiate between independent, assisted, and skilled nursing facilities.
6 List the basic principles covered in the Patient's Bill of Rights and advance directives.
7 Define and spell vocabulary terms.

Performance: On successful completion of this chapter you should be able to:

1 Demonstrate changes in communication techniques used with elderly patients.

VOCABULARY

androgen Any steroid hormone that promotes male characteristics

arteriosclerosis Hardening of the arteries

autonomy The ability to function in an independent fashion

collagen The primary protein of the skin, tendon, bone cartilage, and other connective tissues

costal Pertaining to the ribs

elastin Essential part of elastic connective tissue that when moist is flexible and elastic

hot flashes Flushing of the body caused by blood vessels expanding and then contracting

hyperthermia Greatly increased body temperature

hypothermia Greatly reduced body temperature

impotence Inability to achieve or maintain an erection

incontinence Inability to control excretory functions

informed consent Verbal or written assurance that the patient has had the procedure or treatment explained, including risks, alternatives, and possible outcomes

lacrimation The secretion or discharge of tears

melanin A dark, sulfur-containing pigment normally found in the hair, skin, ciliary body, choroid of the eye, pigment layer of the retina, and certain nerve cells

menopause The phase of life when a woman ceases to menstruate and passes from the reproductive to the nonreproductive stage

mnemonic Improvement of memory by special methods or techniques

myocardium Muscle layer of the heart

nephron units Basic functioning units of the kidney found in the renal pyramids

paranoia A descriptive term limited to the characterization of behavior that is marked by delusions of persecution or grandeur

presbycusis Progressive bilateral perceptive hearing loss occurring with aging

presbyopia Diminution of accommodation of the lens of the eye occurring with aging

senile A pronounced loss of mental, physical, or emotional control in aged people, caused by physical or mental deterioration

tinnitus Ringing or buzzing in the ears

urinary retention Inability to totally empty the bladder

virile Having masculine spirit, strength, vigor, or power

voiding Act of urinating

A report published by the U.S. Census Bureau shows the population of the United States is rapidly graying. More than 33 million Americans were older than 65 in 1994. This represents 12.7% of the population. Approximately 1 in 8 Americans is older than 65. The "oldest old" (people older than 85) are the most rapidly growing age group. It is projected that people older than 65 will represent 13% of the population in 2000 and increase to 20% by 2030. This means by the middle of the next century approximately 60 million people will be older than age 65 (Fig. 39–1).

The aging population will impact all aspects of society. One area in particular will be the greater utilization of health services. To provide better services to the aging consumer it is necessary to understand the aging process, which includes the physical and sensory changes encountered by older people. This knowledge enables the health care professional to recognize the special needs of the aged and to develop effective management and communication skills that will allow us to provide better service to the older client. Through ongoing education regarding the aging process, many of the old stereotype beliefs concerned with aging are disappearing.

OLD STEREOTYPES

Old people are all alike.
Old people are senile.
Most old people are sickly.
Old people are sexless.
Old people cannot learn new things.
Old people are resistant to change.

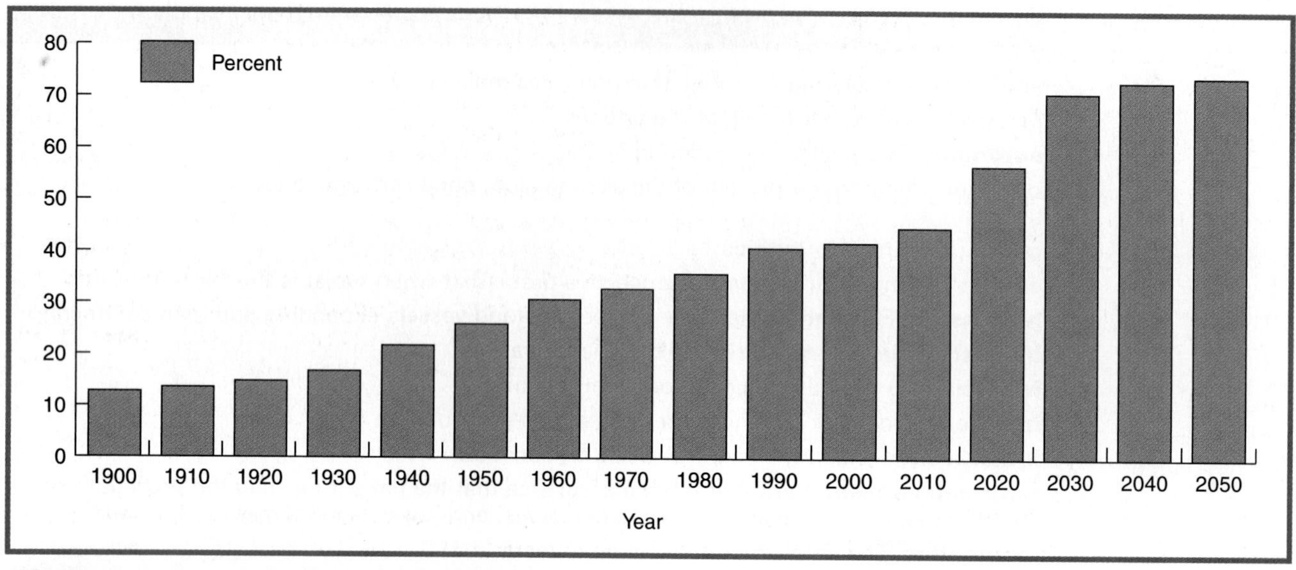

FIGURE 39–1 Percentage of Americans age 65 and older (projected to 2050). (From the American Association of Retired Persons: A Profile of Older Americans. Washington, DC, AARP, 1997.)

Aging is a complex physiologic, psychologic, and social process. Old age is not an illness but a normal life process that people experience in different ways. Lack of exercise, poor nutrition, substance abuse, continual stress, and air pollutants are all factors that cause someone to show the effects of aging decades earlier then someone who has practiced healthy living habits.

As people age they experience changes in their physical appearance and abilities as well as sensory changes in vision, hearing, taste, and smell. These changes do not occur simultaneously nor at the same time in everyone.

APPROXIMATE AGES FOR SENSORY CHANGES

- Vision declines around the mid 40s to 50s.
- Hearing loss begins around 40.
- Taste sensitivity reduction occurs at 55 to 59.
- Smell sensitivity declines after age 70.

These changes are due to the sensory receptors becoming less efficient with age, resulting in the need for increased level of stimuli. As a result, these changes have a profound effect on the individual's ability to interact with his or her environment.

Memory Jogger

1 *Old age is not an illness, it is a _____.*

Changes in Anatomy and Physiology

VISION

By the time a person reaches 50, structural and functional changes in the eye become noticeable. The eyebrow and eyelashes start to gray. The skin around the eyelids wrinkles, and the loss of orbital fat allows the eye to sink deeper into the orbit.

The cornea increases in thickness and has reduced refractive power. There may be the development of a yellow-gray ring (arcus senilis) on the periphery of the cornea. The iris loses pigmentation, and, as a result, most older people appear to have gray-colored eyes.

The lens of the eye continues to grow. As new lens fibers grow, old lens fibers are compressed and pushed to the center, causing the lens to become more dense. The lens becomes flatter, thicker, less elastic, and more opaque. By the age of 70 the lens has tripled in mass. Clouding of the lens causes light rays to scatter, creating glare. Probably everyone has heard the saying "Looking at life through rose-colored glasses." For the aged eye, a more appropriate saying would be "Looking at life through yellow-colored glasses." This is because the lens of the eye progressively yellows with age.

Memory Jogger

 *Functional and structural changes in the eye become noticeable around what age?*

The pupil adjusts to control the amount of light entering the eye. The muscle that causes the pupil to dilate weakens during the aging processes. As a result, there is a reduction in the size of the pupil, limiting the amount of light available to reach the retina.

Tear production normally decreases. Tear glands do not make enough tears or the tears are of poor quality and do not keep the eyes wet enough. Scratchiness, stinging or burning eyes, and excessive tearing are a result of decreased **lacrimation.** The eye becomes red and irritated.

As a result of these changes, several vision problems occur. It becomes increasingly difficult to focus at different distances, there is decrease in the ability to see objects clearly and discriminate color intensity, sensitivity to glare is increased, and sensitivity to light is decreased.

During the 40s and 50s, the ability to focus on detailed objects close at hand changes. This condition is called **presbyopia** (Fig. 39–2). To accommodate this visual decline people will hold printed material at a distance or use bifocal lenses. This may improve the situation, but often fine detail such as lettering on medicine bottles or telephone numbers in a phone book may still be hard to read.

Memory Jogger

3 *What is presbyopia?*

There is a decrease in the ability to refocus quickly from far to near or near to far. Also the ability to follow a moving object is decreased. The loss of peripheral vision is common among older people. Often older people have difficulty reading road signs while driving. The inability to see oncoming cars due to decreased peripheral vision as well as decreased night vision may limit an older person's ability to navigate a car safely.

A decline in visual acuity is related to aging. This means a person is less able to see as clearly as when he or she was younger. Between 20 and 50 there is a slight decline in visual acuity. Between 60 to 80 there is a dramatic change. A visual acuity of 20/50 means a person can see at 20 feet what a person with perfect vision can see at 50 feet. Some states impose restrictions in drivers' licenses for people having this amount of visual acuity.

Memory Jogger

Identify three vision problems resulting from reduction in pupil size.

The yellowing of the lens causes it to act like a filter, making it difficult to distinguish certain color intensities. Blues, greens, and violets, which are considered as having short wavelengths, are hard to differentiate, whereas yellows, reds, and oranges are of longer wavelengths and easier to identify. To understand how objects and color might look though an aging eye, try putting petroleum jelly on a pair of glasses and covering the lens with amber acetate. Then try to identify colors on a paint chart.

The loss in the ability to discriminate closely related colors can affect the older person's ability to judge distances or his or her depth perception. This causes an aging person to become more susceptible to falls and accidents. Stairs become a potential hazard because the edges cannot be seen clearly. Furni-

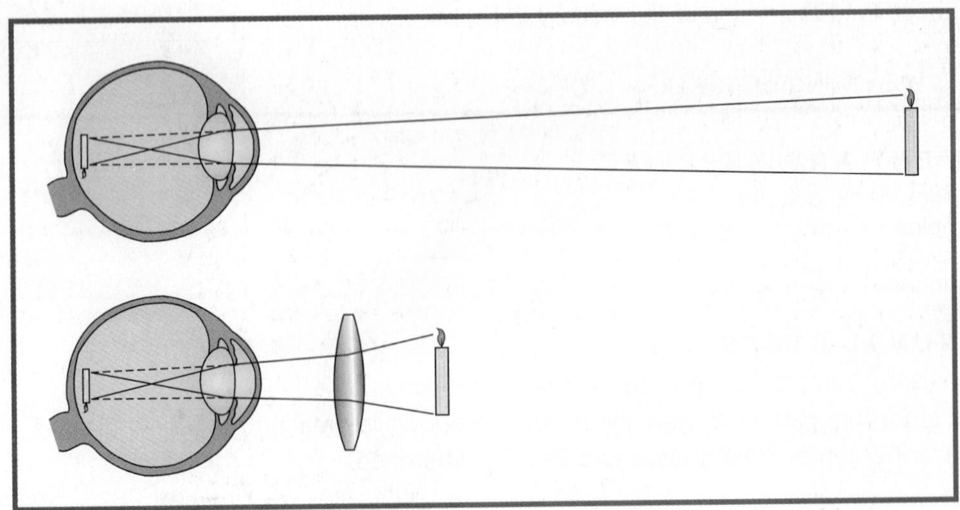

FIGURE 39–2 Presbyopic vision.

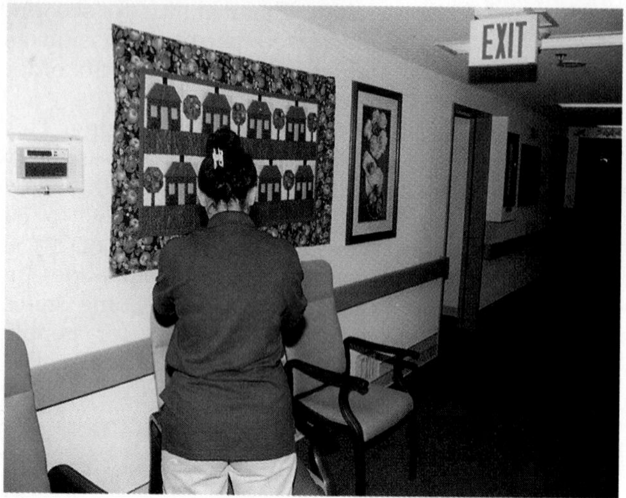

FIGURE 39–3 Creating contrast with color aids in ability to judge distances and in depth perception.

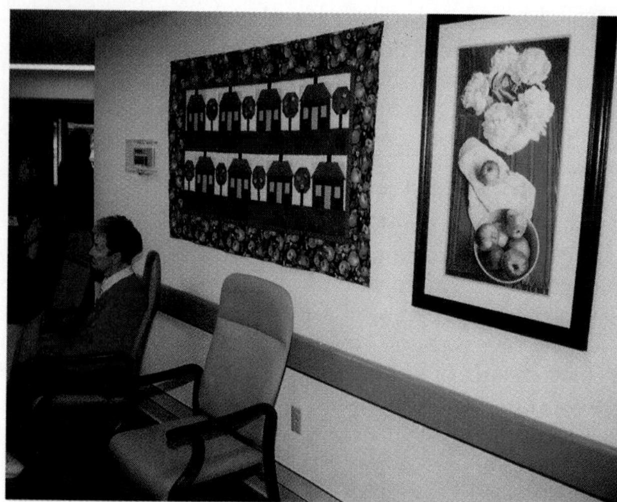

FIGURE 39–4 Colored border shows difference between the walls and floors, which is helpful to someone who has lost the ability to discriminate closely related colors.

ture that blends with the floor could be missed when attempting to sit down. One solution is to create contrast (Fig. 39–3). Use clear warm colors that are three to four steps apart on a value scale. Cool hues should be avoided because they may be perceived as gray. For example, contrast can be created by using a colored border between the wall and the floor (Fig. 39–4). Light switches and doors can be painted to create contrast from walls. Contrast can also be used to distinguish between the vertical risers and the horizontal treads of the stairs (see Procedure 39–1).

PROCEDURE 39–1
The Visually Impaired Older Adult

GOAL

To better understand the needs of the visually impaired.

Project 1: YELLOWING OF THE LENSES OF THE EYES

EQUIPMENT AND SUPPLIES

Yellow glasses or ski goggles
Carpet samples
Paint chip charts
Fabric swatches

PROCEDURAL STEPS

1 Place the carpet samples, paint chips, and fabric swatches on a table.
2 Ask your procedure partner to view the various colors while wearing the yellow glasses.
3 Have him or her remove the glasses and see the difference.

Continued

Project 2: CATARACTS

EQUIPMENT AND SUPPLIES

Low-magnification reading glasses
Vaseline or another form of petroleum jelly
Telephone book
Empty medicine bottles

PROCEDURAL STEPS

1 Smear Vaseline lightly on the outside of the glasses.
2 Ask your partner to find his or her name in the phone book and read the labels on the medicine bottles while wearing the glasses.

Project 3: DEPTH PERCEPTION

EQUIPMENT AND SUPPLIES

Binoculars
Carpet tape (red, yellow, white, and black)

PROCEDURAL STEPS

1 Place the carpet tape on the floor in a zigzag pattern, using approximately 3 feet of each color for each leg of the zigzag.
2 Have the participants walk the zigzag line while looking through the large end of the binoculars.

Older individuals need increasing levels of light illumination for functional vision. An 80-year-old may need three times the amount of light to read than a 20-year-old. Increasing the level of light will not compensate for this visual decline. The reason is the elderly experience an increased sensitivity to glare. Glare is probably one of the most painful experiences for the aging eye. Exposed light bulbs, such as those used in chandeliers, and light from highly reflective surfaces such as glass tables and floors can produce excessive glare. To minimize glare, use evenly distributed or balanced light sources, nonglare surfaces, opalescent lenses, and shielded lamps (Fig. 39–5). Textured sheer draperies can help filter the light.

Memory Jogger

5 *Name the colors that are easier for the elderly to identify.*

The eye decreases in its ability to respond to abrupt changes from light to dark or dark to light. Going from a well-lit waiting room into a dim hallway or negotiating the way down dimly lit aisles in a movie theater could be treacherous to an older person.

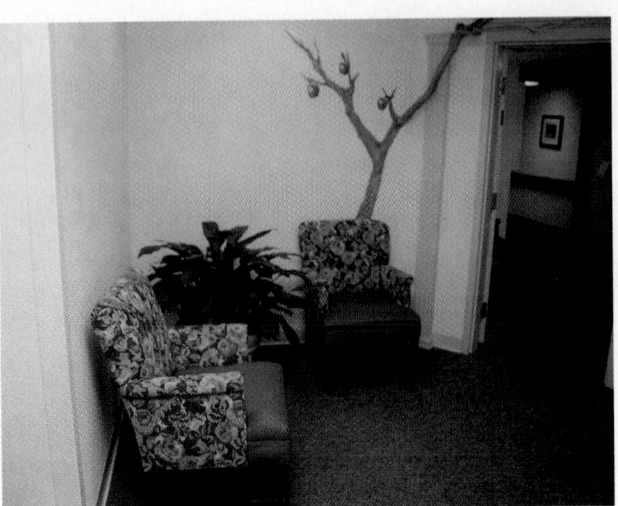

FIGURE 39–5 Balanced light source prevents glare.

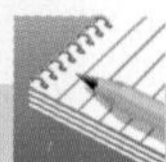

SKILLS AND RESPONSIBILITIES

SUGGESTION FOR HELPING THE VISUALLY IMPAIRED OLDER ADULT

- When escorting an older person, whether he or she is visually impaired or not, allow the client to place his or her hand above your elbow. It is easier for the person to follow your movements. This method also provides a source of support and security (Fig. 39–6).
- Use high levels of evenly distributed glare-free light.
- Ask the pharmacist to use large lettering when labeling medicine bottles.
- Use paper that has a nonglare finish and use large print.
- Make distinct differences (e.g., size of containers) for pills that are similar in size and color.
- When serving food explain what is being served and its location on the plate or table. Use contrast between items on the table. For example, it is hard to differentiate between the edge of a white dish and a white tablecloth (Fig. 39–7).
- Obtain large-print items. Telephones can be purchased that have large dialing buttons. Large-print books can be used at home or made available for patients in waiting rooms. "Talking" books are also available.
- Make hand rails available in bathrooms, by stairs (inside and out), and along dimly lit hallways.
- Avoid clutter, and do not rearrange objects without telling the visually impaired person.
- Avoid using furniture having sharp edges; for example, use coffee tables with rounded edges and chairs with rounded arms for security and push up (Fig. 39–8).

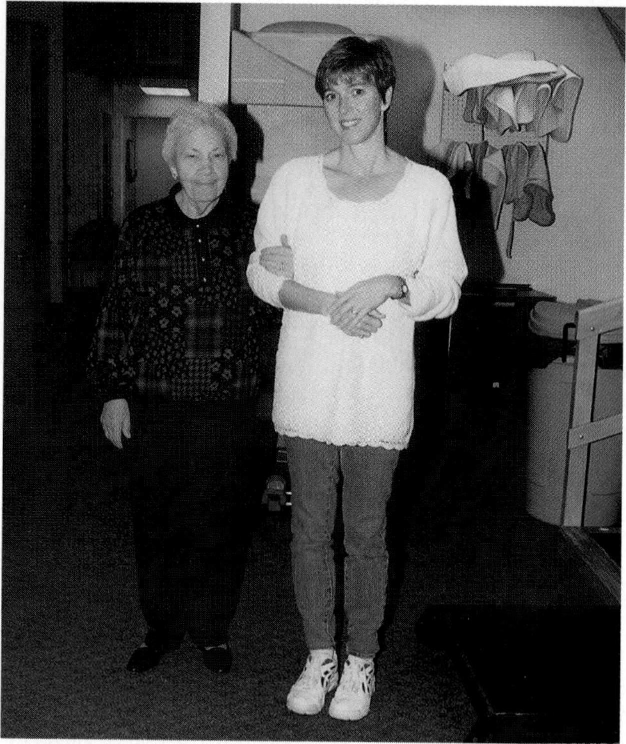

FIGURE 39–6 Allow visually impaired patient to place hand above your elbow for support and security.

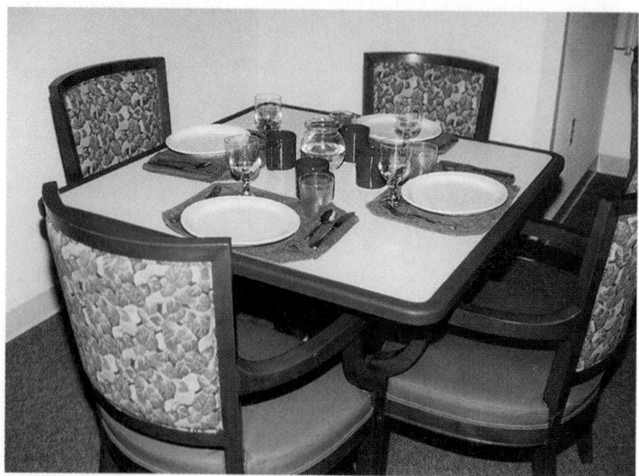

FIGURE 39–7 Contrast between items and table aids the visually impaired.

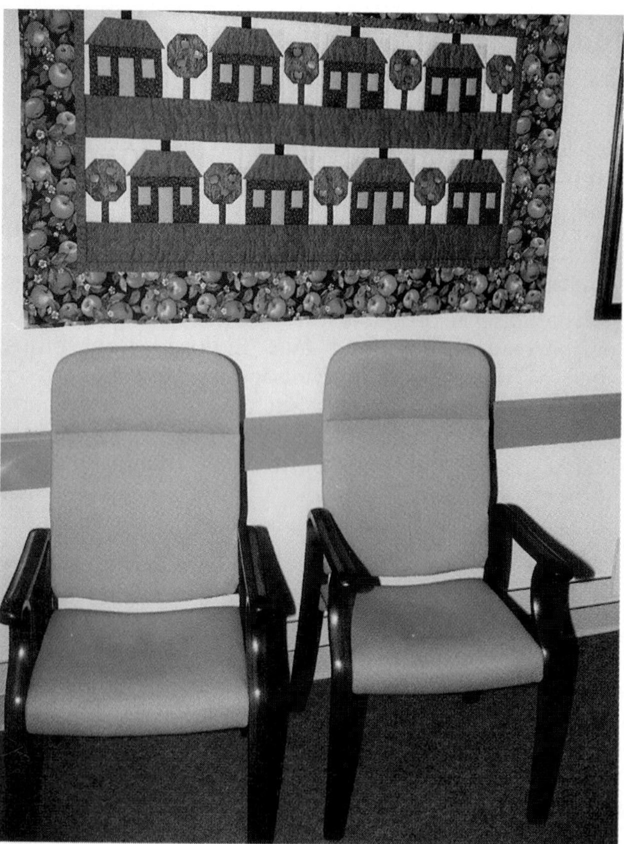

FIGURE 39–8 Chairs have rounded arms for security and push up.

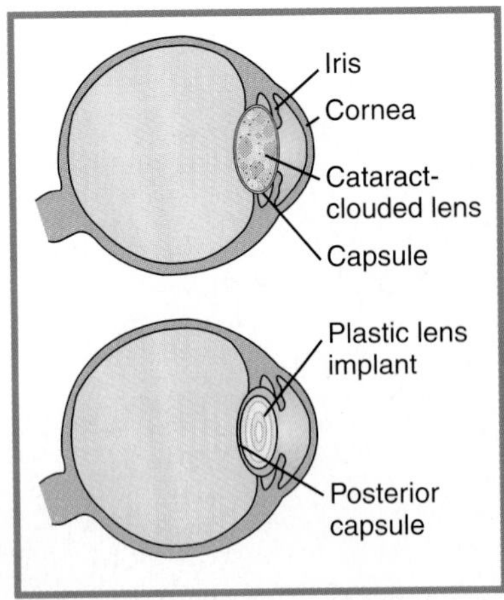

FIGURE 39–9 Lens implant surgery for cataracts.

Cataracts, Glaucoma, and Macular Degeneration

Eye diseases and disorders common in older people are cataracts, glaucoma, and macular degeneration. Cataracts are cloudy or opaque areas in the eye lens that cause blurring of vision. If the cataracts become large, they are removed by surgery (Fig. 39–9). Glaucoma is a result of too much fluid pressure in the eye. The eye does not drain properly, causing fluid pressure to build up and damage the nerve cells. If not treated, glaucoma can cause blindness. The macula is the part of the eye responsible for sharp vision and color. The damage or breakdown of the macula is called macular degeneration. As a result of this breakdown the ability to see fine detail, drive, or read is affected.

Memory Jogger

 *Identity three eye diseases commonly seen in older adults.*

HEARING

Loss of hearing affects the ability to communicate clearly. Imagine not being able to hear the songs you enjoy or the voice of your children or spouse. We depend on hearing to alert us to dangers in the environment, such as the honk of a car horn or the sound of an oncoming train. Hearing loss can produce a profound psychological effect on the aging. Often depression, social withdrawal, and feelings of **paranoia** and isolation result from a decline in hearing ability.

Hearing loss is not as evident as other aging signs such as graying hair or wearing glasses. Often people are less sensitive to a person with a hearing disability because they are not aware of the person's handicap. The older person may not be aware of his or her hearing loss because it has occurred gradually over a long period of time. Lack of attention when being spoken to, inappropriate responses, asking to have statements repeated, and speaking too loudly or too softly are often signs of hearing loss. It is for these reasons an older person may be labeled as confused, inattentive, or even **senile.**

Changes in auditory ability begin around age 30, and by the age of 70 words in a normal conversation are missed. Some people believe hearing loss may not be due to the aging process but is a result of lifelong exposure to environmental noise. Approximately 30% of people 65 to 74 report hearing impairment. This increases to 50% for those older than 80. Women are reported to have a lower percentage of decline.

Presbycusis

Hearing loss that is related to the aging process is termed *presbycusis.* There is the loss of the ability to hear high frequencies and to discriminate sounds or to hear clearly. Parts of a conversation may be missed because the sound of the word goes above the 2000-cycle frequency. When presbycusis occurs, it is because the sensory organs of the ear, particularly the hair cells, have degenerated (see Chapter 31). Often words that sound similar are hard to differentiate. Imagine telling a patient that he needs more "bed" rest and having him interpret this as needing more "dead" rest. More likely than not, he won't get beyond the word "dead."

The consonants such as *g, f, s, sh, t,* and *z* produce high-pitched sounds that are more difficult to hear and differentiate. Low-frequency pitched sounds such as the vowels *a, e, i, o,* and *u* may be more easily heard by people with presbycusis. The inability to hear different frequencies combined with low background noise from groups of people talking, noise from appliances, or busy public places will compromise an older person's ability to hear clearly. Hearing aids increase not only the sound of the human voice but also the background noises resulting in sensory overload.

Sound bounces off hard surfaces such as glass windows, countertops, and furniture, causing an echo effect. Try to carry on a conversation in a quiet area. Use sound-absorbent material such as drapes or upholstered furniture to help soften background noise. High-backed chairs will help shield against unwanted background noise. Additional methods of effective communication with an older person are discussed in Chapter 25. See Procedure 39–2.

PROCEDURE 39-2

The Hearing Impaired Older Adult

GOAL

To better understand the needs of the hearing impaired.

EQUIPMENT AND SUPPLIES

Bag of cotton balls

PROCEDURAL STEPS

1 Ask your partner to pull apart a cotton ball and place one half in each ear. This dampens the sound and the noises all around and simulates hearing loss.

2 Read a section of text aloud to your partner, speaking directly to him or her, and then, while continuing to read, raise the book so that it acts as a barrier between the two of you. Use different voice intonations while you read. Once you have completed the reading, ask your partner to tell you what the reading was about and what was learned.

3 Evaluate the changes in hearing and what was learned by this experience.

Memory Jogger

7 *When can hearing aids result in sensory overload?*

Tinnitus

Another hearing disorder common among older people is **tinnitus.** Tinnitus is characterized by a ringing or buzzing in the ear. It can be caused by impaction with cerumen, an ear infection, use of antibiotics, or a nerve disorder. Tinnitus can cause difficulty in understanding conversational speech and can make sleeping difficult because of the continuous sensation of ringing in the ears. It can be helped by learning behavior modification.

As learned in Chapter 31, an audiologist has a graduate degree in hearing impairment and can identify and measure hearing loss. An otolaryngologist is a physician who specializes in disorders of the ear, nose, throat, and other areas related to the head and neck. An otologist is an ear specialist.

Many products on the market today aid hearing-impaired individuals to function independently. Some telephone companies provide phones that are designed for the hearing impaired at no charge to the customer. Other items may be purchased through catalogues.

TASTE AND SMELL

During the aging process there is a subtle decline in the ability to taste and smell. The taste buds are embedded beneath the surface of the tongue. The number of taste buds decrease. The deterioration and the atrophy of the taste buds are normal and an inevitable consequence of aging. The ability to taste salt and sweet flavors is reduced whereas the ability to detect bitter and sour flavors remains relatively the same. As a result, food tastes bland and unappetizing. Often an older person will add too much salt or sugar to his or her food in an attempt to enhance its flavor. Food becomes less interesting. Weight loss and malnutrition result from poor eating habits.

SUGGESTIONS TO ENHANCE THE DINING EXPERIENCE

- Add different seasonings.
- Vary the texture and color of food to make it more enticing.
- Purchase cookbooks with large print.
- Research finding specially designed eating utensils.
- Consider using devices available to help people who suffer from arthritis. (Retail stores that carry items and devices to assist the arthritic client are available through your local arthritis foundation.)

It is difficult for an older person to detect smells. Not only does this affect his or her ability to enjoy food, but it also exposes the person to environmental dangers. Gas leaks, smoke, and other dangerous odors may go undetected. Eating spoiled food can result in a case of food poisoning, which to an older person could be quite devastating. Checking for gas leaks around stoves and heaters and using smoke alarms reduce some of the danger. Also dating food when it is put in the refrigerator is a good idea.

Memory Jogger

8 *Why is dating food before storing it a good idea?*

MUSCULOSKELETAL SYSTEM

The muscles, bones, and joints of the body support the body, protect the organs, give the body shape, and are responsible for movement. As the body ages, changes occur in muscles, bones, and joints of the body, affecting appearance, strength, and mobility. The amount of change is dependent on diet, exercise, and heredity.

Changes in body composition occur by the age of 75. There is a gradual weight loss, body fat increases by 16%, fluid content decreases by 8%, and the body protein mass (lean body mass) decreases by 15%.

There is a noticeable change in posture and height as people age. Shoulder width decreases and the pelvic and abdominal areas increase, resulting in a "pear shaped" figure. The loss of fat from the face and extremities sharpens the contours of the body. Vertebrae become thinner, intervertebral distances are narrower, and the spinal column compresses, causing the trunk of the body to shorten. The noticeable result is the loss of height. The stooped posture exhibited by some older adults is a result of the compression of the spinal cord, loss of elasticity in the joints and ligaments, and shrinkage of the tendons and muscles. The center of gravity is shifted from the hips to the upper torso (Fig. 39–10).

Vocal cords stiffen and vibrate at a higher frequency. The pitch rises and there is a quaver in the voice that is associated with older speakers. The ability to shout or maintain a monologue on one breath of air decreases.

Memory Jogger

Explain the possible cause for stooped posture of older adults.

Decrease in muscle strength occurs around age 60. The muscle fibers decrease in size and number and are replaced by connective tissue and eventually fat tissue. Loss of motor neurons affect muscular functioning. Older people move more slowly and have less muscular strength and endurance. The amount of atrophy of the muscles depends on the activity level of the individual. As the old saying goes, "If you don't use it, you'll lose it."

The bones are responsible for calcium storage and production of blood cells. They also provide the framework of the body and protect internal organs. Bones are maintained by bone absorption and bone replacement. Bones become more porous and brittle with age because the rate of bone replacement does not keep up with the rate of bone absorption. The incidence of bone fractures increases, and the healing time takes longer. Other factors such a diet deficient in calcium, low levels of vitamin D, lack of exercise, and decreased estrogen levels affect the strength of the bone. Osteoporosis, a condition in which the bones become extremely thin or brittle, is more common in postmenopausal women than in any other group. Arthritis is one of the common physical disorders associated with aging. Broken bones and bone fractures occur at a higher rate in people who have osteoporosis. Sometimes bones break because of the sheer weight of the body on them. Often people say they fell and broke their bone when, in reality, the bone broke, causing them to fall. Weight-bearing exercises, taking calcium supplements, and hormone therapy replacement are used to keep bones from becoming brittle and thin. Alternative medications are now available for persons who cannot have hormone replacement therapy.

The wear and tear of living causes the joints to become worn. The cartilage starts to erode in the joints. The amount of synovial fluid in the joints decreases, leading to varying degrees of stiffness and immobility. This can affect the activities of daily living, such as combing hair or bathing, because of limited range of motion.

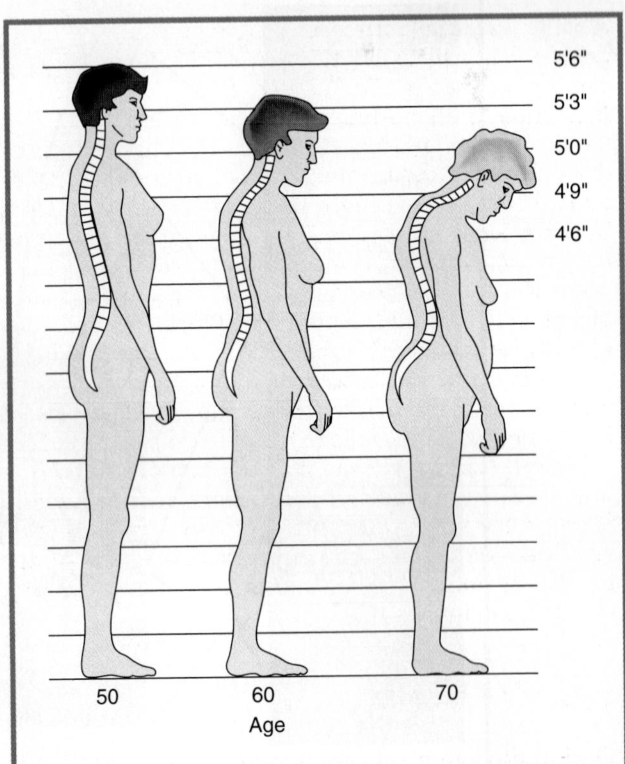

FIGURE 39–10 Typical loss of height associated with osteoporosis and aging.

SKELETAL CHANGES

- Calcium is lost in bones, which causes osteoporosis.
- Cartilage deteriorates.
- Spine shortens, which causes loss of height by 2 to 3 inches.
- Bones in hips widen.
- Shoulders narrow.
- Joints become stiff, rough, and painful.

Memory Jogger

10 *Identify three methods that can help keep bones from becoming brittle and thin.*

INTEGUMENTARY SYSTEM

People spend a considerable amount of money on creams and cosmetics to maintain a youthful appearance. Exposure to ultraviolet light from the sun is the cause of wrinkles, age spots, blotches, and leathery-dry loose skin that we associate with aging. People with fair skin and light hair color are at greater risk from sun damage than people with darker or more olive-colored skin.

The skin is considered the body's first line of protection against infection and is responsible for preventing the loss of body fluid and regulating the body temperature. There are two layers of skin in the integumentary system: the epidermis and the dermis. Below the skin is the subcutaneous tissue. Changes due to the ultraviolet light from the sun or the normal aging process affect these three layers.

The cells in the epidermis reproduce more slowly as people age. This slower regeneration causes the skin to appear thinner. The skin becomes more prone to tearing and blistering. There is an increased risk of infections, the healing process takes longer, and older people are more susceptible to bruising. Because the skin can be easily torn it is important to select an appropriate adhesive when covering a wound or venipuncture site.

The dermis is made of approximately 80% collagen, which gives strength and elasticity to the skin. The number of cells in the dermis that make up the collagen decrease with age. The elastic fibers break down. As a result, the skin appears to sag and wrinkle and when stretched out takes longer to return to its original shape (Fig. 39–11). The glands that secrete oil are located in the dermis layer. They become larger with age, but their function diminishes. Dry skin is one of the most common complaints among older people.

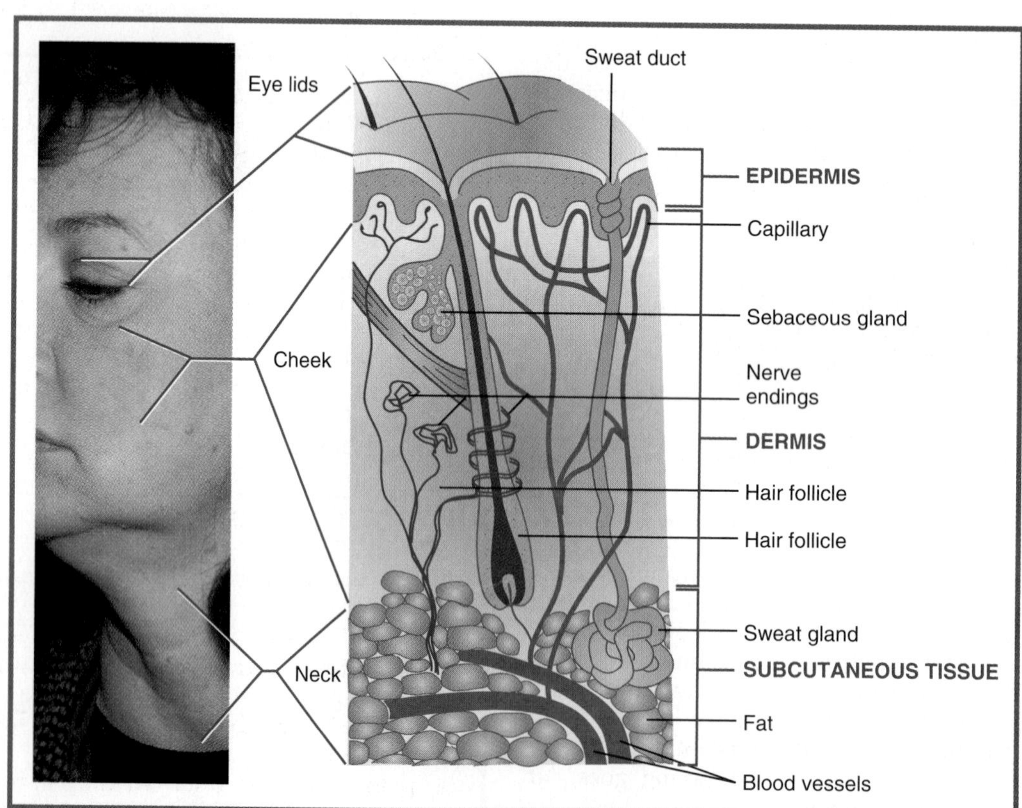

FIGURE 39–11 Anatomy of wrinkles: epidermis breaks down around the eyes, dermis breaks down in the cheek area, and tissue breakdown causes flaccid neck tissue.

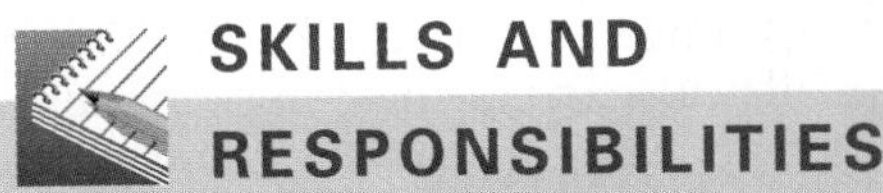

SUGGESTIONS FOR HELPING THE ELDERLY PREVENT AND TREAT DRY SKIN

- Recommend a home humidifier to obtain artificial humidification.
- Advise your elderly patients to bathe less frequently using warm water, NOT hot water.
- Recommend that your patient use a mild, superfatted soap or cleansing cream such as Aveenobar, Oilatum, Basis, or Dove soap.
- Remind the patient to wear protective clothing in cold weather.
- Educate your patient to establish a regimen of using moisturizers for restoration of the epidermal water barrier. Vaseline is an excellent moisturizer.
- Caution your patient to apply creams and moisturizers *after* getting out of the bathtub or shower to decrease the possibility of slipping or falling.

The subcutaneous tissue smooths out the body and is responsible for its insulation. Thinning of the subcutaneous tissue is noticeable in the face and the extremities of the body, the feet, and the hands. These areas become more susceptible to trauma. Fat deposits increase in the abdomen of men and in the abdomen and thighs of women.

Sweat glands and heat and cold sensory receptors are responsible for heat regulation of the body. During the aging process sweat glands decrease in size, number, and function. The body is less able to respond to long exposure to heat or cold. **Hypothermia** occurs when the normal body temperature falls below 95 degrees. People perspire less as they age. As a result, the body temperature becomes too warm when overexposed to conditions of heat. **Hyperthermia** is the result of the body becoming too warm. Heat stroke and heat exhaustion are heat-related illnesses. Any situation in which an older adult is exposed to extremes of cold or heat should be avoided. Make sure there is a blanket available in the examining room if the air conditioning is on. Inquire if the patient is too cold or too hot and take the necessary steps to avoid accidental hyperthermia or hypothermia.

Memory Jogger

11 *Do people perspire more or less as they age?*

Pain receptors are distributed throughout the skin. Because of age-related changes in the receptors the elderly experience an increased threshold to pain. They may not notice a cut or burn as quickly as a younger person would; thus, a burn may become more severe before it is noticed.

Other changes occur in the skin appendages, the nails, and the hair. Hair changes in color, growth, and distribution. Hair grays because of the decreased rate of **melanin** production and the replacement of pigmented hair with nonpigmented hair. Women lose hair on their trunk and have increased facial hair. Men lose their hair because of a predisposed genetic trait. For men, hair on the eyebrows, nose, and ears become courser and longer. Nails of older people take longer to grow and are more brittle. Nails, particularly toenails, thicken as a result of trauma or nutritional causes. Splitting of the nails makes them susceptible to fungal infections.

RESPIRATORY SYSTEM

Around the age of 40 there is a decline in the functioning of the respiratory system. The lungs lose their elasticity owing to changes in **elastin** and **collagen.** They become smaller and flabbier. The alveoli (air sacs) enlarge, their walls become thinner, and there are a reduced number of capillaries. As a result, the effective area for gas exchange is reduced. The chest wall stiffens from osteoporosis of the ribs and vertebrae and calcification of the **costal** cartilage. The respiratory muscles become weaker, making it harder to move air in and out of the lungs. To compensate, older adults rely more on accessary muscles such as the diaphragm. Weakening of the respiratory muscles and the stiffening of the chest wall make it harder to cough deeply enough to clear mucus from the lungs. Older adults also have an increased risk of getting pneumonia.

With age there is a decrease in vital capacity. Vital capacity is the maximum volume of air that is moved in and out of the lungs when a person inhales and exhales as hard as possible. Residual volume, the amount of air left in the lung after a person exhales as hard as possible, increases with age. Pulmonary function tests are used to measure lung volume.

CARDIOVASCULAR SYSTEM

It has been debated if changes in the cardiovascular system are age related or are due to disease. Lifestyle habits such as exercise, diet, and stress control are factors that contribute to the changes that occur in the cardiovascular system. Heart disease is ranked as the number one cause of death among men and women.

Structural changes occur in the heart due to the aging process. Cells of the **myocardium** die and are replaced by fat and connective tissue. This affects the ability of the heart muscle to contract and relax.

TABLE 39-1 Normal Changes of Cardiac Output

Blood Pumped by Resting Heart (quarts per minute)	Maximum Heartbeat During Exercise (beats per minute)
Age 30: 3.6	Age 30: 200
Age 40: 3.4	Age 40: 182
Age 50: 3.2	Age 50: 171
Age 60: 2.9	Age 60: 159
Age 70: 2.6	Age 70: 150

From the American Heart Association.

Cardiac output represents the heart's ability to meet the oxygen requirements of the body. It is defined as the amount of blood pumped by the heart per minute. Recent studies indicate that cardiac output at rest remains stable or slightly declines (Table 39-1).

Heart rate is slower in older persons, and during physical exercise there is a decreased ability to maintain maximum heart rate. The stroke volume (the volume of blood expelled with each heart beat) decreases.

Memory Jogger

 *What does cardiac output represent?*

Arteriosclerosis is considered part of the aging process. The vessel walls thicken and become less elastic due to the calcification and buildup of connective tissue. The ability of the blood vessel to dilate and contract decreases. To maintain an adequate blood supply throughout the body, the heart must work harder to overcome the resistance caused by the stiffened vessels. The diastolic pressure remains the same, but the systolic pressure may increase with age.

URINARY SYSTEM

The function of the urinary system is to rid the body of metabolic waste products and toxic substances. In addition to this, the urinary system regulates acid-base balance and fluid concentration in the body. As the body ages, structural changes in the kidney cause the system to become less efficient.

Between the ages of 40 and 80 the kidney loses about 20% of its mass. The number of functional **nephron units** decreases. There is a reduction in blood flow to the kidney owing to a decrease in cardiovascular efficiency. The reduction of blood flow to the kidney and the decreased number of nephrons cause the kidneys to be less efficient at filtering waste from the blood. This results in a more-diluted, less-concentrated urine. The kidneys require more water to excrete the same amount of waste. Medication takes longer to be removed from the body. Older adults are at an increased risk for toxic levels of medication in the bloodstream because of this reduced filtration rate.

Fibrous connective tissue replaces the smooth muscle and elastic tissue in the bladder. This thickening of the bladder wall decreases the bladder's ability to expand. The bladder's capacity to store fluid comfortably is reduced from 350 to 250 mL. These structural changes in the bladder lead to increased frequency of urination and **urinary retention** after **voiding.** Older adults are at an increased risk for urinary tract infections because of residual urine. Often sleep is interrupted by the need to void during the night. The sensation of bladder fullness is not as quickly recognized by the older brain. Reduced time between awareness of the need to void and involuntary urination can cause anxiety. Often older adults decrease the amount of fluid intake to prevent possible embarrassment. Unfortunately this causes dehydration and an increased risk of urinary infections, which contributes to the possibility of urinary **incontinence.**

Another change is loss of muscle tone in the urethra. Additionally, the pelvic floor muscles in the aging woman relax, owing to decreased estrogen level or previous pregnancy and childbirth.

In spite of these changes, the kidney has great reserve capacity and is still able to function normally. When the system is under stress, problems occur, such as urinary incontinence. Urinary incontinence is the uncontrollable loss of urine. This problem is an emotional one as well as a physical one. To avoid the chance of an embarrassing accident, people with this problem avoid social occasions or doing activities they enjoy. Incontinence is not part of the normal aging process. It can be the result of urinary infections, prostate problems, hormonal changes, disease states such as diabetes, immobility, surgery, and fatigue. Medications such as diuretics, sedatives, and calcium-channel blockers can contribute to incontinence.

Memory Jogger

 *List seven possible causes of urinary incontinence.*

It is reported that 10 million Americans suffer from loss of bladder control. One in 10 persons older than 65 suffers from some form of incontinence. Only 1 of 12 people with incontinence seeks help for this problem. Often people are too embarrassed to admit they have this condition or they believe it is just part of aging. Once the condition is diagnosed by the urologist, pelvic floor muscle exercises, medication, or surgery may be recommended.

GASTROINTESTINAL SYSTEM

One of the first things that comes to mind when thinking about aging and the changes associated with the gastrointestinal system is the loss of teeth. Actually, tooth loss is associated with poor dental hygiene and gum disease rather than age-related change. Enamel on the teeth wears down and the dentin becomes more translucent, but these changes are not significant. With the improvement in dental care and fluoridated water, dental problems will decrease in future generations.

Age does cause a decrease in gastric mobility and gastric secretions. The muscles lose tone, and the regular contractions that move food through the digestive tract become less frequent. Reduction of gastric hydrochloric acid decreases the digestion of calcium, which is needed for bone replacement, and of iron, the mineral needed for red blood cell formation. Secretion of intrinsic factor, a protein that allows vitamin B_{12} to be absorbed, decreases, and this affects the function of the nervous system and the formation of red blood cells and causes excessive fatigue.

The decrease in digestive enzymes produced by the pancreas impairs the utilization of milk products, protein, and fats. The liver decreases in size after age 70. It is still able to perform vital functions, but the time needed to metabolize drugs and alcohol is increased.

One of the problems experienced by the elderly is constipation. Poor eating habits, reduced fluid intake, and some medications such as antidepressants, diuretics, antacids containing aluminum or calcium, and antiparkinsonism drugs contribute to constipation.

REPRODUCTIVE SYSTEM

At approximately age 50, women experience **menopause.** Ovulation and menstruation stop, and they no longer can become pregnant and/or bear children. During this time, some women experience **hot flashes,** which are caused by blood vessels expanding and contracting.

Circulating levels of the female hormones estrogen and progesterone decrease while **androgen** levels increase. The result of this decrease are changes in the genital tract. The vagina diminishes in width and length and becomes less elastic. The cervix, uterus, and ovaries decrease in size. Vaginal secretions decrease; therefore, lubrication diminishes and, in some cases, vaginal dryness may be the result. Bacterial or yeast infections may occur because the vaginal secretions are less acidic. Women who are more sexually active may not experience these effects to the degree that the less active female will. Estrogen replacement therapy can help prevent osteoporosis, heart disease, changes in the vaginal tissue, and vaginal lubrication and lessen the effects of hot flashes. Estrogen cream applied to the vaginal tissue may be prescribed by the physician for help with dryness and thinning of the vaginal tissue. One negative aspect of estrogen replacement therapy is the increased risk of uterine cancer. It is important that the patient discuss the benefits and risks for her individual case with her doctor.

Memory Jogger

14 *Identify the benefits of estrogen replacement therapy.*

Even though sperm production may decline in men older than 50, men remain **virile** well into old age. Men do experience a change in hormonal levels of testosterone, and these changes can affect the prostate gland (Fig. 39–12). The gland enlarges over time and presses down on the urethra, causing difficulty during urination. Surgery may be required to remove excess portions of the gland. Unfortunately, the operation may cause **impotence.** Impotence can be treated by several methods, such as using a vacuum device, self-injection by needle or suppository of medication, penile implants, and oral tablets.

Men do experience some changes in their sexual functioning. It takes longer for the penis to become erect, longer for an orgasm to occur, and longer to recover. Direct stimulation may be required before an erection occurs, and when it does, it may be less firm when compared with how it was when they were much younger.

Some drugs and illnesses can interfere with sexual functioning. Drugs used to control high blood pressure, antihistamines, antidepressants, some stomach acid blockers, diabetes, arthritis, and hardening of the arteries can have an adverse effect on sexual functioning. Often people who have experienced heart surgery or have had heart attacks are concerned about sexual activity. It is important to make patients feel comfortable and not embarrassed to discuss their concerns openly with their physician.

As health care providers, it is important to dismiss old myths that older patients have lost desire and interest in sexual intercourse. Sex at an older age may become more enjoyable than when the participants were younger. Women are more relaxed because the fear of pregnancy is gone. With their children grown and out of the house, couples have more time and privacy. Older people are more experienced and usually can communicate better with one another. At any age, sexuality may be expressed in other forms such as touching, holding, caressing, and, of course, humor. The ability to laugh and share life experiences with one another plays an important role.

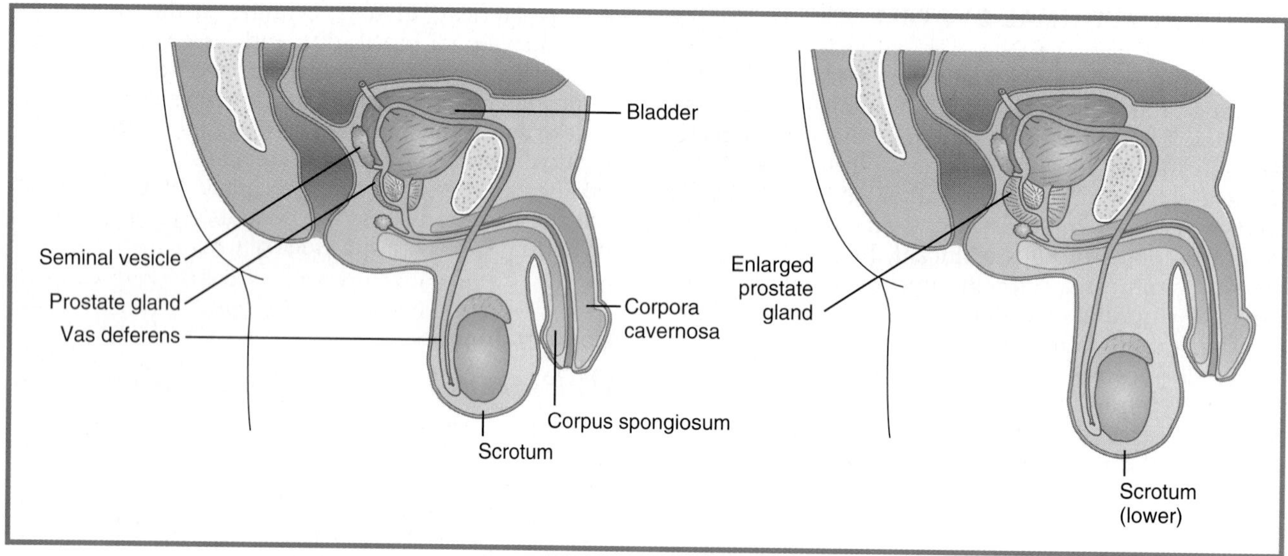

FIGURE 39–12 Comparison of normal prostate (*A*) and enlarged prostate (*B*).

Memory Jogger

Name forms in which sexuality may be expressed other than having sexual intercourse.

INTELLIGENCE AND THE BRAIN

The brain of a person in his or her 50s is different than the brain of a person in his or her 20s. It weighs less, is smaller, and has started to pull away from the sheath or cortical mantle (Fig. 39–13). By the age of 80, the brain has lost about 7% of its weight. Brain cells die and are not replaced because the brain cells do not divide. Cell loss occurs at different rates in different parts of the brain. With age there is a delay in the retrieval of information; but, remember, the older brain has a lot more stored information to sort through before retrieving the needed items. Sometimes aids can be used to help recall information. For example, if a young man and an older man are given a list of words to remember, and then given clues to each word, there is little difference in their ability to recall the words. Therefore, teaching the use of **mnemonic** devices might improve the ability to retrieve information.

Fluid intelligence is the ability to comprehend complex relationships and make inferences. It does not rely on prior learning to perform a task. Crystallized intelligence refers to skills that are learned through education, culture, and life experiences, such as verbal comprehension and numerical skills. Fluid intelligence declines with age, but crystallized intelligence stays the same or increases.

It should not be concluded that senility is an inevitable part of aging. Most men and women remain mentally competent until the end of their lives. Sudden loss of memory, disorientation, and trouble performing the daily tasks of life indicate there is a problem that should be addressed. Other conditions may be the cause of decreased mental capacity. Depression, prescription and over-the-counter medication, alcoholism, and malnutrition may all interfere with mental judgment and motor skills, giving the impression of decreased mental status.

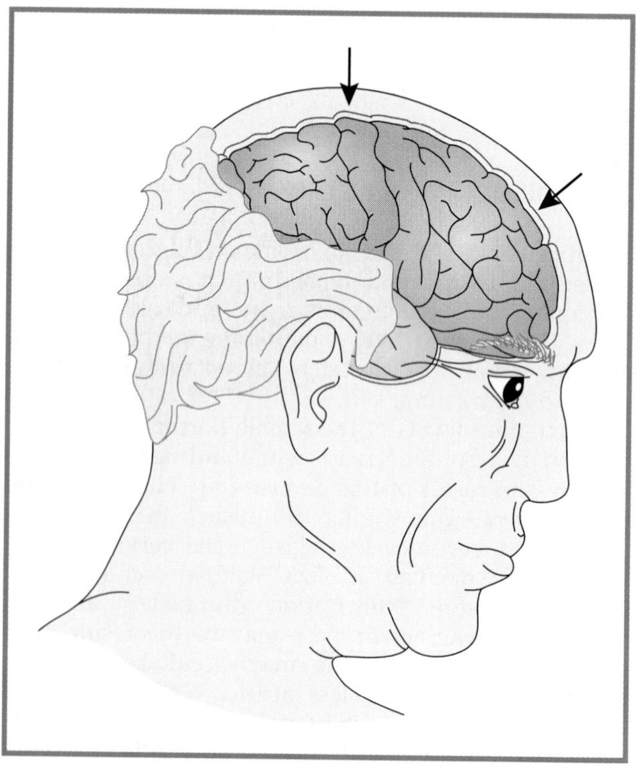

FIGURE 39–13 Shrinking of brain.

The best way to ensure mental functioning in later life is to remain mentally and physically stimulated. Playing a musical instrument, doing community work, hobbies, or reading are all ways to keep mentally active. Research has shown that people can learn new information and skills at any age. Just think of the numbers of older people who have learned how to use computers.

Memory Jogger

 *What is the best way to remain mentally and physically stimulated?*

SLEEP DISORDERS

A good night's sleep is something everyone looks forward to at the end of the day. It is the time the body renews itself to maintain optimum functioning. For older persons, this may be the hardest part of the day.

As a person ages, sleep patterns change. The amount of time spent sleeping may be slightly longer than a younger person, but the quality of sleep decreases. Older people are often light sleepers and experience periods of wakefulness in bed. Rapid eye movement (REM) sleep is the stage of sleep when people experience dreaming. Non-REM sleep is the period of deepest sleep. The amount of time spent in the deepest stages of sleep decreases with age.

Most people have experienced insomnia at some time during their lifetime. Taking longer than 30 to 45 minutes to fall asleep, waking up early, and not being able to fall back to sleep are all signs of insomnia. Sleep that is disturbed or leaves the person feeling tired is not part of the aging process and may indicate some underlying emotional or physical problem. Lack of sleep can result in restlessness, disorientation, thick-speech patterns, and mispronounced words. Often these symptoms are mistaken as signs of dementia. There may be a noticeable increase in the number of daytime naps to counteract the effects of sleep disturbances. Unfortunately, this affects the quality of sleep at night.

Memory Jogger

 *What is the average length of time it takes for a person to fall asleep?*

Other factors that might influence sleep patterns are medications, caffeine, alcohol, depression, and environmental or physical changes.

COMMON SLEEP PROBLEMS IN OLDER ADULTS

- Periodic limb movement disorder (PLMD)—periodic jerking of the legs during sleep interferes with sound sleep.
- Joint and bone pain—pain causes movement, interrupting sound sleep patterns.
- Caffeine and/or monosodium glutamate—these are stimulants and make it difficult to fall asleep.
- Alcohol—alcohol induces drowsiness but increases the number of awakenings.
- **Sleep apnea**—common among overweight individuals, it occurs many times during the night, interrupting sleep.
- Environmental influences—traffic noise, cold or hot bedroom, and lack of privacy tend to cause awakening.
- Boredom—lack of social stimulation contributes to less efficient sleep.
- Depression or anxiety—loss of partner, for example, or moving into new living environment may manifest sleep pattern changes.
- Medications—beta-blockers can cause nightmares, antidepressants increase PDML, and barbiturates may result in nightmares and/or hallucinations.

It is important to be aware of the effect of sleep problems because often these can be confused with dementia. Patients who are experiencing difficulty with sleeping should be encouraged to document their sleeping pattern, napping patterns, medications, diet, exercise patterns, and any events that have resulted in a change of lifestyle and discuss this with their physician. Simple modification of behavioral patterns may resolve the problem. Taking fewer naps, exercising several hours before bedtime, changing eating times, decreasing the amount of alcohol and caffeine ingested, drinking a glass of milk before bedtime, or changing medications or the time that they are taken are all suggestions that might alter the factors responsible for sleep disturbances.

LIVING ARRANGEMENTS

Only 5% of the population older than 65 live in nursing homes. According to information published by the National Institute on Aging most older people live close to their children and are in frequent contact with them. Approximately 80% of men and 60% of women live in family settings (Fig. 39–14).

People prefer to age in place or, in other words, live in their own home environment as long as possible. The reason people are admitted to nursing homes is because they are no longer able to perform

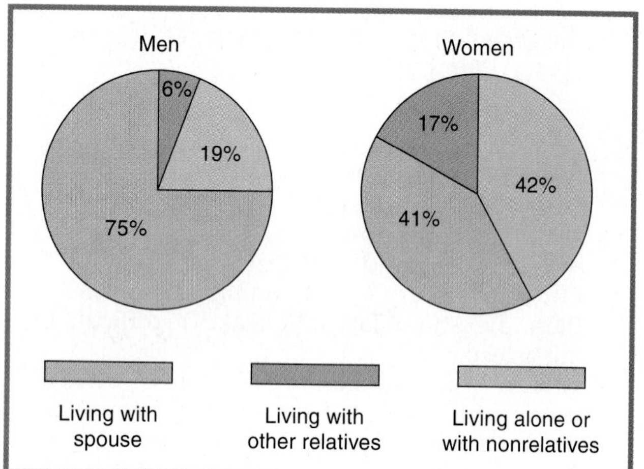

FIGURE 39–14 Living arrangements of persons 65 and older. (Data from U.S. Bureau of the Census.)

activities of daily living, such as bathing, dressing, eating, walking, and maintaining bladder and bowel continence. Instrumental activities are grocery shopping, housekeeping, and money management. Chronic health conditions such as arthritis interfere with the older person's ability to perform these tasks (Fig. 39–15).

There are many resources available that enable seniors to maintain their **autonomy.** Outreach programs, such as Meals-on-Wheels, deliver nutritious meals to the homes of the elderly. The Friendly Visitors Service provides social contact. Senior centers serve as a focal point for many activities and a source of information. Transportation services provide rides to doctor's appointments, day care centers, shopping centers, and community events. Home health agencies provide several types of services, which include personal care, shopping, transportation, and meal preparation. Some home health agencies provide a range of activities from patient education to intravenous therapy, medical-social services, physical speech and occupational therapy, and nutrition and dietary counseling. Advanced technology has allowed people to receive services at home that had formerly been provided at a hospital or physician's office only.

Adult day care centers provide socialization, recreation, meals, and, in some centers, physical therapy, occupational therapy, and transportation (Fig. 39–16). These centers provide supervision for older adults who may be taken care of by family members in the evening but need care during the day. They also serve as a respite for a caregiver.

Senior apartments (shared and congregate housing) provide older persons with a variety of living arrangements. The arrangement may consist of two people sharing a home to apartments designed to meet the special needs of seniors. Continuing-care communities include a full range of care options. These complexes are composed of apartments, assisted-living units, and nursing-care units. Each section of the complex offers services that depend on the functional ability of the resident.

Assisted-living facilities can be retirement homes or board and care homes. These facilities are appropriate for older adults who need assistance with

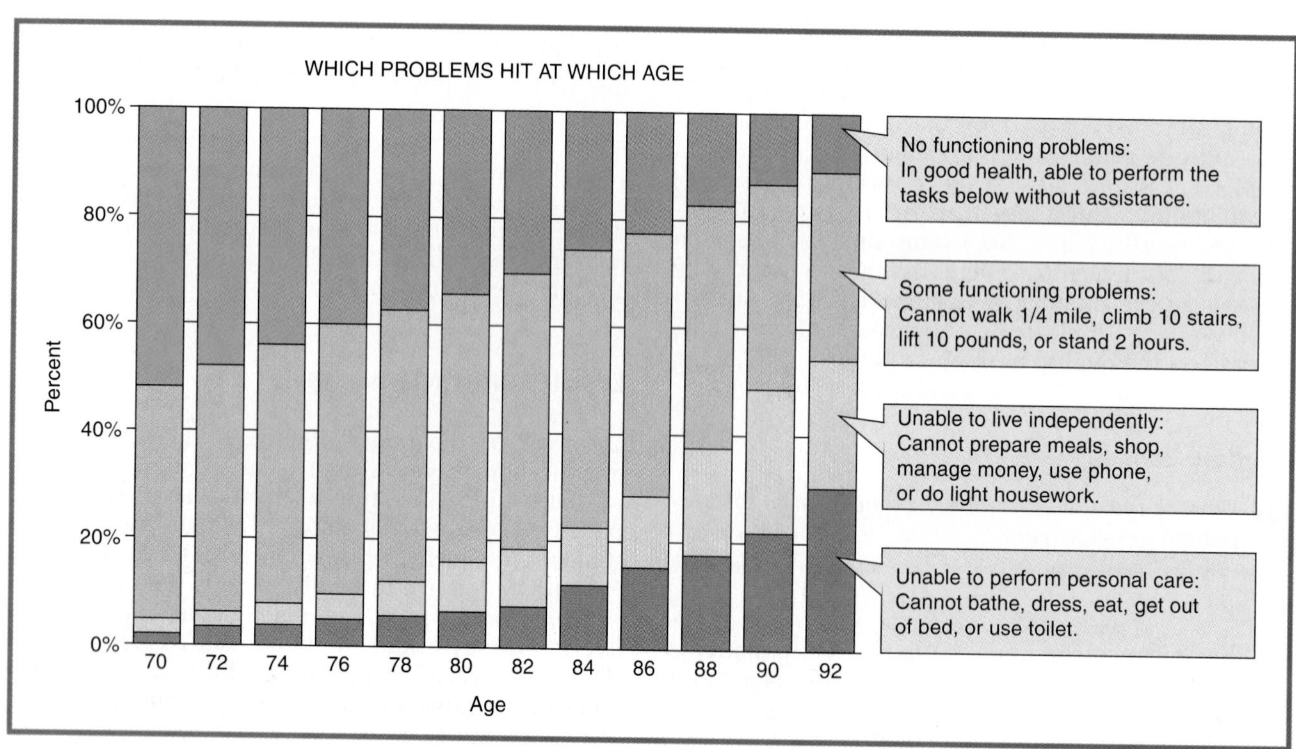

FIGURE 39–15 Problems that arise as we age.

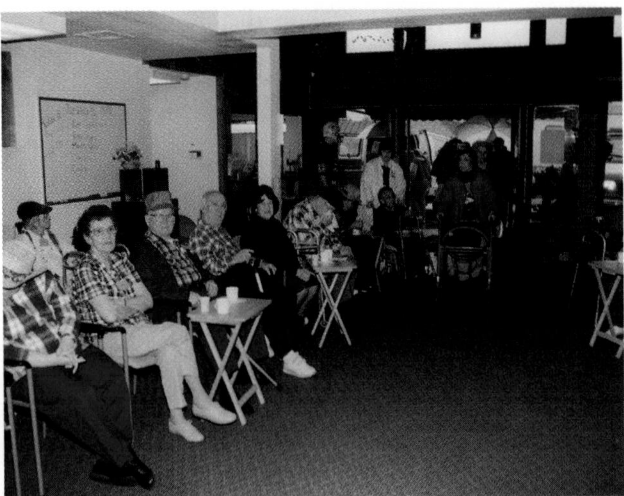

FIGURE 39–16 Adult day care center—a source of activity.

some activities of daily living, such as bathing, dressing, and walking.

Skilled nursing facilities provide 24-hour medical care and supervision. In addition to medical care, residents receive care including physical, personal, occupational, and speech therapy. The objective is to improve or maintain the person's abilities.

Memory Jogger

18 *What is the difference between assisted-living and nursing-care living arrangements?*

The Medical Assistant's Role in Caring for the Older Patient

When elderly patients come into the office it often causes the whole routine to be upset. They need more time, but we have many patients to see so we tend to want to hurry them. This situation can create problems in patient flow management and can lead to personal frustrations. There is really no absolute remedy to the situation, and every office will handle the problem differently. However, the best way to solve this is through office team work.

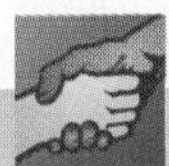

PERSONAL QUALITIES

THE DON'T LIST

DON'T shout if the person appears to be hearing impaired; instead, speak slowly and distinctly.

DON'T use lights that produce glare; instead, use indirect or shielded light

DON'T carry on conversations where there is an excessive amount of background noise.

DON'T use the same vocal tones and mannerisms that you tend to use with young children.

DON'T "patronize" older people; don't talk or act in a way that could be interpreted as condescending.

DON'T "touch" older people more than you would any other person.

DON'T touch older people in a "controlling" way; rather, touch politely and affectionately.

DON'T avoid looking at older people in conversations; eye contact is appropriate when communicating with people of all ages.

DON'T talk *about* an older person when he or she is physically present; talk *with* the older person directly.

DON'T buy into the ageist maxims of our society, such as "You can't teach an old dog new tricks" or "There's no fool like an old fool."

EXAMPLES FOR AN OFFICE SYSTEM TO ACCOMMODATE THE ELDERLY PATIENT

1 Use a different scheduling system to give the elderly patient more time.
2 Have one examination room that is equipped with furniture, magazines, and treatment folders especially designed for the elderly patient (Fig. 39–17).
3 Invite a professional in the management of the elderly patient to visit your office and give an in-service training course to the staff.

Whatever policy is adapted, several changes remain universal in elder care. The primary issue is communication.

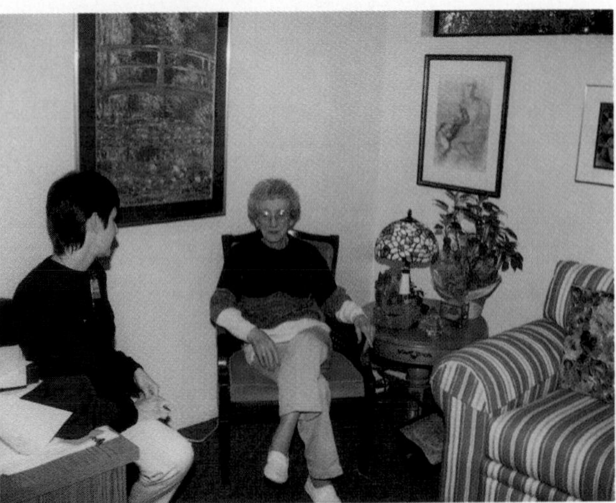

FIGURE 39–17 Elder client waiting room with in-service management offered.

How you communicate with people is often influenced by what you know or don't know about them. Older people are subject to many changes that affect how they are able to communicate with their environment. It is important to recognize these changes and also our personal perception of older people to break down the barriers that prohibit effective communication.

As people age they may encounter a reduction in control over their lives owing to physical disabilities, economic constraints, and institutional living. It is important to enable aging people to maintain their dignity and autonomy. To do this it is necessary to incorporate a positive attitude toward aging by dismissing old myths. The myths that older people are unproductive, senile, sexless, unable to learn or comprehend new ideas, are all the same, and are resistant to change produce a negative attitude toward the aging population. This negative attitude can affect how people interact and communicate with the elderly. Unfortunately, television, greeting cards, films, and cartoons perpetuate these myths.

One particularly disturbing myth is the belief that all older adults lapse into a second childhood. Younger caregivers often use silly and childish phrases when addressing an elderly person. For example the statement, "Honey, drink all of this like a good girl" is demeaning to an older person. Monitor your talk and make sure you are speaking in an appropriate, respectful manner using the correct vocabulary and sentence complexity.

Remember each older person is an individual. Don't talk about an older person when he or she is present. Instead, talk directly to the person. Frequently the older person becomes part of the "third person" syndrome. For example, don't ask the son or daughter who has brought the parent to see the doctor, "What is wrong with your mother today?" Instead ask the mother what is wrong. After all, she *is* the patient. Imagine how the self-esteem of an older person is diminished in these situations.

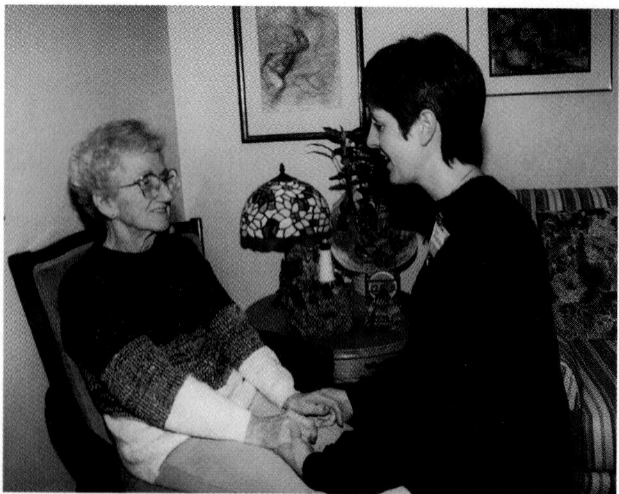

FIGURE 39–18 Good communication skills enhance self-esteem.

Good communication skills dictate the importance of maintaining or enhancing self-esteem (Fig. 39–18). It also is important to listen carefully and to be specific and sincere in responding. When a patient is talking, take time to allow him or her to complete the sentence. Don't finish it for them. Give the patient your full attention rather than continue with multiple tasks while he or she is speaking. Older people may take a little longer to process information. Don't hurry through explanations or questions. A few minutes to review a form will save time on your part in not having to repeat the instructions several times and the patient will feel less angry or apprehensive. Customer service is what keeps patients returning, and in today's health care market customer service is a top priority.

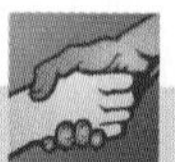

PERSONAL QUALITIES

SUGGESTIONS TO HELP IMPROVE COMMUNICATION SKILLS

- Never approach a visually impaired person without making him or her aware of your presence. Be thoughtful, and identify other people in the room and explain their location.
- Touching or patting someone's hand is a form of communication. It evokes a feeling of comfort and support. It makes the person aware of your presence and aids in getting his or her attention.
- Face the individual to permit maximum use of lip movement and facial expression. Keep on the same level as possible by maintaining a distance of 3 to 6 feet. If using a table, 42 inches is considered the most helpful distance.
- Speak with a slightly louder voice but remember not to raise the pitch of your voice. Don't shout. Shouting causes the facial expressions to be distorted. When speaking louder there is a tendency to furrow the brows and frown. Sadly, this expression can be interpreted as anger, causing the hearing-impaired person to believe you are angry at him or her.
- Speak clearly. Remove objects such as gum, food, or your hand from your mouth. Do not overarticulate because this causes distortion of the mouth and face.
- Speak slowly and pause as necessary. Older people take longer to process information. Be careful not to offend an older listener by "talking down" to him or her.
- Use nonverbal communication such as gestures, facial expressions, and objects to help emphasize a verbal message.
- Beards and mustaches may interfere with facial expressions and prevent the older person from following lip movement and facial cues.
- If repetition of a message is requested, para-

phrase the message or find other words to say the same thing.

- Make sure there is adequate lighting. The light should be above the speaker or facing him. This prevents glare from shining into the eyes of the older person and provides contrast on the speaker's face for greater facial expression.
- Reinforce oral instructions by writing them down.
- Observe gestures and facial expression of the person with whom you are speaking. These cues indicate if he or she is understanding you.
- When leaving a telephone message for an older individual, even if he or she is not hearing impaired, please remember to speak slowly and clearly while leaving the message and repeat it in the same manner. It is hard to interpret a message, and even more difficult to write it down if the message was delivered in a hurried manner. Not all answering machines have a tape that can be replayed.

Many organizations have information available to assist you in educating the senior-aged patient and the immediate family. Besides providing information that could be used within the office, these organizations also have ongoing seminars that you, the patient, and the patient's family may attend. Most of them are a public service.

ORGANIZATIONS THAT PROVIDE INFORMATION

Telephone directories can provide information on services for the elderly
Alzheimer's Association (1-800-272-3900)
American Cancer Society (1-800-227-2345)
American Council of the Blind (1-800-424-8666)—provides referrals to state and other organizations that provide services and equipment for the blind
American Diabetes Association (1-800-232-2472)
American Heart Association (1-800-242-1793)
American Speech-Language-Hearing Association (1-800-638-8255)—offers information on hearing aids or hearing loss and communication problems in older people and provides a list of certified audiologist and speech pathologists
Arthritis Foundation Information Line (1-800-283-7800)—makes referrals to local chapters and provides information
ABLEDATA (1-800-227-0216)—a national database that has information on products for people with disabilities
National Osteoporosis Foundation (1-800-223-9994)
Cancer Information Service (1-800-422-6237)
Eldercare Locator (1-800-677-1116)—run by the National Association of Area Agencies on Aging, the helpline provides information on contacting local chapters that oversee services to the elderly
National Institute on Aging Information Center (1-800-222-2225)—provides information publications on geriatric health issues
National Library Service for the Blind and Physically Handicapped (1-800-424-8567)—provides free of charge books on tapes or record disks and the equipment to play them
National Wheels-on-Meals Foundation (1-800-999-6262)
Hospice Helpline (1-800-658-8898)—provides information about hospice care and makes referrals to local hospices

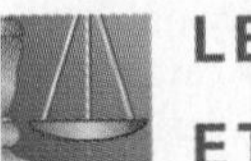

LEGAL AND ETHICAL ISSUES

Patient's Rights and Advance Directives

All patients have the right to know about the medications, treatments, and alternatives available to them. The Patient's Bill of Rights is a document informing the patients of his or her rights. These rights include the right to privacy about personal and medical information and the right to **informed consent,** which holds the physician accountable to clearly explain the advantages and risks of any procedure, tests, or treatments. The patient must give the permission for the medical care and has the right to refuse treatment. The patient has the right to be informed about his or her condition and treatment and the chances of recovery. The patient also has the right to have advance directives explained to him or her. A complete copy of the Patient's Bill of Rights is located in Figure 39–19.

Most states have legal documents available that give people the right to determine what medical procedures they want provided if they become unable to make these decisions. These documents are called *advance directives* and are of two types: a living will and a durable power of attorney for health care. A living will provides written instructions specifying the type of medical care a person wishes to receive in the event they become incapacitated. A durable power of attorney is a written document that names a person (called a proxy) responsible for making medical decisions on a person's behalf if that person is unable to make his or her own treatment decisions. The document provides a list of specific instructions for the proxy to follow. Various issues may be covered in these documents. Do not resuscitate (DNR) orders allow a patient to refuse attempts to restore heartbeat. The patient may decide to withdraw from life-sustaining treatment such

A Patient's Bill of Rights*

1. The patient has the right to considerate and respectful care.

2. The patient has the right to and is encouraged to obtain from physicians and other direct caregivers relevant, current, and understandable information concerning diagnosis, treatment, and prognosis.

Except in emergencies when the patient lacks decision-making capacity and the need for treatment is urgent, the patient is entitled to the opportunity to discuss and request information related to the specific procedures and/or treatments, the risks involved, the possible length of recuperation, and the medically reasonable alternatives and their accompanying risks and benefits.

Patients have the right to know the identity of physicians, nurses, and others involved in their care, as well as when those involved are students, residents, or other trainees. The patient also has the right to know the immediate and long-term financial implications of treatment choices, insofar as they are known.

3. The patient has the right to make decisions about the plan of care prior to and during the course of treatment and to refuse a recommended treatment or plan of care to the extent permitted by law and hospital policy and to be informed of the medical consequences of this action. In case of such refusal, the patient is entitled to other appropriate care and services that the hospital provides or transfer to another hospital. The hospital should notify patients of any policy that might affect patient choice within the institution.

4. The patient has the right to have an advance directive (such as a living will, health care proxy, or durable power of attorney for health care) concerning treatment or designating a surrogate decision maker with the expectation that the hospital will honor the intent of that directive to the extent permitted by law and hospital policy.

Health care institutions must advise patients of their rights under state law and hospital policy to make informed medical choices, ask if the patient has an advance directive, and include that information in patient records. The patient has the right to timely information about hospital policy that may limit its ability to implement fully a legally valid advance directive.

5. The patient has the right to every consideration of privacy. Case discussion, consultation, examination, and treatment should be conducted so as to protect each patient's privacy.

6. The patient has the right to expect that all communications and records pertaining to his/her care will be treated as confidential by the hospital, except in cases such as suspected abuse and public health hazards when reporting is permitted or required by law. The patient has the right to expect that the hospital will emphasize the confidentiality of this information when it releases it to any other parties entitled to review information in these records.

7. The patient has the right to review the records pertaining to his/her medical care and to have the information explained or interpreted as necessary, except when restricted by law.

8. The patient has the right to expect that, within its capacity and policies, a hospital will make reasonable response to the request of a patient for appropriate and medically indicated care and services. The hospital must provide evaluation, service, and/or referral as indicated by the urgency of the case. When medically appropriate and legally permissible, or when a patient has so requested, a patient may be transferred to another facility. The institution to which the patient is to be transferred must first have accepted the patient for transfer. The patient must also have the benefit of complete information and explanation concerning the need for, risks, benefits, and alternatives to such a transfer.

9. The patient has the right to ask and to be informed of the existence of business relationships among the hospital, educational institutions, other health care providers, or payers that may influence the patient's treatment and care.

10. The patient has the right to consent to or decline to participate in proposed research studies or human experimentation affecting care and treatment or requiring direct patient involvement, and to have those studies fully explained prior to consent. A patient who declines to participate in research or experimentation is entitled to the most effective care that the hospital can otherwise provide.

11. The patient has the right to expect reasonable continuity of care when appropriate and to be informed by physicians and other caregivers of available and realistic patient care options when hospital care is no longer appropriate.

12. The patient has the right to be informed of hospital policies and practices that relate to patient care, treatment, and responsibilities. The patient has the right to be informed of available resources for resolving disputes, grievances, and conflicts, such as ethics committees, patient representatives, or other mechanisms available in the institution. The patient has the right to be informed of the hospital's charges for services and available payment methods.

*These rights can be exercised on the patient's behalf by a designated surrogate or proxy decision maker if the patient lacks decision-making capacity, is legally incompetent, or is a minor.

FIGURE 39–19 Patient's Bill of Rights. (© 1992 by the American Hospital Association.)

as the use of respirators or feeding tubes. Both documents must be initiated when the person is competent. These documents may also be changed if the person decides he or she is no longer comfortable with the document as it is written. A copy of the directives should be kept on file as part of the patient's medical record. It is important to check the laws of the state regarding living wills and durable power of attorney because these vary among states.

CRITICAL THINKING

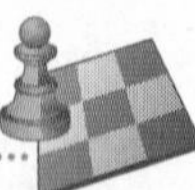

1 Have you any idea how many senators now serving in Congress are older than 65?

2 What are your personal feelings about caring for patients who are 75 and older?

3 Do you ever think about what your needs might be when you are 75 and how you will want these needs taken care of?

4 When was the last time that you voluntarily visited a senior (older than 75) family member?

HOW DID I DO? Answers to Memory Joggers

1. Old age is a normal life process.
2. By the time a person reaches 50 changes in the eyes are noticed.
3. Presbyopia is the inability to focus on detailed objects close at hand.
4. Three vision problems resulting from a smaller pupil are difficulty in focusing at different distances, decrease in the ability to see objects clearly, and difficulty is discriminating color intensity.
5. Yellows, reds, and oranges are easier to identify.
6. Cataracts, glaucoma, and macular degeneration are common in older adults.
7. Hearing aids increase not only the sound of the human voice but also the background noises.
8. Dating food helps in preventing eating of spoiled food, which can cause food poisoning.
9. Stooped posture is a result of the compression of the spinal cord, loss of elasticity in the joints and ligaments, and shrinkage of the tendon muscles.
10. Weight-bearing exercises, taking calcium supplements, and hormone replacement therapy can help keep bones from becoming brittle.
11. People perspire less as they age.
12. Cardiac output represents the heart's ability to meet the oxygen requirements of the body.
13. Urinary infection, prostate problems, hormonal changes, diabetes, immobility, surgery, and fatigue may cause urinary incontinence.
14. Estrogen replacement therapy helps prevent osteoporosis, heart disease, changes in the vaginal tissue; aids in vaginal lubrication; and lessens the effects of hot flashes.
15. Other ways of expressing sexuality are touching, holding, caressing, and humor.
16. Keep mentally and physically stimulated.
17. The average length of time to fall asleep is 30 to 45 minutes.
18. Assisted living is living independently with assistance only when needed. Nursing care is complete care for all of your daily living needs.

Assisting with Office Emergency Procedures

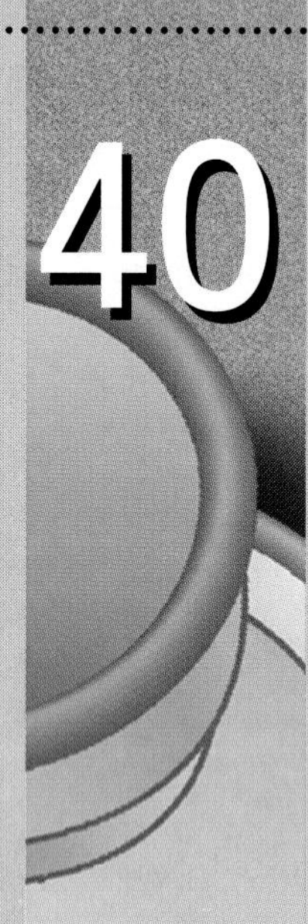

OUTLINE

LEARNING OBJECTIVES

Cognitive: On successful completion of this chapter you should be able to:

1. Describe the medical assistant's responsibilities in an emergency.
2. Recall two resources that can help to make your medical office accident proof.
3. List the basic items that must be included on an emergency cart.
4. Explain the purpose of a defibrillator in an emergency.
5. Recognize a choking victim.
6. Recall the conditions that necessitate the implementation of CPR.
7. List the major symptoms associated with heart attack.
8. Describe the emergency medical care that is usually given to victims of asthma, anaphylactic shock, convulsions, and hemorrhagic shock.
9. State the functions of a poison control center.
10. Define and spell vocabulary terms.

Performance: On successful completion of this chapter you should be able to:

1. Demonstrate triage techniques in a simulated emergency situation.
2. Accurately perform CPR using a simulated mannequin.

VOCABULARY

anaphylaxis Allergic condition caused by an antigen-antibody reaction; may cause shock, bronchoconstriction, airway obstruction, and loss of consciousness

apical pulse Pulse heard over the base (apex) of the heart

convulsion A series of involuntary contractions of the voluntary muscles

cyanosis Blue color of the mucous membranes and body extremities caused by lack of oxygen

diaphragmatic Pertaining to the primary muscle of respiration; separates the thoracic and the abdominal cavities

ecchymosis A hemorrhagic skin discoloration commonly called bruising

epistaxis Nosebleed

insulin shock Shock brought about by too much insulin, too little food, or excessive exercise; when untreated, it can result in death

mediastinum Space in the center of the chest under the sternum

paroxysm The sudden onset of symptoms, such as a spasm or seizure

sublingually Pertaining to under the tongue

syncope Loss of consciousness; fainting

syrup of ipecac A syrup given to induce vomiting

traumatic Pertaining to, resulting from, or causing physical injury or shock

triage To sort or to choose; to determine the priority of need for treatment

venom Poison transmitted through the bite or sting of spiders, snakes, and some insects

First aid is defined as the immediate care given to a person who has been injured or has suddenly taken ill. It includes well-chosen words of encouragement, a willingness to help, a promotion of confidence by the demonstration of competence, and the performance of temporary physical care to alleviate pain or a life-threatening situation. Knowledge of first aid and skill can often mean the difference between life and death, temporary and permanent disability, and rapid recovery and long-term hospitalization.

Frequently, the medical assistant may be responsible for initiating first aid in the office and continuing to administer first aid until the physician or trained medical teams arrive. Every medical assistant should successfully complete a course in cardiopulmonary resuscitation (CPR) and continue to hold a current CPR card as long as employed. Basic knowledge of CPR and life-support skills need to be updated on a regular basis because of recommended changes for procedures as new techniques are developed. Medical assistants should encourage their local medical assisting chapters to offer workshops conducted by physicians and emergency personnel from the community.

There are many acceptable approaches to emergency care. All offices need to establish written policies concerning the handling of medical emergencies. The medical assistant should consult with the physician-employer for his or her preferences in handling emergencies in that particular practice.

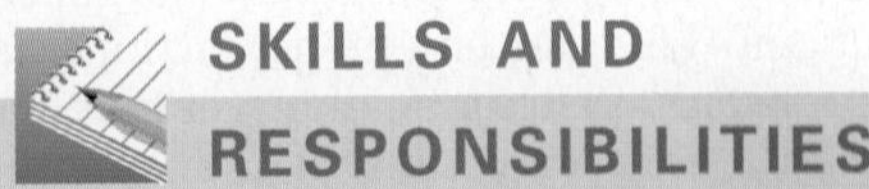

MEDICAL ASSISTANT'S ROLE IN PERFORMING EMERGENCY PROCEDURES

1 Perform only the emergency procedures in which you are trained.
2 If an emergency occurs in the office, notify the physician.
3 If a physician cannot be located, then contact the local emergency medical services team.

Medical assistants do not assume the responsibility of diagnosing but are expected to make decisions based on their medical knowledge. A major goal in emergency care of the injured is to cause no further harm.

In a true emergency, the Good Samaritan law permits anyone to do whatever is reasonably necessary, provided that the care given is within the scope of competence of the person administering first aid. The law holds persons giving emergency care to be responsible for any injury that they cause as a result of their negligence or failure to exercise reasonable care. You, the medical assistant, are limited to the standards of your state laws, and your physician-employer is legally responsible for your mistakes.

Memory Jogger

What is the primary responsibility of the medical assistant in an emergency?

Making the Office Accident Proof

Usually, it is the medical assistant's responsibility to make the office as accident proof as possible. Do not use scatter rugs or delicate chairs, and be sure that floors are not slippery (Fig. 40–1). Keep cupboard doors and drawers closed. Wipe up spills immediately, and pick up dropped objects. All medications should be kept out of sight; dangerous drugs should be kept in locked cupboards. If there are children in the office, keep all sharp objects out of reach. Never leave a seriously ill patient or a restless, depressed, or unconscious patient unattended.

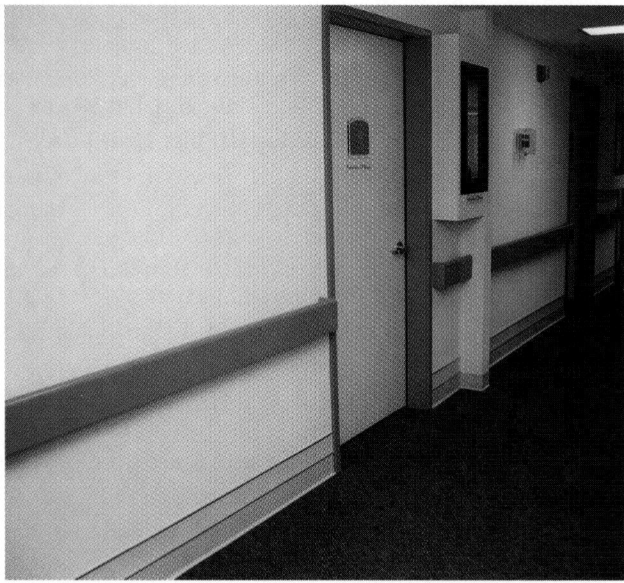

FIGURE 40–1 Keeping office accident proof with doors closed and hallway free of all equipment and unnecessary containers.

Planning Ahead

The office staff should discuss possible emergencies that may occur and have an emergency action plan to be used for rapid, systematic intervention. For instance, local industries may present unique problems that call for very specialized care. Plan for these, and ask the physician's advice on what procedures to follow. If there are several employees, each should be assigned specific duties. Organization and planning make the difference between systematic care for the patient and complete chaos.

Some offices have set up a team management system. This system designates one person to take immediate charge of the patient while another obtains needed materials and calls for assistance.

Memory Jogger

What is the advantage of the team management system?

USING COMMUNITY EMERGENCY SERVICES

Many communities have established an emergency medical services (EMS) system. This system includes an efficient communications network, such as the emergency telephone number 911, well-trained rescue personnel, properly equipped vehicles (Fig. 40–2), an emergency facility that is open 24 hours a day to provide advanced life support, and hospital intensive care for the victims.

There are more than 300 poison control centers in the United States ready to provide emergency information for treating victims of poisonings. Many of the centers have toll-free lines. Some have systems for communicating with deaf persons.

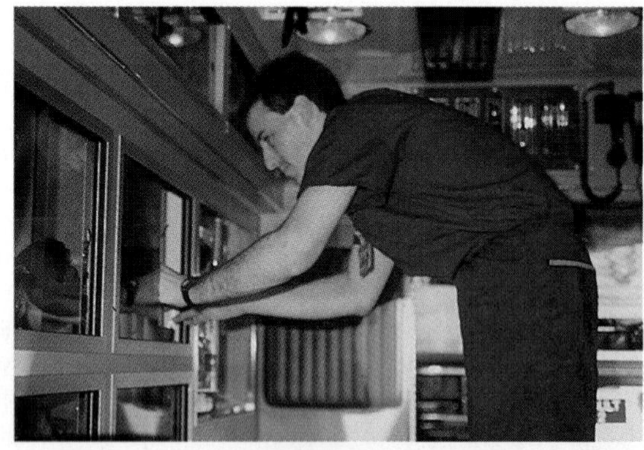

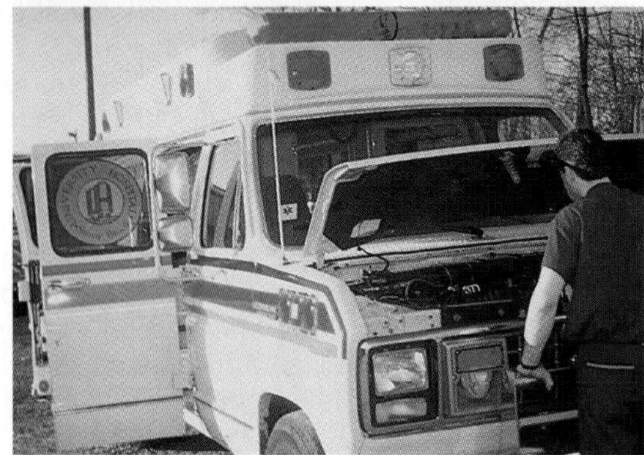

FIGURE 40–2 Emergency medical technicians inspecting ambulance before first run. (From Henry MC, Stapleton ER: EMT Prehospital Care, 2nd ed. Philadelphia, WB Saunders, 1997.)

Every office is required to post a list of local emergency numbers. This list should be in plain sight and should be known to all office personnel. Include on the list the local EMS system, poison control center, ambulance and rescue squad, fire department, and police department numbers.

Memory Jogger

Name the local emergency agencies whose numbers should be posted in the medical office.

Supplies and Equipment for Emergencies

EMERGENCY SUPPLIES

The emergency supplies consist of a properly equipped cart of first-aid items needed for a variety of emergencies (Fig. 40–3). The contents of the cart will vary to some degree, according to the type of emergencies each office encounters. This cart should be kept in an easily accessible place known to all personnel in the office. A firm rule must be made that no one borrows items from the cart. Medication expiration dates must be checked on a routine basis and the cart replenished with fresh supplies after every use.

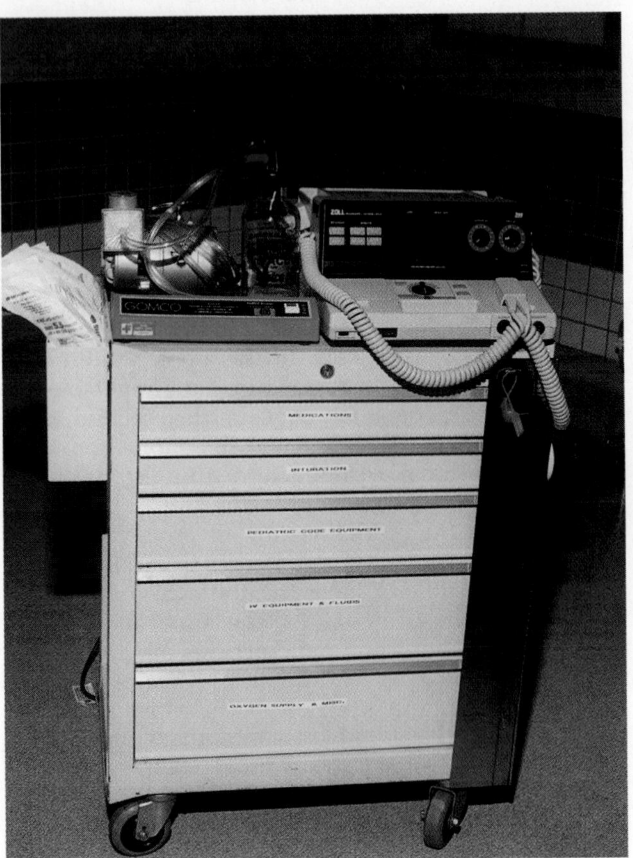

FIGURE 40–3 Office emergency cart with defibrillator. Drawers are marked for easy retrieval of emergency supplies.

BASIC EMERGENCY CART ITEMS

SUPPLIES

Adhesive tape in 1-inch and 2-inch widths
Alcohol (70%) and alcohol wipes
Antimicrobial skin ointment
Cotton balls and cotton swabs
Elastic bandages in 2-inch and 3-inch widths
Gauze pads, 2 × 2- and 4 × 4-inch widths
Gloves, sterile and nonsterile
Hot and cold packs (instant type)
Muslin sling or cravat bandage to be used as a tourniquet
Orange juice
Suction catheters
Sterile dressings (miscellaneous sizes, including two abdominal pads)
Syringes, hypodermic needles, and intravenous equipment in assorted sizes and gauges

MEDICATIONS

Activated charcoal, bottle of 30 to 50 g
Amobarbital (Amytal)
Antihistamine, injectable and oral
Apomorphine
Atropine
Dextrose
Diazepam (Valium)
Digoxin (Lanoxin)
Disposable syringe and needle units
Epinephrine (Adrenalin), injectable (dilution 1:000)
Furosemide (Lasix)
Glucagon
Isoproterenol (Isuprel) aerosol spray
Lidocaine (Xylocaine)
Metaraminol (Aramine)
Spirits of ammonia
Syrup of ipecac

EQUIPMENT

Airways in various sizes
Ambu-bag with assorted sizes of facial masks
Bandage scissors
Blood pressure cuff (pediatric, regular, and large adult sizes)
Bulb syringe
Stethoscope
Flashlight
Portable oxygen tank with regulator and mask
Nasogastric suction unit equipped with tubing
Defibrillator

Epinephrine is a vasoconstrictor used to check hemorrhage. It relaxes the bronchioles, is used to relieve asthmatic **paroxysm,** and is an emergency heart stimulant used to treat shock. Epinephrine should be in a ready-to-use cartridge syringe and needle unit. These are supplied in 1.0-mL cartridges.

Other drugs used are atropine, digoxin (Lanoxin), and lidocaine (Xylocaine). Atropine decreases secretions, increases respiration and heart rates, and is a smooth muscle relaxant. It dilates the pupil of the eye and is a general cerebral stimulant. Atropine relieves gastrointestinal cramps and hypermotility and may also be used to relieve pain locally. Digoxin is a cardiotonic. It is used to treat congestive heart failure and is good for emergency use because it has a relatively rapid action. Lidocaine is used intravenously to decrease heart arrhythmia and as both a local and a topical anesthetic.

Apomorphine is a prompt and effective emetic and is used in cases of poisoning when a stomach pump cannot be employed. **Syrup of ipecac** is also an emetic and one that many physicians recommend be kept on hand in the home for use in emergencies.

Antihistamines are used to counteract the effect of histamine and are used in the treatment of allergic reactions and **anaphylaxis.** Isoproterenol, an antispasmodic, is used in bronchial spasm and is also a cardiac stimulant. Some trade names for this product are Isuprel, Medihaler-Iso, and Norisodrine.

Other medications that may be found on a crash tray are metaraminol (Aramine) (50%, in a prefilled syringe), for severe shock; amobarbital sodium (Amytal) and diazepam (Valium), for convulsions and as sedatives; dextrose and insulin, to treat diabetic patients; and furosemide (Lasix), for congestive heart failure. Glucagon is primarily used to counteract severe hypoglycemic reactions in diabetic patients taking insulin.

Small cans of orange juice, with pull-tab openers, are handy for quick sugar administration in cases of diabetic patients experiencing **insulin shock.**

Most physicians and others involved in emergency care do not recommend a tourniquet because of the danger that may result from incorrect usage. A tourniquet that completely stops blood flow to the point of no measurable pulse is potentially hazardous and should be used very cautiously. It is much better to apply pressure directly over the bleeding area. Today, rather than a tourniquet, a constricting band is employed for the purpose of decreasing lymphatic and superficial venous blood flow for bites by insects and snakes. In these cases, the constricting band is applied just above the bite area.

As more patients come to clinics and physicians' offices to seek emergency care, the medical assistant will need to become even more familiar with specialized equipment on the emergency cart to help save lives. Figure 40–3 shows the outside and the inside of a typical emergency cart. The cart contains numerous locking drawers in which supplies and medicines are kept.

Memory Jogger

When would you use the cans of orange juice on the emergency cart?

DEFIBRILLATORS

The medical assistant who works in a large clinic, in a cardiology office, or in an urgent-care center may be required to assist the team with defibrillation of emergency patients. Defibrillators are instruments that send a massive jolt of electricity into the heart muscle by means of plates or paddles applied to the chest to reestablish the proper rhythm of the heartbeat. One paddle is placed to the right of the upper sternum, and the other is placed just to the left of the nipple, at the apex of the heart.

The office defibrillator is portable and is powered by standard 110-V current or batteries (see Fig. 40–3). The monitor has a nonfading display, and it is possible to freeze the monitor for prolonged viewing. If a permanent record of the victim's heart rate is desired, the machine can make a printed copy.

Memory Jogger

What is the purpose of the defibrillator?

General Rules for Emergencies

When first starting a new job, you should be shown a book of office protocols. In this book should be a section on the accepted steps in handling an office emergency. On the first page of this section there should be a list of emergency telephone numbers. Many offices have a duplicate of this list posted at the telephone locations within the office. This book is considered the guidelines for all procedures done within the office. When an emergency occurs, it may be that you will not have the time to go and look up how the physician wanted this situation handled. You need to know how emergencies are to be handled and this means reading and learning what this book contains and the protocols your employer wants followed. Do not assume that the method used in the last office you worked in is going to be exactly the same in this office. Assuming can cause situations that may be embarrassing or may even cause you to lose your job. *Be certain, read the book!*

When faced with an emergency there are some general rules that are universal.

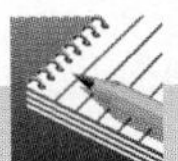

SKILLS AND RESPONSIBILITIES

MEASURES TO TAKE IN EMERGENCY SITUATIONS

- Most importantly, stay calm. Reassure the patient and make him or her as comfortable as possible.
- Survey the situation to determine the nature of the emergency. Decide whether the need is immediate. This decision requires calm judgment and may call for some medical knowledge.
- Examine the scene. Quickly evaluate potential hazards, possible injuries, and any clues that you can determine from the overall appearance of the situation.
- Take immediate steps to remedy the situation. Calmly but firmly give specific instructions to the patient and to other office personnel. Never say, "Will someone call the doctor?" Say, "YOU call the doctor, YOU get a blanket, and YOU get the emergency cart."
- After the emergency is under control, make certain that all the events and the medications used are recorded accurately. Be precise when recording. Have statements of what happened and what events preceded the emergency.
- *Always follow Standard Precautions.* When an emergency occurs, it is impossible to determine the level of infection that you are encountering. A good rule to follow is if it is wet and it isn't yours, don't touch it without protecting yourself. All body fluids must be considered infectious, and the appropriate precautions must be employed.

Memory Jogger

The first and most important rule in emergency situations is ______.

Emergency Management

An emergency can occur at any time to anyone. The office emergency could involve a patient, a co-worker, or the physician. In addition to emergencies that can occur within the office, others might occur outside the office. A person may fall, get hit by a car, or have a heart attack or stroke. Whatever the emergency, documentation becomes an important function in emergency care management.

BASIC INFORMATION THAT NEEDS TO BE COLLECTED

1 Patient's name, address, age, and health insurance information
2 Name and whereabouts of any person with the patient
3 Patient's vital signs and chief complaint
4 Sequence of events, beginning with how trauma occurred, any changes in the patient's overall condition, and any observations you have made regarding the patient's condition
5 Any procedures or techniques performed on the patient
6 If possible, any allergies, medications, or known health conditions

Stay with the patient until you have been relieved of your responsibility by the EMS provider or the physician. Never leave an injured patient alone.

The two primary functions of first aid remain constant. Never do anything that will worsen the situation, and provide the best care you can to correct any life-threatening situation.

Memory Jogger

Name the two primary functions of first aid.

Common Emergencies

FAINTING (SYNCOPE)

One of the most common emergency problems to confront the medical assistant is fainting. **Syncope** is usually caused by lack of oxygen in the blood, with a consequent lack of oxygen to the brain. Before fainting, a person may appear pale; may feel cold, weak, dizzy, or nauseated; and may have numbness of the extremities. Immediately lay the patient flat, with the head lower than the heart. Loosen all tight clothing, and maintain an open airway. Apply a cold washcloth to the forehead. If allowed, pass aromatic spirits of ammonia back and forth under the patient's nostrils, but be careful not to hold the ammonia too close to the nose. Obtain the patient's pulse, respiration rate, and blood pressure, and then report the findings to the physician. Keep the patient in a supine position for at least 10 minutes after consciousness has been regained.

If recovery is not prompt, summon the physician or emergency medical rescue team for transportation to the hospital. Syncope might be a brief episode in the development of a serious underlying illness.

EMERGENCY RESUSCITATION

Breathing may suddenly cease for a variety of reasons, including shock, disease, and trauma. The most obvious sign that breathing has stopped is when the chest is no longer moving. Artificial ventilation must be started immediately, because death may follow within 4 to 6 minutes.

Before beginning assessment of the patient, *put on gloves.* Check the patient responsiveness to determine the level of consciousness. Then check for breath sounds and heartbeat. Now check the airway. When it has been established that CPR must be started as a lifesaving measure, tell someone to call for emergency assistance and then begin the resuscitation procedure.

Establishing the Airway

The airway must be opened by positioning the patient on the back and relieving possible obstruction of the air passage by the tongue. Extreme caution must be used if there is any chance that the patient has suffered a cervical neck injury, as should be assumed in any accident. If neck injury is not suspected, the head is tilted by downward pressure on the forehead and upward pressure under the chin. If neck injury may be present, grasp the angle of the victim's lower jaw without extending the neck.

Resuscitation

Mouth-to-mouth resuscitation is begun if breathing does not follow opening of the airway. Position yourself on the side of the patient's head. One hand should continue pressing on the forehead and should also be turned so that the fingers can hold the nose shut. The other hand should continue lifting the chin upward. Place a CPR mouth barrier (Fig. 40–4) over the patient's face. Place your mouth over the tube in the barrier and give the victim two full breaths. Check for the carotid pulse. If the pulse is present, continue ventilating the lungs every 5 seconds. If the pulse is absent, you must provide artificial circulation in addition to artificial ventilation (see next section).

There are mouth-to-nose and mouth-to-stoma methods for resuscitation of victims with tracheotomies. The reader is referred to the American Red Cross *Standard First Aid Manual* or *American Heart CPR Manual* for specific procedures and precautions. Artificial airways may be inserted by trained personnel to establish or maintain breathing. Airways of various types and sizes should be kept ready on the emergency cart (Fig. 40–5).

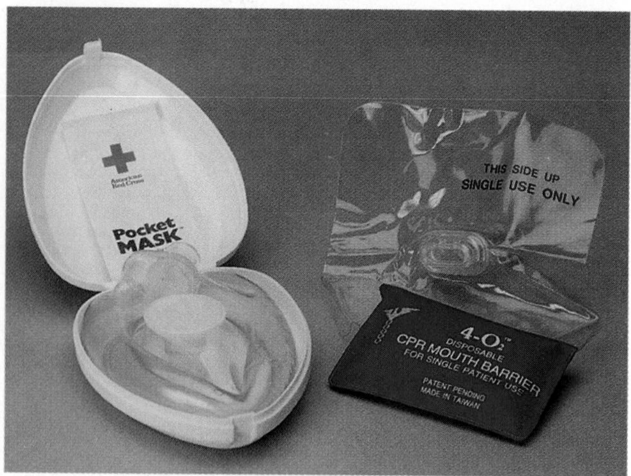

FIGURE 40–4 CPR mouth barriers.

Memory Jogger

 *How often must you ventilate the lungs?*

Cardiopulmonary Resuscitation

Cessation of breathing may be accompanied by a cessation of the heartbeat (cardiac arrest), which is identified by the lack of a pulse. Artificial ventilation must then be accompanied by external (closed) cardiac massage. This is called cardiopulmonary resuscitation, which is the combination of artificial circulation and artificial breathing (see Procedure 40–1).

BASIC ABC STEPS OF CPR

A—airway
B—breathing
C—circulation

When both breathing and pulse stop, the victim has suffered sudden death. There are many causes of sudden death, including choking, drowning, poisoning, suffocation, electrocution, and smoke inhalation. CPR must be started immediately in an attempt to prevent death or permanent damage to body organs, especially the brain.

Because CPR may cause injuries to the ribs, heart, liver, lungs, and blood vessels, it should be performed only by individuals properly trained in the techniques and only if cardiac arrest has occurred. In CPR, the heart is compressed by downward pressure on the sternum, which should cause the blood to circulate. The proper position is for the heel of the one hand to be placed on the sternum, two fingerwidths above the lower notch where the ribs join.

The other hand is placed on top, and the rescuer presses straight down. The sternum will be depressed 1½ to 2 inches with sufficient pressure.

Compressions should be given at a rate of 80 to 100 compressions per minute (15 compressions should take 9 to 11 seconds). Compress down and up smoothly, keeping hand contact with the victim's chest at all times. After every 15 compressions, move back to the mouth, open the airway with the head-tilt/chin-lift, and breathe two full breaths into the victim. After four cycles have been completed, locate and check the carotid pulse, feeling for 5 seconds. Continue CPR until a qualified person can relieve you or until advanced life support is available.

CPR for infants and small children is similar to that for adults, but a few important differences must be remembered. When handling an infant be careful that you do not overextend the head when tilting it back (Fig. 40–5*A*). The infant's neck is so pliable that forceful backward tilting might block breathing passages instead of opening them. With an infant who is not breathing, be certain to cover both the mouth and the nose with your mouth and deliver two slow puffs that are just strong enough to make the chest rise. With a small child, pinch the nose, cover the mouth, and breathe as for an infant. In an infant, check the brachial pulse (see Fig. 40–5*B*) between the elbow and the shoulder. Use only the fingertips at the center of the sternum for compressions on the infant (see Fig. 40–5*C*). Compress the sternum between ½ and 1 inch, at a rate of at least 100 times per minute. Only the heel of one hand is used for compressions on a small child. Depress the sternum 1 to 1½ inches, at a rate of 80 to 100 times per minute. CPR for children older than 8 years of age is the same as that for adults.

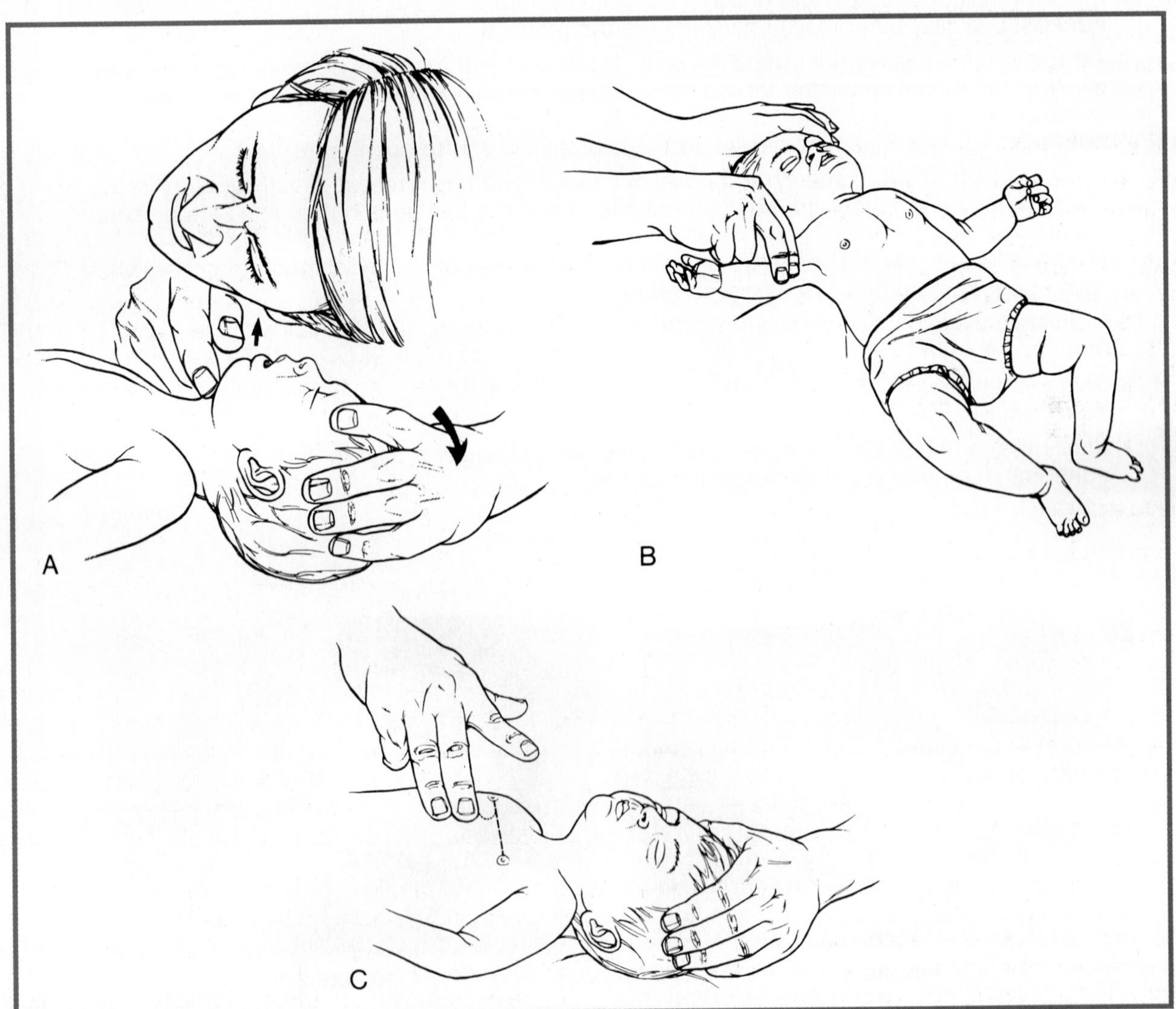

FIGURE 40–5 Modifications necessary for CPR on child. *A,* Chin lift in an infant. *B,* Placement of two fingers over medial aspect of upper arm halfway between elbow and axilla to locate pulse. *C,* To locate correct position for compression in an infant, place your index, middle, and ring fingers of the hand closest to infant's feet adjacent to nipple line and then lift index finger. (From Henry MC, Stapleton ER: EMT Prehospital Care, 2nd ed. Philadelphia, WB Saunders, 1997.)

PROCEDURE 40-1

Performing Cardiopulmonary Resuscitation

GOAL

To restore a victim's breathing and blood circulation when respiration and pulse stop.

EQUIPMENT AND SUPPLIES

Nonsterile gloves (sterile gloves may be preferred)
CPR mouth barrier
American Heart Association–approved mannequin equipped with a printout for demonstration of the proper technique for your instructor.

PROCEDURAL STEPS

(To be performed on an approved mannequin only.)

1 Begin a primary survey. Tap the victim and ask, Are you OK? Wait for victim to respond.
PURPOSE: To determine whether the victim is conscious.

2 Shout for help. Put on gloves. Activate the EMS system.
PURPOSE: To alert other rescue personnel to the problem.

3 Tilt the victim's head and lift the chin. Look, listen, and feel for signs of breathing. Place your ear over the mouth and listen for breathing. Watch the rising and falling of the chest for evidence of breathing (Figure 1).
PURPOSE: To determine whether the victim is breathing and to open the airway.

4 Place the CPR mouth barrier over the victim's mouth and begin rescue breathing by pinching the nose tightly with your thumb and forefinger if none of the signs of breathing are present (Figure 2).
PURPOSE: An airtight seal must be present so that air cannot escape through the nose when you perform mouth-to-mouth resuscitation.

5 Maintain an airtight seal with your mouth on the tube in the barrier that leads to the victim's mouth.

6 Give two full breaths.
PURPOSE: May be sufficient stimulus to initiate breathing by the victim.

7 Check the carotid pulse. If a pulse is felt, continue resuscitation (Figure 3).
PURPOSE: The pulse is easier to feel in this area.

Continued

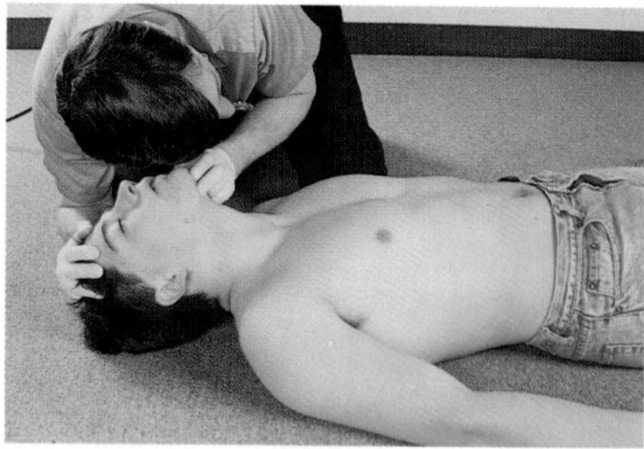

FIGURE 1

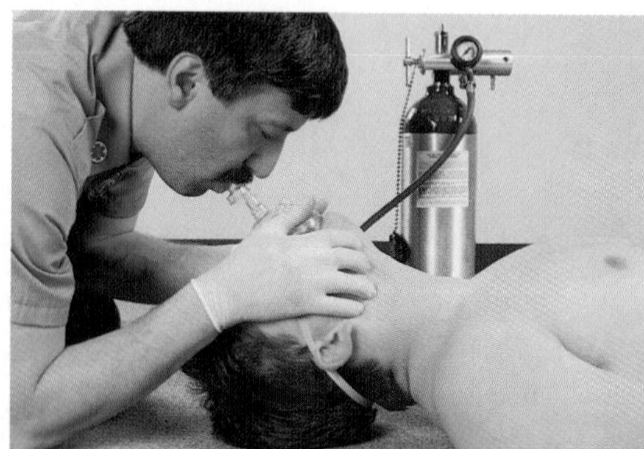

FIGURE 2

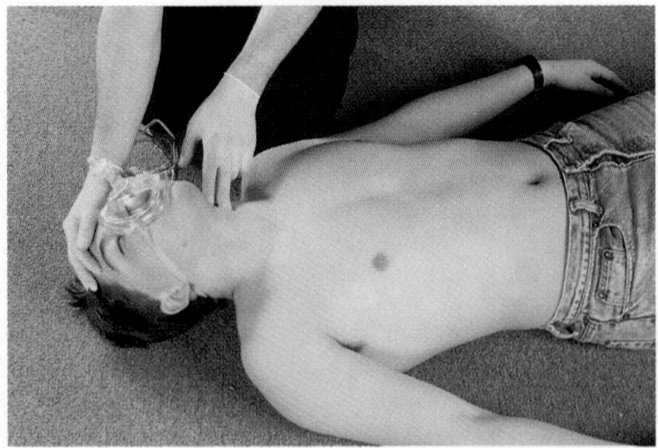

FIGURE 3

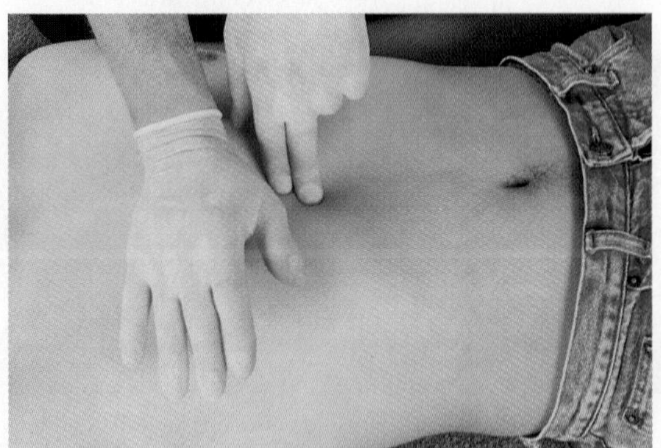

FIGURE 4

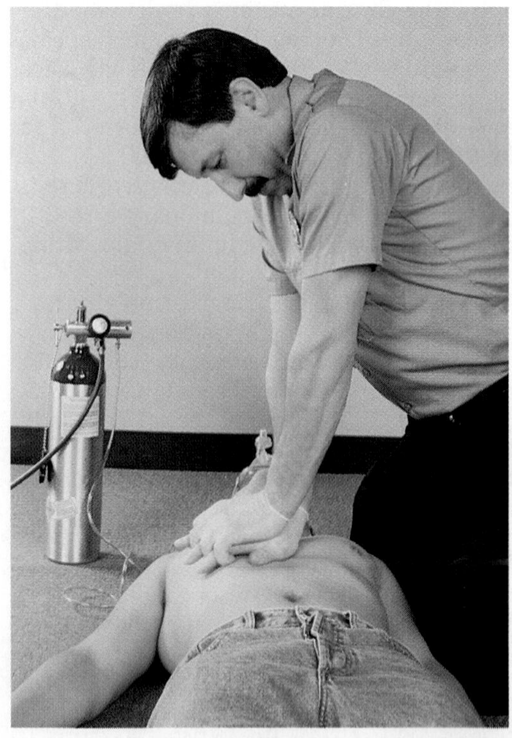

FIGURE 5

8 Continue mouth-to-mouth resuscitation at the rate of approximately one full breath every 5 seconds *if the pulse is present.*

9 Initiate CPR *if there is no pulse.*

10 Kneel at the victim's side opposite the chest. Move your fingers up the ribs to the point where the sternum and the ribs join. Your middle fingers should fit into the area and your index finger should be next to it across the sternum.

11 Place the heel of your hand on the chest midline over the sternum, just above your index finger (Figure 4).

12 Place your other hand on top of your first hand and lift your fingers upward off of the chest (Figure 5).

PURPOSE: This position gives you the most control, allowing you to avoid injuring the victim's ribs as you compress the chest.

13 Bring your shoulders directly over the victim's sternum as you compress downward, and keep you arms straight.

14 Depress the sternum 1½ to 2 inches for an adult victim. Relax the pressure on the sternum after each compression but *do not remove your hands* from the victim's sternum.

PURPOSE: The depth of compression is needed to circulate blood through the heart. Movement of the hands may cause injury to the victim.

15 After performing 15 compressions, open the airway and give two full, slow, breaths.

16 Complete three more cycles of compressions and breaths, ending with 2 breaths. Check for pulse and breathing for 5 seconds. If there is no pulse or breath, resume CPR at the rate of 15 compressions to two breaths. Always start and end each cycle with two full breaths. Continue giving CPR until the EMS relieves you.

CHOKING

Choking is caused by a foreign object, usually food, lodged in the upper airway. Often, exhalation can take place, but inhalation is blocked. Thus, the lungs quickly empty. The choking victim who has food or a foreign object lodged in the throat cannot speak, breathe, or cough. The victim may clutch the neck between the thumb and index finger (Fig. 40–6). This universal distress signal should be viewed as a sign that the victim needs help.

The face pales and turns blue. Eventually, there is loss of consciousness and cardiopulmonary arrest. If the object is not removed, the victim may die within 4 to 6 minutes.

If the victim has good air exchange or only partial obstruction and can speak, cough, or breathe, do not interfere. If the victim cannot speak, cough, or breathe, use the Heimlich maneuver. Give sub**diaphragmatic** abdominal thrusts until the foreign body is expelled or the victim becomes unconscious (Fig. 40–7). If the victim becomes unconscious, position the victim on his or her back and call out for help. Lift the jaw and sweep your finger in the victim's mouth in an attempt to remove the foreign body. Open the airway, and attempt rescue breathing. If you are still unsuccessful in removing the foreign body, use the Heimlich maneuver and give five subdiaphragmatic abdominal thrusts (Fig. 40–8). Repeat the sequence until you are successful. After the obstruction is removed, begin the ABCs of CPR, if necessary.

It is possible to perform the abdominal thrust maneuver on yourself if you are choking and there is no one nearby to help you. Press your fist into your upper abdomen with quick upward thrusts or lean forward and press the abdomen quickly against a firm object such as the back of a chair (Fig. 40–9).

To dislodge a foreign object from an infant, place the victim face down, over your forearm and across your thigh. The head should be lower than the trunk. Next, support the head and neck of the victim with one hand. Using the heel of the other hand, deliver four blows to the back, between the infant's shoulder blades (Fig. 40–10). Place the infant on his or her back, with the head lower than the trunk. Using two or three fingers, deliver four thrusts in the sternum area (Fig. 40–11). Repeat the sequence until the foreign body is expelled or the infant becomes unconscious.

If the infant becomes unconscious, position the infant on his or her back and call out for help. Sweep your finger through the mouth in an attempt to remove the foreign body (Fig. 40–12). Open the airway, and attempt rescue breathing. If you are still unsuccessful in removing the foreign body, perform the sequence of back blows and chest thrusts until you are successful. After the obstruction is removed, begin the ABCs of CPR, if necessary.

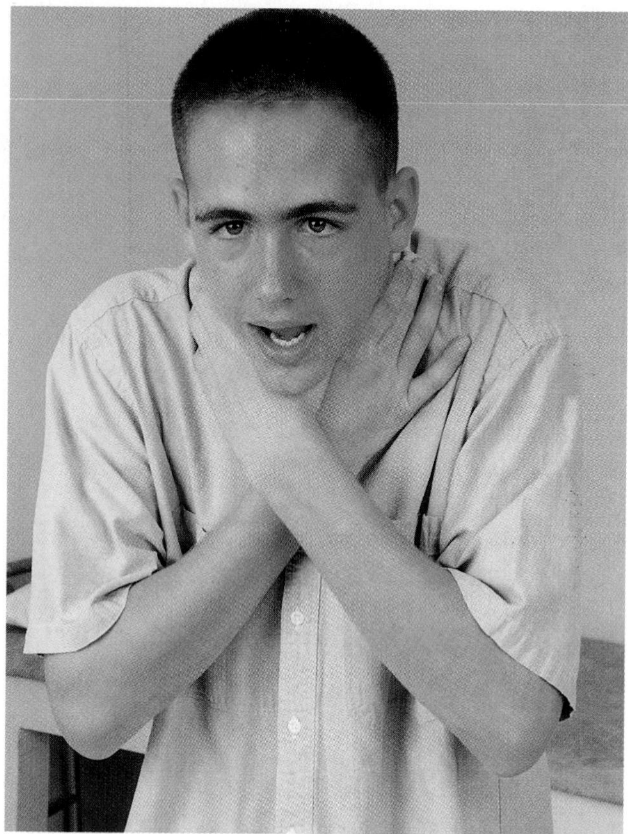

FIGURE 40–6 Universal choking distress signal.

Memory Jogger

Demonstrate the universal distress signal for choking.

CHEST PAIN

Chest pain can be associated with both heart and lung disease, as well as a few other conditions. It can be quite serious; all patients with chest pain are treated as cardiac emergencies until a physician has ruled out this diagnosis. The patient is often sweating and may have a gray, ashen appearance. The lips and fingernails may be blue (a sign of **cyanosis**) (Fig. 40–13). Frequently, the patient is clutching the chest in pain. This pain may radiate from the **mediastinum** down the left arm and up the left side of the neck. The pulse may be rapid and weak. Frequently, there is nausea.

Do not have the patient walk any distance. A wheelchair or a chair with rollers is an excellent method of moving this patient to a quiet room. The patient will probably prefer to have his or her head slightly elevated or even to be in a semi-sitting position. Keep the patient quiet and warm. Loosen all

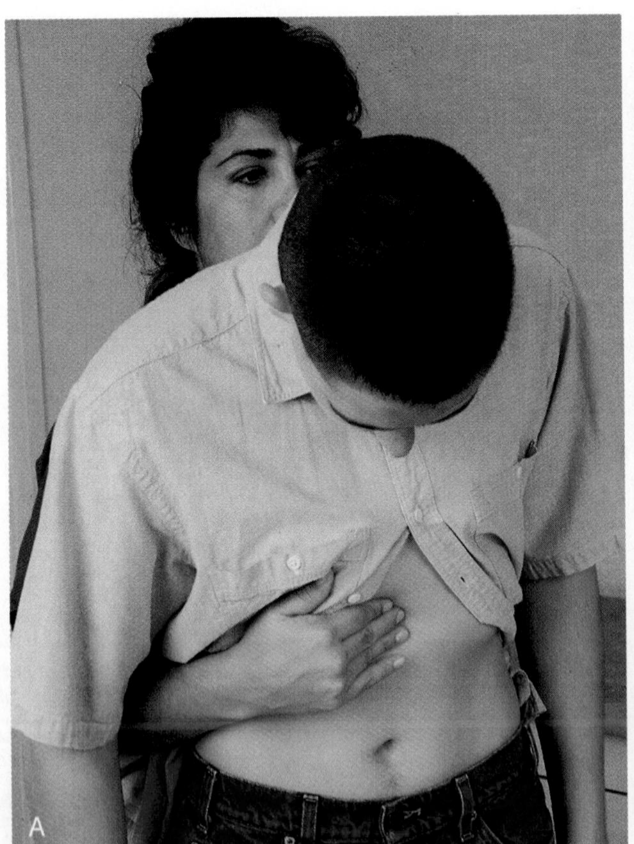

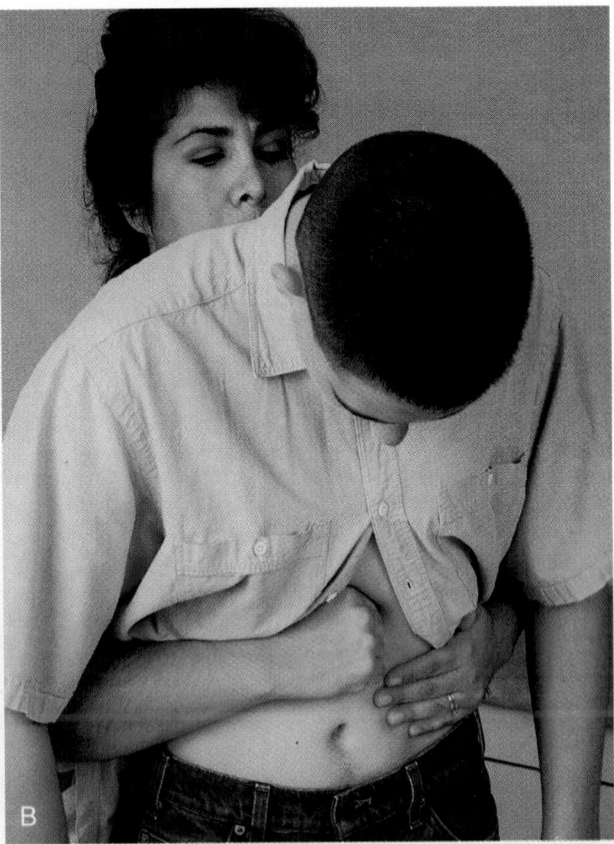

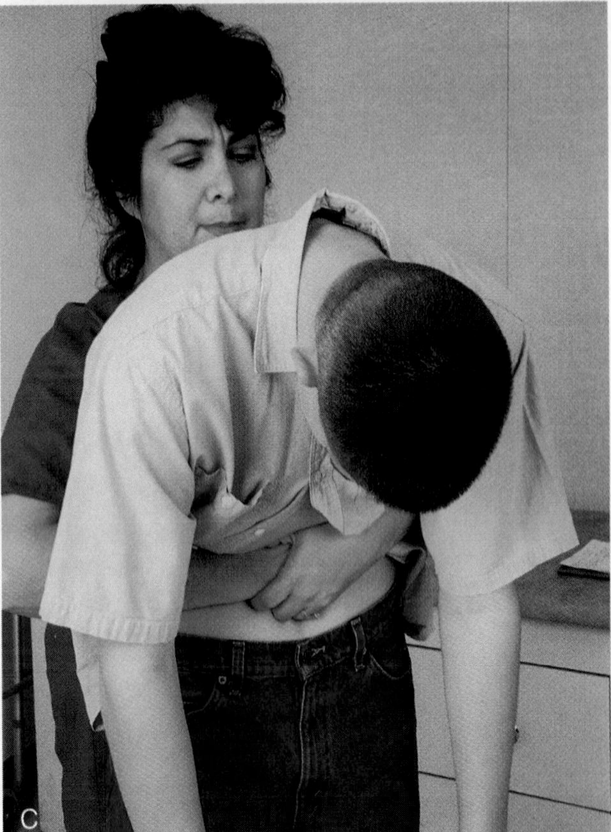

FIGURE 40–7 Heimlich maneuver. *A,* Locate subdiaphragmatic site. *B,* Place heel of one hand against the site. *C,* Place second hand over first hand and give abdominal thrusts.

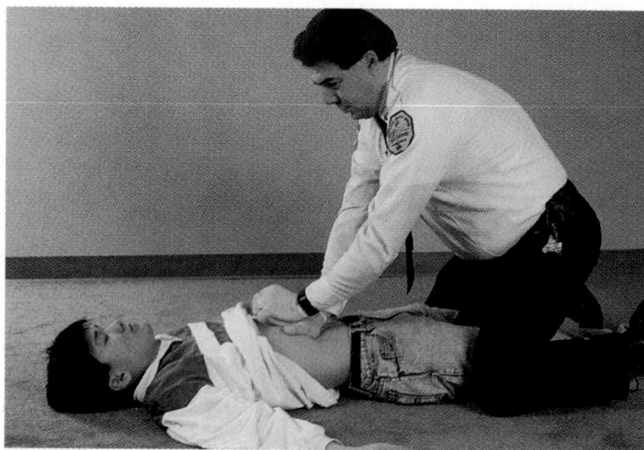

FIGURE 40–8 Performance of Heimlich maneuver in unconscious victim. (From Henry MC, Stapleton ER: EMT Prehospital Care, 2nd ed. Philadelphia, WB Saunders, 1997.)

tight clothing. Record **apical pulse** and radial pulse. Remember, you must use a stethoscope when obtaining an apical pulse. Administer oxygen if the physician has previously given these instructions. *Absolutely no smoking should be allowed by the patient*

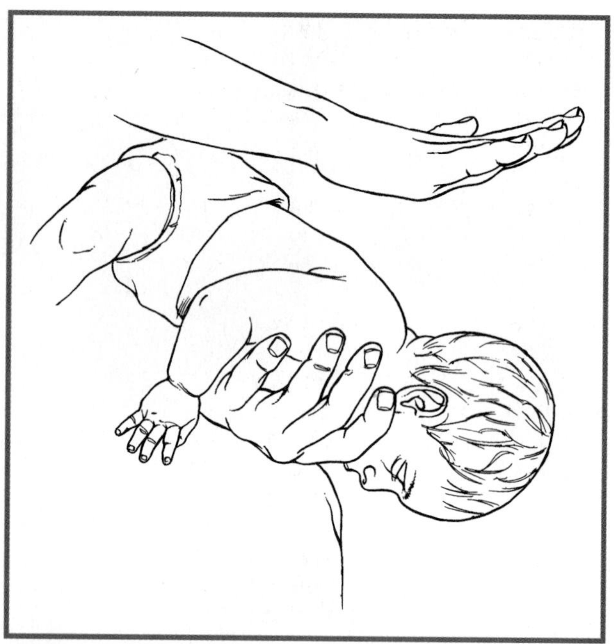

FIGURE 40–10 Back blows administered to infant supported on your arm and thigh. (From Henry MC, Stapleton ER: EMT Prehospital Care, 2nd ed. Philadelphia, WB Saunders, 1997.)

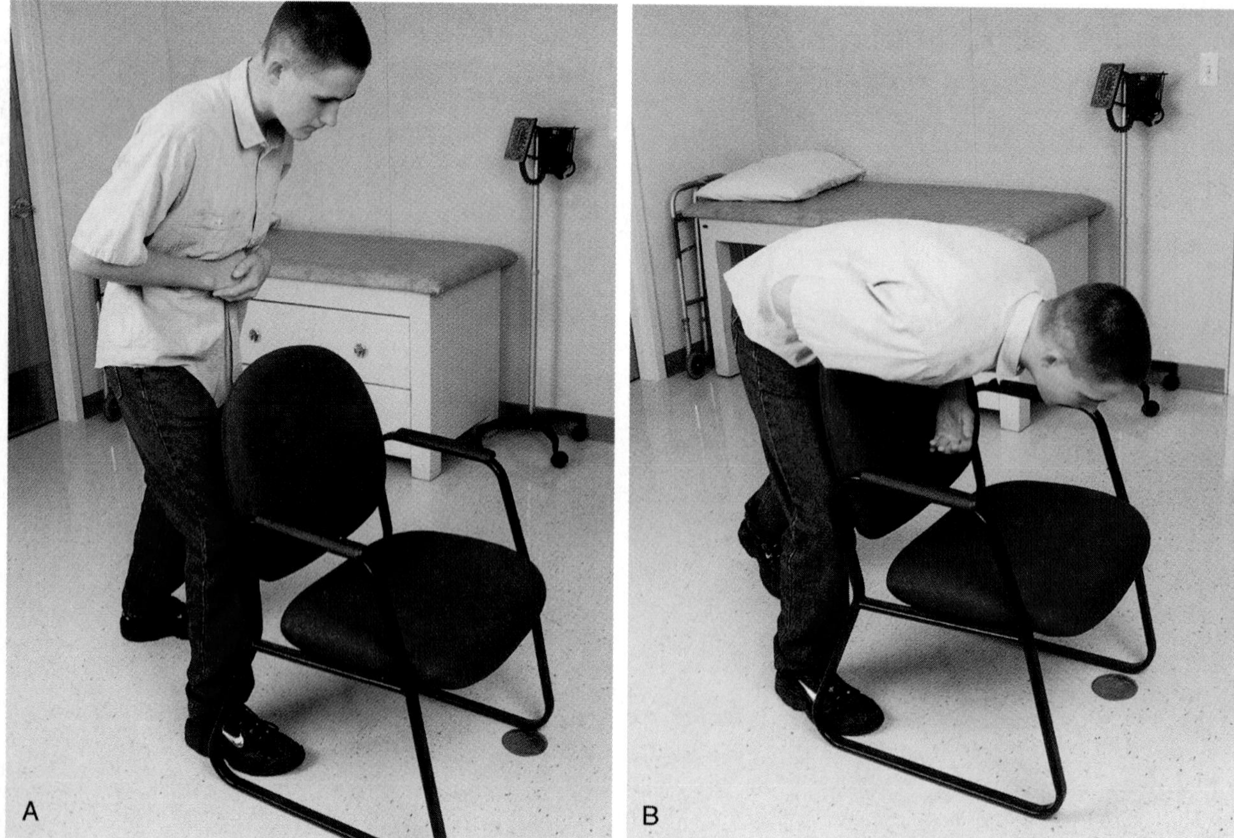

FIGURE 40–9 Self-induced Heimlich. *A,* Press fist into upper abdomen. *B,* Lean forward and press abdomen quickly against a firm object.

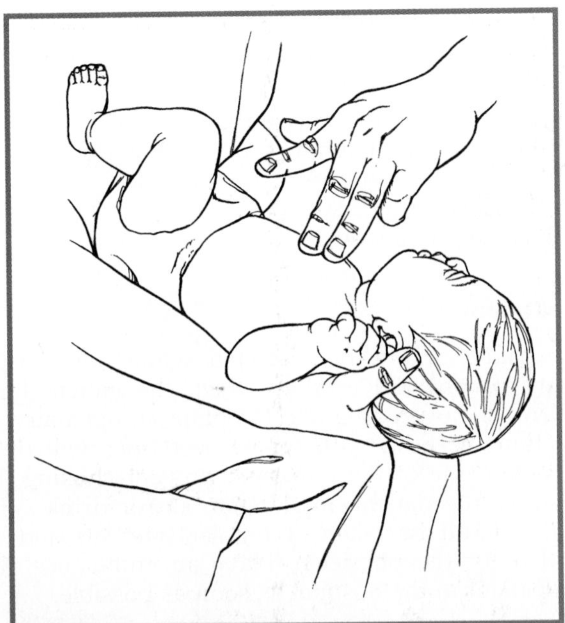

FIGURE 40–11 Chest thrusts administered in same position as cardiac compressions. (From Henry MC, Stapleton ER: EMT Prehospital Care, 2nd ed. Philadelphia, WB Saunders, 1997.)

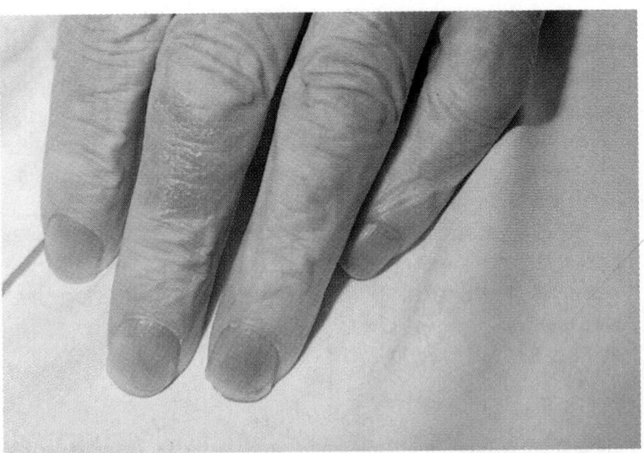

FIGURE 40–13 Cyanosis of nail beds. (From Henry MC, Stapleton ER: EMT Prehospital Care, 2nd ed. Philadelphia, WB Saunders, 1997.)

or by anyone within the vicinity. Bring the emergency cart into the room and open the medication drawer so that the physician is able to quickly prepare the medication(s) needed. This may be epinephrine (Adrenalin), atropine, digitalis, calcium chloride 10%, or morphine. If the patient is conscious, ask him or her about any medication that he or she may be carrying. If this is patient with an established heart disorder, the patient may be carrying nitroglycerin tablets. Nitroglycerin tablets are administered **sublingually,** and you may give them to the patient with the patient's consent (Fig. 40–14). Do not give the patient alcohol, food, or water by mouth without the physician's permission. Do not give spirits of ammonia.

If the physician is in the office or is on the way, connect the patient to the electrocardiograph and

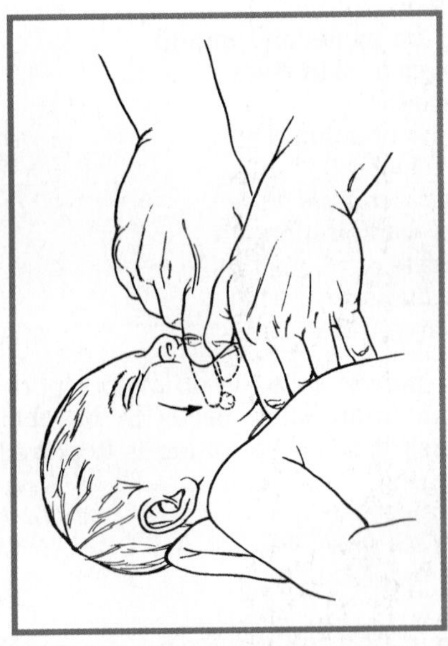

FIGURE 40–12 Finger sweep in infant should be done while maintaining jaw lift. (From Henry MC, Stapleton ER: EMT Prehospital Care, 2nd ed. Philadelphia, WB Saunders, 1997.)

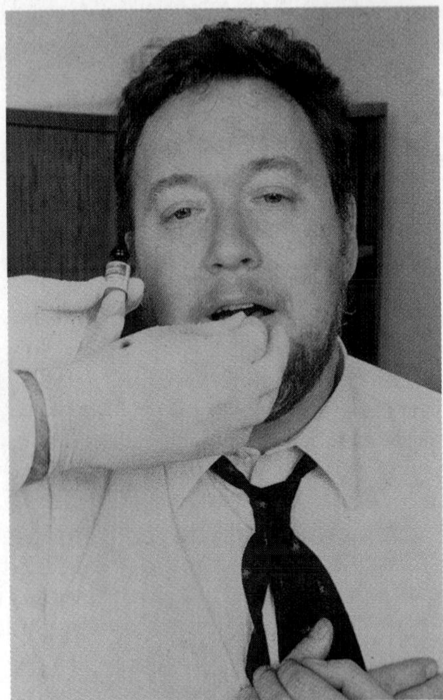

FIGURE 40–14 Nitroglycerin is administered beneath patient's tongue. (From Henry MC, Stapleton ER: EMT Prehospital Care, 2nd ed. Philadelphia, WB Saunders, 1997.)

record a few tracings. Lead II is usually considered to be the monitoring lead. If the physician cannot be reached, call the emergency rescue team. It may be necessary to start mouth-to-mouth resuscitation if the patient is unconscious and there is no evidence of breathing. If chest pain progresses to cardiac arrest, CPR must be performed.

The office staff must remain calm and offer emotional support and reassurance, because all patients with heart disorders are extremely frightened and anxious.

Signs of Heart Attack

A heart attack is caused by a blockage of the coronary arteries so that the blood supply to the heart muscles is stopped. The most common signal of heart attack is an uncomfortable pressure, squeezing, fullness, or pain in the center of the chest, in the mediastinal area. This may spread to the shoulder, neck, jaw, or arms. The pain may not be severe. Other symptoms include

- Sweating
- Nausea
- Indigestion
- Shortness of breath
- Cold and clammy skin
- A feeling of weakness
- Extreme apprehension

Memory Jogger

10 *How are nitroglycerin tablets administered?*

CEREBROVASCULAR ACCIDENT (STROKE)

As learned in Chapter 35, cerebrovascular accident (CVA) is a disorder of the blood vessels serving the brain that results in an impairment of the blood supply to a part of the brain. The term *stroke* is often applied to this problem. This interruption in the normal circulation of blood through the brain leads to a sudden loss of consciousness and some degree of paralysis, which may be temporary or permanent depending on the severity of the oxygen deprivation of the brain cells.

Usually, minor strokes do not produce unconsciousness and the symptoms depend on the location of the hemorrhage and the amount of brain damage. Symptoms of a minor stroke include

- Headache
- Confusion
- Slight dizziness
- Ringing in the ears

This may be followed by minor difficulties in speech, memory changes, weakness of the extremities, and some disturbance of personality. Symptoms of a major stroke include

- Unconsciousness
- Paralysis on one side of the body
- Difficulty in breathing and swallowing
- Loss of bladder and bowel control
- Unequal pupil size
- Slurring of speech

Treatment

The patient should be protected against any further injury or physical exertion. Keep the patient lying down and covered lightly. Maintain an open airway. Position the head so that any secretions will drain from the side of the mouth to prevent choking. Do not give the patient anything to eat or drink. Vital signs should be taken at regular intervals and recorded for the physician. Have an ambulance take the patient to the hospital as soon as possible.

POISONINGS

All poisonings are considered medical emergencies. Poisoning can occur by mouth, absorption, inhalation, and injection. Over-the-counter medications such as acetaminophen, iron tablets, aspirin, or ibuprofen cause the majority of poisoning cases seen in young children. Other typical household poisons include medicines, detergents, cleaners, disinfectants, bleaches, insecticides, ammonia, glues, cosmetics, and poisonous plants (Fig. 40–15). Signs and symptoms of poisoning vary greatly and include

- Open bottles of medicines or chemicals
- Stains on clothing
- Burns on hands and mouth
- Changes in skin color
- Nausea
- Shallow breathing
- Convulsions
- Stomach cramps
- Heavy perspiration
- Dizziness
- Drowsiness
- Unconsciousness

When a person calls the office to report a poisoning, certain information needs to be obtained (see What to Ask When a Poisoning Is Reported).

WHAT TO ASK WHEN A POISONING IS REPORTED

1 The location and the phone number
2 The name of the poison taken
3 How much was taken
4 How long ago the poison was taken

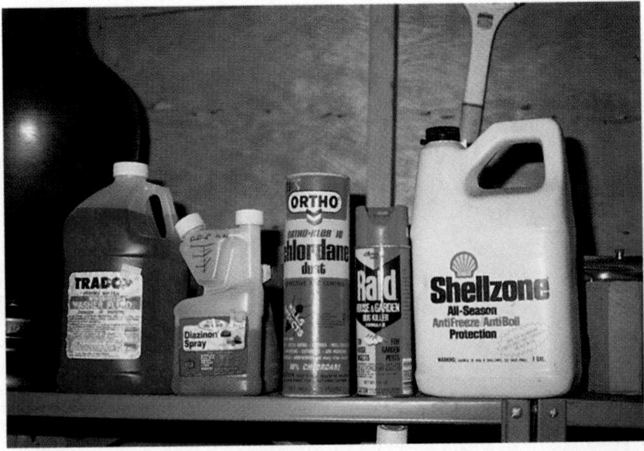

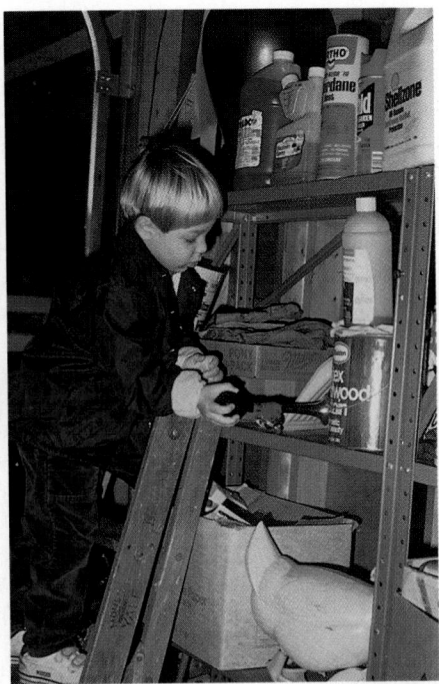

FIGURE 40–15 Hazardous household materials. (From Henry MC, Stapleton ER: EMT Prehospital Care, 2nd ed. Philadelphia, WB Saunders, 1997.)

5 Whether vomiting has occurred
6 The name, weight, and age of the victim
7 Any first aid being given

Instruct the caller *not* to hang up and *not* to leave the victim unattended. Call the local poison control center. Quickly forward all directions to the caller. Tell the caller to bring the container of poison or of vomitus to the office or hospital.

Treatment

Speed is essential in administering first aid in poisonings. In all cases, it is most important to dilute the poison, to induce vomiting (except when the person has swallowed a corrosive poison), and to seek medical attention. Generally, it is safe to try to dilute the poison with 1 or 2 cups of water or milk. It is important to dilute the poison before vomiting is induced. Do not induce vomiting if the victim is unconscious or having a **convulsion.** Do not attempt to induce vomiting when the victim has swallowed a strong corrosive or petroleum product. Give 1 tablespoon of syrup of ipecac with two cups of water to induce dilution of the poison and vomiting. If vomiting does not occur after 20 minutes, repeat the procedure. It may be necessary to make the victim gag to start vomiting. The gag reflex is started by touching the back of the tongue lightly. Encourage the victim to drink fluids until the emesis is reasonably clear. When vomiting has stopped, administer 30 to 50 g of activated charcoal, which absorbs any residual toxic substance and inhibits the absorption of poisons.

Memory Jogger

How can poisoning occur?

ANIMAL BITES

Any animal bite (including human) that breaks the skin should be seen by a physician and reported to the authorities. The animal must be identified and confined for quarantine. The animal should not be killed because a positive rabies identification is almost impossible to make if the animal has been dead for a period of time. Many pet owners will not admit that their pet has bitten a person because they fear that the animal will be killed. Assure them that the health department authorities only want to confine the animal for observation.

Treatment

The bite should be washed thoroughly with soap and water and should be treated as an infected wound would be treated. The victim should be seen by a physician.

INSECT BITES AND STINGS

This type of injury occurs when the insect either bites or stings the victim. **Venom** is injected into the tissue of the victim, which results in a internal body response to a foreign protein. Some of the more common types of bites and stings are those of mosquitoes, bees, wasps, hornets, spiders, fire ants, ticks, and fleas. Bites also can be caused by black widow spiders, brown recluse spiders, and scorpions.

Treatment

Remove the stinger, if there is one, by gently brushing it off or by using forceps or tweezers. Be careful not to squeeze the stinger. This injects more venom into the skin. Place the forceps as close to the skin as possible, not over the stinger sac, and gently remove the stinger. Apply ice in a towel or a plastic bag around the area, to relieve the pain and slow the absorption of the venom. Calamine lotion or a paste of baking soda may be applied to relieve itching. Keep the patient's activities to a minimum to slow down circulation and, thus, the spread of the venom.

If the patient has a history of allergies, especially to insect venom, he or she should be transported to the nearest hospital for immediate care. This patient may experience dyspnea and a decrease in blood pressure. A wet, itchy, swollen rash may occur. The victim may complain of shortness of breath or difficulty in breathing. Sometimes, there is edema of the lips and the face. Difficulty in talking is a sign of edema in the throat. In this situation, there is the possibility of complete airway obstruction. These are signs of a true emergency. Epinephrine and oxygen should be ready for immediate administration on the physician's orders. Antihistamines may be used, as well as cortisone, but the action of these agents is considerably slower than that of epinephrine. If the patient experiences acute anaphylactic shock, death may occur within 1 hour without the intervention of a physician.

SHOCK

Shock is a condition that produces a depressed state of many vital body functions. It is a physiologic reaction resulting from a **traumatic** condition to the body. Shock is often caused by an injury, accident, hemorrhage, illness, surgical operation, or overdose of drugs or by burns, pain, fear, or emotional stress. Shock may be immediate or delayed, mild or severe, and even fatal.

SIGNS OF SHOCK

- Paleness
- Clamminess
- Dilated pupils
- Weak and rapid pulse
- Low blood pressure
- Thirst
- Lethargy
- Feeling of faintness
- Labored breathing

Treatment

Ensure an open airway, and check for breathing and circulation. Place the patient on his or her back, with the legs elevated. Loosen all tight clothing. Cover the patient with a blanket for warmth. Do not move the patient unnecessarily. Fluids may be given by mouth if not contraindicated or if medical care will be delayed for more than 60 minutes. Because there are so many different causes of shock, it is advisable to administer only basic first-aid care and to have the patient transported to the hospital.

Memory Jogger

12 *What are the nine signs of shock?*

ASTHMATIC ATTACK

Asthma is a condition characterized by wheezing, coughing, choking, and shortness of breath resulting from spasmodic constriction of the bronchi in the lungs. Attacks vary greatly. Severe attacks rarely last for more than a few hours, but milder symptoms may persist much longer.

Some asthmatic patients carry respiratory inhalators with them. You may assist them with using their inhalators. A bronchodilator such as epinephrine or aminophylline may be ordered by the physician. Other medications are used to thin the mucus in the air passages so that the patient can clear the lungs more easily.

An asthmatic patient should be warned of the hazards of overstimulation of the body, such as exercise and emotional upsets causing laughing or crying. Explain the importance of relaxation to the patient with asthma.

SEIZURES

Seizures may be idiopathic or as a result of trauma, injury, or metabolic alterations such as hypoglycemia or hypocalcemia. A febrile seizure is transient and occurs with a rapid rise in fever over 101.8° F (38.8° C). Febrile seizures occur in children between 6 months and 5 years of age.

Seizures are frightening to witness, but usually the patient is not suffering, nor is there great danger. Establishing a tranquil environment is an essential component of caring for patients experiencing seizures.

Treatment

Loosen clothing but do not attempt to restrain the patient's movements, except to prevent injury. Remove anything that might be in the way that could cause harm. Always protect the head. Give neither fluids nor medication by mouth. If the patient remains unconscious after the jerking has subsided, position the patient in a semi-prone position to maintain an open airway and to allow drainage of excess saliva. Do not attempt to place anything between the teeth during the convulsion because forcing an object through a tightly clenched mouth may damage the teeth. After the seizure is over, let the patient rest or sleep in a quiet room. Follow the physician's directives and assist in every way that you can. If the physician is not in the office, check the protocol section in the office procedure manual. A general rule is to call 911 for emergency assistance if

- The patient has not regained consciousness within 10 to 15 minutes
- The seizure does not stop within a few minutes
- The patient begins a second seizure immediately after the primary one
- The patient is pregnant
- There are signs of head trauma
- The patient is a known diabetic
- This seizure is expected to be a febrile seizure

ABDOMINAL PAIN

Abdominal pain is any pain or discomfort in the abdomen.

CAUSES OF ABDOMINAL PAIN

- Stress
- Hemorrhage
- Ulcers
- Excessive eating, drinking, or smoking
- Inflammation
- Obstruction
- Tumors

All abdominal pain should be investigated. Severe and persistent abdominal pain, especially when accompanied by fever, should receive medical attention as soon as possible.

Treatment

Treatment varies with the cause of the pain. Keep the patient warm and quiet. Have an emesis basin available. Administer nothing by mouth. Do not apply heat to the abdomen unless so instructed by the physician. Check and record the patient's vital signs.

OBSTETRIC EMERGENCIES

The types of problems found in an obstetrics office are unique to this specialty. Every medical assistant employed in an office where the physician delivers babies should be trained to handle emergencies. The majority of these problems will be presented to you over the telephone. If a physician is in the office, those calls should be transferred to him or her immediately.

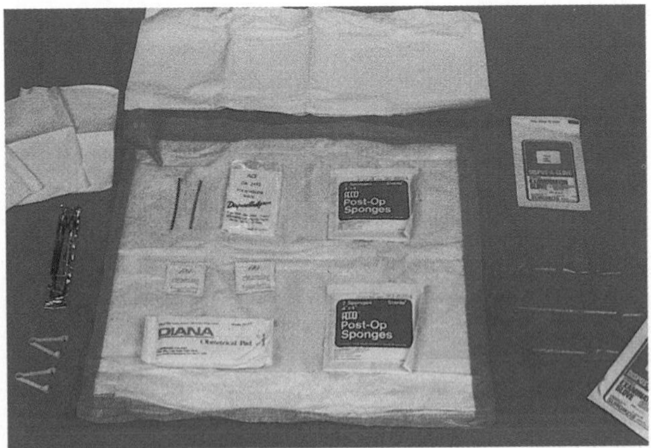

FIGURE 40–16 Emergency obstetrics kit. (From Henry MC, Stapleton ER: EMT Prehospital Care, 2nd ed. Philadelphia, WB Saunders, 1997.)

If a pregnant patient calls to report vaginal bleeding, you must ask some specific questions. Is the bleeding like a menstrual flow or is it a gushing type of hemorrhage? Is it painful or without any pain? If the bleeding is gushing, the patient must be told to lie down immediately while you send for an ambulance. In such a situation, the mother and baby could bleed to death in a matter of a few minutes as the result of pregnancy complications such as a ruptured uterus. If the bleeding is like a normal menstrual flow, have the patient go to bed, with the foot of the bed elevated. Tell her that you will report this to the physician immediately. If the tissue passed is liver-like, it may be a blood clot; white tissue may be fetus. No matter what the appearance of the tissue, have the patient take it with her to the hospital.

If the patient comes to the office and the physician informs you that she is delivering her baby right now, the physician will need an emergency obstetrics kit (Fig. 40–16). Get the kit and prepare to assist immediately. Unwrap the OB kit, being sure to keep sterile items sterile. This kit contains all of the supplies needed for the delivery. If there is time, place the apron and the goggles on the physician for protection against communicable diseases. Assist the physician and offer encouragement and moral support to the mother. Watch the time and record the moment the child takes the first breath as the time of birth.

SPRAINS

In Chapter 37 you learned that a sprain is an acute partial tear of a muscle, a tendon, or a ligament. Sprains may also cause damage to blood vessels and surrounding nerve tissue. The victim may develop edema, ecchymosis, and sharp, radiating pain. It may be difficult to move or bear weight on the injured joint. When sprains are caused by chronic overuse, they typically cause stiffness, tenderness, and soreness.

Treatment

Treatment of sprains entails elevation, mild compression, and immediate application of ice. There is considerable advantage if the ice is applied within 20 to 30 minutes after the injury has occurred. The ice should remain on the part for 24 hours, with the injured area elevated. Reread the application of cold in Chapter 37. After 24 to 36 hours, application of mild heat is usually indicated. The patient may be advised to immobilize the part.

FRACTURES

A fracture is a break or crack in a bone and can result from trauma or disease. Fractures are always very painful, and the patient will have great difficulty in moving the injured part of the body.

Treatment

When a patient with a fracture is brought into the office, the medical assistant should make the patient as comfortable as possible. Place the patient in a position that does not place strain on the area. First aid includes preventing movement of the injured part, elevation of the affected extremity, application of ice, and control of any bleeding. Notify the physician immediately and proceed according to the orders given to you.

BURNS

Burns are among the most frequent cause of injuries in the United States. Burn injuries can result from flame, heat, scalds, electricity, chemicals, or radiation. The extent of the surface area burned, plus the depth and nature of the burn, is directly proportional to the extent of the pain. The skin surface may be reddened, blistered, or charred.

The depth and extent of burns are the major determinants in classifying the severity of a burn. Only second- and third-degree burns are counted when assessing the extent of the burn because first-degree burns do not result in loss of skin function.

Treatment

First aid for burns includes relief of the pain, prevention of infection, and treatment of shock. Burns are extremely painful and dangerous. Bring the emergency cart into the area and open the medication drawer. Next lay out sterile dressings and bandages and a pair of sterile gloves for the physician. Remove loose clothing from the burned area but do not attempt to pick pieces of charred fabric out of the wound site. Stay with the patient and assist the physician in a quiet and efficient manner.

Memory Jogger

Burn pain is directly proportional to ______.

LACERATIONS

Lacerations are a common presentation in the primary care physician's office. A lacerated wound displays a jagged or irregular tearing of the tissues. The severity depends on the mechanism of injury, the site of the injury, the extent of the injury, and the introduction of foreign bodies or contamination into the wound. It is important to consider damage to blood vessels, nerves, bones, joints, and organs within the body cavities.

Treatment

Notify the physician immediately. Have the patient lie down. Keep the patient quiet. Cover the injured area with a sterile dressing; use a dressing that is thick enough to absorb the bleeding. If bleeding persists or is profuse, apply direct pressure to the dressing and also to the area just above the wound. The injured part of the body should be elevated above the level of the victim's heart. Be sure to make an effort to reassure the victim and explain your actions as much as possible. Ask the patient when he or she received the last tetanus shot and record the date in the patient's record. If it has been more than 10 years, the physician will probably want a booster shot given.

Wounds that are not bleeding severely and that do not involve deep tissues should be cleansed. Wash in and around the wound with soap and water to remove bacteria and other foreign matter. If the laceration is extremely dirty, wait for the physician to arrive and tell you how to proceed with the cleansing of the wound. The physician may want to irrigate with sterile normal saline solution and/or rinse the wound thoroughly with clean water and blot dry.

The basic dressing includes a sterile gauze or other absorbent material that is applied directly to the wound. The dressing selected may vary in size and thickness according to the wound. A butterfly closure strip may be used over small lacerations, to hold the edges together. If the wound is superficial and has straight edges, it may be closed with a microporous tape, which eliminates the discomfort of suturing and suture removal as well as some of the potential risks of infected sutures. Figure 40–17

LACERATIONS

What you need to know . . .

It is important to prevent infection and to allow your cut to heal. Call your doctor or return to him or her immediately if any of the "danger signs" occur.

Return for recheck in ______ days
Return for suture removal in ______ days

Danger signs to watch for . . .

1. Increasing pain, swelling, redness, and warmth in the injured area.
2. Pus in or around the cut.
3. Fever greater than 100°F (38°C).
4. Blood soaking through the dressing.

If any of these signs occur, contact your doctor or return to the Emergency Department.

What to do at home . . .

1. Take all medicines exactly as directed.
2. Raise the injured area above your heart level for 1 to 2 days.
3. Keep the wound and bandage clean and dry. For cuts on the face, a bandage is often not necessary. All finger dressings must be changed within 24 hours.
4. Remove the bandage/dressing in 24 hours.
5. After 24 hours, you may shower or bathe. Begin cleaning the wound with clear water twice each day to remove crusting and scabbing. Then apply ointment (Polysporin).
6. Prevent sunburn. Use a sunscreen for 6 months (e.g., Pre-Sun or Eclipse).
7. If you have a private doctor or are a member of an HMO (e.g., Kaiser), you should call for an appointment for your recheck and suture removal. If you can't get an appointment, you are welcome to return here to complete your care.

Please remember . . .

1. The exam and treatment you have just received are not intended to provide complete medical care. You need to call your doctor to schedule a follow-up visit.
2. The X-rays or E.C.G. taken today will be reviewed by a specialist. If there is any change in your diagnosis, we will contact you.

FIGURE 40–17 Laceration educational material for home care of wound.

shows an excellent method of informing patients as to the nature of their injury and of both the office and the home treatment required. If you work in a multicultural community, forms should be printed in different languages for non-English–speaking patients.

Memory Jogger

14 *Describe a lacerated wound.*

NOSEBLEEDS (EPISTAXIS)

Nosebleed, or **epistaxis,** is a hemorrhage usually resulting from the rupture of small vessels within the nose. Nosebleeds can result from injury, disease, strenuous activity, high altitudes, exposure to cold, and overuse of blood-thinning medications such as aspirin.

Treatment

Keep the patient quiet and in a sitting position. Apply direct pressure to the affected nostril by pinching the nose. Continue the pressure for 5 minutes to allow clotting to take place. Repeat if bleeding cannot be controlled, insert a clean pad of gauze into the nostril and notify the physician. If the physician is not available, proceed with standard EMS protocols.

HEMORRHAGES

Bleeding may be external or internal. Those administering first aid can do little about internal bleeding, except to keep the patient quiet and warm to minimize shock and get medical help immediately. External bleeding is not as complex as internal bleeding in that you can frequently see the source of the bleeding. Shock and loss of consciousness may occur from a rapid loss of blood in a short time.

Treatment

There are four practical ways of controlling severe bleeding. The first technique is to use direct pressure over the area by applying a sterile dressing. If blood soaks through the entire pad, do not remove the pad but add additional pads of thick cloth and continue direct pressure. The second method is elevation of the injured part. Elevation uses the forces of gravity to control blood flow. The third method is to apply pressure over the nearest pressure point between the bleeding area and the heart. This compresses the main artery supplying the affected limb. The last resort is the application of a tourniquet. The use of a tourniquet is dangerous and should be used only for a life-threatening hemorrhage. By deciding to use a tourniquet, you have made a decision that the patient will bleed to death without it. In the medical office this decision would be the physician's.

Memory Jogger

15 *What is the first technique used in controlling bleeding?*

HEAD INJURIES

The severity of a head injury can vary greatly. With a head injury, the patient may appear normal; may experience dizziness, severe headache, mental confusion, or memory loss; or may even be unconscious. The loss of consciousness may be brief or prolonged; it may appear immediately or may be delayed. The victim may experience vomiting, loss of bladder and bowel control, and bleeding from the nose, mouth, or ears. The pupils of the eyes may be of unequal diameters.

Treatment

All head injuries must be considered serious. Notify the physician or contact the EMS immediately. Have the victim lie flat. If there is difficulty in breathing, raise the head and shoulders slightly. If there is evidence of neck injury, do not attempt to move the victim, contact the physician and assist with the patient assessment.

Do not administer anything by mouth. Keep the patient warm and quiet. Watch the pupils of the eyes, and record any changes. Obtain the vital signs. Control any hemorrhage. Record the extent and duration of any unconsciousness.

FOREIGN BODIES IN THE EYE

The eye is a delicate organ whose unique structure demands special handling. This kind of emergency is most uncomfortable, and it is often extremely difficult to keep the patient from rubbing the eye. Tell the patient not to touch the eye in any way. If the doctor has given you prior permission, you may put a few drops of ophthalmic topical anesthetic in the eye. The patient will greatly appreciate this and will experience almost immediate relief. The eye may be rinsed with tepid tap water in an attempt to remove the object. Unless the foreign object is clearly visible, do not attempt to search for it or to remove it.

Treatment

The medical assistant should never attempt to remove a foreign body from the cornea. The patient should be placed in a darkened room to wait. Have plenty of tissues available. If there is a contusion and swelling, cold wet compresses will help. If you have been trained to turn an upper eyelid out, then do so gently and search for the foreign body. Be very careful not to place any pressure on the eye. If the foreign body cannot be found, then ask the patient to close the eyes. Cover both eyes with eye pads and hold them in place with a strip of tape until the physician arrives.

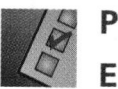

PATIENT EDUCATION

Emergencies can occur in the home, while on vacation, or in the physician's office. Patients need to be instructed in handling an emergency, both by example and through actual instruction. The medical assistant must remain calm, **triage** the situation, call for help, and be prepared to administer appropriate first-aid intervention. This attitude helps the patient learn how to report and handle an emergency. You can give patients brochures that instruct them in home safety.

Accidents are the leading cause of death among children younger than 15 years of age. Even more common are home accidents that cause injuries that do not kill but require hospitalization. More than one-half million of such accidents occur each year. The Children's Bureau of the Department of Health, Education, and Welfare has published pamphlets containing helpful tips on preventing accidents. Child-resistant bottle caps, safer toys, better-educated parents, more responsible toy manufacturers, and government regulations have helped to cut dramatically the number of childhood deaths and injuries. Most states require car safety seats for children younger than 4 years of age or who weigh less than 30 pounds. Parents should be encouraged to use car safety seats, make their homes accident proof, purchase safe toys, become familiar with basic first-aid procedures, and know the local emergency numbers. If you are employed in pediatrics or family practice specialties, you may be called on to educate families in these matters.

Remember to keep your American Red Cross and American Heart Association cards current. Take advantage of community workshops to maintain and extend your skills. Post a list of community safety workshops in an area where it can be seen by patients, and encourage them to attend. Your participation in emergency care workshops and your encouragement to have others participate may help to save lives.

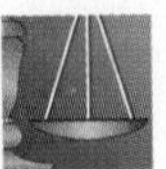

LEGAL AND ETHICAL ISSUES

Most states have enacted Good Samaritan laws to encourage health care professionals to provide medical assistance at the scene of an accident without fear of being sued for negligence. These statutes vary greatly, but all seem to have the intent of protecting the caregiver. It is helpful for the medical assistant to understand the legal responsibilities and the rights of the caregiver. A physician or other health care professional is not legally obligated to give emergency care, regardless of the ethical and moral considerations. Legal liability is limited to gross neglect of the victim or willfully causing further injury to the victim. As a caregiver, you are required to act as a reasonable person and cannot be held liable for personal injury resulting from an act of omission. The Good Samaritan statutes provide for the evaluation of the caregiver's judgment.

If you have never been trained in CPR, you cannot be expected to perform the procedure. However, in many states, a health care provider with CPR training and skills who is present at the scene can be declared negligent if cardiac arrest occurs and he or she does not administer CPR to the victim.

Remember, if the victim is conscious or if a member of his or her immediate family is present, obtain a verbal consent for the emergency care procedure before you begin. Consent is implied if the patient is unconscious and no family member is present.

Many types of emergencies can be handled in the physician's office, and in an emergency situation the patient's life is often determined by the decisions that must be made quickly. You may be called on within the next few minutes to make a decision that could affect the outcome of someone's future. Do you believe that you could make this decision calmly and accurately? If you believe that you could not handle this type of decision making, now is the time to discuss this with your instructor and obtain the necessary help to ensure your ability in handling your first and subsequent emergencies.

CRITICAL THINKING

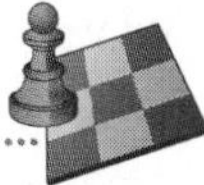

1 How would you triage an emergency situation?

2 Make an emergency phone list for your home telephone.

HOW DID I DO? Answers to Memory Joggers

1 The medical assistant is expected to make decisions based on his or her medical knowledge in an emergency situation.

2 The team management system allows one person to take immediate charge while another obtains needed materials and calls for assistance.

3 Local emergency numbers should include the EMS system, poison control center, ambulance and rescue squad, fire department, and police department.

4 Orange juice is given to diabetic patients experiencing insulin shock.

5 The defibrillator is used to reestablish the proper rhythm of the heartbeat.

6 The first and most important rule is to stay calm.

7 The two primary functions of first aid are never do anything that will worsen the situation and provide the best care you can.

8 Ventilate the lungs every 5 seconds.

9 The universal distress signal is clutching the neck between the thumb and index fingers.

10 Nitroglycerin tables are administered sublingually (under the tongue).

11 Poisoning can occur by mouth, absorption, inhalation, and injection.

12 Signs of shock include paleness, clamminess, dilated pupils, weak and rapid pulse, low blood pressure, thirst, lethargy, a feeling of faintness, and labored breathing.

13 The extent of the surface area burned, plus the depth and nature of the burn, is directly proportionate to the extent of the pain.

14 A lacerated wound displays a jagged or irregular tearing of the tissues.

15 The first technique used in controlling bleeding is direct pressure over the injured area by applying a sterile dressing.

SECTION **9**

Understanding and Performing Diagnostic Orders and Tests

CURRICULUM CONTENT/COMPETENCIES

Chapter 41 Assisting with Diagnostic Imaging and Therapeutic Modalities

- *Prepare and maintain examination and treatment areas*
- *Prepare patient for examinations, procedures, and treatments*
- *Assist with examinations, procedures, and treatments*
- *Recognize and respond to verbal and nonverbal communication*
- *Practice within the scope of education, training, and personal capabilities*
- *Document accurately*

Chapters 42 to 46 Assisting in the Clinical Laboratory

- *Apply principles of aseptic technique and infection control*
- *Collect and process specimens*
- *Perform diagnostic tests*
- *Maintain and dispose of regulated substances in compliance with government guidelines*
- *Comply with quality assurance practices*
- *Document accurately*
- *Screen and follow up patient test results*

Assisting with Diagnostic Imaging and Therapeutic Modalities

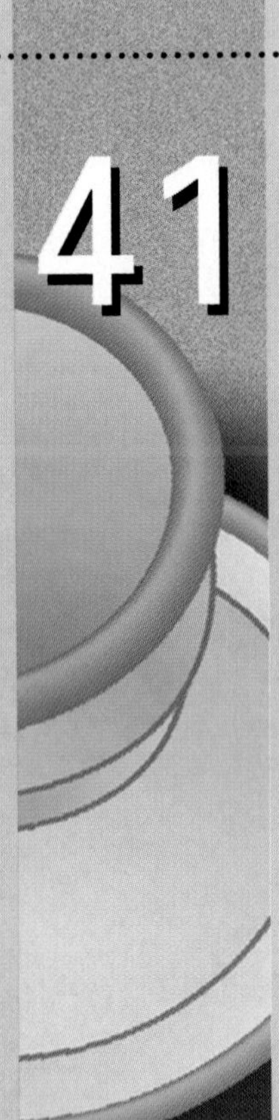

OUTLINE

LEARNING OBJECTIVES

Cognitive: On successful completion of this chapter you should be able to:

1. Explain your role in relation to diagnostic procedures.
2. Identify safety and precautionary measures pertinent to x-ray equipment.
3. State the purpose of contrast media in x-ray procedures.
4. Discuss the various special x-ray diagnostic procedures.
5. Recall the effects of heat on the body and why heat is an important treatment modality.
6. Explain the importance of physical therapy in the treatment of physical disabilities.
7. Compare and contrast passive and active exercising.
8. Recall three theories of pain control.
9. Discuss patient teaching activities for x-ray and therapeutic modalities.
10. Define and spell vocabulary terms.

Performance: On successful completion of this chapter you should be able to:

1. Accurately prepare and assist with an x-ray procedure on a patient.
2. Accurately perform a therapeutic ultrasound diathermy on a patient.
3. Explain to a patient how to use dry or wet heat therapy at home.

VOCABULARY

atrophy Wasting away; decrease in size and substance

claustrophobia Fear of being trapped in enclosed or narrow places

denervation A condition in which the nerve supply has been blocked

extravasated Pertaining to bleeding into the tissues

prostheses Artificial replacements for body parts

quackery Pretense of possessing medical skill

rad A measurement of the actual absorbed dose of radiation

radiation Transfer through space of any form of energy, such as light, heat, or x-rays

rem Method of measuring the amount of radiation absorbed by a patient exposed to x-rays; similar to rad

roentgen Unit used to measure x-ray dosage

Diagnostic Radiology

Diagnostic x-ray procedures allow radiologists to view internal body structures and function. The findings obtained by these procedures help physicians in diagnosis and treatment of diseases. X-rays are produced when electrons traveling at high speed strike certain materials, such as tungsten. X-rays can penetrate most substances and are used to investigate the health condition of certain structures, to therapeutically destroy diseased tissue, and to make photographic images for diagnostic purposes, as in radiography and fluoroscopy.

A radiograph or x-ray film is made by projecting x-rays through organs or structures of the body onto a photographic film. Because some tissue such as bone is more radiopaque than other tissue, such as fat or skin, a shadow is created on the film that is the image of a bone or of a cavity. Today, many special diagnostic x-ray procedures allow for greater observation inside the body.

A contrast medium is a radiopaque substance used in diagnostic radiology. It is sometimes used to allow for a more accurate visualization of internal body structures and tissues in contrast to adjacent structures. Contrast media may be gases (air, oxygen, carbon dioxide), heavy metals (barium sulfate, bismuth carbonate), or organic iodines. These can be administered orally, parenterally, or through an enema. Each contrast medium is specific for the examination of a particular organ, body cavity, or passage. The contrast medium makes the area opaque, allowing for both structural and functional visualization.

RADIOGRAPHIC PROCEDURES USING A CONTRAST MEDIUM AND THE AREAS THAT ARE VISUALIZED

Angiocardiography—heart and large vessels
Angiography—blood vessels
Arteriography—arteries (Fig. 41–1)
Arthrography—joints
Barium enema—lower intestinal tract
Barium swallow—upper gastrointestinal tract (Fig. 41–2)
Bronchography—bronchial tree and lungs
Cholecystography—gallbladder
Hysterosalpingography—uterus and fallopian tubes
Intravenous cholangiography—bile ducts
Intravenous pyelography—renal pelvis, ureters, and bladder
Lymphangiography—lymphatic vessels
Myelography—spinal cord

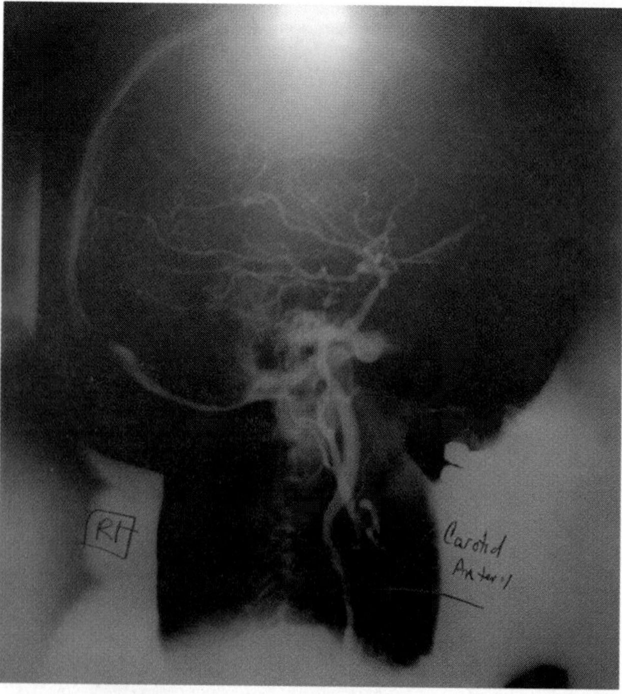

FIGURE 41–1 Arteriography of carotid artery.

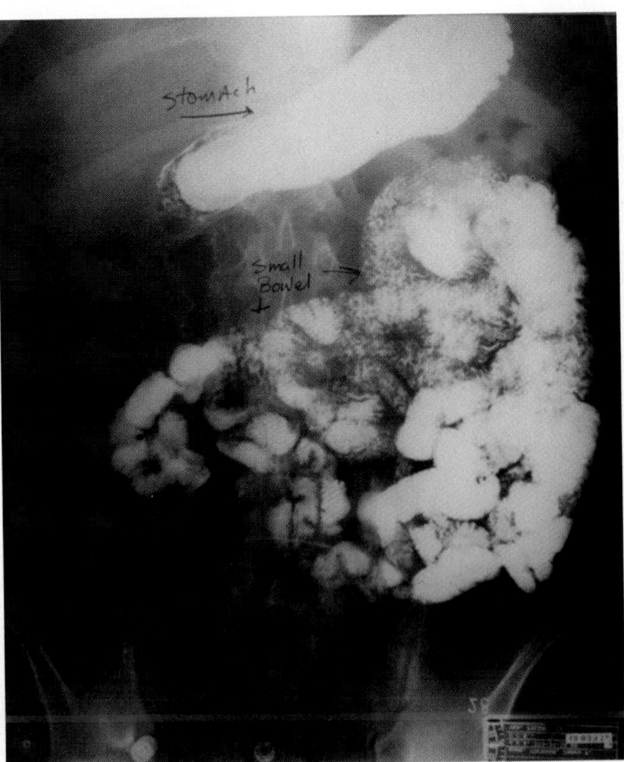

FIGURE 41–2 Barium swallow.

Memory Jogger

 *What is the radiopaque substance used in diagnostic radiology called?*

NUCLEAR MEDICINE

Nuclear medicine is the branch of radiology that uses radioactive compounds, sometimes called "radionuclides" or "isotopes," to trace and evaluate the cause of a health problem. A physician with special training in nuclear medicine will be the specialist who interprets the results of nuclear examinations. Assisting nuclear medicine physicians are trained medical assistants who will position the patient for examination and assist in operating the equipment.

In conventional x-ray imaging, radiation passes through the body from an outside source. Nuclear medicine involves detecting radiation from a radioactive chemical placed within the body or mixed with a sample of blood or urine for laboratory analysis.

In a typical procedure, tiny amounts of radioactive substances are introduced into the patient's body, usually by intravenous injection. The patient is positioned under a large camera. The camera may touch the patient but will not cause discomfort. As the radioactive compounds circulate throughout the body, the camera detects the radiation and translates it into spots of light that expose film. A gamma camera is used to detect the radiation given off by the drug and to convert it into an image that can be photographed or displayed on a television screen. The film, called a scan or scintigram, is then interpreted by the nuclear medicine physician. Nuclear scans provide images that give information about the function and structure of organs and systems.

Memory Jogger

 *How are isotopes used?*

Scans can visualize some organs that cannot be seen on conventional x-ray films.

FREQUENTLY ORDERED SCANS

Bone scan—helps to detect fractures, tumors, and inflammation; used to determine bone growth
Brain scan—often used together with an image of the brain produced by tomography to detect tumors and vascular problems
Liver scan—useful in diagnosing cirrhosis and hepatitis and in detecting tumors and liver abscesses
Lung scan—often done to detect blood clots that have traveled through the bloodstream to the lungs
Thyroid scan—uses radioactive iodine because iodine accumulates in the thyroid; the rate of uptake is an indicator of thyroid function

COMPUTED TOMOGRAPHY

Computed tomography (CT scan) is a radiographic technique that produces a film that represents a detailed cross section of tissue structure. The procedure is painless and requires no special preparation. It is 100 times more sensitive than conventional radiography. Computed tomography uses a narrow beam of x-rays that rotates in a continuous 360-degree motion around the patient to image the body in cross-sectional slices. Detectors positioned at several angles record the x-rays that pass through the body. The rates at which the x-rays are absorbed are detected, and a computer calculates the densities into a picture of the body site on a visual screen. The pictures obtained are very detailed and simulate a three-dimensional appearance (Fig. 41–3).

Memory Jogger

 *Is the CT scan more sensitive than conventional radiography?*

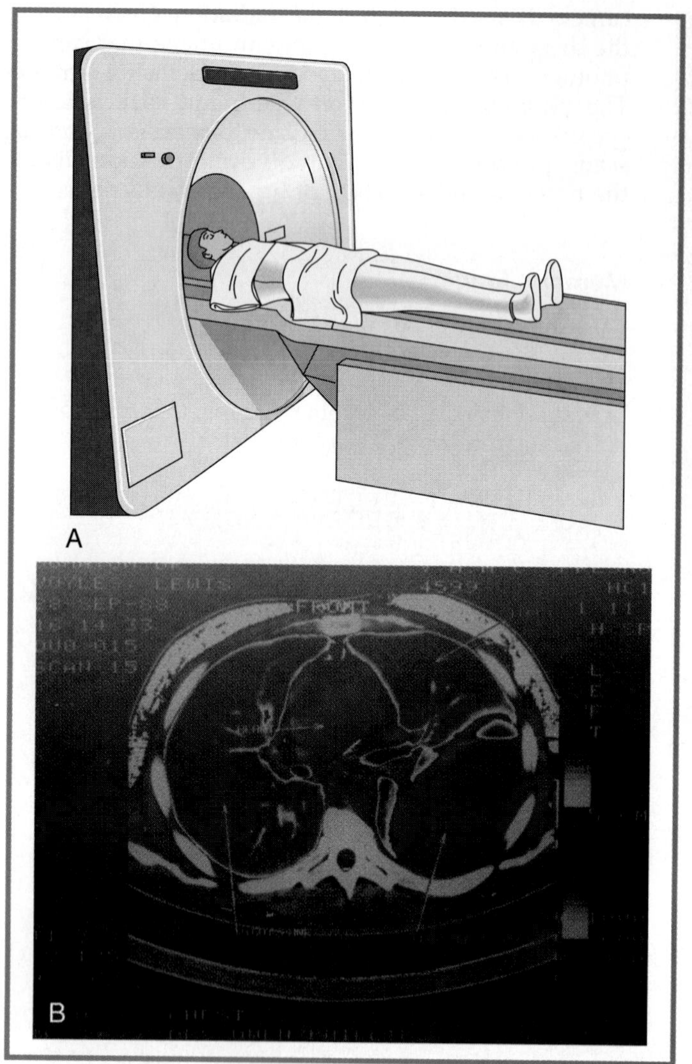

FIGURE 41–3 *A*, Computed tomography (CT) total body scanner. *B*, CT scan.

MAGNETIC RESONANCE IMAGING

Magnetic resonance imaging (MRI) uses a combination of radiowaves and a strong magnetic field to produce images of the soft tissues. It is the method of choice for a growing number of disease processes because of its ability to film soft tissue in multiple planes. MRI is regarded as superior to the CT scan for nervous system and musculoskeletal diseases and is extremely useful in diagnosing cancer and other tumors and masses of the soft tissues. A mild sedative is frequently given before the procedure because many patients experience **claustrophobia** during MRI. The MRI procedure is contraindicated in patients with pacemakers, metallic aneurysm clips, and some metallic **prostheses** (Fig. 41–4).

Memory Jogger

 *Is the CT scan or the MRI believed to be superior in brain imaging?*

FLUOROSCOPY

Fluoroscopy, also called radioscopy, is an x-ray examination that permits both structural and functional visualization of internal body structures. Through the use of a contrast medium, motion of a body part can be viewed. Thus, a physician can observe the action of the esophagus and stomach after a patient swallows a barium mixture. The patient is placed between the x-ray tube and the screen. X-rays pass through the body and project the structures as shadowy images on the screen. The image on the fluoroscope can be recorded on film to produce a permanent record called a photofluorogram.

MAMMOGRAPHY

With the advent of new films and exposure techniques, it is now possible to make an x-ray visualization of breast tissue to detect tumors and to determine the presence of a malignancy. Lesions too tiny to produce symptoms can also be detected. Mammography is performed without the use of a contrast medium. It is discussed in Chapter 33.

STEREOSCOPY

This technique, also called stereoscopic radiography or stereoradiography, uses a special instrument to view films that have been taken at different angles.

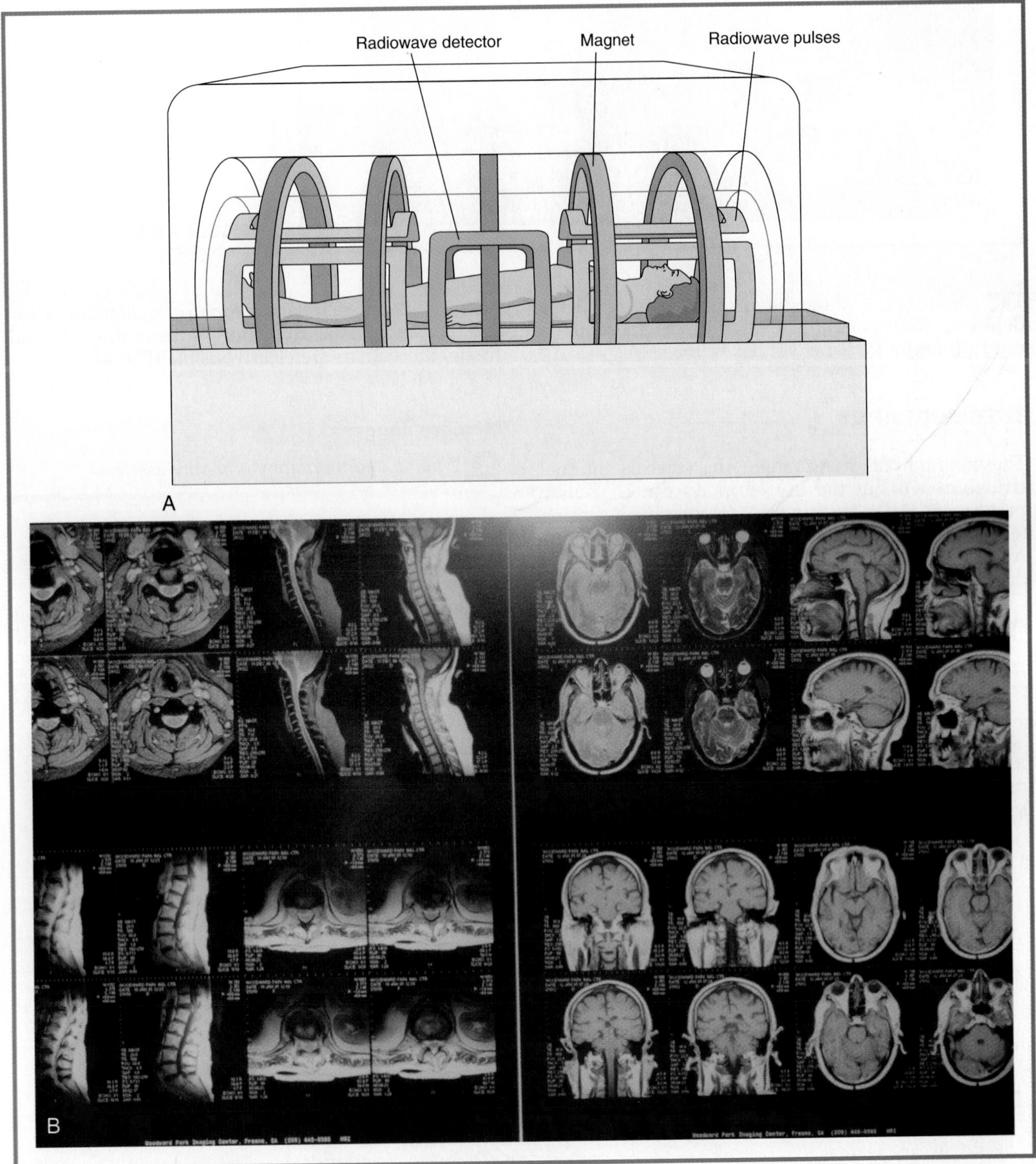

FIGURE 41–4 *A,* Magnetic resonance imaging (MRI) unit. *B,* Magnetic resonance images.

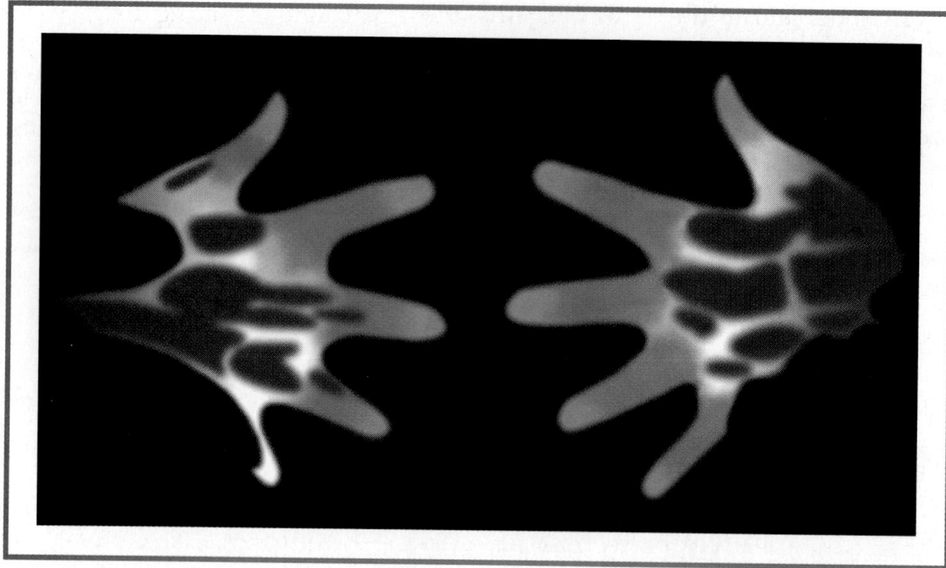

FIGURE 41–5 Normal hand thermogram.

This produces a three-dimensional image having depth as well as height and width. Stereoscopy is used primarily for x-ray studies of the skull.

THERMOGRAPHY

Thermography is a technique that reveals internal structures without the use of x-rays but is usually performed by radiographers. It is a heat-sensing technique used primarily in the detection of tumors. An infrared camera is used to take a photograph that records the variations in skin temperatures. Cool areas appear dark, warm areas are light, and intermediate temperatures show as various shades of gray. Because inflammatory or malignant areas produce more heat than does surrounding normal tissue, these areas are clearly visible (Fig. 41–5).

Memory Jogger

 *When is thermography primarily used?*

ULTRASONOGRAPHY

Ultrasonography is not a radiologic procedure, but it permits visualization of internal structures by the

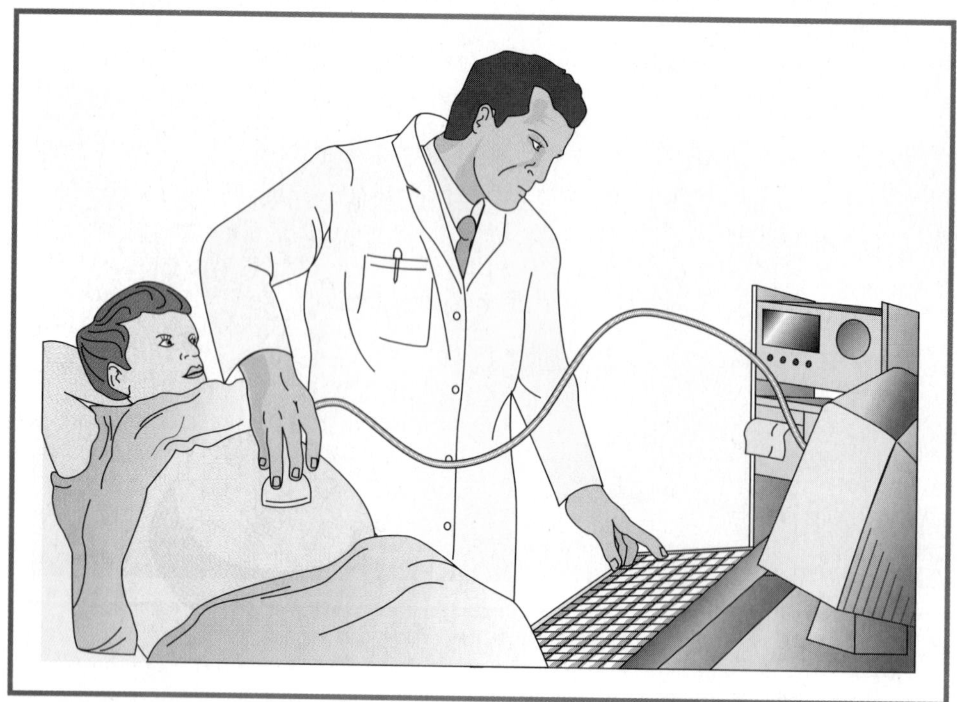

FIGURE 41–6 Obstetric ultrasonography.

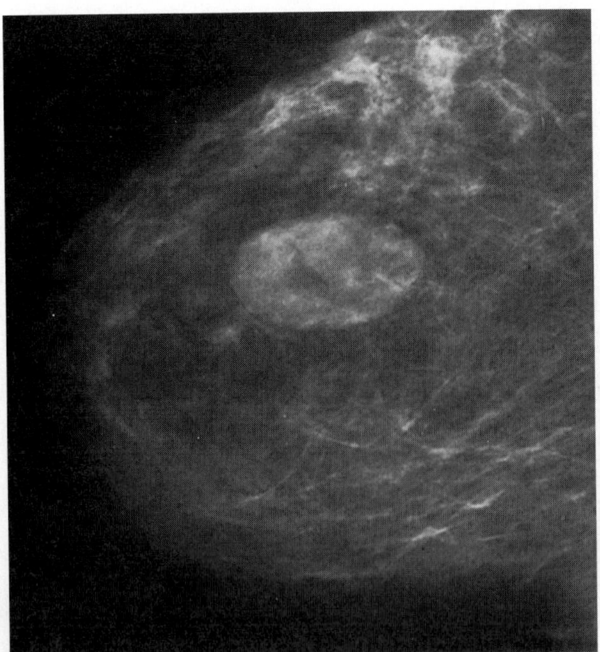

FIGURE 41–7 Xeroradiography showing fibroadenoma of breast. (From Bland KI, Copeland EM: The Breast: Comprehensive Management of Benign and Malignant Diseases, 2nd ed, vol 1. Philadelphia, WB Saunders, 1998.)

use of high-frequency sound waves that echo off the body. An instrument called a transducer, similar to a microphone, is passed over the body part to be examined. It picks up the echoes, which are then displayed on an oscilloscope. The echoes are produced by the sound waves passing through the skin, striking the body part, and bouncing back to the transducer. Because sound waves do not expose the patient to radiation, ultrasound examination is ideal for observing the developing fetus and detecting the presence of multiple fetuses. It is also particularly useful for producing images of soft tissue tumors or lesions in the brain, eyes, abdomen, reproductive organs, and breasts (Fig. 41–6).

XERORADIOGRAPHY

Xeroradiography is a diagnostic x-ray technique in which an image is produced electrically rather than chemically. This permits lower exposure times and radiation of lower energy. The image is made visible with a powder toner similar to that used in a copying machine. The powder image is transferred and is heat fused to a sheet of paper. The process takes only 90 seconds and permits visualization of soft tissues. For this reason, it is most often used to detect lesions or calcifications in the soft tissue of the breast (Fig. 41–7).

FLAT PLATES

X-ray films can also be taken of various body parts without the use of special techniques or the use of a contrast medium. Flat plates are also called plain films. Several x-ray views are usually taken for review by the radiologist. Examples of these are diagnostic x-ray films of the skull, sinuses, chest, abdomen, and bone (Fig. 41–8).

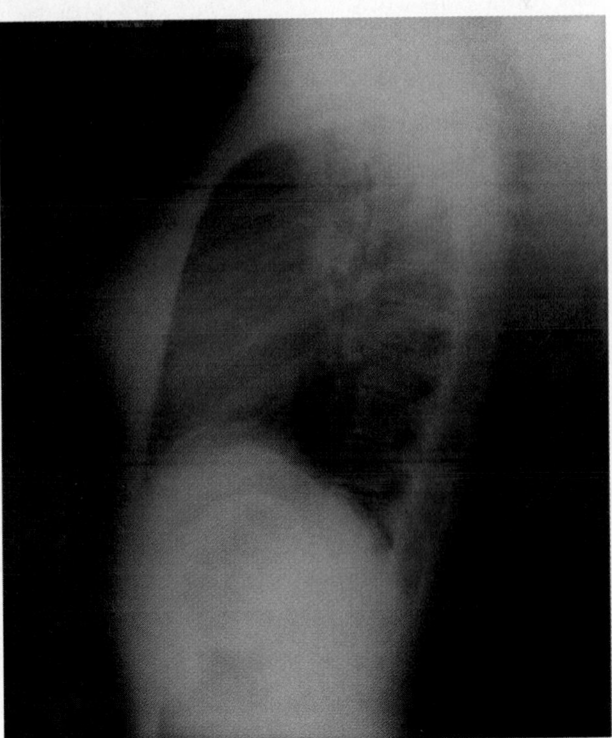

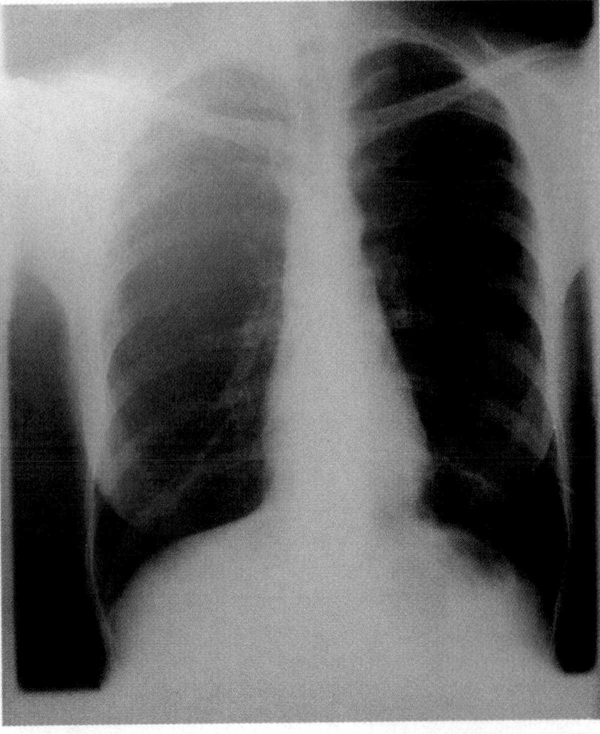

FIGURE 41–8 Chest radiographs.

X-Ray Machine

The x-ray machine consists of tube, table, and control panel. The tube is the part in which the x-rays are produced and then are directed out as an x-ray beam. The entire tube is surrounded by a protective material (lead), except at the point where the rays are emitted. The lead absorbs the radiation like a sponge. The tube is designed to move the entire length of the table. The table is where the patient is positioned for the x-ray study (Fig. 41–9). It is designed to rotate into different positions, as necessary for specific x-ray films. The control panel contains the knobs for operating the tube and the table. It is located behind a lead-lined wall, in another area away from the table and the tube (Fig. 41–10).

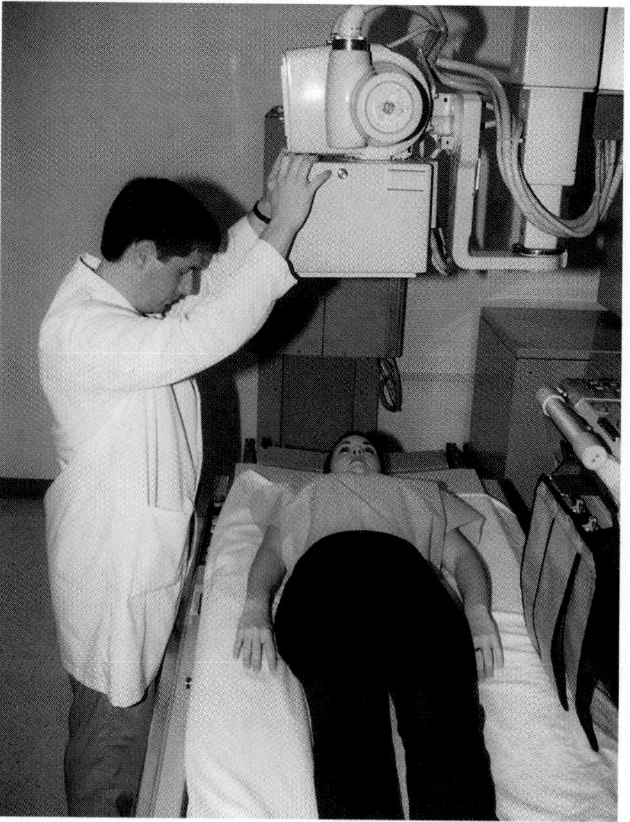

FIGURE 41–9 X-ray machine.

Radiation Hazards and Safeguards

Excessive exposure to radiation can cause both tissue destruction and a variety of ill effects. Harmful effects include temporary or permanent damage to the skin, eyes, and reproductive and blood-forming organs. X-rays may produce harmful effects on the developing embryo and the fetus, causing malformations or death. Overexposure to x-rays produces a variety of symptoms. These include nausea, fatigue, diarrhea, constipation, bleeding, and loss of appetite.

All radiation exposure is cumulative and adds up to a total radiation dosage. The unit that measures this exposure is the **rad, rem,** or **roentgen.** Monitoring devices called dosimeters are worn by persons working near sources of x-rays. These monitors contain special photographic film that is sensitive to radiation and serve as a guide to the amount of radiation to which a person has been exposed. Monitors are submitted periodically for evaluation, and a report of any radiation exposure is maintained on all x-ray personnel (Fig. 41–11).

Radiation exposure can come directly from the x-ray beam or from what is known as scattered radiation. Scattered radiation is the diffusion or deviation of the x-rays that is produced when they pass through a patient or anything in the patient's path. Even though the entire x-ray tube is enclosed in lead, scattered radiation may result from leakage through the tube. To prevent this from happening, all machines must be checked on a regular basis by licensed physicists.

Shielding is of special importance to both patients and personnel. Patients should be protected from unnecessary radiation by using lead aprons to cover the reproductive organs, especially for pregnant patients and all children (see Fig. 41–11). Personnel can obtain additional protection by wearing lead aprons and gloves when assisting. The walls of x-ray rooms are also lined with lead, which absorbs the scattered radiation, protecting all others in the

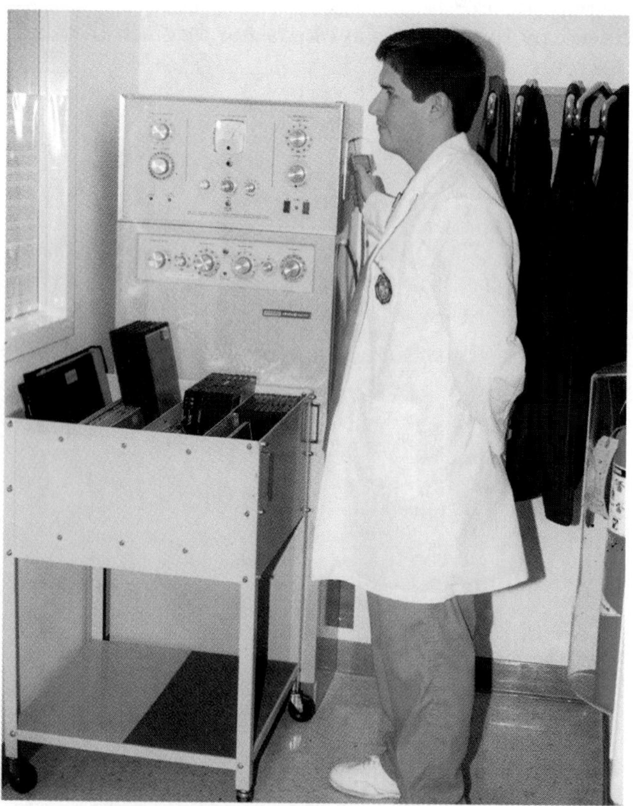

FIGURE 41–10 Control panel of x-ray machine.

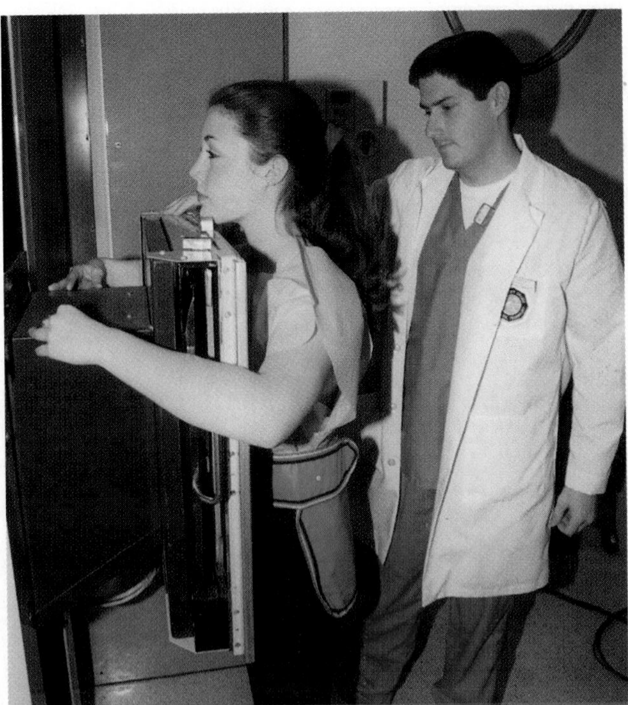

FIGURE 41–11 Technician wearing dosimeter to measure radiation exposure and patient wearing lead apron for protection of reproductive organs.

area. In addition to monitors and shielding, all x-ray personnel should have routine periodic blood cell counts performed to detect the presence of any abnormal or pathologic condition that may result from excessive radiation exposure.

Memory Jogger

6 *How are the reproductive organs of the patient protected during an x-ray procedure?*

The Medical Assistant's Role in Assisting with Radiologic Procedures

There may be occasions when the medical assistant will be called on to assist in the performance of basic x-ray procedures under the physician's supervision, or the physician may train the assistant to take certain x-rays within the office (see Procedure 41–1).

PREPARING THE PATIENT

Preparation of the patient requires a thorough knowledge of the procedure and the ability to communicate all instructions, both written and oral, to the patient to ensure that these instructions are understood. Written instructions are essential, because oral instructions can be easily forgotten. Most physicians use their own printed material or use product literature provided by pharmaceutical companies detailing step-by-step instructions (Fig. 41–12).

Explain the procedure using proper terminology but try to avoid complex descriptions. Encourage the patient to ask questions and discuss any apprehensions. Reinforce the rationale for the x-ray procedure. Many diagnostic x-ray examinations require special preparation by the patient the night before or the morning of the test. Patients may be instructed to eat a low-fat evening meal, not to eat after midnight, to drink plenty of fluids, or take special tablets, laxatives, or enemas.

POSITIONING THE PATIENT

An important responsibility of the medical assistant is the proper positioning of the patient for specific x-ray films. Radiographs are made by directing the x-rays produced by the x-ray tube toward a specific body part. The body part must be positioned correctly between the x-ray film and the x-ray tube (Fig. 41–13). The patient's position is determined by the type of examination required and the specific body part to be visualized. Usually, several views are taken in an attempt to achieve a three-dimensional picture for better diagnosis by the radiologist.

BASIC X-RAY VIEWS, POSITIONS, AND X-RAY BEAM DIRECTION

VIEWS

Anteroposterior (AP) view: The anterior aspect of the body faces the x-ray tube, and the posterior aspect faces the film. The x-ray beam is directed from front to back.

Posteroanterior (PA) view: The posterior aspect of the body faces the x-ray tube, and the anterior aspect faces the film. The x-ray beam is directed from back to front.

Lateral view: The body part is placed on its side. The x-ray beam is directed from one side.

Right lateral (RL) view: The right side of the body faces the film.

Left lateral (LL) view: The left side of the body faces the film.

Oblique view: The body is placed on an angle. The x-ray beam is directed at an angle.

POSITIONS

Supine position: The patient lies on his or her back.

Prone position: The patient lies on his or her abdomen.

THE COLON X-RAY (BARIUM ENEMA)

Your doctor has requested an x-ray examination of your colon (lower bowel). This is a thorough examination of the colon. A special enema (barium) is given that allows the colon to be visible on x-rays.

*****Please Note: This preparation is a laxative. It will empty your colon. Expect to have several loose or liquid bowel movements during the night. Do not be alarmed if you experience cramping and feel some weakness.*

The following preparation is necessary to ensure a satisfactory examination of the colon.

BEGIN DAY BEFORE EXAM DAY

1) Lunch should be a light diet: 1-2 cups soup, 4 Saltines or 1-2 slices bread or toast (butter and jelly OK), 1 serving fruit. May also have: 1 serving cake or up to 3 cookies. Beverage: Any juice, coffee or tea (no milk).

2) Please drink at least one full glass or more of water or clear liquids every 1-2 hours between noon and bedtime (at least six 8 oz. glasses).

3) Thirty minutes before evening meal take Fleet Phospho-Soda. Pour contents (1 1/2 oz.) into one-half glass cool water. Drink, following immediately with one full glass of water.

4) Eat a liquid evening meal (bouillon, strained fruit juice and plain jello). No solid foods. No dairy products (milk, cream or cheese). No carbonated beverages.

5) At 8 PM, take four yellow Fleet Bisacodyl tablets, swallowing tablets whole with a full glass of water. Do not chew or dissolve tablets.

6) Drink nothing after taking the tablets.

7) Eat nothing after the evening meal **(NO BREAKFAST).**

ON THE MORNING OF THE EXAMINATION

1) At least one hour before leaving for your exam use Fleet Bisacodyl Suppository. Remove foil wrap from suppository. Lie on side; insert rounded end of suppository as high as possible in rectum. Wait 15 minutes before evacuating even if urge is strong.

2) On the x-ray table you will be given a barium enema. You will experience a sensation similar to a cleansing enema. It will be only a matter of minutes before you have to go to the bathroom and expel the enema.

3) The radiologist (an x-ray physician specialist) will examine your abdomen by pressing it with his hands and observing the colon with the fluoroscope (television) and x-ray films.

4) When the radiologist has completed his portion of the examination, an x-ray technologist will take some additional films and immediately take you to the bathroom. After you feel you have expelled all of the enema, please have a seat in the hallway and the technologist will take an additional film of your abdomen to visualize your empty bowel.

5) The colon exam will usually require approximately 30 minutes.

Report to your doctor's receptionist the morning of your examination and you will be given a request slip for your x-rays.

We appreciate your cooperation.

FIGURE 41–12 Patient instruction sheet for barium enema.

TERMS TO DESCRIBE THE DIRECTION OF THE X-RAY BEAM

Axillary: The beam is directed toward the axilla (underarm).

Craniocaudal: The x-ray beam is directed downward from head to toe.

Mediolateral: The x-ray beam is directed from the midline toward the side of the body part of which a film is being made.

Memory Jogger

How would you position the patient for a PA view?

EXPOSING X-RAY FILM

X-rays, which can be produced by high-velocity electrons in a vacuum tube, expose (turn black) a sheet of x-ray film. X-rays can also be absorbed by

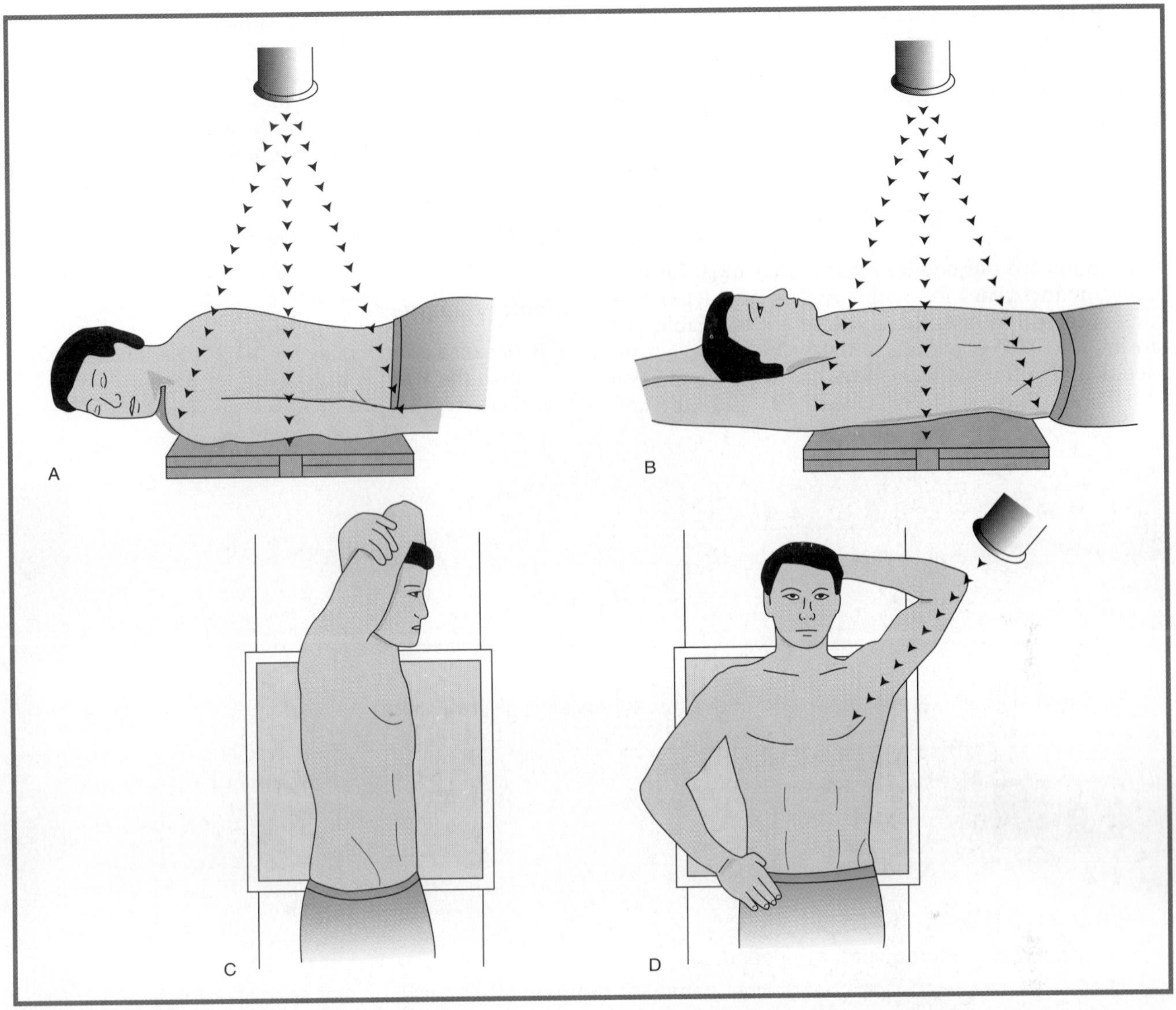

A B C D

FIGURE 41–13 Positioning the patient. *A,* Posteroanterior view. *B,* Anteroposterior view. *C,* Lateral view. *D,* Oblique view.

substances, to a degree relative to the density of that substance. Thus, if part of the body is positioned on a cassette (film holder) and x-rays are directed through it, the rays will be absorbed or scattered by the various substances in the body and will expose the film to varying degrees. The resulting image will show the pattern of substances inside the body. Air, for instance, is least dense and appears as black areas, whereas water, fat, and metal appear increasingly white. Because the human body is made of different materials and is of varying thicknesses, the final image is composed of various degrees of black and white (Fig. 41–14).

PROCESSING X-RAY FILM

Film development takes place in a darkroom. No natural light is permitted in this area. The only arti-

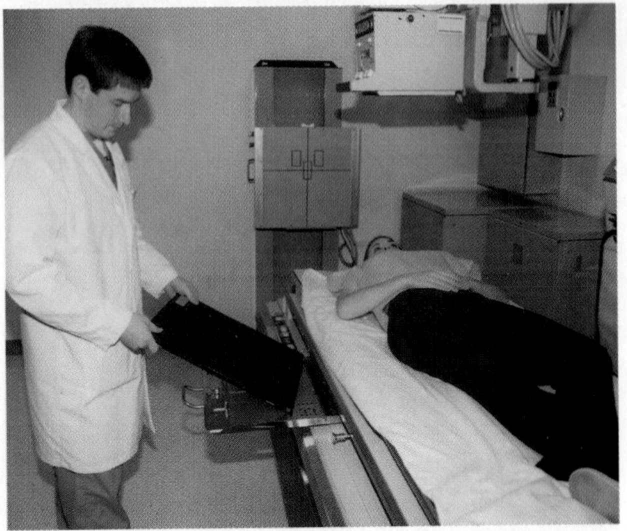

FIGURE 41–14 Insertion of x-ray film cassette.

ficial light used is a specially designed low-wattage bulb that will not expose the film. For x-ray film processing, most modern medical offices use automatic developers, which produce images quickly and automatically.

FILING X-RAY FILMS AND REPORTS

X-ray films are permanent records that must be preserved many years for both medical and legal reasons. Medical assistants are often responsible for storing the patient's films after processing is completed and after the physician has read them. The films are placed in large envelopes, with the patient's name, the patient's number (if used), and the date clearly marked on the outside. These films should be stored in a dry, cool place. In a general practice office, the films are usually kept in a readily accessible area for viewing. X-ray films are the property of the medical office where the films are taken. They do not belong to the patient. Written x-ray reports may be sent out, but the actual films must remain as part of the patient's file.

Memory Jogger

8 *Because patients pay for the x-ray study, do they own the x-ray films?*

PROCEDURE 41-1
Assisting with an X-Ray Examination

GOAL

To assist with an x-ray examination under the supervision of a physician.

EQUIPMENT AND SUPPLIES

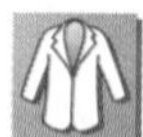 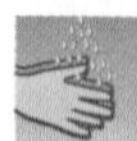

- Physician's order for an x-ray examination
- X-ray machine
- X-ray film and holder
- X-ray darkroom
- X-ray automatic developer or manual processing solutions

PROCEDURAL STEPS

1 Check order and equipment needed.

2 Introduce yourself, and confirm the identity of the patient. Ascertain if any special preparations were employed.
PURPOSE: If special preparations were not followed, the examination may need to be rescheduled.

3 Explain the procedure and load the x-ray cassette into the machine (Figure 1).
PURPOSE: Helps to reassure the patient and alleviates fear and anxiety.

Continued

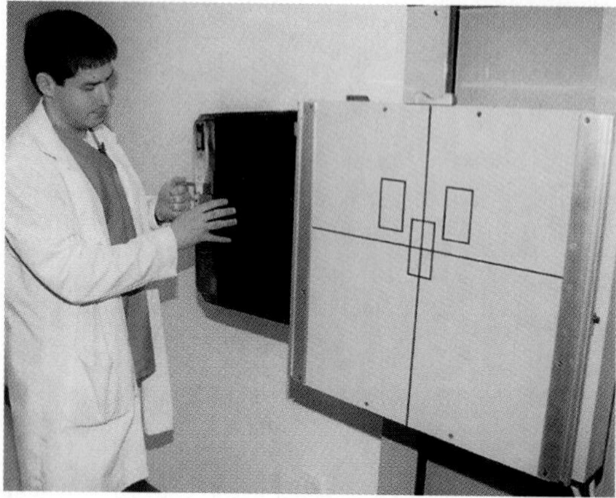

FIGURE 1

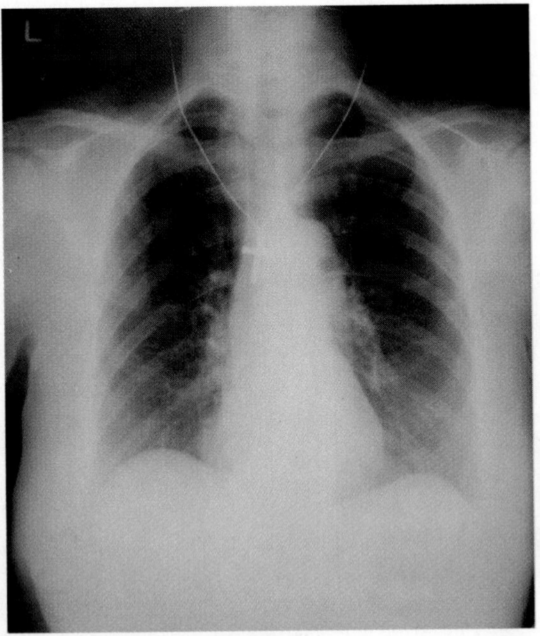

FIGURE 2

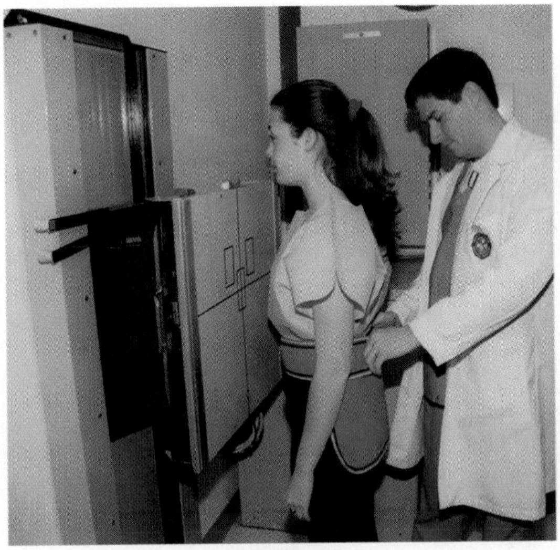

FIGURE 3

4 Check to make certain that the patient has removed all metal objects from the area to be examined.
PURPOSE: Metal objects appear on the film and may obscure the final image (Figure 2).

5 Drape the patient as necessary, and shield the abdominal area (Figure 3).
PURPOSE: Drapes provide warmth, and shields protect the reproductive areas.

6 Position the patient properly, and immobilize the part, if necessary (Figure 4).
PURPOSE: Proper positioning and complete stillness are necessary to achieve a clear, readable radiograph.

7 Adjust and position the camera (Figure 5).

Continued

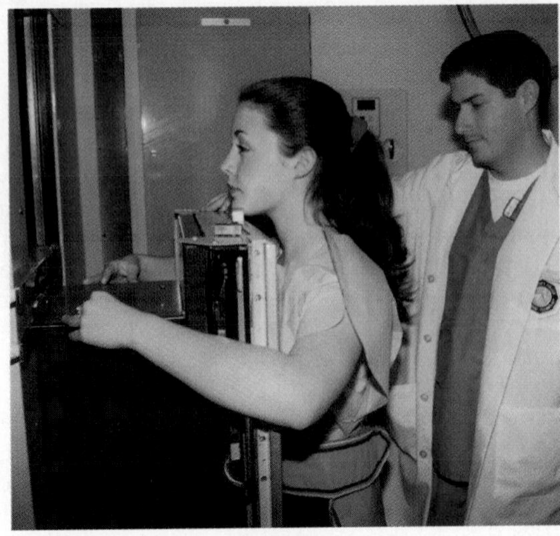

FIGURE 4

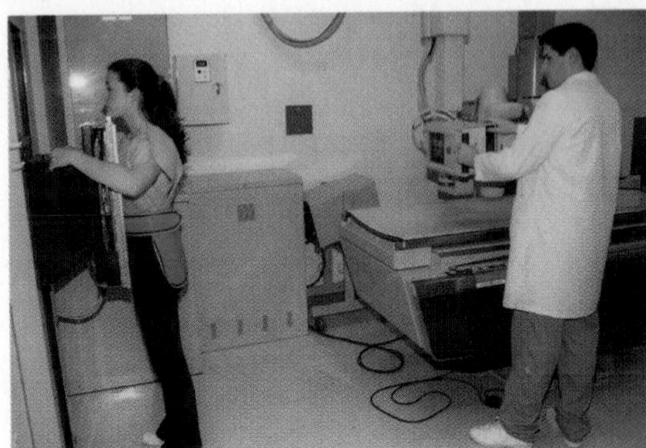

FIGURE 5

PROCEDURE 41–1 (CONTINUED)
Assisting with an X-Ray Examination

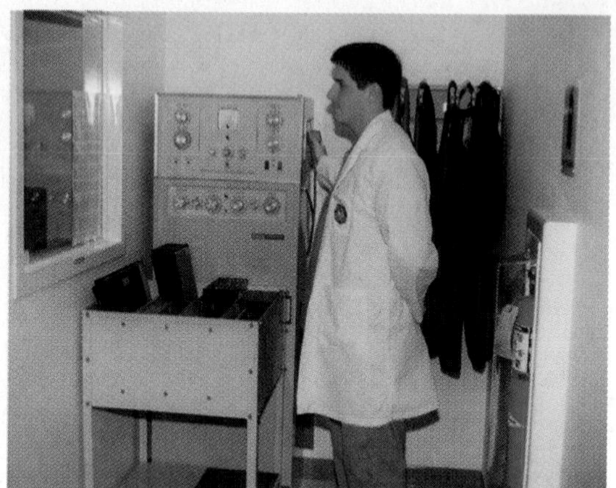

FIGURE 6

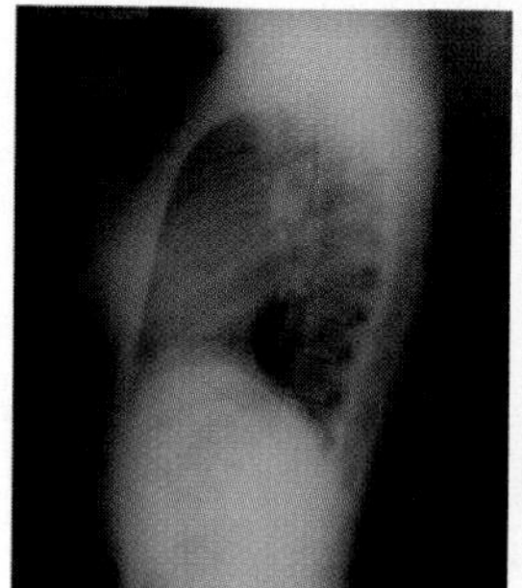

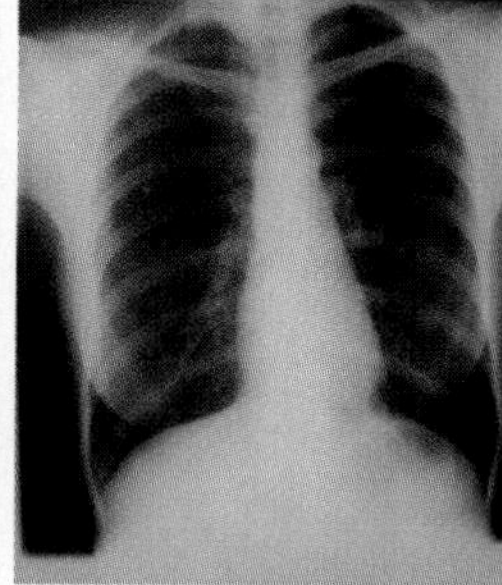

FIGURE 7

8 Stand behind a lead shield during the exposure (Figure 6).
PURPOSE: Lead shields provide protection from scattered radiation.

9 Ask the patient to assume a comfortable position after the examination is completed, and wait until the films are processed.
PURPOSE: In the event that it is necessary to retake an x-ray film, the patient will be readily accessible.

10 Develop the film, using automatic or manual film processing (Figure 7).

11 Dismiss the patient if all films are satisfactory.

12 Place the dry, finished x-ray film in a properly labeled envelope, and file it according to the policies of the office.

13 Record the x-ray examination on the patient's chart, along with the final written x-ray findings.
PURPOSE: A procedure is considered not done until it is recorded.

Therapeutic Modalities

The physical agents, called modalities, include heat, therapy with water, the use of electric currents as a form of physical therapy, and therapeutic exercise.

Heat applications to injured or painful body parts have been used throughout history. Heat therapy is well-practiced, commonsense home treatment easily applied with or without the direction of a physician. You may have had the occasion to apply heat to a swollen, sore body part. Heat is used primarily to improve circulation, minimize pain, and correct or alleviate muscular and joint malfunction.

Physical therapy and therapeutic exercise involve the scientific use of physical measures, devices, and body movement to restore normal function to injured tissues. Physical therapy is a separate profession practiced by physical therapists and physical therapy assistants and aides. The Association of Physical Therapists states that physical therapy treatments should be administered by a trained physical therapist or the treatment should be supervised by a registered physical therapist. Registered physical therapists work mainly in hospitals or in specialized private practices.

Your role may be limited to referring the patient to a physical therapist and explaining preappointment instructions, or, if it is permitted in your area of the United States, you may be able to administer limited physical therapy under the supervision of a physician or a registered physical therapist. Before participating in the physical treatment of patients, it is important for you to know which procedures are permitted by state law to be performed by someone other than a licensed physical therapist.

General Principles of Heat Application

Heat produces local vasodilation and increases circulation. It speeds up the inflammatory process, promotes local drainage, relaxes muscles, and repairs tissue cells. Heat can be applied to relax and relieve pain in a strained muscle; to promote drainage from an abscess or infected area; to relieve tissue congestion and swelling, such as nasal congestion or a localized collection of **extravasated** blood in the tissues; or to improve the repair time of a sprained joint (Fig. 41–15). However, the effects of external heat applications also depend on the following conditions:

- The type of heat used
- The length of time the heat is applied
- The general condition of the patient
- The size of the area needing treatment

Heat can be harmful. Prolonged application of heat increases the secretions of the skin, softening it and lowering its resistance to injury. Extreme heat works adversely by constricting the blood vessels and causing burns. Heat applied too often may increase a patient's tolerance to heat so that the patient may be burned without knowing it. Infants and the elderly are particularly susceptible to burns, so extreme caution must be used when treating them. Infants and patients who cannot report a burning sensation should be evaluated and watched carefully, as should persons with diseases of the cardiovascular, renal, sensorineural, and respiratory systems and those with osteoporosis. In addition, special precautions must be taken with patients with impaired circulation, such as those with diabetes. Because heat can increase the inflammatory process, it should never be applied to the abdomen if appendicitis is suspected. In this instance, heat can rupture the inflamed appendix.

When deciding whether to treat a body part with heat, the following conditions all are generally contraindications. Of course, there may be special conditions, or directions given by the physician, to treat with heat even though one or more of these conditions exist. However, *do not* treat a patient having any of the following conditions until you have specifically discussed the condition with the physician:

- Acute inflammatory conditions: heat should not be used in most acute inflammatory processes for the first 48 hours.
- Severe circulatory problems, such as blockage and bleeding: heat can increase the blockage and cause hemorrhaging.
- The lack of sensation in a body part: there is danger that the patient cannot report burning. A lack of sensation may indicate a lack of circulation in the body part.
- Pregnancy or menstruation: heat can cause uterine contractions and increase menstrual flow.
- Areas containing encapsulated pus and having no drainage: heat increases the inflammatory process, and the encapsulated area could rupture.
- Blisters from hot water bottles, heating pads, skin ointments, or salves previously applied by the patient: heat should not be applied over newly burned skin.
- Scar tissue does not have a normal supply of blood vessels; therefore, heat is not carried away by blood circulation and burns could occur.
- Body areas that may contain malignant tumors: malignant tumor activity may be stimulated by heat.

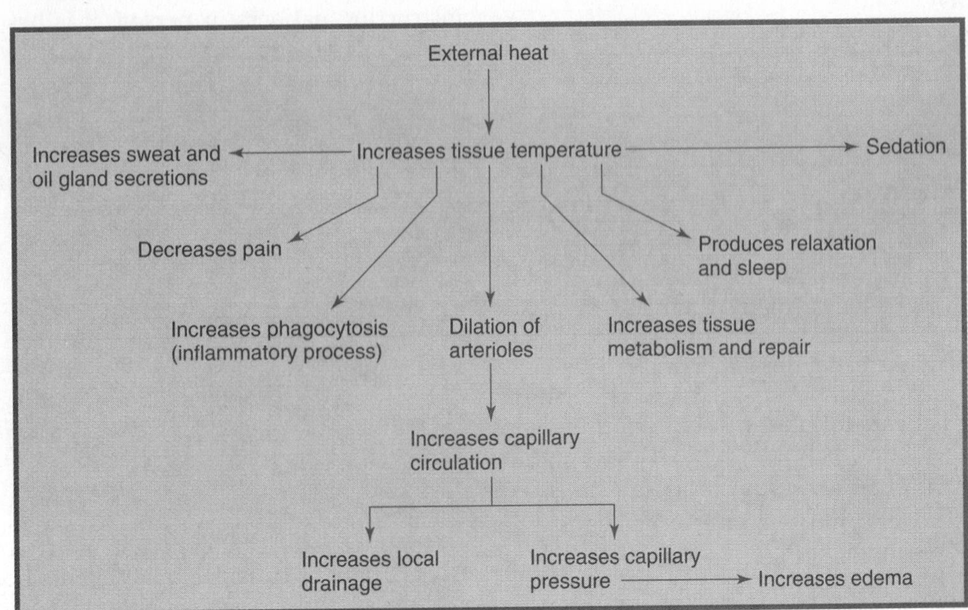

FIGURE 41–15 Body responses to heat application. (Adapted from St. Mary's Hospital, Inc. Russelville, AR.)

- Erythema (redness of the skin) may indicate a blood clot, which could break loose with an increase in circulation caused by application of heat.
- Metal materials: heat concentrates in metal materials, such as metal implants and prostheses. Therefore, patients with internal metal devices should not have those areas treated. To avoid burns, metal objects such as jewelry, watches, hearing aids, hairpins, and metal clips must be removed before treatment. Treatment must be administered on nonmetal tables and chairs.

Memory Jogger

 *The effects of external heat application depend on ______.*

Body parts may be heated to 110° F (44° C) without damage to the tissues. Redness appears because the capillaries become congested with blood at the skin's surface. Continuous heat for more than 20 minutes usually results in the increased circulation carrying away the heat as rapidly as it is applied, and the therapy may lose its effectiveness. Heat applied for more than 1 hour causes the blood vessels to constrict, thereby decreasing the blood supply to the area and adversely affecting the effectiveness of the treatment.

Moist heat penetrates better than dry heat. Moist heat (heat hydrotherapy) may be applied with hot packs and compresses, soaks, or baths.

Dry heat may be applied in the form of hot water bottles or electric heating pads and lamps or by the use of electric current when the treatment of the deeper tissues is necessary.

Memory Jogger

 *What type of heat has better tissue penetration?*

HEAT HYDROTHERAPY

Soaks

With heat hydrotherapy, a body part is immersed gradually into medicated or plain water for approximately 15 minutes at a temperature no greater than 110° F (44° C). The extremities are often treated by this method. Patients can take their own soaks at home, but special instructions in aseptic techniques must be given to the patient if the area being treated is an open wound.

Whirlpool Treatment

This method uses a tank with special equipment that agitates the water to provide gentle massage. It is useful for exercise or to cleanse wounds. The temperature is the same as for any method of heat hydrotherapy.

Paraffin Bath

This is especially useful in treating chronic joint disease. A mixture of seven parts paraffin and one part mineral oil is heated to melting at about 127° F. The patient's body part is dipped into the warm paraffin mixture and removed, and then this is repeated until a thick coat is formed on the body part. The paraffin is left on for about 30 minutes and then is peeled off. It leaves the skin soft, warm, and pliable, with slight erythema (Fig. 41–16).

Hot Moist Compresses

Hot moist compresses are used to increase blood flow to small areas of the body, such as the hands. They may be made at home with soft cloths or a clean washcloth. If hot moist compresses are applied to an open wound in the office, use sterile gauze sponges, a sterile solution, and surgically aseptic conditions. Follow Standard Precautions. Dispose of used materials in a closed container so that personnel and other patients are not in danger of contact with the contaminated materials.

Often, you will be asked to instruct patients on how to apply hot moist compresses at home. Patient instructions for home care should be explicit and simple. The patient should remove all jewelry and should be instructed *not* to apply a hot moist compress if a rash appears or the skin is broken. A plastic covering will help keep in the moisture. A hot water bottle may be used to keep the compress hot. If you are speaking to the patient over the telephone, be sure that the patient writes down the instructions as you read each step. Never assume that the patient knows the correct method. When instructing patients in person, it is best to have preprinted instructions for you to review and give to the patient to take home.

EXAMPLE OF PATIENT INSTRUCTIONS FOR APPLYING HOT COMPRESSES AT HOME

1 Moisten a clean hand towel with warm water.
2 Wring it out.
3 The compress should be warm, not hot.
4 Place the towel directly onto the skin.
5 Cover the towel with plastic to keep in the moist heat.
6 Continue the therapy for the prescribed length of time and the prescribed number of times each day.

Commercially prepared hot moist compresses are packs made of canvas containing a silicon gel, which retains heat (Fig. 41–17). They may be purchased for home use and may be heated in warm water.

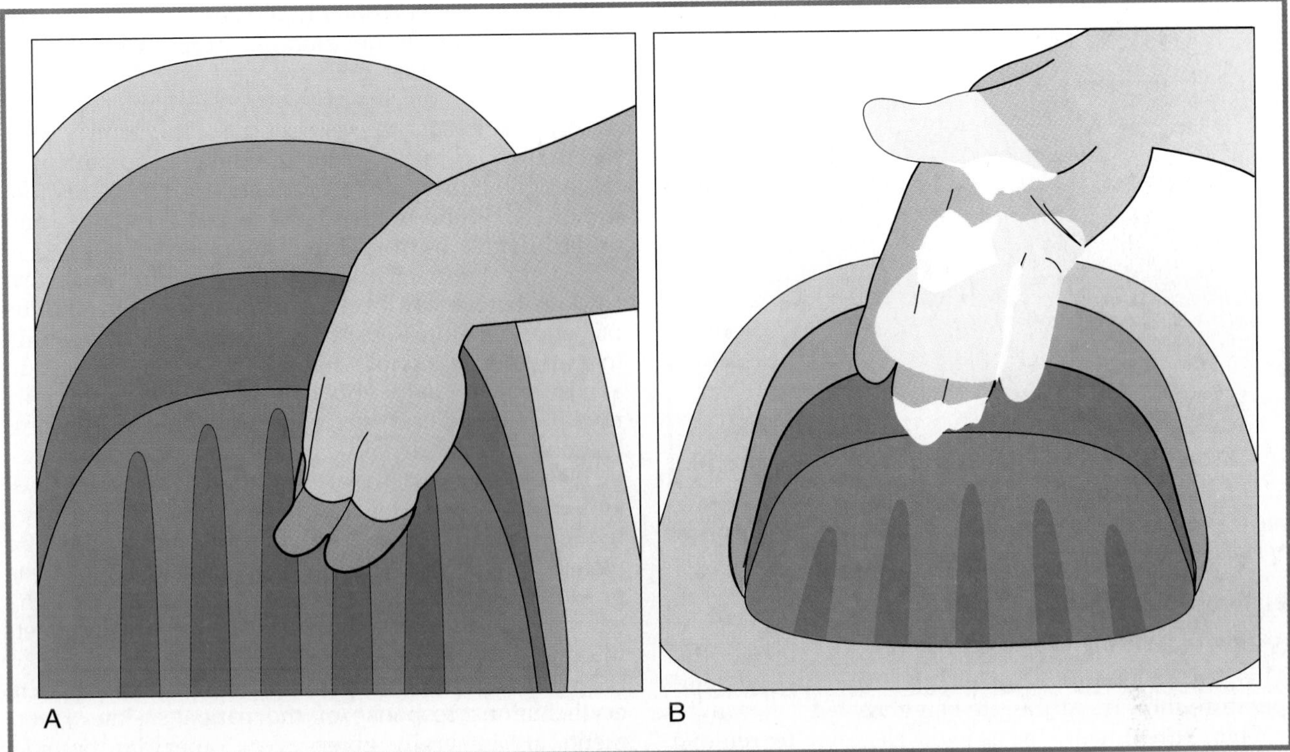

FIGURE 41–16 The paraffin bath is especially helpful for pain relief in patients with arthritis. *A,* The hand is dipped into warm paraffin. If a thicker coating of wax is desired, the hand is dipped again. *B,* The warm paraffin is left on the hand for about 30 minutes and then is peeled off.

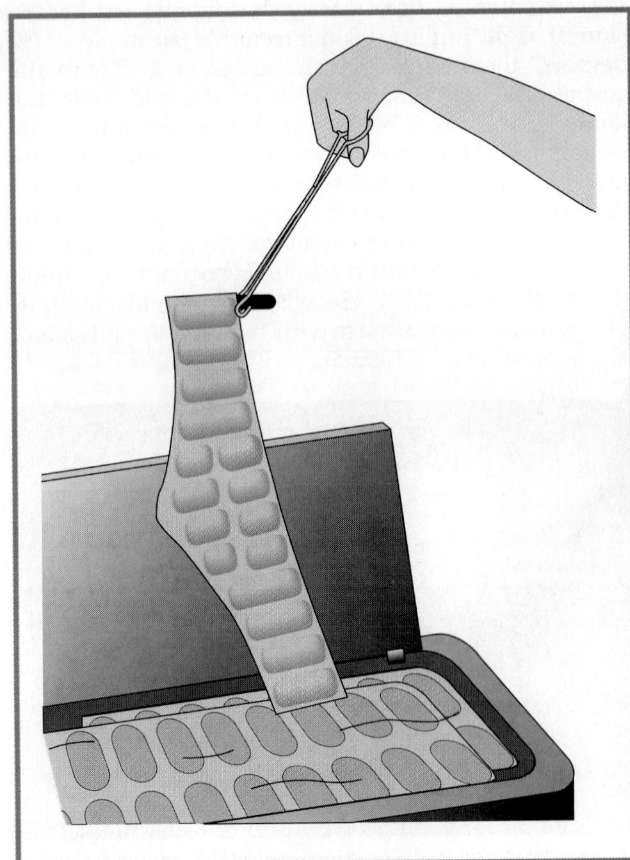

FIGURE 41–17 Commercially prepared hot moist pack made of canvas that contains a silicon gel.

DRY HEAT

Methods of dry heat can produce heat on the superficial skin surfaces or penetrate to the deeper muscle tissues. Heating pads, infrared radiation (heat lamps and hot water bottles), and ultraviolet rays generate heat that can penetrate to a depth of 10 mm. Deeper penetration of heat, produced with high-frequency electric current, is called *diathermy.* Diathermy is derived from the Greek words meaning "heating through."

Heating Pads

The least-complicated method of applying dry heat, heating pads are often used by the patient at home. When giving instructions for use at home, caution the patient that heating pads must not be used near moisture. Instruct the patient to turn the heat control to low or medium (never the high setting) and to keep the pad on the body part only for a prescribed length of time. Heating pads with automatic thermostats are preferred over the older models that do not control the temperature evenly.

Infrared Radiation Lamps

Infrared radiation lamps generate heat within a metal coil element or a special heat-producing electric bulb. This source of energy produces very shallow heat penetration. The penetration is 3 to 5 mm (or 0.1 to 0.2 inch) and depends on the principle of

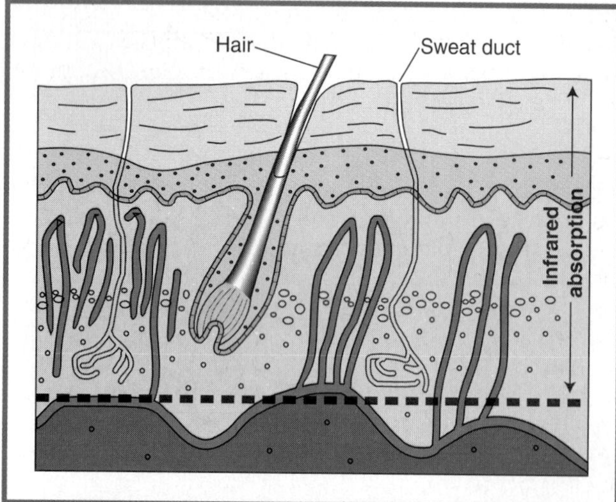

FIGURE 41–18 The broken line indicates the depth of penetration of the infrared rays into the skin.

conduction to warm the deeper tissues (Fig. 41–18). This treatment produces an approximate 1° F temperature increase at the site being treated.

Before treatment, the skin is cleansed to remove any ointments and skin oils. The treatment extends for usually 20 to 45 minutes, according to the physician's instructions. During the course of the treatment, the patient's skin becomes flushed, but a sunburn does not occur. However, if used improperly, the infrared lamp is capable of producing skin burns in exactly the same manner as touching a hot stove or oven. In addition to dry heat treatments, the infrared lamp can be placed above a moist dressing to extend the time of a moist heat treatment.

Maintenance of the infrared lamp is simple. The heating element should be kept in a down position when not in use, to prevent dust from accumulating on the element. The electric connections should be checked and kept in good working condition.

Ultraviolet Radiation

Ultraviolet radiation is produced by the sun, by lamps, or by some types of tanning beds. Ultraviolet radiation is more penetrating than infrared radiation and can cause skin burns or pigmentation changes, resulting in tanning. Ultraviolet rays are also capable of killing bacteria. It is this bactericidal action that makes ultraviolet radiation so useful in therapy. It is effective in treating skin diseases caused by bacteria, such as acne, psoriasis, and ulcerations.

Ultraviolet rays are generated by different types of lamps. One type discharges a current of electricity through certain gases in a quartz tube. The process produces ultraviolet rays with very little heat generation. This lamp is called the *cold quartz lamp* and is most frequently used in the physician's office.

There are two types of cold quartz ultraviolet lamps. One type is used for general body radiation. This energy is very potent, and precautions must be taken to avoid tissue damage from overexposure. The physician must give an exact order in seconds or minutes for the length of exposure and the exact distance between the patient and the lamp. At a distance of 36 inches from the unit to the patient, a first-degree burn can be produced in 30 seconds to 1 minute, a second-degree burn in 1 to 2 minutes, and a third-degree burn in 2 to 4 minutes.

Test the lamp on the patient's forearm for a few seconds before you begin treatment to determine the presence of skin sensitivity. Some patients cannot tolerate any ultraviolet radiation. A history of sun exposure may help you determine this. Ultraviolet rays are considered carcinogenic if their use is prolonged. Certain drugs, especially the sulfonamides, increase the sensitivity of the skin to ultraviolet rays, and treatments should be postponed or the dosage reduced accordingly. Additional precautions include using a towel to cover the genitalia and other areas of the patient's body not being treated. Both the operator and the patient should wear ultraviolet-filtering glasses.

The size of the dose is usually governed by the erythematous response of the patient's skin. Treatments are generally given every other day because 24 hours is not enough time to evaluate the maximum erythematous response of the skin. The penetration of the rays is less than 0.1 mm, and there may be some tanning of the skin. The intensity of the radiation is greatest when the rays strike the skin at right angles (90 degrees). At an angle of 30 degrees, the intensity decreases to 80% (Lambert's cosine law). If the distance from the patient to the lamp is decreased by one half, the strength of the radiation is increased four times (inverse square law). Because of these two factors, it is important that the distance and the angle of the ultraviolet rays are correct and the same for each treatment.

The *portable spot-quartz lamp* is useful when treating small areas (Fig. 41–19). The portable lamp is placed near or in contact with the area to be treated.

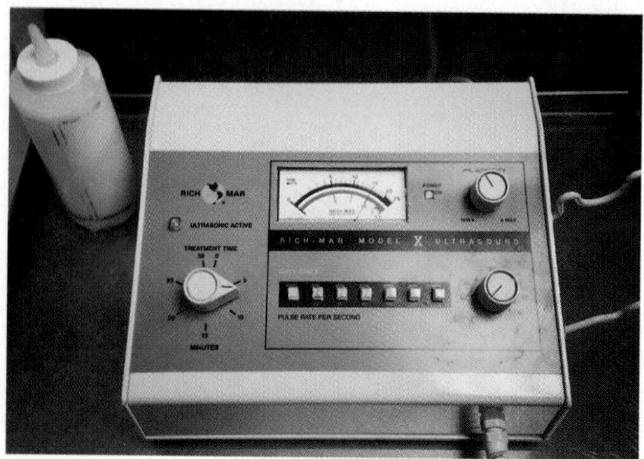

FIGURE 41–19 Ultrasound machine: note output meter and timer.

Practically no heat is generated in the lamp coils; thus skin burns do not occur. The treatment time extends from a few seconds to minutes, depending on the skin condition and the distance between the patient and the lamp. A masking adapter for small areas attaches to the face of the lamp, and a filter (Wood's filter) eliminates the visible light. The glass coils of the lamp must be protected from breakage and must be kept free of dust and soil. They may be cleaned with alcohol.

Hot Water Bottles

These are often used at home without any thought to correct technique. When teaching patients how to use this method at home, caution them to keep the water temperature at or below 125° F (52° C). If the patient is a child, keep the temperature below 115° F (46° C) to prevent burns. A hot water bottle that is less than one half full conforms better to the body and is more comfortable.

HEAT APPLICATION TO DEEPER TISSUES

Three methods of heat application to the deeper tissues are short-wave, microwave, and ultrasound diathermy. All three forms are applied to increase blood flow and speed up metabolism and electrolyte flow across the cell membranes. Treatment is used to stretch and repair tendons, joint capsules, and scars. Treatments usually relieve stiffness of joints, relax muscles, and decrease muscle spasm.

Short-Wave Diathermy

Short-wave diathermy produces energy similar to that emitted by a radio station transmission. This energy penetrates deep into the body tissues and creates heat. The use of short-wave diathermy may be indicated for all types of inflammatory processes (acute, subacute, and chronic). Many patients report pain relief within 36 to 48 hours. Treatments may be prescribed as often as three times a week for 20 to 30 minutes.

Two condenser plates are placed on either side of the body part to be treated. As these high-frequency waves are transmitted through the body from one plate to the other, heat is generated in the tissues. Most short-wave diathermy plates are placed 1 inch from the skin. The dosage panel should be adjusted until a mild heat is felt by the patient. Some patients may believe that if a little warmth produces good results, more heat will be even better. This is not true with short-wave diathermy. Do not increase the volume of energy above the amount ordered by the physician, and carefully explain to the patient that only a gentle warmth is appropriate for effective treatment. Conversely, notify the physician that you need to lower the volume of energy if the amount ordered is too much for the patient. Position the machine so that the patient cannot adjust the controls. If necessary, place a towel on the patient to collect perspiration.

The short-wave diathermy machine must be wiped down after use on each patient. Do not permit the electric cords to tangle. Do not move the machine in any position that will pull the electric cord at any of the connections. The cables leading to the patient electrode plates should not cross one another or touch the patient. Electricity follows the path of least resistance and may flow from one cord to another, thus rerouting the energy away from the area being treated. Almost all machines have spacers on the cables to prevent this. Some machines may require a warm-up period before they can be used in treatment.

Memory Jogger

Short-wave diathermy treatments may be prescribed as often as ________.

Microwave Diathermy

This method uses radar waves. It works on the same principle as microwave ovens used for cooking. Microwaves have a higher frequency and shorter wavelength than radio waves. This mode is the easiest to use (one electrode is placed above the body part to be treated), but it has less penetration than does short-wave diathermy. Microwaves cannot be used over moist dressings or near persons with implanted electronic cardiac pacemakers.

Ultrasound Diathermy

Ultrasound energy is sound energy. The basic principle of ultrasonography is the same as that of sonar, used in oceanography. Ultrasonic waves are concentrated into a narrow beam and are transmitted through a medium in the form of vibrations. The customary sounds that we hear are produced by sound waves vibrating at a rate of 100 to 12,000 cycles per second (hertz). Ultrasound waves vibrate at the rate of 1 million times per second. In therapeutic ultrasound machines, this frequency is created by an electric current passing through an applicator (transducer). In the applicator is a quartz crystal. The current passes through the quartz, causing the quartz to vibrate at an extremely high frequency. When the applicator containing the quartz is brought into contact with the body, the vibrations are transferred and continue through the tissues.

Although the frequency of this vibration is high, the total energy transmitted to the patient is very low. It is normally indicated on an output meter on the machine, in total watts or watts per square centimeter of the applicator element area. Ultra-high-frequency sound waves do not travel through air. The applicator must be held in contact with the body surface and aided with a *coupling agent.* A coupling agent may be either water, lotion, or a gel. If the area of the body to be treated can be immersed in a basin or tank, treatment may be administered under water. For areas of the body that cannot be immersed, gel or lotion is applied to the applicator and to the body part to be treated. The gel or lotion should be water soluble and nonstaining to clothing or skin.

Ultra-high-frequency sound waves cause the tissues to vibrate, which, in turn, vibrates the circulatory system and speeds up circulation. The increased blood flow creates a chemical action in the tissues that has a favorable effect on the body's healing process. All this takes place with little or no heat, and the patient feels no sensation except a little warmth. Because ultrasound waves travel best through water, they penetrate the deep body tissues that have a high water content, such as the muscles. However, because ultrasound waves cannot penetrate and move along tissues that have a low water content, such as bone, the waves are capable of concentrating and bombarding bone and causing damage. Ultrasound treatment must be used very carefully where bones are near the surface of the skin.

Most acute ailments, such as strains, sprains, and torn muscles and tendons, are treated with ultrasound power as low as 0.5 to 1.0 watt/cm^2. Ultrasound treatment is not recommended within the first 48 hours for these acute conditions. During this first 48-hour period, the best treatment is application of cold compresses. Chronic conditions, such as arthritis and osteoarthritis, may be treated at a higher power, 1.5 to 2.5 watts/cm^2. The duration of any treatment varies from 5 to 15 minutes, depending on the physician's instructions (see Procedure 41–2).

Memory Jogger

What is a coupling agent and how is it used?

PROCEDURE 41-2
Assisting with Ultrasound Therapy

GOAL

To apply ultra-high-frequency sound waves to the patient's deep tissues for therapy. (The medical assistant should perform ultrasound therapy only under the supervision of the physician or a registered physical therapist.)

EQUIPMENT AND SUPPLIES

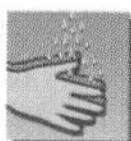

Ultrasound machine
Coupling agent

PROCEDURAL STEPS

1 Prepare your equipment and wash your hands.

2 Confirm the patient's identity.

3 Explain the procedure, and ask the patient to indicate if there is any discomfort.
PURPOSE: To ensure that the patient does not experience any pain or injury.

4 Question the patient for the presence of any internal or external metal objects.

5 Position the patient comfortably, with the area to be treated exposed.

6 Apply a warmed coupling agent liberally over the area to be treated and to the applicator (Figure 1).
PURPOSE: To transmit the sound waves through water or a water-soluble substance.

7 Begin treatment with the intensity control at the lowest setting.

Continued

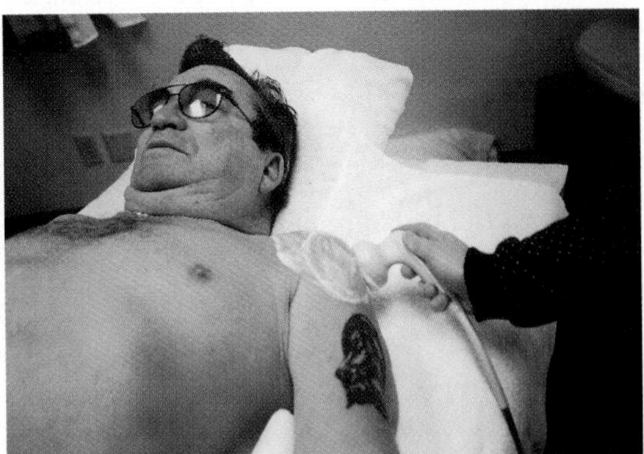

FIGURE 1

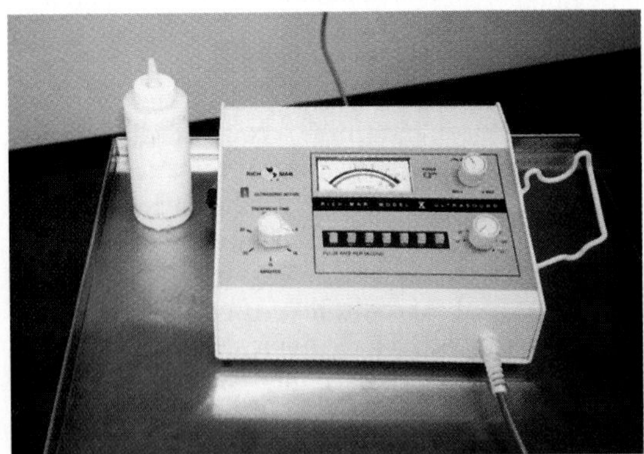

FIGURE 2

8 Set the timer on the machine (Figure 2).
PURPOSE: The timer starts the machine.

9 Increase the intensity control to the ordered amount (Figure 3).

10 Hold the applicator at a 90-degree angle against the patient's skin.
PURPOSE: To ensure close contact.

11 Work the applicator over the area to be treated in a circular fashion, within a radius of 2 inches per second (Figure 4).
PURPOSE: Constant motion prevents hot spots from occurring from excessive ultrasonic waves to one area.

12 If the alternative method of stroking is ordered, move the applicator in short 1-inch strokes so that each stroke overlaps the last stroke by about ½ inch.

13 Keep the applicator moving until the timer sounds. The timer shuts off the machine automatically.

14 Return the intensity control to zero.

15 Remove the coupling agent from the patient and from the applicator with a paper wipe.

16 Assist the patient to the dressing room.

17 Record on the patient's medical record the treatment date, area treated, intensity, duration, and any unusual occurrences or reaction(s) that may have occurred during the treatment.
PURPOSE: A procedure is considered not done until it is recorded.

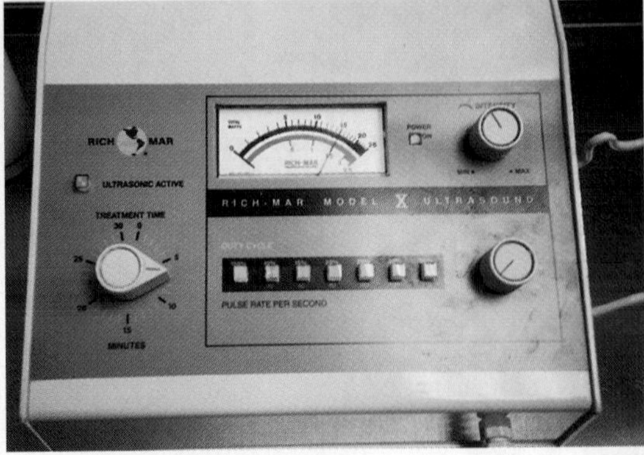

FIGURE 3

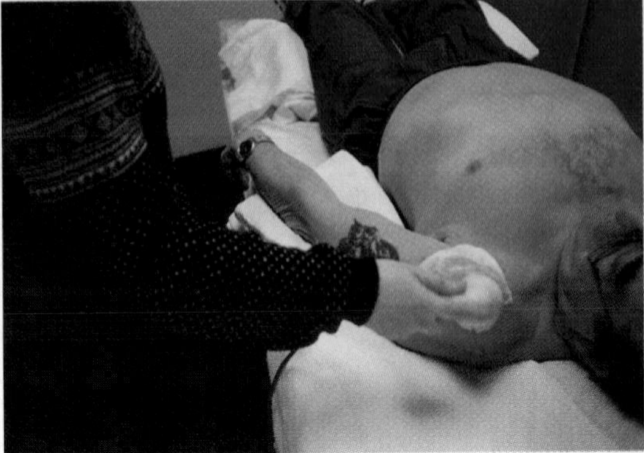

FIGURE 4

Therapeutic Exercise

A therapeutic exercise program is designed to correct specific disabilities of the patient. An exercise program may restore mobility, coordination, and strength to a part or may result in relaxation and relief of tension or pain. Extensive evaluation of the patient's actual physical condition is necessary when exercise therapy is prescribed. This is also a time when a great amount of patient education and encouragement is required. The physical therapist and the physician work together in evaluating the best type of treatment. Often, therapeutic exercise is combined with the heat and heat hydrotherapy treatments.

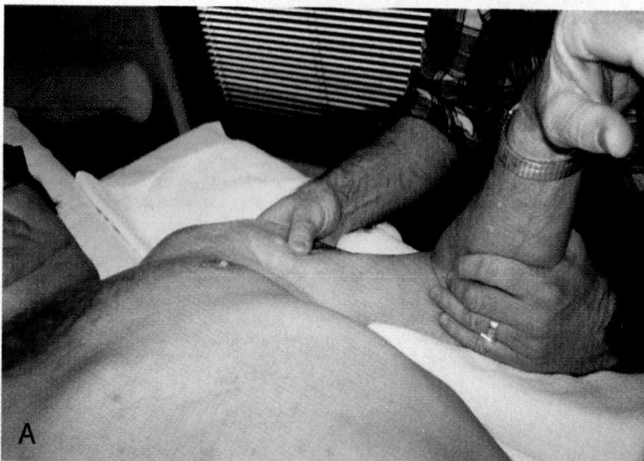

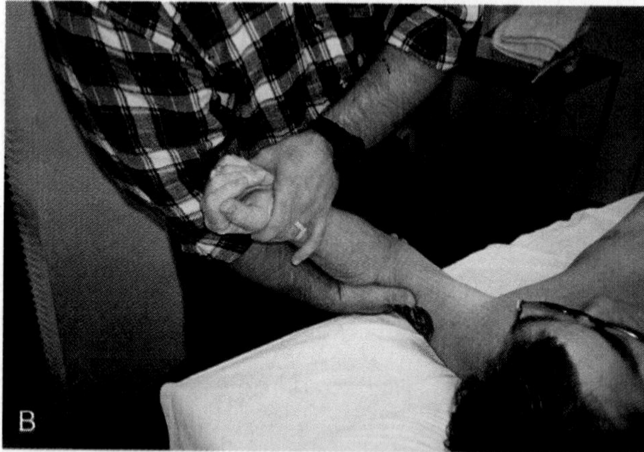

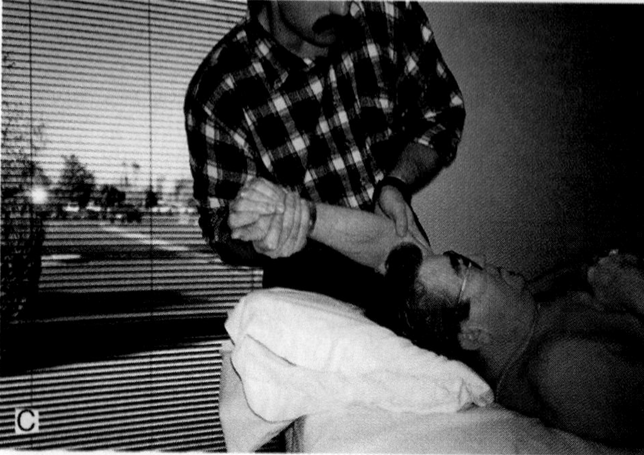

FIGURE 41–20 *A* through *C*, Exercising the shoulder after rotator cuff repair. Note position of hands of the physical therapist for support during passive exercise.

Memory Jogger

Name four possible outcomes in an exercise program.

JOINT MOBILITY

If motion is restricted even for a short time, the joint tissues become dense, hard, and shortened. These changes occur even in normal joints in as short a time as 4 days. It is important to institute joint exercise as soon as possible during therapy. Treatment of joint immobility or disability is accomplished either actively or passively by exercising a joint to its highest degree of possible motion (Fig. 41–20).

Active Exercise

Active exercise is body movement voluntarily initiated and controlled by the patient, although the patient may be assisted by the physical therapist or physical therapist assistant. Active exercise may require specialized equipment, similar to gymnasium equipment. Some devices that are prescribed are stationary bicycles and free weights (Fig. 41–21).

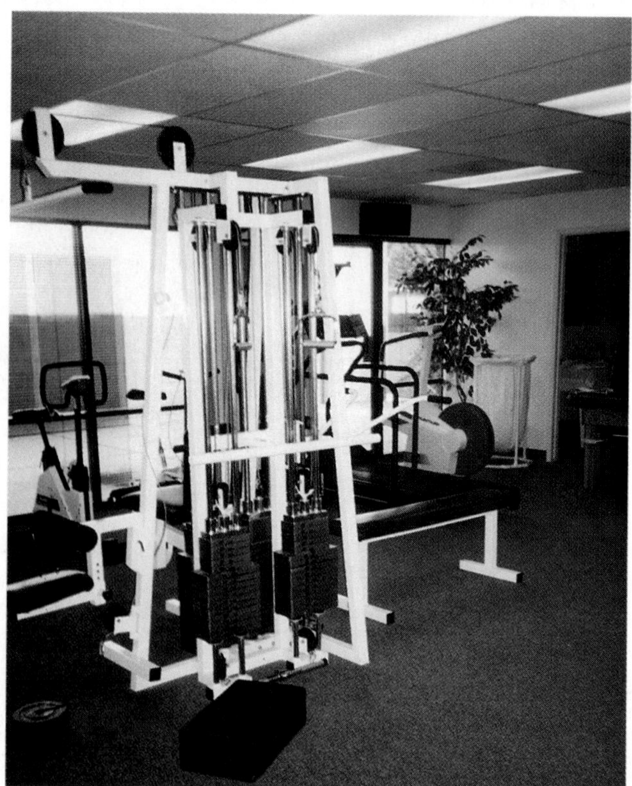

FIGURE 41–21 Active exercise equipment.

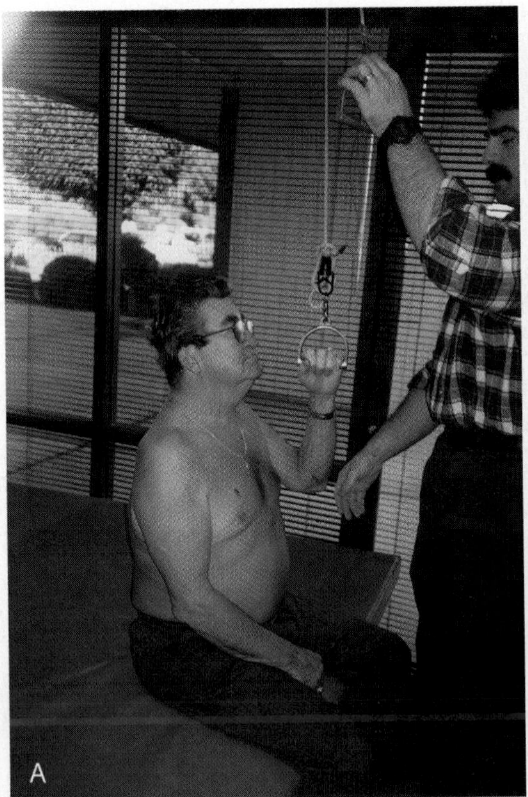

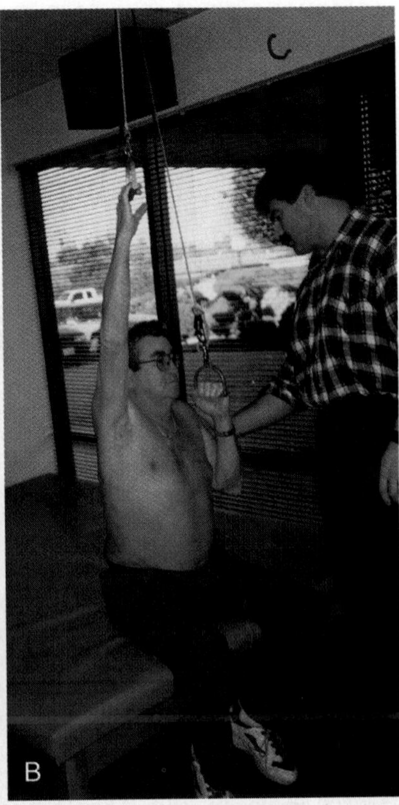

FIGURE 41–22 *A* and *B*, Passive exercise.

Passive Exercise

Passive exercise is moving a body part without the voluntary action of the patient. The movement is performed by someone other than the patient or by the force of a machine (Fig. 41–22).

Range-of-Motion (ROM) Exercises

ROM exercises are specially designed exercises that move each joint of the body through its full range of motion. This form of exercise is discussed in Chapter 37.

MUSCLE TRAINING AND STRENGTH

Muscle training is used to teach patients to gain or regain use of their muscles. This training can involve rehabilitation of muscle control lost as a result of physical trauma or diseases, such as poliomyelitis or cerebral palsy, or learning to use crutches or a wheelchair. Endurance exercises are used in the rehabilitation of the patient whose goal is to return to an active life after a long and debilitating illness or injury.

Electromuscle Stimulators

These are low-voltage machines that create a controlled electric current similar to that coming from an ordinary wall outlet. These low-voltage currents are useful for stimulating the motor and sensory nerves supplying the muscles. Such stimulation provides a passive means of exercising a muscle when a patient cannot activate the muscle voluntarily because of nerve damage. The purpose of the treatment is to revitalize a muscle or prevent **atrophy** of normal muscle.

Small electrode pads are moistened with tap water to increase their contact with the patient's skin. The pads are held by the technician until they are strapped into place. The machine is then operated by passing electric currents into the patient's muscles. The path of the electric current varies, depending on the exact placement of the two pads. As the current is applied to the muscles, the various waves act like the body's own nerves, causing the muscles to contract and relax.

One type of therapeutic current can stimulate and exercise **denervated** muscles and, if applied often enough, maintain a nearly normal muscle tone. Stimulation is also beneficial in retraining a patient to use injured muscles. The current artificially contracts and relaxes the muscles, and the patient is able to remember the feel of moving the body part. This often produces spectacular results and demonstrates to the patient that a muscle is not dead but can be revitalized.

Memory Jogger

14 *What is the primary purpose of the electromuscle stimulator treatment?*

RELIEF OF TENSION AND PAIN

A growing branch of medicine and physical therapy employs exercise to relax the muscles and to provide relief from tension and pain resulting from stress or a wide variety of physical disorders.

Pain Control

Such techniques as relaxation, massage, the application of heat and liniments mechanical electric stimulation, acupuncture, and hypnosis are used for pain control. Mechanical electric stimulation was introduced 100 years ago as an analgesic. It was regarded as **quackery** at that time, even though some patients reported pain relief. Acupuncture, adapted from ancient Chinese techniques, has received wide acceptance during the past few decades. Along with acupuncture, hypnosis has proved helpful in pain relief for many patients. During the past 15 years, the effectiveness of relaxation exercises, heat, and massage for pain relief has been explained scientifically.

There are several theories about pain and its control. The gate theory offers one possible explanation. In 1937, Ronald Melzack and Patrick Wall hypothesized that pain signals can be modified by a hypothetical gate in the spinal cord that opens and closes. Gentle stimulation causes impulses to travel so fast that they rush ahead and close the gate, which keeps the pain signals from reaching the brain.

Since this theory was first proposed, we have learned that our bodies contain morphine-like substances called *cephalins* and *endorphins.* These two analgesic substances are found naturally in the brain and spinal cord and appear to block the transmission of pain signals upward along the spinal cord to the brain. Another discovery is that certain thick sensory fibers extending from tactile receptors in the skin can compete with and suppress the transmission of pain to the brain from the thinner nerve fibers.

The most significant number of chronic pain sufferers seen in the medical office are those with muscle or joint pain such as arthritis, bursitis, and low back pain. All the physical pain control techniques previously mentioned have been useful in treating these conditions. *Intractable pain* is defined as that which cannot be relieved except through the use of addicting drugs or incapacitating sedation. The patient with chronic, prolonged, unrelenting pain becomes a slave to the torment. Indeed, pain may destroy a person's personality or life productivity. Until the last decade, intractable pain was managed by surgical excision of the sensory nerve pathways (pain receptors) to the brain.

For the patient with intractable pain, the electric muscle stimulator can increase blood flow through the area and relieve pain. The TENS-PAC is one type of stimulator that transmits electric stimulation to the patient's nerves by touching the skin (Fig. 41–23) and is called a transcutaneous electric nerve stimulator. Patients can be taught to use this device at home.

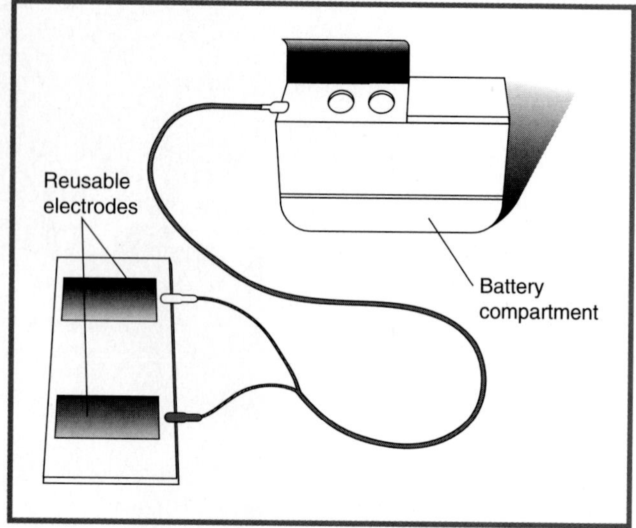

FIGURE 41–23 Small, portable TENS-PAC is prescribed by physicians to help control acute pain.

Massage

Massage is a form of passive exercise that relieves tension and pain. Massage activates the thicker tactile receptors in the skin, which compete with the pain signals. The systematic, therapeutic stroking or kneading of the body or a body part can effectively relieve localized pain as well as pain at a distant site (Fig. 41–24).

The medical assistant is usually not asked to apply therapeutic massages to patients, but you should be familiar with the terminology used.

TERMINOLOGY OF THERAPEUTIC MASSAGES

Effleurage is a stroking movement. In natural childbirth, a light circular stroke of the lower

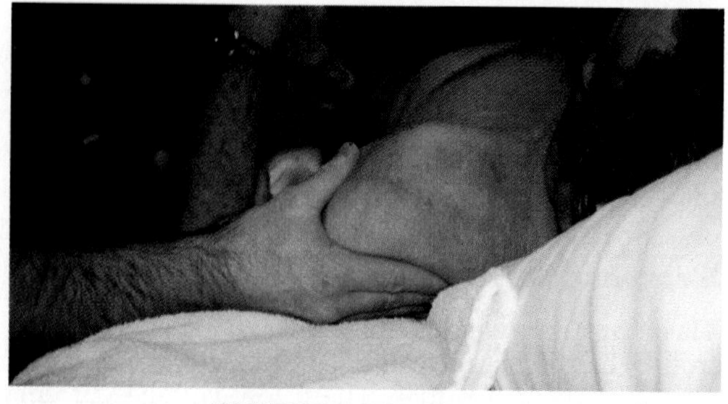

FIGURE 41–24 Massage.

abdomen is done in a rhythm with controlled breathing to aid in the relaxation of the abdominal muscles.

Friction is deep stroking or rubbing that involves deeper tissues. The traditional back rub uses friction.

Pétrissage is a kneading or rolling type of massage with pressing of the muscles. It is also called *foulage.*

Tapotement is a rapidly repeated, light percussion or tapping done with the sides of the hands. It may be called vibratory if it is done with a vibratory instrument or a sound.

Memory Jogger

15 *Is massage considered a form of active or passive exercise?*

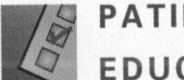

PATIENT EDUCATION

The reasons for patient education can be divided into two categories: to assist you in performing the procedure and to obtain the best possible results. In addition, the informed patient is better prepared to continue with the intervention at home when this is needed. When you work with the physician and the therapist in helping the patient, you become an integral part of the health care team. This type of involvement leads to patient satisfaction and personal achievement.

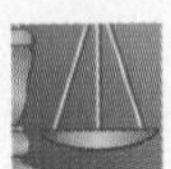

LEGAL AND ETHICAL ISSUES

The procedures described in this chapter are not the basic procedures that the medical assistant will be required to perform when first securing a position in a medical facility. These techniques all involve additional training and practice. Before performing any of the described procedures, it is strongly recommended that you check with your local or state medical assistant organization regarding the laws in your state. Whenever you perform the techniques described in this chapter, you are responsible for the procedures. Remember the following:

1. You must have a written order before doing the procedure.
2. You must follow the procedure as it is ordered.
3. Never advise the patient without permission.
4. Reinforce the instructions given to the patient by the physician or therapist.
5. If you have a concern about the procedure, discuss it with the physician or therapist privately before proceeding with the test.

Always remember, you are *assisting* with this procedure. If you keep this foremost in your mind, you will stay within the law and ethics of your state and your association.

CRITICAL THINKING

1 A patient is pregnant and has fallen and broken her arm. She must have a radiograph and is very concerned about the effects on her unborn child. What might you tell her?

2 You are instructed to massage a patient's leg to relieve a severe leg cramp. What type of massage would you use?

HOW DID I DO? Answers to Memory Joggers

1 A contrast medium is a radiopaque substance used in diagnostic radiology.

2 Isotopes are used to trace and evaluate the cause of a health problem.

3 The CT scan is 100 times more sensitive than the conventional x-ray film.

4 MRI is regarded as superior over the CT scan for all nervous system imaging.

5 Thermography is a heat-sensing technique used primarily in the detection of tumors.

6 A lead apron is used to protect the reproductive organs.

7 The posterior aspect of the body faces the x-ray tube and the anterior aspect faces the film.

8 X-ray films belong to the medical office where the films were taken.

9 Heat application depends on the type of heat used, length of time the heat was applied, general condition of the patient, and size of the area needing treatment.

10 Moist heat penetrates better than dry heat.

11 Short-wave diathermy treatments may be prescribed as often as three times a week for 20 to 30 minutes.

12 A coupling agent may be a gel, lotion, or water. It is used to achieve better contact with the skin.

13 An exercise program may restore mobility, improve coordination, strengthen a body part, or give relaxation and relief of tension and pain.

14 The purpose of the electromuscle stimulator treatment is to revitalize a muscle or prevent atrophy of normal muscle.

15 Massage is a form of passive exercise.

Assisting in the Clinical Laboratory

42

OUTLINE

LEARNING OBJECTIVES

Cognitive: On successful completion of this chapter you should be able to:

1. Discuss your role in coordinating laboratory tests and results.
2. List the 12 departments found in most laboratories.
3. State the safety rules for the laboratory.
4. Identify CLIA's three categories of laboratory testing.
5. Define the objective of quality assurance.
6. Explain quality-control guidelines.
7. List the elements that are included in every laboratory request form.
8. Give five reasons that physicians order laboratory tests.
9. State the medical assistant's responsibilities in specimen collection.
10. Identify the parts of a microscope.
11. Discuss legal and ethical issues in laboratory testing.
12. Define and spell vocabulary terms.

Performance: On successful completion of this chapter you should be able to:

1. Focus a microscope under low power, high power, and oil immersion.

VOCABULARY

aliquot A portion of a well-mixed sample that is removed for testing

antibody An immunoglobulin produced by lymphoid tissue in response to substances interpreted as foreign invaders gaining entry into the body

cerebrospinal fluid Fluid within the subarachnoid space, the central canal of the spinal cord, and the four ventricles of the brain

exudates Fluids with a high concentration of protein and cellular debris that has escaped from the blood vessels and has been deposited in tissues or on tissue surfaces

hematoma A tumor or sac filled with blood that may be the result of trauma; a localized collection of clotted blood caused by a broken vessel

hemolyzed A blood sample in which the red cells have been ruptured

preservatives Substances added to a specimen to prevent deterioration of cells or chemicals in the specimen

quality assurance A law-enforced program that guarantees quality patient care

quality control The operational procedures used to implement the quality assurance program

reference values The listings of accepted ranges for normal values for routine hematology tests

requisition A formal written request from the physician, authorizing a laboratory to perform testing procedures

specimen A sample of body fluid, waste product, or tissue that is collected for analysis

stat Do immediately (from the Latin word *statin,* meaning "at once")

The Laboratory

The laboratory is the place where a **specimen** is tested, analyzed, and evaluated. Precise measurements are made, and the results are then calculated and interpreted. Tests are performed manually (by hand) or through automation (by using specialized instruments).

Medical laboratories are located in either hospitals or nonhospital facilities. Nonhospital facilities include physician's offices, clinics, public health departments, health maintenance organizations, and private reference laboratories. The head of a laboratory is the *pathologist,* a physician specially trained in the nature and cause of disease. The laboratory is divided into various departments, which may include hematology, chemistry, microbiology, specimen collection and processing, blood bank, coagulation, serology, histology, cytology, toxicology, urinalysis, and special chemistry. The laboratory in the physician's office usually performs procedures in urinalysis, hematology, chemistry, and microbiology.

URINALYSIS Urinalysis includes the physical, chemical, and microscopic examination of urine. In the physical examination, the color, transparency, and specific gravity are noted. Chemical analysis is performed to measure levels of glucose, protein, ketones, blood, bilirubin, urobilinogen, nitrites, and pH. Microscopically, the urine is examined for the presence of red, white, and epithelial cells, mucus, casts, crystals, yeasts, parasites, and bacteria.

HEMATOLOGY Whole blood is the specimen used for the majority of the tests performed. The numbers of *leukocytes* (white blood cells), *erythrocytes* (red blood cells), and *thrombocytes* (platelets) are actually counted. Observation is also made of the size, shape, and maturity level of these blood components. The results of these tests are used to diagnose anemias, leukemias, and clotting disorders.

CHEMISTRY Tests are usually performed on *serum,* the liquid part of blood left after a clot has formed. Urine and other body fluids may also be tested. The most common procedures performed measure levels of glucose (to determine blood sugar levels), enzymes (to determine heart damage), and electrolytes (to determine sodium, chloride, potassium, and bicarbonate levels).

MICROBIOLOGY Organisms are grown and identified from blood, urine, sputum, and wound specimens. Susceptibility testing is then performed on these organisms to determine proper antibiotic therapy. Microbiology deals with the study of bacteria, fungi, yeasts, parasites, and viruses.

Memory Jogger

What procedures are usually performed in the physician's office laboratory?

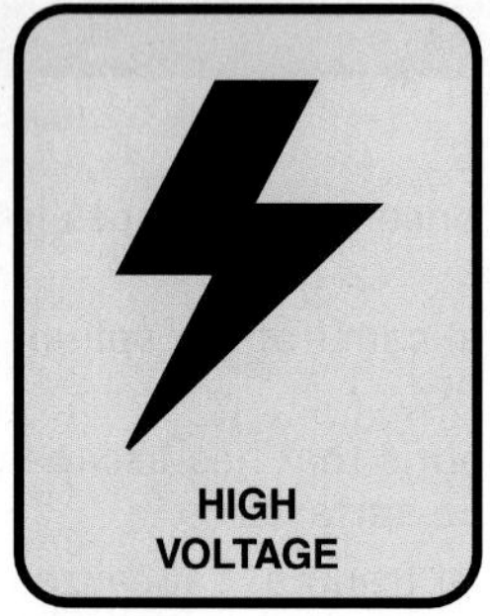

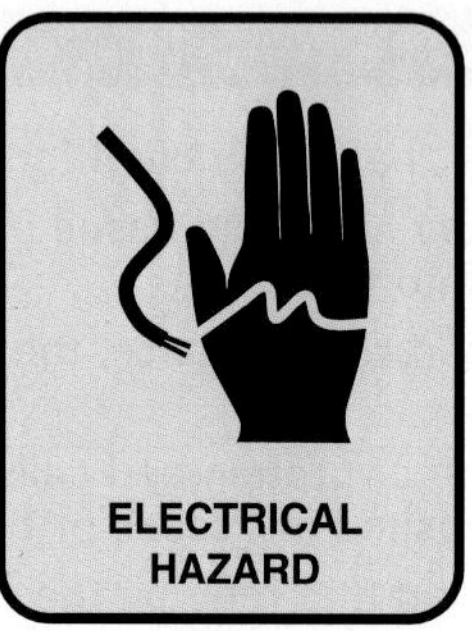

FIGURE 42–1 High voltage and electrical hazard labels. (From Stepp CA, Woods MA: Laboratory Procedures for Medical Office Personnel. Philadelphia, WB Saunders, 1998.)

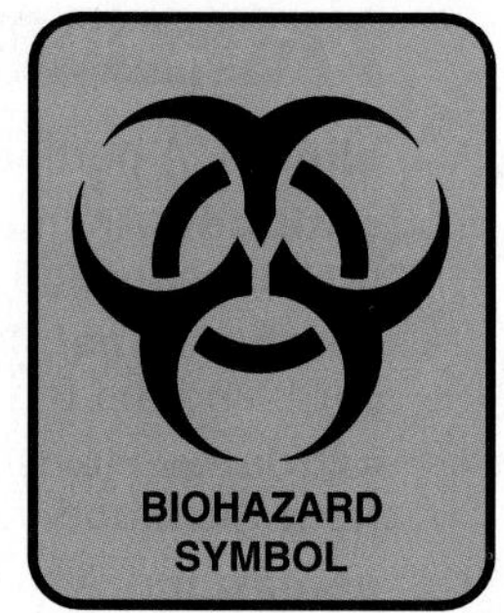

FIGURE 42–3 Biohazard symbol. (From Stepp CA, Woods MA: Laboratory Procedures for Medical Office Personnel. Philadelphia, WB Saunders, 1998.)

Laboratory Safety

Basic safety rules must be observed at all times in the laboratory to avoid personal injury and to prevent equipment damage. Any accident must be reported to the physician or supervisor. Hazards in the laboratory can be classified as either physical, chemical, or biohazard.

PHYSICAL HAZARDS Physical hazards include fires resulting from electrical malfunction or alcohol lamps. Open flames are no longer used in modern laboratories. All personnel must be familiar with the location of fire extinguishers and fire escape routes. Keep all electric equipment in proper repair, and always follow manufacturers' instructions (Fig. 42–1).

CHEMICAL HAZARDS Chemical hazards include contact with corrosives and toxic or carcinogenic substances. Caution should be taken in handling all chemicals and specimens to avoid spills and splashes. Skin or eyes that come into contact with any chemicals must be immediately washed with water for at least 5 minutes (Fig. 42–2).

BIOHAZARDS Biohazards can result from the use of specimens and reagents capable of transmitting disease. Potentially infective biohazard specimens include blood, body tissue biopsy specimens, urine, **exudates,** and bacterial cultures and smears. The laboratory work area must be disinfected before and after each use when dealing with biohazards. Eating, drinking, smoking, or mouth pipetting is not allowed. Gloves and laboratory aprons or coats should be worn. Specimens and any contaminated materials must be disposed of through sterilization or incineration. Hands must be washed before and after every procedure. Extreme caution and common sense are essential at all times in the laboratory. Regulations and precautions must be followed consistently (Fig. 42–3).

LABORATORY RULES

- No eating, drinking, or smoking.
- Keep pens, pencils, and fingers away from mouth and eyes.
- Pull long hair back and up.
- Report all accidents to physician or supervisor.
- Wear laboratory coat or apron.
- Wipe spills and splashes immediately.
- Wash hands before and after every procedure.
- Follow manufacturer's instructions for equipment operation.
- Know the location of all safety equipment and supplies and fire escape routes.
- Wear protective gloves and safety glasses.
- Avoid wearing chains, rings, bracelets, and other loose hanging jewelry.
- Clean work area before and after every procedure.

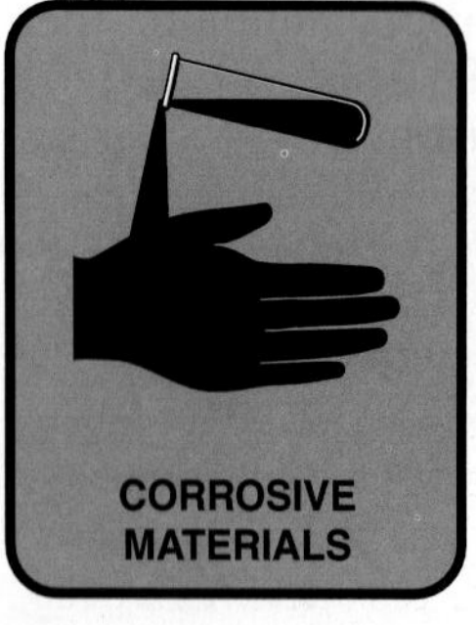

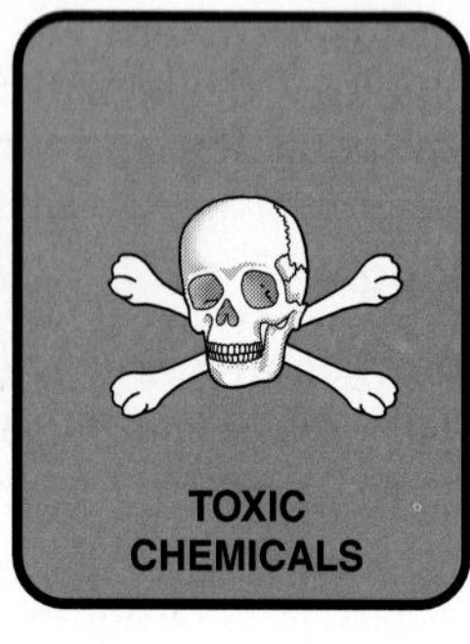

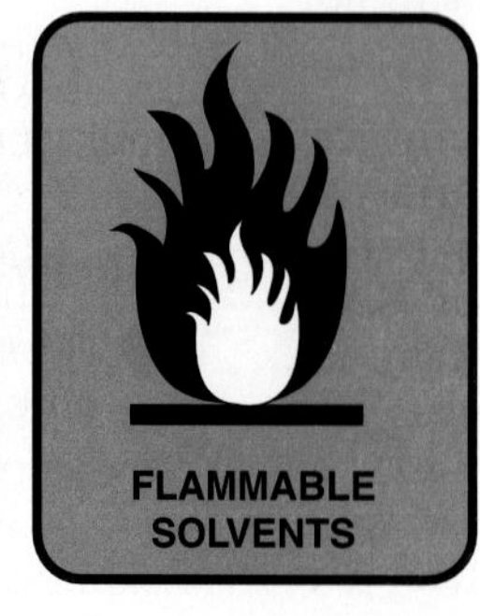

FIGURE 42–2 Chemical hazard warning labels. (From Stepp CA, Woods MA: Laboratory Procedures for Medical Office Personnel. Philadelphia, WB Saunders, 1998.)

- Disinfect or sterilize specimens and materials contaminated with blood or microorganisms.
- Never store food and beverages in laboratory refrigerator.
- Repair malfunctioning equipment immediately.
- Be familiar with appropriate first-aid procedures.
- Properly ground all electric equipment.
- Clearly and accurately label all reagents and solutions.

Memory Jogger

Name the three classifications of laboratory hazards.

CLIA Mandate

In 1988, Congress passed the Clinical Laboratory Improvement Amendments (CLIA '88) to improve the quality of laboratory testing in the United States (Fig. 42–4). The CLIA regulations established three categories of laboratory testing based on the complexity of the testing methods:

1. *Low-complexity test:* Laboratories that perform only this level of testing must apply for a certificate of waiver. There are only nine waived laboratory tests:
   a. Dipstick or tablet reagent urinalysis (nonautomated) for bilirubin, glucose, hemoglobin, ketones, leukocytes, nitrite, pH, protein, specific gravity, and urobilinogen
   b. Fecal occult blood tests
   c. Ovulation testing, using visual color comparison
   d. Urine pregnancy tests using visual color comparison
   e. Erythrocyte sedimentation rate, nonautomated
   f. Hemoglobin by copper sulfate method, nonautomated
   g. Spun microhematocrit
   h. Blood glucose determination with devices approved by the Food and Drug Administration for home use (performed in almost all physician's office laboratories)
2. *Moderate-complexity tests:* This area accounts for approximately 75% of all laboratory tests done in the United States and about 10% of physician's office laboratories.
3. *High-complexity tests:* These include all procedures related to cytogenetics, histopathology, histocompatibility, and cytology (including Papanicolaou testing). These tests are not generally performed in physician's office laboratories.

Laboratories performing moderate- and/or high-complexity tests must meet the CLIA regulations and are subject to unannounced inspections every 2 years. The major components of the CLIA '88 regulations relating to laboratory standards are

- Patient Test Management
- Quality Control
- Quality Assurance
- Proficiency Testing
- Personnel Requirements

Memory Jogger

Name the three categories of laboratory testing identified by CLIA regulations.

QUALITY ASSURANCE

Quality assurance (QA) is the pledge of health care professionals to work to achieve the highest degree of excellence in the health care given every patient. QA is a comprehensive set of policies and procedures developed to ensure the quality of laboratory testing. It includes quality control, personnel orientation, laboratory documentation, knowledge of laboratory instrumentation, and enrollment in a proficiency testing program. QA focuses on establishing a series of operating procedures to produce reliable laboratory results for the benefit of the patient, the physician, and the medical assistant who does the laboratory testing.

These policies benefit the physician by reducing the liability for inaccurate reporting of test results. For a physician to use a laboratory test in diagnosing, the results must be compared with **reference values.** There also must be a way of assessing how well the care given to the patient measures up with the reference values. The QA system enables the laboratory to assess, verify, and document the quality of the test results. This documentation is a way of comparing "what is" with "what should be."

QUALITY CONTROL

The objective of **quality control** in the laboratory is to ensure the *accuracy* of test results while detecting and eliminating error. Physician's office laboratories play a vital part in QA because patient treatment is often based on or reinforced by results of laboratory tests. Mandated by law, quality control programs monitor all aspects of laboratory activity, from specimen collection through the processing, testing, and reporting steps. Programs check supplies, reagents, machinery, personnel, and actual test performance.

HIGHLIGHTS OF CLIA 1988

Purpose of CLIA 1988

In 1988, Congress passed the Clinical Laboratory Improvement Amendments (CLIA 1988) to improve the quality of laboratory testing in the United States. CLIA 1988 consists of federal regulations governing all facilities that perform laboratory tests for health assessment or for the diagnosis, prevention, or treatment of disease. CLIA 1988 includes facilities not previously covered under federal legislation, such as physician's office laboratories (POLs) and nursing homes. The regulations for implementing CLIA, developed by the Department of Health and Human Services (DHHS), consist of four separate sets of rules: laboratory standards, application and user fees, enforcement procedures, and approval of accreditation programs.

Categories of Laboratory Testing

The CLIA regulations establish three categories of laboratory testing based on the complexity of the testing methods:

Low-Complexity Tests: Low-complexity tests are simple procedures, including those that patients can perform at home. Laboratories that perform only low-complexity tests must apply for a certificate of waiver, which exempts them from many of the CLIA oversight requirements. Laboratories with certificates of waiver are still expected to adhere to good laboratory practices, which include following the manufacturer's recommended instructions for each product or testing kit. There are only nine waived laboratory tests:

- Dipstick or tablet reagent urinalysis (nonautomated) for bilirubin, glucose, hemoglobin, ketones, leukocytes, nitrite, pH, protein, specific gravity, and urobilinogen
- Fecal occult blood tests
- Ovulation testing, using visual color comparisons
- Urine pregnancy tests, using visual color comparisons
- Erythrocyte sedimentation rate, nonautomated
- Hemoglobin by copper sulfate method, nonautomated
- Spun microhematocrit
- Blood glucose determination with devices approved by the FDA for home use

Moderate-Complexity Tests: Moderate-complexity tests account for 75 percent of the estimated 10,000 laboratory tests performed in the United States. Examples of moderate-complexity tests performed in the medical office include throat cultures, white blood counts, rapid strep tests, cholesterol, HDL and triglyceride testing with an automated analyzer, Gram staining, urine cultures, pinworm preps, and microscopic analysis of urine sediment.

High-Complexity Tests: High-complexity tests include all procedures related to cytogenetics, histopathology, histocompatibility, and cytology (includes PAP testing). These tests are not usually performed in medical offices; most of these tests are done in laboratories already subject to federal regulation.

Requirements for Moderate- and High-Complexity Testing

Laboratories performing moderate- or high-complexity tests, or both, must meet the CLIA regulations and are subject to unannounced inspections every 2 years by the Department of Health and Human Services. The major components of the CLIA 1988 regulations relating to laboratory standards are listed here:

Patient Test Management: A system must be established to maintain the optimal integrity and identification of patient specimens throughout the testing process and to ensure accurate reporting of results.

Quality Control: To ensure accurate and reliable test results, each laboratory must establish and follow written quality control procedures that monitor and evaluate the quality of each testing process. These include developing a laboratory procedure manual, following the manufacturer's instructions for each product; performing and documenting calibration procedures at least every 6 months and two levels of controls daily; performing and documenting actions taken when problems or errors are identified; and documenting all quality control activities.

Quality Assurance: Each laboratory must establish and follow written policies and procedures to monitor the overall quality of the total testing process.

Proficiency Testing (PT): Proficiency testing is a form of external quality control in which laboratory specimens are prepared by an approved proficiency testing agency. Three times a year, the physician's laboratory must test a shipment of these unknown specimens using the same procedure as for testing a patient's specimen. The results are then forwarded to the proficiency testing agency for evaluation.

Personnel Requirements: The CLIA regulations specify qualifications and responsibilities for personnel for laboratory directors, technical consultants, clinical consultants, and testing personnel. The regulations list specific education and training qualifications for the various positions and also define the responsibilities for the persons who fill these positions. Personnel requirements are most stringent for high-complexity testing.

FIGURE 42-4 Clinical Laboratory Improvement Amendment of 1988 (CLIA '88) regulations. (From Stepp CA, Woods MA: Laboratory Procedures for Medical Office Personnel. Philadelphia, WB Saunders, 1998.)

Without a quality control program, laboratory error is difficult to detect unless the physician would notice test results inconsistent with a patient's history. Undetected laboratory errors may harm patients by delaying appropriate treatment or leading to inappropriate treatment.

Memory Jogger

List the laboratory activities that are monitored by quality control programs.

Quality Control Guidelines

Specially prepared *quality control samples* are tested daily along with patient samples. The results of testing performed on the quality control samples must be within a preestablished range before the patient results can be reported. The quality control samples, called *controls,* are usually supplied with prepackaged kits intended for use in the small laboratory. The controls should be analyzed at specified intervals. For example, positive and negative controls supplied with pregnancy test kits should be performed with each patient specimen. Urinalysis dipsticks (used for chemical examination of urine) should be checked daily and each time a new container is opened. Controls for automated chemistry analyses should be performed at specified intervals during the day. Consistent results of controls ensure constant conditions throughout the testing sequence.

Memory Jogger

Why is it necessary to test prepared quality control samples daily?

Laboratory instrument standardization is important to ensure proper operation and accurate test results. Preventive maintenance prolongs the life of your equipment and reduces breakdowns; it includes daily cleaning and adjusting and replacing parts when necessary. Each instrument should have a log or worksheet to record all changes, including daily maintenance. See the following guidelines for a preventive maintenance program.

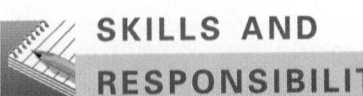

SKILLS AND RESPONSIBILITIES

GUIDELINES FOR A PREVENTIVE MAINTENANCE PROGRAM

- Follow the manufacturer's instructions for calibration of instruments.
- Read and understand instructions for routine instrument care.
- Perform all preventive maintenance provided by manufacturer's instructions.
- Keep all spare parts available for immediate use.
- Record the name, address, and phone number of a contact person for maintenance or repair.
- Create a maintenance form or use the one provided.

Accurate record keeping is one of the key responsibilities of the medical assistant. A variety of forms are available to assist in recording laboratory information. The primary record is the laboratory master log book in which each procedure performed in the physician's office laboratory is entered with dates clearly shown. Every day that patient tests are performed quality-control tests must also be performed. The results of standardization tests and dates when new control vials are begun must be entered along with the expiration dates of the controls. The records must be retained for a period of years, the exact number determined by state laws and CLIA '88 mandate (Fig. 42–5). Employee records must be kept confidential and maintained for 30 years.

EXAMPLE OF WHAT TO INCLUDE IN AN EMPLOYEE RECORD

- employee name and Social Security number
- Hepatitis B virus status
- Copy of *all* results of examinations, medical testing, and follow up necessitated by an exposure incident
- Employer's copy of the examining health care professional's opinion in regard to the exposure

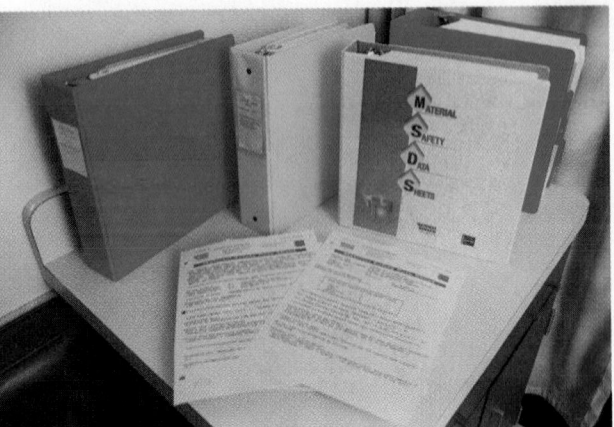

FIGURE 42–5 Material safety data sheets for quality control record keeping.

PERSONNEL REQUIREMENTS

Laboratory tests are performed by professionally trained medical technologists, medical laboratory technicians, and other allied health care personnel. The *medical technologist (MT)* has a bachelor's degree and 1 year of clinical training. The *medical laboratory technician (MLT)* has 1 year of college and 1 year of clinical training. Both become certified by the successful completion of a national certifying examination. In addition to certification, many states monitor laboratory personnel by requiring state licensure.

The medical assistant is a multiskilled professional who is trained to perform administrative and clinical procedures, including basic laboratory testing. Laboratory tests are an essential part of a medical diagnosis, an aid to treatment, and, frequently, a control of medication. Only a physician may request laboratory testing for a patient. You may be responsible for a number of these laboratory testing procedures. To assume this responsibility, you must know the normal range of these tests, proper patient preparation, and the procedure for each. The assistant must carefully follow all laboratory instructions in obtaining and labeling the specimens and sending them to the laboratory. There must be good communication among the patient, the office staff, and the laboratory personnel. The assistant should make patients feel more at ease with these procedures and, thus, elicit more cooperation.

It is the medical assistant's responsibility to alert the physician to any abnormal results or findings. This may be accomplished by either circling or underlining the abnormality in red. Laboratory results are not filed until they are reviewed by the physician. Usually, the assistant contacts the patient concerning reports, follow-up procedures, and office visits.

Memory Jogger

6 *Who can request laboratory testing on a patient?*

SAFETY REQUIREMENTS

Hepatitis B and the acquired immunodeficiency syndrome (AIDS) are a constant threat to the health and safety of clinical laboratory personnel. Hepatitis B and AIDS are both transmitted through exposure to blood and body fluids. Blood and body fluids are the primary substances handled in the laboratory. The Occupational Safety and Health Administration (OSHA) mandated the Bloodborne Pathogens (BBP) Standard, which covers all employees who could be "reasonably anticipated as the result of performing their job duties to face contact with blood and other potentially infectious materials." The BBP Standard requires that the laboratory employer have a written exposure control plan.

EXPOSURE CONTROL PLAN REQUIREMENTS

- Identification of tasks, procedures, and job classification where possible occupational exposure to blood may occur.
- Establishment of methods that protect employees and comply with OSHA regulations.
- Implementation of a vaccination program for hepatitis B virus.
- Provision of training in the proper use of protective equipment regarding bloodborne pathogens.
- Maintainance of records to show compliance with the BBP Standard.

OSHA compliance regulations are grouped into four areas, which are covered in Chapter 26.

In addition to blood and blood products, the BBP Standard includes "other potentially infectious materials" (OPIM). Urine is the only fluid that is not specifically included in OSHA's BBP Standard. Because blood and blood elements are frequently associated with urine, it must be included and considered as a possible source of exposure.

OTHER POTENTIALLY INFECTIOUS MATERIALS

- Semen
- Cerebrospinal fluid
- Pleural fluid
- Amniotic fluid
- Contaminated body fluid
- Human tissue samples
- Hepatitis B virus cultures
- Vaginal secretions
- Synovial fluid
- Pericardial fluid
- Saliva in dental procedures
- Unknown body secretions
- Human immunodeficiency virus (HIV) cultures
- Blood, organs, and tissues from experimental animals

SAFETY GUIDELINES FOR OTHER POTENTIALLY INFECTIOUS MATERIALS

- Handle and process all specimens as if they contain infectious material.
- Wipe the outside of specimen containers with a germicide (see Chapter 26).
- Dispose of all infectious materials following state and federal guidelines.

- Clean up spills using a disinfectant (see Chapter 26).
- Immediately dispose of any chipped or broken glassware in a special disposable container.

Memory Jogger

7 *Is it mandatory for a physician's office laboratory to have a hepatitis B virus immunization program?*

Key to Prevention

There should be absolutely no doubt that hand washing is the key in the prevention of infection (Fig. 42–6). It is the single most effective way of preventing the spread of all infections. Proper hand washing protects you, your patient, and your coworkers because it removes organisms. In the laboratory area it is absolutely required to *wash your hands:*

- When you enter and before leaving this area
- Before and after every patient procedure
- After contact with body fluid even if gloves were worn
- Before and after eating
- Before and after using the rest room

Fire Safety

Fires in the laboratory are not uncommon but are seldom major. Most fires occur in laboratories that use open flames such as Bunsen burners. Every employee working in the laboratory area should be responsible for returning all flammable chemicals to a flameproof cabinet that is located away from all heat sources. If an open flame is to be used, care should be taken to ensure that any loose clothing or long hair does not catch fire. Fire extinguishers should be ready for use at all times and all employees should know how to use them. Fire safety signs should be mounted for quick and easy identification of fire extinguisher, fire escape, and fire alarm (Fig. 42–7).

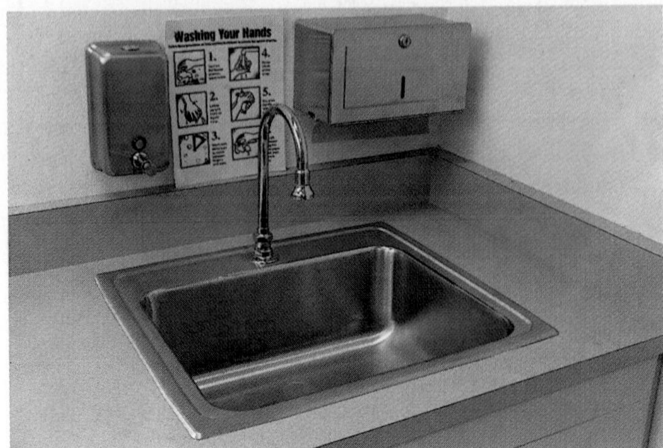

FIGURE 42–6 Sink with soap dispenser. (From Stepp CA, Woods MA: Laboratory Procedures for Medical Office Personnel. Philadelphia, WB Saunders, 1998.)

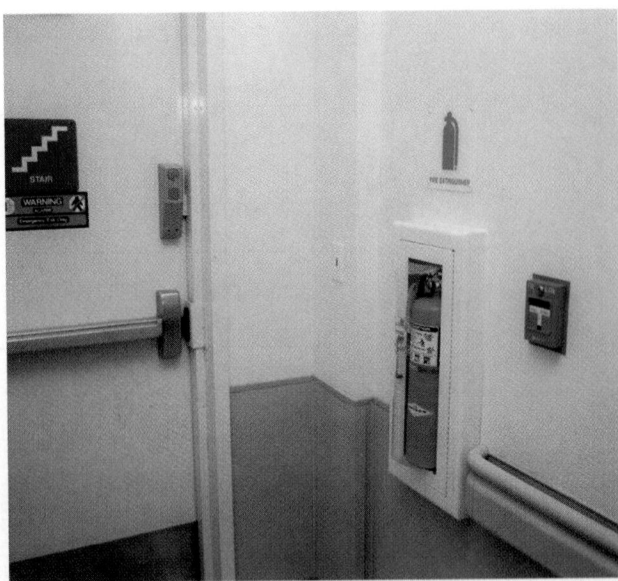

FIGURE 42–7 Fire safety location. Exit, alarm, and extinguisher are clearly labeled and identified.

Laboratory Requests and Reports

A patient's medical record should be maintained in an organized manner to promote easy access to the desired information. There are various methods used when filing laboratory reports in a patient's medical record. Many offices compile records in a set order so that the laboratory report sheets follow entry A and precede entry B. Another method is to use standard-size sheets of a specific color and stagger the reports from the bottom of the sheet upward (Fig. 42–8).

In the source-oriented medical record all like reports are filed in one section. For example, all laboratory reports are together, all surgical reports are together, and all electrocardiographic reports are together. The latest test is on the top, because it is the most important for the patient's current care and treatment.

In the problem-oriented medical record, all test results are entered and recorded in the objective part of the progress notes, preceded by the number and title of the particular problem.

Your responsibility is to make sure that all reports are received for diagnostic tests performed on the patient outside the physician's office. Only after the physician reviews the test results should you file them into the patient's record.

LABORATORY REPORTS

Specimen: BLOOD
Collected: 01/16/97 0840

Result name	Abnormal	Result	Normal Range
WBC		6.8	4.5-11.0 X(10)3
RBC		4.45	4.2-5.4 X(10)6
Hgb		14.0	12-16 g/dL
Hct		40.1	37-47 %
MCV		90.1	81-99 fL
MCH		31.4	28.0-32.0 pg
MCHC		34.9	31.5-35.5 g/dL
RDW		13.0	11.5-14.5 %
Platelet		288	150-400 X(10)3
MPV		8.5	7.4-10.4 fL
Lymph - %		32.3	20-43 %
Mono		6.5	0-8 %
Gran		60.3	51-74 %
Eos		0.9	0-5 %
Baso		0.0	0-1 %
Lymph - Absolute		2.2	1.0-4.7 X(10)3
Mono		0.4	0.1-1.0 X(10)3
Gran		4.1	2.6-8.2 X(10)3
Eos		0.1	< 0.7 X(10)3
Baso		0.0	< 0.2 X(10)3
RBC Morphology		Normal	Normal
WBC Morphology		Normal	Normal

************************ CBC, AUTOMATED DIFFERENTIAL ****************************

************************ METABOLIC STATUS PANEL ********************************

*************************** URINALYSIS ************************************

Thompson, Alexis
Patient

746-25-1111
Number

Dr. Samual Panda, inc.
0000 E. North Avenue
Juno, Maine 99385

FIGURE 42–8 Report record. Blood test results are pink and urine test results are yellow for quick identification.

Lab Services

IMPORTANT
Patient instructions and map on back

PHYSICIAN ORDERS

Patient ______ (Last Name) ______ (First) ___ (M.I.) D.O.B. ______ M ☐ F ☐ Patient SS# ______
Address ______ City ______ Zip ______ Phone # ______
Physician ______
ATTACH COPY OF INSURANCE CARD
Date & Time of Collection: ______ ______
Drawing Facility: ______
Diagnosis/ICD-9 Code ______ (Additional codes on reverse)

☐ 769.00 Abdominal Pain
☐ 285.9 Anemia (NOS)
☐ 414.9 Coronary Artery Disease (CAD)
☐ 250.0 DM (diabetes mellitus)
☐ 780.7 Fatigue/Malaise
☐ 272.0 Hypercholesterolemia
☐ 244.9 Hypothyroidism
☐ 272.4 Hyperlipidemia
☐ 401.9 Hypertension
☐ 465.9 URI (upper respiratory infection)

☐ ROUTINE ☐ PHONE RESULTS TO: # ______
☐ ASAP ☐ FAX RESULTS TO: # ______
☐ STAT ☐ COPY TO: ______

HEMATOLOGY
☐ 1021 CBC, Automated Diff (incl. Platelet Ct.)
☐ 1023 Hemoglobin/Hematocrit
☐ 1020 Hemogram
☐ 1025 Platelet Count
☐ 1150 Pro Time Diagnostic
☐ 1151 Pro Time, Therapeutic
☐ 1155 PTT
☐ 1315 Reticulocyte Count
☐ 1310 Sed Rate/Westergren

URINE
☐ 1059 Urinalysis
☐ 1062 Urinalysis w/Culture if indicated
Urine-24 Hr ______ Spot ______
Ht. ______ Wt. ______
☐ 3033 Creatinine
☐ 3036 Creatinine Clearance (also requires blood)
☐ 3398 Protein
☐ 3096 Sodium/Potassium
☐ Microalbumin 24 Hr ____ Spot ____

SEROLOGY
☐ 8020 ANA (Antinuclear Antibody)
☐ 8040 Mono Spot
☐ 3494 Rheumatoid Factor
☐ 8010 RPR
☐ 5365 Rubella

CHEMISTRY
☐ 5550 Alpha Fetoprotein, Prenatal
☐ 3000 Amylase
☐ 3153 B12/Folate
☐ 3156 Beta HCG, Quantitative
☐ 3321 Bilirubin, Total
☐ 3324 Bilirubin, Total/Direct
☐ 3009 BUN
☐ 3159 CEA
☐ 3348 Cholesterol
☐ 3030 Creatinine, Serum
☐ 3509 Digoxin (recommend 12 hrs., after dose)
☐ 3515 Dilantin
☐ 3168 Ferritin
☐ 3193 FSH
☐ 3066 ▼ Glucose, Fasting
☐ 3061 Glucose, 1° Post 50 g Glucola
☐ 3075 ▼ Glucose, 2° Post Glucola
☐ 3060 Glucose, 2° Post Prandial (meal)
☐ 3049 ▼ Glucose Tolerance Oral GTT
☐ 3047 ▼Glucose Tolerance Gestational GTT
☐ 3650 Hemoglobin, A1C

CHEMISTRY
☐ 5232 HBsAg
☐ 3175 HIV (Consent required)
☐ 3581 Iron & Iron Binding Capacity
☐ 3195 LH
☐ 3590 Magnesium
☐ 3527 Phenobarbital
☐ 3095 Potassium
☐ 3689 Pregnancy Test, Serum (HCG, qual)
☐ 3653 Pregnancy Test, Urine
☐ 3197 Prolactin
☐ 3199 PSA
☐ 3339 SGOT/AST
☐ 3342 SGPT/ALT
☐ 3093 Sodium/Potassium, Serum
☐ 3510 Tegretol
☐ 3551 Theophylline
☐ 3333 Uric Acid

MICROBIOLOGY
Source ______
☐ 7240 Culture, AFB
☐ 7200 Culture, Blood x ______
☐ Draw Interval ______
☐ 7280 Culture, Fungus
☐ Culture, Routine
☐ 7005 Culture, Stool
☐ 7010 Culture, Throat
☐ 7000 Culture, Urine
☐ 7300 Gram Stain
☐ 7355 Occult Blood x ______
☐ 7365 Ova & Parasites x ______
☐ 7400 Smear & Suspension (includes Gram Stain/Wet Mount)
☐ 7060 Rapid Strep A Screen (Negs confir by cult)
☐ 7065 Rapid Strep A Screen only
☐ 7030 Beta Strep Culture
☐ 5207 GC by DNA Probe
☐ 5130 Chlamydia by DNA Probe
☐ 5555 Chlamydia/GC by DNA Probe
☐ 7375 Wright Stain, Stool

Additional Tests ______

PANELS & PROFILES
☐ ✗ 3309 CHEM 12 — Albumin, Alkaline Phosphatase, BUN, Calcium, Cholesterol, Glucose, LDH, Phosphorus, AST, Total Bilirubin, Total Protein, Uric Acid
☐ ▼ 3315 CHEM 20 — Chem 12, Electrolyte Panel, Creatinine, Iron, Gamma GT, ALT, Triglycerides
☐ ▼ 3357 CARDIAC RISK PANEL — Cholesterol, HDL, LDL, Risk Factors, VLDL, Triglycerides
☐ ✗ 3042 CRITICAL CARE PANEL — BUN, Chloride, CO2, Glucose, Potassium, Sodium
☐ 3046 ELECTROLYTE PANEL — Chloride, CO2, Potassium, Sodium
☐ ▼ 3399 EXECUTIVE PANEL — Chem 20, Iron, Cardiac Risk Panel, CBC, RPR, Thyroid Cascade
☐ 5242 HEPATITIS PANEL, ACUTE — HAVIgMAb, HBsAg, HBsAb, HBcAb, HCVAb
☐ ▼ 3355 LIPID MONITORING PANEL — Cholesterol, Triglycerides, HDL, LDL, VLDL, ALT, AST
☐ 3312 LIVER PANEL — Alkaline Phospatase, AST, Total Bilirubin, Gamma GT, Total Protein, Albumin, ALT
☐ ✗ 3083 METABOLIC STATUS PANEL — BUN, Osmolality (calculated), Chloride, CO2, Creatinine, Glucose, Potassium, Sodium, BUN/Creatinine, Ratio, Anion Gap
☐ ✗ 3376 PANEL B — Chem 12, CBC, Electrolyte Panel
☐ ▼ 3382 PANEL D — Chem 20, CBC, Thyroid Cascade
☐ ✗ 3386 PANEL F — Chem 12, CBC, Electrolyte Panel, Thyroid Cascade
☐ ▼ 3391 PANEL G — Chem 20, Cardiac Risk Panel, CBC, Thyroid Cascade
☐ ▼ 3393 PANEL H — Chem 20, CBC, Cardiac Risk Panel, Rheumatoid Factor, Thyroid Cascade
☐ ▼ 3397 PANEL J — Chem 20, Cardiac Risk Panel
☐ 5351 PRENATAL PANEL — Antibody Screen ABO/Rh, CBC, Rubella, HBsAg, RPR
☐ 1059 with Urinalysis, Routine
☐ 1062 with Urinalysis w/Culture if indicated
☐ ✗ 3102 RENAL PANEL — Metabolic Status Panel, Calcium, Phosphorus
☐ 3188 THYROID CASCADE — TSH, Reflex Testing

▼ - patient **required** to fast for 12-14 hours
✗ - patient recommended to fast 12-14 hours

LAB USE ONLY INIT ______
☐ SST ☐ PLASMA
☐ PURPLE ☐ SERUM
☐ YELLOW ☐ SWAB
☐ BLUE ☐ SLIDES
☐ GREEN ☐ DNA PROBE
☐ GREY ☐ B. CULT BTLS
☐ URINE
☐ BLACK
☐ OTHER: ______
REC'V. SPECIMEN: ☐ FROZEN
☐ AMBIENT ☐ ON ICE

Special Instructions/Pertinent Clinical Information ______
Physician's Signature ______ **Date** ______
These orders may be FAXed to: 449-5288
7060-500 (7/96)
LAB

FIGURE 42–9 Laboratory requisition form.

Whenever the physician requests laboratory testing that must be done outside of the office, a written **requisition** for the work must be sent to the laboratory with the patient or with the specimen (Fig. 42–9). These forms are preprinted with the most commonly requested test indicated in logical sequence. Patient information must be complete, accurate, and clearly legible.

EXAMPLE OF INFORMATION USUALLY REQUIRED WHEN SPECIMENS ARE SENT TO THE LABORATORY

- Physician's name, account number, address, and phone number
- Patient's full name, surname first
- Patient's address
- Patient's insurance information
- Patient's age, date of birth, and sex
- Source of specimen
- Date and time of collection
- Specific test(s) requested
- Medications the patient is taking
- Possible diagnosis
- Indication of whether test is **stat** (needed immediately)

Specimen Collection

The medical assistant is responsible for the collection of many different types of specimens. It is important to recognize that all clinical laboratory results are only as good as the specimen received. The most common specimens are blood, urine, and swabs for culture. Less often, feces, gastric contents, **cerebrospinal fluid,** tissue samples, semen, and aspirates, such as synovial fluid or amniotic fluid, are submitted for testing. These specimens are analyzed for levels of many chemicals and drugs, types and numbers of cells present, and the presence of microorganisms.

Instructions for properly obtaining, processing, and preparing a specimen for transporting are usually supplied to the physician's office laboratory by the testing laboratory. If the instructions are not clear or if you have a question regarding a particular collection, the laboratory will answer your question over the phone.

If the specimen is to be mailed, it must be carefully packaged to prevent breakage, damage, or contamination by all persons handling it. Containers of liquid specimens may be wrapped in absorbent material and inserted in unbreakable tubes with safe-top lids. The lids are taped shut so that no leakage occurs if the specimen container breaks. Place all specimens in a second container, such as an impervious bag, for transport. The completed requisition goes inside the outermost wrap. Usually, Styrofoam mailers (Fig. 42–10) are used because they cushion the sample and also provide insulation. Styrofoam inserts can be shaped to fit around the specimen container. A warning label specifying the etiologic agent or biologic specimen is affixed to the outside of the container. The specimen should be given to the laboratory courier or mailed at a post office immediately so that it is not exposed to temperature extremes.

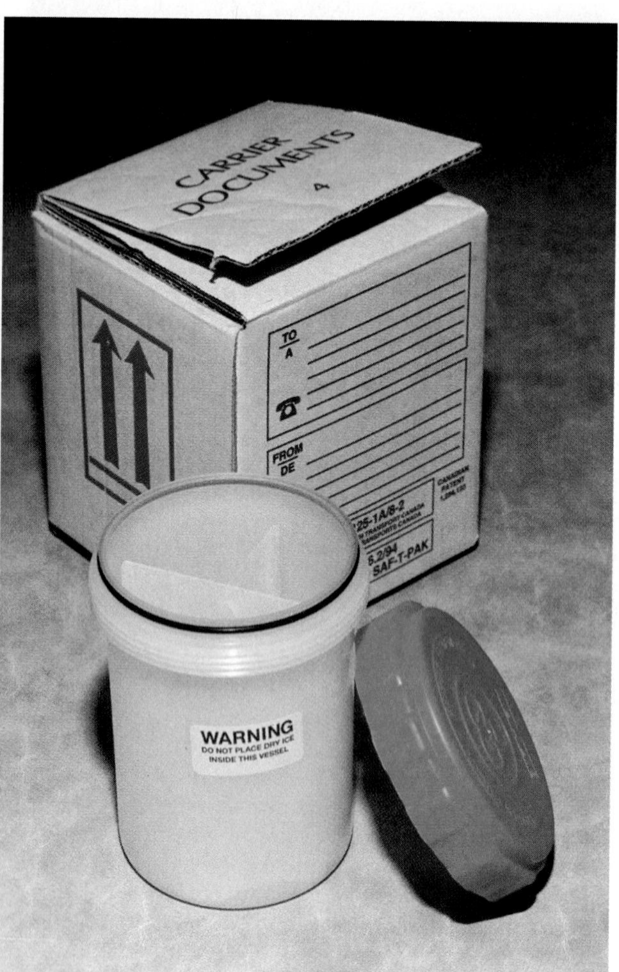

FIGURE 42–10 Specimen mailers.

Memory Jogger

Where is the warning label placed when preparing a biologic specimen for mailing?

RESULTS OF TESTING

The results of these tests done in a reference laboratory are usually returned to the physician on a computerized printout (Fig. 42–11). These testing results, along with other diagnostic testing, patient history, and physical examination, lead the physician to diagnose or rule out a particular disease. Management of the patient's condition may require repeated testing, such as routine glucose level determinations in the diabetic patient. If a patient is receiving medication, the physician may request therapeutic drug monitoring to be certain that the patient is actually taking the medication and to detect possible toxic levels. Patients being given diuretics for the treatment of high blood pressure may need to have their potassium levels checked on a routine basis. Occasionally, the physician may request a test to determine the patient's baseline level, for comparison with the results of future tests.

Screening tests, such as routine urinalysis, are performed to detect hidden disease in otherwise apparently healthy individuals. A urinalysis may reveal the presence of diabetes, liver disease, or pathology of the urinary tract. Some screening tests are required by law in certain states. Persons applying for a marriage license may be required to have a Venereal Disease Research Laboratory (VDRL) test to detect syphilis. A rapid plasma reagin (RPR) test to determine the rubella titer may also be requested. Some states require screening of newborns for hereditary metabolic defects such as phenylketonuria and hypothyroidism. Tests may reveal the extent of disease or degree of damage done to an organ or body system. For example, the measurement of the rise of certain enzymes after a heart attack can indicate the amount of heart damage, whereas the measurement of the level of the HIV **antibody** is an accurate assessment of the risk of AIDS transmission. Repeated testing can allow the physician to follow the course of a disease and assess the effectiveness of the treatment. A person with a diagnosis of leukemia may have daily white blood cell counts performed before receiving chemotherapy.

Agnes Medical

Page: 1

Patient:
Unit#/Acct#:
SEX/DOB:
Patient Phone #:

Physician:

Submitter's Reference #:

CBC, AUTOMATED DIFFERENTIAL

Specimen: BLOOD
Collected: 09/16/97 0838

Result name	Abnormal	Result	Normal Range
WBC		6.3	4.5-11.0 X(10)3
RBC		4.45	4.2-5.4 X(10)6
Hgb		13.6	12-16 g/dL
Hct		41.0	37-47 %
MCV		92.1	81-99 fL
MCH		30.5	28.0-32.0 pg
MCHC		33.1	31.5-35.5 g/dL
RDW		12.8	11.5-14.5 %
Platelet		268	150-400 X(10)3
MPV		8.4	7.4-10.4 fL
Lymph - %		40.8	20-43 %
Mono		7.8	0-8 %
Gran	49.2 L		51-74 %
Eos		1.8	0-5 %
Baso		0.4	0-1 %
Lymph - Absolute		2.6	1.0-4.7 X(10)3
Mono		0.5	0.1-1.0 X(10)3
Gran		3.1	2.6-8.2 X(10)3
Eos		0.1	< 0.7 X(10)3
Baso		0.0	< 0.2 X(10)3

LIPID MONITORING PANEL

Specimen: BLOOD
Collected: 09/16/97 0838

Result name	Abnormal	Result	Normal Range
Cholesterol	242 H		< 200 = Desirable mg/dl 200-239 = Borderline > 240 = High
Triglyceride		146	< 250 mg/dl
ALT/SGPT		19	5-43 IU/L
AST/SGOT		20	9-35 IU/L
HDL Cholesterol	67 H		35.0-80.0 MEAN 60 mg/dl
VLDL		23.4	10-38 mg/dl
LDL Cholesterol	146 H		< 130 Desirable mg/dl 130-159 Borderline-high > 160 High
Chol/HDL		3.6	

Report Status: Complete

FIGURE 42–11 Testing results.

ACHIEVING ACCURATE RESULTS

The importance of specimen collection cannot be overemphasized. If not performed correctly, it can easily lead to inaccurate results. If the tests are to be accurate indicators of the patient's state of health, it is imperative that the concepts of specimen collection be understood and followed exactly.

Using Proper Equipment

The correct specimen must be collected in the correct container; for example, blood may be collected using a vacuum tube system. These tubes are available in a variety of sizes with and without **preservatives** and **anticoagulants.** The tubes are color coded so that the color of the stopper denotes which, if any, additive is present (Fig. 42–12).

The medical assistant should always check the laboratory's specimen requirements manual for any unfamiliar tests. The manual lists all specimen collection information. Any unanswered questions should be resolved by calling the laboratory before collecting the specimen.

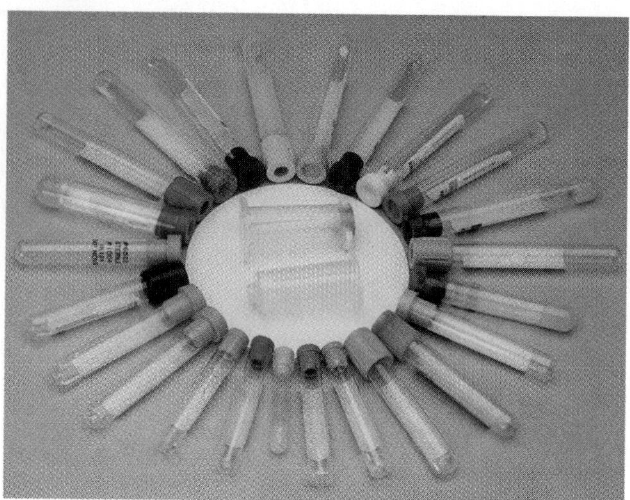

FIGURE 42–12 Vacutainer tubes. Note color-coded tops.

Avoiding Contamination

Care must be taken to avoid contamination of the specimen or the assistant. The correct collection and handling of the specimens used in various microbiology procedures are absolutely essential if the results are to be of any value in the diagnosis of the disease and the treatment of the patient. Expiration dates on swabs, tubes, transport media, and other collection containers should be checked before these items are used.

An improperly handled specimen may become contaminated or may contaminate the surrounding environment. Follow Standard Precautions. All blood and other body fluids from *all* patients should be considered infective.

Providing Sufficient and True Representative Samples

Sufficient samples should be collected for the tests requested by the physician. Amounts may vary based on the methods used. If a report is returned from the laboratory with the term *insufficient sample,* it indicates a request for an additional specimen. Be certain to clarify any questions concerning the previous specimen by calling the laboratory before collecting a new one.

The specimen collected must be a true representative sample. A swab for a wound culture collected from the surface of the wound generally does not yield the same results as one taken from the depths of the wound. A **hemolyzed** blood specimen, or one taken from an atypical area, such as a **hematoma** or the area above an intravenous drop, shows marked differences in many tests. If a large volume of specimen is collected, such as a 24-hour urine or fecal fat specimen, the total volume or weight must be carefully measured and recorded. The specimen must be well mixed before an **aliquot** is removed and submitted for testing.

Proper Handling, Processing, and Storage

The specimen must be handled, processed, and stored according to the instructions, to avoid causing any alterations that would affect test results. Check whether the specimen needs to be kept warm or cool. Specimens such as urine require chilling if the testing is not going to be done immediately. Some cultures or specimens need to be kept at body temperature after collection. *Neisseria* gonococcal cultures and semen analysis are two such examples, because cooling kills the gonococci and sperm. When required, serum must be separated from the cells as soon as possible after the specimen has clotted, to prevent alterations caused by the metabolism of the cells. Specimens for bilirubin testing must be protected from light. Some specimens need to be frozen to prevent chemical constituents from changing. Consult the laboratory specimen requirements to be certain that each specimen is handled and processed properly.

The Microscope

Every medical laboratory is equipped with a microscope. This indispensable instrument is used to view objects too small to be seen with the naked eye (Fig. 42–13). The microscope is helpful in identifying microorganisms in urine sediment and other body fluids. The microscope is employed to evaluate stained blood smears, urine sediment, and microbacterial throat smears and to determine blood cell counts. Because the microscope is an expensive and technical instrument, special care must be taken in its operation, care, and storage.

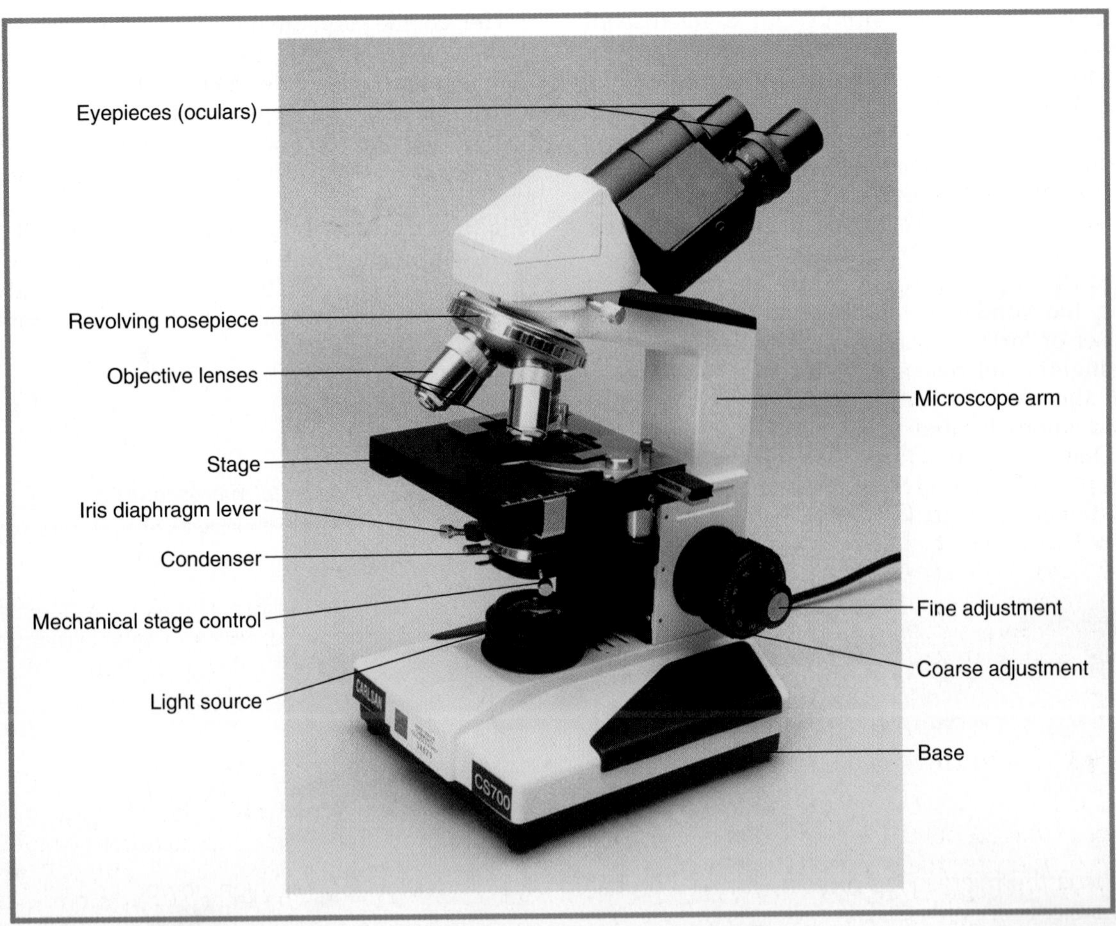

FIGURE 42–13 Parts of a microscope. (Courtesy of CARLSAN Inc., Carlinville, Illinois.)

Microscopes are either *monocular* or *binocular*. A monocular microscope has one eyepiece for viewing, and a binocular has two. The *eyepiece*, or *ocular*, is located at the top of the microscope and contains a lens to magnify what is being seen. The usual magnification is 10 times (10×). The ocular is attached to a barrel or tube that is connected to the microscope *arm*. Under the arm is the *revolving nosepiece*, to which are attached the *objectives*. Most microscopes have three objectives; each has a different magnifying power. The shortest objective has the lowest power (10×). Low power is used to scan the field of interest and then focus on a particular object. Greater detail is observed with the next longest objective, which is high power (40×). The longest objective, oil immersion (100×), allows for the finest focusing of the object.

The arm of the microscope connects the objectives and oculars to the *base*, which supports the microscope and contains its light source. Together, the *condenser* and the *iris diaphragm* direct and regulate the light up through the objective. Just above the base are the focusing knobs. The *coarse adjustment* is used only with low power, and the *fine adjustment* is used with high power and oil immersion. The *stage* of the microscope holds the slide to be viewed.

Memory Jogger

Identify four functions of the microscope in the physician's office laboratory.

Microscopes are very precise and expensive instruments that require careful handling. The amount of routine maintenance depends on the amount of daily use. Dirt is the enemy of the microscope, which must be kept scrupulously clean at all times. The microscope should always be stored in a plastic dust cover when not in use. Lenses should be cleaned before and after each use with lens paper and lens cleaner. Any other type of tissue scratches the lenses or leaves lint residue behind. The use of solvent cleaners, such as xylene, is not recommended on a routine basis because they may loosen lenses. Xylene can be used to remove oil that has dried on the lenses. Oil, makeup, dust, and eye secretions all can obstruct vision through the lens and cause the possible transmission of infection. Finally, the body of the microscope should be dusted with a soft cloth.

The microscope should be placed in a permanent location in the laboratory on a sturdy table in an area where it cannot be bumped. If a microscope must be moved, it should be carried securely, with one hand supporting the base and the other holding the arm. When the microscope is stored, it should be left covered, with the low-power objective in the lowest position. The stage should be centered.

Using a microscope involves focusing and illumination (see Procedure 42–1). Focusing the image is done by moving the objective closer to the specimen, and illumination is accomplished by raising or lowering the condenser and by moving the specimen closer or farther away from the objective.

Focusing the microscope is done through movement of the objective or stage, which is controlled by round knobs located on both side of the microscope. Once you have the specimen in as good a focus as possible, the next step is to use the fine and coarse adjustment focus knob.

The coarse adjustment moves the objective very quickly. This knob is used first to bring the specimen into approximate focus. The fine adjustment focus knob then brings the specimen into precise focus. The fine focus moves the objective more slowly to allow you to zero in on the specimen with greater accuracy.

If the microscope is a binocular scope, it may be necessary to adjust the eyepieces to your own eye span and visual acuity. A gentle push inward or pull outward will adjust the distance between the eyepieces.

Memory Jogger

10 *How do you focus a microscope?*

PROCEDURE 42–1
Using the Microscope

GOAL

To focus the microscope properly, using a prepared slide, under low power, high power, and oil immersion.

EQUIPMENT AND SUPPLIES

Microscope
Lens tissue
Lens cleaner
Slide containing specimen

PROCEDURAL STEPS

1 Wash your hands.
2 Gather the materials needed.
3 Clean the lenses with lens tissue and lens cleaner.
4 Adjust seating to a comfortable height.
5 Plug the microscope into an electric outlet, and turn on the light switch.
6 Place the slide specimen on the stage and secure it.
7 Turn the revolving nosepiece to low power.
8 Carefully raise the stage while observing with the naked eye from the side.
9 Focus the specimen, using the coarse-adjustment knob.
10 Switch to fine adjustment, and focus the specimen in detail.
11 Adjust the amount of light by closing the iris diaphragm and lowering the condenser.
12 Turn the revolving nosepiece between the high-power objective and oil immersion.
13 Place a small drop of oil on the slide.
14 Carefully swing the oil immersion objective into place.
15 Adjust the focus with the fine-adjustment knob.
16 Increase the light by opening the iris diaphragm and raising the condenser.
17 Identify the specimen.

Continued

18 Return to low power.
19 Lower the stage.
20 Center the stage.
21 Remove the slide.
22 Switch off the light and unplug the microscope.
23 Clean the lenses with lens tissue, and remove oil with lens cleaner.
24 Wipe the microscope with a cloth.
25 Cover the microscope.
26 Clean the work area.
27 Wash your hands.

PATIENT EDUCATION

Many testing procedures require that patients be given a specific set of instructions to follow. For example, patients may be required to fast 8 to 12 hours before the collection of blood and urine. They may need to follow a high-carbohydrate diet for several days before a *glucose tolerance test.* The consumption of some foods and medication must be discontinued. The physician will discuss medication alternatives with the patient. Sometimes, it might not be medically advisable to discontinue the medication; this must be noted on the laboratory requisition. The laboratory will then be alerted to the possible drug interferences, and it may be able to use an alternative test method.

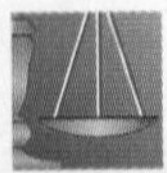

LEGAL AND ETHICAL ISSUES

If disease did not exist there would be little need for clinical laboratories. The fact that the human body is susceptible to disease necessitates the existence of laboratory testing. One cannot anticipate or prevent every health and safety risk, but the risks are greatly reduced when everyone who works in the laboratory setting is conscious of safety guidelines. Use good common sense. If you are in doubt about the safety of a procedure, ask your supervisor. If you are aware of a potential safety problem, report it to the person in charge. Your welfare, the welfare of the patient, and the welfare of your coworkers may depend on your commitment to safety.

CRITICAL THINKING

1 One of your coworkers uses the time in the laboratory to have a cup of coffee and a donut. How would you approach this situation?

2 You need to run a test first thing in the morning and you cannot find the prepackaged control for the test. What would you do?

3 You are unfamiliar with a test that has to be run. What do you do?

HOW DID I DO? Answers to Memory Joggers

1 The physician's office laboratory usually performs procedures in urinalysis, hematology, chemistry, and microbiology.

2 Hazards in the laboratory can be classified as physical, chemical, and biohazard.

3 CLIA regulations established low-complexity, moderate-complexity, and high-complexity testing as the three categories.

4 Quality control programs monitor all aspects of laboratory activity from specimen collection through the processing, testing, and reporting steps.

5 Quality controls are run daily to ensure the accuracy of the test.

6 Only a physician may request laboratory testing for a patient.

7 Yes it is mandatory.

8 A warning label is affixed to the outside of the container.

9 The microscope evaluates stained blood smears, urine sediment, microbacterial throat smears, and blood cell counts.

10 Focusing is done through movement of the objective or stage.

Urinalysis

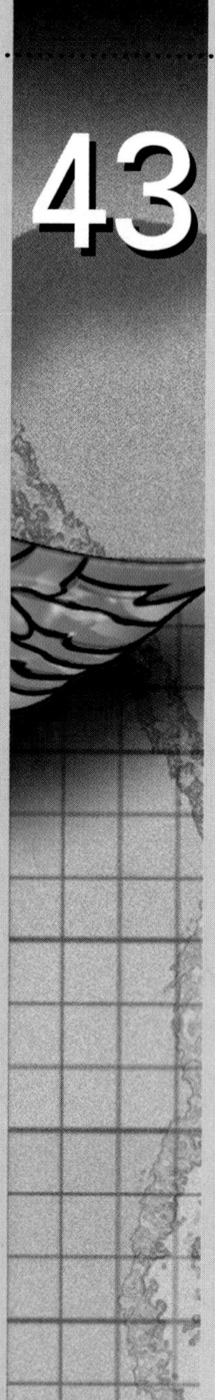

43

OUTLINE

LEARNING OBJECTIVES

Cognitive: On successful completion of this chapter you should be able to:

1 Understand the purpose of routine urinalysis
2 State the five types of urine specimens used.
3 Describe the physiology of urine formation.
4 Describe the tests in the physical and chemical examination of urine.
5 List five materials found in urine sediment microscopically.
6 Define urinary quality control.
7 Spell and define vocabulary terms.

Performance: On successful completion of this chapter you should be able to:

1 Instruct a patient in the collection of a timed urine specimen.
2 Instruct a patient in the collection of a clean-catch midstream urine specimen.
3 Perform a complete urinalysis.
4 Describe the proper use and care of testing equipment.
5 Demonstrate glucose testing using the Clinitest method.
6 Demonstrate the use of precipitation testing for protein in urine.
7 Demonstrate the methods of pregnancy testing.

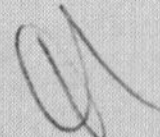

VOCABULARY

anuria Complete suppression of urine formation by the kidney

casts Fibrous or protein materials that are thrown off into the urine in kidney disease

crenate Forming notches or leaflike scalloped edges on an object

enzymatic reaction Chemical reaction controlled by an enzyme

glycosuria Presence of glucose in the urine

hematuria Presence of blood in the urine

human chorionic gonadotropin (hCG) Hormone secreted in large amounts by the placenta during gestation to stimulate the formation of interstitial cells

ischemia Decreased blood flow to a body part or organ, caused by constriction or plugging of the supplying artery

ketones Products of fat metabolism

myoglobinuria Abnormal presence of a hemoglobin-like chemical of muscle tissue in urine, which results in muscle deterioration

phenylalanine Essential amino acid found in milk, eggs, and other foods

proteinuria Excess of serum protein in the urine

void To urinate

A routine *urinalysis* (UA) is one of the more common laboratory examinations used in the diagnosis and treatment of disease. It can be easily and quickly performed. The results of a routine urinalysis can reveal diseases of the bladder or kidneys, systemic metabolic or endocrine disorders such as diabetes, and diseases of the liver, such as hepatitis, cirrhosis, or obstruction of the bile ducts. Urinalysis is routinely performed on all patients undergoing physical examinations and on those entering the hospital for treatment.

Memory Jogger

 *When is routine urinalysis routinely performed?*

Collecting Urine Specimens

Each urine specimen must be properly collected and handled. You should routinely follow Standard Precautions by using nonsterile gloves and other appropriate barrier precautions when handling urine. Most urine specimens collected in the office are *random specimens,* that is, they are collected at different times during the day, in clean but not sterile urine containers. Because the makeup of urine changes constantly, depending on a person's activity, random specimens are used only for routine screening and initial evaluation.

First morning specimens are preferred because they are usually the most concentrated. They are best for pregnancy testing, culturing, and microscopic examination. *Timed specimens* are submitted when more specific information is needed for proper diagnosis. *Two-hour postprandial urine specimens,* collected 2 hours after a meal, are used in diabetic screening and for home diabetic-testing programs. *Twenty-four-hour urine specimens* are collected over a period of 24 hours to give quantitative chemical analysis, such as hormone levels and creatinine clearance rates (a procedure for evaluating the glomerular filtration rate of the kidneys) (Fig. 43–1*A*).

Proper handling of specimens is essential. The chemical and cellular components of urine change if they are allowed to stand at room temperature (Table 43–1). These changes can be avoided by re-

TABLE 43–1 Changes in Urine at Room Temperature

Constituent	Change
Clarity	Becomes cloudy as crystals precipitate and bacteria multiply
Color	May change if pH becomes alkaline
pH	Becomes alkaline as bacteria form ammonia from urea
Glucose	Decreases as bacteria metabolize it
Ketones	Decrease
Bilirubin and urobilinogen	Undergo degradation in light
Blood	May hemolyze. False-positives possible due to bacterial peroxidase
Nitrite	May become positive as bacteria convert nitrate. Can become negative as bacteria metabolize nitrite.
Casts	Lyse or dissolve in alkaline urine
Cells	Lyse or dissolve in alkaline urine
Bacteria	Multiply twofold every 20 minutes
Yeast	Multiply
Crystals	Precipitate as urine cools. May dissolve if pH changes

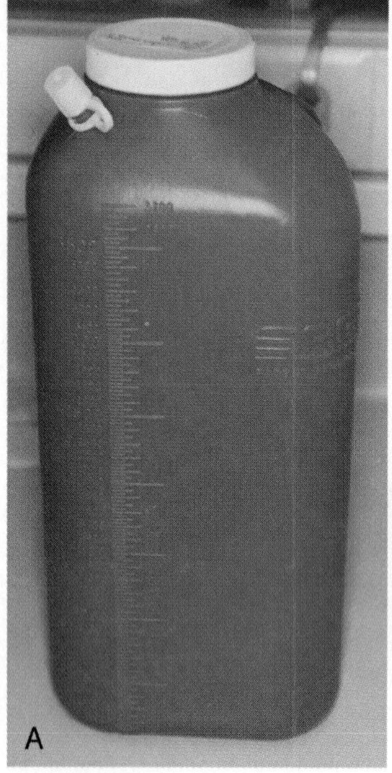

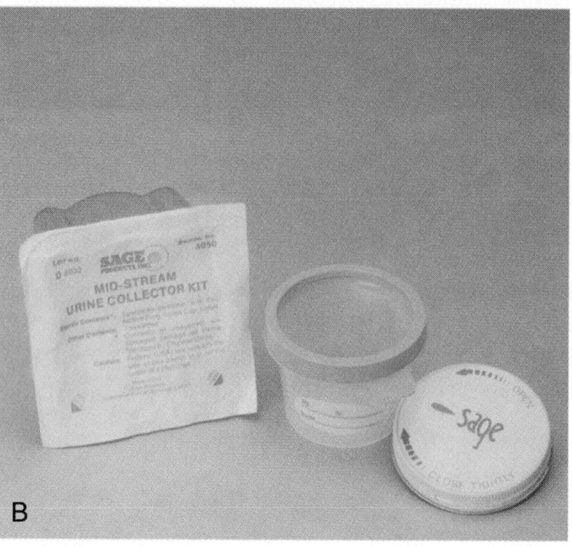

FIGURE 43–1 *A,* Twenty-four-hour specimen container. *B,* Sterile container for midstream specimen.

frigerating the specimen if the analysis cannot be performed within 30 minutes after collection. Occasionally, preservatives must be added.

Routine (random) specimens are collected in nonsterile disposable containers. The container is always labeled with the patient's name before it is given to the patient to use.

A clean-catch midstream specimen may be ordered when the urine is to be cultured or examined for microorganisms. The purpose of the clean-catch technique is to remove microorganisms from the urinary meatus by thoroughly cleansing the area around the meatus and to flush out the distal portion of the urethra. Because the specimen is collected in the medical office by the patient, the medical assistant needs to give complete, understandable instructions to the patient on the method of collection. Failure to do so may mean that the patient will have to return to the office to allow the collection of another specimen. Once the specimen has been collected, it should be tested immediately. If this cannot be done, the specimen should be refrigerated, or a preservative should be added to the specimen. For culturing, urine should be collected by catheterization or the clean-catch method into a sterile container (see Fig. 43–1*B*).

Memory Jogger

2 *What type of urine specimen is best for pregnancy testing, culturing, and microscopic examination? Why?*

CATHETERIZATION

Catheterization is the introduction of a catheter through the urethra into the bladder for the purpose of withdrawing urine (see Chapter 38).

In recent years, the value of catheterization has become increasingly suspect in view of the hazards involved. It is now considered the most prominent cause of nosocomial infections. Therefore, whenever possible, it is recommended that catheterization be avoided. When deemed necessary, it should be performed with careful technique by a fully trained and competent technician. In some states, the medical assistant cannot perform catheterization. Be sure to check your state guidelines regarding the training and the legality of performance.

INSTRUCTING PATIENTS IN COLLECTING A URINE SPECIMEN

Most patients understand the procedure for collecting a routine (random) urine specimen. However, they do need special instructions for collecting a timed specimen and a midstream clean-catch specimen. The following set of instructions is to help you teach patients how to collect urine specimens.

COLLECTING A 24-HOUR SPECIMEN

1 On arising in the morning, **void** into the toilet. Empty your bladder completely. Do not

save this urine. Note exact time, and write it down on the container.

2 Collect all urine voided after this time for exactly 24 hours. Remember that all urine passed at night or during the day in this time period must be saved.

3 Remember to keep the urine cool.

4 At exactly the same time the following morning, urinate completely again. Save this sample. Add it to the collection container. This completes your 24-hour collection.

5 Take all specimens from the 24-hour collection to the medical office, or to the place designated, as soon as possible, maintaining the cool temperature in transit by placing the specimen in a portable cooler or insulated bag.

OBTAINING A CLEAN-CATCH MIDSTREAM SPECIMEN

FEMALE PATIENT

1 Wash hands and remove underclothing.

2 Expose the urinary meatus by spreading apart the labia with one hand (Fig. 43–2*A*).

3 Cleanse each side of the urinary meatus with a front-to-back motion, from the pubis to the anus. Use a fresh cotton ball on each side. (If the midstream specimen kit is used, an antiseptic wipe is provided to cleanse each side of the meatus.)

4 Cleanse directly across the meatus, front-to-back, using a third cotton ball or antiseptic wipe (see Fig. 43–2*A*)

5 Rinse with water to remove traces of the soap used to prevent its entrance into the specimen.

6 Dry the area with a clean cotton ball using front-to-back motion. If a midstream kit has been used, the rinsing and drying procedure can be omitted.

7 Hold the labia apart throughout this procedure.

8 Void a small amount of urine into the toilet (Fig. 43–2*B*).

9 Move the specimen container into position and void the next portion of urine into it. Remember this is a sterile container. Do not put your fingers on the inside of the container (Fig. 43–2C).

10 Remove the cup and void the last amount of urine into the toilet. (This means that the first part and the last part of the urinary flow have been excluded from the specimen. Only the middle portion of the flow is included.)

11 Wipe in your usual manner, redress, and return the sterile specimen to the place designated by the medical facility.

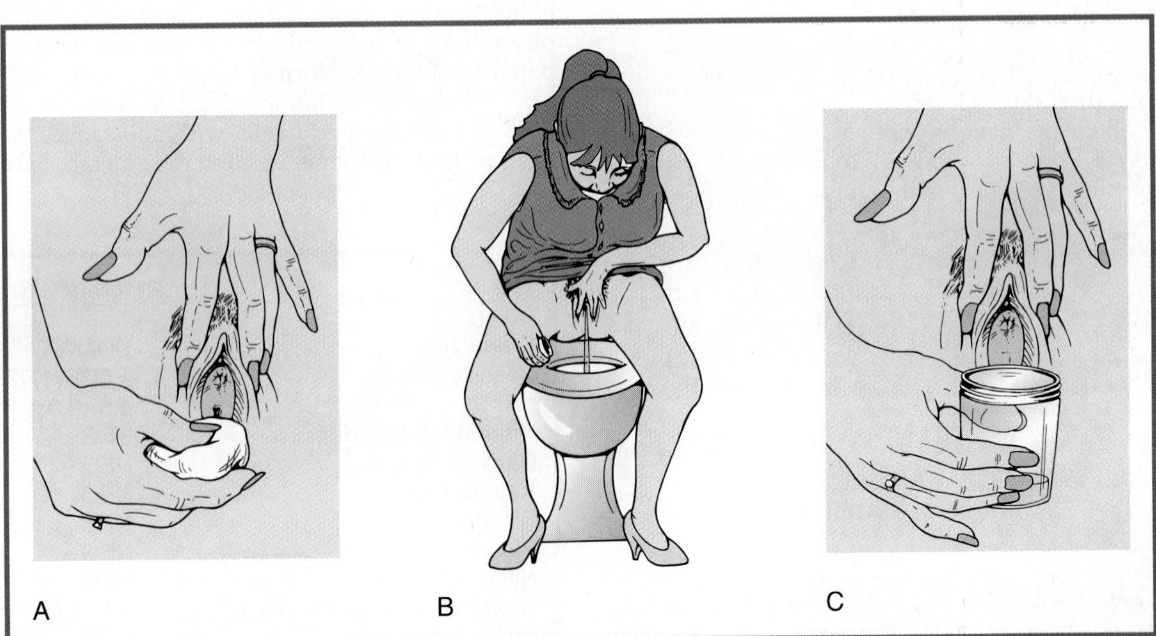

FIGURE 43–2 Procedure for obtaining a clean-catch urine specimen in females. (From Stepp CA, Woods MA: Laboratory Procedures for Medical Office Personnel. Philadelphia, WB Saunders, 1998.)

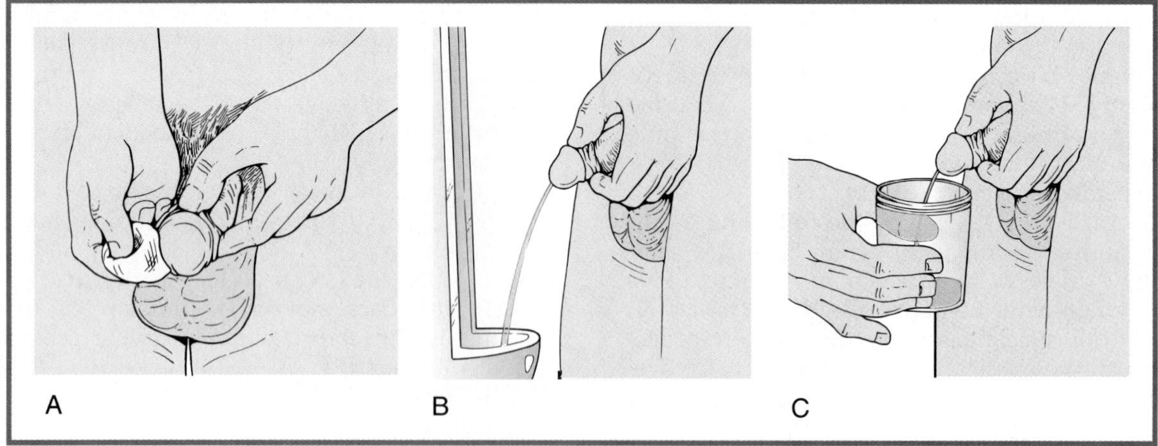

FIGURE 43–3 Procedure for obtaining a clean-catch urine specimen in males. (From Stepp CA, Woods MA: Laboratory Procedures for Medical Office Personnel. Philadelphia, WB Saunders, 1998.)

OBTAINING A CLEAN-CATCH MIDSTREAM SPECIMEN

MALE PATIENT

1 Wash your hands and expose the penis.
2 Retract the foreskin of the penis (if not circumcised).
3 Cleanse the area around the glans penis (meatus) and the urethral opening by washing each side of the glans with a separate cotton ball. If a midstream kit is used, antiseptic wipes are provided (Fig. 43–3*A*).
4 Cleanse directly across the urethral opening using a third cotton ball or antiseptic wipe.
5 If soap and cotton balls are used, rinse with water to remove all traces of soap.
6 Dry the area using a front-to-back motion.
7 Void a small amount of urine into the toilet or urinal (Fig. 43–3*B*).
8 Collect the next portion of the urine in the *sterile* container without touching the inside of the container with hands or penis (Fig. 43–3*C*).
9 Void the last amount of urine into the toilet or urinal.
10 Wipe and redress.
11 Return the specimen to the designated area provided.

GUIDELINES FOR CARING FOR A URINE SPECIMEN OBTAINED AT HOME

- Do not add anything but your urine into the bottle.
- Do not pour out any liquid or powdered preservative from the container.
- If you accidentally spill some of the preservative on you, immediately wash with water and call the testing center or designated laboratory.
- Always keep the collection bottle cool. Refrigerate or keep the bottle in an ice-filled cooler or pail.
- Keep the cap on the container.
- You may find it more convenient to urinate into the smaller container provided and then pour the urine into the larger collection bottle.

Physiology of Urine Formation

To understand the meaning of urinalysis results, it is necessary to have a general understanding of the physiology of urine formation and the normal components of urine. Normal body functions and good health depend on homeostasis. Various organ systems supply the body cells with substances, such as oxygen and nutrients needed for metabolism, and

	Reference Range
Color:	
Character:	Clear
Specific gravity:	1.001–1.035
pH:	4.6–8.0
Protein UA (mg/dL):	NEG
Glucose (mg/dL):	NEG
Ketone (mg/dL):	NEG
Bilirubin (mg/dL):	NEG
Blood/UA (mg/dL):	NEG
Nitrite (mg/dL):	NEG
Urobilinogen (Ehrlich units):	0.1–1.0
White blood cells:	NEG
Red blood cells (per high-power field):	<3

FIGURE 43–4 Normal urine reference range.

TABLE 43–2 Components of the Macroscopic Urinalysis

Physical Property	Chemical Property Measured by Dipsticks
Color	Protein
Clarity	Glucose
Specific gravity	Ketones
Amount*	Bilirubin
Odor*	Blood: intact red blood cells, hemoglobin, myoglobin
Foam*	Nitrite
	Urobilinogen
	Leukocyte esterase
	Specific gravity†
	pH†

* Not always assessed.
† Physical properties measured on dipsticks.

help eliminate the waste products of metabolism, such as carbon dioxide. To function normally, body cells need more than a supply of nutrients and the elimination of waste products. Cells need to exist in a stable internal environment, where the composition of the extracellular fluids is constant. The urinary system functions to maintain this composition and, thus, the physiochemical properties of the internal environment.

Normally, water constitutes about 95% of urine. The other 5% includes dissolved chemicals such as urea, uric acid, creatinine, sodium chloride, calcium, sulfates, phosphates, hydrogen ions, and urochrome. The proportion of water and chemicals varies greatly, depending on the time of day, diet, metabolism, hormones, fluid intake, and nonurine fluid loss. Disease states alter urine volume and change physical, chemical, and microscopic constituents.

A urinalysis consists of a physical, chemical, and microscopic examination. Deviation from normal in any of these three areas assists the physician in the diagnosis and assessment of the patient's condition and treatment regimen (Fig. 43–4).

Memory Jogger

How much of normal urine is water?

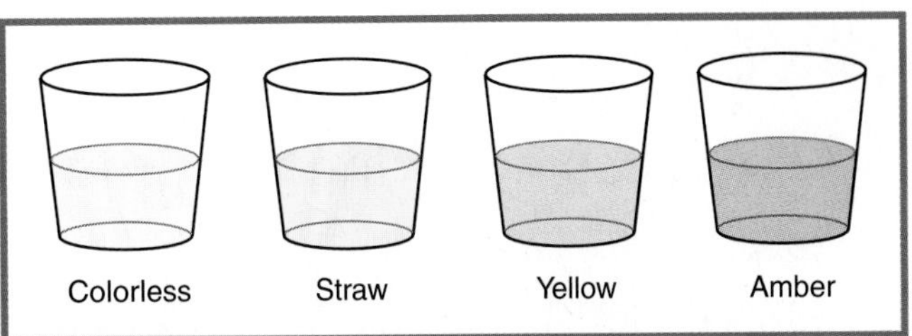

FIGURE 43–5 Colors of normal urine. (From Stepp CA, Woods MA: Laboratory Procedures for Medical Office Personnel. Philadelphia, WB Saunders, 1998.)

Physical Examination of Urine

The first part of a complete urinalysis is the assessment of the physical properties and the measurement of selected chemical constituents of diagnostic importance (Table 43–2).

COLOR AND TURBIDITY

Normal urine color is a shade of yellow ranging from pale straw to yellow to amber (see Procedure 43–1). Color depends on the concentration of the pigment *urochrome* and the amount of water in the specimen. A dilute specimen should be pale, and a more concentrated specimen should be a darker yellow (Fig. 43–5). Variations in color may be caused by diet, medication, and disease. Abnormal colors may be pathologic or nonpathologic (Table 43–3).

Both normal and abnormal urine specimens may range in appearance from clear to very cloudy. Cloudiness may be caused by cells, bacteria, yeast, vaginal contaminants, or crystals. Often, a urine specimen that was clear when voided will become cloudy as it cools when crystals form and precipitate.

Memory Jogger

Are abnormal urine colors always a sign of a pathologic urinary problem?

TABLE 43–3 Urine Colors

Color	Pathologic Cause	Nonpathologic Cause
Straw	Diabetes	Diuretics; high fluid intake (coffee, beer)
Amber	Dehydration	Excessive sweating; low fluid intake
Bright yellow		Carotene, vitamins
Red	Blood, porphyrins	Beets, drugs, dyes
Orange-yellow	Bile, hepatitis	Pyridium (phenazopyridine hydrochloride), dyes, drugs
Greenish yellow	Bile, hepatitis	Senna, cascara, rhubarb
Reddish brown	Old blood, methemoglobin	
Brownish black	Methemoglobin, melanin	Levodopa
Salmon pink		Amorphous urates
White (milky)	Fats, pus	Amorphous phosphates
Blue-green	Biliverdin, infection with *Pseudomonas*	Vitamin B, drugs, dyes

PROCEDURE 43-1

Assessing Urine for Color and Turbidity

GOAL

To assess and record the color and clarity of a urine specimen.

EQUIPMENT AND SUPPLIES

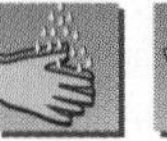

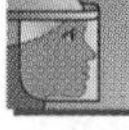

Urine specimen

Centrifuge tube

PROCEDURAL STEPS

1 Wash and dry your hands and apply gloves.

2 Mix the urine by swirling.
PURPOSE: Suspended substances settle when urine stands. If urine is not mixed before assessing appearance, the finding will be incorrect.

3 Label a centrifuge tube if a complete urinalysis is being done.
PURPOSE: If a complete urinalysis is being done, a portion of the specimen will be centrifuged for microscopic examination. The centrifuged specimen must be labeled to avoid specimen confusion.

4 Pour the specimen into a standard-size centrifuge tube.
PURPOSE: Standard-size containers are a better quality control for assessing color and clarity results.

5 Assess and record the color (Fig. 43–5):
- Pale straw
- Yellow
- Dark yellow
- Amber

6 Assess clarity:
- Clear—no cloudiness
- Slightly cloudy—can see light print through tube
- Moderately cloudy—can see only dark print through tube
- Very cloudy—cannot see through tube

7 Clean the work area, remove gloves, and wash your hands.
PURPOSE: Infection control.

8 Record the results in the patient's record.
PURPOSE: A procedure is considered not done until it is recorded.

VOLUME

The amount of urine is rarely measured on a random specimen. With a timed specimen, volume is measured by pouring the entire collection into a large graduated cylinder. Generally, it is not accurate enough to use the markings on the side of the collection container. Once the volume is measured and recorded, a portion of well-mixed specimen, called an *aliquot,* is removed for testing. The remainder is discarded or stored, depending on the preference of the laboratory.

The normal volume of urine produced every 24 hours varies according to the age of the individual. Infants and children produce smaller volumes than adults. The normal adult volume is 750 to 2000 mL in 24 hours, with an average of about 1500 mL. Excessive production of urine is called *polyuria.* It is common in diabetes and certain kidney disorders. *Oliguria* is insufficient production of urine and can be caused by dehydration, decreased fluid intake, shock, or renal disease. The absence of urine production, **anuria,** occurs in renal obstruction and renal failure.

Memory Jogger

Normal adult urine output ranges from ____ to ____ in 24 hours.

FOAM

Normally, the presence of foam is not recorded, but careful observation of this property can be a significant clue to an abnormality. White foam can indicate increased protein (Fig. 43–6). Yellow foam can mean bilirubinuria. Foam is the presence of small bubbles that persist for a long time after the specimen has been shaken; they must not be confused with any bubbles that rapidly disperse.

ODOR

Like foam, odor is not normally recorded but can be an important clue. Normal urine odor is said to be aromatic. Changes in the odor of urine may be due to disease, the presence of bacteria, or diet. The odor of the urine of a patient with uncontrolled diabetes is described as fruity because of the presence of **ketones,** which are the products of fat metabolism. An ammonia smell in the urine can be due to an infection. The bacteria break down the urea in the urine to form ammonia. Infection usually imparts a putrid odor. Foods such as asparagus and garlic can also produce an abnormal odor in the urine.

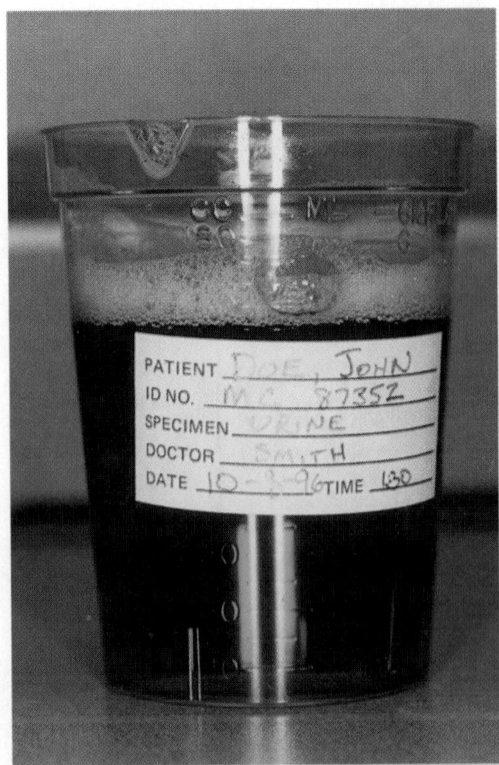

FIGURE 43–6 Dark amber urine with foam indicates possible increased protein and possible hematuria.

SPECIFIC GRAVITY

Specific gravity is the weight of a substance compared with the weight of an equal volume of distilled water. In urinalysis, it is the rough measurement of the concentration, or amount, of substances dissolved in urine. The specific gravity of distilled water is 1. Normal specific gravity of urine ranges from 1.005 to 1.030, depending on the fluid intake of the patient. Most samples fall between 1.010 and 1.025. Urine specific gravity indicates whether the kidneys are able to concentrate the urine and is one of the first indications of kidney disease. The presence of glucose, protein, or x-ray contrast media used in diagnostic studies may also increase the specific gravity of urine. To measure the specific gravity of urine, laboratories use dipstick, urinometer (see Procedure 43–2), or refractometer methods.

The *urinometer* is a sealed glass float with a calibrated paper scale in its stem (Fig. 43–7*A*). With a slight spinning motion, it is placed into a cylinder containing a urine sample and the value is read at the meniscus of the urine. It requires a quantity of urine sufficient to freely suspend the float, usually around 20 to 25 mL. If the sample is insufficient to float the urinometer, use a refractometer (see following) or record as QNS (quantity not sufficient).

The urinometer is fragile, and jarring can cause the paper scale in the stem to shift, resulting in erroneous readings. Occasionally, a damaged urinometer loses its calibration. Thus, the calibration of the urinometer should be checked daily with distilled water. The specific gravity of the distilled water should calibrate at 1.000 at 20° C (room temperature). (For example, if the urinometer reads 1.002 in distilled water, 0.002 must be subtracted from the urine readings. However, it is better to replace the instrument.) For each 3° C that the water temperature measures above 20° C, 0.001 must be added to the reading. For each 3° C that the water temperature measures below 20° C, subtract 0.001 from the reading. Use a laboratory thermometer to determine the water temperature.

The *refractometer* measures the refraction of light through solids in a liquid. The result is called the *refractive index,* which, for our purposes, is the same as specific gravity (Fig. 43–7*B*). The refractometer is both faster and easier to use than the urinometer and requires only a drop of urine. One drop of well-mixed urine is placed under the hinged cover of the instrument, and the value is read directly from a scale viewed through an ocular. The refractometer must be calibrated daily with distilled water.

Memory Jogger

What is specific gravity?

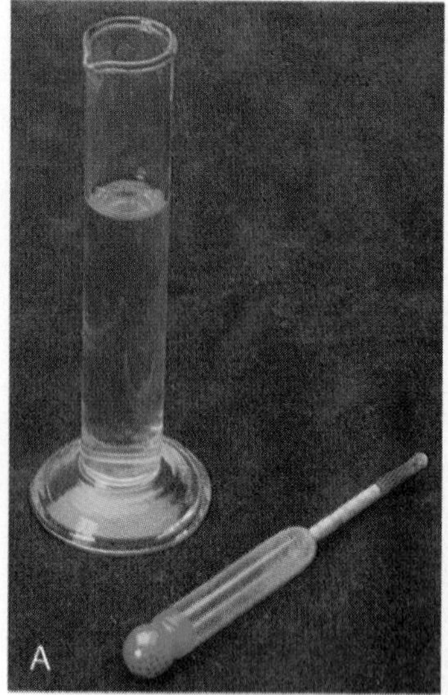

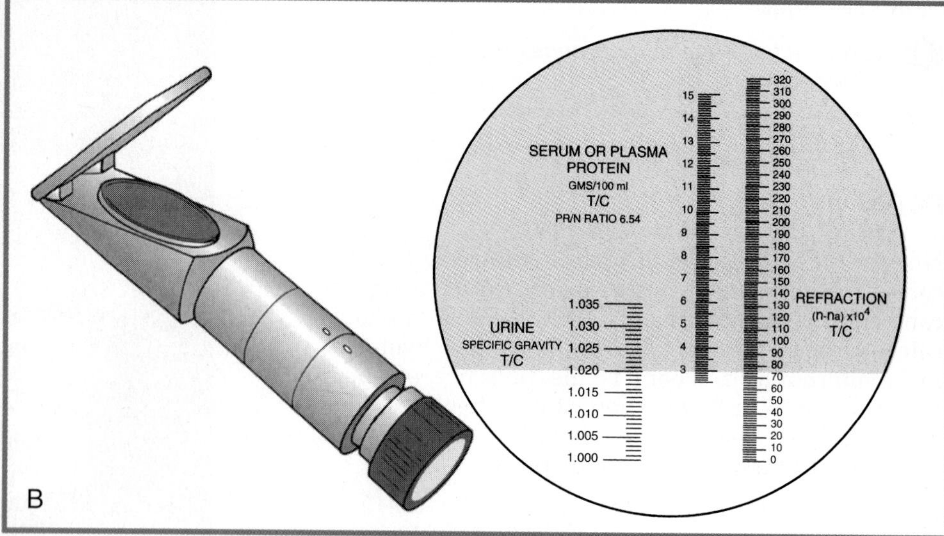

FIGURE 43–7 *A,* Urinometer. *B,* Refractometer. (*B,* from Stepp CA, Woods MA: Laboratory Procedures for Medical Office Personnel. Philadelphia, WB Saunders, 1998.)

PROCEDURE 43–2

Measuring Specific Gravity Using a Urinometer

GOAL

To calibrate the urinometer to perform a quality control check and to obtain duplicate specific gravity readings.

EQUIPMENT AND SUPPLIES

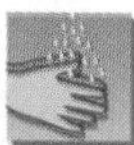
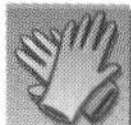
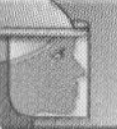

Urine specimen
Distilled water
Urinometer and cylinder

PROCEDURAL STEPS

1 Wash and dry your hands and put on nonsterile gloves and eye protection.

2 Fill the glass cylinder two-thirds full with distilled water at 20° C (room temperature).
PURPOSE: A quantity of 20 to 25 mL is needed to allow the urinometer to float.

3 Read the specific gravity of the distilled water (Figure 1).
PURPOSE: If the urinometer does not read 1.000, a correction factor or a new urinometer is necessary.

4 Allow the specimen to come to room temperature if it was refrigerated.
PURPOSE: Specific gravity measured by the urinometer is temperature dependent.

5 Mix the specimen well by swirling.

6 Pour the specimen into the clean glass cylinder to two-thirds to three-fourths full (Figure 2).
PURPOSE: A sufficient sample must be present to allow the urinometer to float freely.

7 Remove any foam using filter paper (Figure 3).

Continued

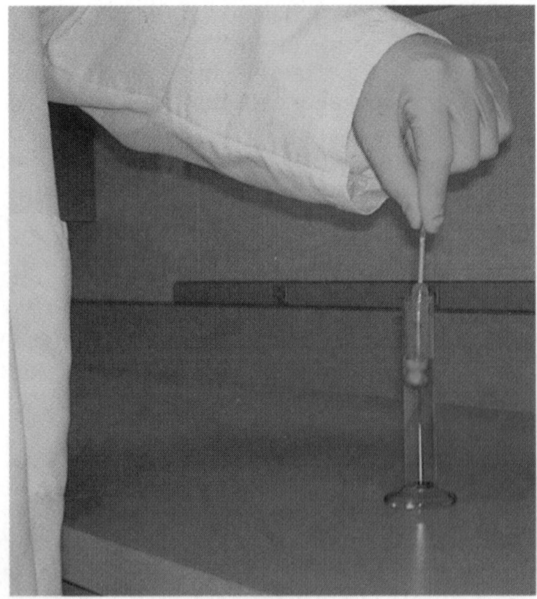

FIGURE 1

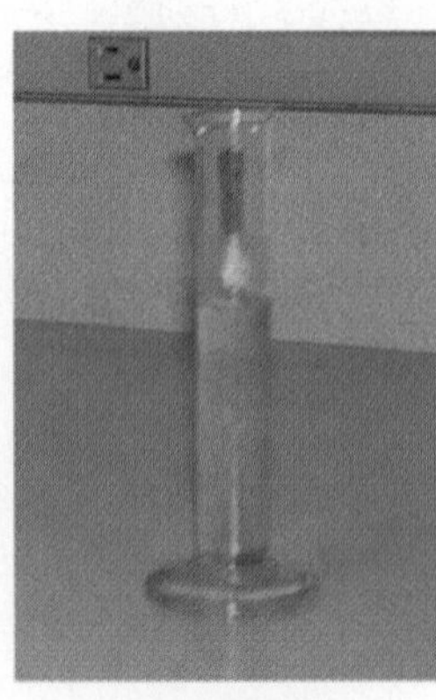

FIGURE 2

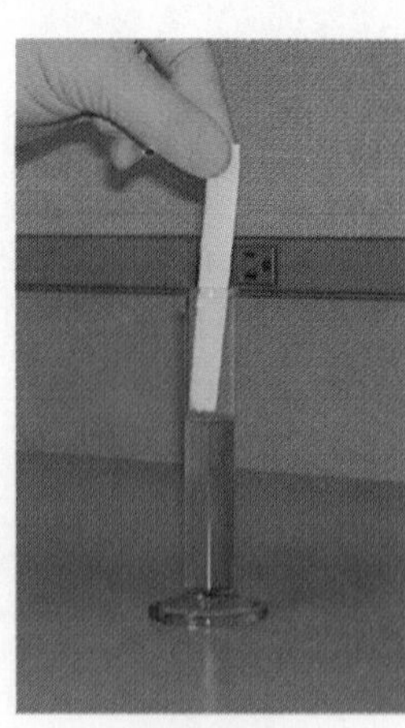

FIGURE 3

8 With the cylinder on a level surface, gently insert the urinometer in the specimen with a spinning motion (Figure 4).

9 While the urinometer stops rotating in the specimen, read the lower curve of the meniscus, at eye level (Figure 5*).
PURPOSE: For accurate results, the urinometer must be read at eye level. Adjust your line of vision to the urinometer: do not hold the cylinder in your hand.

10 Clean and dry the equipment, and return it to proper storage.
PURPOSE: Urine salts dried on the equipment cause erroneous readings in later tests.

11 Clean the work area. Wash your hands.

12 Record the results on the laboratory form or in the patient's record.
PURPOSE: A procedure is considered not done until it is recorded.

*From Stepp CA, Woods MA: Laboratory Procedures for Medical Office Personnel. Philadelphia, WB Saunders, 1998.

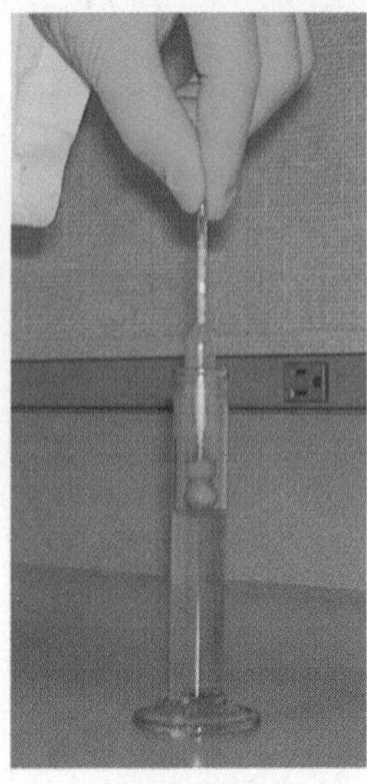

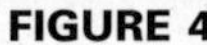

FIGURE 4

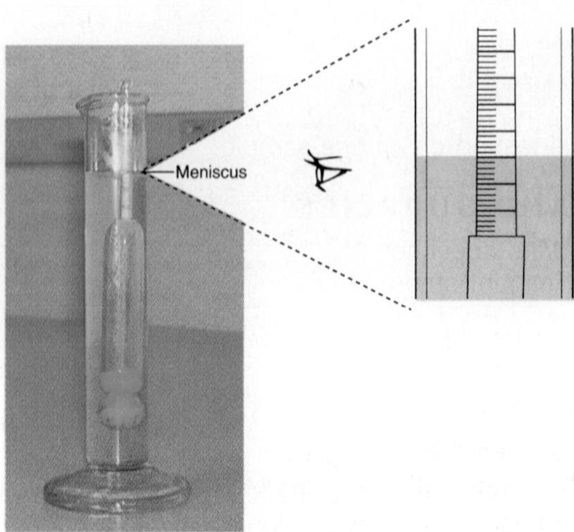

FIGURE 5

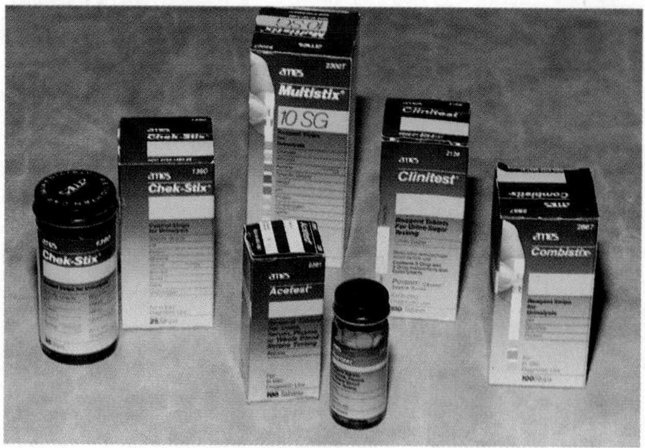

FIGURE 43–8 Examples of reagent strips.

Chemical Examination of Urine

Tests can be performed on urine to detect the presence of certain chemicals that can provide valuable information to the physician. In certain situations, these chemical test results can be critical to the diagnosis.

Reagent strips (dipsticks) are the most widely used technique of detecting chemicals in the urine (see Procedure 43–3) and are available in a variety of types (Fig. 43–8). Reagent strips are plastic strips to which one or more pads containing chemicals are attached. Tests are available for pH, specific gravity, vitamin C, leukocytes, protein, ketones, glucose, blood, bilirubin, nitrite, urobilinogen, phenylketones, and others. The presence or absence of these chemicals in the urine provides information on the status of carbohydrate metabolism, liver and kidney function, and the acid-base balance of the patient.

These reagent strips are designed to be used once and then discarded. The directions for each strip are located in the package, and these instructions must be followed exactly to obtain accurate results. A color-comparison chart is located on the label of the container. In addition to reagent strips, various tablet tests are available. Quality controls are also available to ensure reliable test results.

All strips and tablets must be kept in tightly closed containers and should only be removed immediately before testing. Reagents should be stored in a cool, dry area.

pH

The pH is a measurement of the degree of acidity or alkalinity of the urine. A urine specimen with a pH of 7 is neutral (Fig. 43–9). Less than 7 is acid, and greater than 7 is alkaline. Normal, freshly voided urine may have a pH range of 5.5 to 8.0. Urinary pH varies with an individual's metabolic status, diet, drug therapy, and disease. Colors on the pH reagent pad usually range from yellow-orange for an acid pH to green-blue when the pH is alkaline.

Memory Jogger

The measurement of urinary pH determines ________.

PROCEDURE 43–3

Testing Urine with Chemical Reagent Strips

GOAL

To perform chemical testing on a urine sample.

EQUIPMENT AND SUPPLIES

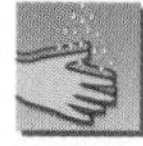

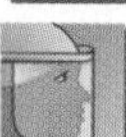

Urine specimen
Reagent strips
Timer

PROCEDURAL STEPS

1 Wash and dry your hands. Put on nonsterile gloves and eye protection.
PURPOSE: Infection control.

Continued

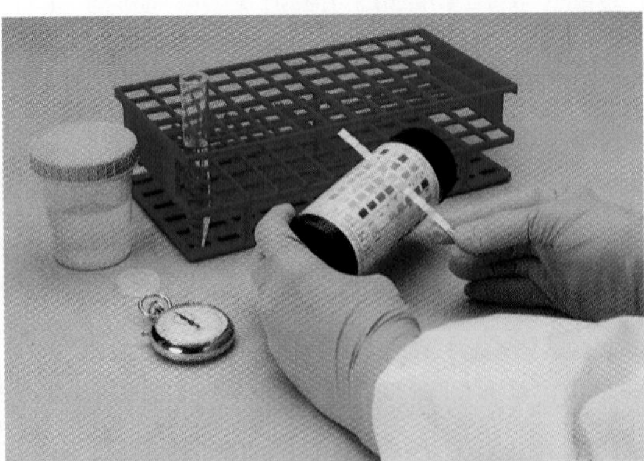
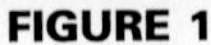

FIGURE 1

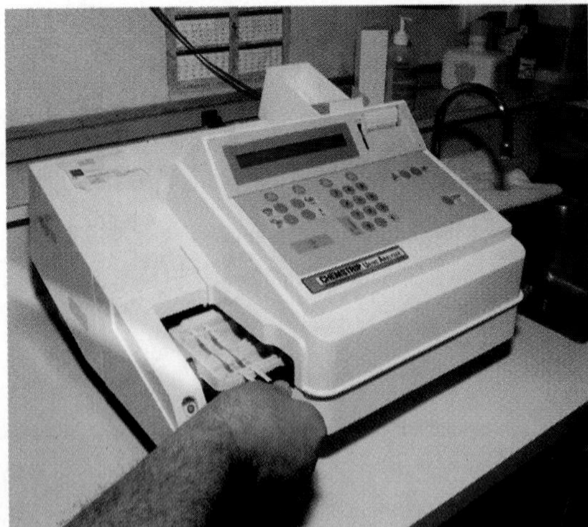

FIGURE 2

2 Check the time of collection, the container, and the mode of preservation.
PURPOSE: Proper specimen identification and screening of specimens for appropriate collection containers and collection procedures prevents testing of inappropriate specimens.

3 If the specimen has been refrigerated, allow it to warm to room temperature.
PURPOSE: Certain tests are temperature dependent. Testing of cold specimens may cause false-negative results.

4 Check the reagent strip container for expiration date.
PURPOSE: Do not use expired reagents.

5 Remove the reagent strip from the container. Hold it in your hand, or place it on a clean paper towel. Recap the container tightly.
PURPOSE: Test strips are sensitive to moisture and must be stored in tightly sealed containers. Contamination from chemical residues on countertops can affect results.

6 Compare nonreactive test pads with the negative color blocks on the color chart on the container.
PURPOSE: Discolored pads have not been properly stored and must not be used for testing.

7 Thoroughly mix the specimen by swirling or inverting.
PURPOSE: If settling occurs, certain elements may not be detected.

8 Following manufacturer's directions, note the time, and simultaneously dip the strip into the urine and remove.
PURPOSE: Tests are time dependent. Positive tests result in darkening with time.

9 Quickly remove the excess urine from the strip.
PURPOSE: Excess urine on the strip, or prolonged dipping time, affects test results.

10 Hold the strip horizontally. At the exact time, compare the strip with the appropriate color chart on the reagent container (Figure 1).
PURPOSE: Holding the strip horizontally prevents runover from one test pad to another and prevents interference from the mixing of chemicals in the test pads.

11 Read the concentration. Reagent strips with automated reaction readings are available as an alternative to manual reading. Automation gives more consistent results, because it eliminates timing and color perception as variables (Figure 2).
PURPOSE: Timing is critical.

12 Clean the work area, remove your gloves, and wash your hands.
PURPOSE: Infection control.

13 Record the results in the patient's record.
PURPOSE: A procedure is considered not done until it is recorded.

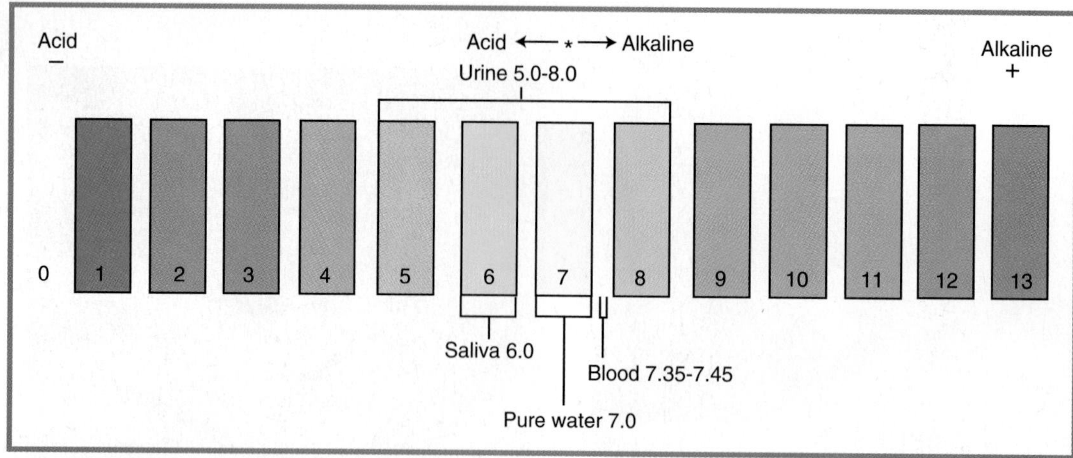

FIGURE 43-9 pH scale. (From Stepp CA, Woods MA: Laboratory Procedures for Medical Office Personnel. Philadelphia, WB Saunders, 1998.)

GLUCOSE

Glucose is filtered at the glomerulus, but under normal conditions most of it is reabsorbed by the tubules. The minute quantities normally present are not detected by strips and tablets. Detectable **glycosuria** occurs whenever the renal tubules cannot reabsorb the filtered glucose load. A positive glucose finding is common in urine from diabetic patients and may be the first indication of the disease.

The reagent-strip glucose testing method is **enzymatic.** It detects only glucose; in other words, it is *specific* for glucose. None of the other sugars that can occur in urine are detected by the reagent strips. A copper reduction test is commonly used to screen and confirm existing glucose and other sugars present in urine (see Procedure 43–4). Colors on the reagent strip range from green (low concentration of glucose) to brown (high concentration of glucose).

PROCEDURE 43-4

Testing Urine for Glucose Using Copper Reduction (Clinitest)

GOAL

To perform confirmatory testing for glucose in the urine using the Clinitest procedure for reducing substances.

EQUIPMENT AND SUPPLIES

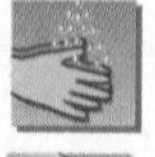
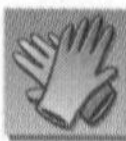

Urine specimen
Clinitest tablet, tube, and dropper
Distilled water
Test tube rack
Color chart
Timer

PROCEDURAL STEPS

1 Wash and dry your hands and put on nonsterile gloves and eye protection.

2 Holding a Clinitest dropper vertically, add 10 drops of distilled water and then 5 drops of urine to a Clinitest tube.
PURPOSE: Holding the dropper vertically prevents altering the size of the drops.

Continued

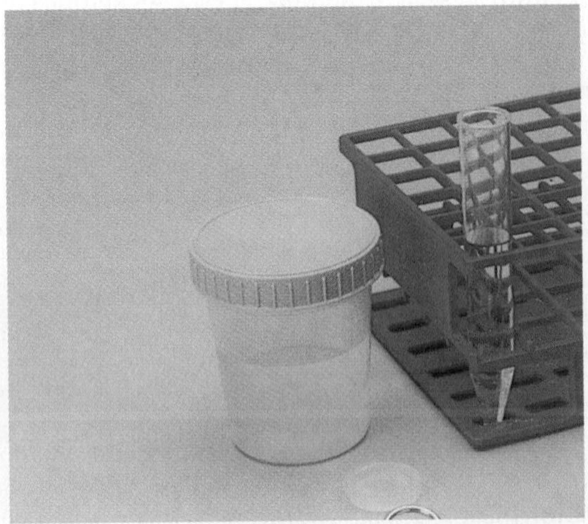
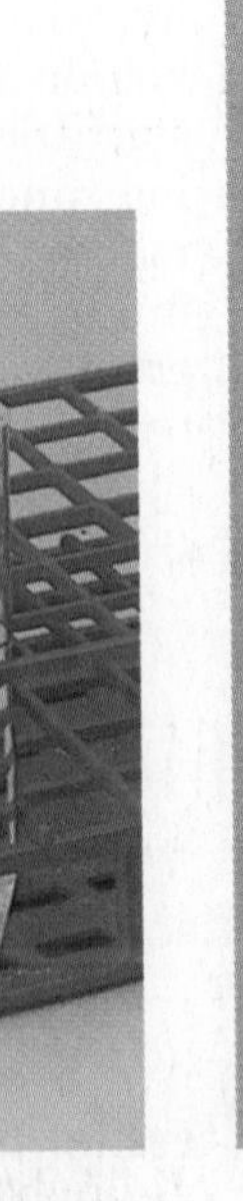

FIGURE 1

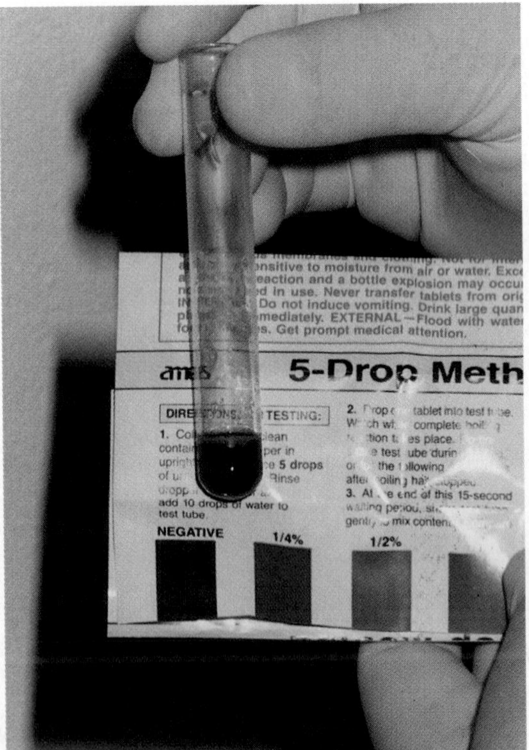

FIGURE 2

3 Place the prepared tube into the rack (Figure 1).
PURPOSE: The tube will become too hot to hold when the tablet is placed into the tube.

4 With dry hands, remove a Clinitest tablet from the bottle by pouring the tablet into the bottle cap.
PURPOSE: Clinitest tablets react with moisture and became caustic. Handling tablets with moist hands could result in hydroxide burns.

5 Tap the tablet into the test tube, and recap the container.

6 Observe the entire reaction to detect the rapid pass-through phenomenon. (See step 9.)
PURPOSE: If pass-through occurs but is not detected, the reading will be falsely low.

7 When boiling ceases, time exactly 15 seconds; then gently shake the tube to mix the entire contents.

8 Immediately compare the color of the specimen with the five-drop color chart, and record your findings (Figure 2).
PURPOSE: Color darkens with time. For accurate results, time carefully.

9 If an orange color briefly develops during the reaction, rapid pass-through has occurred, and the test must be repeated using the two-drop color chart.

10 Clean the work area, remove gloves, and wash hands.
PURPOSE: Infection control.

11 Record the results:
- Negative—Clear
- Trace—Slightly cloudy
- 1+—Can see light print through tube
- 2+—Can see dark print through tube
- 3+—Cannot see through tube
- 4+—Large, fluffy precipitate forms and settles, on standing

PURPOSE: A procedure is considered not done until it is recorded.

PROTEIN

Protein in the urine in detectable amounts is called **proteinuria** and is one of the first signs of renal disease. We normally excrete a small amount of protein every day, but our testing procedures are designed to detect only pathologic levels in the urine (see Procedure 43–5). Proteinuria may be light to heavy, constant, or sporadic. It may be affected by posture. In orthostatic proteinuria, protein is excreted only when the patient is in an upright position. Generally, first morning specimens from these patients are negative, but protein is found in urine passed throughout the day. Proteinuria is a common finding in pregnancy. It is almost always present after heavy exercise. Colors on the protein reagent pad usually range from yellow for negative to yellow-green or green for positive.

KETONES

Ketone bodies are the end product of fat metabolism in the body. Acetoacetic acid, acetone, and beta-hydroxybutyric acid are collectively referred to as ketone bodies, or ketones. *Ketonuria* is common in starvation, low-carbohydrate diets, excessive vomiting, and diabetes mellitus. Because ketones evaporate at room temperature, urine should be tested immediately, or the specimen should be tightly covered and refrigerated if not tested promptly. Color reactions on the strip range from pink to maroon

PROCEDURE 43–5

Testing Urine for Protein Using the Sulfosalicyclic Acid (SSA) Precipitation Test

GOAL

To perform the sulfosalicylic acid (SSA) precipitation test for the presence of protein in the urine.

EQUIPMENT AND SUPPLIES

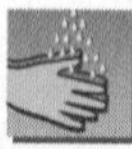

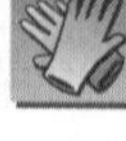

- Urine specimen
- 3% sulfosalicylic acid
- Centrifuge tube and centrifuge
- Test tube and rack
- Dropper

PROCEDURAL STEPS

1 Wash and dry your hands. Put on nonsterile gloves and eye protection.

2 If the urine is cloudy, filter the specimen or use a centrifuged specimen.
PURPOSE: If the urine is already turbid (cloudy), the test will be difficult to interpret.

3 In a clear test tube, mix equal volumes of urine and 3% SSA.

4 Observe for cloudiness and record:
- Negative—Clear
- Trace—Slightly cloudy
- 1+—Can see light print through tube
- 2+—Can see dark print through tube
- 3+—Cannot see through tube
- 4+—Large, fluffy precipitate forms and settles on standing

PURPOSE: This result gives a rough estimation of the protein concentration of the urine.

5 Clean the work area, remove gloves and face protection, and wash hands.
PURPOSE: Infection control.

6 Record the results in the patient's chart.
PURPOSE: A procedure is considered not done until it is recorded.

when ketones are present. *Acetest* reagent tablets provide an alternative to strip testing.

BLOOD

The presence of blood in the urine may indicate infection or trauma to the urinary tract or bleeding in the kidneys. The blood test pad on the reagent strip reacts with three different blood constituents: intact red blood cells, hemoglobin from red blood cells, and myoglobin, a hemoglobin-like molecule that transports oxygen in muscle tissue.

Hematuria is the presence of intact red blood cells in urine. The color reaction on the reagent strip ranges from yellow through green to dark green when hematuria is present. Hematuria can be due to irritation of the ureters, bladder, or urethra. It is also a common finding in cystitis and in persons passing kidney stones.

Hemoglobinuria is the presence of hemolyzed red blood cells. True hemoglobinuria is rare. It occurs as the result of intravascular red blood cell destruction and can be caused by transfusion reactions, malaria, drug reactions, snake bites, and severe burns. **Myoglobinuria** occurs when muscle tissue is damaged or injured, such as in crushing injuries, myocardial infarctions, and contact sports. Muscular dystrophy patients often exhibit myoglobinuria. Hemoglobinuria cannot be distinguished from myoglobinuria by strip testing.

BILIRUBIN AND UROBILINOGEN

Bilirubin is a product of the breakdown of hemoglobin. Hemoglobin is released from old red blood cells and is gradually converted to bilirubin in the liver and then further to urobilinogen in the intestines. Bilirubin is a bile pigment not normally found in urine. Its presence in urine is one of the first signs of liver disease or other disease in which the liver may be involved, such as infectious mononucleosis.

Bilirubinuria can occur even before jaundice or other symptoms of liver disease are evident. It is the result of liver cell damage or obstruction of the common bile duct by stones or neoplasms (tumors). Excessive bilirubin colors the urine yellow-brown to greenish orange. Because direct light causes decomposition of bilirubin, urine samples must be protected from light until testing is complete. *Ictotest* tablets (Ames Company) are more sensitive to bilirubin than are the strips and are often easier to interpret when the urine is highly colored.

Urobilinogen is normally present in urine in small amounts. Increases are seen when there is increased red blood cell destruction and in liver disease. When there is total obstruction of the bile duct, no urobilinogen is formed in the intestines, none is reabsorbed into the circulation, and, hence, none is present in the urine. Strip methods cannot detect a decrease in urobilinogen. The reagent strip for positive testing results in color changes from cream through dark mauve.

NITRITE

Nitrite occurs in urine when bacteria break down nitrate. A positive nitrite test indicates a urinary tract infection. However, not all bacteria are able to reduce nitrate to nitrite. Negative nitrite tests can also occur when bacteria are insufficient or when the urine has not incubated in the bladder long enough for the reaction to occur. *Escherichia coli,* the organism that causes the majority of urinary tract infections, is nitrite positive. False-positive results can occur if a specimen is allowed to sit at room temperature and contaminating bacteria multiply. False-negative results occur if the bacteria further metabolize the nitrite they have produced. Any shade of pink on the reagent strip indicates a positive test.

Memory Jogger

 *What causes nitrite to occur in urine?*

LEUKOCYTES

Leukocytes occur in urine in infections of the urinary tract. They can also be contaminants from the vagina. The *leukocyte esterase test* on reagent strips detects intact and lysed polymorphonuclear white blood cells. However, it does not detect mononuclear white blood cells, which are occasionally present during infections. The test does not react with the small numbers of white blood cells found in normal urine. On the reagent strip the leukocyte reading goes from pale lavender to lavender to dark purple.

SPECIFIC GRAVITY

Reagent strips are available that report specific gravity by the use of colored pads. The individual test pads on the strip give readings every 0.005 on the specific gravity scale from 1.000 to 1.030.

PHENYLKETONES

Phenistix are reagent strips used to detect the presence of phenylketones in the urine. This condition is called *phenylketonuria* (PKU). In this genetically inherited disorder, the body is unable to properly metabolize the nutrient **phenylalanine.**

As high levels of the phenylketones accumulate in

the bloodstream, mental retardation occurs. Phenylketonuria is easily treated by limiting dietary intake of phenylalanine in childhood. Because individuals who are properly treated for the disease do not suffer mental retardation, early detection is very important.

ASCORBIC ACID (VITAMIN C)

Ascorbic acid normally is not found in urine in quantities large enough to interfere with chemical urine tests. However, in persons who habitually consume large quantities of vitamin C, the urine levels of ascorbic acid may affect results of nitrite, glucose, bilirubin, and occult blood tests. Strips are available to detect interfering levels of the drug. If an elevated level is found, the patient should be instructed to discontinue vitamin C intake for 24 hours, and then another urine specimen should be collected for testing.

Microscopic Examination of Urine Sediment

The microscopic examination of urine consists of categorizing and counting cells, casts, crystals, and miscellaneous constituents of the sediment obtained when a measured portion of urine is centrifuged (see Procedure 43–6). The clear upper portion of the specimen is called the supernatant. It is poured off, and a drop of the well-mixed sediment is examined under a microscope. This part of the urinalysis gives the physician information about the course and progress of renal disease and detects the presence of infection.

Memory Jogger

9 *What does the microscopic examination of urine consist of?*

CASTS

Casts are formed when protein accumulates and precipitates in the kidney tubules and is washed into the urine. The protein takes on the size and shape of the tubules, hence the term *casts.* Casts are cylindric, with flat or rounded ends, and are classified according to the substances observed in them. Certain types of casts are associated with renal pathologic conditions; others are physiologic and are generally caused by strenuous exercise.

Casts are counted and reported under low-power magnification, but occasionally high-power magnification is needed to identify the type. Because casts tend to migrate to the edges of the coverslip, this area should be examined closely. Casts dissolve in alkaline urine on standing; therefore, examination of a fresh urine specimen is very important.

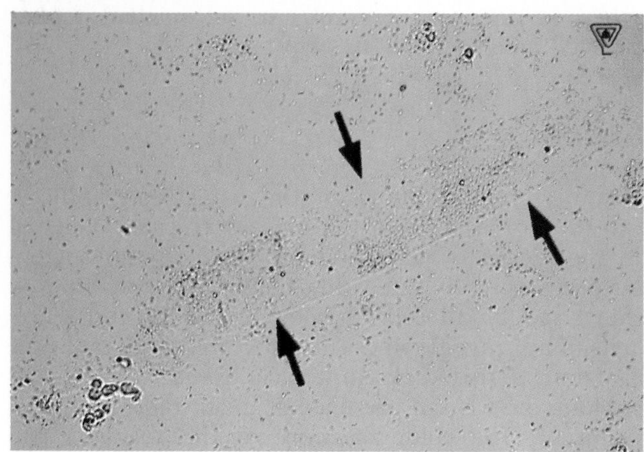

FIGURE 43–10 Hyaline casts. (From Stepp CA, Woods MA: Laboratory Procedures for Medical Office Personnel. Philadelphia, WB Saunders, 1998.)

Hyaline casts are pale, transparent cylindric structures that have rounded ends and parallel sides. Hyaline casts will be missed entirely if subdued light is not used. They are formed when urine flow through individual nephrons is diminished. They can be found in kidney disease but can also be found in urine specimens of normal subjects who have exercised heavily. Occasionally, hyaline casts have granular or cellular inclusions. *White blood cell casts* are hyaline casts that contain leukocytes. White blood cells usually have a multilobed nucleus, which differentiates them from renal tubular epithelial cells, which have single, round nuclei. White blood cell casts are seen in pyelonephritis (Fig. 43–10).

Finely and coarsely granular casts may be due to exercise but, when present in increased numbers, may indicate renal disease. On close examination, granular casts show a hyaline matrix with coarse or fine granular inclusions. The granules are thought to

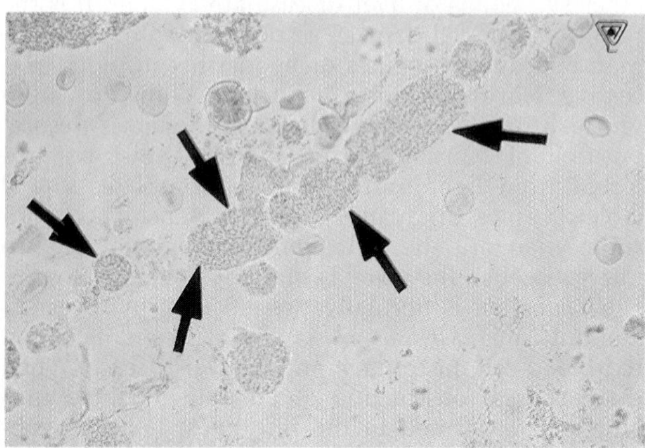

FIGURE 43–11 Granular casts. (From Stepp CA, Woods MA: Laboratory Procedures for Medical Office Personnel. Philadelphia, WB Saunders, 1998.)

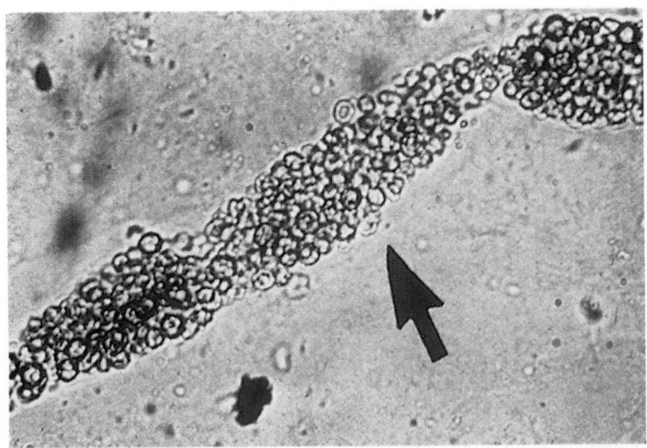

FIGURE 43-12 Red blood cell casts. (From Stepp CA, Woods MA: Laboratory Procedures for Medical Office Personnel. Philadelphia, WB Saunders, 1998.)

be due to protein aggregation or degeneration of cellular inclusions (Fig. 43-11).

Red blood cell casts are always pathologic and highly diagnostic. Red blood cell casts occur in glomerulonephritis. They are hyaline casts with embedded red cells, and their presence indicates damage to the glomerular membrane. They may appear brown as a result of the color of the red blood cells present (Fig. 43-12).

Renal tubular epithelial cell casts contain embedded renal tubular epithelial cells. These casts are easily confused with white blood cell casts, particularly if the cells have started to degenerate. Renal tubular epithelial cell casts are found when there is excessive damage. Causes are shock, renal ischemia, heavy-metal poisoning, certain allergic reactions, and nephrotoxic drugs (Fig. 43-13).

Waxy casts are rarely seen. They appear as glassy, brittle, smooth, homogeneous structures. They are usually yellowish, have cracks or fissures, and have squared or broken ends. They are considered to be degenerated cellular casts and are found in severe renal disease (Fig. 43-14).

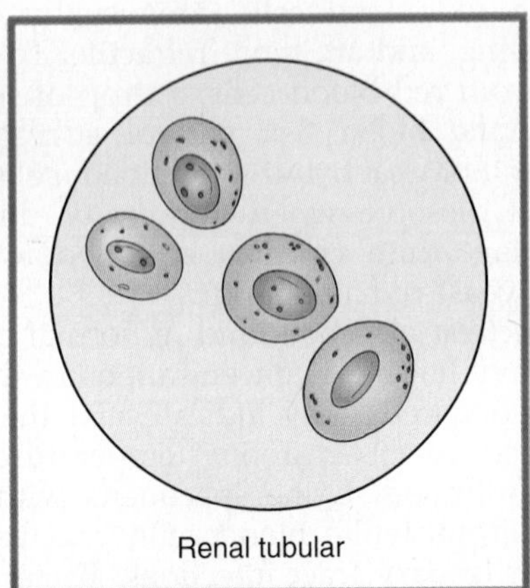

FIGURE 43-13 Renal tubular casts. (From Stepp CA, Woods MA: Laboratory Procedures for Medical Office Personnel. Philadelphia, WB Saunders, 1998.)

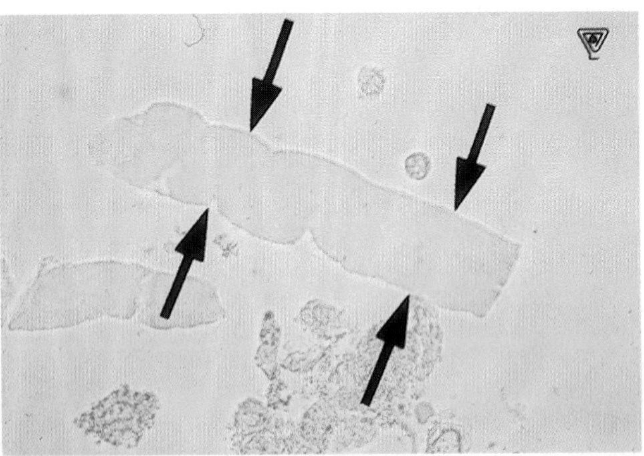

FIGURE 43-14 Waxy casts. (From Stepp CA, Woods MA: Laboratory Procedures for Medical Office Personnel. Philadelphia, WB Saunders, 1998.)

Occasionally, more than one type of cell will be found in a single cast. Mixed cellular casts have been reported. Absolute identification of the cell types present may be difficult. Be as specific as possible.

CELLS

Cells that are found in urine include epithelial cells, which are derived from the lining of the genitourinary tract. Other cells in urine include red blood cells and white blood cells from the bloodstream. Cells are classified and counted under high-power magnification.

Red blood cells may enter the urinary tract at any point where there is inflammation or injury. They may be found in normal urine in small numbers, usually less than 1 to 2 per high-power field. Persistent hematuria should be investigated. Red blood cells are pale, round, nongranular, and flat or biconcave (Fig. 43-15). They are smaller than white blood cells and have no nucleus. In hypotonic, or dilute,

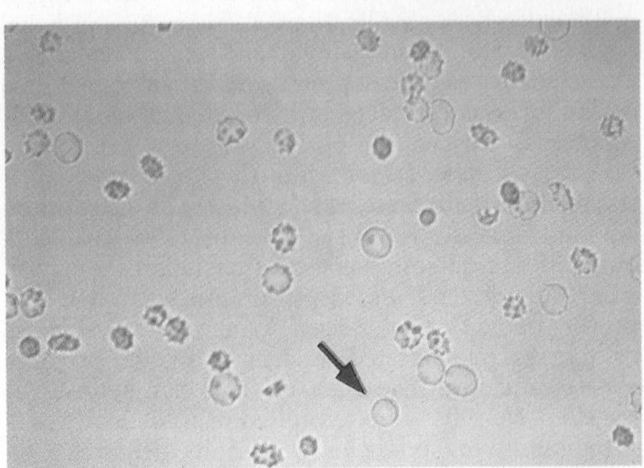

FIGURE 43-15 Red blood cells in urine. (From Stepp CA, Woods MA: Laboratory Procedures for Medical Office Personnel. Philadelphia, WB Saunders, 1998.)

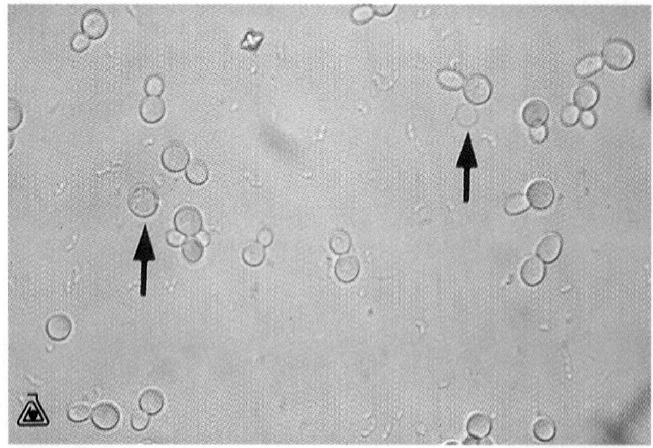

FIGURE 43-16 Yeast in urine. (From Stepp CA, Woods MA: Laboratory Procedures for Medical Office Personnel. Philadelphia, WB Saunders, 1998.)

urine, they swell and burst. In hypertonic, or concentrated, urine, they may crenate and wrinkle. When they crenate, they can be mistaken for white blood cells, because the wrinkled surface makes them appear granular. They are often confused with yeast (Fig. 43–16), oil droplets, and droplets of lens cleaner.

White blood cells may occasionally be found in normal urine, but increased numbers, usually greater than 5 cells per high-power field, are associated with inflammation or contamination of the specimen during collection. White blood cells are larger than red blood cells, have a granular appearance, and usually contain a multilobed nucleus, although nuclear detail may not be evident.

Renal tubular or round epithelial cells are somewhat larger than white blood cells, are round to oval, and have a single, large, oval and sometimes eccentric nucleus. A few may be found in normal urine specimens, but their presence in increased numbers indicates tubular damage.

Transitional epithelial cells line the urinary tract from the renal pelvis to the upper portion of the urethra. They vary from slightly larger than a round epithelial cell to smaller than a squamous epithelial cell. They are round to oval and may have a tail. Occasionally, two nuclei are seen. When transitional cells are present in large numbers, a pathologic condition may exist.

Squamous epithelial cells line the lower portion of the genitourinary tract. When present in large numbers in females, they usually indicate vaginal contamination. Squamous epithelial cells are large, flat, irregular cells and are easily recognized under low-power magnification. They have a single, small, round, centrally located nucleus and often occur in sheets or clumps. Because of their flat nature, the edges of the cells are often rolled or folded.

In identifying epithelial cells, it is helpful to remember the appearance of eggs; round epithelial cells resemble hard-boiled eggs that have been cut in half. Transitional forms resemble poached eggs, and squamous cells resemble fried eggs with large, runny whites.

Memory Jogger

 *Cells are classified and counted under what microscopic power?*

CRYSTALS

Crystals are common in urine specimens, particularly if they have been allowed to cool. Cooling causes the solid crystals to precipitate out of the urine. The presence of most crystals is not clinically significant unless they are found in large numbers in patients with kidney stones. Occasionally, pathologic crystals are found. Identification of crystals begins with the determination of the pH of the urine. From there, one looks at color, shape, and refractility. Often, a history of drug intake is helpful. Consult Table 32–5 for nonpathologic and pathologic urine crystals. It is not always possible to identify crystals without additional chemical testing (Fig. 43–17).

Memory Jogger

 *Are crystals commonly found in urine specimens?*

MISCELLANEOUS FINDINGS

Oval fat bodies are formed when renal tubular epithelial cells or macrophages absorb fats. The fat droplets contained in the cells vary in size and are quite refractile. Oval fat bodies are characteristic of the nephrotic syndrome.

Yeast in urine may indicate vaginal contamination or infection of the urine with yeast. It is common in the urine of diabetic patients. Yeasts are easily confused with red blood cells, are usually oval, may show budding, and are more refractile. To differentiate yeast from red blood cells, a drop of sediment is placed on the blood test pad of a reagent strip. Yeast does not react, but red blood cells do. Red blood cells dissolve when a drop of dilute acetic acid (regular white vinegar) is added to the sediment. The yeast remains intact.

A few *bacteria* may be found in normal urine specimens. Heavy bacterial concentrations in the absence of white blood cells may indicate that the specimen was allowed to sit at room temperature and the bacteria multiplied. Urine specimens with a putrid odor, numerous white blood cells, and bacteria are common in urinary tract infections. Bacteria may be rods or cocci and are identified under high-power magnification.

Sperm are often found in the urine specimens of

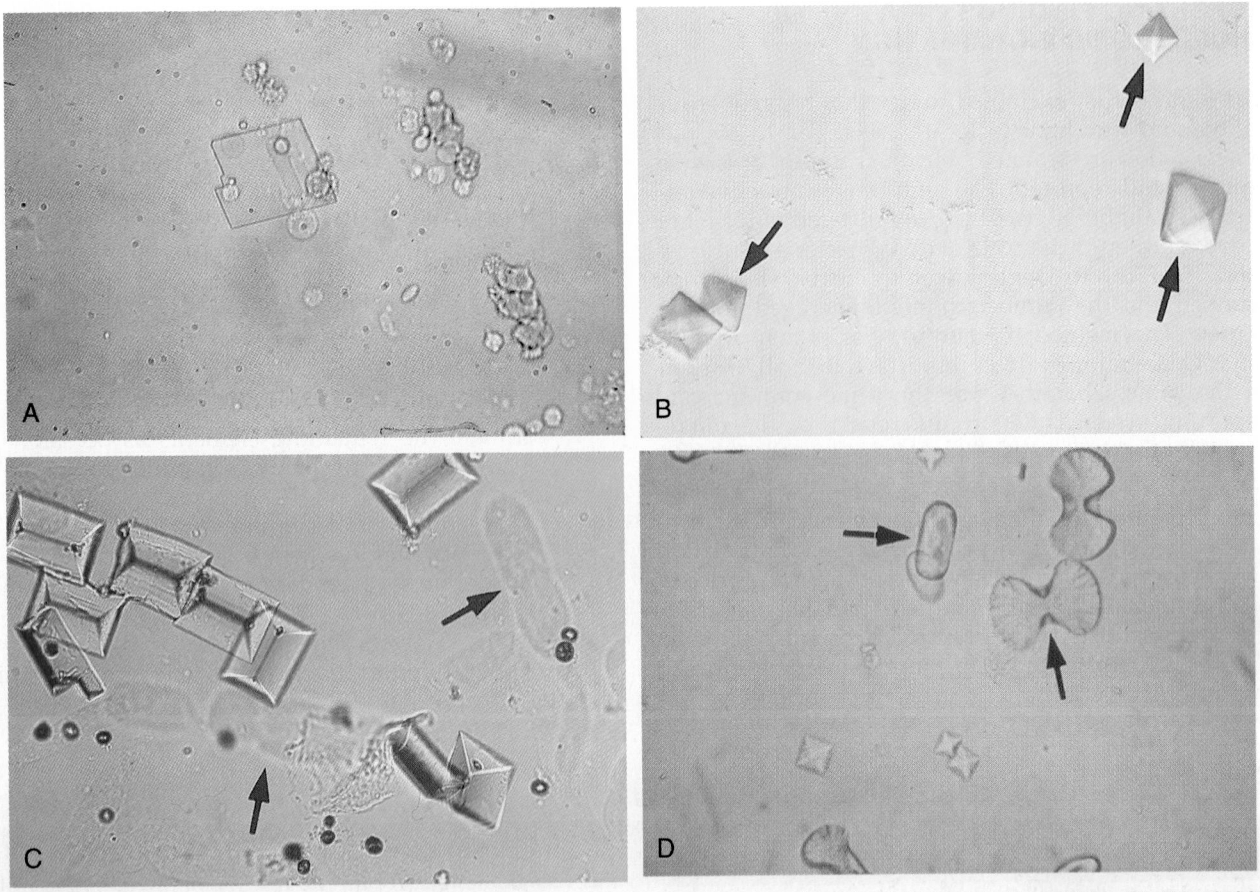

FIGURE 43–17 Crystals in urine *A,* Cholesterol, *B,* Calcium oxalate, *C,* Triple phosphate. *D,* Sulfonamide. (From Stepp CA, Woods MA: Laboratory Procedures for Medical Office Personnel. Philadelphia, WB Saunders, 1998.)

both males and females. In the latter, their presence represents vaginal contamination of the specimen. Sperm usually have pointed, oval heads and long threadlike tails. They may be motile in fresh urine.

The most commonly encountered parasite in urine is *Trichomonas vaginalis* (Fig. 43–18). It is usually a vaginal contaminant but may also be found in urine specimens from males. When urine is fresh and warm, the trichomonas may be motile. *Trichomonas* organisms are pear-shaped protozoa with four flagella. They are larger than round epithelial cells but smaller than squamous cells. *Trichomonas* organisms die when the specimen is cooled.

Mucous threads can be found in most urine specimens. They appear as pale, irregular, thready structures with tapered ends. Beginners often confuse hyaline casts and mucous threads. Increased numbers are seen in inflammation and when there has been contamination of the specimen with vaginal contents (Fig. 43–19).

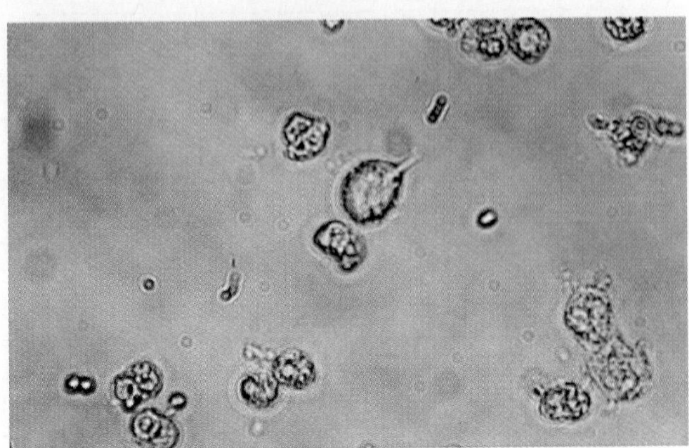

FIGURE 43–18 *Trichomonas* in urine. (From Stepp CA, Woods MA: Laboratory Procedures for Medical Office Personnel. Philadelphia, WB Saunders, 1998.)

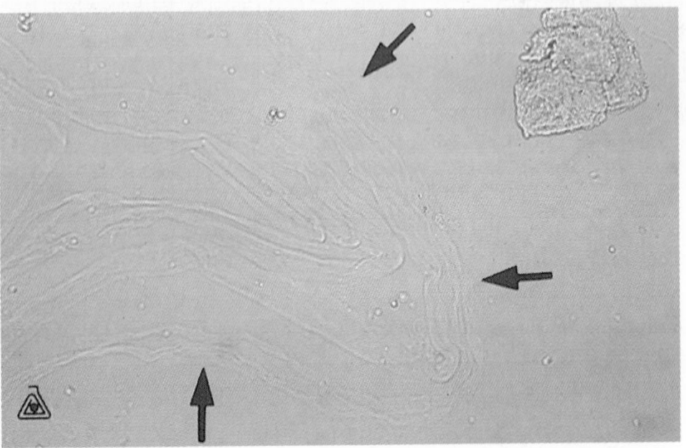

FIGURE 43–19 Mucous threads in urine. (From Stepp CA, Woods MA: Laboratory Procedures for Medical Office Personnel. Philadelphia, WB Saunders, 1998.)

REPORTING FINDINGS OF A MICROSCOPIC EXAMINATION

The slide is first examined under the low-power objective and low light to locate casts. Ten to 15 low-power fields are scanned, and the number of casts is counted and reported. The high-power objective and increased light is used to identify red and white blood cells, epithelial cells, yeasts, bacteria, and crystals. Ten to 15 high-powered fields should be scanned and the number counted, averaged, and reported. The method of counting varies considerably among laboratories. It is important that all workers in the same laboratory use the same counting and reporting systems. Report the results of the microscopic examination as follows (Table 43–4):

1. Separately total the numbers for each element counted, and then average. (Casts, white blood cells, red blood cells and the three categories of epithelial cells are counted, totaled, and averaged.) Casts, white blood cells, and red blood cells are reported using numerical ranges based on the average:

0	10–20
0–1	20–30
1–2	30–40
2–5	40–50
5–10	>50

   Epithelial cells are reported as occasional, few, moderate, or many, according to the following:
   0
   0–3 = occasional
   3–6 = few
   6–12 = moderate
   12 = many
2. Estimate the remaining elements as occasional, few, moderate, or many, according to the following:
   Occasional—not seen in every field
   Few—covers less than a quarter of the field
   Moderate—covers approximately half of the field
   Many—covers the entire field
   Do not report fibers, hair, talc granules, oil droplets, and other artifacts.

TABLE 43–4 Calculating a Microscopic Urinalysis

	Per Low-Power Field		Per High-Power Field							
Field	Casts	Mucus	WBC	RBC	Squamous Epithelial	Transitional Epithelial	Round Epithelial	Bacteria	Crystals	Other
1	0	Few	16	1	1	0	0	Moderate (rods)	Calcium oxalate—few Uric acid—few	—
2	1 hyaline	Few	32	0	3	0	0	Many	Calcium oxalate—few	Yeast
3	1 coarse granular	Moderate	21	2	3	0	0	Many	Calcium-oxalate—few	Yeast
4	1 coarse granular	Few	12	1	5	0	1	Moderate	Uric acid—few	—
5	0	Few	25	0	4	0	0	Many	—	—
Total	1 hyaline 2 coarse granular	Few	106	4	16	0	1	Many	Calcium oxalate—few Uric acid—few	Yeast
Average	0.2 hyaline 0.4 coarse granular	Few	21.2	0.8	3.2	0	0.2	Many	Calcium oxalate—few Uric acid—few	Yeast
Report	0-1 hyaline 0-1 coarse granular	Few	20–30	0–1	Few	0	Occasionally	Many (rods)	Calcium oxalate—few Uric acid—few	Yeast

PROCEDURE 43-6
Analyzing Urine Microscopically

GOAL

To perform a microscopic examination of urine to determine the presence of normal and abnormal elements.

EQUIPMENT AND SUPPLIES

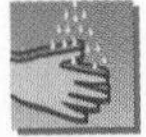

- Urine specimen
- Centrifuge tube
- Centrifuge
- Disposable pipette
- Microscope slide and coverslip
- Microscope
- Permanent marker

PROCEDURAL STEPS

1 Wash and dry your hands. Put on face protection and nonsterile gloves.
PURPOSE: Infection control.

2 Gently mix the urine specimen.
PURPOSE: If the urine is not well mixed, elements that have settled to the bottom of the specimen container will be missed.

3 Pour 10 mL of urine into a labeled centrifuge tube and cap the tube.

4 Place the tube in the centrifuge (Figure 1).

5 Place another tube containing 10 mL of water in the opposite cup.
PURPOSE: For proper operation, centrifuges must be carefully balanced. If not properly balanced, damage to the instrument can occur.

6 Secure the lid, and centrifuge for 5 minutes or for the time specified for your instrument.
PURPOSE: Timing varies based on the speed and the size of the centrifuge head.

Continued

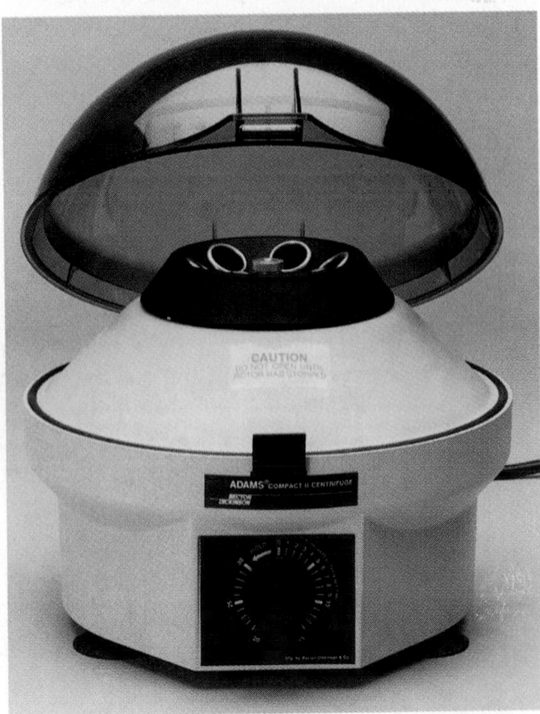

FIGURE 1

PROCEDURE 43-6 (CONTINUED)
Analyzing Urine Microscopically

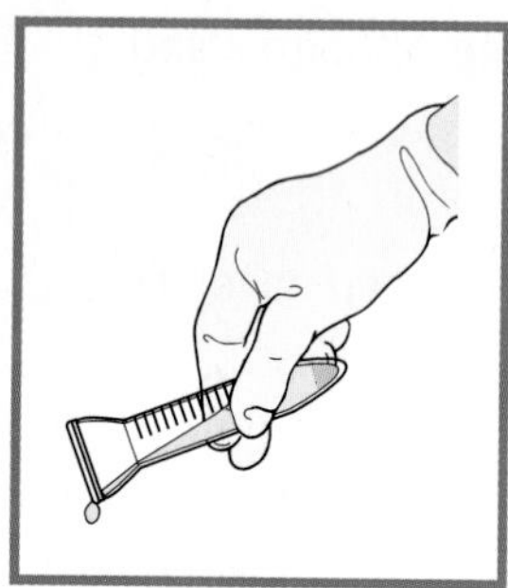

FIGURE 2*

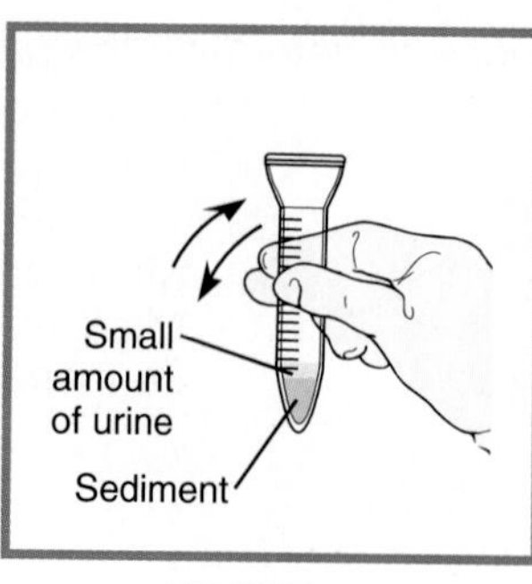

FIGURE 3*

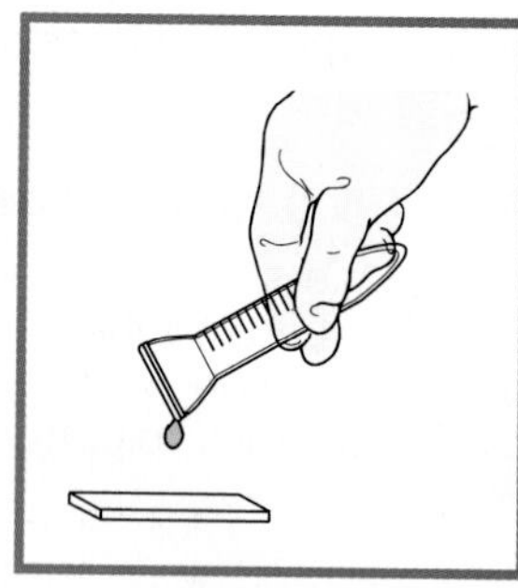

FIGURE 4*

7 Remove the tube from the centrifuge after the instrument has come to a full stop.

8 Pour off the clear supernatant from the top of the specimen by inverting the centrifuge tube over the sink drain (Figure 2*).

9 Prevent the loss of sediment down the drain.
PURPOSE: The sediment is what you will examine under the microscope.

10 Thoroughly mix the sediment by grasping the tube near the top and rapidly flicking it with the fingers of the other hand until all sediment is thoroughly resuspended (Figure 3*).
PURPOSE: Elements centrifuge at different rates. Failure to completely mix the entire sediment will cause errors in quantification.

11 Transfer one drop of sediment to a clean, labeled slide (Figure 4*).

12 Place a clean coverslip over the drop, and place the slide on the microscope stage. Remove face protection.

13 Focus under low power, and reduce the light.
PURPOSE: Mucus and casts are easily missed if reduced light is not used. Constant focusing helps locate them.

14 First, scan the entire coverslip for abnormal findings.
PURPOSE: Casts tend to migrate to the edges of the coverslips.

15 Examine five low-power fields. Count and classify each type of cast seen, if any, and note mucus if present.
PURPOSE: Choose five fields so that one is selected from each corner of the coverslip and the last one is chosen from the middle of the coverslip. If you move to an area and there is nothing there, record a zero.

16 Switch to high-power magnification, and adjust the light.
PURPOSE: As magnification increases, more light is needed.

17 In five high-power fields, count the following elements: red blood cells, white blood cells, and round, transitional, and squamous epithelial cells.

18 In the same five fields, report the following as few, moderate, or many: crystals (identify and report each type seen separately), bacteria (identify as rods or cocci), sperm, yeast, and parasites.
PURPOSE: These three terms are more easily and universally understood than are exact numbers.

Continued

*From Stepp CA, Woods MA: Laboratory Procedures for Medical Office Personnel. Philadelphia, WB Saunders, 1998.

19 Average the five fields, and report the results. Do not remove the slide from the microscope until the physician has verified the results.

20 Clean up the work area, remove face protection and gloves, and wash hands.

21 Record the verified results in the patient's chart.
PURPOSE: A procedure is considered not done until it is recorded.

INTERPRETATION OF URINE CULTURES

Interpretation of urine cultures is performed by estimating the number of colonies and determining if one or more organisms are growing. Urine culture must be performed on a clean-catch urine specimen (see Procedure 43–7). The number of bacteria present in the urine can be estimated by counting the colonies that grow out after 24 hours of incubation (i.e., colony count). For example, if 30 colonies are counted on the medium and a 0.001-mL calibrated inoculating loop was used, the bacterial count is 30,000 per milliliter of urine. The number of colonies is multiplied by 1000, because only 1/1000 mL of urine was cultured. Usually, an infection is indicated when the *colony count* is over 100,000 bacteria per milliliter of urine.

After the organisms have been counted and isolated from the culture, they can then be identified by various means. Growth characteristics can be observed visually. Agglutination kits and biochemical strip tests are also available for identification of the isolated organisms (Fig. 43–20).

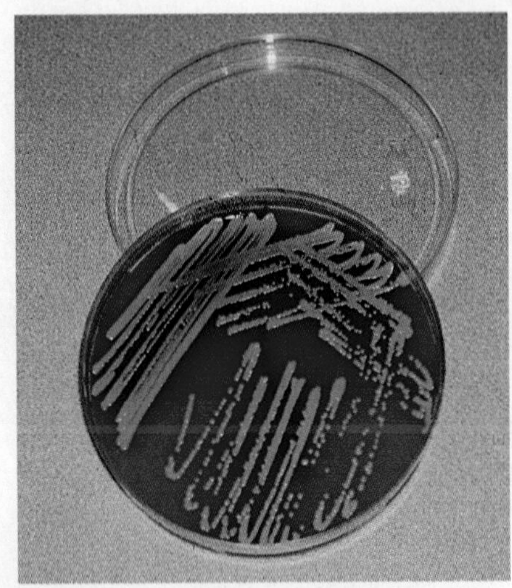

FIGURE 43–20 *Escherichia coli* urinary culture showing more than 100,000 colony-forming units.

Memory Jogger

When counting cells, how many high-power fields should be scanned?

PROCEDURE 43–7
Collecting a Clean-Catch Urine Specimen for Culture or Analysis

GOAL

To collect a contaminant-free urine sample for culture or analysis using midstream clean-catch technique.

EQUIPMENT AND SUPPLIES

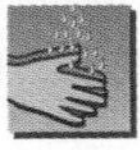

Sterile container with lid
Antiseptic towelettes
Set of written instructions

Continued

PROCEDURE 43-7 (CONTINUED)
Collecting a Clean-Catch Urine Specimen for Culture or Analysis

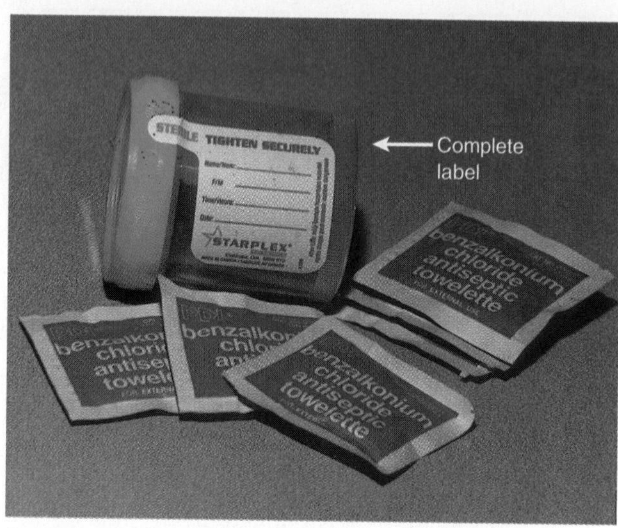

FIGURE 1

PROCEDURAL STEPS

1 Label the container and give the patient the supplies (Figure 1).
PURPOSE: Labeling the container avoids possible mixup of specimens.

2 Explain the instructions to adult patients or to the guardians of child patients.
PURPOSE: Instructions must be understood if they are to be followed. By talking to the patient, you can determine if the patient understands. (Follow instructions given at the beginning of this chapter.)

Quality Control

Quality control is a method of checking reagents, procedures, and personnel to ensure that results are accurate. Many commercially prepared products are available for use in both macroscopic and microscopic testing programs. Check in the procedure manual or the Material Safety Data Sheets book, and follow the protocols accurately. Quality control tests must be recorded and kept according to Occupational Safety and Health Administration and Clinical Laboratory Improvement Amendment regulations.

Pregnancy Testing

Medical assistants are often asked about the use of the home pregnancy tests now on the market. These tests are based on the same principles used in the kit methods most often used in laboratories. All the tests detect the presence of human chorionic gonadotropin (hCG) present in urine during pregnancy. The tests vary considerably in their sensitivity. Some of the home tests are able to detect hCG in urine as early as 9 days after a missed period. Other tests are more sensitive but are not available for home testing. The major drawback to the home test kits is their lack of positive and negative controls, which are supplied with the kits used in the laboratories. However, the home tests do show good agreement with the laboratory methods now in use.

A variety of home pregnancy tests are available in pharmacies. These urine assays for hCG are usually based on some type of enzyme assay procedure, which is usually simple. In spite of clearly written instructions, these tests have high false-positive and false-negative rates due to problems in technique and failure to use an adequate sample. The tests are somewhat expensive, and a physician will need to have the test repeated when the patient is first seen for a prenatal visit. The medical assistant should be familiar with these home tests, their techniques, and their shortcomings. You can be a great help in providing reliable consumer information and in encouraging patients to obtain proper testing and prenatal care.

After pregnancy begins, the hCG levels in serum double every few days. This rapid rise occurs for approximately 7 weeks and then begins to slow. It is during this period that many women request a pregnancy test. The Wampole One-Step HCG is one such test that can be performed by using urine or serum (see Procedure 43–8). It is used routinely in many physicians' office laboratories.

PROCEDURE 43-8
Performing a Pregnancy Detection Test

GOAL

To perform a pregnancy testing of urine using the Wampole (Cranbury, New Jersey) method.

EQUIPMENT AND SUPPLIES

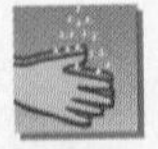
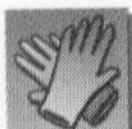
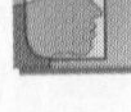

- Urine specimen
- Pregnancy test kit
- Clean test slide
- Disposable mixing sticks
- Wampole One-Step HCG test
- Droppers

PROCEDURAL STEPS

1 Wash and dry hands. Put on face protection and nonsterile gloves.

2 Prepare the testing equipment.

3 Collect the needed specimen. If urine is to be used, collect approximately 0.250 mL in a clean container (Figure 1).

4 Label the handle of the absorbent device or conjugate tube with the patient's name and control number.

5 Remove stopper from the conjugate tube. Discard the stopper (Figure 2*).
PURPOSE: To prevent possible contamination.

6 With a disposable specimen dispenser, draw specimen to the 0.250-mL calibration line and expel specimen into the conjugate tube (Figure 3*).
PURPOSE: To ensure accurate test results, specimen amount must be exact.

Continued

*From Stepp CA, Woods MA: Laboratory Procedures for Medical Office Personnel. Philadelphia, WB Saunders, 1998.

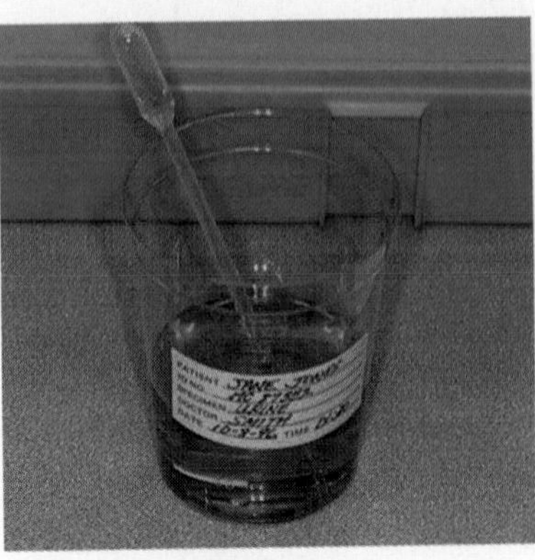

FIGURE 1

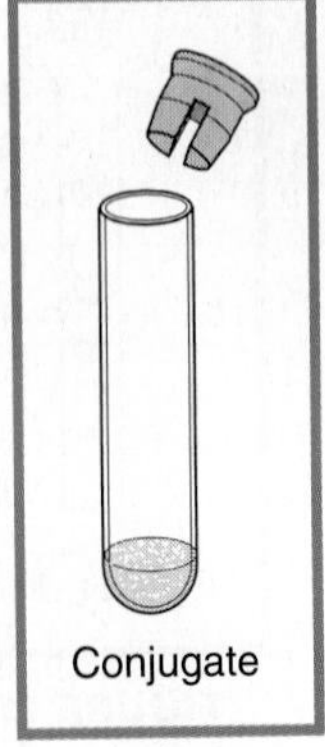

FIGURE 2

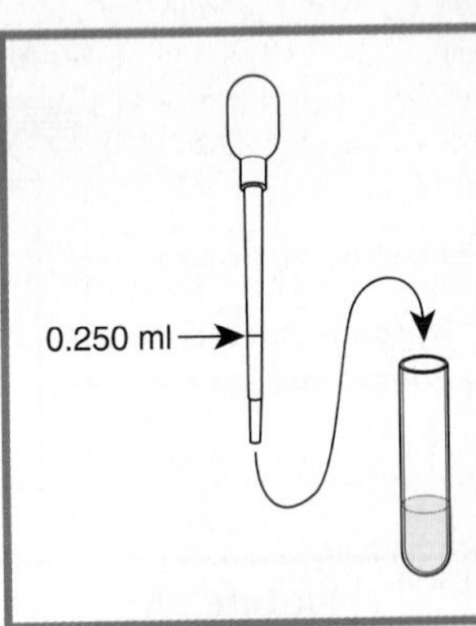

FIGURE 3

PROCEDURE 43–8 (CONTINUED)

Performing a Pregnancy Detection Test

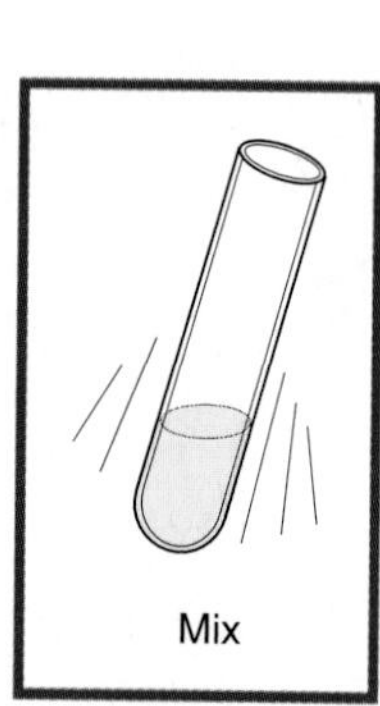

FIGURE 4

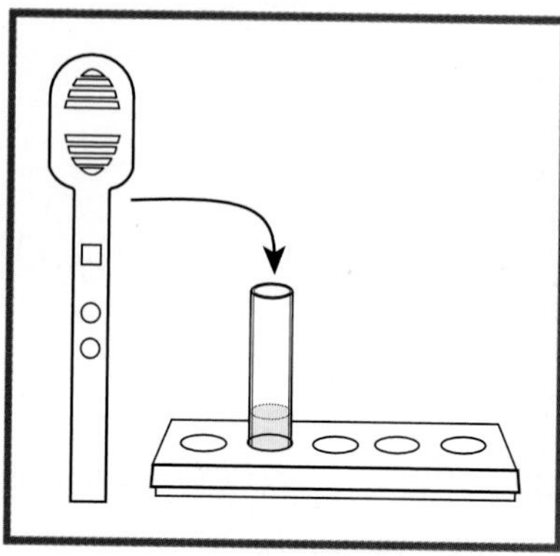

FIGURE 5

7 Mix briefly with a side-to-side motion to reconstitute the conjugate. Do not turn the tube upside down. Vortexing is not required or recommended. The mixture will appear cloudy (Figure 4*).

8 Place the conjugate tube into the work station (Figure 5*).

9 Place a labeled absorbent device into the conjugate tube.
PURPOSE: To ensure proper identification of the test.

10 Read the reactions after 5 minutes for urine and 7 minutes for serum specimens. The absorbent device must be left in the conjugate tube when reading results.
PURPOSE: Removing the device may alter the test results.

11 To read the results, compare the color development in the three reaction zones (Figure 6*A**). If the pink-rose color in the sample reaction zone is darker than the negative control zone, the test result is *positive* (Figure 6*B**). If the pink-rose color in the sample reaction zone is equal to the color in the negative control zone, the test result is *negative* (Figure 6*C**).

Continued

*From Stepp CA, Woods MA: Laboratory Procedures for Medical Office Personnel. Philadelphia, WB Saunders, 1998.

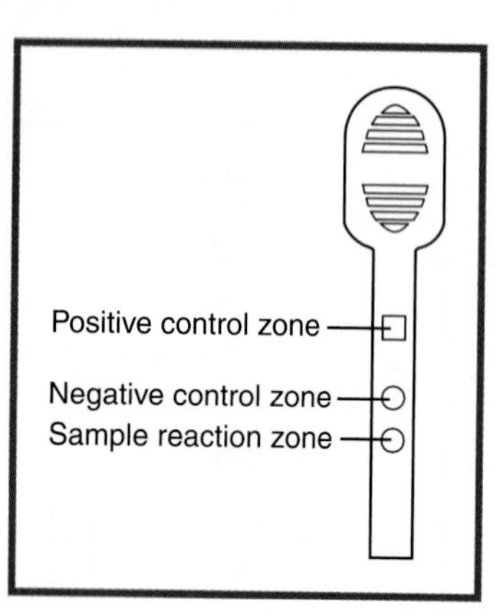

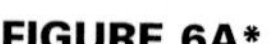

FIGURE 6A*

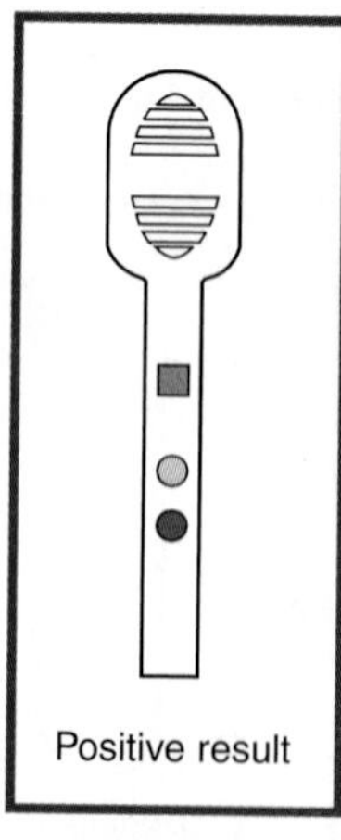

FIGURE 6B*

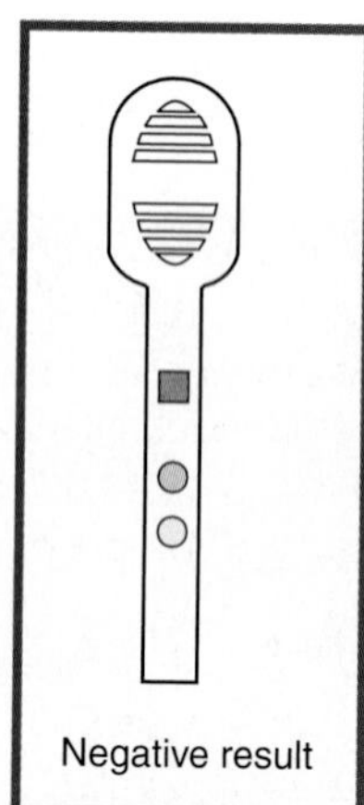

FIGURE 6C*

12 Dispose of all used testing equipment in proper biowaste container. Clean area. Remove gloves and face protection, and wash hands.
PURPOSE: Consider each component that comes in contact with specimen to be potentially infectious.

13 Record test results.
PURPOSE: A procedure is not considered done until it is recorded.

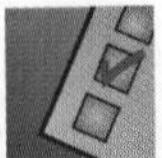

PATIENT EDUCATION

Frequently it will be the medical assistant who will be called on to explain to the patient collection techniques. Patients want to do the procedure correctly but often lack the knowledge of urinary terminology and are embarrassed to or don't know how to ask questions regarding the cleaning of the genital area. When explaining a urinary collection procedure, use lots of pictures and words that the patient understands. As you talk to them in terms that they know, the patient will also feel comfortable in telling you or asking you pertinent details that may have a definite impact on the treatment of the problem.

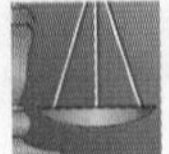

LEGAL AND ETHICAL ISSUES

Like all other procedures, the test is only as valid as the specimen and the procedure performed on that specimen. You, as the physician's agent, are responsible for that validity when you instruct the patient and when you perform the test.

The medical assistant who is responsible for office laboratory testing must clearly understand the basic concepts of laboratory medicine. To do this, you must stay current with the rapid technologic advances in laboratory medicine and assist in the establishment of a protocol of the tests best suited to your physician/employer.

You have the responsibility for properly collecting specimens and accurately testing them. The office laboratory can provide a real challenge and the opportunity to work with the physician in promoting and improving the health of the patient.

CRITICAL THINKING

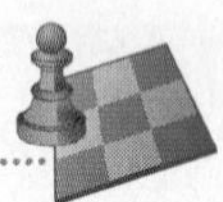

1. Prepare an educational folder that will
   a. Instruct a patient in the collection of a timed/24-hour urine specimen.
   b. Instruct a patient in the collection of a clean-catch midstream urine specimen.
2. You have just done a pregnancy test on a friend of yours and she is very excited to know the results. She tells you that she will not tell the doctor that you told her. What would you do?

HOW DID I DO? Answers to Memory Joggers

1. Urinalysis is routinely performed on all patients undergoing physical examinations and on entering the hospital for treatment.
2. First morning specimens are best for pregnancy, culturing, and microscopic examination.
3. Normally, water constitutes about 95% of urine.
4. Abnormal colors are not always pathologic.
5. Normal adult urine volume is 750 to 2000 mL in 24 hours.
6. Specific gravity is the weight of a substance compared with the weight of an equal volume of distilled water.
7. The pH is a measurement of the degree of acidity or alkalinity of the urine.
8. Nitrite occurs in urine when bacteria break down nitrate.
9. Microscopic examination of urine consists of categorizing and counting cells, casts, crystals, and miscellaneous constituents of sediment.
10. Cells are classified and counted under high-power magnification.
11. Crystals are common in urine.
12. *Ten to 15 high-power fields should be scanned.*

Venipuncture

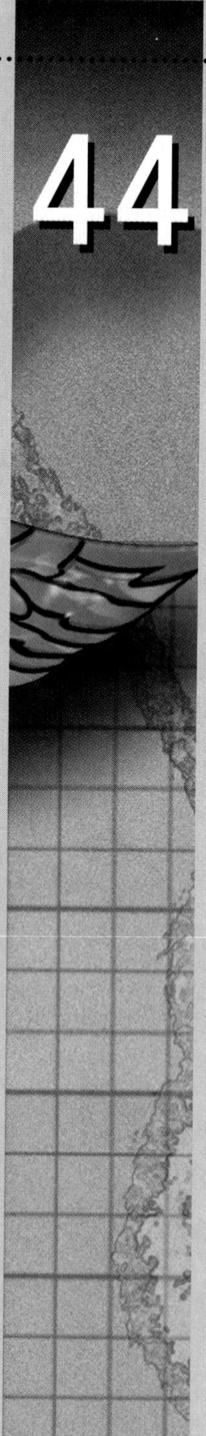

OUTLINE

LEARNING OBJECTIVES

Cognitive: On successful completion of this chapter you should be able to:

1 Explain the medical assistant's responsibility in a venipuncture procedure.

2 Describe the equipment used for obtaining a venous sample by syringe method, evacuated tube method, and butterfly draw method.

3 Identify the anticoagulant that prevents coagulation.

4 List the color-coded tubes by use and purpose.

5 Differentiate between a pipette and a Unopette.

6 Explain the medical assistant's patient responsibility.

7 Define and spell vocabulary terms.

Performance: On successful completion of this chapter you should be able to:

1 Accurately collect a blood specimen by venipuncture using a syringe.

2 Accurately collect a blood specimen by venipuncture using an evacuated tube.

3 Accurately collect a blood specimen by hand or wrist venipuncture using the butterfly needle.

4 Assemble the appropriate supplies; collect a capillary blood specimen suitable for testing, using fingertip puncture technique; and correctly complete each step of the procedure in proper order.

VOCABULARY

antecubital The area in front of and at the bend of the elbow

bifurcation The point of forking or separating into two branches

cyanotic Pertaining to a bluish discoloration of the skin and mucous membranes

hemolysis Pertaining to the breakdown of red blood cells and the release of hemoglobin into the plasma

heparin Naturally occurring antithrombin factor that prevents intravascular clotting

invasive Pertaining to a procedure in which a body cavity is entered or tissue pierced

lumen The open space within a blood vessel in which the blood travels

morphology The study of the form, structure, and size of organisms, organs, tissues, and cells

syncope Fainting; a brief loss of consciousness

tourniquet A device used to compress an artery or a vein

Through the centuries, blood has fascinated and awed humans. Early myths about blood became a basis for sacrificial religious ceremonies, medical practices, and even poetry. Although these ancient beliefs about blood have, for the most part, disappeared, some still remain to frustrate modern medical procedures. In certain religions, taking blood samples is forbidden because it is believed that vital spirits needed to keep the body alive might be removed with the blood. Another primitive belief is that blood cannot be replaced once it is removed from the body.

Collection of Blood Specimens

The most common method of obtaining blood for hematology testing is by venipuncture (phlebotomy). In a venipuncture the blood is taken directly from a superficial vein. The vein is punctured with a needle, and the blood is collected in either a syringe or a tube. A venipuncture is a safe procedure when performed by a trained professional, but the procedure must be performed with care. You should routinely use appropriate Standard Precautions when handling blood specimens. The good condition of the veins must also be preserved. Much practice is required to become skilled and confident in the technique of venipuncture.

Generally, veins in the forearm or the elbow (**antecubital** area) are used for venipunctures (Fig. 44–1). The puncture site should be carefully selected after inspecting both arms. Alternative sites may be indicated if the area is cyanotic, scarred, bruised, edematous, or burned. You may use veins on the lower forearm, the back of the hand, or the wrist. Use foot or ankle veins only if the patient has good

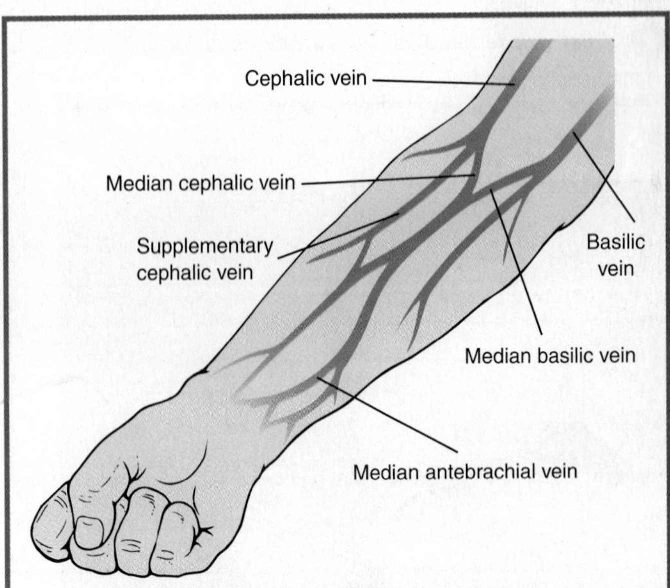

FIGURE 44–1 Veins of the forearm. (From Stepp CA, Woods MA: Laboratory Procedures for Medical Office Personnel. Philadelphia, WB Saunders, 1998.)

circulation in the legs and you have received permission from your supervisor or the physician.

Performing a venipuncture involves several important steps with which you must be thoroughly familiar before attempting the procedure. The first step is to select the proper method for venipuncture (syringe or evacuated tube). Next, the patient must be prepared for the procedure. Patient preparation is followed by the actual venipuncture and specimen collection. The final step is care of the puncture site before discharging the patient.

Memory Jogger

 *When would you look for an alternative venipuncture site?*

SYRINGE METHOD

When veins are very small or fragile, the syringe method of venipuncture may be used. The equipment required includes a sterile syringe and hypodermic needle, tourniquet, 70% alcohol, sterile gauze, and a blood-collecting tube (Fig. 44–2). Laboratories use disposable needles and syringes. The needle and syringe must be assembled carefully to maintain sterility. Do not touch the tips of either the needle or syringe, and do not uncap the needle until just before the actual puncture. Needles of 20 to 23 gauge are used for venipunctures. The needle should be inspected to make a certain that it is sharp and smooth. The syringe plunger should be checked for free movement and should be left completely pushed into the barrel so that no air remains in the syringe.

Memory Jogger

 *What gauge needles are usually used for venipuncture?*

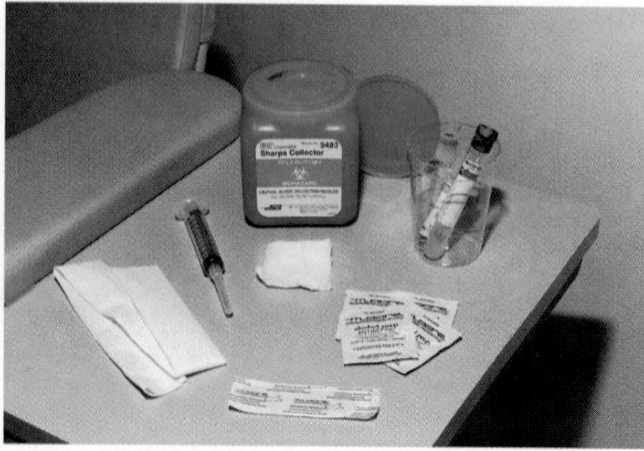

FIGURE 44–2 Syringe method equipment.

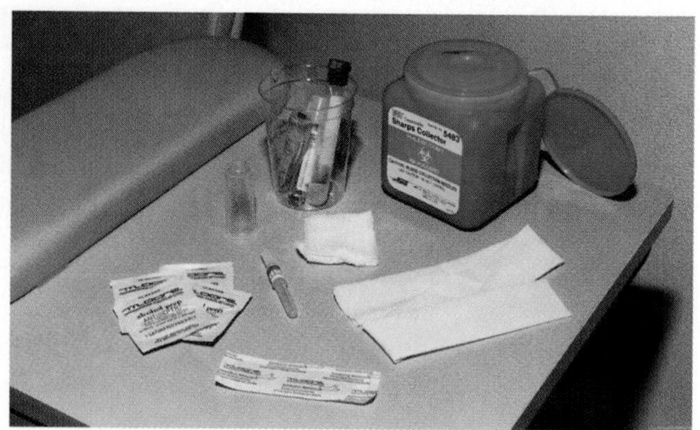

FIGURE 44–3 Evacuated tube method equipment.

EVACUATED TUBE METHOD

The evacuated tube (Vacutainer) system is the most common collection system in use. It consists of evacuated tubes of various sizes, with color-coded tops indicating tube contents (Table 44–1), sterile disposable double-ended needles of different lengths and gauges, and a reusable plastic adapter that holds the needle and guides the tube (Figs. 44–3 and 44–4). Both pediatric- and adult-size adapters and tubes are available. The needle has two sharp ends. The short end is fitted into the adapter, and the long end is used to puncture the vein. After the vein is entered, the tube is pushed onto the needle in the adapter and blood is drawn into the tube by vacuum. When the tube is full, it can be replaced by another tube.

Memory Jogger

 *Which end of the evacuated needle fits into the adapter?*

Several tubes of blood can be collected using a variety of color-coded tubes with a single venipuncture. Tubes containing ethylenediaminetetraacetic acid (EDTA) anticoagulant additive are recommended for use when doing hematology studies.

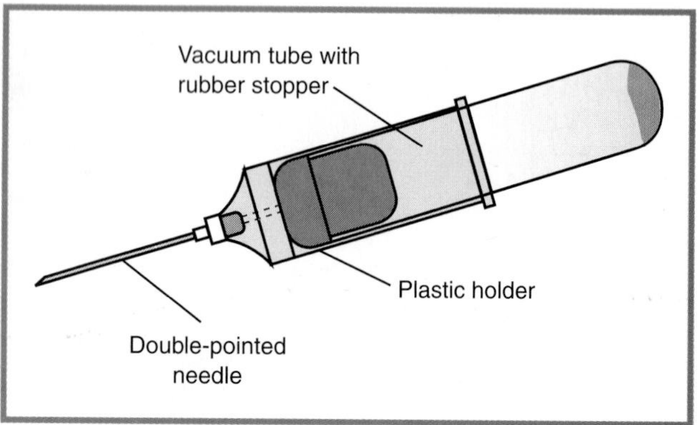

FIGURE 44–4 Evacuated tube system.

TABLE 44–1 List of Common Stoppers, Additives, and Laboratory Uses

Vacutainer Colors*	Color	Hemogard Colors†	Additive/Additive Function§	Laboratory Use‡·§	Optimum Volume/Minimum Volume
Adult Tubes					
Yellow		Yellow	Sodium polyanetholsulfonate (SPS); prevents blood from clotting and stabilizes bacterial growth	Blood or body fluid cultures	5 mL/NA
Red		Red	None	Serum testing; chemistry studies, blood bank, serology	10 mL/NA
Red/gray (marbled)		Gold	None, but contains silica particles to enhance clot formation	Serum testing	10 mL/NA
Light blue		Light blue	Sodium citrate; removes calcium to prevent blood from clotting	Coagulation testing	4.5 mL/4.5 mL
Green		Green	Heparin (sodium/lithium/ammonium); inhibits thrombin formation to prevent clotting	Chemistry testing	10 mL/3.5 mL
Green/gray (marbled)		Light green	Lithium heparin and gel for plasma separation	Plasma determinations in chemistry studies	2 mL/2 mL
Yellow/gray (marbled)		Orange	Thrombin	Stat serum demonstrations in chemistry studies	2 mL/2 mL
Lavender		Lavender	Ethylenediaminetetraacetic acid (EDTA); removes calcium to prevent blood from clotting	Hematology testing	7 mL/2 mL
Gray		Gray	Potassium oxalate/sodium fluoride; removes calcium to prevent blood from clotting; fluoride inhibits glycolysis	Chemistry testing especially glucose/alcohol levels	10 mL/10 mL
Royal blue		Royal blue	Sodium heparin (also sodium EDTA); inhibits thrombin formation to prevent clotting	Chemistry trace elements	7 mL
Pediatric Tubes					
Red		Red			2 mL/NA; 3 mL/NA; 4 mL/NA
Lavender		Lavender			2 mL/0.6 mL; 3 mL/0.9 mL; 4 mL/1 mL
Green		Green			2 mL/2 mL
Light blue		Light blue			2.7 mL/2.7 mL

*Stopper colors are based on Becton-Dickinson Vacutainer tubes.

†Hemogard closures provide a protective plastic cover over the rubber stopper as an additional safety feature.

‡Sterile needles come in a variety of lengths and gauges (bore or opening size). Needles are also made to fit the evacuated tube holder by screwing in or by attaching to the tips of syringes. Most evacuated tube needles have a rubber sleeve to prevent blood from dripping into the holders when tubes are changed; these are called multiple-sample needles. The open end of the needle containing the point has a slanted side (bevel), which must be facing up when the needle is inserted into the vein. Needle positioning is very important in drawing blood. The angle of entry in relation to the skin surface should be 15 degrees. The most common needle size for adult venipuncture is 21 gauge.

§Additives, additive functions, and laboratory uses are the same for both pediatric and adult tubes.

From Rodak BF: Diagnostic Hematology. Philadelphia, WB Saunders, 1995.

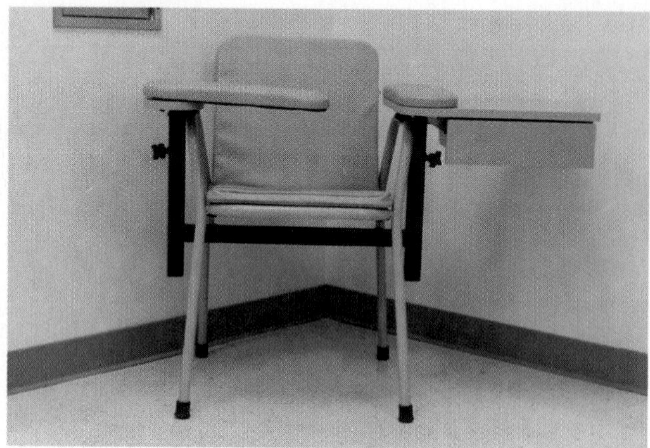

FIGURE 44–5 Venipuncture chair.

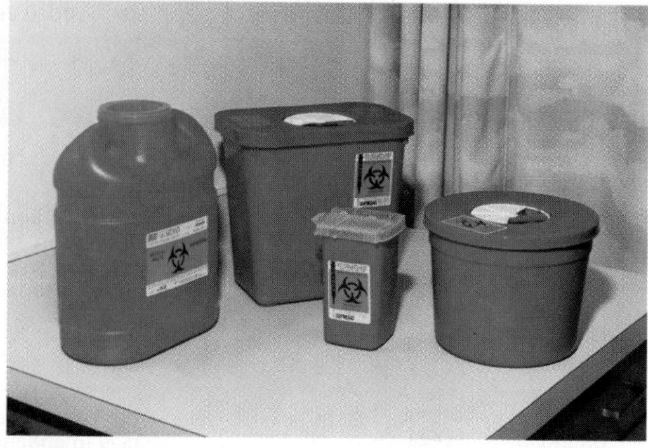

FIGURE 44–7 Needle disposal biological waste containers.

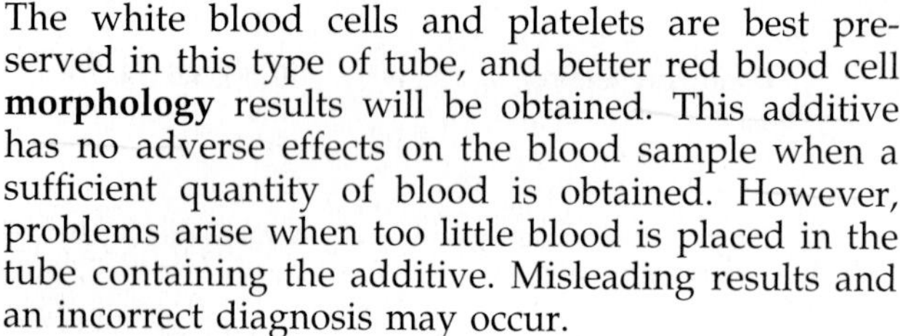

The white blood cells and platelets are best preserved in this type of tube, and better red blood cell **morphology** results will be obtained. This additive has no adverse effects on the blood sample when a sufficient quantity of blood is obtained. However, problems arise when too little blood is placed in the tube containing the additive. Misleading results and an incorrect diagnosis may occur.

PATIENT PREPARATION

Proper patient preparation begins with identification of the patient and a brief explanation of the procedure to minimize anxiety. The patient should be lying down or seated in a chair.

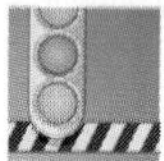

Safety Alert: Never have the patient standing or sitting on a high stool.

Special venipuncture chairs are available with adjustable arm rests and a locking safety mechanism that prevents the patient from falling should fainting occur (Fig. 44–5). (See Chapter 40 for the first-aid procedure for fainting.)

All necessary supplies should be within easy reach. When using the evacuated tube method, you should have extra tubes available in case you encounter a bad vacuum. The **tourniquet** should be flat, broad, and elastic (Fig. 44–6). Blood pressure cuffs may be used. They can be easily inflated or deflated during the procedure, if necessary.

Alcohol from a dispenser or individual packets is used for most collections. For designated sterile collections, individually packaged povidone-iodine (Betadine) swabs are used. Specimens for testing for blood alcohol levels are collected using benzalkonium chloride as the antiseptic. Alcohol may not be used for this collection, because it could interfere with the results of the test.

Needle disposal units should be available. Used needles should not be recapped, because this is the most probable cause of accidental needlesticks. Present guidelines for needle disposal recommend that the used needle be removed directly into the needle disposal unit, without cutting or recapping (Fig. 44–7).

Keep your supplies clean and in order. The expiration dates of the evacuated tubes should be checked to be certain that outdated supplies are removed from use. Restock supplies as they are used (Fig. 44–8).

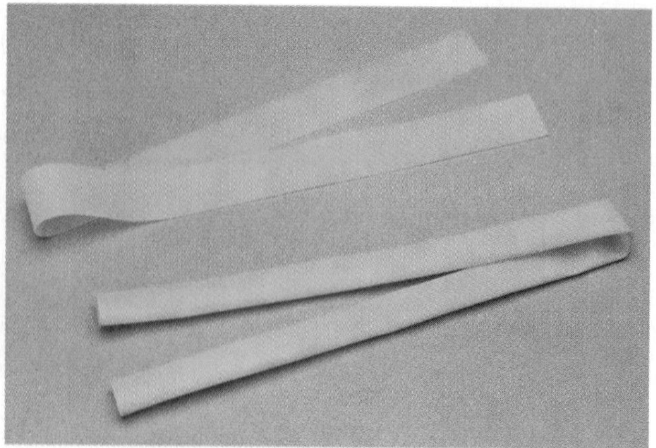

FIGURE 44–6 Examples of tourniquets.

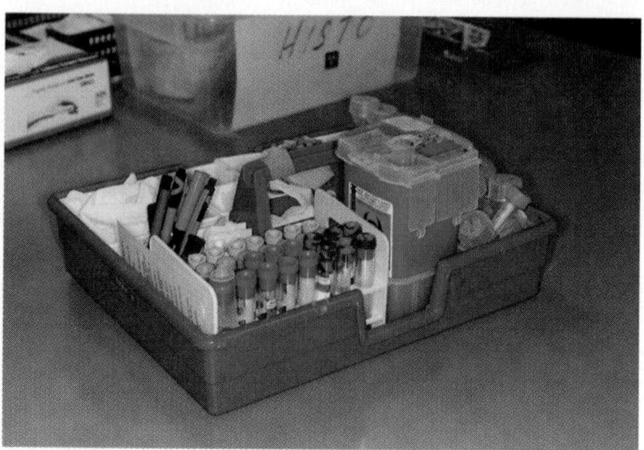

FIGURE 44–8 Well-stocked venipuncture tray.

Memory Jogger

What is used to prep the skin when drawing blood for blood alcohol levels?

SPECIMEN COLLECTION

The patient's arm is fully extended and supported. A tourniquet is applied to the arm, 3 to 4 inches above the elbow, to make the veins more prominent by slowing blood flow. The puncture site is located by gently pressing on the veins with your fingertips. This will determine the direction of the vein and its approximate size and depth. The area around the puncture site is cleansed with alcohol and sterile gauze. The site is then allowed to air dry or is blotted dry with sterile gauze. *Do not fan or blow dry the puncture site.*

The syringe or assembled Vacutainer system is held in one hand, at a 15- to 30-degree angle to the arm. The needle is bevel up and pointing in the same direction as the vein. The skin and vein are entered with one smooth motion until the needle is in the **lumen** of the vein. The blood is obtained by gently pulling back on the plunger with the other hand while holding the syringe and needle motionless. When using the Vacutainer method, place two fingers at the end of the holder and, with your thumb, push the tube into the adapter. Release the tourniquet as soon as blood begins to fill the tube or to flow into the syringe. When you have obtained the required amount of blood, place a dry sterile gauze pad over the puncture site and remove the needle from the vein. Never apply pressure on the needle site until the needle is completely removed from the vein.

Large, heavy arms often have veins that are difficult to palpate and usually require that the needle be inserted at an angle between 40 and 90 degrees (Fig. 44–9). If you miss the vein, do not probe for the vein with the inserted needle because you may rupture red blood cells and cause the release of tissue clotting factors. If you feel uncomfortable about this draw, ask for assistance.

Memory Jogger

What is the correct location for placing the tourniquet when you plan to do an antecubital draw?

CARE OF THE PUNCTURE SITE

Apply pressure to the puncture site for a few minutes. You may have the patient elevate the arm at this time to prevent oozing of blood. If you have used the syringe method, the blood must be transferred to a tube at this time. Gently insert the needle through the rubber stopper of a vacuum tube. The vacuum inside will draw the required amount of blood into the tube. For tubes that contain additives, gently invert the tube eight to ten times to mix (Fig. 44–10).

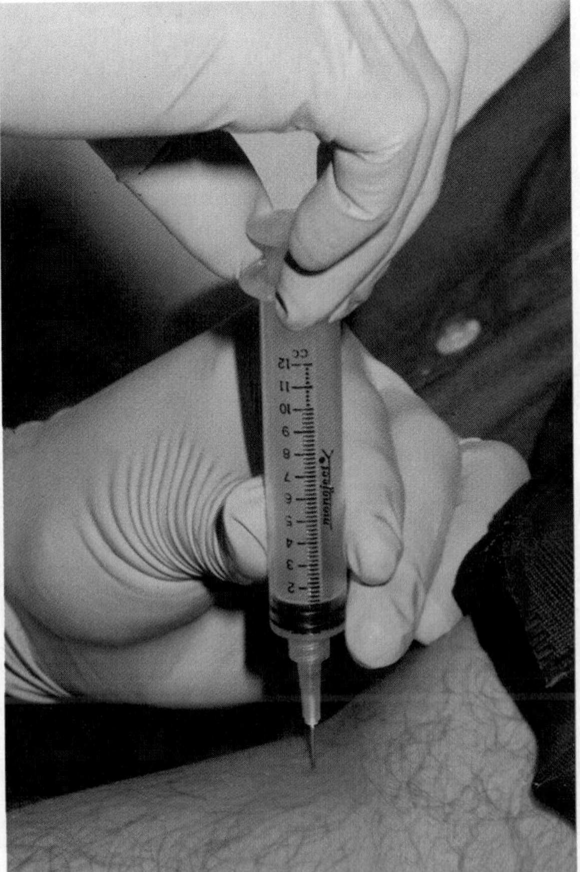

FIGURE 44–9 Obesity draw at increased angle.

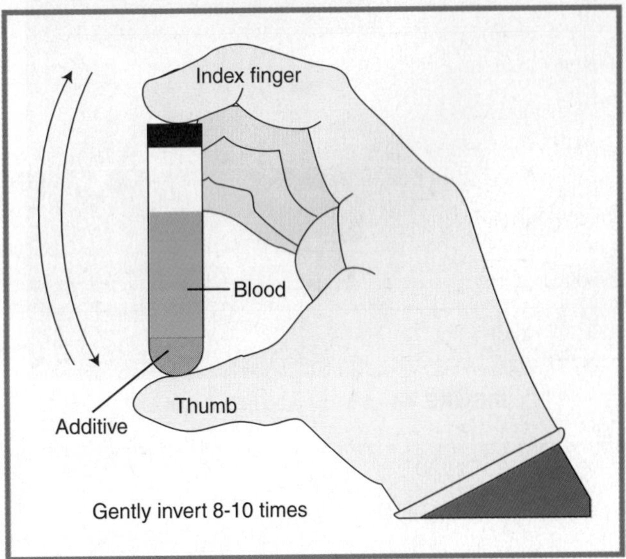

FIGURE 44–10 Method of gently inverting tube.

Safety Alert: When transferring blood from the syringe to the vacuum tube, observe extreme caution to avoid needlesticks.

Check the puncture site and apply a hypoallergenic bandage over several layers of folded gauze to the puncture site. Advise the patient to remove the bandage in about 30 minutes. In some laboratories bandaging the puncture site is not done because bandages tend to irritate the skin and leave a sticky residue. Check your procedure manual or consult with the physician to determine the accepted method.

Memory Jogger

How many times do you gently invert blood sample tubes that have additives added?

NEEDLE DISPOSAL

If the syringe method was used for venipuncture, discard the needle and syringe into the designated biohazard sharps container immediately. Do not place it on any surface, and never recap it. If the evacuated tube system was used, place the needle in the proper slot of a biohazard sharps container and turn it counterclockwise until it unscrews from the evacuated tube holder (Fig. 44–11). If the needle refuses to separate from the holder, discard the entire unit into the biohazard container.

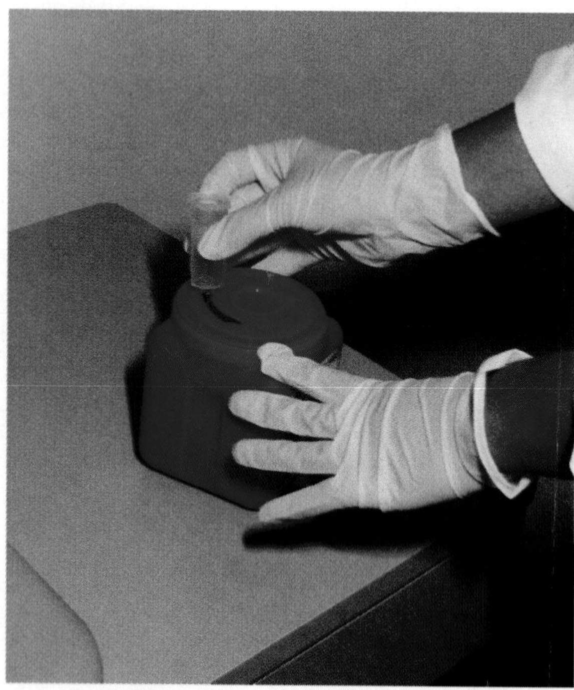

FIGURE 44–11 Needle separation unit.

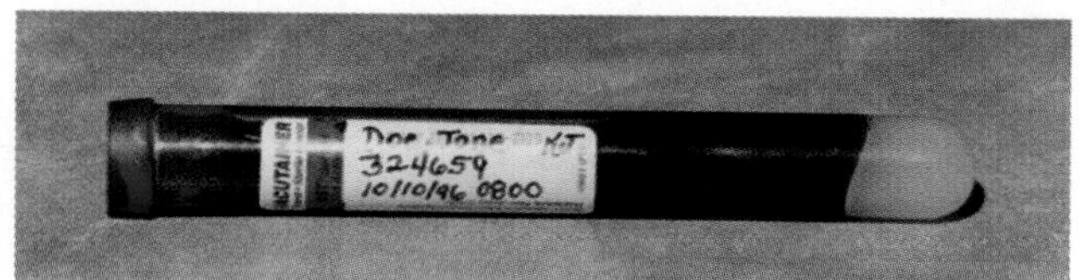

FIGURE 44–12 Labeled specimen.

SPECIMEN HANDLING

Label the specimen, complete the laboratory requisition, and forward the blood specimen to the appropriate place. The importance of accurate labeling of the blood specimen cannot be overemphasized. Improper identification of a specimen can cause serious consequences and may even cause physical detriment to the patient. One of the easiest ways to avoid this situation is to label the specimen immediately after it is obtained (Fig. 44–12).

GLOVE REMOVAL

Gloves should be removed carefully so as to not allow any fluid contaminant to become airborne from the surface of the gloves. This is best done by grasping one glove at the wrist and pulling it inside out and off of the hand (Fig. 44–13*A*). Now with the removed glove in the palm of the still-gloved hand, slip your nongloved fingers under the second glove at the wrist (see Fig. 44–13*B*) and pull it off of the hand (see Fig. 44–13C). You will end up with one glove inside of the other and the contaminated surfaces will be to the inside (see Fig. 44–13*D*). Avoid "snapping" the gloves as you remove them. Place the contaminated gloves in a biohazardous waste container but *not* in the sharps container (see Fig. 44–13*E*). Wash your hands and dry them thoroughly.

Memory Jogger

How do you dispose of your used gloves?

Text continued on page 892

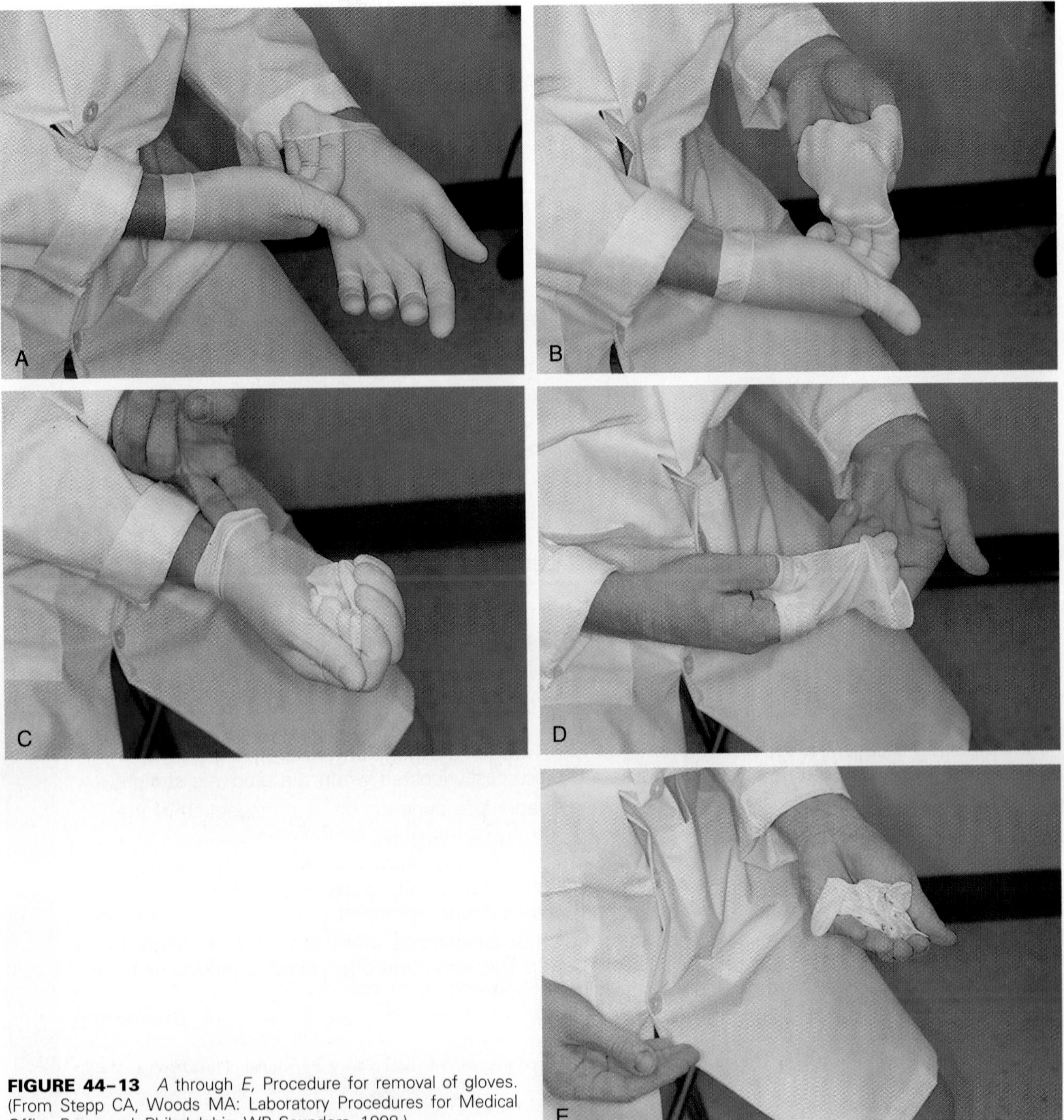

FIGURE 44–13 *A* through *E*, Procedure for removal of gloves. (From Stepp CA, Woods MA: Laboratory Procedures for Medical Office Personnel. Philadelphia, WB Saunders, 1998.)

PROCEDURE 44-1

Collecting a Venous Blood Sample Using the Syringe Method

GOAL

To collect a venous blood specimen.

EQUIPMENT AND SUPPLIES

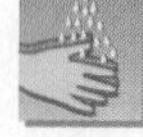
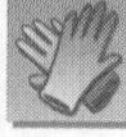
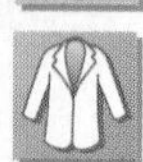
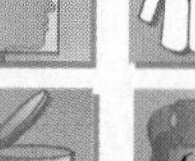
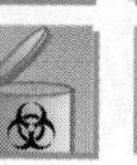
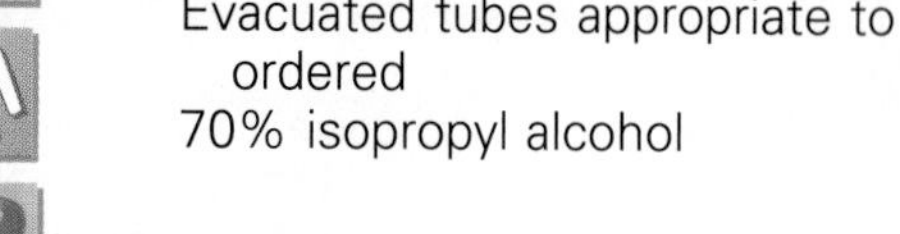

Needle, syringe with 21- or 22-gauge needle
Evacuated tubes appropriate to tests ordered
70% isopropyl alcohol
Sterile gauze pads
Tourniquet
Nonallergenic tape
Permanent marking pen

PROCEDURAL STEPS

1 Check the requisition form to determine the tests ordered. Gather the correct tubes and supplies that you will need.
PURPOSE: Allows for proper specimen collection.

2 Wash and dry your hands, and put on face protection and nonsterile gloves.
PURPOSE: Infection control.

3 Identify the patient and explain the procedure.
PURPOSE: Ascertains patient identity, and explanations help gain the patient's cooperation.

4 Assist the patient to sit with the arm well supported in a slightly downward position.
PURPOSE: Veins of the antecubital fossa are more easily located when the elbow is straight.

5 Assemble equipment: Choice of syringe and needle size depends on your inspection of the patient's veins. Attach the needle to the syringe. Keep the cover on the needle.

6 Apply the tourniquet around the patient's arm 3 to 4 inches above the elbow. The tourniquet should never be tied so tightly that it restricts blood flow in the artery (Figure 1*).
PURPOSE: The tourniquet is used to make the veins more prominent.

7 Select the venipuncture site by palpating the antecubital space, and use your index finger to trace the path of the vein and to judge its depth. The vein most often used is the median cephalic, which lies in the middle of the elbow (Figure 2).

Continued

*All figures from Stepp CA, Woods MA: Laboratory Procedures for Medical Office Personnel. Philadelphia, WB Saunders, 1998.

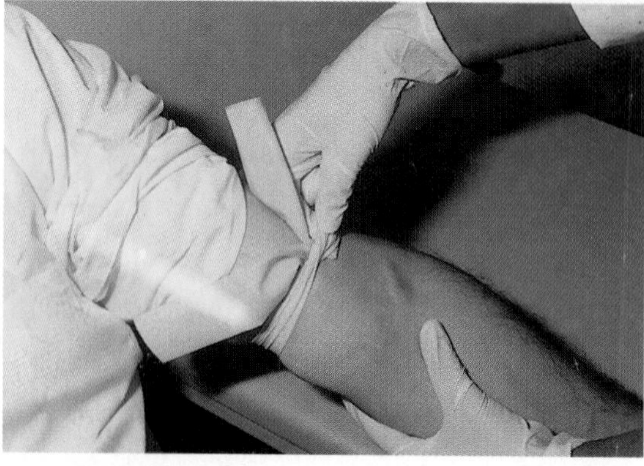

FIGURE 1

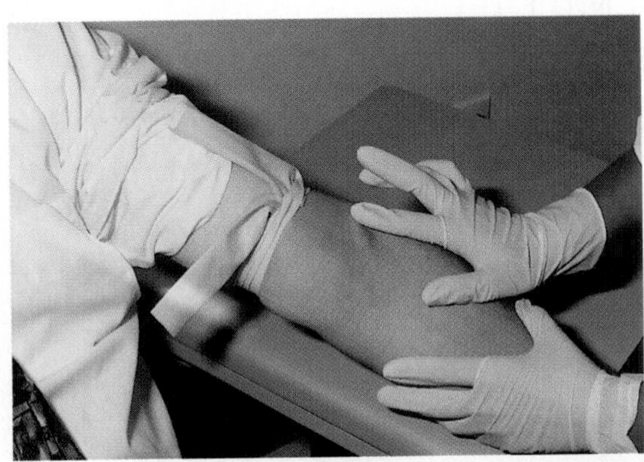
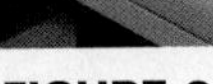

FIGURE 2

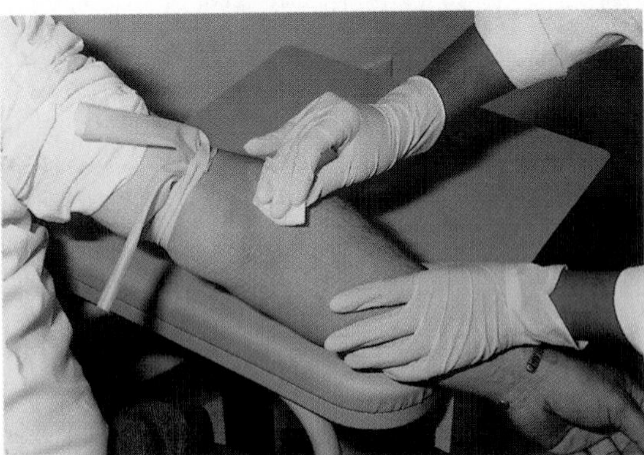

FIGURE 3

PURPOSE: The index finger is most sensitive for palpating. Do not use the thumb, because it has a pulse of its own, which may confuse you.

8 Ask the patient to open and close his or her hand several times.
PURPOSE: Clenching the fist produces engorgement of the vein.

9 Cleanse the site, starting in the center of the area and working outward in a circular pattern (Figure 3).

10 Dry the site with a sterile gauze pad.
PURPOSE: The circular pattern helps avoid recontamination of the area. Puncturing a wet area stings and can cause hemolysis of the sample.

11 Remove the needle sheath.

12 Hold the syringe in your dominant hand. Your thumb should be on top and your fingers underneath.

13 Grasp the patient's arm with the nondominant hand while using your thumb and forefinger to draw the skin taut over the site to anchor the vein.
PURPOSE: Failure to anchor the vein makes puncturing more difficult and painful and may result in a missed vein.

14 Insert the needle through the skin and into the vein with the bevel of the needle up, aligned parallel to the vein, at a 15-degree angle, rapidly, and smoothly (Figure 4).
PURPOSE: The sharpest point of the needle is inserted first.

15 Slowly pull back the plunger of the syringe with the nondominant hand. Make sure that you do not move the needle after entering the vein. Allow the syringe or tube to fill to optimum capacity (Figure 5).

Continued

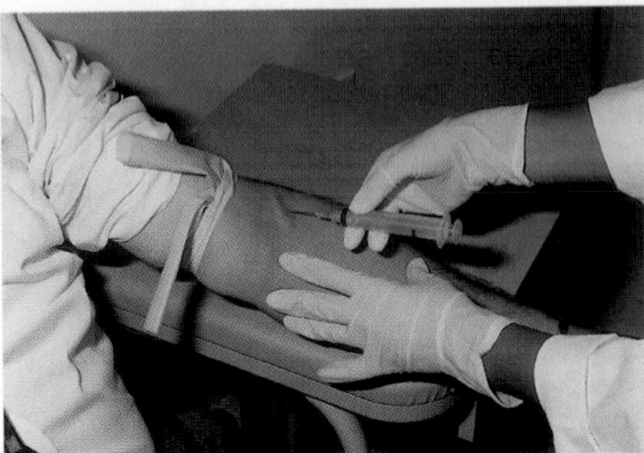

FIGURE 4

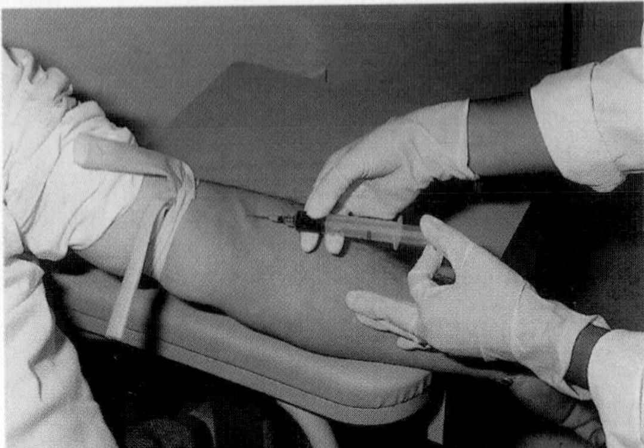

FIGURE 5

PROCEDURE 44-1 (CONTINUED)

Collecting a Venous Blood Sample Using the Syringe Method

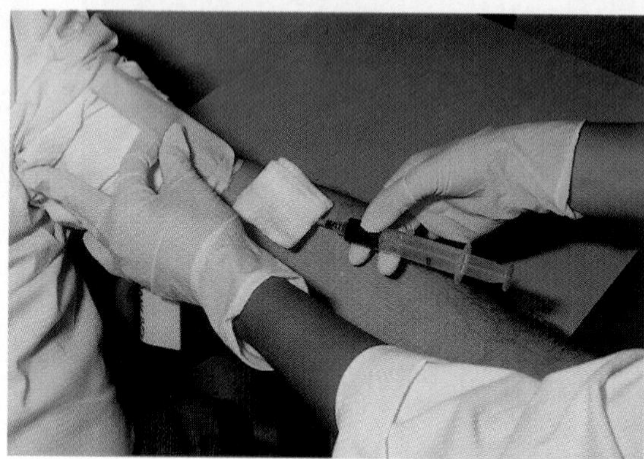

FIGURE 6

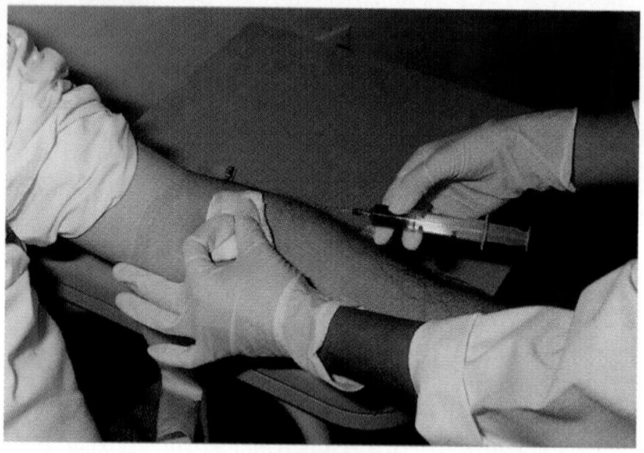

FIGURE 7

16 Release the tourniquet when venipuncture is complete. It must be released before the needle is removed from the arm (Figure 6).

PURPOSE: Removal of the tourniquet releases pressure on the vein and helps prevent blood from getting into adjacent tissues and causing a hematoma.

17 Place sterile gauze over the puncture site at the time of needle withdrawal (Figure 7).

18 Instruct the patient to apply direct pressure on the puncture site with sterile gauze. The patient may elevate the arm.

PURPOSE: Direct pressure is the best method to stop bleeding. Elevating the arm above the heart also stops bleeding.

19 Transfer the blood to a tube. Gently invert tubes to mix anticoagulants and blood. *Label tubes with the patient's name, the date, and the time* (Figure 8).

PURPOSE: Prevents clotting of blood. Vigorous mixing may cause hemolysis.

Continued

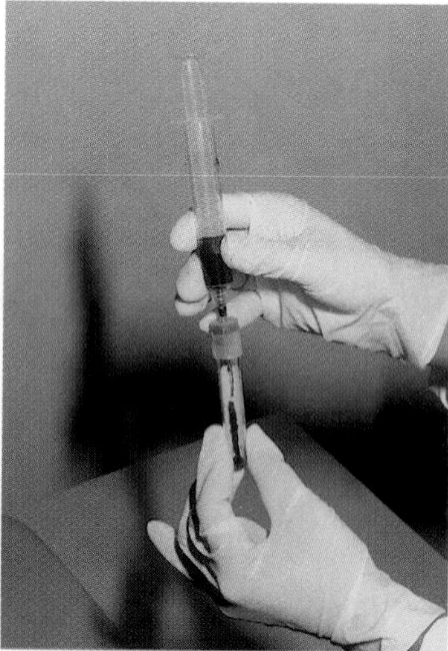

FIGURE 8

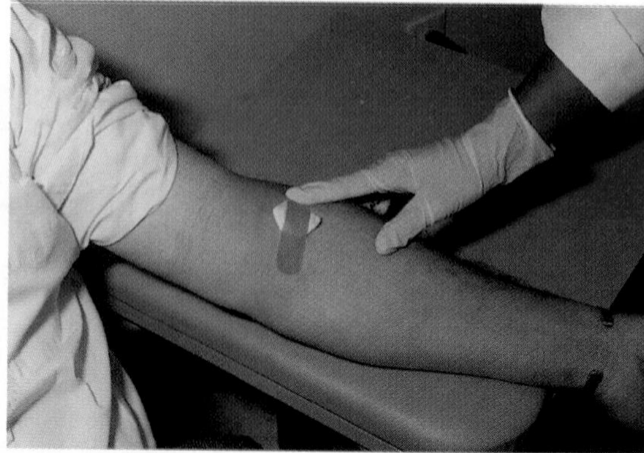

FIGURE 9

20 Check the puncture site for bleeding.

21 Apply a hypoallergenic bandage (Figure 9).

22 Dispose of the needle safely. Allow it to drop directly into the disposal unit without touching it with your fingers. Do not recap used needles.
PURPOSE: Most accidental needlesticks occur when a needle is being recapped. Report any accidents to your supervisor or the physician.

23 Clean the work area, remove gloves and face protection, and wash your hands.
PURPOSE: Infection control.

24 Complete the laboratory requisition form, and route the specimen to the proper place. Record the procedure in the patient's record.
PURPOSE: A procedure is considered not done until it is recorded.

PROCEDURE 44-2
Collecting a Venous Blood Sample Using the Evacuated Tube Method

GOAL
To collect a venous blood specimen.

EQUIPMENT AND SUPPLIES

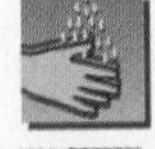

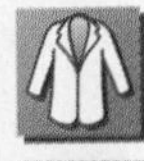
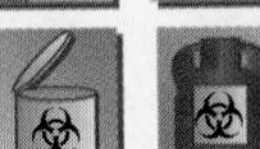

Vacutainer needle, adapter, and proper tubes for requested tests
70% isopropyl alcohol
Sterile gauze pads
Tourniquet
Nonallergenic tape
Permanent marking pen

PROCEDURAL STEPS

1 Check the requisition form to determine the tests ordered. Gather the correct tubes and supplies that you will need.
PURPOSE: Allows for proper specimen collection.

2 Wash and dry your hands, and put on face protection and nonsterile gloves.
PURPOSE: Infection control.

3 Identify the patient and explain the procedure.
PURPOSE: Ascertains patient identity, and explanations help gain the patient's cooperation.

4 Assist the patient to sit with the arm well supported in a slightly downward position.
PURPOSE: Veins of the antecubital fossa are more easily located when the elbow is straight.

5 Assemble equipment: Choice of needle size depends on your inspection of the patient's veins. Attach the needle to the Vacutainer holder. Keep the cover on the needle.

Continued

PROCEDURE 44-2 (CONTINUED)

Collecting a Venous Blood Sample Using the Evacuated Tube Method

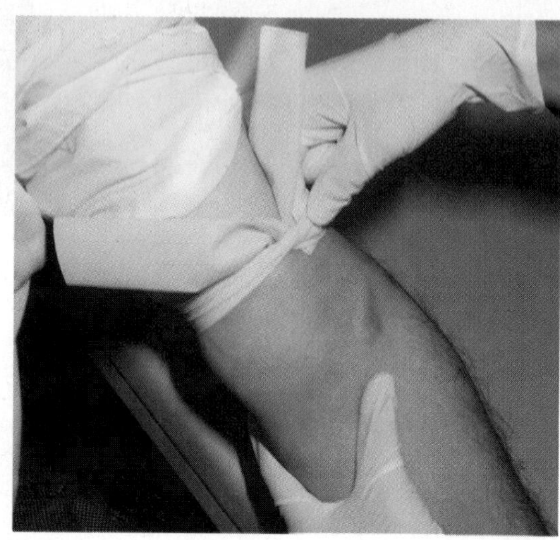

FIGURE 1

6 Apply the tourniquet around the patient's arm 3 to 4 inches above the elbow. The tourniquet should never be tied so tightly that it restricts blood flow in the artery (Figure 1).
PURPOSE: The tourniquet is used to make the veins more prominent.

7 Select the venipuncture site by palpating the antecubital space, and use your index finger to trace the path of the vein and to judge its depth. The vein most often used is the median cephalic, which lies in the middle of the elbow (Figure 2).
PURPOSE: The index finger is most sensitive for palpating. Do not use the thumb, because it has a pulse of its own, which may confuse you.

8 Ask the patient to open and close his or her hand several times.
PURPOSE: Clenching the fist produces engorgement of the vein.

9 Cleanse the site, starting in the center of the area and working outward in a circular pattern (Figure 3).

10 Dry the site with a sterile gauze pad.
PURPOSE: The circular pattern helps avoid recontamination of the area. Puncturing a wet area stings and can cause hemolysis of the sample.

Continued

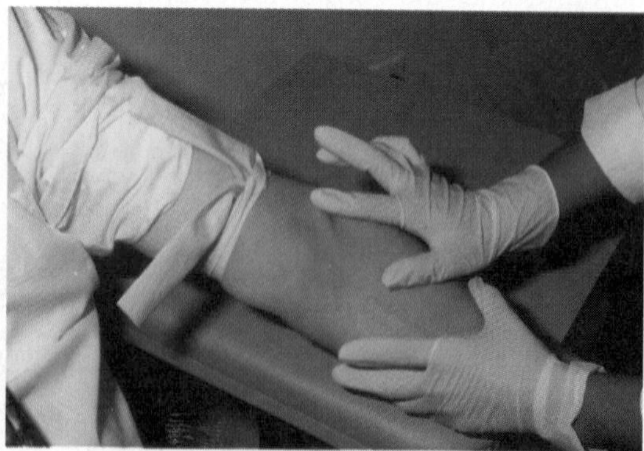

FIGURE 2

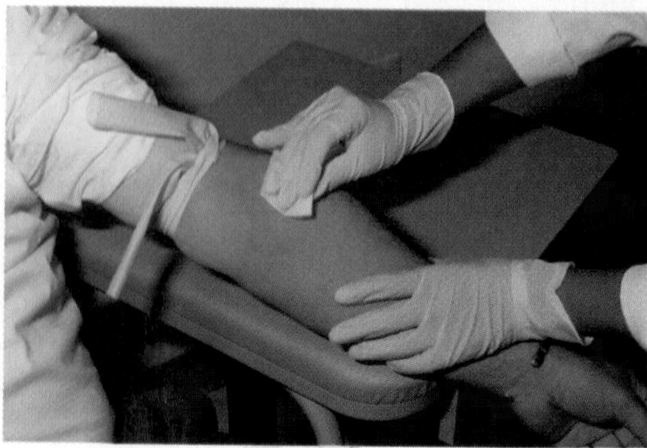

FIGURE 3

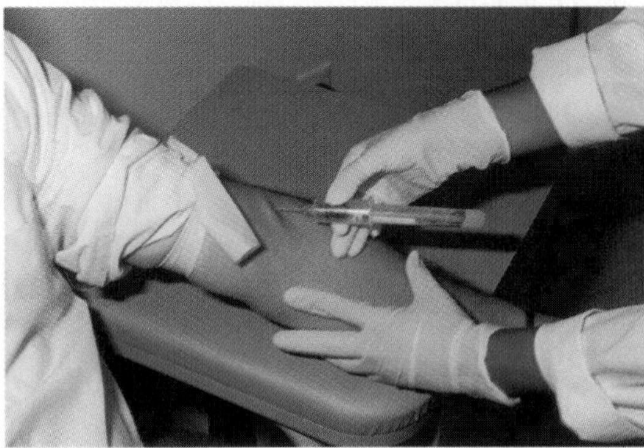
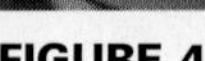

FIGURE 4

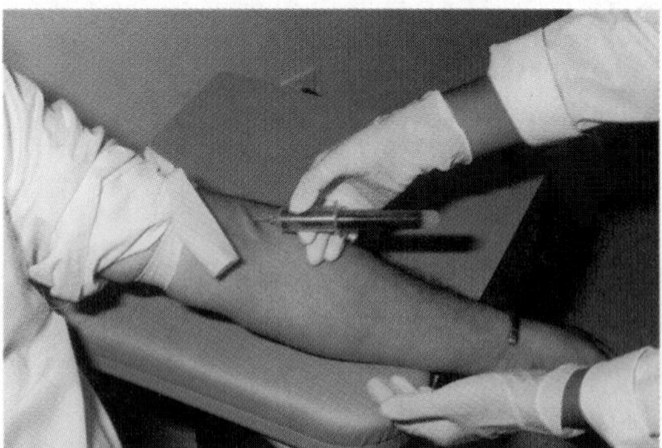

FIGURE 5

11 Remove the needle sheath.

12 Hold the Vacutainer assembly in your dominant hand. Your thumb should be on top and your fingers underneath.

13 Grasp the patient's arm with the nondominant hand while using your thumb and forefinger to draw the skin taut over the site, to anchor the vein.

PURPOSE: Failure to anchor the vein makes puncturing more difficult and painful and may result in a missed vein.

14 Insert the needle through the skin and into the vein with the bevel of the needle up, aligned parallel to the vein, at a 15-degree angle, rapidly, and smoothly (Figure 4).

PURPOSE: The sharpest point of the needle is inserted first.

15 Place two fingers on the flanges of the Vacutainer holder and, with the thumb, push the tube onto the needle inside the holder. Make sure that you do not move the needle after entering the vein. Allow the tube to fill to optimum capacity (Figure 5).

16 Remove the Vacutainer tube from the adapter before removing the needle from the vein (Figure 6).

PURPOSE: A nontraumatic venipuncture produces the most reliable results. Proper tube filling ensures the correct ratio of blood to additive. Removal of the tube from the holder before removal from the vein prevents any excess blood from dripping from the tip of the needle onto the patient.

17 Release the tourniquet when venipuncture is complete. *It must be released before the needle is removed from the arm.*

PURPOSE: Removal of the tourniquet releases pressure on the vein and helps prevent blood from getting into adjacent tissues and causing a hematoma.

18 Place sterile gauze over the puncture site at the time of needle withdrawal (Figure 7).

Continued

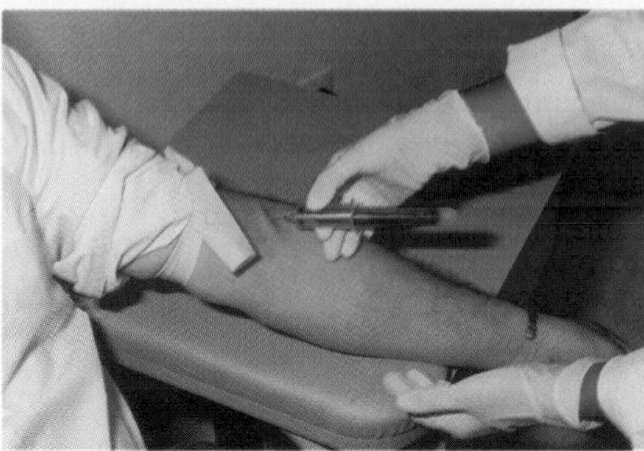

FIGURE 6

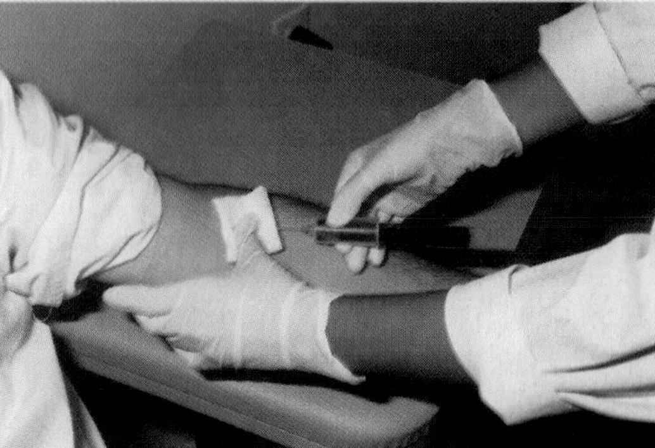

FIGURE 7

PROCEDURE 44–2 (CONTINUED)
Collecting a Venous Blood Sample Using the Evacuated Method

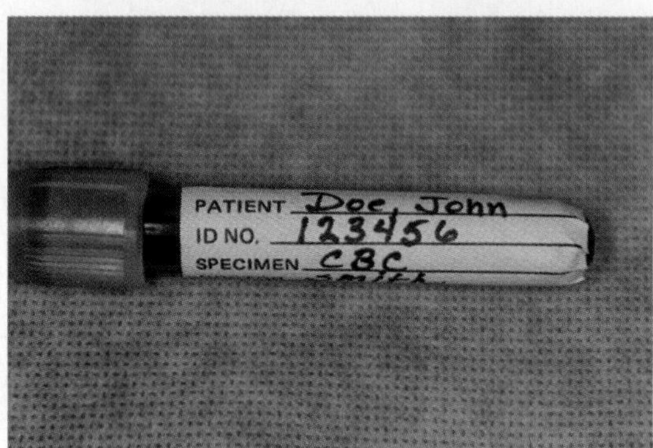

FIGURE 8

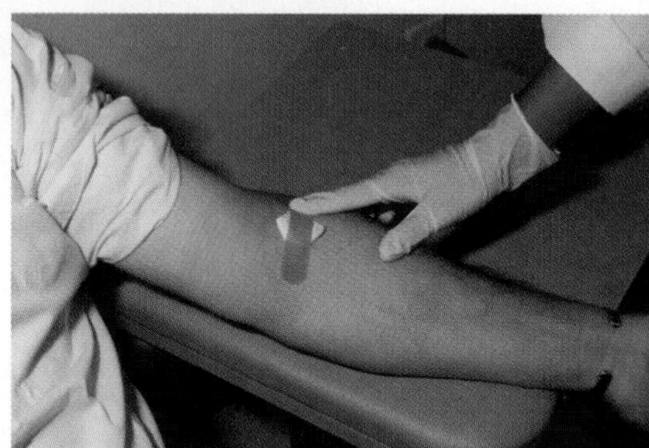

FIGURE 9

19 Instruct the patient to apply direct pressure on the puncture site with a sterile gauze pad. The patient may elevate the arm.
PURPOSE: Direct pressure is the best method to stop bleeding. Elevating the arm above the heart also stops bleeding.

20 Gently invert tubes to mix anticoagulants and blood. *Label tubes with the patient's name, the date, and the time* (Figure 8).
PURPOSE: Prevents clotting of blood. Vigorous mixing may cause hemolysis.

21 Check the puncture site for bleeding.

22 Apply a hypoallergenic bandage (Figure 9).

23 Dispose of the needle safely. Allow it to drop directly into the disposal unit without touching it with your fingers. Do not recap used needles.
PURPOSE: Most accidental needlesticks occur when a needle is being recapped. Report any accidents to your supervisor or the physician.

24 Clean the work area, remove gloves and face protection, and wash your hands.
PURPOSE: Infection control.

25 Complete the laboratory requisition and route to the proper place. Record the procedure in the patient's record.
PURPOSE: A procedure is considered not done until it is recorded.

USING A BUTTERFLY NEEDLE

An infant or small child or adults with debilitated arm veins may require hand or wrist draws. When you are attempting to obtain this sample, the butterfly needle may prove to be the method of choice. This small needle, sometimes referred to as a winged infusion set, is equipped with small "wings" on either side of the 23-gauge needle, giving it the appearance of a butterfly.

When using a butterfly set, the butterfly device with a multiple Luer-Lok adapter is preferred because it locks securely to the needle tube. This adapter can be attached directly to an evacuated tube holder. Carefully select the small-volume pediatric tubes in which to place the collections because the large volume tubes may create too great a vacuum pressure on the vein and cause it to collapse, or they can cause **hemolysis** of the specimen. You may find that using the syringe method is the method of choice. Prepare the patient in the same manner as for the regular draw.

Memory Jogger

Why is it advisable to place blood drawn with a butterfly needle set into pediatric tubes?

PROCEDURE 44-3

Performing a Butterfly Draw Using a Hand Vein

GOAL

To accurately obtain the venous sample from a hand vein using the butterfly method.

EQUIPMENT AND SUPPLIES

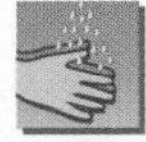

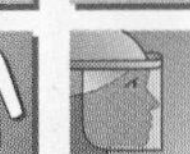
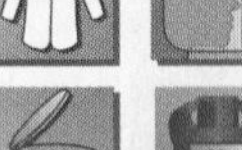
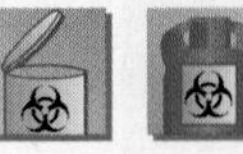

Tourniquet
Alcohol pads or other antiseptic preps
Gauze pads
Butterfly needle set
Appropriate pediatric tubes arranged in the order of the draw or Luer-Lok syringe
Sharps disposal container
Nonallergenic bandage
Permanent marking pen

PROCEDURAL STEPS

1 Check the requisition and gather the appropriate tubes for the needed tests. Assemble the balance of your supplies.
PURPOSE: Efficiency in preparation.

2 Wash your hands, and put on face protection and gloves.
PURPOSE: Infection control.

3 Prepare your patient as for an antecubital draw.

4 Remove the butterfly device from the package and stretch it slightly.
PURPOSE: To keep the tube from recoiling.

5 Attach the butterfly device to the syringe (Figure 1) or evacuated tube holder (Figure 2).

6 Seat the first tube into the evacuated tube holder.

7 Apply a tourniquet to the patient's wrist, just proximal to the wrist bone.

8 Hold the hand in your nondominant hand with the fingers lower than the wrist.
PURPOSE: This position help in identifying the veins and draw site.

9 Select a vein and cleanse the site at the **bifurcation.**

10 Using your thumb, pull the patient's skin taut over the knuckles.

11 With the needle at a 10- to 15-degree angle, bevel up, align it with the vein.

Continued

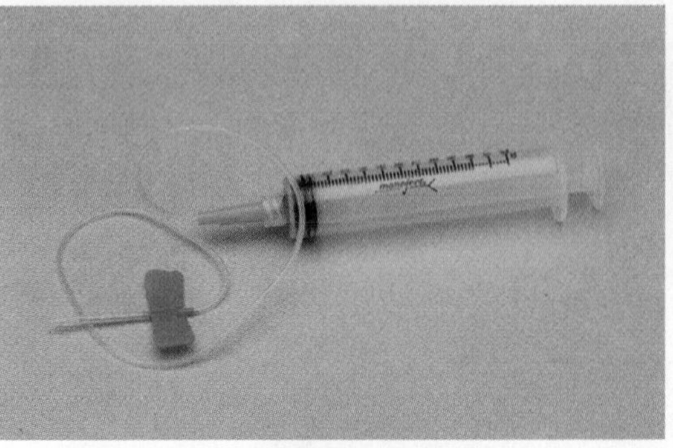

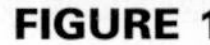
FIGURE 1

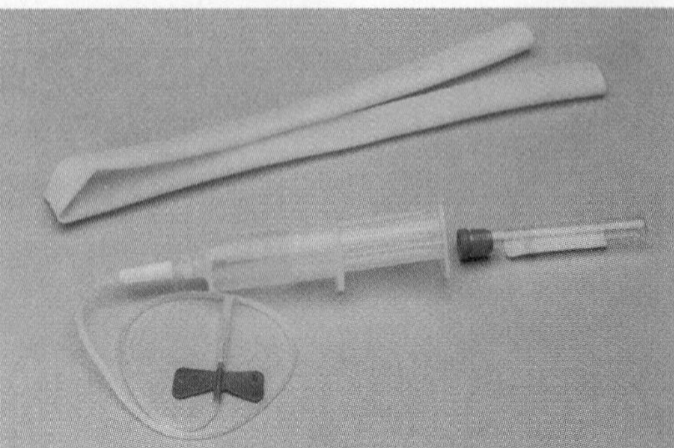

FIGURE 2

PROCEDURE 44-3 (CONTINUED)

Performing a Butterfly Draw Using a Hand Vein

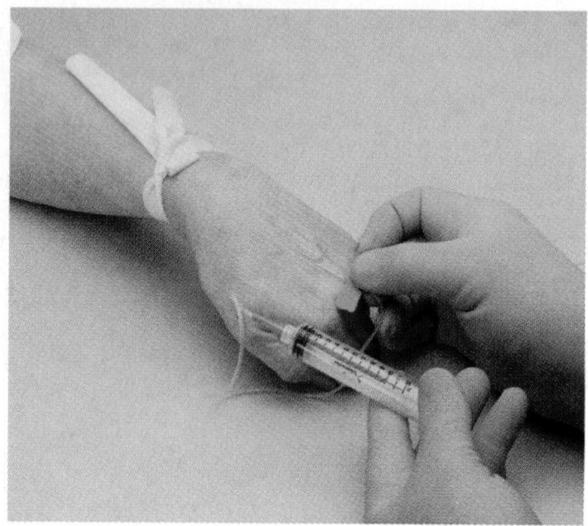

FIGURE 3

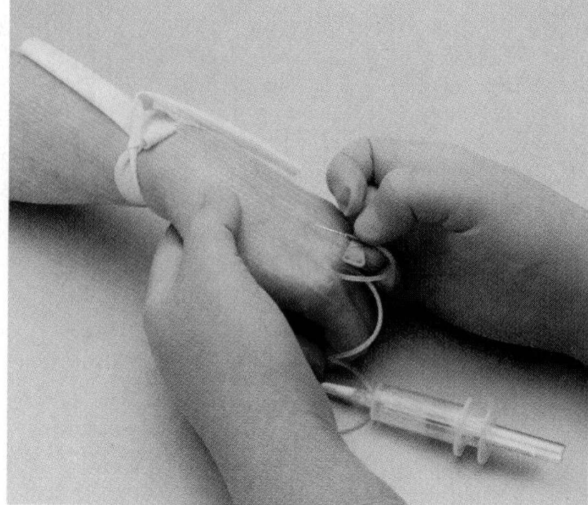

FIGURE 4

12 Insert the needle gently by threading it up the lumen of the vein.
PURPOSE: So that it will not twist out of the vein if you let go of the needle (Figures 3 and 4).

13 Push the blood collecting tube onto the end of the holder (Figure 5) or draw blood into the syringe (Figure 6). Note the position of the hands while drawing the blood.

14 Release the tourniquet when the blood appears in the tube.

15 Always keep the tube and the holder in a downward position so that the tube will fill from the bottom up.

16 Place a gauze pad over the puncture site and gently remove the needle.

17 Complete the procedure as you would for a antecubital draw; see Procedure 44-2, steps 19 through 25.

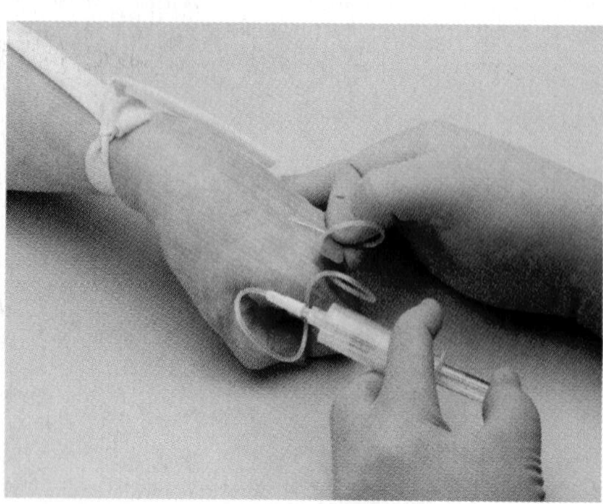

FIGURE 5

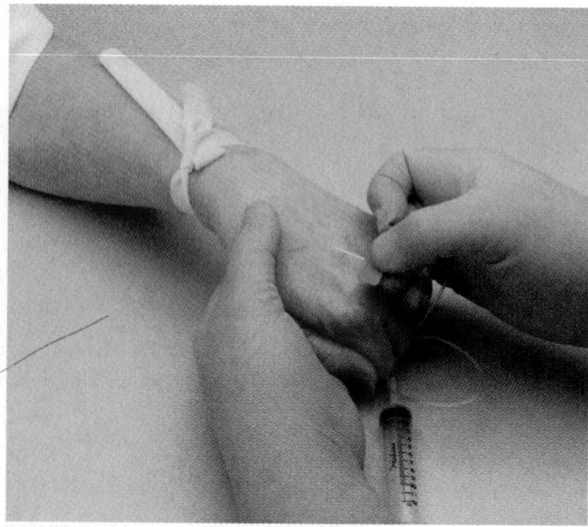

FIGURE 6

POSSIBLE BLOOD COLLECTION COMPLICATIONS

Failure to obtain blood can be the result of a number of factors. Determining the cause of the problem may help you to decide whether you will be successful on the second attempt. The first issue before you is to remain calm so that you can think clearly, systematically determining the possible cause of the problem.

A *hematoma* is a large, painful bruised area at the puncture site caused by blood leaking into the tissue, which causes the tissue around the puncture site to swell. The most frequent causes are (1) when the needle goes completely through the vein and the needle bevel is only partially in the vein and (2) when insufficient pressure is applied to the puncture site after the needle has been removed. If a hematoma forms, discontinue the procedure stat, apply pressure to the area for a minimum of 3 minutes, and then apply an ice pack to the area. Notify the physician and observe the site to determine if bleeding has stopped. An incident report will need to be completed and recorded in the patient's record.

Table 44–2 lists some probable solutions. As a general rule, it is wise to limit yourself to two attempts to obtain blood from any one patient. If you fail on the second attempt, ask the patient if he or she would prefer having someone else try or if it would be better to come back at another time. This maneuver lets the patient feel that he or she is in control of the situation. Everyone fails to obtain a needed blood sample at one time or another, so do not feel that you are a failure. Very likely, you will be the one who will be able to obtain a blood sample from another patient after your coworker has tried and failed.

In addition to the complications listed in Table 44–2, there are four other situations that you must consider when preparing to obtain a blood sample:

1. The number of times blood has been drawn from this patient in the past 24 hours
2. The relationship between the volume of blood needed and the age of the patient
3. The overall health of the patient
4. The procedure to follow if the patient refuses to allow you draw blood

These are concerns that should be answered by the physician and may be answered in the office policy and procedures manual. If you cannot find a formal procedure covering these four points, talk to the physician and see that these procedures are written out, approved by the physician, and placed in the office policy and procedures manual.

Memory Jogger

If the patient develops a hematoma, what do you do?

TABLE 44–2 Managing Blood Draw Complications

Possible Complication	Strategies
Burned area	Must be avoided, because these areas are prone to infection
Convulsions	Stay calm. *Remove the needle;* then help guide the patient to the floor, protecting him or her from injury. Call for help.
Damaged/scarred veins or infected areas	Look for an alternative site; *Do not* draw blood from scarred or infected areas.
Edema	Avoid the area; look for an alternative site.
Hematoma	Adjust the depth of the needle or remove the needle and apply pressure.
Intravenous (IV) therapy/ blood transfusion sites	Blood samples should not be drawn from an arm that is also the site for IV infusion or blood transfusion owing to the dilution factor.
Mastectomy	*Do not* draw blood from the site of the mastectomy, because mastectomy surgery causes lymphostasis, which may produce false results.
Nausea	Place a cold cloth on the patient's forehead, give the patient a basin, in case of vomiting, and instruct him or her to take deep breaths. Alert the physician.
No blood	Manipulate the needle slightly, or remove the Vacutainer and perform the blood draw again using a syringe or butterfly set-up.
Petechiae	Loosen the tourniquet, because this complication usually results from the tourniquet being in place for longer than 2 minutes.
Syncope (fainting)	Position the patient's head between the knees (if in a sitting position). Check and record the patient's pulse, blood pressure, and respiration rate, and continue to observe the patient. *Never leave the patient unattended.*

Modified from Stepp CA, Woods MA: Laboratory Procedures for Medical Office Personnel. Philadelphia, WB Saunders, 1998.

MICROCAPILLARY BLOOD COLLECTION

Capillaries are small blood vessels connecting the small arterioles to the small venules. The capillary puncture is an efficient means of collecting a blood specimen when only a small amount of blood is required or when a patient's condition makes venipuncture difficult.

Patient Preparation

In adults and children, the usual puncture site is the ring finger, but capillary blood can be obtained from

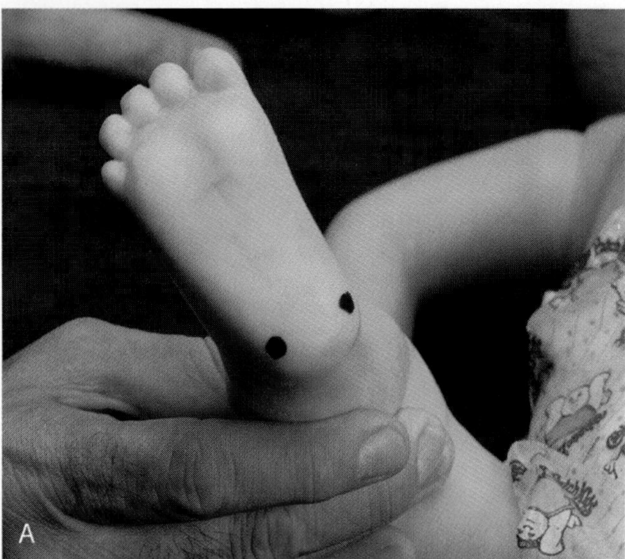

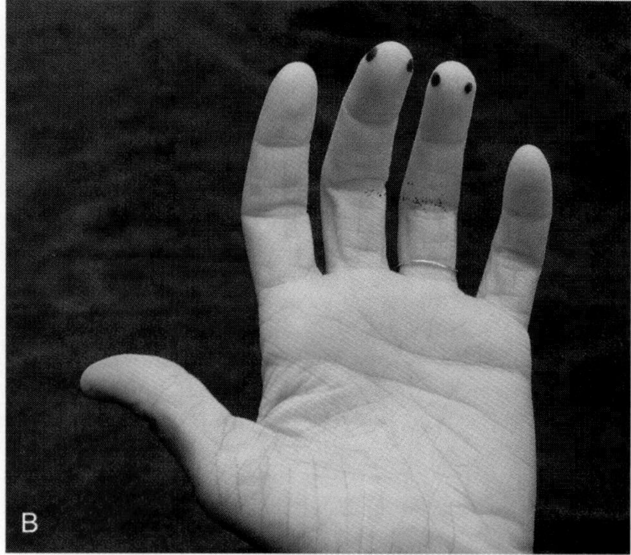

FIGURE 44–14 *A* and *B*, Capillary puncture sites on fingers and heel.

the middle finger or heel (Fig. 44–14). The puncture is made at the tip and slightly to the side of the finger.

The puncture site must be prepared by gentle massaging or placing the finger in warm water. This will increase blood circulation and allow a good flow of blood. The site is cleansed with 70% alcohol and wiped with a dry sterile gauze pad.

Collecting the Specimen

The patient's hand is held in a lateral position, with the skin near the puncture site pulled taut. A sharp-pointed blade called a lancet is used. Capillary punctures may also be performed using semiautomated devices such as the Autolet (Fig. 44–15). The puncture is performed in one quick, smooth motion. The lancet should puncture the site to a depth of 3 to 4 mm. The first drop of blood is wiped away because it contains tissue liquid and would dilute any results. The second and following drops are used. The finger is massaged to increase blood flow. Squeezing the finger should be avoided, because this will force tissue fluid to dilute the blood. Samples must be collected quickly to avoid clotting. For this reason, it is important to assemble all equipment needed before performing the capillary puncture (Fig. 44–16).

Pipetting the Blood

Blood must be diluted before blood cells can be counted microscopically because the cellular elements of blood are so concentrated. Blood-diluting pipettes are used to dilute the blood with a diluting

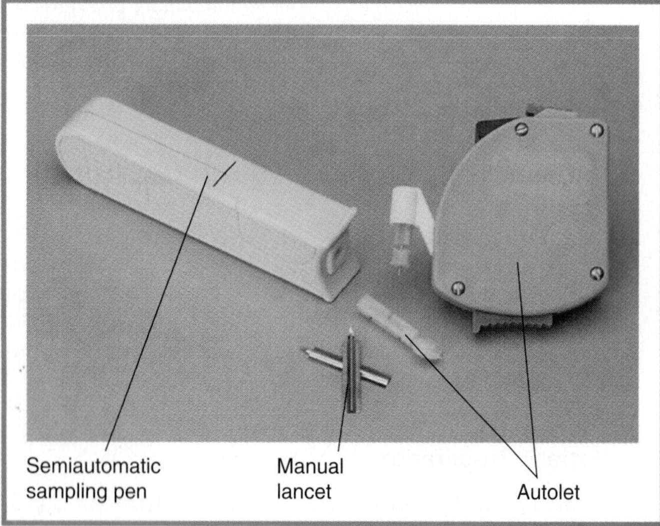

FIGURE 44–15 Blood sampling devices.

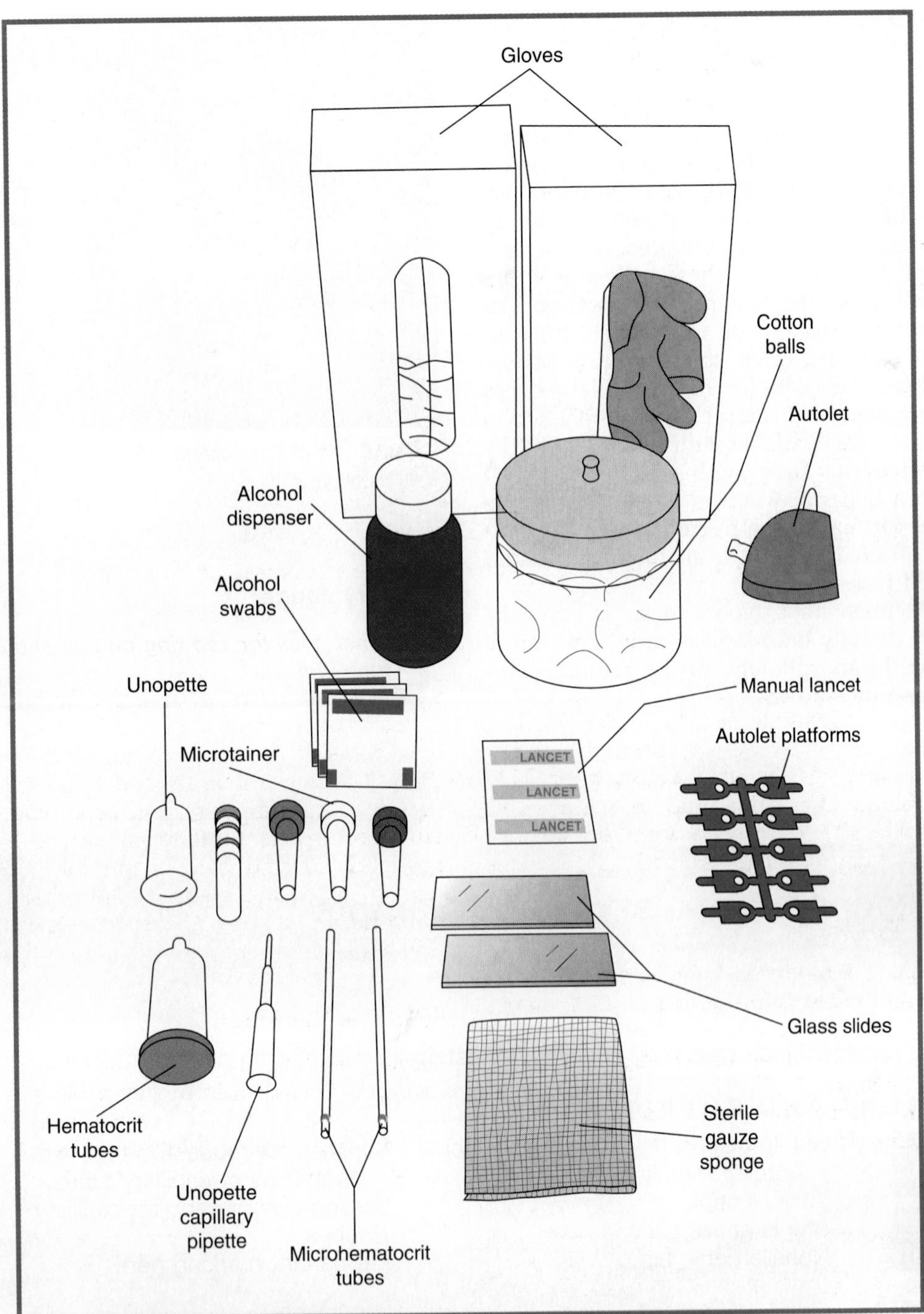

FIGURE 44–16 Capillary puncture supplies.

fluid, to manually perform leukocyte, erythrocyte, and thrombocyte counts. Blood is collected in glass blood-diluting pipettes, self-filling disposable pipettes, or capillary tubes or on glass slides.

Self-filling and self-measuring disposable micropipette systems are also available for counting leukocytes, erythrocytes, and platelets. The Unopette system consists of a disposable self-filling diluting pipette and a plastic reservoir prefilled with a precise amount of diluting fluid. These collection tubes allow for easy measuring, color-coding, stoppering, centrifugation, and storage of the blood samples. The collection caps are often shaped like a scoop, which eliminates the need for microcapillary tubes when collecting the blood sample (Fig. 44–17).

Capillary tubes are available with and without the anticoagulant **heparin.** Tubes with a red ring around one end contain heparin, whereas those with a blue ring are nonheparinized. The microhematocrit specimen can be collected directly from the finger using the heparinized tubes.

The best specimen for a blood smear is capillary blood smeared directly onto a glass slide. The smear is stained, and the morphology of the cellular components can then be studied.

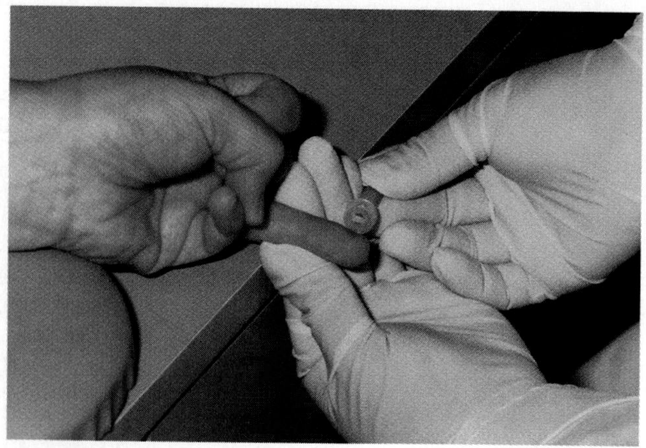

FIGURE 44–17 Unopette. Note that the collection cap is shaped like a scoop.

Memory Jogger

What does the red ring on one end of the capillary tube indicate?

PROCEDURE 44-4
Collecting a Capillary Blood Sample

GOAL

To collect a capillary blood specimen suitable for testing, using fingertip puncture technique.

EQUIPMENT AND SUPPLIES

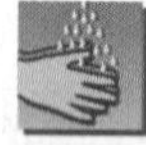

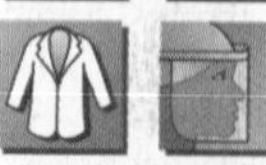
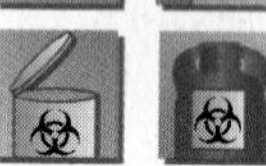

Sterile disposable manual lancet or Autolet with Autolet platforms
70% alcohol
Sterile gauze pads
Nonallergenic tape
Supplies for requested test (e.g., Unopettes or capillary tubes)
Sealing clay or caps for capillary tubes
Permanent marking pen

PROCEDURAL STEPS

1 Read requisition and gather all of the needed supplies.
PURPOSE: Efficiency.

2 Wash and dry your hands. Put on face protection and nonsterile gloves.

3 Explain the procedure to your patient.
PURPOSE: Explanations help gain the patient's cooperation.

Continued

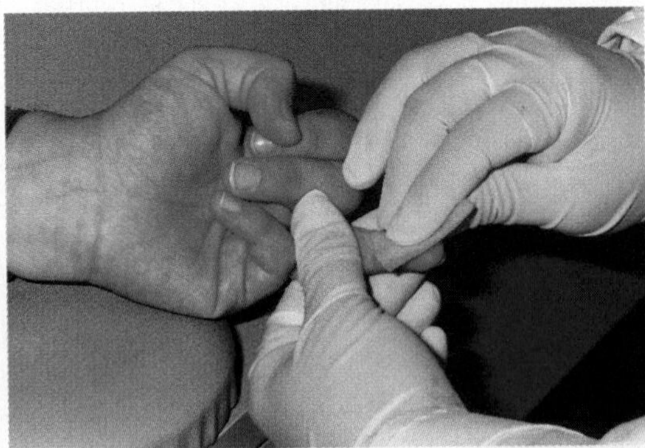

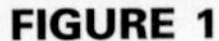

FIGURE 1

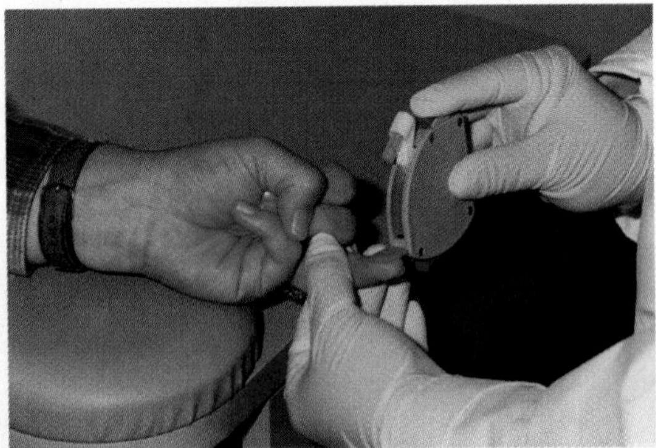

FIGURE 2

4 Assemble the needed materials, based on the physician's requisition.
PURPOSE: Once the skin has been punctured, the collection must proceed as rapidly as possible so the blood does not clot before the entire specimen has been collected.

5 Select a puncture site (side of middle finger of nondominant hand, outer edge of ear lobe, medial or lateral curved surface of the heel or the great toe for an infant).
PURPOSE: The nondominant hand may have fewer calluses. The side of the finger is less sensitive, and the skin is usually not as thick.

6 Milk, or very gently rub, the finger along the sides.
PURPOSE: This promotes circulation. If the finger is very cold, you may immerse it in warm water or moisten it with warm towels.

7 Clean the site with alcohol, and dry it with sterile gauze (Figure 1).
PURPOSE: Puncturing wet skin is painful and can hemolyze the specimen.

8 Grasp the patient's finger on the sides near the puncture site, with your nondominant forefinger and thumb.
PURPOSE: Firmly holding the site allows control of the puncture.

9 Hold the lancet at a right angle to the patient's finger, and make a rapid, deep puncture on the patient's fingertip (Figure 2).
PURPOSE: Lancets are designed to puncture at a depth of 3 to 4 mm, which is sufficient to obtain the required drops of blood.

10 Wipe away the first drop of blood (Figure 3).
PURPOSE: The first drop of blood contains tissue fluid.

Continued

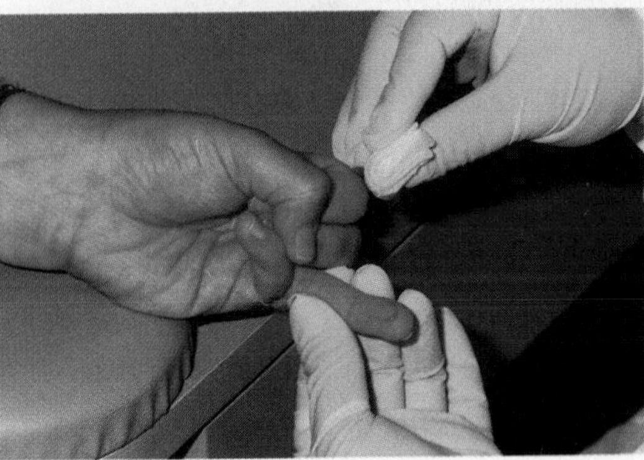

FIGURE 3

PROCEDURE 44-4 (CONTINUED)

Collecting a Capillary Blood Sample

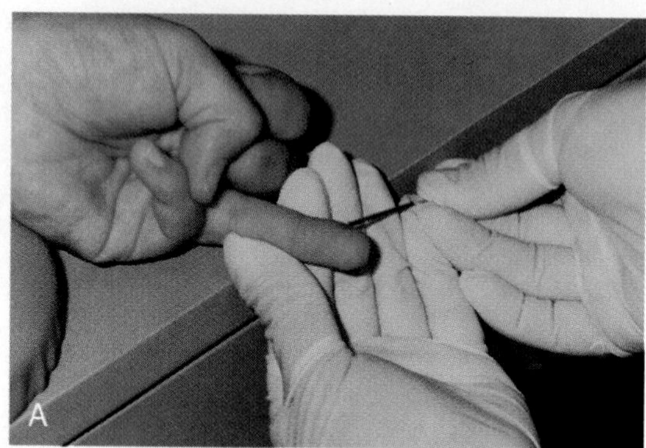

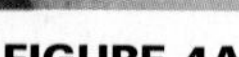

FIGURE 4A

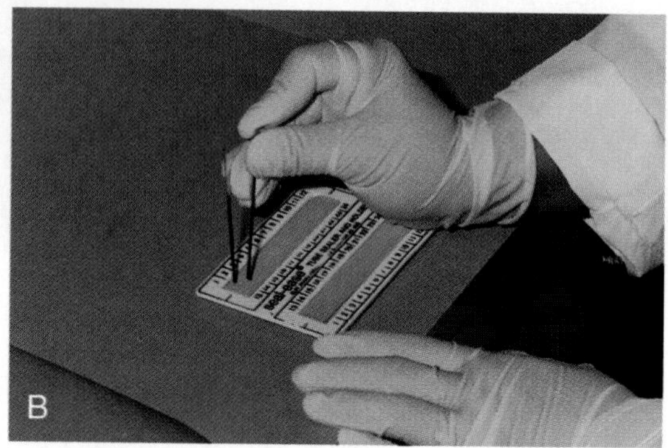

FIGURE 4B

11 Apply gentle pressure to cause the blood to flow freely.
PURPOSE: Squeezing liberates tissue that dilutes the blood and causes inaccurate results.

12 Collect blood samples.

- **a.** Express a large drop of blood, fill capillary tubes (Figure 4*A*), and seal the end of the tube in clay (Figure 4*B*).
- **b.** Wipe the finger with a clean sterile gauze pad, and fill a Unopette (Figure 5).

13 Apply pressure to the site with clean sterile gauze (Figure 6).

14 Label all samples and requisitions correctly, and forward them to the laboratory for testing.

15 Check the patient for bleeding, and apply a nonallergenic bandage if indicated.

16 Dismiss the patient.

17 Dispose of used materials in proper containers.

18 Clean the work area. Remove face protection and gloves. Wash your hands.
PURPOSE: Infection control.

19 Record the procedure in the patient's record.
PURPOSE: A procedure is considered not done until it is recorded.

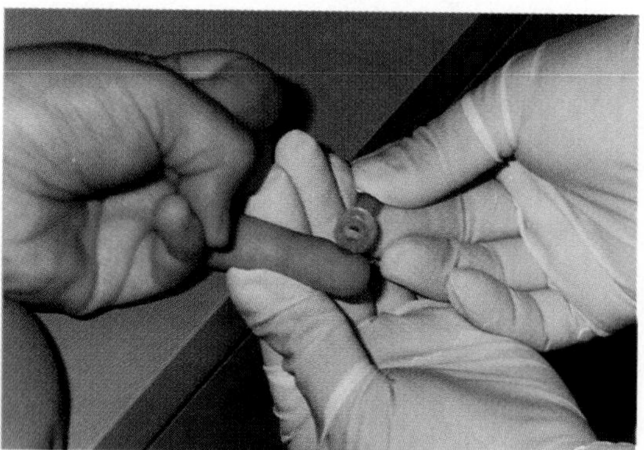

FIGURE 5

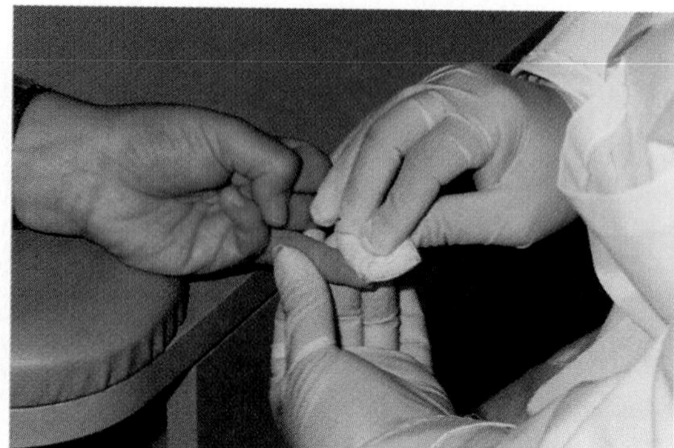

FIGURE 6

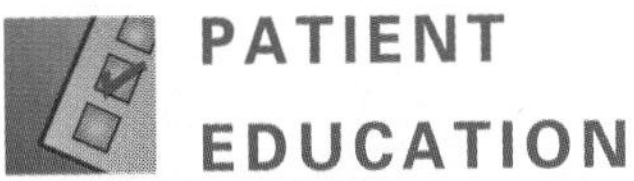

PATIENT EDUCATION

When working as a phlebotomist, the medical assistant must maintain a professional attitude and still be sympathetic to the fears and apprehensions of the patient. By establishing an environment that encourages the patient to relax, the amount of pain and discomfort experienced by the patient during the drawing procedure is kept to a minimum.

If the patient has a positive attitude, you need to provide little explanation about the procedure. Often, the patient can help you by telling from which site the last blood sample was successfully drawn. It is wise to follow the patient's suggestion in choosing the site for the removal of the blood specimen. When a patient is allowed to become an active participant in the procedure, he or she remains more relaxed, talkative, and confident in your expertise as a phlebotomist.

This atmosphere can change dramatically when the patient has had an unpleasant experience and associates pain and hurt with venipuncture. Such a patient usually is ill at ease, nervous, and apprehensive. When confronted with this scenario, you need to make every effort to perform the procedure quickly, efficiently, and effectively. Once the blood has been drawn and the patient has relaxed, you then will have an opportunity to help the patient develop a positive attitude.

If your patient has a history of **syncope** when blood is drawn, or if you suspect that this patient may faint during the procedure, have the patient lie down. Assemble your equipment and alert the physician before beginning the procedure. This type of professional care may help the patient get through the procedure without a traumatic effect.

Always remember to identify your patient and explain what you are going to do. Answer any questions the patient may have, and perform a skilled venipuncture before anxiety is allowed to set in.

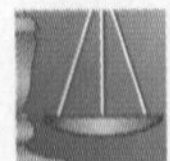

LEGAL AND ETHICAL ISSUES

Venipuncture and microcapillary blood collection are **invasive** procedures in which a sterile needle or a lancet is inserted through the skin. Because the skin is penetrated, drawing blood becomes a surgical procedure and is subject to the laws and regulations of surgery. When performing venipuncture, the rules and regulations must be enforced and there are no deviations from them. Be sure to follow the procedures as written and also become familiar with the regulations and standards established by local and state agencies, as well as the Clinical Laboratory Improvement Amendment of 1988 and OSHA Occupational Safety and Health Administration regulations.

CRITICAL THINKING

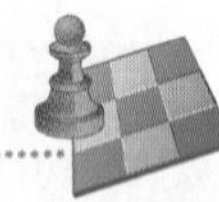

1 The patient tells you that she is afraid of needles and faints at the sight of her own blood. She refuses to have a venipuncture performed. What would be your response?

2 While performing a venipuncture procedure with the patient seated in a venipuncture chair, you notice that the patient is becoming pale and is perspiring. What steps would you take regarding the specimen and the patient's safety?

HOW DID I DO? Answers to Memory Joggers

1. Alternative sites may be indicated if the area is cyanotic, scarred, bruised, edematous, or burned.
2. Needles of 20 to 23 gauge are used for venipunctures.
3. The short end is fitted into the adapter.
4. Specimens for testing for blood alcohol levels are collected using benzalkonium chloride as the antiseptic.
5. A tourniquet is applied to the arm 3 to 4 inches above the elbow.
6. For tubes that contain additives, gently invert tube 8 to 10 times to mix.
7. Place the contaminated gloves in a biohazardous waste container, not in the sharps container.
8. Pediatric tubes are used because the volume in large tubes may create too great a vacuum pressure on the vein.
9. If a hematoma occurs, discontinue the procedure stat, apply pressure to the site for 3 minutes, place an ice pack on the area, and notify the physician.
10. Tubes with a red ring around one end contain heparin.

Assisting in Hematology and Serology

45

OUTLINE

LEARNING OBJECTIVES

Cognitive: On successful completion of this chapter you should be able to:

1. Identify the tests included in a complete blood cell count.
2. Describe the composition and function of blood.
3. Explain the purpose of a microhematocrit.
4. Describe hemoglobin.
5. Explain the purpose of a differential cell count.
6. Explain the methods of evaluating blood cells.
7. Understand the purpose of an erythrocyte sedimentation rate.
8. Explain the purpose for lipid testing.
9. Describe diabetes mellitus and glucose testing.
10. Discuss the Blood Safety Act.
11. Spell and define vocabulary terms.

Performance: On successful completion of this chapter you should be able to:

1. Accurately perform a microhematocrit.
2. Determine the level of hemoglobin present in a given blood sample.
3. Fill a Unopette capillary pipette and transfer to a Unopette reservoir, correctly completing each step in proper order.

4 Fill a hemacytometer chamber and correctly complete each step of the procedure in the proper sequence.
5 Using the filled hemacytometer, count and calculate a manual white or red blood cell count to a minimum performance level of 200 WBC/mm^3 and 50,000 RBC/mm^3.
6 Prepare and stain a blood smear, using Wright's stain, completing each step in proper sequence.
7 Perform a differential cell count, red blood cell examination, and platelet estimation to a minimum performance level of 90% accuracy.
8 Using an EDTA blood specimen, determine a sedimentation rate using the Wintrobe method to a minimum performance level of 1 mm.
9 Follow manufacturer's directions and accurately determine a patient's cholesterol level.
10 Secure a capillary blood sample and determine the ABO and Rh grouping of the sample with 100% accuracy.

VOCABULARY

analyte Any component in blood or other body fluid that can be measured

anemia Condition in which there is a reduction in the number of circulating red blood cells per cubic millimeter of blood

centrifuge Laboratory machine used to separate particles of different densities within a liquid by spinning them at very high speed

enzymes Proteins produced by living cells, which act as a catalyst, increasing the rate at which a chemical reaction occurs

eosin Any of the synthetic dyes used to stain tissues blue and yellow for microscopic identification

erythrocytes Red blood cells

hemolytic disease A group of diseases in which the characteristic feature is the breakdown of red blood cells and the release of hemoglobin into the plasma

hormones Chemical substances secreted by endocrine glands and carried through the blood to specific designated targets

leukemia Malignancy of the blood-forming cells in the bone marrow

leukocytes White blood cells

morphology The study of the form, structure, and size of organisms, organs, tissues, and cells

phagocytosis The process by which certain cells surround, engulf, and ingest microorganisms and cellular debris

plasma The liquid portion of the blood when only the cells have been removed

polycythemia vera Condition of unknown origin that is characterized by a marked increase in total blood volume, red blood cells, white blood cells, platelets, and hemoglobin

serum Liquid portion of blood that remains after the clotting proteins and cells have been removed

thrombocytes Clotting cells in the blood, also known as platelets

toxemia Distribution throughout the bloodstream of poisonous products of bacteria

urea End product of protein metabolism after ammonia is broken down by the liver; a systemic osmotic diuretic found in urine

Hematology

Hematology is the study of blood. The average body holds 10 to 12 pints of blood. The heart rotates the blood through the circulatory system more than a thousand times every day. There are more than 70,000 miles of passageways, most narrower than a human hair, that carry blood throughout the body.

The blood is contained in a closed system of vessels, of which the largest is the aorta and the smallest are the capillaries. The capillaries are only one cell layer thick, and these thin permeable walls allow certain substances to move back and forth between the blood vessels and the surrounding tissue. The blood contains more than 25 trillion cells, and every second the body replaces 8 million old red blood cells with 8 million new red blood cells.

Besides supplying body cells with their needed nutrients and oxygen, the blood also carries away carbon dioxide and **urea,** which are the waste products of normal cell activity. If the blood did not carry away the carbon dioxide and urea, these wastes would accumulate and cause cell damage and possibly **toxemia.** Carbon dioxide is carried in the blood to the lungs, where it is exhaled as part of normal breathing. The blood carries urea to the kidneys where, along with other body wastes, it is excreted in the urine. The blood also distributes **enzymes, hormones,** and other chemicals that the body needs for control and regulation of body activities. In addition, the blood functions to maintain the body at a uniform temperature, to keep other body fluids in a state of pH balance, and to carry the hormones from the secreting gland to the tissues where they are needed.

Memory Jogger

How much blood does the average body hold?

The hematology section of the laboratory deals with the *counting* of red blood cells, white blood cells, and platelets; *differentiating* white blood cells on a stained smear; *measuring* the percentage of red blood cells in blood (hematocrit); and *determining* the oxygen-carrying capacity of the blood (hemoglobin).

The *complete blood cell count (CBC)* is the most frequent laboratory procedure ordered on blood. It gives a fairly complete look at the components of blood and can provide a wealth of information concerning a patient's condition. The CBC routinely includes the tests shown under Complete Blood Cell Count Procedure.

COMPLETE BLOOD CELL COUNT PROCEDURE

Red blood cell count
White blood cell count
Hemoglobin determination
Hematocrit determination
Differential white blood cell count
Estimation of platelet numbers
Red blood cell morphology (size and shape)

BLOOD COMPOSITION, FUNCTION, AND FORMATION

Whole blood is composed of formed elements suspended in a clear yellow liquid portion called **plasma.** Plasma makes up about 55% of the blood by volume. The remaining 45% consists of the formed elements, which are the **erythrocytes** (red blood cells), **leukocytes** (white blood cells), and **thrombocytes** (platelets).

Blood is the vital circulating fluid of the body and has been referred to as the river of life. It is a transportation system bringing numerous substances of nourishment to all the cells of our body for growth, function, and repair and, in turn, carrying waste products away for disposal. In addition, blood functions to maintain the body at a uniform temperature; to keep the other body fluids in a state of equilibrium between alkalinity and acidity; and to carry hormones from the various glands to distant tissues where they are needed.

The cellular elements are produced and mature in the bone marrow, spleen, and lymph nodes. Then, they are released into the bloodstream. These cellular elements all have special functions.

The erythrocytes transport oxygen from the lungs to the body cells and carry carbon dioxide away from the cells, back to the lungs to be exhaled. They are disc-shaped cells that have two concave sides and no nucleus. Their main constituent is the red pigment hemoglobin, which is composed of iron and protein. Hemoglobin actually carries the oxygen and carbon dioxide throughout the body. The life span of an erythrocyte is about 120 days. Then the cell is broken down, and the wastes are stored in the liver. The iron is reused for new red blood cell formation, and the protein is converted into a bile pigment.

The prime function of the leukocyte is to protect the body against infection and disease. The five types of leukocytes are classified into granular and agranular groups. The granular leukocytes are called *polymorphonuclear* leukocytes and include the neutrophils, eosinophils, and basophils. They are characterized by their heavily granulated cytoplasm and segmented nuclei. The *agranular* leukocytes are the lymphocytes and monocytes, both of which have clear cytoplasm and a solid nucleus.

Thrombocytes (platelets) play a vital role in initiating the clotting process of blood. Humans cannot survive for long without the continuous flow of blood nourishing the tissues and protecting the body from disease. That is why an injury to a vessel could be disastrous if it resulted in the loss of too much blood. When a vessel is injured, thrombocytes adhere to each other and the edges of the injury and form a plug that becomes a blood clot. As the plug forms, a group of blood proteins called clotting factors form a net of fibers around and through the platelet plug. This blood clot soon retracts and stops the loss of blood. Hemophilia is one disease that involves impaired clotting factors.

Plasma is a highly complex liquid that is involved in the structure and function of the blood cells. Plasma is also the carrier for the formed elements and other substances such as proteins, carbohydrates, fats, hormones, enzymes, mineral salts, gases, and waste products. Plasma is composed of about 90% water, 9% protein, and 1% various other chemical substances. When the plasma proteins and other components are used up during the clotting process, the remaining liquid is called **serum.**

Memory Jogger

 *Identify the four primary elements in blood.*

COLLECTION OF BLOOD SPECIMENS

For most hematology tests, an adequate blood sample can be obtained from capillaries by finger puncture. If a larger sample is required, blood can be obtained from a vein by venipuncture. To perform a complete blood cell count, venous blood is collected in a tube containing an *anticoagulant* that prevents clotting. Adding an anticoagulant results in a whole blood sample. When a blood specimen has had anticoagulant added, the liquid portion is plasma. When a blood specimen is collected without an anticoagulant, it forms a clot and the liquid portion remaining is serum.

Memory Jogger

 *Is a tube anticoagulant needed when obtaining blood for hematologic study?*

MICROHEMATOCRIT

The microhematocrit (Hct) is a measurement of the percentage of packed red blood cells in a volume of blood. The test is based on the principle of separating the cellular elements from the plasma. The separation process is speeded up by centrifugation. Two or three drops of blood are collected in two capillary tubes and are placed in a specially designed microhematocrit **centrifuge** (Fig. 45–1; see Procedure 45–1).

After centrifugation, the red blood cells will be at the bottom of the tube, the white blood cells and platelets in the center, and the plasma on top. From this separation, the microhematocrit is determined by comparing the concentration of red blood cells with the total volume of the whole blood sample.

The percentage is read by placing the tubes on a special microhematocrit reader. Some microhematocrit centrifuges have a built-in reading scale that reads calibrated capillary tubes. Microhematocrits should be performed in duplicate, and the average of the two results reported.

The microhematocrit is a commonly performed test requested by physicians separately or as part of the complete blood cell count. Because it is a simple procedure requiring only a small amount of blood, it is an ideal test for following the progress of patients.

Memory Jogger

 *How much blood is needed to do a microhematocrit?*

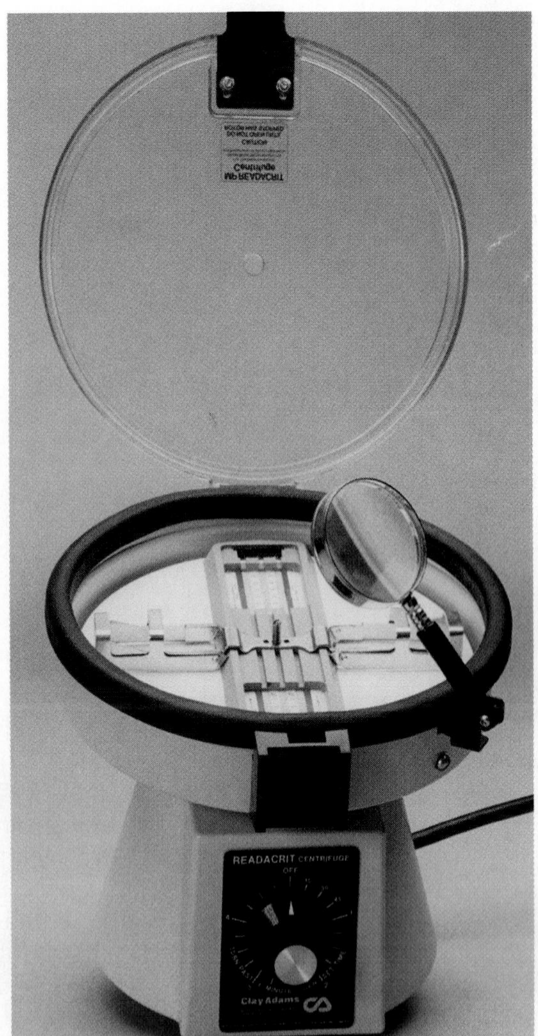

FIGURE 45–1 Centrifuge with capillary tube placement indications.

The normal values vary with the sex and age of the patient (Table 45–1). The values range from a low of 36% in women to a high of 52% in men. Low microhematocrit readings can indicate **anemia** or the presence of bleeding in a patient; high readings may be caused by dehydration or a condition such as **polycythemia vera.** Values can be influenced by physiologic or pathologic factors, as well as by collection techniques.

TABLE 45–1 Hematocrit Reference Values

Age/Gender	Hct Value (%)
Neonate	44–64
Infant	
1 month of age	35–49
6 months of age	30–40
Child, 1–10 years of age	35–41
Adult	
Men	42–52
Women	36–45

From Stepp CA, Woods MA: Laboratory Procedures for Medical Office Personnel. Philadelphia, WB Saunders, 1998.

PROCEDURE 45-1

Performing a Microhematocrit

GOAL

To accurately perform a microhematocrit

EQUIPMENT AND SUPPLIES

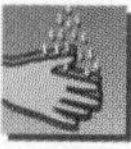 
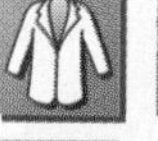
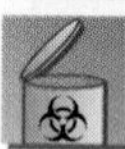

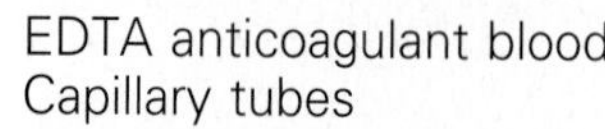

EDTA anticoagulant blood
Capillary tubes
Sealing clay
Centrifuge

PROCEDURAL STEPS

1 Wash and dry your hands. Put on face protection and nonsterile gloves.

2 Assemble the materials needed.

3 Fill two plain (blue-tipped) capillary tubes three fourths full with well-mixed EDTA anticoagulant blood.
PURPOSE: Duplicates should always be done as a means of quality control.

4 Plug the dry end of each tube with a sealing clay.
PURPOSE: Sealing the wet end may result in loss of the plug and the sample during centrifugation.

5 Place the tubes opposite each other in the centrifuge, with sealed ends securely against the gasket. Note tube arrangement in Figure 45-1.
PURPOSE: The centrifuge must always be balanced to avoid damage. If the clay ends of the capillary tubes are not outermost against the gasket, the sample will spin out of the tubes.

6 Note the numbers on the centrifuge slots and record them.
PURPOSE: The sample must be identified throughout the entire procedure.

7 Secure the locking top, fasten the lid down, and lock.
PURPOSE: If the locking top is not firmly in place during the spinning cycle, the tubes will come out of their slots and break. The lid is always locked during centrifugation for safety purposes, to avoid aerosols or broken glass from being ejected.

8 Set the timer, and adjust the speed as needed.
PURPOSE: The prescribed time is between 3 and 5 minutes. Check the manufacturer's instructions for time and speed.

9 Allow the centrifuge to come to a complete stop. Unlock the lids.

10 Remove the tubes immediately.
PURPOSE: Tubes left in the centrifuge will show altered results, as the red blood cell layer spreads horizontally.

11 Determine the microhematocrit values, using one of the following methods:
a Centrifuge with built-in reader using calibrated capillary tubes.
1) Position the tubes as directed by manufacturer's instructions.
2) Read both tubes.
3) The average of the two results is reported.
4) The two values should not vary by more than 2%.
b Centrifuge without built-in reader.
1) Carefully remove the tubes from the centrifuge.
2) Place a tube on the microhematocrit reader.

Continued

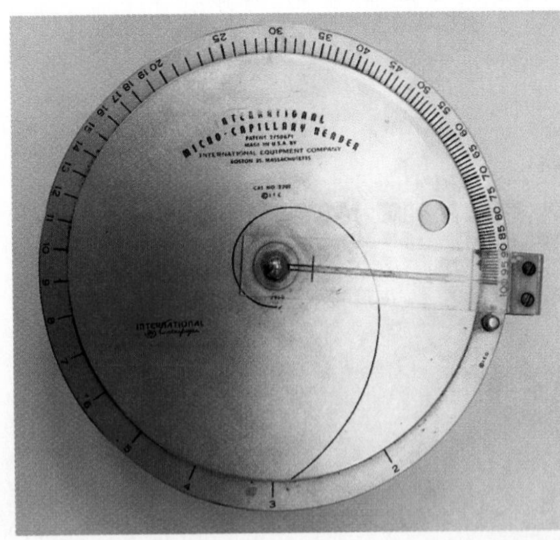

FIGURE 1

3) Align the clay–red blood cell junction with the zero line on the reader. Align the plasma meniscus with the 100% line. The value is read at the junction of the red cell layer and the buffy coat (Figure 1).*
4) Read both tubes.
5) The average of the two results is reported.
6) The two values should not vary by more than 2%.

12 Dispose of the capillary tubes in a biohazard container.

13 Clean the work area and properly dispose of all biohazard materials. Remove gloves and face protection and wash your hands.

14 Record the results in the patient's medical record.
PURPOSE: A procedure is not considered done until it is charted.

*From Stepp CA, Woods MA: Laboratory Procedures for Medical Office Personnel. Philadelphia, WB Saunders, 1998.

HEMOGLOBIN

The hemoglobin (Hgb) determination is a rough measure of the oxygen-carrying capacity of the blood. Determining hemoglobin concentration can be performed as part of the complete blood cell count or as an individual test (see Procedure 45–2). Many methods of determining hemoglobin concentration have been used throughout the years. One widely used hemoglobin measurement method is for *cyanmethemoglobin.* A sample of whole blood is diluted in *Drabkin reagent,* which breaks down (lyses) red cells, releasing the hemoglobin into the solution. The chemicals in the reagent react with the released hemoglobin to form the pigment cyanmethemoglobin, which can be measured by using a photometer.

The normal hemoglobin value varies throughout life. Values are normally quite high at birth, decline during childhood, and then increase through the teens until the adult levels are reached (Table 45–2). Values range from a low of 12.5 g/dL in women to a high of 17.5 g/dL in men. The various factors that affect the hemoglobin level include age, sex, diet, altitude, and disease.

Memory Jogger

5 *What are the value ranges for hemoglobin?*

TABLE 45–2 Hemoglobin Reference Values

Age/Gender	Hgb Level (g/dL)
Neonate	17–23
Infant (2 months of age)	9–14
Adult female	12–16
Adult male	15–18

From Stepp CA, Woods MA: Laboratory Procedures for Medical Office Personnel. Philadelphia, WB Saunders, 1998.

PROCEDURE 45-2

Obtaining a Hemoglobin Count

GOAL

To accurately determine the level of hemoglobin present in a blood sample using the hemoglobinometer method.

EQUIPMENT AND SUPPLIES

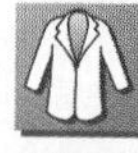
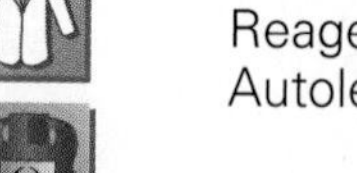

Hemoglobinometer
Reagent applicators
Autolet or blood lancet
Alcohol preps
Gauze squares

PROCEDURAL STEPS

1 Wash and dry hands.
PURPOSE: Infection control.
2 Collect and assemble all equipment and supplies needed.
3 Explain the procedure to the patient.
4 Put on gloves.
5 Prepare the clipped chamber by slightly offsetting the cover slide to expose the chamber slide surface.
6 Examine the fingers and choose the site to be used to obtain the blood sample.
PURPOSE: The site to be used must be free of trauma, calluses, and scarring.
7 Clean the site with alcohol or other recommended antiseptic preparation.
8 Perform a capillary puncture and obtain the blood sample.
9 Wipe away the first drop of blood (Figure 1).
PURPOSE: This drop may contain tissue fluid.
10 Place one large drop of blood on the chamber slide. Do not touch the slide with the finger (Figure 2).
PURPOSE: Contact of the slide with the skin may alter your results.
11 Agitate the blood with a reagent stick until the blood appears shiny or transparent. This takes about 45 seconds.
PURPOSE: To ensure action of anticoagulation.

Continued

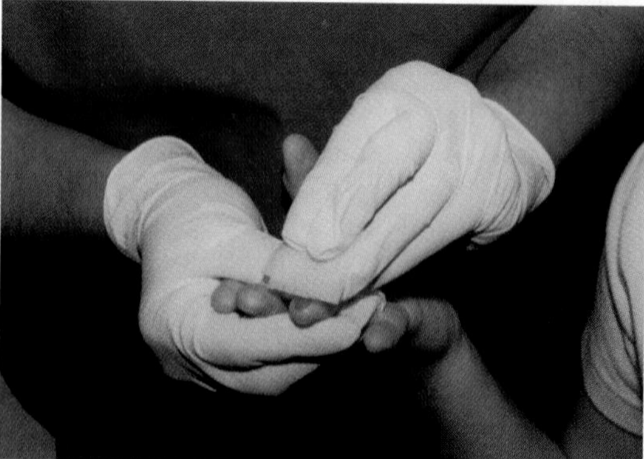

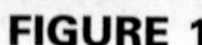
FIGURE 1

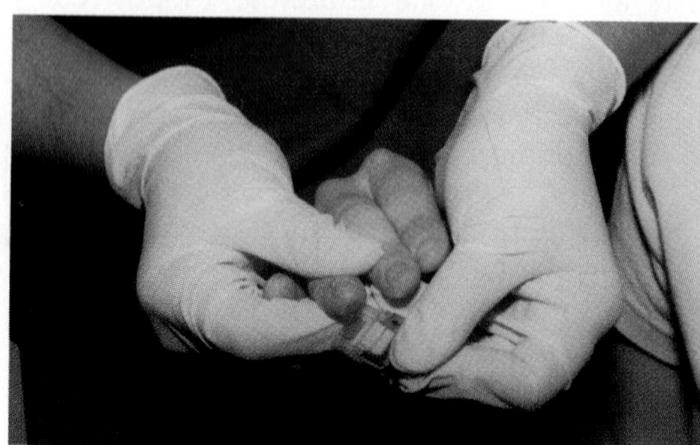

FIGURE 2

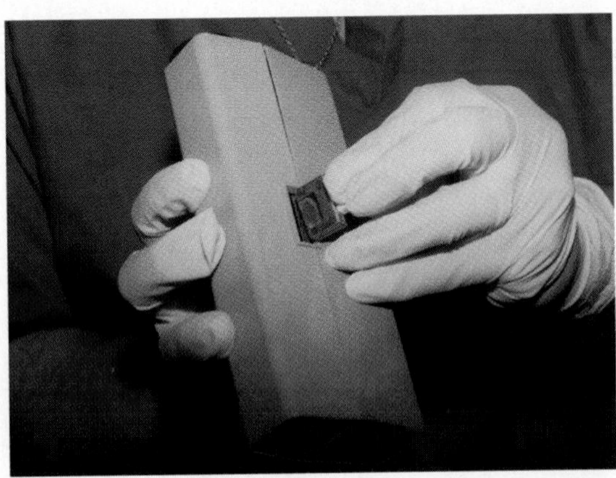

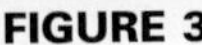

FIGURE 3

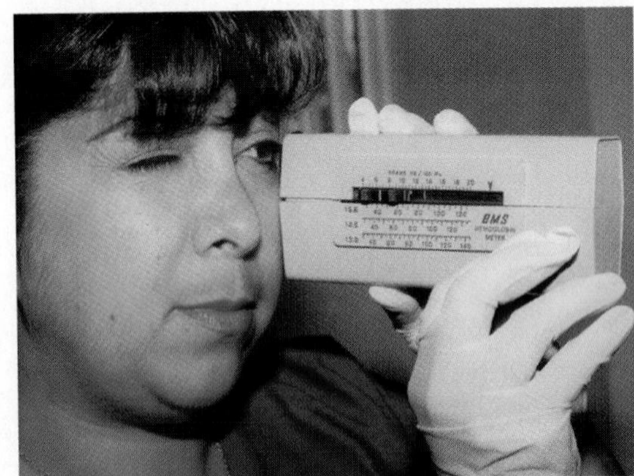

FIGURE 4

12 Close the chamber and insert the chamber into the hemoglobinometer (Figure 3).

13 Hold the device horizontally at eye level and turn on the light at the base of the unit with the left hand (Figure 4).

14 Visualize the split green field through the viewer and with the right hand move the slide adjustment until there is no visible difference between the two hemispheres in the viewer.

15 Read the scale on the right side of the instrument. Your reading will be in grams of hemoglobin per 100 ml of blood.

16 Dispose of the biohazard waste in correct containers, and properly clean the hemoglobinometer chamber and work area. Return equipment to proper storage location.

17 Remove gloves and wash hands.
PURPOSE: Infection control.

18 Record the test results in the patient's medical record.
PURPOSE: A procedure is considered not done until it is recorded.

RED BLOOD CELL COUNT

The red blood cell count is a commonly performed procedure and is part of the complete blood cell count (Table 45–3). It approximates the number of circulating red blood cells. The function of red blood cells is to transport oxygen to the tissues. The condition in which this oxygen-carrying capacity of the blood is below normal is called anemia. The red blood cell count is usually decreased in anemia. Increases are found in people with dehydration, polycythemia vera, or severe burns and in people who live at high altitudes, as an adaptation to the lower oxygen content of the air.

The normal values for red blood cell counts range from 4 million to 6 million cells/mm^3. Red blood cell counts are usually higher in males than in females.

Memory Jogger

6 *What is the normal value range for red blood cells per cubic millimeter?*

WHITE BLOOD CELL COUNT

The white blood cell count is one of the most frequently requested hematology tests. It gives an approximation of the total number of leukocytes in circulating blood. The count is performed to aid the physician in determining if an infection is present. It may also be used to follow the course of a disease and to determine if the patient is responding to treatment.

The normal white blood cell count varies with age. It is higher in newborns and decreases throughout life. The average adult range is between 4500 and 12,000 cells/mm^3. Many factors affect the white blood cell count. Elevation in white blood cells is called *leukocytosis*. Physiologic increases in the white blood cell count are seen in pregnancy, stress, anesthesia, exercise, and exposure to temperature extremes and after treatment with corticosteroids. Pathologic causes of leukocytosis include many bacterial infections, leukemia, appendicitis, and pneumonia. A decrease in the white blood cell count is called *leukopenia*. This condition may be caused by viral infections or by exposure to radiation, certain chemicals, and drugs.

TABLE 45–3 Reference Ranges for a Complete Blood Count

<table>
<tr><th rowspan="2">Test</th><th rowspan="2">Neonates</th><th rowspan="2">Infants (6 mo)</th><th rowspan="2">Children</th><th colspan="2">Adults</th></tr>
<tr><th>Men</th><th>Women</th></tr>
<tr><td>RBCs</td><td>4.8–7.1 million/mm^3</td><td>3.8–5.5 million/mm^3</td><td>4.5–4.8 million/mm^3</td><td>4.5–6.0 million/mm^3</td><td>4.0–5.5 million/mm^3</td></tr>
<tr><td>Hematocrit (Hct)</td><td>44–64%</td><td>30–40%</td><td>35–41%</td><td>42–52%</td><td>36–45%</td></tr>
<tr><td>Hemoglobin (Hgb)</td><td>17–21 g/dL</td><td>10–15 g/dL</td><td>11–16 g/dL</td><td>15–18 g/dL</td><td>12–16 g/dL</td></tr>
<tr><td>RBC Indices</td><td></td><td></td><td></td><td></td><td></td></tr>
<tr><td>MCV</td><td>96–108 μm</td><td></td><td></td><td colspan="2">82–98 μm</td></tr>
<tr><td>MCH</td><td>32–34 pg</td><td></td><td></td><td colspan="2">26–34 pg</td></tr>
<tr><td>MCHC</td><td>31–33 g/dL</td><td></td><td></td><td colspan="2">31–37 g/dL</td></tr>
<tr><td>WBCs</td><td>9000–30,000/mm^3</td><td>6000–16,000/m^3</td><td>5000–13,000/mm^3</td><td colspan="2">4000–11,000/mm^3</td></tr>
<tr><td>Differential WBC count</td><td></td><td></td><td></td><td></td><td></td></tr>
<tr><td>Neutrophils</td><td>≥45% by 1 week of age</td><td>32%</td><td>60% for children 2 years of age and older</td><td colspan="2">50–65%</td></tr>
<tr><td>Bands</td><td>—</td><td>—</td><td>—</td><td colspan="2">0–7%</td></tr>
<tr><td>Eosinophils</td><td>—</td><td>—</td><td>0–3%</td><td colspan="2">1–3%</td></tr>
<tr><td>Basophils</td><td>—</td><td>—</td><td>1–3%</td><td colspan="2">0–1%</td></tr>
<tr><td>Monocytes</td><td>—</td><td>—</td><td>4–9%</td><td colspan="2">3–9%</td></tr>
<tr><td>Lymphocytes</td><td>≥41% by 1 week of age</td><td>61%</td><td>59% for children 2 years of age or older</td><td colspan="2">25–40%</td></tr>
<tr><td>Platelets</td><td>140,000–300,000/mm^3</td><td>200,000–473,000/mm^3</td><td>150,000–450,000/mm^3</td><td colspan="2">150,000–400,000/mm^3</td></tr>
</table>

From Stepp CA, Woods MA: Laboratory Procedures for Medical Office Personnel. Philadelphia, WB Saunders, 1998.

Memory Jogger

How can a white blood cell count aid the physician?

METHODS OF COUNTING RED AND WHITE BLOOD CELLS

Manual Counts

Both the red blood cell count and the white blood cell count approximate the number of these circulating cells in the blood. These cellular elements are very concentrated in the blood. Therefore, the blood must be diluted for these cells to be counted microscopically. Blood-diluting pipettes and diluting fluids are used for this purpose. The counts are then performed using the diluted blood, a counting chamber called a *hemacytometer,* a hemacytometer coverslip, and a microscope.

Unopettes

Manual counts using blood-diluting pipettes and diluting fluid should not be performed by medical assistants. This type of testing is usually done in a formal laboratory by a licensed laboratory technician or technologist. A simpler and less error-prone method for performing manual counts is done by using a prefilled reservoir containing a premeasured diluting-fluid unit such as the Unopette (see Procedure 45–3). This unit comes equipped with a capillary pipette and pipette shield. Unopettes are available for counting erythrocytes, leukocytes, and platelets (Fig. 45–2). Package inserts contain detailed instructions that, when correctly followed, result in a more accurate dilution than with the blood-diluting pipettes.

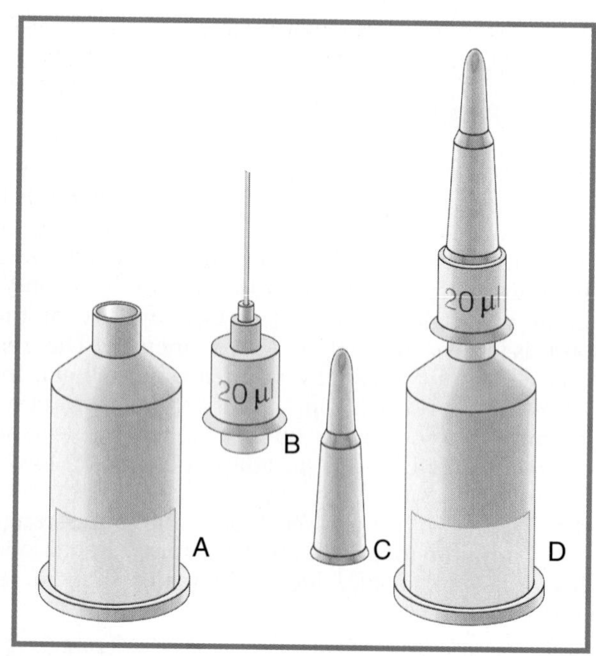

FIGURE 45–2 Components of a disposable blood-diluting unit, such as the Unopette system. *A,* A prefilled reservoir, containing premeasured diluting fluid, is sealed with a diaphragm. *B,* A capillary pipette with overflow chamber and capacity marking. *C,* A pipette shield. *D,* Assembled unit. (From Stepp CA, Woods MA: Laboratory Procedures for Medical Office Personnel. Philadelphia, WB Saunders, 1998.)

PROCEDURE 45-3

Filling a Unopette

GOAL

To properly fill a Unopette pipette with blood and to transfer the sample to a Unopette reservoir.

EQUIPMENT AND SUPPLIES

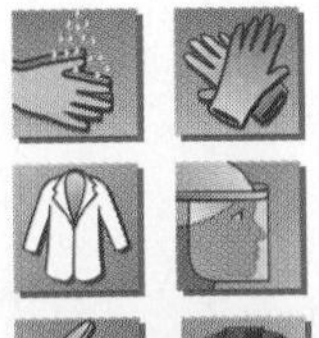

Unopette unit: capillary pipette, pipette shield, reservoir
EDTA anticoagulant blood
Gauze squares
Test tube rack

PROCEDURAL STEPS

1 Wash and dry your hands, and put on face protection and nonsterile gloves.
PURPOSE: Infection control.

2 Remove a Unopette reservoir from the storage container, and recap the container tightly.
PURPOSE: The container is humidified. Loss of the humid conditions will allow evaporation, and the remaining Unopettes will give inaccurate results.

3 Use the pipette shield to puncture the diaphragm of the Unopette reservoir. The hole must be large enough to allow the pipette to enter freely.
PURPOSE: If the hole is too small, loss of a portion of the sample can occur when the pipette is inserted into the reservoir (Figure 1).*

4 Remove the pipette shield.

5 Hold the pipette nearly horizontal.

6 Place the tip of the pipette into a well-mixed tube of blood, and allow the pipette to fill by capillary action until blood reaches the end of the pipette. It will stop by itself (Figure 2).

Continued

*Figures from Stepp CA, Woods MA: Laboratory Procedures for Medical Office Personnel. Philadelphia, WB Saunders, 1998.

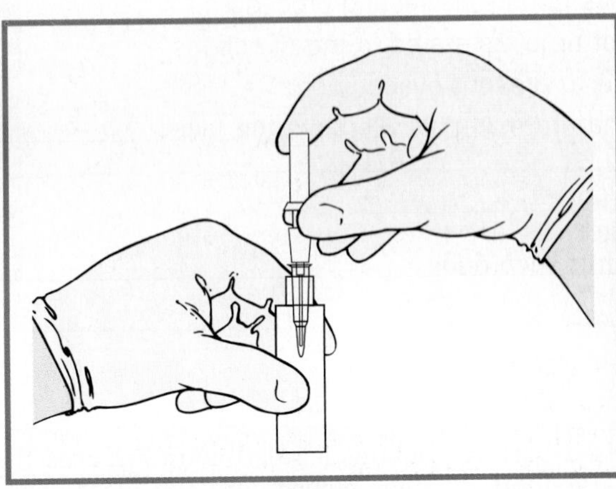

FIGURE 1

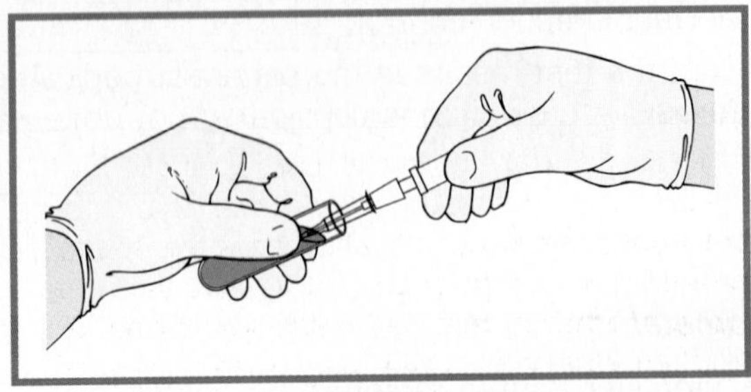

FIGURE 2

PROCEDURE 45-3 (CONTINUED)
Filling a Unopette

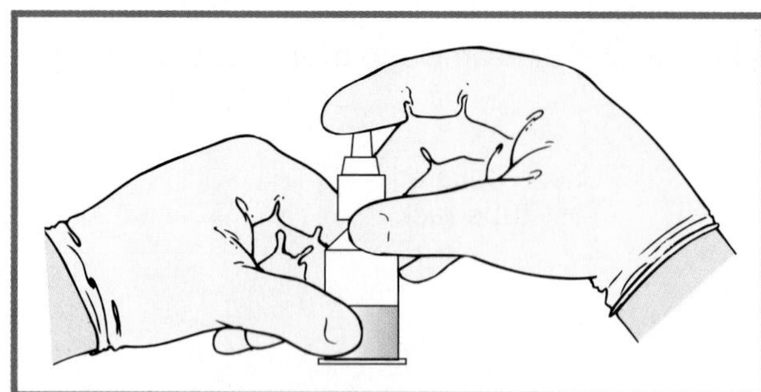

FIGURE 3

FIGURE 4

7 Place a finger over the hole in the end of the pipette to prevent loss of any sample, and carefully wipe the outside of the pipette with gauze to remove all traces of blood (Figure 3).
PURPOSE: Blood on the outside of the pipette will enter the reservoir and give inaccurate results.

8 Squeeze the reservoir with one hand.

9 While holding your index finger over the hole in the top of the pipette, insert the pipette into the reservoir and seat it firmly in place with a twisting motion.
PURPOSE: Squeezing the reservoir before inserting the pipette is necessary. It creates a vacuum, which will draw the sample into the reservoir:

10 Release the pressure on the reservoir, and remove your finger from the top of the pipette. The sample will be drawn into the reservoir.

11 Gently squeeze and release the reservoir several times to rinse all blood from the pipette into the reservoir. Liquid should rise to the overflow chamber but should not be forced out of the top of the pipette.
PURPOSE: The capillary pipette is calibrated to contain an amount of blood. It must be rinsed several times with the diluting fluid to ensure that all of the sample has been delivered into the reservoir.

12 Mix the contents of the Unopette gently by inversion or by rolling between the palms of your hands (Figure 4).

13 Identify the Unopette.
PURPOSE: The sample must be identifiable at all times during the testing procedure.

14 Allow the Unopette to sit for the specified amount of time, as stated in the directions.

15 Place the shield on the top of the prepared Unopette to prevent evaporation.

16 Clean the work area by properly disposing of all biohazard materials. Remove the face protection and gloves and wash your hands.
PURPOSE: Infection control.

17 Record the test results in the patient's medical record.
PURPOSE: A procedure is considered not done until it is recorded.

Hemacytometer

The hemacytometer is used to count the cellular elements of the blood. It is a heavy glass slide that, when viewed from the top, has two raised platforms surrounded by depressions on three sides. Each raised surface contains a ruled counting area that is marked off by lines etched into the glass. The depressions surrounding these platforms are called moats. The raised areas and depressions form an H. A special hemacytometer coverslip of uniform thick-

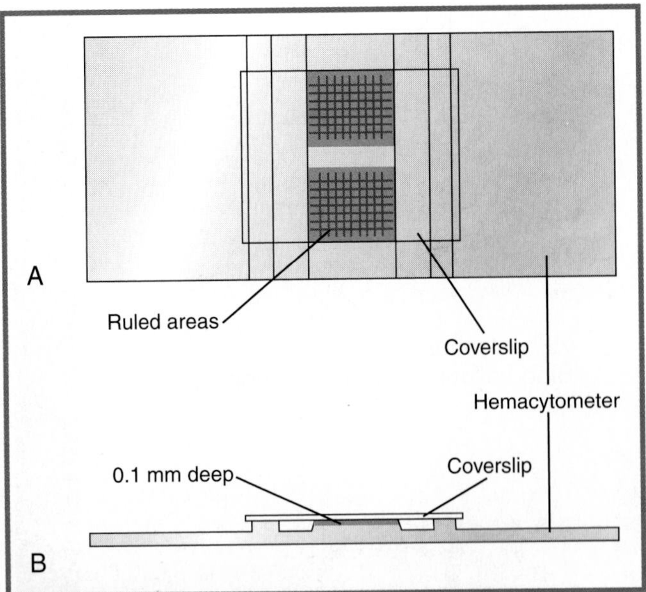

FIGURE 45–3 Hemacytometer: top (*A*) and side (*B*) views. The blood sample should fill the shaded areas when the chamber is properly filled.

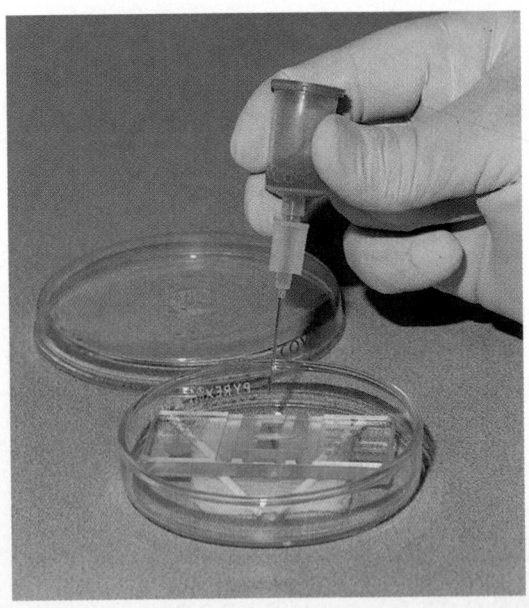

FIGURE 45–5 Charging a counting chamber using a Unopette system. (From Stepp CA, Woods MA: Laboratory Procedures for Medical Office Personnel. Philadelphia, WB Saunders, 1998.)

ness is used. The coverslip is positioned on the hemacytometer so that it covers the ruled areas, confines the fluid in the chamber, and regulates the depth of the fluid. The depth of the fluid in the most commonly used *Neubauer-type* hemacytometer is 0.1 mm with the coverslip in place (Fig. 45–3).

Each ruled area of the counting chamber consists of a large 3-mm³ square. This area, in turn, is divided into nine equal squares, each of which is 1 mm². The white blood cell counting area consists of the four large corner squares labeled "W" (Fig. 45–4).

The center squares are used to count the red blood cells. Each center square is subdivided into 25 smaller squares. Only the 4 corner and center squares within the large center square are used to count red blood cells (Fig. 45–4).

After the coverslip has been positioned, the hemacytometer is filled, or *charged*. This is accomplished by touching the tip of the diluting pipette or Unopette to the point where the coverslip and the raised platform meet (Fig. 45–5). The fluid will flow by capillary action into one side of the hemacytometer. The opposite side is also filled (see Procedure 45–4).

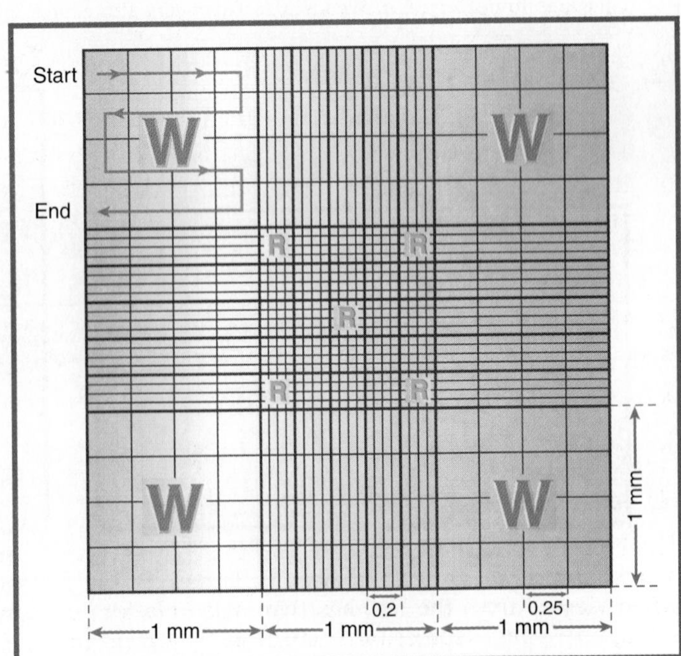

FIGURE 45–4 Arrangement of counting squares. (From Stepp CA, Woods MA: Laboratory Procedures for Medical Office Personnel. Philadelphia, WB Saunders, 1998.)

PROCEDURE 45-4

Charging (Filling) a Hemacytometer

GOAL

To fill the hemacytometer for a manual cell count.

EQUIPMENT AND SUPPLIES

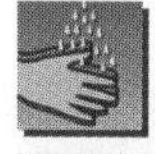
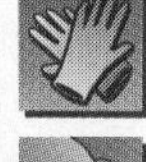
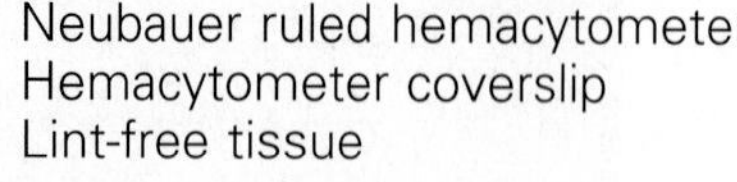
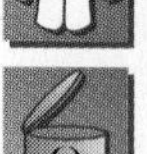

Neubauer ruled hemacytometer
Hemacytometer coverslip
Lint-free tissue
70% alcohol
Blood-diluting pipette or Unopette

PROCEDURAL STEPS

1 Wash and dry your hands. Put on face protection and nonsterile gloves.
PURPOSE: Infection control.

2 Clean the hemacytometer and coverslip with 70% alcohol and lint-free tissue, and thoroughly dry.
PURPOSE: Dirt, fingerprints, grease, or lint interferes with filling and counting.

3 Align the coverslip on the chamber.

4 Convert to dropper assembly by withdrawing the pipette from the reservoir and reseating it securely in reverse position. (Figure 1*).

5 To clean the capillary bore, invert the reservoir and gently squeeze the sides, expelling two drops from the well-mixed pipette or Unopette.
PURPOSE: Diluent in the calibrated stem contains no cells and must be discarded before filling the chamber of the hemacytometer.

6 Touch the tip of the pipette to the edge of the coverslip in the loading area of the chamber (Figure 2).

Continued

*Figures from Stepp CA, Woods MA: Laboratory Procedures for Medical Office Personnel. Philadelphia, WB Saunders, 1998.

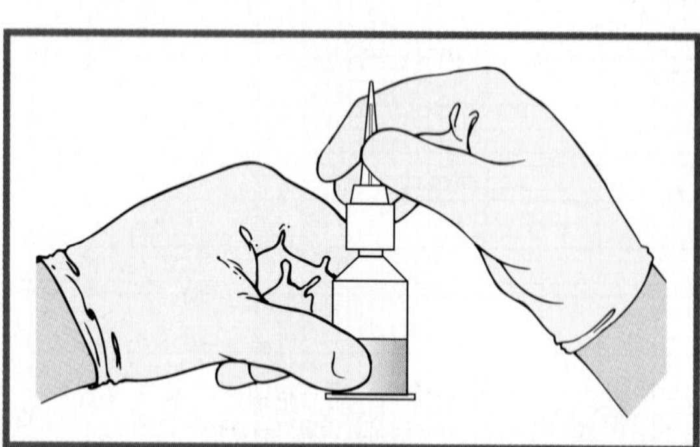

FIGURE 1

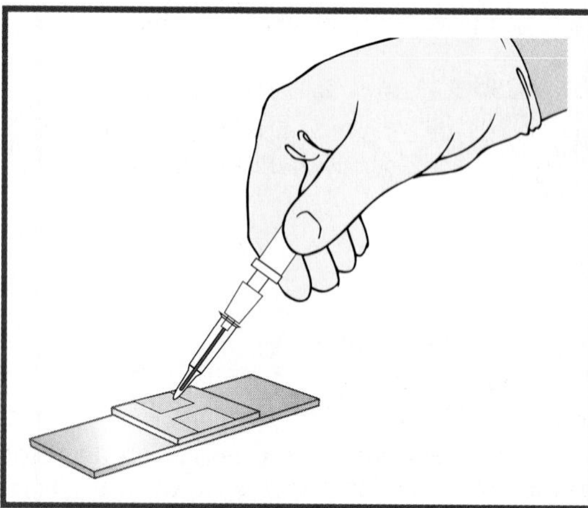

FIGURE 2

7 Controlling the flow with the finger on the pipette or by gentle squeezing of the Unopette, fill the chamber in one smooth motion.
PURPOSE: Chamber fills by capillary action. If the pipette is not touching the edge of the coverslip, the chamber will not fill properly.

8 Stop filling when the ruled area is full, and do not overfill.

9 Fill both sides of the hemacytometer.

10 Allow the chamber to sit undisturbed for 1 or 2 minutes so that the cells settle, but do not allow the sample to dry.
PURPOSE: Once the cells have settled in the chamber, the counting procedure is easier. Drying contracts the sample and elevates the count.

11 Clean the work area by properly disposing of all biohazard materials.
PURPOSE: Infection control.

12 Record the testing results in the patient's record.
PURPOSE: A procedure is not considered done until it is recorded.

Counting

The hemacytometer is placed on the microscope. White blood cell counts are observed under the 10× objective, and red blood cells are counted under the 40× objective. A counting pattern of left to right and right to left is used to ensure that cells are counted only once. Counts should begin in the upper left corner square. All cells within the squares are counted. Only cells touching top and left boundary lines are counted (Fig. 45–6; see Procedure 45–5).

PROCEDURE 45–5
Counting Cells in the Neubauer Ruled Hemacytometer

GOAL

To properly focus a hemacytometer, to locate the appropriate areas to count, and to direct your field of vision through the chamber in the proper manner while counting cells.

EQUIPMENT AND SUPPLIES

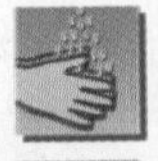
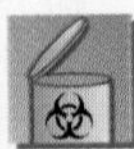
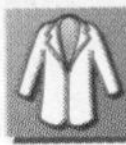

Properly filled hemacytometer (see Procedure 45–4)
Microscope
Hand tally counter

PROCEDURAL STEPS

1 Wash and dry your hands.
PURPOSE: Infection control.

2 Place the hemacytometer on the lowered microscope stage under low-power magnification.
PURPOSE: The thick chamber will not fit under the objective unless the stage is lowered.

3 Center the ruled area over the opening in the stage.

Continued

PROCEDURE 45–5 (CONTINUED)

Counting Cells in the Neubauer Ruled Hemacytometer

4 Reduce the light intensity by closing the diaphragm and lowering the condenser.
PURPOSE: The unstained cells require reduced light for counting.

5 Raise the stage carefully while watching from the side to be certain that the objective lens does not hit the coverslip.
PURPOSE: The chamber or the microscope lens can easily be damaged by improper focusing techniques.

6 Focus and center the correct area (top left large W square for counting white blood cells), using the coarse adjustment and mechanical stage simultaneously.
PURPOSE: You will be moving through several planes of focus. When you see the chamber moving through the ocular lens, you will know that you are in approximate focus and will be able to locate the lined area easily.

7 Adjust the light until the cells are easily visible.
PURPOSE: Too much light will prevent you from visualizing the cells.

8 Count white blood cells under low power, by depressing the hand tally once for each cell seen (Figure 1*).
- a Begin in the top row, on the far left.
- b Count the top row, moving visually from left to right.
- c Count all cells within the boundaries of the square, and also cells touching the top and the left-hand lines of the square.
- d Do not count cells touching the right-hand lines or the bottom lines of the square.
- e When you come to the end of the top row, drop to the second row.
- f Count the second row, moving visually from right to left.
- g Continue counting in this zigzag pattern, ending at the bottom left small square.

PURPOSE: Using the same sequence when counting helps you to count all cells that should be counted and to avoid counting cells twice or missing them entirely.

9 When you have finished counting a large square, record the number.

10 Return the tally to zero, move to the next large square, and begin to count.
PURPOSE: You need to know the total cells counted in each square individually to determine if the chamber was filled correctly. An unevenly filled hemacytometer voids the count.

Continued

*Figures from Stepp CA, Woods MA: Laboratory Procedures for Medical Office Personnel. Philadelphia, WB Saunders, 1998.

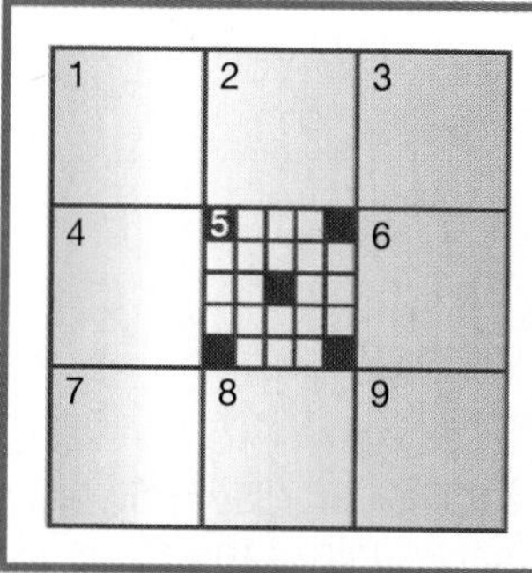

FIGURE 1

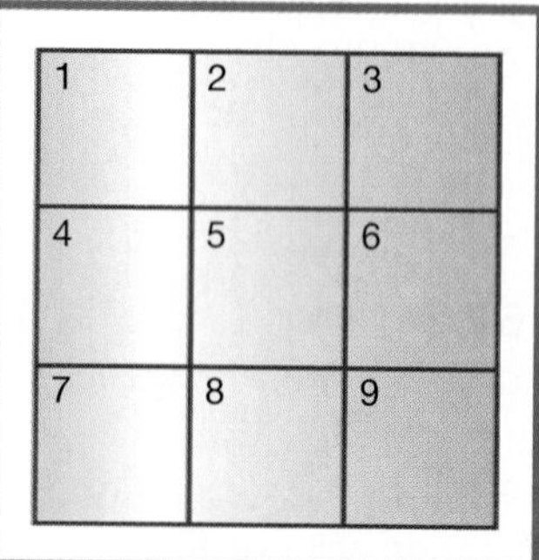

FIGURE 2

11 Switch to high power, and focus with the fine adjustment for counting red blood cells (top left R square).

12 Locate the remaining squares to be counted, and determine the number of cells in each. For white blood cells, the counts from each square should vary by no more than 10 cells. For red blood cells, the numbers should vary by no more than 20 cells. Greater variation indicates an unevenly filled hemacytometer (Figure 2). In such cases, the chamber should be cleaned and refilled.

13 Total the cells counted in all four squares for white blood cells and in five squares for red blood cells.

14 Count the second side of the chamber in the same manner.

15 Average the counts from both sides.

16 Calculate the results:
- For red blood cells: average times 10,000
- For white blood cells: average times 50

17 Record the results in the patient's medical record.
PURPOSE: A procedure is considered not done until it is recorded.

18 Clean the work area. Wash your hands.

Calculations

Calculations for a red blood cell count are determined by counting both sides of the hemacytometer and obtaining an average. This number is then multiplied by 10. For white blood cell counts, the average of the two sides is multiplied by 50.

Memory Jogger

8 *How do you calculate the number of red blood cells and white blood cells in a blood sample?*

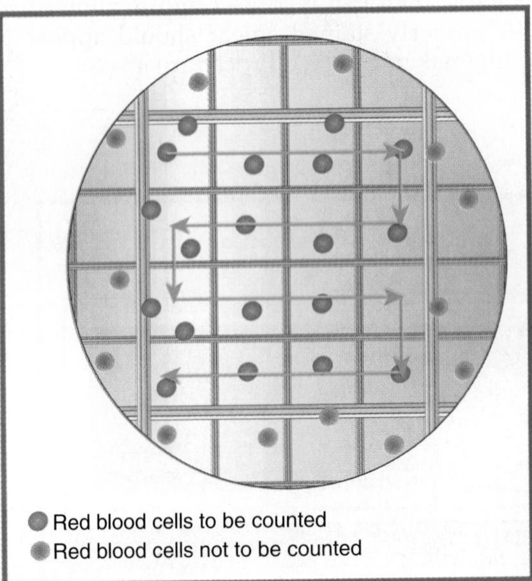

FIGURE 45–6 Neubauer counting chamber. (From Stepp CA, Woods MA: Laboratory Procedures for Medical Office Personnel. Philadelphia, WB Saunders, 1998.)

Automation

Blood cell counts may be performed manually in the physician's office or by an automated counter. Current availability of many different types of instruments has made it possible for the physician's office to become fully automated. The modern instruments range from relatively simple, inexpensive counters to the very complex and expensive machines. The automated cell counter provides accurate results and does not require a technologist to operate.

Most of the automated cell counters operate by first diluting the cells in a fluid that conducts an electric current. Then, these diluted cells pass through a special narrow opening in the machine. The passing cells interrupt the flow of current, and each interruption is counted. Some machines use a laser beam instead of an electric current (Fig. 45–7).

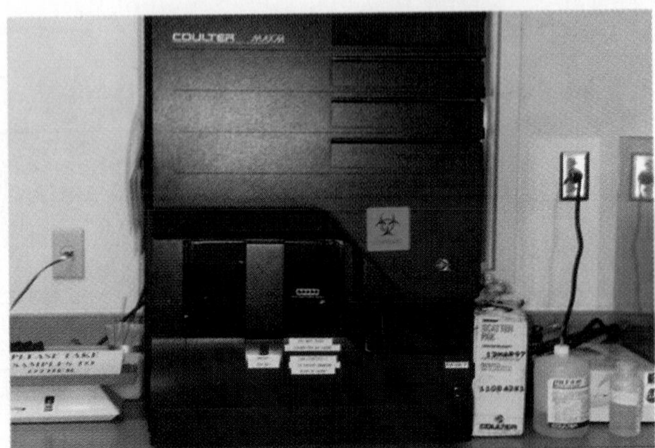

FIGURE 45–7 Automated cell counter. (Courtesy of Coulter Corp., Los Angeles, California 90026.)

Automation improves the accuracy of cell counting and results in greater efficiency. In addition, automation reduces the frequency of handling the individual blood specimen and decreases the risk of exposure to bloodborne pathogens, such as the hepatitis B virus or the human immunodeficiency virus.

DIFFERENTIAL CELL COUNT

Preparation of Blood Smears

A blood smear enables you to view the cellular components of the blood in as natural a state as possible. The morphology of the leukocytes, erythrocytes, and platelets can be studied. Their size, shape, and maturity can be evaluated. Examining a blood smear is part of a complete blood cell count.

A blood smear is prepared by spreading a drop of blood on a clean glass slide. The slides must be free of dust and grease. The best specimen for a blood smear is capillary blood that has no anticoagulant added. EDTA anticoagulant blood can be used, provided the smear is made within 2 hours of collection.

There are several methods of spreading the drop of blood on the slide that result in a good smear. One method is to place a small drop of blood one-half inch from the right end of a glass slide. The end of a second glass spreader slide is placed in front of the drop of blood at an angle of 30 to 35 degrees. The spreader slide is brought back into the drop until the blood spreads along the edge of the spreader slide. This is done with a quick but smooth gliding motion. The spreader slide is then pushed to the left with a quick, steady motion, spreading the blood across the slide.

A good smear should cover one half to three fourths of the slide. It should show a gradual transition from a thick to a thin end with a feathered edge. It should have a smooth appearance with no ridges, holes, lines, streaks, or clumps (Fig. 45–8). The cells should be distributed evenly on microscopic examination.

After the smear has been made, it should be allowed to dry. The slide should be propped up to dry with the thick end down. Do not blow on the slide to dry it. This can cause artifacts in the red blood cells from the moisture in your breath. Once dry, the slide is labeled in the thick portion of the smear by writing the patient's name in the dried blood film. If slides with frosted ends are used, the label can be written on the frosted end.

After labeling, the slide is fixed in *methanol,* which preserves and prevents changes or deterioration of the cellular components. Many of the quick stains available on the market contain the fixative in the stain.

Memory Jogger

A good smear should cover ______ of the slide.

Staining of Blood Smears

The stains commonly used for examination of blood cells are called *polychromatic* because they contain dyes that will stain various cell components different colors. These stains usually contain *methylene blue,* a blue stain, and **eosin,** a red-orange stain. These stains are attracted to different parts of the cell. Thus, the cells and their structures are more easily visualized and differentiated. The most commonly used differential blood stain is *Wright's stain.*

Wright's stain is applied to the slide for 1 to 3 minutes. A buffer is added on top of the stain, and it is mixed by gently blowing until a green metallic sheen appears. This usually takes 2 to 4 minutes. The slide is then gently rinsed and is allowed to air dry. A properly stained smear should appear pinkish to the naked eye (see Procedure 45–6).

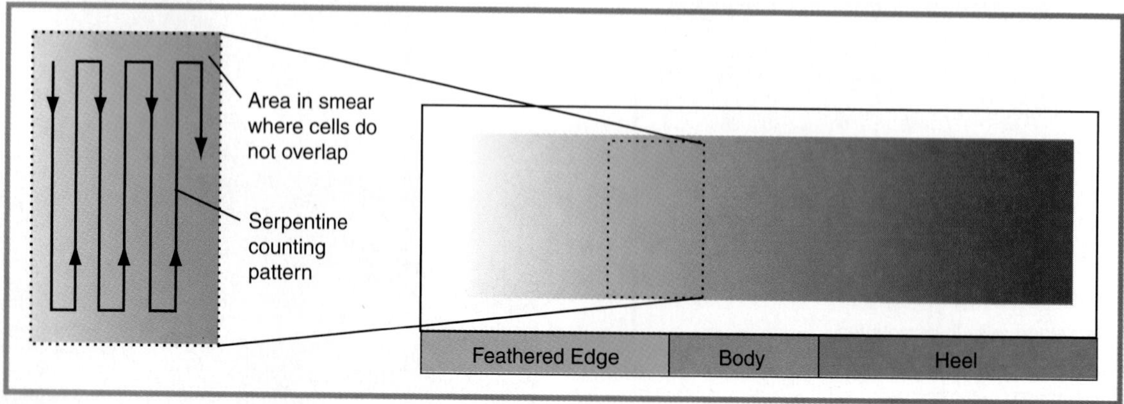

FIGURE 45–8 Serpentine (winding) pattern used to count cells. (From Stepp CA, Woods MA: Laboratory Procedures for Medical Office Personnel. Philadelphia, WB Saunders, 1998.)

PROCEDURE 45-6

Preparing a Smear Stained with Wright's Stain

GOAL

To prepare and stain a slide that meets the criteria for the performance of a differential examination.

EQUIPMENT AND SUPPLIES

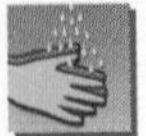
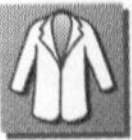

Clean glass slides
Transfer pipette or capillary tube
Wright stain materials
EDTA anticoagulant blood specimen

PROCEDURAL STEPS

1 Wash and dry your hands. Put on face protection and nonsterile gloves.
PURPOSE: Infection control.

2 Assemble the materials needed.

3 Mix the blood specimen.

4 Dispense a small drop of blood onto a slide, about ½ to ¾ inch from the right end. Use a transfer pipette or capillary tube (Figure 1*).

5 Hold one side of this slide with your nondominant hand.

6 Place the spreader slide in front of the drop of blood at an angle of 30 to 35 degrees. Use your dominant hand (Figure 2).
PURPOSE: An angle of 30 to 35 degrees makes a smear with a good feathered edge.

7 Pull back the spreader slide into the drop of blood, and allow the blood to spread to the edges of the slide (Figure 3).

Continued

*Figures from Stepp CA, Woods MA: Laboratory Procedures for Medical Office Personnel, Philadelphia, WB Saunders, 1998.

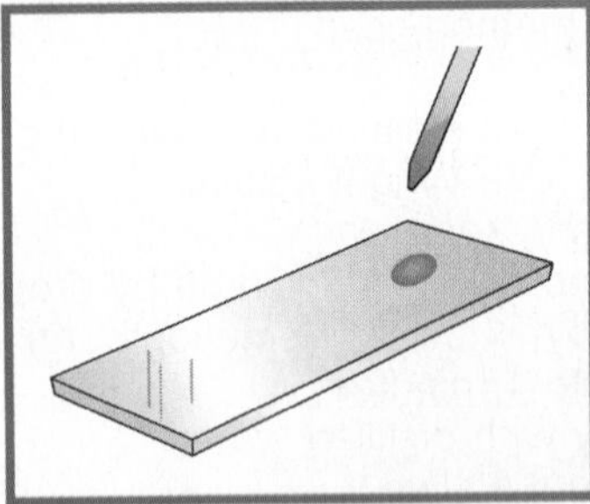

FIGURE 1

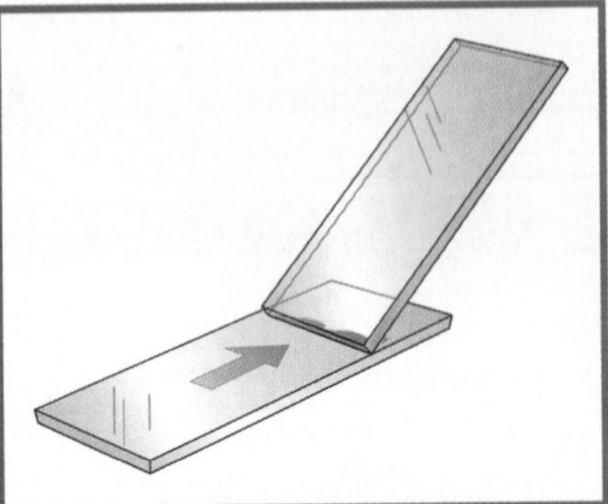

FIGURE 2

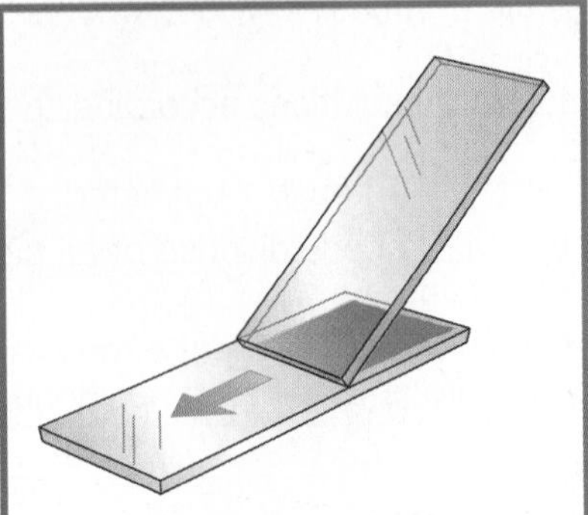

FIGURE 3

PROCEDURE 45-6 (CONTINUED)

Preparing a Smear Stained with Wright's Stain

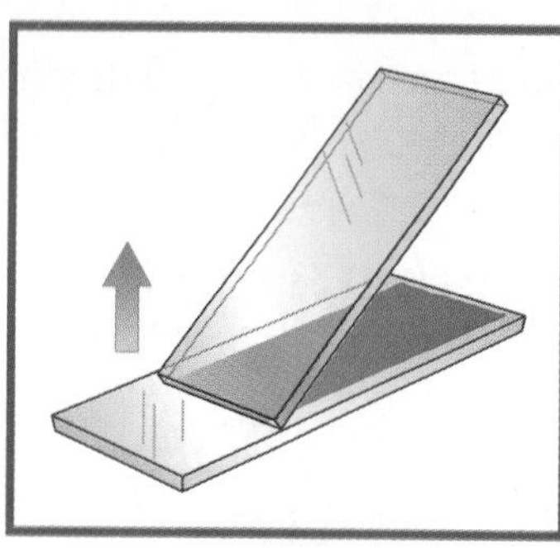
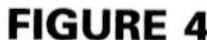

FIGURE 4

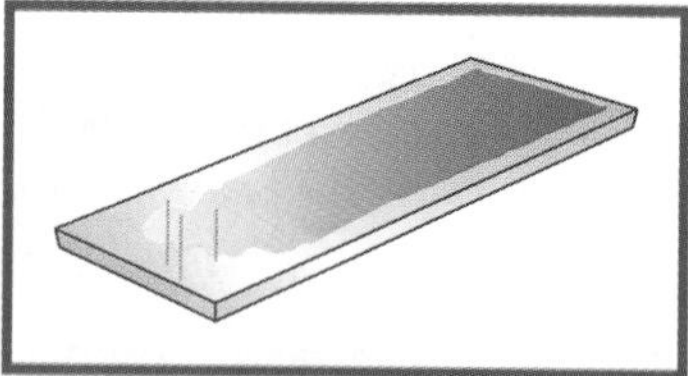

FIGURE 5

8 Push the spreader slide forward with a quick smooth motion, maintaining the same angle throughout (Figure 4).
PURPOSE: If the motion is not smooth, ridges will occur in the smear.

9 Rapidly but gently wave the slide to accelerate the drying process.

10 Stand the slide with the thick end down, and allow the slide to complete drying (Figure 5).
PURPOSE: If the thick end is up, the undried portion of the blood may run down into the dry thin area and ruin the smear.

11 Label the slide when it is dry. Use a pencil, and write the name in the thick end of the smear.
PURPOSE: Pencil will scratch the name into the smear and will not wash off in the staining process.

12 Stain according to method used.
Two-step method:
a Place the smear on a staining rack, with the blood side up.
b Flood the smear with Wright's stain.
c Wait for 1 to 3 minutes.
d Add an equal amount of buffer, drop by drop, on top of the Wright stain.
e Blow gently, and mix the two solutions until a green metallic sheen appears. This should appear within 2 to 4 minutes.
f Rinse thoroughly with distilled water.
g Drain water from the slide.
h Wipe the back of the smear with gauze.
i Stand the smear to dry.
Quick stain:
a Place the smear into solutions according to the manufacturer's instructions (Figure 6*A* through *D*).
b Proceed with steps *f* through *i* just listed.

13 Clean the work area. Properly dispose of all biohazard materials. Remove face protection and gloves. Wash your hands.

14 Record the test results in the patient's medical record.
PURPOSE: A procedure is considered not done until it is recorded.

Continued

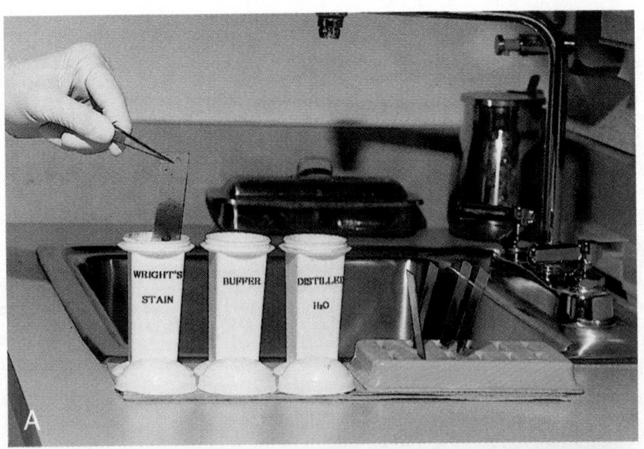
WRIGHT'S STAIN
BUFFER
DISTILLED H2O
A

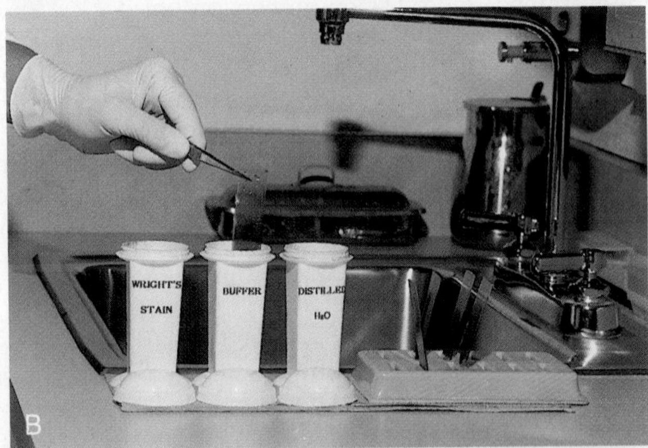
WRIGHT'S STAIN
BUFFER
DISTILLED H2O
B

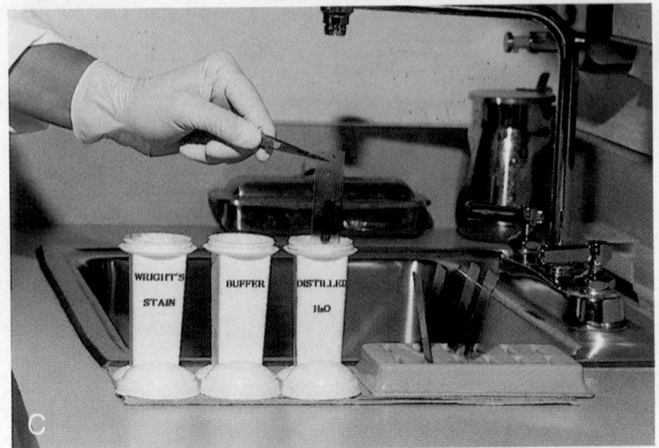
WRIGHT'S STAIN
BUFFER
DISTILLED H2O
C

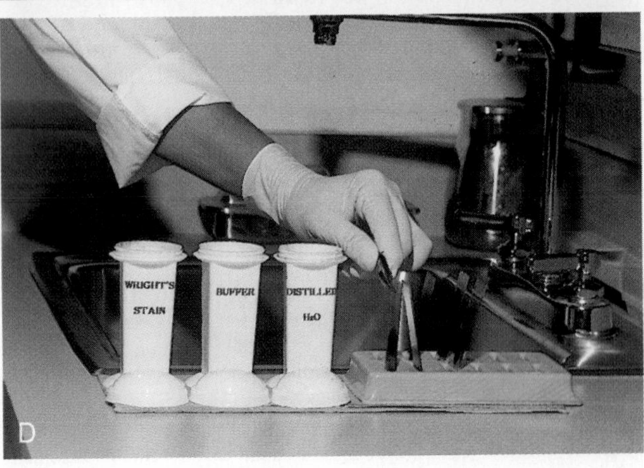
WRIGHT'S STAIN
BUFFER
DISTILLED H2O
D

FIGURE 6

Identification of Normal Blood Cells

Much useful information can be gathered from the microscopic identification and evaluation of blood cells in a stained smear. A great deal more information can be acquired from the observation of these blood cells than from actual cell counts. Blood smears can impart more knowledge than any other laboratory test.

The features of blood cells that you will observe and evaluate are cell size, nuclear appearance, and cytoplasmic characteristics. The results of observing these three features will allow for cell identification, although much practice is required to be able to recognize and classify all the blood cells that may be seen in various disease states.

Cells are examined under the oil-immersion objective. The light should be bright to facilitate the visualization of colors and small structures. The slide is examined near the feathered end of the smear, where the cells are barely touching each other and are easiest to identify.

Red blood cells are the most numerous of the cellular elements. They are biconcave discs that have no nuclei. The red cells should appear pinkish tan, as a result of the staining of the hemoglobin within the cells (Fig. 45–9).

Thrombocytes, or *platelets,* are the smallest of the cellular elements. They may be round or oval. No nucleus is present, because the platelet is just a fragment of cytoplasm from a large bone marrow cell. They stain blue.

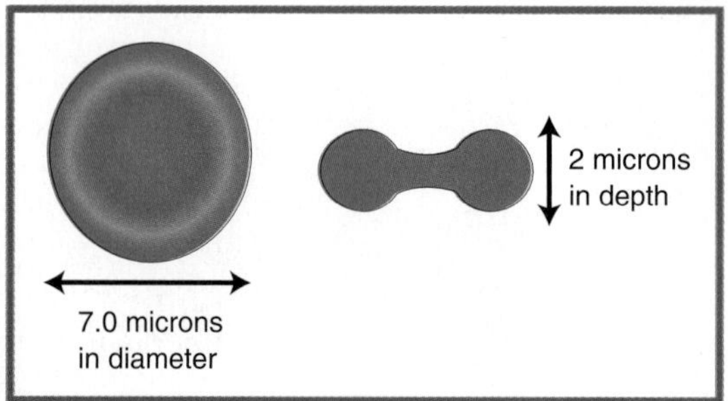

FIGURE 45–9 Red blood cell morphology. (From Stepp CA, Woods MA: Laboratory Procedures for Medical Office Personnel. Philadelphia, WB Saunders, 1998.)

Leukocytes are the largest of the normal circulating blood cells (Table 45–4). Each of the five types has a characteristic appearance. The granulocytes include neutrophils, eosinophils, and basophils. Granulocytes contain distinctive granules in their cytoplasm and may have segmented nuclei. The agranulocytes include lymphocytes and monocytes. They have few, if any, granules and nonsegmented nuclei. The nuclei of the leukocytes should appear purple, and their cytoplasm may vary from pink to blue or blue-gray. *Neutrophils* are known by a variety of names, including *polymorphonuclear neutrophils, segmented neutrophils, polys,* and *segs* (Fig. 45–10). They are the most numerous white blood cells in circulation in adults. They are produced in the bone marrow, are released into the circulation, and eventually enter

TABLE 45–4 Characteristics of Leukocytes

	Granulocytes				Agranulocytes	
	Neutrophil Segmented (mature)	Neutrophil Band (immature)	Eosinophil	Basophil	Lymphocyte	Monocyte
Cell size	10–15 μm	10–15 μm	10–15 μm	10–15 μm	6–15 μm	12–20 μm
Nucleus shape	2–5 lobes connected by threadlike filaments	Band or U-shaped	Bilobed or band	Slightly segmented, granular, or band	Round or oval	Round, indented, or superimposed lobes
Nucleus structure	Coarse	Coarse	Coarse	Obscured by granules	Smudged, lumpy, or clumped	Brainlike convolutions or folded
Cytoplasm amount	Abundant	Abundant	Abundant	Abundant	Scant	Abundant
Cytoplasm color	Colorless to light pink	Colorless to light pink	Colorless to light pink	Colorless to light pink	Sky blue to dark blue	Dull gray to blue-gray
Cytoplasm inclusions	Many tiny tan, pink, or red-purple granules	Many tiny tan, pink with increased red-purple granules	Large rounder oval red to red-orange granules	Large, coarse blue-black granules	None to few round red-purple granules	Ground glass appearance, fine red-purple granules, rare blue granules

From Stepp CA, Woods MA: Laboratory Procedures for Medical Office Personnel. Philadelphia, WB Saunders, 1998.

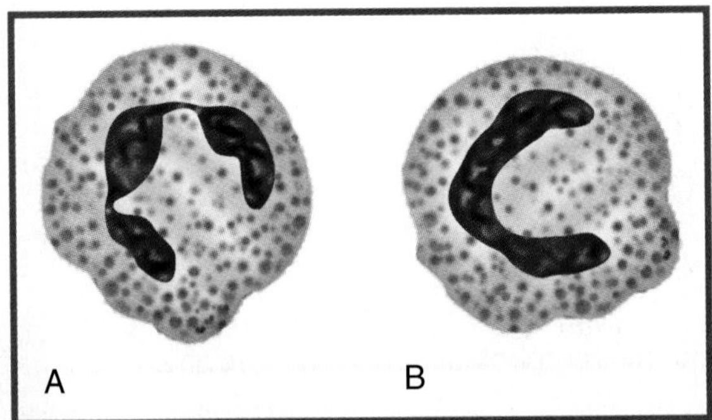

FIGURE 45–10 Neutrophilic cells. *A*, Segmented. *B*, Band. (From Stepp CA, Woods MA: Laboratory Procedures for Medical Office Personnel. Philadelphia, WB Saunders, 1998.)

tissue to fight off invading microorganisms by engulfing them **(phagocytosis).** Many types of bacterial infections stimulate increased production of neutrophils.

Memory Jogger

10 *How can you identify a granulocyte?*

The *segmented neutrophil* nucleus is segmented into two to five lobes that are connected by a strand. The nucleus stains a dark purple. The cytoplasm is pale pink and contains fine pink or lilac granules.

An immature form of the neutrophil is called a *band,* or *stab.* Instead of having a segmented nucleus, where the lobes are separated by a thin filament, the band has an unsegmented nucleus shaped like a horseshoe. The staining is the same as in the segmented neutrophil. An increase in bands is termed a *shift to the left* and is seen in infections such as bacterial meningitis, pneumonia, appendicitis, strep throat, and abscesses and in chronic granulocytic leukemia. The nucleus of the *eosinophil* is divided into two or three lobes that stain purple. The cytoplasm stains pink and contains large round or oval red-orange granules. Eosinophils are phagocytic and are associated closely with allergies such as hay fever and with asthma, as well as with certain parasitic infestations such as trichinosis, amebiasis, and schistosomiasis. The nucleus of the *basophil* is segmented and stains light purple. The large dark blue-black granules contain histamine, which is a part of the allergic response. Little is known about the function of basophils.

Lymphocytes are the second most numerous white blood cell in adults. In children, they are usually the most numerous. Their nucleus is usually oval or round and smooth. It stains purple. The cytoplasm stains blue. Lymphs, as they are commonly called, are responsible for the recognition of foreign antigens and the production of circulating antibodies for immunity to disease. Increased numbers of lymphocytes are found in most viral diseases; in some bacterial infections such as syphilis, brucellosis, tuberculosis, and typhoid and paratyphoid fevers; in leukemias; and in young children who are actively making antibodies. In many viral infections, stimulated or reactive lymphocytes, called *atypical lymphs,* are found. These are common in infectious mononucleosis.

Monocytes are the largest white blood cell in the circulation. The nucleus may be oval, indented, or horseshoe shaped. The cytoplasm stains a dull gray-blue and may contain *vacuoles,* which appear as clear spaces in the cytoplasm filled with fluid or air. Monocytes are called macrophages and ingest bacteria and the debris of cellular breakdown. They are increased in certain viral infections such as hepatitis and mumps; rickettsial infections such as Rocky Mountain spotted fever; and bacterial infections such as brucellosis, tuberculosis, and typhoid.

Memory Jogger

What are the names that are given to immature neutrophils?

Differential Examination

A specific area of the stained smear must be examined when doing the differential count. This area must be where the red blood cells are touching but are not clumped when viewed microscopically. After you have located an appropriate area under low power, focus under oil immersion. The differential examination consists of counting and classifying 100 consecutive white blood cells while moving in a specific winding pattern through the smear (see Procedure 45–7). This pattern must be followed to avoid counting the same cells twice. A tally is kept of the cells observed on a *differential cell counter* (Fig. 45–11).

Normal values vary with age. Many disease states alter the ratios of the different types of leukocytes.

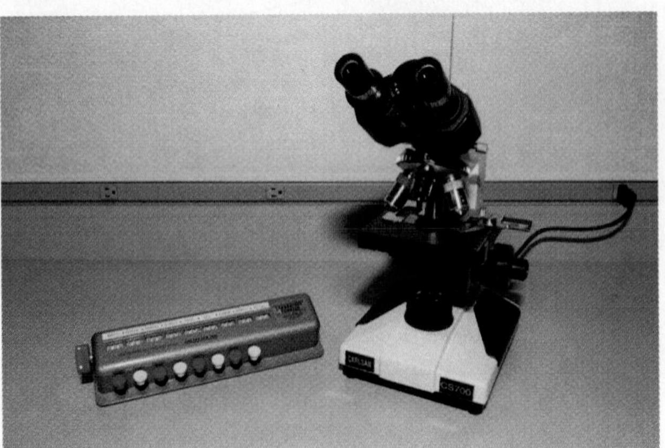

FIGURE 45–11 Microscope with counting tray. (Courtesy of Carlsan, Inc., Carlinville, IL 62626.

PROCEDURE 45-7
Performing a Differential Examination of a Smear Stained with Wright's Stain

GOAL

To perform a differential cell count, evaluate the red blood cell morphology, and estimate the number of platelets.

EQUIPMENT AND SUPPLIES

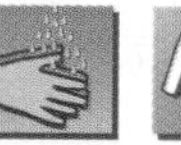
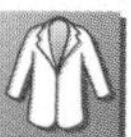
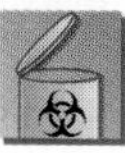

Microscope
Immersion oil
Lens tissue
Lens cleaner

PROCEDURAL STEPS

1 Wash and dry your hands.
PURPOSE: Infection control.

2 Assemble the materials needed.

3 Clean the microscope with lens tissue and lens cleaner.
PURPOSE: Dirty optical surfaces interfere with viewing.

4 Place the slide on the stage, with the smear facing up.
PURPOSE: If the slide is face down, you will not be able to focus under oil immersion.

5 Locate an area of the smear where the red blood cells barely touch each other or slightly overlap, using the low-power objective.
PURPOSE: If the slide is too thick, the cells will be crowded, small, and difficult to evaluate. If the slide is too thin, the cells will be very far apart and will show the effects of excessive flattening.

6 Focus under oil immersion with the fine-adjustment knob and increased light.

7 Count 100 consecutive white blood cells in a winding pattern, identifying each cell encountered (Figure 1*).

Continued

*From Stepp CA, Woods MA: Laboratory Procedures for Medical Office Personnel. Philadelphia, WB Saunders, 1998.

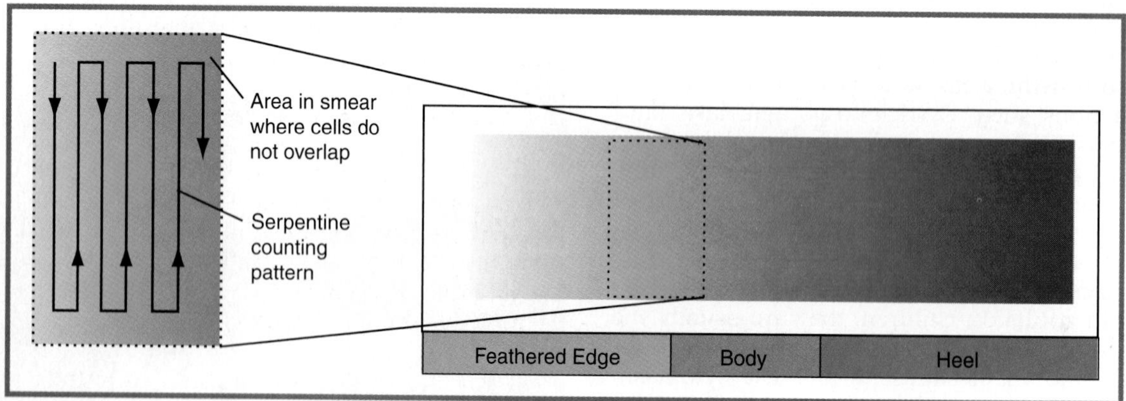

FIGURE 1

8 Record each white cell on the differential cell counter by depressing the appropriate key for each cell.
PURPOSE: The differential examination must proceed systematically, to avoid missing cells or counting any cell twice.

9 Evaluate the red blood cells observed in 10 fields. Record any variations in
- Size—microcytosis, macrocytosis, anisocytosis
- Shape—poikilocytosis, ovalocytosis, target cells, sickle cells, etc.
- Content—normochromic or hypochromic

PURPOSE: The red blood cell evaluation gives the physician important information about the red blood cell population and is an important tool in the assessment of anemias and red blood cell diseases.

10 Count the platelets in 10 fields, obtain an average, and multiply that average by 15,000 to give an estimate of the platelet count. The normal platelet count is 150,000 to 400,000/mm^3. Report the count as normal, decreased, or increased.
PURPOSE: Platelet numbers can be a clue to bleeding disorders.

11 Clean the microscope with lens tissue and lens cleaner.

12 Clean the work area and properly dispose of all materials. Wash your hands.
PURPOSE: Infection control.

13 Record the testing results in the patient's record.
PURPOSE: A procedure is considered not done until it is recorded.

Red Blood Cell Morphology

After determining the differential cell count, the red blood cells are observed and evaluated. Normally, stained red blood cells are the same size and shape and are well filled with hemoglobin. Any variations from the normal state are reported (Fig. 45–12).

Size

Normal-sized red blood cells are known as *normocytic.* If the cells are larger than normal, they are *macrocytic;* if smaller, they are *microcytic.* The condition in which different sizes of red blood cells are present is called *anisocytosis.*

Shape

Normal red blood cells are round or slightly oval. Cells may be shaped like sickles, targets, crescents, or burrs. *Poikilocytosis* is a significant variation in the shape of the red blood cells.

Content

A red blood cell with the normal amount of hemoglobin is called *normochromic.* Pale-staining cells are *hypochromic* and have less hemoglobin than normal.

Memory Jogger

What are the red blood cell variations that must be reported?

Platelet Observation

Platelets, or thrombocytes, are formed in the bone marrow by *megakaryocytes.* As megakaryocytes mature, platelets are shed from the cytoplasm and are released into the circulation, where they function in coagulation. When damage to a vessel occurs, platelets form a plug at the site, and eventually a fibrin clot seals the leak. On a stained smear, the morphology of the platelets is observed for any abnormalities. They are small and irregularly shaped and may vary considerably in size. The average number of platelets seen in 10 to 15 fields is reported. The normal platelet count is 150,000 to 400,000/mm^3. An increase in platelets is called *thrombocytosis,* and a decrease is called *thrombocytopenia.*

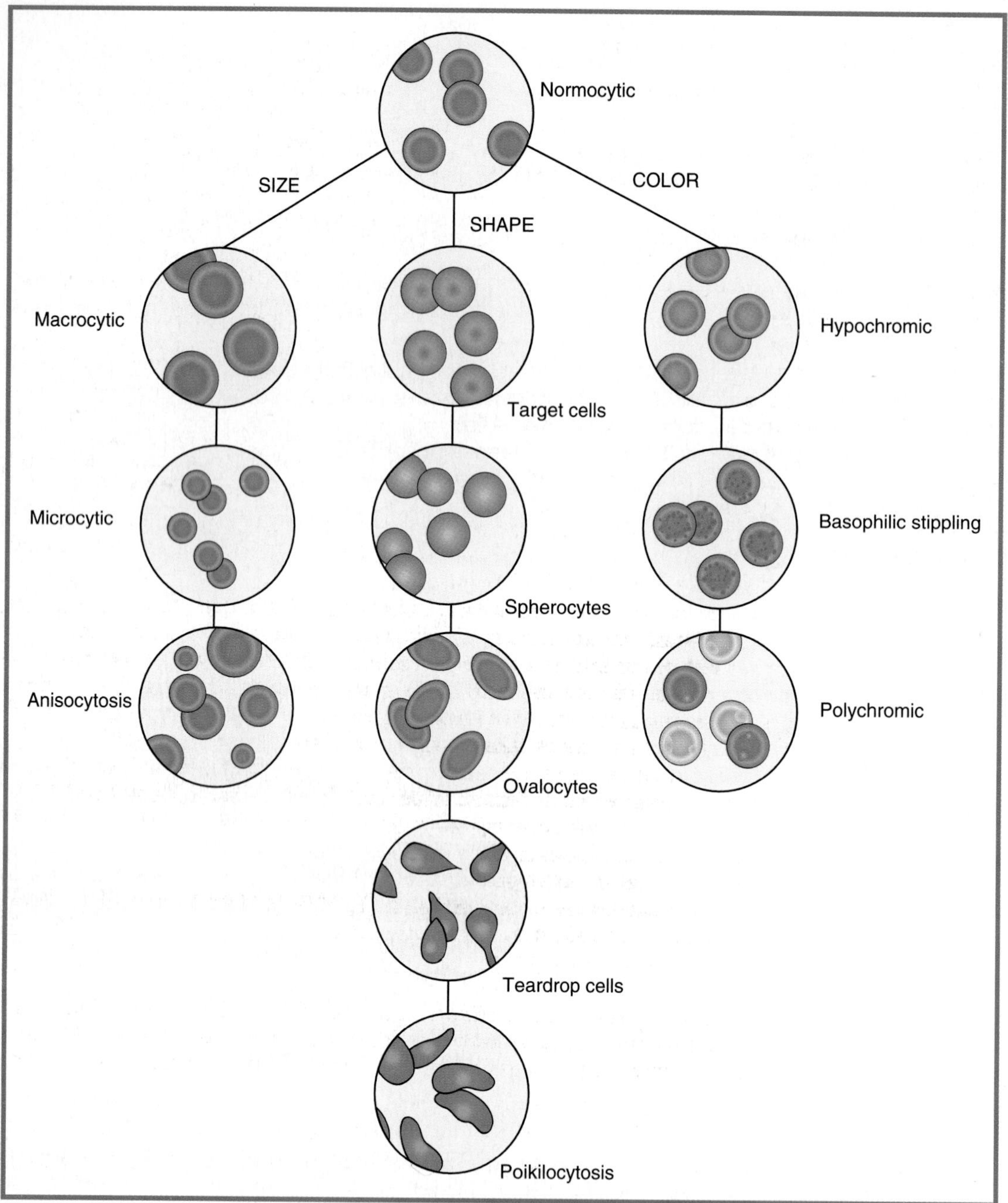

FIGURE 45–12 Abnormal erythrocytes. (From Stepp CA, Woods MA: Laboratory Procedures for Medical Office Personnel. Philadelphia, WB Saunders, 1998.)

ERYTHROCYTE SEDIMENTATION RATE

The erythrocyte sedimentation rate (ESR) is a laboratory test that measures the rate at which erythrocytes gradually separate from plasma and settle to the bottom of a specially calibrated tube. The number of these red blood cells that fall in 1 hour is the result. The test is not specific for a particular disease but is used as a general indication of inflammation. Increases are found in such conditions as acute and chronic infections, rheumatoid arthritis, tuberculosis, hepatitis, cancer, multiple myeloma, rheumatic fever, and lupus erythematosus.

Normal values vary slightly with age and sex (Table 45–5). Only increased ESR rates are significant.

Several methods of measuring the erythrocyte sedimentation rate are used, including *Wintrobe, Westergren,* and *Landau-Adams.* All these methods are based on the same principle and differ only in the amounts of blood needed and the tube size and calibration used (see Procedure 45–8).

The Wintrobe method is commonly used. It con-

TABLE 45-5 ESR Reference Values

	Wintrobe Method (mm/hour)	Westergren Method (mm/hour)
Men	0–10	≤50 years of age: 0–15 >50 years of age: 0–20
Women	1–20	≤50 years of age: 0–20 >50 years of age: 0–30

From Stepp CA, Woods MA: Laboratory Procedures for Medical Office Personnel. Philadelphia, WB Saunders, 1998.

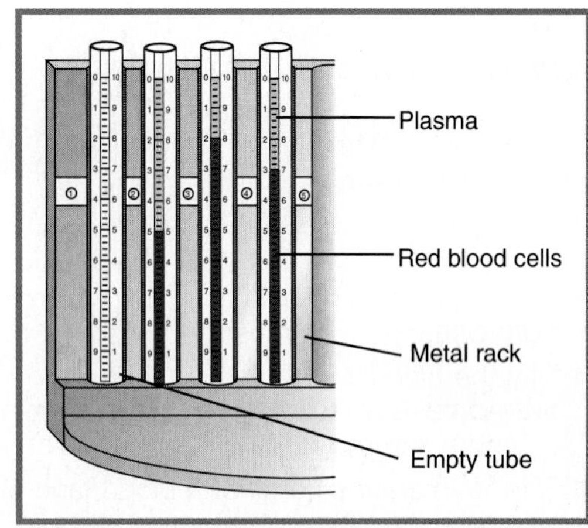

FIGURE 45-13 Wintrobe sedimentation rate system. (From Stepp CA, Woods MA: Laboratory Procedures for Medical Office Personnel. Philadelphia, WB Saunders, 1998.)

sists of a Wintrobe tube that is graduated from 0 to 100 mm and a specially designed Wintrobe rack, which holds the tube in a vertical position. A long-tipped *Pasteur pipette* is used to fill the Wintrobe tube with 100 mL of blood to the zero mark on the tube. The tube is placed in the Wintrobe rack for 1 hour. At the end of 1 hour, the level on the tube to which the erythrocytes have fallen is measured. The rate is recorded in millimeters per hour (mm/h) (Fig. 45-13).

Many factors can affect the ESR. The tube must be totally filled with blood and must not contain air bubbles. The tube must be allowed to sit in a vertical position undisturbed for a full hour. Minor degrees of tilting may increase the sedimentation rate; careful timing is important. Jarring or vibrations from nearby machinery will falsely increase the ESR.

Testing must be performed within 2 hours after the blood has been collected.

Memory Jogger

How do you correctly record an ESR?

PROCEDURE 45-8

Determining a Sedimentation Rate by the Wintrobe Method

GOAL

To properly fill a Wintrobe tube and observe and record the findings of an erythrocyte sedimentation rate, using the Wintrobe method.

EQUIPMENT AND SUPPLIES

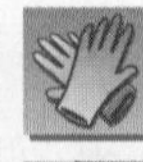
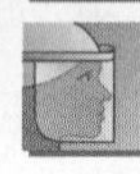

- EDTA anticoagulant blood specimen
- Wintrobe tube
- Wintrobe rack
- Timer
- Pasteur pipette
- Bulb

PROCEDURAL STEPS

1 Wash and dry your hands. Put on face protection and nonsterile gloves.
PURPOSE: Infection control.

2 Assemble the materials needed.

Continued

PROCEDURE 45-8 (CONTINUED)

Determining a Sedimentation Rate by the Wintrobe Method

3 Check the leveling bubble of the Wintrobe rack.
PURPOSE: The rack must be horizontal to ensure that the tube is vertical.

4 Mix the blood well.
PURPOSE: Cells settle when the specimen stands, and blood must always be well-mixed before sampling.

5 Fill the Pasteur pipette with blood, and insert the tip of the pipette to the bottom of the Wintrobe tube.

6 Fill the Wintrobe tube to the 0 mark by squeezing the bulb of the pipe.

7 Slowly remove the pipette from the tube while keeping the tip of the pipette below the level of the blood.
PURPOSE: If the tip of the pipette is above the level of the blood, bubbles will be trapped in the tube and will invalidate the test.

8 Place the tube in a numbered slot in the Wintrobe rack, and set the timer for 1 hour. The tube must be in a vertical position and free from all vibration.
PURPOSE: Jarring will increase the sedimentation rate.

9 Measure the distance the erythrocytes have fallen after 1 hour. The ESR scale measures from 0 at the top to 100 at the bottom. Each line is 1 mm (Figure 1*).

10 Clean the work area and properly dispose of all biohazard materials. Remove face protection and gloves and wash your hands.

11 Record the findings in the patient's medical record.
Remember: The ESR is reported in millimeters per hour.
PURPOSE: A procedure is considered not done until it is recorded.

---

*From Stepp CA, Woods MA: Laboratory Procedures for Medical Office Personnel. Philadelphia, WB Saunders, 1998.

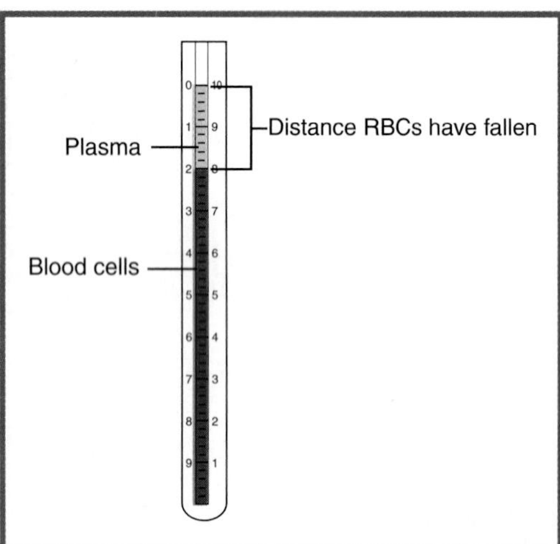

FIGURE 1

LIPID TESTING

Lipid tests are used in assessing body fats, which are found in the body. Lipid tests include cholesterol, triglyceride, high-density lipoprotein (HDL), and low-density lipoprotein (LDL) levels. Both diet and genetic factors play a part in the concentration of body fats, which are synthesized in the liver and stored in adipose tissue. Lipid tests can be used to calculate cardiac risk factors based on sex and age and have become a popular component of the routine physical examination.

The most common coronary heart disease is arteriosclerosis, hardening of the arteries. This condition is often caused by the accumulation of fatty deposits on the wall of the coronary arteries (atherosclerosis), which leads to obstruction of normal blood flow (see Chapter 29).

Cholesterol may be monitored at home through over-the-counter testing devices and is frequently done in the physician's office as a reference guide in cholesterol management. The tests involve a capillary puncture, placing a blood-saturated testing strip into the measuring device, and reading the results in the LED window. The physician may have a standard set of protocols for you to follow when the test results indicate a high blood cholesterol level (see Procedure 45–9).

Memory Jogger

What do lipid tests include?

PROCEDURE 45-9

Determining Cholesterol Level Using a ProAct Testing Device

GOAL

To accurately perform and and report a ProAct test for cholesterol level.

EQUIPMENT AND SUPPLIES

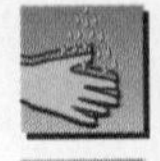

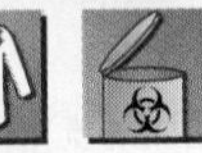

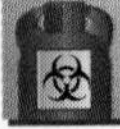

- ProAct testing device
- Lithium heparin capillary tube and capillary pipettor
- Lancets and lancet device
- Sterile gauze
- Alcohol preps
- Biohazard waste container
- Biohazard sharps container

PROCEDURAL STEPS

1 Reread the physician's order and assemble all the supplies and equipment needed to complete the test.

2 Wash your hands and put on gloves.
PURPOSE: Infection control.

3 Explain the procedure to the patient.

4 Load the lancet device with a sterile lancet.

5 Examine the patient's index and ring fingers and pick a puncture site.
PURPOSE: Puncture site must be free of trauma.

6 Cleanse the chosen puncture site with alcohol and allow the site to air dry.

7 Puncture the site and wipe away the first drop of blood with a sterile gauze square.
PURPOSE: The first drop of blood may contain tissue fluid.

Continued

PROCEDURE 45-9 (CONTINUED)

Determining Cholesterol Level Using a ProAct Testing Device

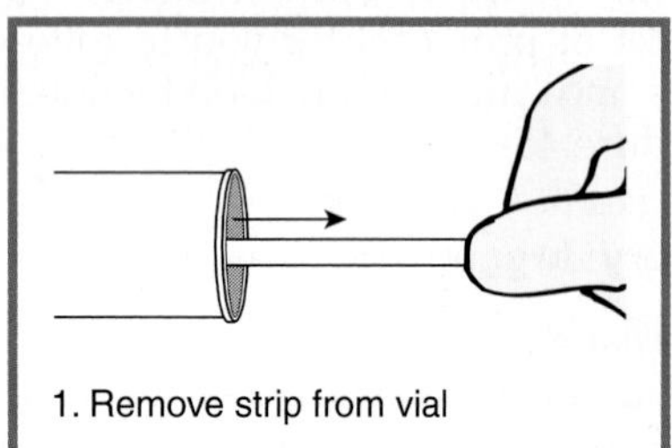

1. Remove strip from vial

FIGURE 1

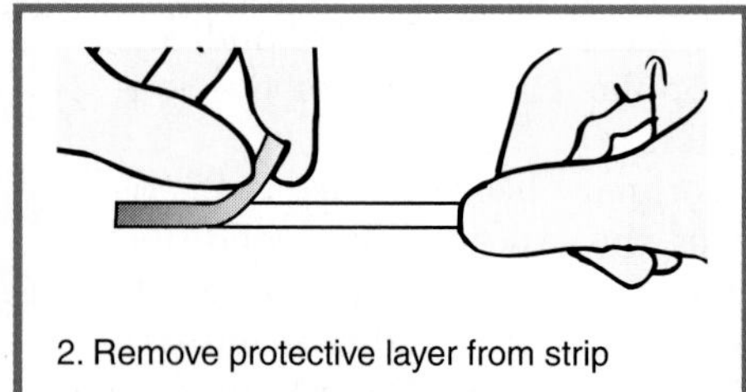

2. Remove protective layer from strip

FIGURE 2

8 Hold the capillary tube horizontally by the colored end of the tube, and allow the tube to fill. Do not allow air bubbles to enter the tube; if this occurs, discard the capillary tube and continue drawing the sample with a new tube.
PURPOSE: Air bubbles may cause erroneous test results.

9 Give the patient a clean gauze square and ask the patient to apply pressure to the puncture site.

10 Remove a cholesterol testing strip from the container and close the container immediately (Figure 1*).
PURPOSE: Closing the container will avoid possible exposure of the unused strips.

11 Remove the foil protecting the test area of the strip and place the strip on a dry, hard, flat surface (Figure 2).

12 Attach the capillary tube filled with blood to the pipettor.

13 Squeeze the plunger of the pipettor completely to allow a drop of blood to form at the end of the capillary tube.

14 Allow the drop of blood to fall onto the center of the red mesh application zone. Make sure that the tip of the capillary tube does not touch the test strip and that all blood is dispensed (Figure 3).
PURPOSE: Strip must be saturated with blood to obtain best testing results.

Continued

*Figures from Stepp CA, Woods MA: Laboratory Procedures for Medical Office Personnel. Philadelphia, WB Saunders, 1998.

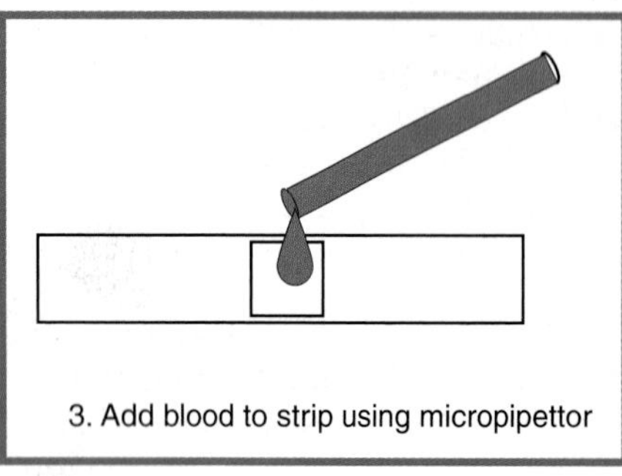

3. Add blood to strip using micropipettor

FIGURE 3

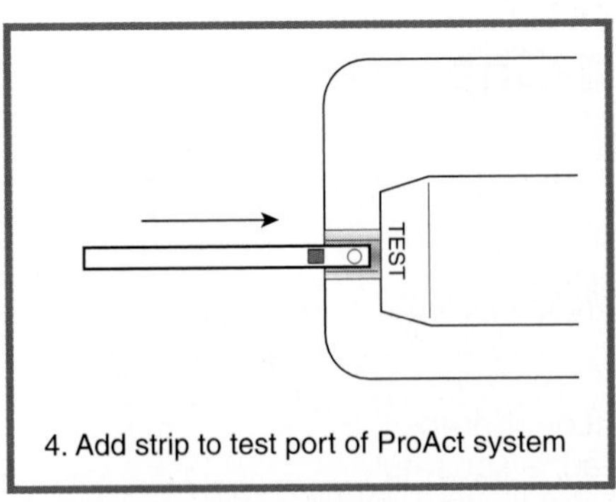

4. Add strip to test port of ProAct system

FIGURE 4

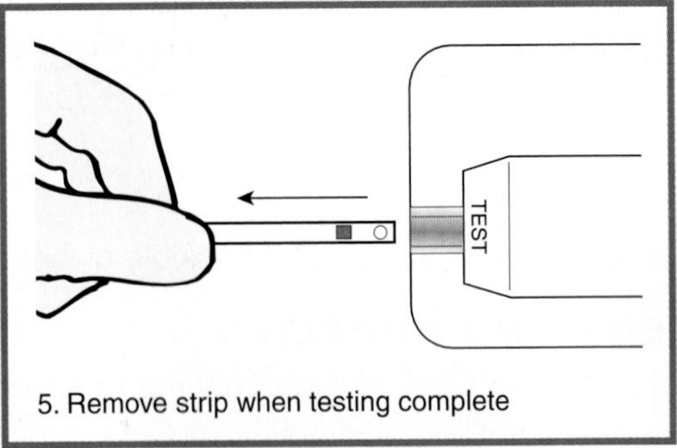

5. Remove strip when testing complete

FIGURE 5

15 Allow the sample to soak into the red mesh for 3 to 15 seconds.

16 Insert the cholesterol strip into the test port. The ProAct device will count down approximately 160 seconds (Figure 4).

17 Remove the capillary tube from the pipettor and discard it in a biohazard container.
PURPOSE: Infection control.

18 When the measurement time is completed, REMOVE STRIP will appear in the LED display window. Remove the used test strip and the test result will appear on the display (Figure 5).

19 Examine the test area of the used testing strip for uneven color development before discarding it into the biohazard waste container.
PURPOSE: If the color appears mottled, the test may not be valid and it is advisable that you repeat the entire testing process.

20 Discard all biohazard testing waste in appropriate containers, clean the testing area, remove gloves, and wash your hands.
PURPOSE: Infection control.

21 Record the test results in the patient's medical record.
PURPOSE: A procedure is not considered done until it is recorded.

BLOOD GLUCOSE

Glucose is used as a fuel by many of the cells within the body; under normal circumstances, it is the only substance used by the brain. Maintenance of blood glucose levels within the normal range is vitally important to the homeostasis of the acid–base balance of the human body. Understanding the importance of glucose helps in understanding the reason why glucose is the most frequently tested **analyte** (see Procedure 45–10).

Elevated blood glucose levels are most often associated with diabetes mellitus but may also indicate pancreatitis, endocrine disorders, and/or chronic renal failure. Diabetes mellitus is a disorder of carbohydrate metabolism that results in elevated blood and urine glucose levels secondary to the inability of the pancreas to produce sufficient insulin.

To check the patient for possible diabetes mellitus, the physician may request a blood glucose tolerance test. For this test, the fasting patient receives an adequate carbohydrate meal of 100 g of glucose by mouth. This is usually given to the patient as a drink that is similar to a sweet fruit punch. The amount may be adjusted according to the patient's weight. If the glucose level does not exceed 100 g/dL at the onset of the testing period or 180 g/dL 1 hour after the ingesting of the glucose drink, the patient is believed to have a normal glucose level. If the blood glucose level exceeds 200 g/dL, glucose will escape into the urine because the renal tubules are no longer able to absorb the excessive amount present in the glomerulus.

PROCEDURE 45-10
Performing a Blood Glucose Accu-Chek Test

GOAL

To accurately perform a blood test for possible diabetes mellitus.

EQUIPMENT AND SUPPLIES

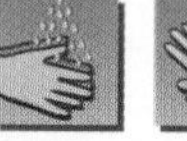

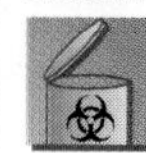
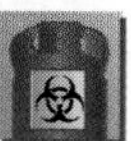

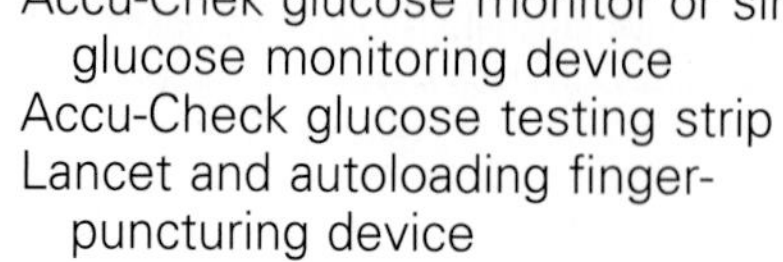

Accu-Chek glucose monitor or similar glucose monitoring device
Accu-Check glucose testing strip
Lancet and autoloading finger-puncturing device
Alcohol preps
Gauze squares

PROCEDURAL STEPS

1 Reread the physician's order and collect the necessary equipment and supplies needed to complete the testing procedure.

2 Wash your hands and put on gloves.
PURPOSE: Infection control.

3 Ask the patient to wash his or her hands in warm soapy water, then to rinse them in warm water, and dry them completely.
PURPOSE: Warming the fingers may increase blood peripheral blood flow.

4 Check the patient's index and ring fingers and select the site for puncture.
PURPOSE: Site of puncture must be free of trauma.

5 Turn on the Accu-Chek monitor by pressing the ON button (Figure 1*).

6 Make sure the code number on the LED display matches the code number on the container of testing strips.
PURPOSE: If code numbers do not match, the device must be reprogrammed with the new code for the test results to be valid.

7 Remove a testing strip from the vial and immediately replace the vial cover.
PURPOSE: Vial must be closed to protect unused strips from possible contamination.

8 Check the strip for dicoloration by comparing the color of the round window on the back of the testing strip with the designated "unused" color chart provided on the test strip vial label.
PURPOSE: This will establish the validity of the testing procedure.
Do not touch the yellow test pad or round window on the back of the strip when handling the strip.

9 When the test strip symbol begins flashing in the lower right-hand corner of the display screen, insert the test strip into the designated testing slot until it locks into place. When the test strip is inserted correctly, the arrows on the test strip will be facing up and pointing toward the monitor (Figure 2).

10 Cleanse the selected site on the patient's fingertip with the alcohol wipe and allow the finger to air dry.

11 Perform the finger puncture and wipe away the first drop of blood.
PURPOSE: There may be tissue fluid present in the first drop of blood.

12 Apply a large hanging drop of blood to the center of the yellow testing pad (Figure 3).
a *Do not touch the pad with the patient's finger.*
b *Do not apply a second drop of blood.*

Continued

*Figures from Stepp CA, Woods MA: Laboratory Procedures for Medical Office Personnel. Philadelphia, WB Saunders, 1998.

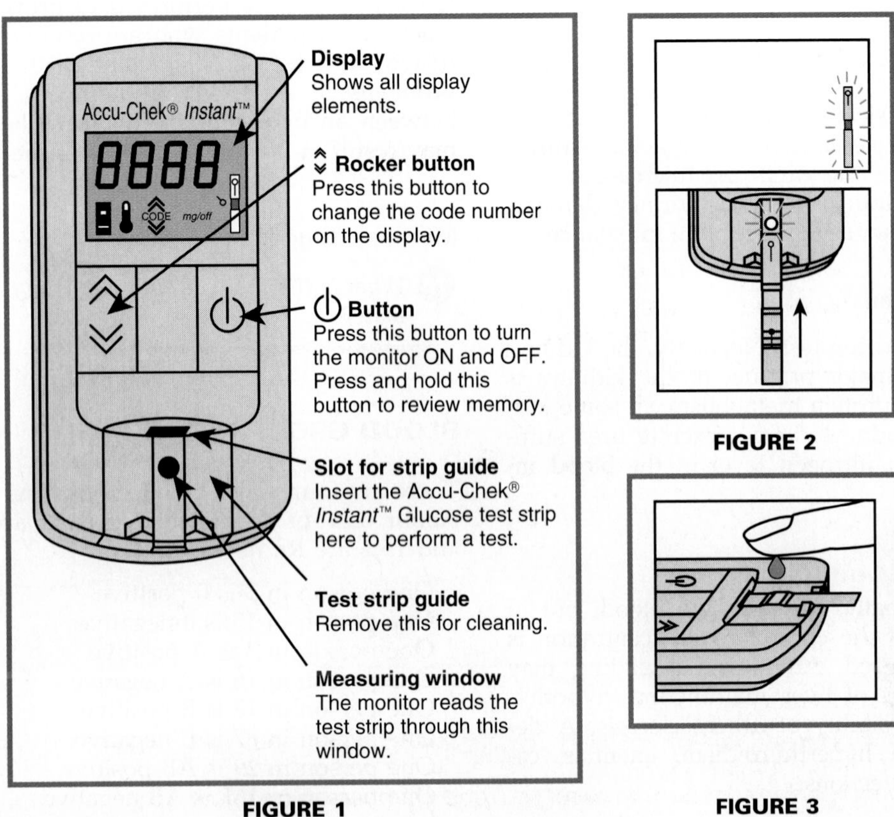
Accu-Chek® Instant™
8888
CODE mg/off
Display
Shows all display elements.
Rocker button
Press this button to change the code number on the display.
Button
Press this button to turn the monitor ON and OFF. Press and hold this button to review memory.
Slot for strip guide
Insert the Accu-Chek® Instant™ Glucose test strip here to perform a test.
Test strip guide
Remove this for cleaning.
Measuring window
The monitor reads the test strip through this window.

FIGURE 1

FIGURE 2

FIGURE 3

c *Do not smear the blood with your finger.*
d *Be certain the yellow test pad is saturated with blood.*

13 Give the patient a gauze square to hold securely over the puncture site.

14 The monitor will automatically begin the measurement process as soon as it senses the drop of blood.

15 Read the test result when it is displayed in the display window in milligrams per deciliter.

16 Turn off the monitor by pressing the "O" button.

17 Discard all biohazard waste into the proper waste containers.
PURPOSE: Infection control.

18 Clean the work area, remove gloves, and wash your hands.

19 Record the testing results in the patient's medical record.
PURPOSE: A procedure is considered not done until it is recorded.

Memory Jogger

 *How does the body use glucose?*

OTHER BLOOD CHEMISTRY TESTS

Often the physician may order a *panel* or *profile* on a patient. Some tests relate to a particular organ or system. Cardiac, liver, and thyroid profiles are common. Panels may include 20 or more tests relating to a number of different body systems and are performed on sophisticated automated machinery and provide maximum information with minimum sample and cost.

Serum Calcium

Calcium is essential in the formation of bone tissue, in muscular activity, and in blood coagulation. When there is a deficiency of calcium, tetany occurs. This condition is characterized by a twitching of muscle fibers and tetanic convulsions. An increase in serum calcium level is found in hyperparathyroidism, multiple myeloma, and some respiratory diseases.

Uric Acid

This test is used basically to aid in the diagnosis of gout, a metabolic disease marked by acute arthritis and inflammation of the joints. An increase in uric acid levels is also found in severe kidney damage, toxemias of pregnancy, and electrolyte imbalance.

Blood Urea Nitrogen

This is a kidney function test. Normally, the kidneys excrete urea. This major product of the kidneys is the end product of protein metabolism. In some kidney diseases, the kidneys do not excrete urea sufficiently, so the urea nitrogen level in the blood increases.

Cholesterol

Cholesterol is normally found in the blood, but in some disease states the cholesterol concentration is increased or decreased. An elevated reading may aid in the diagnosis of liver malfunction, hypothyroidism, and a possibility of atherosclerosis. A decrease is found in hyperthyroidism, anemias, cachexia, and acute infections.

Serology

Serologic testing provides information about past or present infections by antigen–antibody reactions. Most serologic testing done in the physician's office is done with individual testing kits. Whenever you will be performing a serologic test, the first step is to review the package insert provided by the manufacturer. The review will provide valuable information about the test, the principle on which the test is based, the reagents and equipment required, proper specimen collection techniques, preparation requirements, test procedures, and any precautions or warnings that pertain to the procedure. In addition, the inserts provide information regarding quality control, the interpretation of results, limitations of the procedure performance characteristics, and references.

Examples of tests that may be done include serum pregnancy tests, testing for infectious mononucleosis, slide-agglutination testing for rheumatoid arthritis factor, and enzyme-linked immunosorbent assays for acquired immunodeficiency syndrome, human immunodeficiency virus, and rubella.

Immunohematologic Testing

The major reason for performing immunohematologic tests is to prevent problems caused by incompatibility of blood types. Compatibility testing (crossmatching) is performed to prevent transfusion reactions in patients who are receiving blood transfusions and to identify potential Rh incompatibility problems in expectant mothers. Rh incompatibility between an expectant mother and the unborn child may result in hemolytic disease of the newborn.

Memory Jogger

What is the first step in performing all serologic tests?

BLOOD GROUPING

There are four major blood groups: A, B, O, and AB. About 85% of these blood groups are Rh positive and 15% are Rh negative.

One person in 3 is 0 positive.
One person in 15 is 0 negative.
One person in 3 is A positive.
One person in 16 is A negative.
One person in 12 is B positive.
One person in 67 is B negative.
One person in 29 is AB positive.
One person in 167 is AB negative.

DETERMINATION OF ABO GROUP

The determination of ABO blood groups is a simple test that can easily be performed. The test detects the presence of A or B antigens on red blood cells based on the presence or absence of agglutination with a known antiserum (Table 45–6).

When the antigen on the patient's red blood cells corresponds to the antibody, agglutination occurs. If the corresponding antigen is not present on the cells, no agglutination will occur.

EXAMPLES OF BLOOD AGGLUTINATION

- Type A blood will agglutinate in the presence of anti-A antiserum but will not agglutinate in the presence of anti-B antiserum.
- Type B blood will agglutinate in the presence of anti-B antiserum but not in the presence of anti-A antiserum.
- Type O blood will not agglutinate in the presence of anti-A antiserum or anti-B antiserum.
- Type AB blood will agglutinate in the presence of both anti-A antiserum and anti-B antiserum (Procedure 45–11).

Memory Jogger

What determines ABO blood groups?

TABLE 45-6 Blood Compatibility

Recipient Blood*		Compatible with
RBC Antigen	***Plasma antibodies***	***Donor Types†***
Type O (no antigens)	Anti-A and anti-B	O
Type A (type A antigen)	Anti-B	O and A
Type B (type B antigen)	Anti-A	O and B
Type AB (type AB antigen)	None	O, A, B, and AB

*Patients with type AB blood are considered to be *universal recipients.*
†Patients with type O blood are considered to be *universal donors.*
From Stepp CA, Woods MA: Laboratory Procedures for Medical Office Personnel. Philadelphia, WB Saunders, 1998.

PROCEDURE 45-11
Determining ABO Group Using a Slide Test

GOAL

To accurately determine a patient's ABO group using the slide test technique.

EQUIPMENT AND SUPPLIES

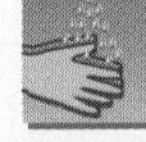

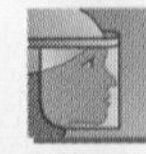
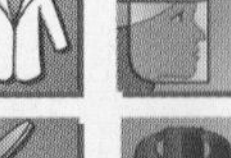
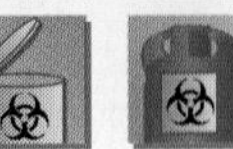

- Glass slide with frosted ends
- Anti-A and anti-B serum (Figure 1*)
- Applicator sticks
- Lancet and automatic finger puncture device
- Alcohol preps
- Sterile gauze squares
- Laboratory marking pen or pencil

PROCEDURAL STEPS

1 Reread the physician's orders and assemble all of the supplies and equipment needed to complete the testing procedure.

Continued

*Figures from Stepp CA, Woods MA: Laboratory Procedures for Medical Office Personnel. Philadelphia, WB Saunders, 1998.

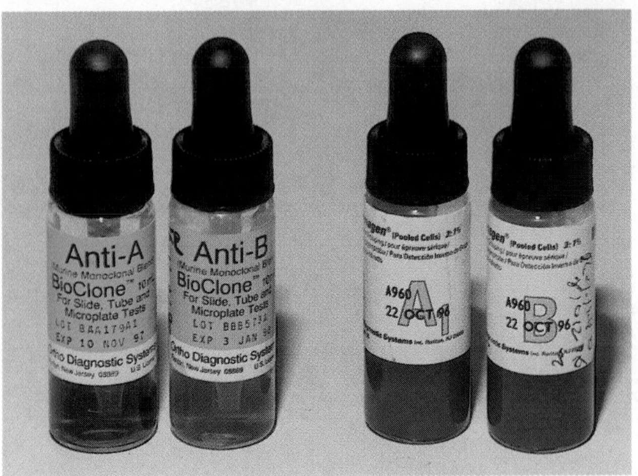

FIGURE 1

PROCEDURE 45-11 (CONTINUED)

Determining ABO Group Using a Slide Test

2 Wash your hands and put on face protection and gloves.
PURPOSE: Infection control.

3 Explain the procedure to the patient.

4 Label the slides in the frosted area with the patient's name.
PURPOSE: To ensure proper identification of testing results.

5 Place 1 drop of anti-A serum on slide #1, 1 drop of anti-B serum on slide #2, and 1 drop of anti-A and anti-B on slide #3.

6 Select the puncture site and perform a finger puncture procedure.

7 Wipe away the first drop of blood.
PURPOSE: The first drop of blood may contain tissue fluid.

8 Place one large drop of blood on each of the three prepared slides.

9 Cover the puncture site with a sterile gauze square and instruct the patient to apply gentle pressure to the site.

10 Mix the antiserum and blood thoroughly, using a clean applicator stick for each slide. The mixture should be spread over an area measuring approximately 20 × 40 mm.

11 Read and interpret the results of the reaction for all slides (Figure 2).

12 Discard all biohazard testing waste in the appropriate container.
PURPOSE: Infection control.

13 Clean the testing area.

14 Record the testing results in the patient's medical record.
PURPOSE: A procedure is not considered done until it is recorded.

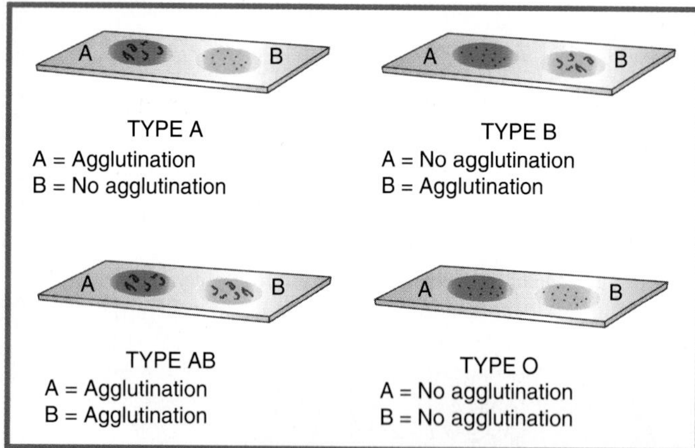

FIGURE 2

DETERMINATION OF THE RH FACTOR

The determination of Rh type is also a simple test that can be performed with a minimum amount of equipment. This test detects the presence of D antigens on the surface of the red blood cells based on the presence or absence of agglutination with anti-D antiserum. When the D antigen is present, agglutination occurs when the anti-D antiserum is reacted with the red blood cells. If the D antigen is not present, no agglutination will occur. Rh-positive blood will agglutinate in the presence of anti-D antiserum but not in the presence of the Rh control. Rh-negative blood will not agglutinate in the presence of anti-D antiserum nor will it agglutinate in the presence of the Rh control (Procedure 45–12).

PROCEDURE 45-12
Determining Rh Factor Using the Slide Method

GOAL

To accurately determine the presence or absence of anti-D agglutinations.

EQUIPMENT AND SUPPLIES

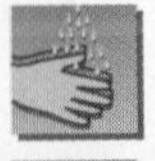

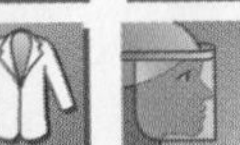
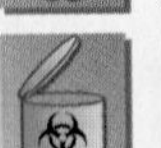
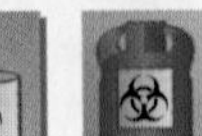

- Two glass slides with frosted ends
- Anti-D serum (Figure 1*)
- Applicator sticks
- Lancet and automatic finger puncture device
- Alcohol preps
- Sterile gauze squares
- Laboratory marker or pencil

PROCEDURAL STEPS

1 Check the physician's order and assemble all of the equipment and supplies needed to complete the testing procedure.

Continued

*Figure from Stepp CA, Woods MA: Laboratory Procedures for Medical Office Personnel. Philadelphia, WB Saunders, 1998.

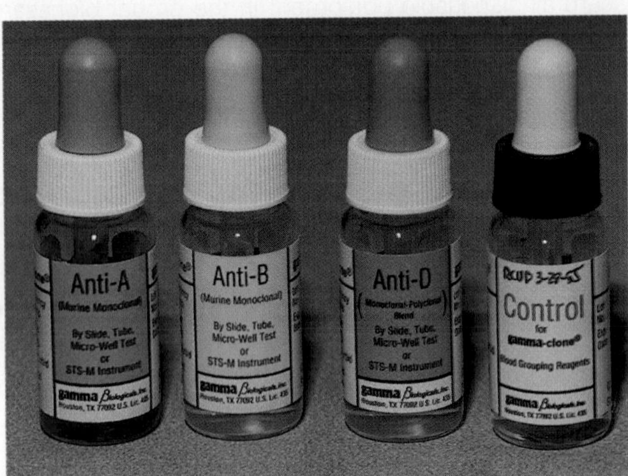

FIGURE 1

PROCEDURE 45-12 (CONTINUED)

Determining Rh Factor Using the Slide Method

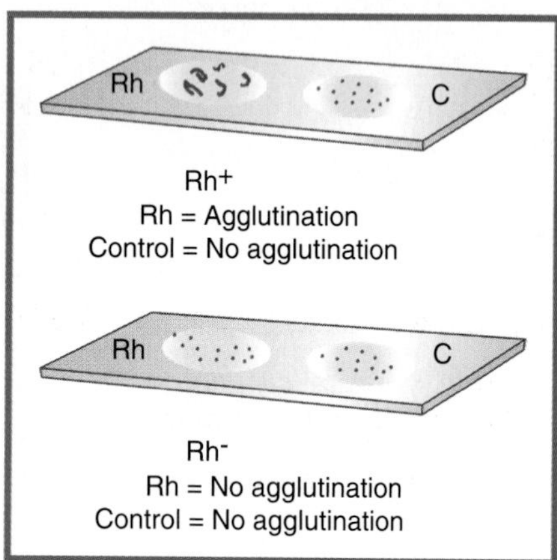

FIGURE 2

2 Wash your hands and put on face protection and gloves.
PURPOSE: Infection control.

3 Label one slide "D" and one slide "C".
PURPOSE: To differentiate between the anti-D slide and the control slide.

4 Place 1 drop of anti-D serum on the "D" slide.

5 Place 1 drop of the appropriate control reagent on the "C" slide.

6 Perform a capillary puncture to secure a blood specimen.

7 To each slide, add 2 drops of the patient's blood.

8 Thoroughly mix the blood with the anti-D serum, using a clean applicator stick for each slide, and spread the reaction mixture over an area measuring approximately 20 × 40 mm on each slide.

9 Read the results immediately (Figure 2).
PURPOSE: Drying of the reaction mixture must not be confused with agglutination.

10 Discard all disposable equipment in the proper biohazardous waste containers.

11 Clean area. Remove gloves and wash your hands.
PURPOSE: Infection control.

12 Record the testing results in the patient's medical record.
PURPOSE: A test is considered not done until it is recorded.

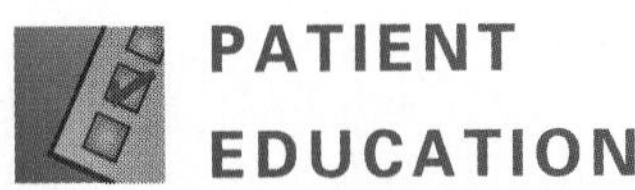

PATIENT EDUCATION

Depending on the type of medical office that you work in, you may never have the occasion to assist with the procedures discussed in this chapter. However, you will likely be present when patients are advised that these tests are necessary, so you may be in the position to answer the patient's questions about these procedures. By fully understanding the methods used and the testing process, you will be able to help the patient gain an understanding of the procedures and to offer reassurance. It is important to remember that through knowledge comes acceptance and understanding.

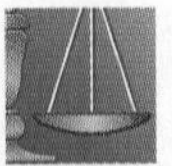

LEGAL AND ETHICAL ISSUES

In 1991, many states adopted the Blood Safety Act, which requires physicians to provide patients with information concerning blood transfusion options. This information is given before surgery and before any medical procedure in which there is a possibility that blood transfusion may be necessary. Physicians are also required to note on each patient's medical record that a written summary was given to the patient. As the physician's agent, you share this responsibility. If this is needed for a particular patient, it is the responsibility of every member of the health care team to see to it that this information is supplied to the patient, noted on the chart, and initialed. The written summary has been formally prepared. Copies of it can be requested from the state department of health services.

Be sure to follow the procedures established by your employer and the regulations of your state. If the blood sample drawn is for drug level studies, serology evaluations, or human immunodeficiency virus determinations, the procedure must be performed exactly as the law dictates. Courts of law require absolute adherence to procedures and complete and exact documentation of the chain of events for collecting, handling, and analyzing the specimen. Skin preparation for a blood alcohol level test must be done with povidone-iodine (Betadine) rather than alcohol because the alcohol could falsely elevate the blood alcohol level. Many states have statutes that specify exactly how, when, and under what circumstances this testing can be done. You can find out the regulations for your state by requesting a copy of the legislation from the state hospital association, the state police headquarters, or a state congressman.

Memory Jogger

18 *When is it necessary to give the patient information regarding blood safety?*

CRITICAL THINKING

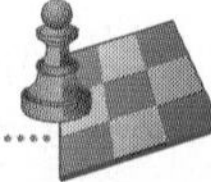

1 Why are red blood cells counts usually higher in men than in women?

2 After referring to Chapter 29, explain the purpose of keeping a cholesterol level within normal values.

3 If a woman is Rh negative and pregnant, why is it important to know the Rh factor of the unborn child's father?

HOW DID I DO? Answers To Memory Joggers

1 The average body holds 10 to 12 pints of blood.

2 Plasma, erythrocytes, leukocytes, and thrombocytes are the four elements of blood.

3 Yes, the collection tube must contain an anticoagulant.

4 Two or three drops of blood are collected.

5 Hemoglobin values range from a low of 12.5 g/dL to a high of 17.5 g/dL.

6 Normal values for red blood cells range from 4 to 6 million cells/mm^3.

7 The white blood cell count assists the physician in determining if an infection is present.

8 Calculations for a red blood cell count are determined by counting both sides of the hemacytometer and obtaining an average.

9 A good smear should cover one half to three fourths of the slide.

10 Granulocytes contain distinctive granules in their cytoplasm.

11 Neutrophils are also known as polys and segs.

12 Red blood cells are evaluated by their size, shape, and content.

13 ESR is recorded in millimeters per hour.

14 Lipid tests include cholesterol, triglyceride, high-density lipoprotein, and low-density lipoprotein levels.

15 Glucose is used as fuel in the body.

16 The first step is to review the package insert provided by the manufacturer.

17 The test detects the presence of A and B antigens on red blood cells.

18 Blood safety information must be given to the patient before surgery and before any medical procedure in which there is the possibility of a blood transfusion.

Assisting in Microbiology

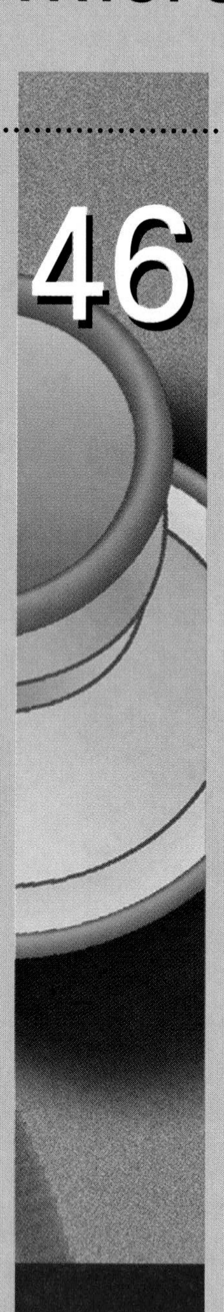

OUTLINE

LEARNING OBJECTIVES

Cognitive: On successful completion of this chapter you should be able to:

1. List the classifications of microorganisms.
2. Cite the morphologic differences of bacteria.
3. Describe the differences between viruses and bacteria.
4. Cite examples of disease for each of the microorganism classifications.
5. Identify elements needed for microorganism growth.
6. Cite the protocols for specimen collection.
7. Describe the different growth media used for culturing.
8. Compare rapid culture with standard culture growth methods.
9. Discuss legal and ethical issues in laboratory testing.
10. Define and spell vocabulary terms.

Performance: On successful completion of this chapter you should be able to:

1. Identify bacteria through microscopic viewing.
2. Inoculate media for culture.
3. Prepare direct smears and indirect smears from culture.
4. Examine stained smears for the presence of microorganisms.
5. Perform a rapid culture.
6. Secure a collection for pinworms.
7. Perform slide agglutination testing for infectious mononucleosis.

VOCABULARY

agar A substance extracted from algae and used in the laboratory to grow cultures of bacteria and other microorganisms.

agglutination The clumping together of particles (antigens and antibodies) resulting from their interaction with specific antibodies (or antigens); used in laboratory tests for blood typing and many other pathologic tests.

antibody Immunoglobulin produced by lymphoid tissue in response to substances interpreted as foreign invaders gaining entry into the body

arthropod vector Member of a phylum of the animal kingdom that includes the arachnids, crustaceans, and insects that can serve as a means of parasitic infestation

asepsis Condition of being free of infection or infectious materials

colony The visible growth on a culture plate, usually resulting from a single type of bacteria

disease A definite pathologic process having a descriptive set of signs and symptoms

hemolysis Pertaining to the destruction of red blood cells and the release of hemoglobin into the plasma

infection Invasion and multiplication of microorganisms in body tissues causing injury and damage to the tissues

inoculate To place a specimen in a culture medium to allow it to grow so that it can be identified

in vitro Pertaining to a biologic reaction that occurs in an artificial environment, usually within a test tube

microorganisms Microscopic living organisms (also called *microbes*)

mordant A chemical (Gram's iodine) used to make the primary stain adhere to the cells it stains

nosocomial Pertaining to the spread of infection among patients, staff, and visitors at a given institution such as a hospital, school, or prison

pathogens Disease-causing microorganisms

reference laboratory A large laboratory that accepts specimens from smaller laboratories to perform tests not done by smaller laboratories

screening test Laboratory tests done on large numbers of people to detect occult diseases

spore Thick-walled reproductive cell formed within bacteria and capable of withstanding unfavorable environmental conditions

toxin Poisonous protein substance produced by some plants, animals, and pathogenic bacteria that builds up in the body as the microorganisms multiply

Microbiology is the study of microorganisms, including bacteria, fungi, viruses, rickettsiae, mycobacteria, and parasites. Microbiology became a science in its own right with the work of such men as Louis Pasteur, Robert Koch, Joseph Lister, and many others. Pasteur was a French chemist who in about 1837 was asked by wine makers to try to find out what was turning their wine sour. He discovered that it was a microorganism. This led him to work in other microbiologic areas. He perfected a treatment that prevented rabies in persons bitten by rabid animals, and later he discovered the means for controlling anthrax, a disease of sheep.

After many years of research, medical microbiology now includes many classifications of disease-producing organisms. Viruses are the smallest known microorganisms and were not discovered until the powerful electron microscope was developed.

The main objective of microbiologic procedures is to identify the organisms responsible for illness so that the physician can properly treat the patient. In addition, responsibilities include preventing **nosocomial** infections and assisting with infection control in the physician's office laboratory and in the society the physician's office laboratory serves. Microbiologic procedures may be performed in the physician's office or in the microbiology department of a medical **reference laboratory.**

Microbes that cause disease are called pathogens. The study of **pathogens** and their effects on the defense systems of the body is complex. Many factors determine the role of microbes in disease, the identification of microbes in the laboratory, and the ability of the body to maintain or recover health.

Memory Jogger

Define microbiology *and cite the organisms covered.*

Classifications of Microorganisms

Microorganisms are almost everywhere. The only places that are free of microorganisms are the insides of sterilized containers; inside fresh, unbruised fruits; and in certain internal body organs and tissues. Organs and tissues that do not connect with the outside by means of mucus-lined membranes are, in the normal state, free from all living microorganisms.

Microbes range from being visible to the naked eye, such as the tapeworm, to being visible only with the use of a microscope (e.g., bacteria and yeasts), to being so small that they are visible only with the use of the electron microscope (viruses). Microorganisms are classified in five major classifications. Some, such as bacteria, have subclassifications.

CLASSIFICATIONS OF MICROORGANISMS

Bacteria
Fungi
Mycobacteria
Viruses
Parasites

BACTERIA

The study of bacteria is called *bacteriology*. Bacteria are one-celled plant microorganisms. There are numerous ways of identifying bacteria, including their morphology (form and structure), their ability to retain certain dyes, their growth in different physical

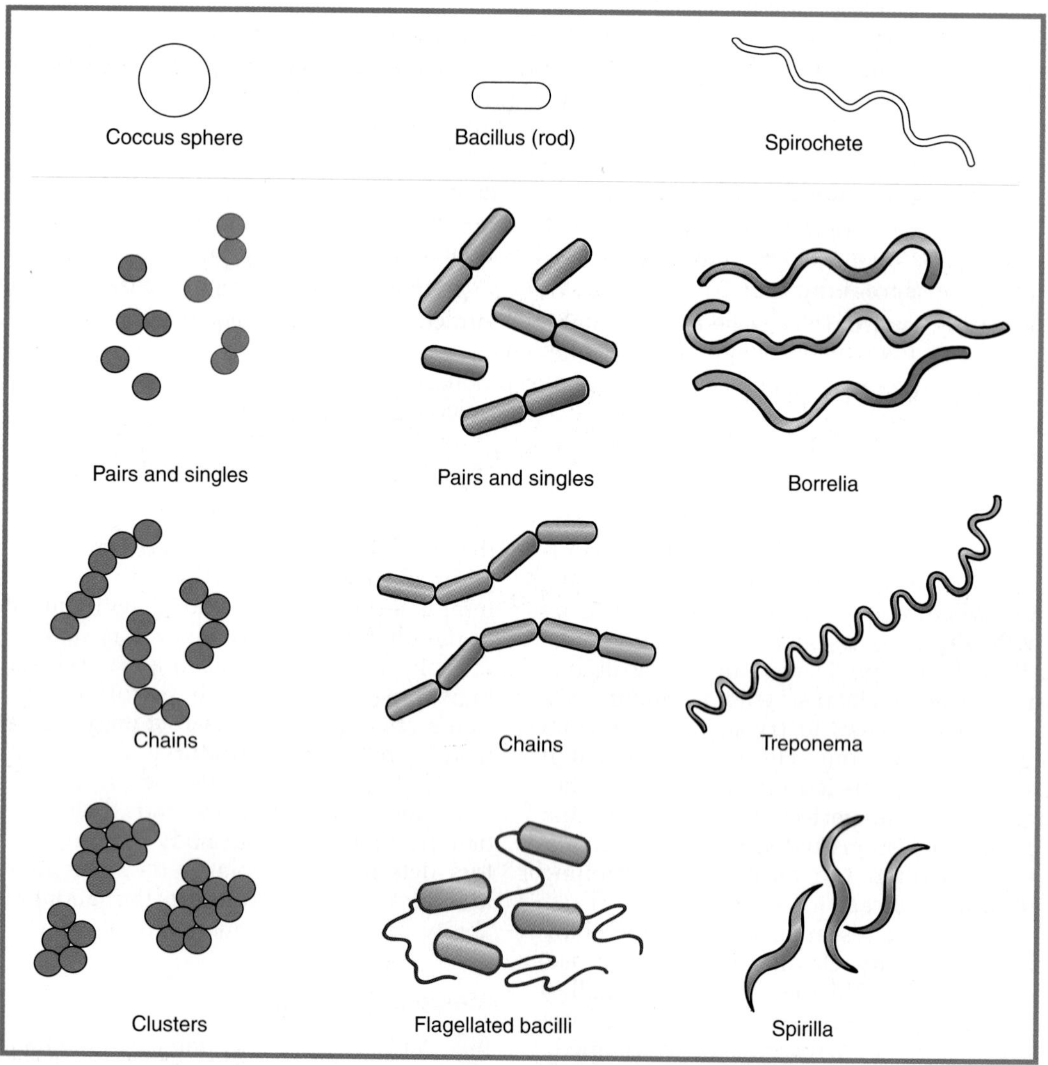

FIGURE 46–1 The three basic shapes of bacteria. (From Stepp CA, Woods MA: Laboratory Procedures for Medical Office Personnel. Philadelphia, WB Saunders, 1998.)

environments, and the results of certain biochemical reactions.

Bacteria (singular, bacterium), like plants, have cell walls, but, unlike plants, they lack chlorophyll. Usually, pathogenic bacteria grow best at 98.6° F (37° C), in a moist, dark environment. A bacterial **infection** can be spread by any means of transmission. Bacteria live and reproduce in nutrients supplied by the body or in a laboratory culture medium, which is an **agar** preparation that simulates the body's environment. Because bacteria are the most commonly encountered pathogens, most of the laboratory procedures performed in the medical office deal with the isolation and identification of these microbes.

Humans host a variety of bacteria, both harmful and harmless, at all times. The skin, respiratory tract, and gastrointestinal tract are inhabited by a great variety of harmless bacteria, called *normal flora*. They are beneficial and protect the human host by aiding in metabolism and interfering with the harmful bacteria that may gain entrance. An infection occurs when bacteria occurring naturally in one part of the body invade another part of the body and become harmful. When this occurs, the normal flora are considered *opportunistic;* that is, they cause infection. When one type of flora that is normal to one area invades another area, it becomes pathogenic. One common example is *cystitis,* a urinary tract infection caused by contamination with *Escherichia coli,* a bacterium that is normal flora in the intestine.

Pathogenic bacteria can be transmitted from person to person by many mechanisms, including direct contact (by means of airborne infections, contact with animals, or transmission by insects) and indirect contact (through drinking water or food products or on inanimate objects). Another example is the bacterium *Staphylococcus epidermidis,* normally found on the surface of the skin. When bacteria of this type invade the body, as through a cut, an infection usually results.

Memory Jogger

What are normal flora and where in the human body are they located?

Bacteria may be classified by *morphology* (size and shape). Spherical bacteria are called *cocci,* rod-shaped bacteria are called *bacilli,* and those shaped like threads are called *spirilla* or *spirochetes.* If any of these groups grow in pairs, the prefix *diplo* is used, as in *diplococci;* if in chains, the prefix *strepto* is used, as in *streptococci.* If they grow in clusters, like grapes, the prefix *staphylo* is used, as in *staphylococci* (Fig. 46–1).

Different kinds of bacteria tend to affect the various organs of the body in different ways, producing a **disease** with specific symptoms and effects (Tables 46–1 and 46–2).

Memory Jogger

What are the major morphologic classifications of bacteria?

TABLE 46–1 Selected Diseases Caused by Bacilli and Spirilla

Disease	Organism	Description	Transmission	Symptoms	Tests/ Specimens	Prevention and Immunization
Tuberculosis	*Mycobacterium tuberculosis*	Acid-fast beaded bacilli	Inhalation	Pulmonary: cough, hemoptysis, sweats, weight loss. May affect other systems	Sputum for culture; x-ray; skin tests	BCG vaccine
Urinary tract infections	*Escherichia coli, Proteus* sp., *Klebsiella* sp., *Pseudomonas aeruginosa*	Gram-negative bacilli	Ascends urethra; catheterization	Cystitis: frequency, burning bloody urine. Pyelonephritis: flank pain, fever	Clean-catch urine for culture and analysis	Good personal hygiene; always wipe from front to back
Syphilis	*Treponema pallidum*	Spirochete	Sexually; congenitally	*Primary:* painless sore. *Secondary:* generalized rash involving palms and soles of feet. *Congenital:* birth defects	Blood for serologic tests: VDRL, RPR, FTA-ABS	Avoidance of infected persons; use of condoms
Lyme disease	*Borrelia*	Spirochete	Tick bite	Fever, joint pain, red annular rash	Swab for culture	Eliminating animal vectors

Table continued on following page

TABLE 46–1 Selected Diseases Caused by Bacilli and Spirilla *Continued*

Disease	Organism	Description	Transmission	Symptoms	Tests/ Specimens	Prevention and Immunization
Cholera	*Vibrio cholerae*	Gram-negative spirillum	Fecal contamination of food and water (warm climates)	Severe vomiting and diarrhea; dehydration	Stool for culture	Cholera vaccine; boiling water; cooking foods
Legionnaires' disease	*Legionella pneumophila*	Gram-negative bacillus (stains poorly with usual methods)	Grows freely in water (air conditioning systems)	Pneumonia-like symptoms	Sputum; blood	Isolation
Tetanus (lockjaw)	*Clostridium tetani*	Gram-positive spore-forming bacilli, anaerobic	Open wounds, fractures, punctures	Toxin affects motor nerves; muscle spasms, convulsions, rigidity	Blood	DPT in childhood; T or Td every 10 years
Gas gangrene	*Clostridium perfringens*	Gram-positive spore-forming bacilli, anaerobic	Wounds	Gas and watery exudate in infected wound	Swab, aspirate of wound for culture	Proper wound care
Botulism	*Clostridium botulinum*	Gram-positive spore-forming bacilli, anaerobic	Improperly cooked canned foods	Neurotoxin affects speech, swallowing, vision; paralysis of respiratory muscles, death	Contaminated food; blood	Botulinus antitoxin; boil canned goods 20 minutes before tasting or eating
Diphtheria	*Corynebacterium diphtheriae*	Gram-positive bacilli, club-shaped	Respiratory secretions	Sore throat, fever, headache, gray membrane in throat	Swabs; Gram's stain, culture; Schick test for immunity	DPT in childhood
Whooping cough	*Bordetella pertussis*	Gram-negative bacilli	Respiratory secretions	Upper respiratory tract symptoms; high-pitched crowing whoop	Swabs for culture	DPT in childhood
Typhoid and paratyphoid fevers	*Salmonella* sp.	Gram-negative bacilli	Contaminated food, water, poor hygiene; carriers	Fever, headache, diarrhea, toxemia, rose spots on skin	Stool for culture	Typhoid/para-typhoid A and B vaccine
Plague	*Yersinia pestis*	Gram-negative bacilli	Via flea bite from infected rodents	Fever and chills, delirium, enlarged, painful lymph nodes	Sputum for culture; blood	Vaccine available; rodent control
Nonspecific vaginitis	*Gardnerella vaginalis,* with anaerobes	Gram-variable bacillus	Sexual	Vaginal irritation itching, fishy-smelling malodorous discharge	Swab; wet prep for "clue cells"	Avoidance of infected persons; good personal hygiene

BCG vaccine, bacille Calmette-Guérin vaccine; VDRL, Venereal Disease Research Laboratory; RPR, rapid plasma reagin (test); FTA-ABS, fluorescent treponemal antibody absorption (test); DPT, diphtheria-pertussis-tetanus (vaccine); T, tetanus (toxoid); Td, tetanus and diphtheria (toxoids).
Courtesy of Kathleen Moody.

Chlamydia and Mycoplasma

Chlamydia are *obligate* parasites (unable to survive without a host) and the smallest of all bacteria. They are important because of their role in sexually transmitted disease (STD). *Chlamydia trachomatis* is the most frequent cause of pelvic inflammatory disease and is considered the most prevalent STD today. Flies can carry *Chlamydia trachomatis* and cause trachoma, the leading cause of infectious blindness (Table 46–3).

TABLE 46–2 Common Diseases Caused by Cocci

Disease	Organism	Description	Transmission	Symptoms	Specimens	Tests
Pneumonia	*Streptococcus pneumoniae*	Gram-positive cocci in pairs	Direct contact, droplets	Productive cough, fever, chest pain	Sputum; bronchoscopy secretions	Culture, Gram stain
Strep throat	*Streptococcus pyogenes* (group A strep)	Gram-positive cocci in chains	Direct contact, droplets, fomites	Severe sore throat, fever, malaise	Direct swab	Direct agglutination; culture, WBC and differential
Wound infection, abscesses, boils	*Staphylococcus aureus*	Gram-positive cocci in clusters	Direct contact, fomites, carriers; poor hand washing	Area red, warm, swollen; pus; pain; ulceration or sinus formation	Deep swab; aspirate of drainage	Culture and sensitivity (aerobic and anaerobic)
Staphylococcal food poisoning	*Staphylococcus aureus*	Gram-positive cocci in clusters	Poor hygiene and improper refrigeration of foods	Vomiting, abdominal cramps, diarrhea	Suspected food, stool	Culture
Toxic shock	*Staphylococcus aureus*	Gram-positive cocci in clusters	Use of absorbent packing materials (e.g., tampons, nasal packs)	Fever, headache, nausea, vomiting, delirium, low blood pressure	Swab, blood	Culture and serology
Gonorrhea	*Neisseria gonorrhoeae*	Gram-negative cocci in pairs; intracellular in WBC	Sexually transmitted	*Females:* pelvic pain, discharge. May be asymptomatic *Males:* urethral drip, pain on urination	Swab of cervix, urethra; rectal and pharyngeal swabs in homosexuals	Gram stain; culture
Meningococcal meningitis	*Neisseria meningitidis*	Gram-negative diplococci	Respiratory tract secretions	High fever, headache, projectile vomiting, delirium, neck and back rigidity, convulsions, petechial rash	Nasopharyngeal swabs, cerebrospinal fluid, blood	Gram stain; culture; cell counts and chemistries

WBC, white blood cells.
Courtesy of Kathleen Moody.

TABLE 46–3 Diseases Caused by *Rickettsia, Chlamydia,* and *Mycoplasma*

Disease	Organism	Transmission	Symptoms	Tests/Specimens
Rocky Mountain spotted fever	*Rickettsia rickettsii*	Tick bite	Headache, chills, fever, characteristic rash on extremities and trunk	Blood for serologic tests; skin biopsy for direct fluorescent microscopy
Typhus	*Rickettsia prowazekii*	Tick bite	Fever, rash, confusion	Blood for serology
Atypical pneumonia	*Mycoplasma pneumoniae*	Respiratory secretions	Fever, cough, chest pain	Blood, sputum
Nongonococcal urethritis and vaginitis	*Chlamydia trachomatis*	Sexual	May be asymptomatic	Swabs for culture and serologic testing
Inclusion conjunctivitis, pneumonia		Congenital	Severe conjunctivitis in newborns Afebrile pneumonia in newborns	

Courtesy of Kathleen Moody.

TABLE 46–4 Selected Fungal Diseases

Disease	Organism	Predisposing Conditions and Transmission	Symptoms	Tests/Specimens
Thrush (oral yeast); *Candida* (vaginal yeast)	*Candida* species (yeast)	Oral: during birth; other: following antibiotic therapy, oral birth control, severe diabetes	White, cheesy growth	Swab for KOH prep, culture
Athlete's foot, jock itch, ringworm (tinea)	Several species of dermatophytes (skin fungi)	Opportunist; direct contact; clothing; prolonged exposure to moist environment	Hair loss, thickening of skin, nails; itching; red, scaly patches	Skin scraping for KOH prep; skin, hair for culture
Histoplasmosis	*Histoplasma capsulatum*	Inhalation of dust contaminated with bird or bat droppings	Mild, flu-like to systemic	Serologic
Cryptococcosis	*Cryptococcus neoformans*	Contact with poultry droppings	Cough, fever, malaise; can become systemic	Sputum culture
Sporotrichosis	*Sporothrix schenckii*	Farmers, florists, people exposed to soil	Skin lesions that spread along lymphatics; can become systemic	Cerebrospinal fluid culture, India ink direct examination, scrapings; serologic

KOH, potassium hydroxide.
Courtesy of Kathleen Moody.

FUNGI

Mycology is the study of fungi and the diseases they cause. Fungi (singular, fungus) are larger than bacteria and have rigid cell walls. They are vegetable organisms and include yeasts and molds. Fungi are present in the soil, air, and water, but only a few species cause disease. Fungi thrive in warm, moist, dark places. They are transmitted by direct contact with infected persons, by prolonged exposure to a moist environment, or by inhalation of contaminated dust or soil. Fungal infections may be quite superficial, affecting only the skin, hair, or nails. However, some fungi can penetrate the tissues of the internal body structures and produce serious diseases of the mucous membranes, heart, lungs, and other organs. Fungal infections are resistant to antibiotics used in the treatment of bacterial infections and must be treated with drugs active against the unusual cell walls of this organism. Examples of fungal diseases are *ringworm, athlete's foot* (tinea pedis), *thrush* (oral candidiasis), *histoplasmosis, coccidioidomycosis,* and *blastomycosis.*

Diagnosis is usually based on the culturing or testing of skin scrapings, hair samples, or samples of sputum or mucous membranes (Table 46–4).

Memory Jogger

Describe the environment in which fungi thrive.

MYCOBACTERIA

Mycobacteria have been important agents of disease throughout the world since before the time of recorded history. There are 54 species of *Mycobacterium,* and 14 of these cause diseases in humans. *Mycobacterium tuberculosis* is the cause of tuberculosis.

World Health Organization reports indicate that tuberculosis has been increasing in new active cases in the United States for the past decade. The increase is partly related to decreased resistance caused by new virulent strains of diseases such as human immunodeficiency virus (HIV) infection and the acquired immunodeficiency syndrome and to the introduction of new, more drug-resistant strains of tuberculosis brought to the United States by immigrants from underdeveloped countries.

VIRUSES

Viruses are the smallest infectious microorganisms. New and increasingly destructive viruses are being discovered and have caused the creation of a special area within microbiology called *virology* (the study of viruses and their effects).

Viruses can be seen with the electron microscope. Each virus is an organism made up of a nucleic acid core covered with a coating of protein; but the nucleic acid core of the virus is unique because it has either ribonucleic acid (RNA) or deoxyribonucleic acid (DNA) but never both. All other organisms have both RNA and DNA, which together form pairs of chromosomes that contain all the genetic codes necessary for protein synthesis and reproduction. Viruses, on the other hand, have a complete set of hereditary factors in half the number of chromosomes and, therefore, can reproduce only within living cells and only after a living host cell's enzymes dissolve the outer protein coating. A virus enters a host cell, and the host's enzymes wash away the virus's outer coating. Then the virus's nucleic acid is released into the cell's cytoplasm, where it mixes, and the virus is able to replicate itself. Once infected, the parasitized host cells die, while the multiplying viruses continue to swarm from the dying cells to invade and attack new cells and tissues.

Viruses cause many clinically significant diseases in humans. Unfortunately, most viral diseases can be treated only symptomatically, that is, for the symptom and not the infective cause. Viruses cannot be grown on artificial culture media and cannot be destroyed by antibiotic drugs. General antibiotics are ineffective in preventing or curtailing viral infections, and even the few drugs that are effective against some specific viruses have limitations because viruses often produce different types of infections in host cells (Table 46–5).

Viruses can be treated easily in the external environment. Widely used chemicals such as chlorine (bleach), iodine, phenol, and formaldehyde easily and effectively destroy viruses on surfaces and objects coming into contact with the infected patient. These agents, however, are too toxic to be used internally. Viral diseases are transmitted by direct contact, insects, blood transfusion, contamination of food or water, and inhalation of droplets expelled by coughing or sneezing.

TABLE 46–5 Viral Diseases

Disease	Transmission	Symptoms	Tests	Prevention
Smallpox	Direct contact; fomites	Vesicles on entire body, including soles and palms		Eradicated (vaccine is still available)
Herpes 1 (cold sores, fever blisters)	Direct contact; fomites	Recurrent painful blisters on lips, mouth	Serologic	Avoid contact with active lesions
Herpes 2 (genital)	Sexual contact	Recurrent painful blisters on labia, penis, rectum	Serologic	Avoid sexual contact with persons having active lesions
Infectious mononucleosis	Direct and airborne	Sore throat, fever, malaise, lymph gland involvement; hepatitis, enlarged spleen	Blood for Monospot	Avoid direct contact with known cases
Influenza	Droplet and fomites	Fever, body aches, cough		Immunization for old, young, debilitated
Warts	Direct and indirect contact	Circumscribed outgrowths on skin; most common on hands and feet		
Rabies	Contact with saliva of infected animal (dog, cat, skunk, fox, bat are usual)	Fever, uncontrollable excitement, spasms of throat, profuse salivation	Animal's brain tissue examined for Negri bodies	Vaccine available. Vaccinate pets
Mumps	Direct contact	Pain, swelling of salivary glands, fever	Acute and convalescent titers	MMR* vaccine
Measles	Direct contact; droplets	Fever, nasal discharge, red eyes; Koplik's spots, rash	Serologic	MMR vaccine
Rubella	Direct contact; droplets. Congenital	Rash, swollen lymph glands; causes severe birth defects	Serologic	MMR vaccine
Common cold	Direct; droplets; fomites	Headache, fever, runny nose, congestion		Good hygiene (hand washing)
Hepatitis A (infectious hepatitis)	Fecal-oral; contaminated food and water	Nausea, fever, weakness, loss of appetite, jaundice	Serologic	Good hygiene (hand washing)
Hepatitis B (serum hepatitis)	Blood and blood products; accidental needle sticks	Similar to hepatitis A, but more severe	Serologic	Vaccine is available. Avoid contact with blood from infected persons
AIDS	Sexual; drug abuse (needles); blood and body fluids	Poor immunity, resulting in disseminated viral, fungal, and protozoan infections; Kaposi's sarcoma	Serologic	Avoid casual sexual contact. Use extra caution when drawing and/or handling specimens
Polio	Direct contact; carriers. Enter via mouth	Fever, headache, stiff neck and back, paralysis of muscles		Trivalent oral polio vaccine (TOPV)

*Measles, mumps, rubella.
Courtesy of Kathleen Moody.

Some of the more than 50 known viral diseases include the common cold, smallpox, chickenpox, influenza, poliomyelitis, measles, mumps, German measles, cold sores, shingles, viral hepatitis, rabies, infectious mononucleosis, croup, viral encephalitis, yellow fever, and HIV infection.

Memory Jogger

 *How is the nucleic acid core of the virus unique?*

PARASITES

Parasitology includes the study of all parasitic organisms that live on or in the human body. Some types may cause little or no injury to the body, whereas other parasites can cause serious illness, even death, if not treated. Parasites are transmitted by ingestion during the infective stage, direct penetration of the skin by infective larvae, and inoculation by an **arthropod vector.** It is not possible to identify a parasite accurately on the basis of a single test or specimen. Most parasites are identified in urine, sputum, tissue fluids, or tissue biopsy samples.

There are about 70 species of parasites that commonly infect the human body. Some of the more frequently found organisms include *Entamoeba hystolytica,* which causes amoebic dysentery; *Giardia lamblia,* found in contaminated drinking water; *Trichomonas vaginalis,* a common sexually transmitted organism; and *Cryptosporidium,* which is known to cause diarrheal disease in immunodeficient individuals (Table 46–6).

Memory Jogger

 *Cite the types of samples used to identify most parasites.*

TABLE 46–6 Diseases Caused by Protozoa and Other Parasites

Disease	Organism	Transmission	Symptoms	Tests/Specimens
Malaria	*Plasmodium* sp. (protozoa)	Bite of the *Anopheles* mosquito	Chills, fever (cyclic)	Blood: examination of stained film for parasites
Toxoplasmosis	*Toxoplasma gondii* (protozoa)	Fecal contamination (cat litter); congenitally	Febrile illness, rash; congenital: jaundice, enlarged liver and spleen, brain abnormalities	Skin test
Amebic dysentery	*Entamoeba histolytica* (protozoa)	Fecal contamination of food and water	Bloody diarrhea, cramping, fever	Stool for O & P
Giardiasis	*Giardia lamblia* (protozoa)	Common in intestinal tract, opportunist; contaminated surface water	Asymptomatic to severe diarrhea and abdominal discomfort	Stool for O & P; intestinal biopsy; string test
Interstitial plasma cell pneumonia	*Pneumocystis carinii*	Widely prevalent in animals. Occurs in debilitated persons, immunosuppressed; common in AIDS	Pneumonia-like	Biopsy
Trichinosis	*Trichinella spiralis* (roundworm)	Ingestion of undercooked pork, bear meat	Nausea, fever, diarrhea, muscle pain and swelling, edema of face	Biopsy; blood tests
Tapeworm	*Taenia* sp.	Undercooked meats (beef and pork)	Abdominal discomfort, diarrhea, weight loss	Stool for O & P
	Diphyllobothrium latum	Undercooked fish; common among Norwegians, Japanese	As above, may become anemic	Stool for O & P
Pinworm	*Enterobius vermicularis* (roundworm)	Fecal-oral	Severe rectal itching, restlessness, insomnia	Scotch tape applied to perianal region for ova
Scabies	Itch mite: *Sarcoptes scabiei*	Direct contact; clothing, bedding	Nocturnal itching; skin burrows	Skin scrapings for parasites
Lice	*Pediculus humanus; Pthirus pubis* (crabs)	Direct contact; clothing, bedding, furniture (can transmit other diseases via bite)	Intense itching; skin lesions	Finding adult lice or eggs (nits) on body or hair

O & P, ova and parasites.
Courtesy of Kathleen Moody.

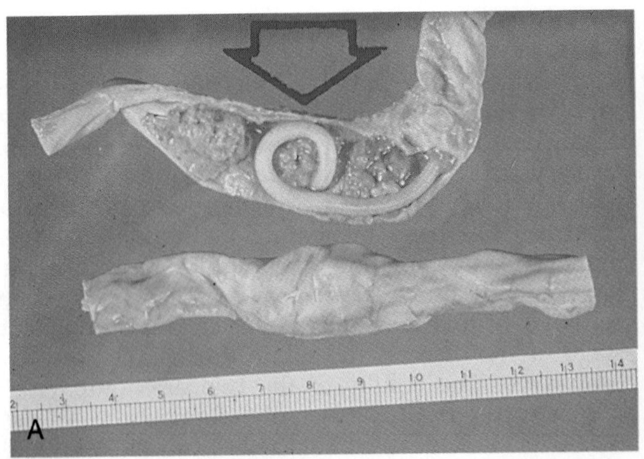

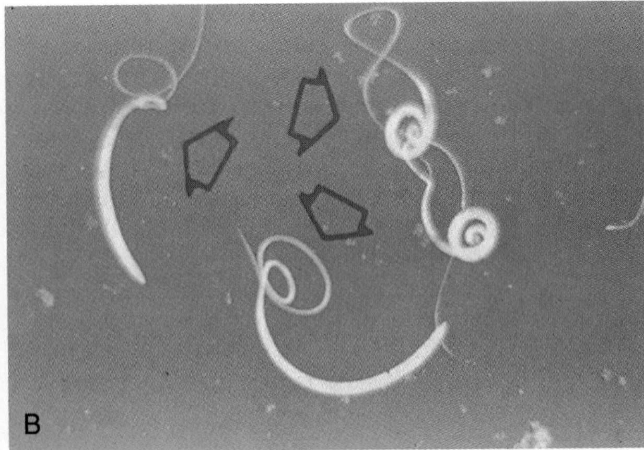

FIGURE 46-2 *A,* Roundworms. *B,* Whipworms. (From Stepp CA, Woods MA: Laboratory Procedures for Medical Office Personnel. Philadelphia, WB Saunders, 1998.)

Helminths

Helminths are animal parasites called worms. Helminths live upon or within another living organism and nourish themselves at the expense of the host organism. They may live in animals or humans and are usually transmitted through the soil or by infected clothing or fingernails, contact with infected persons, or contaminated food or water. Helminths go through the same life cycle as other worms. The adult worm lays eggs (ova). The ova develop into larvae. Larvae grow into adult worms, which lay eggs, and the cycle begins again. Diagnosis is usually based on microscopic examination of feces for ova and parasites and on the patient's signs and symptoms (Fig. 46-2).

Protozoa

Protozoa (singular, protozoon) are single-celled parasitic animals ranging in size from microscopic to macroscopic (visible to the naked eye). They are present in moist environments and in bodies of water such as lakes and ponds. Protozoa are transmitted through contaminated feces, food, or drink. Some pathogenic protozoa inhabit the bloodstream, whereas others inhabit the intestines and genital tract. Diagnosis is usually based on the patient's signs and symptoms and on microscopic examination of stool and blood (see Table 46-6).

Rickettsiae

Rickettsiae (singular, rickettsia) are microscopic parasites that are insect borne and fever producing. They are transmitted from rodents or other animals to humans by the bites of lice, fleas, ticks, and mites. These parasites attack the linings of small blood vessels. Usually, diagnosis is based on the patient's signs and symptoms and on blood testing (see Table 46-3). Rickettsial diseases include Rocky Mountain spotted fever, typhus, and tick fever. They may be prevented by using insecticides, vaccines, and antibiotics (see Table 46-3).

Conditions That Favor Growth

Most pathogens prefer a fluid nutrient environment and an atmosphere full of oxygen. Pathogens that thrive in oxygen are called *aerobes.* Aerobes grow best when specific conditions are present.

CONDITIONS FAVORABLE TO THE GROWTH OF AEROBES

- Oxygen
- Moisture (water)
- Nutrients from a living source, called a host (sometimes at the expense of the host) or from dead or decaying material
- Temperature of 98.6° F or 37° C
- Darkness
- Neutral to slightly alkaline pH environment

Other pathogens prefer an environment without oxygen. These organisms are referred to as *anaerobes.* Anaerobes thrive in the dark, damp, warm, airless places inside the body. For example, the anaerobic bacterial pathogen *Clostridium tetani* causes tetanus (lockjaw). Found in the soil or street dust, it is dormant and protected by a hard coating in what is called the **spore** stage. However, once inside human tissue, the protective spore becomes a living bacterium that releases a **toxin.** The puncture wound that closes over and blocks out air (oxygen) is the perfect medium for growth. The bacterium rapidly multiplies and spreads through the bloodstream, causing the disease. In the same family of spore-forming bacteria is *Clostridium perfringens*, which causes gas gangrene. The cycle is the same as for tetanus, except the infection is localized and often necessitates the amputation of a limb. Gas gangrene can result from contaminated surgical wounds. The third in this group of rod-shaped, spore-forming bacilli (bacteria) is *Clostridium botulinum*. This organism grows in the oxygenless atmosphere of canned goods; when the can is opened, released toxins cause the disease known as botulism. Organisms that produce spores and release toxins are extremely dangerous.

Memory Jogger

What are aerobes?

Collection of Specimens

Medical assistants are often called on to collect specimens for the identification of possible microorganisms. A microbiology specimen must contain as few contaminants as possible and must be composed of material from the actual site of the infection. The specimen is most often contaminated by normal flora (bacteria) from the site of collection, such as normal skin flora from a wound site. Wound swabs should be taken from the depths of the wound; surface organisms may not be the true cause of the infection.

An improperly collected or transported specimen can severely limit the speed, dependability, and quality of the information needed by the physician in prescribing treatment. Before collecting or preparing the bacteriologic specimen for transport, you should be certain that you are familiar with the specimen requirements of the reference laboratories and the physician's office laboratory protocols for collection techniques. Most reference laboratories provide the proper specimen collection apparatus and instructions to the physician's office laboratory on request without charge. Specimens that are improperly collected or transported may be rejected by the reference laboratory, which may cause a hardship to the patient and slow down the treatment process.

EXAMPLES OF PROTOCOLS FOR BACTERIOLOGIC SPECIMEN COLLECTION

- Optimal collection times
- Sufficient sample
- Proper equipment and procedure
- Type of specimen collected

OPTIMAL COLLECTION TIMES

Knowledge of the optimal collection times is necessary for the best chance of recovering the causative organisms or collecting positive serologic specimens. Urinary tract infections are best diagnosed from the first specimen voided in the morning, because the specimen has been incubating in the bladder overnight. In addition, this specimen is most likely to have a high number of microorganisms. Blood for serologic testing is usually collected during the acute stage of the disease and again during the convalescent stage. The results of the two are compared; a rise in **antibody** titer is usually diagnostic.

SUFFICIENT SAMPLE

A sufficient sample must be obtained to perform all tests requested. For example, in cases of suspected mycobacterial infection, which causes tuberculosis, the physician may order a sputum specimen to be collected for a Gram stain, acid-fast stain, and acid-fast culture for aerobes and anaerobes. The patient must be instructed to collect at least 10 mL of a first morning sputum specimen.

PROPER EQUIPMENT AND PROCEDURES

The proper collection containers, media, and procedures must be used. These include sterile, nonbreakable containers with tight-fitting lids; polyester (not cotton) swabs; appropriate transport media and containers for aerobic and anaerobic cultures (Fig. 46–3); and the immediate inoculation of swabs for gonococcus cultures onto prewarmed modified Thayer-Martin agar. If possible, obtain specimens for culture before antibiotics are given. This is particularly important for throat and gonococcus cultures. If an antibiotic has been given, note it on the requisition and send the specimen to the laboratory immediately for inoculation into the media. Even small amounts of the antibiotic interfere with the culture.

Memory Jogger

What often contaminates a microbiology specimen?

Memory Jogger

Recall the bacteriologic specimen collection protocols.

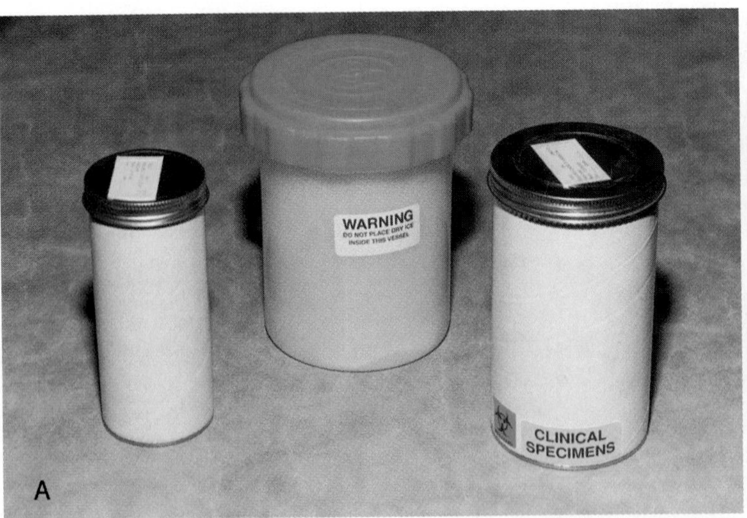

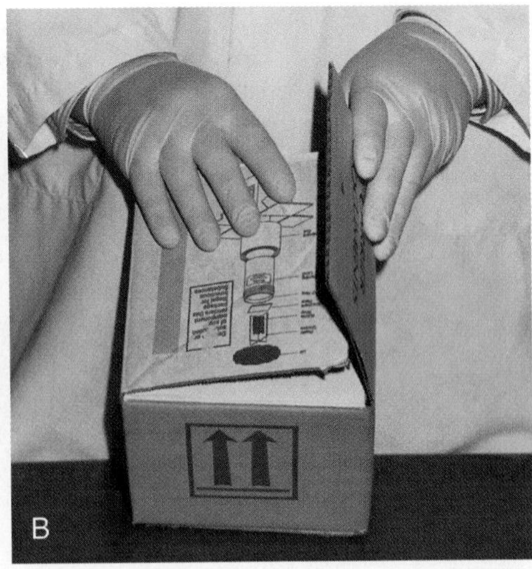

FIGURE 46–3 *A,* Appropriate containers for transport. *B,* Appropriate packaging for transport.

Microbiology Procedures

Some physicians prefer to perform some of the simple screening procedures in their offices and refer the more complex tests to **reference laboratories.** Others collect specimens in the office and send all of them to larger laboratories for analysis. The basic microbiology procedures most frequently encountered in the physician's office laboratory include preparation of direct smears; staining; microscopic examination of smears, wet preps, and potassium hydroxide (KOH) preps; **screening tests** for strep throat and infectious mononucleosis; and screening for urinary tract infections. Many types of tests are available in kit form. The kits supply all needed reagents and most equipment (Fig. 46–4). Directions for the entire test procedure are contained in the kits and must be followed carefully. Known controls are also included to ensure accurate testing. To perform microbiologic procedures in the office, the following equipment is needed: a microscope, an incubator, a staining rack and materials, slides, culture media, inoculation loops, a Bacti-cinerator, and sterile supplies for specimen collection.

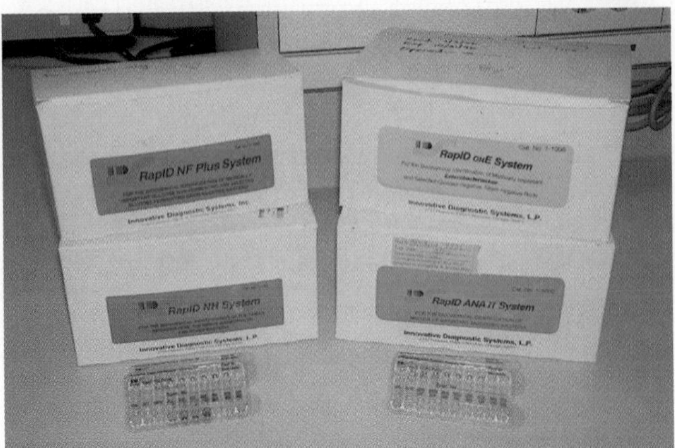

FIGURE 46–4 Rapid biochemical test kits. (From Stepp CA, Woods MA: Laboratory Procedures for Medical Office Personnel. Philadelphia, WB Saunders, 1998.)

PREPARATION OF SMEARS

A smear is made on a glass slide and is stained and examined under the microscope. A direct smear is made from a swab of the infected area; a culture smear is taken from a single cluster of organisms (**colony**) growing on a plate of solid media or in a tube of liquid broth, using a loop. The material must be applied thinly or the resulting smear is too thick to study under the microscope. Slides should be labeled before the infectious material is applied. This prevents possible incorrect labeling and contamination of hands with infectious organisms. Smears are dried, heat fixed, and stained.

Staining

Most bacteria are so small and possess so little color that they are difficult to observe. Staining allows the microorganisms to be clearly seen under the microscope. The Gram stain is used most often. This staining procedure consists of applying a sequence of dye, **mordant,** decolorizer, and counterstain to the bacteria. The dyes are taken up differently according to the chemical composition of the cell walls. This serves to classify organisms according to their reactions to the stain and separates them into gram positive, which stain purple, and gram negative, which stain red.

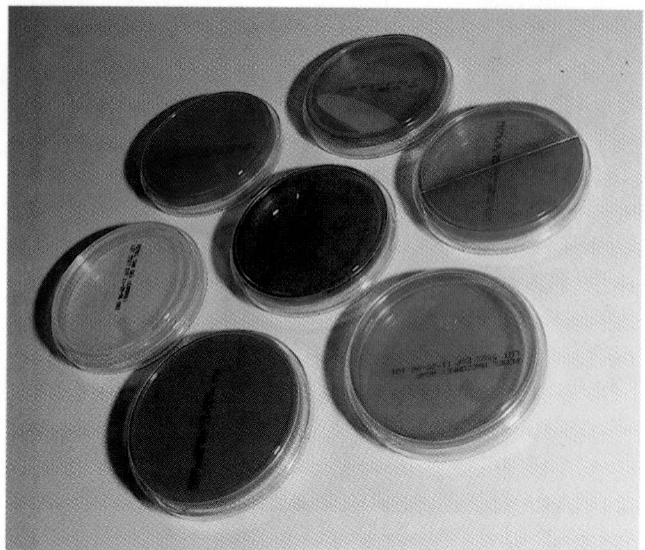

FIGURE 46–5 Media used in cultures. (From Stepp CA, Woods MA: Laboratory Procedures for Medical Office Personnel. Philadelphia, WB Saunders, 1998.)

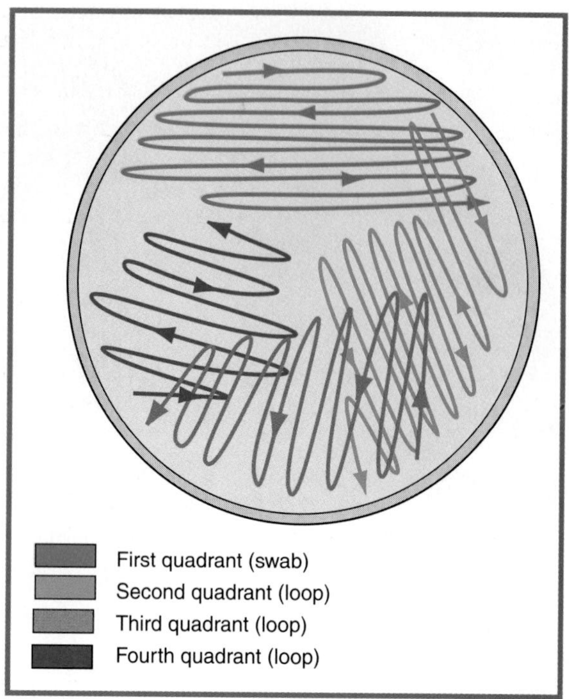

FIGURE 46–6 Basic streaking pattern. (From Stepp CA, Woods MA: Laboratory Procedures for Medical Office Personnel. Philadelphia, WB Saunders, 1998.)

Types of Media

A variety of growth media is available to promote the optimum growth of microorganisms. A growth medium may be liquid, semisolid, or solid. Liquid broth can be solidified by adding agar, a seaweed extract. The agar broth may come in tubes or plates, also called Petri dishes. Media can be selective or nonselective. Selective media allow the growth of specific bacteria while inhibiting the growth of others. Eosin methylene blue (EMB), MacConkey, and Thayer-Martin are examples of selective media. Nonselective media support the growth of most bacteria. Generally, this medium is blood agar. This contains sheep blood and tryptic soy broth (TSB). These media have undergone extensive quality control testing for both sterility and appropriate reactions with certain organisms. An expiration date appears on each tube or plate. The used containers are autoclaved and then disposed of.

Blood agar is used for performing throat cultures. The organism that causes strep throat (*Streptococcus*) is able to use the red blood cells in the agar for growth. This growth results in a detectable change in the medium called **hemolysis.** For urine cultures, two types of media are used: EMB or MacConkey and blood agar. The organism *Escherichia coli* is commonly isolated from urine (Fig. 46–5).

Memory Jogger

10 *What would be your choice of medium for a throat culture?*

Cultures

To **inoculate** a culture, a swab or loop is passed lightly over the surface of an agar medium in a zigzag pattern (Fig. 46–6). Broths are inoculated by

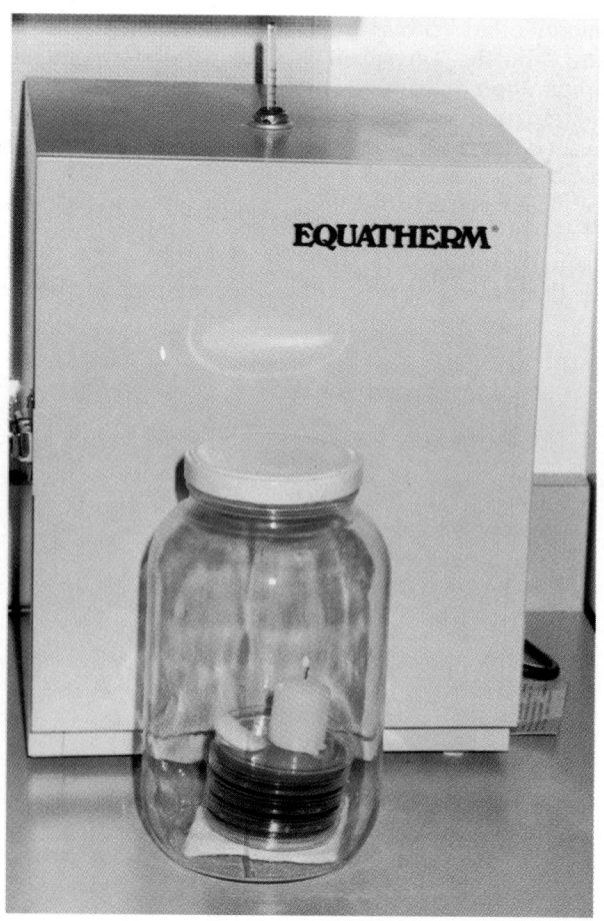

FIGURE 46–7 Candle jar used as incubator.

swirling the swab or loop in them. The inoculated tubes or plates are incubated at 37° C for 24 hours and are then examined for growth. (See Procedures 46–1 through 46–4.)

Some organisms require a high concentration of carbon dioxide (CO_2) for growth. Transport plates of chocolate agar or Thayer-Martin agar have a CO_2-generating tablet that is placed in a well in the plate immediately after inoculation. Without this special atmosphere, organisms such as *Neisseria gonorrhoeae,* which causes gonorrhea, would die. The plate is then placed into the incubator or, alternatively, in a sealed jar with a lighted candle. The burning of the candle generates CO_2 (Fig. 46–7).

Text continued on page 959

PROCEDURE 46–1
Inoculating a Blood Agar Plate for Culture of Strep Throat

GOAL

To inoculate a blood agar plate for culture of strep throat.

EQUIPMENT AND SUPPLIES

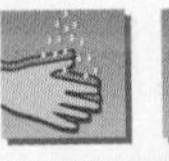

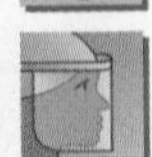
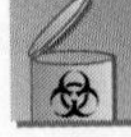

- Blood agar plate
- Bacitracin disk or strep A disk
- Bacti-cinerator
- Inoculating loop
- Permanent marker
- Swab from patient's throat (see Procedure 30–3)
- Forceps

PROCEDURAL STEPS

1 Wash and dry your hands. Glove and apply face protection.
PURPOSE: Infection control.

2 Remove the swab from the container. Grasp the plate by the bottom (media side), and lift the cover, or lift the cover while the plate is on the table.
PURPOSE: To make handling the plate easier and to prevent contamination of the plate.

3 Roll the swab down the middle of the top half of the plate, then use the swab to streak the same half of the plate. Dispose of the swab properly (Figure 1*).
PURPOSE: Rolling the swab ensures contact with the surface of the agar.

Continued

*Figures from Stepp CA, Woods MA: Laboratory Procedures for Medical Office Personnel. Philadelphia, WB Saunders, 1998.

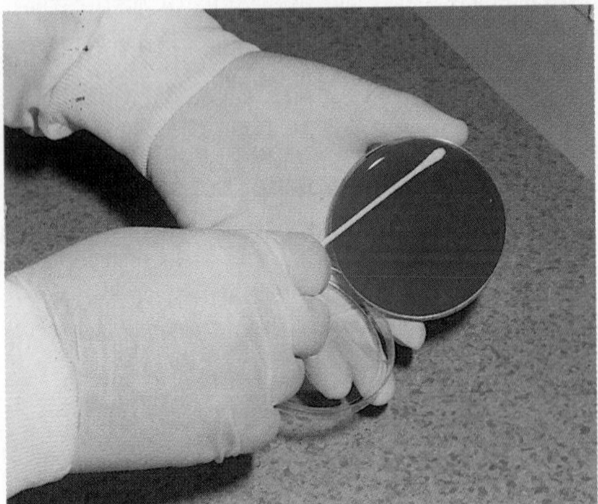

FIGURE 1

PROCEDURE 46-1 (CONTINUED)
Inoculating a Blood Agar Plate for Culture of Strep Throat

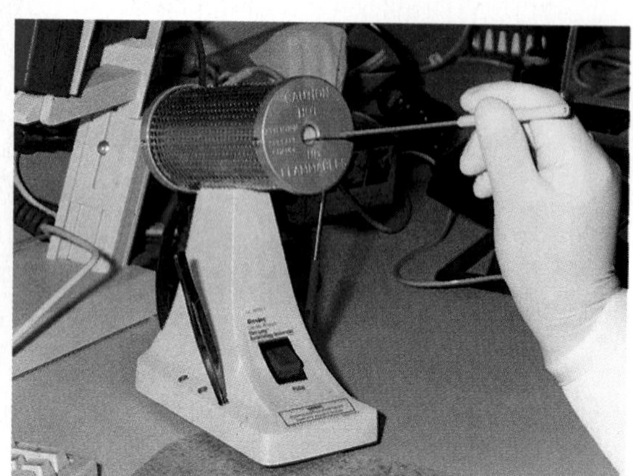

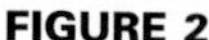

FIGURE 2

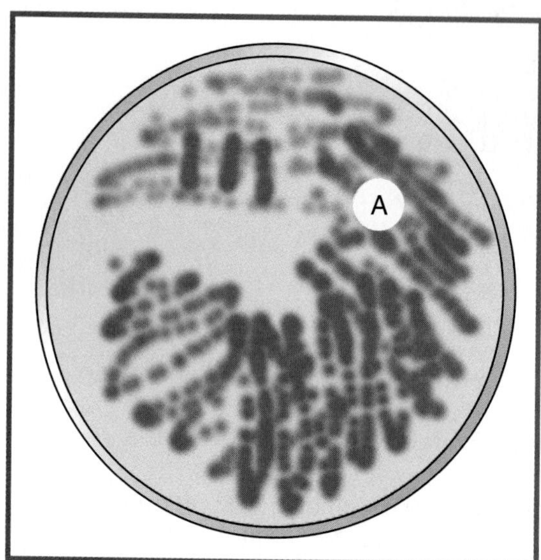

FIGURE 3

4 Sterilize the loop in the Bacti-cinerator, and allow it to cool (Figure 2).
PURPOSE: Loops must be sterilized before and after use, to prevent cross-contamination of specimens.

5 Streak for isolation of colonies in the third and fourth quadrants, using the loop. Use the loop to make three slices in the agar in the area of heavy inoculum. Sterilize the loop (Figure 3).
PURPOSE: Isolated colonies are needed for observation of colony morphology. The agar is sliced where the disk is to be placed, to allow for detection of subsurface hemolysis.

6 Sterilize the forceps and remove one disk from the vial. Place the disk on the agar between the cuts. Sterilize the forceps.
PURPOSE: Group A beta-hemolytic streptococci are presumptively identified by their sensitivity to the disk.

7 Label with permanent marker the agar side of the plate with the patient's name and identification number and the date.
PURPOSE: Labeling the agar side of dish prevents mixing up specimens.

8 Place the plate in the incubator, with the agar side of the plate on the top.
PURPOSE: Placing the plate with the agar side up prevents accumulation of moisture on the surface of the agar.

9 Record all information in the patient's medical record.
PURPOSE: A procedure is not considered done until it is recorded.

10 Incubate for 24 hours and then examine. Incubate negative cultures for an additional 24 hours.
PURPOSE: Some hemolysis patterns are not well defined after 24 hours of growth.

11 Clean the work area and properly dispose of all biohazard waste.

12 Remove your gloves and wash your hands.

PROCEDURE 46-2

Streaking Plates for Quantitative Cultures

GOAL

To inoculate two plates with urine, using quantitative streaking methods.

EQUIPMENT AND SUPPLIES

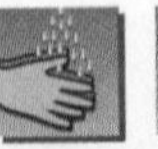

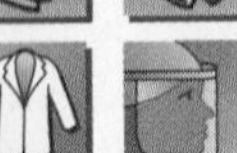
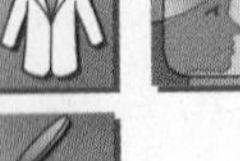
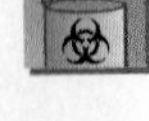

Urine specimen
Bacti-cinerator
Calibrated inoculating loop
Blood agar plate or biplates, which are plates having both blood agar and either EMB or MacKintex in a single plate

PROCEDURAL STEPS

1 Wash and dry your hands. Glove and apply face protection.
PURPOSE: Infection control.

2 Mix the urine specimen thoroughly by swirling.
PURPOSE: Microorganisms settle to the bottom of the specimen when the specimen is allowed to stand.

3 Sterilize the calibrated loop, cool, and dip the tip into the specimen.
PURPOSE: The loop must be allowed to cool, or the heat will destroy the microorganisms as the loop comes into contact with the urine specimen, resulting in falsely low colony counts on the culture. Urine on the shaft of the loop will run down the shaft and increase the size of the specimen deposited on the plate, resulting in a falsely elevated colony count on the culture.

4 Deposit the specimen on the plate, as indicated in Figure 1 in Procedure 46–1. Use the loop to streak as shown in Figure 3 in Procedure 46–1.
PURPOSE: Careful streaking of the plates is necessary for an accurate estimate of the organisms present.

5 Inoculate the second plate in the same manner.

6 Label the bottom of the plates with the patient's name and identification number and the date.
PURPOSE: Labeling the bottom of the plates prevents mixing up of the specimens.

7 Record all information in the patient's medical record.

8 Place the plates in the incubator, with the agar sides of the plates facing up.

9 Incubate for 24 hours, then identify organisms.

10 Clean the work area, dispose of all biohazard waste, remove gloves, and wash your hands.

11 Record procedure in patient's medical record.
PURPOSE: A procedure is not considered done until it is properly recorded.

PROCEDURE 46–3
Preparing a Direct Smear or Culture Smear for Staining

GOAL
To prepare a smear for staining from a clinical specimen or from a culture medium.

EQUIPMENT AND SUPPLIES
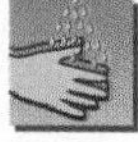

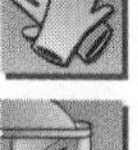
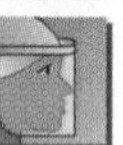
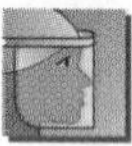
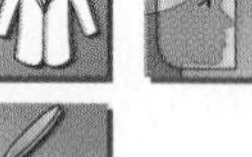

Clean glass slides
Permanent marker
Bacti-cinerator
Saline solution
Specimen

PROCEDURAL STEPS
Direct Smear

1 Wash and dry your hands. Glove and put on face protection.

2 Label the slide with a permanent marking pen.
PURPOSE: Other labels are destroyed in the staining process.

3 Prepare a thin smear by rolling the swab on the slide. Make certain that all areas of the swab touch the slide (Figure 1).
PURPOSE: Rolling the swab ensures that all parts of the swab come in contact with the slide so that the organisms collected are deposited on the slide. Thin smears are needed for evaluation.

4 Allow the smear to air dry. Do not wave it or heat-dry it.
PURPOSE: Waving the slide spreads pathogens. Overheating organisms distorts them.

5 Hold the slide with the smear up. Heat-fix the slide using a Bacti-cinerator. Check the heating process by touching the slide to the back of the hand (Figure 2). The slide should feel warm,

Continued

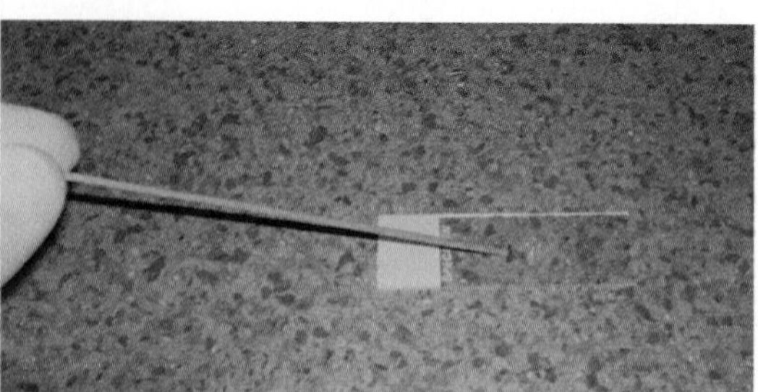
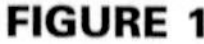

FIGURE 1

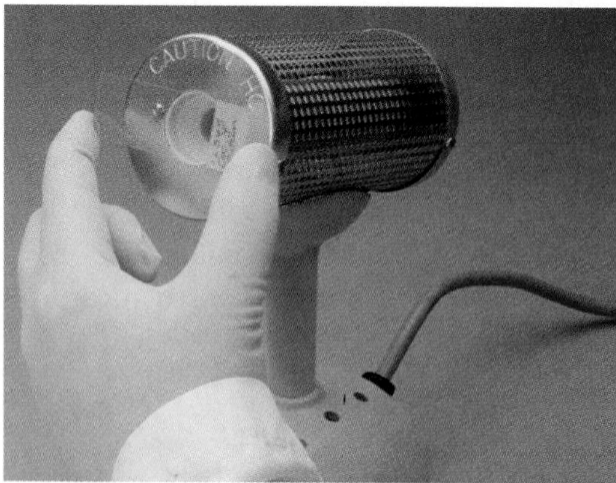

FIGURE 2

not hot. Check it often by touching the back of the slide to the back of the hand. Cool the slide.
PURPOSE: Heat-fixing causes materials to adhere to the slide.

Culture Smear

1 Wash and dry your hands. Glove yourself and don face protection.
2 Identify the colonies to be stained by circling them on the back of the plate and numbering them with a permanent marker. Label the slide accordingly.
PURPOSE: This allows accurate identification of colonies.
3 Apply a small drop of saline solution to the slide, using a loop.
PURPOSE: Liquid is needed to emulsify the colony. Large drops require a longer drying time.
4 Touch, with a sterile loop, only the top of the colony chosen. Transfer the material picked up to the appropriate area of the slide, and spread it in a circular motion to the size of a dime. Repeat for each colony chosen.
PURPOSE: Only a small amount of colony is needed for staining.
5 Allow the smear to air dry.
6 Heat-fix the smear.
7 Properly dispose of all biohazard materials and clean the work area.
8 Remove gloves and wash your hands.

PROCEDURE 46-4
Staining a Smear with Gram Stain

GOAL

To stain a slide, using Gram stain, so that the organisms present are colored appropriately (neither overcolorized nor too strongly decolorized).

EQUIPMENT AND SUPPLIES

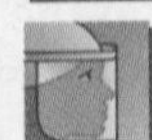
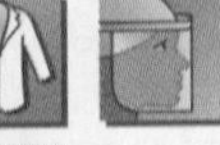
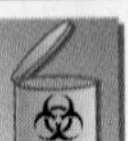

Gram stain reagents
Staining rack
Forceps
Wash bottle of water
Prepared smear for staining
Absorbent paper

PROCEDURAL STEPS

1 Wash and dry your hands. Glove and put on face protection.
PURPOSE: Infection control.
2 Place the slide face up on a level staining rack.
PURPOSE: If the slide is face down, the organisms will not be stained. If the rack is uneven, the stain will run off the slide surface.

Continued

PROCEDURE 46-4 (CONTINUED)
Staining a Smear with Gram Stain

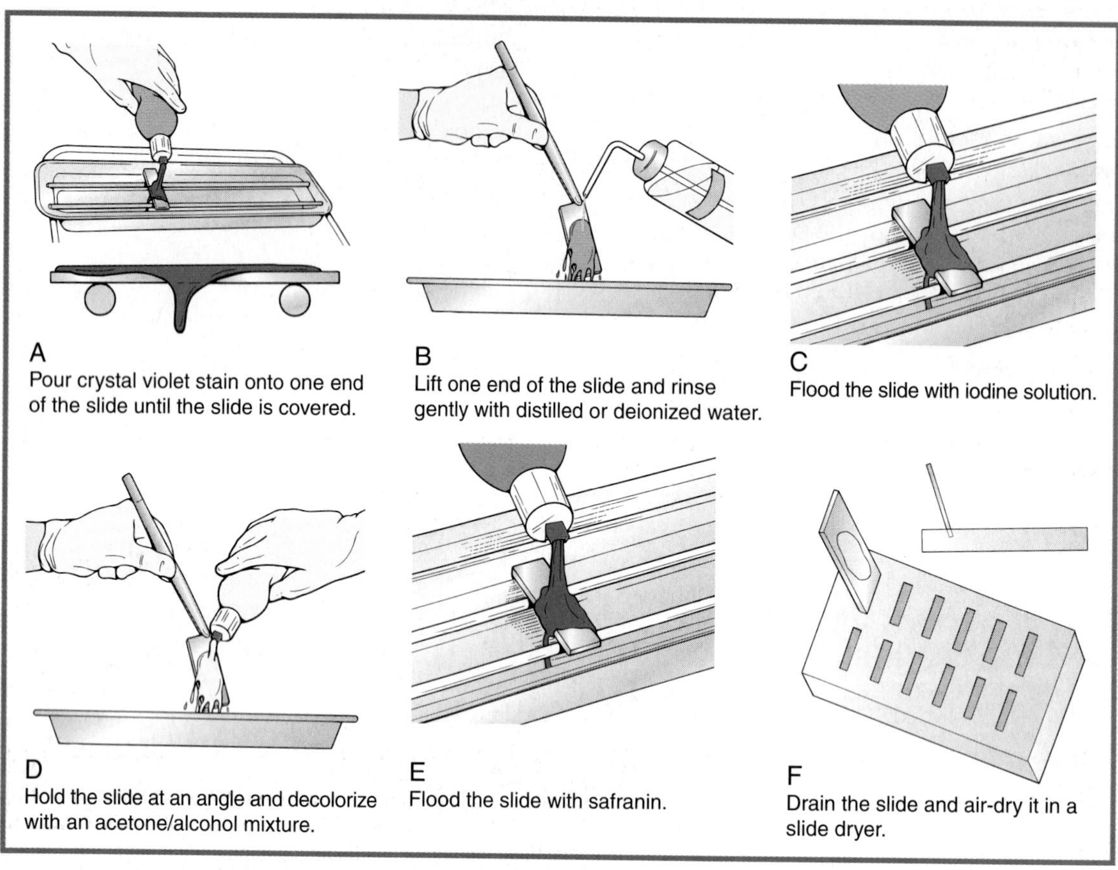

A
Pour crystal violet stain onto one end of the slide until the slide is covered.

B
Lift one end of the slide and rinse gently with distilled or deionized water.

C
Flood the slide with iodine solution.

D
Hold the slide at an angle and decolorize with an acetone/alcohol mixture.

E
Flood the slide with safranin.

F
Drain the slide and air-dry it in a slide dryer.

FIGURE 1

3 Flood the slide with crystal violet. Time for 30 seconds. Figure 1* shows the entire staining process.
PURPOSE: Crystal violet is the primary stain and colors everything purple.

4 Flood the stain off with a sharp stream of water from the wash bottle. With forceps, tip the slide to remove the water.
PURPOSE: Using forceps keeps your fingers clean.

5 Flood the slide with Gram's iodine (mordant). Time for 30 seconds.
PURPOSE: Gram's iodine causes the stain to set in the organisms that are gram positive.

6 Flood the iodine off with water. Grasp the slide with forceps, and hold it nearly vertical.

7 Decolorize by running the decolorizer (alcohol) down the slide until the smear stops, giving off purple stain in all but the thickest portions (about 10 seconds).
PURPOSE: This is the critical step. The decolorizer removes stain from the organisms that are gram-negative.

Continued

*From Stepp CA, Woods MA: Laboratory Procedures for Medical Office Personnel. Philadelphia, WB Saunders, 1998.

8 Rinse the slide with water, and return it to the staining rack.

9 Flood the slide with safranin, and time for 30 seconds.
PURPOSE: Safranin is the counterstain and stains red everything that decolorized.

10 Rinse the slide well with water.

11 Wipe off the back of the slide with an alcohol tissue.
PURPOSE: The back of the slide is cleaned to remove traces of stain, which make examination of the smear difficult.

12 Blot the slide dry between sheets of absorbent paper.

13 Clean the work area. Remove gloves and wash your hands.

14 Record the procedure in the patient's record.
PURPOSE: A procedure is not considered done until it is properly recorded.

ANTIMICROBIAL SENSITIVITY TESTING

Isolating the infectious agent from a patient is only the first step in successful treatment. Most bacteria exhibit resistance to antimicrobial agents. These patterns of resistance are continuously changing; therefore, they cannot be predicted.

Shifting patterns of resistance require testing of individual bacteria against the appropriate antimicrobial agent.

HOW TO DEFINE THE APPROPRIATE ANTIMICROBIAL AGENT

- Demonstrates the most activity against the infectious agent
- Has the least toxicity to the patient
- Has the least impact on the normal flora of the body
- Has the desired pharmacologic characteristics
- Is the most economical

The clinical microbiology laboratory can only recommend antimicrobial agents based on their **in vitro** activity. The final therapeutic outcome is the decision of the physician. The physician bases this decision on numerous factors, including the test results, the physical examination, and the knowledge of the patient. The expertise of a pharmacologist can be very helpful in choosing the most effective antimicrobial agent for the patient.

Whenever you are inoculating specimens, **asepsis** must be strictly observed to ensure safety and good results.

RAPID CULTURE METHODS

Physician's office laboratories are permitted to perform many rapid culture tests. The tests used in a particular laboratory depend on the number of tests performed per month and the amount of refrigerator space available for storage. Dry media tests have a long shelf life, do not require refrigeration, and occupy little incubator space. Some types of test kits contain small screw-top vials of media on paddles. The vials are self-standing for growth in any conventional incubator and do not require refrigeration before use. The long plastic containers can be used in their own incubator or in a conventional incubator. They must be refrigerated until ready to be used. The rapid culture methods offer presumptive identification of most organisms. Further specialization and sensitivity testing require additional materials, equipment, and procedures. Rapid tests are designed to give the physician a positive indication of the problem so that treatment may be instituted. For a differential or a specific diagnosis, the physician may need additional test results.

Memory Jogger

What form of rapid culture kits have a long shelf life?

INTERPRETATION OF THROAT CULTURE

Group A beta-hemolytic streptococci (*Streptococcus pyogenes*) cause septic sore throat and are capable of producing severe complications if not diagnosed and treated. Complications include scarlet fever, rheumatic fever, and glomerulonephritis. Group A beta-hemolytic streptococci may be identified by placing an antibiotic (bacitracin) disk on a streaked plate and observing inhibition of any bacterial growth after 24 hours of incubation (Fig. 46–8). Complete clearing of the agar around the colonies indicates beta-hemolysis.

Several slide and tube tests have been developed for the detection of group A streptococci directly from throat cultures. The tests can be performed while the patient waits. The patient's throat is swabbed, the swab is placed in a tube, reagents are added at timed intervals, and a liquid extract is expressed from the swab onto a slide. Reagents are added and mixed. The slide is gently rocked and then examined for agglutination after a specified time. **Agglutination** indicates the presence of group A streptococci. The entire procedure can be performed in approximately 15 minutes (see Procedure 46–5).

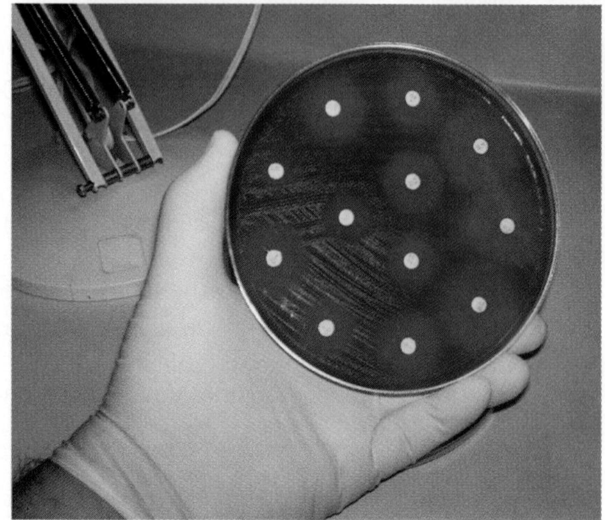

FIGURE 46–8 Group A beta-*Streptococcus* kit. Note disks placed for identification.

PROCEDURE 46–5
Performing a Rapid Strep Test

GOAL

To properly prepare a slide for microscopic identification of group A beta-hemolytic streptococci.

EQUIPMENT AND SUPPLIES

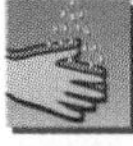

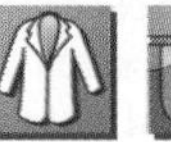
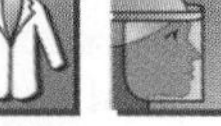
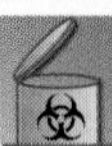

- Directigen Test kit of Strep A
- Timer or wristwatch with sweep second hand
- Throat swab specimen (see Procedure 30–3)

PROCEDURAL STEPS

1 Collect all supplies and equipment needed to perform the test. Bring all reagents and reaction disks to room temperature (minimum of 30 minutes).

2 Wash and dry your hands. Put on gloves and face protection.
PURPOSE: Infection control.

3 Position all bottles vertically, and dispense reagents slowly as free-falling drops. Avoid reagent contact with your eyes because the reagent is an irritant (Figure 1).

4 Add 3 drops of reagent 1 to an extraction tube. This solution is pink.

5 Add 3 drops of reagent 2 to the same tube. The solution should turn yellow.

6 Place the specimen swab in the tube, twirling the swab in the mix.

7 Let stand for exactly 1 minute.

Continued

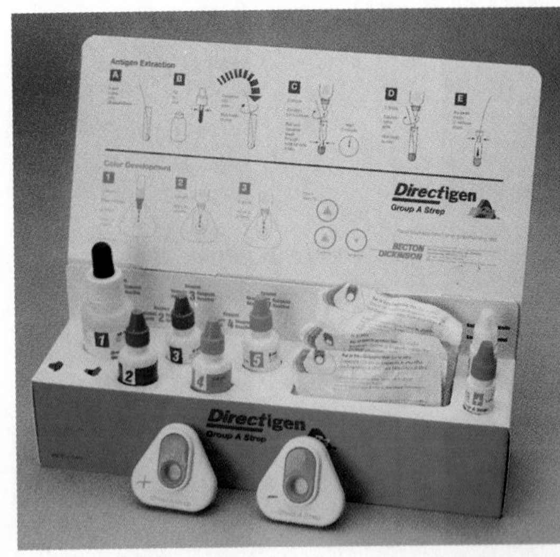

FIGURE 1

8 Add 3 drops of reagent 3 to the same tube, again twirling the swab in the tube to mix. This solution should be pink.

9 Express the liquid from the swab by squeezing the tube with the thumb and forefinger and rotating the swab as it is withdrawn. The liquid must be thoroughly removed from the swab. Best results are achieved when the liquid reaches or exceeds the line on the tube.

10 Discard the swab in a biohazard waste container.

11 Remove the reaction disk from the pouch and place it on a dry, flat surface.

12 Pour the entire contents of the tube into the reaction disk.

13 Read the test results when the entire end of assay window turns red (5 to 10 minutes).

14 Properly dispose of all contaminated waste.
PURPOSE: Items contacting samples are considered potentially infectious.

15 Clean work area, remove gloves, and wash your hands.
PURPOSE: Infection control.

16 Record the test results in the patient's medical record.
PURPOSE: A procedure is considered not done until it is properly recorded.

TESTING FOR PINWORMS

Enterobius vermicularis, commonly called a pinworm, is a parasite that primarily infests young children. Humans are infected by ingestion of mature eggs via hand-to-mouth transfers, feces-contaminated fingers, or feces-contaminated foods or liquids or by inhaling eggs in air currents from infected areas. The eggs hatch in the small intestine, with the females migrating out of the anus, usually at night, to deposit the eggs. The eggs adhere to the skin, perianal hairs, sleeping garments, and other clothing items. This results in itching of the anal area, whereby the eggs come in contact with the hands and fingernails of the host.

In children, specimens are best collected late at night or early in the morning before a bowel movement, urination, or bathing. Petroleum jelly–impregnated paraffin swabs or cellulose tape may be used to collect the eggs deposited by the adult worm during the night. Diagnosis is based on laboratory detection of the eggs in fecal smears.

If the parent does not feel comfortable in obtaining the needed specimen, instruct the parent to bring the child to the office as soon as he or she awakens in the morning. Advise the parent to not change the child's clothing or change the child's diaper before coming to the office but bring the child immediately upon waking. When the child arrives, have all of the needed supplies ready to use and do the procedure immediately (see Procedure 46–6).

PROCEDURE 46-6

Performing a Cellulose Tape Collection for Pinworms

GOAL

To obtain a rectal sample using cellulose tape for the purpose of testing for pinworm eggs.

EQUIPMENT AND SUPPLIES

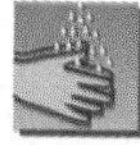

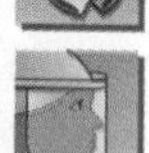
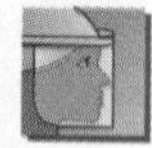
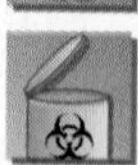

Glass slide
Clear cellulose tape
Wooden tongue depressor
Toluene
Microscope
Gauze or cotton balls

PROCEDURAL STEPS

Ask the patient to assist you with this procedure.

1 Gather and prepare supplies and equipment needed for obtaining the specimen.
   a. Place a strip of cellulose tape on a glass slide, starting ½ inch from one end and running toward the same end. Continuing around this end lengthwise. Tear off the strip so that it is even with the other end (Figure 1*). *Note:* Do not use Magic transparent tape; use regular clear cellulose tape.
   b. Place a strip of paper measuring ½ × 1 inch between the slide and the tape at the end where the tape is torn flush. This will be the specimen labeling area.

   As soon as the child arrives, place the child with the attending parent in the prepared examination room.

2 Wash hands, glove, and apply face protection.
   PURPOSE: Infection control.

3 Remove the clothing and diaper from the child and lay the child in a prone position, over the parent's lap, with the buttocks in a superior plane.

4 To obtain the perianal sample, first peel back the tape on the slide by gripping the label (Figure 2). With the tape looped (adhesive side outward) over a wooden tongue depressor

Continued

*Figures from Stepp CA, Woods MA: Laboratory Procedures for Medical Office Personnel. Philadelphia, WB Saunders, 1998.

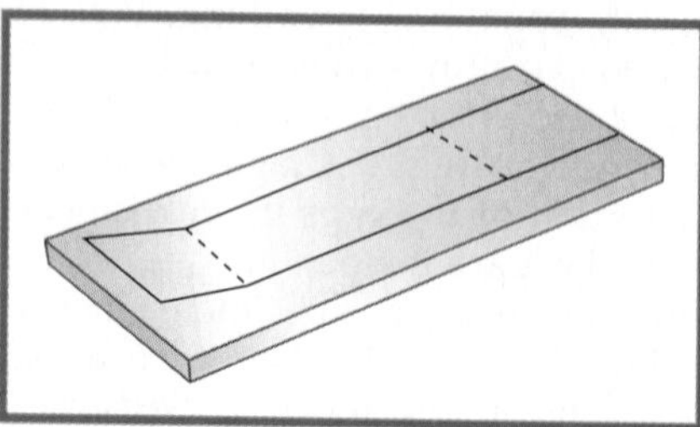

FIGURE 1

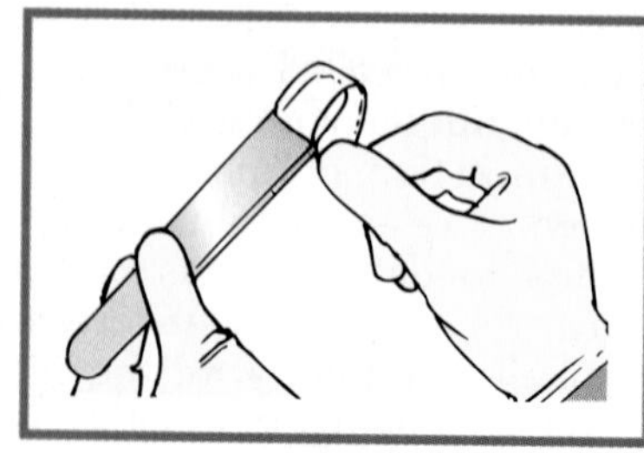

FIGURE 2

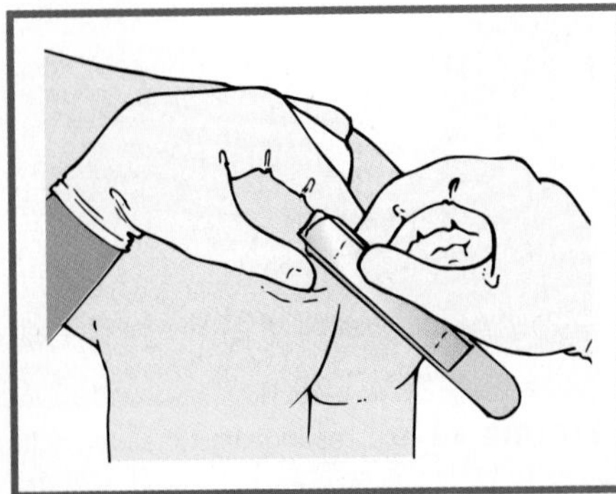

FIGURE 3

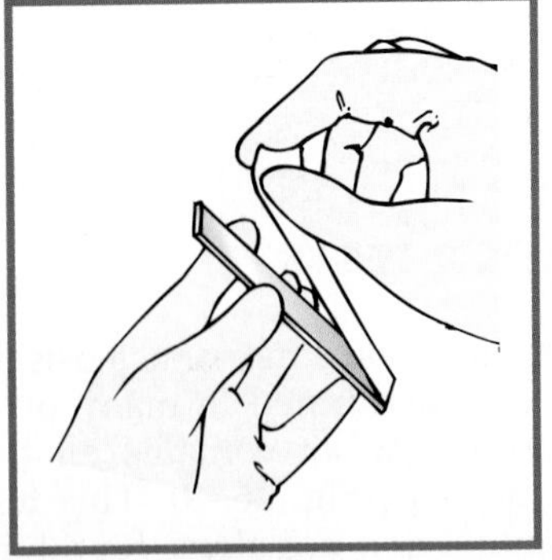

FIGURE 4

that is held against the slide and extended about 1 inch beyond it, press the tape firmly against the right and left anal folds (Figure 3).

5 Spread the tape back on the slide, adhesive side down (Figure 4).

6 Smooth the tape using a cotton ball or gauze square (Figure 5).

7 Write the patient's name and date on the slide label.

8 Advise the parent that the child can be dressed or assist with dressing the child if needed.

Testing the Sample

9 Lift one side of the tape and apply 1 drop of toluene before pressing the tape back down on the glass slide.
PURPOSE: This will clear the specimen so that any eggs will be visible.

10 Place the prepared slide under the microscope's low-power objective and examine it under low illumination (Figure 6).

11 Report and record your findings in the patient's record as a positive result if pinworm eggs were visualized and a negative result if no eggs were seen.

12 Dispose of all biohazard waste, clean the work area, remove gloves, and wash your hands.

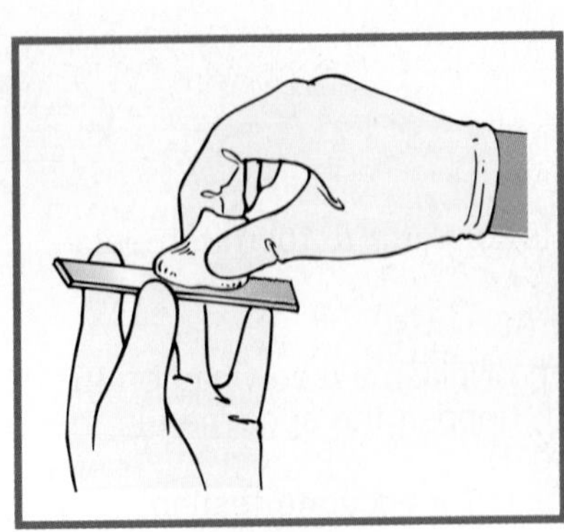

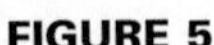

FIGURE 5

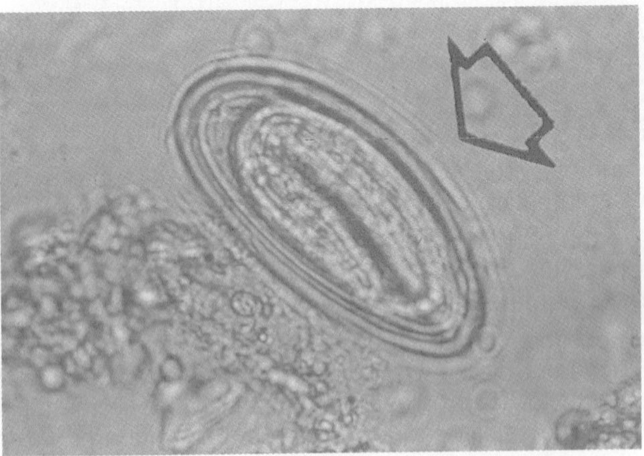

FIGURE 6

Memory Jogger

 *Recall how humans are infected with pinworms.*

SLIDE AGGLUTINATION TESTS

The screening test for infectious mononucleosis is included here because it is performed in many physician's office laboratories. The kit contains all the supplies and reagents needed (Fig. 46–9). This test is an example of agglutination reactions found in many testing procedures. In agglutination tests, antigen-coated red cells (or latex particles) and antibodies are combined in a test tube or on a microscopic glass slide. The test suspension is rocked or mixed for a specified amount of time and is observed for the presence of clumping. The visible clumps indicate a positive test. Known positive and negative controls are run at the same time as the patient's sample to ensure qualitative control. (See Procedure 46–7).

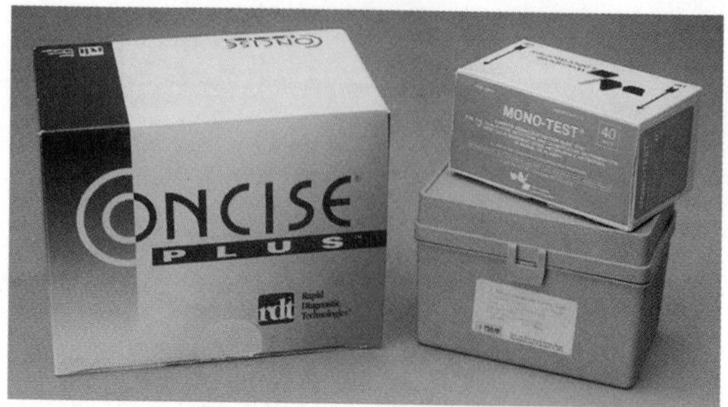

FIGURE 46–9 Testing kits for slide agglutination.

PROCEDURE 46–7

Mono-Test for Infectious Mononucleosis

GOAL

To perform and interpret a slide test for infectious mononucleosis.

EQUIPMENT AND SUPPLIES

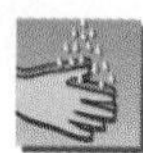  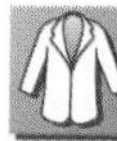 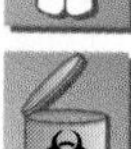

Mono-test kit
Blood specimen (serum or plasma)

PROCEDURAL STEPS

1 Wash and dry your hands. Glove and put on face protection.
PURPOSE: Infection control.

2 Remove the test kit from the refrigerator, and allow the reagents to warm to room temperature. Check the expiration date of the kit.
PURPOSE: Outdated or cold reagents do not react as expected.

3 Fill a disposable capillary tube to the calibration mark with serum or plasma (see Chapter 45 for collection of blood). Using the rubber bulb included in the kit, deposit the specimen in the first circle of the clean glass slide also provided in the kit (Figure 1).
PURPOSE: The capillary tube measures the exact amount of sample for accurate testing.

4 Place one drop of negative control in the second circle and one drop of positive control in the third circle (Figure 2).
PURPOSE: Known controls ensure that reagents are functioning properly.

Continued

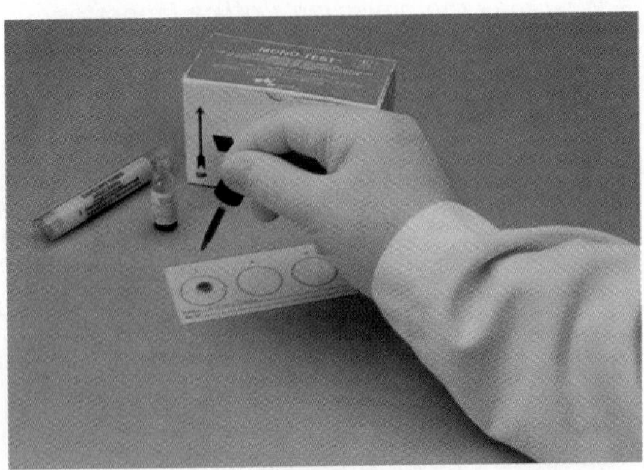

FIGURE 1

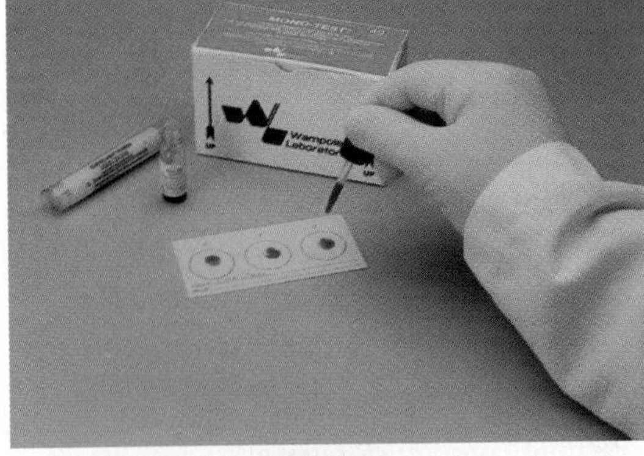

FIGURE 2

5 Thoroughly mix the Mono-Test reagent by rolling the bottle gently between the palms of the hands. Squeeze the enclosed dropper to mix all the contents of the bottle.
PURPOSE: Reagent red blood cells settle on standing and must be mixed before use.

6 Hold the dropper in a vertical position, and add one drop of Mono-Test reagent to each area of the slide. Do not touch the dropper to the slide.
PURPOSE: Holding a dropper vertically ensures delivery of the same size drop. If the dropper touches other materials, it becomes contaminated, and results will be inaccurate.

7 Using separate stirrers, quickly and thoroughly mix each area, spreading each area out to 1 inch in diameter.
PURPOSE: Failure to use a clean stirrer for each area would invalidate the test because of cross-contamination.

8 Rock the slide gently for exactly 2 minutes; observe immediately for agglutination. A dark background is best for viewing.
PURPOSE: Timing is always important.

9 Interpret the test results, and record them. Agglutination is positive, and no agglutination is negative.

10 Clean the work area. Remove gloves, and wash your hands.

11 Record the test results in the patient's medical record.
PURPOSE: A procedure is not considered done until it is properly recorded.

COLLECTION OF SEMEN

Semen analysis is usually performed for fertility studies and after vasectomies to establish the effectiveness of the vasectomy. The patient is advised to refrain from intercourse for 2 to 4 days before the sample is collected. Instruct the patient to collect the total specimen in an opaque glass container. Masturbation or coitus interruptus may be employed as methods of obtaining the specimen, but if the latter is used, great care must be taken to collect the entire ejaculate. Condoms should never be employed, because the latex has definite spermicidal qualities. The cap of the container must be tightly closed, with the patient's name, the date, and the time of ejaculation written on the label. The specimen must be kept at body temperature and must be delivered to the laboratory within 3 hours after collection.

Memory Jogger

 *Why should condoms never be employed when collecting semen for analysis?*

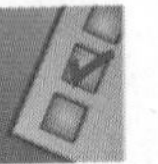

PATIENT EDUCATION

Microorganisms such as bacteria, viruses, fungi, and parasites are responsible for most human diseases.

Patient education plays an important role in helping the patient and the patient's family to control the spread of infection.

The following is a list of teaching topics that will help you in educating the patient in infection control:

- An explanation of the patient's type of infection—bacterial, viral, fungal, or parasitic
- How infection spreads
- Normal barriers to infection
- Risk factors for infection
- Patient preparation for cultures and serologic, hematologic, and imaging tests, as necessary
- The patient's role in specimen collection
- Hand washing, proper storage and cleaning of personal items, and disposal of contaminated supplies

Explain to the patient that infection does not always occur at the entry site; for example, measles can be transmitted through the respiratory tract or through the conjunctivae by touching an affected patient and then rubbing the eye.

Reinforce the need for strict adherence to the prescribed antimicrobial therapy by pointing out the possible complications of noncompliance, such as relapse or systemic involvement. Explain to the patient that inadequate drug therapy (not taking the medication as prescribed) may cause the infection to worsen and spread.

Above all, *always listen to the patient;* be sure that the questions asked are answered. Don't try to answer questions that you are unsure of. Notify the physician of the patient's concerns so that the doctor can include the answers and explanations in the patient's consultation.

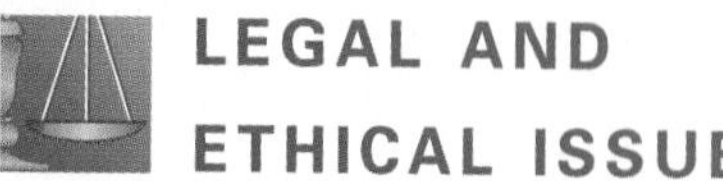

LEGAL AND ETHICAL ISSUES

Maintaining a laboratory in the office increases the physician's liability. By testing patients' specimens in the office, the physician assumes responsibility for the interpretation and accuracy of the results. As the person in the office who runs the tests and notes the results on the patient's chart, it is your responsibility to maintain optimal accuracy in the testing results. A *quality assurance* (QA) program for physician's office laboratories may reduce the risks involved and still allow the patient to benefit from the convenience of office testing.

Physician's office laboratories that have established QA programs, with written policies and procedures that govern their laboratory testing and ensure that these policies are implemented, are in compliance. If the office where you are employed does not have laboratory guidelines, suggest developing testing guidelines.

Memory Jogger

14 *Why may the physician's office laboratory increase the physician's liability?*

CRITICAL THINKING

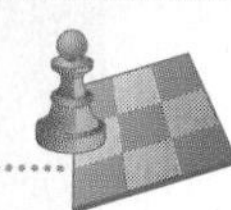

1 Is rickets caused by the parasite *Rickettsia?* Use outside references to substantiate your answer.

2 A child's parents are irate when told that their 5-year-old child probably has pinworms and a specimen will need to be obtained for confirmation. How would you handle the situation?

3 Why is it important for the physician's office laboratory to develop and maintain testing guidelines?

HOW DID I DO? Answers to Memory Joggers

1 Microbiology is the study of microorganisms including bacteria, fungi, viruses, rickettsiae, mycobacteria, and parasites.

2 The skin, respiratory tract, and gastrointestinal tract are inhabited by harmless bacteria called natural flora.

3 Morphologic classification of bacteria include cocci, bacilli, and spirilla.

4 Fungi thrive in warm, moist, and dark environments.

5 The nucleic acid core of the virus is either RNA or DNA but never both.

6 Most parasites are identified in urine, sputum, tissue fluids, or tissue biopsy samples.

7 Pathogens that thrive in oxygen are called aerobes.

8 Microbiology specimens are most often contaminated by normal flora from the site of collection.

9 Protocols for bacteriologic specimen collection include optimal collection times, sufficient sample, proper equipment and procedures, and the type of specimen collected.

10 Blood agar is the medium of choice for throat cultures.

11 Dry media tests have a long shelf life and do not require refrigeration.

12 Humans are infected with pinworms by ingestion of mature eggs, feces-contaminated fingers, feces-contaminated foods and liquids, and inhalation of eggs in the air current.

13 Condoms should never be used because the latex has definite spermicidal qualities.

14 By testing patient's specimens, the physician assumes responsibility for the interpretation and accuracy of the results.

Notes

SECTION 10

Advanced Clinical Care Techniques

CURRICULUM CONTENT/COMPETENCIES

Chapter 47: Nutrition and Exercise

- *Project a professional image.*
- *Adapt communications to individual's ability to understand*
- *Practice within the scope of education, training, and personal capabilities*
- *Instruct individuals according to their needs*

Chapters 48 and 49: Pharmacology Applications

- *Apply principles of aseptic technique and infection control*
- *Prepare and administer medications and immunizations*
- *Maintain confidentiality*
- *Document accurately*

Chapters 50 to 52: Assisting with Surgical Procedures

- *Apply principles of aseptic technique and infection control*
- *Comply with quality assurance practices*
- *Maintain and dispose of regulated substances in compliance with government guidelines*
- *Maintain supply inventory*
- *Evaluate and recommend equipment and supplies*

Nutrition and Exercise

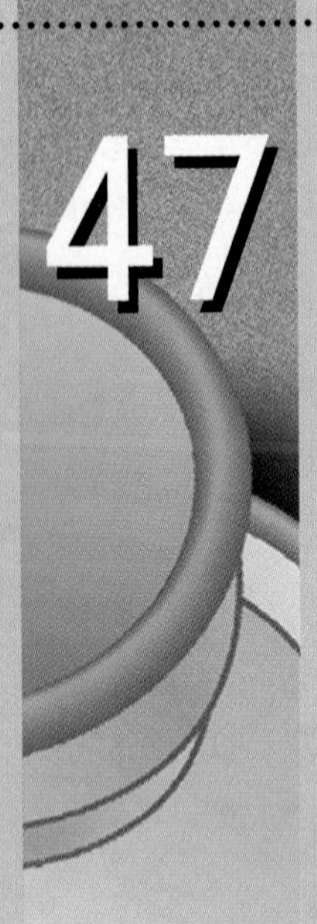

OUTLINE

LEARNING OBJECTIVES

Cognitive: On successful completion of this chapter you should be able to:

1 Describe normal nutrition.
2 List the six areas of the Food Guide Pyramid.
3 Discuss the meaning of "recommended dietary allowance."
4 Calculate the caloric value of carbohydrates, fats, and proteins.
5 Differentiate between vitamins and minerals.
6 Describe the role of carbohydrates in the daily diet.
7 Explain the need for minerals in the diet.
8 Outline the three phases of prescribing a diet.
9 Recognize possible eating disorders.
10 Understand the role that exercise plays in good health.
11 Define and spell vocabulary terms.

Performance: On successful completion of this chapter you should be able to:

1 Read and interpret food labels.
2 Measure body fat using the caliper method.

VOCABULARY

amino acids Twenty organic compounds that form the chief constituents of protein and are used by the body to build and repair tissues

anorexia nervosa An emotional disorder characterized by a refusal to eat and an altered physical self-image

bulimia Abnormal increase in hunger characterized by binge eating and self-induced vomiting

calorie The amount of heat necessary to raise the temperature of 1 g of water 1° C or a pint of water 4° F.

cholesterol Substance produced by the liver found in plant and animal fats, such as saturated oils, egg yolk, and milk, that can produce fatty deposits in the blood vessels

carbohydrates Chemical substances, including sugars, glycogen, starches, dextrins, and celluloses, that contain only carbon, oxygen, and hydrogen

deficiencies Conditions caused by a below-normal intake of a particular substance

diabetes mellitus Disorder of carbohydrate metabolism caused by underproduction of insulin and characterized by excessive urinary output and weight loss

dietitian Person with a bachelor's degree in foods and nutrition who is concerned with the maintenance and promotion of health and the treatment of diseases through diet

digestion Process of converting food into chemical substances that can be used by the body

endogenous Produced within or caused by factors within the organism

exogenous Produced outside or caused by factors outside the organism

fats Adipose tissues of the body that serve as an energy reserve

hydrogenated Combined with, treated with, or exposed to hydrogen

obesity An excessive accumulation of body fat (usually defined as more than 20% above the recommended body weight)

proteins Organic compounds occurring in plants and animals that contain the major elements carbon, hydrogen, oxygen, and nitrogen and the amino acids essential for life maintenance

turgor Resistance of the skin to being grasped between the fingers and released; refers to normal skin tension

Now more than ever, the public wants to know about the food it eats and how food affects health. Tremendous progress in the improvement of the general health of Americans has occurred over the past century, and an increase in longevity has resulted from the control of preventable disease through better nutrition. Factors that affect one's health include proper care and functioning of all body organs, good diet, and a sound mental attitude. It is generally agreed that good nutrition is one of the most important environmental factors that affect the health of an individual, a community, or a nation.

Good health is the state of emotional and physical well-being that is determined, to a large extent, by a person's diet. We are, quite literally, what we eat, because the food we consume is used to build and repair every part of our bodies. Consequently, it is important that the food choices we make are based on sound information and knowledge. A person who is well nourished is usually more alert in every way and emotionally better balanced. The well-nourished person is also better able than the poorly nourished individual to ward off infections.

The physician, the medical assistant, and the dietitian all are closely involved in the nutritive care of the patient. The physician prescribes the diet, and, ideally, the dietitian instructs the patient in how to follow it. If professional aid is not available, the medical assistant may be asked to discuss the diet with the patient, answer questions, and explain certain aspects of the modifications involved. Occasionally, patients may hesitate to ask the physician details about the diet, or questions may arise after the patient leaves the office. Such concerns typically include methods of preparation, sources of information, and interpretation of labels. The medical assistant is the one the patient turns to for answers. Consequently, the assistant should be able to answer basic questions on normal nutrition and should have a fundamental knowledge of the diets that physicians prescribe most often.

Nutrition and Dietetics

Nutrition refers to all the processes involved in the intake and utilization of nutrients. *Nutrients* are the organic and inorganic chemicals in food that supply the energy and raw materials for cellular activities. *Metabolism* refers to the cellular activities that occur inside and outside the cells. **Digestion** is a series of reactions occurring in the mouth, stomach, and small intestine that result in reducing large food molecules into simple absorbable forms such as amino acids, fatty acids, glucose, and glycogen. These absorbed nutrients are then carried by the bloodstream to all parts of the body, where they are metabolized.

The term *nutrition* is also used to indicate nutritional status, or the condition of the body resulting from the utilization of the essential nutrients available to the body. Public interest in nutrition has increased in recent years owing to the growing concern about physical fitness.

Dietetics is the practical application of nutritional science to individuals. It is the combined science and art of feeding individuals or groups under different economic or health conditions according to the principles of nutrition and management. The **dietitian** is the individual concerned with the promotion of good health through proper diet and with the therapeutic use of diet in the treatment of disease.

FOOD

Food is any material that meets the nutritive requirements of an organism for the maintenance of growth and physical well-being. To be classified as a food, a substance must perform one or more of three basic functions in the body: (1) provide a source of fuel or energy; (2) supply nutrients to build and repair tissues; and (3) supply nutrients to regulate body processes (Table 47–1). Most foods supply both fuel and nutrients; however, no one food supplies all the nutrients required for proper metabolism. Consequently, a combination of different foods is necessary. With a little planning, a well-balanced diet supplying all the body's needs can be obtained. **Deficiencies** in a diet or an inadequate diet results in malnutrition and may lead to a variety of diseases. Good nutrition is particularly critical for pregnant women, young children, and the elderly, because malnutrition during these time periods may result in physical and/or mental retardation.

Memory Jogger

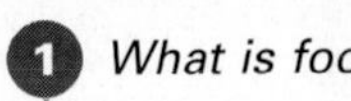

1 *What is food?*

ENERGY

Every action of the body, whether voluntary or involuntary, requires energy. Even when asleep, the body still needs a source of energy to keep the heart beating, the lungs breathing, and other vital organs functioning. The involuntary activities of digestion and respiration also require energy even though they are not consciously controlled. *Basal metabolism* is the term used for this energy expenditure when the body is at rest.

There are basically two energy sources available to the body: **exogenous** and **endogenous.** When the quantities of food (exogenous) consumed are insufficient to furnish the required fuel, the body begins to break down its fat reserves (endogenous) in an attempt to supply the necessary energy. Generally, it is desirable for the daily food intake to equal the total energy needs of the body (number of calories needed for both voluntary and involuntary activities).

A patient is generally thought of as being overweight or underweight when his or her present weight is compared with the accepted national averages of desired weight for a given height. **Obesity** may be due to one of these two origins: exogenous, involving excessive caloric intake in relation to the expenditure of calories, or endogenous, involving certain endocrine imbalances.

Quantities of energy are expressed in units of heat energy called calories. A **calorie** (cal) is the amount of heat needed to raise the temperature of 1 g of water 1° C. Because this unit represents a relatively small amount of energy and metabolism involves much larger quantities of energy, the large calorie (Cal), or kilocalorie (kcal), is commonly used. A *kilocalorie* is defined as the amount of heat required to raise the temperature of 1 kg of water 1° C. Of the seven food constituents (carbohydrates, proteins, fats, water, minerals, vitamins, and fiber), only carbohydrates, proteins, and fats are capable of furnishing the body with energy. Carbohydrates and proteins yield 4 kcal/g, whereas 1 g of fat provides 9 kcal.

Determining energy needs can be done by using the Harris-Benedict formula.

EXAMPLE OF USING THE HARRIS-BENEDICT FORMULA

Males: $(5 \times \text{height}) + (13.7 \times \text{weight} + 660) - (6.8 \times \text{age}) = \text{kcal/d}$

Females: $(1.8 \times \text{height}) + (9.6 \times \text{weight} + 655) - (4.7 \times \text{age}) = \text{kcal/d}$

Height should be expressed in inches, current weight in kilograms, and age in years.

Example: A 20-year-old woman weighs 110 pounds and is 5 feet 2 inches (62 inches) tall; thus, $(1.8 \times 62) + (9.6 \times 50 + 655) - (4.7 \times 20) = 1152.6$ kcal/d.

The amount of energy needed by a given individual varies considerably according to activity level and basal requirements; however, most adults, between 20 and 40 years of age, require 1800 to 3300 kcal/d.

TABLE 47–1 Food and Nutrition Board, National Academy of Sciences—National Research Council Recommended Dietary Allowances* Revised 1989

Designed for the maintenance of good nutrition of practically all healthy people in the United States

Age (y) or Condition	Weight† (kg)	Weight† (lb)	Height† (cm)	Height† (in)	Protein (g)	Fat-Soluble Vitamins: Vitamin A (μg RE)‡	Vitamin D (μg)§	Vitamin E (μg α-TE)‖	Vitamin K (μg)	Water-Soluble Vitamins: Vitamin C (mg)	Thiamin (mg)	Riboflavin (mg)	Niacin (mg NE)¶	Vitamin B_4 (mg)	Folate (μg)	Vitamin B_{12} (μg)	Minerals: Calcium (mg)	Phosphorus (mg)	Magnesium (mg)	Iron (mg)	Zinc (mg)	Iodine (μg)	Selenium (μg)
INFANTS																							
0.0–0.5	6	13	60	24	13	375	7.5	3	5	30	0.3	0.4	5	0.3	25	0.3	400	300	40	6	5	40	10
0.5–1.0	9	20	71	28	14	375	10	4	10	35	0.4	0.5	6	0.6	35	0.5	600	500	60	10	5	50	15
CHILDREN																							
1–3	13	29	90	35	15	400	10	6	15	40	0.7	0.8	9	1.0	50	0.7	800	800	80	10	10	70	20
4–6	20	44	112	44	24	500	10	7	20	45	0.9	1.1	12	1.1	75	1.0	800	800	120	10	10	90	20
7–10	28	62	132	52	28	700	10	7	30	45	1.0	1.2	13	1.4	100	1.4	800	800	170	10	10	120	30
MALES																							
11–14	45	99	157	62	45	1000	10	10	45	50	1.3	1.5	17	1.7	150	2.0	1200	1200	270	12	15	150	40
15–18	66	145	176	69	59	1000	10	10	65	60	1.5	1.8	20	2.0	200	2.0	1200	1200	400	12	15	150	50
19–24	72	160	177	70	58	1000	10	10	70	60	1.5	1.7	19	2.0	200	2.0	1200	1200	350	10	15	150	70
25–50	79	174	176	70	63	1000	5	10	80	60	1.5	1.7	19	2.0	200	2.0	800	800	350	10	15	150	70
51+	77	170	173	68	63	1000	5	10	80	60	1.2	1.4	15	2.0	200	2.0	800	800	350	10	15	150	70
FEMALES																							
11–14	46	101	157	62	46	800	10	8	45	50	1.1	1.3	15	1.4	150	2.0	1200	1200	280	15	12	150	45
15–18	55	120	163	64	44	800	10	8	55	60	1.1	1.3	15	1.5	180	2.0	1200	1200	300	15	12	150	50
19–24	58	128	164	65	46	800	10	8	60	60	1.1	1.3	15	1.6	180	2.0	1200	1200	280	15	12	150	55
25–50	63	138	163	64	50	800	5	8	65	60	1.1	1.3	15	1.6	180	2.0	800	800	280	15	12	150	55
51+	65	143	160	63	50	800	5	8	65	60	1.0	1.2	13	1.6	180	2.0	800	800	280	10	12	150	55
PREGNANT					60	800	10	10	65	70	1.5	1.6	17	2.2	400	2.2	1200	1200	320	30	15	175	65
LACTATING																							
1st 6 mo					65	1300	10	12	65	95	1.6	1.8	20	2.1	280	2.6	1200	1200	355	15	19	200	75
2nd 6 mo					62	1200	10	11	65	90	1.6	1.7	20	2.1	260	2.6	1200	1200	340	15	16	200	75

From Poleman CM, Peckenpaugh NJ: Nutrition Essentials and Diet Therapy, 6th ed., Philadelphia, WB Saunders, 1991, inside cover.

*The allowances, expressed as average daily intakes over time, are intended to provide for individual variations among most normal persons as they live in the United States under usual environmental stresses. Diets should be based on a variety of common foods to provide other nutrients for which human requirements have been less well defined. See text for detailed discussion of allowances and of nutrients not tabulated.

†Weights and heights of reference adults are actual medians for the U.S. population of the designated age, as reported by NHANES II.

‡Retinol equivalents. 1 retinol equivalent = 1 μg retinol or 6 μg β-carotene.

§As cholecalciferol, 10 μg cholecalciferol = 400 IU of vitamin D.

‖α-Tocopherol equivalents. 1 mg d-α tocopherol = 1 α-TE.

¶1 NE (niacin equivalent) is equal to 1 mg of niacin or 60 mg of dietary tryptophan.

Memory Jogger

 *Identify the two energy sources available to the body.*

Food Guide Pyramid

In 1992, to reflect the new dietary guidelines that called for more consumption of grains and less consumption of meat, sweets, and fats, the Food Guide Pyramid was introduced by the United States Department of Agriculture (Fig. 47–1). The pyramid is divided into six sections. The largest sections are those foods that should be consumed in the largest quantities. The grain group, the largest section, was placed at the bottom of the pyramid and the sweets and fats group, the smallest section, was at the top to emphasize the difference in importance between the two groups in the diet. The Food Guide Pyramid shows how the proportions of each basic food group contribute to a balanced diet.

Two symbols, a circle and a triangle, are used on the pyramid. The circle indicates fat that occurs naturally or is added, and the triangle indicates sugar that is added. These symbols show how fat and sugar, even though they come mainly from fats, oils, and sweets, can occur naturally or be added to foods in the five basic food groups.

Explaining this food pyramid to patients will encourage healthful eating habits. When people eat a

KEY
Fat (naturally occurring and added)
Sugars (added)
These symbols show fats, oils, and added sugars in foods.
Fats, Oils, and Sweets
Use sparingly
Milk, Yogurt, and Cheese Group
2–3 servings
Meat, Poultry, Fish, Dry Beans, Eggs, and Nuts Group
2–3 servings
Vegetable Group
3–5 servings
Fruit Group
2–4 servings
Bread, Cereal, Rice, and Pasta Group
6–11 servings
CEREAL
WHAT IS THE FOOD GUIDE PYRAMID?
The Pyramid is an outline of what to eat each day. It's not a rigid prescription, but a general guide that lets you choose a healthful diet that's right for you. The Pyramid calls for eating a variety of foods to get the nutrients you need and, at the same time, the right amount of calories to maintain a healthy weight.
The Pyramid also focuses on fat, because most American diets are too high in fat, especially saturated fat.

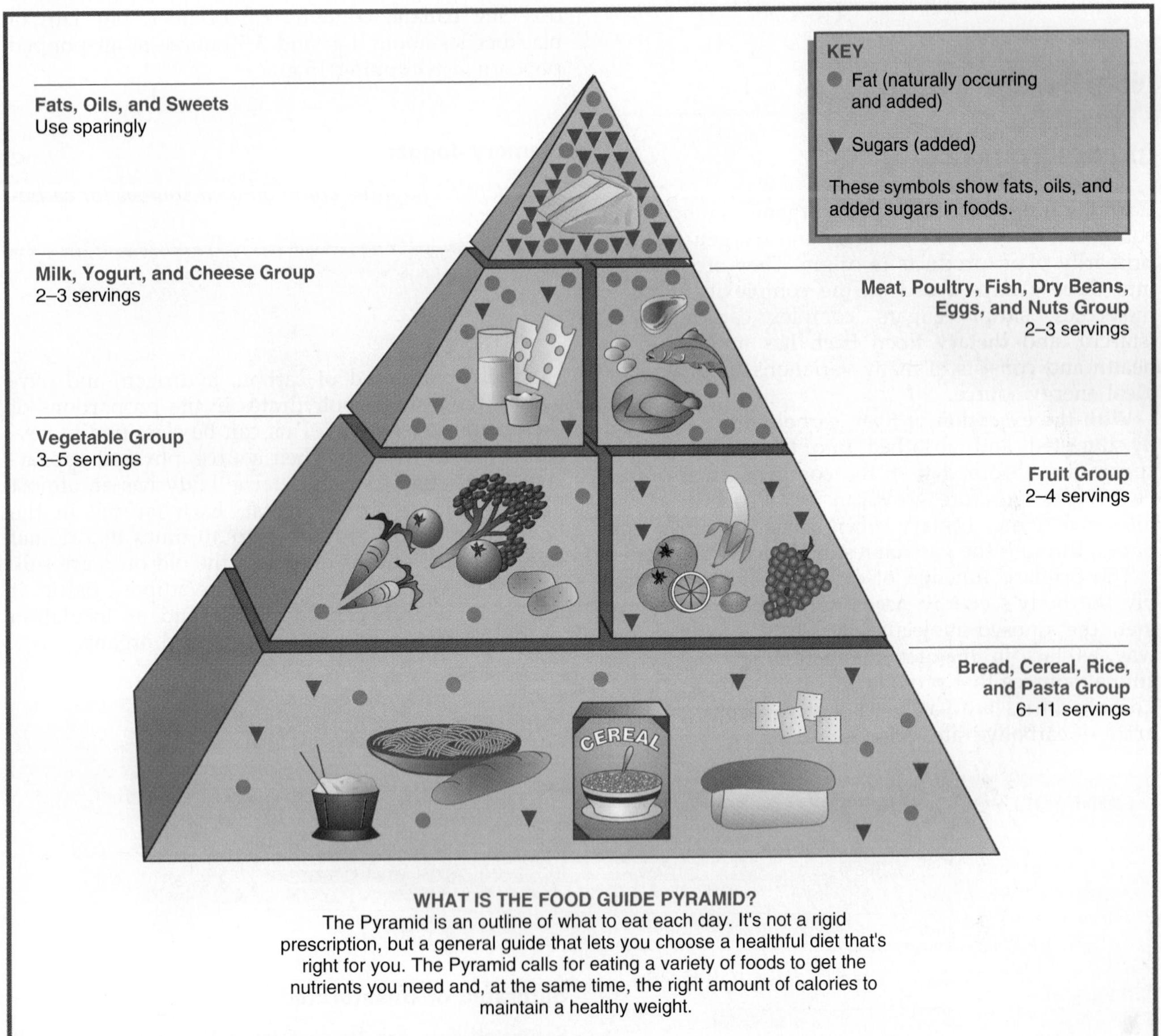

FIGURE 47–1 Food guide pyramid. (From U.S. Department of Agriculture.)

healthful diet, they feel better, are more energetic, and have a more positive outlook on life. Some patients have never been educated in nutrition and do not know how to plan a balanced healthy diet for themselves or their families. Placing the Food Guide Pyramid Poster near the scale in the office may be a reminder to patients or may act as a point of interest to prompt questions regarding a nutritional diet.

Good nutrition is a balance between protein, vitamins, minerals, and fiber, with little fat, sodium, sugar, and alcohol. The energy intake must be balanced with the energy output.

Memory Jogger

Name the two symbols used in the Food Guide Pyramid and how they are used.

Nutrients

CARBOHYDRATES

Carbohydrates are chemical organic compounds composed of carbon, hydrogen, and oxygen and are primarily plant products in origin. They are divided into three groups based on the complexity of their molecules: simple sugars, complex carbohydrates (starch), and dietary fiber. Each has a function in health and consists of many variations. They are the ideal energy source.

With the exception of fiber, carbohydrates are easily digested and absorbed into the body. Simple sugars are absorbed first; the complex sugars must be processed before they can be absorbed in the intestinal tract. Dietary fiber is indigestible and passes through the gastrointestinal tract unchanged.

The primary function of carbohydrates is to supply the body's energy needs. Once these needs are met, the unused molecules are handled the same way as fats in maintenance action. There are no animal sources that provide adequate carbohydrates. Carbohydrates are easily converted to energy. One gram of carbohydrate yields 4 kcal.

COMMON FOOD SOURCES

- *Cereal grains:* rice, wheat, corn, oats, barley, and buckwheat
- *Vegetables:* green leafy vegetables, seeds, and dried peas and beans
- *Sweets:* table sugar, molasses, and maple and corn syrups

Dietary fiber is commonly called *roughage.* It is defined as the portion of the plant eaten that cannot be digested or absorbed. It is classified by its water solubility; it adds bulk to the intestinal tract; and it is beneficial for normal gastrointestinal functioning. Water-soluble fiber found in oat bran, fruits, and vegetables helps to lower cholesterol; and insoluble fiber, which is found in whole grains and beans, is known to help prevent colon cancer and seems to reduce heart attack risk. In 1998, Harvard University researchers completed a 6-year study of nearly 44,000 middle-aged men and found that diets high in roughage reduced heart disease risk independent of the amount of fat in the diet.

Although most nutritionists recommend a diet that includes 20 to 35 g of fiber a day (the equivalent of two large bowls of wheat bran cereal), the average American consumes only half that much. Yet the Harvard group estimates that every 10-g increase in fiber could decrease a person's chances of having a heart attack by about 20%.

Sneaking fiber into the diet isn't that difficult to do: One banana contains 2 g of fiber; one cup of blackberries about 4 g; and 3.5 ounces of air-popped popcorn, a whopping 15 g.

Memory Jogger

Identify the three common food sources for carbohydrates.

FATS

Fats, also composed of carbon, hydrogen, and oxygen, differ from carbohydrates in the proportions of each of these elements. Fats can be classified in several different ways: by their source, physical appearance, or chemical structure. The body has an almost limitless capacity to store fat. Each fat cell in the body can balloon to more than 10 times its original size, and new ones grow when the old ones are full. When fat is stored in the body as adipose tissue, it acts as a reserve energy supply and as insulation and padding for the body and its vital organs.

COMMON FOOD SOURCES

- *Animal fats:* dairy products, meat, fish, and eggs
- *Vegetable oils:* corn, olives, avocados, cottonseed, nuts, and beans

Saturated or Unsaturated

Saturated fats are those fatty acids that contain all the hydrogen possible. They are usually from animal sources and are solid at room temperature. Examples of saturated fats are lard, butter, meat fat, and **hydrogenated** fats. The main exceptions are coconut and palm oils, which are of plant origin but exceptionally high in saturated fat. Hydrogenated vegetable oils (shortening) are also saturated fats. Unsaturated fatty acids can take on more hydrogen under the proper conditions. They are found in plants and are usually liquid at room temperature. Examples are the oils from corn and safflower. Some fats, such as those of the soft-type margarine, are partially hydrogenated. That is, an unsaturated fat is treated so that it takes up a predetermined quantity of hydrogen, resulting in a product that exhibits properties of both a saturated and an unsaturated fat. These fats are usually soft at room temperature.

Cholesterol

Cholesterol is a lipid commonly found in saturated fat. It is also manufactured within the body. The confusion between good and bad fat stems from the distinction between the fat in food and the fat in our bodies. The good fats in our diet are polyunsaturated and monounsaturated fats. The bad dietary fats are cholesterol and saturated fats. The fat in our bodies is divided into two categories. The good fat is high-density lipoprotein (HDL); the bad fats are low-density lipoprotein (LDL) and very low-density lipoprotein (VLDL). The HDL and the LDL levels can often be successfully changed through diet. The secret is to understand what the different types of lipids are, what the numbers mean, and how a person improves a lipid profile in an effort to reduce the risk of developing heart disease (Fig. 47–2).

Fats make up 35% to 40% of the total calories in the American diet. Because fats supply 9 kcal/g, they are the most concentrated source of energy in our diet. Nutritionists and epidemiologists believe that decreasing dietary fat to 30% would decrease the risk of developing cancer, especially of the colon, breast, and prostate.

MAJOR FUNCTIONS OF FAT

- Provide a source of energy
- Carry fat-soluble vitamins A and D
- Supply fatty acids essential for growth and life
- Slow down emptying time of the stomach, thus increasing the satiety value of the diet

CORONARY HEART DISEASE RISK AND YOUR LIPID PROFILE

Everyone has heard about the connection between high levels of cholesterol and coronary heart disease, which accounts for about 500,000 deaths a year in the United States. As a health-conscious consumer, you're naturally concerned about your cholesterol level. But if you're like most other people, you find the language about cholesterol and other "lipids" – fatty substances in the body – confusing.

Here's a quick guide to help you understand what the different types of lipids are, what the numbers mean, and what you can do to improve your lipid profile in an effort to reduce your risk of developing heart disease.

1. ***Look at your different lipid levels, and check your risk.*** Lipid levels are expressed as milligrams of lipid per deciliter of blood (mg/dL). The symbols used with these numbers are explained below.

■ **Total Cholesterol** – Everyone should know his or her total cholesterol level, which provides a rough estimate of heart disease risk. Cholesterol is transported through the bloodstream by lipoprotein (lipid plus protein) carriers. Total cholesterol level includes the amount of cholesterol carried by HDL (high-density lipoprotein) and LDL (low-density lipoprotein), as well as a small amount carried by very-low-density lipoprotein. This measurement, however, does not give a specific value for each lipoprotein. The total cholesterol test is used to screen for heart disease risk or to monitor general progress in those on a special diet or medication for high cholesterol.

What's your total cholesterol level?	Desirable	<200 mg/dL
	Borderline high	200–239 mg/dL
	High-risk	≥240 mg/dL

■ **HDL Cholesterol** – HDL-C is known as the "good" cholesterol because higher HDL levels are generally associated with lower risk for heart disease. HDL-C is believed to take excess cholesterol away from coronary arteries. The more HDL cholesterol you have, the better. Everyone should know his or her HDL cholesterol number.

What's your HDL cholesterol level?	Desirable	≥35 mg/dL

■ **LDL Cholesterol** – LDL-C is known as the "bad" cholesterol because too much LDL in the blood is associated with blockage of the arteries in the heart. LDL cholesterol is calculated in those who have a high total cholesterol level or other risk factors for heart disease.

What's your LDL cholesterol level?	Desirable	<130 mg/dL
	Borderline high	130–159 mg/dL
	High-risk	≥160 mg/dL

■ **Triglyceride** – Triglyceride is a lipid that helps store fat in the body. High triglyceride levels can cause inflammation of the pancreas, and elevated levels of triglyceride may play a role in heart disease risk.

What's your triglyceride level?	Desirable	<250 mg/dL

2. ***Review your lipid tests with your physician.*** Assessing heart disease risk is a process that should be performed under your doctor's guidance. Together you can develop your personal plan for action. Some patients, such as those with high total cholesterol, hypertension, or coronary heart disease (among other patient groups), should have a complete lipoprotein profile, which includes determinations of total cholesterol, HDL-C, triglyceride, and LDL-C.

3. ***Make changes that can improve your lipid profile to help reduce your risk of heart disease.***

FIGURE 47–2 Cholesterol/lipid profile. (© 1991 HealthScan, Inc.)

Memory Jogger

How can fats be classified?

Antioxidants

Cholesterol has been high on the list of dietary villains for years and has been thought to be a serious contributor to the development of heart disease. Recent studies indicate that the problem may not lie with the cholesterol itself, but in the way in which it reacts with oxygen (or oxidizes) in the bloodstream. Our bodies have developed mechanisms to protect us against toxins created by oxidation, by utilizing, the antioxidant vitamins E and C and beta carotene, but their amounts are not always sufficient. When there are enough antioxidants circulating in the blood, cholesterol is prevented from oxidizing. Without enough, the opposite is true and then the damage to arteries begins.

In addition to lowering the cholesterol intake, increasing the dietary intake of antioxidants may prove to be a great help. Increasing the dietary intake of antioxidants should not be difficult because many fruits, vegetables, and certain seasonings contain naturally occurring antioxidants.

ANTIOXIDANT FOOD LIST

VITAMIN C

Peppers (green or red)	Oranges	Brussels sprouts
Strawberries	Tangerines	Broccoli
Lemons	Black currants	Cabbage
Grapefruit	Raspberries	Cauliflower

VITAMIN E

Wheat germ	Almonds	Oatmeal
Chick peas	Hazelnuts	Rye flour
Soya beans	Sunflower seeds	

CAROTENOIDS (INCLUDING BETA-CAROTENE)

Carrots	Broccoli	Apricots
Kale	Sweet potatoes	Pumpkin
Mustard greens	Winter squash	Spinach
Cantaloupe		

MIXED ANTIOXIDANTS

Nutmeg	Thyme	Wheat bran
Rosemary	Wine	Rice
Cloves	Green tea	Pepper
Oregano	Sesame	

PROTEINS

Proteins are very large, complex molecules. They are composed of units known as **amino acids,** which are the materials that our bodies use to build and repair tissues. It is in the form of amino acids that proteins are absorbed into the system and metabolized. There are 20 amino acids, of which 8 are essential in the adult for normal growth and maintenance of tissues. These 8 essential amino acids must come from food.

Proteins are classified according to whether they contain all essential amino acids in good proportion to one another. A *complete protein* is one that contains a well-balanced mixture of all 8 essential amino acids. If it is the only source of protein in the diet, it will support life and normal growth. A *partially complete protein* is one that supplies an imbalanced mixture of essential amino acids. If it is the sole protein source, it will maintain life but will not support normal growth. An *incomplete protein* will support neither life nor normal growth. It must not be the sole protein source, for it is missing, or extremely low in, one or more of the essential amino acids.

PROTEIN FOOD SOURCES

- *Complete proteins:* meat, fish, poultry, eggs, and dairy products
- *Partially complete proteins:* grains and vegetables
- *Incomplete proteins:* corn and gelatin

Fortunately, most foods have a mixture of proteins that supplement each other. Because there is little, if any, storage of amino acids in the body, it is important that a source of protein be included at each meal. If incomplete or partially complete proteins are used, attempts should be made to balance them. That is, a protein deficient in one amino acid should be eaten with one that is high in the same amino acid.

Vegetarianism has become increasingly popular, and many different forms exist. Some vegetarians consume no red meats but will eat fish and poultry. Some include eggs and/or dairy products in their diets. Others (classified as vegans) consume no animal proteins at all, relying solely on vegetable foods for protein. Those who eat some animal protein in the form of fish, eggs, and milk are generally not at risk nutritionally. Vegetarians must include a variety of foods to ensure the nutritional adequacy of their diets. To supply sufficient protein, vegetables that complement each other must be eaten together. Vegetarians must compensate for the deficiencies in their diets by properly combining foods to get the correct proportion of amino acids. This is customarily done in the diets of different cultures. For example, in Mexico, beans are combined with rice, and in Middle Eastern countries, wheat bread is combined with cheese.

The recommended intake of proteins is 0.8 g/kg

of weight, and at least one third should be obtained from complete proteins. However, if the individual is a strict vegetarian, as already mentioned, care must be taken to balance the proteins consumed.

The average American diet is 12% to 15% protein. Protein deficiency is the most common form of malnutrition that exists throughout the world.

FUNCTIONS OF PROTEIN

- Builds and repairs body tissue
- Aids in the body's defense mechanisms against disease
- Regulates body secretions and fluids
- Provides energy

Memory Jogger

 *Recall the recommended daily intake of protein.*

VITAMINS (MICRONUTRIENTS)

Vitamins are organic substances occurring in minute quantities in plant and animal tissues that are essential for specific metabolic functions or reactions to proceed normally. Vitamins are classified as body regulators and do not supply calories in our diets. Rather, they function as catalysts and help or allow metabolic reactions to proceed. Originally, they were lettered or numbered as they were discovered. However, as they have been identified chemically, they have been given more specific names. In many cases, their chemical names are as well known as their letter designations.

VITAMINS

- Regulate the synthesis of bones, skin, glands, nerves, brain, and blood
- Aid in the metabolism of protein, carbohydrates, and fats
- Prevent nutritional deficiency diseases
- Provide for good health at all ages

Vitamins are divided into two groups: fat soluble (A, D, E, and K) and water soluble (C and the B complex). There is no good evidence that large intakes of vitamins are useful in the healthy individual; however, deficiencies of a vitamin cause illness. Vitamins will not cure a disease or illness other than one caused by the lack of that nutrient. For example, vitamin C will not cure bleeding gums unless the condition is specifically caused by a lack of ascorbic acid, the chemical name for vitamin C. It should also be noted that toxic symptoms from excessive ingestion of vitamins A and D are proven clinically to exist, and large intakes of some water-soluble vitamins may cause adverse effects (Table 47–2).

There is still extensive research being done regarding the role vitamins play in disease prevention and treatment. We are continuously hearing statements regarding the use of vitamin B, C, and E and their possible use in preventing or correcting disorders; for example, vitamin C to prevent the common cold, vitamin E to help fight cancer, and vitamin B to aid in Alzheimer's disease.

MINERALS (ELECTROLYTES)

Minerals are inorganic chemical elements that make up about 4% of body weight. Of the many that are used by the body, only 14 are believed to be essential. Of those, allowances have been established for only 6. Most minerals are required in relatively small amounts, but even so, they are absolutely essential for life (Table 47–3).

Minerals contribute to the body's water–electrolyte balance and acid–base balance. The largest proportion of inorganic elements is found in the skeleton. Minerals present in the largest amount include sodium, potassium, calcium, chlorine, phosphorus, and magnesium. Those present in very small amounts, the *trace elements,* include iron, zinc, copper, selenium, chromium, manganese, iodine, and fluorine.

The minerals that are needed only in trace amounts seem either to behave as part of hormone or enzyme systems or to work with vitamins in various metabolic reactions throughout the body. For example, iodine is part of the thyroid hormone *thyroxine,* and another hormone, *insulin,* has zinc as part of its structure. Cobalt, on the other hand, is an essential part of the vitamin B_{12} molecule.

Like vitamins, these minerals can be obtained from common foods in a well-balanced diet. With the exception of iodine and iron, mineral deficiencies are rare in the average American diet.

Memory Jogger

 *Name the six minerals present in the body in the largest amount.*

WATER

Water is all too often overlooked when nutritional status is evaluated. Yet the body is approximately 80% water and can survive longer without food than it can without water.

Text continued on page 982

TABLE 47–2 Vitamin Facts

Vitamin	U.S. RDA*	Best Sources	Functions	Deficiency Symptoms†	Toxic?	Processing Tips	Did You Know?
A (carotene)	5000 IU/d	Yellow or orange fruits and vegetables, green leafy vegetables, fortified oatmeal, liver, dairy products	Formation and maintenance of skin, hair and mucous membranes; helps us see in dim light; bone and tooth growth.	Night blindness, dry and scaly skin, frequent fatigue	Yes, in high doses, but beta-carotene is nontoxic.	Serve fruits and vegetables raw and keep covered and refrigerated. Steam veggies; broil, bake, or braise meats.	Low-fat and skim milks are often fortified with vitamin A, which is removed with the fat.
B_1 (thiamine)	1.5 mg/d	Fortified cereals and oatmeals, meats, rice and pasta, whole grains, liver	Helps body release energy from carbohydrates during metabolism; growth and muscle tone.	Heart irregularity, fatigue, nerve disorders, mental confusion	No, high doses are excreted by the kidneys.	Don't rinse rice or pasta before and after cooking. Cook in minimal water.	Pasta and breads made of refined flours have B_1 added because it is lost in the milling process.
B_2 (riboflavin)	1.7 mg/d	Whole grains, green leafy vegetables, organ meats, milk and eggs	Helps body release energy from protein, fat, and carbohydrates during metabolism.	Cracks in corners of mouth, rash, anemia	No toxic effects reported.	Store foods in containers that light cannot enter; cook vegetables in minimal water; roast or broil meats.	Most ready-to-eat cereals are fortified with 25% of the U.S. RDA for B_2.
B_6 (pyridoxine)	2 mg/d	Fish, poultry, lean meats, bananas, prunes, dried beans, whole grains, avocados	Helps build body tissue and aids in metabolism of protein.	Convulsions, dermatitis, muscular weakness, skin cracks, anemia	Long-term megadoses may cause nerve damage in hands and feet.	Serve fruits raw or cook for shortest time in little water; roast or broil meats.	Because B_6 aids in use of protein in the body, the need for B_6 increases with protein intake.
B_{12} (cobalamin)	6 μg/d	Meats, milk products, seafood	Aids cell development, functioning of the nervous system, and the metabolism of protein and fat.	Anemia, nervousness, fatigue, and, in some cases, neuritis and brain degeneration	No toxic effects reported.	Roast or broil meat and fish.	Vegetarians who do not eat any animal products may need a supplement.
Biotin	0.3 mg/d	Cereal/grain products, yeast, legumes, liver	Involved in metabolism of protein, fats, and carbohydrates.	Nausea, vomiting, depression, hair loss, dry, scaly skin	No toxic effects reported.	Storage, processing, and cooking do not appear to affect this vitamin.	Biotin deficiency is extremely rare in the United States.

Folate (folacin, folic acid)	0.4 mg/d	Green leafy vegetables, organ meats, dried peas, beans, and lentils	Aids in genetic material development and involved in red blood cell production.	Gastrointestinal disorders, anemia, cracks on lips	Some evidence of toxicity in large doses.	Store vegetables in refrigerator and steam, boil, or simmer in minimal water.	Deficiencies can occur in premature infants and pregnant women.
Niacin	20 mg/d	Meat, poultry, fish, enriched cereals, peanuts, potatoes, dairy products, eggs	Involved in carbohydrate, protein, and fat metabolism.	Skin disorders, diarrhea, indigestion, general fatigue	Nicotinic acid form should be taken only under doctor's care.	Roast or broil beef, veal, lamb and poultry. Cook potatoes in minimal water.	Niacin is formed in the body by converting an amino acid found in proteins.
Pantothenic acid	10 mg/d	Lean meats, whole grains, legumes, vegetables, fruits	Helps in the release of energy from fats and carbohydrates.	Fatigue, vomiting, stomach stress, infections, muscle cramps	No toxic effects reported.	Eat fruits and vegetables raw.	It is believed some pantothenic acid is produced in the gastrointestinal tract.
C (ascorbic acid)	60 mg/d	Citrus fruits, berries, and vegetables—especially peppers	Essential for structure of bones, cartilage, muscle and blood vessels. Also helps maintain capillaries and gums and aids in absorption of iron.	Swollen or bleeding gums, slow wound healing, fatigue/depression, poor digestion	Intakes of 1 g or more can cause nausea, cramps, and diarrhea.	Do not store or soak fruits and vegetables in water. Refrigerate juices and store only 2 to 3 days.	Smokers may benefit from an increased intake of vitamin C.
D	400 IU/d	Fortified milk, sunlight, fish, eggs, butter, fortified margarine	Aids in bone and tooth formation; helps maintain heart action and nervous system.	In children: rickets and other bone deformities. In adults: calcium loss from bones.	High intakes may cause diarrhea and weight loss.	Storage, processing and cooking do not appear to affect this vitamin.	Sunlight starts vitamin D production in the skin.
E	30 IU/d	Fortified and multigrain cereals, nuts, wheat germ, vegetable oils, green leafy vegetables	Protects blood cells, body tissue and essential fatty acids from harmful destruction in the body.	Muscular wasting, nerve damage, anemia, reproductive failure	Relatively nontoxic.	Store in air-tight containers away from light.	Most fortified cereals have 40% of the RDA.
K	‡	Green leafy vegetables, fruit, dairy and grain products	Essential for blood clotting functions.	Bleeding disorders in newborns and those on blood-thinning medications	Not toxic as found in food.	Store in containers away from light.	Vitamin K is also formed by bacteria in the colon.

*For adults and children older than 4. IU, international units; mg, milligrams, μg, micrograms.

†Many of the symptoms outlined under this heading can also be attributed to problems other than vitamin deficiency. If you have these symptoms and they persist, consult your doctor.

‡There is no U.S. RDA for vitamin K; however the Recommended Dietary Allowance is 1 $\mu g/kg$ of body weight.

Information for this chart was obtained from the Food and Drug Administration, the American Institute for Cancer Research, and the United States Department of Agriculture/Human Nutrition Information Service. Shaded vitamins are fat-soluble; non-shaded vitamins are water-soluble.

TABLE 47–3 Minerals

Functions	Sources	Deficiency Symptoms	Toxicity Symptoms
	Mineral and Elemental Symbol: Calcium (Ca^{2+})		
Helps muscles to contract and relax, thereby helping to regulate heartbeat Plays a role in the normal functioning of the nervous system Aids in blood coagulation and the functioning of some enzymes Helps build strong bones and teeth May help prevent hypertension	Primarily found in milk and milk products; also found in dark green, leafy vegetables, tofu and other soy products, sardines, salmon with bones, and hard water	Poor bone growth and tooth development, leading to stunted growth and increased risk of dental caries, rickets (bowing of legs) in children, osteomalacia (soft bones) and osteoporosis (brittle bones) in adults, poor blood clotting, and possible hypertension	Kidney stones
	Mineral and Elemental Symbol: Chloride (Cl^-)		
Involved in the maintenance of fluid and acid–base balance Provides an acid medium, in the form of hydrochloric acid, for activation of gastric enzymes	Major source is table salt (sodium chloride); also found in fish and vegetables	Disturbances in acid–base balance, with possible growth retardation, psychomotor defects, and memory loss	Disturbances in acid–base balance
	Mineral and Elemental Symbol: Magnesium (Mg^{2+})		
Helps build strong bones and teeth Activates many enzymes Participates in protein synthesis and lipid metabolism Helps regulate heartbeat	Raw, dark green vegetables, nuts and soybeans, whole grains and wheat bran, bananas and apricots, seafoods and coffee, tea, cocoa, and hard water	Rare but in disease states may lead to central nervous system problems (confusion, apathy, hallucinations, poor memory) and neuromuscular problems (muscle weakness, cramps, tremor, cardiac arrhythmia)	Drowsiness, weakness, and lethargy and in severe toxicity skeletal paralysis, central nervous system depression, respiratory depression, and ultimately coma and death
	Mineral and Symbol: Phosphorus (PO_4)		
Helps build strong bones and teeth Present in the nuclei of all cells Helps in the oxidation of fats and carbohydrates (energy metabolism) Aids in maintaining the body's acid–base balance	Milk and milk products, eggs, meats, legumes, whole grains, soft drinks (used to make the "fizz")	Rare but with malabsorption can cause anorexia, weakness, stiff joints, and fragile bones	Hypocalcemic tetany (muscle spasms)
	Mineral and Elemental Symbol: Potassium (K^+)		
Plays a key role in fluid and acid–base balance Transmits nerve impulses and helps control muscle contractions and promotes regular heartbeat Needed for enzyme reactions	Apricots, bananas, oranges, grapefruit, raisins, green beans, broccoli, carrots, greens, potatoes, meats, milk and milk products, peanut butter and legumes, molasses, coffee, tea, cocoa	May cause impaired growth, hypertension, bone fragility, central nervous system changes, renal hypertrophy, diminished heart rate, and death	Hyperkalemia (excess potassium in the blood) with cardiac function disturbances

TABLE 47–3 Minerals *Continued*

Functions	Sources	Deficiency Symptoms	Toxicity Symptoms
Mineral and Elemental Symbol: Sodium (Na^{+})			
Plays a key role in the maintenance of acid–base balance Transmits nerve impulses and helps control muscle contractions Regulates cell membrane permeability	Salt (sodium chloride) is the major dietary source; minor sources occur naturally in foods such as milk and milk products and several vegetables	Hyponatremia (too little sodium in the blood)	May cause hypertension, which can lead to cardiovascular diseases and renal (kidney) disease; in the form of salt tablets, can cause gastric irritation
Mineral and Elemental Symbol: Chromium (Cr^{3+})			
Activates several enzymes Enhances the removal of glucose from the blood	Liver and other meats, whole grains, cheese, legumes, and brewer's yeast	Weight loss, abnormalities of the central nervous system, and possible aggravation of diabetes mellitus	Inhibited insulin activity
Mineral and Elemental Symbol: Copper (Cu^{2+})			
Aids in the production and survival of red blood cells Part of many enzymes involved in respiration Plays a role in normal lipid metabolism	Shellfish—especially oysters—liver, nuts and seeds, raisins, whole grains, and chocolate	Anemia, central nervous system problems, abnormal electrocardiograms, bone fragility, impaired immune response; may be a factor in failure to thrive in premature infants	In Wilson's disese and Huntington's chorea (both hereditary diseases), copper accumulation causes neuron and liver cell damage
Mineral and Elemental Symbol: Fluorine (F^{-})			
Helps the formation of solid bones and teeth, thereby reducing incidence of dental caries, and may help prevent osteoporosis	Fluoridated water (and foods cooked in fluoridated water), fish, tea, gelatin	Increased susceptibility to dental caries	Fluorosis and mottling of teeth
Mineral and Elemental Symbol: Iodine (I^{-})			
Helps regulate energy metabolism through being part of thyroid hormones Essential for normal cell functioning, helps to keep skin, hair, and nails healthy	Primarily from iodized salt, also found in saltwater fish, seaweed products, vegetables grown in iodine-rich soils	Goiter, cretinism in infants born to iodine-deficient mothers, with accompanying mental retardation and diffuse central nervous system abnormalities	Little toxic effect in individuals with normal thyroid gland functioning
Mineral and Elemental Symbol: Iron (Fe^{3+})			
Essential to the formation of hemoglobin, which is important for tissue respiration and ultimately growth and development Part of several enzymes and proteins in the body	Heme sources: organ meats—especially liver, red meats, and other meats Nonheme sources: iron-fortified cereals, dark green leafy vegetables, legumes, whole grains, blackstrap molasses, dried fruit, and foods cooked in iron pans	Iron-deficiency anemia and possible alterations that impair behavior	Idiopathic hemochromatosis, which can lead to cirrhosis, diabetes mellitus, skin pigmentation, arthralgias (joint pain), and cardiomyopathy

Table continued on following page

TABLE 47–3 Minerals *Continued*

Functions	Sources	Deficiency Symptoms	Toxicity Symptoms
	Mineral and Elemental Symbol: Manganese (Mn^{2+})		
Needed for normal bone structure, reproduction, normal functioning of cells and the central nervous system A component of some enzymes	Nuts, whole grains, vegetables and fruits, coffee, tea, cocoa, and egg yolks	None observed in humans	Iron-deficiency anemia through inhibiting effect on iron absorption; pulmonary changes, anorexia, apathy, impotence, headaches, leg cramps, and speech impairment; in advanced stages of toxicity resembles Parkinson's disease
	Mineral and Elemental Symbol: Selenium (Se)		
Part of an enzyme system Acts as an antioxidant with vitamin E to protect the cell from oxygen	Protein-rich foods (meat, eggs, milk), whole grains, seafood, liver and other meats, egg yolks, and garlic	Keshan disease (a human cardiomyopathy) and Kashin-Bek disease (an endemic human osteoarthropathy)	Physical defects of the fingernails and toenails and hair loss
	Mineral and Elemental Symbol: Zinc (Zn^{2+})		
Plays a role in protein synthesis Essential for normal growth and sexual development, wound healing, immune function, cell division and differentiation, and smell acuity	Whole grains, wheat germ, crabmeat, oyster, liver and other meats, brewer's yeast	Depressed immune function, poor growth, dwarfism, impaired skeletal growth and delayed sexual maturation, acrodermatitis	Severe anemia, nausea, vomiting, abdominal cramps, diarrhea, fever, hypocupremia (low blood serum copper), malaise, fatigue

From Poleman CM, Peckenpaugh NJ: Nutrition Essentials and Diet Therapy, 6th ed. Philadelphia, WB Saunders, 1991, pp 128–129. Data from Garrison RH, Somer E: The Nutrition Desk Reference. New Canaan, CT, Keats Publishing, 1985; Griffeth HW: Complete Guide to Vitamins, Minerals and Supplements. Tucson, AZ, Fisher Books, 1988.

FUNCTIONS OF WATER

- Plays a key role in the maintenance of body temperature
- Acts as a solvent and the medium for most biochemical reactions
- Acts as the vehicle for transport of substances such as nutrients, hormones, antibodies, and metabolic waste
- Acts as a lubricant for joints and mucous membranes

Approximately two thirds of the total body weight is water. It is lost daily from the body in urine, feces, sweat, and expiration. Extensive water losses due to diarrhea, vomiting, burns, or perspiration can lead to electrolyte losses that result in life-threatening imbalances.

Most of the daily requirements for water are satisfied by ingested fluids and foods because all food contains some water. Vegetables and fruits are more than 80% water and meats are 40% to 60% water. The recommended daily allowance of water for an adult is 2 L, which is about 64 ounces.

To aid in the prevention of cancer, the American Cancer Society advises the following nutritional guidelines:

AMERICAN CANCER SOCIETY NUTRITIONAL GUIDELINES

- Eat more high-fiber foods such as fruits, vegetables, and whole grain cereals.
- Eat plenty of dark green and deep yellow fruits and vegetables rich in vitamins A and C.
- Eat plenty of broccoli, cabbage, Brussels sprouts, kohlrabi, and cauliflower.
- Be moderate in consumption of salt-cured, smoked, and nitrite-cured foods, such as bacon and smoked sausage.
- Cut down on total fat intake from animal sources and fats and oils.
- Avoid obesity.
- Be moderate in consumption of alcoholic beverages.

Therapeutic Nutrition

Although a majority of patients are treated medically without using a therapeutic diet, there are some illnesses and diseases that can be cured and patients whose recovery can be facilitated by the use of a special diet. An example of this is **diabetes mellitus.** The patient's lifestyle and background must be taken into consideration, and certain adjustments may need to be made to ensure the patient's full cooperation. The closer the special diet is to a normal one, the fewer changes the person will need to accept, and the easier it will be for the patient to adhere to the diet. It is easier to be certain that the patient's diet supplies adequate amounts of the essential nutrients if a regular diet pattern is used as a baseline.

MODIFYING A DIET

The normal diet can be modified with regard to the following features (or combination thereof) to create a therapeutic diet:

- Consistency
- Caloric level
- Levels of one or more nutrients
- Bulk
- Spiciness
- Levels of specific foods

In general, the normal diet is modified by restricting foods that are sources of the nutrient involved. Except for the nutrient in question, the recommended daily allowances can usually be met. However, if several restrictions are ordered for the same patient, a nutrient supplement may be necessary (Fig. 47–3).

SOFT OR LIGHT DIET Foods with roughage are eliminated (no raw fruits or vegetables). No strongly flavored or gas-forming vegetables are allowed (onions, beans, broccoli, and cauliflower). In many cases, spices are limited. Often this diet is used after surgery to place less strain on the gastrointestinal system.

MECHANICAL SOFT DIET A regular diet in which the food is either chopped, ground, or pureed, depending on the degree of texture change required. No foods or spices are restricted. This diet may be used after dental or oral surgery.

LIQUID DIET There are two types of liquid diets. The clear liquid diet includes only broth soups, tea, coffee, and gelatin. In some cases, apple juice and cranberry juice may be allowed. The full liquid diet includes all foods allowed on a clear liquid diet plus milk, custards, strained cream soups, refined cereals, egg nogs, milkshakes, and all juices. This diet may be indicated as part of the preparation process for diagnostic testing or for the first several days after major surgery.

HIGH- OR LOW-FIBER DIET Bulk or residue is changed when treating problems of the colon or large bowel. In some cases, high-residue diets are ordered; in others, low-residue diets. In either case, foods high in cellulose are considered to be high in residue because the body does not digest this carbohydrate well and a residue is left in the colon. In some instances, a low-residue diet is distinguished

WHAT COUNTS AS A SERVING?

Food Group	Food and Quantity
Bread, cereal, rice, and pasta	1 slice bread 1 oz ready-to-eat cereal 1/2 c cooked cereal, rice, or pasta
Vegetable	1 c raw leafy vegetables 1/2 c other vegetables—cooked or raw 3/4 c vegetable juice
Fruit	1 medium apple, banana, or orange 1/2 c chopped, cooked, or canned fruit 3/4 c fruit juice
Milk, yogurt, and cheese	1 c milk or yogurt 1 1/2 oz natural cheese 2 oz process cheese
Meat, poultry, fish, dry beans, eggs, and nuts	2–3 oz cooked lean meat, poultry, or fish 1/2 c cooked dry beans or 1 egg counts as 1 oz lean meat 2 tbsp peanut butter or 1/3 c nuts counts as 1 oz meat

FIGURE 47–3 What counts as a serving? (From Nutrition and Your Health: Dietary Guidelines for Americans, 4th ed. Washington, DC, U.S. Department of Agriculture and U.S. Department of Health and Human Services, 1995.)

from a low-fiber diet. In this case, a low-fiber diet eliminates those foods with a high-cellulose content and a low-residue diet restricts milk, in addition to fiber content. Either diet should supply all the nutrients needed; however, if milk is restricted drastically, the calcium level must be watched carefully.

BLAND DIET A bland diet restricts those dietary components that are classified as gastrointestinal irritants. Such a diet limits any foods that are chemically (e.g., caffeine, pepper, chili, nutmeg, and alcohol) or mechanically (high-fiber) irritating. No fried foods or highly concentrated sweets are included. Gas-forming vegetables belonging to the onion and cabbage family are also eliminated. The diet is commonly used for problems occurring in the gastrointestinal tract (such as ulcers). The bland diet should supply sufficient nutrients for the individual to meet the recommended daily allowances, unless fruits and vegetables are eliminated (in which case, a supplement may be necessary).

ELIMINATION DIET Diets that modify the levels of specific foods are most frequently used to treat allergies of various kinds. There are two basic elimination-type regimens. A simple elimination diet removes only one or two foods that are suspected of causing the allergy. The Rowe elimination diet involves a more extensive program. Using this method, the basic diet consists of a few hypoallergenic foods such as rice cereal, apples, pears, carrots, sweet potatoes, lamb, and milk substitutes. If no allergic reaction is observed, single food-family groups are added slowly in periods of about 10 days. In children, the most common allergies are to chocolate, wheat, eggs, and milk. In some cases, it may be difficult to meet the recommended daily allowances for all nutrients. When this situation occurs, supplements should be ordered.

PRESCRIBING A DIET

Because there are so many different types of therapeutic diets, it is frequently impossible for the physician to stay abreast of all the restrictions and other considerations involved. For this reason, the physician will often rely on either a local dietitian or a nutritional consultant to plan the therapeutic diet and instruct patients on the modifications they should follow.

Basically, diet therapy involves a problem-solving process. First, data concerning the nutritional status of the patient must be collected. This information is generally accumulated by a variety of health care professionals (headed by the physician), including, in some cases, medical assistants, and is expanded and coordinated by the registered dietitian. The second step is the planning phase, during which the collected data are analyzed, the nutrition-related problems are delineated, and the possible solutions are outlined. The proposed dietary measures are then implemented as a planned dietary program. Last, the program, or diet being used, is evaluated in terms of the medical problem to determine whether the nutrition-related disorder is being or has been corrected. If necessary, the entire process is repeated. At all times, it is preferable to involve the patient as much as possible to maximize results and maintain long-term dietary modifications.

If it is not feasible to use professional dietetic assistance, the physician may wish to use a service offered by some firms that develop diets, printed with the physician's name on them, that can be given to the patient. Numerous pharmaceutical or medical suppliers also supply diet lists, which usually are used as additional advertising for the products of the manufacturer (Figs. 47–4 and 47–5). If such diets are employed, the information must be as

NUMBER OF SERVINGS REQUIRED FOR DIFFERENT CALORIE LEVELS

Calorie Level (Common Individuals in Group)	About 1600 Many women, older adults	About 2200 Children, teen girls, most men, active women	About 2800 Teen boys, active men
Grain Products Group Servings	6	9	11
Vegetable Group Servings	3	4	5
Fruit Group Servings	2	3	4
Milk Group Servings	2–3*	2–3*	2–3*
Meat and Beans Group Servings	2 (5 oz total)	2 (6 oz total)	3 (7 oz total)
Total Fat (g)	53	73	93

*Women who are pregnant or breast-feeding, teenagers, and young adults to age 24 need 3 servings.

FIGURE 47–4 Number of servings required for different calorie levels. (From Nutrition and Your Health: Dietary Guidelines for Americans, 4th ed. Washington, DC, U.S. Department of Agriculture and U.S. Department of Health and Human Services, 1995.)

A FEEDING GUIDE FOR CHILDREN

What you teach your child about food will last a lifetime. Weight Watchers, a leader in good nutrition, has developed this guide to help get you and your child off to a good start. Starting now on the road to healthy eating can lead your child to a healthier lifestyle as an adult. This is a guide to a basic diet. Fats, desserts, and sauces will contribute additional kilocalories to meet the needs of the growing child.

	1 Year Old		2–3 Years Old		4–6 Years Old		7–Puberty		
Food	**Portion sizes**	**No. of servings**	**Portion sizes**	**No. of servings**	**Portion sizes**	**No. of servings**	**Portion sizes**	**No. of servings**	**Comments**
Milk	1/2 cup	4–5	1/4–3/4 cup	4–5	1/4–3/4 cup	3–4	1 cup	3	The following may be substituted for one-half cup of liquid milk: 1/2–3/4 oz. cheese 1/4–1/2 cup yogurt 2 1/2 tbsp. non-fat dry milk powder
Meat and meat equivalents	1/4–1 oz. (2–4 tbsp.)	1	1–2 oz.	2	1–2 oz.	2	2–3 oz.	3	The following may be substituted for 1 oz. of meat, fish, poultry: 4–5 tbsp. cooked legumes 1 egg 2 tbsp. peanut butter
Fruit and vegetable		4–5		4–5		4–5		4–5	
Vegetables: Cooked	1–2 tbsp.		2–3 tbsp.		3–4 tbsp.		1/2 cup		Include one green leafy or yellow vegetable, e.g., spinach, broccoli, carrots, winter squash
Vegetables: Raw	1–2 tbsp.		few pieces		few pieces		1/2 cup		
Fruit: Canned	2–4 tbsp.		2–4 tbsp.		4–6 tbsp.		1/2 cup		Include one vitamin C-rich fruit or juice per day
Fruit: Raw	2–4 tbsp. (chopped)		1/2–1 small		1/2–1 small		1 med.		
Fruit: Juice	2–4 oz.		3–4 oz.		4 oz.		4 oz.		
Grains and grain products	1/2 slice	3	1/4–1 slice	3	1 slice	4	1 slice	6	The following may be substituted for one slice of bread: 1/2 cup cooked cereal 1/2 cup spaghetti or other pasta 1/2 cup rice 5 saltines Whole grain products provide additional bulk to the diet

FIGURE 47–5 Children's dietary needs. (Courtesy of Weight Watchers International, Inc.)

clear and concise as possible so that the patient is not confused or discouraged.

It is important that the patient return home with written instructions after leaving the office. Many questions will arise after the diet has first been introduced in the office. A written list is the easiest method of answering these questions.

Reading Food Labels

In 1995, the U.S. Department of Agriculture required that all food products contain a nutritional fact label (Fig. 47–6). These labels are usually on the back of the package and are a source of nutrition information and provide facts on the nutrients within the labeled can or package. When planning or implementing a designated diet, the food label can be used as a valuable source of information (see Procedure 47–1). Every label must include

- Individual serving size
- Number of servings per container
- Total calories
- Calories derived from fat content
- Percentage of daily value (percentage of daily nutrient requirements in serving)

PROCEDURE 47-1

Patient Education: Reading Food Labels

GOAL

To accurately explain the nutritional labeling of food products to the patient.

EQUIPMENT AND SUPPLIES

One each of four candy bars: Snickers, Twix, Healthy Choice, Fat Free Fruit Bar
Pencil and paper

PROCEDURAL STEPS

1. Explain what you are going to talk about to the patient. Be sure to include reasons why this label is a valuable source of nutritional information in diet planning.
2. Using the labels on each candy bar, point out the nutritional information.
   PURPOSE: Using actual labels assists in learning.
3. Give the patient pencil and paper to write down the serving size of each type of candy bar.
   PURPOSE: Writing something down helps memory retention.
4. Together compare similarities and differences.
5. Next have the patient write down the caloric amount for each.
   PURPOSE: Writing assists in learning.
6. Compare similarities and differences.
   PURPOSE: Comparing the results completes the learning activity.
7. Write down the percentage of fat, total and saturated and unsaturated.
8. Compare similarities and differences.
9. Together analyze the nutritional level of each.
10. Discuss any new information that was learned.
    PURPOSE: Patient feels part of the learning experience and senses your genuine interest in the learning experience.
11. Ask the patient if he or she will use this information when shopping and how will it will be implemented into the shopping and diet planning.
    PURPOSE: Method to evaluate the learning experience.

NUTRITION FACTS

Serving size 1 1/4 cup (30 g)
Servings per container about 16

Amount per serving	Cereal	Cereal with 1/2 cup skim milk
Calories	110	160
Calories from fat	0	0
	% Daily value**	
Total fat 0 g*	**0%**	**0%**
Saturated fat 0 g	**0%**	**1%**
Cholesterol 0 mg	**0%**	**1%**
Sodium 270 mg	**11%**	**14%**
Total carbohydrate 26 g	**9%**	**11%**
Dietary fiber less than 1 g	**0%**	**0%**
Sugars 3 g		
Other carbohydrate 22 g		
Protein 2 g		
Vitamin A	0%	6%
Vitamin C	10%	10%
Calcium	0%	15%
Iron	50%	50%
Thiamin	25%	25%
Niacin	25%	25%
Vitamin B_6	25%	25%
Folate	25%	25%
Vitamin B_{12}	25%	30%

*Amount in cereal. One half cup skim milk contributes an additional 40 calories, less than 5 mg cholesterol, 65 mg sodium, 6 g total carbohydrate (6 g sugars) and 4 g protein.
**Percent daily values are based on a 2,000 calorie diet. Your daily values may be higher or lower depending on your calorie needs:

	Calories:	2000	2500
Total fat	Less than	65 g	80 g
Saturated fat	Less than	20 g	25 g
Cholesterol	Less than	300 mg	300 mg
Sodium	Less than	2400 mg	2400 mg
Total carbohydrate		300 g	375 g
Dietary fiber		25 g	30 g

Calories per gram:
Fat 9 • Carbohydrate 4 • Protein 4

FIGURE 47–6 Nutritional facts label.

INGREDIENT LABEL

INGREDIENTS: COOKED WHITE RICE, WATER, COOKED CHICKEN TENDERLOINS, GREEN BEANS, CARROTS, RED PEPPERS, BROWN SUGAR. CONTAINS LESS THAN 2% OF MODIFIED FOOD STARCH, MUSTARD (VINEGAR, MUSTARD SEED, SALT, SPICES, TURMERIC), DIJON MUSTARD (WATER, MUSTARD SEED, DISTILLED VINEGAR, SALT, WHITE WINE, CITRIC ACID, TARTARIC ACID, SPICES), HONEY, MALTODEXTRIN (FROM CORN), SALT, EGG YOLK SOLIDS, SODIUM PHOSPHATE, VINEGAR POWDER (MALTODEXTRIN, MODIFIED FOOD STARCH, VINEGAR SOLIDS), XANTHAN GUM FLAVORS, SPICES, LEMON JUICE CONCENTRATE

FIGURE 47–7 Ingredient label. (Courtesy of Weight Watchers International, Inc.)

HOW TO USE NUTRITION FACTS

Start with serving size information that is listed in both household and metric units. The serving size is uniform across product lines so that you can easily compare the nutritional qualities of similar foods.

KEY TO UNDERSTANDING SERVING SIZE

g = grams (about 28 g = 1 ounce)
mg = milligrams (1000 mg = 1 g)

The amounts of each nutrient in the food is expressed in two ways: in terms of weight per serving and as a percentage of the daily value. By using the percentage of daily values, you can easily determine whether a food contributes a lot or a little of a particular nutrient. But if you eat more or less than the serving size on the label, you will need to adjust the amounts of nutrients accordingly.

Keep in mind that the percentage of daily values is based on the amount of food usually eaten in 1 day. The goal is to choose foods that together give you about 100% a day.

INGREDIENT LABELING

The ingredient list also can help you learn more about the foods you eat. A list of ingredients is required on almost all foods, even standardized ones such as mayonnaise and bread. Ingredients are listed in descending order of weight. That helps you get an idea of the proportion of an ingredient in a food (Fig. 47–7).

Also, artificial colors have to be named in the ingredient list; they no longer can be stated as "color added." The total percentage of juice in juice drinks must be declared so that you can see exactly how much juice is in the product.

The front label is where manufacturers often place statements describing the nutritional qualities of their product. The government has set strict conditions under which statements such as low fat, cholesterol free, or good source of fiber can be used as part of the front label (Fig. 47–8).

NUTRIENT CLAIMS Examples include "low fat," "high fiber," "reduced calories," and "cholesterol free." Some of these claims make a comparison to the "regular" version of the food or a similar food. For example, a *reduced-fat* claim on a jar of Italian salad dressing means the food has at least 25% less fat than regular Italian salad dressing. A *light* Italian salad dressing has at least 50% less fat or one third fewer calories than the regular one.

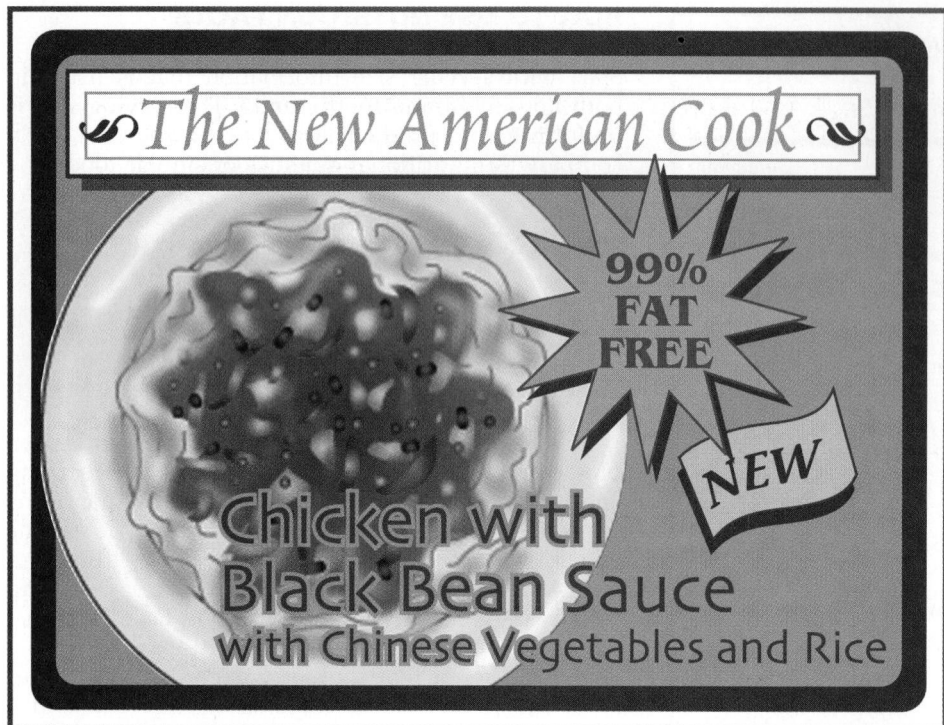

FIGURE 47–8 Front claim label.

Other claims show that a food is high or low in a nutrient. For example, *low-fat* Italian salad dressing has 3 g of fat or less per 2-tablespoon (30-g) serving and *fat-free* Italian salad dressing has less than 0.5 g of fat per serving (Fig. 47–9).

HEALTH CLAIMS The Food and Drug Administration now allows claims linking a nutrient or food to the risk of a disease or health-related condition. Only health claims supported by scientific evidence are allowed.

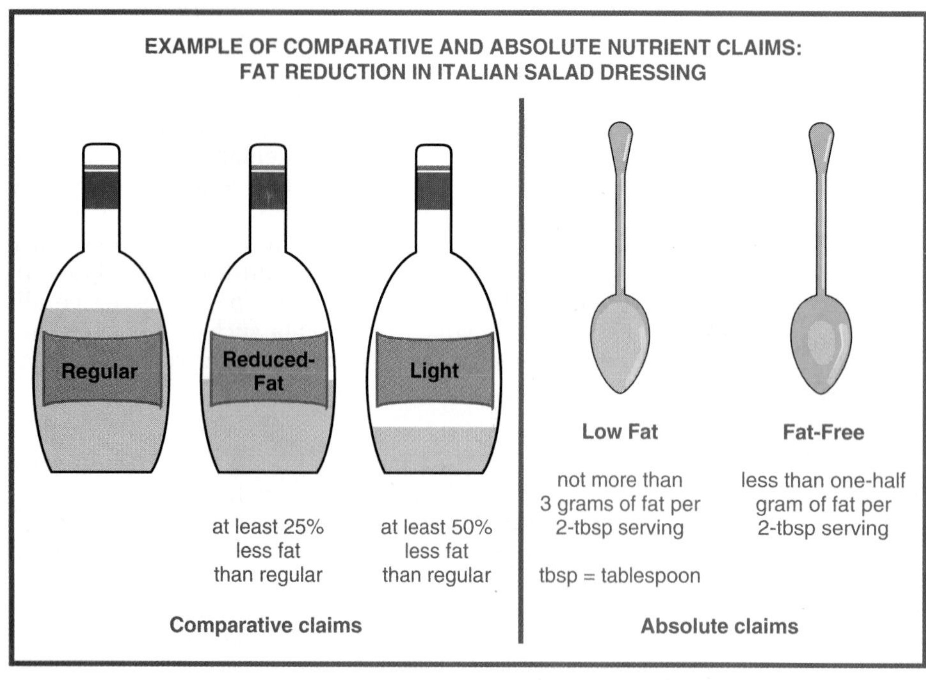

FIGURE 47–9 Comparative versus absolute nutrient claims.

Organic Foods Production Act

In 1990 the U.S. Department of Agriculture proposed that rules be established regarding the labeling of food that was "organically grown." Since then, it has been working on establishing regulations to validate the fast-growing organic food industry. These regulations state that food with the organic label must have been grown without the use of any chemical pesticides, herbicides, or fertilizers. It also prohibits the use of hormones in seed preparation.

In addition to the regulations that will regulate the growing of fruits and vegetables, there are also regulations in regards to meat, poultry, and milk. As with plants, the use of all hormones is prohibited during any phase of the animal's growth or in the preparation of the product for consumption. Milk that carries the organic label will have no added vitamins or chemicals and the regulations of preparation will be closely monitored.

This means that the consumer will get the benefit of natural growth and preparation and will be sure there is a set standard followed.

Nutritional Level Assessment

During the physician's examination of the patient, an assessment is made regarding the patient's nutritional status. The physician considers the patient's age, height and weight, type of body frame, overall health status, recent changes in weight, diet and exercise habits, and lifestyle, culture, and educational level. In addition to this information, the physician will check the turgor of skin, calculate body mass, and assess percentage of body fat.

CALCULATING BODY MASS

To determine how healthy the patient's weight level is, the physician may want you to calculate the patient's body mass. To do this you first must obtain the weight and height of the patient. The height must be converted into inches. Then, using the nomogram in Figure 47–10, measure the mass. To do this, angle the edge of a piece of paper or a ruler from the patient's weight (on the left) to the pa-

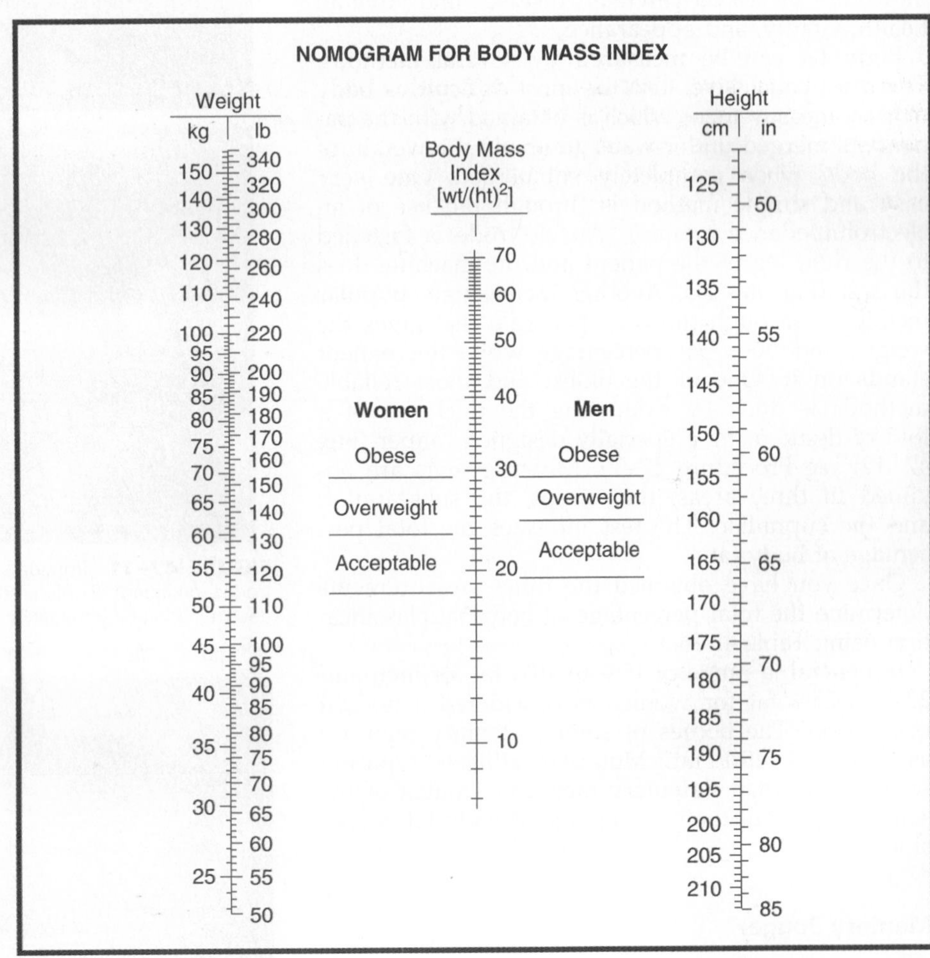

FIGURE 47–10 Nomogram for body mass index.

tient's height (on the right). Then read the risk where the edge crosses the center line. If the risk is anything other than acceptable, it may indicate a need for dietary modifications. This will have to be decided by the physician when all of the information on the patient is evaluated.

Body-Fat Measurement

The location of body fat is very important. Studies conducted in the United States and in Sweden indicate that the body has two different fat stores: one at the hips and the other in the abdomen. Fat at the hips, which is more common in women and more difficult to lose, is primarily stored for special purposes, such as to provide extra energy during pregnancy and nursing. Abdominal fat, which is easier to lose, seems to be more dangerous to overall health. Measure the waist and hips of the patient and correlate the waist-to-hip ratio (the bigger the belly, the higher the ratio). Normal ratios are less than 0.75 in women and are 0.9 to 0.95 in men.

At the physician's request, the medical assistant may be asked to perform body fat measurements on a patient. The percentage of body fat may be an indicator of cardiovascular disease and overall health, vitality, and appearance.

Body fat can be measured by several methods. The most conclusive, also the most difficult, is body density measurement which is obtained with the patient submerged under water to obtain the weight of the body when completely submerged. One very easy and simple method is through the use of an electroimpedance monitor. An electrode is fastened to the right leg of the patient and the machine does the rest (Fig. 47–11). Another increasingly popular method is through the use of a scale that gives the weight and body fat percentage while the patient stands on it. One of the oldest and most reliable methods is done by evaluating the thickness of a fold of tissue using a specially designed caliper (Fig. 47–12; see Procedure 47–2). Measurements are obtained in three areas, the triceps, the subscapular, and the suprailiac. The test indicates the total percentage of body fat.

Once you have obtained the three measurements determine the total percentage of body fat classification using Table 47–4.

In general, a range of 15% to 19% fat for men and 22% to 25% fat for women is considered a normal body level. The bodies of some sedentary men are as much as 40% fat. Muscular athletes typically weigh more than sedentary men and women of the same height, but their percentage of body fat is considerably lower.

Memory Jogger

8 *Identify four methods for obtaining body-fat percentages.*

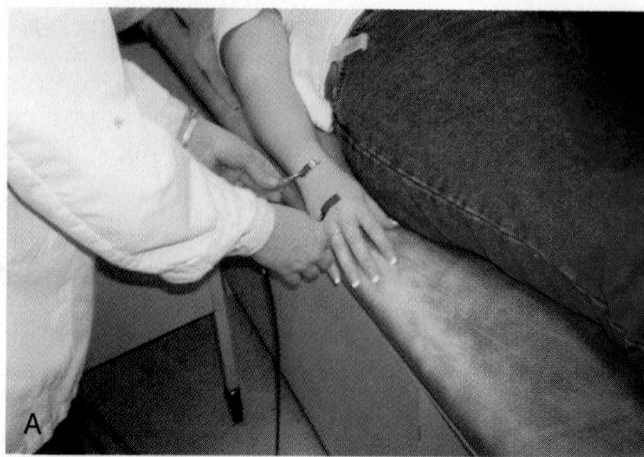

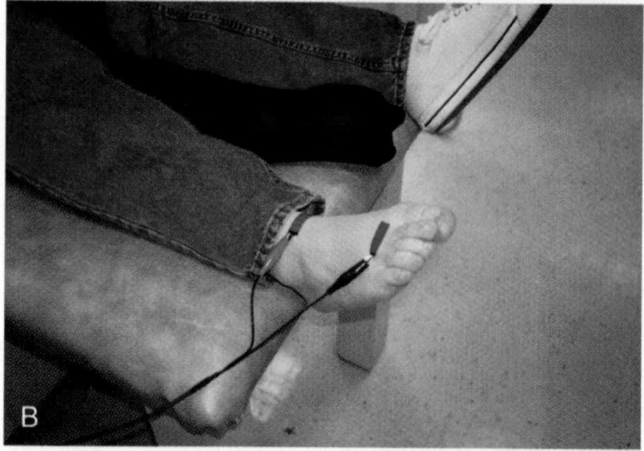

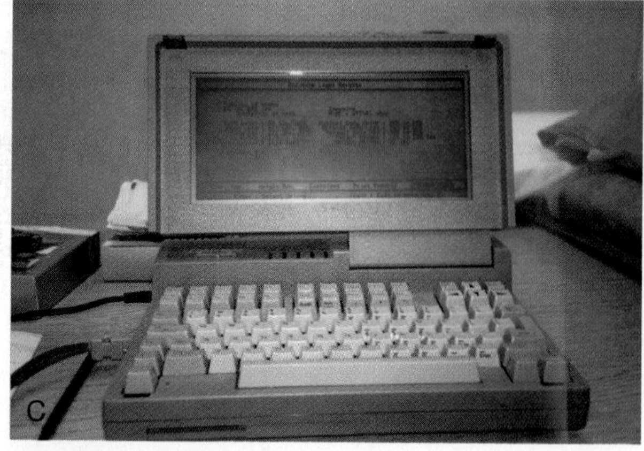

FIGURE 47–11 Impedance monitor fat readout. *A,* Place electrodes on hand. *B,* Place electrodes on foot. *C,* Read body fat determination on impedance monitor.

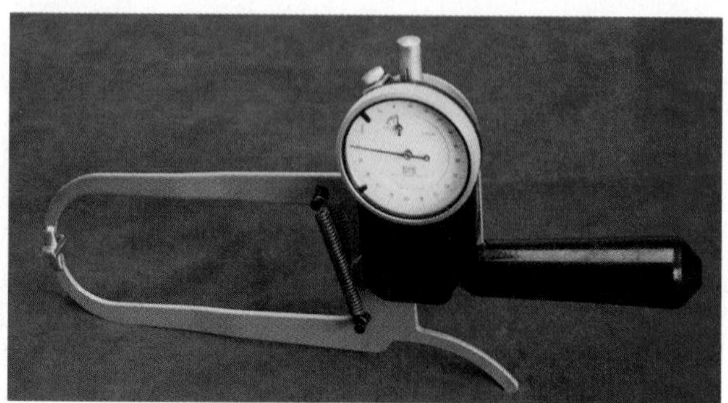

FIGURE 47–12 Fat-fold calipers.

PROCEDURE 47-2

Determining Fat-Fold Measurements

GOAL

To accurately determine and record a measurement of body fat.

EQUIPMENT AND SUPPLIES

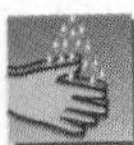

Fat-fold body calipers

Pencil and paper

PROCEDURAL STEPS

1 Read the directions before you begin.

2 Gather the equipment and supplies needed to complete the procedure.

3 Identify the patient.
PURPOSE: To make sure that you have the right patient.

4 Explain the procedure to the patient.
PURPOSE: To provide assurance to the patient.

5 Using the triceps of the upper arm, grasp the skinfold with thumb and index finger. Make sure that the fold is in a parallel angle by keeping the thumb and index finger in line with one another. Be sure you do not grasp muscle tissue or pinch too tightly (Figure 1).
PURPOSE: Best site to start with because it is the easiest to obtain.

6 Place calipers over the fold and measure.

Continued

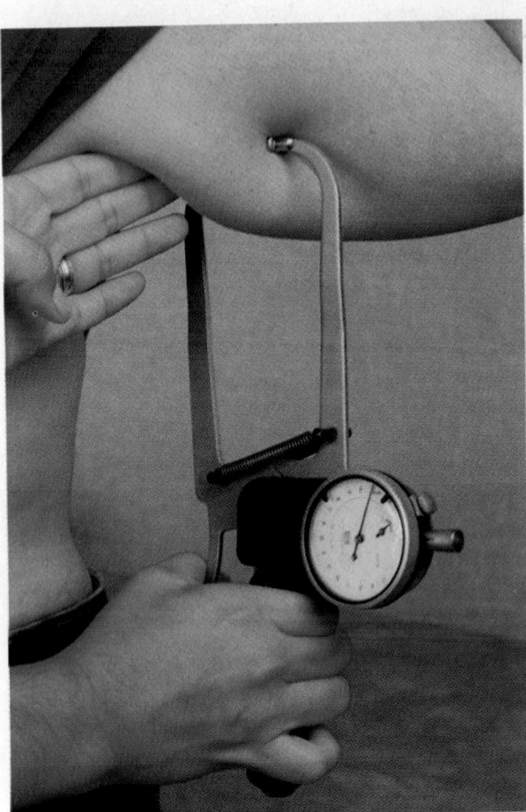

FIGURE 1

PROCEDURE 47-2 (CONTINUED)
Determining Fat-Fold Measurements

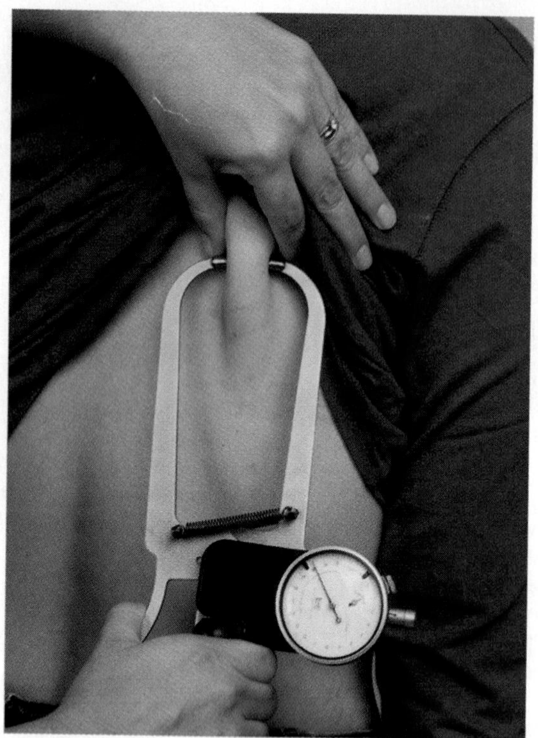

FIGURE 2

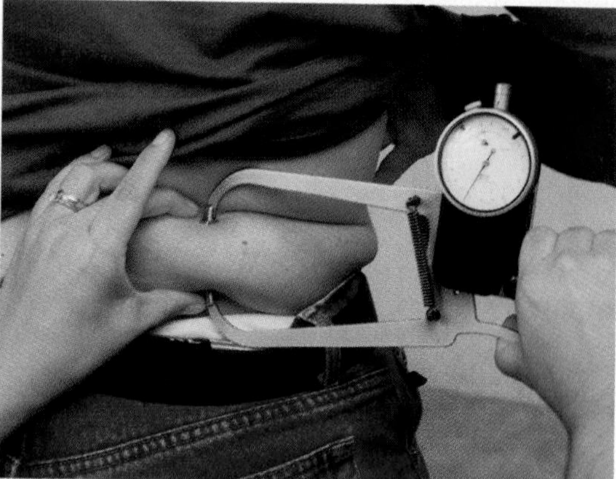

FIGURE 3

7 Record the measurement.

8 Using the subscapular located beneath the shoulder blade, obtain your second measurement (Figure 2).

9 Record the measurement.

10 Using the suprailiac area located immediately superior to the fanning of the hip bone, obtain your third measurement (Figure 3).

11 Record the measurement.

12 Determine total percent of body fat using chart in text.

13 Record the calculations in the patient's medical record.
PURPOSE: A procedure is considered not done until it is recorded.

14 Return equipment to its proper place.

15 Wash your hands.
PURPOSE: Infection control.

TABLE 47-4 Body Fat Classification

Classification	Triceps	Scapular	Abdomen	Total
Male				
Lean <7%	<7 mm	<8 mm	<10 mm	<25 mm
Acceptable 7%–15%	7–13 mm	8–15 mm	10–20 mm	25–48 mm
Overfat >15%	>13 mm	>15 mm	>20 mm	>48 mm
Female				
Lean <12%	<90 mm	<7 mm	<7 mm	<23 mm
Acceptable 12–25%	9–17 mm	7–14 mm	7–15 mm	23–46 mm
Overfat >25%	>17 mm	>14 mm	>15 mm	>46 mm

Eating Disorders

Eating disorders are defined as any eating behavior pattern that can lead to a health problem. The two problems that cause the most serious health risks are **anorexia nervosa** and **bulimia.** These disorders can damage all of the body systems and cause death. They are found most frequently in adolescent and young adult women (Table 47–5).

Anorexia nervosa is characterized by self-induced starvation. These individuals usually have a type A personality, are in their early to mid 20s, and fear becoming grossly overweight if they allow themselves to eat. As a result, they will lose an excessive amount of weight, become extremely malnourished, and will die without medical intervention. The first phase of treatment is to establish an immediate level of nourishment to the body systems, which is done intravenously or by nasogastric tube feedings. Then the patient will need psychotherapy to alleviate depression and to be assisted in forming a positive self-image.

Bulimia is sometimes referred to as binging and purging disorder. This behavior pattern can occur when an individual is slightly overweight, diets, but fails to achieve the expected results. Psychologically the person believes that self worth is related to being thin. Usually the pattern begins with some form of stress that upsets the individual, and the person will find consolation in eating an outrageous amount of food. The eating binge is followed by self-induced punishment in the form of vomiting, using laxatives and enemas, excessive exercise, and food abstinence. Most bulimic individuals want help and will make attempts to get into treatment programs. The program must be a combination of medication, psychotherapy, and nutritional counseling. The goal is to establish healthy eating patterns and to develop an improved self image.

Memory Jogger

9 *State the major characteristic of anorexia nervosa and bulimia.*

TABLE 47-5 Common Diet-Related Disorders

Disorder	Major Dietary Components	Corrective Dietary Measures
Allergies	Wide variety of foods are possible allergens: wheat, milk, eggs, chocolate most common	Eliminate or restrict food sources of allergen
Anemia	Deficiency of iron, vitamin B_{12}, or folacin	Increase amount of deficient nutrient
Anorexia nervosa	Starvation; fear of becoming fat; altered body image	High-calorie diet, psychotherapy, behavior modification
Atherosclerosis	High cholesterol, high saturated fat, excessive calories	Control calories, decrease total fat in diet to 30% to 35% of calories, change to more unsaturated fats, lower cholesterol content of diet, stress complex carbohydrates rather than simple sugars
Bulimia	Binge eating, self-induced vomiting	Regular diet; behavior modification, psychotherapy
Cancer of the colon	Low fiber	Increase dietary fiber, increase fluids
Cirrhosis of the liver	Excessive ingestion of alcohol or nutrients such as iron, lead, vitamin A or D	Reduce dietary level of excessive nutrient or substance
Constipation/diverticulosis	Poor fiber intake, poor fluid intake	Increase dietary fiber and fluids
Diabetes mellitus	Obesity, excessive sugar consumption	Control calories and carbohydrates
Hypertension	Obesity, high salt intake	Control calories, decrease sodium intake
Obesity	Excessive calorie intake, inadequate physical activity	Decrease calories, increase activity; behavior modification, group therapy

Exercise

Exercise is defined as physical exertion for the maintenance or improvement of health or for the correction of a physical handicap. Although most Americans say they know about the benefits of exercise, more than 60% of American adults do not get the recommended amount of physical activity. In fact, 25% are not active at all and nearly half of all American youths 12 to 21 years of age are not vigorously active on a regular basis and physical activity declines during adolescence.

A well-balanced diet is only one half of the fitness balancing act. Adequate exercise and sufficient rest are the other half of the equation needed to ensure good health. Like special diets, exercise programs must be approved for each individual by the physician. It is the physician who will determine the patient's exercise needs and tolerance levels to safeguard the patient from overexertion and stress.

BENEFITS OF EXERCISE

- Increases self-esteem
- Improves mood
- Boosts energy
- Strengthens heart
- Strengthens muscles
- Burns calories
- Improves cholesterol levels
- Relieves stress
- Lowers risk of heart disease, hypertension, and diabetes
- Prevents bone loss
- Decreases risk of some cancers

There are many forms of exercise available. Some patients may find that it is best to go to a gym and develop a formal program of physical fitness. Others may purchase home exercise equipment that will enable them to exercise in privacy. Many will feel that getting out in the fresh air and walking is the best form of exercise.

WALKING FOR EXERCISE

- Begin with only 5 minutes a day.
- Work up to 10 minutes after 1 or 2 weeks.
- Add 5 more minutes at biweekly intervals after that.
- When walking, always swing your arms freely.
- Wear comfortable walking shoes.

All of these are acceptable because all have one thing in common, physical activity. Each individual should find the outlet that brings enjoyment and enrichment to his or her life. It is not the form of exercise that is important, just the fact that the person is participating in physical activity.

Regular exercise improves circulation and muscle tone along with relieving tension and emotional stress. People who have followed an exercise routine regularly find that they experience a better outlook on life, have more energy, and feel better about themselves.

If you are working with a patient who cannot engage in a full physical exercise program, you can suggest range of motion exercising. These exercise patterns are designed to improve circulation and promote muscle tone by putting each joint through its full range. Patients with disabilities such as partial paralysis, arthritis, bursitis, and musculoskeletal deformities may be helped with these exercises.

Memory Jogger

What is the primary purpose of exercise?

Developing the Right Habits

Americans have gone through a remarkable revolution in their ideas about aging. Many people exude remarkable vitality at a time in life that would have been unimaginable to their grandparents. Scientists also have learned that age is not just measured by the calendar. It is now known that the most feared part of aging, that dreaded slide into frailty and dependence, has more to do with biology than chronology. A person's biology, in turn, is shaped by his genetic makeup, which cannot be controlled, and his lifestyle which can be controlled. We can influence and control our biologic age by the way we conduct our life. Years can be added to our active life with the right kinds of habits. There are components of a lifestyle that can delay and even reverse many maladies that we too often assume are the inevitable result of old age.

HINTS FOR A HEALTHFUL LIFESTYLE

- **Eat right.** While appetite declines with age, many nutritional needs increase. Get five daily servings of fruits and vegetables, plus generous portions of whole grains, beans, and dairy products.
- **Protect your immune system.** Eat whole grains, green leafy vegetables, seafood, lean meats, and moderate amounts of vegetable oils to get vitamins E and B_6, and the trace mineral zinc. Your body will be able to fight infections and chronic disease.
- **Keep your bones strong.** Drink milk and eat cheese and yogurt for calcium. If you get little

direct sunlight, be sure your daily supplement gives you vitamin D, which helps your body absorb calcium more effectively.

- **Be regular.** Try to eat 20 to 35 g of fiber a day to keep your digestive system active and healthy. Good fiber sources are fruits and vegetables, oats, beans, and wheat-bran cereals.
- **Watch your vision.** Eat citrus fruits, tomatoes, and orange, yellow, and green vegetables to get the antioxidant power of vitamin C and the carotenoids. Cataract formation is just one of the damaging effects of oxidation in the body.
- **Reduce your risk of heart disease and cancer.** Limit your intake of saturated fats in fatty meat, cheese, butter, and partially hydrogenated fats (*trans*-fatty acids) found in many margarines and commercial baked goods.
- **Maintain your body weight.** It is harder to keep off the pounds as you age because your muscle tissue tends to decline and with it, your ability to use all the energy in foods. So our bodies store that energy as fat, and that can hasten the onset of diabetes, heart disease, arthritis, and other problems.
- **Exercise, exercise, exercise!** Inactivity hastens the aging process and exercise does the opposite. Mix aerobic exercises like walking and swimming with simple stretch-training exercises to build and strengthen muscle tissue. Try to incorporate three half-hour sessions of each into your weekly schedule.

From USDA Human Nutrition Research Center on Aging, Boston, MA

PATIENT EDUCATION

You may be called on to discuss a diet plan with a patient. It is extremely important to have a thorough knowledge of diet therapy to talk with the patient in a convincing manner. The patient must understand the diet and the rationale behind its use. If the patient feels uneasy or has many unanswered questions, he or she may be less motivated to follow a diet plan. You can be a very valuable asset to the physician, the dietitian, and the patient.

When talking to patients about a diet, the following may be helpful:

- Use charts and diagrams to illustrate diets.
- Consider the patient's dietary likes and dislikes.
- Remember ethnic and cultural foods are important.
- Allow the patient to play an active role in the learning process.
- Suggest local support groups that can help in diet maintenance.

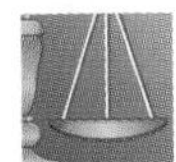

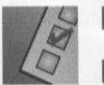

LEGAL AND ETHICAL ISSUES

Always remember that you are not a doctor, nor are you a dietitian. Follow the doctor's instructions, and if the patient has questions that you are not sure of, *always* ask the physician for his or her advice in handling the question. If your workplace employs a registered dietitian, refer questions involving meal patterns and food selection changes to him or her. When seeking advice in the field of nutrition and exercise programs, direct patients to someone who is a qualified expert.

CRITICAL THINKING

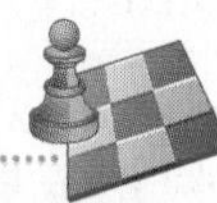

1 You are asked to assist a patient who is a vegetarian with a 1500-calorie diet to assist her in maintenance of her diabetes. How do you plan on doing this?

2 A close friend of your sister is visiting at your home and you hear her tell your sister that she is using ipecac and Ex-Lax after every meal and secretly exercising for 3 hours at night after the rest of the family is asleep. She also tells your sister that she is 5′6″ tall and determined not to weigh over 100 pounds at graduation. What do you do?

HOW DID I DO? Answers to Memory Joggers

1. Food is any material that meets the nutritive requirements of an organism for the maintenance of growth and physical well-being.
2. The two energy sources available to the body are exogenous and endogenous.
3. The circle is used to indicate fat, and the triangle is used to indicate sugar.
4. Carbohydrates are found in cereal grains, vegetables, and sweets.
5. Fats are classified by their source, their physical appearance, and their chemical structure.
6. The recommended daily intake of proteins is 0.8 g/kg of body weight, and one third should be from complete proteins.
7. The largest quantity minerals are sodium, potassium, chlorine, calcium, phosphorus, and magnesium.
8. Four ways to obtain the percentage of body fat are body density measurement, electroimpedance, weight/body-fat scale, and caliper measurement.
9. Anorexia nervosa is characterized by self-induced starvation, and bulimia is characterized by binging and purging.
10. The primary purpose of exercise is physical exertion for the maintenance or improvement of health or for the correction of a physical handicap.

Applying the Principles of Pharmacology

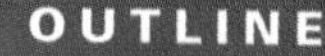

Mary Agnes Taylor, RN

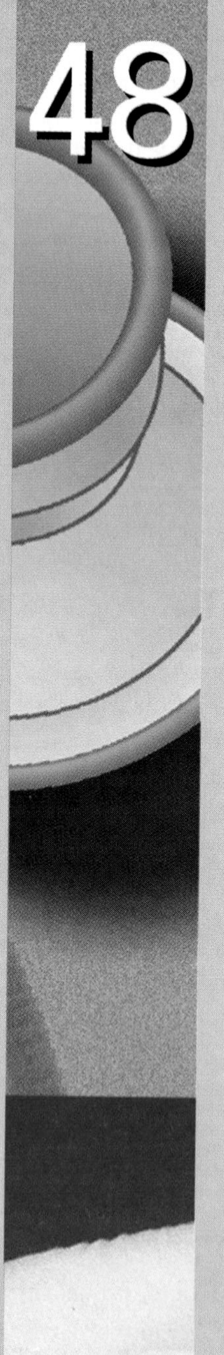

OUTLINE

LEARNING OBJECTIVES

Cognitive: On successful completion of this chapter you should be able to:

1. Spell and define the words listed in the Vocabulary.
2. Differentiate between a drug's generic name and trade name.
3. Cite the dangers of using over-the-counter drugs.
4. List the information needed in each part of a prescription.
5. Cite the Drug Enforcement Agency (DEA) regulations for the storage of controlled or regulated substances.
6. List the DEA regulations for prescription drugs under each of the five schedules of the Controlled Substance Act.
7. Define the major types of drug dependency.
8. Cite the clinical uses of drugs.
9. Recall the five steps that describe the fate of a drug in the human body.
10. Cite factors that influence the effect of a drug in the body.
11. Describe the use of the *Physician's Desk Reference.*

Performance: On successful completion of this chapter you should be able to:

1. Calculate the correct dose for administration.
2. Calculate the correct dose for administration using two systems of measurement.
3. Calculate the correct pediatric dose when only an adult medication is available.
4. Calculate the correct pediatric dose for administration using body weight.

VOCABULARY

alkalosis A disorder characterized by excess base condition

antidote Agent that neutralizes a poison or its effect

cardiotonic Increasing contractility of the heart

colloidal Pertaining to a gluelike substance

controlled substance Drugs that are regulated by the federal government (Drug Enforcement Agency)

enteric-coated Drug formulation in which tablets are coated with a special compound that does not dissolve until the tablet is exposed to the fluids of the small intestine

generic Drugs that are not protected by trademark

ions Electrically charged particles

lumen Space within a vessel or tube

nomogram Representation by graphs, diagrams, or charts of the relationships between numeric variables

orphan drugs Group of drugs that at one time were used in medical treatments but due to misuse or discovery of side effects have been removed from market (ex: Phen-phen).

over-the-counter drugs Medications sold without a prescription

parenteral Denoting any medication route other than the gastrointestinal (oral)

permeability Ability to allow solutions to pass through a membrane

psychosomatic Disorders that have a physiologic component but are thought to originate in the mind of the patient

synergism Joint action of agents that results in a combined effect that is greater than the effects of the individual components

Pharmacology is the broad science that deals with the origin, nature, chemistry, effects, and uses of drugs. *Clinical pharmacology* deals with the biologic effects a drug has when used as a medical treatment. It covers the actions of a drug in the body over a period of time, including the biologic effects a drug has on the patient; how it is used as a medical treatment; the rate at which body tissues absorb a drug; where a drug is distributed or localizes in the tissues; the chemical changes of the drug that occur in the body; the specific effects a drug has on the body; the route by which a drug is excreted; and, finally, *toxicity,* which is a drug's poisonous effect.

As a result of the rapid, technical advances in drug therapy and biochemistry, the importance of how the body deals with a drug is now emphasized more than the specific effects that a drug has on the body. As a medical assistant, you should have a general understanding of the types of drugs that are available. For every drug that you administer, you should know the functional changes that each drug brings about in the body. That is, you should know the drug's *effect* and how the body absorbs, uses, and eliminates the drug, which is the fate of a drug. With the advent of new drugs, you will continually need to update your knowledge of the specific drugs used in your particular practice. Your role as the person responsible for administering medications and instructing patients on drug administration may change from time to time, but you must always assist the physician, and sometimes the pharmacist, in providing safe drug therapy for the patients.

Memory Jogger

Define pharmacology.

Drug Sources

Some drugs have been used since ancient times. Dating back to 2000 BC, written recipes using opium, castor oil, alcohol, and iron have been found on Egyptian papyrus and Sumerian clay tablets. In medieval times, drugs derived from plants included belladonna (used to treat gastrointestinal disorders), ipecac (used to induce vomiting), and digitalis (used in the treatment of cardiac disorders). The South American Indians have used quinine for reducing fevers and curare, a skeletal muscle relaxant, as a paralyzing poison for centuries.

Today, pharmacology has become a science, in which the drug industry is able to isolate and manufacture synthetically the chemical components of drugs in a form purer than the naturally occurring counterpart. The development of pure drugs enables the administration of drugs to be exact, establishing dose–response relationships, that is, knowing exactly how much of a particular drug is needed to bring about a desired effect.

Drugs can be obtained from the leaves, seeds, sap, stem, or root of certain plants. For example, digitalis is an extract from the leaf of the purple foxglove

(*Digitalis purpurea*). *Alkaloids* are the organic compounds extracted from plants and, in pure medicinal form, are quite potent. Morphine sulfate and atropine sulfate are examples. *Glycosides* contain a sugar and one or more active ingredients that are extracted from plants such as digoxin. Other products of plants include *oils*, such as castor oil, a fixed oil, and volatile oils, such as peppermint and clove. *Gums* are used as soothing lotions or suspending agents.

Animals are another natural drug source and often supply replacement hormones for human therapy. Insulin is a hormone extracted from the cells of the beef or pork pancreas; and thyroid extract is obtained from the thyroid glands of animals.

Minerals also supply a wide variety of natural drugs, such as sodium chloride, potassium, and iron supplements.

Most drugs produced today are manufactured in pharmaceutical laboratories. They are made of chemical substances and are pure drugs. These are identical to the naturally occurring drugs or created as entirely new substances. Scientists can now create genetically engineered medications, such as interferon, which can be used in the treatment of cancer.

Drug Names

A single drug may have up to three names: chemical, generic, and trade. The chemical name represents the drug's exact formula. The chemical name of the analgesic acetaminophen is *N*-(4-hydroxyphenyl). Acetaminophen is the generic name. One of its trade names is Tylenol. All drugs have a **generic** or nonproprietary (official) name assigned to them. This name is much simpler than the chemical name, and it is not protected by copyright. The majority of generic drugs are therapeutically equivalent. The trade or brand name is assigned by the manufacturer and is protected by copyright. The use of generic names is encouraged over trade names to avoid confusion. Drugs are also classified by their use. For example Advil is a brand name of the generic drug ibuprofen, which is classified as an analgesic and an anti-inflammatory agent.

Any U.S. pharmaceutical company that develops a new drug is given a 17-year patent on the drug. It is not until this patent time expires that other companies may manufacture the drug and sell it under their own brand names. Therefore, there are many brand names for each generic drug.

Memory Jogger

Identify the three names given to a drug.

Food and Drug Administration Regulation

The Food and Drug Administration (FDA) is an agency of the United States Department of Health and Human Services. It makes mandatory the testing of all drugs before release to the public. Testing includes toxicity tests in laboratory animals, then clinical studies in a controlled group of voluntary patients. A manufacturer must prove not only the safety of a drug but also its effectiveness. A drug that is safe but cannot be proved to have an advantageous effect on the human body will not be approved by the FDA. When all the phases of the preclinical and clinical studies pass investigation, the FDA will approve a new drug for marketing. Only one of 10 new drugs ever reaches the clinical testing phase. Very few new drugs reach the consumer. After approval, a manufacturer must continue to demonstrate a drug's effectiveness and safety and must submit reports whenever unexpected adverse reactions are discovered. If there is evidence that an approved drug no longer appears safe or effective, the FDA may suspend or withdraw the drug from manufacture and distribution.

DRUG QUALITY AND STANDARDIZATION

Manufacturing standards are established by the FDA to ensure the proper identity, strength, purity, and quality of drugs shipped in interstate commerce, which includes nearly all the drugs that are encountered in the medical office.

STANDARDS FOR MANUFACTURERS

- Identify every drug by a particular color, form, shape, size, and label.
- Produce every dose at the same tested strength.
- Produce the exact formula approved by the FDA.
- Use ingredients that are free from contaminants and of the highest quality.

DISPENSING DRUGS

There are two methods of dispensing drugs: **over-the-counter** (OTC) and by prescription (Table 48–1). Over-the-counter drugs are available to the public for self-medication. These drugs have been approved by the FDA and are considered safe for patients to use without the physician's advice.

The medical assistant who is directly involved in patient care should have an understanding of some

TABLE 48–1 Prescription Drugs Dispensed in U.S. Community Pharmacies, New and Refill Prescriptions—All Strengths (1998, Most Frequently Prescribed)

Manufacturer's Abbreviation	Drug Label	Manufacturer's Abbreviation	Drug Label
PY	Acetaminophen/cod #3 Table 1	PY	Carbamazepine 200-mg tablet
WZ	Hydrocodone/Apap 5/500 tablet	G7	Macrobid 100-mg capsule
BS	Trimox 500-mg capsule	GG	Cimetidine 400-mg tablet
WY	Premarin 0.625-mg tablet	GI	Lanoxin 0.25-mg tablet
EX	Ibuprofen 800-mg tablet	MS	Vasotec 5-mg tablet
WR	Albuterol 90-μg inhaler	EX	Medroxyprogesterone 2.5 mg
BS	Veetids 500-mg tablet	LE	Potassium CL 10-mEq capsule
AT	Prilosec 20-mg capsule	AB	Biaxin 500-mg tablet
LM	Cotrim DS tablet	ZL	Doxycycline 100-mg capsule
BS	Cephalexin 500-mg capsule	PY	Diphenhydramine 50-mg capsule
PY	Propoxy-N/APAP 100–650 tablet	LY	Humulin 70/30 vial
WY	Prempro 0.625/2.5-mg tablet	MS	Zocor 20-mg tablet
BS	Trimox 250-mg/5-mL suspension	TH	Cipro 500-mg tablet
EX	Ibuprofen 600-mg tablet	OT	Ortho Tri-Cyclen 28 tablet
GG	Atenolol 50-mg tablet	EN	Coumadin 2-mg tablet
GG	Naproxen 500-mg tablet	UP	Xalatan 0.005% eye drops
SC	Claritin 10-mg tablet	DC	Levoxyl 50-μg tablet
BS	Glucophage 500-mg tablet	NK	Novolin 70/30 U100 Insulin
WZ	Hydrocodone/APAP 7.5/750 tablet	BG	Tussin DM Syrup
WZ	Furosemide 40-mg tablet	BS	Cephalexin 250-mg capsule
UA	Acetaminophen 500-mg tablet	VZ	Orasone 5-mg tablet
BS	Pravachol 20-mg tablet	SC	Vanceril inhaler
SK	Paxil 20-mg tablet	KN	Vicodin 5/500 tablet
MS	Vasotec 10-mg tablet	MS	Mevacor 20-mg tablet
GG	Glyburide 5-mg tablet	UP	Deltasone 20-mg tablet
LY	Prozac 20-mg pulvule	CP	Lotensin 10-mg tablet
RU	Carisoprodol 350-mg tablet	CP	Lotensin 20-mg tablet
GG	Metoprolol 50-mg tablet	NY	Cyclobenzaprine 10-mg tablet
RU	Ferrous sulfate 325-mg tablet	GG	Alprazolam 0.25-mg tablet
GG	Hydrochlorothiazide 25-mg tablet	UP	Deltasone 10-mg tablet
MC	Ultram 50-mg tablet	LY	Humulin R 100-U/mL vial
PF	Norvasc 5-mg tablet	PY	Lorazepam 1-mg tablet
MS	Pepcid 20-mg tablet	BS	Trimox 125-mg/5-mL suspension
WY	Premarin 1.25-mg tablet	OT	Ortho-Cyclen 28 tablet
GG	Triameterene/HCTZ 50/25 capsule	GX	Pseudoephedrine 60-mg tablet
DC	Levoxyl 100-μg tablet	GG	Lonox tablet
GI	Lanoxin 0.125-mg tablet	GG	Phentermine HC 30-mg capsule
BS	Trimox 250-mg capsule	LV	One touch test strips
WZ	Furosemide 20-mg tablet	NA	Promethazine VC syrup
PD	Lipitor 10-mg tablet	PF	Glucotrol XL 5-mg tablet
WY	Triphasil-28 tablet	BG	Aspirin 325-mg tablet EC
NY	Amitriptyline HCL 25-mg tablet	OT	Ortho-Novum 7/7/7-28 tablet
NA	Promethazine/codeine syrup	GI	Nix 1% creme rinse liquid
PF	Zoloft 50-mg tablet	GG	Fiorpap tablet
RU	Tri-Vit/Fluoro 0.25-mg drops	MS	Fosamax 10-mg tablet
LM	Sulfamethoxazole w/tmp suspension	OQ	Captopril 25-mg tablet
PD	Dilantin 100-mg kapseal	WZ	Estradiol 1-mg tablet
GG	Ibuprofen 400-mg tablet	AB	Erythrocin 250-mg filmtab
BG	Non-ASA 160-mg/5-mL elixir	TZ	Prevacid 30-mg capsule
PF	Zithromax 250-mg tablet	SC	Claritin-D 12-hour tablet
AB	Erythrocin 500-mg filmtab	ZL	Verapamil 240-mg tablet
RN	Azmacort inhaler	PD	Nitrostat 0.4-mg sublingual tablet
NA	Triamcinolone AC 0.1% cream	BS	Sumycin 250-mg capsule
BB	Diazepam 5-mg tablet		
LY	Humulin N 100U/mL vial		
FF	Octicair otic suspension		
GG	Triamterene/HCTZ 37.5/25 capsule		
AL	Tobradex eye drops		
WR	Albuterol sulf 2-mg/5-mL syrup		
MR	Allegra 60-mg capsule		
GG	Atenolol 25-mg tablet		
NY	Amitriptyline HCL 50-mg tablet		
GG	Triamterene/HCTZ 75/50 tablet		

From www.National Association of Retail Druggists.com.

basic facts regarding OTC drugs. Patients are better informed about their personal health care and want to be active participants in health care decisions. They need facts to make informed choices when using OTC preparations. Most OTC preparations are safe if used as directed on the package; however, patient education contributes greatly to the safe and correct usage. The number of prescription drugs that have been granted OTC status is constantly increasing, and as the list of OTC drugs increases so does the need for consumer education. Examples of prescription drugs that now have OTC status include vaginal creams such as Monistat 7 for the treatment of yeast infections; Benadryl for allergic reactions; Motrin as an anti-inflammatory agent; and Dimetapp for upper respiratory tract disorders.

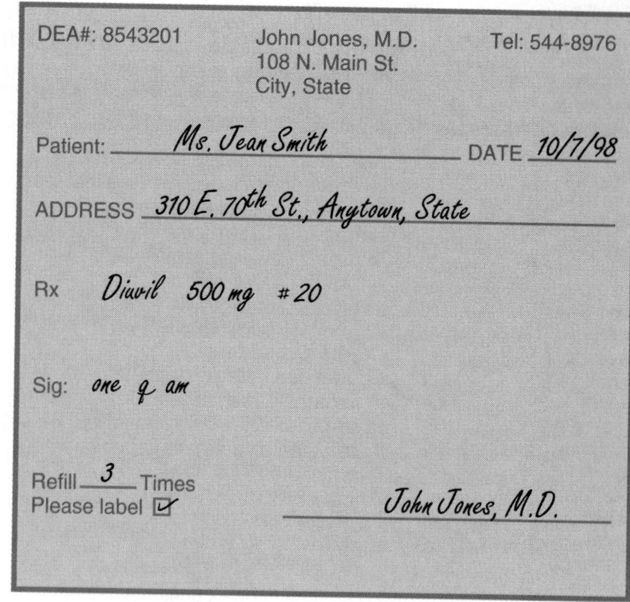
DEA#: 8543201
John Jones, M.D.
108 N. Main St.
City, State
Tel: 544-8976

Patient: Ms. Jean Smith DATE 10/7/98

ADDRESS 310 E. 70th St., Anytown, State

Rx Diuril 500 mg #20

Sig: one q am

Refill 3 Times
Please label ☑
John Jones, M.D.

FIGURE 48–1 A sample prescription.

Memory Jogger

What are the two methods of dispensing drugs?

Prescription Drugs

Federal law makes drugs that are dangerous, powerful, or habit-forming illegal to use except under a physician's order. A *prescription* is an order written by the physician for the compounding or dispensing and administration of drugs to a particular patient. Sometimes an order may be written for the medical assistant on the patient's medical record; however, most often it is a written order on a prescription blank for the pharmacist to fill. A prescription must be given, and signed, by the physician or the order cannot be carried out.

FOUR PARTS OF A PRESCRIPTION

- *Superscription:* Patient's name and address, the date, and the symbol Rx (for the Latin *recipe,* meaning "take")
- *Inscription:* Names and quantities of the ingredients
- *Subscription:* Directions for compounding. Prescription writing is not as complicated for the physician as in earlier times because pharmaceutical manufacturers prepare most medications ready for dispensing or administration. Rarely will a pharmacist have to compound or mix a medication.
- *Signature:* Directions for the patient. It is usually preceded by the symbol Sig: (for the Latin *signa,* meaning "mark"). This is where the physician indicates what instructions are to be put on the label to tell the patient how, when, and in what quantities to use the medication.

Prescription directions may be in English or Latin. Medical terminology and abbreviations are used. It is easier to write *tab. 1 tid c̄ aq pc* than one tablet three times each day with water after meals. A typical prescription is shown in Figure 48–1.

Memory Jogger

Name the four parts of a prescription.

The medical assistant does not write prescriptions but must know prescription terms and abbreviations to communicate with the physician and the pharmacist and to administer medications by written order. The more common terms and abbreviations are listed in Table 48–2.

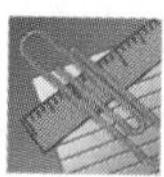
Project: Write a sentence using as many abbreviations as possible.

Prescription Pads

The prescription pads that the physician uses are kept in a designated area that is out of view of the public. It is wise to only have one or two pads in use at a time because these pads are small and substance abusers can easily steal a single prescription or an entire pad. To assist in quantity control measures, handle these pads with care and follow the suggested guidelines.

TABLE 48–2 Common Prescription Abbreviations

Abbreviation	Meaning	Abbreviation	Meaning	Abbreviation	Meaning
a.a.	of each	MTD	maximum tolerated dose	sub-q.	subcutaneous
a.c.	before meals	NPO	nothing by mouth	$\overline{ss}$	one-half
ad lib.	as desired	noct.	at night	stat.	immediately
agit.	shake, stir	N/S	normal saline	t.i.d.	three times a day
a.m.	morning	O_2	oxygen	tinct.	tincture
amp.	ampule	OD	overdose	TO	telephone order
a.u.	each ear	OD	right eye	tus.	cough
a.d.	right ear	OS	left eye	U	unit
a.s.	left ear	OU	both eyes	vag.	vagina
aq.	water	OTC	over-the-counter (drugs)	ves.	bladder
b.i.d.	twice a day	p.c.	after meals	VO	verbal order
$\bar{c}$	with	PL	placebo	W/O	water in oil
cap.	capsule	p.m.	afternoon	cm	centimeter
DC	discontinue	PMI	patient medication instruction	mcg, µg	microgram
D.E.A.	Drug Enforcement Administration	per os	by mouth	mg	milligram
dil.	dilute	p.r.	per rectum	Gm, g	gram
disp.	dispense	pulv.	powder	kg	kilogram
ext.	extract	q.	every	cc	cubic centimeter
F.D.A.	Food and Drug Administration	q.d.	every day	ml	milliliter
fl.	fluid	q.h.	every hour	L	liter
h	hour	q.2h	every 2 hours	gr	grain
h.s.	at bedtime	q.3h	every 3 hours	dr	dram
inj.	injection	q.4h	every 4 hours	oz	ounce
IM	intramuscular	q.i.d.	four times a day	lb	pound
ID	intradermal	q.m.	every morning	♏	minim
IV	intravenous	q.n.	every night	gtt	drops
med.	medicine	q.o.d.	every other day	t, tsp	teaspoon
meq.	milliequivalent	q.s.	quantity sufficient	T, tbs	tablespoon
MLD	minimum lethal dose	R	rectal	C	cup, Celsius
mn.	midnight	℞	"take thou"	pt	pint
MO	mineral oil	S, Sig	give the following directions	qt	quart
MOM	milk of magnesia	$\bar{s}$	without	gal	gallon
MS	morphine sulfate	SC	subcutaneous	F	Fahrenheit

GUIDELINES FOR SAFEGUARDING PRESCRIPTION PADS

- Keep all prescription pads except for the one in use in a designated locked drawer or cabinet.
- Always return the pad that is being used to the designated area, usually the physician's desk.
- Never ask the physician to presign a prescription blank.
- Do not use the back of a prescription blank as note paper.
- Always mutilate a voided prescription before discarding it in the common trash.

Prescription pads may be ordered tinted for easy detection of erasures or correction fluid usage and in colored ink that cannot be reproduced. The pads should be sequentially numbered with the number preprinted on the blanks because this will make a missing blank more quickly discovered. Each prescription blank should have a no-carbon duplicate attachment to provide a permanent record of all prescriptions written. This duplicate is kept in the patient's medical record. Many physicians are now having the words "NOT VALID FOR SCHEDULE II OR III DRUGS" printed in an ink-wash design through the center of every prescription blank. This means that a separate prescription pad that is kept for only writing Schedule II or III drugs will be used when ordering these drugs. This pad will be the only pad that will contain the preprinted physician's DEA registration number.

Memory Jogger

Explain the reason for ordering prescription pads in colored ink on tinted paper.

CONTROLLED SUBSTANCES

Before the first law regulating the sale of foods and drugs in the United States was enacted in 1906, the consumer did not know the actual ingredients of foods and drugs. Cough medications contained excessive amounts of codeine. Vitamin and mineral supplements contained high levels of alcohol. A popular soft drink contained cocaine as its active ingredient. Over the years, more than 50 pieces of legislation have been enacted to control the dispensing and administration of drugs. Today, narcotics and various other substances are controlled and regulated by the Drug Enforcement Agency (DEA), a branch of the Justice Department.

The DEA regulates drugs under five schedules of controlled substances, known as Schedules I, II, III, IV, and V. Drugs are listed under a particular schedule based on their abuse potential and medical usefulness. These schedules not only list the drugs regulated by each category but also address regulations concerning the writing, telephoning, and refilling of prescriptions and the storage and maintenance of drugs. Every medical practice should have a copy of the controlled substances regulations. The medical assistant may secure this list from a regional office of the DEA. It is also important to be on the DEA's mailing list to receive updates as drugs are added, deleted, or moved from one schedule to another.

SCHEDULE I Schedule I includes substances that have no accepted medical use and a high potential for abuse. The possession of these drugs is illegal. Drugs included in this schedule are heroin, lysergic acid diethylamide (LSD), marijuana, mescaline, and peyote. Also included in Schedule I are drugs that are classified as **orphan drugs**.

SCHEDULE II Schedule II includes various narcotics such as opium, the opium derivatives (e.g., morphine), and the synthetic opium derivatives (e.g., synthetic morphine and methadone); stimulants, such as cocaine and amphetamines; and the commonly abused depressant barbiturates. To write these prescriptions, a physician must have a special license (DEA number). The prescription form required for Schedule II drugs varies from state to state. It is essential for the medical assistant to know the state's legal requirements. In California, the prescription must be entirely handwritten by the physician on Federal Triplicate Order Forms imprinted with the DEA number or with the DEA number written in by the physician. These prescriptions must be filled within 72 hours and may not be refilled. In an emergency, a physician may telephone a Schedule II order to the pharmacist. However, the amount of the drug must be limited, and the physician must furnish to the pharmacy, within 72 hours, a written, signed prescription for the drug prescribed. If these drugs are kept in the medical office, they must be stored under lock and key and routinely counted and inventoried. The law requires that a dispensing record be kept on file for 2 years (or as otherwise specified by state law) and be subject to inspection by the DEA. The record must include the following:

Full name and address of the patient
Date of order
Name, dosage form, and quantity of the drug
Method (administered or dispensed)

SCHEDULE III Schedule III includes the lesser abused combination drugs that contain limited quantities of codeine, narcotic substances, or amphetamine-like substances. The physician must handwrite the prescription, but a DEA number is not required. Refills, up to five in any 6-month period, are allowed, but they must be indicated on the original prescription order. When changes or additions are made by telephone, the physician must directly communicate with the pharmacist, and a written prescription order confirming the telephone request should be forwarded to the pharmacist as soon as possible.

SCHEDULE IV Schedule IV includes the minor tranquilizers and hypnotics that have a lesser potential for abuse. Prescriptions may be handwritten by the medical assistant under the physician's direction, but the physician must sign them. Up to five refills are allowed within a 6-month period. Requests for refills may be telephoned to the pharmacist by the medical assistant under order of the physician, but the physician should record the order on the patient's medical record. Schedule IV drugs include meprobamate (Equanil), chlordiazepoxide (Librium), diazepam (Valium), flurazepam (Dalmane), chloral hydrate, and the nonnarcotic analgesic propoxyphene (Darvon).

SCHEDULE V Schedule V includes miscellaneous mixtures containing limited amounts of narcotic drugs. Prescription orders and refills are the same as for Schedule IV drugs. Examples are most cough medications containing codeine and some drugs used for gastrointestinal disorders, such as the combination product Donnagel and diphenoxylate (Lomotil). In addition, all inventory records require the physician's name, address, DEA registration number, date of inventory, and the signature of the person taking the inventory.

SAFETY ISSUES

All **controlled substances** must be stored in a safe or immovable locked cabinet. Prescription forms should be kept out of areas that are used by patients and preferably secured in an area that prohibits unauthorized or illegal use. The DEA Prescription Form 222 and the state triplicate forms also need to be kept in a locked area. Because of the increase in office thefts, many offices do not keep controlled substances in the office. If there is a loss of drugs, it must be reported to the regional DEA office and local law enforcement authorities immediately.

Memory Jogger

 *How long must a dispensing record be kept on file?*

The expiration dates of medications must be checked on a regular basis, before administration, and a medication is properly discarded if its date has expired.

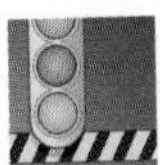

Safety Alert: A drug cannot be given or dispensed to a patient after its expiration date.

ACCEPTED METHODS FOR DISCARDING SMALL QUANTITIES

- Liquids and ointments may be rinsed down the drain.
- Powders should be mixed with water and then flushed down the drain.
- Tablets and capsules should be flushed down the toilet.
- Vials and ampules are opened and their contents poured down the drain.

As an added safety precaution, *two* employees should be present when drugs are destroyed, and both should sign and date the list of destroyed substances.

PREGNANCY CATEGORIES

The FDA, recognizing that the use of any medication has potential of causing birth defects, has established five categories indicating the level of the possibility of risk to the developing fetus. Information regarding the pregnancy category of any drug is found in the drug information literature, which is in the drug package, on the container, or in all approved drug references. It is very important for the medical assistant to ask women of child-bearing age if they might be pregnant.

Memory Jogger

 *What is the purpose of the pregnancy categories?*

Drug Abuse

Any drug from aspirin to alcohol may be misused or abused. Today, there is a tremendous increase in the use of illegal and legal drugs. Nationally, treatment programs are available everywhere for people in all walks of life. Programs include detoxification, rehabilitation, and long-term rehabilitation maintenance. Medical assistants may frequently encounter patients who are misusing or abusing drugs. It is important for you to be alert to the symptoms of drug dependence and to notify the physician when you suspect a patient, or co-worker, of having a problem with drug or alcohol dependency.

Drug misuse is the improper use of common drugs that can lead to dependence or toxicity. Examples of persons with chronic dependencies include people who cannot have a bowel movement unless they take a laxative; those who have used nasal decongestants for so long that they cannot breathe without the use of nasal sprays; or those who take so many antacids that they suffer systemic metabolic alkalosis.

Drug abuse is the self-administration of a drug continually or periodically that could result in addition (physical dependence). Drinking alcohol and cigarette smoking are examples of once-accepted behaviors. Both of these substances might be abused depending on the culture or beliefs of society.

Drug dependency is the inability to function unless under the influence of a substance. *Psychologic dependency* is the compulsive craving for the effects of a substance. *Habituation* is a form of psychologic and physiologic dependency. In this case, a person forms a habit of using a substance even to the detriment of physical health and well-being. Drinking coffee and soft drinks that contain caffeine and smoking cigarettes are common examples of habituation. *Physical dependency* is a person's need for a substance to avoid physical discomfort. This type of dependency occurs when abused substances produce biochemical changes, usually in the nervous system tissues. Discontinuing a substance that causes physical dependency creates the withdrawal syndrome. *Addiction* is a term that is being replaced by the term *dependency.* Regardless of the type of drug abused, it will have two effects on the person: acute and chronic. The acute effect is what the person feels when *intoxicated,* or directly under the influence of a particular substance. The chronic effects include the temporary or permanent physical and mental changes that result from long-term abuse.

The medical assistant often is called on to answer patient questions concerning drug abuse and problems. The medical assistant should read and keep up to date on the drug-related issues of society. Pamphlets and agency referral names should be available for patients. Patient concerns and questions regarding drug abuse should also be conveyed to the physician.

Memory Jogger

 *What are the three forms of drug dependency?*

Drug Interactions with the Body

The study of pharmacology used to focus on the *desired effect* a drug has on the human body, that is, the so-called end result. Now, knowledge of what happens to a drug while it is in the body (i.e., the *fate* of the drug) is as important as the drug's effect. This shift is valuable because it is known that different patients may react to the same dose of a drug in very different ways and that the same patient may react to the same dose of a drug differently at various times. Simply knowing the effect of a drug does not ensure the safety of the patient.

USES OF DRUGS

Drugs may be called pharmaceuticals, medicines, or medications. As a form of therapy (i.e., the treatment of disease by medicines), drugs occupy a prominent position. However, drugs also are used for other than therapeutic purposes.

EXAMPLES OF USES OF DRUGS

- *Therapeutic:* Used to cure a disease (e.g., antibiotics used to treat bacterial infections)
- *Palliative:* Used to relieve the symptoms of a disease (e.g., pain relievers and **cardiotonics**)
- *Preventive:* Used to prevent a condition (e.g., dimenhydrinate (Dramamine) for motion sickness)
- *Replacement:* Used to replace or supplement what the body is not producing (e.g., insulin for the diabetic)
- *Diagnostic:* Used to aid in the diagnosis of a disease or condition (e.g., contrast media used in radiography examinations)

Generally, therapeutic drugs either eradicate foreign substances from the body, such as antibiotics destroying pathogens, or interfere with or enhance the functioning of the patient's own cells, tissues, or organs. This action always has the potential to be dangerous to the body. However, the object of *rational drug therapy* is to control the degree of interference and to bring about the desired effect without any adverse, or *untoward,* effects.

Most drugs that affect the body tissues either bring about stimulation (increased activity) or depression (decreased activity). Some drug reactions are much more complicated: a drug may increase activity at the cellular level, which, in turn, decreases the activity of a particular organ, or vice versa. For example, a drug may decrease the nerve impulse transmission of certain cells in the heart, resulting in an increased heart rate. Some drugs stimulate one area of the body while depressing another. Morphine depresses the cough mechanism yet increases the mechanism that causes vomiting. Epinephrine (adrenalin) decreases (constricts) the openings of the blood vessels yet increases (dilates) the opening of the bronchial tubes.

Although most drugs can ultimately be classified as stimulants or depressants of some area of the body (especially the central nervous system), it is important to know how and where a drug affects the body, as well as what the drug does. Many drugs bring about the same effect, but in different ways from different parts of the body. For example, many drugs reduce blood pressure. Some act by depressing or stimulating central nervous system sites, some by relaxing the smooth muscle in the vessels in the heart, and others by decreasing the total fluid volume in the tissues. The end result, or effect, of all these methods is the same—a decreased blood pressure. However, each method is very different. Pain can be relieved by drugs acting in different ways at different sites. Some pain relievers act by relaxing smooth muscle spasms (antispasmodics); others block sensory nerve impulses to an area (local anesthesia); and still others dull the general senses of a patient so that an awareness of pain is lost (analgesics or general anesthesia).

People differ greatly in their reactions to drugs. Knowledge of how and where a drug produces its effect helps the physician to know which type of drug to use and when two or more drugs may be used for a more advantageous effect called **synergism** or synergistic effect. For example, treating a hypertensive patient with two drugs may be more effective than therapy with just one drug.

THE FATE OF DRUGS

By knowing what happens to the drug in the body, we can know the *onset* of a drug's activity (beginning), when the action is likely to peak, the minimal amount of drug needed (therapeutic dose), and the *duration* of a particular drug's activity. All these facts help to determine the dosage form, amount, route, and frequency of administration of medications.

PHARMACOKINETIC TERMS

- *Absorption*—how a drug is absorbed into the body's circulating fluids, which depend on the route by which it is administered.
- *Distribution*—how a drug is transported from the site of administration to the various points in the body
- *Action*—what changes the drug causes once it has reached its destination
- *Biotransformation or Metabolism*—how the drug is inactivated, including the time it takes for a drug to be detoxified and broken down into byproducts
- *Excretion or Elimination*—the route by which a drug is excreted, or eliminated, and the amount of time such a process requires

mal human cells. Research scientists continue to look for differences between cancer cells and normal cells to enable them to apply the principle of selected toxicity in cancer treatment. Most of the anticancer drugs in use today are not selectively toxic, and normal human cells are also poisoned by the cancer drugs.

Both drugs that have a selective affinity for cells and those that bind with enzymes can be counteracted by administering large amounts of the natural substances with which the drugs compete. This process is known as administering an **antidote** to a drug that may be acting as a poison.

Some drugs alter the function of cells by affecting the physical properties of the cell membrane rather than altering the biochemical processes within the cell itself. This is especially true of drugs that affect nerve cells, such as anesthetics and alcohol. A change in the cell membrane changes the **permeability** of the membrane, which, in turn, changes the flow of **ions** in and out of the cells. This change in ion flow changes the polarity (opposite effects at two extremities, the two extremities being inside and outside the cell membrane) on which nerve pulses are conducted and produces general sleep or stupor.

Biotransformation (Metabolism) of Drugs

This is the process by which drugs are converted into harmless byproducts. These byproducts are then more easily eliminated by the kidneys. Most drugs are broken down by the enzyme activity of the liver. The ability to break down the chemical components of a drug varies among individuals. Factors that determine this ability include age, the presence of other drugs, and liver disease. In some patients on long-term drug therapy, a drug may overstimulate the enzyme activity of the liver. This results in a too rapid destruction of the drug, and the patient has to take larger and larger doses for the drug to be effective. This situation is called *tolerance.*

Excretion (Elimination) of Drugs

The kidneys are the most important route for the elimination of drugs. Most drugs are filtered out of the circulation, broken down into harmless particles, and then excreted in the urine. Because the kidneys are so important in the elimination of drugs from the body, drug therapy must be carefully monitored in patients with kidney disease or malfunction. Drugs are also eliminated through the sweat glands and saliva and in bile. Exhalation, another mechanism for drug elimination, is the basis for measuring alcohol concentrations in the blood by the breathalyzer test. Drugs may be eliminated through the milk glands of the lactating mother, which means a woman breastfeeding a child has to be extremely careful about taking medications.

FACTORS THAT INFLUENCE THE EFFECT OF A DRUG

As stated earlier, different people react to the same dose of medication in different ways, and the same patient can react to the same dose of the same drug differently on various occasions. The following factors are important in determining the correct medication for a patient.

Body Weight

A person's weight has a direct relationship with the effects of medication. Basically, the same dosage has a greater effect on a person who weighs less and a lesser effect on a patient who weighs more. Manufacturers of adult medications calculate dosages based on a normal adult weight (approximately 150 pounds). Sometimes, the physician will adjust the dosage to better suit the patient's body size. Pediatric medications are designed for the body weight or body surface area of children. If adult medications are used for children, the correct dosage must be calculated and adjusted for the child's body weight.

Age

In the newborn and the very elderly, age has its greatest effect on the body's response to a drug. This usually has to do with immature or deteriorating body systems. In addition, both groups are particularly sensitive to drugs that affect the central nervous system and to toxicity. Dosage calculations for these two groups must be carefully decided, and therapy usually begins with very small doses.

Sex

Drugs may affect men and women differently. As previously mentioned, the pregnant woman has to be extremely cautious, when taking medications, to avoid damage to the developing fetus. In addition, some drugs have side effects that can stimulate uterine contractions, causing premature labor and delivery. Intramuscular medications are absorbed faster by men. Because women have a higher body fat content and a musculature with less blood supply, intramuscular drugs remain in their tissues longer than in men's tissues.

Time of Day

Diurnal means during the day or time of light. Diurnal body rhythms play an important part in the effects of some drugs. Sedatives given in the morning will not be as effective as when administered before bedtime, because the central nervous system is more stimulated and more resistant to the effects of the drug. Corticosteroid administration is preferred in the morning because it best mimics the body's natural pattern of corticosteroid production and elimination. Diuretics are best administered in the morning to reduce the need for the patient to get up during the night to void.

Pathologic Factors

Patients may adversely respond to drugs in the presence of liver or kidney disease because the body will not be able to detoxify and excrete chemicals properly. Drugs may also produce liver or kidney pathology, and patients may need monitoring. In patients with liver or kidney disease, some drugs may cause unconsciousness or death. Patients with other diseases or disorders may react quite differently than expected. Therefore, a thorough medical history is always required before administering medications. Even temporary pain and fever may alter the expected effect of a drug.

Immune Responses

The presence of a drug can stimulate a patient's immune response, and the patient will develop antibodies to a particular chemical. If the same drug is again administered, the patient will have an allergic reaction to the drug, ranging from a mild reaction to a serious respiratory and circulatory emergency.

Psychologic Factors

People may respond differently to a drug because of the way they feel about the drug. If a patient believes in the therapy, even a *placebo* (sugar pill or sterile water thought to be a drug) may help or bring about relief. A patient's personality can affect whether he or she will be cooperative in following the directions for a particular drug, and a patient's negative mind set, or mental attitude, can reduce an expected response to a drug.

Tolerance

Tolerance is the phenomenon of reduced responsiveness to a drug. *Congenital tolerance* is an inborn resistance. *Acquired tolerance* occurs after taking a particular drug for a period of time. *Cross tolerance* occurs when a patient acquires a tolerance to one drug and becomes resistant to other similar drugs. *Physical dependence* often accompanies tolerance. The body becomes so adapted to the presence of the drug that it cannot function properly without it. To withdraw the drug is to throw the body out of its equilibrium, causing the well-known withdrawal syndrome.

Accumulation

When a drug is taken too frequently to allow for proper elimination, it accumulates in the tissues. The result is a more intense effect and a longer duration. Accumulation can cause overdose, toxicity, and **alkalosis**. Proper dosage and timing of administration are the best prevention of drug accumulation.

Idiosyncrasy

Occasionally, a person reacts to a drug in a manner that is unexpected and peculiar to that individual only. An idiosyncrasy may manifest in many different ways, such as a hypnotic drug keeping a person awake, acting as a stimulant to this person rather than as a depressant. Usually, these reactions cannot be explained.

Memory Jogger

List the factors that influence the effect of a drug.

CLASSIFICATIONS OF DRUG ACTIONS

Clinical pharmacology is a complex subject. To make the subject easier, drugs are classified according to their actions on the body (e.g., diuretics or emetics). Drugs may also be classified according to the body system that they affect (e.g., drugs acting on the cardiovascular system). The following is a glossary of terms describing some basic drug actions. As you read some of the examples, remember that a drug classified as one type of agent may have other uses and actions on other systems of the body. For example, a drug classified as a diuretic may also be an antihypertensive drug, and a vasodilator may also be a respiratory antispasmodic. It takes time to understand not only the basic classification of a particular drug but also the many secondary uses and effects it has on the human body.

These are just a few examples of the different classifications of medications. Remember to research and review all medications prior to their administration.

Adrenergic

Action: constricts blood vessels, narrows the **lumen** of a vessel
Examples: epinephrine: phenylephrine (Neo-Synephrine)
Primary Use: Stop superficial bleeding, raise and sustain blood pressure, and relieve nasal congestion

Analgesic

Action: lessens the sensory function of the brain
Examples: nonnarcotic: aspirin; acetaminophen (Tylenol); ibuprofen (Advil, Motrin); narcotic: me-

peridine (Demerol); hydrocodone (Vicodin); propoxyphene (Darvon)
Primary Use: Pain relief

Anesthetic

Action: produces insensibility to pain or the sensation of pain
Examples: bupivacaine (Marcaine); lidocaine (Xylocaine)
Primary Use: local or general anesthesia

Antianxiety

Action: reduces anxiety and tension
Examples: chlordiazepoxide (Librium); diazepam (Valium); alprazolam (Xanax)
Primary Use: produces calmness and releases muscle tension

Antibiotic

Action: kills or inhibits the growth of microorganisms
Examples: cefaclor (Ceclor); tetracycline (Acromycin); amoxicillin (Augmentin)
Primary Use: treatment of bacterial invasions and infections

Anticholingergic

Action: parasympathetic blocking agent, reduces spasm in smooth muscle
Examples: scopolamine; atropine sulfate
Primary Use: dry secretions

Anticoagulants

Action: delays or blocks the clotting of blood
Examples: heparin; warfarin sodium (Coumadin)
Primary Use: treatment of blood clots

Antidepressant

Action: treats depression
Examples: fluoxetine (Prozac); imipramine pamoate (Tofranil); amitriptyline (Elavil)
Primary Use: mood elevator

Antiemetic

Action: acts on hypothalamus center in the brain
Examples: prochlorperazine (Compazine); trimethobenzamide (Tigan); metoclopramide (Reglan)
Primary Use: prevent and relieve nausea and vomiting

Antiepileptic (Anticonvulsant)

Action: reduces excessive stimulation of the brain
Examples: phenytoin (Dilantin); phenobarbital; carbamazepine (Tegretol)
Primary Use: epilepsy and other convulsive disorders

Antifungal

Action: slows or retards the multiplication of fungi
Examples: miconazole (Monistat); nystatin (Mycostatin); amphotericin B
Primary Use: treat systemic or local fungal infections

Antihistamine

Action: counteracts the effects of histamine by blocking action in tissues; may be used to inhibit gastric secretions
Examples: brompheniramine maleate (Dimetane); chlorpheniramine (Chlor-Trimeton); diphenhydramine (Benadryl); promethazine (Phenergan); cimetidine (Tagamet); ranitidine (Zantac)
Primary Use: relief of allergies; prevention of gastric ulcers

Antihypertensive

Action: blocks nerve impulses that cause arteries to constrict; or slows heart rate decreasing its contractility; or restricts the hormone aldosterone in the blood
Examples: atenolol (Tenormin); doxazosin mesylate (Cardura); metoprolol (Lopressor); methyldopa (Aldomet)
Primary Use: reduce and control blood pressure

Antiinflammatory

Action: acts as an antiinflammatory or antirheumatic
Examples: nonsteroidal (NSAIDs): ibuprofen (Advil, Motrin); naproxen (Naprosyn). Steroidal: dexamethasone (Decadron); prednisone (Cortisone)
Primary Use: treatment of arthritic and other inflammatory disorders

Antineoplastic

Action: inhibits the development of and destroys cancerous cells
Examples: interferon alfa-2a (Roferon-A); hydroxyurea (Hydrea); cyclophosphamide (Cytoxan); fluorouracil (Adrucil)
Primary Use: cancer chemotherapy

Antispasmodic

Action: relieves or prevents spasms from musculoskeletal injury or inflammation
Examples: methocarbamol (Robaxin); carisoprodol (Soma)
Primary Use: sport injuries

Antitussive (Cough Suppressant)

Action: inhibits the cough center
Examples: narcotic: codeine sulfate; nonnarcotic: dextromethorphan (Romilar, Robitussin DM)
Primary Use: temporarily suppresses a nonproductive cough; reduces the thickness of secretions

Bronchodilator

Action: relaxes the smooth muscle of the bronchi
Examples: aminophylline (Aminophyllin); theophylline (Theo-Dur); epinephrine (Adrenalin, Sus-Phrine); albuterol (Ventolin, Proventil); isoproterenol (Isuprel)
Primary Use: treat asthma, bronchospasm; promotes bronchodilation

Cathartic (Laxative)

Action: increases peristaltic activity of the large intestine
Examples: magnesium hydroxide (milk of magnesia); bisacodyl (Dulcolax); casanthranol (Peri-Colace); psyllium hydrophilic muciloid (Metamucil)
Primary Use: increases and hasten bowel evacuation (defecation)

Contraceptive

Action: inhibits conception
Examples: medroxyprogesterone acetate (Depo-Provera); norgestrel (Ovrett); ethinyl estradiol and ethynodiol diacetate (Demulen 1/35)
Primary Use: family planning

Decongestant

Action: relieves local congestion in the tissues
Examples: ephedrine or phenylephrine (Neo-Synephrine); pseudoephedrine (Sudafed); oxymetazoline (Afrin)
Primary Use: relief of nasal and sinus congestion due to common cold, hay fever, or upper respiratory tract disorders

Diuretic

Action: inhibits the reabsorption of sodium and chloride in the kidneys
Examples: hydrochlorothiazide (Dyazide, Esidrix, HydroDiuril); furosemide (Lasix); triamterene (Dyrenium)
Primary Use: increases urinary output, decreases blood pressure

Expectorant

Action: increases secretions and mucus from the bronchial tubes
Examples: diphenhydramine (Benylin); guaifenesin guaiacolate (Fenesin, Robitussin)
Primary Use: upper respiratory tract congestion

Hemostatic

Action: controls bleeding, a blood coagulant
Examples: phytonadione, vitamin K (Konakion); absorbable hemostatics, such as Gelfoam and Surgicel, are applied directly to a wound.
Primary Use: control of acute or chronic blood-clotting disorder; formation of absorbable, artificial clot

Hypnotic (Sedative)

Action: induces sleep and lessens the activity of the brain
Examples: secobarbital (Seconal); flurazepam (Dalmane); tamazepam (Restoril)
Primary Use: insomnia; lower doses sedate

Hormone Replacement

Action: replaces or compensates hormone deficiency
Examples: chlorpropamide (Diabinese); insulin (Humulin); levothyroxine sodium (Synthroid); estrogen (Premarin)
Primary Use: maintenance of adequate hormone levels

Miotic

Action: causes the pupil of the eye to contract
Examples: carbachol (Isopto Carbachol); isoflurophate (Floropryl); pilocarpine (Isopto Carpine)
Primary Use: counteract pupil dilation

Mydriatic (Anticholinergic)

Action: dilates the pupil of the eye
Examples: atropine sulfate (Isopto Atropine)
Primary Use: ophthamologic examinations

Narcotic

Any of a group of drugs that depress the central nervous system and cause insensibility or stupor. Natural narcotics include the opium group (codeine phosphate, morphine sulfate). Synthetic narcotics include meperidine (Demerol), methadone (Dolophine), pentazocine (Talwin), and propoxyphene HCl (Darvon).

Sympathetic Blocking Agent (Sympatholytic)

Action: blocks certain functions of the adrenergic nervous system

Examples: propranolol (Inderal); metaprolol (Lopressor); phentolamine (Regitine); prazosin (Minipress)
Primary Use: treating cardiovascular conditions

Approaches to Studying Pharmacology

A pharmaceutical glossary could be endless. Many terms are combinations of the condition to be treated with the prefix *anti* (e.g., antianginal, antianxiety, antiarrhythmic, anticoagulant, anticonvulsant, antidiarrheal).

Notice how these names emphasize the drug's effect (use) rather than its action in the body. More recent classifications, such as *parasympathomimetic* and *cholinesterase inhibitors,* describe the pharmacologic action rather than the therapeutic use. However, both viewpoints are necessary for a more complete understanding of drugs and what they do in the human body.

Of course no one can remember all there is to know about clinical pharmacology. Even if you did one day, there would be more to learn the next. The number of new drugs being introduced into use far exceeds the number of older drugs being replaced or discontinued. Thus, the number of drugs available for clinical use grows beyond the possible knowledge of one person. Therefore, numerous resources are necessary for study and review of the details concerning particular drugs.

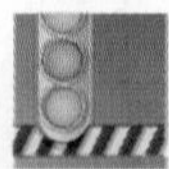

Safety Alert: Remember, when in doubt, look it up before you use a drug.

REFERENCE MATERIALS

A good pharmacology textbook is handy for studying the principles and concepts of each drug classification. There are several comprehensive editions available in bookstores. The physician's office will have materials available. In addition, reference and cross-reference books that are updated annually or periodically should be available for easy reference. Most references list drug information in the following sequence:

1. *Action:* How the drug acts in the body.
2. *Indication:* The conditions for which the drug is used.
3. *Side Effects:* An effect on the body other than the one(s) for which the drug is given.
4. *Adverse Effects:* An effect on a tissue or organ system other than the one being sought by the administration of a medication.
5. *Precautions:* Actions necessary because of special conditions of the patient, drug, or environment that need to be considered for the drug to be successful or not harmful.
6. *Contraindications:* Conditions that make the administration of a drug improper or undesirable.
7. *Toxic Effects:* The poisonous effects and symptoms of toxicity.
8. *Dosage and Administration:* The usual route, dosage, and timing for administering the drug.

Memory Jogger

List the eight items of information that should be known about each medication.

Package Inserts

Every drug package contains an insert describing all the significant aspects of using the drug, including information on the chemical formulation of the drug and clinical studies. The information on the inserts is controlled by the FDA.

Physician's Desk Reference (PDR)

This reference book is published annually by the Medical Economics Company, Inc. (Oradell, NJ). For physicians who subscribe to *Medical Economics Magazine,* it is provided free. Copies can be purchased through the publisher or in local bookstores. Supplements are published throughout the year. This reference contains information on approximately 2500 drugs, and the product descriptions are identical to the package inserts. The drug manufacturers pay for this space, so the *PDR* could be called the yellow pages of the drug industry.

The book's sections are color-coded and cross-referenced for easy use. The various sections allow you to begin searching for information concerning a drug from any starting point. You can start with the usage, classification, generic name, manufacturer's name, or trade name of a drug or what the drug looks like. There is a special photographic section for visual product identification (Fig. 48–2). Once you know which drug you want to study, the product information section lists the actual package insert information alphabetically, first by the manufacturer, then by the brand name.

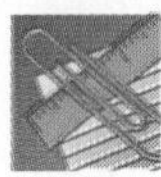

Project: Practice the different ways of researching the different drugs in the PDR.

Text continued on page 1016

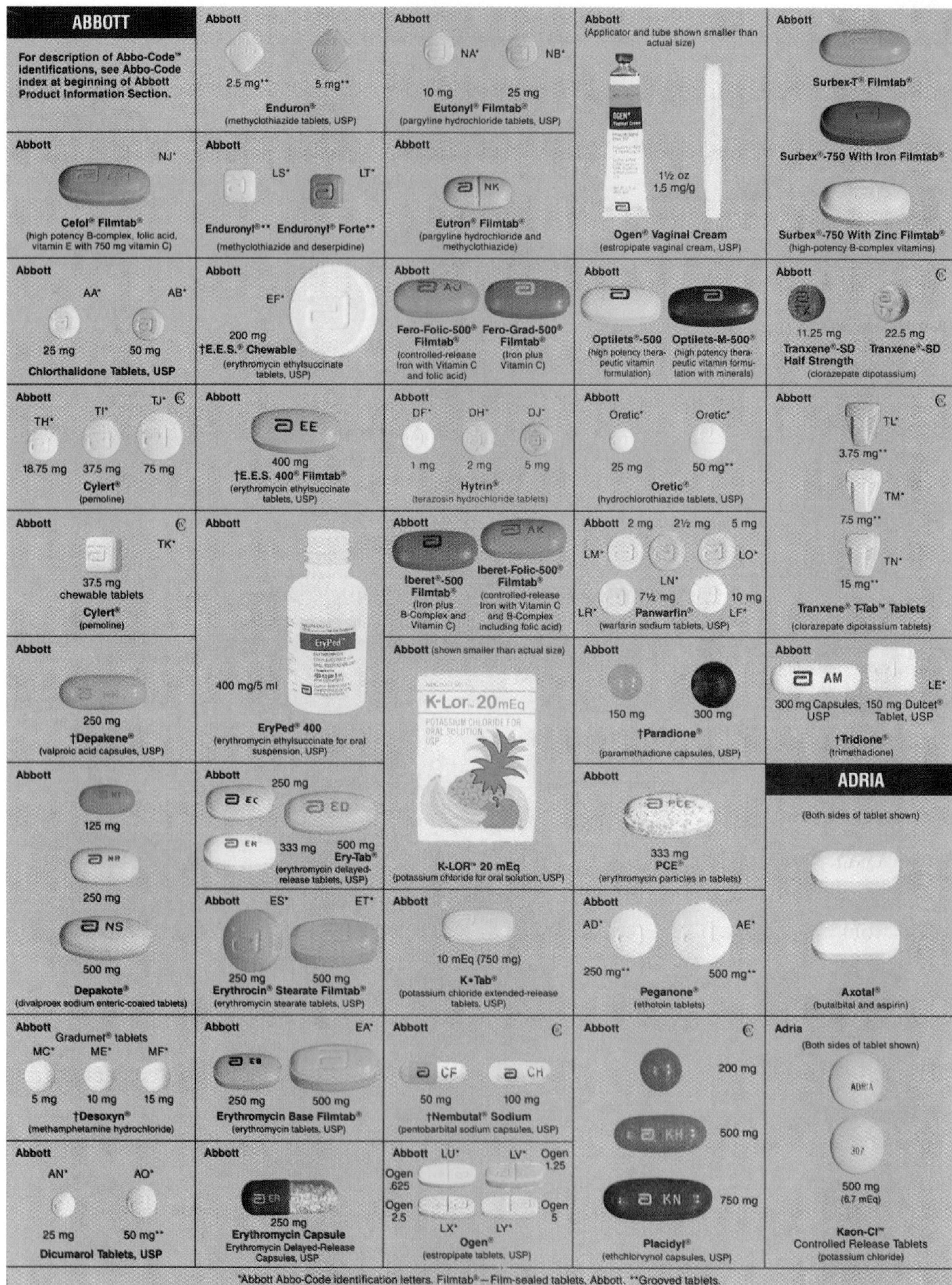

FIGURE 48–2 Example of product identification page from *Physician's Desk Reference*. (From Physician's Desk Reference, Oradell, NJ, Medical Economics, 1998.)

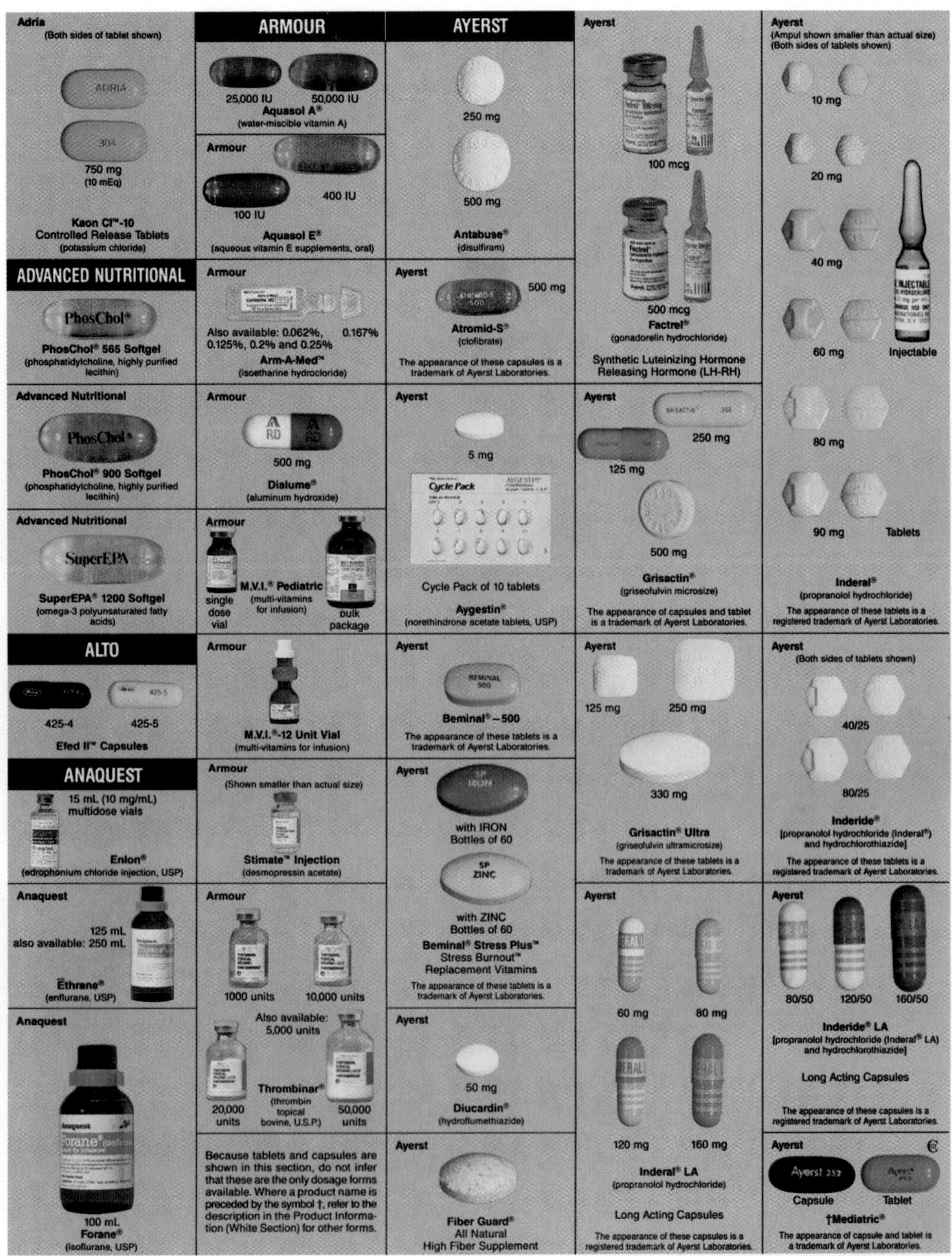

FIGURE 48–2 *Continued*

Illustration continued on following page

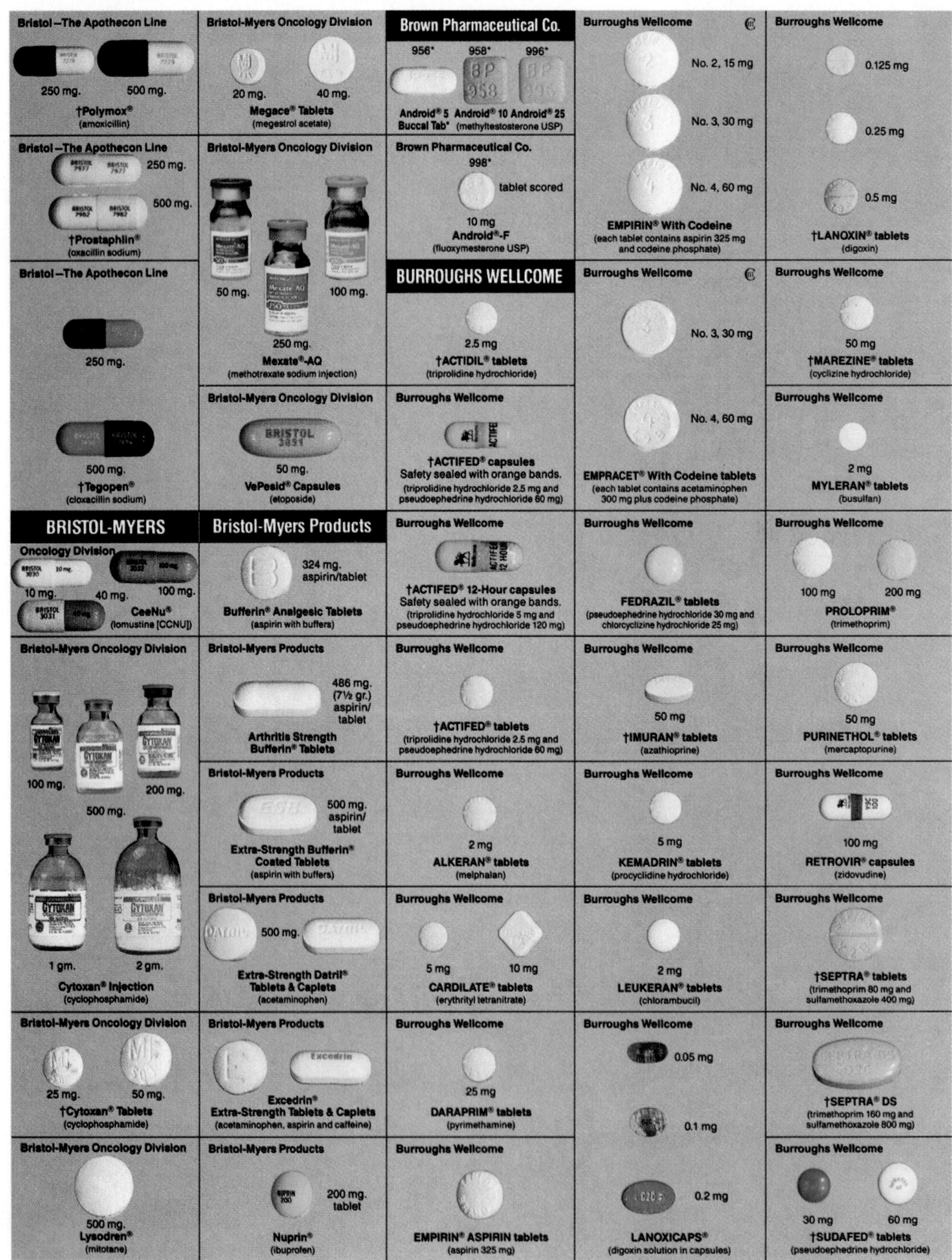

FIGURE 48–2 *Continued*

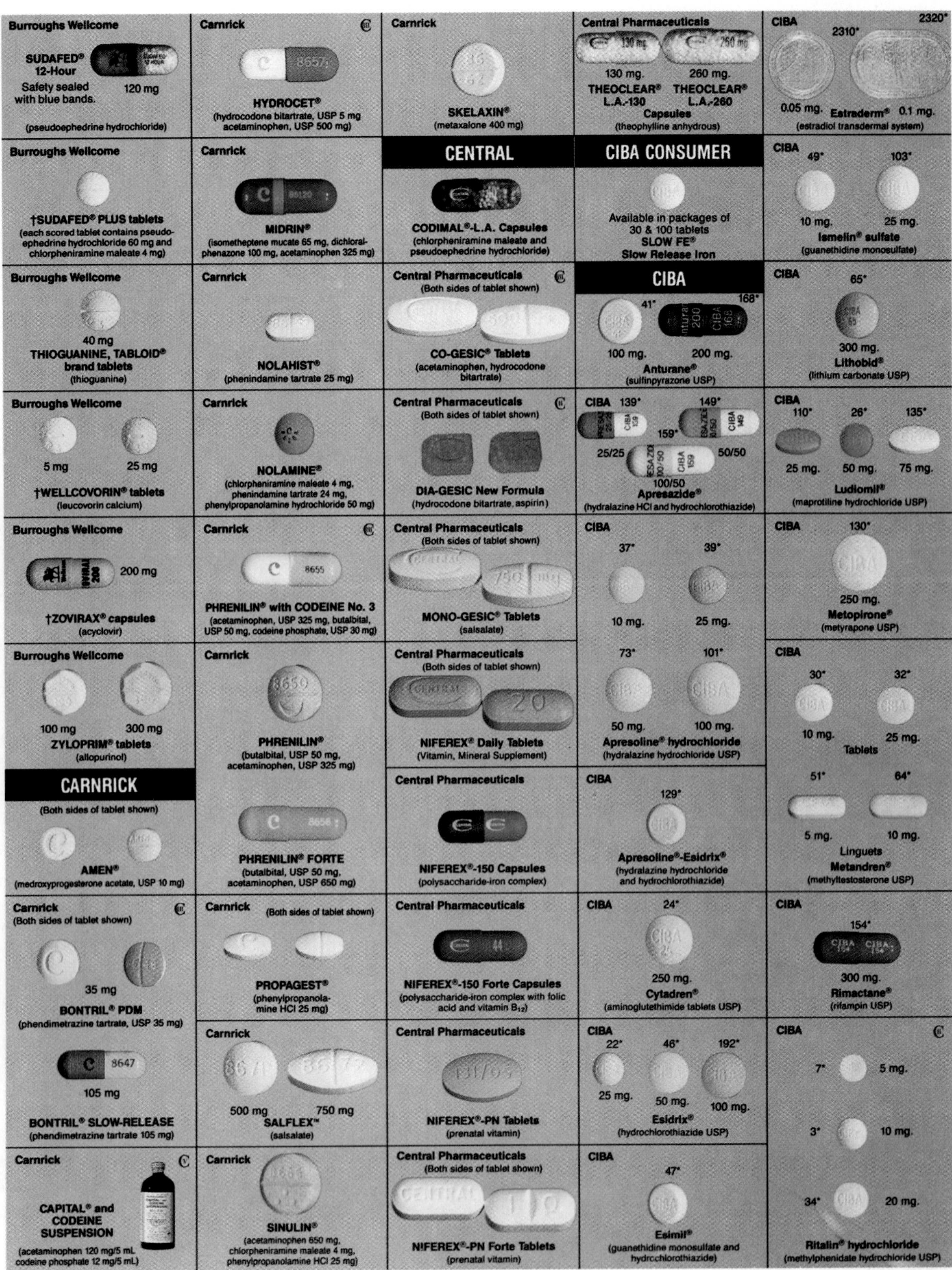

FIGURE 48–2 *Continued*

The American Hospital Formulary

This reference is published by the American Society of Hospital Pharmacists (Bethesda, MD) and is available by subscription. The information is contained in a two-volume set, with four to six supplements added each year. Generic names are listed, and it is divided into sections based on drug actions.

The U.S. Pharmacopeia (USP)

This publication was first printed in 1820, and new editions are still published every 5 years. England and Canada each publish similar volumes. The *Pharmacopeia* is usually not an appropriate reference purchase for the medical office.

The U.S. Pharmacopeia/National Formulary (USP/NF)

This reference is the official source of drug standards for the United States. The *Pharmacopeia* was just recently combined with the *National Formulary*, which lists the chemical formulas for all accepted drugs. This new combined reference lists and describes all the approved medications that are considered useful and therapeutic in the practice of medicine. Single drugs rather than combined products (compound mixtures) are listed. If a drug name is the same as the official name in this volume, the drug will have the initials USP after it (e.g., digitoxin, USP).

LEARNING ABOUT DRUGS

The study of pharmacology is difficult, at best. However, there are a few ways you can make it easier.

First, take opportunities to observe the use of drugs in patient care. Studying about epinephrine (Adrenalin) becomes more meaningful when you see how its cardiovascular actions get a patient through an anaphylactic episode. This is more memorable than any textbook.

Second, concentrate on the most important drugs in each classification. For example, learn about digitalis (cardiovascular), morphine (narcotic analgesic), epinephrine (autonomic nervous system blocker), and atropine (anticholinergic). As you expand your knowledge to other drugs in each classification, you will easily understand new drugs by noting the similarities and differences between them and the basic, important drugs you studied first.

Third, learn about a drug's primary action and use and then expand your knowledge to its other actions and uses. Soon, you will be able to name the drug that is usually indicated for a particular condition. Then, by knowing a drug's secondary effects, you will be able to understand what side effects are likely to occur during the use of the drug. More important, you will be aware of the contraindications for the drug (conditions that make the use of the drug improper or undesirable). Knowledge of the drug's actions will also enable you to predict what toxic reactions could occur from overdose.

It is hoped that pharmacology will always remain exciting and interesting to you as you work with patients and the other members of your team and that you will continue to assess and evaluate new drugs as their administration becomes your responsibility.

Calculating Drug Dosages for Administration

The correct dosage of a medication may depend on the patient's age, weight, or state of health or on what other drugs the patient may be taking. Often, the physician will order a medication in a dosage that is different from that of the medications you stock. The difference may be in the system of measurement, the strength, or the form. There are formulas and mathematical tables of conversion for calculating the correct dosage of medication to be administered. Let's look at how you arrive at the correct calculation, one step at a time.

MATHEMATICAL EQUIVALENTS

You may need to review some basics of arithmetic before you begin to tackle drug calculations. You must thoroughly understand the addition, subtraction, multiplication, and division of fractions and decimals; the relationship of decimals and fractions; and how they are converted from one to the other. In addition, you need to review how decimals and percentages are converted back and forth. Table 48–3 provides some examples of these relationships.

TABLE 48–3 Mathematical Equivalents

Percentage	Decimal	Fraction	Ratio
25%	0.25	1/4	1:4
50%	0.5	1/2	1:2
60%	0.6	3/5 (6/10)	3:5
0.5%	0.005	1/200	1:200
0.1%	0.001	1/1000	1:1000
85%	0.85	17/20	17:20
1%	0.01	1/100	1:100

The table shows that a fraction is, in another sense, a ratio. For example, ¼ (a fraction) is the same as the ratio 1:4 (one to four). If there is one apple and four oranges, then the number of apples that you have is ¼ the number of oranges, and the ratio of apples to oranges is 1:4. Now, divide the numerator 1 by the denominator 4 (a fraction is also an automatic division problem waiting to be solved):

$$4\overline{)1.00}\quad 0.25$$

The act of dividing a fraction results in a decimal number. Decimal numbers can then be converted to percentages by moving the decimal two spaces to the right:

$$0.25 = 25.0\%,\quad \text{commonly written } 25\%$$

Now, we can see all the relationships of Table 48–3. Using the example of apples and oranges, you can see that 1 is 0.25, or 25%, of 4. Therefore, the number of apples is 0.25, or 25%, of the number of oranges. If you need to review any of these concepts, please stop now and practice these steps of arithmetic. To go on without this background could be very frustrating as you attempt to understand problems in dosage calculations.

RATIO AND PROPORTION

We have just reviewed that *ratio* is one way of expressing a fraction, or division problem, and shows the relationship of the numerator to the denominator. The comparison of two ratios is called a *proportion.* A proportion is written as follows:

$$\frac{4}{16} = \frac{1}{4} \quad \text{or} \quad 4:16 :: 1:4$$

This is read as 4 divided by 16 equals 1 divided by 4, or four is to 16 as 1 is to 4. What we are saying here is that both ratios have the same proportions and are equal to one another even though the numbers are different. This is the key to calculating drug dosages. The physician's order for a medication may be a ratio different from that of the medication that is in stock. We will then compare the ordered ratio to the available ratio (what we have in stock) to find the correct proportion to administer. However, before going on, there is more background material that we need to know.

The preceding proportion example has all the answers in it; there is nothing to solve. In calculating dosages, we use mathematical proportions, but with one element unknown. We must solve for that unknown, or x. For example:

$$\frac{4}{16} = \frac{1}{x}$$

Always in a proportion, we solve the problem by *cross-multiplication.* Do not confuse this with plain multiplication. If you see an equal sign (=) between two fractions, you know this is an equation to be *cross-multiplied.*

$$\frac{4}{16} = \frac{1}{x}$$

Now cross-multiply:

$$4 \times x = 16 \times 1$$

Therefore:

$$4x = 16$$

We know what $4x$ equals, but next we must find what $1x$, or x, equals. To find the value of x, we must find a way to leave x (or $1x$) alone on one side of the equation. We can change $4x$ to $1x$ by dividing the number 4 by itself:

$$4x \div 4 = 1x$$

But what we do on one side of an equation, we must do on the other side, or the equation will not be equal anymore. Therefore, we divide 16 by 4:

$$16 \div 4 = 4$$

The answer is $x = 4$. Let's put it all together now:

$$\frac{1}{x} = \frac{4}{16}$$

$$4 \times x = 16 \times 1$$

$$4x = 16$$

$$\frac{4x}{4} = \frac{16}{4}$$

$$x = 4$$

We take the answer 4 and replace the x with it in the ratio. We have solved for x.

$$\frac{4}{16} = \frac{1}{4}$$

CALCULATING DOSAGES

When calculating dosages, a standard set of formulas is used (see Procedures 48–1 through 48–4). These formulas employ certain specific terms. Every drug has a *strength* (potency) and a *dosage unit (amount)*. The strength is the quantity of the drug held together in a particular form. The amount (volume) is what contains the drug. It may be a solid form, such as a tablet, or a liquid form, such as 1 milliliter (mL) of injectable physiologic saline. In liquids, the drug strength is often called the *solute*. The solute is dissolved in an amount called the *solvent*. It is important to understand which measurements pertain to the strength (potency) of a drug and which pertain to the unit of dosage (form, volume, or amount). For example, a vial of injectable material may read 500 mg/mL. This means there are 500 mg (strength) of drug in every milliliter (amount) of liquid. When an oral medication reads 5 gr, it means that there are 5 grains (strength) in every tablet (amount). Let's use these two examples and the proportion formula previously reviewed to work out two problems: (1) filling a syringe and (2) administering tablets.

Problem 1

Order: Give 250 mg of a drug.
Available: A vial marked 500 mg/mL.
Standard Formula:

$$\frac{\text{Available strength}}{\text{Ordered strength}} = \frac{\text{Available amount}}{\text{Amount to give}}$$

Problem: Given the strength of the drug needed, the amount of fluid to be withdrawn must be determined.

We will set up a proportion with the three known quantities: (1) the strength of the drug in the vial, (2) the unit of fluid in which that strength is contained, and (3) the strength of the drug the physician wishes to be administered to the patient.
Apply the problem to the standard formula:

$$\frac{500 \text{ mg}}{250 \text{ mg}} = \frac{1 \text{ mL}}{x \text{ mL}}$$

$$500 \times x = 250 \times 1$$

$$500x = 250$$

$$\frac{500x}{500} = \frac{250}{500}$$

$$x = \frac{1}{2} \text{ mL} = 0.50 \text{ mL}$$

Solution: Administer 0.50 mL of the drug.

Problem 2

Order: Give 10 gr (grains) of a drug.
Available: A bottle with tablets labeled 5 gr each.
Standard Formula:

$$\frac{\text{Available strength}}{\text{Ordered strength}} = \frac{\text{Available amount}}{\text{Amount to give}}$$

Problem: Given the strength of the drug needed, the number of tablets to be administered must be determined.

We will set up a proportion with the three known quantities: (1) the strength of the drug in each tablet, (2) the unit amount that is one tablet, and (3) the strength of the drug the physician wishes to be administered to the patient.
Apply the problem to the standard formula:

$$\frac{5 \text{ gr}}{10 \text{ gr}} = \frac{1 \text{ tablet}}{x(\text{no. of tablets})}$$

$$5 \times x = 10 \times 1$$

$$5x = 10$$

$$\frac{5x}{5} = \frac{10}{5}$$

$$x = 2 \text{ tablets}$$

Solution: Administer 2 tablets.

Use the *standard formula* for any type of calculation. You may be using strengths that are measured in International Units (IU), as with insulin or penicillin; grams; milligrams; grains; or percentages. The forms in which drugs may be prepared include cubic centimeters (cc) or milliliters (mL), minims, drops, drams, ounces, pints, gallons (for making up diluted stock solutions from concentrated solutions, such as with alcohol and hydrogen peroxide), or spoonfuls. Follow the steps previously shown, and, above all, discipline yourself to write down each step with complete calculations. This is the only way to ensure maximum accuracy and the safety of your patients. If you have difficulty with the calculation, or the answer does not seem quite right, ask the physician to check your calculation. A double check is always preferred.

PROCEDURE 48–1

Calculating the Correct Dosage for Administration

GOAL

To calculate the correct dosage amount and choose the correct equipment when the physician orders 2.4 million IU of (penicillin G benzathine) (Bicillin) to be administered to a patient.

EQUIPMENT AND SUPPLIES

Premixed syringes of Bicillin in the following two strengths are available:
0.6 million IU/syringe
1.2 million IU/syringe

PROCEDURAL STEPS

1 Read the order in quiet surroundings to make sure that you fully understand it.
2 Using pencil and paper, write out the order.
3 Examine the drug labels to see what strengths and amounts are available.
4 Write down the standard formula.
PURPOSE: To eliminate the chances of error, orders should never be carried out unless the calculations are completed in writing.
5 Rewrite the formula, replacing the unknown values with the known quantities. The unknown *x* will be the amount of the drug to give.
6 Work the proportion problem by cross-multiplying to solve for *x*.
7 State your answer by filling in the blanks, as follows:
To administer 2.4 million IU of Bicillin, I would select ____________ of the premixed syringes labeled ____________.

SYSTEMS OF MEASUREMENT

Sometimes, the physician will order a medication in a strength that is totally different from the one on the label of the vial or bottle. For example, the physician may order one grain of a drug, but the available dosage form is in milligrams. Before you can use the ratio and proportion formulas to arrive at the amount to administer, you first must convert to one system or the other. The best way is to convert to the measurement system that is on the label (what is available). After all, that is the system you will have to use. Dosage calculations would be easier if pharmacology dealt with just one system of measurement. Unfortunately, there are three: the metric system, the apothecary system, and the household system.

The *metric system* of weights and measures is now used throughout the world as the primary system for weight (mass), capacity (volume), and length (area). In the United States, it is used for scientific work, including most pharmaceuticals. However, some medication forms still use the older apothecary system, which necessitates learning the two systems and the relationships (conversions) between the two. A few hints about each system follow.

The metric system of weights and measures is a decimal system, which means that it uses the base ten (10). Each higher measure is 10 times the measure at hand; each lower, $\frac{1}{10}$ the measure. The fraction is always written as a decimal, and the number precedes the letters designating the actual measure. Thus, 1 and a half liters would be written 1.5 L (Table 48–4). The cubic centimeter (cc) and the milliliter (mL) are interchangeable. In the metric system, 1 cc is a measurement of area, and an area this size holds exactly 1 mL ($\frac{1}{1000}$ of a liter) of fluid (volume). In fact, if you were to weigh 1 mL of water contained in 1 cc of area under certain conditions of temperature and barometric pressure, it would also

TABLE 48–4 Abbreviations and Symbols for Selected Weights and Measures

Apothecary System				Metric System	
	♏	Min. (M.)	minim	g	gram
	℈	scr	scruple	L	liter
	ʒ	dr	dram	cc	cubic centimeter
fl	ʒ	f dr	fluid dram	mL	milliliter
	℥	oz	ounce		
fl	℥	fl oz	fluid ounce		
	O	pt	pint		
	C	gal	gallon		
		gr	grain		

weigh exactly 1 gram (g). In the metric system, these three basic units of measurement are convertible from one to the other.

With the *apothecary system,* the basic unit of weight is the grain (gr), and the basic unit of volume is the minim. As in the metric system, these two units are related: the grain is based on the weight of a single grain of wheat, and the minim is the volume of water that weighs one grain. Either Roman or Arabic numerals may be used, but it is not proper to use them together in the same prescription. Either symbols or abbreviations are used; for example, one and a half drams might be written ʒiss or dr 1½. The number follows the symbol or abbreviation. Table 48–5 compares the units of weight and volume in the metric and the apothecary systems. Fluid ounces is used to differentiate liquids from solid weight.

The household system is used in most American households. This system of measurement is important for the patient at home who has no knowledge of the metric or apothecary systems. The basic measure of weight is the pound; the basic measure of volume, the drop. The household drop is equal to the apothecary minim, so these two systems are sometimes easily interchangeable. Both the household and the apothecary systems use the terms *dram* and *ounce* as units of measurement, so always be sure of which system you are using. Medications are not measured in household weights, but many prescriptions contain directions using the household measurements of volume. Liquid oral medications are taken by the drop, teaspoon, or tablespoon and are supplied in bottles labeled in ounces or pints. Tables 48–6 and 48–7 show the household system of measurement (note that there are some apothecary equivalents).

TABLE 48–5 Approximate Equivalents for Some Commonly Used Measures

			Liquid Measure	
Grains	Grams	Milligrams	*Apothecary*	*Metric*
15	1.0	1000	1 quart	1000 mL (cc)
10	0.6	600	1 pint	500 mL
7½	0.5	500	8 fl oz	250 mL
5	0.3	300	7 fl oz	200 mL
4½	0.25	250	3.5 fl oz	100 mL
3	0.2	200	1 fl oz	30 mL
2	0.12	120	4 fl d	15 mL
1½	0.1	100	2.5 fl d	10 mL
1	0.06	60	2 fl d	8 mL
¾	0.050	50	1 fl d	4 mL
½	0.030	30	45 M.	3 mL
⅜	0.025	25	30 M.	2 mL
¼	0.015	15	15 M.	1 mL
⅙	0.010	10	12 M.	0.75 mL
⅛	0.008	8	10 M.	0.6 mL
1/10	0.006	6	8 M.	0.5 mL
1/12	0.005	5	5 M.	0.3 mL
1/20	0.003	3	4 M.	0.25 mL
1/30	0.002	2	3 M.	0.2 mL
1/60	0.001	1	1.5 M.	0.1 mL
1/100	0.0006	0.6	1 M.	0.06 mL
1/120	0.0005	0.5	.75 M.	0.05 mL
1/150	0.0004	0.4	.5 M.	0.03 mL
1/200	0.0003	0.3		
1/250	0.00025	0.25		
1/300	0.0002	0.2		
1/400	0.00015	0.15		
1/500	0.00012	0.12		
1/600	0.0001	0.1		

Weight conversions; 1 lb = 0.45 kg; 1 kg = 2.2 lb; 10 lb = 4.5 kg; 10 kg = 22 lb; 30.0 g = 1 oz; 15.0 g = 4 d; 7.5 g = 2 d; 4 g = 1 d; 4 g = 60 grains; Domestic equivalents: 1 teaspoon = 5 mL (cc) = 1 fl d; 1 tablespoon = 15 mL = .5 fl oz; 1 measuring cup = 250 mL = 8 fl oz; 4 measuring cups = 1000 mL = 1 quart.

TABLE 48-6 Household Equivalents

60 gtt	=	1 t or tsp		
3 t or tsp	=	1 T		
180 gtt	=	1 T	=	½ oz
2 T	=	1 oz	=	6 t or tsp
360 gtt	=	2 T		
1 oz	=	30 cc or 30 ml		
6 oz	=	1 tcp		
8 oz	=	1 C or 1 glass		
2 C	=	1 pt	=	16 oz
2 pt	=	1 qt	=	32 oz
4 C	=	1 qt	=	32 oz
4 qt	=	1 gal	=	128 oz

TABLE 48-7 Common Household Measures

60 drops*	1 teaspoon
1 dash	Less than ⅛ teaspoon
3 teaspoons	1 tablespoon
2 tablespoons	1 ounce
4 ounces	1 juice glass
6 ounces	1 teacup
8 ounces	1 glass or cup
16 tablespoons or 8 ounces	1 measuring cup
2 cups	1 pint
2 pints	1 quart
4 quarts	1 gallon

*Drop (gtt) = approximate liquid measure depending on kind of liquid measured and the size of the opening from which it is dropped.

PROCEDURE 48-2

Calculating the Correct Dosage for Administration Using Two Systems of Measurement

GOAL

To choose the correct system of measurement and calculate the correct dosage amount when the physician orders 120 mg of a drug to be administered to a patient. (Tablet label reads 1 gr each.)

EQUIPMENT AND SUPPLIES

Tablets labeled 1 gr (grain) each
Standard mathematical formula:

$$\frac{\text{Available strength}}{\text{Ordered strength}} = \frac{\text{Available amount}}{\text{Amount to give}}$$

Conversion equivalent: 1 gr = 60 mg

PROCEDURAL STEPS

1 Read the order in quiet surroundings to make sure that you fully understand it.

2 Using pencil and paper, write out the order.

3 Examine the drug labels to see what strengths and amounts are available.

4 Convert the ordered system of measurement to the system of measurement on the label.

5 Write down the standard formula.
PURPOSE: To eliminate the chances of error, orders should never be carried out unless the calculations are completed in writing.

6 Rewrite the formula, replacing the unknown values with the known quantities and using the system of measurement on the label. The unknown *x* will be the amount of the drug to give (amount to give).

7 Work the proportion problem by cross-multiplying to solve for *x*.

8 State your answer by filling in the blank, as follows:
To administer 120 mg of a drug from tablets labeled 1 gr (grain) each, I would give ________ tablet(s).

PEDIATRIC DOSE CALCULATIONS

As noted earlier in the chapter, there is no perfect system for converting adult medications to proper pediatric dosages. In most cases, children are not able to tolerate adult medications, because a child's metabolism is very unstable compared with that of an adult. When it is necessary to administer an adult medication to a child, the following formulas are accepted. Calculating dosage in this manner is permitted only under the direct order and supervision of the physician.

Fried's Law

This calculation is for children younger than 1 year of age and is based on the age of the child in months compared with a child 12½ years old. The calculation assumes that an adult dose would be appropriate for a child aged 12½ years (150 months).

$$\text{Pediatric dose} = \frac{\text{Child's age in months}}{\text{150 months}} \times \text{Adult dose}$$

Young's Rule

Young's rule is for children older than 1 year of age.

$$\text{Pediatric dose} = \frac{\text{Child's age in years}}{\text{Child's age in years} + 12} \times \text{Adult dose}$$

Clark's Rule

This rule is based on the weight of the child. This system is much more accurate, because children of any age can vary greatly in size and body weight. Clark's rule uses 150 pounds (70 kg) as the average adult weight and assumes that the child's dose is proportionately less. The formula is

$$\text{Pediatric dose} = \frac{\text{Child's weight in pounds}}{\text{150 pounds}} \times \text{Adult dose}$$

West's Nomogram

West's nomogram calculates the body surface area of infants and young children. Many physicians use

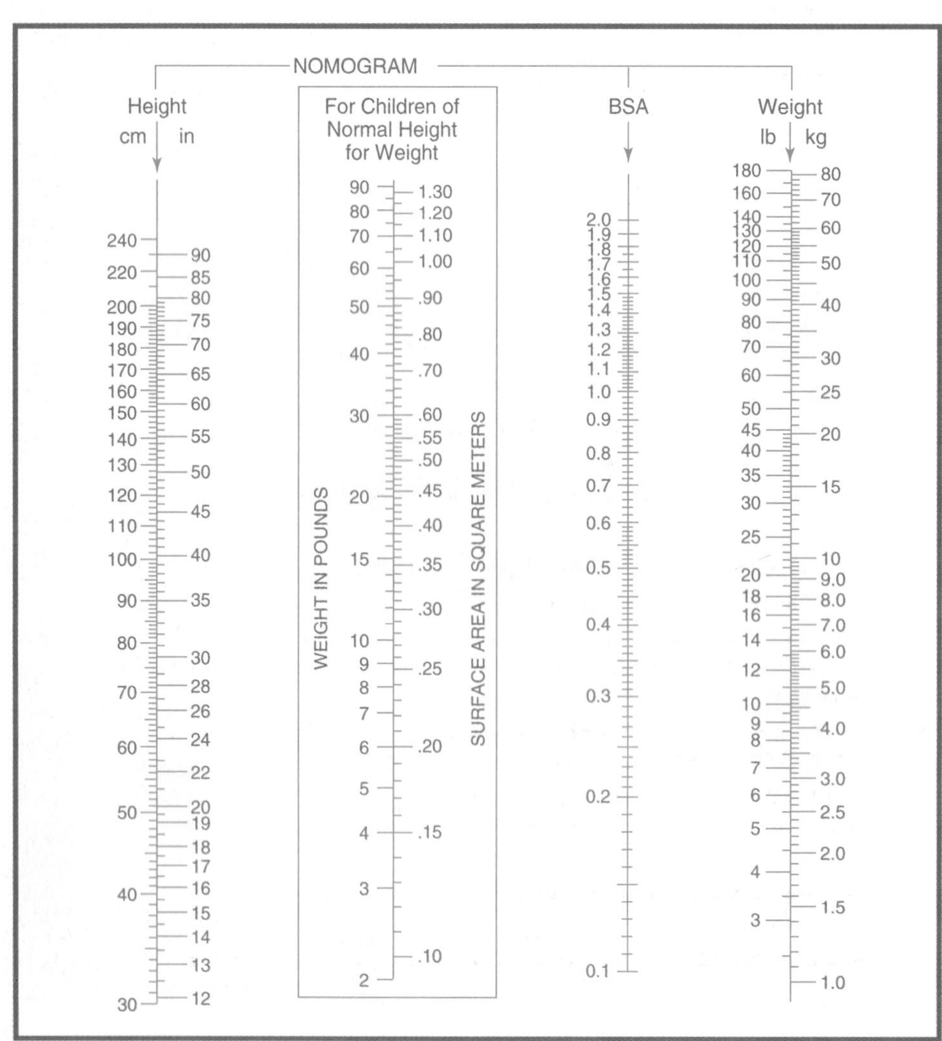

FIGURE 48–3 West's nomogram for estimation of body surface area. (From Behrman RE, Vaughan VC III: Nelson Textbook of Pediatrics, 13th ed. Philadelphia, WB Saunders, 1987.)

the **nomogram** because even a small miscalculation could be critical, especially when a child is ill, underweight, or overweight (Fig. 48–3).

Pediatric dose

$$= \frac{\text{Basic surface of child (in m}^2\text{)}}{1.73} \times \text{Adult dose}$$

You need complete mastery in calculating dosages, whether they be for children or adults. Until you master the arithmetic, the accurate placement of the decimal point, converting equivalents from one system to another, and the use of the ratio and proportion formula for every type of calculation, you must practice problems in dosages and solutions with someone who can check your work. Mastery of dosage calculations may take some time and much practice, but as with any other skill, you can achieve it if you take the time to understand the basics first, then advance to the concepts of ratio and proportion and, finally, to the calculation of specific drugs and solutions.

PROCEDURE 48–3

Calculating the Correct Dosage for a Child When Only an Adult Medication Is Available

GOAL

To calculate the correct dosage amount for a 90-pound child using Clark's rule when the adult dosage is 250 mg.

EQUIPMENT AND SUPPLIES

Adult dosage 250 mg/mL
Clark's rule:

$$\text{Pediatric dose} = \frac{\text{Child's weight in pounds}}{150}$$

Standard mathematical formula:

$$\frac{\text{Available strength}}{\text{Ordered strength}} = \frac{\text{Available amount}}{\text{Amount to give}}$$

PROCEDURAL STEPS

1 Read the order in quiet surroundings to make sure that you fully understand it.

2 Using pencil and paper, write out the order.

3 Examine the drug labels to see what strengths and amounts are available.

4 Write down Clark's rule.
PURPOSE: To eliminate the chances of error, orders should never be carried out unless the calculations are completed in writing.

5 Using Clark's rule, replace the unknown values with the known quantities. The unknown *x* will be the pediatric strength ordered (pediatric dose).

6 Write down the standard formula.
PURPOSE: To eliminate the chances of error, orders should never be carried out unless the calculations are completed in writing.

7 Rewrite the formula, replacing the unknown values with the available quantities and the pediatric strength just determined. The unknown *x* will be the amount of the drug to give (amount to give).

8 Work the proportion problem by cross-multiplying to solve for *x*.

9 State your answer by filling in the blank, as follows:
To administer an adult medication labeled 250 mg/mL to a 90-pound child, I will give ______________ mL.

PROCEDURE 48-4

Calculating the Correct Dosage for Administration Using Body Weight

GOAL

To calculate correct dosage by using body weight method.
Ordered: Zovirax capsules 5 mg/kg every 8 hours for 7 days for a patient who has a diagnosis of herpes zoster. The patient weighs 132 pounds. The capsules are labeled 50 mg = 1 capsule.
Weight: 2.2 lb = 1 kg

EQUIPMENT AND SUPPLIES

Capsules labeled 50 mg/kg
Balance scale
Formula for conversion of pounds to kilograms
Standard math formula:

$$\frac{\text{Available strength}}{\text{Ordered strength}} = \frac{\text{Available amount}}{\text{Amount to give}}$$

Paper and pencil

PROCEDURAL STEPS

1 Read the order in quiet surroundings to make sure that you fully understand it.
2 Write out the order.
3 Examine the drug label to check the strength and amount.
4 Convert the patient's weight from pounds to kilograms.
5 Write down the standard formula.
PURPOSE: To eliminate the chances of error.
6 Rewrite the formula, replacing the unknown values with the known quantities. The unknown *x* will be the amount of the drug to give.
7 Work the problem by cross-multiplying to solve for *x*.
8 State your answer by filling in the blank as follows:
To administer 5 mg/kg of body weight of Zovirax from capsules labeled 50 mg each, I would give ______________ capsule(s).

Charting

All medications must be charted as they were written by the physician. For parenteral medications the site of injection should be included in the charting. In addition, the patient's immediate reaction to the medication, if any, should be noted.

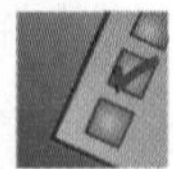

PATIENT EDUCATION

It is important to the patient to be aware of the effects a drug may have and should have on his or her system. Good communication is the key to a well-informed, confident, compliant patient. With this in mind, you should approach the following issues:

1. Ask the patient if she is pregnant.
2. Preassess the patient for any adverse effects, such as allergy or drug-to-drug or drug-to-food interactions.
3. Observe the patient for any adverse effects that might occur immediately after the administration of a medication in the office. Inform the patient of a possible adverse reaction to the medication at home and give specific instructions of how to deal with this emergency.
4. Discuss with the patient how the prescribed drug is to be appropriately administered by the patient.
5. Reassess that the patient is taking the medication properly.

6. Provide comfort, encouragement, and guidance to patients to ensure their understanding, safety, and cooperation while being on drug therapy.
7. Answer any questions asked. Remember if you are not certain of the answer, consult the prescribing physician.

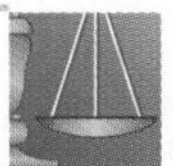

LEGAL AND ETHICAL ISSUES

The medical assistant who prepares and administers medications is ethically and legally responsible for his or her own actions. Under the law, you are required to be licensed, registered, or authorized by a physician to administer medications. Laws vary from state to state. Therefore, it is essential that you become familiar with the laws in the state of your employment before giving medications. Legislation in some states gives physicians broad authority to delegate responsibility for giving medications. The medical assistant acts as the "agent" of the physician. The assistant is responsible and accountable for the acts performed and may be subject to penalty in case of default.

Regardless of the differences in state authorization laws, the courts will not permit the carelessness of health care workers to go unpunished, especially when such actions result in the harming or death of the patient. Under the law, those administering medications are expected to be familiar with the drugs administered and the effects that they might have on a patient. It is your responsibility to be aware of the drugs that your physician prescribes. Make it a habit to look up and check any drug that you are not familiar with. Despite differences in the duties of drug administration assigned to you by your physician, the following considerations are your ultimate responsibility:

- To be informed about the drugs that you administer
- To review the legal requirements for controlled substances
- To ensure that a drug being used is correct in its order, dosage, route, time, and use

Answers to Procedures 48–1 through 48–4

PROCEDURE 48–1

To administer 2.4 million IU of Bicillin, I would select two of the premixed syringes labeled 1.2 million IU per syringe.

PROCEDURE 48–2

To administer 120 mg of a drug from tablets labeled 1 gr each, I would give two tablets.

PROCEDURE 48–3

To administer an adult medication labeled 250 mg/mL to a 90-pound child, I would give 0.6 mL.

PROCEDURE 48–4

To administer Zovirax, 5 mg/kg of body weight from capsules labeled 50 mg each, I would give a patient weighing 132 pounds two capsules (100 mg).

CRITICAL THINKING

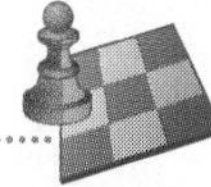

1 You suspect that a patient waiting to see the physician is "under the influence." How would you handle the situation?

2 How would you determine from the diabetic patient the following:
a. Plans for eating three meals a day
b. How and when the patient would make sure oral hypoglycemics were taken

HOW DID I DO? Answers to Memory Joggers

1. Pharmacology is the study of the origin, nature, chemistry, effects, and uses of drugs.
2. Classification name, generic name, and brand name
3. Methods of dispensing are over-the-counter and prescription.
4. Superscription, inscription, subscription, and signature
5. Colored ink cannot be reproduced and tinted paper make detection of erasures or correct fluid usage easy.
6. Dispensing record must be kept for 2 years.
7. Pregnancy categories indicate the level of possible risk to the developing fetus.
8. Psychologic dependency, habituation, physical dependency
9. Fate of a drug includes absorption, distribution, action, biotransformation, and excretion.
10. Parenteral route
11. Body weight, age, sex, time of day, pathologic factors, immune response, psychologic factors, tolerance, cumulation, and idiosyncrasy
12. Action, indication, side effects, adverse effects, precautions, contraindications, toxic effects, dosage, and administration

REFERENCES

Clark J, Queener S, Karb V: Pocket Guide to Drugs. St. Louis, CV Mosby, 1986
Kee J, Hayes E: Pharmacology: A Nursing Process Approach, 2nd ed. Philadelphia, WB Saunders, 1997
Physician's Desk Reference, 51st ed. Oradell, NJ, Medical Economics, 1997
Reynard A, Smith C: Textbook of Pharmacology. Philadelphia, WB Saunders, 1992
Woodrow R: Essentials of Pharmacology for Health Occupations, 2nd ed. New York, Delmar Publishers, 1992

Administering Medications

Mary Agnes Taylor, RN

49

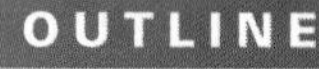

OUTLINE

LEARNING OBJECTIVES

Cognitive: On successful completion of this chapter you should be able to:

1. Spell and define the words listed in the Vocabulary.
2. List six factors of patient assessment that may influence whether you should continue with an order to administer a drug.
3. State two situations in which it may be your responsibility to further assess an ordered drug before administering it.
4. State two environmental factors that would contraindicate the administration of a medication.
5. Recall the "three befores" and the "six rights."
6. List the basic solid and liquid oral dosage forms and give an example of each.
7. For each of the five mucous membrane sites, cite the methods for administering medications.
8. Differentiate among the nine types of topical medications.
9. For each parenteral method, list the preferred needle gauges and lengths and the usual syringe size.
10. State the risks of using reusable injection equipment and three advantages of disposable injection equipment.
11. List the contraindications for administering a parenteral drug in any particular site.
12. Locate the anatomic landmarks for each intramuscular injection site.
13. List the special considerations of anatomy when administering injectable medications to infants and small children.
14. Recall the Centers for Disease Control and Prevention standards.

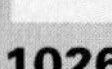

Performance: On successful completion of this chapter you should be able to:

1 Fill a syringe using sterile (aseptic) technique.
2 Demonstrate giving an intradermal injection.
3 Demonstrate giving a subcutaneous injection.
4 Demonstrate giving an intramuscular injection.
5 Demonstrate giving a Z-track intramuscular injection.
6 Demonstrate the application of a transdermal patch.
7 Instruct a patient in the use of an oral medication.
8 Instruct a patient in the use of a rectal medication.
9 Instruct a patient in the use of a vaginal medication.
10 Instruct a patient in the use of a inhaler.

VOCABULARY

allergy immunotherapy Administering repeated injections of diluted extracts of the substance that cause the allergy, also called *desensitization*

ampule Small (usually a single-dose) glass container of medication prepared for parenteral administration

aspirate To withdraw fluid by negative pressure; pulling up on the plunger of the syringe after inserting the needle to check for blood

hermetically sealed Sealed so no air is allowed to enter

induration An abnormally hard spot or place

radical mastectomy Complete surgical removal of the breast, the surrounding muscles, and the lymph glands

sublingual Under the tongue

sustained or time-released Pertaining to medications that are manufactured to release their action over a period of time

topical Applied to a certain area of the skin and affecting only that area

vesiculation Formation of blister-like elevations on the skin

vial A small bottle, usually made of glass

viscosity The quality of being thick and gluelike and of lacking the capability of easy movement

volatile Referring to an explosive substance's capacity to vaporize at a low temperature

wheal Localized area of edema on the body's surface

Drug therapy has become one of the most significant aspects of patient care and one of the most significant responsibilities that a physician may delegate to a medical assistant. The medical assistant who is asked to administer medications must have a thorough understanding of the scientific principles of drug therapy and the confidence and assurance to follow through with the physician's request. Chapter 48 is an introduction to how drugs interact with the body, the basic routes of administration, and the standard formulas for dosage calculation. This chapter builds on the last, developing the specific skills of patient assessment and drug administration. Most of the drugs administered in the medical office will be by injection (parenterally). Most oral medications will be filled by prescription and will be started by the patient at home. Occasionally, the medical assistant may be required to instill drops into a patient's eyes, ears, or nose or may be called on to insert a rectal suppository.

No matter what type of medications are to be administered, the order must come from the physician. If the physician delegates drug administration to you as part of your job, it must be allowable under state laws. Every state has a medical practice act that will define whether a medical assistant can administer drugs under the supervision of a physician. Some states allow medical assistants to administer only certain types of medications; some prohibit medical assistants from giving injections. Information concerning the scope of practice for medical assistants in your particular state should be obtained from your local government or medical society. You should know what the law states and how your duties fit into that law.

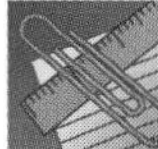

Project #1: Obtain a copy of your state's regulations for medical assistants. Review the scope of practice for medication administration.

Drug Therapy Assessment

Although medications may be given only under the direct order and supervision of the physician, you are a part of the assessment and problem-solving processes in the care of the patient. In medicine, assessment never ends and never is it the responsibility of just one person. A physician gives the order to administer medication to a patient based on a medical assessment, but you also must continue to assess the patient and the patient's environment as you follow through with the order. The physician depends on you to be alert to changes or new information that could result in a condition or consequence that would make the use of a drug improper or undesirable. Before giving any medication, you should assess the patient, the drug, and the environment.

PATIENT ASSESSMENT

Assessment of the patient includes the patient's history and current status. As you are about to act on a physician's order, you, too, should mentally review factors that may influence whether you continue with the order or return to the physician for further clarification.

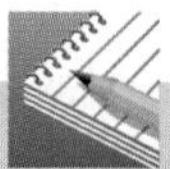

SKILLS AND RESPONSIBILITIES

FACTORS THAT INFLUENCE THE ADMINISTERING OF DRUGS

- Are there any conditions that may contraindicate the use of the drug or the dosage ordered?
- Do you have special knowledge of any other drug use (a dependency or the use of prescription or over-the-counter drugs) that may contraindicate the completion of the medication order?
- Does the patient have any allergies to drugs of this type or to certain foods or animals that may indicate that this drug will produce a similar allergic effect?
- Are the patient's age, height, and weight correct for the dosage ordered?
- Is there a reason that the route chosen for administration may not be desirable? For example, an injection may be ordered for a particular site. However, you notice there is an injury at the site that would contraindicate its use for an injection.

Patient assessment does not end with the administration of the drug. Observe patients carefully for drug reactions that may follow injectable medications. Patients receiving penicillin (a drug with a high incidence of allergic response) or **allergy immunotherapy** must remain in the office for 20 to 30 minutes in case of acute anaphylactic reaction. Acute anaphylactic reaction can result in respiratory failure and circulatory collapse within minutes if not reversed with epinephrine. Lesser allergic reactions include hives, swelling, and itching. An antihistamine, such as diphenhydramine (Benadryl), may need to be administered (see Chapter 40).

DRUG ASSESSMENT

Drug assessment includes evaluation of the drug and the dosage ordered. No medication should be administered without a written order. If you are to administer a medication by verbal order, be sure to have the physician sign or write the order on the patient's medical record as soon as possible. If there is doubt about a particular order, written or verbal, *do not* give the drug until you are sure that it is what the physician intends. If you still have doubts, confidentially and politely request that the physician personally administer the drug. Remember you assume the responsibility if you do not understand an order but administer the drug anyway.

You must also evaluate the drug's appropriateness. For example, you have a patient who is a diabetic and the physician orders Ornade. You know that Ornade is a time-released antihistamine and that Orinase is an oral hypoglycemic. Never hesitate to question a misinterpretation or possible mistake on a drug order. So many drugs sound and are spelled alike that mistakes are possible. If you do not know the details of the drugs you are administering, you will not be able to assess their appropriateness and, therefore, support the physician and safeguard the patient.

Know the appropriate dosages. The standard abbreviations for dosages may not be clearly written, and you may need to know whether the order was for a minim (M.) or for a milliliter (mL). Because there are 15 to 16 minims in a milliliter, to guess or not to know the appropriate dosage, in this case, could result in a patient receiving 15 times the desired amount, or $\frac{1}{15}$ the necessary amount. Either way, harm may come to a patient from an irresponsible act on your part.

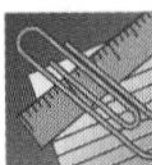

Project #2: Review the standard abbreviations for weights and measures.

ENVIRONMENT ASSESSMENT

The patient's surroundings could determine an order's inappropriateness. The patient may become hysterical or uncooperative about receiving the medication, or the patient's family may protest the use of the drug. A patient may come to the office for a weekly drug treatment, but the physician may not be present. Drugs should not be administered to patients, even on order, if there is not someone present who cannot only administer emergency first aid but also reverse acute anaphylactic reactions with injectable epinephrine. The medical assistant cannot inject epinephrine without an order. In the absence of a physician, there would be no one to give that order in an emergency.

The environment must be safe for drug administration. Be sure that the patient is comfortable and protected from further injury. If a patient is to receive an injection, make sure to place the patient in a position that best exposes the site and protects the patient from injury in case he or she faints or has a drug reaction. If the patient is to take an oral medication with water, be sure that he or she is seated in a position that will prevent choking. Because any medication is potentially dangerous to a patient, there also must be emergency drugs, readily available, to counteract any adverse effects that might occur immediately after the administration of a medication. Emergency drugs should be in injectable form for rapid effect. Typically, emergency carts include adrenergics, such as epinephrine; anticholinergics, such as atropine; bronchodilators; and histamine blockers.

The entire process of administering medications should be completed in quiet surroundings and with concentration. When you are preparing and administering a medication, do not do anything else, including talking. The process requires organized and concise movements and involves the "three befores" and the "six rights."

THE "THREE BEFORES"

Before administering any drug, check the label for the correct drug choice and dosage three times:

1 *Before* removing the drug from the shelf—make sure you start with the right medication and dosage.
2 *Before* pouring or preparing the drug—a double check while you work.
3 *Before* returning the drug to the shelf—a third check. Drugs are returned to the shelf before you leave the medication room to administer the medication to the patient.

THE "SIX RIGHTS"

Before you leave the medication room, take the time to say yes to the following six questions.

Do I have the

1 *Right patient?* Check the name on the patient's chart. (Before administering the drug, you will again check, by greeting the patient by name, to be sure that you have the right person.)
2 *Right drug?* Compare the written drug name with the label of the container that you are using. Does it seem appropriate? Know the medications that you are using. Never prepare medications from a bottle with a damaged label. READ THE LABEL THREE TIMES. Compare the written order with the strength labeled on the container. If the ordered strength is not available, you will have to give more or less, depending on the situation.
3 *Right dose?* Compare the written dosage order with the amount of drug that you prepare (number of tablets, quantity of solution). (Drug calculation formulas are located in Chapter 48.) READ THE LABEL THREE TIMES.
4 *Right time?* Should the medication be given now? Is it the correct time of day? Is it the correct time in a series of administrations? Is it the correct time in the body cycle?
5 *Right route?* Can the patient receive this medication by the route ordered? Is the particular drug available for the route ordered? Is the route an appropriate one?
6 *Right documentation?* Did I enter it on the patient's record? Was my entry precise and accurate? Did I initial the entry?

Memory Jogger

Why is it important to read the medication label three times?

Calculating Drug Dosages for Administration

The medical assistant who prepares and administer medications is ethically and legally responsible for his or her own actions. The dose of medication that is administered to the patient must be absolutely correct. In the preceding chapter, basic arithmetic was reviewed and the procedures for calculating dosages were given. If the review of dose calculations is necessary, please refer to Chapter 48.

Memory Jogger

The patient is to receive 250 mg of Duricef oral suspension. If the label reads 125 mg/5 mL, how much will you give the patient?

Drug Forms and Administration

As discussed in Chapter 48, the chosen route of drug administration determines whether the drug will have an effect and, often, the intensity of the effect. A drug prepared for one route but administered by another route may not have any effect at all or may potentially be dangerous. Each route requires different dosage forms.

SOLID ORAL DOSAGE FORMS

The basic forms are tablets, capsules, powders, and lozenges (troches). Pills are rarely manufactured today, but many people mistakenly call tablets "pills" (Fig. 49–1).

TABLETS AND CAPLETS Tablets are compressed powders or granules that, when wet, break apart in the stomach, or in the mouth if they are not swallowed quickly. Tablets may be *sugar* coated to taste better, or *enteric* coated to resist the acid action of the stomach. Some tablets are coated with a volatile liquid that is meant to dissolve in the mouth, such as an antacid tablet. Caplets are oblong-like capsules.

CAPSULES Capsules are gelatin coated and dissolve in the stomach, or they may be coated with substances that protect them from the acid action of the stomach. Timed- or **sustained-release** capsules are designed to dissolve at different rates, over a period of time, to reduce the number of times a patient has to take a medication.

POWDERS Powders are no longer popular. Effervescent antacids and laxatives are now being manufactured in the form of a large tablet or granules.

LOZENGES (TROCHES) Lozenges are flattened discs that are dissolved in the mouth for coating the throat.

Oral Administration

Make sure the patient has enough water to transport the drug to the stomach. Make sure that the patient is able to swallow the medication. It may be helpful to place the medication on the back part of the tongue. If a patient has difficulty in swallowing or is very young, you may crush and mix the solid form in a soft food, such as applesauce, provided that the food does not interact with the drug. Enteric-coated tablets or timed-release capsules should never be crushed or dissolved. If your patient has been vomiting or is nauseated, an alternative route might be necessary.

Memory Jogger

What is the difference between capsules and tablets?

LIQUID AND ORAL DOSAGE FORMS

Many types of liquid forms are available. They differ mainly in the type of substance used to dissolve the drug: water, oils, or alcohol.

SOLUTIONS Solutions are drug substances contained in a homogeneous mixture with a liquid. Several types are

- *Syrups:* Solutions of sugar and water, usually containing flavoring and medicinal substances. Cough syrups are the most common.
- *Aromatic waters:* Aqueous solutions containing **volatile** oils such as oil of spearmint, peppermint, or clove.
- *Liquors:* Solutions that contain a nonvolatile material, such as alcohol, as the solute.

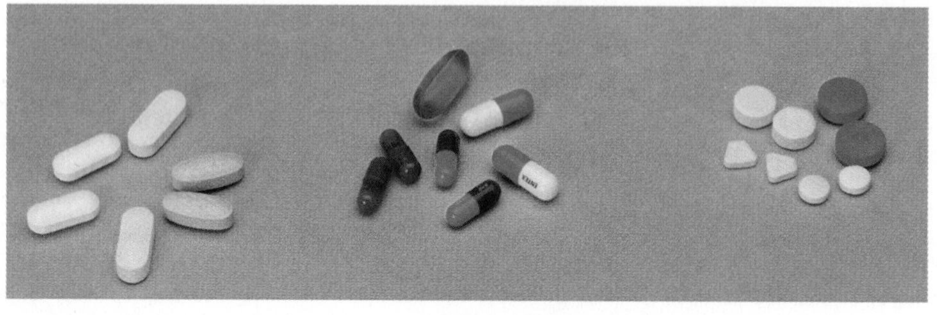

FIGURE 49–1 *Left to right,* Caplets, capsules, and tablets.

SUSPENSIONS Suspensions are insoluble drug substances contained in a liquid. Examples are

- *Emulsions:* Mixtures of oil and water that improve the taste of otherwise distasteful products such as cod liver oil.
- *Gels and magmas:* Minerals suspended in water. Minerals settle; therefore, products containing minerals must be shaken before use. Milk of magnesia is an example.

ALCOHOL SOLUTIONS A drug substance can be mixed with alcohol to enhance the drug's properties. Examples are:

- *Fluid extracts:* Combinations of alcohol and vegetable products that are more potent than tinctures. For example, belladonna fluid extract has a higher percentage of the powdered belladonna leaf than does tincture of belladonna.
- *Tinctures:* An alcoholic preparation of a soluble drug or chemical substance, usually from plant sources. An example is tincture of belladonna. A less potent example is tincture of benzoin and tincture of iodine, which are applied externally.
- *Extracts:* Very concentrated combinations of vegetable products and alcohol or ether that are evaporated until a syrupy liquid, solid mass, or powder is formed. Extracts are many times stronger than the crude drug itself.
- *Elixirs:* Aromatic, alcoholic, sweetened preparations. Elixir of phenobarbital is one example; the alcoholic cough medicines, terpin hydrate with codeine and plain elixir of codeine, are two more. Elixirs differ from tinctures in that they are sweetened. They should be used with caution in patients with diabetes or a history of alcohol abuse. Some pediatric medications retain the name of elixir although they no longer contain alcohol.

Oral Administration

If the drug is not intended to coat the oral cavity or throat, liquid medications may be followed by a quantity of water. Use a straw for fluid iron preparations, acids, and certain other minerals to avoid staining the teeth. Then rinse the mouth with water. Liquid medications are not recommended for patients who are too weak to pour the liquid and to hold it steady in the spoon. Liquid medications are ideal for children. Solid drugs should not be administered to children until they reach the age when they can safely swallow a solid drug form without the danger of aspirating the drug. Always remain with the patient until you are certain that the medication has been totally swallowed.

MUCOUS MEMBRANE FORMS

Some mucous membranes are selected for their ability to absorb medication for a systemic effect. The most commonly used areas are the gums, cheeks (buccal), under the tongue (sublingual), rectum, and the respiratory mucosa (inhalation). Nasal, ophthalmic, rectal, and vaginal preparations may also be applied to these mucous membranes for their localized effects.

Rectal Administration

The rectal mucosa provides a rapid absorption even though the surface of the rectum is small. Drugs are absorbed directly into the bloodstream, without being altered as they would be by the digestive processes, and without irritation to the patient's gastric mucosa. Rectal medications are useful if the patient is nauseated, vomiting, or unconscious. Manufacturers supply rectal medications in the form of gelatin or cocoa butter–based suppositories, which melt in the warmth of the rectum and release the medication, or in the form of enemas. Suppositories may be used to soften the stool or stimulate evacuation of the bowel; enemas are used to cleanse and evacuate.

The best time to administer a rectal drug intended for a systemic effect is after a bowel movement or enema. The patient should be cautioned to remain lying down for 20 to 30 minutes to prevent accidental evacuation of the drug by a bowel movement or elimination of the enema. Suppositories intended to treat constipation, of course, are administered to bring about bowel evacuation. The patient should be instructed to insert the suppository about 2 inches above the rectal sphincter muscles; a little mineral oil or vegetable oil may be used as lubrication. If suppositories are individually wrapped in foil, make sure the patient knows that the foil is the wrapper and is not part of the treatment.

Vaginal Administration

Vaginal suppositories, tablets, creams, and fluid solutions are used to treat local infections. Irrigating solutions (douches) may be used as anti-infectives. Creams and foams are available as local contraceptives. Vaginal instillation is most effective if the patient remains lying down; many preparations are therefore prescribed at bedtime. The patient may need to wear a pad to absorb drainage. Liquid medications can be applied to tampons and inserted for a period of time; then a pad is usually not needed. Solid suppositories and tablets may be lubricated or moistened with water and inserted by hand or with an applicator. Creams are instilled with applicators. Prepackaged, disposable irrigation kits are available for douching.

In addition to prescription douches, many over-the-counter preparations are now marketed. Advise your patients that vaginal secretions have their own wash-effect that is antiseptic. Frequent douching can remove the secretions and change the acidity of the vaginal canal, resulting in infection caused by either normal flora or invading bacteria. When instructing patients, confirm that the patient can differentiate the urinary meatus from the vaginal orifice and the rectum. Mistakes could result in vaginal infections or in damage or infection to the urinary tract. A simple drawing and explanation may be required.

Inhalation

Inhalation drugs are supplied in the form of droplets, vapors, or gas. Because of the large surface area and the rich blood supply of the respiratory membranes, the respiratory tract absorbs medications more rapidly than any other mucous membrane. Inhalation can be used to produce a local effect, such as with medications to liquefy bronchial secretions or to dilate the bronchi to bring relief to asthmatic or emphysemic patients. In addition, inhalation may be used for systemic effects, such as with oxygen and general anesthesia. Most inhalant substances do spill over into the bloodstream, however, and caution must be taken not to bring about cardiac irregularities and central nervous system side effects. Hand-held inhalers or metered-dose inhalers (MDIs) are very common today. Each brand is different, and the patient needs to read the package insert carefully for proper use of the inhaler (Table 49–1).

TABLE 49–1 Correct Use of a Metered-Dose Inhaler

1. Insert the medication canister using the plastic holder.
2. Shake the inhaler well before using. Remove cap from mouthpiece.
3. Breathe out through the mouth. Open mouth wide and hold the mouthpiece 1–2 inches from the mouth. Do *not* put mouthpiece in the mouth unless using a spacer. Discuss techniques with the health care provider.
4. With mouth open, take a slow, deep breath through mouth and at same time push the top of the medication canister once.
5. Hold breath for a few seconds; exhale slowly through pursed lips.
6. If a second dose is required, wait 2 minutes and repeat the procedure by first shaking the canister in the plastic holder with the cap on.
7. If the inhaler has not been used recently or when it is first used, "test spray" before administering the metered dose.
8. If a glucocorticoid inhalant is to be used with a bronchodilator, wait 5 min before using the inhaler containing the steroid.
9. Teach client to monitor pulse rate.
10. Caution against overuse, because side effects and tolerance may result.
11. Teach client to monitor amount of medication remaining in the canister.
12. Instruct client to avoid smoking.
13. Teach client to do daily cleaning of the equipment:
    a. Wash hands.
    b. Take apart all washable parts of equipment and wash with warm water.
    c. Rinse.
    d. Place on clean towel and cover with another clean towel to air dry.
    e. Store in clean plastic bag when *completely* dry. Having two sets of washable equipment makes this process much easier!

From Kee JL, Hayes ER: Pharmacology: A Nursing Process Approach, 2nd ed. Philadelphia, WB Saunders, 1997.

Oral Administration

Mouth and throat agents come in the form of sprays, swabs, sublingual tablets, and buccal tablets. The mouth and throat membranes may be treated locally with antiseptics for oral hygiene and local infections, with anesthetics for relief of pain, and with astringents that form a protective film over the mucous membranes. The patient may have to gargle, or the area may be painted or sprayed. To paint or spray the throat, first look for the area of inflammation to be treated. Otherwise, the part needing treatment may be missed entirely. Avoid touching the posterior pharynx (back of the throat); this causes gagging and possibly vomiting.

Sublingual tablets are placed under the tongue, where they are rapidly absorbed into the bloodstream by the rich supply of capillaries. Sublingual absorption is systemic and bypasses the acids in the stomach, which may inactivate the medication. Nitroglycerin, used for treating the chest pains of angina pectoris, is one of these medications. Patients should not chew or swallow sublingual medications. The patient should be instructed not to smoke, eat, or drink during administration of these drugs.

Buccal tablets are placed between the cheek and the upper molars. The same rules of sublingual administration apply to buccal administration.

Nasal Administration

Nose drops, nasal sprays, and tampons are used for their localized effect, but, like the inhalation drugs, they may spill over into the bloodstream, causing a change in the heart rate, an increase in blood pressure, or central nervous system stimulation. Nasal medications are commonly used for blocked nasal passages (decongestants) and nosebleeds (hemostatics). Nose drops should be instilled with the patient's head tilted back. Then the patient should be instructed to tilt the head forward to distribute the medication properly. Short, quick breaths will help spread the solution. Any medication spilling down the throat should be expectorated; swallowing nasal preparations can result in systemic side effects.

Nasal sprays are designed for administration with the patient's head upright. Be sure that the spray tip is centered in the nostril and not against the side of the nasal cavity. Nasal decongestant sprays are often misused by patients. Be sure to teach the patient not to exceed the amount or frequency ordered by the physician. If too much is used, these drugs can dry the mucosa and make congestion worse.

Topical Forms

With a few exceptions, **topical** drugs are local in their effect. Most drugs applied to the skin cannot be absorbed into the bloodstream (unless there is a break in the skin). However, large amounts of a drug left on the skin for a long time can be absorbed and cause systemic poisoning. For example, the previous use of hexachlorophene soaps on hospitalized infants caused toxic reactions and even infant deaths. Now this drug is banned from use in nonprescription soaps and lotions. Oil-based substances have a better chance of being absorbed through the skin than do substances that are water based. Skin medication forms include lotions, liniments, ointments, compresses, creams, and patches.

LOTIONS Often used to control itching, lotions are applied by dabbing with a soft cloth, cotton ball, or tongue blade. Calamine is an example. Rubbing will increase the itching or irritation. The medical assistant should wear gloves. Some lotions are used to relieve congestion and pain in muscles and joints. In these cases, the application is covered with a thick cloth to retain heat. It is said that these lotions and heat dilate the superficial blood vessels, thus drawing blood to the surface and away from the congested parts. However, this is controversial. Many believe that the effects of these lotions are limited to the skin surface where the medication is applied.

LINIMENTS Liniments (emulsions) have a higher portion of oil than do lotions, and volatile active ingredients may be added. Liniments are often used to protect dried, cracked, or fissured skin.

OINTMENTS Ointments are semisolid medications containing bases such as petrolatum and lanolin, or nongreasy bases. Ointments are applied to dry, scaly areas with little or no hair and can exert a prolonged effect. They are used in small amounts and are applied with firm strokes to avoid increasing itchiness. Ointments that stain clothing should be covered. An ointment should be removed from a jar or tube with a tongue blade to prevent contamination of the remaining medication.

SOAKS, COMPRESSES, AND WET DRESSINGS These aqueous solutions of substances with mild astringent properties have a soothing, cooling, antipyretic effect when applied to blistered and oozing areas. Bandages may be soaked in the solution, then applied to the patient, or the patient's extremity may be immersed in the solution and then wrapped in cloth. Plastic wrap can be applied over the bandage or cloth, or the wet dressing can rest on a plastic-covered surface until the air dries the bandage. If the solution contains a dye, the patient should be advised that the treatment will stain clothing or bedding.

HOT SOAKS AND COMPRESSES Hot compresses are used to treat abscesses and cellulitis. Extreme care must be taken to avoid burning the patient. Hot soaks are applied for up to 20 minutes; after this amount of time, circulation to a part reaches maximum flow and dissipates heat as fast as the compress can create it.

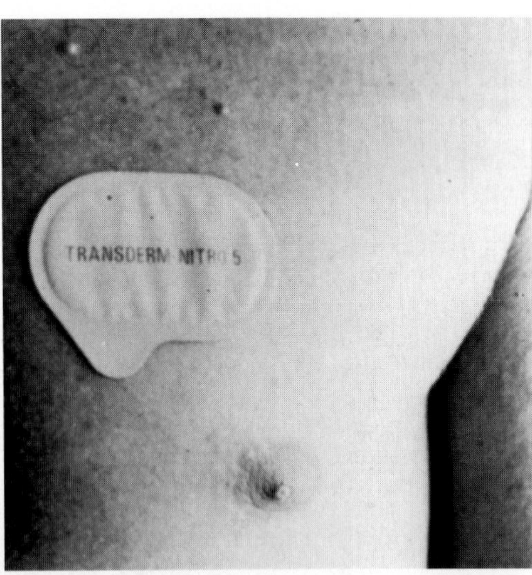

FIGURE 49–2 Transdermal patch (e.g., Transderm-Nitro). (Courtesy of Summit Pharmaceutical.) (From Kee JL, Hayes ER: Pharmacology: A Nursing Approach, 2nd ed. Philadelphia, WB Saunders, 1997.)

CREAMS Creams contain active ingredients incorporated into emulsions that vanish when they are rubbed into the skin.

THE TRANSDERMAL PATCH Certain medications can be absorbed slowly through the skin to create a constant, time-released systemic effect. The nitroglycerin patch is particularly useful for patients with frequent attacks of angina. Hormone patches, mainly estrogen, can also be absorbed slowly through the skin, providing the needed hormonal levels to women. With dermal patches, drugs can be administered in a time-released manner for up to 3 days. The date and time the patch was applied should be written on the patch as well as documented in the patient's record (Fig. 49–2).

EAR DROPS AND IRRIGATIONS Topical ear medications have a local effect and come in the form of drops and irrigations. Medications are instilled into the ear canal to treat infections, reduce inflammation, and bring about local anesthesia. Drops should be instilled with the patient lying down on the unaffected side. Ear drops are supplied in small bottles, with a dropper attached to the cork or cap. The bottle should be held in the hand for a few minutes to warm the solution to body temperature. Drops that are too cold or too warm can cause pain or dizziness. If the contents need mixing, roll the bottle between the palms; do not shake. The patient should lie still for 15 to 30 minutes to allow the medication to coat the ear canal and to be absorbed. Cotton ear plugs should not be used unless specifically ordered. In addition, ear irrigations are performed with the patient sitting; in infants, the patient should be supine (Fig. 49–3).

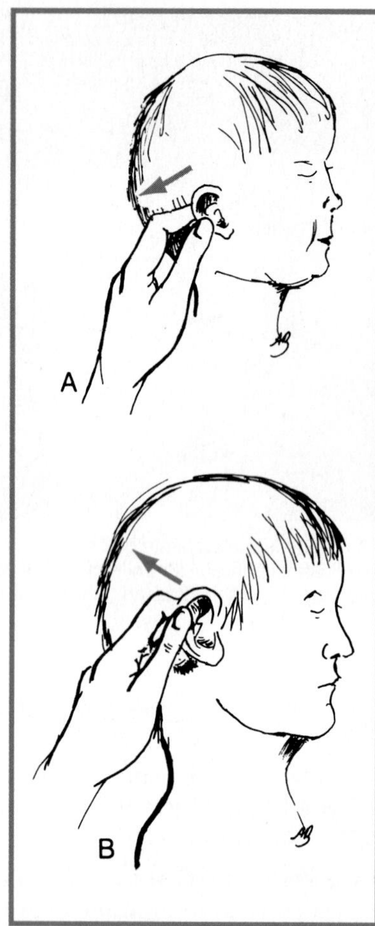

FIGURE 49–3 To facilitate administration of ear drops, straighten the external ear canal by pulling down on the auricle in children (*A*) or by pulling up and back in adults (*B*). (From Kee JL, Hayes ER: Pharmacology: A Nursing Approach, 2nd ed. Philadelphia, WB Saunders, 1997; Courtesy of Summit Pharmaceutical.)

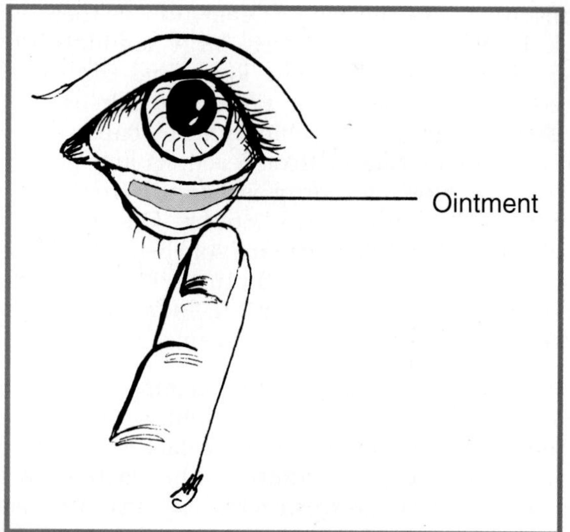

FIGURE 49–4 To facilitate administration of eye ointment, squeeze strip of ointment, about ¼ inch, onto conjunctival sac. (From Kee JL, Hayes ER: Pharmacology: A Nursing Approach, 2nd ed. Philadelphia, WB Saunders, 1997.)

EYE DROPS, OINTMENTS, AND IRRIGATIONS Drug forms for medicating the eye are sterile. Eye solutions come in dropper bottles; ointments are supplied in small tubes. Drops and ointments should not be applied to the sensitive cornea of the eye. Tips of the dropper and the tube must not touch any portion of the eye or eyelid. Drugs instilled into the eye are generally absorbed slowly and affect only the area in contact. However, some medications can act systemically if improper administration techniques are used. If a medication is allowed to flow into the lacrimal system, it can travel

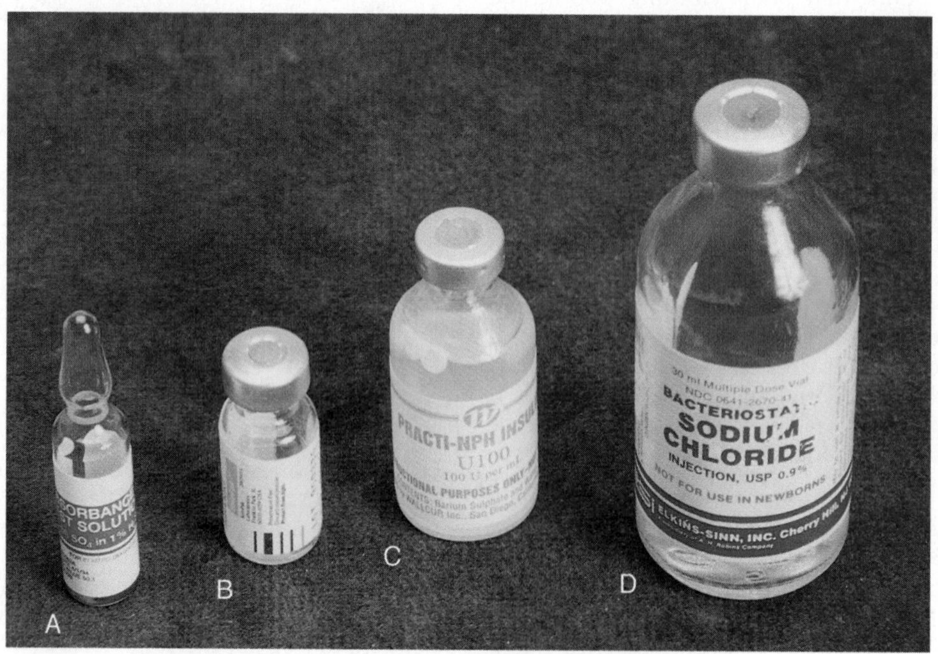

FIGURE 49–5 *A*, Ampule. *B*, Single-dose vial. *C* and *D*, Multidose vials.

down into the nasal cavity and can be absorbed into the circulatory system. To avoid this, you should apply pressure to the inner angle (inner canthus) of the eye with a tissue immediately after instillation of the medication onto the lower eyelid. Eye drops and ointments are placed between the eyeball and the lower lid (Fig. 49–4). To teach the patient to self-administer eye drops, demonstrate how to hold back the head, open the eye wide, and let the drops fall into the lower portion of the eye. Tell the patient not to worry if the drops run onto the face; the solution is harmless.

Parenteral Medication Forms

Injectable medications must be sterile and in liquid form. The medications may come in an ampule, a single-dose vial, a multi-dose vial, or a prefilled syringe (Fig. 49–5). The drug is usually in a solution that is minimally irritating to human tissues, such as physiologic saline or sterile water, and may contain a preservative or a small amount of antibiotic to prevent bacterial growth in the **vial.** All injectable medications are dated. Before use, check the expiration date, and examine the solution for possible deterioration. A parenteral medication is administered with a sterile syringe and needle.

AMPULE An **ampule** is a small **hermetically sealed** glass flask, usually containing a single dose of medication. Ampules have a neck with a weak point that is broken just before use. To open an ampule:

1. Gently tap the top of the ampule with your fingers to settle all the medication to the bottom portion of the flask (Fig. 49–6).
2. Wipe the neck of the ampule clean with alcohol (Fig. 49–7).
3. It may be necessary to use a small file provided by the manufacturer to score an ampule at the breaking point to facilitate easier breaking.
4. Sharply tap the top so that the top breaks away from you.
5. If the top does not snap off easily, it may be necessary to bend it off. Hold each half of the ampule between your thumbs and fingers, in front of you and above waist level.
6. Snap your wrists toward your body to break the neck of the ampule in two (Fig. 49–8). You will hear a pop because the ampule is vacuum sealed. The glass is designed not to shatter, and the medication will not spill out. Without touching the sides, a syringe and needle unit is inserted into the ampule, and the medication is withdrawn into the syringe.

SINGLE-DOSE VIAL A single-dose vial is a small bottle with a rubber stopper through which you insert a sterile needle to withdraw the single dose of medication inside. Before a sterile syringe and needle unit can be introduced into the solution, the rubber stopper must be wiped in a circular motion with alcohol or another suitable disinfectant.

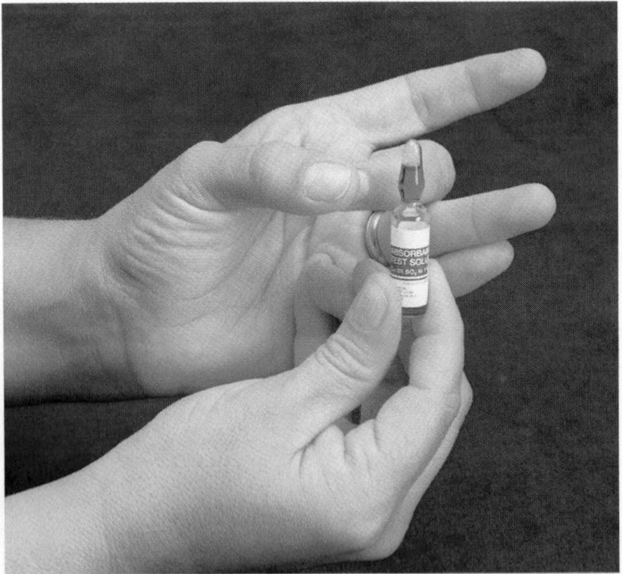

FIGURE 49–6 Glass ampule being tapped and showing the weak point at the neck, indicating the breaking point.

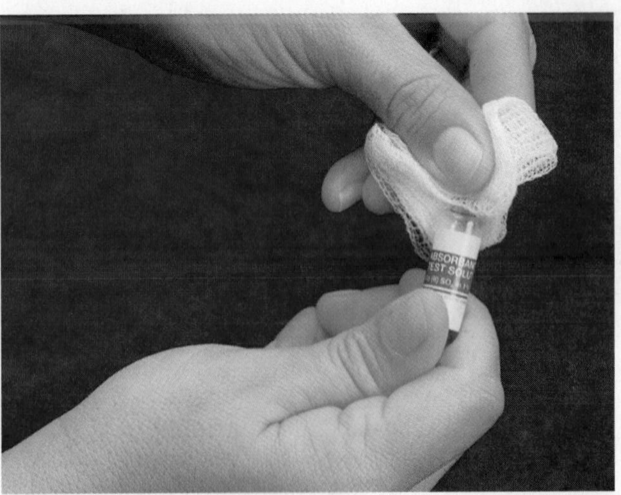

FIGURE 49–7 Wipe the neck of the ampule with alcohol prep.

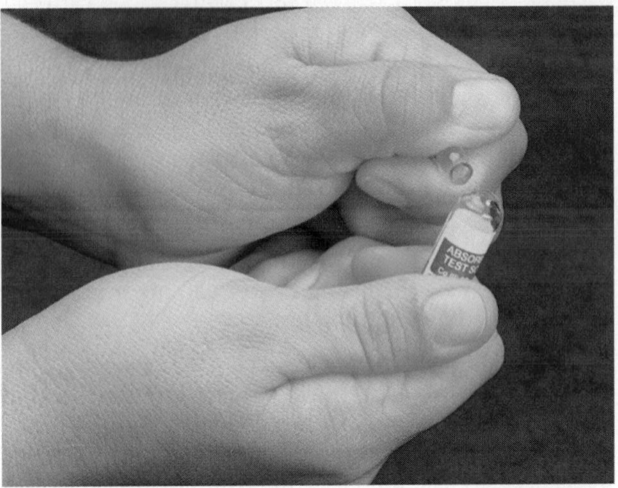

FIGURE 49–8 Snap off neck of vial.

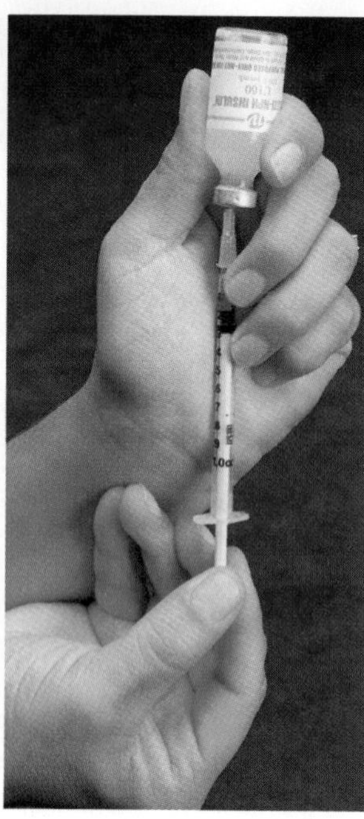

FIGURE 49–9 Filling a syringe from a multiple-dose vial. Keep the syringe at eye level.

MULTIDOSE VIAL A multidose vial is a bottle with a rubber stopper that contains enough medication for multiple injections (Fig. 49–9). A vial may contain 30 mL of a drug. If the usual dosage is 0.5 mL, the bottle contains enough medication for 60 injections. Vials vary greatly in size, from 2 mL to 100 or more doses. Because multidose vials are entered more than once, extreme caution must be taken every time a needle is inserted into the medication. Contamination could cause very serious infections in future patients. If at any time, you feel that an error has been made or you suspect possible contamination, discard the vial. Never return unused medication to the vial. Learn to withdraw fluids to the correct mark. If you have more medication than you need in the syringe, eject the excess after you remove the unit from the vial. However, remember, your employer will not tolerate excessive waste of drugs due to imprecise withdrawing of medications for injection.

Vials are vacuum sealed. Each time you withdraw medication from a vial, you must first replace the portion of withdrawn medication with the same portion of air. Not enough replaced air will make it difficult to withdraw the medication; too much replaced air will force the medication into the syringe without your pulling on the plunger to withdraw it.

PREFILLED SYRINGE A prefilled syringe is a sterile disposable syringe and needle unit packaged by the manufacturer with a single dose of medication inside and ready to administer.

CARTRIDGE INJECTION SYSTEM A cartridge injection system is a prefilled syringe and needle that is loaded into a metal or plastic (Fig. 49–10) cartridge for administration. The prefilled syringes are purchased by the box, and the same cartridge-loader is used over and over.

The technique for using a closed injector system (Fig. 49–11*A*) is described below.

METHOD OF LOADING

1. Hold the injector in a vertical position with the plunger rod in one hand.
2. Grasp the ribbed top section of the injector with the other hand and turn it clockwise until it stops. At this time the arrow on the assembly will be on the "OPEN" position (Fig. 49–11*B*).
3. Continue to hold the injector in the same position, open and pointing up, and insert the sterile medication cartridge with the needle attached into the open end (Fig. 49–11*C*).
4. Turn the ribbed top section of the injector counterclockwise until it is tight and the arrow points to the "CLOSE" position (Fig. 49–11*D*).
5. Engage the plunger rod into the threads of the cartridge plunger of the sterile medication cartridge (Fig. 49–11*E*).
6. Rotate the plunger clockwise until resistance is felt, which indicates that the system is now secure.

METHOD OF ADMINISTRATION

Follow the same steps as for an injection with a conventional syringe and needle assembly.

1. Select the site for the injection and prepare the site.
2. Remove the needle sheath by grasping it securely, then twist it and pull it free from the needle (Fig. 49–11*F*).
3. Insert the needle at the correct angle into the prepared injection site.

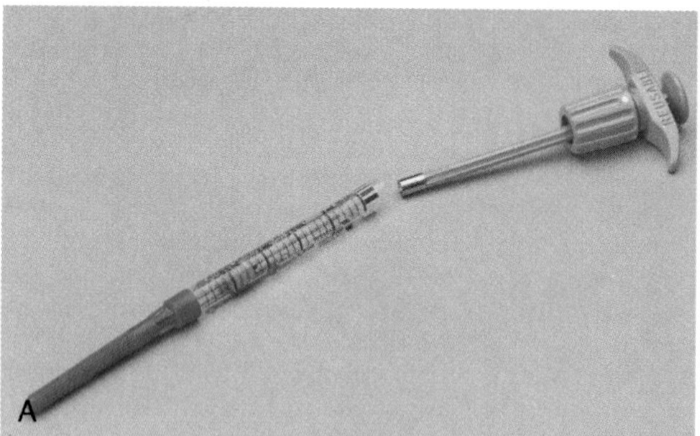

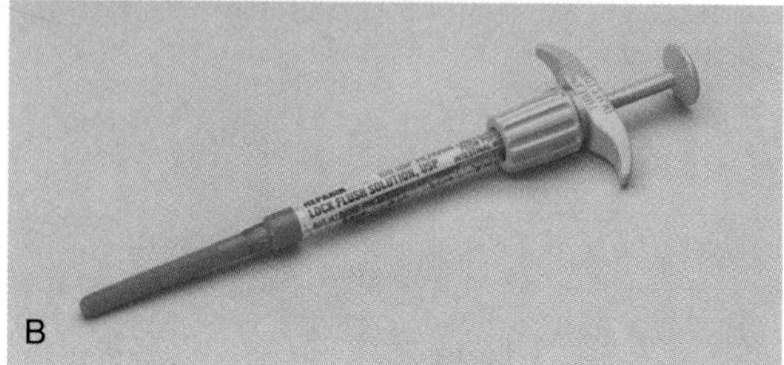

FIGURE 49–10 *A*, The parts of the closed injection system. *B*, Assembled closed injection system.

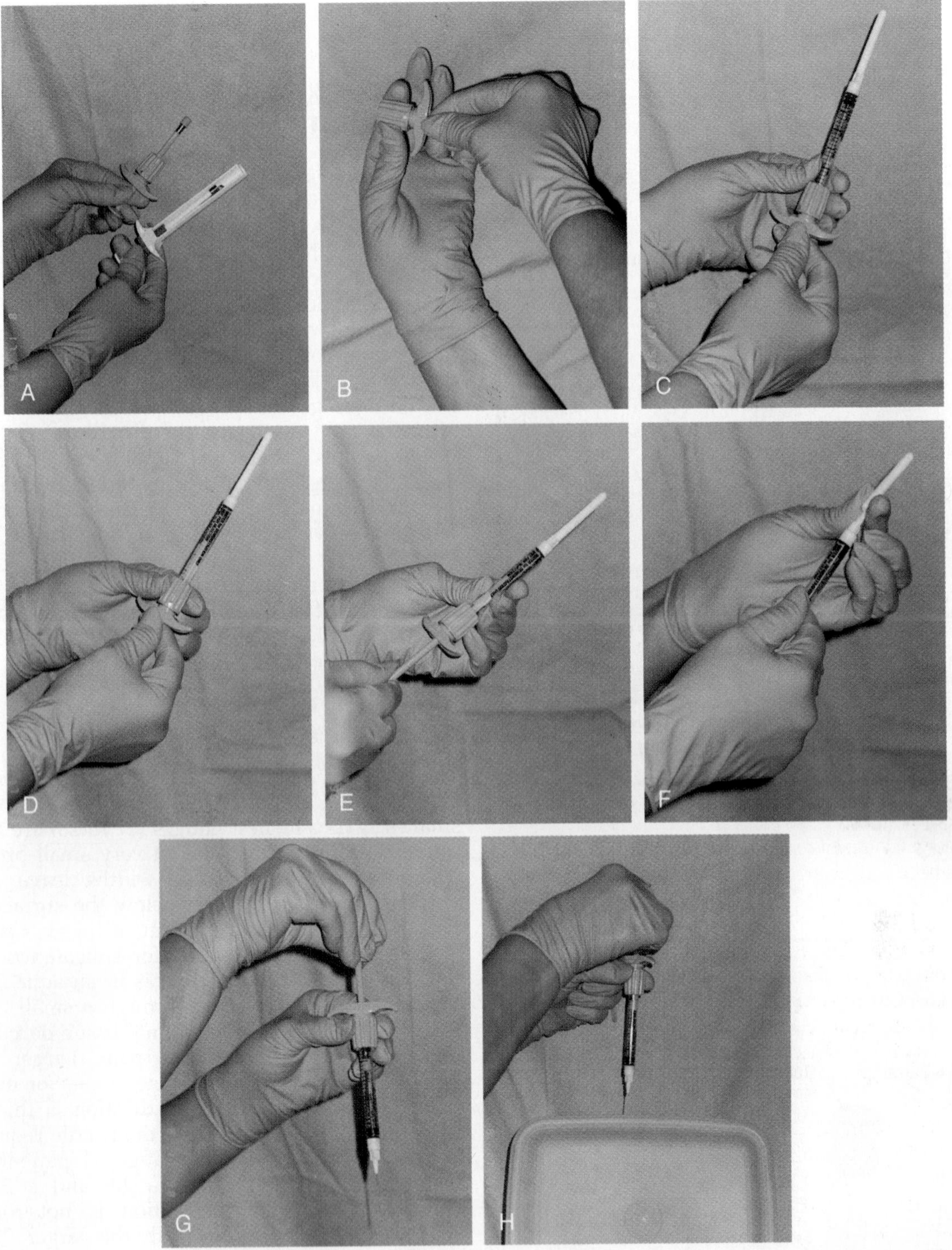

FIGURE 49–11 The closed injection system. See text for details.

4. Aspirate if necessary by gently pulling back on the plunger.
5. With a steady, even push on the plunger, inject the medication.
6. Remove the needle and perform any postinjection site care that is indicated.

DISMANTLING THE SYSTEM

1. Hold the system in the reverse vertical position, needle down, plunger rod up.
2. Twist the plunger rod counterclockwise until it is free from the plunger in the medication cartridge (Fig. 49–11*G*).
3. Place the injector system, needle down, over a biohazard sharps container and loosen the ribbed top section by turning it counterclockwise. The cartridge will fall into the sharps container when it is free from the injector (Fig. 49–11*H*).

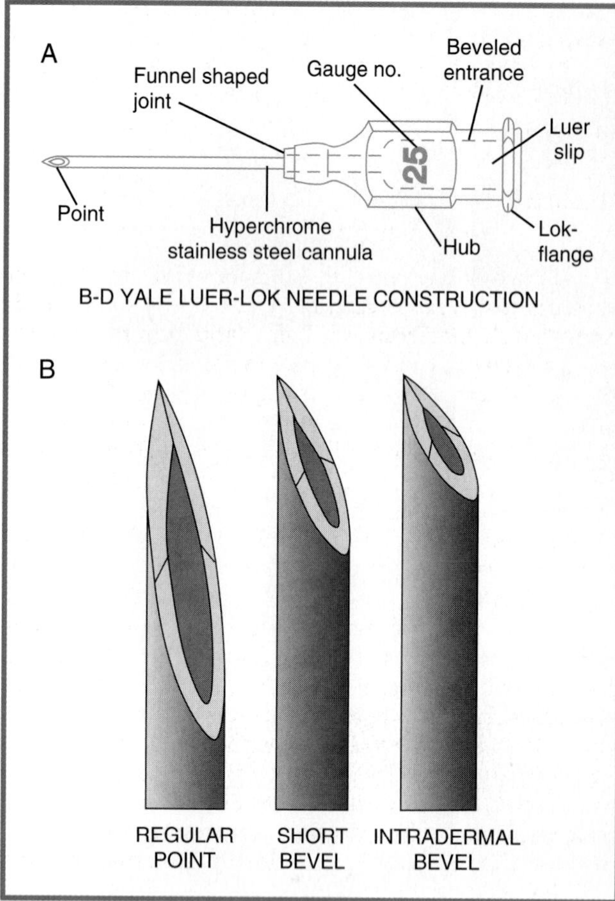

FIGURE 49–12 *A,* The construction of a hypodermic needle. *B,* Needle points.

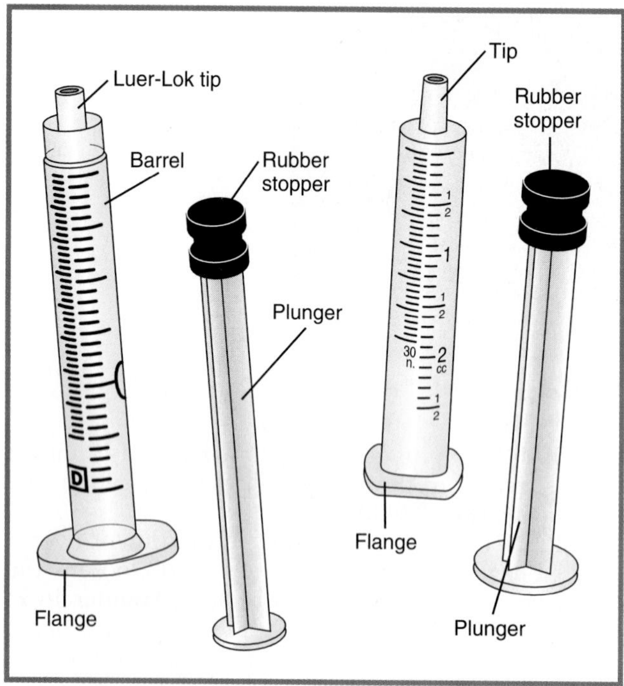

FIGURE 49–13 Parts of a syringe.

4. The injector system is reusable. DO NOT DISCARD.

PARENTERAL MEDICATION EQUIPMENT

Both syringes and needles are manufactured in countless varieties for specific purposes and, sometimes, for specific medications. For example, there is a special syringe for insulin. Also, there is a special syringe unit for diabetics to use for self-injecting.

Hypodermic needles are manufactured in many lengths and widths, depending on the depth needed and the **viscosity** of the medication to be injected. Needles may be purchased separately or as part of a needle–syringe unit. Figure 49–12 shows the construction of a needle and the three common types of needle points. There are some facts to remember about the construction of a hypodermic needle. The Becton Dickinson Company states the size of the needle is governed by four factors: safety, rate of flow, comfort of the patient, and depth of penetration. There are three standard dimensions: length, outside diameter of the cannula, and wall thickness. Regular needles are measured for length from where the cannula joins the hub to the tip of the (needle) point.

Needle Gauge

The width of a needle is called its *gauge,* and needle gauges range in size from 14 (the largest) to 28 (the smallest). The smallest gauges (27 to 28) are used for intradermal injections when a very small opening is desired. These fine needle widths leave a small amount of medication just below the surface of the skin, with a minimum amount of injury. Gauges 25 and 26 are commonly used for subcutaneous injections. With a medication that is in an aqueous solution and is easily injected through a small opening, these two gauges cause minimal tissue damage, and the patient experiences less pain. Larger needles (gauges 20 to 23) are usually necessary for intramuscular injections when the medication is thick, such as penicillin, or the length of the needle requires the extra support of a thicker gauge. A patient cannot feel the difference between a 20- and a 22-gauge needle. In fact, the medication is not forced as strongly into the tissues with the larger 20-gauge needle as with the 22-gauge one, and the patient actually experiences less pain. Needles larger than 20 gauge are not used for drug therapy. They are mostly used for venipuncture, blood donations, and blood transfusions.

Needle Length

The choices of needle lengths vary from ⅜ inch to 4 inches, depending on the area of the body to be injected and the route (depth) used. Intradermal injections require only the short ⅜-inch needle. Needles that are ½ or ⅝ inch long are used for subcuta-

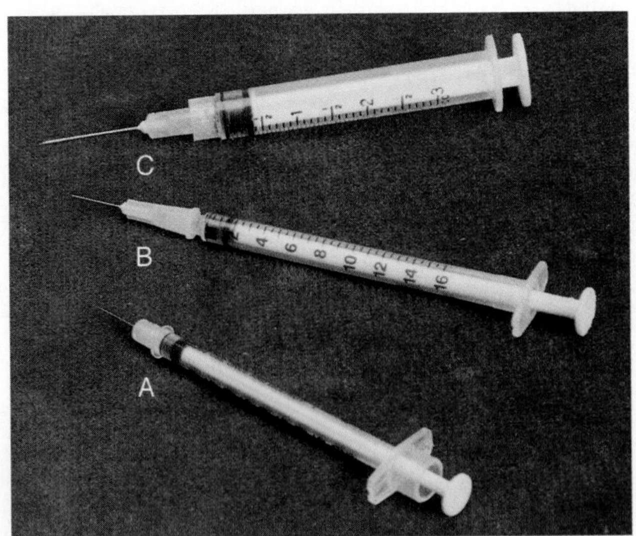

FIGURE 49–14 *A,* Insulin syringe. *B,* Tuberculin syringe. *C,* Regular (3-mL) syringe.

neous injections. Longer needles are necessary for depositing drugs intramuscularly. The choice of a 1-inch, 1½-inch, 2-inch, 2½-inch or 3-inch length depends on both the muscle being used and the size of the patient.

Syringes

Figure 49–13 illustrates the construction of a 3.0-mL and a 5.0-mL syringe. The parts of a syringe are its barrel, calibrated scale(s), plunger, and tip. *Regular* syringes that hold up to 3.0 mL are usually calibrated with two scales: mL (cc) and minims. Larger *regular* syringes are calibrated in milliliters only (Fig. 49–14*A*). The *tuberculin* syringe is used for small quantities of drug, because it holds only up to 1.0 mL of injectable material (see Fig. 49–14*B*). The *insulin* syringe is calibrated in units specifically for diabetic use (see Fig. 49–14*C*).

Most syringes and needles are disposable, the advantages being the prevention of cross-infection, equipment that has not been damaged by use, and freedom from the duties of autoclaving and sterilization. Disposable needles are coated with silicon and are extremely smooth and sharp. Disposable units are packaged in sealed, rigid plastic containers or in peel-apart paper wrappers. Both have an internal, rigid plastic sheath protecting the needle. Both individual needles and syringe–needle units are color coded for easy identification. Do not attempt to cut expenses by purchasing inferior or unknown brands of needles or syringes. Table 49–2 and Figure 49–15

TABLE 49–2 Needle and Syringe Sizes for Injections

Route	Gauge	Length	Syringe
Intradermal	27–28	⅜ in	Tuberculin
Subcutaneous	25–26	½, ⅝ in	2 mL; tuberculin; insulin
Intramuscular	20–23	1–3 in	2–5 mL

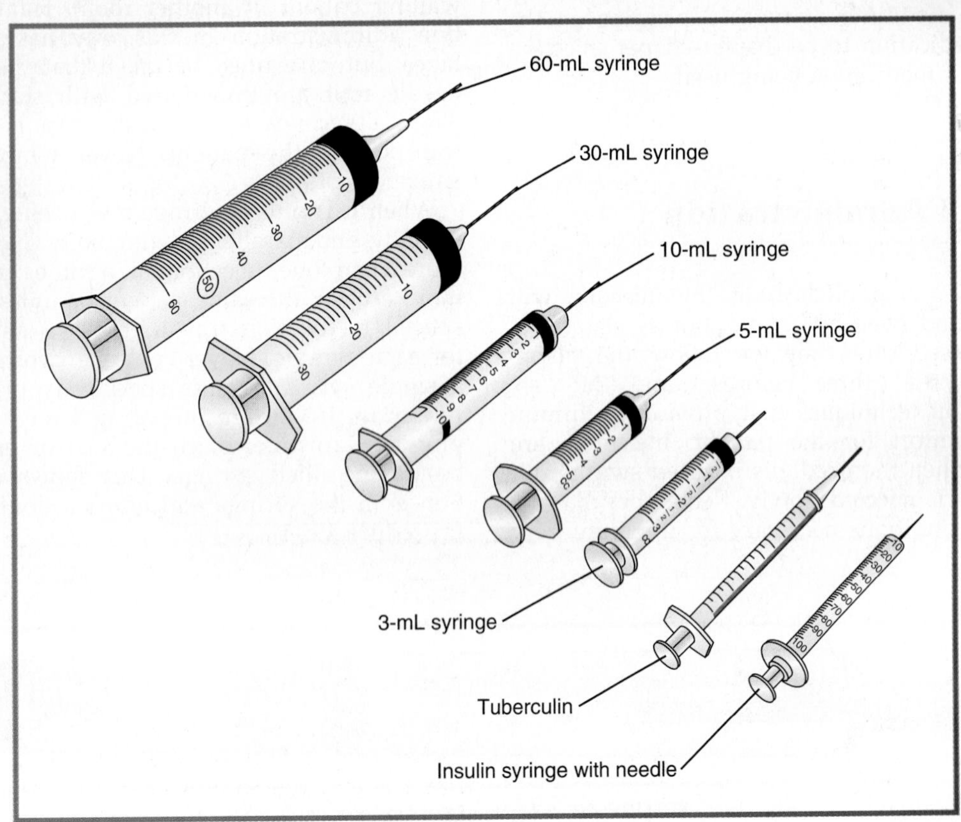

FIGURE 49–15 Various sizes of disposable syringes.

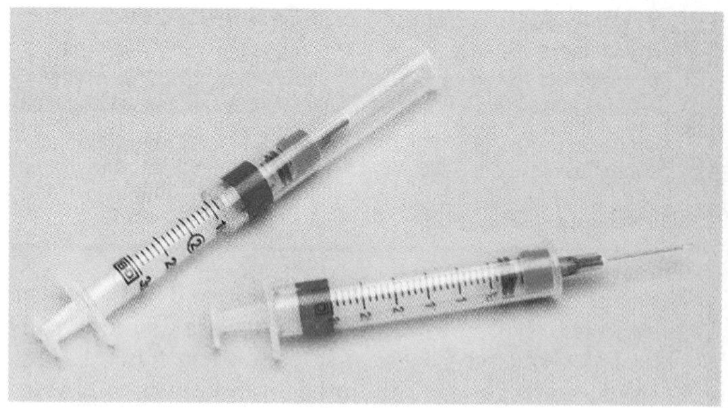

FIGURE 49–16 Disposable syringe with retractable needle cover.

summarize the needle and syringe sizes used for injections.

With the establishment of Standard Precautions and the danger of needle sticks, a syringe with a retractable needle cover has been developed (Fig. 49–16).

Needleless Syringes

Today with all of the concerns regarding needle sticks, proper disposing of needles, and cross-contamination of individuals through needle misuse, the public concerns have been to find a method of injecting medication without the use of a needle. One of the possible answers is the injector pen (Fig. 49–17). There are different types depending on the amount of medication to be dispensed per injection and the type of medication being used.

Parenteral Administration

With practice, giving medications by injection will become easy and even automatic, but as stated before and stressed often, always follow the physician's orders, the "three befores," and the "six rights." Develop techniques that provide maximum safety and comfort for the patient. Injections are least painful when the needle is inserted swiftly and the medication is injected slowly. Remember that the same aseptic conditions necessary for minor surgery are necessary whenever you penetrate the protective skin barrier.

Injections are not given near bones or blood vessels. Injections should never be given in an area where there is scar tissue, a change in skin pigmentation or texture, or excess tissue growth such as a mole or a wart. The point of injection should be as far as possible from any major nerve, and the site selected should be capable of holding the amount of medication that is injected. Never inject into an arm from which the lymph nodes have been removed (as after a **radical mastectomy**), because the medication cannot be absorbed into the bloodstream.

Make certain that all materials are ready for use. Many offices have a central room where medications are prepared. The medication is then taken to the waiting patient in another room. Handling medication administration in this way has many advantages, but care must be taken that the syringe and needle unit are transported with sterile technique. After a syringe is filled, the cap is replaced for transport to the patient. Never wrap a needle in gauze or cotton.

When carrying a syringe and needle, hold it horizontally and parallel to your body. Never transport more than one injection at a time, unless two or more are for the same patient or unless you have a special medication tray that has a named position for each syringe. Never combine two medications in a single syringe unless specifically ordered by the physician. If you are preparing a medication for the physician to give, place the vial or empty ampule beside the filled syringe. This shows what medication is in the syringe and offers a double check (see Procedure 49–1).

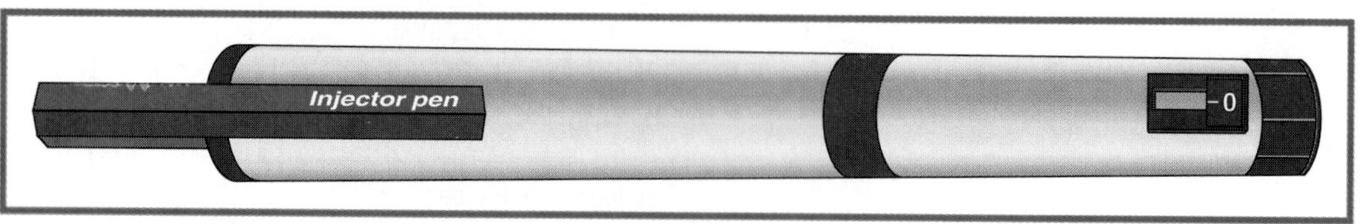

FIGURE 49–17 Needleless injector pen.

PROCEDURE 49-1
Filling a Syringe

GOAL
To fill a syringe with 1.5 mL of sterile water from a multipurpose vial, using sterile technique.

EQUIPMENT AND SUPPLIES
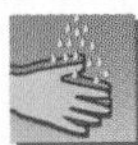

A vial or ampule containing the material to be injected
Antiseptic sponges
A sterile needle and syringe unit
A written order, including the drug name, strength, and route

PROCEDURAL STEPS
1 Read the order and choose a correct vial of medication.
PURPOSE: To check the medication the first of three times.

2 Choose the correct syringe and needle size, depending on the site and the quantity of medication to be injected (Figure 1).

3 Wash your hands.

4 Compare the order to both the name of the drug on the vial of medication and the amount to be withdrawn in the syringe.
PURPOSE: To check the medication the second of three times.

5 Gently agitate the medication by rolling the vial between your palms (Figure 2).
PURPOSE: To mix any medication that may have settled.

6 Check the quality of the medication and the expiration date.
PURPOSE: Medications may become contaminated or outdated.

Continued

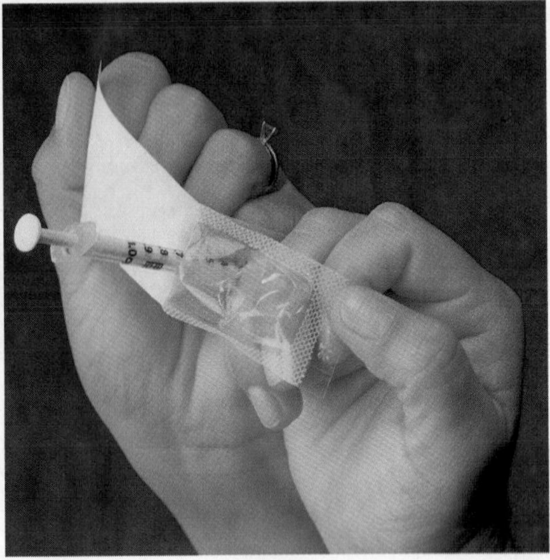

FIGURE 1

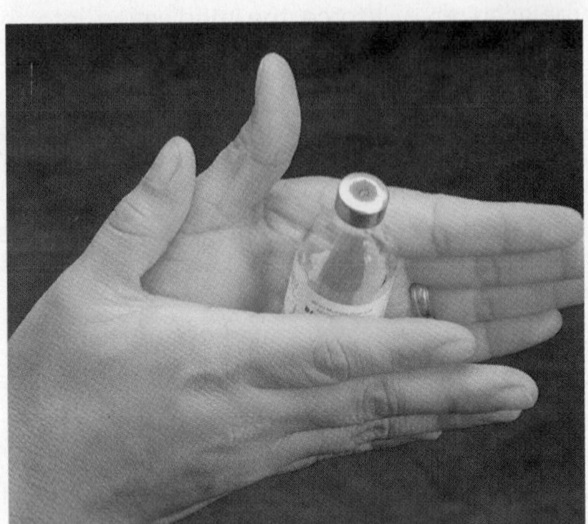

FIGURE 2

PROCEDURE 49–1 (CONTINUED)

Filling a Syringe

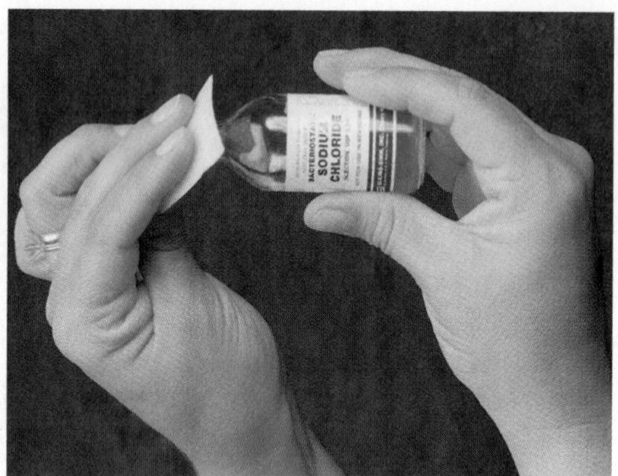

FIGURE 3

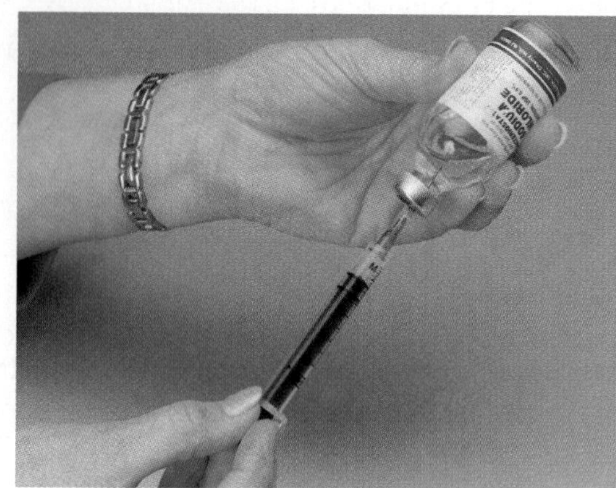

FIGURE 4

7 Cleanse the rubber stopper of the vial with the antiseptic sponge, using a circular motion (Figure 3).

8 Set down the vial. (You may hold the vial in the palm of your minor hand while you continue, if you do not contaminate the rubber stopper.)

9 Take the needle–syringe unit and remove the cap from the plastic protective case, or peel away the protective wrapper.

10 Remove the syringe.

11 Grasp the plunger and draw up an amount of air equal to the amount of medication ordered.
PURPOSE: Not enough replaced air will make it difficult to withdraw the medication; too much replaced air will force the medication into the syringe without your pulling on the plunger to withdraw it.

12 Grasp the plastic sheath covering the needle between two fingers on the posterior side of your minor hand, and pull the syringe out of the sheath with your major hand.
PURPOSE: To keep the sheath sterile for replacing it on the needle for transportation to the patient. The sheath may not be placed on a nonsterile surface or touched near its opening.

13 If you are not already holding the vial with the sheath in your minor hand, pick up the vial with the same hand that is holding the empty sheath, being careful not to touch the sheath to any nonsterile surface.

14 Turn the vial upside down without touching the rubber stopper.

15 Fully insert the needle into the center of the rubber stopper with your major hand.

16 Inject the air in the syringe into the vial.

17 Slowly pull back on the plunger until the proper amount of medication is withdrawn.
PURPOSE: Withdrawing medication rapidly will cause air bubbles to form in the syringe (Figure 4).

18 While the needle is still in the vial, check that there are no air bubbles in the syringe.
PURPOSE: Air bubbles displace medication, and the patient will not receive the proper amount of medication.

19 If there are air bubbles, slip the fingers holding the vial down to grasp the vial and syringe as a single unit.
PURPOSE: This frees your major hand.

Continued

20 With your free hand, tap the syringe until the air bubbles dislodge and float into the tip of the syringe.

21 Gently expel these tiny air bubbles through the needle, then continue withdrawing the medication.

22 Withdraw the needle from the vial, and replace the sheath over the needle without the needle touching the sides of the sheath.

23 Return the medication to the shelf or the refrigerator, checking that you have the correct drug and dosage.
PURPOSE: This is the third of the "three befores" of drug checking.

24 Clean the area.

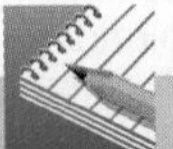

SKILLS AND RESPONSIBILITIES

INTERACTION WITH A PATIENT WHEN GIVING AN INJECTION

1 Use a professional approach and tell the patient what you are going to do.
2 Small talk can keep the patient's mind off the procedure.
3 Never tell a patient that it will not hurt; you may destroy your credibility.
4 Make the patient as comfortable as possible, and allow for privacy.
5 Never allow the patient to stand during the procedure.
6 Keep the equipment out of the patient's sight as much as possible.
7 Wear gloves and other blood and body-fluid protection barriers.

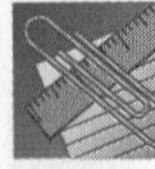

Project #3: Role-play the medical assistant and explain the reason for an injection.

DESTRUCTION OF USED SYRINGES AND NEEDLES

Follow guidelines in Chapter 26. After giving an injection, dispose of the syringe, needle, and gloves by placing them into a closed container immediately (Fig. 49–18). The cap should not be replaced on the needle, and the needle should not be cut or broken.

REUSABLE SYRINGES

Reusable syringes are not recommended; however, there are some medications that must be administered in glass syringes. If you must use reusable syringes, the Centers for Disease Control and Prevention requires that needles be discarded in a puncture-resistant rigid container immediately. Reusable glass syringes should be thoroughly rinsed in cold water after use and soaked in a 10% bleach solution or commercial recommended soak. Syringes should be wrapped and sterilized.

INTRAMUSCULAR INJECTIONS

Intramuscular injections are given into the muscle when (1) drugs will irritate the subcutaneous tissues, (2) a more rapid absorption is desired, or (3) the

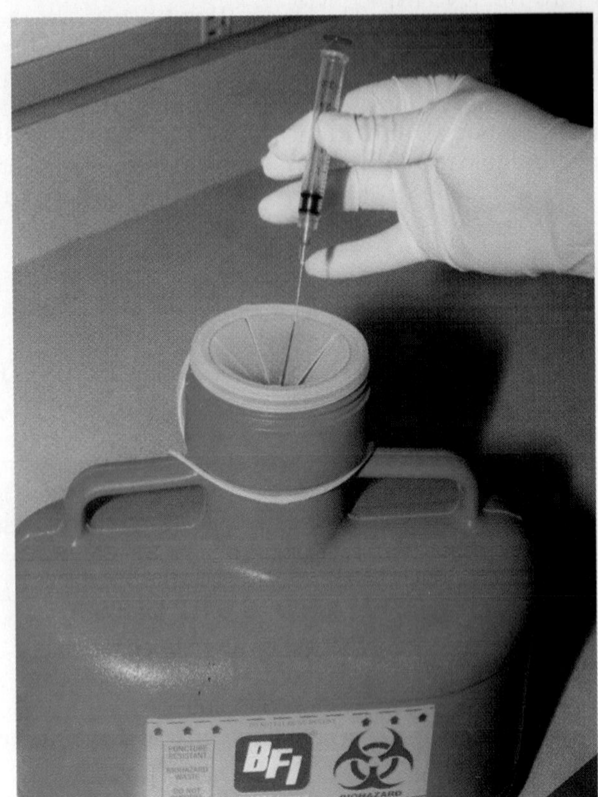

FIGURE 49–18 A rigid puncture-resistant, disposable container into which needle/syringe units are placed immediately after use.

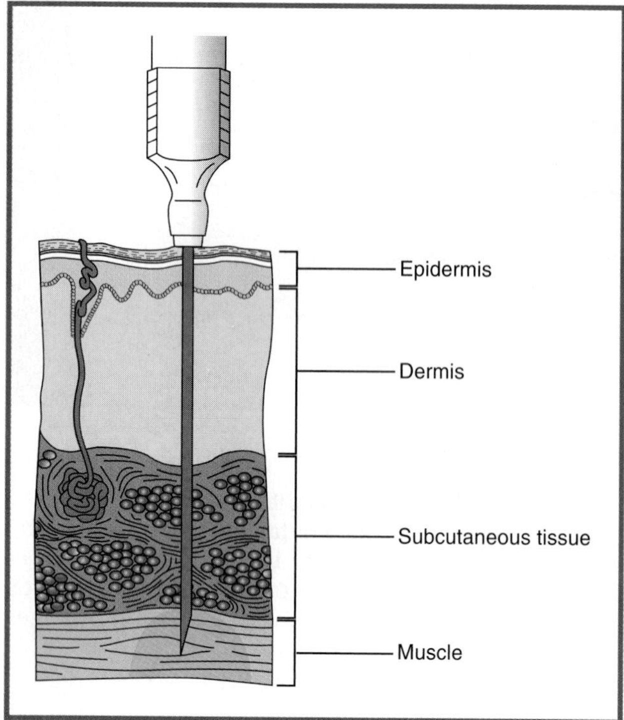

FIGURE 49–19 Anatomic illustration of the intramuscular injection. Note that the needle is inserted at a 90-degree angle and deposits the medication into the large central part of the muscle.

TABLE 49–3 Types of Injections

Method	Drug Amount	Sites	Examples
IM	Adult, 1–2 mL	Deltoid	Epinephrine (Adrenalin)
	Adult, 2–5 mL	Vastus lateralis	Penicillin
		Dorsogluteal, ventrogluteal	Meperidine (Demerol)
	Child, 1–2 mL	Vastus lateralis, ventrogluteal	Penicillin
IM, Z	As above	Dorsogluteal, ventrogluteal	Irritating drugs
SC	Adult, 0.1–2.0 mL	Deltoid	Insulin
		Thigh	Vaccines
		Abdomen	Toxoids
	Child, 0.5 mL	Deltoid	Vaccines
		Thigh, abdomen	Toxoids
ID	Adult and child, 0.1–0.5 mL	Forearm	Tuberculin test, skin tests

volume of the medication to be injected is large. The angle of insertion is 90 degrees (Fig. 49–19), and the preferred sites are the *gluteus medius, vastus lateralis, deltoid, and ventrogluteal muscles* of the adult (Fig. 49–20). It is believed that some intramuscular injections are not given with a long enough needle, and medications may, therefore, be deposited into the upper adipose (fatty) tissue by error. Fatty tissue does not absorb medications well, and the medication may remain at the site of the injection. Be certain to select needles that are long enough, especially for obese patients.

When locating a site for an intramuscular injection, expose the site so that you are able to visualize and palpate the landmarks correctly. Table 49–3 lists the sites as well as the criteria for choosing one site over another (see Procedure 49–2).

PROCEDURE 49-2

Giving an Intramuscular Injection

GOAL

To inject 2 mL of medication into the muscle, using a needle and syringe of the correct size, as directed by the physician.

EQUIPMENT AND SUPPLIES

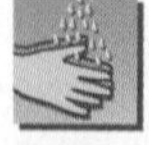

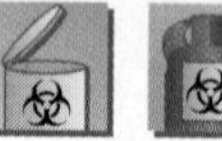

A vial or ampule containing the material to be injected
Antiseptic sponges
A sterile needle and syringe unit
A written order, including the patient's name, when to give the drug, the route of administration, and the name and strength of the drug

Continued

PROCEDURAL STEPS

1 Wash your hands. Follow Standard Precautions. Glove yourself with nonsterile gloves.

2 Select the correct medication from the shelf or the refrigerator.
PURPOSE: Some medications must be refrigerated.

3 Read the label to be sure that you have the right drug and the right strength.
PURPOSE: One medication may be manufactured and prepackaged in different strengths; for instance, a particular drug may be available in vials of both 250 mg/mL and 500 mg/mL.

4 Warm refrigerated medications by gently rolling between your palms.

Continued

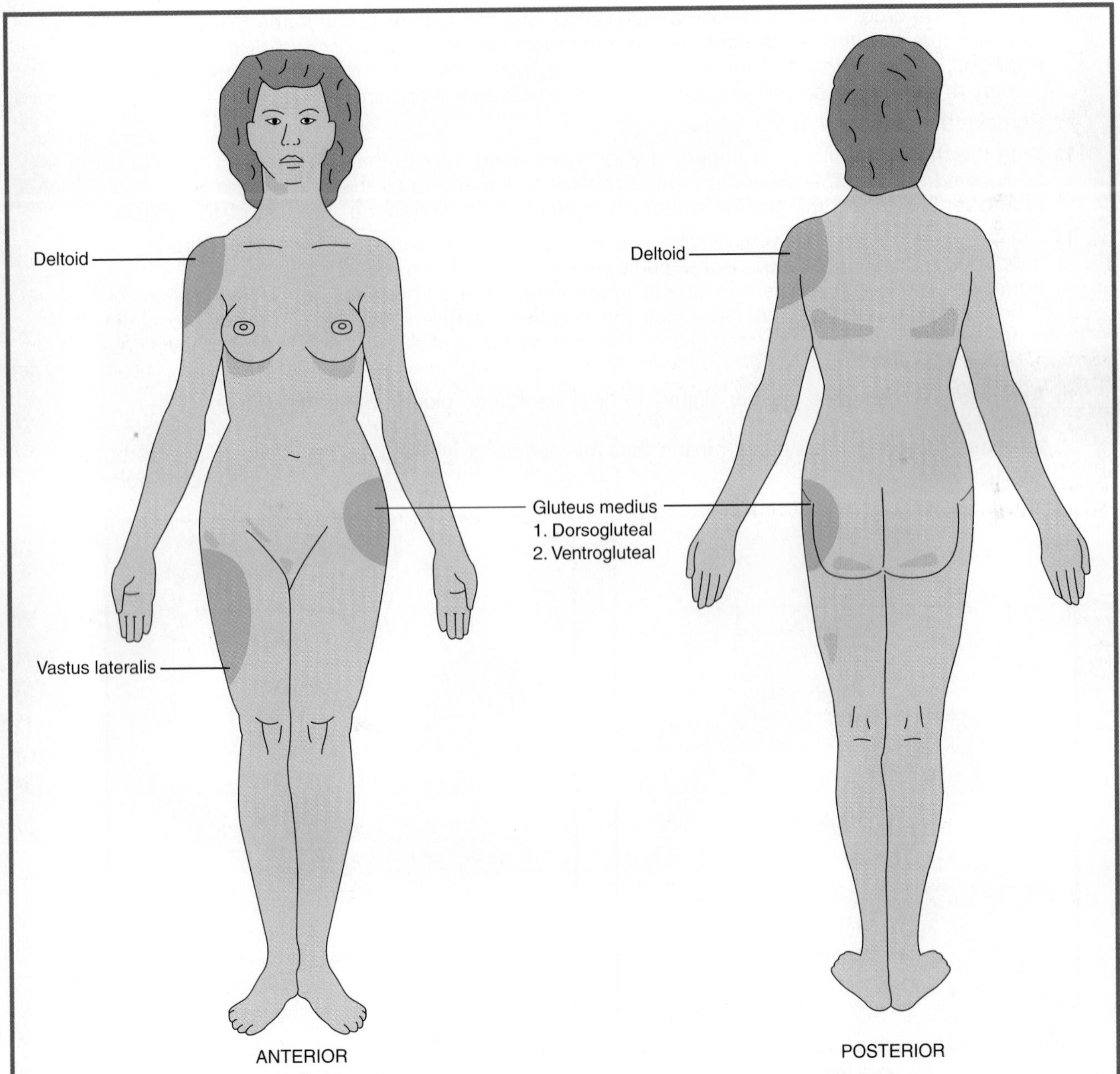

FIGURE 49–20 The muscles commonly used for intramuscular injection.

PROCEDURE 49-2 (CONTINUED)

Giving an Intramuscular Injection

5 Prepare the syringe, calculating the right dose.

6 Transport the medication to the patient.

7 Greet and identify the patient by name.
PURPOSE: To be sure that you have the right patient.

8 Position the patient comfortably.

9 Expose the site.

10 Cleanse the patient's skin with the antiseptic sponge, using a circular motion, moving outward from the center (Figure 1).

11 Compare the order with the prepared medication, and the patient to the name on the order, to make sure that this is the right time to administer the drug.
PURPOSE: This is the last of the six checks to be made before administering a medication. If there is any doubt, do not proceed. Check first with the physician.

12 Remove the sheath from the needle.

13 With the thumb and first two fingers of your minor hand, spread the skin tightly at the site to be injected or pinch a large portion of the muscle at the site to be injected (Figure 2).
PURPOSE: Smoothing the skin by stretching or pinching facilitates the insertion of the needle.

14 Grasp the syringe as you would a dart, and with one swift movement, insert the entire needle up to the hub, at a 90-degree angle into the muscle (Figure 3).
PURPOSE: The depth of the injection is determined by the choice of needle length, not by how far you insert the needle. Once the needle is at the tissue layer, do not move the needle while injecting the medication. Being in as far as the hub helps to keep the needle in one place.

15 **Aspirate:** Withdraw the plunger slightly to be sure that no blood enters the syringe (Figure 4).
PURPOSE: Blood in the syringe means that the needle is in a blood vessel and is not in the

Continued

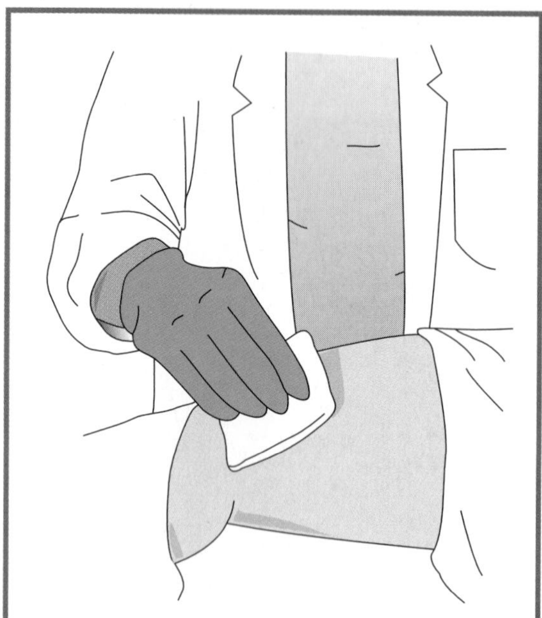

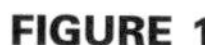

FIGURE 1

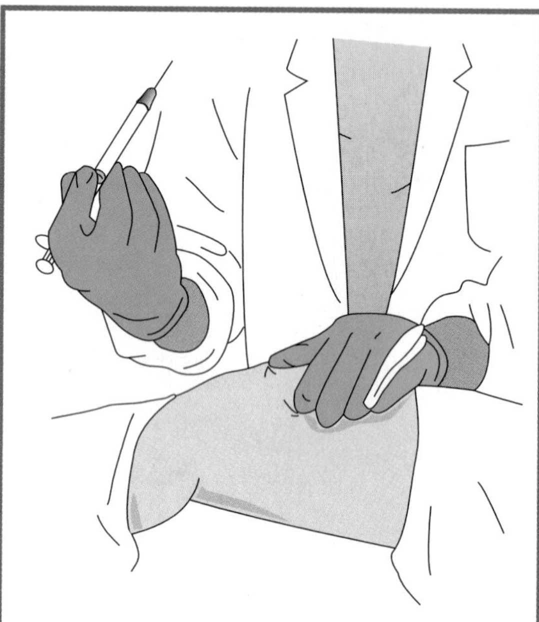

FIGURE 2

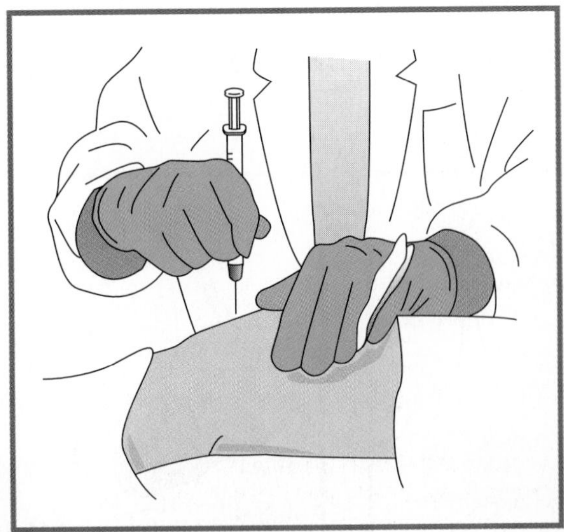

FIGURE 3

muscle tissue. You may *not* administer an intramuscular medication by the intravenous route.

16 If blood appears, immediately withdraw the syringe, and compress the injection site with the sponge.

17 Begin again with step 1.
PURPOSE: Blood is now mixed with the medication, and the medication is considered contaminated. Blood may interact with the drug and may be irritating to the intramuscular tissues.

18 If no blood appears in the syringe, push in the plunger slowly and steadily until all medication has been administered (Figure 5).
PURPOSE: A rapid injection may tear the muscle tissue.

Continued

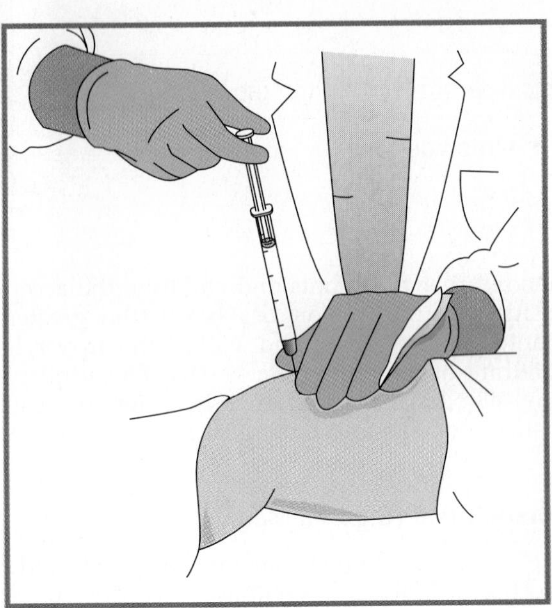

FIGURE 4

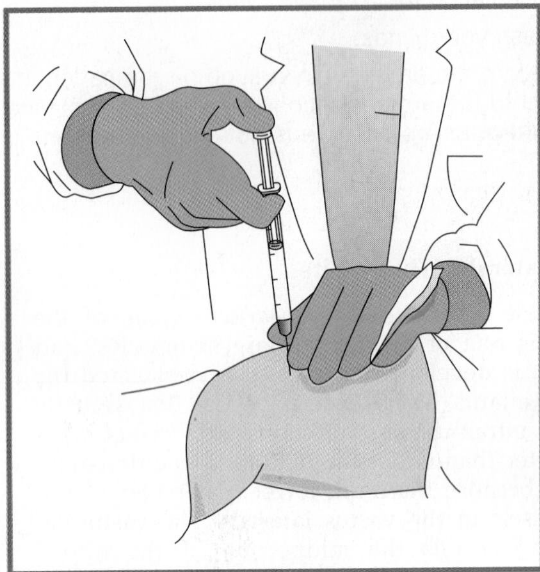

FIGURE 5

PROCEDURE 49-2 (CONTINUED)

Giving an Intramuscular Injection

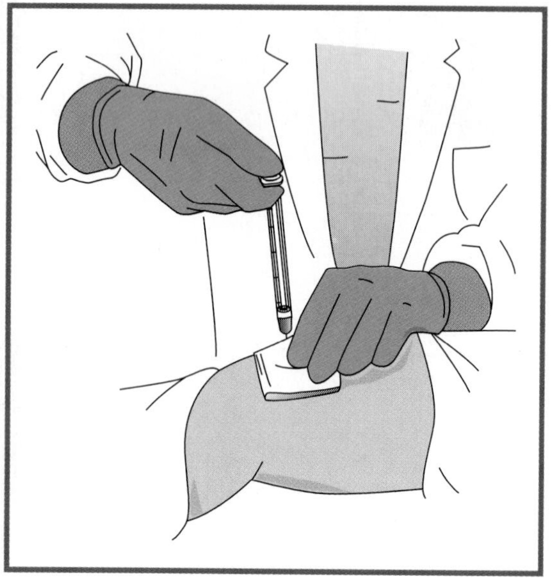

FIGURE 6

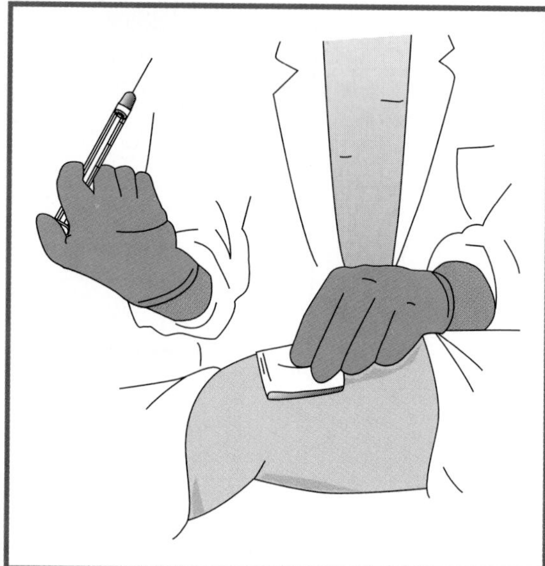

FIGURE 7

19 Cover the area with the sponge, and withdraw the needle at the same angle of insertion (Figure 6).

20 Gently massage the site with the antiseptic sponge.
PURPOSE: Massage helps to increase absorption and to decrease pain (Figure 7).

21 Make sure that your patient is comfortable and safe.

22 Dispose of the needle and syringe.

23 Observe the patient for any adverse reaction. You may need to keep the patient under observation for 20 to 30 minutes.

24 Wash your hands.

25 Record the drug administration on the patient's medical record, and on the required DEA record if the medication is a controlled substance.
PURPOSE: A procedure is not considered done until it is recorded.

Vastus Lateralis (Thigh) Site

This muscle is part of the *quadriceps group* of the thigh. It is one of the body's largest muscles, and because it is developed at birth, it is considered the safest for infants. Many experts believe that as a site for adult intramuscular injections, the vastus lateralis is better than either the deltoid or the dorsogluteal sites because there are fewer major nerves and blood vessels in the vastus lateralis. The vastus lateralis muscle fills the midportion of the upper, outer thigh. In the adult, it can be located from one hand's width below the proximal end of the *greater trochanter* to one hand's width above the top of the *patella* (knee cap). Wyeth Laboratories has recommended that for infants and children, the acceptable position of this region lies below the greater trochanter of the femur and within the upper lateral quadrant of the thigh (Fig. 49–21). The adult patient may sit or lie supine, but it is easier to locate the vastus lateralis with the patient lying down.

Dorsogluteal (Gluteus Medius) Site

This is the traditional site for deep intramuscular injections. However, complications due to sciatic nerve injury are frequent enough that experts are suggesting that this site be abandoned and replaced with the vastus lateralis and ventrogluteal sites. The

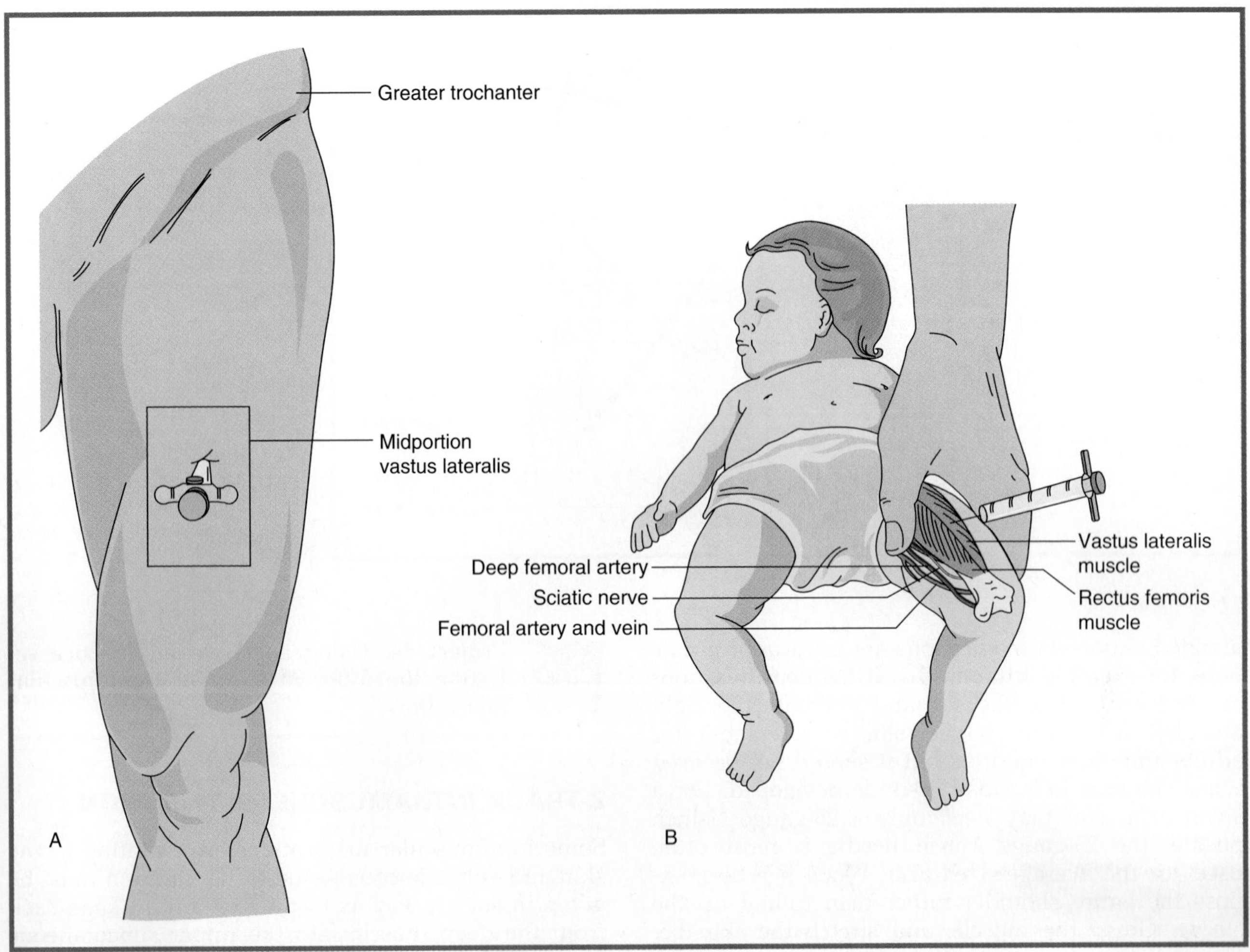

FIGURE 49–21 The vastus lateralis muscle is the preferred site for intramuscular injections in infants and children. *A,* Site selection for adults. *B,* Site selection for infants and children.

dorsogluteal site continues to be popular, and it is still acceptable for adults if care is taken to locate the exact site. It is recommended that this site *not* be used for infants. The patient must lie in the prone position. To relax the muscles, the toes should be pointing inward. To locate the site, draw an imaginary diagonal line starting at the *greater trochanter* of the femur, across the buttocks, to the posterior spine of the ilium. Palpate these bony prominences to make certain that you are at the correct site. The injection is made into the gluteus medius muscle several inches below the iliac crest (Fig. 49–22).

Ventrogluteal (Gluteus Medius) Site

Although considered safe, this site is not used as frequently as the others. This technique uses a larger mass of the gluteus medius muscle than when using the dorsogluteal site. The area is free of major nerves and blood vessels, and it is considered safe for both infants and adults (Fig. 49–23). All types of intramuscular medications can be injected here, including the thick oily preparations. To locate the site, place your right palm on the patient's greater trochanter, then put your index finger on the anterior iliac spine, and spread your middle finger back as far as possible from your index finger, trying to touch the crest of the ilium. The center of the triangle formed by your index and middle fingers is the site for the injection. Choose the hand that is the opposite of the patient's side, that is, use your left hand to palpate the patient's right ventrogluteal site and your right hand to palpate the patient's left side. For a child, you will need a 1-inch needle, whereas in an obese adult patient, you may need a 2½-inch needle to reach the depth of the muscle.

Deltoid Site

The deltoid muscle, the muscular cap of the shoulder, is located at the top of the upper, outer arm. The muscle mass is somewhat limited, so it cannot hold a large volume of medication. This triangular muscle is located between the acromion and deltoid tuberosities and fills an area approximately two fingerbreadths below the acromion process (Fig. 49–24). The major nerves and blood vessels located in the posterior portion of the arm must be

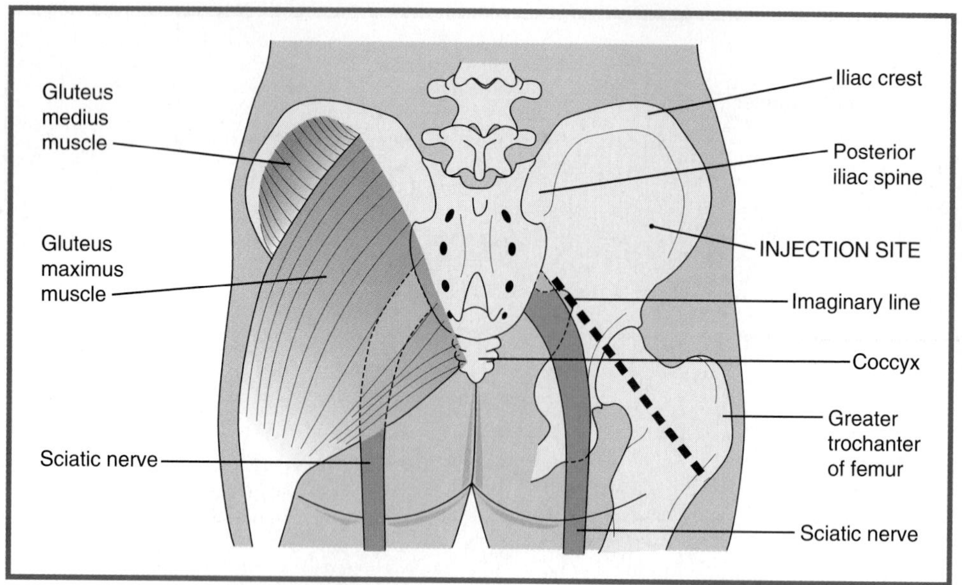

FIGURE 49–22 The dorsogluteal (gluteus medius) site is still preferred by many physicians.

avoided. Aqueous medications are most appropriate here, for example, vitamin B_{12}. If frequent injections are ordered, rotate the site and alternate the right and left arm. The deltoid site is acceptable for adults and older children, but it should not be used when the muscle is small or underdeveloped. For a small arm, you may need only a 25-gauge ⅝-inch needle; the 23-gauge 1-inch needle is most often used for the average-sized arm. When injecting, expose the entire shoulder rather than rolling up the sleeve. Grasp the muscle, and stretch the skin before injecting the medication. The patient may be seated or lying down.

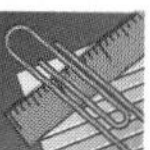

Project #4: Using a classmate, practice selecting the different sites for intramuscular injections.

Z-TRACK INTRAMUSCULAR INJECTION

Some intramuscular medications are irritating to the skin and subcutaneous tissues. The injection must be given in such a way as to prevent any leakage back from the deep muscle into the upper subcutaneous layers. The Z-track method displaces the upper tissue laterally before the needle is inserted (Fig. 49–25).

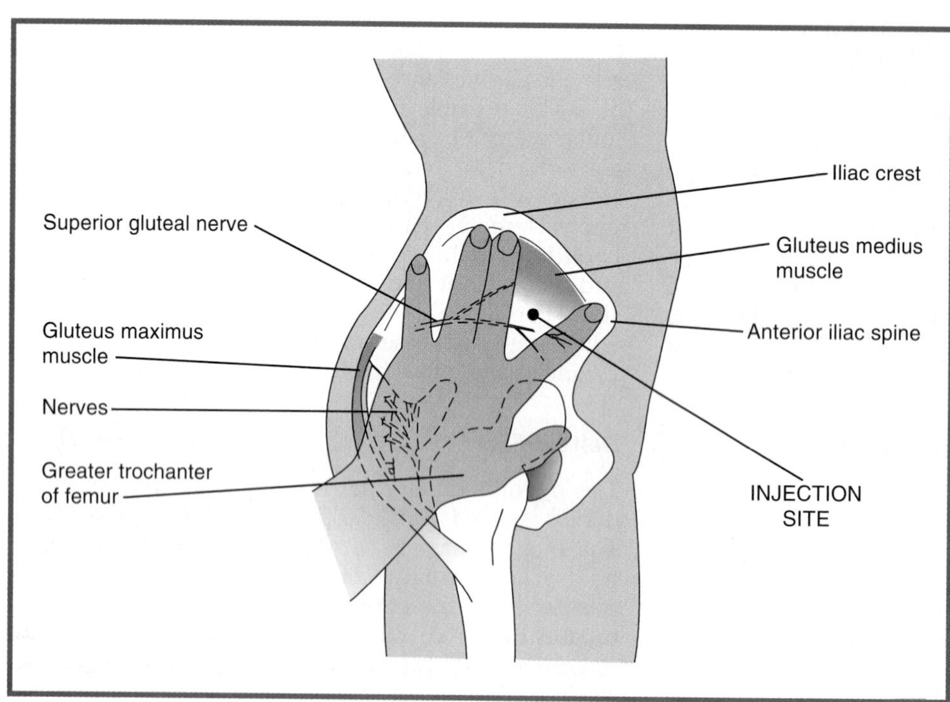

FIGURE 49–23 The ventrogluteal site can be used for most intramuscular injections.

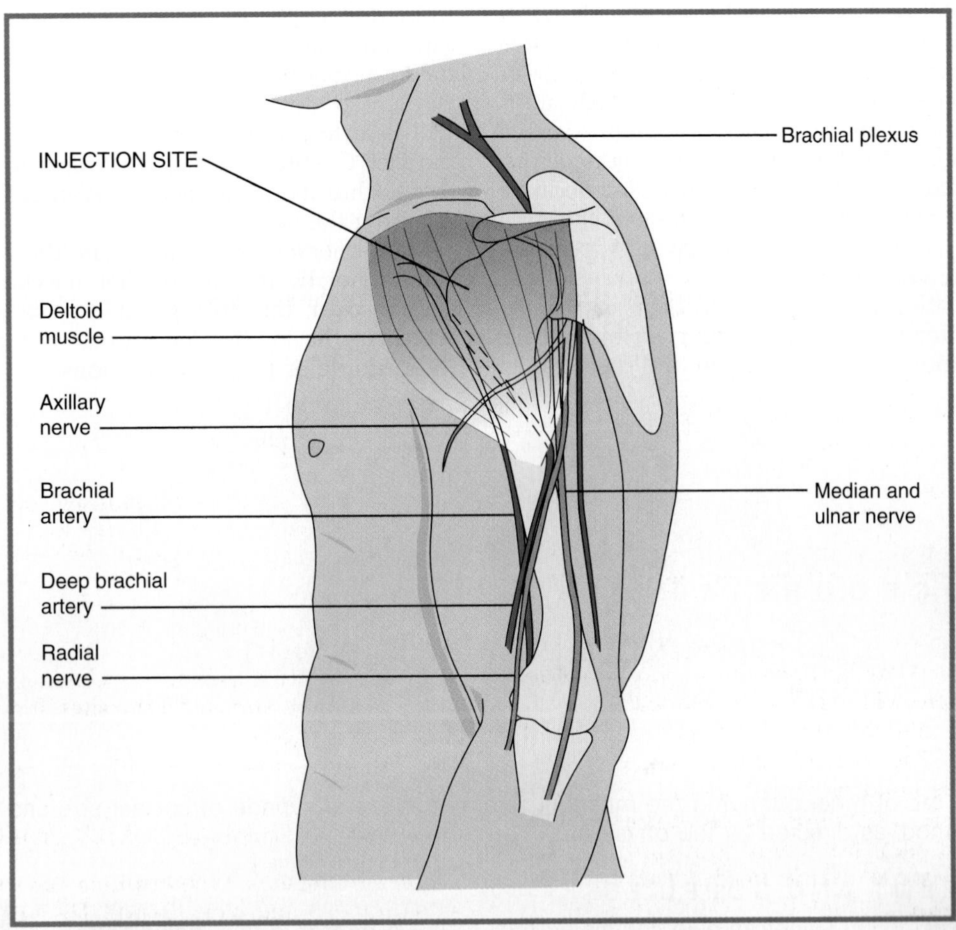

FIGURE 49–24 The deltoid muscle site is used for both intramuscular and subcutaneous injections. It is not recommended for infants because the muscle is not developed until later in childhood.

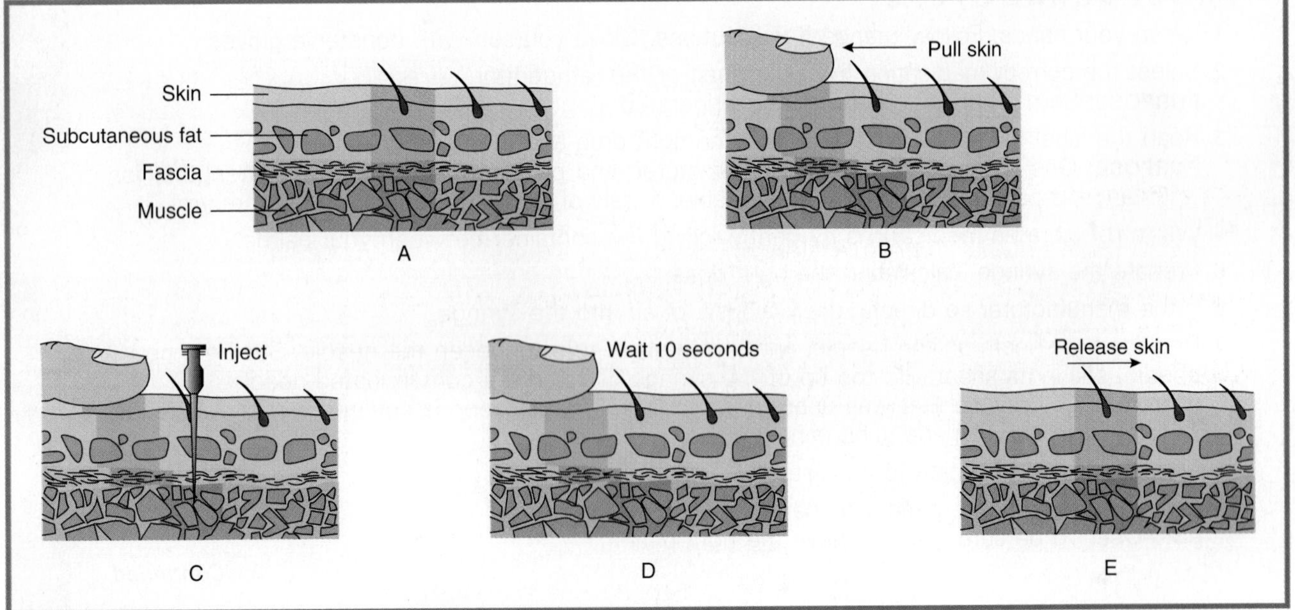

FIGURE 49–25 The Z-track method of intramuscular injection is used when medications are irritating to subcutaneous tissues. This technique helps prevent the medication from leaking into the subcutaneous tissues.

The skin is pulled to one side before the tissue is grasped for the injection (see Procedure 49–3). After the needle is withdrawn, the tissue is released, with the needle track to one side of where the medication is deposited in the muscle. The medication cannot leak out. These medications are always injected into the gluteus medius muscle of the buttocks. Because the medication is so irritating to the tissues, the needle should be changed after withdrawing the medication from the vial.

Some medications require the injection of 0.5 mL of air after an injection. This air will clear the needle of the medication and will prevent the medication from flowing back along the track of the injection. This air can be pulled into the syringe after the medication has been drawn in. Because the syringe is pointed downward during the injection, the air will float to the other end of the syringe and will be the last to enter the tissue. Wait a few seconds before withdrawing the needle. Wait 10 seconds before releasing the skin.

Many medications that require the Z-track method should not be massaged after injection; just hold a sponge over the area for a few seconds. Walking will help the medication absorb. Use alternate sides for multiple or frequent injections.

PROCEDURE 49-3

Giving a Z-Track Intramuscular Injection

GOAL

To inject 1 mL of medication into the muscle using a needle and syringe of correct size and the Z-track method, as directed by the physician.

EQUIPMENT AND SUPPLIES

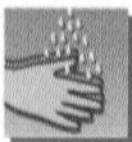

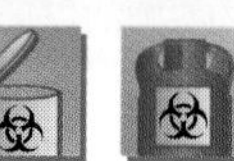

A vial or ampule containing the material to be injected
Antiseptic sponges
A sterile needle and syringe unit
A written order, including the patient's name, when to give the drug, the route of administration, and the name and strength of the drug

PROCEDURAL STEPS

1 Wash your hands. Follow Standard Precautions. Glove yourself with nonsterile gloves.

2 Select the correct medication from the shelf or the refrigerator.
PURPOSE: Some medications must be refrigerated.

3 Read the label to be sure that you have the right drug and the right strength.
PURPOSE: One medication may be manufactured and prepackaged in different strengths; for instance, a particular drug may be available in vials of both 250 mg/mL and 500 mg/mL.

4 Warm refrigerated medications by gently rolling the container between your palms.

5 Prepare the syringe, calculating the right dose.

6 If the manufacturer so directs, draw 0.5 mL of air into the syringe.

7 Replace the sheath on the needle, and give a slight turn to loosen the needle. Secure a new needle, still in its sheath, to the tip of the syringe. Discard the contaminated needle.
PURPOSE: The needle that was used to withdraw the medication is covered with a substance irritating to the skin and subcutaneous tissues.

8 Transport the medication to the patient.

9 Greet and identify the patient by name.
PURPOSE: To be sure that you have the right patient.

Continued

10 Position the patient comfortably.

11 Expose the site.

12 Cleanse the patient's skin with the antiseptic sponge, using a circular motion, moving outward from the center.

13 Compare the order with the prepared medication, and the patient with the name on the order, to make sure that this is the right time to administer the drug.
PURPOSE: This is the last of the six checks to be made before administering a medication. If there is any doubt, do not proceed. Check first with the physician.

14 Remove the sheath from the needle.

15 Pull the skin to one side and hold it firmly in place. If the skin is slippery, use a dry gauze sponge to hold the skin in place.
PURPOSE: Displacing the skin prevents irritating medications from leaking back to the surface.

16 Grasp the syringe as you would a dart, and with one swift movement, insert the entire needle up to the hub, at a 90-degree angle into the muscle.
PURPOSE: The depth of the injection is determined by the choice of needle length, not by how far you insert the needle. Once the needle is at the tissue layer, do not move the needle while injecting the medication. Being in as far as the hub helps to keep the needle in one place.

17 Aspirate: Withdraw the plunger slightly to be sure that no blood enters the syringe.
PURPOSE: Blood in the syringe means that the needle is in a blood vessel and not in the muscle tissue. You may *not* administer an intramuscular medication by the intravenous route.

18 If blood appears, immediately withdraw the syringe, and compress the injection site with the sponge.
PURPOSE: To minimize bleeding and bruising.

19 Begin again with step 1.
PURPOSE: Blood is now mixed with the medication, and the medication is considered contaminated. Blood may interact with the drug and may be irritating to the intramuscular tissues.

20 If no blood appears in the syringe, push in the plunger slowly and steadily until all medication has been administered.
PURPOSE: A rapid injection may tear the muscle tissue.

21 Wait a few seconds, then cover the area with the sponge, and withdraw the needle at the same angle of insertion. Wait 10 seconds, then release the skin.

22 If the manufacturer recommends it, gently massage the site with the antiseptic sponge.
PURPOSE: Massage helps to increase absorption and to decrease pain.

23 Make sure your patient is comfortable and safe.

24 Dispose of the needle and syringe.

25 Observe the patient for any adverse reaction. You may need to keep the patient under observation for 20 to 30 minutes.

26 Wash your hands.

27 Record the drug administration on the patient's medical record, and on the required DEA record if the medication is a controlled substance.
PURPOSE: A procedure is not considered done until it is recorded.

SUBCUTANEOUS INJECTIONS

Subcutaneous injections are given just under the skin, into the fatty areolar layer called *adipose tissue* (Fig. 49–26; see Procedure 49–4). Smaller doses of less irritating drugs are given by this method. The angle of insertion is 45 degrees; however, heparin and insulin are usually administered at a 90-degree angle. The deltoid area is an injection site; however, the abdomen, thigh, and upper back may be used (Fig. 49–27). When multiple or frequent injections are ordered, the sites must be rotated. It is best to keep a rotation record.

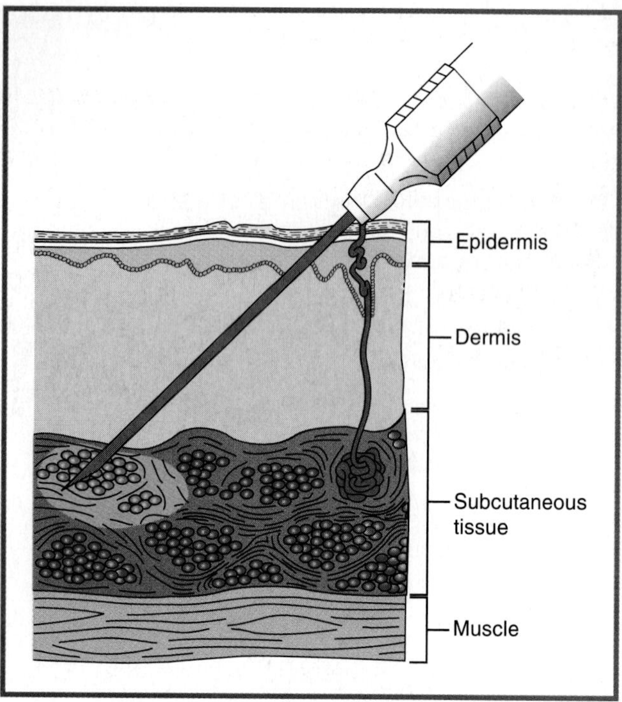

FIGURE 49–26 The subcutaneous injection is administered with a needle smaller and shorter than that used for the intramuscular injection. This method is used for small amounts of nonirritating medications in aqueous solution. It is injected at a 45-degree angle (at a 90-degree angle for insulin and heparin). The most common site is the deltoid region of the upper arm.

PROCEDURE 49–4

Giving a Subcutaneous Injection

GOAL

To inject 0.5 mL of medication into the subcutaneous tissue using a needle and syringe of correct size, as directed by the physician.

EQUIPMENT AND SUPPLIES

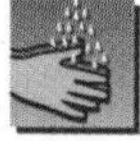
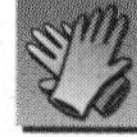
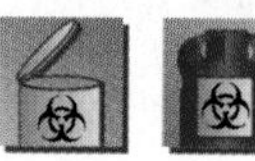

A vial or ampule containing the material to be injected
Antiseptic sponges
A sterile needle and syringe unit
A written order, including the patient's name, when to give the drug, the route of administration, and the name and strength of the drug

PROCEDURAL STEPS

1. Wash your hands. Follow Standard Precautions. Glove yourself with nonsterile gloves.
2. Select the correct medication from the shelf or the refrigerator.
   PURPOSE: Some medications must be refrigerated or stored under special conditions.
3. Read the label to be sure that you have the right drug and the right strength. Perform any necessary dose calculations.
   PURPOSE: One medication may be manufactured and prepackaged in different strengths. For instance, a particular drug may be available in vials of both 250 mg/mL and 500 mg/mL.
4. Warm refrigerated medications by gently rolling the container between your palms.
5. Prepare the syringe, withdrawing the right dose.
6. Transport the medication to the patient.

Continued

7 Greet and identify the patient by name.
PURPOSE: To be sure that you have the right patient.

8 Position the patient comfortably.

9 Expose the site.

10 Cleanse the patient's skin with the antiseptic sponge, using a circular motion, moving outward from the center.

11 Compare the order with the prepared medication, and the patient with the name on the order, to be sure that this is the right time to administer the drug.
PURPOSE: This is the last of the six checks to be made before administering a medication. If there is any doubt, do not proceed. Check first with the physician.

Continued

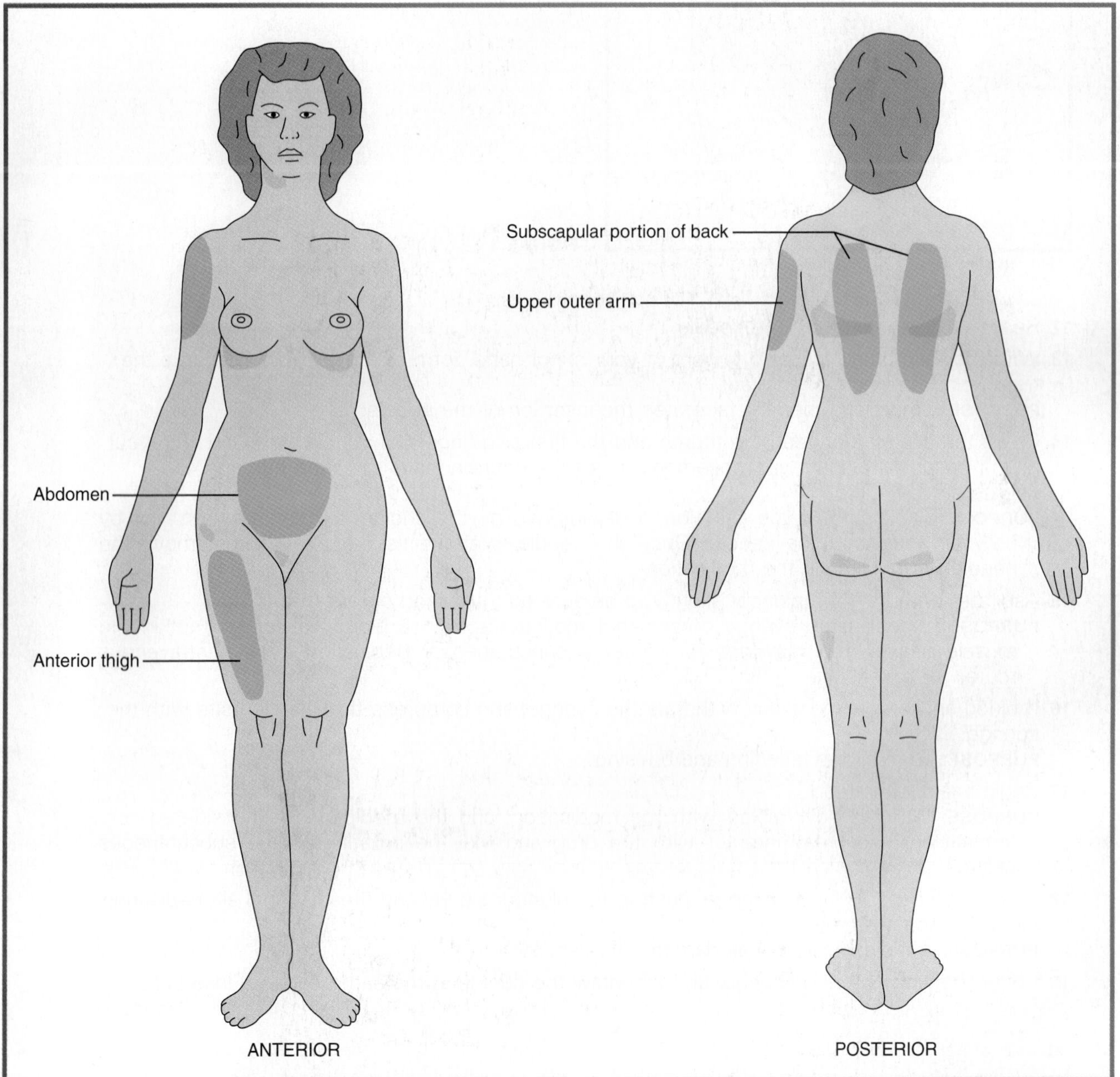

FIGURE 49–27 Areas of the body commonly used for subcutaneous injections.

PROCEDURE 49-4 (CONTINUED)

Giving a Subcutaneous Injection

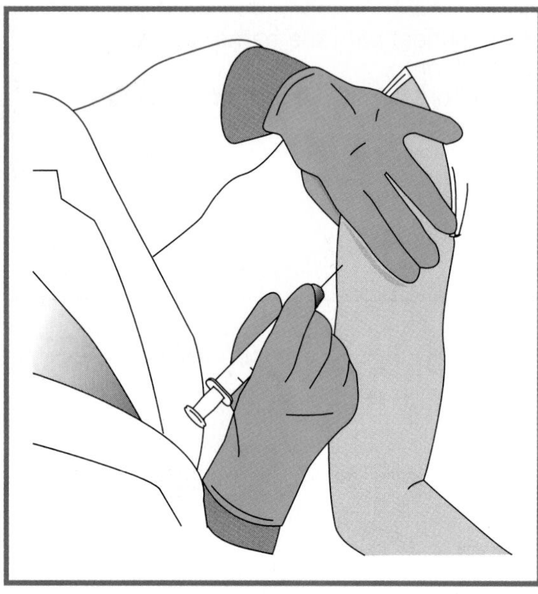

FIGURE 1

12 Remove the sheath from the needle.

13 With the thumb and first two fingers of your minor hand, form a skin fold by picking up the tissue or by pulling the skin taut.
PURPOSE: Smoothing the skin facilitates the insertion of the needle.

14 Grasp the syringe between the thumb and the first two fingers of your major hand with your palm up, and with one swift movement, insert the entire needle up to the hub at a 45-degree angle (Figure 1).
PURPOSE: The depth of the injection is determined by the choice of needle length, not by how far you insert the needle. Once the needle is at the tissue layer, do not move the needle while injecting the medication.

15 Aspirate: Withdraw the plunger slightly to be sure that no blood enters the syringe.
PURPOSE: Blood in the syringe means that the needle is in a blood vessel and not in the muscle tissue. You may *not* administer a subcutaneous medication by the intravenous route.

16 If blood appears, immediately withdraw the syringe, and compress the injection site with the sponge.
PURPOSE: To minimize bleeding and bruising.

17 Begin again with step 1.
PURPOSE: Blood is now mixed with the medication, and the medication is considered contaminated. Blood may interact with the drug and may be irritating to the subcutaneous tissues.

18 If no blood appears in the syringe, push in the plunger slowly and steadily until all medication has been administered.
PURPOSE: A rapid injection may damage the tissues.

19 Cover the area with the sponge, and withdraw the needle at the same angle of insertion.

Continued

20 Gently massage the site with the antiseptic sponge.
PURPOSE: Massage helps to increase absorption and to decrease pain.

21 Make sure that your patient is comfortable and safe.

22 Dispose of the needle and syringe.

23 Observe the patient for any adverse reaction. You may need to keep the patient under observation for 20 to 30 minutes.

24 Wash your hands.

25 Record the drug administration on the patient's medical record, and on the required DEA record if the medication is a controlled substance.
PURPOSE: A procedure is not considered done until it is recorded.

Memory Jogger

5 *What is the needle and syringe size selected for a subcutaneous injection?*

INTRADERMAL INJECTIONS

Intradermal injections differ from subcutaneous injections in that they are given *within the skin,* not under the skin layer (Fig. 49–28; see Procedure 49–5). When they are correctly administered, a small **wheal** (elevation) (Fig. 49–29) is raised on the skin. A very short needle and a small gauge are used. The angle of insertion is 15 degrees, almost parallel to the skin surface. The best site of injection is the center of the forearm, but the upper chest and back areas are used (Fig. 49–30). An area with minimum hair is preferred. Most intradermal injections are skin tests for allergies and screening for diseases, such as tuberculosis. When intradermal injections are given properly, **vesiculation** forms immediately at the site of the injection. **Induration** will follow if there is an allergic reaction.

Memory Jogger

6 *What size needle and syringe did you select for an intradermal injection?*

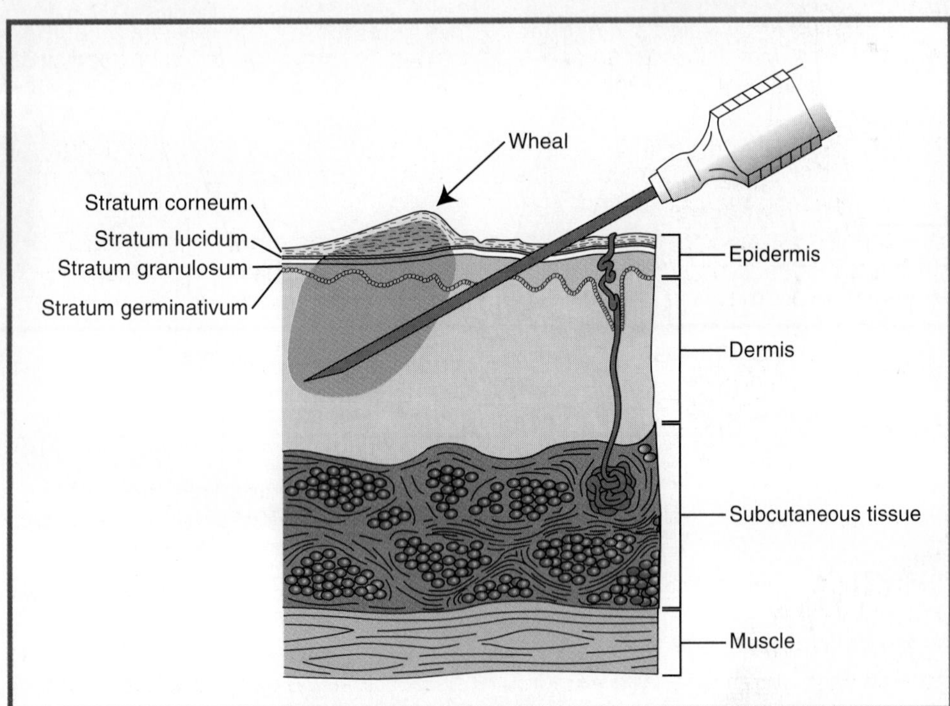

FIGURE 49–28 The intradermal injection is administered just under the epidermis. The drug is dispersed into an area where many nerves are present; thus, it causes momentary burning or stinging. Minute amounts of medication are injected. This method is used to test for allergies, drug sensitivities, and susceptibility to some diseases.

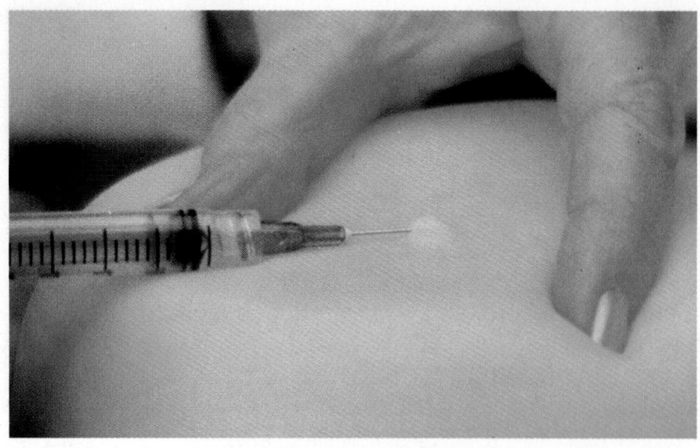

FIGURE 49–29 An intradermal injection with a wheal present. *Note:* Gloves should be worn.

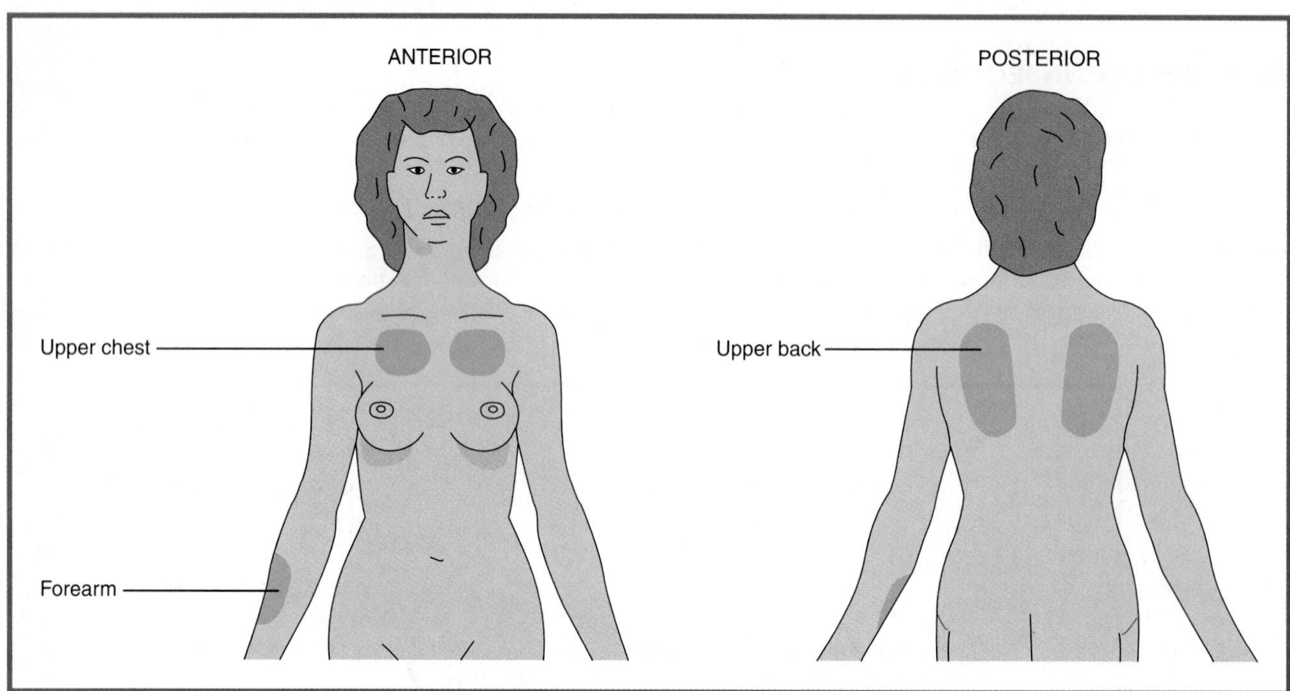

FIGURE 49–30 Sites recommended for intradermal injections.

PROCEDURE 49-5

Giving an Intradermal Injection

GOAL

To inject 0.1 mL of medication into the skin using a needle and syringe of correct size, as directed by the physician.

EQUIPMENT AND SUPPLIES

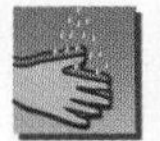

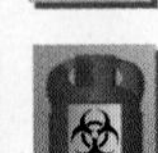
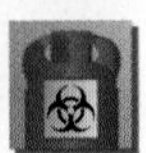

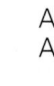

A vial or ampule containing the material to be injected
Antiseptic sponges
A sterile needle and syringe unit
A written order, including the patient's name, when to give the drug, the route of administration, and the name and strength of the drug

PROCEDURAL STEPS

1 Wash your hands. Follow Standard Precautions. Glove yourself with nonsterile gloves.

2 Select the correct medication from the shelf or the refrigerator.
PURPOSE: Some medications must be refrigerated.

3 Read the label to be sure that you have the right drug and the right strength.
PURPOSE: One medication may be manufactured and prepackaged in different strengths; for instance, an allergen may be available in 1 : 1000, 1 : 100, or 1 : 10 dilutions.

4 Warm refrigerated medications by gently rolling the container between your palms.

5 Prepare the syringe, withdrawing the right dose.

6 Transport the medication to the patient.

7 Greet and identify the patient by name.
PURPOSE: To be sure that you have the right patient.

8 Position the patient comfortably.

9 Locate the antecubital space, then find a site several fingerwidths down the inner aspect of the forearm.

10 Cleanse the patient's skin with an antiseptic sponge, using a circular motion, moving outward from the center.

11 Allow the antiseptic to dry.
PURPOSE: Because the injected drug is deposited so near the skin surface, the antiseptic could interact with the drug.

12 Compare the order with the prepared medication, and the patient with the name on the order to be sure that this is the right time to administer the drug.
PURPOSE: This is the last of the six checks to be made before administering a medication. If there is any doubt, do not proceed. Check first with the physician.

13 Remove the sheath from the needle.

14 With the thumb and first two fingers of your minor hand, stretch the skin taut.
PURPOSE: Stretching the skin facilitates the insertion of the needle.

15 Grasp the syringe between the thumb and first two fingers of your major hand, palm down, with the needle bevel upward.

Continued

PROCEDURE 49-5 (CONTINUED)

Giving an Intradermal Injection

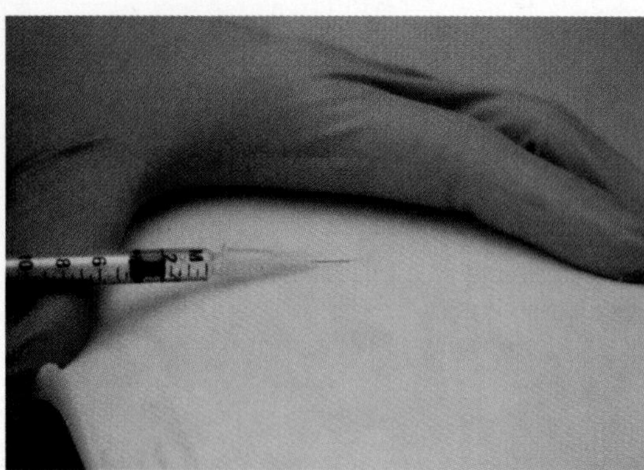

FIGURE 1

16 At a 15-degree angle, carefully insert the needle through the skin about ⅛ inch, keeping the needle visible through the skin (Figure 1).

17 Turn the syringe 180 degrees to turn the bevel downward.
PURPOSE: To prevent the medication from breaking through the skin by the force of the injection.

18 Slowly and steadily inject the medication. A wheal should appear.
PURPOSE: A rapid injection may force the substance through to the surface.

19 After administering all of the medication, withdraw the needle.

20 Do not massage.
PURPOSE: Massaging will interfere with the intended results.

21 Make sure that your patient is comfortable and safe.

22 Dispose of the needle and syringe.

23 Observe the patient for any adverse reaction. You may need to keep the patient under observation for 20 to 30 minutes.

24 Wash your hands.

25 Record the drug administration and any reactions that occurred at the site of the injection on the patient's medical record.

26 If the injection site needs to be read (TB skin test), be sure to tell the patient when to return to the office.
PURPOSE: A procedure is not considered done until it is recorded.

INFANTS AND CHILDREN

Injecting infants and small children requires some special considerations. The choice of a site is based on muscular development, as well as the absence of major nerves and blood vessels. The most popular site for intramuscular injection is the vastus lateralis muscle (lateral thigh). Other sites are avoided for the following reasons:

- Infants do not have well-developed deltoid muscles.
- The sciatic nerve is proportionately larger in the infant.
- The gluteus medius is not well developed until the child is walking.

The best policy is to ask the physician to show you just where to inject. Any site selected for infants and children has a greater margin for error because the muscles are smaller than the muscles of the adult.

Infants should be restrained by another assistant or the parent to avoid injury. If the child is old enough to understand, be honest and explain that the injection may "sting" for a minute, but that it is important to hold very still. Obtain assistance when giving an injection to an uncooperative child. You may keep the fact that the child is to receive an injection from the child until the last minute, but always let the child know. After the injection, praise the child for being helpful; show appreciation and reassurance. If you do this, the child will remember more than just the "hurt" of the needle and will trust in you, the physician, and health care in general. Many children like to have an adhesive bandage applied after the injection as a badge of bravery. Do not give any syringe to a child for play.

Memory Jogger

7 *List three reasons for selecting the vastus lateralis muscle for injections in children.*

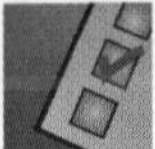

PATIENT EDUCATION

It is extremely important that a patient be instructed about how to take a medication and why he or she is taking it. Ideally, the patient is informed by the physician, but the medical assistant should be prepared to reinforce the physician's information to the patient or explain parts of the information that the patient did not understand. When the patient does not understand the need for the medication or the directions regarding how to take it, there is a greater risk of the medication being taken incorrectly. As a result, the physician's orders will not be carried out. The patient should fully understand the type of medication, its route of administration, its desired effect, and the side effects that need to be reported if they occur.

If a patient is given a diuretic in the office, he or she needs to know what the immediate effect is going to be. This helps the patient to understand the urgency and polyuria that he or she will experience within a relatively brief period of time. When a pain medication is given, the patient should have full knowledge so that the possibility of personal injury can be avoided.

Emphasis should be placed on instructing the patient to take all of the medication prescribed. Many times, if a prescription is not completed, the treatment objectives are altered. Patients should also be instructed to take their medication in the time sequence prescribed. This keeps the optimum level of the drug circulating in the bloodstream.

When sample medications are dispensed in the office to the patient, the package contains inserts that can be helpful in educating the patient. If there are certain parts of the inserts that the patient is especially to remember, highlight this information for quick reference. If the physician has specific written instructions for the patient to follow, read over the form with the patient before giving it to him or her.

Always remember that the more the patient knows and understands about how to take the medication and why it is prescribed, the greater the chances are that the drug treatment will be successful.

This would also be a good time to suggest that the patient check the status of medications at home. The National Association of Retail Druggists recommends that the medicine cabinet be checked once a month to determine the age and quality of medications. At that time dispose of any medications falling under the following guidelines:

1. Medicines for past illnesses.
2. Any expired medicines, unidentified medications, or medications that are more than 2 years old.
3. Hydrogen peroxide that no longer bubbles or has changed color, ointments or salves that have separated or are crumbly, vinegar-smelling aspirins, antiseptic solutions that are cloudy or have a solid residue on the bottom, and any medicine of unsure quality.

The association also suggests the following:

1. Keep medicines stored away from light, heat, air, and moisture.
2. Use medicine from the original container until it is completely used or expired.
3. Do not combine medicines from several containers.
4. Keep medicine locked away from children.
5. Make sure that child-proof medicine caps are used properly.

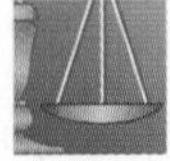

LEGAL AND ETHICAL ISSUES

The medical assistant must be extremely knowledgeable when given the responsibility of administering medications in the physician's office. When the physician has written an order for the medication, follow it exactly. If you have a question about the order, ask for clarification before you proceed with the order. It is advisable to give a medication only after the order is written in the patient's chart. This helps eliminate errors and possible omissions in the medication therapy. Legal responsibilities include the prevention of error by carefully following safe practice procedures in pouring and administering drugs. Memorize the "six rights." Any person administering a drug must know the possible serious complications related to the drug and watch for side effects of the medication. The assistant must demonstrate compliance with the laws governing medications and their administration. Precise charting of the administration of medications cannot be overemphasized.

The administration of drugs also involves ethical principles. The patient always come first; and with that foremost in mind, you cannot risk giving an incorrect medication. There is no chance for a "slight" error because any such error may result in a patient's death. If an error is made, it must be reported immediately to the physician so that measures can be taken to help the patient. It is difficult to admit that a mistake has been made, but it is *absolutely* necessary. For that reason, be sure to double-check your calculations with a co-worker or the physician.

Errors in medication administration can cause serious problems for the patient. Errors should be reported and charted as soon as discovered. To whom the error was reported, any action taken, and observations of the patient should be included.

HOW DID I DO? Answers to Memory Joggers

1. Reading the label before, during, and after pouring the drug is a triple check that you have the right drug.
2. The patient will receive 10 mL of Duricep oral suspension.
3. Capsules are coated with gelatin and tablets are not.
4. For intramuscular injection, the needle gauge is 20 to 23, length is 1 to 3 inches, and the syringe is 2 to 5 mL.
5. For subcutaneous injections, the needle is 25 to 26 gauge and ½ to ⅝ inches long. The syringe may be 2 mL, tuberculin or insulin.
6. The intradermal injection uses a 27- to 28-gauge needle, ⅜ to ½ inch long with a tuberculin syringe.
7. The gluteus medius and the deltoid muscles are not well developed. There is greater danger of hitting the sciatic nerve.

CRITICAL THINKING

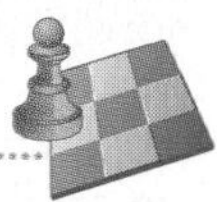

1 The physician has written an order for a medication that you cannot clearly read. He is now with another patient. What will you do?

2 You are about to administer a prescribed medication to a patient. The patient says that you are mistaken, that you have the wrong drug. What will you do?

3 You are giving instructions to the patient about taking his antibiotic prescription. His wife states, "Oh, I always save some of his prescription to take when I have an infection. Then I do not have to go to the doctor myself." What is your response to them?

REFERENCES

Clark J, Queener S, Karb V: Pocket Guide to Drugs. St. Louis, CV Mosby, 1986

Kee J, Hayes E, Pharmacology: A Nursing Process Approach, 2nd ed. Philadelphia, WB Saunders, 1997

Physician's Desk Reference, 51st ed. Oradell, NJ, Medical Economics, 1997

Reynard A, Smith C: Textbook of Pharmacology. Philadelphia, WB Saunders, 1992

Rice J: Pharmacology for Medical Assisting. Philadelphia, Delmar Publishers, 1989

Woodrow R: Essentials of Pharmacology for Health Occupations, 2nd ed. New York, Delmar Publishers, 1992

Preparing for Surgery

Mary Jane McClain, RN, BS, CNOR

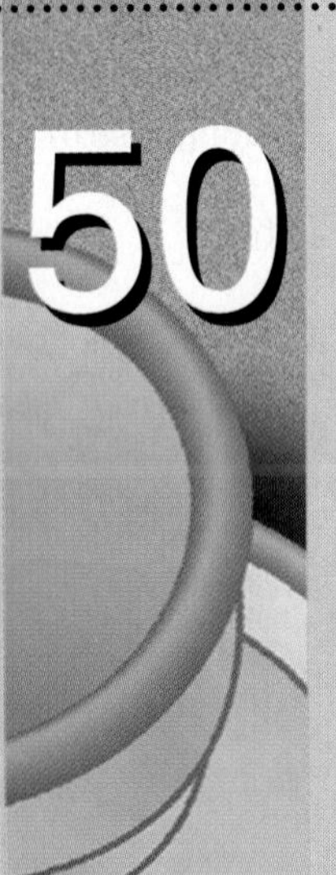

OUTLINE

LEARNING OBJECTIVES

Cognitive: On successful completion of this chapter you should be able to:

1 Define and spell the words in the Vocabulary.
2 Identify by name the instruments used in minor surgery procedures.
3 Identify types of sutures and surgical needles.

VOCABULARY

abrasion Rubbing or scraping of the skin or mucous membrane (e.g., a skinned knee)

abscess Localized collection of pus that may be located under the skin or deep within the body that causes tissue destruction

approximation Act or process of drawing together skin or wound edges

biopsy Small sample of tissue excised from the body for diagnostic or therapeutic purposes

cannula Rigid tube that surrounds a blunt trocar or a sharp, pointed trocar inserted into the body; when withdrawn, fluid may escape from the body through the cannula, depending on where it is inserted

caustic Substance that burns or destroys organic tissue by chemical action

curettage Act of scraping a body cavity with a surgical instrument, such as a curette

cyst Sac of fluid or semisolid material located in or under the skin

debridement Surgical removal of damaged, diseased, or contaminated tissue until healthy tissue is exposed

dilatation Opening or widening the circumference of a body orifice with a dilating instrument

diluent Substance, such as water, that renders a drug or a solution less potent

dissect To cut or separate tissue with a cutting instrument or scissors

fascia Sheet or band of fibrous tissue located deep in the skin that covers muscles and body organs

fistula Abnormal, tubelike passage within the body tissues

lesion Wound, sore, ulcer, tumor, or any traumatic tissue damage that causes a lack of tissue continuity or a loss of function

lumen Open space, such as within a blood vessel, the intestine, the inside of a needle, or an examining instrument

obturator Metal rod with a smooth rounded tip that is placed into hollow instruments to decrease destruction of the body tissues during insertion

parenteral Any medication route other than the alimentary canal

paroxysm Sudden turn or amplification of symptoms such as a spasm or seizure

patency Open condition of a body cavity or canal

polyps Tumors with stems, frequently found on mucous membranes

stylus Metal probe that is inserted into or passed through a catheter, needle, or tube used for clearing purposes or to facilitate passage into a body orifice

suppuration Production of purulent material (pus) from a wound

Minor surgery is surgery that is restricted to the management of minor problems and injuries. Almost all medical assistants are expected to glove and assist with the preparation of the sterile field and the patient. A few are expected to assist with outpatient surgical procedures that were once performed in the hospital. Although these more difficult operations may involve complete gowning and gloving with surgical masks and caps, the next two chapters limit discussion and descriptions to the routines necessary to prepare for and assist in minor surgery only. This chapter includes a discussion of surgical supplies and instruments, the care and handling of instruments, and the different types of surgical sutures and needles. It prepares you for the following chapters in which specific minor surgical procedures and care of the patient are presented.

A complete understanding of minor surgery procedures includes material presented in preceding chapters, specifically, Chapter 26, Infection Control. You are urged to refer to this previous chapter while reading the following chapters.

Surgical Supplies

When minor surgery is routinely performed, the medical office is usually designed to include a changing room and a minor surgery room that is separate from the other examining rooms. The larger surgery centers are frequently designed to include recovery rooms and family waiting areas. The minor surgery room should be near a workroom with a sink and an autoclave, if the room does not have its own. It should be easy to clean or decontaminate, and it should be uncluttered to allow easy movement and minimal dust collection. In addition to the operating table, equipment should include a clock with a second sweep, an operating light, sitting

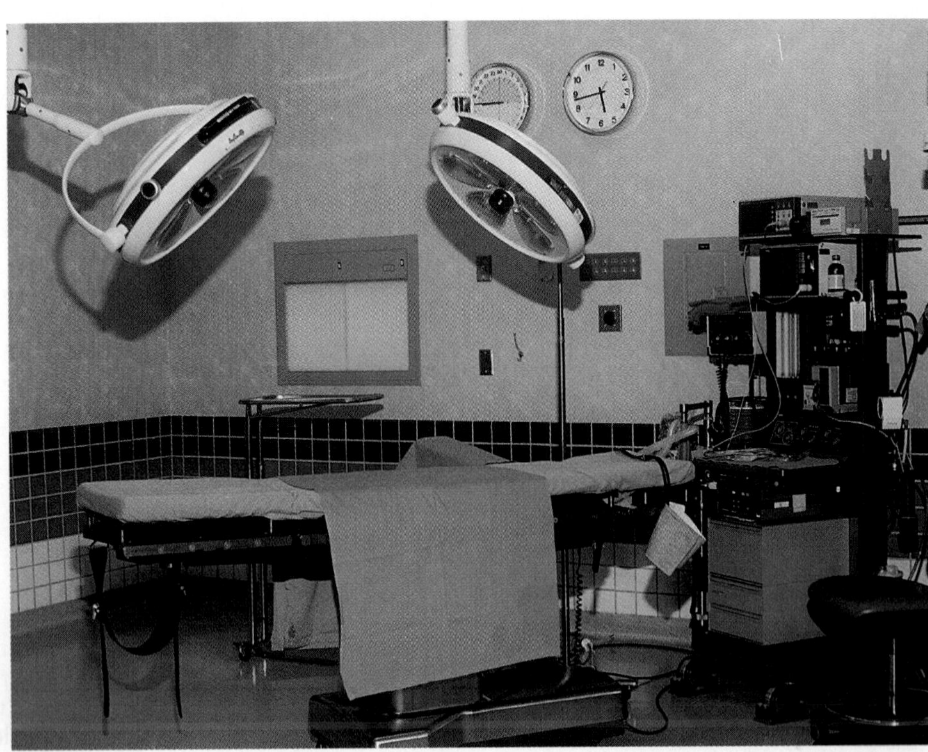

FIGURE 50–1 Operating room and equipment. (Courtesy of Fresno Surgery Center, Fresno, CA.)

stools, and a Mayo stand (Fig. 50–1). Cabinets with countertops are necessary to serve as a side or back table during the surgery. All surgical supplies are stored in these cabinets. Supplies used in this room should not be used elsewhere, and supplies used elsewhere should not be brought into this room.

Memory Jogger

 *What equipment should be included in an operating room in addition to the operating table?*

Surgical Solutions and Medications

Treatment room supplies include standard solutions and medications that are used in minor surgery and dressing changes. Although the solutions and medications listed here are basic, every practice has preferred items and methods of applying them. Many of these items are used by the medical assistant. Others are used by the physician only, but the medical assistant is responsible for their care and supply.

Sterile water is kept in two forms. Multiple-dose vials are used for injectable distilled water and as a **diluent** for medications. Larger containers of sterile water are used for rinsing instruments that have been in a chemical disinfectant solution.

Sterile physiologic saline solution (0.9%) is also stocked in two sizes. The small multiple-dose vial is used for injection. A larger-size container of saline is used for rinsing and irrigating wounds. These high-quality, commercially prepared products can be purchased from a medical supply company.

Memory Jogger

 *What are two surgical purposes for sterile water and for sterile physiologic saline?*

Povidone-iodine (Betadine) is currently the preferred skin antiseptic. Isopropyl alcohol 70% was the antiseptic choice in the past. Neither of these products is sporicidal. Betadine does not cause the allergic problems of the earlier tincture of iodine and is used in several different ways: as a skin preparation for surgery, as a surgical hand scrub, for saturating dressings, and as a topical ointment.

DuraPrep is an iodine and alcohol surgical solution that is used as a skin antiseptic. It provides long-lasting microbial action against a broad spectrum of microbes.

Surgical soap, such as Betadine Scrub and Hibiclens (chlorhexidine gluconate), is used for hand scrubbing, for the patient's skin preparation before surgery, and before the application of an antiseptic.

Hydrogen peroxide (H_2O_2) in a 3% solution is used as a mild antiseptic. It kills by its oxidizing power. The mechanical action creates bubbles when applied to a skin **abrasion** or wound and has a

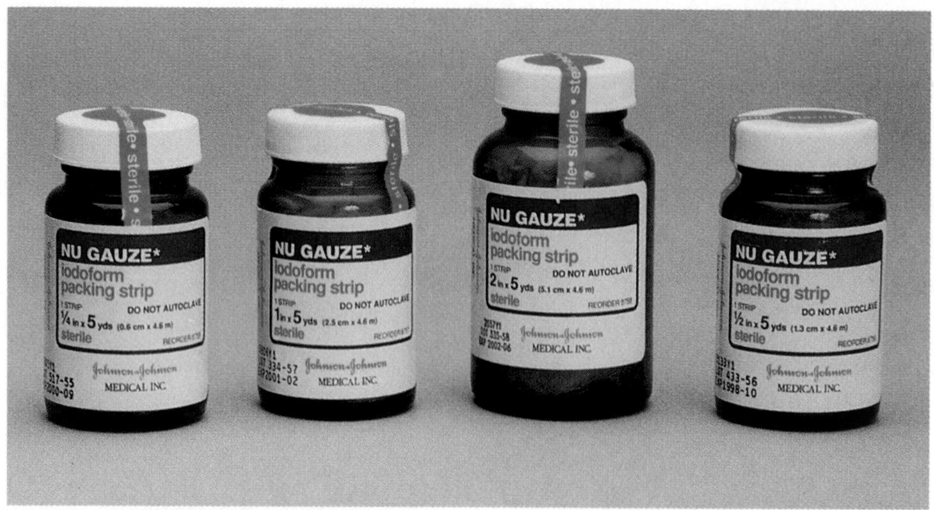

FIGURE 50–2 Iodoform gauze. (Courtesy of Johnson & Johnson Medical, Inc., Arlington, TX.)

cleansing action. It is used in irrigations and **debridement** and is nonirritating.

Lidocaine (Xylocaine) and Sensorcaine are local anesthetics, and there are many others. Local anesthetics are purchased in multiple-dose vials of 30 to 50 mL. When highly vascular areas are involved, anesthetics with epinephrine may be used. Epinephrine causes vasoconstriction at the site, which keeps the anesthetic in the tissues longer, prolonging its effect. It also minimizes local bleeding. Epinephrine may tend to maximize swelling at the operative site and distort close **approximation** of the wound edges; it is not generally used on the extremities. Epinephrine must be used with caution in patients with a history of heart disease.

Epinephrine (Adrenalin) 1:1000 is a vasoconstrictor used to control hemorrhage, asthmatic **paroxysm,** and shock. It is also used to counter allergic reactions. Administration can be topical, by inhalation, by injection, or **parenteral.**

Memory Jogger

 *Describe the systemic effect of epinephrine.*

Tincture of benzoin is applied as a protective coating over ulcers and abrasions. It is used under adhesive tape to increase holding power and to decrease skin sensitivity to the tape. Tincture of benzoin is supplied in spray cans as well as in solution for painting on the skin with an applicator.

Ethyl chloride is used as a skin anesthetic (topical). It is a highly volatile liquid that is sprayed on the skin. It evaporates so quickly that the tissue is immediately cooled and numbed. It has a very short duration. It is sometimes referred to as "freezing" the skin.

Formalin, 10% solution, is used to preserve excised tissue for specimens, such as those taken in **biopsy** or for histology studies.

Aromatic spirits of ammonia is supplied in bottles or in small glass ampules covered with cotton gauze to prevent injury when they are crushed to open. It was most commonly used for fainting, but studies have shown that the danger of damage to the respiratory system far outweighs any advantages for certain patients.

Vaseline (petroleum jelly or petrolatum) is used to impregnate gauze squares or strips. It is packaged and sterilized by commercial manufacturers.

Iodoform gauze strips are slender strips of gauze, ¼ to 2 inches wide, impregnated with iodoform (96%) iodine and contained within sterile bottles. They may be used to pack an **abscess,** acting as a wick to draw out the infection and as a local antibacterial agent (Fig. 50–2).

Silver nitrate ($AgNO_3$) is available in solution or coated on applicator sticks. It is a **caustic** and is applied topically. It must be kept in lightproof brown containers. The most commonly used strength is 20%. The applicator sticks are convenient for touching an oral or nasal **lesion.** Silver nitrate may be used to promote the healing process after surgery. This is not the same solution that is used in eyes.

Memory Jogger

 *What is the use of iodoform gauze strips?*

Additional Supplies

Certain pieces of equipment are frequently used in minor surgery. An electrosurgical unit (ESU) is used to cauterize blood vessels and incise tissue with an electric current. Fiberoptic lights cables and cords attached to scopes and headlights supply an intense light to a small area. Wound drains (Penrose drain), are rubber drains sometimes used in a wound at the end of a surgical procedure if the wound is filled with fluid or is oozing or may need draining.

Surgical sponges are used to absorb blood and protect tissues during surgery. They also may be used to wipe blood or other debris from the instruments. The 4 × 4-inch gauze square (i.e., sponge) is used in most minor surgeries.

Syringes and needles are used to inject local anesthetics, to aspirate fluids from a wound, and to irrigate wounds.

Instruments are fundamental to the performance of diagnostic procedures and patient treatments. With the growth of urgent care centers and an increase in outpatient surgery, the medical assistant now must care for and use a greater variety of surgical instruments.

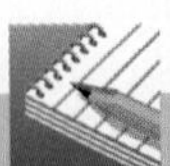

SKILLS AND RESPONSIBILITIES

BEING FAMILIAR WITH SURGICAL INSTRUMENTS

The administrative medical assistant must properly spell the names of instruments when transcribing medical dictation as well as purchase and inventory them by name. The clinical medical assistant must know which instruments are used for each procedure to package them for sterilization and set-up and to assist the physician during surgery or an examination.

Identifying Surgical Instruments

Instruments have clearly identifiable parts and can be visually differentiated from one another (see Procedure 50–1). The basic components are the handle, the closing mechanism, and the part that comes into contact with the patient, commonly called the jaws. Many instruments may be ordered straight or curved, depending on the operator's preference

Instruments have either ring handles (finger rings) or spring handles (sometimes called thumb-handled or thumb grasp). The instruments with a ring handle are scissors. Tweezers are listed under spring-handled instruments. Some instruments have a hinge type of mechanism called a box lock. A ring-handled forceps is shown in Figure 50–3*A*. An instrument with a box-lock mechanism is shown in Figure 50–3*B*, and a spring-handled thumb forceps is pictured in Figure 50–3*C*.

Ratchets resemble gears and are located just below the ring handles. Ratchets are used to lock an instrument into position. Most ratchets can be closed at three or more positions, depending on the thickness of the tissue or materials being grasped. An example of an instrument with a ratchet closing mechanism is shown in Figure 50–4.

The inner surfaces of the jaws on some instruments have ridged teeth called serrations, and both ring-handled and thumb-type instruments may have them. These serrations may be crisscross, horizontal, or lengthwise (Fig. 50–5). Serrations prevent small

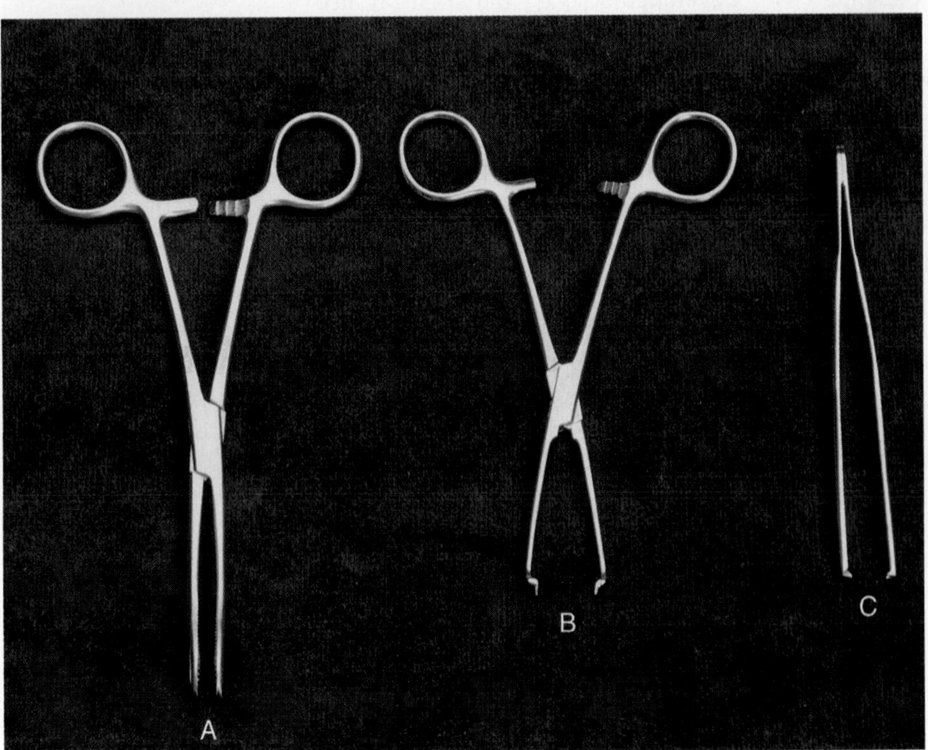

FIGURE 50–3 *A,* Ring-handle forceps. *B,* Box-lock hinge forceps. *C,* Spring-handle thumb forceps.

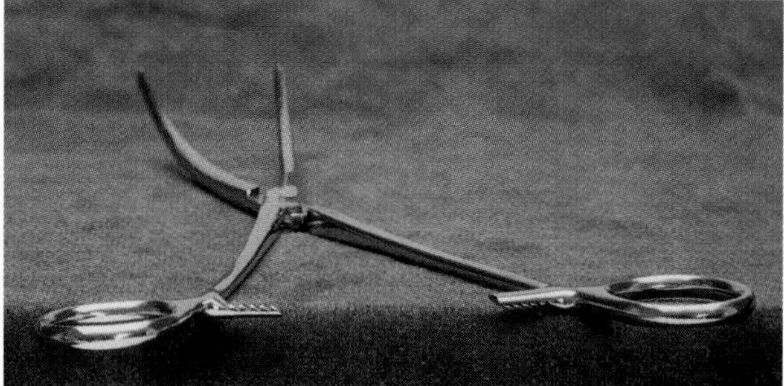

FIGURE 50–4 Instrument with ratchet closing mechanism.

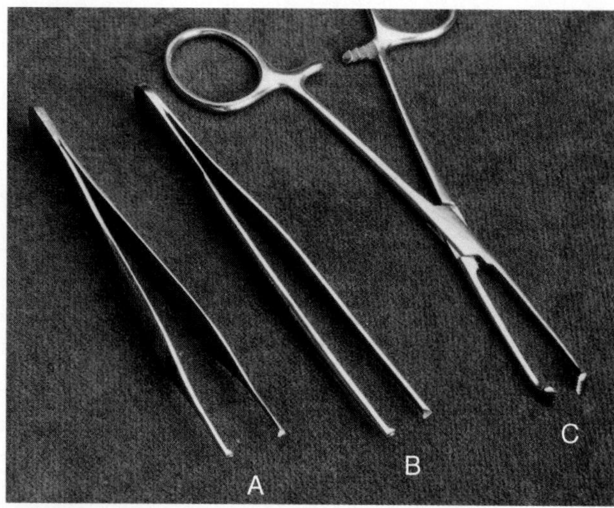

FIGURE 50–6 *A*, Mouse-toothed jaws. *B*, Rat-toothed jaws. *C*, Teeth of Allis tissue forceps.

blood vessels and tissue from slipping out of the jaws of the instrument.

Jaws may be plain tipped or mouse toothed (Fig. 50–6*A*). If the tooth is large, the tip may be called rat toothed (see Fig. 50–6*B*) rather than mouse toothed. Toothed instruments are usually called tissue forceps and are identified by the number of intermeshing teeth (e.g., 1 × 2, 2 × 3, 3 × 4). Figure 50–6*C* shows part of an Allis tissue forceps. Because this forceps is used to grasp delicate soft tissues, the teeth are finer, shallower, and more rounded; others may be sharper and deeper. Still others have sharp hooklike single or double teeth, such as the tenaculum and vulsellum. Usually, the tenaculum has a single sharp hook on each jaw. The vulsellum has a double hook that resembles the fangs of a snake. Toothed instruments commonly have ratchets for locking into towels or human tissues.

An instrument is usually named for its use (e.g., splinter forceps, for removing splinters) or after the person(s) who developed it (e.g., Mayo-Hegar needle holder). Many general instruments are identified by the part of the body where they are used (e.g., rectal speculum and nasal speculum).

There are thousands of surgical instruments, and there are great variations in their names. The same instrument may carry two or three different names, depending on the physician or the part of the country. A physician may ask for a clamp or a forceps when a Kelly hemostat is wanted, and you will need to know what a clamp or forceps means in each case. As in building words from word parts, if you train yourself to recognize the distinctive parts of instruments, and the reasons for each part, you will quickly build a working knowledge of hundreds of instruments.

Memory Jogger

How are instruments usually named?

Classifications of Surgical Instruments

Surgical instruments are generally classified according to their use, and most belong to one of four groups:

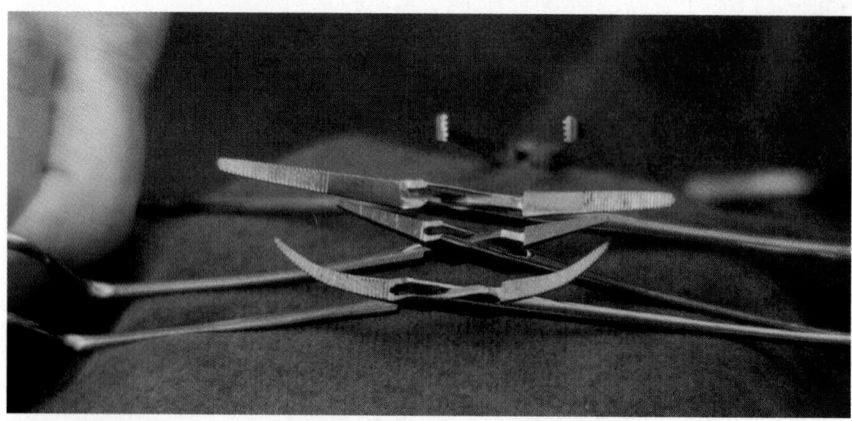

FIGURE 50–5 Instruments with serrations.

- Cutting
- Grasping
- Retracting
- Probing and Dilating

CUTTING AND DISSECTING INSTRUMENTS

These are cutting, incising, scraping, punching, and puncturing instruments. Included are scissors, scalpels, chisels, elevators, curettes, punches, drills, and needles. Instruments with a sharp blade or surface can cut, scrape, or dissect.

Bandage scissors (Fig. 50–7*A*)
- Probe tip is blunt.
- Easily inserted under bandages with relative safety.
- Used to remove bandages and dressings.

Operating scissors (surgical scissors) (Fig. 50–7*A* through *F*)

Metzenbaum ("Metz") scissors (Fig. 50–7*B*)
- Most frequently used length is 5¼ inches.
- Used to cut and **dissect** tissue.

Mayo scissors (Fig. 50–7*C* and *D*)
- Have curved or straight blade tips.
- Used to cut and dissect fascia and muscle.
- Straight Mayo scissors may be used as suture scissors.

Iris scissors (Fig. 50–7*E* and *F*)
- Usual length is 4 inches.
- Have curved or straight blade tips.
- Straight tips usually used for suture removal.

Gauze shears
- Have sharp blades and large ring handle.
- Used to cut gauze, tubing, and adhesive.

Littauer stitch or suture scissors
- Blade has beak or hook to slide under sutures.
- Used to remove sutures.

Bone rasp (Fig. 50–7*G* and *H*)
- Flat or curved, serrated, or sharp.
- Used to smooth the surface of the bone.

Scalpel handle (Fig. 50–8*A* through *C*)
- No. 3 is the standard handle.
- No. 3L and No. 7 are used in deeper cavities.

Scalpel blades (Fig. 50–8*D* through *G*)
- No. 15 is commonly used.
- Nos. 10, 11, and 12 are used for specialty incisions.

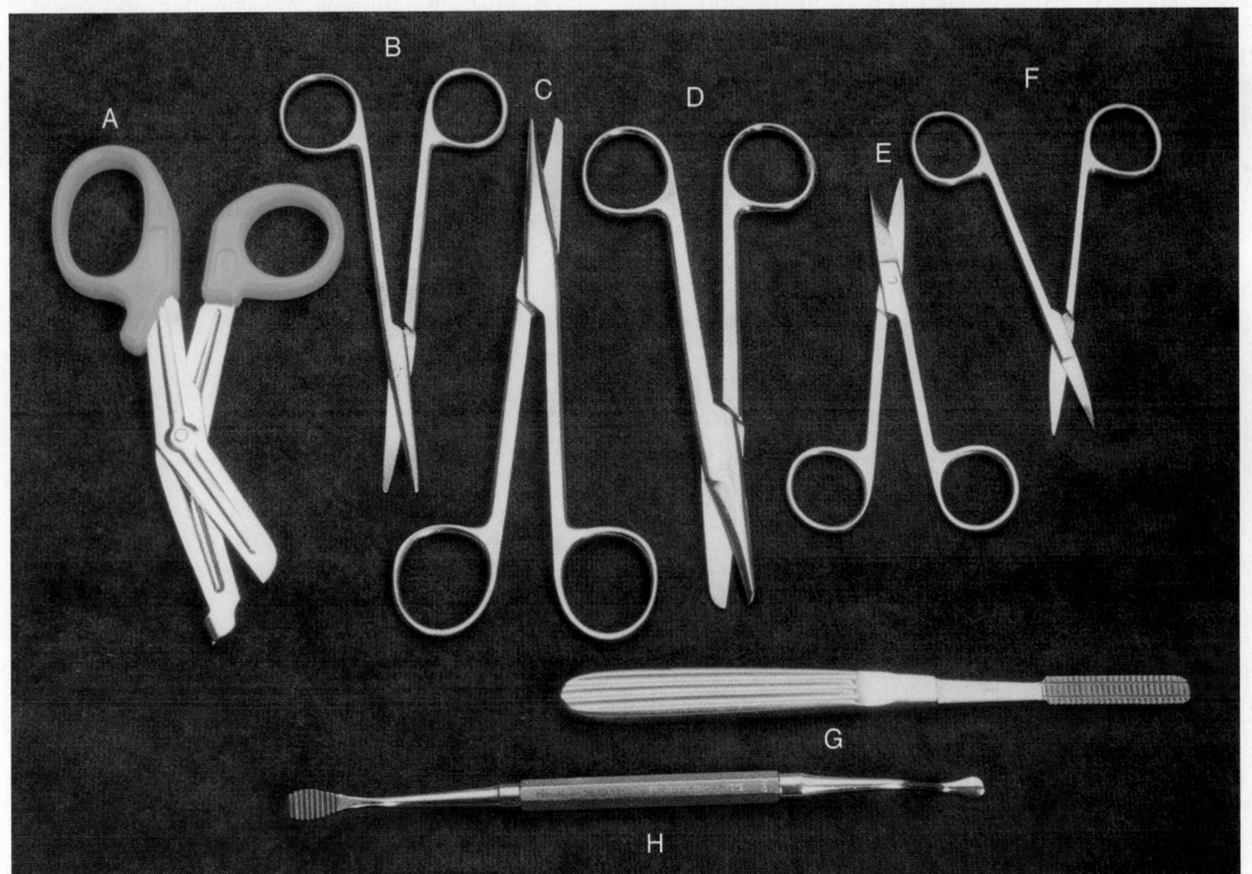

FIGURE 50–7 Operating scissors. *A*, Bandage scissors. *B*, Metzenbaum ("Metz") scissors. *C*, Curved Mayo scissors. *D*, Straight Mayo scissors. *E*, Straight iris scissors. *F*, Curved iris scissors. *G*, Bone rasp, single ended. *H*, Bone rasp, double ended.

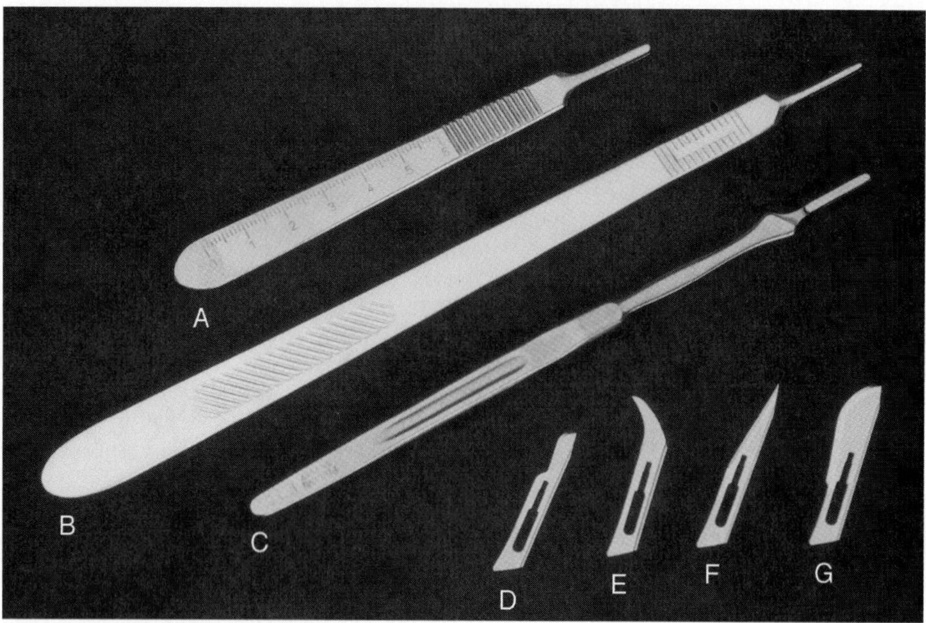

FIGURE 50–8 *A,* No. 3 scalpel blade. *B,* No. 3 long scalpel handle. *C,* No. 7 scalpel handle. *D,* No. 15 blade. *E,* No. 12 blade. *F,* No. 11 blade. *G,* No. 10 blade.

GRASPING AND CLAMPING INSTRUMENTS

Clamping instruments are used for many different tasks. Many have a sharp tooth or teeth and are used to retract, hold, and manipulate human **fascia.** The most common clamping instruments are the hemostats, which were originally designed to stop bleeding or to clamp severed blood vessels. Other clamping instruments are used to grasp other instruments or sterilized materials. Sometimes hemostats and the other clamping instruments are used interchangeably.

Hemostat forceps (Fig. 50–9*A* and *B*)

- Jaws may be fully or partially serrated, without teeth.
- Used to clamp small vessels or hold tissue.
- Mosquito forceps are smaller and used for very small vessels.

Needle holders (Fig. 50–9*C* and *D*)

- Jaws are shorter and look stronger than hemostat jaws.
- Jaws may be serrated or may have a groove in the center.
- Used to firmly grasp a suture needle.
- Manufactured in different lengths.

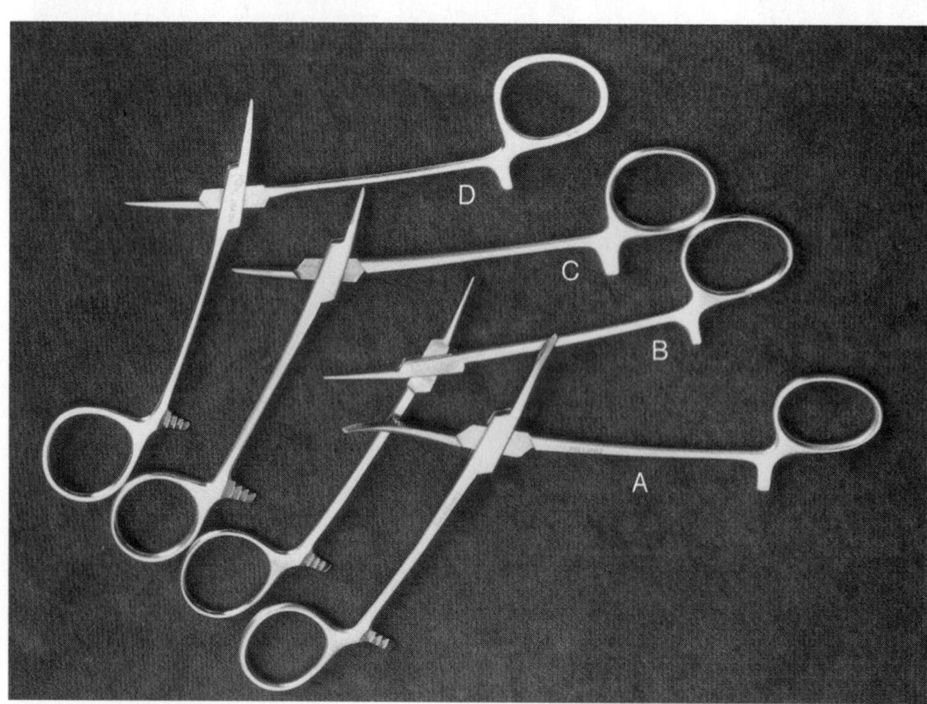

FIGURE 50–9 *A,* Kelly hemostat forceps. *B,* Mosquito hemostat forceps. *C,* Needle holder. *D,* Smooth-tip needle holder.

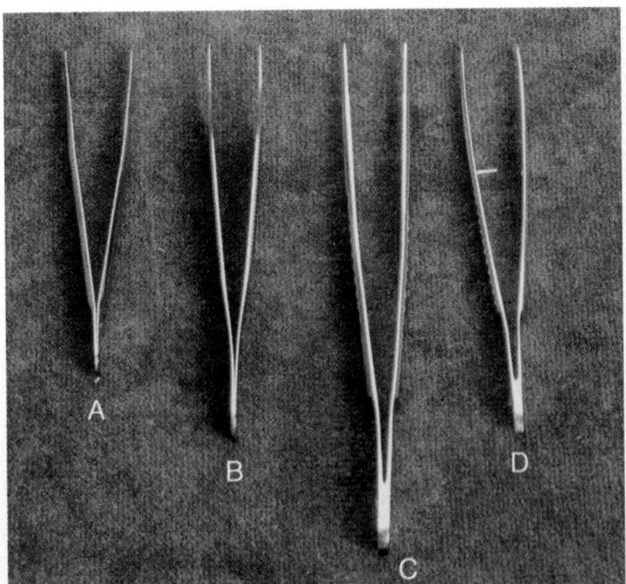

FIGURE 50–10 *A,* Splinter forceps. *B,* Smooth Adson forceps. *C,* Long plain-tip forceps. *D,* Short plain-tip tissue forceps.

Splinter forceps (Fig. 50–10*A*)

- Design and construction vary.
- Fine tip for foreign object retrieval.
- Used to grasp foreign bodies embedded in skin.

Smooth Adson forceps (Fig. 50–10*B*)

- Same use as the Adson thumb forceps.

Plain thumb (dressing) forceps (Fig. 50–10*C*)

- Manufactured in lengths from 4 to 12 inches.
- Have varying types of serrated jaws but no teeth.
- Used to insert packing into or remove objects from deep cavities.

Towel forceps (towel clamp) (Fig. 50–11*A* through *D*)

- Have very sharp or atraumatic hooks.
- Are various lengths from 3 to 6½ inches.
- May be used to grasp and retract tissue.
- Used to hold drapes in place during surgery.

Allis tissue forceps (Fig. 50–12*A*)

- Available in different lengths and jaw widths.
- Is less traumatic to tissue, teeth are not as sharp.
- Used to grasp tissue, muscle, or skin surrounding a wound.

Transfer forceps (Fig. 50–12*B* through *E*)

- Many sizes and lengths are available.
- Sterile transfer forceps may be used to arrange items on sterile tray.

Adson thumb forceps (Fig. 50–13*A* and *B*)

- Usually in 4-inch lengths.
- Shaped differently from plain and toothed forceps.
- Manufactured with or without teeth.
- Used to grasp tissue and in suturing.

Bayonet forceps (Fig. 50–13*C, D,* and *E*)

- Manufactured in different lengths.
- Smooth tipped.
- Used to insert packing into or remove objects from nose and ear.

Plain-tip tissue forceps (Fig. 50–13*F*)

- Manufactured in different lengths.
- Atraumatic to tissue.
- Same use as the toothed tissue forceps.

Toothed tissue forceps (Fig. 50–13*G*)

- Manufactured in 4- to 18-inch lengths.
- Pincher grip.
- Same use as Allis tissue forceps.

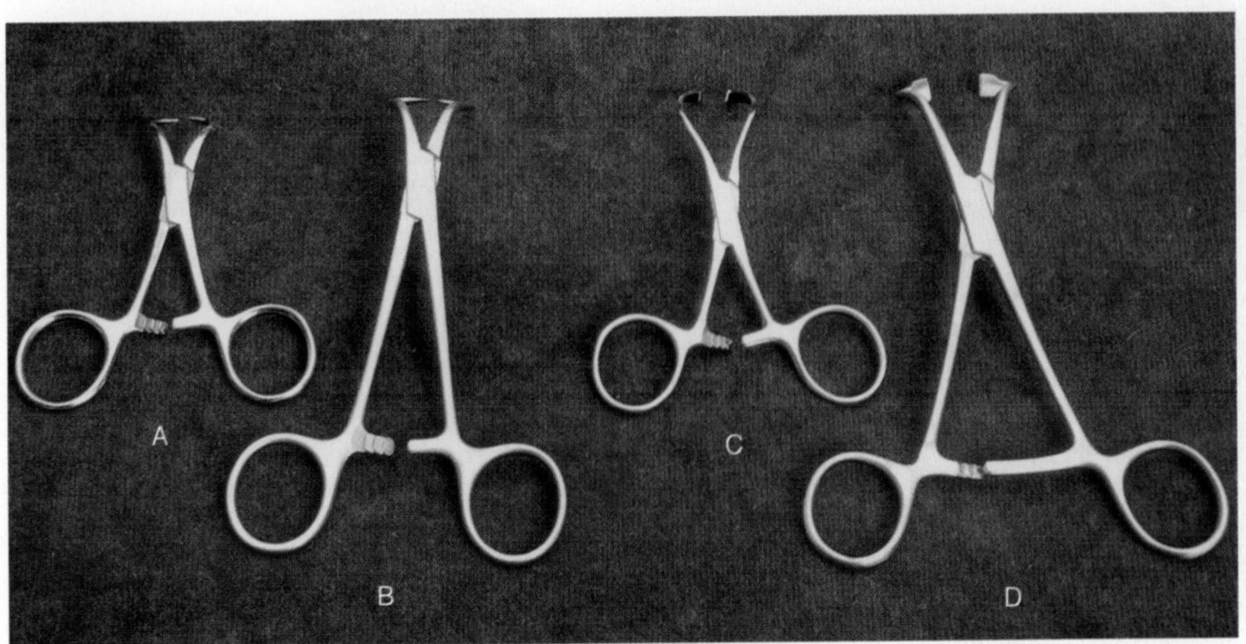

FIGURE 50–11 *A,* Small sharp towel forceps. *B,* Large sharp towel forceps. *C,* Small atraumatic towel forceps. *D,* Large atraumatic towel forceps.

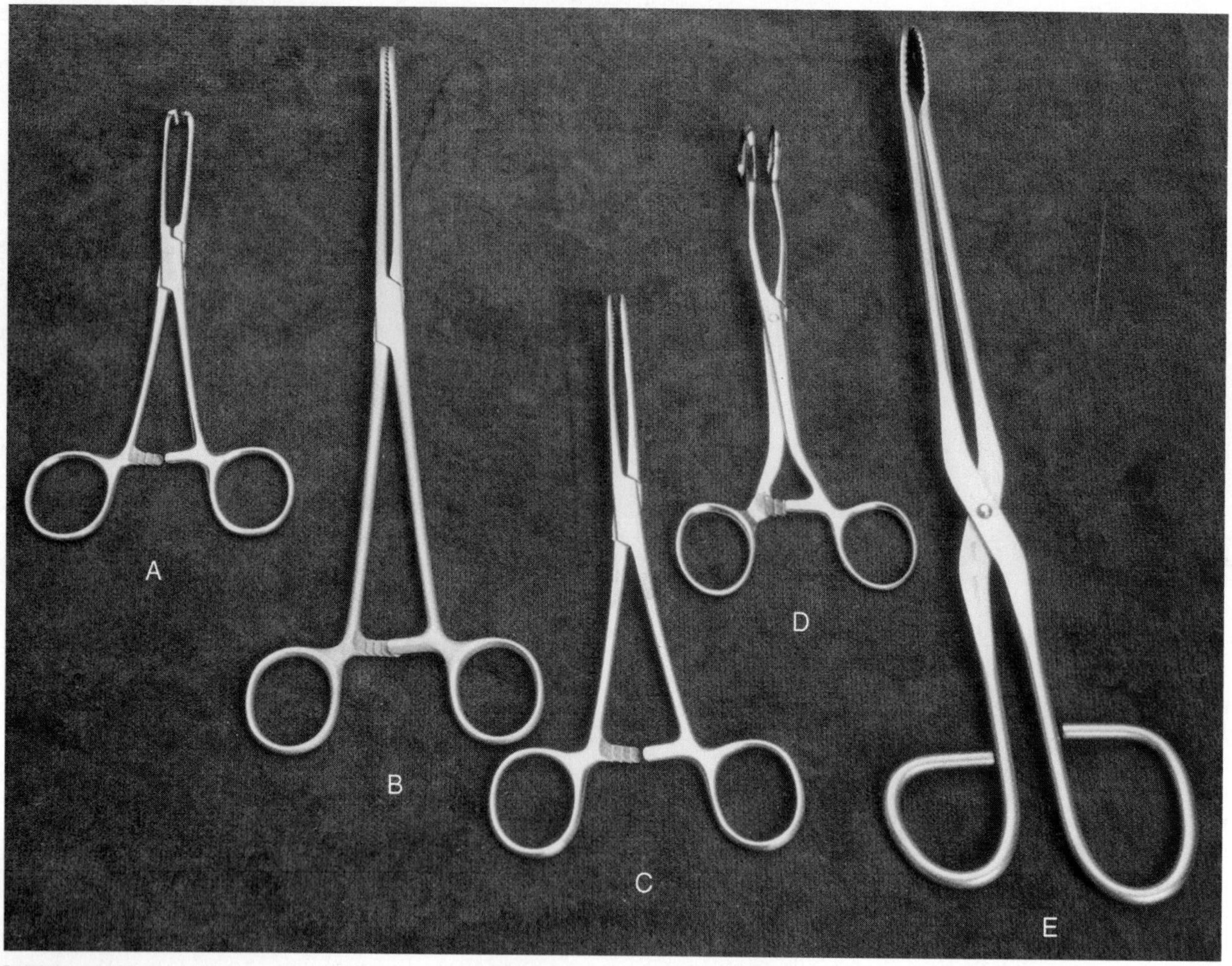

FIGURE 50–12 *A,* Allis forceps. *B,* Foerster sponge forceps. *C,* Straight transfer forceps. *D,* Short transfer forceps. *E,* Long transfer forceps.

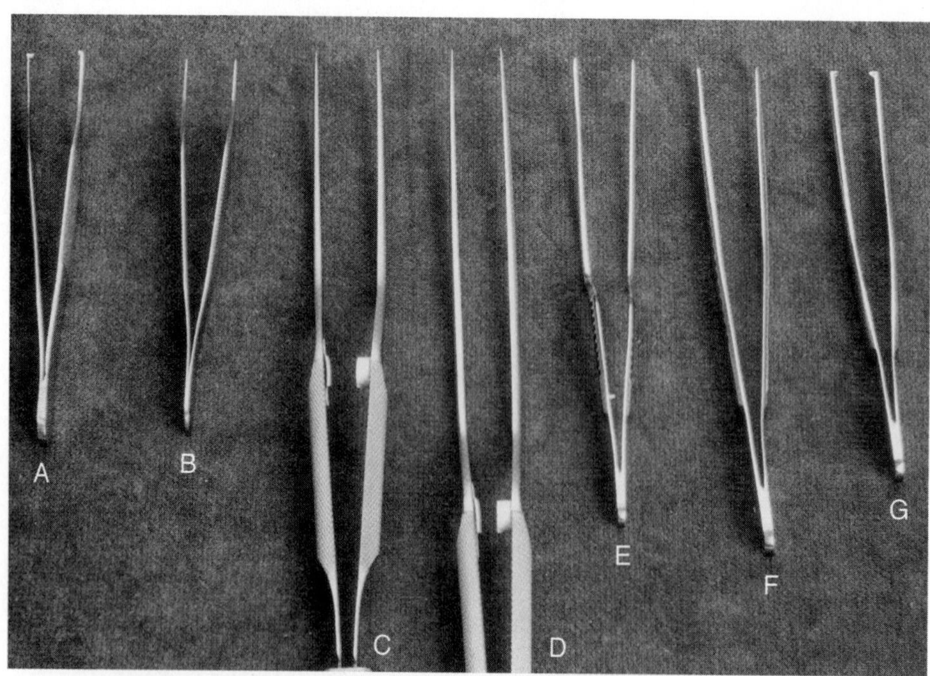

FIGURE 50–13 *A,* Toothed Adson forceps. *B,* Smooth Adson forceps. *C,* Medium long bayonet forceps. *D,* Long bayonet forceps. *E,* Short bayonet forceps. *F,* Plain-tip tissue forceps. *G,* Toothed tissue forceps.

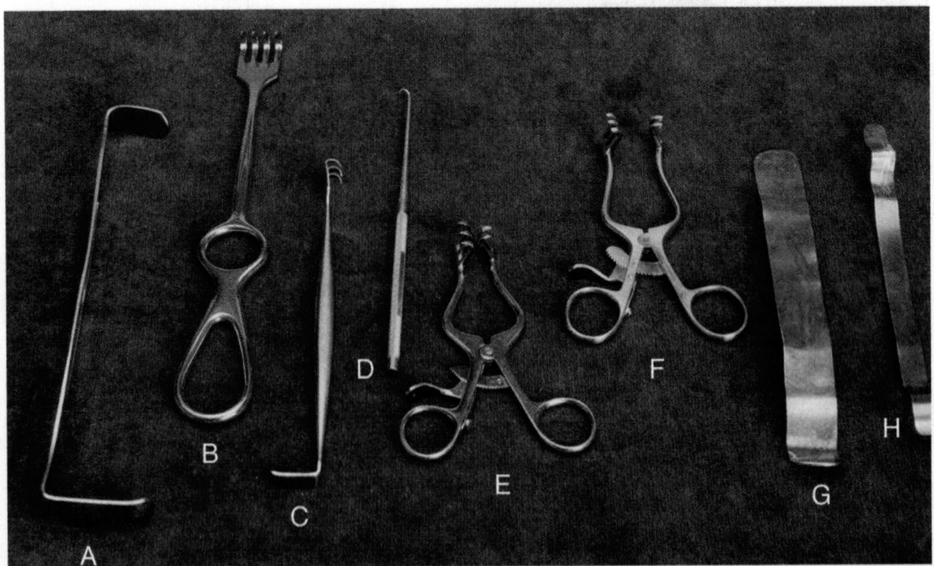

FIGURE 50–14 *A*, Army-Navy retractor. *B*, Four-prong rake retractor. *C*, Senn retractor. *D*, Single skin hook. *E*, Sharp 3/2 Weitlaner retractor. *F*, Dull 3/2 Weitlaner retractor. *G*, Wide Crile (ribbon) retractor. *H*, Narrow Crile (ribbon) retractor.

RETRACTORS

Retracting instruments hold tissue away from the surgical wound (incision). Depending on physician preference, skin hooks and Senn retractors are used to retract during most minor surgical procedures. These retractors are hand held and used for skin retraction. The Army-Navy hand-held retractor is used for deeper wounds. The medical assistant is required to hold it in place. A self-retaining retractor, a Weitlaner, holds itself in place and remains extended by mechanical means.

Army-Navy (Service) retractor (Fig. 50–14*A*)
- Used to retract small incisions.

Four-prong rake retractor (Fig. 50–14*B*)
- Pronged end may be sharp or dull.
- Manufactured in different lengths.

Senn retractor and skin hook (Fig. 50–14*C* and *D*)
- Used to retract small incisions or to secure a skin edge for suturing.
- Flat end is a blunt retractor.
- Three-prong end may be sharp or dull.

Weitlaner retractor (Fig. 50–14*E* and *F*)
- Used to retract incisions.
- Self-retaining.
- Available with sharp or blunt teeth.
- Available in different lengths.

Crile malleable (ribbon) retractor (Fig. 50–14*G* and *H*)
- Used to hold back margins of large wounds and connective tissue or organs from the surgeon's viewing field.

PROBES AND DILATORS

These instruments are used for both surgery and examinations. Probes may be used to search for a foreign body in a wound or to enter a **fistula.** Dilators are used to stretch a cavity or opening for examination or before inserting another instrument to obtain a tissue specimen.

Probes (Fig. 50–15*A* through *C*)
- Length ranges from 4 to 12 inches, available with or without bulbous tip.
- May be smooth or have a grooved director.
- Used to find foreign bodies embedded in dermal tissue.

Trocars and obturators (Fig. 50–15*D* through *G*)
- Consist of a sharply pointed **stylus (obturator)** contained in a **cannula** (outer tube).
- Available in various sizes.
- Used to withdraw fluids from cavities or for draining and irrigating with a catheter.

Specula (Fig. 50–16*A* through *D*)
- Most common dilator used.
- Valves are spread apart, dilating the opening.
- Used to open or distend a body orifice or cavity.

Nasal specula (Fig. 50–16*A* and *B*)
- Valves can be spread to facilitate viewing.
- An applicator or snare can be introduced through the valves.
- Used to spread the nostrils for examination.

SPECIALTY INSTRUMENTS

Although all instruments fall under the same four categories as the surgical instruments just discussed, the remaining instruments are organized into specialty groupings. Presenting the instruments in this manner makes it easy to see how the instruments relate to particular examinations. In addition to recognizing the name and usage of each instrument, you must organize and set out the instruments

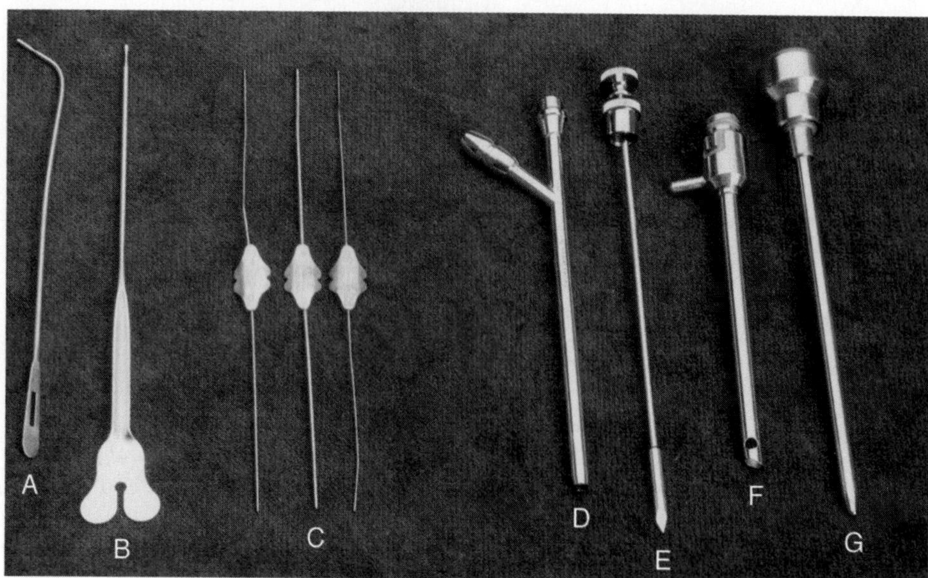

FIGURE 50–15 *A,* Probe. *B,* Grooved director. *C,* Lacrimal duct probes. *D,* Double-ended cannula. *E,* Sharp trocar. *F,* Cannula. *G,* Blunt-tip obturator.

needed for each particular examination on what is called a tray set-up.

Gynecology

Foerster sponge forceps (Fig. 50–17*A*)
- Used in the same way as the dressing forceps.
- Tips are round and serrated.

Placenta forceps (Fig. 50–17*B*)
- Used to remove tissue from the uterus.

Bozeman uterine dressing forceps (Fig. 50–17*C*)
- Used to swab the area or apply medication.
- Designed to hold sponges or dressings.
- Capable of reaching the cervix and vagina easily.

Endocervical curette (Fig. 50–17*D*)

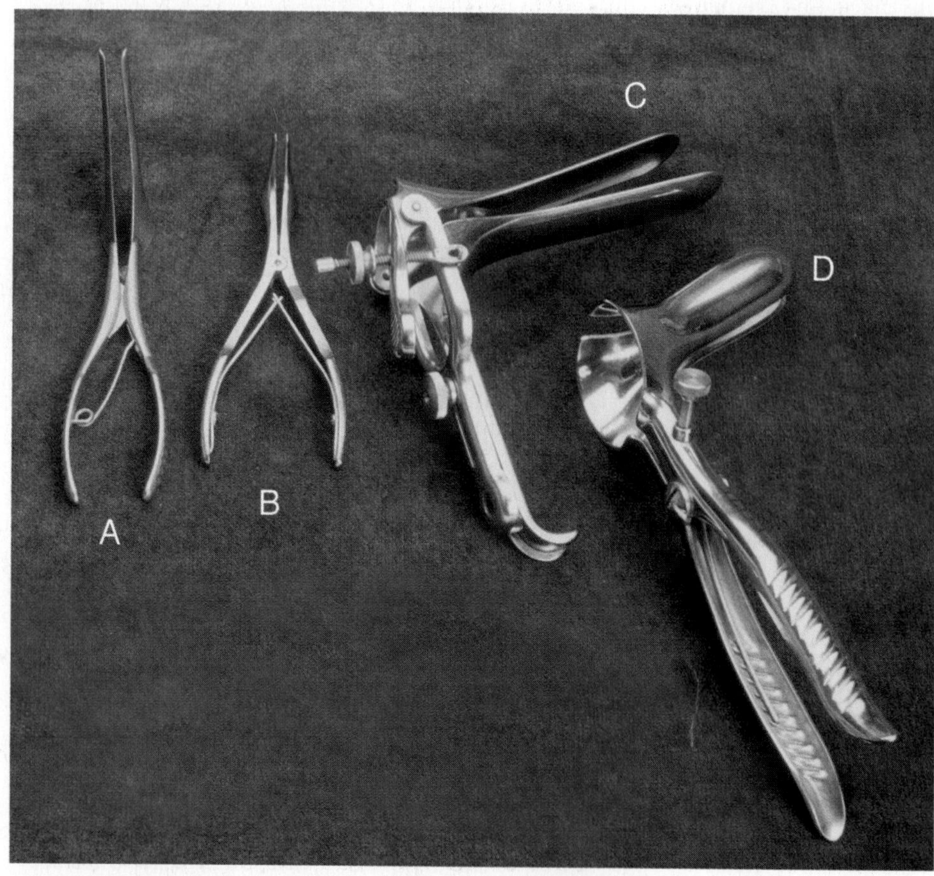

FIGURE 50–16 *A,* Long nasal speculum. *B,* Short nasal speculum. *C,* Graves vaginal speculum. *D,* Anal speculum, self-retaining.

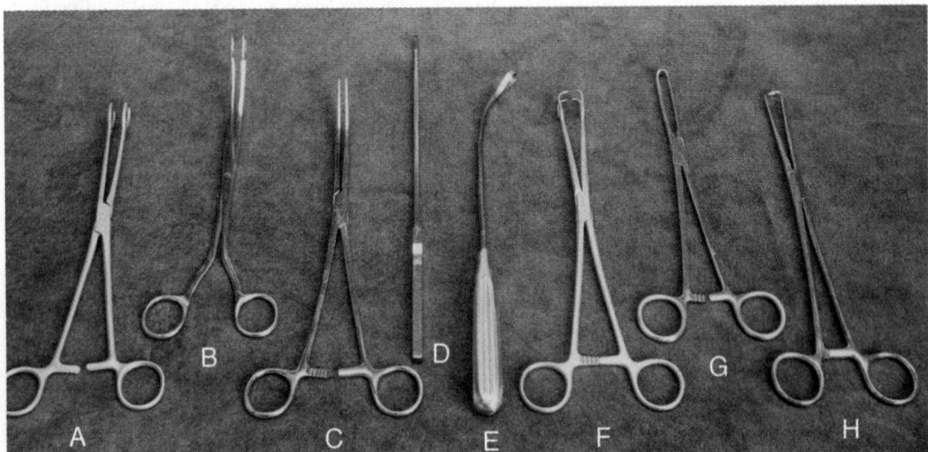

FIGURE 50–17 *A,* Foerster sponge forceps. *B,* Placenta forceps. *C,* Bozeman uterine dressing forceps. *D,* Endocervical curette. *E,* Sims uterine curette. *F,* Schroeder uterine vulsellum forceps. *G,* Long Allis forceps. *H,* Schroeder uterine tenaculum forceps.

- Smaller than the uterine curette.
- Used the same as the uterine curette.

Sims uterine curette (Fig. 50–17*E*)
- Used to remove **polyps,** secretions, and bits of placental tissue.
- Manufactured in several sizes.
- Hollow and spoon-shaped, used for scraping.

Schroeder uterine vulsellum forceps (Fig. 50–17*F*)
- Used to hold tissue (such as cervix) while obtaining a tissue specimen, or to lift the cervix to view the fornix.

Long Allis forceps (Fig. 50–17*G*)
- Same as Allis forceps.
- Used in deeper body cavities.

Schroeder uterine tenaculum forceps (Fig. 50–17*H*)
- Used in the same way as the vulsellum forceps.
- Have very sharp, pointed tips.

Hegar uterine dilators (Fig. 50–18*A*)
- Used to dilate the cervix for **dilatation** and **curettage.**
- Available in sets.
- Double or single ended.

Sounds (Fig. 50–18*B*)
- Used to check the **patency** of the cervical os or the urethral meatus.

Ophthalmology and Otolaryngology

Krause nasal snare (Fig. 50–19*A*)
- Has a wire loop at the tip that can be tightened.
- Used to remove polyps from the nares.

Metal tongue depressor (Fig. 50–19*B*)
- Used to depress the tongue for oral examinations.

Hartmann "alligator" ear forceps (Fig. 50–17*C* and *D*)
- Have a 3-½ inch shaft and is made in a variety of styles.
- Action of the jaw is similar to that of an alligator's jaw.
- Used to remove foreign bodies or polyps.

Laryngeal mirror (Fig. 50–19*D*)
- Made in various sizes.
- May have a nonfogging surface.
- Used for examination of the larynx and postnasal area.

Ivan laryngeal metal applicator (Fig. 50–19*E*)
- Holds cotton in place with its roughened end.
- Used to swab or sponge throat or postnasal tissue.
- Six to 9 inches long with curved end for use in throat or postnasal areas.

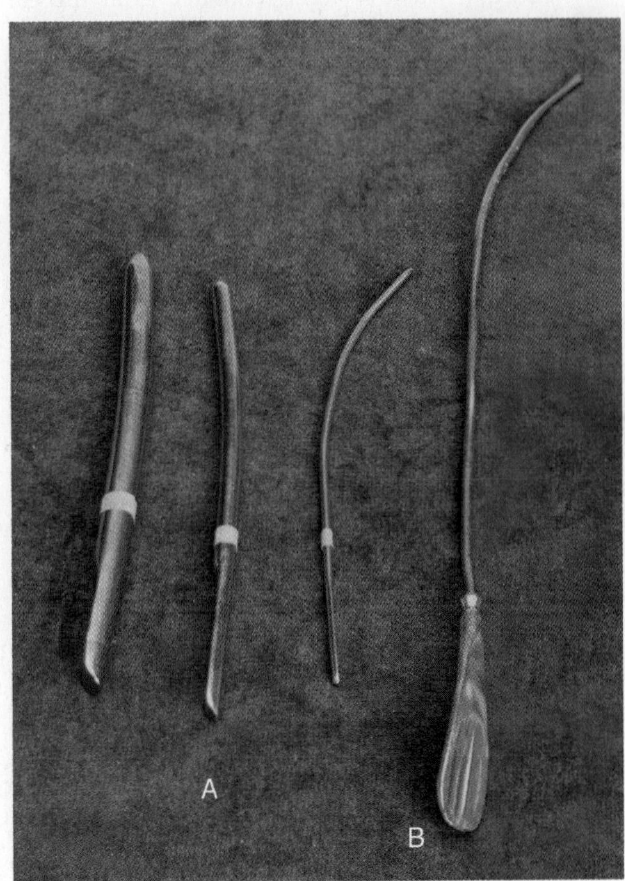

FIGURE 50–18 *A,* Uterine dilators. *B,* Sims uterine sounds.

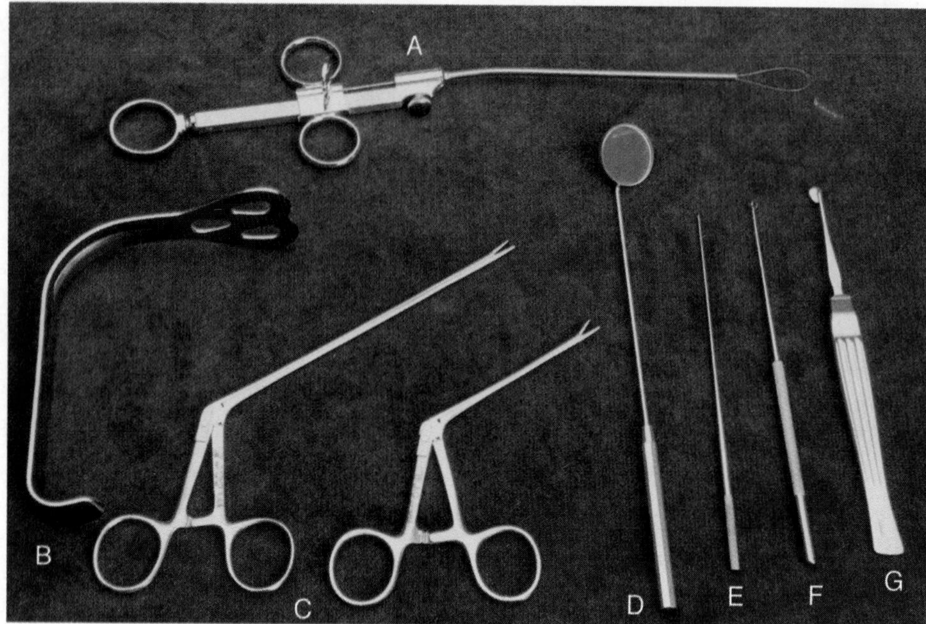

FIGURE 50–19 *A,* Krause nasal snare. *B,* Metal tongue depressor. *C,* Long and short alligator forceps. *D,* Laryngeal mirror. *E,* Ivan metal applicator. *F,* "Buck" ear curette. *G,* Sharp ear dissector.

Foreign body eye spud
- Used to remove foreign bodies imbedded in the eye.

Buck ear curette (Fig. 50–19*F*)
- Made with sharp or blunt scraper ends.
- Manufactured in various sizes.
- Used to remove foreign matter from the ear canals.

Sharp ear dissector (Fig. 50–19*G*)
- Used to remove debris from the ear canal.

Biopsy

Cervical biopsy forceps (Fig. 50–20*A*)
- Available with or without teeth.
- Used to obtain specimens for diagnostic examination.

Rectal biopsy punch (Fig. 50–20*B*)
- Manufactured with interchangeable stems.
- Available in different lengths and styles.
- Used through a proctoscope or sigmoidoscope.

Silverman biopsy needle
- Manufactured with a split cannula.
- Works on the same principle as an obturator.
- Stylus is removed, and cannula is inserted to retrieve specimen.
- Needle biopsy can eliminate the need for surgical incision.

Abscess needle
- Used to withdraw fluids or **suppuration** (pus) from a **cyst** or abscess.
- Usually are disposable.

Genitourinary

Brown-Buerger cystoscope, sheath, and obturator
- Used to visually examine the urethra and bladder.

Catheter guide (Fig. 50–21*A*)
- Metal device.
- Used with extreme caution.
- Used by the physician when it is impossible to insert a catheter by normal means.

Foley catheter (Fig. 50–21*B*)
- Manufactured in sizes 8 to 32 French.
- Manufactured with a double rubber lining toward the tip.
- After insertion, sterile solution is injected into the inner lining (inflating the balloon), to hold it in the bladder.
- Used as an indwelling catheter.

Robinson catheter (Fig. 50–21*C*)
- Soft rubber urethral catheter in sizes 8 to 32 French.
- The higher the number, the smaller the **lumen.**
- Inserted into the bladder for drainage or to obtain a specimen.

12-mL Luer-Lok syringe (Fig. 50–21*D*)
- Used for injecting amounts greater than 5 mL.

Colon-Rectal

Sigmoidoscope (Fig. 50–22*A* and *B*)
- Used to internally view the anus, rectum, and colon.
- Manufactured rigid or flexible.
- Used with a fiberoptic light source; may use photography or video set-up.

Memory Jogger

6 *Name the four major instrument classifications.*

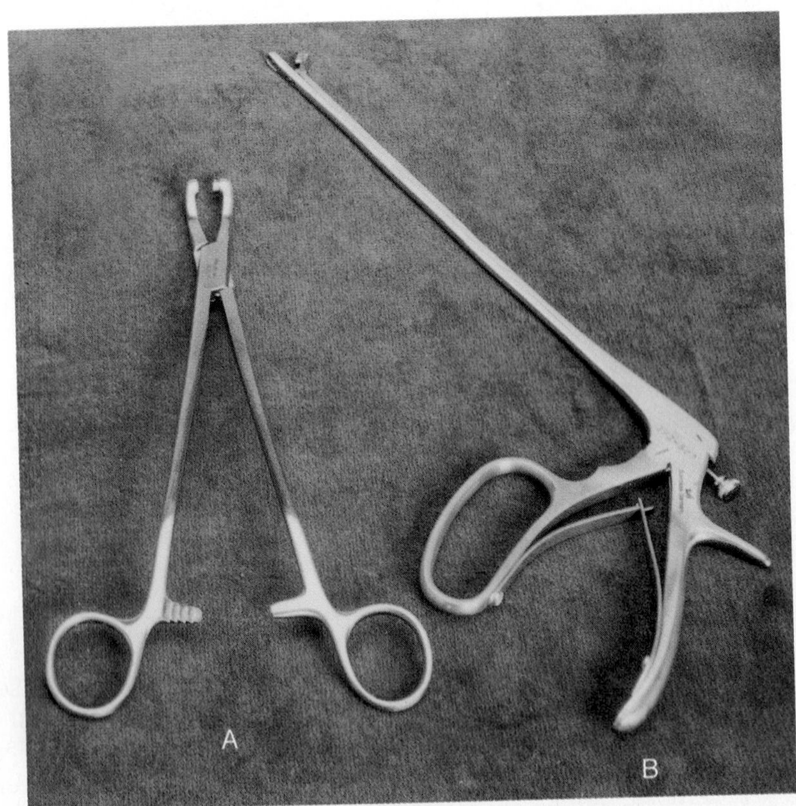

FIGURE 50–20 *A*, Cervical biopsy forceps. *B*, Rectal biopsy punch.

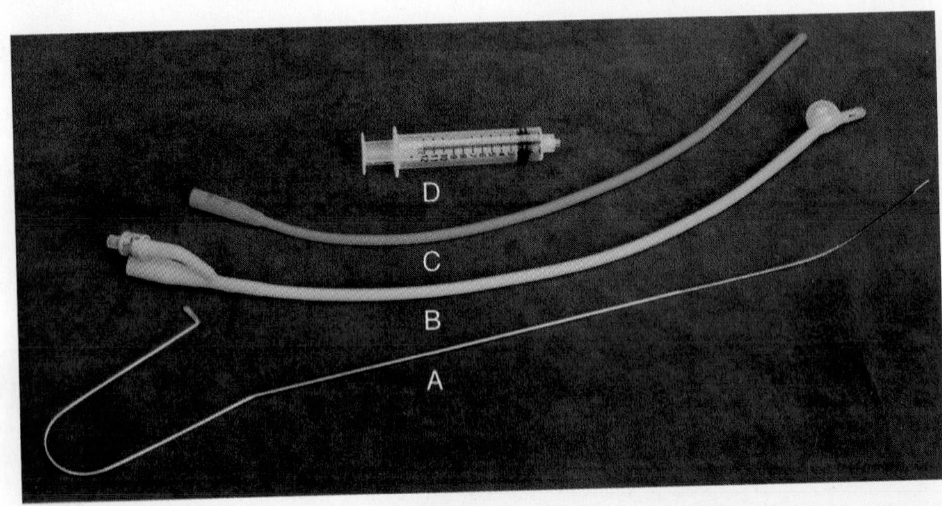

FIGURE 50–21 *A*, Metal catheter guide. *B*, Foley catheter with inflated balloon. *C*, Red Robinson catheter. *D*, 12-mL Luer-Lok syringe.

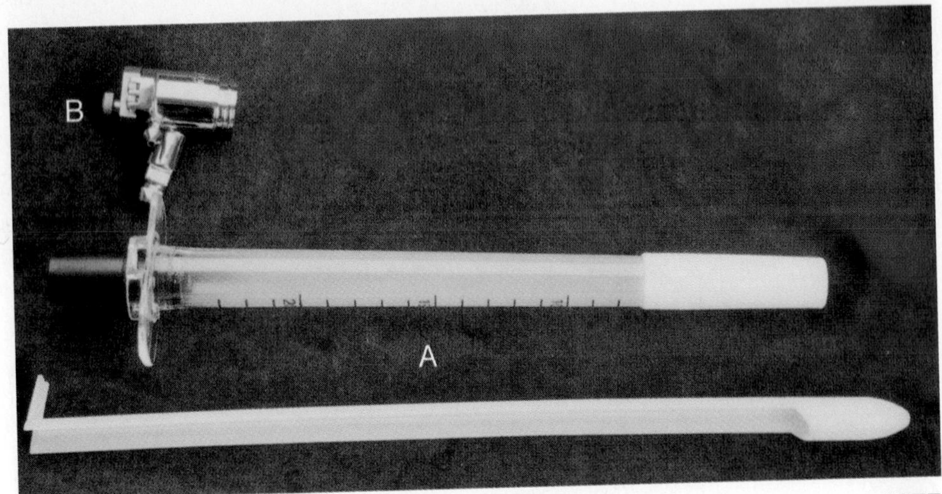

FIGURE 50–22 *A*, Rigid disposable sigmoidoscope. *B*, Nondisposable lens and light.

PROCEDURE 50-1

Identifying Surgical Instruments

GOAL

To identify, correctly spell, and determine the use(s) of standard office instruments or those selected by your instructor.

EQUIPMENT AND SUPPLIES

Curved hemostat
Straight hemostat
Dressing (thumb) forceps
Paper and pencil
Scalpel and blade
Dissecting scissors
Towel clamp
Vaginal speculum
Bandage scissors
Allis tissue forceps

PROCEDURAL STEPS

1 Look for the following parts that determine usage: box-lock, serrations, finger rings, cutting edge, noncutting edge, thumb type, teeth ratchets, and electric attachments.
PURPOSE: To determine the combination of features and parts for each instrument.

2 Consider the general classification of the instrument: cutting and dissection, grasping and clamping, retracting, or probing and dilating.
PURPOSE: The clue to the name of the instrument may be found by determining the classification.

3 Carefully examine the teeth and serrations.
PURPOSE: The clue to the name of the instrument may be found by determining its distinctive parts.

4 Look at the length of the instrument to determine the area of the body for which it is used.
PURPOSE: The clue to the name of the instrument may be found by determining where it can reach.

5 Try to remember whether the instrument was named for a famous physician, university, or clinic.
PURPOSE: Many instruments are named for the inventor.

6 If the instrument is a pair of scissors, look at the points and determine whether they are sharp-sharp, sharp-blunt, or blunt-blunt.

7 Carefully compare the instrument with similar instruments that you know, to determine whether it is in the same category or has the same name.
PURPOSE: The clue to the name of an instrument may be found with the knowledge you already have.

8 Write, with correct spelling, the complete name of each instrument, including its category and usage.

Care and Handling of Instruments

Because instruments are expensive and the physician's skill is dependent on the quality of the instruments, the medical assistant must properly care for each instrument to maximize its life and ensure that every part is in safe, working order.

Most instruments are made of fine-grade stainless steel. The term *stainless* is usually taken too literally. Although stainless steel does resist rust and keeps a fine edge and tip longer, even the best stainless steel may develop water spots and stains, especially if water with a high mineral content is used. Proper hardness and flexibility are important. Inexpensive instruments may be too brittle or too soft. Mistreatment of chrome-plated instruments can cause minute breaks in the finish, which may become a source of contamination or may tear the surgeon's gloves.

Instruments should be carefully examined when they are purchased. Scissors should be tested to see if they shear the full length of the blades completely to the tip. This can be checked by cutting a piece of cotton. If the scissors cut cleanly and do not chew at any point, even at the tip, they are functioning correctly. Teeth and serrations should be checked to see if they intermesh completely and if the jaws are even on the sides and tip. Each instrument should be felt over its entire surface for any rough areas that may tear or snag the surgeon's gloves. Boxlocks and hinges must work freely but should not be too loose. Thumb- and spring-handled instruments must have the correct tension and meet evenly at the tips.

Under no circumstances should instruments be bundled together or allowed to become entangled. Avoid mixing stainless steel instruments with others made of different metals. This may cause electrolysis and may result in etching. Even mixing stainless steel with chrome-plated instruments is best avoided. If an instrument is accidentally dropped, it may be permanently damaged. If scissors are dropped with the blades partially open, there may be a nick at the point at which the blades cross. Do not leave ratchets closed. Do not leave an instrument clamped onto material such as a drape or gauze.

Reserve a special place after the surgical procedure to receive contaminated instruments. This is usually a basin of water or a disinfectant solution placed in the sink within reach of the assistant (countertop). If a metal basin is used, it is advisable to place a small towel on the bottom of the basin to prevent damage to the instruments as they are placed or dropped in the solution. Never allow blood or other coagulable substances to dry on an instrument. If immediate cleaning is not possible, they should be rinsed well and placed in a cold water solution with a blood solvent and mild detergent. The detergent increases the wetting ability of the water, allowing the instrument surfaces to be better exposed to the solution. It is best to use a detergent that has a neutral pH. It should be low sudsing and easy to rinse off. Each manufacturer of the various disinfectants and blood solvents recommends the correct dilution and time of immersion for its product. Always follow the manufacturer's instructions.

Memory Jogger

What is the purpose of the detergent when washing instruments?

On completion of the surgical procedure, the receiving basin for the instruments is transferred from the surgical area to the cleaning and sterilization room. It is important to remove used instruments from the patient's view as soon as possible.

Separate the various types of instruments. Sharp instruments should be carefully handled to prevent damage to cutting edges or possible injury to the person sanitizing them. Rubber and plastic items are easily punctured and often discolor metals. Some plastic and rubber goods should not be soaked too long because they will discolor. Plastics may become porous and lose their glossy surface. Wash, sanitize, and sterilize surgical packs without delay. The instruments must be ready for the next scheduled procedure or any emergency. Surgical packs should be processed daily at a designated time, depending on the practice and surgical schedule of the facility.

Commercially prepared disposable packs are available for most minor surgical procedures. They are timesavers and convenient because they can eliminate linen laundering and supply autoclaving. One disadvantage may be high cost. Available packs include towel packs, skin prep packs, irrigation sets, suture sets, suture removal sets, catheterization sets, biopsy sets, and shave prep packs. Other types can be especially made for each office.

Disposable Surgical Drapes

Disposable surgical drapes are available in several different materials and sizes and may contain an opening (fenestration) for the operative site. A special incisional drape has an adhesive backing around the opening to prevent slippage (Fig. 50–23). This clear incisional drape adheres to the patient's cleansed skin and remains taped to the area throughout the procedure. The skin incision is made with the scalpel through the adhesive drape. Disposable drapes are rapidly replacing the use of autoclaved linen towels in the medical office.

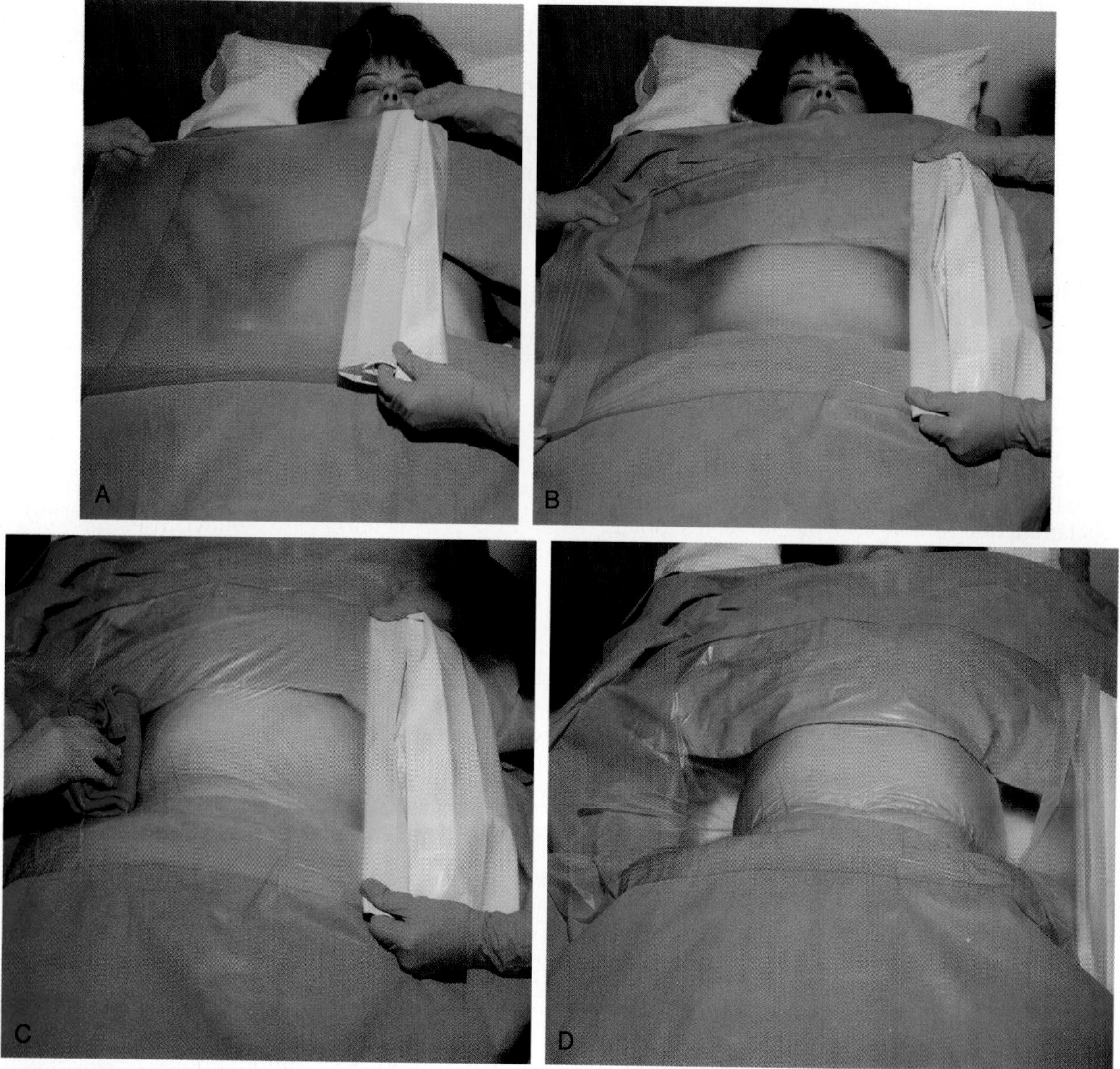

FIGURE 50–23 *A,* Application of adhesive-backed drape. *B,* Adhesive backing of drape removed. *C,* Drape secured with sterile towel. *D,* Ready for the incision.

Sutures

The word "suture" is used as both a noun and a verb. As a noun, it refers to a surgical stitch or to the material used. As a verb, it refers to the act of stitching. Sutures were used as long ago as 2000 BC. History does not record the first surgical operations and the use of sutures, but ancient medical writings do make reference to using sinews and strings to tie off blood vessels and control bleeding.

Modern surgery and the use of sutures began in 1865, when Lister developed antisepsis and the disinfection of suture materials. Many kinds of materials have been used over the centuries, including precious metals, horse hair, animal tendons, and cotton and linen cord. Most of the improvements in suture materials and techniques have occurred in the past 50 years.

A suture may also be used as a ligature. This is a strand of suture material used to tie off a blood vessel or to strangulate tissue. A ligature may be tied around a skin growth and left there until the growth is strangulated and falls off. If a ligature is used to tie off an internal tubular structure, it must last permanently or long enough for the structure itself to disintegrate. To "ligate" means to apply a ligature.

TYPES OF SUTURES

Sutures may be classified as either absorbable or nonabsorbable. Many different materials are avail-

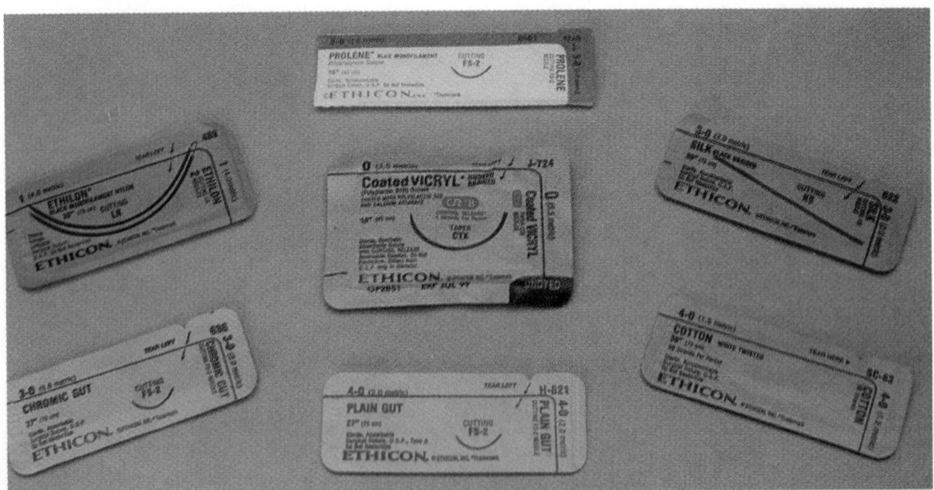

FIGURE 50–24 Suture packets labeled according to size, type, length, and type of needle point and shape.

able, each having its advantages and disadvantages. The following are commonly used suture materials in minor surgery procedures (Fig. 50–24).

Absorbable Suture

The absorbable suture dissolves and is absorbed by the body's enzymes during the healing process. Surgical catgut is used in tissue that heals rapidly. It is obtained from sheep, cattle, or pig intestine. It is packaged in an alcohol solution to keep it pliable. Dipping the suture strands in sterile saline solution helps to rinse the alcohol before using.

- Plain catgut is used in tissues that heal most rapidly, such as mucous membrane and subcutaneous tissues.
- Chromic catgut is coated with chromic salts, which delays its absorption rate to up to 80 days.
- Vicryl is a synthetic absorbable suture made of polyglactin. It may take 11 weeks to be absorbed.

Nonabsorbable Suture

Nonabsorbable suture either is left in the body (where it becomes imbedded in scar tissue) or is removed when healing is complete. It is frequently used in minor surgical procedures performed in the medical office because the majority of the suturing required is superficial and in areas where sutures can be removed after healing has taken place.

- Silk is used because it is strong and easy to tie. It is treated with a coating to prevent tissue drag and flaking.
- Surgical cotton is not as strong as silk but has the same applications. The use of cotton has diminished through the years with the use of polyester fiber.
- Polyester fiber suture is one of the strongest sutures along with surgical steel. These fine filaments are braided and have great tensile strength.
- Stainless steel is the strongest suture and is well tolerated by the body. It is difficult to handle and can be easily contaminated during a procedure. The end of the wire suture is controlled by the medical assistant while the surgeon sutures. It can be hand held, or a small hemostat can be applied to the end while suturing. Surgical staples are used. They are also made of stainless steel or titanium and are available in different sizes. They are used on skin, nerves, blood vessels, and small structures and are applied with clip appliers (Fig. 50–25).
- Nylon suture is strong and has a high degree of elasticity. It is primarily used for skin closure. Owing to its elasticity and stiffness, many knots must be used, and these knots tend to untie if placed incorrectly.

Memory Jogger

8 *How are sutures classified?*

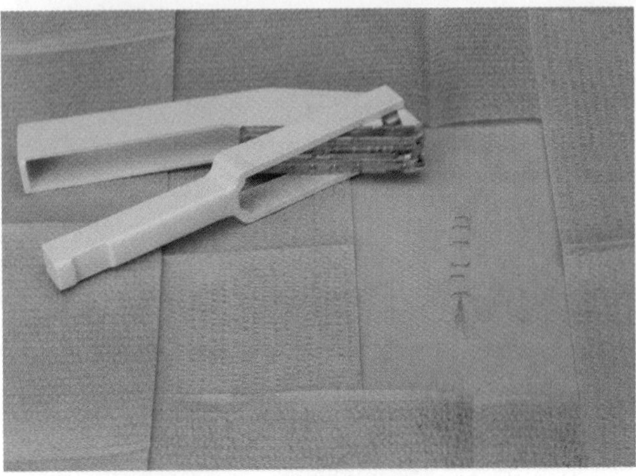

FIGURE 50–25 Disposable skin stapler.

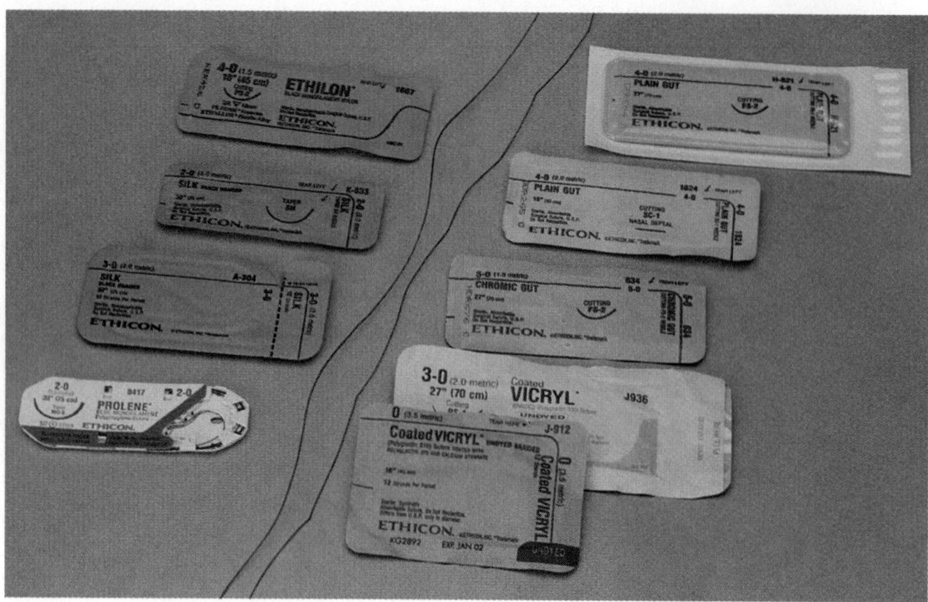

FIGURE 50–26 Suture packets (and opened suture strands) with and without needles.

SUTURE SIZING AND PACKAGING

The diameter of the suture strand determines its size; for instance, 2-0 is thinner than size 0. Size 0 is thinner than size 2. Sutures as thin as size 11-0 and as thick as size 7 are available. The sizes from 2-0 to 6-0 are the most frequently used in the medical office. The length of the suture may vary. Strands are precut in 18-, 24-, 54-, and 60-inch lengths (Fig. 50–26).

Memory Jogger

Which is the smallest (thinnest) diameter suture, 2-0 or 0?

Needles

Surgical needles are chosen according to the area in which they are to be used and the depth and width of the desired suture. They are classified according to the shape and by the type of point, shaft, and eye (Fig. 50–27). The shape of a needle may be straight or curved. Straight needles are not easily manipulated and are used on the skin. A curved needle allows the surgeon to penetrate the surface and then back up again on the other side. The sharper the curve of the needle, the deeper the surgeon can pass the needle. The point of a needle can be a taper or a cutting edge. A taper is used on delicate tissues. The cutting edge needle is used on the skin. It lacerates the skin as the needle is passed through. This is advantageous on the tougher tissues, such as connective tissue.

The needle can have an eyelet or can be eyeless. Atraumatic needles do not have an eyelet. These cause the least amount of tissue trauma as they are passed through the tissues. Manufacturers supply the suture strands with the suture needle attached in peel-apart sterile disposable packages. These may be obtained single-individual packed or multipacked sutures. The suture materials used in the medical office are prepackaged atraumatic and disposable. The most common needle type for minor skin repair is the curved, cutting-edged, atraumatic needle.

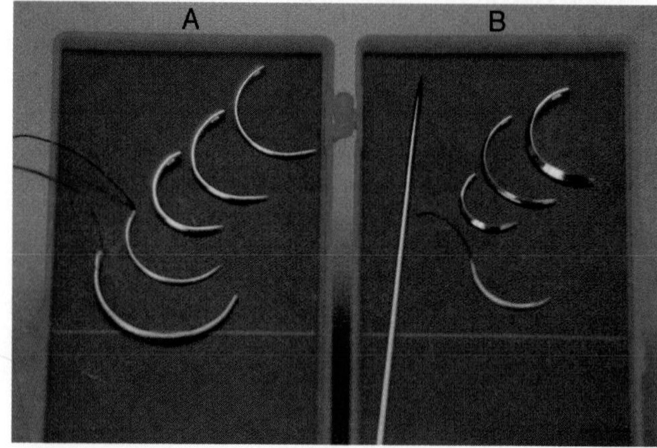

FIGURE 50–27 Surgical needle shapes. *A*, Taper point. *B*, Cutting point.

Memory Jogger

10 *What is the most common needle type for minor skin repair?*

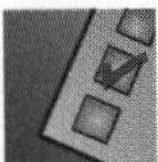

PATIENT EDUCATION

Patients may have questions concerning the instruments the surgeon is using. The medical assistant can assist the patient by answering his or her curious or anxious questions to help alleviate any fears. Explaining the surgical procedure and what to expect afterward helps make the procedure easier to perform and encourages the patient to follow the physician's advice and orders.

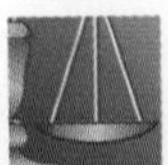

LEGAL AND ETHICAL ISSUES

When surgical procedures are to be performed in the medical office, awareness of legal responsibilities is imperative. The medical assistant must know what procedure is to be performed and whether the patient has been informed regarding the procedure. In the surgical setting, the medical assistant must realize the full extent of his or her role as the "patient's advocate" and the "physician's agent."

Confirm the fact that the physician has explained the procedure to the patient and that the patient fully understands all aspects of the procedure that will be performed. This means that when the patient signs the consent for surgery, he or she is fully informed. Increasing the patient's understanding ensures greater compliance with the presurgical preparations, the surgical procedure, and the postsurgical care.

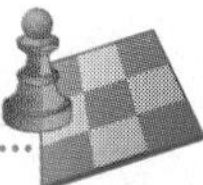

CRITICAL THINKING

1 Who do you think is responsible for making certain that all consent forms are signed before treatment?

2 If an instrument is dropped during a procedure, and there isn't a duplicate available, what do you do?

3 Why is it recommended that office surgery be done in a special room and not in one of the regular examination rooms?

HOW DID I DO? Answers to Memory Joggers

1 Equipment should include a clock with a sweep second-hand, an operating light, stools to sit on, and a Mayo stand.

2 Sterile water—diluent for medications and rinsing instruments. Saline—injections and rinsing and irrigating.

3 Epinephrine causes vasoconstriction, minimizes local bleeding, maximizes site swelling, and distorts approximation of the wound edges.

4 Iodoform gauze strips are used to pack an abscess.

5 Instruments are named for their use or after the person who developed them.

6 Cutting, grasping, retracting, and probing and dilating.

7 Detergent increases the wetting ability of the water.

8 Sutures are classified absorbable or nonabsorbable.

9 The thinnest is 2-0.

10 A curved, cutting-edged, atraumatic needle.

Surgical Methods

51

Mary Jane McClain, RN, BS, CNOR

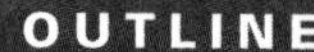

OUTLINE

LEARNING OBJECTIVES

Cognitive: On successful completion of this chapter you should be able to:

1 Define and spell the terms in the Vocabulary.
2 Define concepts of "aseptic technique."
3 List safety precautions for electrosurgery.
4 List safety precautions for laser surgery.

Performance: On successful completion of this chapter you should be able to:

1 Perform surgical hand scrub.
2 Demonstrate the open-glove method.
3 Demonstrate sterile gloving with closed-glove method.

VOCABULARY

coagulum A blood clot
don To put on sterile gown and gloves
fomites Any substance that adheres to and transmits infectious material
microsurgery Surgery performed under a microscope using very small instruments
pedunculated Having a stemlike connecting part
photocoagulation Clotting of blood with light
plume Carbon and steam byproducts from the electrical surgical unit or laser
slough Shedding away of dead tissue cells

There are so many different minor surgical procedures and set-ups, and each physician–medical assistant team has individual preferences. We cannot cover all minor surgical procedures or even list all the specific items that may be used for a specific technique. The following procedures are merely composites of acceptable practices in minor surgical techniques. Once you know these basics, with a little background information you will be able to assist with any minor surgical procedure.

Minor surgery may be used to remove a mass, small tumor, or bone spur (overgrowth of bone). These lesions may be caused by a variety of reasons and may cause a problem with the patient's activities of daily living. An incision is made after the application of local anesthetic. A basic set-up with sterile instruments, drapes, and suture is used.

Aseptic Technique

There is no mystery about aseptic technique. Handling sterile items requires a degree of dexterity and vigilance, but it is really a matter of concentration, with planned movements and steps.

Although the procedures outlined in this chapter and the next are for minor surgery, all the sterile techniques of major surgery must be observed. To have a sound knowledge of sterility and sterile technique, start with the following analogy:

Everything sterile is white, everything that is not sterile is black, and there is no gray.

Sterile surfaces must not come into contact with nonsterile surfaces. Honesty is important. An incomplete or incorrect step may lead to serious wound contamination and postoperative infection.

Memory Jogger

 *State the basic analogy of sterile technique.*

PERSONNEL

Hands and hair are two of the greatest sources of contamination. With practice, you will learn to know what may be touched with the hands and what must be touched with only sterile gloved hands. Hair that is allowed to fall free over the shoulders and forward will give off a cloud of bacteria. It must be contained back and off the shoulders.

FUNDAMENTAL RULES

- Remember that air currents carry bacteria, so body motions and talking over a sterile field should be kept to a minimum.
- Sterile team members face each other.
- Always keep the sterile field in your line of vision. Never turn your back on a sterile field or wander away from the sterile field.
- Nonsterile persons do not reach over a sterile field.

Memory Jogger

 *Identify the two greatest sources of contamination.*

THE STERILE FIELD

A sterile field is any sterile surface on which sterile items are placed. In surgery, a sterile field is created by draping sterile towels, prepackaged or from autoclaved packs, over a Mayo stand or table. A sterile field is also the draped surgical site after the patient's skin has been prepped and draped for a surgical procedure.

CORRECT STERILE FIELD TECHNIQUES

- Sterile field towels and sterile table drapes are fanfolded so that they may be unfolded easily by lifting one edge.
- If an entire set-up is in a single package and is double wrapped, the wrappings can be left underneath as the sterile table drape.
- Sterile tables are sterile only at table height.

- Any item below your waist level must be considered contaminated.
- A 1-inch edge around the entire sterile field is considered not sterile.
- The edges of all wrappers, packs, and towels are considered not sterile.
- The sides of containers are considered not sterile.
- Sterile goods must not be allowed to come into contact with the 1-inch margin around the sterile field, the edges of wrappers, or the sides of containers.
- If the sterility of an item is questionable, consider the item contaminated.

Memory Jogger

 *Why are sterile towels and sterile table drapes fanfolded?*

MOISTURE

Moisture carries bacteria from a nonsterile surface to a sterile surface. Therefore

- A sterile field placed on a drop of moisture results in the contamination of the field.
- Spills contaminate a sterile field.
- Sterile wrapped and packaged items must remain dry.
- Polylined sterile drapes can prevent wicking.

Preparing Sterile Packs

Surgical packs must be prepared the day before the procedure or at least in enough time for the pack to be dry and cool for the surgical procedure (see Chapter 26):

- Before closing the pack to be autoclaved, take a count on at least two separate occasions of the items required for the procedure. Use a procedure file card for guidance.
- If the items are numerous, label the pack with the name of the procedure rather than the individual contents.
- Instruments can be arranged on the sterile field in their sequence of use with sterile gloved hands.
- If disposable sterile towels and drapes are not used, you may autoclave linen towels. These towels must be approved for use and should be 100% cotton and properly woven for steam permeability. One or two fanfolded in a package are commonly used.
- In many cases, an entire set-up may be autoclaved in one pack (instruments, sponges, dressings, suture materials, syringes, and needles); however, you must be certain that the pack is not so thick that it prevents steam circulation to all the parts of the pack.
- Sterility indicators should be placed in the very middle of large packs to indicate whether proper sterilization has occurred through the pack.
- In case of contamination, it is always best to have more than one pack ready for every procedure.

Memory Jogger

 *Why is it best to have more than one pack ready for every procedure?*

Surgical Asepsis

Surgical asepsis is defined as the destruction of organisms before they enter the body. This technique is used for any procedure that invades the body's skin or tissues, such as surgery or injections. Any time the skin or mucous membrane is punctured, pierced, or incised (or will be, during a procedure), surgical aseptic techniques are practiced. The surgical hand wash (scrub) must be used. Everything that comes into contact with the patient should be sterile, such as gowns, drapes, instruments, and the gloved hands of the surgical team. Minor surgery, urinary catheterizations, injections, and some specimen collections (e.g., blood and biopsy specimens) are performed using surgical aseptic technique.

Because it is not possible to sterilize your hands, the goal of the hand scrub is to reduce skin bacteria by the use of mechanical friction, special surgical soaps, and running water. Normally, there are two types of bacteria on your skin:

- *Transient bacteria*—These are surface bacteria that are introduced by **fomites** and remain with you a short time.
- *Resident bacteria*—These are found under fingernails, in hair follicles, in the openings of the sebaceous glands, and in the deeper layers of the skin.

Resident bacteria in the deeper skin layers come to the surface with perspiration, which is why sterile gloves are used in addition to the surgical scrub. Some agencies recommend that you scrub for a specific number of minutes. Others count the number or scrub strokes. Follow the guidelines of your employer and take periodic cultures from your scrubbed hands to determine whether your technique is effective.

Memory Jogger

 *State the goal of the hand scrub.*

TABLE 51–1 How to Distinguish Between Medical and Surgical Asepsis

	Medical Asepsis	Surgical Asepsis
Definition	Destruction of organisms *after* they leave the body	Destruction of organisms *before* they enter the body
Purpose	Prevent reinfection of the patient. Avoid cross-infection from one person to another	Care for open wounds. Use in surgery
Technique	Universal blood and body-fluid precautions Isolation techniques	Sterile technique
Procedure	Clean objects are kept from contamination Clean gloves and clean barriers used Objects disinfected as soon as possible after contact with the patient	Objects must be sterile Sterile gloves and articles used Objects must be sterilized before contact with the patient
When used	For examinations that do not involve open wounds or breaks in the skin or mucous membranes but do involve patient blood or body fluids. Isolating infected persons from others	Surgery, biopsy, wound treatment, insertion of instruments into sterile body cavities
Hand wash technique	Hands and wrists washed for 1 to 2 minutes; soap, water, and plenty of friction used to remove oil and microorganisms from fingers Hands held downward, running water allowed to drain off fingertips; hands dried with paper towels	Hand and forearms scrubbed for 3 to 10 minutes; surgical soap, running water, friction, and sterile brush used; fingernails must be cleaned Hands held up, under running water, to drain off elbows; hands dried with sterile towels

The Hand Scrub

As stated in Chapter 26, there are two types of asepsis: medical and surgical. The purpose of both the medical and the surgical hand washing techniques is infection control. However, there are differences between the two (Table 51–1). The surgical hand wash is the same as the medical hand wash with the exception of several adaptations, which are described in Procedure 51–1. Gloving and gowning are described in Procedures 51–2 through 51–4.

Text continued on page 1104

PROCEDURE 51–1
Hand Scrubbing for Assisting with Surgical Procedures

GOAL

To scrub your hands with surgical soap, using friction, running water, and a sterile brush to sanitize your skin before assisting with any procedure that requires surgical asepsis.

EQUIPMENT AND SUPPLIES

Sink with foot or arm control for running water
Surgical soap in a dispenser
Towels
Nail file or orange stick
Sterile brush

PROCEDURAL STEPS

1 Remove all jewelry.
PURPOSE: Jewelry harbors bacteria and is not permitted in surgical asepsis.
2 Inspect your fingernails for length and your hands for skin breaks.
3 Turn on the faucet and regulate the water to a comfortable temperature.

Continued

PROCEDURE 51–1 (CONTINUED)
Hand Scrubbing for Assisting with Surgical Procedures

4 Keep your hands upright and held at or above waist level (Figure 1).
PURPOSE: Water running from the nonscrubbed area above the elbow down to the hands will drag bacteria back onto the hands. All areas below the waist are considered contaminated during all surgical procedures.

5 Clean your fingernails with a file, discard it, and rinse your hands under the faucet without touching the faucet or the insides of the sink basin (Figure 2).

6 Allow water to run over your hands, apply acceptable solution, lather while holding your fingertips upward, and remember to rub between the fingers (Figures 3 and 4).
PURPOSE: The surfaces of the fingers have four sides.

7 Wash wrists and forearms while holding your hands above waist level (Figures 5 and 6). Rinse arms and forearms without touching the faucet or the insides of the sink basin.
PURPOSE: Always keep away from the contaminated faucet and basin.

Continued

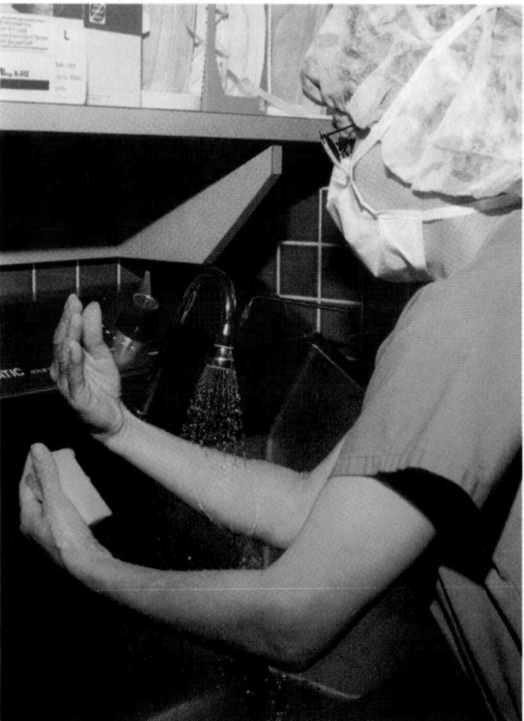

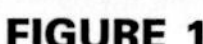

FIGURE 1

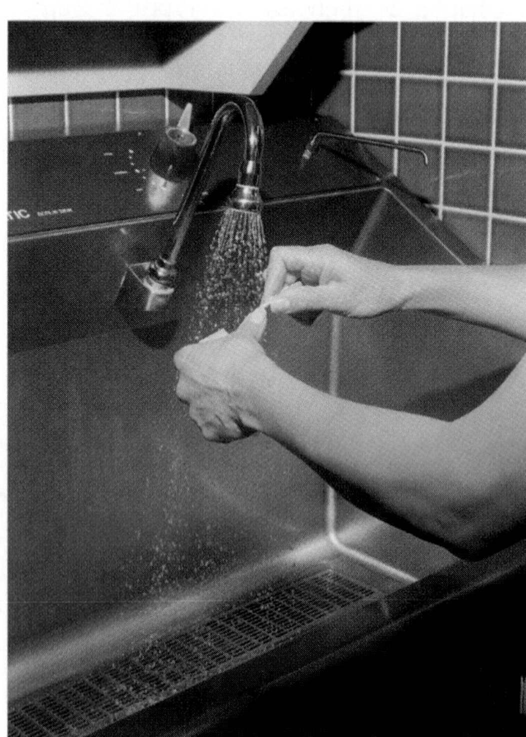

FIGURE 2

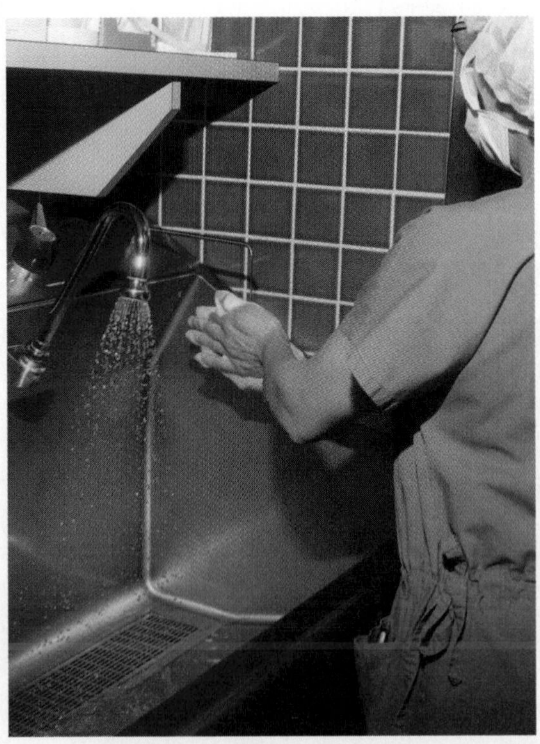

FIGURE 3

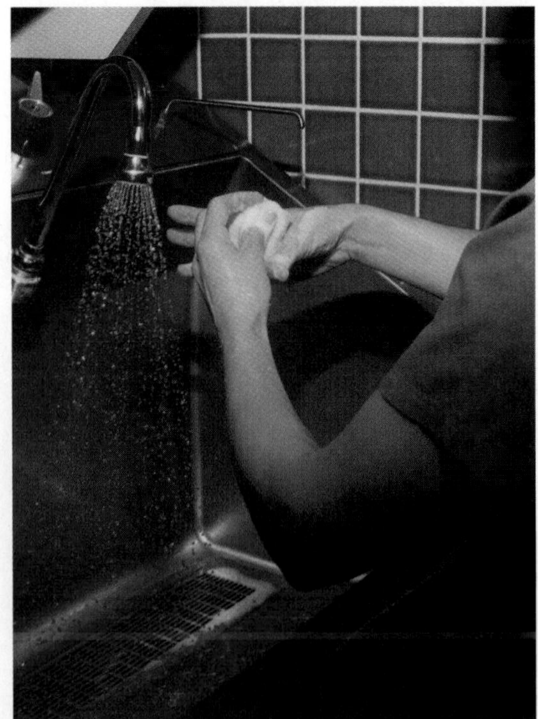

FIGURE 4

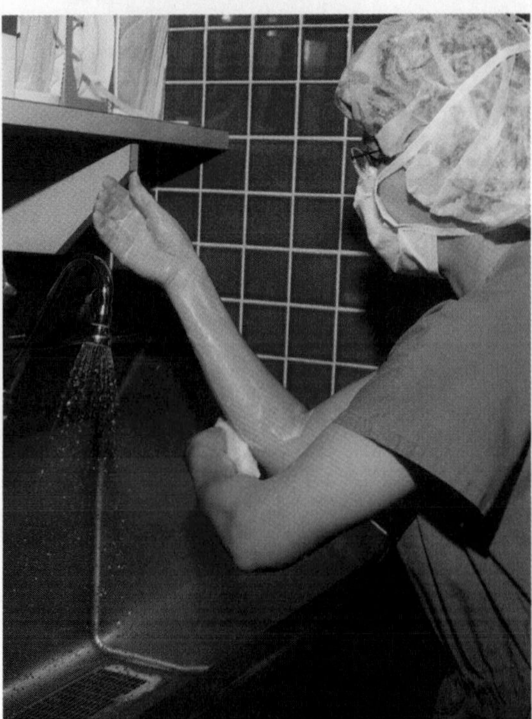

FIGURE 5

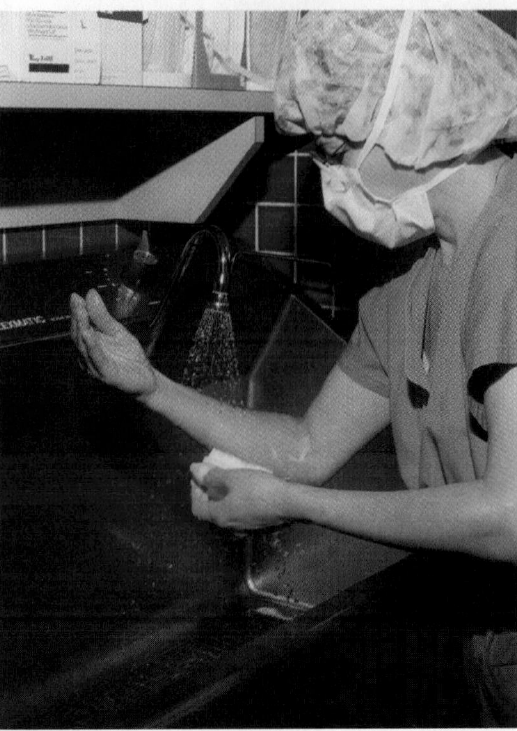

FIGURE 6

Continued

PROCEDURE 51–1 (CONTINUED)

Hand Scrubbing for Assisting with Surgical Procedures

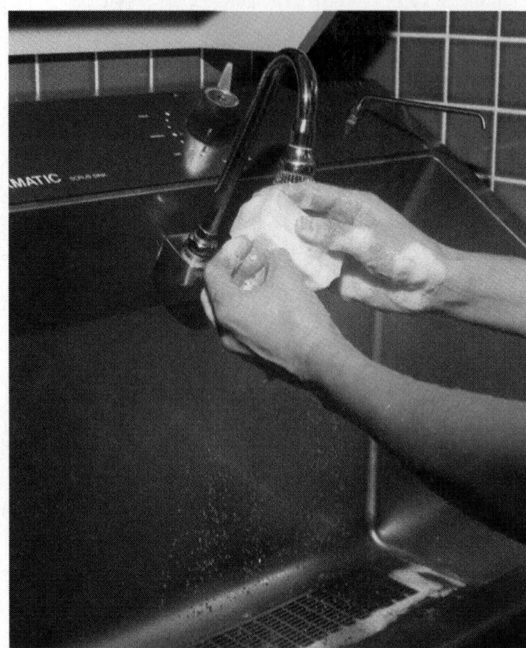

FIGURE 7

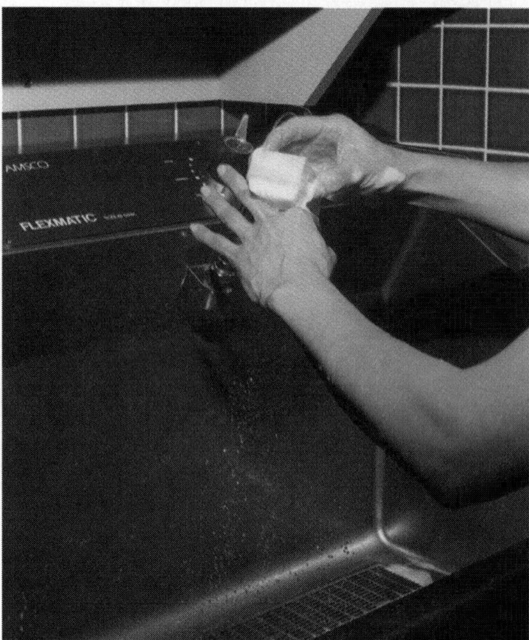

FIGURE 8

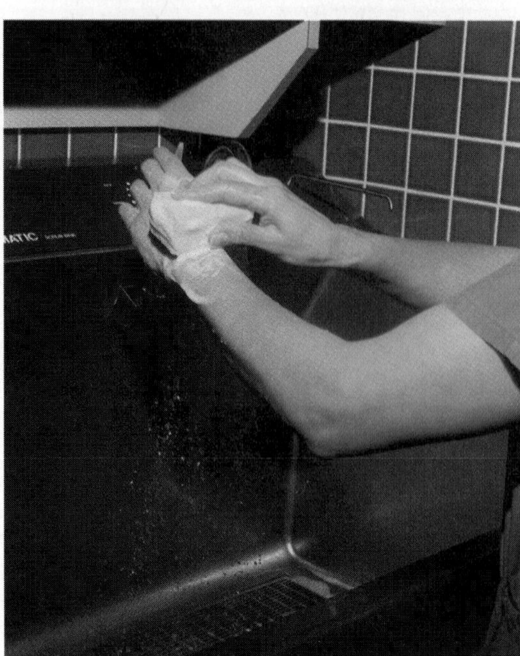

FIGURE 9

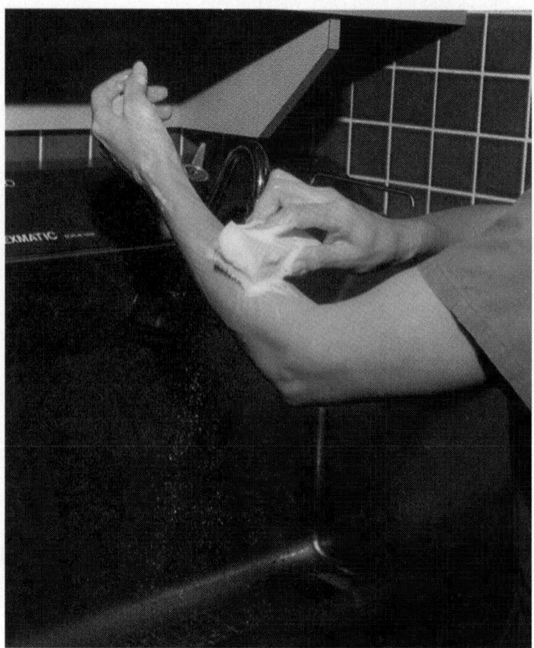

FIGURE 10

Continued

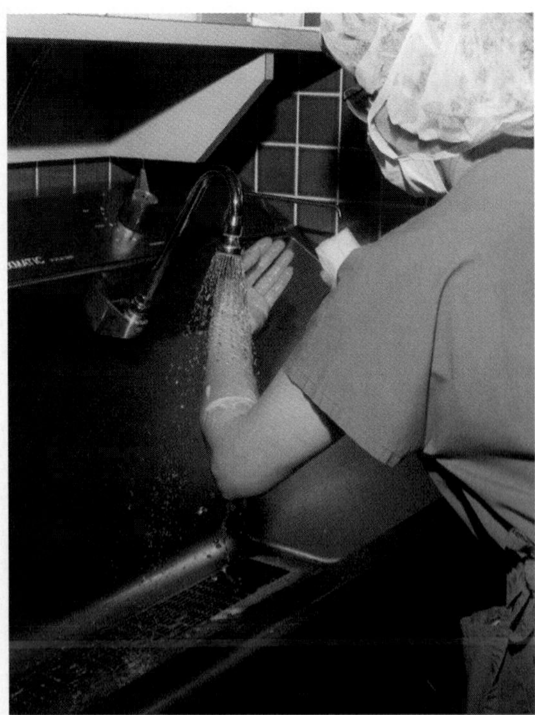

FIGURE 11

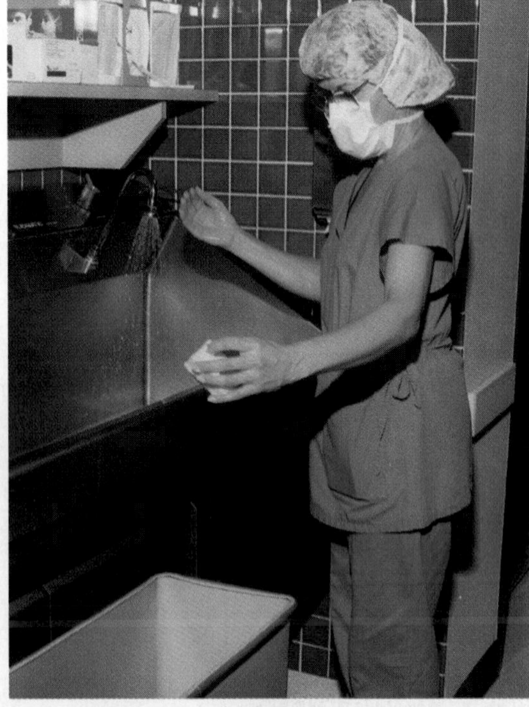

FIGURE 12

8 Apply more solution and repeat the scrub on the other side, remembering to wash and use friction between each finger with a firm, circular motion (Figures 7 and 8).

9 Scrub all surfaces with a brush, being careful not to abrade your skin. The second washing process should take at least 3 minutes (Figures 9 and 10).

10 Rinse thoroughly, keeping your hands up and above waist level. Discard scrub brush (Figures 11 through 13).

Continued

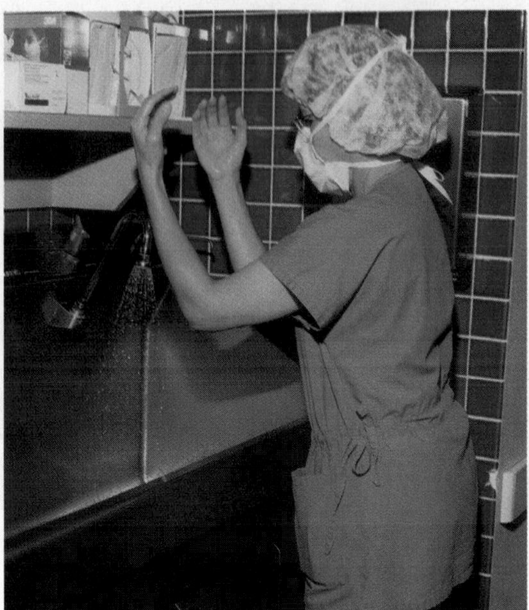

FIGURE 13

PROCEDURE 51–1 (CONTINUED)
Hand Scrubbing for Assisting with Surgical Procedures

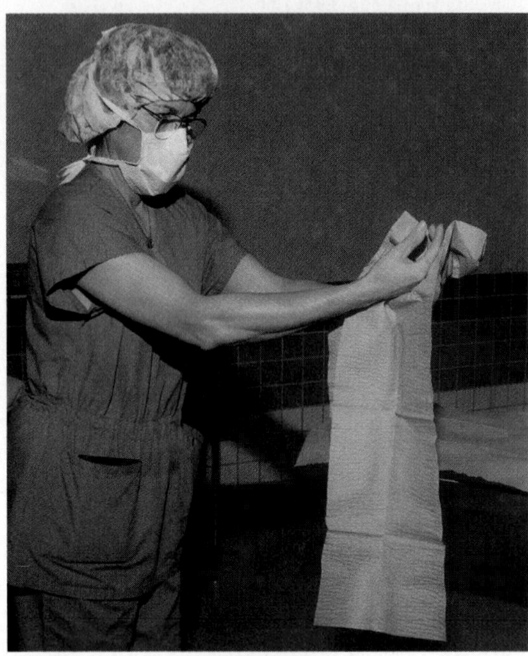

FIGURE 14

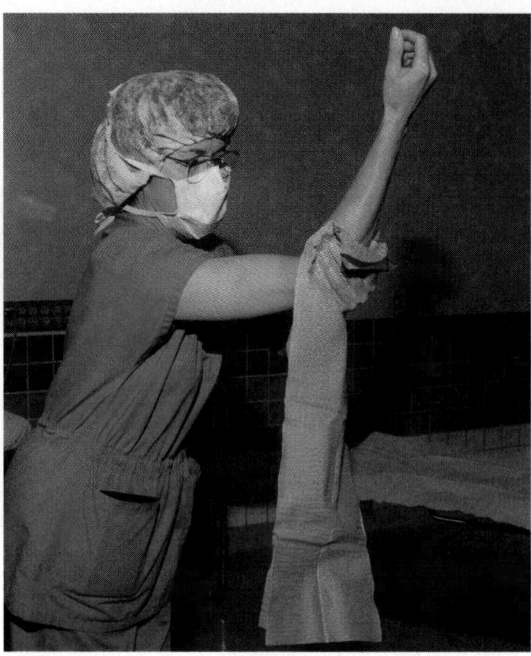

FIGURE 15

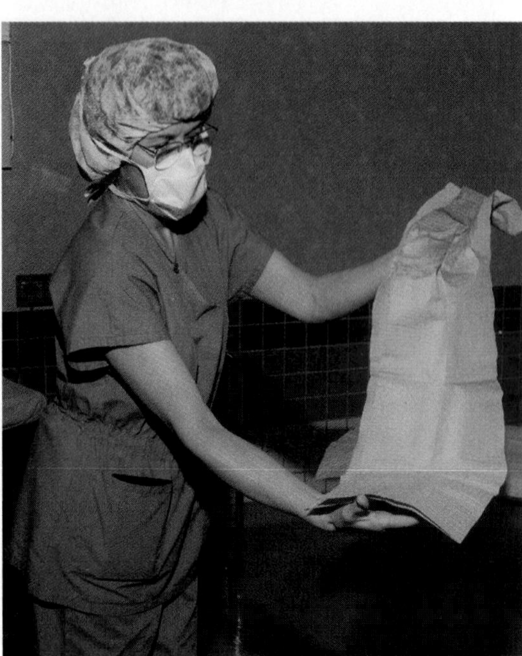

FIGURE 16

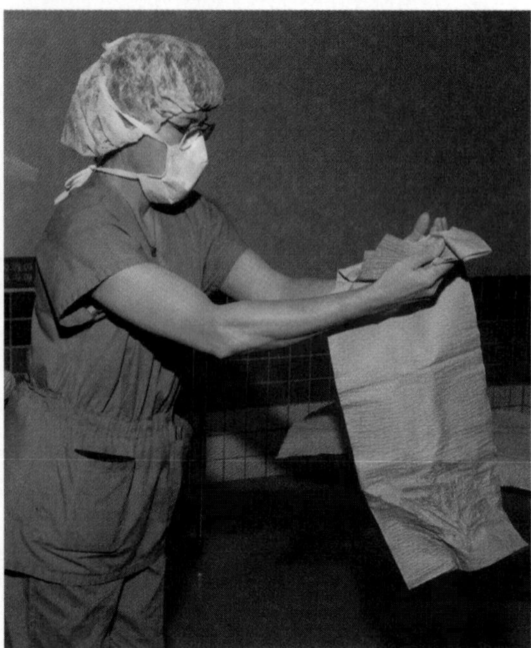

FIGURE 17

Continued

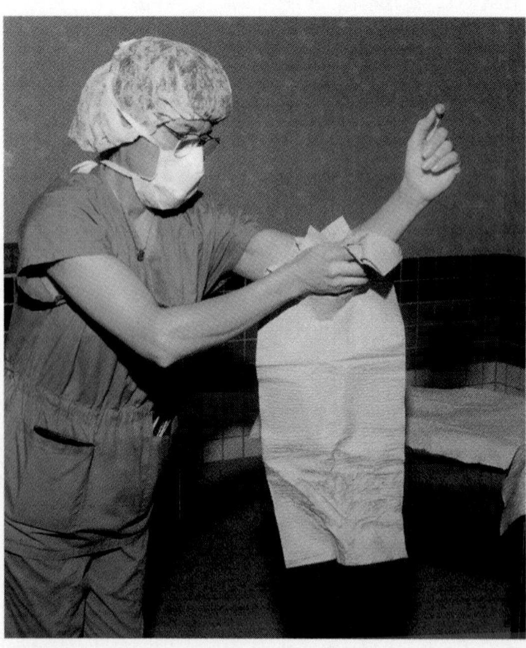

FIGURE 18

11 Turn off the faucet with the foot or forearm lever, if available.
PURPOSE: To separate the clean hand(s) from the contaminated faucet handle(s).

12 Dry your hands with a sterile towel (Figures 14 and 15). Use opposite end of towel for other hand (Figures 16 and 17).
PURPOSE: To keep your clean hands from touching the part of the towel that comes into contact with your forearms, which are not as clean as your hands. If you are to gown and glove for a procedure, you will be required to use a sterile towel.

13 Using a patting motion, continue to dry the forearms (Figure 18). Discard towel and keep your hands up and above the waist level (Figures 19 and 20).

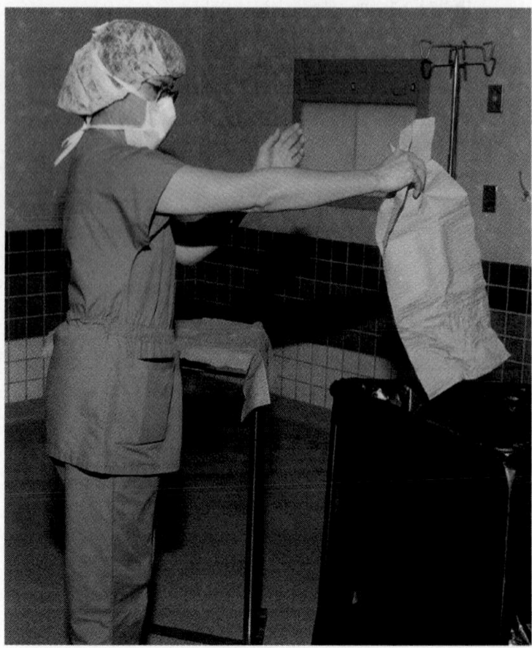

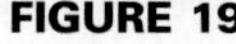

FIGURE 19

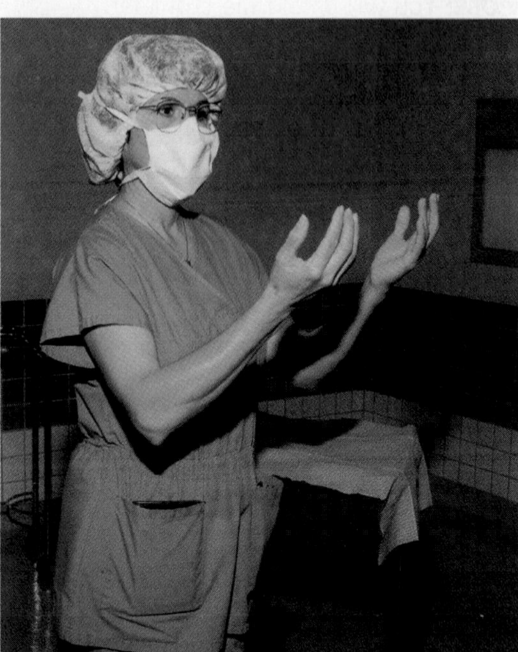

FIGURE 20

PROCEDURE 51-2
Gloving Using the Open-Glove (Without a Gown) Method

GOAL

To apply your own sterile gloves before performing sterile procedures.

EQUIPMENT AND SUPPLIES

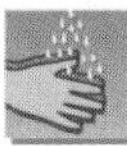

A pair of packaged sterile gloves in your size

PROCEDURAL STEPS

1 Open your glove pack. Remember, a 1-inch area around the perimeter of the glove wrapper is considered not sterile.
PURPOSE: The open glove pack is a sterile field.

2 Perform the surgical hand scrub.

3 Dry your hands well.
PURPOSE: Gloves do not slide easily over moist hands.

4 Glove your major hand first.
PURPOSE: This will set up your major hand to do the more difficult step, which is to apply the second glove.

5 With your minor hand, pick up the glove for your major hand with your thumb and forefinger, grabbing the top of the folded cuff, which is the inside of the glove (Figure 1).
PURPOSE: The inside of the glove will be next to your skin and is considered not sterile.

6 Lift the glove up and away from the sterile package.
PURPOSE: Movement over a sterile field must be kept to a minimum.

7 Hold your hands away from you, and slide your major hand into the glove (Figure 2).

8 Leave the cuff folded (Figure 3).
PURPOSE: You will unfold the cuff later.

9 With your gloved major hand, pick up the second glove by slipping your gloved fingers under the cuff so that your gloved hand only touches the outside of the second glove (Figure 4).
PURPOSE: Sterile surfaces must always touch sterile surfaces.

10 Slide your second hand into the glove, without touching the exterior of the glove or any part of your hand (Figures 5 through 7).

Continued

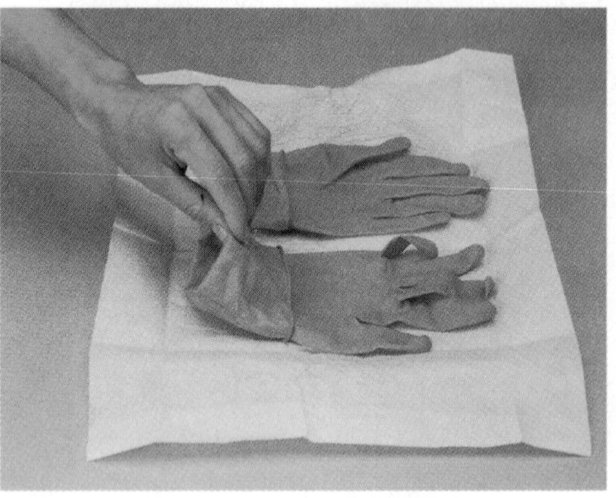

FIGURE 1

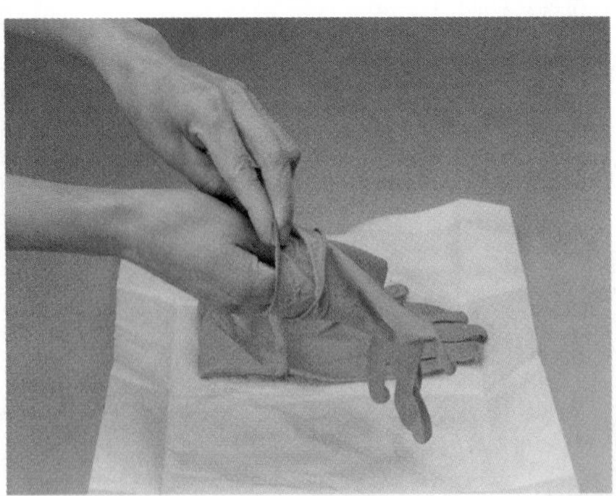

FIGURE 2

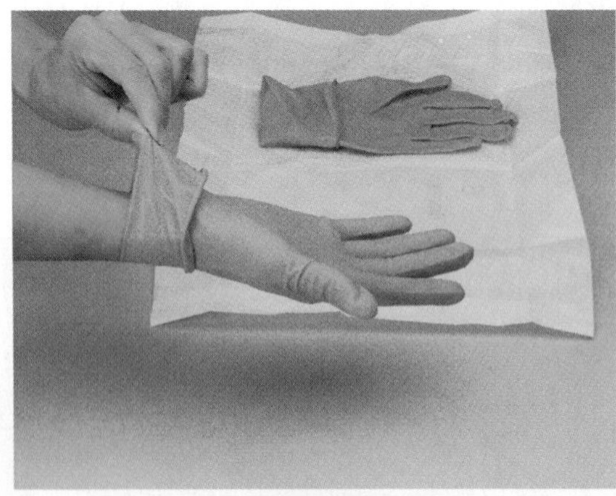

FIGURE 3

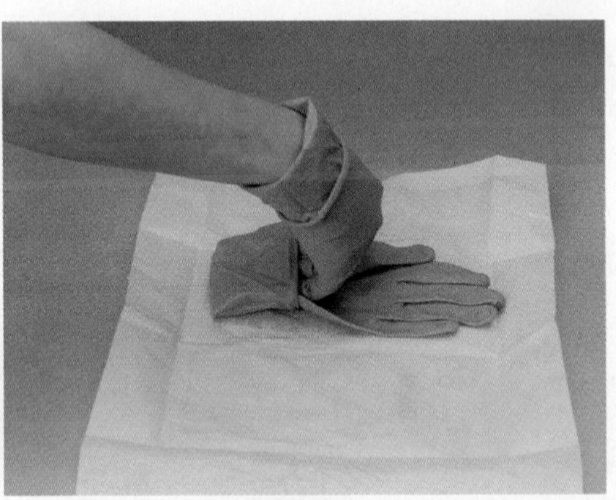

FIGURE 4

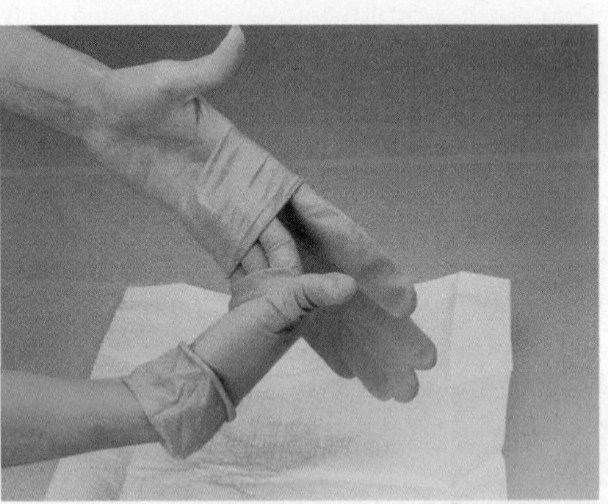

FIGURE 5

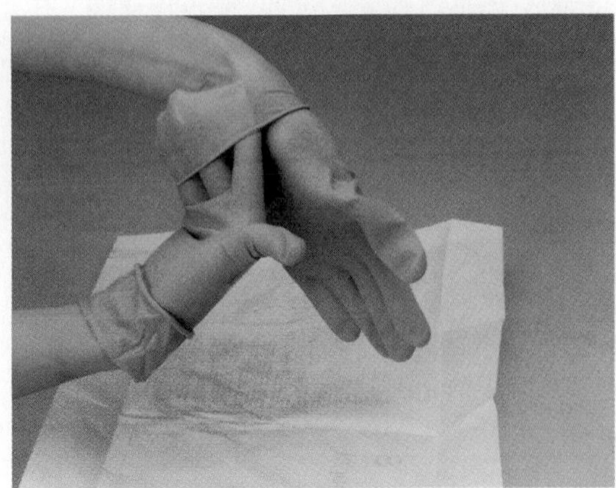

FIGURE 6

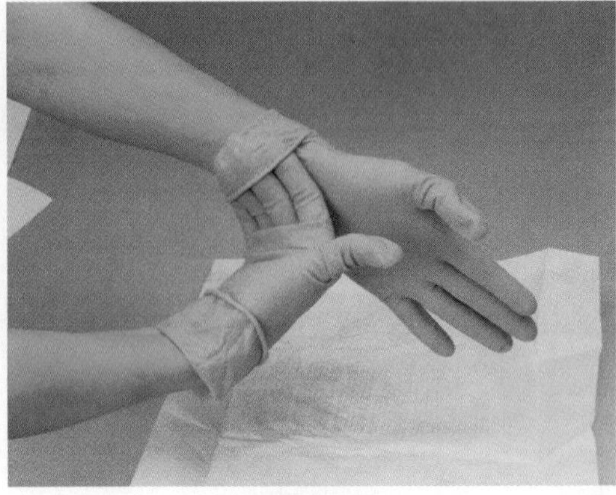

FIGURE 7

Continued

PROCEDURE 51-2 (CONTINUED)

Gloving Using the Open-Glove (Without a Gown) Method

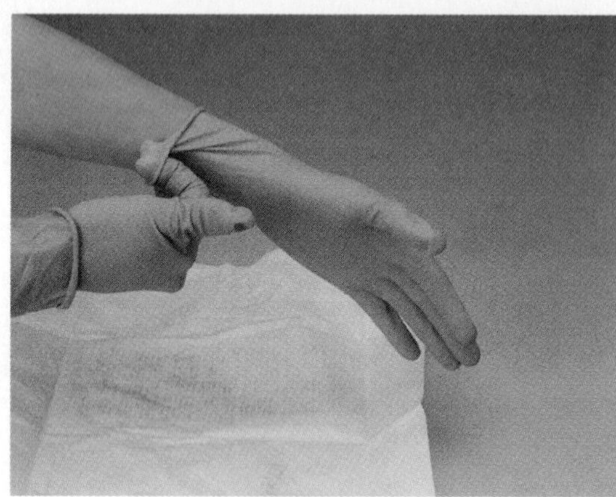

FIGURE 8

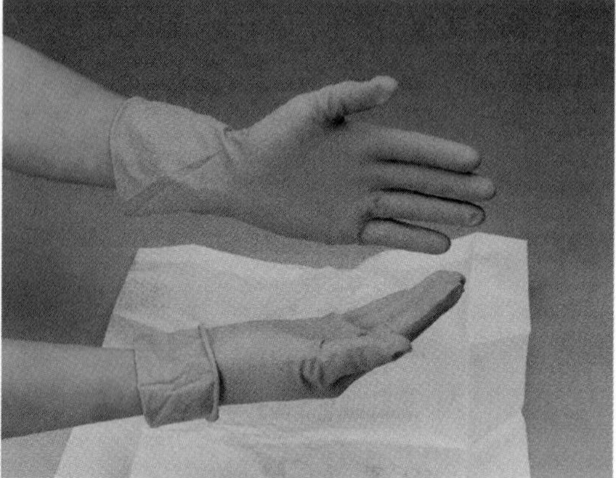

FIGURE 9

11 Still holding your hands away from you, unroll the cuff by slipping the fingers up and out. Stay away from your bare arm (Figure 8).

12 Now, slip your gloved fingers up under the first cuff and unroll it, using the same technique (Figures 9 through 11).

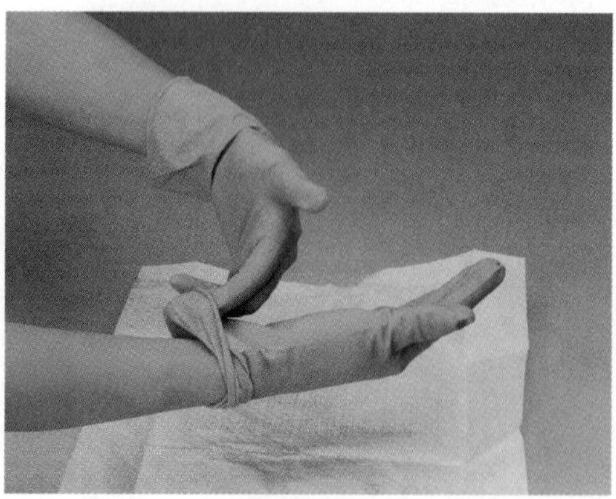

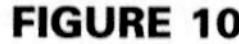

FIGURE 10

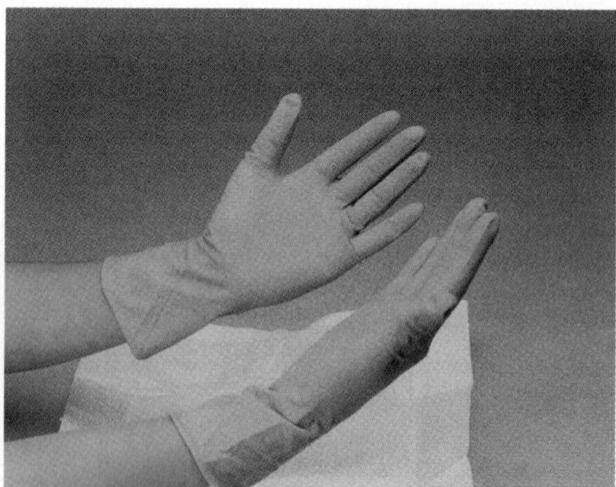

FIGURE 11

PROCEDURE 51–3

Gowning with a Sterile Gown

GOAL

To **don** a sterile gown before assisting with a surgical procedure.

EQUIPMENT AND SUPPLIES

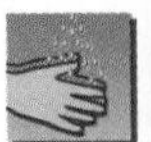 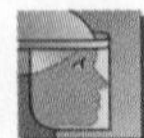

Sterile gown and gloves (opened on a counter or Mayo stand, in an opened area to dress)

Note: A mask and goggles and hair cover are worn.

PROCEDURAL STEPS

1 Scrub, using aseptic technique. Remember to keep hands up and above waist level (Figure 1).
PURPOSE: Protect the patient from your resident bacteria.

Continued

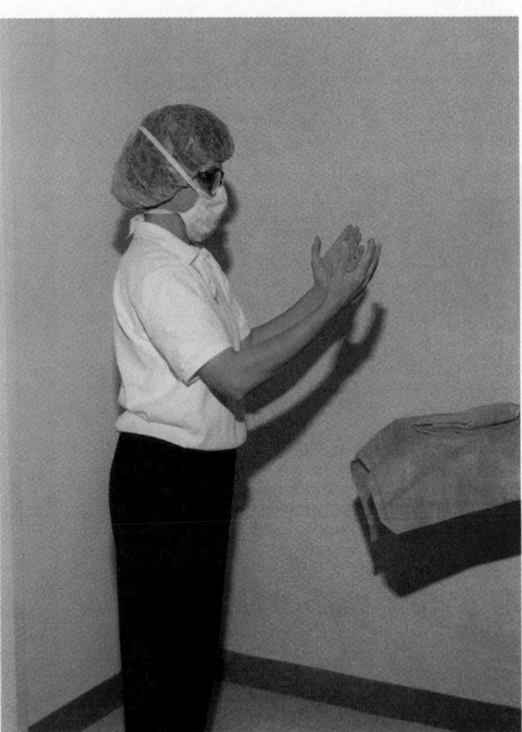

FIGURE 1

PROCEDURE 51-3 (CONTINUED)
Gowning with a Sterile Gown

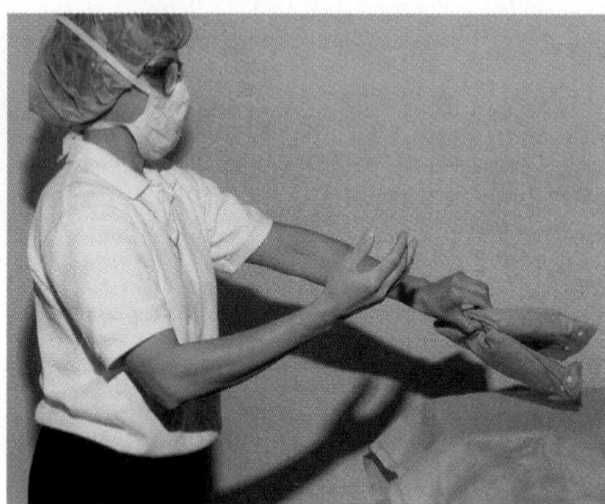
FIGURE 2

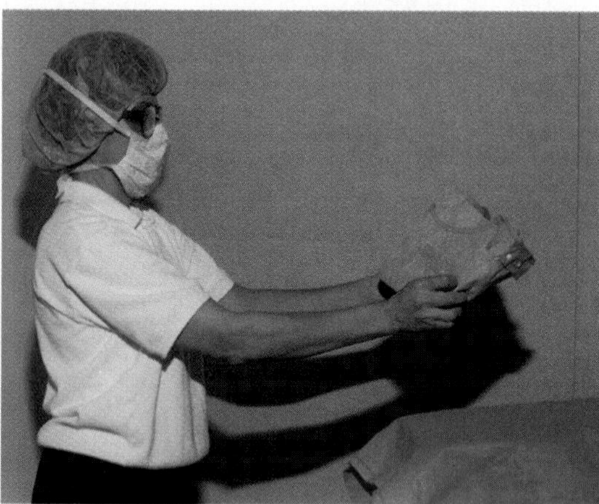
FIGURE 3

2 Grasp the sterile gown by the collar and gently lift it from the sterile gown wrapper (Figures 2 and 3).

PURPOSE: The sterile gown will not be contaminated by the edges of the wrapper.

3 Hold the gown away from your body. Allow it to gently unfold, grasping only the inside of the gown (Figures 4 and 5).

PURPOSE: Only the inside of the gown touches you; the outside of the gown must remain sterile.

Continued

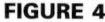

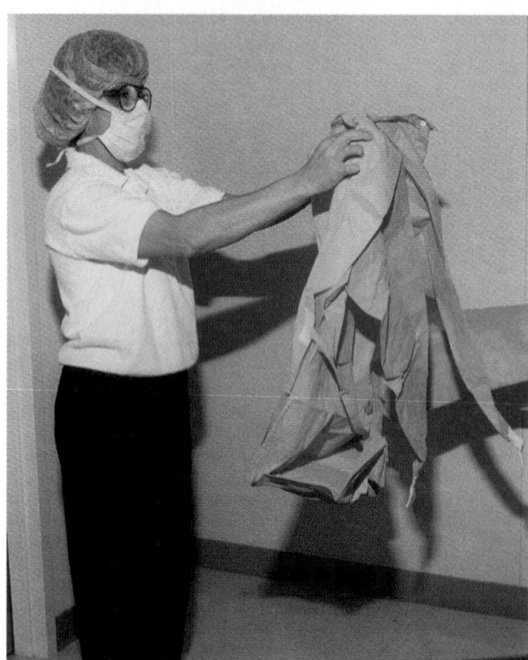
FIGURE 4

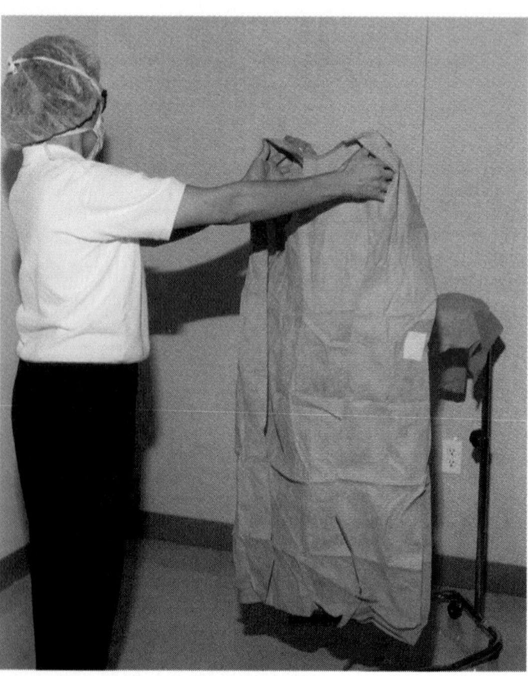
FIGURE 5

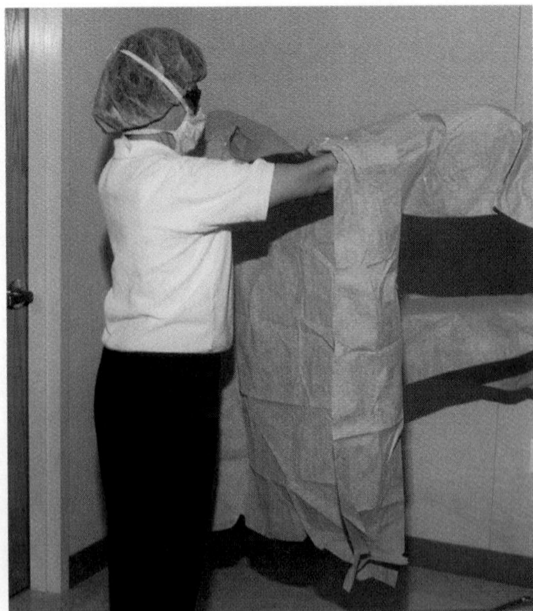

FIGURE 6

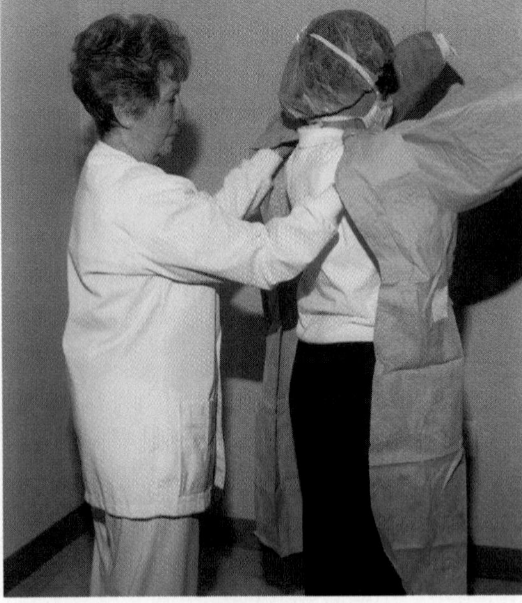

FIGURE 7

4 Slip your hands into the sleeve openings. Remember to touch only the inside of the gown (Figure 6).
PURPOSE: Keep the outside of the gown sterile and away from contaminants.

5 The hand and forearms are advanced only to the edge of the gown cuff.
PURPOSE: The hands are kept covered to avoid contamination of the gown.

6 The circulating assistant touches only the inside of the gown, pulling the gown over the scrub assistant's shoulders (Figure 7).

7 The waistline and neck ties are tied (Figures 8 and 9).
PURPOSE: The gown is fastened to prevent contamination from a flapping gown while applying sterile gloves.

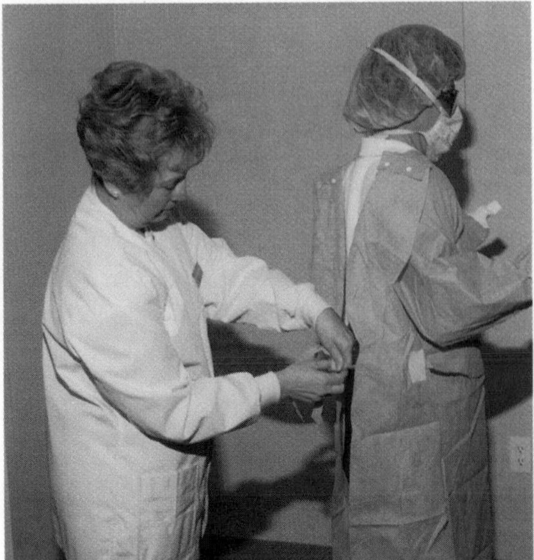

FIGURE 8

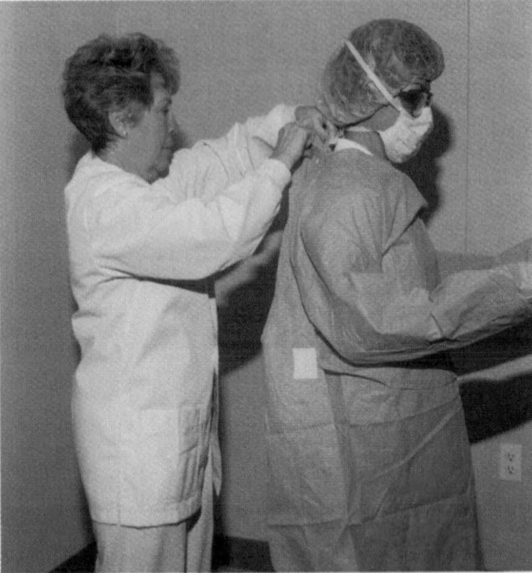

FIGURE 9

PROCEDURE 51-4

Gloving Using the Closed-Glove Method (with a Sterile Gown)

GOAL

To apply sterile gloves while dressed in a sterile gown before assisting with a surgical procedure.

EQUIPMENT AND SUPPLIES

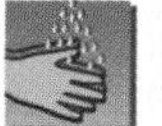
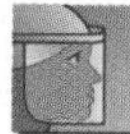

Sterile gloves, opened on a sterile field

Note: A mask, goggles, hair cover, and a sterile gown are worn. The gloves are applied with the hands covered by the sterile gown to avoid contamination.

PROCEDURAL STEPS

1 Glove your minor hand first.
PURPOSE: The major hand does the most difficult step, which is to apply the first glove.

2 Lift the glove with your major hand, and use your thumb and forefinger to grasp the top of the folded cuff (Figure 1). Remember, your hands are covered with the sterile gown sleeves.
PURPOSE: Movement over a sterile field must be kept to a minimum.

3 Place the glove in the palm of your minor hand, with glove fingers pointing to elbows (Figure 2).
PURPOSE: Your bare hand will only touch the inside of the glove as it slides into the glove.

4 Grasp the inside of the cuff with your fingers and gently stretch the glove cuff (Figure 3).
PURPOSE: Sterile surfaces touch only sterile surfaces.

5 Pull the glove over your hand as you push through the gown cuff (Figures 4 through 6).
PURPOSE: Your bare hand touches only the inside of the glove.

6 Gently slide your fingers in the glove (Figure 7).

7 With your minor gloved hand, slip your fingers under the cuff of the second glove (Figure 8).
PURPOSE: Sterile items touch only sterile items.

Continued

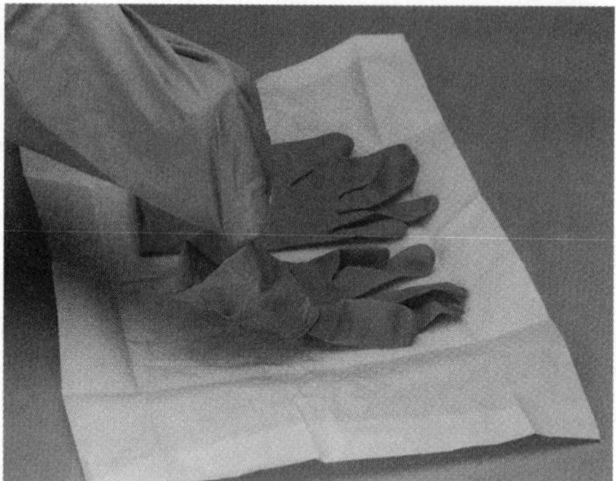

FIGURE 1

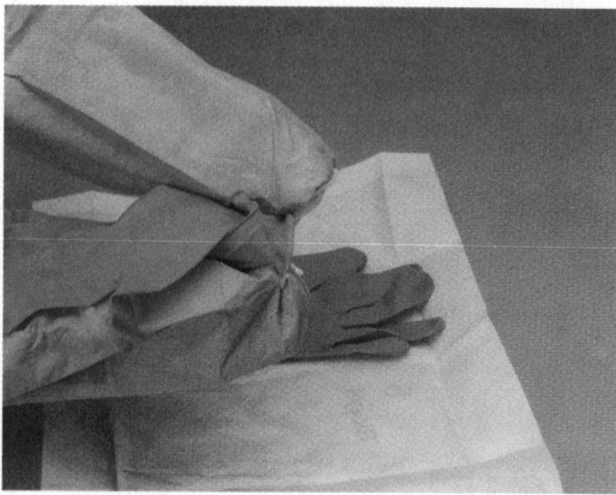

FIGURE 2

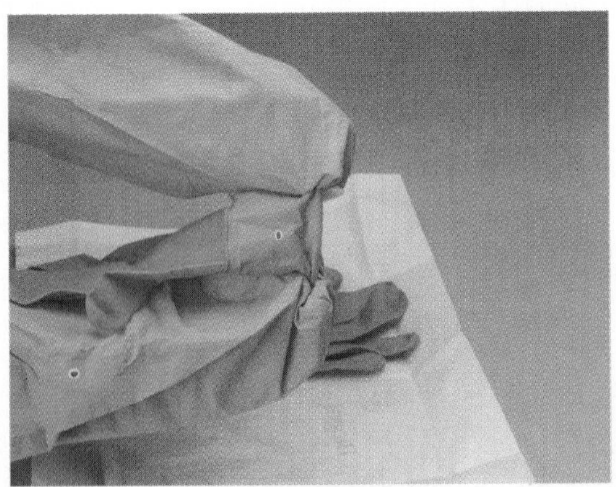

FIGURE 3

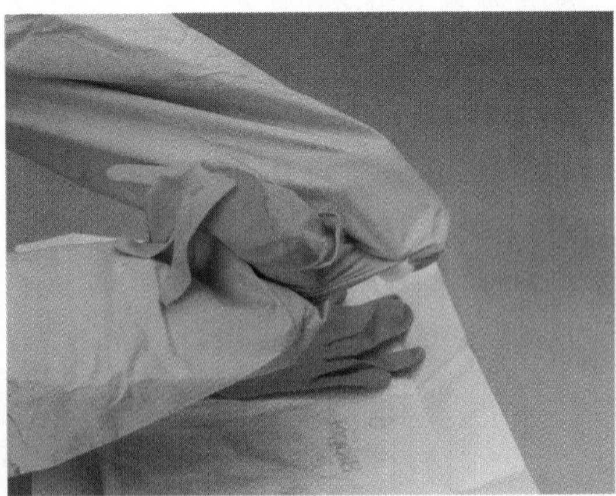

FIGURE 4

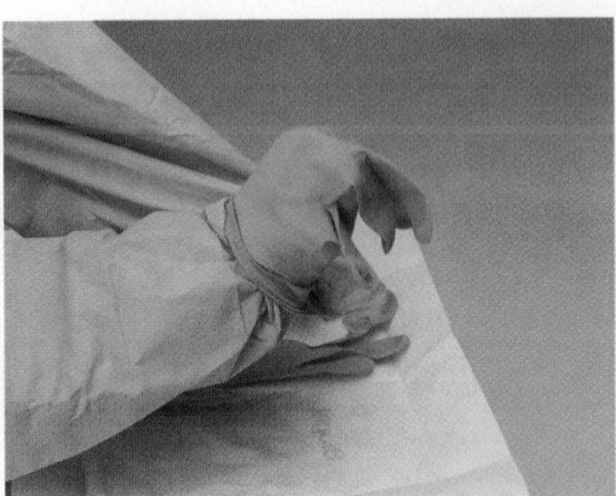

FIGURE 5

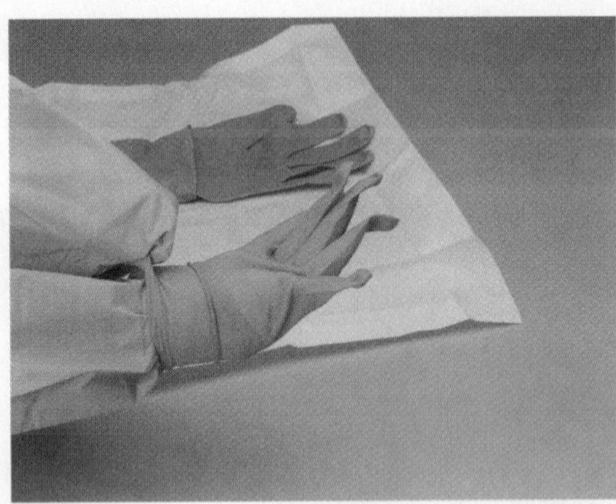

FIGURE 6

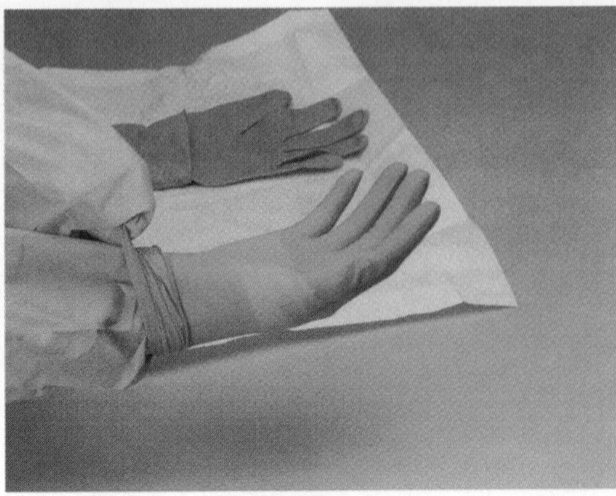

FIGURE 7

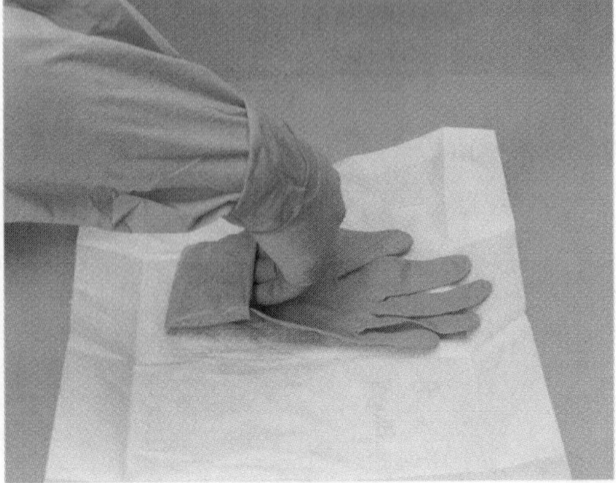

FIGURE 8

Continued

PROCEDURE 51–4 (CONTINUED)

Gloving Using the Closed-Glove Method (with a Sterile Gown)

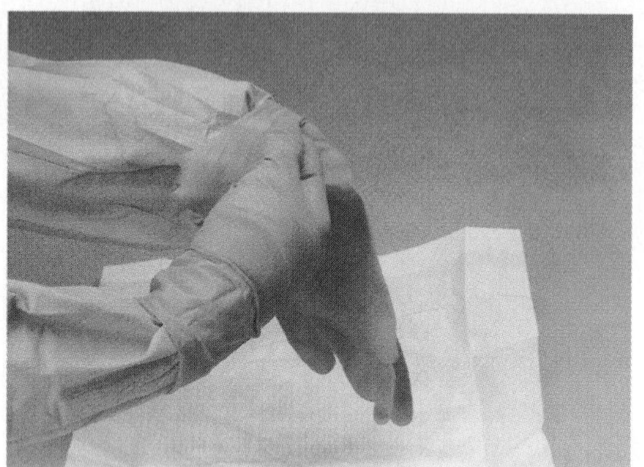

FIGURE 9

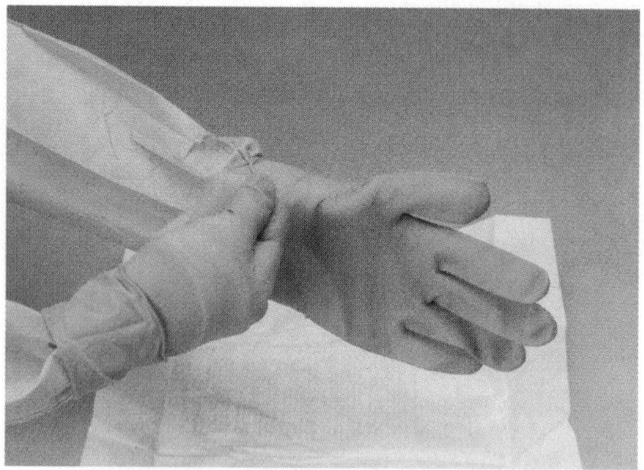

FIGURE 10

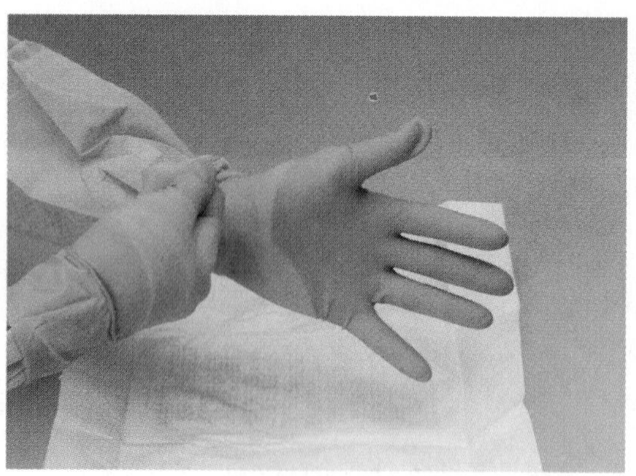

FIGURE 11

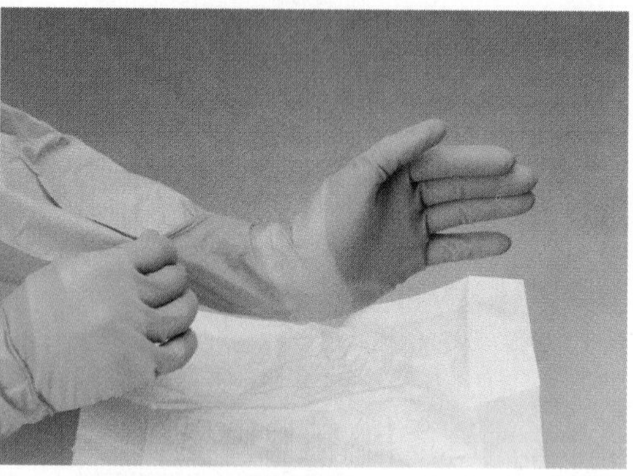

FIGURE 12

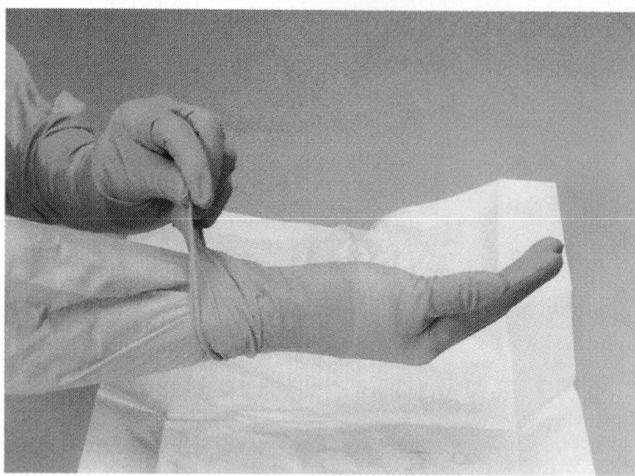

FIGURE 13

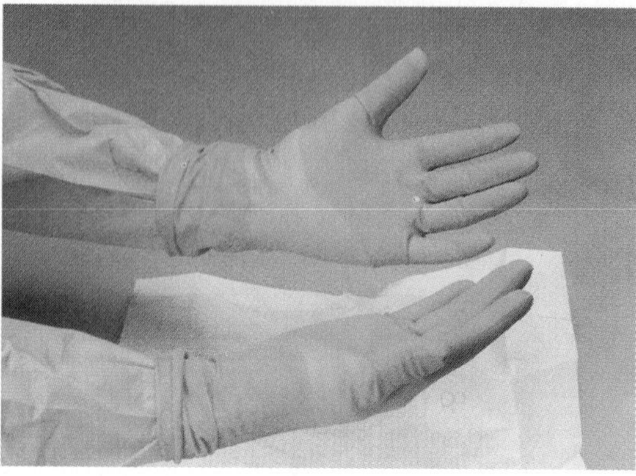

FIGURE 14

Continued

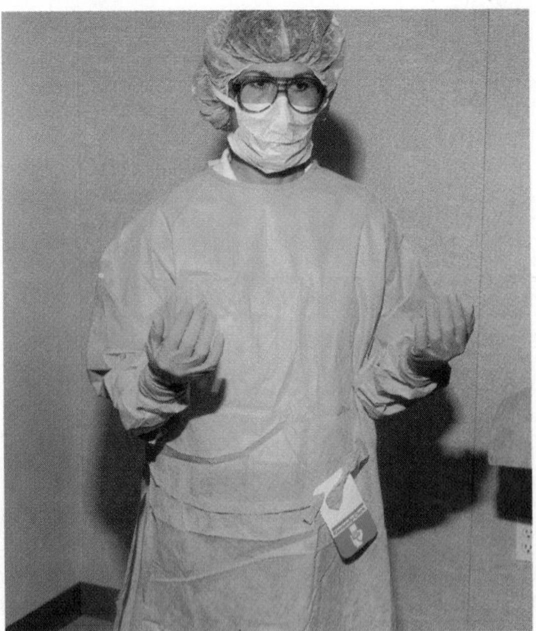

FIGURE 15

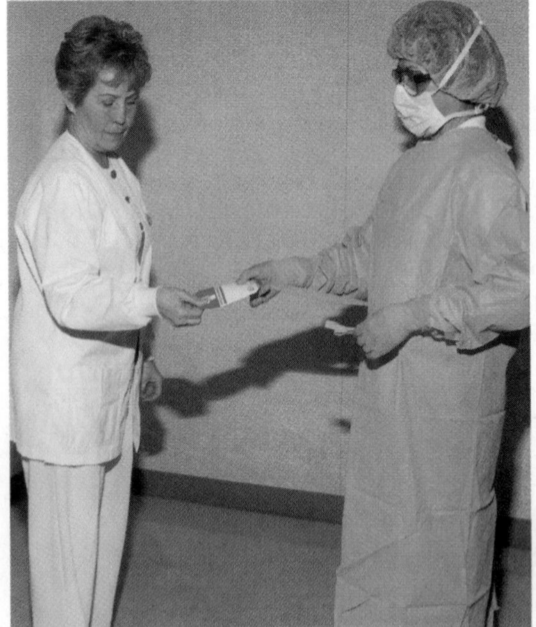

FIGURE 16

8 Follow steps 3, 4, 5, and 6 for the second glove (Figures 9 through 12).

9 The cuffs may now be adjusted (Figures 13 and 14).

10 The outside sterile gown ties may now be tied with the circulator's assistance (Figures 15 to 18).

11 The circulator grasps the red part of the tag by the corner (Figures 17 and 18).
PURPOSE: This will be discarded after the scrub assistant is able to fasten the waist ties. Nonsterile areas do not touch sterile areas.

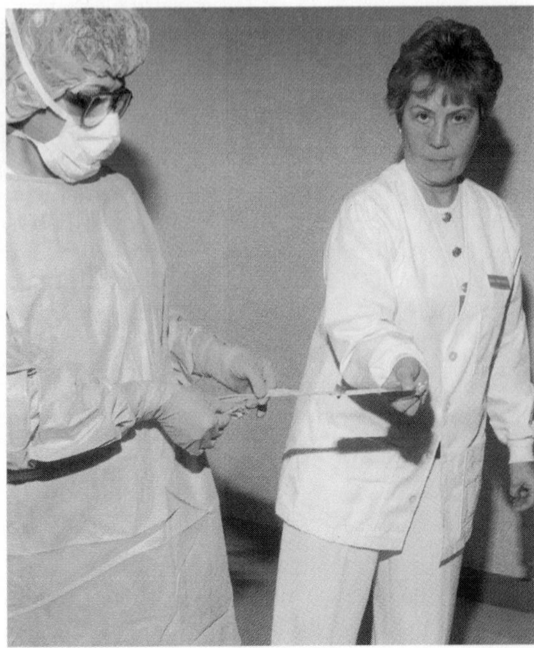

FIGURE 17

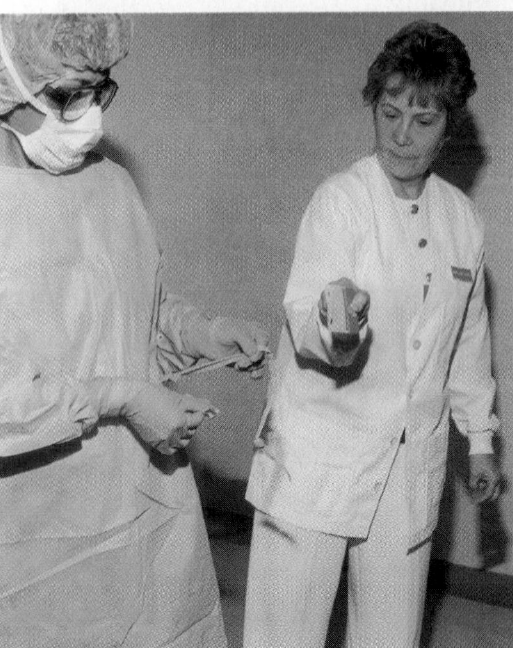

FIGURE 18

Surgical Procedures

ELECTROSURGERY

Electrosurgery is also known as electrocautery. The electrosurgical unit (ESU) uses a high-frequency current to coagulate blood vessels and cut tissue (Fig. 51–1). The electric current comes in contact with tissue and blood cells, exploding them and producing carbon and steam products. This process also seals the cells and any blood vessels. Cellular oozing and vascular bleeding can be kept to a minimum. Electrosurgery may be used to destroy granulations and small polyps. It is sometimes used to destroy the stem of a **pedunculated** growth. It also provides hemostasis and helps to minimize the polyp's growth.

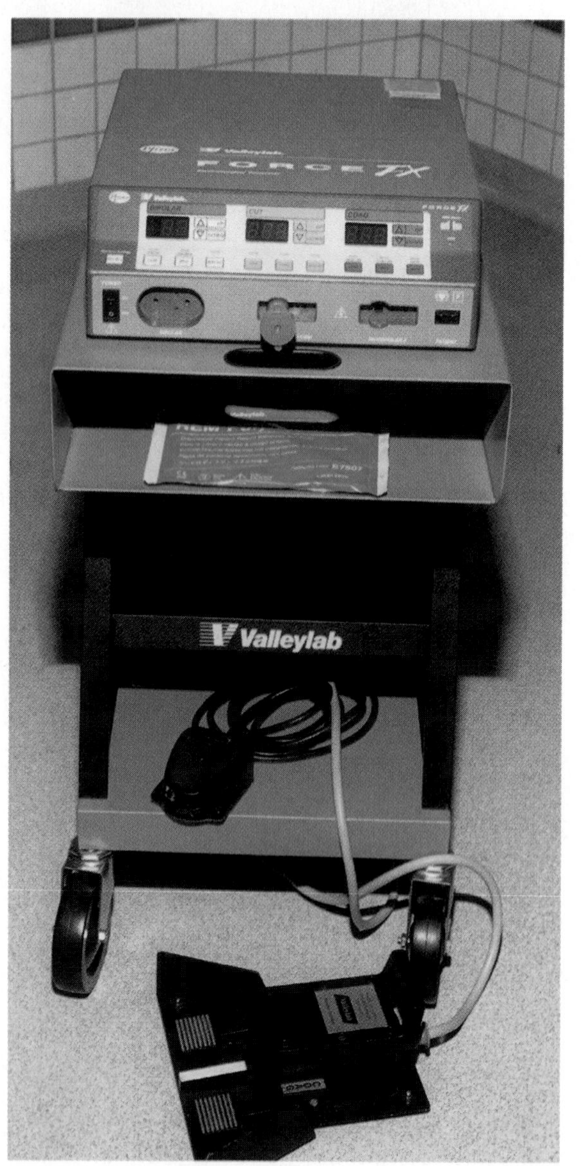

FIGURE 51–1 Electrosurgical unit with foot control. (Courtesy of Valley Lab, Inc., Fresno, CA.)

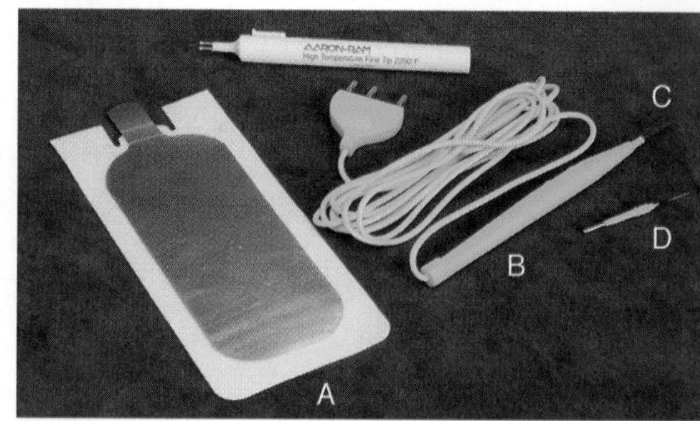

FIGURE 51–2 Electrosurgical unit components. *A,* Grounding pad. *B,* Pencil with cord and blade tip. *C,* Flat blade tip. *D,* Needle tip.

The necessary components are the electrosurgical unit's power source, the grounding cable and pad, and the active electrode (pencil with tip and cord). Pencil tips are disposable and are used according to the type of procedure being performed. There are a variety of types and sizes. The two most commonly used are the needle and flat tips (Fig. 51–2).

The pencil is held by the surgeon; when the tissue is touched with the pencil tip, the electric current is activated by a switch on the pencil or foot pedal. The electric current proceeds from the machine through the cord and pencil and into the tissues.

Memory Jogger

Identify the primary use of electrocautery.

TYPES OF CURRENT

MONOPOLAR CURRENT When monopolar is used, the ESU is activated and the electric current is transmitted to the patient through the pencil tip. The current travels through the tissue or blood vessel seeking a return path to the ESU. The electric circuit path is completed through the grounding pad, which should always be used.

BIPOLAR CURRENT The electric circuit is conducted between the two tips of the active electrode. A bipolar forceps is used. A grounding pad is not needed with a bipolar current.

SAFETY

Safety is critical when electrocautery is used in surgery. The medical assistant should know proper grounding techniques and ignitable skin prep solution precautions. Flammable prep solutions, alcohol, or alcohol-based solutions should not be allowed to pool around the patient but should be dried to avoid any possible igniting of the drapes. Proper placement of the grounding pad is important. The patient's skin should always maintain uniform contact with the pad's surface or serious harm can result to the patient.

Disposable pads are available. They consist of a foil plate imbedded in a pregelled foam pad that has an adhesive to hold the pad securely in place. Reusable nondisposable pads consist of a metal plate with a permanently attached grounding cable. The reusable pad must be coated with a specifically designated conductive gel and must be sufficiently coated and spread evenly to avoid drying out during surgery. Skin burns can occur at site application.

IMPORTANT TIPS ABOUT THE GROUNDING PAD

- Place the pad as close to the operative site as possible.
- Do not allow the pad to gap or tent on the patient's skin.
- Apply to fleshy areas (patient's thigh).
- Avoid bony prominences or areas where the flesh is fragile and thin.
- Avoid areas with excess body hair. The hair may act as an insulator between the pad and the patient.
- Always inspect the pad, the cable, and the patient's skin before and after application.
- Ask the patient if he or she has any metal implants or pacemaker. Avoid placing it near or over these implants. Electric current should not be used around metal.

Never store or place solutions on top of the ESU. Fluid spills could cause an electrical short circuit. Always follow the manufacturer's directions for safe use.

Patient Care

Anesthesia is usually used with electrocautery. The surgeon decides the type and amount used according to the procedure and site. Ethyl chloride, a topical freezing agent, is sometimes used. Care should always be taken when using this because it is a flammable agent. Electrosurgery causes the tissue to form a grayish white **coagulum.** The tissue sloughs within 1 or 2 weeks, depending on the depth and the size of the area treated. When the **slough** has completely separated, healthy tissue appears underneath. There may be a slight grayish discharge from the site.

After the treatment, the physician will decide whether an antiseptic and/or a dressing is needed. If the treatment area is small and superficial, only an adhesive bandage may be needed to protect the area from trauma or for cosmetic reasons. The patient should be instructed to keep the area dry and clean and to protect it from more trauma and infection. A follow-up appointment and treatment may be needed depending on the initial cause for surgery.

Care of the Equipment

Breaks in the electric circuit can occur in damaged grounding cables and the power unit. If there is a break in an electric circuit, electricity will find another path back to the power unit. All cables should be inspected for breaks or frays before and after use. The power unit should be inspected by a qualified engineer on a regular basis. Any damage must be corrected immediately. Disposable tips and pencil handles with cords are thrown away after one-time patient use. Always read the manufacturer's instructions for equipment that you must maintain.

LASER SURGERY

Laser is the acronym for *l*ight *a*mplification by *s*timulated *e*mission of *r*adiation. These light waves were first used in medicine with the treatment of diseases of the retina. Their application was later expanded to **photocoagulation** therapy and then to thermal vaporization, coagulation, and ablation of tissue.

Lasers are used in the following types of surgery: ophthalmic, genitourinary, gynecologic, orthopedic, neurologic, laryngologic, otologic, rhinologic and sinus, vascular, thoracic, and gastrointestinal. Laser equipment is found in hospitals, surgery centers, and medical offices.

Types of Lasers

Examples of different types of lasers are argon, carbon dioxide, holmium, neodymium:yttrium-aluminum-garnet (Nd:YAG), and excimer.

Components

The laser has five basic components: the laser head, excitation source, ancillary components, control panel, and delivery system. The excitation source can be electricity, flash lamps, chemicals, radio waves, or another laser source. The laser head has the substance or active medium that produces the photons that generate the laser light. It can be a gas (argon or CO_2), a crystal (Nd:YAG), a solid (Nd: YAG), or a liquid (a tunable dye). Ancillary components are other laser parts that are used to help produce laser energy. Delivery systems can be an articulating arm or a fiber system (cord) or tip. This device conducts the laser energy from the laser to the target area.

Laser Safety

The laser key should be accessible to authorized persons only. The medical assistant must be trained to operate the laser before assisting with the surgery. Proper instruments are needed for some lasers.

A smoke **(plume)** evacuator is necessary for use with the CO_2 laser. The filter must be monitored for use, and proper disposable procedures are important. Always check the cords and foot pedal and connections to the laser. A proper fire extinguisher (Halon) must be available that will not damage the laser's internal components.

Training is essential concerning moving and storing of the laser. Preventive maintenance records should be kept. Patient education is important to help diminish any anxiety associated with the surgery and to assist with patient compliance during the healing period.

Laser Hazards

Laser light destroys tissue and, if improperly handled, can harm not only the patient but also the physician and you. The dangers of the laser include (1) burns, (2) fire, (3) inhalation of plume, and (4) electrical hazards related to high-wattage equipment. A full laser safety program should be completed before assisting in laser procedures.

Assisting with Laser Surgery

Planning becomes very important when high technology tools are used in surgical procedures. You should have specific training regarding the type of laser to be used, accessory equipment for operating the laser, and safety intervention. The CO_2 laser beams reflect off any shiny instrument surfaces. Protective supplies such as wet sponges and towels should be available. A smoke evacuator and suction should be available to eliminate any plume and debris that accumulate from the lasering process. Warning signs should be posted on entry doors. Goggles are required for the patient and the operative team members.

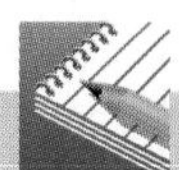

SKILLS AND RESPONSIBILITIES

THE MEDICAL ASSISTANT'S FUNCTION DURING LASER SURGERY

- Observe the surgical field through safety goggles for possible contamination.
- Keep wet sponges ready.
- Remove any ignitable item from the CO_2 laser beam's path.
- Assist with the suctioning of plume so the surgeon has a clear visual field.
- Have a basin of sterile water and a filled irrigating syringe ready. It may be necessary to cool thermally involved tissue or to extinguish any inadvertent heating of supplies.
- Watch each application of the laser beam and anticipate any need for protective supplies, special equipment, or instruments.

Memory Jogger

List four dangers of laser usage.

MICROSURGERY

Microsurgery involves the use of the operating microscope in many types of surgical procedures. One of its major uses is in ophthalmologic surgery. It is also used in otologic, rhinologic and sinus, laryngologic, neurosurgical, microvascular, gynecologic, and genitourinary procedures. Basic operational knowledge and care of the microscope is necessary.

Components

The basic components are the light source, oculars, (eyepieces), lenses, and microscope cord. Accessory pieces consist of assistant and observer lenses, cameras, video recorders, television monitors, and still photography printers. These are all valuable for documentation and teaching the patient and the assistant to understand the disease and surgical procedure.

Disposable drapes and handle covers are available for use during surgical procedures.

Care of the Equipment

Storage and handling of the microscope and its parts is very important. Lenses and cords should be carefully inspected before and after each use. Microinstruments are delicate and expensive. Care when handling and cleaning these instruments is essential. Always inspect these fine instruments. They may easily be bent, hooked, dulled, sprung, or damaged in some way.

ENDOSCOPIC SURGERY

A telescope or long tube with an optical system and a light source is used to examine a hollow organ or cavity, such as the urinary bladder, bronchus, larynx, colon, stomach, uterus, abdomen, the knee, wrist, and shoulder joints, and many more parts of the body. Direct visualization is necessary for diagnostic purposes or to perform a surgical operative procedure.

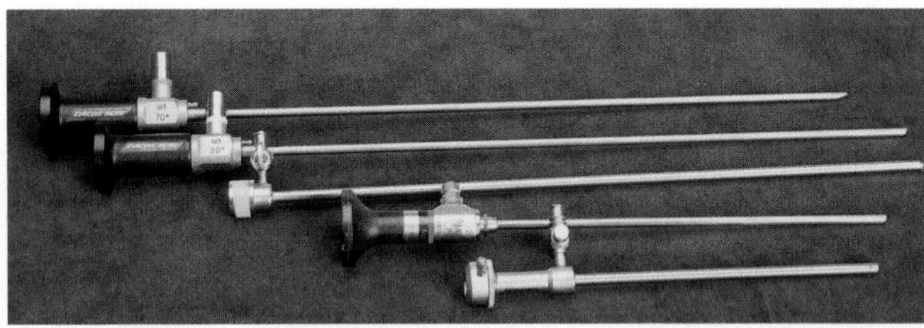

FIGURE 51–3 Endoscopes with cannulas.

Types of Scopes

The scopes may be rigid, semirigid, or flexible. An example of a rigid scope is a laparoscope or hysteroscope. Colonoscopes, bronchoscopes, and gastroscopes are flexible scopes. The many types of scopes (Fig. 51–3) are all delicate and expensive and are made in a variety of diameters and lengths based on the patient and procedural requirements. They may be direct or angled scopes ranging from 0 to 120 degrees (Fig. 51–4).

Memory Jogger

8 *Name the three types of scopes.*

Accessory Equipment

Accessory equipment used with endoscopic surgery may include a fiberoptic light cable or cord, the light source, irrigator for solution and suction, a camera (still photography or video) and power source, video monitor, printer, or video cassette recorder for documentation.

Care of the Equipment

Scopes are fragile and expensive. They must be handled and stored with care. The fiberoptic light cable or cords consist of hundreds of glass fibers. It is important to protect them from being bent, dropped, kinked, squashed, or smashed. Light sources can be very hot. Extreme caution must be used. They must be kept out of contact with the patient, any person's skin, or flammable material. All equipment must be checked before and after use. Always follow manufacturer's recommendations for use, care, and maintenance of equipment.

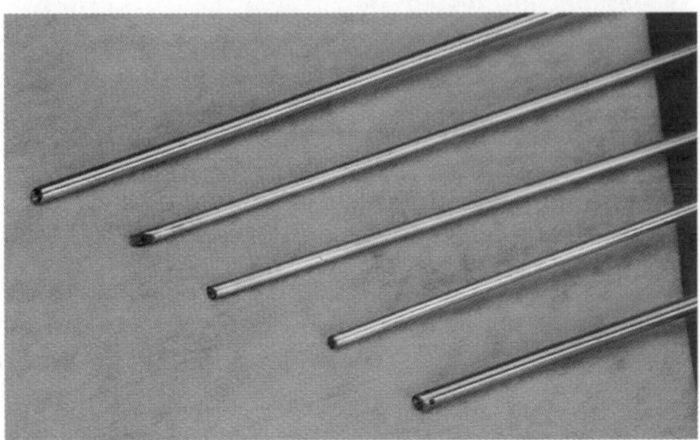

FIGURE 51–4 Endoscopy scope tips with different angles.

CYSTOSCOPY

The bladder, ureters, and prostate gland are viewed with a cystoscope inserted into the bladder. The bladder is distended with the use of continuous irrigation solution (sterile water). The surgeon can examine, make diagnoses, sample tissue, and perform surgery using the cystoscope. A local anesthetic is used when the procedure is done in the medical office.

Components

A rigid or flexible cystoscope, a cystoscopy cannula and obturator, a fiberoptic light cable or cord, a light source, and sterile irrigation fluid are used for the procedure. The cystoscope is made in different angles to offer particular angles of view: forward, right-angle, lateral, and forward oblique. The scope is used with its cannula, designed with an irrigation stopcock. The cystoscopy cannula protects the patient and cystoscope in the urethra and bladder. The patient is placed in lithotomy position. A cystoscopy bed with knee or ankle stirrups is usually used. The "cysto" bed has a drainage drawer with a screen that is extended during the procedure to filter drainage. Photographs may be taken by adding the necessary equipment.

Memory Jogger

9 *What procedures can the surgeon do with the cystoscope?*

Care of the Equipment

The cystoscope is a delicate, expensive instrument. Care should be taken to avoid scratching the lens or bending the shaft of the scope. Storage and handling of the scope, light cable, and light source are very important. Proper care of the photography equipment, if used, should be followed.

The medical assistant sets up the sterile instruments and table and checks all equipment before and after the procedure. It is important to monitor the patient, the irrigation fluids, and the sterile field. Decontamination and resterilization of instruments and scope are done after surgery.

SIGMOIDOSCOPY

A sigmoidoscopy is performed to examine the rectum and sigmoid colon. It may be performed to confirm a diagnosis or to obtain a specimen.

Components

The sigmoidoscope may be rigid or flexible with a fiberoptic light source and air insufflator (Fig. 51–5). Irrigation and suction are sometimes used. The necessary photography equipment may be added for documentation and teaching purposes.

Care of the Equipment

The sigmoidoscope is delicate and fragile. Immediate cleaning and resterilization are essential. Always use care when handling and storing the scope and its accessories.

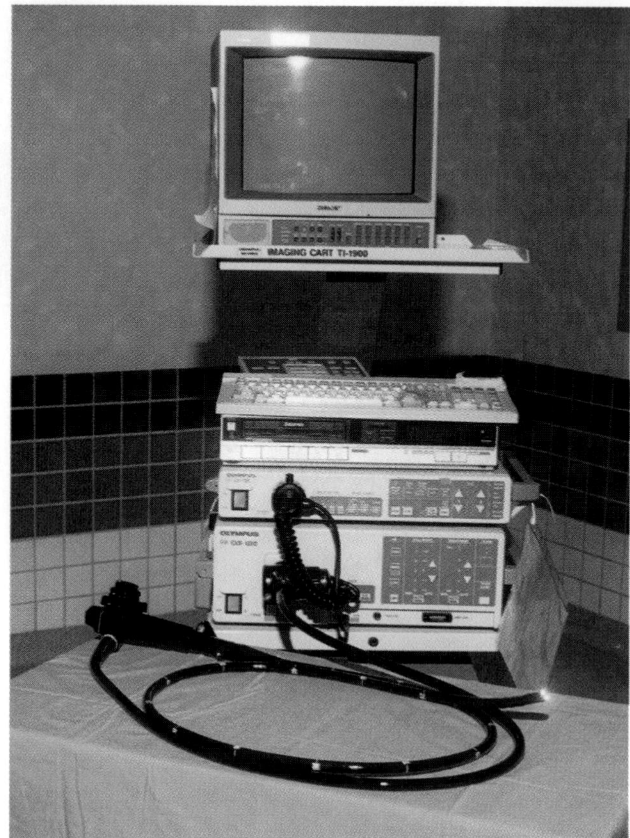

FIGURE 51–5 Flexible colonoscope with video set-up.

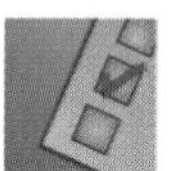

PATIENT EDUCATION

The medical assistant's duty may include calling the patient the day before surgery to confirm the surgical procedure and appointment time. Explaining the procedure and what to expect during and after surgery will prepare the patient and calm any fears or concerns. Lying still during surgery is important, and eating a light, well-balanced meal the night before should be encouraged. Bathing before coming to the office will help reduce the amount of bacteria on the skin, and wearing comfortable loose clothing is recommended.

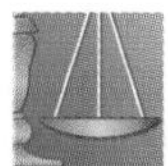

LEGAL AND ETHICAL ISSUES

Many minor surgical procedures previously performed in the hospital are now being done in the medical office, surgery center, or clinic. As insurance companies continue to recognize the cost-effectiveness of performing minor surgical procedures in these settings, the role of the medical assistant continues to increase.

The medical assistant must practice perfect aseptic technique. A break in technique may invite infection and possible legal action. It is the medical assistant's duty to protect the patient. A self-commitment to adhere strictly to aseptic technique and correct immediately any violation is a major responsibility for the medical assistant.

Memory Jogger

Why must the medical assistant practice perfect aseptic technique?

CRITICAL THINKING

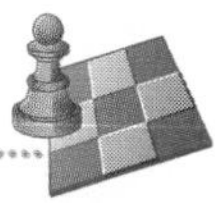

1 What might be some of a patient's concerns when he or she is facing surgery? How might you help a patient?

2 You must prepare the surgical procedure room for a minor procedure. List what you would do.

3 One of your responsibilities is to protect the patient. What do you think this entails doing?

HOW DID I DO? Answers to Memory Joggers

1. Everything sterile is white, everything that is not sterile is black, and there is no gray.
2. Hands and hair.
3. They may be unfolded easily by lifting one edge.
4. In case of contamination.
5. To reduce skin bacteria by use of mechanical friction, special soaps, and running water.
6. To coagulate blood vessels and cut tissue.
7. Dangers include burns, fire, inhalation of plume, and electrical hazards.
8. Scopes may be rigid, semirigid, and flexible.
9. Examination, diagnosis, and surgery.
10. To avoid possible legal action and to protect the patient.

Assisting with Surgical Procedures

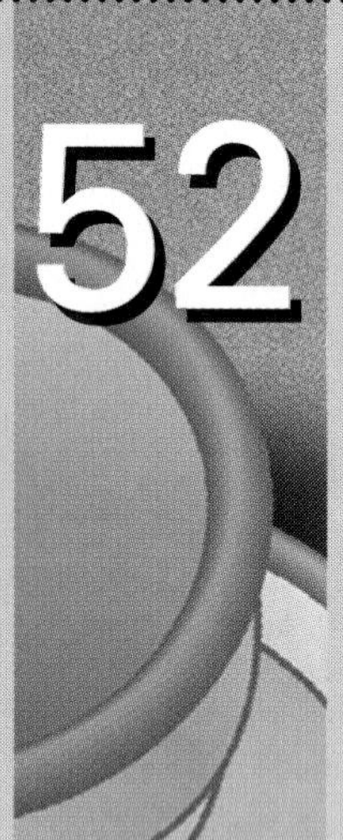

Mary Jane McClain, RN, BS, CNOR

OUTLINE

LEARNING OBJECTIVES

Performance: On successful completion of this chapter you should be able to:

1. Transfer sterile instruments.
2. Prepare a patient's skin for minor surgery.
3. Open a sterile linen pack.
4. Open and add a sterile pack to a sterile field.
5. Add sterile items in a peel-back wrapper to a sterile field.
6. Assist with a minor surgical procedure.
7. Assist with suturing.
8. Assist with suture removal.
9. Bandage the injured site.
10. Define and spell vocabulary terms.

VOCABULARY

approximated When wound or skin edges are brought together

hematoma Localized collection of clotted blood caused by a broken vessel

irrigation Flushing out of a cavity or wound with a solution

lesion Wound, sore, ulcer, tumor, or any traumatic tissue damage that causes a lack of tissue continuity or a loss of function

Minor surgery is restricted to the management of minor problems and injuries. Most medical assistants are expected to glove and assist with the preparation of the sterile field and the patient. The following are acceptable procedures and techniques for assisting with minor surgery in the medical office, clinic, and outpatient surgery center. Individual practices and preferences may modify some of the following procedures described.

Procedural File

Keeping a card file for each procedure and listing the preferences of each physician in the office helps in the preparation for surgery. It is particularly helpful for complicated procedures and for procedures that are seldom performed. Color-code the 5 × 8-inch cards for each physician, and keep the information current. The cards contain information essential to proper preparation for surgery (see Procedure Card File).

PROCEDURE CARD FILE

- Preoperative instructions
- Preoperative and operative medications
- Universal blood and body fluid precautions, listing specific protection barriers (goggles, masks, gowns, aprons, and gloves) to be worn by the surgeon and the assistants (see Chapter 26)
- Glove sizes
- Prep solution and shaving instructions
- Patient position
- Sterile packs, instruments, sutures, and equipment
- Syringe and needle sizes
- Postoperative instructions and the routine number of days for a follow-up appointment

A more detailed procedures manual should be developed by the medical assistant and the physician. The procedures should be reviewed at regular intervals for revision and development.

Memory Jogger

 *What is the purpose for a procedure card file?*

Handling Equipment

When two medical assistants work with the surgeon, one serves as the circulating assistant and the other as the scrub assistant. The scrub assistant scrubs with the surgical scrub and gloves for the procedure. During the procedure, the scrub assistant receives only sterile items, monitors the sterile field, and passes instruments and supplies to the surgeon.

The circulating assistant wears nonsterile gloves, opens sterile supplies before and during the procedure, helps position the patient for the procedure, performs the scrub prep on the patient, and handles all nonsterile equipment in the room during the procedure. Before every surgery, the team members review which universal blood and body fluid precautions (goggles, masks, and special procedures) are necessary for the procedure. After the procedure, the scrub assistant assists the surgeon with the bandage and cleans, washes, and sanitizes the room and used instruments for resterilization. The circulating assistant assists the patient with dressing as needed and escorts the patient to the receptionist for a follow-up appointment.

If you are the single assistant, you must do all of these functions. The sequence in which you carry out the required functions is vital. If you do not follow the proper sequence, you will find yourself in sterile gloves without any sterile packs opened or with a nonsterile item to retrieve, or you may find that the surgeon is waiting and you cannot work because you do not have your gloves on. It is very important to learn sterile aseptic technique step-by-step—how to get from the beginning to the end. Table 52–1 outlines the chronologic steps for the assistant who must function as both the circulating and the scrub assistant.

Memory Jogger

 *Describe the role of the circulating assistant.*

TABLE 52–1 Preparation for Minor Surgery: Single-Assistant Preparation

1. Wash your hands; gather all supplies.
   Sterile side (Mayo tray): two towel packs, skin prep pack, patient drape pack, instrument pack, miscellaneous pack(s), three glove packs, masks, goggles, aprons or gowns
   Nonsterile side (side counter): syringes, suture material, anesthesia solutions, additional sponges, dressings, bandages, transfer forceps, waste basin, waste receptacle, nonsterile gloves, masks, goggles, aprons, or gowns
2. Escort patient into the room.
3. Greet and converse with patient.
4. Position patient on table.
5. Wash your hands.
6. Open first towel pack.
7. Open skin prep pack.
8. Pour soap and antiseptic solutions.
9. Expose the site to be prepped.
10. Scrub with the surgical hand wash.
11. Glove and arrange prep items within sterile field.
12. Place sterile towels at skin scrub boundaries.
13. Prep the patient's skin.
14. Discard skin prep materials.
15. Discard gloves; wash your hands.
16. Open table drape pack on Mayo stand to create sterile field.
17. Open instrument pack(s), and transfer instruments to sterile field. Add sterile syringe unit.
18. Add sterile items as requested.
19. Physician joins you and converses with the patient.
20. Open physician's glove pack (physician now gloves).
21. Open patient drape pack (physician now drapes the surgical site).
22. Cleanse and hold up anesthesia vial for physician to withdraw anesthesia with sterile syringe (physician will now administer the anesthesia).
23. Repeat surgical hand wash; reglove with a new glove pack.
24. Arrange sterile field instruments and other materials for safety and in sequence; check instrument condition.
25. Unwind suture materials; load the first suture into the needle holder.
26. Place two gauze sponges at the site.
27. Assist with the procedure.*
   For physician—pass instrument; maintain field; anticipate needs; cut sutures.
   For patient—retract tissue; sponge blood from wound; apply bandage; and care for specimen.
28. Escort patient to recovery area.
29. Record and prepare specimens.
30. Clean the room; clear materials; discard gloves.
31. Chart the procedure on the medical record.
32. Help the patient to prepare to leave the office.
33. Disinfect and sterilize equipment at first available time.

*By law, the assistant may not clamp tissue, place sutures, or alter body tissues in any way.

When you are the circulating assistant, you must be able to transfer a sterile item from the autoclave or transfer a sterile package to the sterile team or field (see Procedure 52–1). This must be done with sterile gloves or a sterile transfer forceps.

Sterile transfer forceps must be autoclaved and kept sterile in a peel-pack or linen wrap package. The package is opened properly, and only the ring handles are touched with the hands. The tips of the forceps should always remain pointing down toward the floor. If the tips are turned upward, any solution it may encounter will run onto the nonsterile area and then back down over the sterile end when the tips are turned down again, thus contaminating the forceps. Once the sterile forceps have been used to transfer a sterile item or set up a minor procedure, the sterile forceps must be removed and not used again.

PROCEDURE 52–1
Transferring Sterile Instruments

GOAL

To move sterile items on a sterile field or transfer sterile items to a gloved team member.

EQUIPMENT AND SUPPLIES

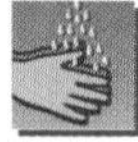

- A sterile item to move or transfer
- A pair of packaged sterile gloves
- A sterile wrapped transfer forceps
- A Mayo stand set-up with a sterile field and sterile instruments

Continued

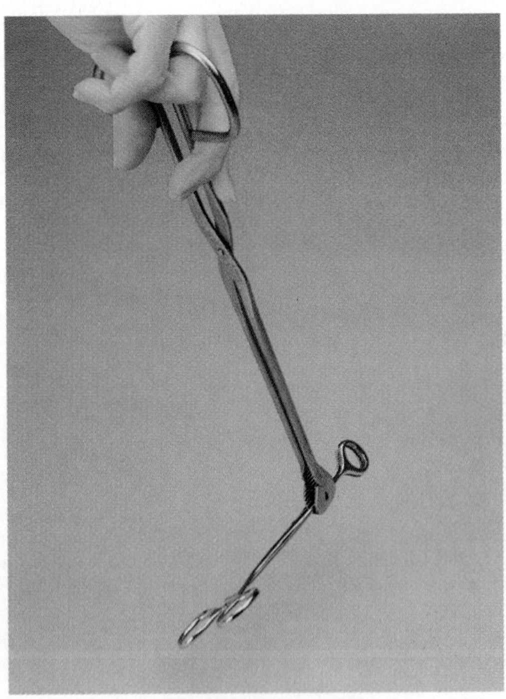

FIGURE 1

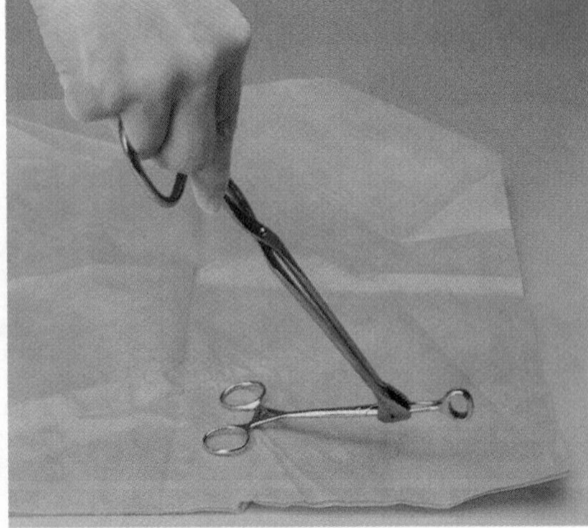

FIGURE 2

PROCEDURAL STEPS

1 Wash your hands and dry them carefully.
PURPOSE: Water on your hands makes gloving difficult.

2 Put on sterile gloves or open a package containing a sterile transfer forceps.

3 Using aseptic technique, handle sterile forceps by ring handle only. Always point forceps tips down (Figure 1).
PURPOSE: If the tips are turned upward, any solution encountered will run onto the nonsterile area and then back down over the sterile end when the tips are turned down again, thus contaminating the forceps.

4. Grasp an item on the sterile field with your sterile gloved hand or the sterile forceps, points down, and move it to its proper position for the procedure (Figure 2).
PURPOSE: Sterile items touch only sterile items.

5. Or, transfer an instrument from the autoclave to the sterile field.

6. Remove the transfer forceps after one-time use.

Assisting the Physician

The physician is ultimately responsible for the patient; however, the medical assistant is responsible for ensuring that everything the assistant and the physician use in the care of the surgical patient is accounted for, ready for use, and prepared in a safe and sterile manner. A surgical conscience is the practice of good aseptic technique and demands that breaks in aseptic technique be corrected immediately without regard to delays or embarrassment.

Every team has preferences regarding the sequence that the team follows concerning the routines of minor surgery. Once a routine is established, it should be followed in every case. Sample set-ups for various types of minor surgery are provided in Table 52–2.

TABLE 52–2 Sample Minor Surgery Set-ups

Procedure	Side Counter	Sterile Field	Comments	Postoperative Care
Suture repair	Local anesthetic, dressings and bandages, splints or guards, tape, drape, gloves, sterile physiologic saline	Syringe and needle, hemostats (3), scissors, sponges, suture material and needle, tissue forceps or skin hook, needle holder	If an emergency patient arrives in the office with a pressure dressing over a laceration, do not remove the pressure dressing until the physician is ready to suture. If the patient's pressure cloth *must* be removed, have ample sterile dressings ready to apply immediately. Ask the patient the possible length, depth, and exact location of the laceration. Usually there is limited cleansing of a wound because of the bleeding. If not, let the physician instruct you on the necessary cleansing.	Frequently, clean lacerations in a moderately protected area will not be dressed but left open. The patient will be instructed to keep the area clean and dry. Some lacerations may be closed with adhesive strips. These are becoming increasingly popular, because they reduce the chance of infection and do not leave suture scars.
Needle biopsy	Specimen bottle with sufficient fixative or preserving solution, laboratory form and label, local anesthetic, gloves	Biopsy needle, syringe and needle, sponges	A biopsy is the examination of tissue removed from the living body. Biopsies are usually done to determine whether a growth or swelling is malignant or benign; however, it may be done as a diagnostic aid in other diseases or infections. A needle biopsy may be done by aspiration with a needle and syringe or by a special biopsy needle. The specimen is then sent to a pathologist for either a cytologic or histologic examination.	Usually there is no special dressing required after a needle biopsy. A Band-Aid is often sufficient.
Cyst removal	Local anesthetic, disinfectant (skin prep), laboratory form, dressing (size depends on site), gloves, drape, specific bottle with sufficient fixative or preserving solution	Kelly hemostats (2 straight and 2 curved), dressing forceps (2), suture and needle, scissors s/s or s/b, dissector (physician's choice), skin hook, syringe and needle, knife handle with blade No. 11 or No. 15, tissue forceps (2), Allis forceps, needle holder, sponges	A sebaceous cyst is a benign retention cyst of a sebaceous gland containing fatty substance of the gland. It is also called a *wen.* They may occur any place on the body, with the exception of the palms of the hands and the soles of the feet. They are more common on the neck and shoulder; and because they are frequently the source of irritation, they are removed. Ordinarily, the cyst is attached only to the skin and moves freely over the underlying tissue. For cosmetic reasons, the physician will make the incision on the natural skin crease lines.	See suture repair above or apply a small dressing depending on size of incision.

Preparation and Care of the Patient

Whether minor surgery is the result of an unforeseen accident or a planned, elective procedure, the patient needs psychological care as well as physical care. The patient facing any surgical procedure suffers from fear of pain, fear of disfigurement, and often the fear of cancer being discovered. An injured patient may feel anxious about the medical bills or loss of employment. Because surgery is a frightening and dehumanizing experience, the medical assistant must take the time, both preoperatively and at the time of surgery, to help the patient through these fears and anxieties. The best method is to help the patient talk about the procedure or voice any concerns or misgivings.

Questions should be answered directly, but you should answer only those questions that are within your scope of experience and the policies of the office. If you cannot answer a question, assure the patient that you will relay the question to the physician before the procedure. Do not forget to relay the message. What may seem to be a minor or unimportant question to you may be very frightening to the patient. A good technique is to write down the question in the patient's presence and then give it to the physician. The minor surgery room can look very frightening to the patient, so unless the patient is sedated, try to make conversation with the patient while you prepare for the physician's arrival.

The physical preparation may involve obtaining blood and urine samples for tests the day before surgery, completing forms and consents, and gathering a current history concerning any recent illnesses or medications and allergies. Before the day of surgery, preoperative instructions may include a shave prep, cleansing enemas, food intake restrictions, special bathing, and a sedative medication.

On the day of surgery, the patient's vital signs are recorded, and the patient is assisted in undressing, if necessary, and then is asked to empty his or her bladder. Keep the patient on schedule but never appear to rush the process.

Memory Jogger

List three procedures that are done to the patient on the day of surgery.

Preoperative Instructions

When planning office surgery, certain procedures should be followed before the time of the appointment.

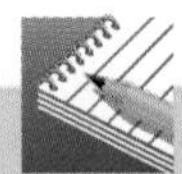

SKILLS AND RESPONSIBILITIES

PROCEDURES TO FOLLOW BEFORE THE SCHEDULED SURGERY

- Have the necessary consent forms ready to sign.
- Give the patient all the necessary preoperative instructions, such as medications to be used and special skin cleansing.
- Instruct the patient to bring a relative or friend to drive him or her home after the surgery.
- When appropriate, instruct the patient to wear special clothing that is easily removed and can be worn over bulky dressings or a cast.
- Instruct the patient to leave jewelry and other valuables at home.
- Call the patient the day before the surgery to confirm any special instructions.

Positioning the Patient

Have the patient disrobe sufficiently to completely expose the surgical area. There is much risk of contamination in performing the procedure while either you or the patient is holding back clothing that may slide into the area where the physician is working. Clothing may also act as a tourniquet or may make it difficult to apply a proper dressing or bandage. The patient's clothing may also be stained with the skin disinfecting solution or may prevent a large area from being treated properly.

It is equally important to position the patient as comfortably as possible. An uncomfortable position can be held for only a limited time, and the patient will have to move, often in the middle of a procedure. If not comfortable, the patient's muscles may stiffen or ache after the surgery. If bandaging is applied to an area with the patient in an awkward position, the bandage may bind or improperly fit when the patient assumes a normal position. When deciding on the correct patient position, consider where you and the physician will stand or sit, where the instruments will be placed, and where other needed equipment will be. If the patient has an open wound, or has a wound that will need **irrigation,** wear nonsterile gloves to assist the patient into position for the procedure. If there is active and profuse bleeding, a gown and gloves should be worn. If there is danger of blood and body fluid contamination to your face, wear goggles and a mask.

The Skin Prep

The human skin is a reservoir of bacteria and cannot be sterilized. Resident organisms cannot be completely removed or destroyed. Transit bacteria can also be harmful, and all care must be given to cleanse the patient's skin of bacteria as much as possible. Cleansing the patient's skin before surgery with surgical soap and an antiseptic is called a skin prep (see Procedures 52–2 and 52–3). A good skin prep eliminates the transference of harmful organisms to the incision site. The skin prep is performed by a gloved assistant. Sometimes the patient may be instructed to repeatedly cleanse the surgical area with bacteriostatic or antiseptic soap several days before the surgery. The medical assistant or physician may need to shave the surgical area before the skin prep. Disposable skin prep trays and razors are available.

PROCEDURE 52-2

Pouring a Sterile Solution into a Container on a Sterile Field

GOAL

As a circulating assistant, pour a sterile solution into a stainless-steel bowl or medicine glass that is sitting at the edge of a sterile field.

EQUIPMENT AND SUPPLIES

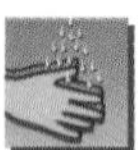

A sterile bottle of solution
A stainless-steel bowl or medicine glass
A sterile field
A sink or waste receptacle

Note: A medicine glass or bowl on the sterile field should be near one edge of the field and the perimeter of the 1-inch barrier.

PROCEDURAL STEPS

1 Wash your hands and dry them carefully.
PURPOSE: Moisture on your hands may cause the bottle to slip from your hand.

2 Read the label.
PURPOSE: Always read the label before and after administering any solution or medication.

3 Place your hand over the label and lift the bottle. *Note:* If the container has a double cap, set the outer cap on the counter inside up, then proceed.

4 Lift the lid of the bottle straight up, and then slightly to one side, and hold the lid in your minor hand facing downward.
PURPOSE: Air currents carry contaminants that could settle on the inside of the lid.

5 Pour away from the label (Figure 1).
PURPOSE: Spills down the side of the bottle stain or make the label unreadable.

6 If the container does not have a double cap, pour off a small amount of the solution into a waste receptacle.
PURPOSE: To rinse any contaminants off the bottle lip. *Note:* If the container has a double cap, skip this step and proceed to step 7.

Continued

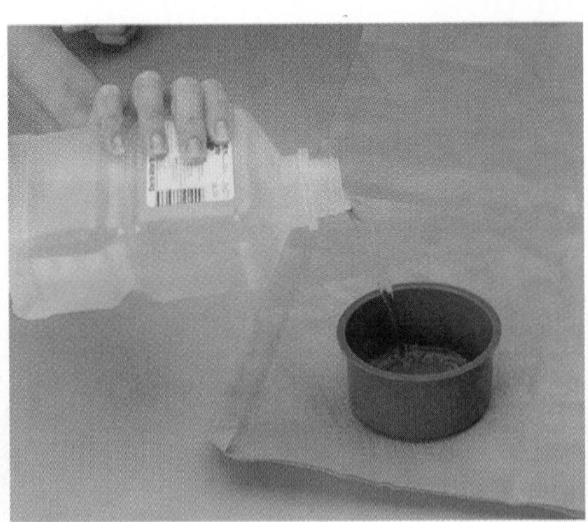
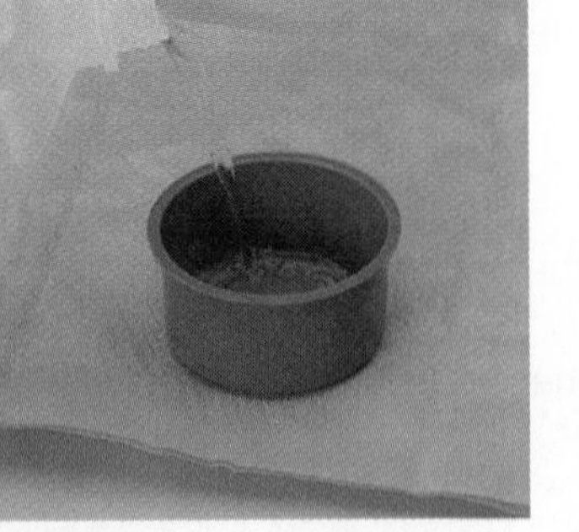

FIGURE 1

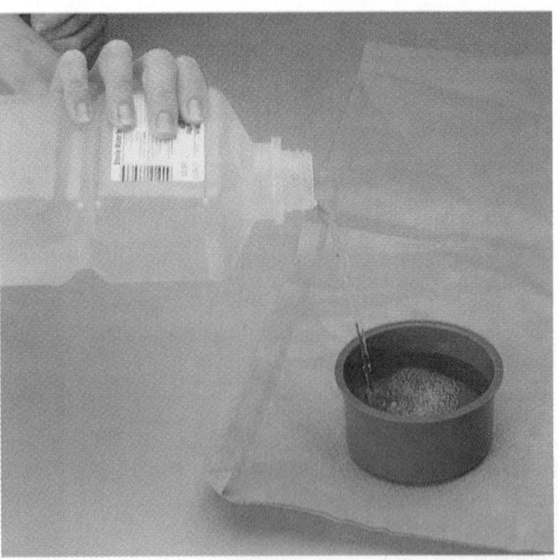

FIGURE 2

7 Pour away from the label, into the bowl, without allowing any part of the bottle to touch the bowl (Figure 2).
PURPOSE: The bottle exterior is not sterile.

8 Tilt the bottle up to stop the pouring while it is still over the bowl.
PURPOSE: Solutions spilled on the sterile field may contaminate the field.

9 Remove the bottle from over the sterile field.
PURPOSE: Motion over a sterile field should be kept to a minimum.

10 Replace the cap(s) off to the side, away from the sterile field.

PROCEDURE 52-3
Preparing a Patient's Skin for Surgery

GOAL
To prepare the patient's skin for a surgical procedure to reduce the risk of wound contamination.

EQUIPMENT AND SUPPLIES
A disposable skin prep kit or an autoclave skin prep containing

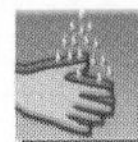

- Gauze sponges
- Cotton-tipped applicators
- Antiseptic soap
- Sterile gloves
- Two small stainless-steel bowls
- Antiseptic
- *Optional:* Cotton balls, nail pick, scrub brush
- A waste receptacle

Continued

PROCEDURE 52-3 (CONTINUED)

Preparing a Patient's Skin for Surgery

PROCEDURAL STEPS

1 Wash your hands and dry them carefully. Follow Universal Precautions.
PURPOSE: Moisture on your hands contaminates the pack.

2 Open your skin prep pack.

3 Arrange the items with sterile gloved hands.
PURPOSE: The skin prep is a sterile field.

4 Add the surgical soap and antiseptic solutions to the two bowls.

5 Instruct the patient of scrub procedure.
PURPOSE: To ensure cooperation and keep the patient comfortable.

6 Expose the site. Use a light if necessary.

7 Glove, using aseptic technique.
PURPOSE: To protect the patient from your resident bacteria.

8 Place two sterile towels at the edges of the area to be scrubbed.
PURPOSE: The area must be scrubbed up to the sterile towels, which will be beyond the opening of the surgical drape when the drape is applied.

9 Start at the incision site, and begin washing with the antiseptic soap on a gauze sponge in a circular motion, moving from the center to the edges of the area to be scrubbed (Figures 1 and 2).
PURPOSE: Circular motion from inside to outside drags contaminants away from the incision site.

10 After one complete wipe, discard the sponge, and begin again with a new sponge soaked in the antiseptic solution.
PURPOSE: After one circular sweep, the sponge is now contaminated with skin bacteria and debris. When you return to the incision site for the next circular sweep, you must use sterile material.

11 Repeat the process, using sufficient friction for 5 minutes (or follow office policy for the length of time required for a particular prep).

12 Dry the area, using the same circular technique with dry sponges. The area may be dried by blotting with a third sterile towel.

13 Check that no solutions are pooling under the patient.
PURPOSE: The solution will irritate or burn the skin.

Continued

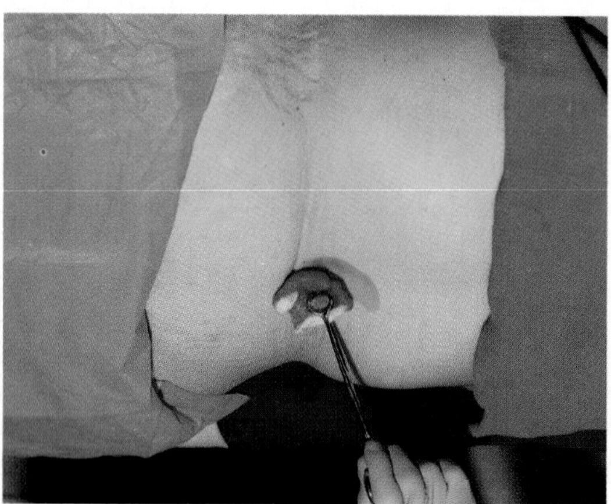

FIGURE 1

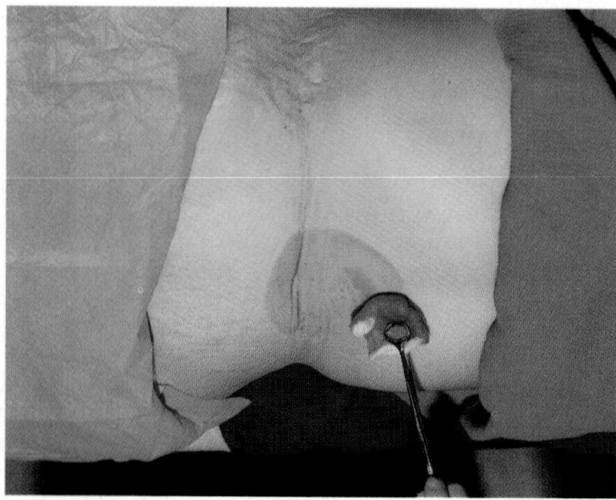

FIGURE 2

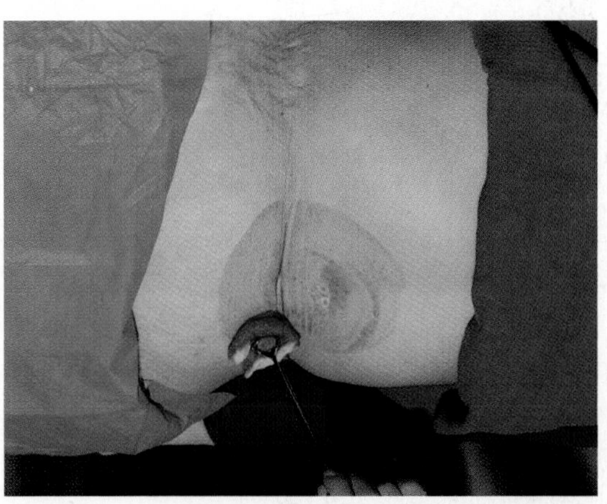

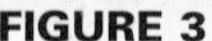

FIGURE 3

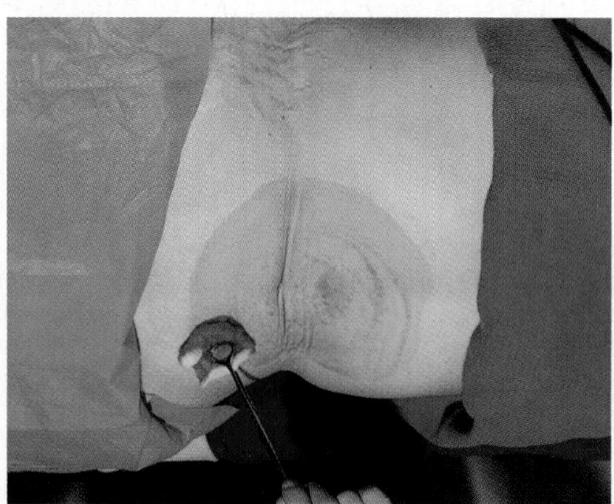

FIGURE 4

14 Paint on the antiseptic with the cotton-tipped applicators or gauze sponges, using the same circular technique and never returning to an area that has already been painted (Figures 3 through 5).

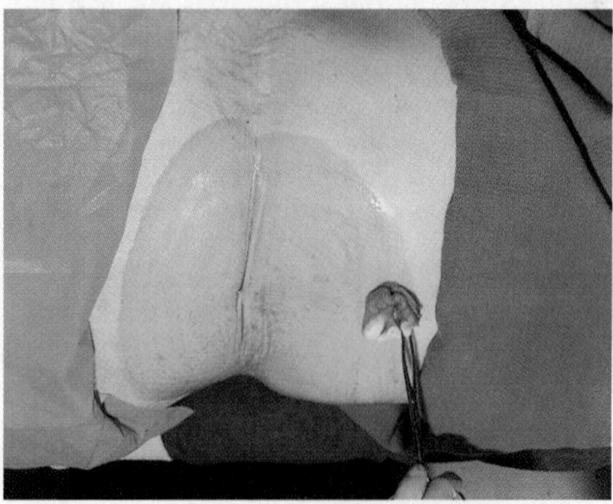

FIGURE 5

Surgical Routines

After receiving an assignment to assist in a minor surgical procedure, study the physician preference card to review the procedure and note the materials that are needed. Next, prepare the room and gather the supplies to be used. Sterile supplies are opened just before the procedure. Opened materials that have been exposed longer than an hour, due to some delay, must be considered unsterile. Supplies should not be placed where they can be knocked over or dropped. Wrapped sterile supplies that fall to the floor must not be used. Once supplies are opened, a team member should stay in the room to monitor them. The circulating assistant opens the packs, beginning with the pack that provides the sterile surface for the remaining sterile items (see Procedures 52–4, 52–5, and 52–6).

The Mayo tray is usually prepared as soon as the scrub assistant is gloved and ready to manage the sterile field.

Drapes, towel packs, additional sponge packs, and other sterile packages are stacked on the side or back table. Items from this table may be added, if needed, during the procedure. A basin or trash bucket for waste is placed nearby for use during the surgery.

The scrub assistant sorts and places the scalpels, hemostats, scissors, tissue forceps, and retractors on the sterile field according to their sequence and frequency of use (Fig. 52–1). Scalpels and sharp instruments should be conspicuously placed so that they do not accidentally harm a team member. If the scrub assistant has not previously prepped the patient, the circulating assistant now performs the patient skin prep. The circulating assistant opens the drape pack. The physician enters the room and

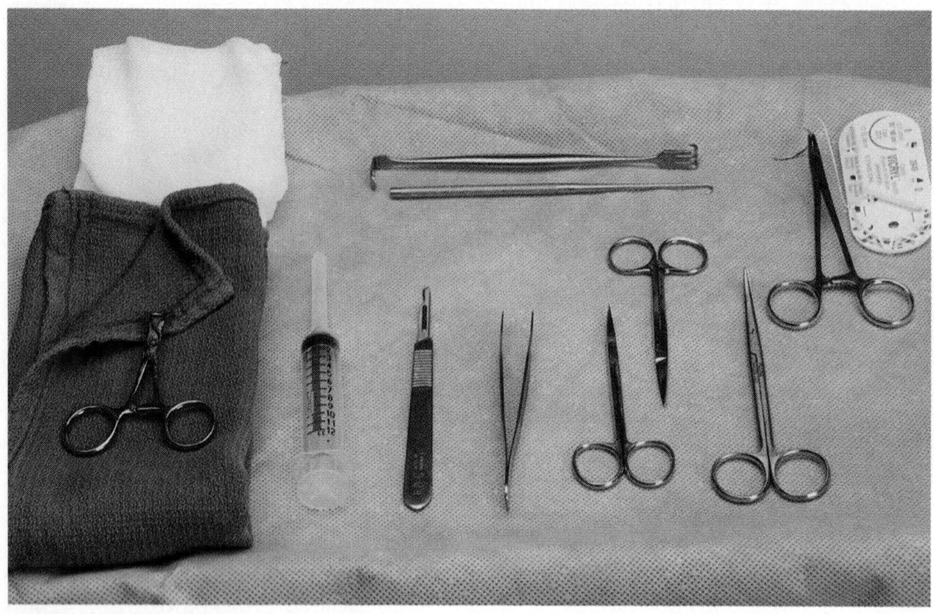

FIGURE 52–1 Surgical set-up on sterile Mayo stand.

gloves. The physician drapes the patient with towels or a fenestrated drape as the scrub assistant hands the drapes, one at a time. In many offices, the scrub assistant alone drapes the site. Once the site is draped, the Mayo stand is positioned below the site and the scrub assistant stands opposite the physician over the patient. The circulating assistant cleans the vial of anesthesia medication with an alcohol swab and holds the vial (with the label visible to read) for the scrub assistant or the physician. The scrub assistant or physician lifts the syringe from the sterile field and withdraws the appropriate amount of anesthesia medication into the syringe. The physician administers the anesthesia medication, after reading the label. The scrub assistant places a sponge on the patient, next to the wound site, for sponging blood at the time of the first incision or to sponge an open injury as the first step of the procedure (see Procedure 52–7). Local anesthesia medication is administered either directly into the **lesion** or into the tissues surrounding the site to be incised. After the local anesthesia has taken effect, the physician begins the procedure.

During the procedure, the scrub assistant must protect the sterile field from contamination, notify the physician if there is a break in sterile technique, dispose of soiled sponges into the waste receptacle, and anticipate the surgeon's need for instruments and hand pass instruments. The physician may verbally request instruments or may use hand signals (Fig. 52–2). As the team works together over time, the physician may not need to give any signals.

Instrumentation is logical; if the physician requests a suture, then scissors will be needed to cut the suture strand (see Procedure 52–8). In case of sudden hemorrhage from a bleeding vessel, the physician will need a hemostat. In gaining experience, the assistant watches, listens, and learns to judge what will be needed or performed next. Pass instruments with a firm and purposeful motion so that the physician will not have to look up. Wait until you feel the physician grasp the instrument, so it will not drop onto the patient or to the floor. Pass instruments so that you and the physician are protected from injury. Pass the scalpel blade down. Hold all instruments by their tips, and pass the handle ends into the physician's palm or fingers. Avoid painful slapping of the instruments into the surgeon's hand. Correct passing produces a faint, gentle "snap" as it contacts the gloved hand.

If a specimen is collected during the procedure, it is placed in a sterile glass or basin. Do not remove the specimen from the sterile field until the physician gives the order. He or she may want to examine it again during the procedure.

Memory Jogger

 *Identify the scrub assistant's responsibilities during the surgical procedure.*

Completion of the Surgical Procedure

At the conclusion of the procedure, the physician will begin the wound closure. The techniques and methods of tissue closure vary greatly, and it would be impossible to describe or illustrate all of them. There are two basic methods of suturing: the continuous (running) placement of a single strand and the interrupted suture, in which each knot is placed and tied independently, so that if one breaks, the others keep the wound closure intact (Fig. 52–3). The ma-

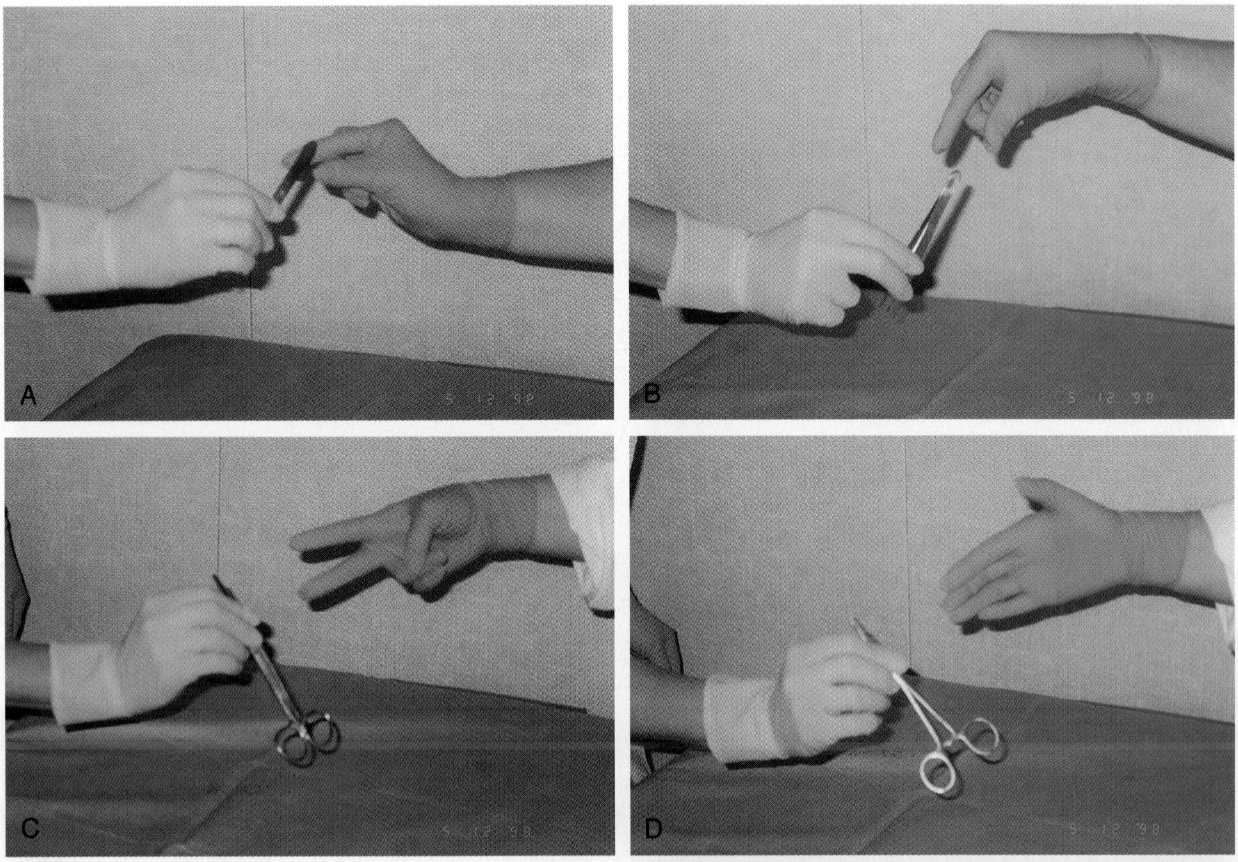

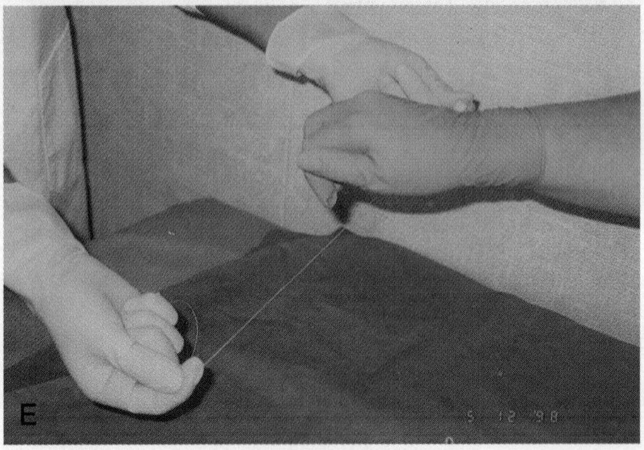

FIGURE 52–2 *A*, Hand signal for scalpel. *B*, Hand signal for forceps. *C*, Hand signal for scissors. *D*, Hand signal for clamp. *E*, Hand signal for free suture pass (free tie).

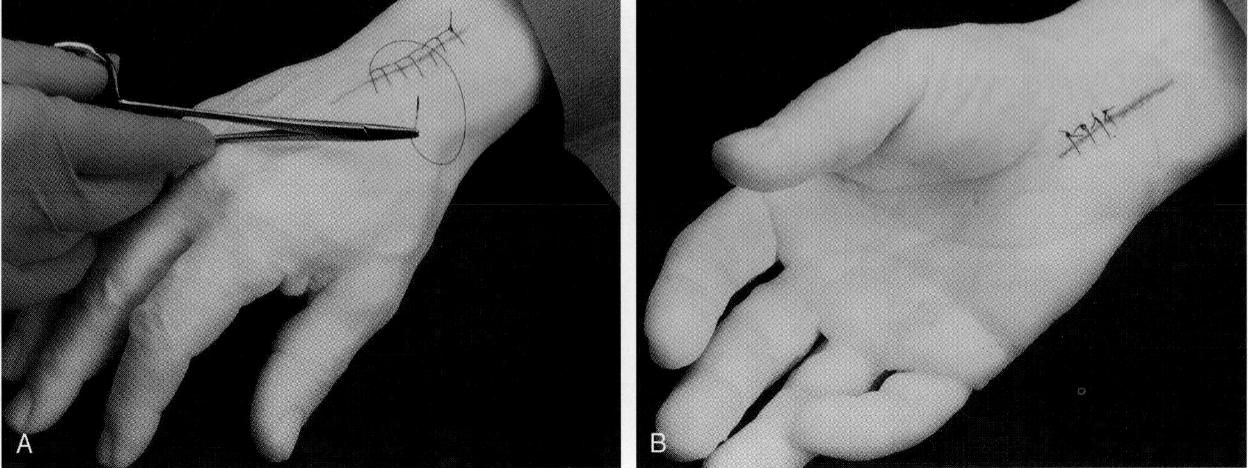

FIGURE 52–3 *A*, Continuous (running) suture placement. *B*, Interrupted suture placement.

jority of skin closures in the medical office are limited to the interrupted technique.

The scrub assistant mounts the suture and needle in the needle holder and passes the unit to the physician. As the physician closes the wound, the scrub assistant assists by cutting the suture and sponging the site. The physician places the first interrupted suture at the midpoint of the incision. Then, each side of the first suture is mentally divided in half again, and the next two sutures are placed at each of these midpoints. The rest of the sutures are placed by the same technique of mentally dividing the remaining suture line in half until the length of the wound edge is totally **approximated.**

After the skin closure, the wound site is cleaned with wet and dry sponges. This may be done by the surgeon or the scrub assistant. Care must be taken not to disturb the wound edges or the sutures. Next, sterile dressings are placed over the incision and the drapes are removed. Lift the drapes directly off the patient with minimum movement so as not to disturb the dressing or stir up the air currents. The circulating assistant or the surgeon then applies the bandage and tape to the dressing. Do not take away your Mayo stand with instruments until the patient has left the room or the surgeon instructs you. If there is an unexpected contamination of the wound site during the dressing application, more materials will be needed from the sterile field.

Memory Jogger

Why is the Mayo stand with instruments left in place until the patient has left the surgery room?

Text continued on page 1132

PROCEDURE 52-4

Opening a Sterile Pack That Will Serve as the Sterile Field

GOAL

To open a sterile pack that contains a table drape, using correct aseptic technique.

EQUIPMENT AND SUPPLIES

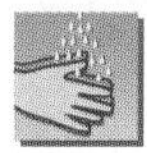

A sterile pack (autoclaved linen or disposable) that will serve as a sterile table drape or field.
A Mayo stand or countertop
Disinfectant and gauze sponges

PROCEDURAL STEPS

1 Check that the Mayo stand or counter top is dust free and clean. If it is not, clean with 70% alcohol or another disinfectant and towel.

Continued

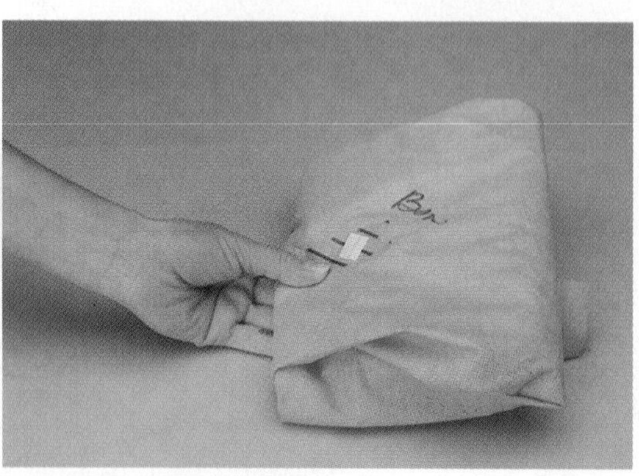

FIGURE 1

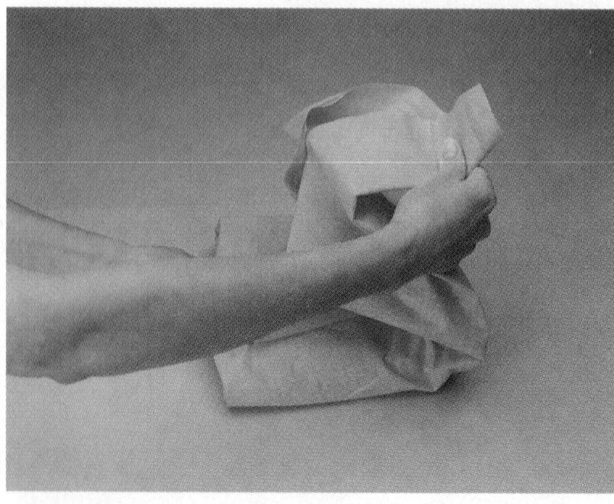

FIGURE 2

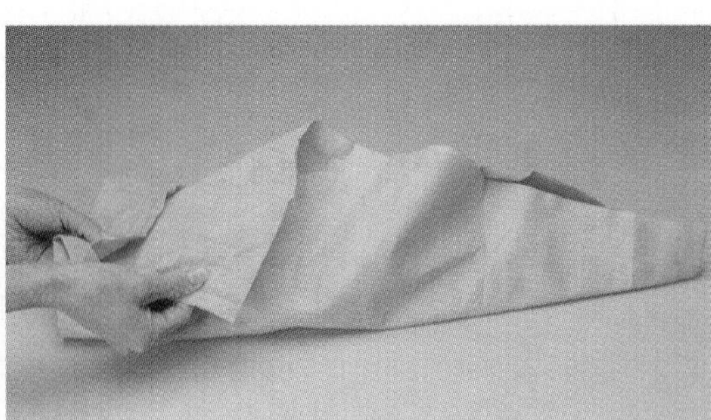

FIGURE 3

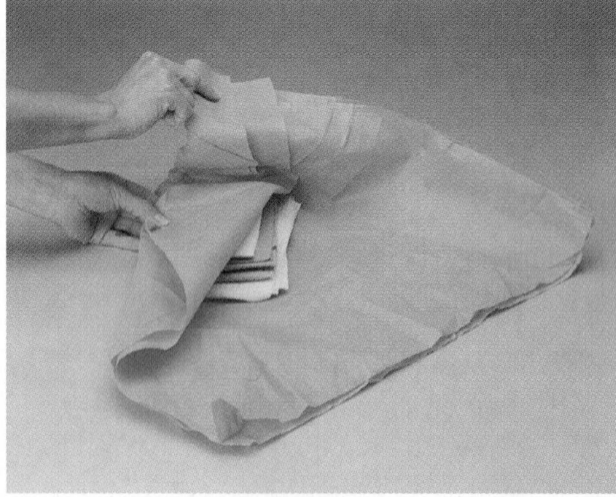

FIGURE 4

PURPOSE: Although some areas cannot be sterile, steps must be taken to keep contamination to a minimum.

2 Wash your hands and dry them carefully.
PURPOSE: Moisture on your hands contaminates the pack.

3 Place the sterile pack on the Mayo stand or countertop and read the label.
PURPOSE: Most medical offices have a limited supply of autoclaved packs. To open a wrong package could mean not having enough sterile supplies for a different procedure.

4 Check the expiration date (Figure 1). If using an autoclaved pack, check the indicator tape for color change.
PURPOSE: An expired pack is not considered sterile. Autoclave indicator tape changes color after the sterile processing cycle.

5 Position the package so that the outer envelope flap is face up and at the top as you look at the package.
PURPOSE: This positions the pack for correct opening, using aseptic technique.

6 Open the first flap away from you (Figure 2).
PURPOSE: Otherwise, you will be reaching over a sterile field for the other three flaps.

7 Pull away the two side flaps, one at a time. Be careful to lift each flap by reaching under the small folded-back tab and without touching the inner surface of the pack or its contents (Figures 3 and 4).

8 Pull the last flap toward you by its tab, exposing the towel (Figure 5).

9 You now have a sterile drape as a sterile field to work from and for the distribution of additional sterile supplies and instruments (Figure 6).

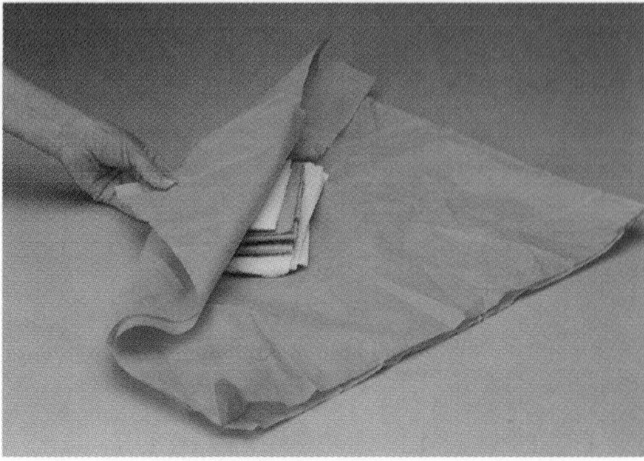

FIGURE 5

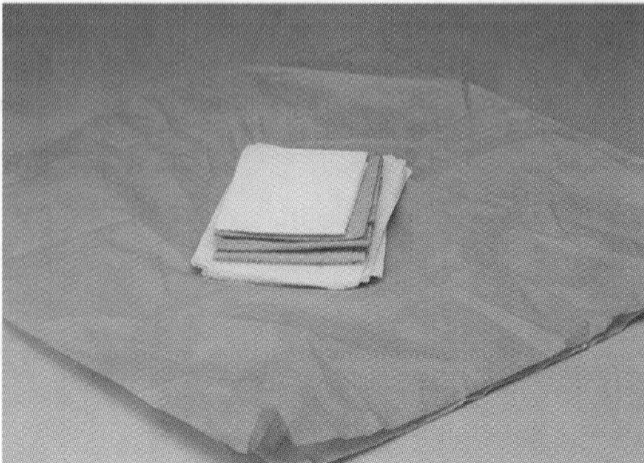

FIGURE 6

PROCEDURE 52-5
Opening a Sterile Pack to Add Its Contents to a Sterile Field

GOAL
As a circulating assistant, add instruments from sterile pack to a sterile field, using correct aseptic technique.

EQUIPMENT AND SUPPLIES
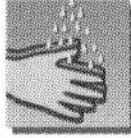

An autoclaved pack that contains at least three sterile items

A Mayo stand set-up with a sterile field or an opened sterile wrapper

PROCEDURAL STEPS
1 Wash your hands and dry them carefully.
PURPOSE: Moisture on your hands contaminates the pack.

2 Position the pack on the palm of your minor hand so that the outer envelope flap is face up and at the top as you look at the package (Figure 1).
PURPOSE: This positions the pack for correct opening, using aseptic technique.

3 Check the expiration date and indicator tape.
PURPOSE: Always check for sterility.

4 Open the first flap away from you (Figure 2).

5 Pull away the two side flaps. Be careful to lift each flap by reaching under the small folded-back tab and without touching the inner surface of the pack or its contents (Figure 3).

6 The last flap is pulled toward you by its tab, exposing the contents (Figure 4).

7 By closing your open palm, grasp the items through the cloth at the ends (if it is an instrument).
Note: To make this possible, all items must be autoclaved in the same direction.

Continued

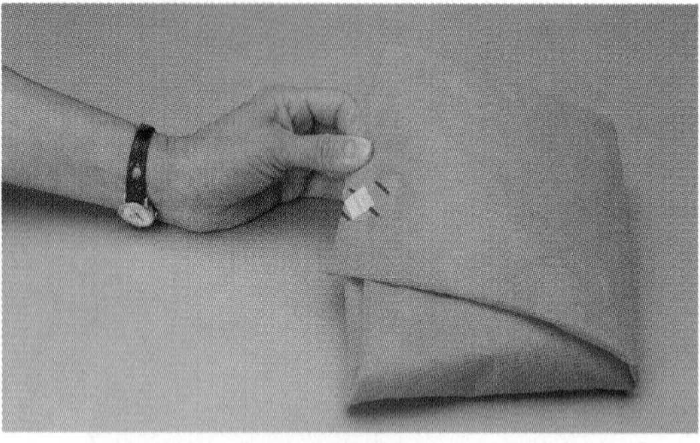

FIGURE 1

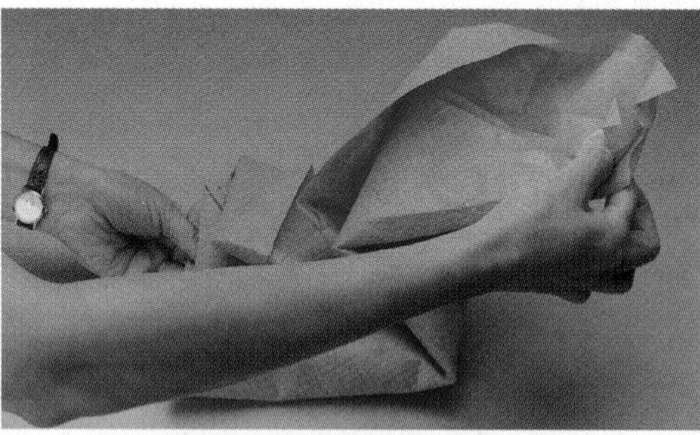

FIGURE 2

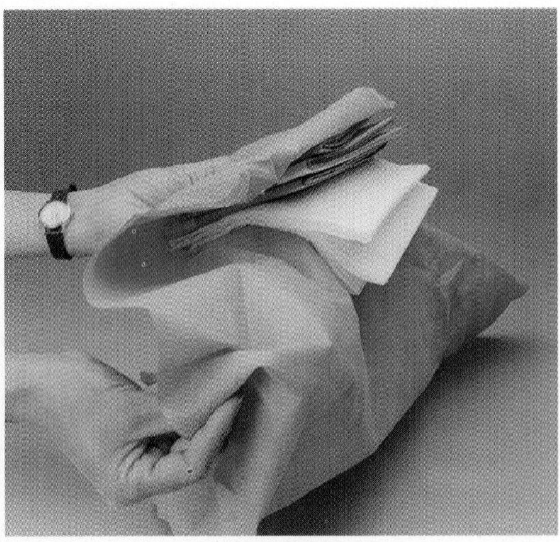

FIGURE 3

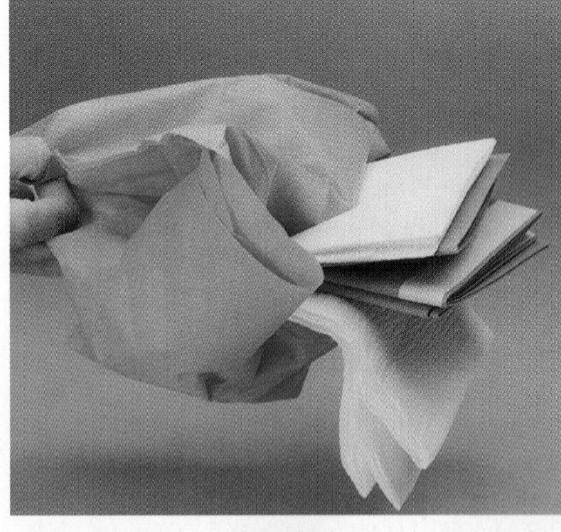

FIGURE 4

8 Hold the four flaps around your wrist with your major hand (Figure 5).
PURPOSE: All parts of the four flaps are now considered not sterile. Do not allow them to touch any part of the instruments or the sterile field.

9 Place the items onto the field. If they are instruments, handles should be first.
PURPOSE: To avoid damaging the fine tips.

10 Do not reach over the sterile field, yet place the instruments inside the perimeter of the 1-inch margin.
PURPOSE: The 1-inch perimeter around the sterile field is considered not sterile.

11 Or, hand the items to a gloved team member.

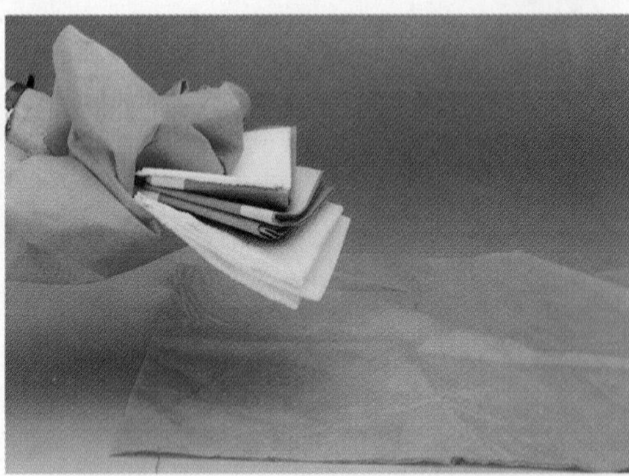

FIGURE 5

PROCEDURE 52-6

Adding Sterile Items in a Peel-Back Wrapper to a Sterile Field

GOAL

To add the contents of a sterile pack, such as syringes, needles, and suture materials, to the sterile field, using correct sterile technique.

EQUIPMENT AND SUPPLIES

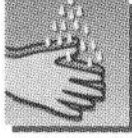

A Mayo stand set-up with a sterile field

A package containing suture material

PROCEDURAL STEPS

1 Wash your hands and dry them carefully.
PURPOSE: Moisture on your hands contaminates the pack.

2 Hold the package in your hand and read the label.
PURPOSE: Most medical offices have a limited supply of items. To open a wrong package could mean not having enough supplies for a different procedure.

3 Check for sterility and expiration date.
PURPOSE: All items must be sterile.

4 Hold the package, and grab a peel-away edge in each hand (Figure 1).

5 Open by peeling the two flaps apart. Keep the flaps away from the sterile item by holding them outward. The item should be protruding between the peel-back flaps (Figures 2 and 3).
PURPOSE: The edges of a sterile package are considered not sterile.

6 Continue to peel with a snap of the hands to "pop" the items out of the package and onto the sterile field from a distance of 8 to 12 inches. Do not reach over the field, yet place the item inside the perimeter of the 1-inch margin (Figures 4 through 6).

Continued

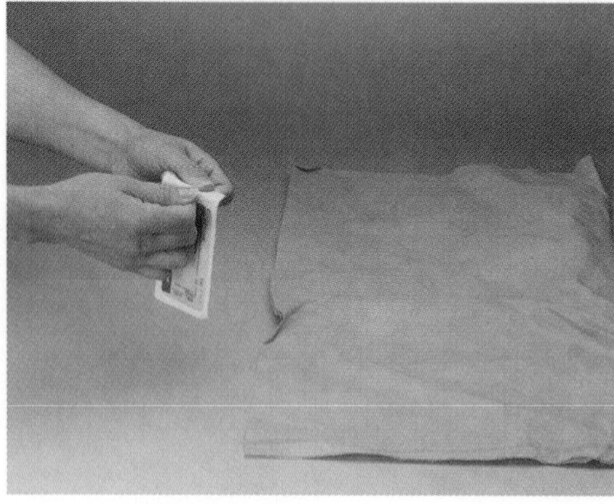

FIGURE 1

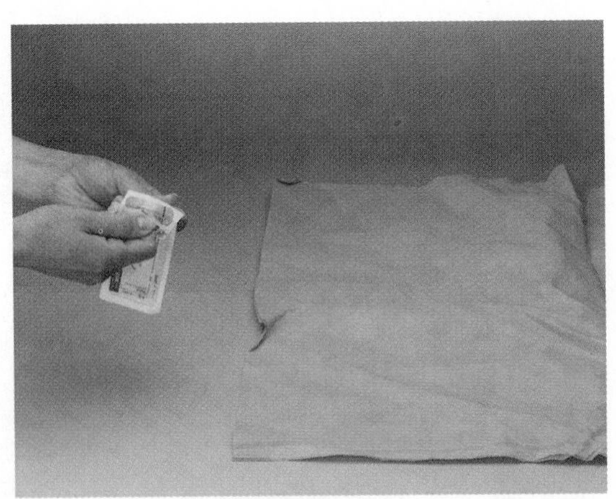

FIGURE 2

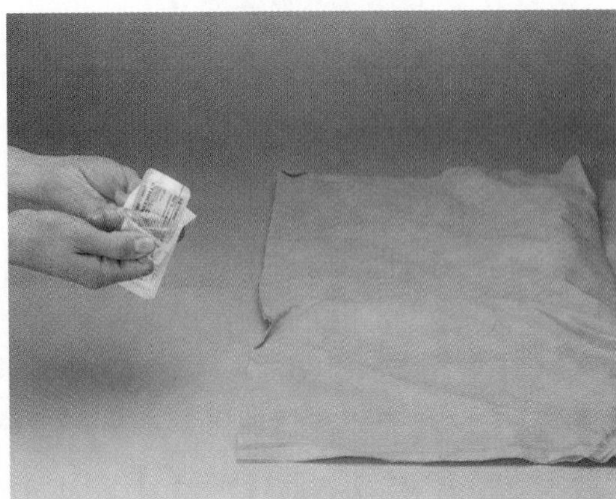

FIGURE 3

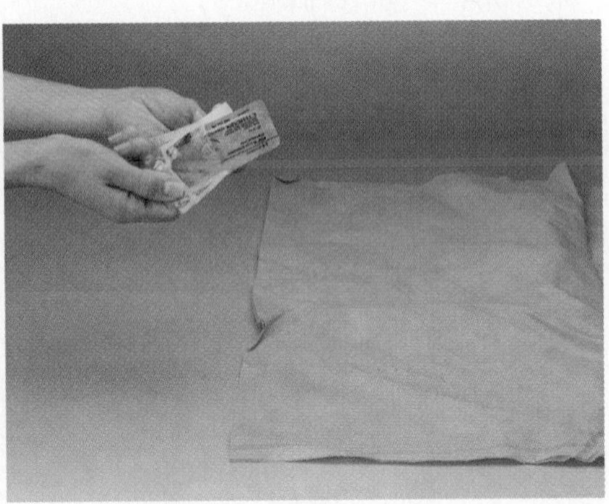

FIGURE 4

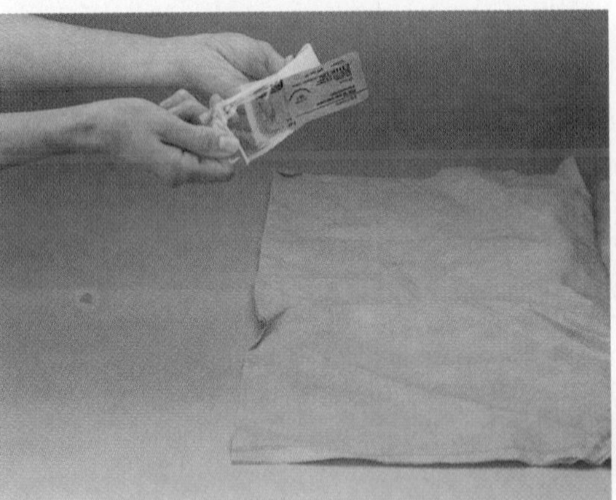

FIGURE 5

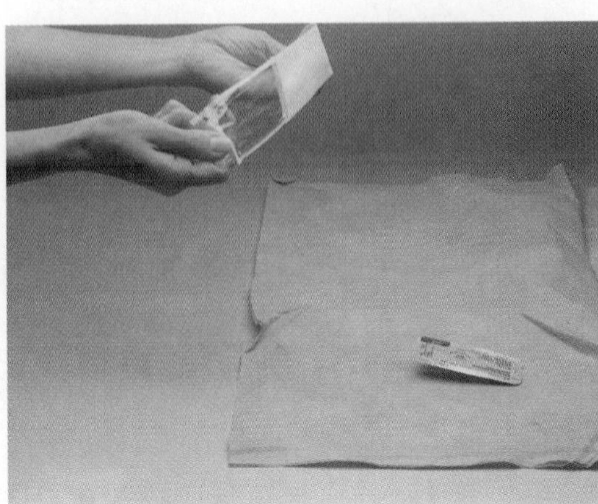

FIGURE 6

PROCEDURE 52-7
Assisting During the Minor Surgical Procedure

GOAL

To maintain the sterile field and to pass instruments in a prescribed sequence during a surgical procedure that involves the making of a surgical incision and the removal of a growth.

EQUIPMENT AND SUPPLIES

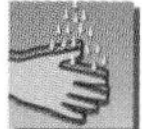
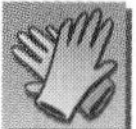

An open patient drape pack on the side counter
A Mayo stand covered with a sterile drape
Packaged sterile gloves (two pairs)
A needle and syringe for anesthesia medication
A vial of local anesthetic medication
One medicine glass or small bowl
A scalpel handle and a No. 15 blade
An Allis tissue forceps
One skin retractor
Three hemostats
A supply of gauze sponges
A waste receptacle

PROCEDURAL STEPS

1 Wash your hands. Dry thoroughly.
PURPOSE: Gloving is difficult with moist hands.

2 Glove, using aseptic technique. Set up the sterile field with instruments and supplies, in the sequence to be used (Figure 1).

3 Remove your gloves. Read the label of the local anesthetic medication and pour the medication in a medicine glass (Figure 2).
PURPOSE: The vial of local anesthetic medication cannot be held after both team members are gloved.

4 Glove, using aseptic technique, and prep the patient's skin with surgical soap and antiseptic solution. Instruct the patient of prep procedure.
PURPOSE: Infection control and to ensure the patient's cooperation.

5 Scrub, using the surgical hand wash procedure. Follow Universal Precautions.

Continued

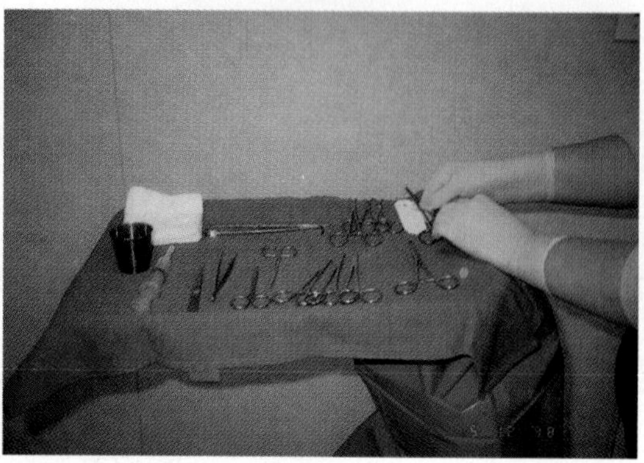

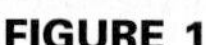
FIGURE 1

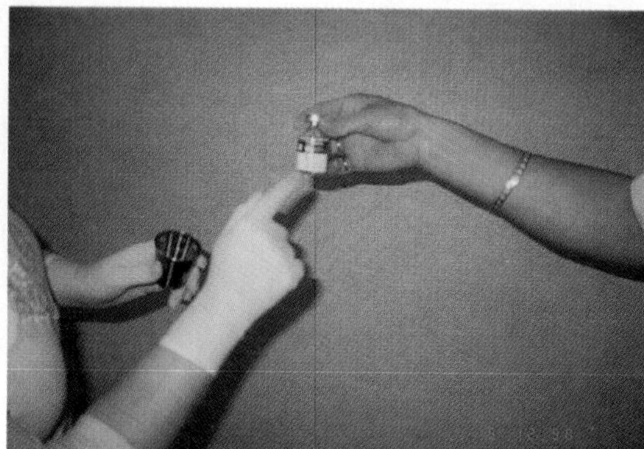

FIGURE 2

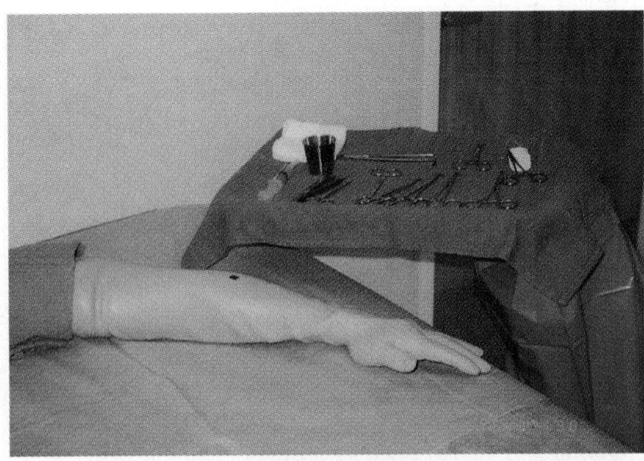

FIGURE 3

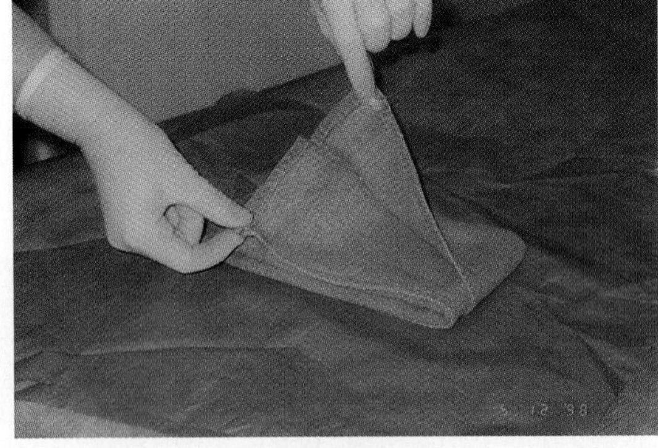

FIGURE 4

6 Dry your hands thoroughly.

7 Glove, using aseptic technique.

8 Position the Mayo stand near the patient and the operative site (Figure 3).
PURPOSE: Motion over a sterile field should be kept to a minimum.

9 Lift the patient drape from the open pack without touching the drape to any of the pack edges.
PURPOSE: The 1-inch perimeter around the sterile field is considered nonsterile.

10 Grasp the patient drape by holding one edge or corner in each hand (Figure 4).

11 Drape the surgical site without touching any part of the patient or the operating area with your gloved hands (Figure 5).

12 The surgeon injects the local anesthesia, after looking at the empty vial on the counter and confirming the type, strength, and expiration date. *Note:* The surgeon may drape the patient while you glove.
PURPOSE: Everyone should read the medication label before using or dispensing a medication.

13 Position yourself across the surgeon. Arrange the sterile field. Check instrument placement condition (Figure 6).

Continued

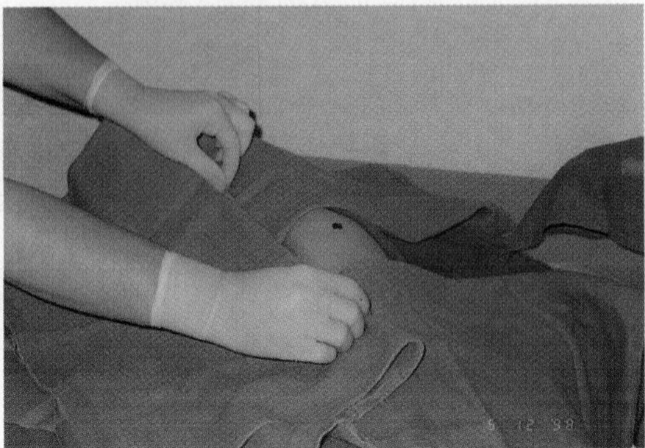

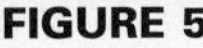

FIGURE 5

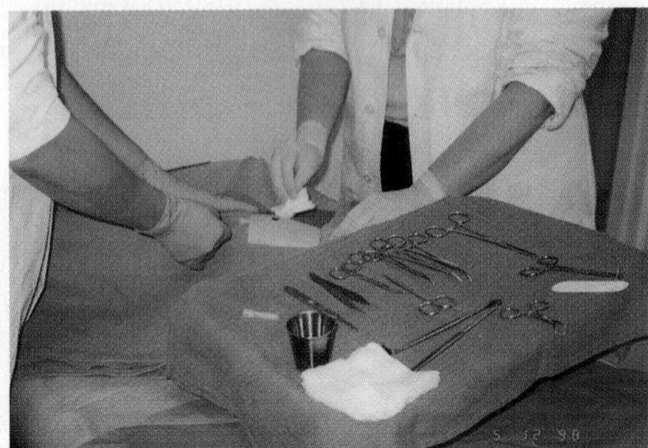

FIGURE 6

PROCEDURE 52-7 (CONTINUED)
Assisting During the Minor Surgical Procedure

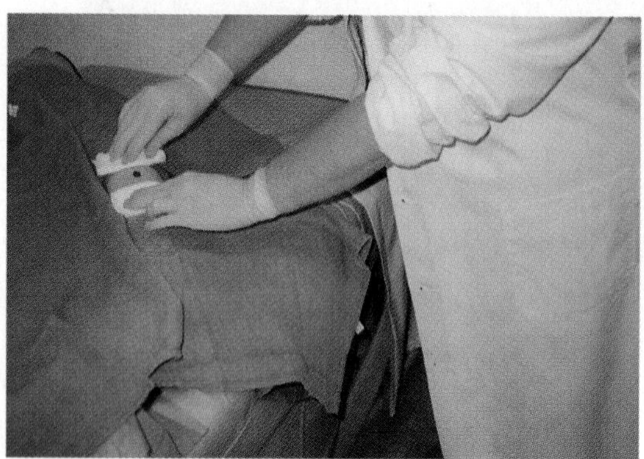

FIGURE 7

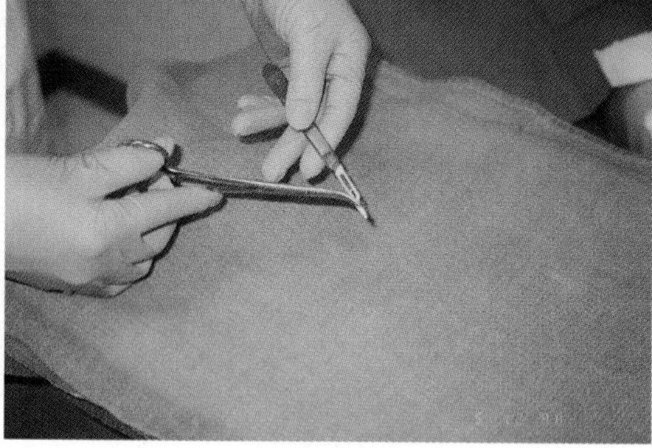

FIGURE 8

14 Place two sponges on the patient, next to the wound site (Figure 7).

15 Grasp the scalpel blade with a hemostat and mount the scalpel blade onto the scalpel handle. Keep all sharp equipment conspicuously placed on the sterile field (Figure 8).
PURPOSE: Sharp instruments that are not clearly visible may injure a team member.

16 Pass the scalpel, blade down, to the surgeon or he or she will reach for it himself or herself. The surgeon will take the scalpel with the thumb and forefinger in the position ready for use (Figure 9).
PURPOSE: To protect the surgeon and yourself from injury.

17 Grasp an Allis tissue forceps by the tips, and pass it to the surgeon to grasp a piece of the tissue to be excised (Figure 10).

18 Pass the handles into the surgeon's open palm with a firm and purposeful motion. A gentle "snap" is heard as it contacts the surgeon's gloved hand.
PURPOSE: The surgeon will not have to look up to receive the instrument.

19 Dispose of soiled sponges, using the waste receptacle.

Continued

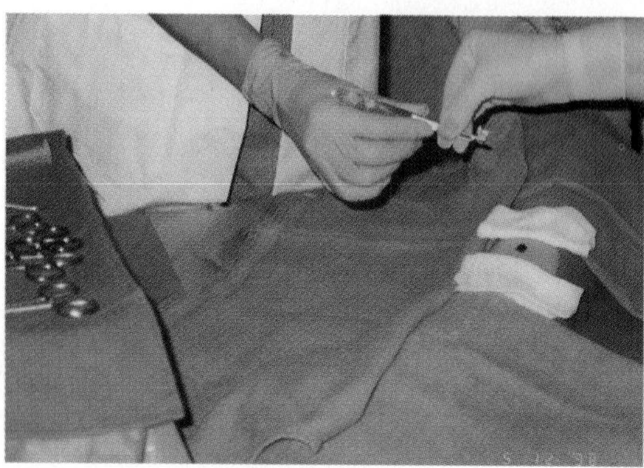

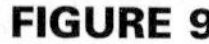

FIGURE 9

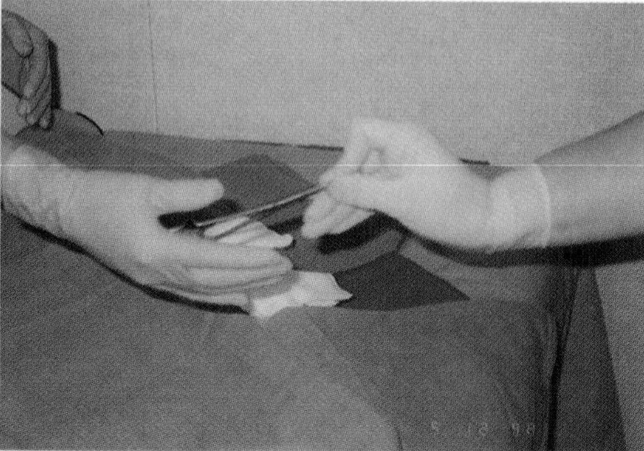

FIGURE 10

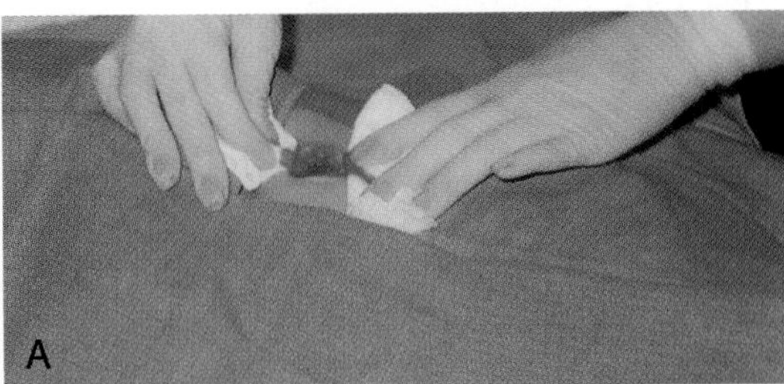

FIGURE 11A

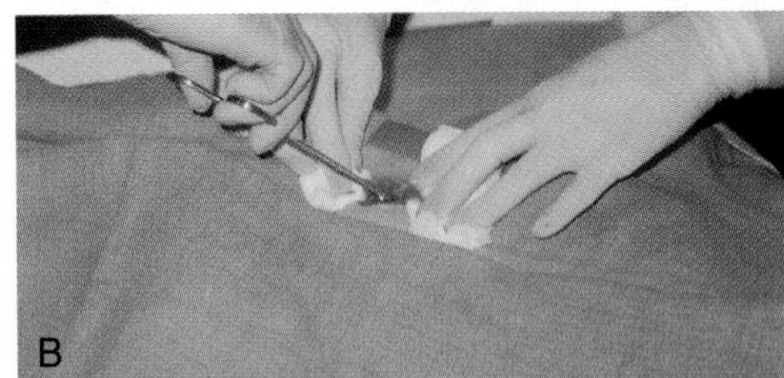

FIGURE 11B

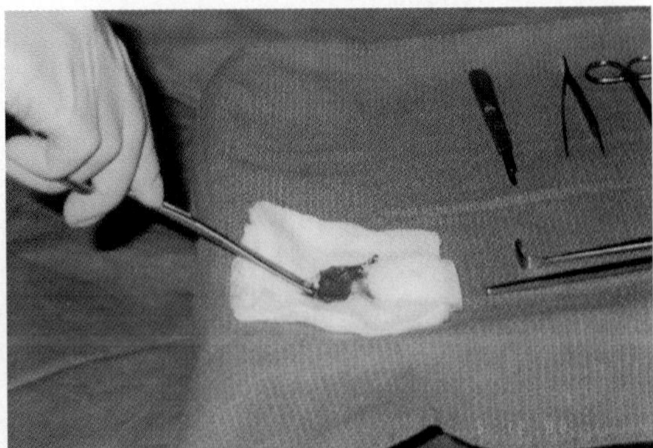

FIGURE 12

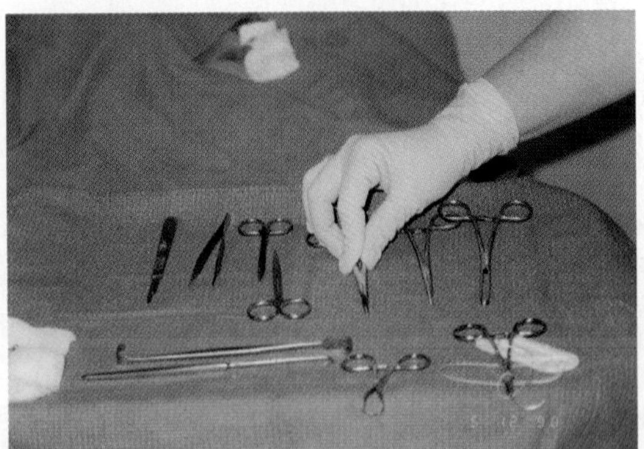

FIGURE 13

20 Hold clean sponges in your hand, to pass or sponge the wound, as needed (Figure 11).

21 Safely position the specimen (if any) where it will not be disturbed on the sterile field (Figure 12).

22 If there is a bleeding vessel, or if a hemostat is requested, pass the hemostat in the manner described in steps 17 and 18.

23 Receive instruments, and place them on the sterile field (Figure 13).

24 Continue to sponge blood from the wound site.
PURPOSE: A clear sterile field expedites the procedure.

25 Retract the wound edge, as needed, with a skin retractor.

26 Continue to monitor the sterile field and assist the surgeon as needed.

27 Pass the surgeon the suture to close the wound (Figure 14).

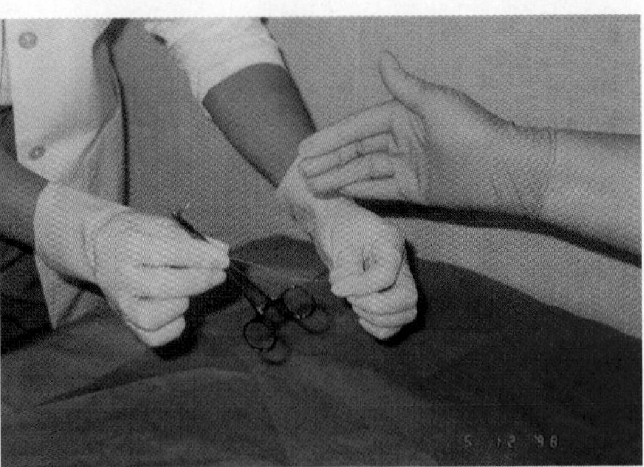

FIGURE 14

PROCEDURE 52-8

Assisting with Suturing

GOAL

To assist the surgeon in wound closure, using sterile technique.

EQUIPMENT AND SUPPLIES

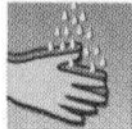 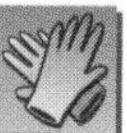

A sterile field on a Mayo stand
Surgical scissors
Suture material
Sterile gloves
Needle holder
Gauze sponges

PROCEDURAL STEPS

Note: This procedure may be a continuation of Procedure 52–7. If done independently, you must perform the surgical scrub and glove before beginning step 1.

1 Hold the curved needle point in your minor hand, 4 to 5 inches over the sterile field (Figure 1).
PURPOSE: Always work over a sterile field.

2 With the needle holder, clamp the suture needle at the upper third of its total length (Figure 2).
PURPOSE: Clamping in the middle weakens and may distort the shape of the needle. Clamping too near the thread may cause the suture to detach from the needle. Clamping at the lower third of the needle damages the needle point.

3 With your major hand, hold the needle holder halfway down its shaft, at the box-lock, with the suture needle point up.

Continued

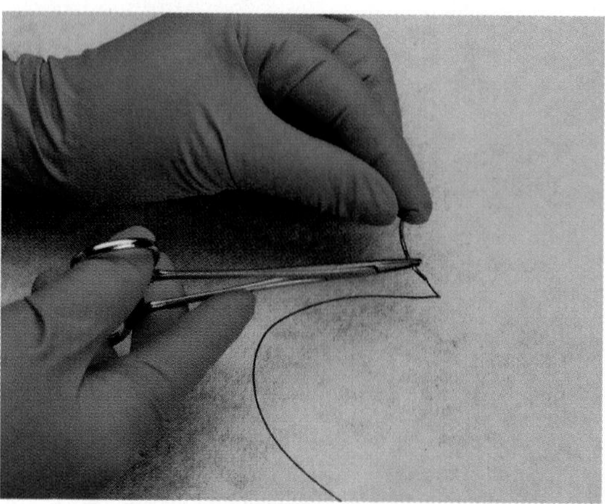

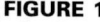

FIGURE 1

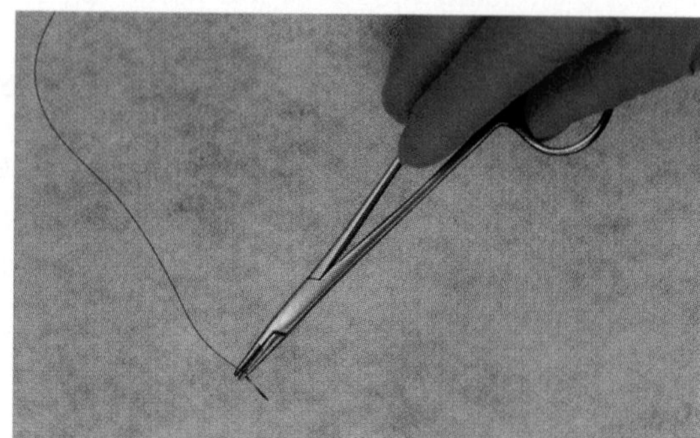

FIGURE 2

Postsurgical Routines

CLEANING AND DISINFECTING AFTER SURGERY

While the circulating assistant escorts the patient from the room, the scrub assistant clears the sterile field. Universal blood and body fluid precautions must be followed. The scrub assistant should not remove his or her gloves until all contaminated materials are removed and cared for. Sharp items are placed in separate basins, and all instruments are taken to the clean-up area. Disposable items are properly placed in trash cans and sharps containers, and the linen is placed in the linen hamper. The room should be checked for any blood spills or

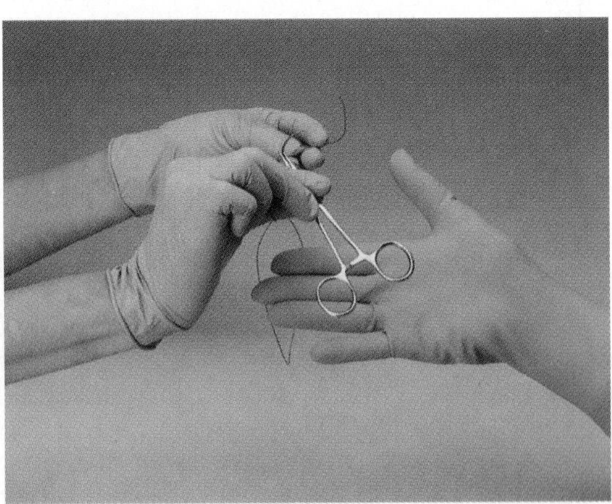

FIGURE 3

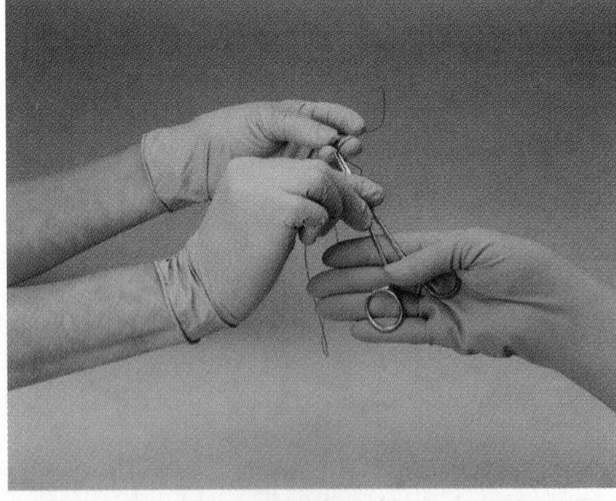

FIGURE 4

4 With your minor hand, hold the suture strand, and pass the needle holder into the surgeon's hand (Figures 3 and 4).

5 Pick up the surgical scissors with your major hand and a gauze sponge with your minor hand.

6 After the surgeon has placed a closure suture, knots it, and holds the two strands taut, cut both suture strands in one motion. Cut between the knot and the surgeon, at the length requested, about ⅛ inch.

PURPOSE: Too long a suture may irritate the patient during recovery, and too short a suture may untie during recovery.

7 Gently blot the closure once with the gauze sponge in your minor hand.

PURPOSE: Rubbing or friction may damage the wound edges.

8 If additional strands of suture are needed, repeat the process.

other contamination. Remove the contaminated gloves and wash your hands.

Use clean gloves to decontaminate, sanitize, and disinfect the room. The used instruments and linens are washed and resterilized for future use. Label any specimens, and prepare them for transport to the laboratory. Documentation of the procedure is done by the physician and the medical assistant on the patient's medical record.

POSTOPERATIVE INSTRUCTIONS AND CARE

The patient is given time to rest after the surgery. If a sedative was administered, make certain that the patient is sufficiently recovered to avoid injury after the surgery or during the journey home. If the patient has been given a topical or local anesthetic medication, explain to the patient that the anesthesia medication will wear off and that there may be discomfort at the operative site. Check with the physician if pain medication has not been prescribed. If medication has been prescribed, review the purpose of the medication, and the directions for use, with the patient and his or her companion. Before the patient leaves the office, a follow-up appointment should be made.

Postoperative care extends for the total recovery period, not just for the time of immediate care before the patient leaves the office. Most medical assistants are responsible for teaching patients to care for themselves at home after the surgical experience. Because it is well known that the concentrative powers of the postoperative patient are diminished after the stress of surgery, instructions should be in writing. They should be simple in style and easily understood by the patient and the caregiver at home. These instructions can be preprinted forms for each type of surgery or a general form with boxes checked for whichever postoperative instructions apply to a particular patient.

EXAMPLES FOR PRINTED INSTRUCTIONS ON PHYSICIAN'S LETTERHEAD STATIONERY

- Whether or not to elevate a limb
- Limitations of exercise or food intake
- Whether or not to bathe

- How to apply hot or cold compresses, if needed
- How to recognize and care for drainage, if a wound drain is in place
- Whether or not to change dressings
- What types of complications necessitate the patient calling the office
- The medications prescribed and their purposes
- When to return to work or school
- The time to call and report in for the next day
- The date and time of the next appointment

Explain to the patient the importance of calling the office if there are any questions or untoward changes. If the patient does not call within the next 24 hours, you should call the patient. Many patients tend to "ride it out" or say they did not want to disturb you. Never allow the postoperative patient to leave the office without the physician's knowledge and approval.

Memory Jogger

6 *For how long does the postoperative care extend?*

POSTOPERATIVE RETURN VISITS

If the healing process is a long one or if the wound becomes wet or infected, the patient may return for a dressing change. Notify the physician immediately. Check the patient's medical record, and follow the physician's instructions carefully. Follow Universal Precautions. Wear gloves and other protection barriers as appropriate. Place the patient in a comfortable position, explain what you will be doing, and adequately expose the area to be redressed. Try to obscure the wound site from the patient's vision, and do not reveal any unpleasant reactions by either comment or facial expression. If at any time you determine that the wound may be infected, stop and have the physician examine it.

The reusable Ace bandage may be cut off or rerolled depending on the physician's preference. The medical assistant may reroll the bandage with gloved hands as it is taken off the patient. Because microorganisms are carried by the air currents, keep the bandage close to the patient. Do not allow it to flap loosely as you work.

Tape applied directly to the patient's skin is not a good dressing immobilizer. If tape is used, always keep it to a minimum. If there is tape holding a dressing in place, always remove it by pulling toward the wound. If it is adhering to a hairy area of the body, lift the outer tape edge with one hand and slowly and gently separate the underlying hair and skin from the tape with the thumb of your other hand. Peel the skin from the bandage, not the bandage from the skin. Never rapidly "rip" tape from the body. The patient's skin may be injured. If the tape is not irritating to the patient, it may be advisable to leave the tape in place until total healing has taken place.

After the physician examines the wound, the medical assistant will either apply a new dressing or remove the patient's sutures, as directed (see Procedure 52–9).

PROCEDURE 52–9
Removing Sutures

GOAL

To remove sutures from a healed incision, using sterile technique and without injury to the closed wound.

EQUIPMENT AND SUPPLIES

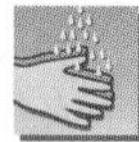

Suture removal pack containing:
- Suture removal scissors
- Gauze sponges
- Thumb dressing forceps

Steri-Strips or Band-Aids
Skin antiseptic

Continued

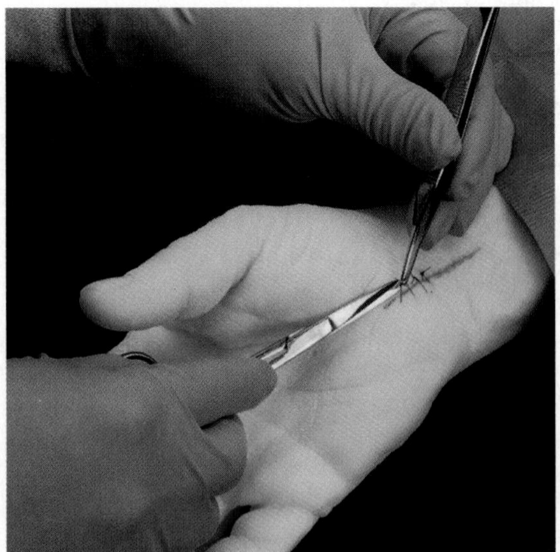

FIGURE 1

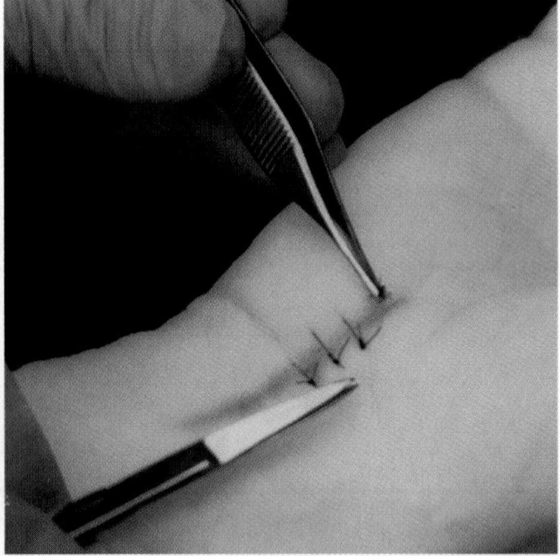

FIGURE 2

PROCEDURAL STEPS

1 Assemble necessary supplies.

2 Wash and dry your hands. Follow Universal Precautions.

3 Open the suture removal pack.

4 Instruct patient of procedure and to lie or sit still during procedure.
PURPOSE: To ensure cooperation during the procedure.

5 Place dry towels under the patient area.

6 Position patient comfortably and support the area.

7 Place a gauze sponge next to the wound site.
PURPOSE: To place the removed sutures.

8 Grasp the knot of the suture with the dressing forceps, without pulling.

9 Cut the suture at skin level (Figure 1).

10 Lift, do not pull, the suture toward the incision and out with the dressing forceps (Figure 2).

11 Place the suture on the gauze sponge, and check that the entire suture strand has been removed.
PURPOSE: Suture fragments left in a wound may cause irritation and/or infection and may prolong the healing process.

12 If there is any bleeding, blot the area with a new gauze sponge before continuing.

13 Continue in the same manner until all the other sutures have been removed.

14 Remove the gauze sponge with the sutures on it.

15 The surgeon may apply Steri-Strips or a Band-Aid for added support, strength, and protection.

16 The patient is instructed to keep the wound edges clean and dry and not place excessive strain on the area.

Wounds

A wound is an interruption in the continuity of the internal or external body tissues.

TYPES OF WOUNDS

A wound may be intentional (such as surgery) or accidental and open or closed (Fig. 52–4). An open wound is one with an outward opening where the skin is broken, causing the underlying tissues to be exposed. A closed, or nonpenetrating, wound does not have an outward opening, but the underlying tissues are damaged, as in a **hematoma** or contusion (bruise). Closed wounds are usually the result of a blow or a violent jar or shock (concussion) to the body. An aseptic (clean) wound is not infected with pathogens. Septic wounds are infected with pathogens.

Open wounds may be classified according to the appearance of their openings. An incised wound has a clean edge and is made with a cutting instrument. An incised wound may be the result of intentional surgery, an accident, or a knife wound. A lacerated wound has torn or mangled tissues and is made by a dull or blunt instrument. The penetrating, or puncture, wound is caused by a sharp, slender object such as a needle or ice pick and passes through the skin into the underlying tissues. A perforating wound is a penetrating wound that passes through to a body organ or cavity.

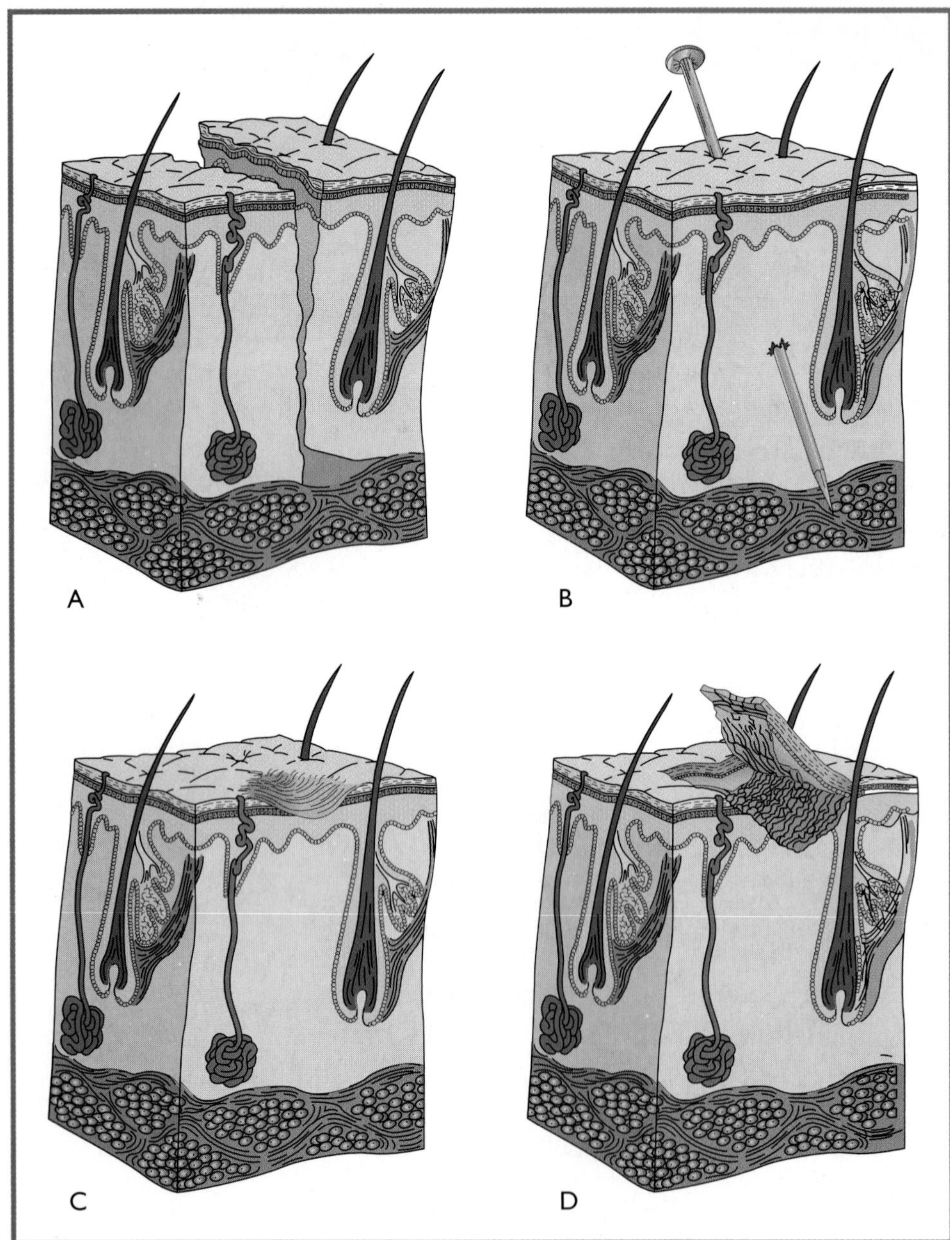

FIGURE 52–4 Types of wounds. *A,* Laceration—jagged, irregular breaking or tearing of tissues, usually caused by a sharp blow to the body. *B,* Puncture—skin is pierced by a pointed object, such as pin, nail, splinter, or bullet. *C,* Abrasion—superficial wound, scraping of the skin. *D,* Avulsion—tissue forcibly torn or separated, caused by accidents.

Memory Jogger

 *Name the different types of wounds.*

WOUND HEALING

All wounds go through a healing, or repair, process that has three phases. The first phase (lag) is the period when the blood vessels contract to control hemorrhage and blood platelets form a network in the wound that acts like glue to plug the wound. After a complex series of chemical reactions, a substance called fibrin is released into the wound that begins clotting. The fibrin continues to collect red blood cells, and the clot becomes a scab. About 12 hours later, special white blood cells arrive at the site to clear away debris and bacteria. Within 1 to 4 days, the fibrin threads contract and pull the edges of the wound together under the clot or scab.

The second phase (proliferation) is the wound healing and new growth period and lasts from 5 to 20 days. It is during this phase that the tissues repair themselves. New cells form, and the wound continues to contract and seal. If the wound is a clean surgical incision, complete contraction usually

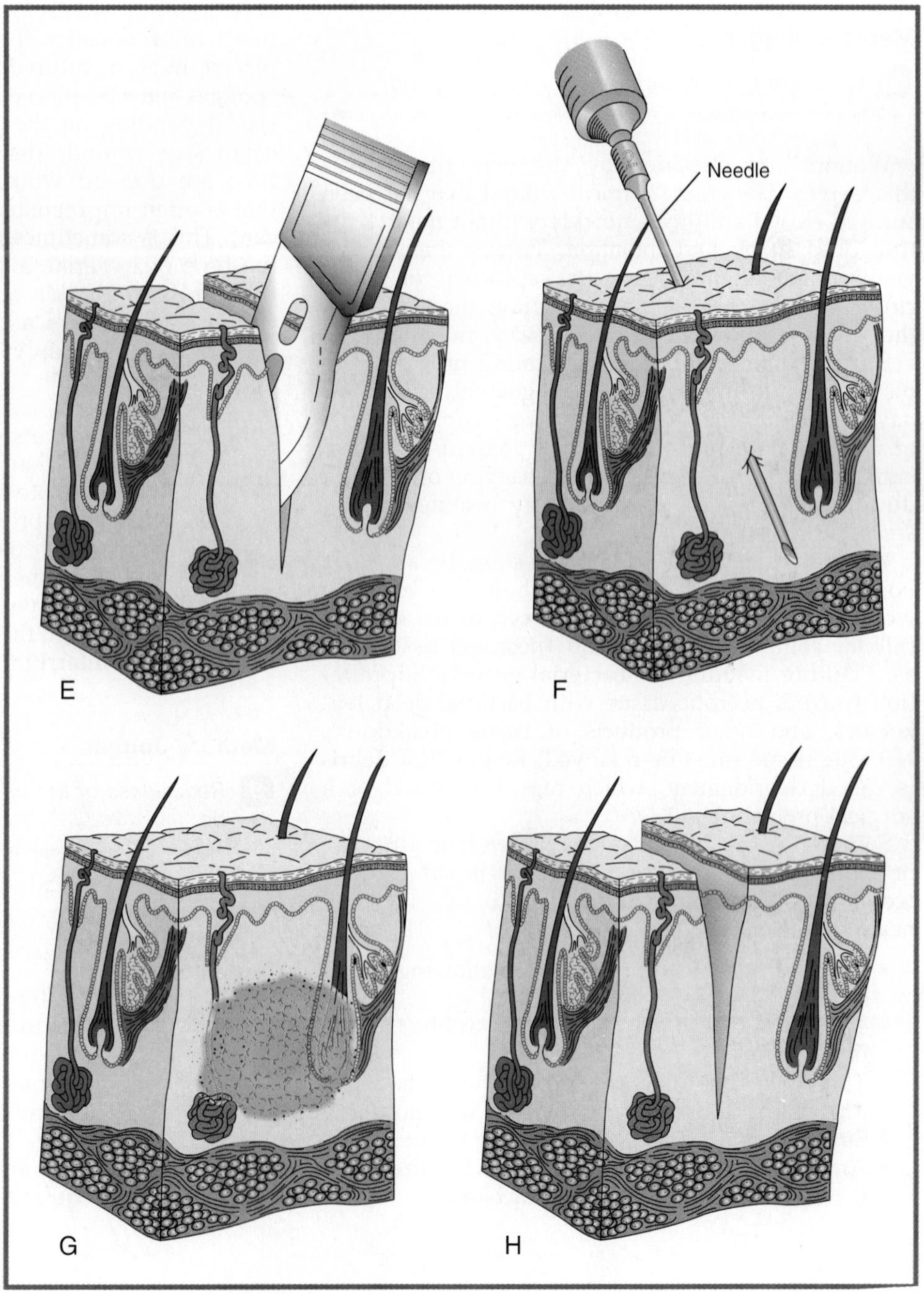

FIGURE 52–4 *Continued* *E,* Surgical incision—a neat, clean cut. *F,* Hypodermic puncture—injection under the skin. *G,* Contusion—closed nonpenetrating wound in which blood from broken vessels accumulates in tissues. *H,* Incision—neat, clean cut from sharp objects, such as glass, knives, or metal.

takes place during this phase; and there is little scarring or permanent fibrous tissue (cicatrix) formation.

The third phase (remodeling) occurs from the 21st day on. Whereas the clean, shallow wound may contract in the first two phases, large or mangled wounds require the time and cellular activity of this third phase to build a bridge of new tissue to close the gap of the wound. The cells produce a fibrous protein substance called collagen (connective tissue) that gives the wounded tissues strength and forms scar tissue. Scar tissue is not true skin; it is usually very strong, but it cannot stand the tension of the normal skin because it lacks elasticity. Scar tissue is also devoid of normal blood supply and nerves.

Memory Jogger

 *What are the three phases of wound healing?*

Wounds are classified by the way they repair themselves. The clean, surgical wound that has been sutured closed and heals quickly without much scarring does so by first intention. Tissues that are severely damaged, are purposely kept open, or fail to close are said to heal by granulation (healing from the bottom up), which is called second intention.

Several factors influence the healing process. People who are young and in good general health and have adequate nutrition heal more rapidly. Adequate protection and rest to the injured area also enhances the healing process. Destruction or reinjury during the second phase can delay healing and increase scarring.

Wounds are susceptible to infection because the normal skin barrier is broken. If there is debris in a wound as a result of the breakdown of the various cellular components, this dead (necrotic) tissue acts as a culture medium for bacterial growth. Suppuration (pus) is necrotic tissue with bacteria, dead leukocytes, and other products of tissue breakdown. Necrotic tissue must be removed. Removal of debris is called debridement, which may be natural or a surgical procedure.

Sometimes the physician may prefer no dressing or bandage on small wounds. This is called open wound healing. Some advantages to open wound healing are

- There are strong arguments for allowing air to freely circulate in the wound.
- The wound is not irritated or rubbed by a dressing or bandage.
- The wound stays dry, which inhibits bacterial growth, resulting in less chance of infection.
- Sutures stay dry and hold together better.
- Any preexisting infection remains localized and is not spread by the dressing or bandage.

Dressings and Bandages

DRESSINGS

A dressing is a sterile covering placed over a wound to

- Protect the wound from injury and contamination
- Maintain a constant pressure
- Hold the wound edges together
- Control bleeding
- Absorb drainage and secretions
- Hide temporary disfigurement

A dressing usually consists of a strip of lubricated mesh or a nonstick Telfa pad or a clear dressing placed over a sutured wound (Fig. 52–5). Gauze sponges may be placed over the nonadhering material, depending on the physician's preference. Body cavities or wounds that need to remain open for a time are dressed with long, thin packing material that is often impregnated with an antiseptic or lubricant. This is sometimes called packing. Regardless of the type of material, a good dressing must be effective and comfortable and must remain in place. If the dressing covers a hairless area, it may be anchored with tape only but no tape may touch the wound.

Frequently, small, clean lacerations may be closed with special adhesive strips called Steri-Strips. These strips reduce the chance of infection and do not leave suture scars. Steri-Strips are used on areas of the body that are protected from movement and stress. They are often used on the face. Because they are a suture replacement, only the physician should place them. The physician places the Steri-Strips onto the wound in the sequence and at the same intervals as in interrupted sutures (Fig. 52–6).

Memory Jogger

 *Regardless of the material, a good dressing must be _____?*

BANDAGES

Dressings are usually held in place by bandages. Bandages also help to maintain even pressure, support the affected part, and keep the wound free from injury or contamination. Bandages can be gauze, cloth, or elastic cloth rolls and are bound by clips, tape, or tying. Dressings and bandages frequently appear easy and simple to apply; however, special skill is required to apply a functional dress-

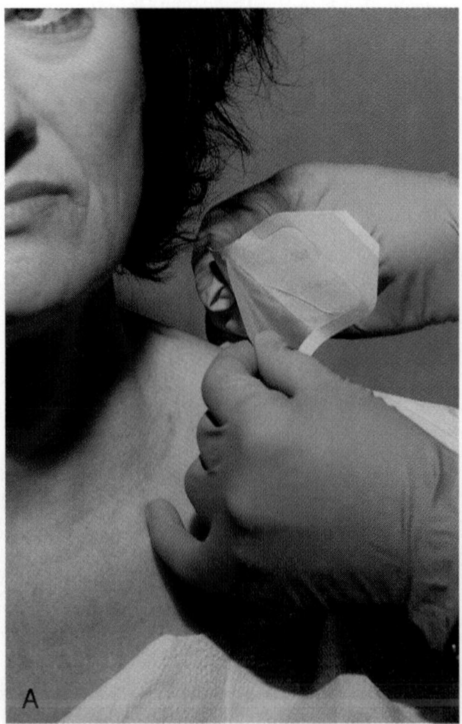

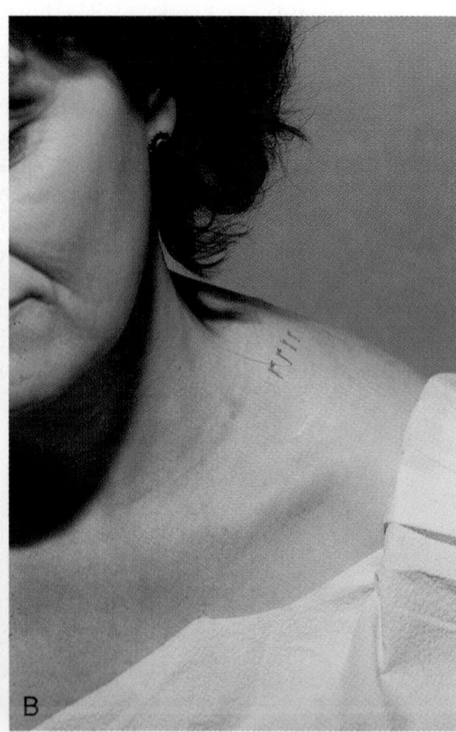

FIGURE 52–5 *A,* Placing a clear dressing on a sutured wound. *B,* Clear dressing placed over a sutured wound.

ing that serves the purpose for which it is intended. Bandages that are too loose fall off. Those that are too tight may further harm the patient. Patients do not feel that good medical care has been given if bandages are messy or uncomfortable. Swelling may occur after a dressing and bandage are applied, and the patient may need a dressing change sooner than scheduled.

Plain gauze roller bandage is seldom used. It is difficult to handle because it must be applied with reverse spiral turns if the area is uneven. It has no elasticity and tends to bind. Because it does not adhere to itself, it is also more likely to slip. Wrinkled crepe-type bandages (e.g., Kling) are preferred because they adhere to the various shapes of the body as well as to themselves (Fig. 52–7*A*). Roller bandages are not applied without a dressing.

Plain elastic cloth bandage (e.g., Ace [see Fig. 52–7*B*]) or elastic roller cloth with adhesive backing

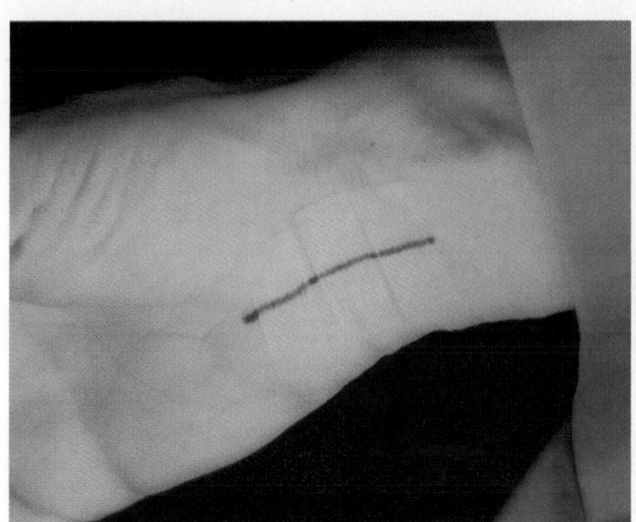

FIGURE 52–6 Steri-Strips on a wound.

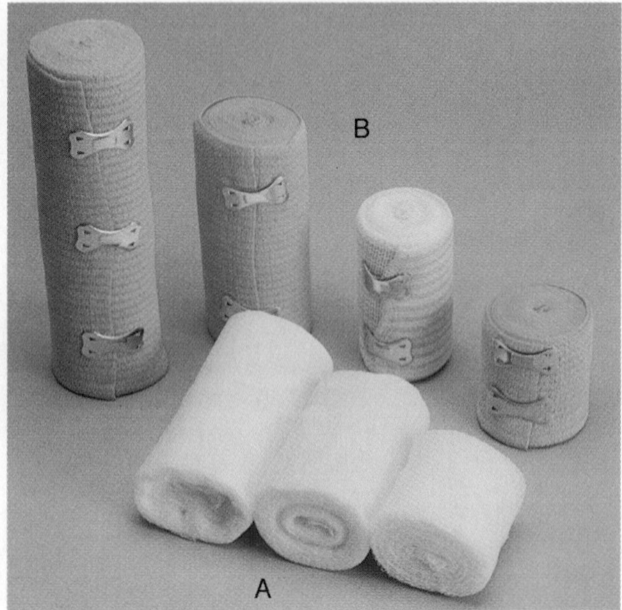

FIGURE 52–7 *A,* Kling bandages. *B,* Roller bandages.

makes a flexible and secure cover. When applying Ace elastic roller bandage as a pressure bandage, especially to the lower limbs, it is essential to keep the bandage consistent in spacing and tension to ensure even pressure. Even and gentle pressure stimulates circulation and healing. Uneven pressure causes constriction points that can create pressure sores and ulcers. Roller bandages are usually applied from the distal to the proximal part of the area. Bandaging can remain even and snug if it is wrapped from a smaller to a larger circumference. Elevate the limb while you are bandaging, and work with the roller facing upward, close to the patient's skin. This technique is more likely to keep the tension consistent, and you will be less likely to drop the roll (Fig. 52–8). Common bandaging techniques are shown in Figures 52–9 through Figure 52–11.

Adhesive bandages are commercially prepared elastic bandages, commonly called Band-Aids. They are available in various shapes to fit the various body parts. Small circular bandages are called "spots."

Seamless tubular gauze bandage, with or without elastic, is superior material for covering round surfaces, such as fingers and toes. It can be used as either a dressing or a bandage. Tubular bandage is

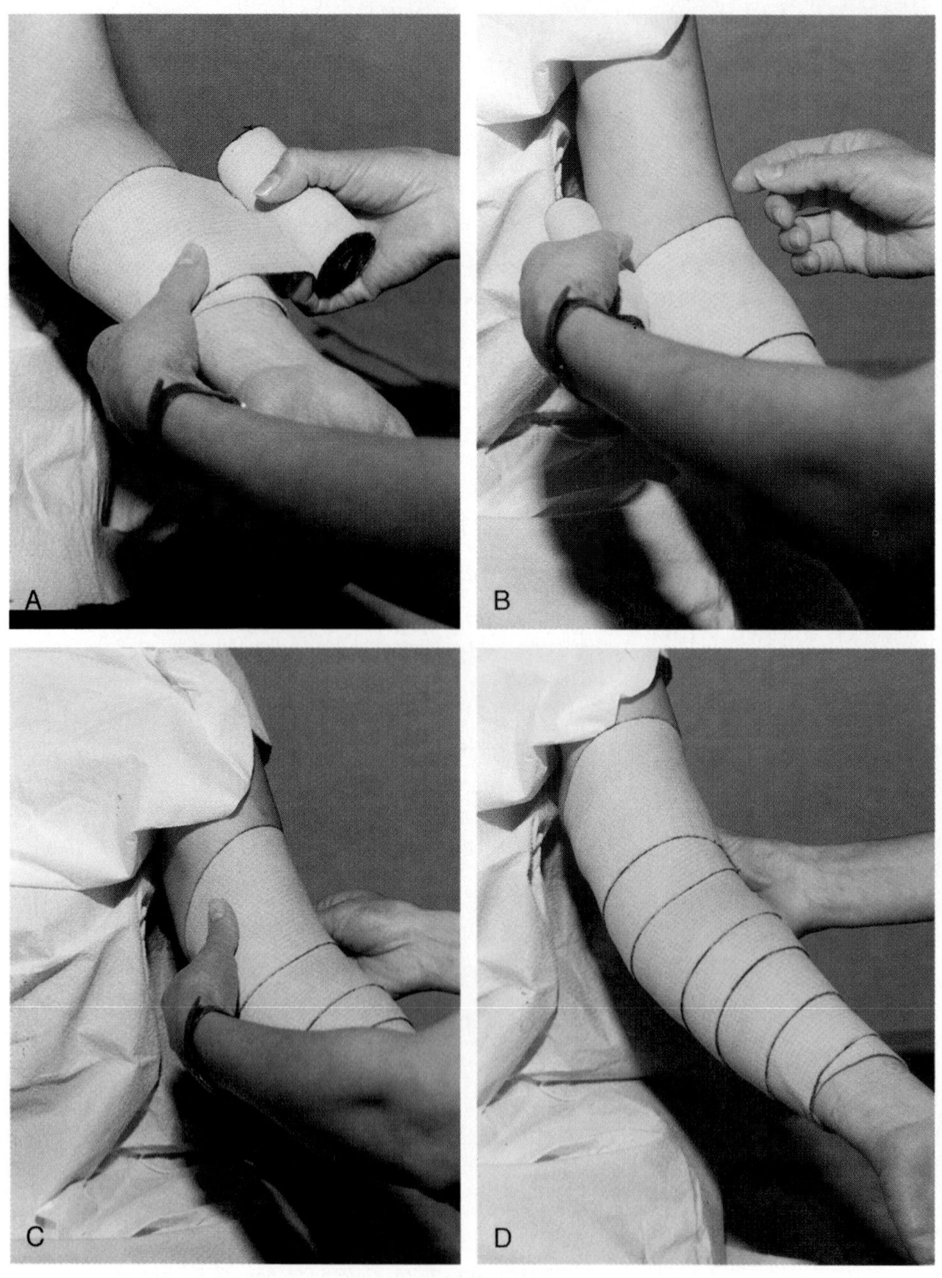

FIGURE 52–8 *A,* Applying a roller bandage to the forearm. Start at distal point. *B,* Keep the roll close to the patient and keep it upward. *C,* Maintain tension and spacing consistently even. *D,* Roller bandage applied to forearm.

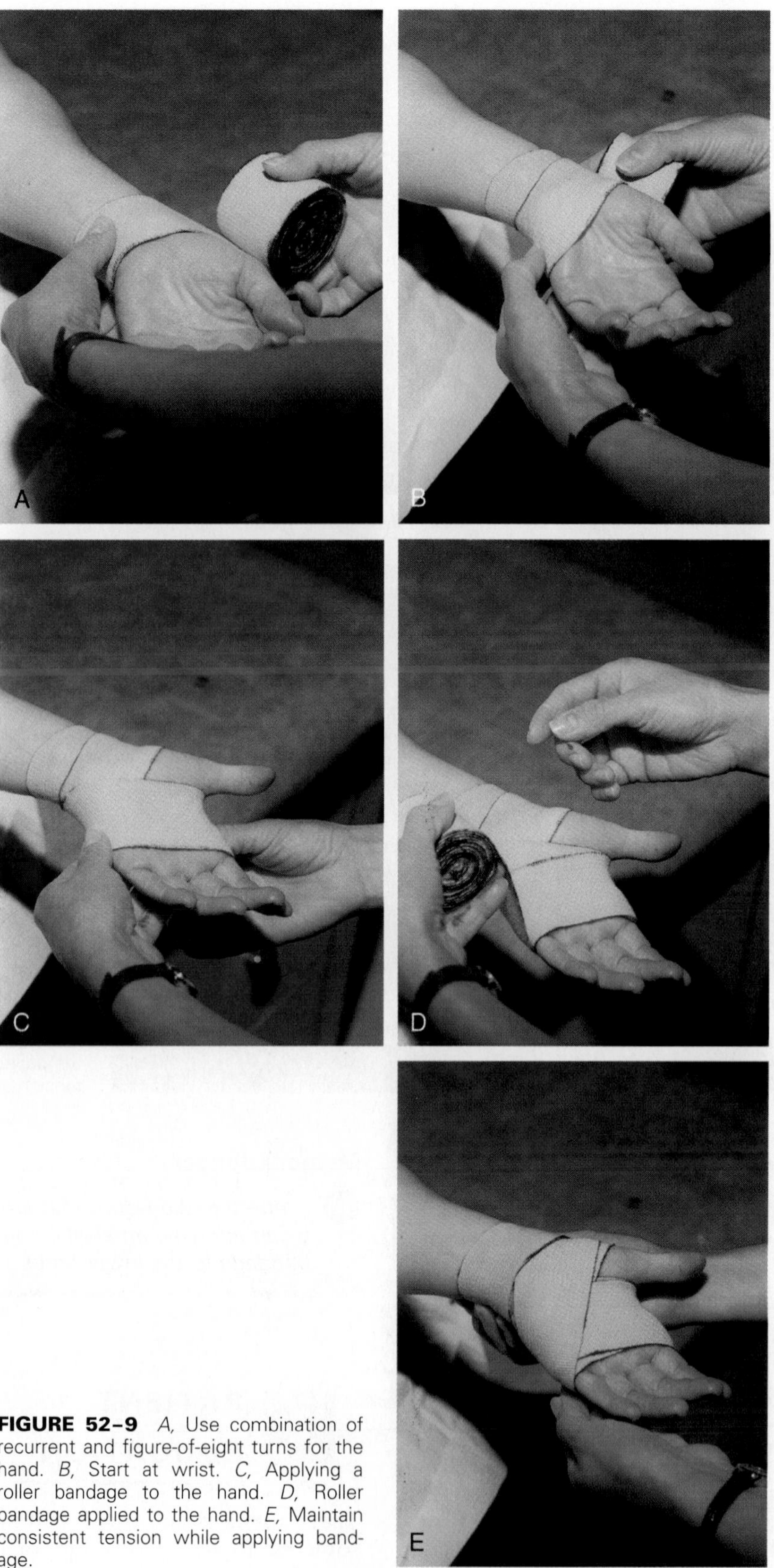

FIGURE 52–9 *A,* Use combination of recurrent and figure-of-eight turns for the hand. *B,* Start at wrist. *C,* Applying a roller bandage to the hand. *D,* Roller bandage applied to the hand. *E,* Maintain consistent tension while applying bandage.

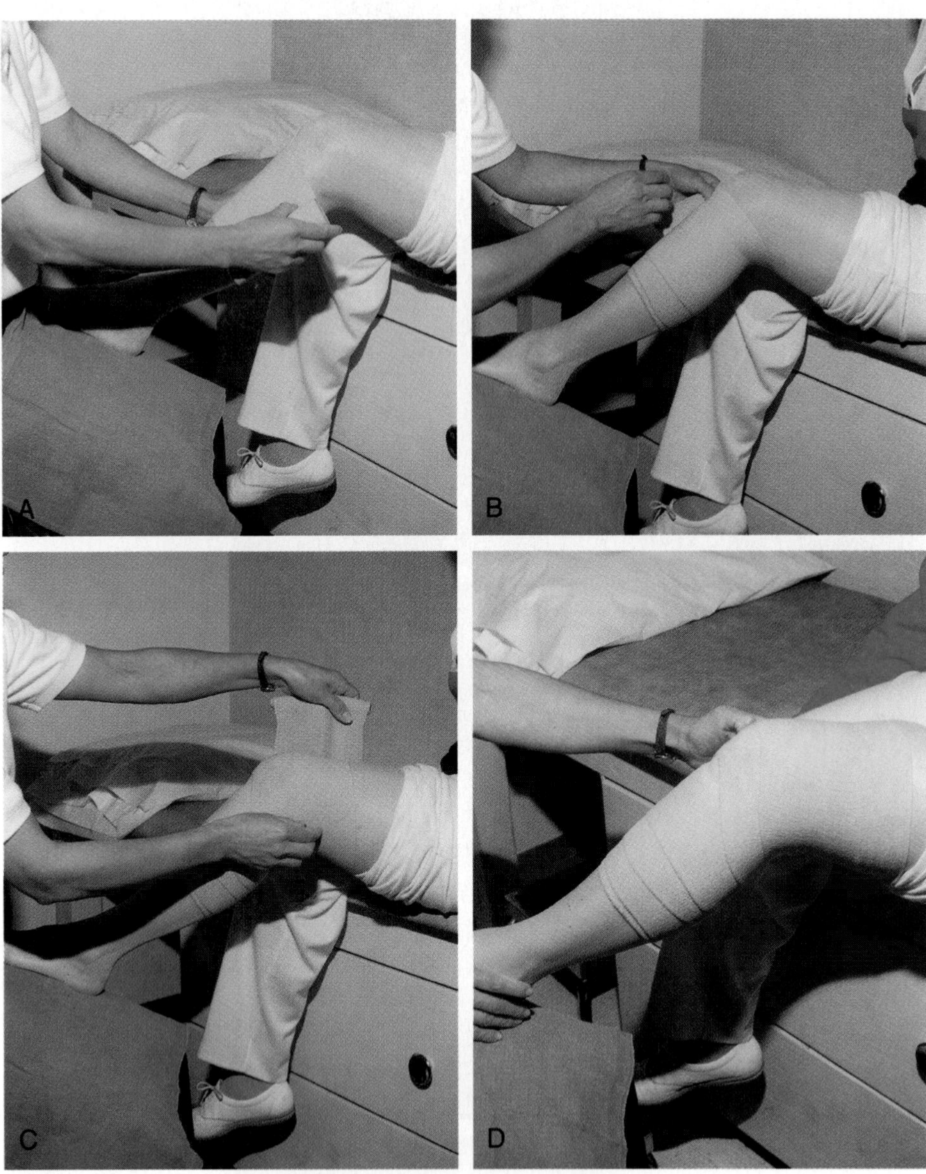

FIGURE 52–10 *A,* Applying a 6-inch roller bandage to the leg. *B,* Start at the distal point. Support patient's foot. *C,* Keep roll close to the patient. *D,* Maintain consistent tension and spacing.

applied with a cagelike applicator. Work with the cutting channel of the applicator facing toward the patient. You may start in the middle of the area to be dressed and anchor the dressing, if there is one, with a small piece of tape. Hold the applicator in the dominant hand, and control the tension flow with your fingers as the applicator is gradually rotated and the material slides off. Tubular dressings may be applied with or without slight pressure. Beyond the tip of the bandaged part, give the applicator a full half-turn, place the applicator again over the part, and repeat the process. Be very careful not to create a tourniquet effect when you reverse the applicator. When the desired thickness of the bandage is reached, cut the gauze and anchor the final dressing with tape (Fig. 52–12). This lightweight gauze should not be used as a stockinet under a cast. Patients should be advised to call the physician's office if there is any problem with the dressing.

Memory Jogger

Name the two issues that are absolutely essential when applying an elastic bandage as a pressure bandage to the lower limbs.

PATIENT EDUCATION

The patient is informed that he or she may need someone to accompany him or her home. There will be a bandage applied after surgery, and it must be kept clean and dry. There may be pain, and pain medication may be ordered by the physician. An appointment is given for a return visit and examination.

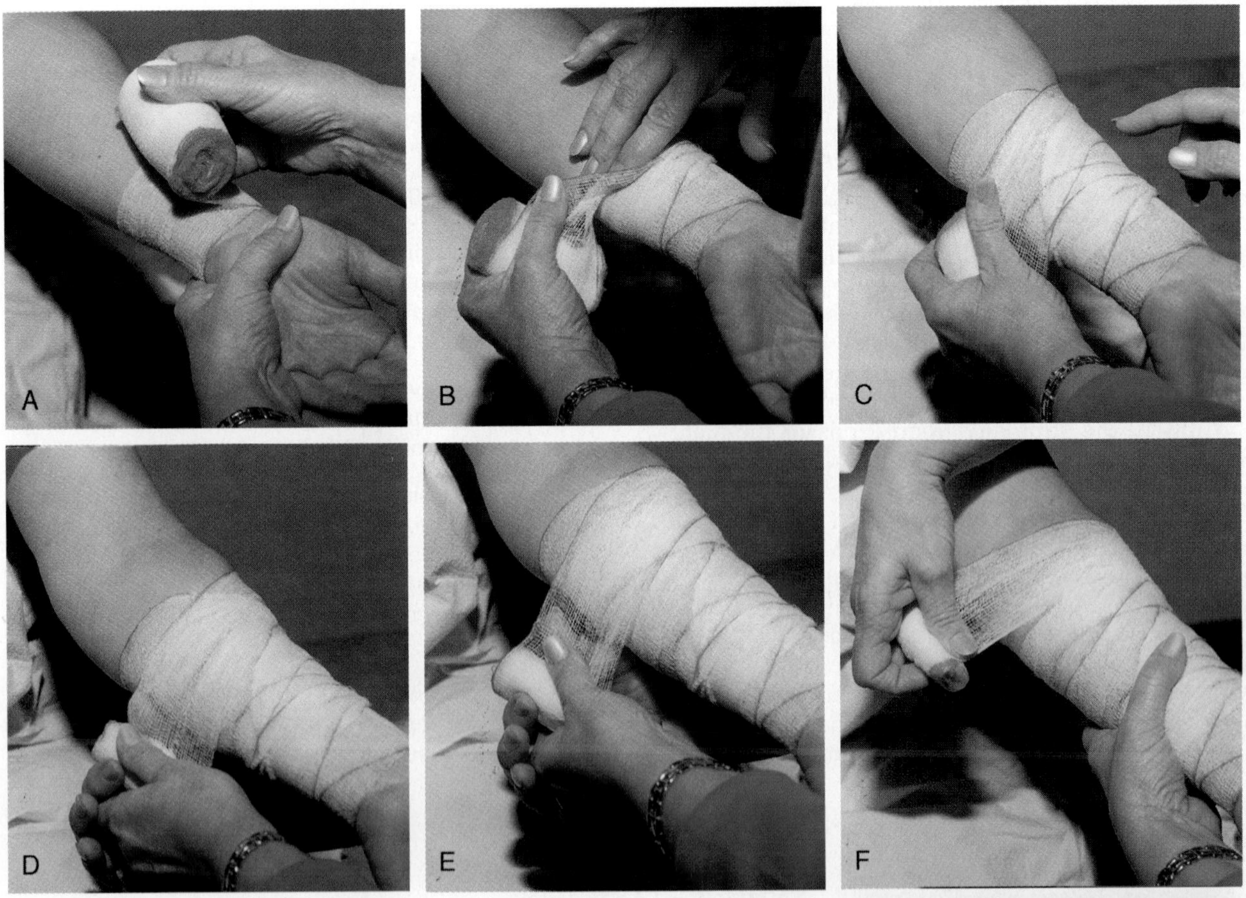

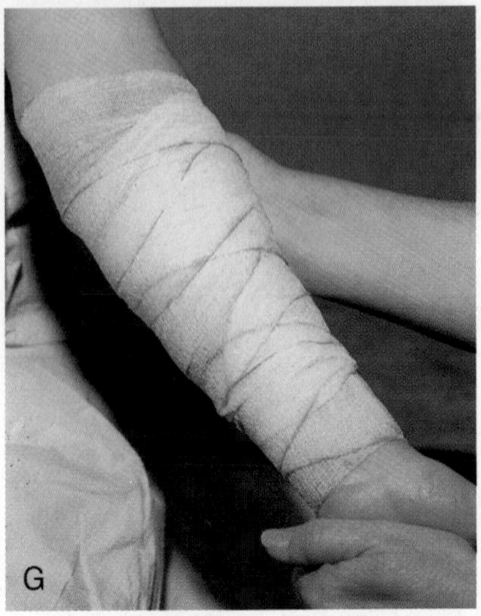

A

B

C

D

E

F

G

FIGURE 52–11 *A,* Applying a reverse spiral bandage. *B,* Start at distal point. *C,* Keep the roll close to the patient and keep it upward. *D,* Combination recurrent and twisting of bandage turns used for the forearm. *E,* Maintain tension and spacing consistently even. *F,* Continue combination of turns up the forearm. *G,* Reverse spiral bandage applied to forearm.

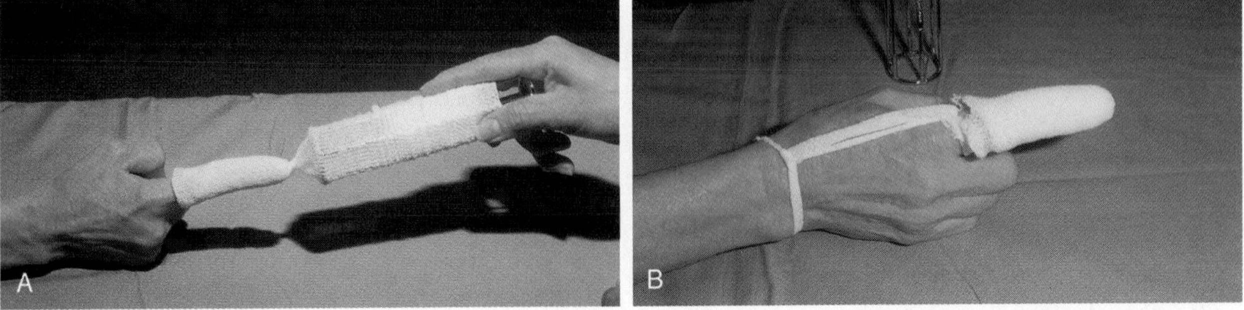

FIGURE 52–12 *A,* Tube gauze applied with even tension, twisting at fingertip before applying next layer. *B,* Tube gauze bandage applied and secured at wrist.

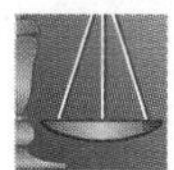

LEGAL AND ETHICAL ISSUES

The medical assistant must check that the patient has signed a minor surgery consent form. This means that the patient understands and consents to all aspects of the surgical procedure and is truly informed. Legal action can occur when complications arise from failure to complete procedure and consent forms. If the surgery to be performed is a sterilization procedure for birth control, it is essential to follow the stipulated regulations of the state in which you are employed. A waiting period is usually required.

The surgical procedure is expedited when the patient is given instructions and knows what to expect. The patient's fears are alleviated. This encourages patient cooperation during surgery, and the patient is inclined to follow instructions and advice after surgery.

When the physical and psychological needs of the patient are met, one can be assured that the patient has sufficient information to be comfortable before, during, and after a surgical procedure. Meeting such needs is one of the truly rewarding aspects of medical assisting.

CRITICAL THINKING

1 What type of personality traits are necessary for a scrub assistant?

2 Do you think that all medical assistants can be taught to be circulating assistants? Why?

3 If given the opportunity, would you like to work in surgery? Do you feel you have the personality traits to make a good surgical assistant?

HOW DID I DO? Answers To Memory Joggers

1 The procedure card file helps in the preparation for surgery.

2 The circulating assistant opens sterile supplies before and during surgery, helps position the patient for the procedure, performs the scrub prep on the patient, handles all nonsterile equipment during surgery, and assists the patient with dressing after the procedure.

3 The patient's vital signs are recorded, the patient is assisted in undressing, and the patient is asked to empty his or her bladder.

4 The scrub assistant protects the sterile field from contamination, notifies the physician if there is a break in sterile technique, disposes of soiled sponges into the waste receptacle, anticipates the surgeon's need for instruments, and hand passes instruments.

5 In case there is an unexpected contamination of the wound site during the dressing application, more materials will be needed from the sterile field.

6 Postoperative care extends for the total recovery period.

7 Intentional, accidental, open, closed

8 Phase one = lag phase
Phase two = proliferation phase
Phase three = remodeling

9 A good dressing must be effective, comfortable, and remain in place.

10 It is essential to keep the bandage consistent in spacing and tension.

APPENDIX A

Combining Forms in Medical Terminology*

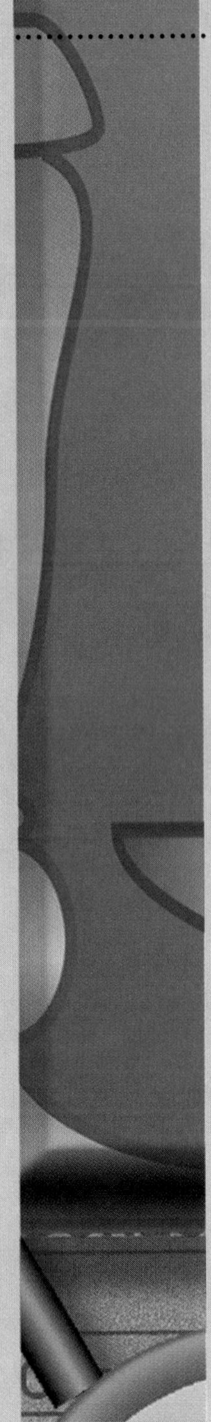

The following is a list of combining forms encountered frequently in the vocabulary of medicine. A dash or dashes are appended to indicate whether the form usually precedes (as *ante-*) or follows (as *-agra*) the other elements of the compound or usually appears between the other elements (as *-em-*). Following each combining form, the first item of information is the Greek or Latin word, or both a Greek and a Latin word, from which it is derived. Those words that are not printed in Greek characters are Latin. Information necessary to an understanding of the form appears next in parentheses. Then the meaning or meanings of the word are given, followed where appropriate by reference to a synonymous combining form. Finally, an example is given to illustrate the use of the combining form in a compound English derivative.

a- *α-* (*n* is added before words beginning with a vowel) negative prefix. Cf. in-[3]. *a*metria

ab- *ab* away from. Cf. apo-. *ab*ducent

abdomin- *abdomen, abdominis*. *abdomin*oscopy

ac- See ad-. *ac*cretion

acet- *acetum* vinegar. *aceto*meter

acid- *acidus* sour. *acid*uric

acou- *ἀκούω* hear. *acou*esthesia. (Also spelled acu-)

acr- *ἄκρον* extremity, peak. *acro*- megaly

act- *ago, actus* do, drive, act. re*act*ion

actin- *ἀκτίς, ἀκτῖνος* ray, radius, Cf. radi-. *actin*ogenesis

acu- See acou-. osteo*acu*sis

ad- *ad* (*d* changes to *c, f, g, p, s,* or *t* before words beginning with those consonants) to. *ad*renal

aden- *ἀδήν* gland. Cf. gland-. *aden*oma

adip- *adeps, adipis* fat. Cf. lip- and stear- *adip*ocellular

aer- *ἀήρ* air. an*aer*obiosis

aesthe- See esthe-. *aesthe*sioneurosis

af- See ad-. *af*ferent

ag- See ad-. *ag*glutinant

-agogue *ἀγωγός* leading, inducing. galact*agogue*

-agra *ἄγρα* catching, seizure, pod*agra*

alb- *albus* white. Cf. leuk-. *albo*cinereous

alg- *ἄλγος* pain. neur*alg*ia

all- *ἄλλος* other, different, *all*ergy

alve- *alveus* trough, channel, cavity. *alve*olar

---

*Compiled by Lloyd W. Daly, A.M., Ph.D., Litt.D., Allen Memorial Professor of Greek, University of Pennsylvania. *In* Dorland's Pocket Medical Dictionary, 21st ed. Philadelphia, W. B. Saunders Co., 1968.

amph- See amphi-. *amph*eclexis
amphi- ἀμφί (*i* is dropped before words beginning with a vowel) both, doubly. *amphi*celous
amyl- ἄμυλον starch. *amyl*osynthesis
an-[1] See ana-. *an*agogic
an.-[2] See a-. *an*omalous
ana- ἀνά (final *a* is dropped before words beginning with a vowel) up, positive, *ana*phoresis
ancyl- See ankyl-. *ancyl*ostomiasis
andr- ἀνήρ, ἀνδρός man. gyn*andr*oid
angi- ἀγγεῖον vessel. Cf. vas-. *angi*emphraxis
ankyl- ἀγκύλος crooked, looped, *ankyl*odactylia. (Also spelled ancyl-)
ant- See anti-. *ant*ophthalmic
ante- *ante* before. *ante*flexion
anti- ἀντί (*i* is dropped before words beginning with a vowel) against, counter. Cf. contra-. *anti*pyogenic
antr- ἄντρον cavern. *antr*odynia
ap-[1] See apo-. *ap*heter
ap-[2] See ad-. *ap*pend
-aph- ἅπτω, ἀφ- touch. dys*aph*ia. (See also hapt-)
apo- ἀπό (*o* is dropped before words beginning with a vowel) away from, detached. Cf. ab-. *apo*physis
arachn- ἀράχνη spider. *arachn*odactyly
arch- ἀρχή beginning, origin. *arch*enteron
arter(i)- ἀρτηρία elevator (?), artery. *arteri*osclerosis, peri*arter*itis
arthr- ἄρθρον joint. Cf. articul-. syn*arthr*osis
articul- *articulus* joint. Cf. arthr-. dis*articul*ation
as- See ad-. *as*similation
at- See ad-. *at*trition
aur- *auris* ear. Cf. ot-. *aur*inasal
aux- αὔξω increase. enter*auxe*
ax- ἄξων or *axis* axis. *ax*ofugal
axon- ἄξων axis. *axon*ometer
ba- βαίνω, βα- go, walk, stand. hypno*ba*tia
bacill- *bacillus* small staff, rod. Cf. bacter-. antino*bacil*losis
bacter- βακτήριον small staff, rod. Cf. bacill-. *bacter*iophage
ball- βάλλω, βολ- throw. *ball*istics. (See also bol-)
bar- βάρος weight. pedo*bar*ometer
bi-[1] βίος life. Cf. vit-. aero*bi*c
bi-[2] *bi-* two (see also di-[1]). *bi*lobate
bil- *bilis* bile. Cf. chol-. *bil*iary
blast- βλαστός bud, child, a growing thing in its early stages. Cf. germ-. *blast*oma, zygoto*blast.*
blep- βλέπω look, see. hemia*blep*sia
blephar- βλέφαρον (from βλέπω; see blep-)eyelid. Cf. cili-. *blephar*oncus
bol- See ball-. em*bol*ism
brachi- βραχίων arm. *brachi*ocephalic
brachy- βραχύς short. *brachy*cephalic
brady- βραδύς slow. *brady*cardia
brom- βρῶμος stench. podo*brom*idrosis
bronch- βρόγχος windpipe. *bronch*oscopy
bry- βρύω be full of life. em*bry*onic
bucc- *bucca* cheek. disto*bucc*al
cac- κακός bad, abnormal. Cf. mal-. *cac*odontia, arthro*cace*. (See also dys-)
calc-[1] *calx, calcis* stone (cf. lith-), limestone, lime. *calci*pexy
calc-[2] *calx, calcis* heel. *calc*aneotibial
calor- *calor* heat. Cf. therm-. *calor*imeter
cancr- *cancer, cancri* crab, cancer. Cf. carcin-. *cancr*ology. (Also spelled chancr-)
capit- *caput, capitis* head. Cf. cephal*decapit*ator
caps- *capsa* (from *capio;* see cept-) container. en*capsu*lation
carbo(n)- *carbo, carbonis* coal, charcoal. *carbo*hydrate, *carbon*uria
carcin- καρκίνος crab, cancer. Cf. cancr-. *carcin*oma
cardi- καρδία heart. lipo*cardi*ac
cary- See kary-. *cary*okinesis
cat- See cata-. *cat*hode
cata- κατά (final *a* is dropped before words beginning with a vowel) down, negative. *cata*batic
caud- *cauda* tail. *caud*ad
cav- *cavus* hollow. Cf. coel-. con*cave*
cec- *caecus* blind. Cf. typhl-. *cec*opexy
cel-[1] See coel-. amphi*cel*ous
cel-[2] See -cele. *cel*ectome
-cele κήλη tumor, hernia. gastro*cele*
cell- *cella* room, cell. Cf. cyt-. *cell*iferous
cen- κοινός common. *cen*esthesia
cent- *centum* hundred. Cf. hect-. Indicates fraction in metric system. [This exemplifies the custom in the metric system of identifying fractions of units by stems from the Latin, as centimeter, decimeter, millimeter, and multiples of units by the similar stems from the Greek, as hectometer, decameter, and kilometer.] *centi*meter, *centi*pede
cente- κεντέω puncture. Cf. punct-. entero*cente*sis
centr- κέντρον or *centrum* point, center. neuro*centr*al
cephal- κεφαλή head. Cf. capit-. en*cephal*itis
cept- *capio, -cipientis, -ceptus* take, receive. re*cept*or
cer- κηρός or *cera* wax. *cer*oplasty, *cer*omel
cerat- See kerat-. a*cerat*osis
cerebr- *cerebrum. cerebr*ospinal
cervic- *cervix, cervicis* neck. Cf. trachel-. *cervic*itis
chancr- See cancr-. *chancr*iform
cheil- χεῖλος lip. Cf. labi-. *cheil*oschisis
cheir- χείρ hand. Cf. man-. macro*cheir*ia. (Also spelled chir-)
chir- See cheir-. *chir*omegaly
chlor- χλωρός green. a*chlor*opsia
chol- χολή bile. Cf. bil-. hepato*chol*angeitis
chondr- χόνδρος cartilage. *chondr*omalacia
chord- χορδή string, cord. peri*chord*al
chori- χόριον protective fetal membrane. endo*chori*on
chro- χρώς color. poly*chro*matic
chron- χρόνος time. syn*chron*ous
chy- χέω, χυ- pour. ec*chy*mosis
-cid(e) *caedo, -cisus* cut, kill. infanti*cide*, germi*cid*al
cili- *cilium* eyelid. Cf. blephar-. super*cili*ary
cine- See kine-. auto*cine*sis
-cipient See cept-. in*cipient*
circum- *circum* around. Cf. peri-. *circum*ferential
-cis- *caedo, -cisus* cut, kill. ex*cis*ion
clas- κλάω, κλασ- break. cranio*clas*t
clin- κλίνω bend, incline, make lie down. *clin*ometer
clus- *claudo, -clusus* shut. Maloc*clus*ion
co- See con-. *co*hesion
cocc- κόκκος seed, pill. gono*cocc*us
coel- κοῖλος hollow. Cf. cav-. *coel*enteron. (Also spelled cel-)
col-[1] See colon-, *col*ic
col-[2] See con-. *col*lapse
colon- κόλον lower intestine. *colon*ic
colp- κόλπος hollow, vagina. Cf. sin-. endo*colp*itis
com- See con-. *com*masculation
con- *con-* (becomes co- before vowels or *h;* col- before *l;* com- before *b, m,* or *p;* cor- before *r*) with, together. Cf. syn-. *con*traction
contra- *contra* against, counter. Cf. anti-. *contra*indication
copr- κόπρος dung. Cf. sterco-. *copr*oma
cor-[2] κόρη doll, little image, pupil. iso*cor*ia
cor-[1] See con-. *cor*rugator
corpor- *corpus, corporis* body. Cf. somat-. intra*corpor*al
cortic- *cortex, corticis* bark, rind. *cortic*osterone
cost- *costa* rib. Cf. pleur-. inter*cost*al
crani- κρανίον or *cranium* skull. peri*crani*um
creat- κρέας, κρεατ- meat, flesh. *creat*orrhea
-crescent *cresco, crescentis, cretus* grow. ex*crescent*

cret-[1] *cerno, cretus* distinguish, separate off. Cf. crin-. dis*crete*

cret-[2] See -crescent. ac*cret*ion

crin- κρίνω distinguish, separate off, secrete. Cf. cret-[1]. endo*crin*ology

crur- *crus, cruris* shin, leg. brachio*crur*al

cry- κρύος cold. *cry*esthesia

crypt- κρύπτω hide, conceal. *crypt*orchism

cult- *colo, cultus* tend, cultivate. *cult*ure

cune- *cuneus* wedge. Cf. sphen-. *cune*iform

cut- *cutis* skin. Cf. derm(at)-. sub*cut*aneous

cyan- κύανος blue. antho*cyan*in

cycl- κύκλος circle, cycle. *cycl*ophoria

cyst- κύστις bladder. Cf. vesic-. nephro*cyst*itis

cyt- κύτος cell. Cf. cell-. plasmo*cyt*oma

dacry- δάκρυ tear. *dacry*ocyst

dactyl- δάκτυλος finger, toe. Cf. digit-. hexa*dactyl*ism

de- *de* down from. *de*composition

dec-[1] δέκα ten. Indicates multiple in metric system. Cf. dec-[2]. *dec*agram

dec-[2] *decem* ten. Indicates fraction in metric system. Cf. dec-[1]. *dec*ipara, *dec*imeter

dendr- δένδρον tree. neuro*dendr*ite

dent- *dens, dentis* tooth. Cf. odont-. inter*dent*al

derm(at)- δέρμα, δέρματος skin. Cf. cut-. endo*derm*, *derma*titis

desm- δεσμός band, ligament. syn*desm*opexy

dextr- *dexter, dextr-* right-hand. ambi*dextr*ous

di-[1] *di-* two. *di*morphic. (See also bi-[2])

di-[2] See dia-. *di*uresis.

di-[3] See dis-. *di*vergent.

dia- διά (*a* is dropped before words beginning with a vowel) through, apart. Cf. per-. *dia*gnosis

didym- δίδυμος twin. Cf. gemin-. epi*didym*al

digit- *digitus* finger, toe. Cf. dactyl-. *digit*igrade

diplo- διπλόος double. *diplo*myelia

dis- *dis-* (*s* may be dropped before a word beginning with a consonant) apart, away from. *dis*location

disc- δίσκος or *discus* disk. *disc*oplacenta

dors- *dorsum* back. ventro*dors*al

drom- δρόμος course. hemo*drom*ometer

-ducent See duct-. ad*ducent*

duct- *duco, ducentis, ductus* lead, conduct. ovi*duct*

dur- *durus* hard. Cf. scler-. in*dur*ation

dynam(i)- δύναμις power. *dynam*oneure, neuro*dynami*c

dys- δυσ- bad, improper. Cf. mal-. *dys*trophic. (See also cac-)

e- *e* out from. Cf. ec- and ex-. *e*mission

ec- ἐκ out of. Cf. e- *ec*centric

-ech- ἔχω have, hold, be. syn*ech*otomy

ect- ἐκτός outside. Cf. extra-. *ect*oplasm

ede- οἰδέω swell. *ede*matous

ef- See ex-. *ef*florescent

-elc- ἕλκος sore, ulcer. enter*elc*osis. (See also *helc-*)

electr- ἤλεκτρον amber. *electr*otherapy

em- See en-. *em*bolism, *em*pathy, *em*phlysis

-em- αἷμα blood. an*em*ia. (See also hem(at)-)

en- ἐν (*n* changes to *m* before *b*, *p*, or *ph*) in, on. Cf. in-[2]. *en*celitis

end- ἔνδον inside. Cf. intra-. *end*angium.

enter- ἔντερον intestine. dys*enter*y

ep- See epi-. *ep*axial

epi- ἐπί (*i* is dropped before words beginning with a vowel) upon, after, in addition. *epi*glottis

erg- ἔργον work, deed. en*erg*y

erythr- ἐρυθρός red. Cf. rub(r)-. *erythr*ochromia

eso- ἔσω inside. Cf. intra-. *eso*phylactic

esthe- αἰσθάνομαι, αἰσθη- perceive, feel. Cf. sens-. an*esthe*sia

eu- εὐ good, normal. *eu*pepsia

ex- ἐξ or *ex* out of. Cf. e-. *ex*cretion

exo- ἔξω outside. Cf. extra-. *exo*pathic

extra- *extra* outside of, beyond. Cf. ect- and exo-. *extra*cellular

faci- *facies* face. Cf. prosop-. brachio*faci*olingual

-facient *facio, facientis, factus, -fectus* make. Cf. poie-. cal*efacient*

-fact- See facient-. arte*fact*

fasci- *fascia* band. *fasci*orrhaphy

febr- *febris* fever. Cf. pyr-. *febr*icide

-fect- See -facient. de*fect*ive

-ferent *fero, ferentis, latus* bear, carry. Cf. phor-. ef*ferent*

ferr- *ferrum* iron. *ferr*oprotein

fibr- *fibra* fibre. Cf. in-[1]. chondro*fibr*oma

fil- *filum* thread. *fil*iform

fiss- *findo, fissus* split. Cf. schis-. *fiss*ion

flagell- *flagellum* whip. *flagell*ation

flav- *flavus* yellow. Cf. xanth-. ribo*flav*in

-flect- *flecto, flexus* bend, divert. de*flect*ion

-flex- See -flect-. re*flex*ometer

flu- *fluo, fluxus* flow. Cf. rhe-. *flu*id

flux- See flu-. af*flux*ion

for- *foris* door, opening. per*for*ated

-form *forma* shape. Cf. -oid. ossi*form*

fract- *frango, fractus* break. re*fract*ive

front- *frons, frontis* forehead, front. naso*front*al

-fug(e) *fugio* flee, avoid. vermi*fuge*, centri*fug*al

funct- *fungor, functus* perform, serve, function. mal*funct*ion

fund- *fundo, fusus* pour. in*fund*ibulum

fus- See fund-. dif*fus*ible

galact- γάλα, γάλακτος milk. Cf. lact-. dys*galact*ia

gam- γάμος marriage, reproductive union. a*gam*ont

gangli- γάγγλιον swelling, plexus, neuro*gangli*itis

gastr- γαστήρ, γαστρός stomach. cholangio*gastr*ostomy

gelat- *gelo, gelatus* freeze, congeal. *gelat*in

gemin- *geminus* twin, double. Cf. didym-. quadri*gemin*al

gen- γίγνομαι, γεν-, γον- become, be produced, originate, or γεννάω produce, originate. cyto*gen*ic

germ- *germen, germinis* bud, a growing thing in its early stages. Cf. blast-. *germ*inal, ovi*germ*

gest- *gero, gerentis, gestus* bear, carry. con*gest*ion

gland- *glans, glandis* acorn. Cf. aden-. intra*gland*ular

-glia γλία glue. neuro*glia*

gloss- γλῶσσα tongue. Cf. lingu-. tricho*gloss*ia

glott- γλῶττα tongue, language. *glott*ic

gluc- See glyc(y)-. *gluc*ophenetidin

glutin- *gluten, glutinis* glue. ag*glutin*ation

glyc(y)- γλυκύς sweet. *glyc*emia, *glycy*rrhizin. (Also spelled gluc-)

gnath- γνάθος jaw. ortho*gnath*ous

gno- γιγνώσκω, γνω- know, discern. dia*gno*sis

gon- See gen-. amphi*gon*y

grad- *gradior* walk, take steps. retro*grad*e

-gram γράφω, γραφ- + -μα scratch, write, record. cardio*gram*

gran- *granum* grain, particle. lipo*gran*uloma

graph- γράφω scratch, write, record. histo*graph*y

grav- *gravis* heavy. multi*grav*ida

gyn(ec)- γυνή, γυναικός woman, wife. andro*gyn*y, *gynec*ologic

gyr- γῦρος ring, circle. *gyr*ospasm

haem(at)- See hem(at)-. *haem*orrhagia, *haemat*oxylon

hapt- ἅπτω touch. *hapt*ometer

hect- ἑκτ- hundred. Cf. cent-. Indicates multiple in metric system. *hect*ometer

helc- ἕλκος sore, ulcer. *helc*osis

hem(at)- αἷμα, αἵματος blood. Cf. sanguin-. *hem*angioma, *hemat*ocyturia. (See also -em-)

hemi- ἡμι- half. Cf. semi-. *hemi*ageusia

hen- εἷς, ἑνός one. Cf. un-. *hen*ogenesis

hepat- ἧπαρ, ἥπατος liver. gastro*hepat*ic

hept(a)- ἑπτά seven. Cf. sept-[2]. *hept*atomic, *hepta*valent

hered- *heres, heredis* heir. *hered*oimmunity

hex-[1] ἕξ six. Cf. sex-. *hex*yl-. An *a* is added in some combinations.

hex-[2] ἔχω, ἐχ- (added to σ becomes ἑξ-) have, hold, be. cac*hexy*

hexa- See hex-[1]. *hexa*chromic

hidr- ἱδρώς sweat. hyper*hidr*osis

hist- ἱστός web, tissue. *hist*odialysis

hod- ὁδός road, path. *hod*oneuromere. (See also od- and -ode[1])

hom- ὁμός common, same. *hom*omorphic

horm- ὁρμή impetus, impulse. *horm*one

hydat- ὕδωρ, ὕδατος water. *hydat*ism

hydr- ὕδωρ, ὑδρ- water. Cf. lymph-. achlor*hydr*ia

hyp- See hypo-. *hyp*axial

hyper- ὑπέρ above, beyond, extreme. Cf. super-. *hyper*trophy

hypn- ὕπνος sleep. *hypn*otic

hypo- ὑπό (*o* is dropped before words beginning with a vowel) under, below. Cf. sub-. *hypo*metabolism

hyster- ὑστέρα womb, uterus. colpo*hyster*opexy

iatr- ἰατρός physician. pedi*atr*ics

idi- ἴδιος peculiar, separate, distinct. *idi*osyncrasy

il- See in-[2,3]. *il*linition (in, on), *il*legible (negative prefix)

ile- See ili- [ile- is commonly used to refer to the portion of the intestines known as the ileum]. *ile*ostomy

ili- *ilium* (*ileum*) lower abdomen, intestines [ili- is commonly used to refer to the flaring part of the hip bone known as the ilium]. *ili*osacral

im- See in-[2, 3]. *im*mersion (in, on), *im*perforation (negative prefix)

in-[1] ἴς, ἰνός fiber. Cf. fibr-. *in*osteatoma

in-[2] *in* (*n* changes to *l*, *m*, or *r* before words beginning with those consonants) in, on. Cf. en-. *in*sertion

in-[3] *in-* (*n* changes to *l*, *m*, or *r* before words beginning with those consonants) negative prefix. Cf. a-. *in*valid

infra- *infra* beneath. *infra*orbital

insul- *insula* island. *insul*in

inter- *inter* among, between. *inter*carpal

intra- *intra* inside. Cf. end- and eso-. *intra*venous

ir- See in-[2, 3]. *ir*radiation (in, on), *ir*reducible (negative prefix)

irid- ἶρις, ἴριδος rainbow, colored circle. kerato*irido*cyclitis

is- ἴσος equal. *is*otope

ischi- ἰσχίον hip, haunch. *ischi*opubic

jact- *iacio, iactus* throw. *jact*itation

ject- *iacio, -iectus* throw. in*ject*ion

jejun- *ieiunus* hungry, not partaking of food. gastro*jejun*ostomy

jug- *iugum* yoke. con*jug*ation

junct- *iungo, iunctus* yoke, join. con*junct*iva

kary- κάρυον nut, kernel, nucleus. Cf. nucle-. mega*kary*ocyte. (Also spelled cary-)

kerat- κέρας, κέρατος horn. *kerat*olysis. (Also spelled cerat-)

kil- χίλιοι one thousand. Cf. mill-. Indicates multiple in metric system. *kil*ogram

kine- κινέω move. *kine*matograph. (Also spelled cine-)

labi- *labium* lip. Cf. cheil-. gingivo-*labi*al

lact- *lac, lactis* milk. Cf. galact-. gluco*lact*one

lal- λαλέω talk, babble. glosso*lal*ia

lapar- λαπάρα flank. *lapar*otomy

laryng- λάρυγξ, λάρυγγος windpipe. *laryng*endoscope

lat- *fero, latus* bear, carry. See -ferent. trans*lat*ion

later- *latus, lateris* side. ventro*later*al

lent- *lens, lentis* lentil. Cf. phac-. *lent*iconus

lep- λαμβάνω, ληπ- take, seize. cata*lep*tic

leuc- See leuk-. *leuc*inuria

leuk- λευκός white. Cf. alb-. *leuk*orrhea. (Also spelled leuc-)

lien- *lien* spleen. Cf. splen-. *lien*ocele

lig- *ligo* tie, bind. *lig*ate

lingu- *lingua* tongue. Cf. gloss-. sub*lingu*al

lip- λίπος fat. Cf. adip-. glyco*lip*in

lith- λίθος stone. Cf. calc-[1]. nephro*lith*otomy

loc- *locus* place. Cf. top-. *loc*omotion

log- λέγω, λογ- speak, give an account, *log*orrhea, embryo*log*y

lumb- *lumbus* loin. dorso*lumb*ar

lute- *luteus* yellow. Cf. xanth-. *lute*oma

ly- λύω loose, dissolve. Cf. solut-. kerato*ly*sis

lymph- *lympha* water. Cf. hydr-. *lymph*adenosis

macr- μακρός long, large. *macr*omyeloblast

mal- *malus* bad, abnormal. Cf. cac- and dys-. *mal*function

malac- μαλακός soft. osteo*malac*ia

mamm- *mamma* breast. Cf. mast-. sub*mamm*ary

man- *manus* hand. Cf. cheir-. *man*iphalanx

mani- μανία mental aberration. *mani*graphy, klepto*mania*

mast- μαστός breast. Cf. mamm-. hyper*mast*ia

medi- *medius* middle. Cf. mes-. *medi*frontal

mega- μέγας great, large. Also indicates multiple (1,000,000) in metric system. *mega*colon, *mega*dyne. (See also megal-)

megal- μέγας, μεγάλου great, large. acro*megal*y

mel- μέλος limb, member. sym*mel*ia

melan- μέλας, μέλανος black. hippo*melan*in

men- μήν month. dys*men*orrhea

mening- μῆνιγξ, μήνιγγος membrane. encephalo*mening*itis

ment- *mens, mentis* mind. Cf. phren-, psych-, and thym-. de*ment*ia

mer- μέρος part. poly*mer*ic

mes- μέσος middle. Cf. medi-. *mes*oderm

met- See meta-. *met*allergy

meta- μετά (*a* is dropped before words beginning with a vowel) after, beyond, accompanying. *meta*carpal

metr-[1] μέτρον measure. stereo*metr*y

metr-[2] μήτρα womb. endo*metr*itis

micr- μικρός small. photo*micr*ograph

mill- *mille* one thousand. Cf. kil-. Indicates fraction in metric system. *mill*igram, *mill*ipede

miss- See -mittent. intro*miss*ion

-mittent *mitto, mittentis, missus* send. inter*mittent*

mne- μιμνήσκω, μνη- remember. pseudo*mne*sia

mon- μόνος only, sole. *mon*oplegia

morph- μορφή form, shape. poly*morph*onuclear

mot- *moveo, motus* move. vaso*mot*or

my- μῦς, μυός muscle. inoleio*my*oma

-myces μύκης, μύκητος fungus. myelo*myces*

myc(et)- See -myces. asco*mycet*es, strepto*myc*in

myel- μυελός marrow. polio*myel*itis

myx- μύξα mucus. *myx*edema

narc- νάρκη numbness. topo*narc*osis

nas- *nasus* nose. Cf. rhin-. palato*nas*al

ne- νέος new, young. *ne*ocyte

necr- νεκρός corpse. *necr*ocytosis

nephr- νεφρός kidney. Cf. ren-. para*nephr*ic

neur- νεῦρον nerve. esthesio*neur*e

nod- *nodus* knot. *nod*osity

nom- νόμος (from νέμω deal out, distribute) law, custom. taxo*nom*y

non- *nona* nine. *non*acosane

nos- νόσος disease. *nos*ology

nucle- *nucleus* (from *nux, nucis* nut) kernel. Cf. kary-. *nucle*ide

nutri- *nutrio* nourish. mal*nutri*tion

ob- *ob* (*b* changes to *c* before words beginning with that consonant) against, toward, etc. *ob*tuse
oc- See ob-. *oc*clude
ocul- *oculus* eye. Cf. ophthalm-. *ocul*omotor
-od- See -ode[1]. peri*od*ic
-ode[1] ὁδός road, path. cath*ode*. (See also hod-)
-ode[2] See -oid. nemat*ode*
odont- ὀδούς, ὀδόντος tooth. Cf. dent-. orth*odont*ia
-odyn- ὀδύνη pain, distress. gastr*odyn*ia
-oid εἶδος form. Cf. form. hy*oid*
-ol See ole-. cholester*ol*
ole- *oleum* oil. *ole*oresin
olig- ὀλίγος few, small. *olig*ospermia
omphal- ὀμφαλός navel. peri*omphal*ic
onc- ὄγκος bulk, mass. hemat*onc*ometry
onych- ὄνυξ, ὄνυχος claw, nail. an*onych*ia
oo- ᾠόν egg. Cf. ov-. peri*oo*thecitis
op- ὁράω, ὀπ- see. erythr*op*sia
ophthalm- ὀφθαλμός eye. Cf. ocul-. ex*ophthalm*ic
or- *os, oris* mouth. Cf. stom(at)-. intra*or*al
orb- *orbis* circle. sub*orb*ital
orchi- ὄρχις testicle. Cf. test-, *orchi*opathy
organ- ὄργανον implement, instrument. *organ*oleptic
orth- ὀρθός straight, right, normal. *orth*opedics
oss- *os, ossis* bone. Cf. ost(e)-. *oss*iphone
ost(e)- ὀστέον bone. Cf. oss-. en*ost*osis, *oste*anaphysis
ot- οὖς, ὠτός ear. Cf. aur-. par*ot*id
ov- *ovum* egg. Cf. oo-. syn*ov*ia
oxy- ὀξύς sharp. *oxy*cephalic
pachy(n)- παχύνω thicken. *pachy*derma, myo*pachyn*sis
pag- πήγνυμι, παγ- fix, make fast. thoraco*pag*us
par-[1] *pario* bear, give birth to. primi*par*ous
par-[2] See para-. *par*epigastric
para- παρά (final *a* is dropped before words beginning with a vowel) beside, beyond. *para*mastoid
part- *pario, partus* bear, give birth to. *part*urition
path- πάθος that which one undergoes, sickness. psycho*path*ic
pec- πήγνυμι, πηγ- (πηκ- before τ) fix, make fast. sym*pec*tothiene. (See also pex-)
ped- παῖς, παιδός child. ortho*ped*ic
pell- *pellis* skin, hide. *pell*agra
-pellent *pello, pellentis, pulsus* drive. re*pellent*
pen- πένομαι need, lack. erythrocyto*pen*ia
pend- *pendeo* hang down. ap*pend*ix
pent(a)- πέντε five. Cf. quinque-. *pent*ose, *penta*ploid
peps- πέπτω, πεψ- (before σ) digest. brady*peps*ia
pept- πέπτω digest. dys*pept*ic
per- *per* through. Cf. dia-. *per*nasal
peri- περί around. Cf. circum-. *peri*phery
pet- *peto* seek, tend toward. centri*pet*al
pex- πήγνυμι, πηγ- (added to σ becomes πηξ-) fix, make fast. hepato*pex*y
pha- φημί, φα- say, speak. dys*pha*sia
phac- φακός lentil, lens. Cf. lent-. *phac*osclerosis. (Also spelled phak-)
phag- φαγεῖν eat. lipo*phag*ic
phak- See phac-. *phak*itis
phan- See phen-. dia*phan*oscopy
pharmac- φάρμακον drug. *pharmac*ognosy
pharyng- φάρυγξ, φαρυγγ- throat. glosso*pharyng*eal
phen- φαίνω, φαν- show, be seen. phos*phen*e
pher- φέρω, φορ- bear, support. peri*pher*y
phil- φιλέω like, have affinity for. eosino*phil*ia
phleb- φλέψ, φλεβός vein. peri*phleb*itis
phleg- φλέγω, φλογ- burn, inflame. adeno*phleg*mon
phlog- See phleg-. anti*phlog*istic
phob- φόβος fear, dread. claustro*phob*ia
phon- φωνή sound. echo*phon*y
phor- See pher-. Cf. -ferent. exo*phor*ia
phos- See phot-. *phos*phorus
phot- φῶς, φωτός light. *phot*erythrous
phrag- φράσσω, φραγ- fence, wall off, stop up. Cf. sept-[1]. dia*phrag*m
phrax- φράσσω, φραγ- (added to σ becomes φραξ-) fence, wall off, stop up. em*phrax*is
phren- φρήν mind, midriff. Cf. ment-. meta*phren*ia, meta*phren*on
phthi- φθίνω decay, waste away. ophthalmo*phthi*sis
phy- φύω beget, bring forth, produce, be by nature. noso*phy*te
phyl- φῦλον tribe, kind. *phyl*ogeny
-phyll φύλλον leaf. xantho*phyll*
phylac- φύλαξ guard. pro*phylac*tic
phys(a)- φυσάω blow, inflate. *phys*ocele, *phys*alis
physe- φυσάω, φυση- blow, inflate. em*physe*ma
pil- *pilus* hair. e*pil*ation
pituit- *pituita* phlegm, rheum. *pituit*ous
placent- *placenta* (from πλακοῦς) cake. extra*placent*al
plas- πλάσσω mold, shape. cine-*plas*ty
platy- πλατύς broad, flat. *platy*rrhine
pleg- πλήσσω, πληγ- strike. di*pleg*ia
plet- *pleo, -pletus* fill. de*plet*ion
pleur- πλευρά rib, side. Cf. cost-. peri*pleur*al
plex- πλήσσω, πληγ- (added to σ becomes πληξ-) strike. apo*plex*y
plic- *plico* fold. com*plic*ation
pne- πνοιά breathing. traumato*pne*a
pneum(at)- πνεῦμα, πνεύματος breath, air. *pneum*odynamics, *pneumat*othorax
pneumo(n)- πνεύμων lung. Cf. pulmo(n)-. *pneumo*centesis, *pneumon*otomy
pod- πούς, ποδός foot. *pod*iatry
poie- ποιέω make, produce. Cf. -facient. sarco*poie*tic
pol- πόλος axis of a sphere. peri*pol*ar
poly- πολύς much, many. *poly*spermia
pont- *pons, pontis* bridge. *pont*ocerebellar
por-[1] πόρος passage. myelo*por*e
por-[2] πῶρος callus. *por*ocele
posit- *pono, positus* put, place. re*posit*or
post- *post* after, behind in time or place. *post*natal, *post*oral
pre- *prae* before in time or place. *pre*natal, *pre*vesical
press- *premo, pressus* press. *press*oreceptive
pro- πρό or *pro* before in time or place. *pro*gamous, *pro*cheilon, *pro*lapse
proct- πρωκτός anus. entero*proct*ia
prosop- πρόσωπον face. Cf. faci-. di*prosop*us
pseud- ψευδής false. *pseud*oparaplegia
psych- ψυχή soul, mind. Cf. ment-. *psych*osomatic
pto- πίπτω, πτω- fall. nephro*pto*sis
pub- *pubes, puber, puberis* adult. ischio*pub*ic. (See also puber-)
puber- *puber* adult. *puber*ty
pulmo(n)- *pulmo, pulmonis* lung. Cf. pneumo(n)-. *pulmo*lith, cardio*pulmon*ary
puls- *pello, pellentis, pulsus* drive. pro*puls*ion
punct- *pungo, punctus* prick, pierce. Cf. cente-. *punct*iform
pur- *pus, puris* pus. Cf. py-. sup*pur*ation
py- πύον pus. Cf. pur-. nephro*py*osis
pyel- πύελος trough, basin, pelvis. nephro*pyel*itis
pyl- πύλη door, orifice. *pyl*ephlebitis
pyr- πῦρ fire. Cf. febr-. galacto*pyr*a
quadr- *quadr-* four. Cf. tetra-. *quadr*igeminal
quinque- *quinque* five. Cf. pent(a)-. *quinque*cuspid
rachi- ῥαχίς spine. Cf. spin-. encephalo*rachi*dian
radi- *radius* ray. Cf. actin-. ir*radi*ation
re- *re-* back, again. *re*traction
ren- *renes* kidneys. Cf. nephr-. ad*ren*al
ret- *rete* net. *ret*othelium
retro- *retro* backwards. *retro*deviation
rhag- ῥήγνυμι, ῥαγ- break, burst. hemor*rhag*ic
rhaph- ῥαφή suture. gastror*rhaph*y
rhe- ῥέω flow. Cf. flu-. diar*rhe*al

rhex- ῥήγνυμι, ῥηγ- (added to σ becomes ῥηξ-) break, burst. metror*rhex*is

rhin- ῥίς, ῥινός nose. Cf. nas-. basi*rhin*al

rot- *rota* wheel. *rot*ator

rub(r)- *ruber, rubri* red. Cf. erythro-. bili*rub*in, *rubr*ospinal

salping- σάλπιγξ, σάλπιγγος tube, trumpet. *salping*itis

sanguin- *sanguis, sanguinis* blood. Cf. hem(at)-. *sanguin*eous

sarc- σάρξ, σαρκός flesh. *sarc*oma

schis- σχίζω, σχιδ- (before τ or added to σ becomes σχισ-) split. Cf. fiss-. *schis*torachis, rachi*schis*is

scler- σκληρός hard. Cf. dur-. *scler*osis

scop- σκοπέω look at, observe. endo*scop*e

sect- *seco, sectus* cut. Cf. tom-. *sect*ile

semi- *semi-* half. Cf. hemi-. *semi*flexion

sens- *sentio, sensus* perceive, feel. Cf. esthe-. *sens*ory

sep- σήπω rot, decay. *sep*sis

sept-[1] *saepio, saeptus* fence, wall off, stop up. Cf. phrag-. naso*sept*al

sept-[2] *septem* seven. Cf. hept(a)-. *sept*an

ser- *serum* whey, watery substance. *ser*osynovitis

sex- *sex* six. Cf. hex-[1]. *sex*digitate

sial- σίαλον saliva. poly*sial*ia

sin- *sinus* hollow, fold. Cf. colp-. *sin*obronchitis

sit- σῖτος food. para*sit*ic

solut- *solvo, solventis, solutus* loose, dissolve, set free. Cf. ly-. dis*solut*ion

-solvent See solut-. dis*solvent*

somat- σῶμα, σώματος body. Cf. corpor-. psycho*somat*ic

-some See somat-. dictyo*some*

spas- σπάω, σπασ- draw, pull. *spas*m, *spas*tic

spectr- *spectrum* appearance, what is seen. micro*spectro*scope

sperm(at)- σπέρμα, σπέρματος seed. *sperm*acrasia, *spermat*ozoon

spers- *spargo, -spersus* scatter. di*spers*ion

sphen- σφήν wedge. Cf. cune-. *sphen*oid

spher- σφαῖρα ball. hemi*spher*e

sphygm- σφυγμός pulsation. *sphygm*omanometer

spin- *spina* spine. Cf. rachi-. cerebro*spin*al

spirat- *spiro, spiratus* breathe. in*spirat*ory

splanchn- σπλάγχνα entrails, viscera. neuro*splanchn*ic

splen- σπλήν spleen. Cf. lien-. *splen*omegaly

spor- σπόρος seed. *spor*ophyte, zygo*spor*e

squam- *squama* scale. de*squam*ation

sta- ἵστημι, στα- make stand, stop. genesi*sta*sis

stal- στέλλω, σταλ- send. peri*stal*sis. (See also stol-)

staphyl- σταφυλή bunch of grapes, uvula. *staphyl*ococcus, *staphyl*ectomy

stear- στέαρ, στέατος fat. Cf. adip-. *stear*odermia

steat- See stear-. *steat*opygous

sten- στενός narrow, compressed. *sten*ocardia

ster- στερεός solid. chole*ster*ol

sterc- *stercus* dung. Cf. copr-. *sterc*oporphyrin

sthen- σθένος strength. a*sthen*ia

stol- στέλλω, στολ- send. dia*stol*e

stom(at)- στόμα, στόματος mouth, orifice. Cf. or-. ana*sto*mosis, *stomat*ogastric

strep(h)- στρέφω, στρεπ- (before τ) twist. Cf. tors-. *streph*osymbolia, *strep*tomycin. (See also stroph-)

strict- *stringo, stringentis, strictus* draw tight, compress, cause pain. con*strict*ion

-stringent See strict-. a*stringent*

stroph- στρέφω, στροφ- twist. ana*stroph*ic. (See also strep(h)-)

struct- *struo, structus* pile up (against). ob*struct*ion

sub- *sub* (*b* changes to *f* or *p* before words beginning with those consonants) under, below. Cf. hypo-. *sub*lumbar

suf- See sub-. *suf*fusion

sup- See sub-. *sup*pository

super- *super* above, beyond, extreme. Cf. hyper-. *super*motility

sy- See syn-. *sy*stole

syl- See syn-. *syl*lepsiology

sym- See syn-. *sym*biosis, *sym*metry, *sym*pathetic, *sym*physis

syn- σύν (*n* disappears before *s*, changes to *l* before *l*, and changes to *m* before *b*, *m*, *p*, and *ph*) with, together. Cf. con-. myo*syn*izesis

ta- See ton-. ec*ta*sis

tac- τάσσω, ταγ- (τακ- before τ) order, arrange. a*tac*tic

tact- *tango, tactus* touch. con*tact*

tax- τάσσω, ταγ- (added to σ becomes ταξ-) order, arrange. a*tax*ia

tect- See teg-. pro*tect*ive

teg- *tego, tectus* cover. in*teg*ument

tel- τέλος end. *tel*osynapsis

tele- τῆλε at a distance. *tele*ceptor

tempor- *tempus, temporis* time, timely or fatal spot, temple. *tempor*omalar

ten(ont)- τένων, τένοντος (from τείνω stretch) tight stretched band. *ten*odynia, *tenon*itis, *tenont*agra

tens- *tendo, tensus* stretch. Cf. ton-. ex*tens*or

test- *testis* testicle. Cf. orchi-. *test*itis

tetra- τετρα- four. Cf. quadr-. *tetra*genous

the- τίθημι, θη- put, place. syn*the*sis

thec- θήκη repository, case. *thec*ostegnosis

thel- θηλή teat, nipple. *thel*erethism

therap- θεραπεία treatment. hydro*therap*y

therm- θέρμη heat. Cf. calor-. dia*therm*y

thi- θεῖον sulfur. *thi*ogenic

thorac- θώραξ, θώρακος chest. *thorac*oplasty

thromb- θρόμβος lump, clot. *thromb*openia

thym- θυμός spirit. Cf. ment-. dys*thym*ia

thyr- θυρεός shield (shaped like a door θύρα). *thyr*oid

tme- τέμνω, τμη- cut. axono*tme*sis

toc- τόκος childbirth. dys*toc*ia

tom- τέμνω, τομ- cut. Cf. sect-. appendec*tom*y

ton- τείνω, τον- stretch, put under tension. Cf. tens-. peri*ton*eum

top- τόπος place. Cf. loc-. *top*esthesia

tors- *torqueo, torsus* twist. Cf. strep-. ex*tors*ion

tox- τοξικόν (from τόξον bow) arrow poison, poison. *tox*emia

trache- τραχεῖα windpipe. *trache*otomy

trachel- τράχηλος neck. Cf. cervic*trachel*opexy

tract- *traho, tractus* draw, drag. pro*tract*ion

traumat- τραῦμα, τραύματος wound. *traumat*ic

tri- τρεῖς, τρία or *tri-* three. *tri*gonid

trich- θρίξ, τριχός hair. *trich*oid

trip- τρίβω rub. en*trip*sis

trop- τρέπω, τροπ- turn, react. sito*trop*ism

troph- τρέφω, τροφ- nurture. a*troph*y

tuber- *tuber* swelling, node. *tuber*cle

typ- τύπος (from τύπτω strike) type. a*typ*ical

typh- τῦφος fog, stupor. adeno*typh*us

typhl- τυφλός blind. Cf. cec-. *typhl*ectasis

un- *unus* one. Cf. hen-. *un*ioval

ur- οὖρον urine. poly*ur*ia

vacc- *vacca* cow. *vacc*ine

vagin- *vagina* sheath. in*vagin*ated

vas- *vas* vessel. Cf. angi-. *vas*cular

vers- See vert-. in*vers*ion

vert- *verto, versus* turn. di*vert*iculum

vesic- *vesica* bladder. Cf. cyst-. *vesic*ovaginal

vit- *vita* life. Cf. bi-[1]. de*vit*alize

vuls- *vello, vulsus* pull, twitch. con*vuls*ion

xanth- ξανθός yellow, blond. Cf. flav- and lute-. *xanth*ophyll

-yl- ὕλη substance. cacod*yl*

zo- ζωή life, ζῷον animal. micro*zo*aria

zyg- ζυγόν yoke, union. *zyg*odactyly

zym- ζύμη ferment. en*zym*e

APPENDIX B

Common Abbreviations, Acronyms, and Symbols

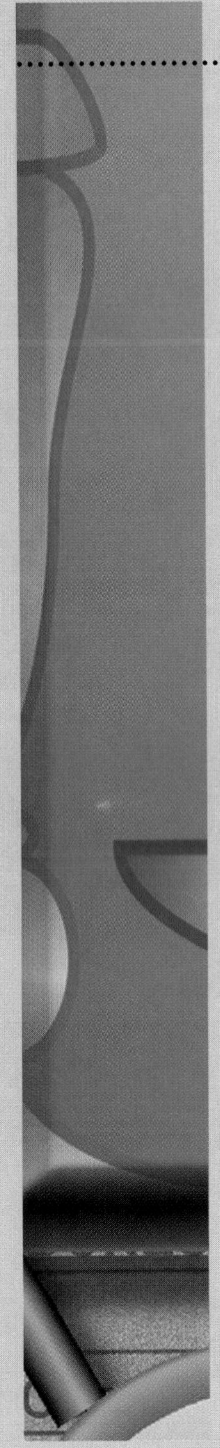

abd abdomen
a.c. before meals
ad lib as desired
$AgNO_3$ silver nitrate
A/KA above knee amputation
Anesth anesthesia
A & P anterior and posterior, auscultation and percussion
ASCVD arteriosclerotic cardiovascular disease
ASHD arteriosclerotic heart disease
A & W alive and well

BE barium enema
BID twice a day
B/KA below knee amputation
BM bowel movement
BMR basal metabolic rate
BP blood pressure
BPH benign prostatic hypertrophy
BUN blood urea nitrogen
Bx biopsy

C centigrade
Ca calcium
CA carcinoma
cal calorie
CBC complete blood count
cc cubic centimeter
CCU Coronary Care Unit
CHF congestive heart failure
cm centimeter
CNS central nervous system
CO_2 carbon dioxide
COPD chronic obstructive pulmonary disease
CPR cardiopulmonary resuscitation
C/S cesarean section
CSF cerebrospinal fluid
CT computed tomography
CVA cerebrovascular accident
cysto cystoscopy

D & C dilatation and curettage
disch discharge
DJD degenerative joint disease
DM diabetes mellitus
DNA deoxyribonucleic acid
DOA dead on arrival
DOB date of birth
DPT diphtheria, pertussis, tetanus
DR delivery room
Dx diagnosis

ECG electrocardiogram
EDC estimated date of confinement
EEG electroencephalogram
EENT eye, ear, nose, and throat
EKG electrocardiogram
ENT ear, nose, and throat
EOM extraocular movements
ER emergency room
EUA examination under anesthesia
expl lap exploratory laparotomy

F female
Fa or F Fahrenheit
FB foreign body
FBS fasting blood sugar
FH family history
FHT fetal heart tones
FS frozen section
FTG full thickness graft
FU follow up
FUO fever of unknown origin
Fx fracture

GB gallbladder
GE gastroenterology
GI gastrointestinal
g gram
GP general practitioner
GTT glucose tolerance test
gtt drops
GU genitourinary
GYN gynecology

HCl hydrochloric acid
HCVD hypertensive cardiovascular disease
Hgb hemoglobin
hs at bedtime
Hx history

ICU Intensive Care Unit
I & D incision and drainage
IM intramuscular
inj injection
int & ext internal and external
I & O intake and output
IP inpatient
IPPB intermittent positive pressure breathing
IT inhalation therapy
IUD intrauterine device
IV intravenous
IVP intravenous pyelogram

K potassium
KJ knee jerk
KUB kidney, ureter, and bladder

L left
L & A light and accommodation
lat lateral
LLQ left lower quadrant
LMP last menstrual period
LOM limitation of motion
LUQ left upper quadrant

M male
MH marital history
MRI magnetic resonance imaging
MS multiple sclerosis

NB newborn
NP neuropsychiatric
NPN nonprotein nitrogen
N.P.O. nothing by mouth
N & V nausea and vomiting

OB obstetrics
O.C. oral contraceptive
OD overdose
O.D. right eye
OP outpatient
O.R. operating room
O.S. left eye
O.U. both eyes

Path pathology
PBI protein bound iodine
p.c. after meals
PCCU Postcoronary Care Unit
Peds pediatrics
PERRLA pupils equal, round, regular, react to light and accommodation
PFT pulmonary function test
PH past history
PID pelvic inflammatory disease
PKU phenylketonuria
PMR paramedic run
PND paroxysmal nocturnal dyspnea
PO by mouth (per os)
PROM premature rupture of membranes
pro time prothrombin time
prn when needed
Psych psychiatry
pt patient
PT physical therapy
PU peptic ulcer
Px physical examination

q every
qd every day
qh every hour
QID four times a day
qn every night
qns quantity not sufficient

R right
Ra radium
R.A. rheumatoid arthritis
RBC red blood cell
REM rapid eye movement
RHD rheumatic heart disease
R/O rule out
ROS review of systems
R.R. recovery room
Rx prescription

SH social history
sig directions
SMR submucous resection
SOB shortness of breath
stat immediately
STG split thickness graft
subq subcutaneous
SWD short wave diathermy

T temperature
T & A tonsillectomy & adenoidectomy
tab tablet
TB tuberculosis
TIA transient ischemic attack
TID three times a day
TPR temperature, pulse, respiration
TUR transurethral resection

UA urinalysis
UCHD usual childhood diseases
UR utilization review

URI	upper respiratory infection
UTI	urinary tract infection
VA	visual acuity
VD	venereal disease
VDRL	Venereal Disease Research Laboratory
VS	vital signs
Wass	Wassermann
WBC	white blood cell
WDWN	well developed and well nourished
WF	white female
WM	white male
WNL	within normal limits

Symbols

$\bar{a}$	before
$\overline{aa}$	of each
$\bar{c}$	with
$\bar{p}$	after
$\bar{s}$	without
ss	one half
↓	decreased
↑	increased
>	greater than
<	less than
℃	birth
−	negative
+	positive
±	negative or positive (indefinite)
♂	male
♀	female
μ	micron
†	death
♏	minim
ʒ	dram
℥	ounce

APPENDIX C

Resources

Professional Organizations

American Association of Medical Assistants
20 North Wacker Drive, Suite 1575
Chicago, IL 60606

American Association for Medical Transcription
PO Box 576187
Modesto, CA 95357

Professional Secretaries International
10502 NW Ambassador Drive
PO Box 20404
Kansas City, MO 64195-0404

Registered Medical Assistant
710 Higgins Road
Park Ridge, IL 60068

Office Materials

Colwell Company
275 Kenyon Road
Champaign, IL 61820

Control-o-Fax
Box 778
Waterloo, IA 50704
(800) 344-7777

Patient Care Systems
16 Thorndal Circle
Darien, CT 06820

VISIrecord Systems
160 Gold Star Boulevard
Worcester, MA 01606

Bibbero Systems, Inc.
1300 N. McDowell Boulevard
Petaluma, CA 94954

Glossary

abetting Encouraging or supporting

abrasion Rubbing or scraping of the skin or mucous membrane (e.g., a skinned knee)

abscess A localized collection of pus that may be located under the skin or deep within the body causing tissue destruction

absorption The passage of the products of digestion from the gastrointestinal tract into the blood and lymphatic vessels and the tissue cells

abstract A written summary of the key points of a book, paper, or case history

academic degree A title conferred by a college, university, or professional school on completion of a program of study

accelerating Causing to act or move faster

access Freedom to obtain or make use of

accommodation Adjustment of the eye for seeing various sizes of objects at different distances

account A single financial record

account balance The debit or credit balance remaining in an account

accounting equation Assets = Liabilities + Proprietorship (Capital)

accounts payable Debts incurred and not yet paid

accounts receivable Amounts owed to the creditor (physician)

accounts receivable control A summary of unpaid accounts

accounts receivable ledger The combined record of all patient accounts

accounts receivable ratio A formula for measuring how fast outstanding accounts are being paid

accounts receivable trial balance A method of determining that the journal and the ledger are in balance

accrual basis of accounting Income is recorded when earned, and expenses are recorded when incurred

acute Having a rapid onset and severe symptoms; usually subsiding within a relatively short period of time

adhesions Fibrous scar tissue that clings to the surface of adjoining tissue sometimes forming an unwanted union of two surfaces

adipose Pertaining to fatty tissue

adjustment column An account column, sometimes included to the left of the balance column, that is used for entering discounts

administering Instilling a drug into the body of a patient

administrative Having to do with management duties; in medical assisting, refers to all "front office" activities

administrative law Regulations set forth by government agencies

advocate A person who pleads the cause of another

agar A substance extracted from algae and used in the laboratory to grow cultures of bacteria and other microorganisms

age analysis A procedure for classifying accounts receivable by age from the first date of billing

agenda A list of the specific items under each division of the order of business that is to be presented at a business meeting

agglutination The clumping together of particles (antigens and antibodies) resulting from their interaction with specific antibodies (or antigens); used in laboratory tests for blood typing and many other pathologic tests

albumin A water-soluble, heat-coagulable protein

albuminuria The abnormal presence of albumin in the urine

alignment The state of being in the correct relative position

aliquot A portion of a well-mixed sample that is removed for testing

allegation A statement of what a party to a legal action will undertake to prove

allergens Substances that are capable of producing an allergic reaction

allocation Apportioned for a specific purpose or person

alphabetic filing Any system that arranges names or topics according to the sequence of letters in the alphabet

alphanumeric Filing systems made up of combinations of letters and numbers

amblyopia Reduction or dimness of vision with no apparent organic cause; often referred to as lazy eye syndrome

ampule A small (usually a single dose) glass container of medication prepared for parenteral administration

analgesic A drug that will relieve pain without loss of consciousness

analyte Any component in blood or other body fluid that can be measured

anaphylaxis An allergic condition caused by an antigen/antibody reaction; may cause shock, bronchoconstriction, airway obstruction, and loss of consciousness

ancillary Subordinate; auxiliary

ancillary diagnostic services Services that support patient diagnoses (e.g., laboratory or x-ray, specialists, or surgery)

androgen Any steroid hormone that promotes male characteristics

anemia Condition in which there is a reduction in the number of circulating red blood cells per cubic millimeter of blood

anesthetic Agent that causes loss of sensation with or without loss of consciousness

angina pectoris Acute pain in the chest resulting from decreased blood supply to the heart muscle

annotating To furnish with notes, which are usually critical or explanatory

anomaly(ies) Marked deviation(s) from normal; congenital deformity(ies) as a result of faulty development of the fetus

anorexia Lack or loss of appetite for food

anoxia Severe hypoxia; absence of oxygen in inspired gases or in arterial blood

antecubital The area in front of and at the bend of the elbow

anthrax An acute infectious disease caused by a bacillus. Humans contract the disease from animal hair, hides, or waste matter

antibody An immunoglobulin produced by lymphoid tissue in response to substances interpreted as foreign invaders gaining entry into the body

antipruritic An agent that will prevent or relieve itching

antiseptic Pertaining to a substance that renders microorganisms harmless

anuria Complete suppression of urine formation by the kidney

anus The opening of the rectum on the body surface

aphonia Loss of the ability to speak

aphrodisiacs Drugs that cause sexual arousal

apical pulse Pulse heard over the base (apex) of the heart

apnea Absence or cessation of breathing

appease To make peaceful or quiet

applications Software programs designed to perform specific tasks

appraisal Setting a value on, or judging as to quality

approximate To bring wound or skin edges together

approximation The act or process of drawing together skin or wound edges

arbitration The hearing and determination of a cause in controversy by a person or persons either chosen by the parties involved or appointed under statutory authority

arbitrator A neutral person chosen to settle differences between two parties in controversy

arrhythmia Abnormal or irregular heart rhythm

arteriosclerosis Hardening and thickening of the walls of the arteries

arthropod vector A member of a phylum of the animal kingdom that includes the arachnids, crustaceans, and insects that can serve as a means of parasite infestation

artificial insemination The introduction of semen into the vagina or cervix by artificial means

asepsis Condition of being free from infection or infectious materials

aspirate To withdraw fluid by negative pressure; pulling up on the plunger of the syringe after inserting the needle to check for blood

aspirating To withdraw in by suction

assault An intentional, unlawful *attempt* of bodily injury to another by force or threat

assignment of benefits Statement authorizing the insurance company to pay benefits directly to the physician

asymptomatic Showing no symptoms

ataxia Failure or irregularity of muscle actions and coordination

atelectasis Collapsed or airless state of the lung

atherosclerosis Common type of arteriosclerosis in which deposits of yellow plaques form on the interior walls of the arterioles

atria Upper chambers of the heart

atrioventricular (AV) node Part of the conductive system located between the atria and the ventricles near the septum that receives the impulses from the sinoatrial node and sends them down the bundles of His and the bundle branches

atrophy Wasting away; decrease in size and substance

attenuated Weakened, or change in, virulence of a pathogenic microorganism

audiologist An allied health professional specializing in evaluation of hearing function, detection of hearing impairment, and the determination of the anatomical site of impairment

auditory ossicles The three small bones of the middle ear responsible for converting air conduction to bone conduction

augment To make greater (larger) or more effective (intense)

aura A peculiar sensation preceding the appearance of more definite neurological disturbance

auscultation The act of listening for sounds within the body, normally with a stethoscope

authority The quality of being in command

autocratic Ruling with unlimited authority

autonomy The ability to function in an independent fashion

avocational Pertaining to a subordinate occupation or a hobby

back up A tape or floppy disk for storage of files to prevent their loss in the event of hard disk failure

back-space key Key at upper right of keyboard with left arrow that deletes characters as it is struck

bacteria Single-celled microscopic organisms

balance The difference between the debit and credit totals

balance column The account column on the far right that is used for recording the difference between the debit and credit columns

balance sheet A financial statement for a specific date that shows the total assets, liabilities, and capital of the business

barrier A factor that restricts free movement

battery A willful and unlawful use of force or violence upon the person of another

beneficiary The person receiving the benefits of an insurance policy

benign Not cancerous, not recurrent

bibliography A list of the works that are referred to in a text or that were consulted by the author in producing a text

biennially Occurring every 2 years

bifurcates Divides into two branches

bifurcation The point of forking or separating into two branches

bilirubin Orange-colored pigment in bile; accumulation leads to jaundice

biophysical Pertaining to the science dealing with the application of physical methods and theories to biological problems

biopsy Excision of a small sample of living tissue from the body for diagnostic or therapeutic purposes

birthday rule The rule governing the hierarchy of coordination of benefits

blepharitis Inflammation of the glands and lash follicles along the margin of the eyelids

body language Gestures and mannerisms that influence communication

bolus The mass of food, made ready by mastication, that enters the esophagus as one swallows

bookkeeping The recording part of the accounting process

bounding pulse Pulse characterized by increased tension

bradycardia A slow heartbeat; a pulse below 60 beats per minute

bradypnea Respirations that are regular in rhythm but slower than normal in rate

bronchiectasis Dilation of the bronchi and bronchioles associated with secondary infection or ciliary dysfunction

bruit Abnormal sound or murmur heard on auscultation of an organ, vessel, or gland

bundle of His Atrioventricular bundle of impulse-conducting fibers in the myocardium

cancer Any cellular tumor or neoplastic disease in which there is a transformation of normal body cells into malignant cells

candid Frank; straightforward

cannula A flexible tube that surrounds a sharp, pointed trocar inserted into the body; when the trocar is withdrawn, fluid escapes from the body through the cannula

capital purchase The purchase of a major item of furniture or equipment

capitation System of payment in which providers are paid a fixed per capita fee for each enrolled patient, not dependent on the services rendered

caption A heading, title, or subtitle under which records are filed

cardiac arrest Total cessation of a functional heartbeat

cardiomyopathy Disease of the myocardium that is caused by a primary disease of the heart muscle

cardiotonic Increasing tonicity of the heart

carrier Unaffected person who can transmit infection to another person

cash basis of accounting Income is recorded when received, and expenses are recorded when paid

cash flow statement A financial summary for a specific period that shows the beginning balance on hand, the receipts and disbursements during the period, and the balance on hand at the end of the period

cash payment journal A record of all cash paid out

cassette A magnetic tape wound on two reels and encased in a plastic or metal container; *microcassette* A very small cassette tape that may be used in a handheld dictating unit

casts Fibrous or protein material molded to the shape of the part in which it has accumulated and thrown off into the urine in kidney disease

categorically Applied to a limited classification; placed in a specific division of a system of classification

catheter Thin flexible tube inserted into the body to permit introduction or withdrawal of fluid

catheterization The act of passing a tube through the body for removing fluids or injecting them into body cavities

caustic A substance that burns or destroys organic tissue by chemical action

caustic remark Biting wit

caustics Substances that corrode or eat away tissues

CD-ROM Compact disk–read only memory

censure The act of blaming or condemning sternly

centrifuge Laboratory machine used to separate particles of different densities within a liquid by spinning them at very high speed

cerebrospinal fluid Fluid within the subarachnoid space, the central canal of the spinal cord, and the four ventricles of the brain

cerumen A waxy secretion in the ear canal; commonly called *ear wax*

ceruminous Pertaining to the waxy secretion of the glands of the external auditory canal; commonly called ear wax

cervical spatula Wooden instrument designed to remove cervical secretions from the cervical os and from the cervical cuff; used to obtain secretions for the Papanicolaou test

cervical vertebrae The upper seven bones of the spinal column; the skeleton of the neck

cervix The narrow lower end of the uterus, sometimes called the *neck of the uterus*

chalazion A small eyelid mass resulting from inflammation of a meibomian gland

chancre Primary lesion of syphilis occurring at the site of entry of the infection

chemotherapy The treatment of disease using chemical agents

chief complaint Reason for patient seeking medical care

cholangiogram The film obtained by x-ray examination of the bile ducts, using a radiopaque dye as a contrast medium

cholecystogram The film obtained by x-ray examination of the gallbladder, using a radiopaque dye as a contrast medium

cholera An acute, infectious, bacillus-caused disease involving the entire bowel; *chicken cholera*—cholera that affects chickens

choroid The middle, vascular layer of the eye containing many blood vessels and brown pigment that serves to reduce reflection when it falls on the retina

chronic Persisting for a long period of time and showing little change

chronic bronchitis Recurrent inflammation of the membranes lining the bronchial tubes

chronologic In the order of time

cilia Hairlike projection from the surface of a cell; provides locomotion in free unicellular organisms

circumcision Surgical removal of the foreskin

circumvention Going around or avoiding

cirrhosis A disease of the liver that causes impairment in the metabolism of nutrients and the detoxification of poisons absorbed from the intestines

claim A demand to the insurer by the insured person for the payment of benefits under a policy

clarity The quality or state of being clear; the state of being clear or lucid

claustrophobia Fear of being trapped in enclosed or narrow places

clinical Pertaining to actual observation and treatment of patients

clitoris Small, elongated erectile body situated above the urinary meatus at the superior point of the labia minora

coagulable Capable of being formed into clots

coagulum A blood clot

coding Converting verbal descriptions of diseases, injuries, and procedures into numeric and alphanumeric designations

cognitive Pertaining to the operation of the mind process by which we become aware of perceiving, thinking, and remembering

co-insurance/copayment A policy provision by which both the insured person and the insurer share in a specified ratio of the expenses resulting from an illness or injury

coitus Sexual union between male and female; also known as intercourse

collagen A strong, fibrous, insoluble protein found in connective tissue; the primary protein of the skin, tendon, bone cartilage, and other connective tissues

collection ratio A formula for measuring the effectiveness of the billing system

collodion A preparation of cellulose nitrate that when applied to the skin dies to form a strong, thin, transparent film

colloquialisms Expressions that are acceptable and correct in ordinary conversation or informal speeches but unsuitable for formal speech or writing

colony The visible growth on a culture plate, usually resulting from a single bacterium

colostomy An artificial opening (stoma) created in the large intestine and brought to the surface of the abdomen for the purpose of evacuating the bowels

colostrum Thin, yellow, milky fluid secreted by the mammary gland a few days before and after delivery

coma An unconscious state from which the patient cannot be aroused

communicable Capable of being transmitted from one person to another

comorbidity A preexisting condition that will, because of its presence with a specific principal diagnosis, cause an increase in length of hospital stay by at least one day in approximately 75% of the cases

compensatory damages General or special damages without specific monetary value

complication A condition that arises during the hospital stay that prolongs the length of stay by at least one day in approximately 75% of the cases

compression The state of being pressed together

compulsory Obligatory; enforced

computer A machine that is designed to accept, store, process, and give out information

concise Expressing much in a brief form

concurrently Occurring at the same time

cones Structures found in the retina that make the perception of color possible

confidential Containing information that requires authorization for disclosure

congenital Present at and existing from birth

congruency The quality of agreeing

conjunctiva Delicate membrane lining of the eyelids and covering of the eyeball

conjunctivitis Inflammation of the conjunctiva

consultation report A report of the findings of the consulting physician to be sent to the referring physician

contagious Transmitted readily from one person to another by direct or indirect contact

contamination The act of soiling, staining, or polluting; especially the introduction of infectious materials or germs that produce disease

contingent Dependent on or conditioned by something else

continuation pages The second and following pages of a letter

continuity The quality or state of being continuous

contract law Enforceable promises

controlled substance Drugs that are regulated by the federal government (Drug Enforcement Agency)

conversely Reversed in order

convulsion A series of involuntary contractions of the voluntary muscles

coordination of benefits The provision in an insurance contract that limits benefits to 100% of the cost

copay A flat fee payable by the insured in most health maintenance organization plans

copulation Sexual intercourse

cornea Clear, transparent anterior covering of the eye

correlation A mutual relationship

costal Pertaining to the ribs

CPT-4 manual *Current Procedural Terminology* manual

CPU Central processing unit; the part of a computer system that processes information

creatinine Nitrogenous waste from muscle metabolism excreted in urine

credit The record of a payment received

credit balance The amount of advance payment or overpayment on an account (amount of receipts exceeding amount of charges)

credit column The account column to the right of the debit column that is used for entering funds received

crenate The formation of notches or leaflike scalloped edges on an object

crepitation Dry, crackling sound or sensation produced by the grating of the ends of a fractured bone

crossover claim A claim for benefits under both Medicare and Medicaid

cryosurgery The technique of exposing tissue to extreme cold to produce a well-defined area of cell destruction

culminate To reach a high or decisive point

curettage The act of scraping a body cavity with a surgical instrument, such as a curette

cursor A symbol appearing on the monitor that shows where the next character to be typed will appear

cursor-control keys Keys that have an arrow pointing up, down, left, or right that are used to move a cursor

cyanosis Bluish discoloration of the skin, extremities, and mucous membranes caused by a decreased level of oxygen transported to cells

cyanotic Pertaining to a bluish discoloration of the skin and mucous membrane

cyst A sac of fluid or semisolid material located in or under the skin

cytology Biologic science devoted to the study of cell morphology

daily journal The book in which all transactions are first recorded; the book of original entry, or general journal

daisy wheel A printing element made of plastic or metal used on some typewriters and impact printers that derives its name from its shape, which is like that of a daisy

database A collection of related files that serves as a foundation for retrieving information

debit The record of a charge or debt incurred

debit column The account column on the left that is used for entering charges

debridement Surgical removal of damaged, diseased, or contaminated tissue until healthy tissue is exposed

deceptive Misleading; having the power to deceive

deductible A statement in an insurance policy that the insuring company will pay the expenses incurred after the insured person has paid a specified amount

defecation Elimination of wastes and undigested food, as feces, from the rectum

defibrillator Apparatus used to produce a brief electroshock to the heart through electrodes placed on the chest wall

delirium An acute, reversible organic mental syndrome characterized by reduced ability to maintain attention to external stimuli

democratic Relating to social equality

demographics Relating to the statistical characteristics of populations, such as births, marriages, mortality, and health

denervation A condition in which the nerve supply has been blocked

deposition Oral testimony taken from a party or witness to the litigation and is not limited to parties named in the lawsuit

dermatophyte A fungal parasite that grows in or on the skin

diagnosis Concise technical description of the cause, nature, or manifestations of a condition or problem. *Initial:* physician's temporary impression sometimes called a *working diagnosis. Final:* Conclusion the physician reaches after evaluating all findings, including laboratory and other testing results

diaphoresis Profuse perspiration

diaphragmatic Pertaining to the primary muscle of respiration that separates the thoracic and the abdominal cavities

diaphysis Portion of the long bone between the ends enclosing the medullary cavity

dictation The process of recording the spoken word onto a storage medium from which a printed copy will be produced

diction Choice of words to express ideas, especially with regard to correctness, clearness, or effectiveness

digestion The process of converting food into chemical substances that can be used by the body

dilatation Opening or widening the circumference of a body orifice with a dilating instrument

diluent A substance, such as water, that renders a drug or a solution less potent

diplopia Double vision

direct filing system A filing system in which materials can be located without consulting an intermediary source of reference

disability The condition resulting from illness or injury that makes an individual unable to be employed

disbursements Money (funds) paid out

disbursements journal A summary of amounts paid out

discernible A difference that can be seen between two or more things

discounts Subtractions from the patient's balance

discretion Quality of being discreet, tactful, or prudent

discrimination Different treatment on a basis other than individual merit

disease A definite pathologic process having a descriptive set of signs and symptoms

disinfection Destruction of pathogenic organisms by chemical or physical means

disk A magnetic surface that is capable of storing computer programs that sometimes is flexible (floppy disks) and sometimes is hard (hard disks)

disk drives Devices that load a program or data stored on a disk into a computer

dispensing Giving of drugs, in some type of bottle, box, or other container, to the patient. (Under the Controlled Substances Act of 1970, the definition of "dispense" includes the administering of controlled substances.)

disruption A breaking down or upset

dissect To cut or separate tissue with a cutting instrument or scissors

dissection The process of cutting apart or separating tissues for anatomic study

disseminate To broadcast or spread over a considerable area

don To put on

dot matrix printer An impact printer that forms characters using patterns of dots

draft A preliminary outline or writing that the author expects to amend or revise

dysmenorrhea Painful menstruation

dysphagia Difficult or painful swallowing

dyspnea Difficult or painful breathing

dysuria Difficult or painful urination

ecchymosis A skin discoloration produced by a hemorrhagic area, bluish black in color; also known as a bruise

edema Intracellular accumulation of excess fluid; swelling between the layers of tissue

editing The process of examining text to determine accuracy and clarity

ejaculation Ejection of the seminal fluid from the male urethra

elastic pulse Pulse with regular alterations of weak and strong beats without changes in cycle

elastin Essential part of elastic connective tissue that when moist is flexible and elastic

electrodesiccation The destructive drying of cells and tissue by means of short high-frequency electrical sparks

electrolyte Chemical substance that when dissolved, dissociates into electrically charged particles and is capable of conducting an electric current; essential to the normal function of cells

electronic billing The submission of a claim via computer to computer

electronic mail (E-mail) Communications transmitted via computer using a telephone modem

elimination Discharge from the body of indigestible materials and of waste products of body metabolism

emancipated minor A person under legal age who is self-supporting and living apart from parents or a guardian

embryology The science or study of the development of living organisms during the embryonic stage

empathy Intellectual and emotional awareness of another person's thoughts, feelings, and behavior

emphysema Pathologic accumulation of air in the tissues or organs

endorsement To express approval publicly and definitely

endorser Person who signs his or her name on the back of a check for the purpose of transferring title to another person

***enter* key** Key that performs the same function as the return key on a typewriter

enunciation The act of pronouncing words distinctly

enzymatic reaction A chemical reaction controlled by an enzyme

enzymes Proteins produced by living cells that act as a catalyst, increasing the rate at which a chemical reaction occurs

eosin Any of the synthetic dyes used to stain tissues blue and yellow for microscopic identification

eosinophil Granular leukocyte that increases in number in allergic conditions

epigastric Medial area of the abdominal cavity located between the umbilical area and the diaphragm

epiphyses Ends of the long bone, which are wider than the shaft of the bone

epistaxis Nosebleed

eradicated Wiped out or cancelled

erythema Redness of the skin caused by congestion of the capillaries in the skin layers

erythrocytes Red blood cells

erythropoietin Substance released from the kidney and liver that promotes red blood cell formation

essential hypertension Elevated blood pressure of unknown cause that develops for no apparent reason; sometimes called *primary hypertension*

established patient A patient who has received care from the physician within the past 3 years or other specified period

estrogen Female sex hormone secreted primarily by the ovary

ethics A set of moral principles or values

ethnic Pertaining to large groups of people classed according to cultural origin or background

etiology Classifying a claim according to the cause of the disorder

eustachian tube Narrow tube leading from the middle ear to the pharynx

exacerbation Aggravation of symptoms or increased severity of a disease

excoriation Scratch or similar abrasion to the skin

exemplary Serving as a warning

exophthalmia Pertaining to an abnormal protrusion of the eyes

exophthalmometer Instrument used to measure the pressure in the central retinal artery

expediency A situation requiring haste or caution

expendable Concerning supplies or equipment that is normally used up or consumed in service

expert witness Professional who belongs to a certifying or qualifying organization and who is called to testify in court

expulsion Act of expelling or forcing out

externship The practice of receiving employment experience in qualified health care facilities under the cooperative supervision of the medical staff and the program instructor as part of the educational curriculum

extracurricular Relating to those activities that form part of the life of students but are not part of the courses of study

extravasated Pertaining to bleeding into the tissues

exudate(s) Fluid with a high concentration of protein and cellular debris that has escaped from blood vessels and has been deposited in tissues or on tissue surfaces

fallopian tubes The tubes that capture the expelled ova and transport them to the uterus; usual location of fertilization; also called the *oviducts*

familial Occurring in or affecting members of a family more than would be expected by chance

fascia A sheet or band of fibrous tissue that covers muscles and body organs

feces Body waste discharged from the intestine; also called stool or excreta

fee profile Compilation of a physician's fees over a given period of time

fee schedule Compilation of preestablished fee allowances for given services or procedures

fee splitting Sharing a fee with another physician, laboratory, or drug company not based on services performed

feedback Letting people know how you feel about them at a given moment

felony A crime of a graver nature than one designated as a misdemeanor; generally, an offense punishable by imprisonment in a penitentiary

fenestrated drape A surgical drape or cover that has a prepared opening

fimbriae Fringelike border found on the distal part of the fallopian tube

fiscal agent An organization under contract to the government as well as some private plans to act as financial representative in handling insurance claims from providers of health care; also referred to as **fiscal intermediary**

fiscal intermediary An organization that handles claims from hospitals, nursing facilities, intermediate and long-term care facilities, and home health agencies

fissures Narrow slits or clefts in the abdominal wall

fistula Any abnormal, tubelike passage within the body tissue, usually between two internal organs

fixative Agent used in preserving a histologic or pathologic specimen to maintain its normal structure

flagged Using something to signal or attract attention

flagging A way of bringing attention to a blank space for possible correction in a transcribed page (also called tagging, carding or marking)

flatus Gas expelled through the anus

floppy disk (diskette) A thin disk (diskette) of magnetic material capable of storing a large amount of information

flourishing Achieving success

fonts Sets of printing type that are of one size and style

footnotes Comments placed at the bottom of a page that would be distracting if placed within the main text

format Shape, size, and general makeup of a publication, such as a resumé; to magnetically create tracks on a disk where information will be stored; to initialize a disk

fovea centralis A small pit in the center of the retina that is considered the center of clearest vision

freestanding emergency center An emergency facility not associated with a hospital

frequency Excessive need to urinate

fringe benefit A benefit granted by an employer that involves a money cost but does not affect the basic wage rates of employees

fundus Part of the uterus between the junctions of the fallopian tubes

gait Manner or style of walking

galley proofs Printer's proofs taken from composed type before page composition

gangrene The death of body tissue due to loss of nutritive supply, followed by bacteria invasion and putrefaction

general journal The book of original entry in bookkeeping

genetic Pertaining to the branch of biology dealing with heredity and variation among related organisms

germicides Agents that destroy pathogenic organisms

gestation Period of development from fertilization until birth

gesture The use of motions as a means of expression

ghost surgery A situation in which a patient has consented to have surgery done by one surgeon but, without the patient's knowledge or consent, the surgery is actually performed by another surgeon

glioma A neoplasm of the supporting structure of nervous tissue in the brain

glomerulonephritis Disease that interferes with the basic functions of the kidneys

glycosuria The presence of glucose in the urine

goniometer Instrument for measuring muscle angles

group policy A policy that covers a group (e.g., all employees of one company) under a master contract

group practice The provision of services by a group of at least three practitioners

grouper Computer software program that is used by the fiscal intermediary in all cases to assign discharges to the appropriate DRGs using the following information abstracted from the inpatient bill: patient's age, sex, principal diagnosis, principal procedures performed, and discharge status

guarding The act of physically protecting a specific part of the body from another person's touch

hard copy The readable paper copy or printout of information

hardware Computer components that perform four main functions

harmonious All parts are agreeably related or in accord

harmony Having an atmosphere of cordiality

HCFA Health Care Financing Administration; the authority that administers Medicare

HCPCS Acronym for HCFA's Common Procedure Coding System, used in determining Medicare fees

health maintenance organization (HMO) An organization that provides comprehensive health care to an enrolled group for a fixed periodic payment

Helicobacter pylori A gram-negative spiral bacterium that causes gastritis and pyloric ulcers in humans

hematocrit The volume percentage of erythrocytes in whole blood

hematoma Tumor or sac filled with blood that may be the result of trauma; a localized collection of clotted blood caused by a broken vessel

hematuria The presence of blood in the urine

hemiplegia Paralysis of one side of the body

hemodialysis Type of kidney dialysis where an artificial kidney machine is used to cleanse the blood

hemoglobin A protein found in erythrocytes that transports molecular oxygen in the blood

hemolysis Pertaining to the breakdown of red blood cells and the release of hemoglobin into the plasma

hemolytic disease A group of diseases in which the characteristic feature is the breakdown of red blood cells and the release of hemoglobin into the plasma

hemolyzed A blood sample in which the red cells have been ruptured

hemoptysis Coughing and spitting of blood as a result of bleeding in the respiratory tract

heparin A naturally occurring antithrombin factor that prevents intravascular clotting

hereditary Transmitted from parent to offspring; genetically determined

hermetically sealed Sealed so no air is allowed to enter; or plugging of the supplying artery

hertz (Hz) Unit of frequency equal to one cycle per second

histologist One who specializes in the study of the minute structure, composition, and function of the tissues

homeostasis Ability of the body systems to maintain relatively constant conditions in the internal environment; internal adaptation and change in response to environmental factors

hordeolum Inflammation of one or more sebaceous glands of the eyelid; often called a stye

hormones Chemical substances secreted by endocrine glands and carried through the blood to specific designated targets

hot flashes Flushing of the body caused by blood vessels expanding and then contracting

human chorionic gonadotropin (hCG) Hormone secreted by the female when pregnant; a hormone secreted in large amounts by the placenta during gestation to stimulate the formation of interstitial cells

hydrocephaly Enlargement of the cranium caused by abnormal accumulation of cerebrospinal fluid within the cerebral system

hyperpnea Increased rate of respiration

hypertension High blood pressure (systolic pressure consistently above 160 mm Hg and diastolic pressure above 90 mm Hg)

hyperthermia Greatly increased body temperature

hyperventilation Abnormally prolonged and deep breathing usually associated with acute anxiety or emotional tension

hypogastric Medial area of the abdominal cavity located below the umbilical area and above the pubic bone

hypotension Blood pressure that is below normal (systolic pressure below 90 mm Hg and diastolic pressure below 50 mm Hg)

hypothermia Greatly reduced body temperature

hysterectomy Surgical removal of the uterus

ICD manual *International Classification of Diseases* manual

ileocecal valve The valve guarding the opening between the ileum and cecum; also called the ileocolic valve

immunology Science that deals with the phenomena and causes of immunity and immune responses

impartiality The quality of treating or affecting all equally

impotence Inability to achieve or maintain an erection

in balance Total ending balances of patient ledgers equal total of accounts receivable control

in vitro Pertaining to a biologic reaction that occurs in an artificial environment, possibly in a test tube

incontinence Inability to control excretory functions

indemnity A benefit paid by an insurer for a loss insured under a policy

indicator strip A charted strip that is inserted into the dictation unit and on which the dictator marks the beginning and end point of each document and any corrections to be made

indirect filing system A filing system in which an intermediary source of reference, such as a card file, must be consulted to locate specific files

individual policy A policy usually held by a person who does not qualify for a group policy

induration An abnormally hard spot or place

infarction Area of tissue that has died because of lack of blood supply

infection Invasion and multiplication of microorganisms in body tissues causing injury and damage to the tissues

infectious Capable of causing infection

inflection Change in pitch or loudness of the voice

informed consent A consent, verbal or written, in which there is understanding of what treatment is to be undertaken and of the risks involved, why it should be done, and alternative methods of treatment available (including no treatment) and their attendant risks

infraction Breaking the law, a minor offense of the rules

ingestion The taking of food, drugs, etc., into the body by mouth

innovation Act of introducing something new or novel

inoculate To place a specimen in a culture medium to allow it to grow so that it can be identified

input Information entered into and used by the computer

insidious Diseases that come on in an symptomatic manner; of gradual and subtle development

insubordination Refusing to submit to authority

insulin shock Shock brought about by too much insulin, too little food, or excessive exercise; when untreated, can result in death

integral Essential; being an indispensable part of a whole

interaction A two-way communication

intercom (intercommunication system) A direct telephone line from one station to another

intermittent Coming and going at intervals, not continuous

intermittent pulse Pulse in which beats are occasionally skipped

intrinsic Inward; indwelling

invasive A procedure in which a body cavity is entered or tissue pierced

inventory A list of articles in stock, with the description and quantity of each

invoice A paper describing a purchase and the amount due

invulnerable Incapable of being injured or harmed

ion An electrically charged particle

iris Circular pigmented membrane behind the cornea, perforated by the pupil

irregular pulse Pulse that varies in force and frequency

irrigation The cleansing of a cavity or wound with water or other fluids to treat inflammation or infection

ischemia Decreased bloodflow to a body part or organ, caused by constriction

ischemic Refers to a temporary deficiency of blood supply to a tissue or organ

jaundice A yellowness of the skin and mucous membranes caused by deposition of bile pigment; not a disease but a symptom of a number of diseases, especially liver disorders

keratin A very hard, tough protein found in hair, nails, and epidermal tissue

keratinocytes Any one of the skin cells that synthesizes keratin

keratitis Inflammation of the cornea of the eye

keratolytic A substance that causes the shedding of skin cells at regular intervals

keyboarding The process of entering characters into the memory of a word processor

kyphosis Abnormally increased convex curve of the thoracic spine; also called *hunchback*

labia majora Two folds of adipose tissue that extend from the mons pubis to the perineum in the female

labia minora Two thin folds of epithelial tissue between the labia majora and the opening of the vagina

lacrimal sac Sac located over the upper, outer corner of the eye that secretes tears

lacrimation The secretion or discharge of tears

laissez faire Management style of "hands off" when dealing with employees

laryngoscopy Visual examination of the voice box area through an endoscope equipped with a light and mirrors for illumination

latent Describing the seemingly inactive time between the exposure of tissue to an injurious agent and the time that response signs and symptoms begin to appear

legend Heading or title of a figure

lens Transparent, biconvex body separating the posterior chamber and the vitreous body of the eye

lesion A wound, sore, ulcer, tumor, or any traumatic tissue damage that causes a lack of tissue continuity or a loss of function

letter-quality printer A printer that resembles a typewriter and that may be either mechanical or electronic

leukemia A malignancy of the blood-forming cells in the bone marrow

leukocytes White blood cells

leukoderma White patches on the skin

liability Subject to some adverse action

ligation Something that binds

ligation The process of tying off something to close it, usually a blood vessel, during surgery. The ties are called ligatures

listening An active process of receiving information and examining one's reaction to the messages received

litigation Contest in a court of justice for the purpose of enforcing a right

litigious Tending to engage in lawsuits

living will A document in which an individual expresses wishes regarding medical treatment at or near the end of life

lordosis Forward curvature of the lumbar spine

lubricant Water-soluble substance used on the glove when the rectum or vaginal cavity is examined

lumen An open space, such as within a blood vessel, the intestine, or an examining instrument

luxation Total dislocation of the bone from the joint

main memory Section of the computer where information and instructions are stored

major diagnostic category (MDC) Broad clinical category that is differentiated from all others based on body system involvement and disease etiology

maker (of a check) Any individual, corporation, or legal party who signs a check or any type of negotiable instrument

maladies Diseases or disorders of the body

malaise Feeling of uneasiness or discomfort

malfeasance The doing of an act that is wholly wrongful and unlawful

malignant Growing worse, resisting treatment, threatening to produce death

malpractice Professional misconduct, improper discharge of professional duties, or failure to meet the standard of care by a professional that results in harm to another

mammary glands Breasts

mandated Having a formal order from a superior to an inferior source

mandatory In the nature of a mandate or command; obligatory

manipulation Moving or exercising a body part by an externally applied force

manipulative Treating or operating with the hands in a skillful manner

manuscript Written or typewritten document, as distinguished from printed copy

masking To obscure or diminish a sound with the presence of another sound of different frequency

mastication The act of chewing

matrix Something in which something else originates, develops, takes shape, or is contained; a base upon which to build

maturation Physical and mental development process from beginning to maximum growth

mediastinal Pertaining to the space in the center of the chest under the sternum

mediastinum The space in the center of the chest under the sternum, containing the heart, great vessels, esophagus, and trachea

medically indigent Able to take care of ordinary living expenses but cannot afford medical care

medullary cavity Inner portion of the bone that contains the bone marrow

medulloblastoma A tumor composed of embryonic cells in the medulla oblongata

melanin A dark, sulfur-containing pigment normally found in the hair, skin, ciliary body, choroid of the eye, pigment layer of the retina, and certain nerve cells

member physician A physician who has agreed to accept the contracts of an insurer; this usually includes accepting the insurance benefits as payment in full

menarche Onset of the menstrual cycle

meningioma A hard vascular tumor invading the dura and skull

menopause The phase of life when a woman ceases to menstruate and passes from the reproductive to the nonreproductive stage; biologic end of the reproductive cycle of the female; also called *climacteric*

menstruation Cyclic shedding of the lining (endometrium) of the uterus

metabolic Referring to the processes concerned with the disposition of nutrients absorbed into the blood after digestion

meticulous Extremely careful of small details

microcephaly Small size of the head in relation to the rest of the body

microfilming Photographic records in reduced size on film

microorganism An organism of microscopic or ultramicroscopic size (also called *microbe*)

microsurgery Surgery performed under a microscope using very small instruments

micturition Act of voiding or urinating

millennia Thousands of years (*mille* = thousands)

misdemeanor A crime less serious than a felony

misfeasance The improper performance of a lawful act

mnemonic Improvement of memory by special methods or techniques

modem Acronym for modulator demodulator; a device that enables data to be transmitted over telephone lines

monitor To listen to a matter transmitted by telephone as a third party; a device used to display computer-generated information; a video screen; a CRT

monograph Learned treatise on a small area of knowledge; a written account of a single thing or class of things

mons pubis Fat pad that covers the symphysis pubis

mons veneris The rounded, elevated area overlying the symphysis pubis that is covered with hair after puberty

mordant A chemical (Gram's iodine) used to make the primary stain adhere to the cells it stains

morphology The study of the form, structure, and size of organisms, organs, tissues, and cells

motivation Process of inciting a person to some action or behavior

mouse Pointing device that controls the cursor

multiparous Pertaining to women who have had two or more pregnancies

murmur Abnormal sound heard when auscultating the heart that may or may not be pathologic

myocardial Pertaining to the middle layer of the walls of the heart muscle

myocardium Muscle layer of the heart

myoglobinuria Abnormal presence of a hemoglobin-like chemical of muscle tissue in urine, which is a sign of muscle deterioration

myringotomy Surgical process performed to relieve pressure and allow fluid drainage from the middle ear

mysticism The experience of seeming to have direct communication with God or ultimate reality

mythology A branch of knowledge that deals with the interpretation of myths

nebulization Treatment by a spray

necrosis The morphologic changes indicative of cell death caused by enzymatic degradation

negligence The doing of some act that a reasonable or prudent physician would not do, or the failure to do some act that such a person would or should do

negotiable Legally transferable to another party

neophyte A new convert or novice

neoplasm Abnormal new mass of tissue that serves no purpose; often cancerous

nephron units Basic functioning units of the kidney found in the renal pyramids

new patient A patient who has not received any professional services from the physician in the past 3 years or other specified period

nitrogenous waste Product of metabolism that if left to accumulate may become toxic

nits Eggs of the louse

nocturia Night-time urination

nodule Small lump, lesion, or swelling felt when palpating the skin

nominal Existing in name only

nomogram Representation by graphs, diagrams, or charts of the relationships between numerical variables

noncommittal Not revealing any specific attitude or opinion

nonconsensual Not having received consent

nonfeasance The failure to do something that should have been done

non-par Nonparticipating provider

nonparticipating provider A physician who does not accept assignment under Medicare or the Blue Plans

no-show A person who fails to keep an appointment without giving advance notice of that failure

nosocomial Pertaining to the spread of infection among patients, staff, and visitors inside of a given institution such as a hospital, school, or prison

NSAIDs Nonsteroidal antiinflammatory drugs; nonnarcotic analgesics that do not belong to the steroid group of drugs; drugs that have antiinflammatory, antipyretic, and analgesic effects

numeric filing The filing of records, correspondence, or cards by number

objective Something toward which effort is directed; an aim or end of action

objective information Perceptible to the external senses (e.g., conclusions reached by a physician after listening to body sounds with a stethoscope)

obliteration To remove from existence; destroy

observation An inference from what has been seen or heard

obturator A metal rod with a smooth rounded tip that is placed into hollow instruments to decrease destruction of the mucous membrane during insertion

occult Hidden; not visible with the eye alone

office policy manual An informational guide for employees.

oliguria Sudden drop in urine volume

onychomycosis Fungus of the nail bed

opaque Impervious to light rays; neither translucent nor transparent

ophthalmologist Physician specializing in the diagnosis and treatment of disorders of the eye

optic disc Region at the back of the eye where the optic nerve meets the retina; considered the blind spot of the eye because it contains only nerve fibers and no rods or cones and thus is insensitive to light

optic nerve Second cranial nerve that carries impulses for the sense of light

optician One who can translate, fill, and adapt ophthalmic prescriptions, products, and accessories and who does not need to be licensed

optometrist Professional trained to examine the eyes and prescribe eyeglasses to correct irregularities in vision

oral hygiene Proper care of mouth and teeth resulting in clean teeth and an absence of unpleasant breath.

orbit Bony cavity containing the eyeball and its associated structures

order of business List of the different divisions of business in the order in which each is to be addressed at a business meeting

organ of Corti Located within the cochlear duct; contains special sensory receptors for hearing

orientation The determination or adjustment of one's intellectual or emotional position with reference to circumstances

orthopnea Breathing in an upright position

orthopneic Pertaining to breathing in an upright or straight position

orthostatic (postural) hypotension Temporary fall in blood pressure when a person rapidly changes from a recumbent position to a standing position

otalgia Pain in the ear; an earache

otitis media Inflammation of the middle ear

otosclerosis Formation of spongy bone in the labyrinth of the ear, often causing the auditory ossicles to become fixed and unable to vibrate when sound enters the ears

OUTfolder A folder used to provide space for the temporary filing of materials

OUTguide A heavy guide that is used to replace a folder that has been temporarily moved from the filing space

outliers (atypical cases) Cases involving an extremely long stay (day outlier) or extraordinarily high costs (cost outlier) when compared with most discharges classified in the same DRG

output Information that is processed by the computer and transmitted to a monitor, printer, or other device

ovaries Pair of almond-shaped organs located at the distal end of the fallopian tubes that are responsible for the production and release of ova and a large percentage of the female hormones

overaccentuate Greatly emphasize

over-the-counter drugs Medications sold without a prescription

overutilization Excessive use

oviducts The pair of tubes in the female that carry the egg from the ovary to the uterus; fallopian tubes

packing slip An itemized list of objects in a package

palliative A substance that alleviates or eases a painful situation without curing it

pallor Lack of color; pale skin

pandemic Affecting the majority of the people in a country or a number of countries

par Participating provider

paradox A statement that seems to be contradictory and yet is perhaps true

paranoia A descriptive term limited to the characterization of behavior that is marked by delusions of persecution or grandeur

paresthesia An abnormal sensation of burning, prickling, or stinging

parlance Manner or mode of speech

paroxysm Sudden turn or amplification of symptoms such as a spasm or seizure

paroxysmal A sudden recurrent spasm of symptoms

participating provider A physician who accepts assignment under Medicare or the Blue Plans

parturition Act or process of giving birth to a child

patency The open condition of a body cavity or canal

pathogens Disease-causing microorganisms

pathologic Altered or caused by disease

payables Amounts owed to others

payee Person named on a draft or check as the recipient of the amount shown

payer Person who writes a check in favor of the payee

pediatrician A physician who specializes in the care of children

pedunculated Having a stemlike connecting part

peer review organization (PRO) An entity that is composed of a substantial number of licensed doctors of medicine and osteopathy engaged in the practice of medicine or surgery in the area, or an entity that has available to it the services of a sufficient number of physicians engaged in the practice of medicine or surgery, to ensure the adequate peer review of the services provided by the various medical specialties and subspecialties

pejorative Having negative connotations; a depreciatory word

perception A mental image

percussion The act of striking a part of the body with short, sharp blows as an aid in diagnosing the condition of the underlying parts by the sound obtained

perfusion The passing of a fluid through spaces

pericardium Sac that surrounds the heart

periodicals Journals published with a fixed interval (greater than 1 day) between its issues or numbers

periphery The external surface or boundary of a body

peristalsis The wavelike movement by which the gastrointestinal tract moves food downward

peritoneal dialysis A type of dialysis where fluid is injected through a catheter into the abdomen to remove waste products

perjured testimony Telling what is false when sworn to tell the truth

permeability Ability to allow solutions to pass through a membrane

permeable To pass or soak through

personal inventory A complete summary of pertinent information about oneself

petechiae Small, purplish hemorrhagic spots on the skin

petty cash fund A fund maintained from which to pay small unpredictable cash expenditures

phagocytosis The engulfing of microorganisms, other cells, and foreign particles by phagocytes

phagocytosis The process by which certain cells surround, engulf, and ingest microorganisms and cellular debris

phenylalanine An essential amino acid found in milk, eggs, and other foods

philosophy The general laws that furnish the rational explanation of anything

phlegm Expectorated matter; saliva mixed with discharges from the respiratory tract

phonetic Alteration of ordinary spelling that better represents the sounding of a word

photocoagulation Clotting of blood with light

physical impairment A lessening of physical capabilities

pitch The vibratory frequency of a tone or sound

placenta The vascular structure that develops within the uterus during pregnancy and through which a fetus receives nourishment

placenta Vascular structure that develops within the uterus during pregnancy and through which the fetus receives nourishment

plasma The liquid portion of the blood when only the cells have been removed

pleural Pertaining to a two-layer serous membrane that encapsulates the lungs

plume Carbon and steam byproducts from the electrical surgical unit or laser

polycythemia vera Condition of unknown origin that is characterized by a marked increase in total blood volume, red blood cells, white blood cells, platelets, and hemoglobin

polyps Tumors on stems frequently found in the mucosal lining of the colon

POMR Problem-oriented medical record

portfolio A set of documents either bound in book form or loose in a folder

posting The act of transferring information from one record to another

power of attorney A legal statement in which a person authorizes another person to act as his or her attorney or agent. The authority may be limited to the handling of certain procedures. The person authorized to act as the agent is known as an *attorney in fact*

practitioner One who practices a profession

preamble An introductory portion; a preface

preauthorization Permission by the insurance carrier obtained prior to giving certain treatment to a patient

precepts Practical rules guiding behavior or technique

preexisting condition A physical condition of an insured person that existed prior to the issuance of the insurance policy

premium The periodic payment required to keep a policy in force

prenatal Period of time between conception and birth

prepaid plan A plan that provides all covered services to a policyholder for payment of a monthly fee

presbycusis Progressive bilateral perceptive hearing loss occurring with age

presbyopia Diminution of accommodation of the lens of the eye occurring with aging

prescribe To issue a prescription for the patient; to direct, designate, or order use of a remedy

present illness Amplification of the chief complaint, usually written in chronologic sequence with dates of onset

preservatives Substances added to a specimen to prevent deterioration of cells or chemicals in the specimen

principal diagnosis That condition that after study is determined to be chiefly responsible for occasioning the admission of the patient to the hospital

principal procedure One that was performed for definitive treatment rather than for diagnostic or exploratory purposes, or one necessary to take care of a complication. It is that procedure most related to the principal diagnosis

printout The output from a printer, also called *hard copy*

privileged communication Information disclosed to a physician during the relationship between physician and patient that is confidential and should not be revealed without the express consent of the patient, unless required to do so by law

probationary Pertaining to a trial or a period of trial to ascertain fitness for a job

procrastination The intentional putting off of doing something that should be done

professional courtesy Reduction or absence of fee to professional associates

professional standards review organization (PSRO) A group of physicians working with the government to review cases for hospital admission and discharge under government guidelines; sometimes referred to as peer review

proficiency Competency as a result of training and practice

progesterone Female hormone that plays a major part in the menstrual cycle

progress notes Records of patient visits, telephone calls, progress, and treatment that are inserted into the patient's chart

pronunciation The act or manner of pronouncing words

proofreading Checking a document for spelling, sentence structure, punctuation, capitalization, style, and format

Prospective Payment Assessment Commission (ProPAC) A 15-member commission of independent experts with experience and expertise in the provision and financing of health care who are appointed to review and provide recommendations on the annual inflation factor, DRG recalibration, and new and existing medical and surgical procedures and services

prostheses Artificial replacements for body parts

proteinuria An excess of serum protein in the urine

protozoa Primitive animal organisms, each of which consists of a single cell

provider One who provides medical service (e.g., a physician)

prudent Marked by wisdom or circumspection

pruritus Itching

psoriasis Usually chronic, recurrent skin disease marked by bright red patches covered with silvery scales

psychosocial Pertaining to or involving both the psychic (behavior) and communal activity

ptosis Drooping of the upper eyelid

public domain The realm embracing property rights that belong to the community at large and that are subject to appropriation by anyone

puerperal fever The fever that accompanies an infection of the birth canal following delivery of a child; childbed fever

puerperium The period between childbirth and the return of the uterus to its normal size

pulmonary consolidation Process of the lungs becoming solidified as they fill with exudates in pneumonia

pulse deficit Difference between the apical pulse and the radial pulse

pulse pressure Difference between the systolic and the diastolic blood pressures (greater than 30 points or less than 50 points is considered normal)

punitive Inflicting punishment

purulent Consisting of or containing pus

pustule A raised pus-filled area or sac

putrefaction Decomposition of animal matter that results in a foul smell

pyemia The presence of pus-forming organisms in the blood

pyuria Pus in the urine

quackery Pretense of possessing medical skill to cure disease

quality assurance A law-enforced program that guarantees quality patient care

quality control The operational procedures used to implement the quality assurance program

rabies An acute infectious disease of the nervous system caused by a virus, usually communicated to humans through animal bite

rad A measurement of the actual absorbed dose of radiation

radiation Transfer through space of any form of energy, such as light, heat, or x-rays

radical mastectomy The complete surgical removal of the breast, the surrounding muscles, and the lymph glands

rales Abnormal or crackling chest sounds that occur during the inspirational portion of ventilation

random access memory (RAM) The computer's temporary memory that stores data and programs that are input

rapport Relationship of harmony and accord between patient and physician

reabsorption The act or process of absorbing again, as the absorption by the colon of the fluids already secreted into the gastrointestinal tract

read-only memory (ROM) Memory that can be altered only by changing the physical structure of the computer chip and that is used to store information that is essential to the operation of the computer

receipts Money received

receivables Amounts owing from others

reciprocity A mutual exchange of privileges

reconciliation (of bank statement) The process of proving that the bank statement and the checkbook balance are in agreement

recruitment The supplying of new members or help

rectum The distal portion of the large intestine located between the sigmoid colon and the anus

reduction Correction of a fracture, dislocation, or hernia

reentry student One who has been away from formal education or employment for several years and who is now preparing to reenter the workplace

reference laboratory A large laboratory that accepts specimens from smaller laboratories to perform tests not done by the smaller lab

reference values The listings of accepted ranges for normal values for routine hematology tests

reflux A return or backward flow

refraction Deviation of light produced by the eye and resulting in the focusing of images upon the retina

regional Pertaining to a region or territory; local

rehabilitation Restoration of normal form and function after injury or illness

rem Method of measuring the amount of radiation absorbed by a patient exposed to x-rays; similar to rad

remission A lessening in the severity of a disease or symptoms

remittent fever Fever in which temperature fluctuates greatly but never falls to the normal level

renin An enzyme produced in the kidney that helps in the regulation of blood pressure

reprints Reproductions of printed matter

reputable Honorable; having a good reputation

requisition A formal written request from the physician authorizing a laboratory to perform testing procedures

res ipsa loquitur The thing speaks for itself

resident A graduate and licensed physician receiving training in a specialty in a hospital

residual Urine left in the bladder after urination

respondeat superior Let the master answer

response Something constituting a reply or reaction

responsible person One who is responsible for payment, usually the patient if an adult

résumé A *selective* summary of one's education and employment record tailored to the position being sought

rete mucosum The innermost layer of the epidermis (*rete* = network of nerves or vessels)

retention The inability to empty the bladder

retention schedule A listing of dates until which records are to be kept, based on statutes of limitation, tax regulations, and other factors

retina Innermost layer of the eye composed of light-sensitive neurons

revoke To annul by recalling or taking back

rheumatic endocarditis Disease associated with hemolytic streptococci in the inside lining of the heart, valves, and great vessels

rheumatic fever Delayed sequela of an upper respiratory tract infection caused by the group A hemolytic *Streptococcus*

rhonchi Rattling noises in the throat that may resemble snoring; continuous dry rattling in the throat or bronchial tube due to partial obstruction

rider A legal document that modifies the protection of a policy

rods Structures located in the retina of the eye and forming the light-sensitive elements

roentgen Unit used to measure x-ray dosage

rural Pertaining to the country, as distinguished from a city or town

saliva Liquid secreted into the mouth by the salivary gland; moistens the mouth and starts the digestion of starches

salutation Expression of greeting (e.g., *good morning*)

sanitization Reducing the number of microorganisms to a level that is relatively safe

scanner An input device that converts printed matter into a computer-readable format

sclera Tough white, outer layer of the eyeball, covering about five sixths of its surface; white part of the eye that forms the orb

sclerotherapy Injection of sclerosing solutions in the treatment of hemorrhoids, varicose veins, or esophageal varices

scoliosis Lateral deviation in the normal vertical curve of the spine

screen The act of determining to whom a telephone call is to be directed

screening test A laboratory test done on large numbers of people to detect occult diseases

sebaceous gland An oil-secreting gland of the skin

seborrhea Excessive discharge of sebum from the sebaceous glands forming greasy scales or cheesy plugs on the body

sebum A fatty secretion of the sebaceous glands

secondary hypertension Elevated blood pressure due to another condition

self-concept A mental picture of one's self

semen Thick, whitish secretion containing spermatozoa

seminar A group of students meeting regularly and informally with a professor to discuss ideas and problems

senility A pronounced loss of mental, physical, or emotional control in aged people, caused by physical or mental deterioration

septicemia Presence of pathogenic microorganisms in the blood

sequential Succeeding or following in order or as a result; **sequentially** Following one another in an orderly plan

serous Thin, watery, serum-like drainage

serum Liquid portion of blood that remains after the clotting proteins and cells have been removed

service benefit plan A plan that agrees to pay for certain surgical and medical services and that is not restricted to a fee schedule

sheath The covering surrounding the axon of the nerve cell that acts as an electrical insulator to speed the conduction of nerve impulses

shelf filing A system that uses open shelves (rather than cabinets) for storing records

sinoatrial (SA) node Pacemaker of the heart located in the right atrium

sinus arrhythmia Irregular heartbeat originating in the sinoatrial node (pacemaker)

site A designated place or point

slough To shed dead tissue cells

socioeconomic Relating to a combination of social and economic factors

software The programming necessary to direct the hardware of a computer system; computer programs

sole community hospital (SCH) Those hospitals that, by reason of factors such as isolated location, weather conditions, travel conditions or absence of other hospitals are the sole source of inpatient hospital services reasonably available to individuals in a geographic area

solo private practice One physician practicing alone

specimen A sample of body fluid, waste product, or tissue that is collected for analysis

spermatozoa The mature male sex cells or germ cells

spores Thick-walled reproductive cells formed within bacteria and capable of withstanding unfavorable environmental conditions

stat Do immediately (from the Latin word *statin,* meaning "at once")

stat report An immediate report (from the Latin *statim,* meaning "at once")

statement A request for payment

statement of income and expense A summary of all income and expenses for a given period

statute of limitations The time limit within which an action may legally be brought upon a contract

statutory body A part of the legislative branch of a government

steepling Upward position of hands together with fingertips touching

stent Device used to prevent the lumen of the vessel from closing after angioplasty

sterilization Complete destruction of all forms of microbial life

stertorous Describing a deep snoring sound that occurs with each inspiration

stethoscope An instrument for listening to sounds within the body

stridor Shrill, harsh respiratory sound heard during inhalation in laryngeal obstruction

stroke A sudden loss of consciousness and/or paralysis caused by extreme trauma or injury to an artery in the brain

stylus A metal probe that is inserted or passed through a catheter, needle, or tube; used for clearing purposes or to facilitate passage into a body orifice

subject filing Arranging records alphabetically by names of topics or things rather than by names of individuals

subjective information Findings perceptible only by the affected person (the patient) (e.g., pain experienced in a specific area under certain circumstances)

sublingual Under the tongue

sublingually Pertaining to under the tongue

subluxation Partial dislocation of the bone from the joint

subpoena A writ commanding a person to appear in court

subscriber A person named as principal in an insurance contract

subscripts Symbols or numbers written immediately below another character

subsidize To aid or promote something (such as a private enterprise) with public money

substantiated Having been established as true by proof of competent evidence; verified

superbill A combination charge slip, statement, and insurance reporting form

superscripts Symbols or numbers written immediately above another character

suppurative Formation and/or discharge of pus

suspend To debar temporarily from a privilege

suspension The act of interrupting or discontinuing temporarily, but with an expectation or purpose of resumption

swine erysipelas A contagious disease affecting young swine in Europe

symptoms Any indication of disease felt by the patient

syncope Brief loss of consciousness; fainting

synergism Joint action of agents that results in a combined effect that is greater than the effects of the individual components

synopsis A summary of the main points of a longer text

synovial Pertaining to synovia, which is a clear fluid found in the joint cavities that facilitates smooth, painless movement

syphilitic chancre The primary sore of syphilis

syrup of ipecac A syrup given to induce vomiting

tab The projection on a file folder or guide on which the caption is written

tachycardia Fast heartbeat

tachypnea Respirations that are regular in rhythm but faster than normal in rate

Tax Equity and Fiscal Responsibility Act (TEFRA) Signed into federal law in 1982; contains provisions for major changes in Medicare reimbursement

tedious Tiresome because of length or dullness

telecommunications The science and technology of communication by transmission of information from one location to another via telephone, television, or telegraph

teller A bank employee who is assigned the duty of waiting on the bank's customers

tenacious Stubbornly unyielding; sticking together

thallium scan Intravenous administration of a radioisotope that localizes calcium in the myocardium in areas referred to as "cold spots" thus pinpointing the site of occlusions of coronary arteries

third-party check A check written to the order of the person offering payment and unknown to the payee, who is a third party in the process

third-party payer Someone other than the patient, spouse, or parent who is responsible for paying all or part of the patient's medical costs

thready pulse Pulse that is scarcely perceptible

thrombocytes Clotting cells in the blood, also known as platelets

tickler (file) A chronologic file used as a reminder that something must be taken care of on a certain date

tinnitus Ringing in the ears; a symptom of labyrinthitis, eighth cranial nerve damage, or cerebral arteriosclerosis

topical Applied to a certain area of the skin and affecting only that area

tort An act that brings harm to a person or damage to property, caused negligently or intentionally

tourniquet A device used to compress an artery or a vein

toxemia Distribution throughout the bloodstream in the body of poisonous products of bacteria

toxin A poisonous protein substance produced by some plants, animals, and pathogenic bacteria that builds up in the body as the microorganisms multiply

transaction The occurrence of a financial event or condition that must be recorded

transcription Listening to recorded dictation and translating it into written form

transection A cross section, division by cutting transverse

transillumination Inspection of a cavity or organ by passing light through its walls

transmitter The part of a telephone into which one speaks

trauma Physical injury or wound caused by an external force or violence

traumatic Pertaining to, resulting from, or causing physical injury or shock

treason A crime against the United States

treatise Systematic exposition or argument in writing

trespass To exceed the bounds of what is lawful, right, or just

triage Responding to requests for immediate care and treatment after evaluating the urgency of the need and prioritizing the treatment; to sort or to choose; to determine the priority of need for treatment

trial balance A method of checking the accuracy of accounts

triglyceride Neutral fat that is the usual storage form of lipids in the human body

umbilicus Depressed scar on the abdomen marking the site of entry of the umbilical cord; also called the navel

unequal pulses Difference felt between right and left radial and/or femoral pulse counts

uniform hospital discharge data set (UHDDS) A minimum data set required to be collected for each Medicare patient on discharge

unit Each part of a name that is used in indexing

urban Characteristic of or pertaining to a city or town

urea End-product of protein metabolism after ammonia is broken down by the liver; a systemic osmotic diuretic found in urine

uremia Toxic renal condition characterized by an excess of urea, creatinine, and other nitrogenous end-products in the blood

urethral meatus External opening to the urinary system

urgency Sudden, compelling desire to urinate and the inability to control the release of urine

urinary retention Inability to totally empty the bladder

usual, customary, and reasonable A formula for determining medical insurance benefits payable

uterus Pear-shaped organ located in the pelvic cavity between the bladder and the rectum and attached to the cervix; holds the fetus during pregnancy

vagina Collapsible muscular tube extending from the vaginal opening to the cervix in the female

vaginal speculum Instrument used to expand the vaginal orifice and allow the physician to examine the vagina and cervix or to obtain a cytologic specimen for the Papanicolaou test

Valsalva's maneuver Occurs when one strains to defecate and urinate, uses the arms and upper trunk muscles to move up in bed, or strains during laughing, coughing, or vomiting. The maneuver causes a trapping of blood in the great veins, preventing it from entering the chest and right atrium, and may cause heart attack and death

vascular Pertaining to blood vessels or indicative of a copious blood supply

vasectomy Sterilization procedure for the male

venereal Due to or propagated by sexual intercourse

venom A poison transmitted through the bite or sting of spiders, snakes, and some insects

ventricles Lower chambers of the heart

vertigo Sensation of rotation or movement; dizziness

vesiculation Formation of blister-like elevations on the skin

viability State or quality of being able to live after birth

viable Able to sustain life

vial A small bottle, usually glass

virile Having masculine spirit, strength, vigor, or power

virulency Exceedingly pathogenic, noxious, or deadly

virulent Exceedingly pathogenic, noxious, or deadly

viscosity The quality of being gluelike and lacking the capability of easy movement

vitiligo A loss of pigment in areas of the skin

vitreous Glasslike or hyaline fluid found inside the eye

vivisection Operation or cutting on a living animal for research purposes

void To urinate

volatile Referring to an explosive substance's capacity to vaporize at a low temperature

vulva The external female genitalia, which begins at the mons pubis and terminates at the anus

weight (DRG) An HCFA-derived figure intended to reflect the relative resource consumption of each DRG. The payment rate is multiplied by the appropriate DRG weight to determine the reimbursement amount for each patient

wheal A localized area of edema on the skin that is usually accompanied by itching

word processing System used to process written communications

zygote Cell resulting from the union of the male and female sex cells

Index

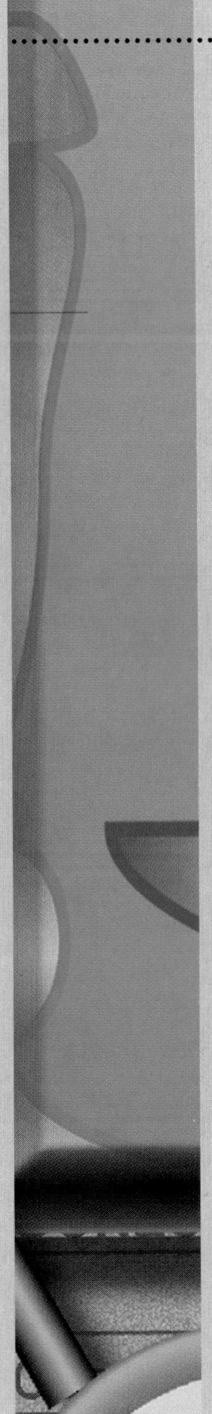

Note: Page numbers in *italics* refer to illustrations; page numbers followed by (t) refer to tables.